Paller and Mancini - Hurwitz Clinical Pediatric Dermatology

Paller and Mancini - Hurwitz Clinical Pediatric Dermatology

A Textbook of Skin Disorders of Childhood and Adolescence

SIXTH EDITION

Amy S. Paller, MD
Walter J. Hamlin Professor and Chair of Dermatology
Director, Skin Biology and Disease Resource-Based Center
Northwestern University Feinberg School of Medicine
Professor of Pediatrics
Ann & Robert H. Lurie Children's Hospital of Chicago
Chicago, Illinois
USA

Anthony J. Mancini, MD
Professor of Pediatrics and Dermatology
Northwestern University Feinberg School of Medicine
Head, Division of Pediatric Dermatology
Director, Fellowship Training Program
Ann & Robert H. Lurie Children's Hospital of Chicago
Chicago, Illinois
USA

ELSEVIER

Elsevier
3251 Riverport Lane
St. Louis, Missouri 63043

PALLER AND MANCINI – HURWITZ CLINICAL PEDIATRIC DERMATOLOGY, SIXTH EDITION ISBN: 978-0-323-54988-2

Notices

Knowledge and best practice in this field are constantly changing. As new research and experience broaden our understanding, changes in research methods, professional practices, or medical treatment may become necessary.

Practitioners and researchers must always rely on their own experience and knowledge in evaluating and using any information, methods, compounds or experiments described herein. Because of rapid advances in the medical sciences, in particular, independent verification of diagnoses and drug dosages should be made. To the fullest extent of the law, no responsibility is assumed by Elsevier, authors, editors or contributors for any injury and/or damage to persons or property as a matter of products liability, negligence or otherwise, or from any use or operation of any methods, products, instructions, or ideas contained in the material herein.

Previous editions copyrighted 2016, 2011, 2006, 1993 and 1981.

Library of Congress Control Number: 2020948302

Content Strategist: Charlotta Kryhl
Content Development Specialist: Kathleen Nahm
Content Coordinator: Reina Carmellite F. Cabusao
Project Manager: Janish Paul
Designer: Renee Duenow
Marketing Manager: Aly Abrams

Printed in China

Last digit is the print number: 9 8 7 6 5 4 3 2 1

Dedication

We again dedicate the text to our families,
whose ongoing patience, encouragement, support,
and personal sacrifice enabled us
to complete this project:
To Etahn, Josh, Max, Laura, and Ben, and
to Nicki, Mallory, Christopher, Mackenzie, and
Alexander: thank you.

We also dedicate this sixth edition
to Sidney Hurwitz, MD,
the epitome of a role model in academic
pediatric dermatology.

Preface

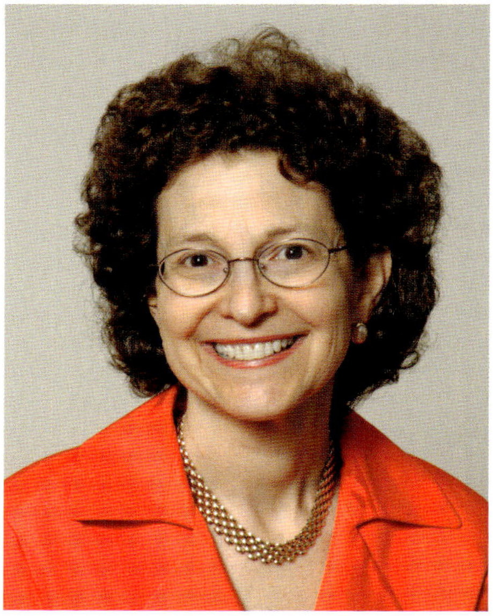

Amy S. Paller, MD

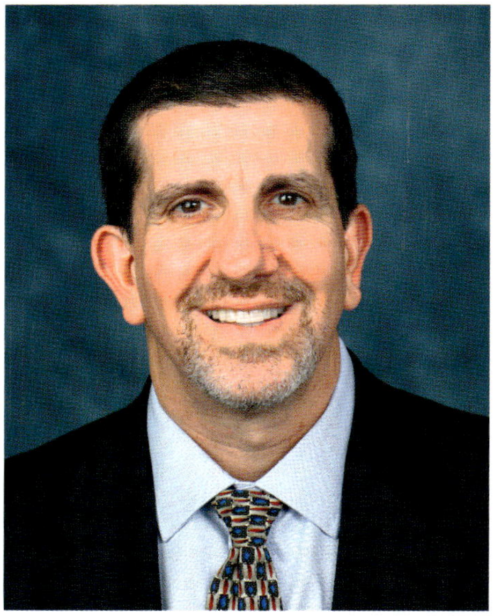

Anthony J. Mancini, MD

We were truly honored when initially asked to consider updating *Hurwitz Clinical Pediatric Dermatology*. Dr. Hurwitz was a true icon of our specialty and one of its founding fathers. We have advanced this text to be evidence based but full of our tips for the diagnosis and treatment of pediatric skin diseases in the four editions since Dr. Hurwitz "passed the baton" after writing the first and second editions. In this Paller/Mancini text, we have maintained the focus on educating and enlightening pediatricians, dermatologists, family practitioners, medical students, residents, fellows, nurses, and other allied pediatric care providers with a book that is practical, relevant, and user friendly in both its online and paper formats.

What lies between these covers will be familiar but with many additions. The field of pediatric dermatology has continued to expand since our last edition. The molecular bases for many established skin diseases continue to be elucidated, and several new disease and syndrome associations have been described. The therapeutic armamentarium for cutaneous disease has broadened, with many new forms of pathogenesis-based therapy available for patients, including through new classes of drugs. We have strived to maintain a book that represents a balance between narrative text, useful tables, and vivid clinical photographs.

Several new features have been added to this sixth edition, including a downloadable e-book with the printed edition and more than 350 new clinical images. We have updated the sections on atopic dermatitis, psoriasis, connective tissue diseases, and autoinflammatory disorders to reflect our growing armamentarium of new medications. Our sections on the ichthyoses, hair and ectodermal dysplasias, genetic blistering disorders, and mosaic gene disorders have grown based on so many new discoveries of underlying causes. New directions, such as the use of stem cell and cell therapy, as well as recombinant protein, for treating epidermolysis bullosa are also mentioned.

Our discussion of treatment for pediatric head lice reflects the multitude of new therapy options, and we have expanded the discussion of viral exanthematous diseases, including the resurgence in measles infections and the broadened scope of manifestations related to infection with human herpesviruses and enteroviruses. There are expanded discussions of mycoplasma-associated disorders and updated sections on congenital syphilis, toxoplasmosis, and pediatric melanoma. A discussion of congenital Zika virus infections has been added, as have expanded discussions of therapy for infantile hemangiomas, newer approaches for other vascular tumors and malformations, and the expanding spectrum of genetic mutations and clinical presentations of vascular disorders and syndromes. We have expanded the discussions of pediatric vasculitides, as well as factitial disorders and delusional infestation in children.

Several new tables have been added or updated in this edition, including the evaluation of suspected neonatal infection with herpes simplex virus, a discussion of monitoring for comorbidities in psoriasis, new classifications for ectodermal dysplasias and epidermolysis bullosa that focus on a molecular basis, fixed-dose combination therapies for acne vulgaris, contraindications to combined oral contraceptives, clinical features of polycystic ovary syndrome, the RASopathies, gene polymorphisms and pigmentation, the epidermal necrolysis classification, diagnostic criteria for hemophagocytic lymphohistiocytosis, an update on the contemporary classification of pediatric histiocytoses, consensus-derived PHACES syndrome criteria, the updated ISSVA classification of vascular anomalies, updated treatment recommendations for herpes simplex virus infections, revised Jones criteria for acute rheumatic fever, and features of juvenile dermatomyositis.

As with our last edition, the references have again been extensively updated in our companion online edition, leaving only some excellent reviews and landmark articles to allow for more complete textual content for our readers of the print version.

We continue to be indebted to several individuals, without whom this work would not have been possible. First and foremost, we thank Dr. Sidney Hurwitz, whose vision, dedication, and enthusiasm for the specialty of pediatric dermatology lives on as a legacy in this text, initially published in 1981. We are indebted to Teddy Hurwitz, his wife, who entrusted to us the ongoing tradition of this awesome project; to Dr. Alvin Jacobs, a "father" of pediatric dermatology, who kindled the flame of the specialty in both of us through his teaching at Stanford; to Dr. Nancy B. Esterly, the "mother" of pediatric dermatology, whose superb clinical acumen and patient care made her the perfect role model for another female physician who yearned to follow in her footsteps; and to Dr. Alfred T. Lane, who believed in a young pediatric intern and mentored him through the process of becoming a mentor himself.

We are also indebted to the staff at Elsevier, most notably Charlotta Kryhl, Melissa Rawe, Kathleen Nahm, and Janish Paul, who worked tirelessly through this edition to again meet the many demands of two finicky academicians; to our patients, who continue to educate us on a daily basis and place their trust in us to provide them care; to the clinicians who referred many of the patients seen in these pages; to our pediatric dermatology fellows (especially Dr. Ayelet Ollech), nurses, and office staff (especially Melissa Jones and Giuliana Wells), who contributed enormously through assistance with literature searches and the taking and archiving of our many clinical photographs; and to our families, whose understanding, sacrifice, support, and unconditional love made this entire endeavor possible.

Contents

1 An Overview of Dermatologic Diagnosis and Procedures

Accurate diagnosis of cutaneous disease in infants and children is a systematic process that requires careful inspection, evaluation, and some knowledge of dermatologic terminology and morphology to develop a prioritized differential diagnosis. The manifestations of skin disorders in infants and young children often vary from those of the same diseases in older children and adults. The diagnosis may be obscured, for example, by different reaction patterns or a tendency toward easier blister formation. In addition, therapeutic dosages and regimens often differ from those of adults, with medications prescribed on a "per kilogram" (/kg) basis and with liquid formulations.

Nevertheless, the same basic principles that are used to detect disorders affecting viscera apply to the detection of skin disorders. An adequate history should be obtained, a thorough physical examination performed, and, whenever possible, the clinical impression verified by appropriate laboratory studies. The easy visibility of skin lesions all too often results in a cursory examination and hasty diagnosis. Instead, the entire skin should be examined routinely and carefully, including the hair, scalp, nails, oral mucosa, anogenital regions, palms, and soles, because visible findings often hold clues to the final diagnosis.

The examination should be conducted in a well-lit room. Initial viewing of the patient at a distance establishes the overall status of the patient and allows recognition of distribution patterns and clues to the appropriate final diagnosis. This initial evaluation is followed by careful scrutiny of primary and subsequent secondary lesions in an effort to discern the characteristic features of the disorder.

Although not always diagnostic, the morphology and configuration of cutaneous lesions are of considerable importance to the classification and diagnosis of cutaneous disease. A lack of understanding of dermatologic terminology commonly poses a barrier to the description of cutaneous disorders by clinicians who are not dermatologists. Accordingly, a review of dermatologic terms is included here (Table 1.1). The many examples to show primary and secondary skin lesions refer to specific figures in the text that follows.

Configuration of Lesions

A number of dermatologic entities assume annular, circinate, or ring shapes and are interpreted as ringworm or superficial fungal infections. Although tinea is a common annular dermatosis of childhood, there are multiple other disorders that must be included in the differential diagnosis of ringed lesions, including pityriasis rosea, seborrheic dermatitis, nummular eczema, lupus erythematosus, granuloma annulare, annular psoriasis, erythema multiforme, erythema annulare centrifugum, erythema migrans, secondary syphilis, sarcoidosis, urticaria, pityriasis alba, tinea versicolor, lupus vulgaris, drug eruptions, and cutaneous T-cell lymphoma.

The terms *arciform* and *arcuate* refer to lesions that assume arc-like configurations. Arciform lesions may be seen in erythema multiforme, urticaria, pityriasis rosea, bullous dermatosis of childhood, and sometimes epidermolysis bullosa simplex.

Lesions that tend to merge are said to be *confluent*. Confluence of lesions is seen, for example, in childhood exanthems, *Rhus* dermatitis, erythema multiforme, tinea versicolor, and urticaria.

Lesions localized to a dermatome supplied by one or more dorsal ganglia are referred to as *dermatomal*. Herpes zoster classically occurs in a dermatomal distribution.

Discoid is used to describe lesions that are solid, moderately raised, and disc shaped. The term has largely been applied to discoid lupus erythematosus, in which the discoid lesions usually show atrophy and dyspigmentation.

Discrete lesions are individual lesions that tend to remain separated and distinct. *Eczematoid* and *eczematous* are adjectives relating to inflamed, dry skin with a tendency to thickening, oozing, vesiculation, and/or crusting; although atopic dermatitis is a classic eczematous disorder, other examples of eczema are contact, nummular, and dyshidrotic forms.

Grouping and clustering are characteristic of vesicles of herpes simplex or herpes zoster, insect bites, lymphangioma circumscriptum, contact dermatitis, and bullous dermatosis of childhood.

Guttate or drop-like lesions are characteristic of flares of psoriasis in children and adolescents that follow an acute upper respiratory tract infection, usually streptococcal.

Gyrate refers to twisted, coiled, or spiral-like lesions, as may be seen in patients with urticaria and erythema annulare centrifugum.

Iris or target-like lesions are concentric ringed lesions characteristic of erythema multiforme. The classic "targets" in this condition are composed of a central dusky erythematous papule or vesicle, a peripheral ring of pallor, and then an outer bright red ring.

Keratosis refers to circumscribed patches of horny thickening, as seen in seborrheic or actinic keratoses, keratosis pilaris, and keratosis follicularis (Darier disease). *Keratotic* is an adjective pertaining to keratosis and commonly refers to the epidermal thickening seen in chronic dermatitis and callus formation.

The *Koebner phenomenon* or *isomorphic response* refers to the appearance of lesions along a site of injury. The linear lesions of warts and molluscum contagiosum, for example, occur from autoinoculation of virus from scratching; those of *Rhus* dermatitis (poison ivy) result from the spread of the plant's oleoresin. Other examples of disorders that show a Koebner phenomenon are psoriasis, lichen planus, lichen nitidus, pityriasis rubra pilaris, and keratosis follicularis (Darier disease).

Lesions in a linear or band-like configuration appear in the form of a line or stripe and may be seen in epidermal nevi, Conradi syndrome, linear morphea, lichen striatus, striae, *Rhus* dermatitis, deep mycoses (sporotrichosis or coccidioidomycosis), incontinentia pigmenti, pigment mosaicism, porokeratosis of Mibelli, or factitial dermatitis. In certain genetic and inflammatory disorders, such linear configurations represent the lines of Blaschko, which trace clones of embryonic epidermal cells and, as such, represent a form of cutaneous mosaicism. This configuration presents as a linear pattern on the extremities, wavy or S-shaped on the lateral trunk, V-shaped on the central trunk, and varied patterns on the face and scalp.

Text continued on p. 7

Table 1.1 Glossary of Dermatologic Terms

Lesion	Description	Illustration	Examples
PRIMARY LESIONS			
The term *primary* refers to the most representative, but not necessarily the earliest, lesions; it is distinguished from the cutaneous features of secondary changes such as excoriation, eczematization, infection, or results of previous therapy.			
Macule	Flat, circumscribed change of the skin. It may be of any size, although this term is often used for lesions <1 cm. A macule may appear as an area of hypopigmentation or as an area of increased coloration, most commonly brown (hyperpigmented) or red (usually a vascular abnormality). It is usually round but may be oval or irregular; it may be distinct or may fade into the surrounding area.	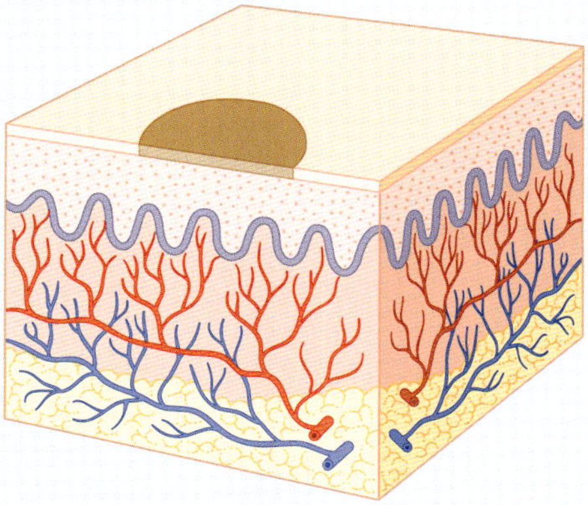	Ephelides; lentigo (see Fig. 11.45); flat nevus (see Fig. 9.1); and tinea versicolor (see Fig. 17.40)
Patch	Flat, circumscribed lesion with color change that is >1 cm in size.	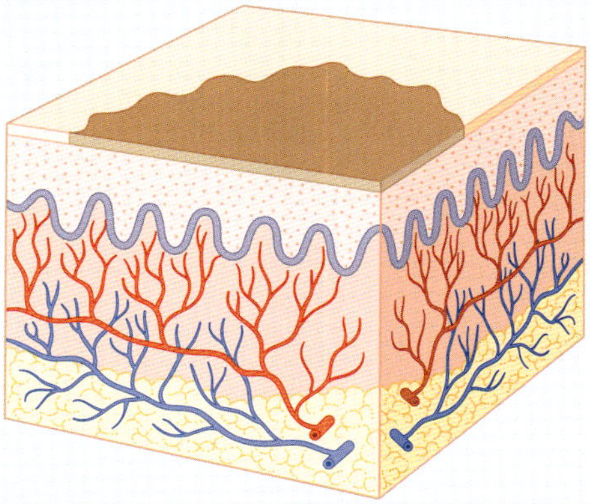	Congenital dermal melanocytosis (see Fig. 11.65); port wine stain (see Fig. 12.63); nevus depigmentosus (see Fig. 11.24); larger café-au-lait spot (see Fig. 11.49); and areas of vitiligo (see Figs. 11.2–11.10)
Papule	Circumscribed, nonvesicular, nonpustular, elevated lesion that measures <1 cm in diameter. The greatest mass is above the surface of the skin. When viewed in profile, it may be flat topped, dome shaped, acuminate (tapering to a point), digitate (finger-like), smooth, eroded, or ulcerated. It may be covered by scales, crusts, or a combination of secondary features.	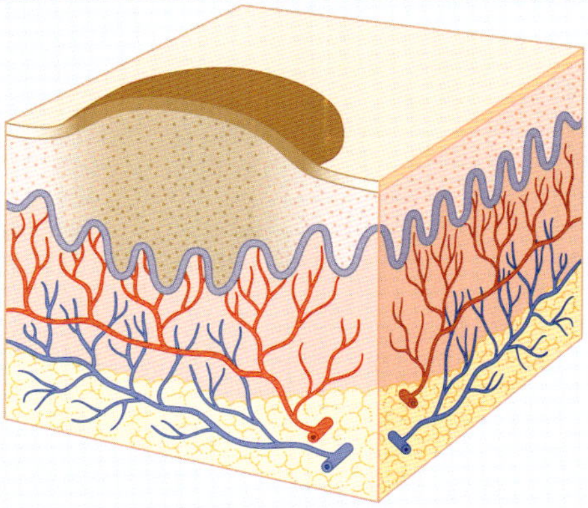	Elevated nevus (see Fig. 9.4); verruca (see Fig. 15.20); molluscum contagiosum (see Fig. 15.40); perioral dermatitis (see Fig. 8.23); and individual lesions of lichen planus (see Fig. 4.54)
Plaque	Broad, elevated, disk-shaped lesion that occupies an area of >1 cm. It is commonly formed by a confluence of papules.	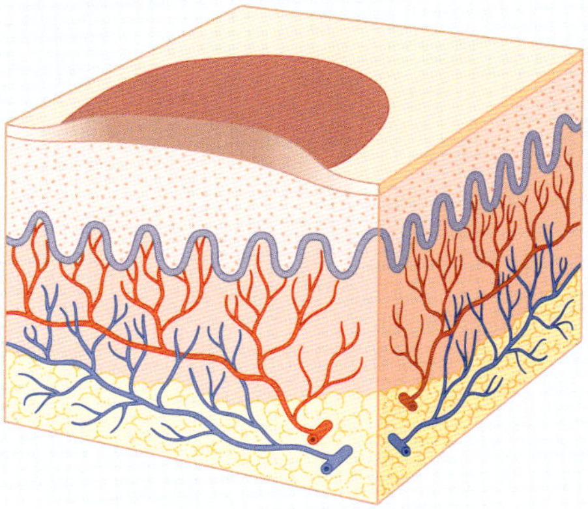	Psoriasis (see Fig. 4.6); lichen simplex chronicus (neurodermatitis, see Fig. 3.43); granuloma annulare (see Fig. 9.62); nevus sebaceus (see 9.43–9.46); and lesions of lichen planus (see Fig. 4.55)

Table 1.1 Glossary of Dermatologic Terms (Continued)

Lesion	Description	Illustration	Examples
Nodule	Circumscribed, elevated, usually solid lesion that measures 0.5–2 cm in diameter. It involves the dermis and may extend into the subcutaneous tissue with its greatest mass below the surface of the skin.	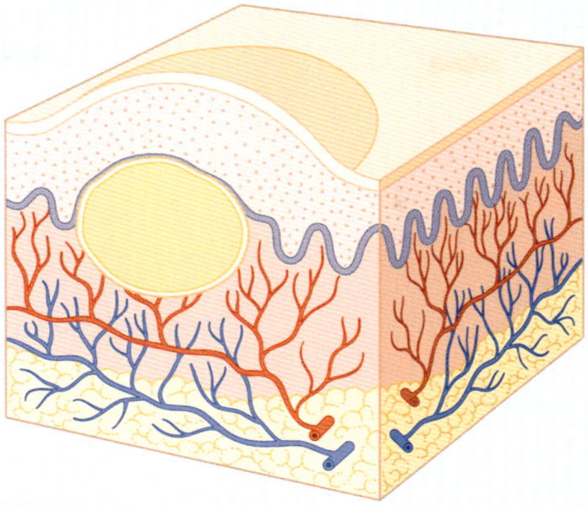	Erythema nodosum (see Fig. 20.45); pilomatricoma (see Figs. 9.50 and 9.51); subcutaneous granuloma annulare (see Fig. 9.64); and nodular scabies (see Figs. 18.9 and 18.10)
Tumor	Deeper circumscribed solid lesion of the skin or subcutaneous tissue that measures >2 cm in diameter. It may be benign or malignant.	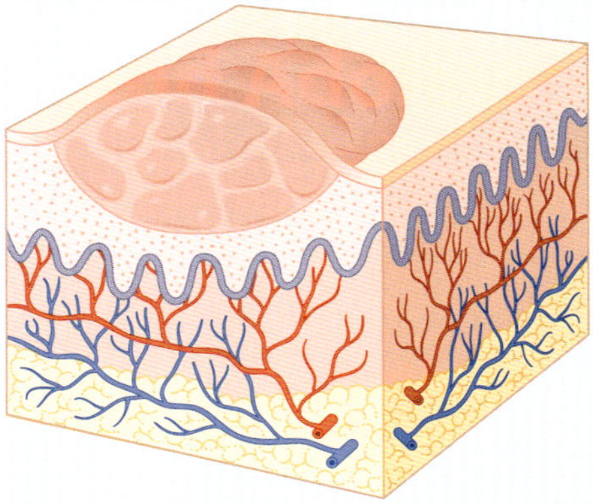	Deep hemangioma (see Fig. 12.8) and plexiform neurofibroma (see Fig. 11.56)
Wheal	Distinctive type of elevated lesion characterized by local, superficial, transient edema. White to pink or pale red, compressible, and evanescent, they often disappear within a period of hours. They vary in size and shape.	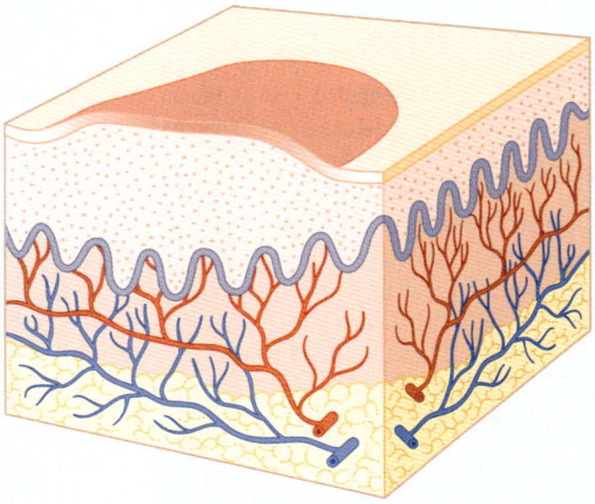	Darier sign of mastocytosis (see Fig. 9.59); urticarial vasculitis (see Fig. 21.15); and various forms of urticaria (see Figs. 20.2–20.7)
Vesicle	Sharply circumscribed, elevated, fluid-containing lesion that measures ≤1 cm in diameter.	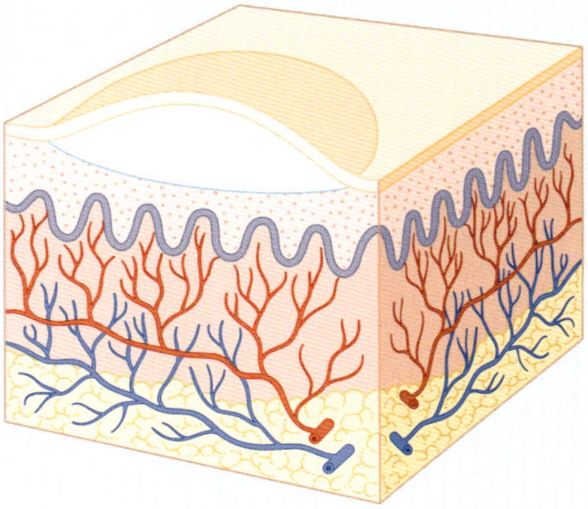	Herpes simplex (see Figs. 15.8 and 15.12); hand-foot-and-mouth disease (see Fig. 16.32); pompholyx (see Fig. 3.47); varicella (see Fig. 16.1); and contact dermatitis (see Fig. 3.65, *B*)

Continued on following page

Table 1.1 Glossary of Dermatologic Terms (Continued)

Lesion	Description	Illustration	Examples
Bulla	Larger, circumscribed, elevated, fluid-containing lesion that measures >1 cm in diameter.	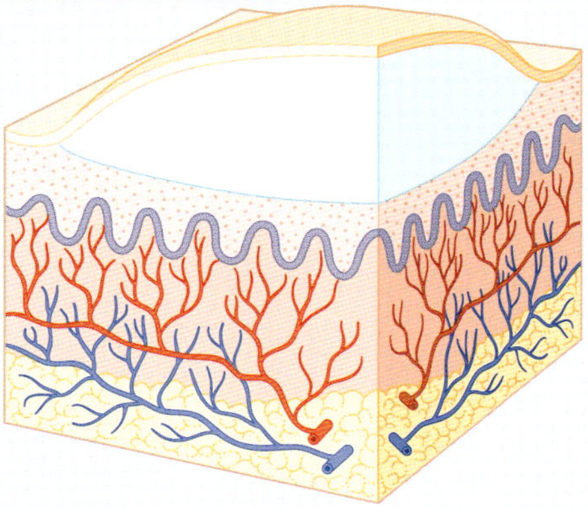	Blistering distal dactylitis (see Fig. 14.22); bullous pemphigoid (see Fig. 13.33); chronic bullous disease of childhood (see Fig. 13.37); bullous flea bite reaction (see Figs. 18.33 and 18.34); and epidermolysis bullosa (see Fig. 13.4)
Pustule	Circumscribed elevation <1 cm in diameter that contains a purulent exudate. It may be infectious or sterile.	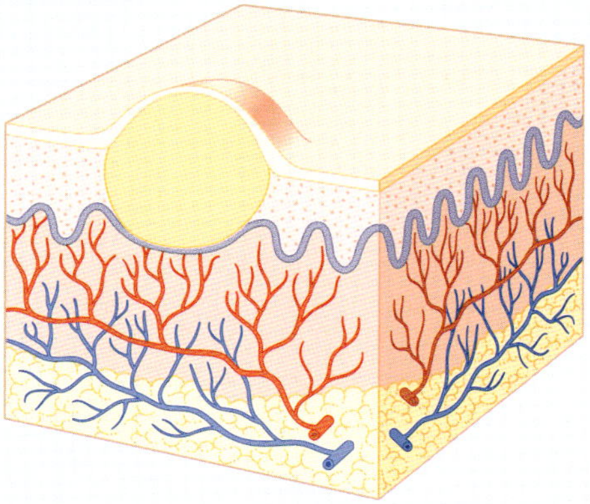	Folliculitis (see Fig. 14.11); transient neonatal pustular melanosis (see Fig. 2.22); pustular psoriasis (see Fig. 4.30); and neonatal cephalic pustulosis (see Fig. 2.16), neonatal *S. aureus* pustulosis (see Fig. 2.21), and infantile acropustulosis (see Fig. 2.24)
Abscess	Circumscribed, elevated lesion >1 cm in diameter, often with a deeper component and filled with purulent material.	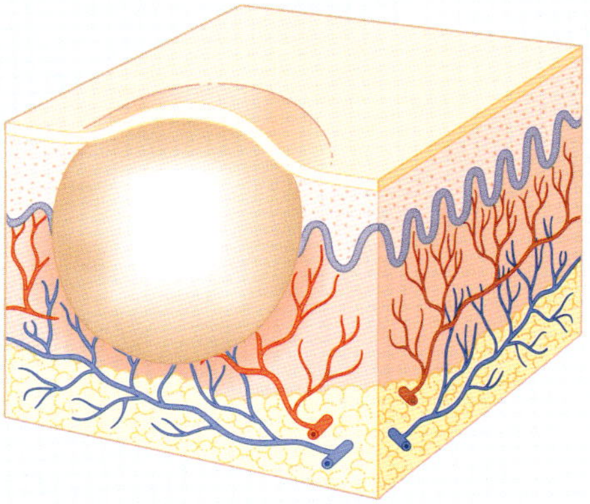	Staphylococcal abscess (in a neonate, see Fig. 2.5; in a patient with hyperimmunoglobulinemia E, see Fig. 3.41)
OTHER PRIMARY LESIONS			
Comedone	Plugged secretion of horny material retained within a pilosebaceous follicle. It may be flesh colored (as in closed comedone or whitehead) or slightly raised brown or black (as in open comedone or blackhead). Closed comedones, in contrast to open comedones, may be difficult to visualize. They appear as pale, slightly elevated, small papules without a clinically visible orifice.		Acne comedones (see Figs. 8.3 and 8.4) and nevus comedonicus (see Fig. 9.47)
Burrow	Linear lesion produced by tunneling of an animal parasite in the stratum corneum.		Scabies (see Fig. 18.3) and cutaneous larva migrans (creeping eruption, see Fig. 18.41)
Telangiectasia	Persistent dilation of superficial venules, capillaries, or arterioles of the skin.		Spider angioma (see Fig. 12.97); periungual lesion of dermatomyositis (see Figs. 22.26 and 22.29); CREST syndrome (see Fig. 22.45); and focal dermal hypoplasia (see Fig. 6.18)

Table 1.1 Glossary of Dermatologic Terms (Continued)

Lesion	Description	Illustration	Examples
SECONDARY LESIONS			
Secondary lesions represent evolutionary changes that occur later in the course of the cutaneous disorder. Although helpful in dermatologic diagnosis, they do not offer the same degree of diagnostic aid as that afforded by primary lesions of a cutaneous disorder.			
Crust	Dried remains of serum, blood, pus, or exudate overlying areas of lost or damaged epidermis. Crust is yellow when formed by dried serum, green or yellowish-green when formed by purulent exudate, and dark red or brown when formed by bloody exudative serum.	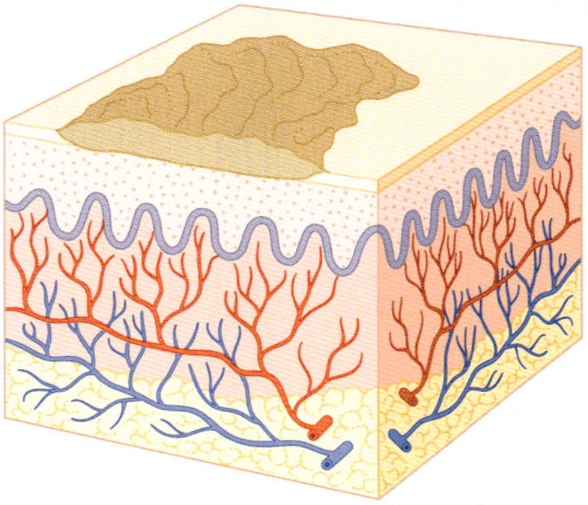	Herpes simplex (see Fig. 15.5); weeping eczematous dermatitis (see Fig. 3.1); and dried honey-colored lesions of impetigo (see Fig. 14.1)
Scale	Formed by an accumulation of compact desquamating layers of stratum corneum as a result of abnormal keratinization and exfoliation of cornified keratinocytes.	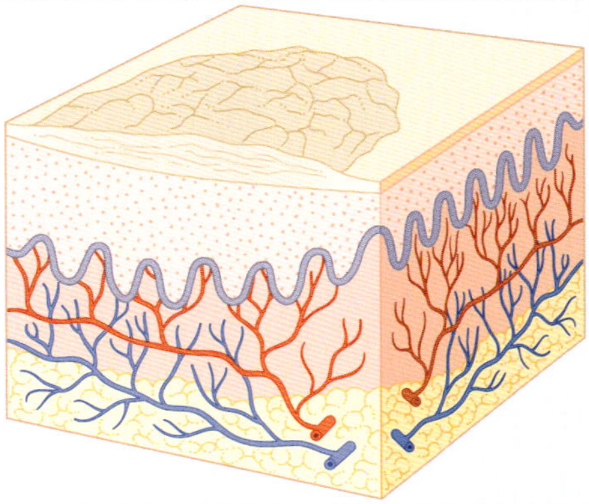	Seborrheic dermatitis (greasy and yellowish, see Fig. 3.3); psoriasis (silvery and mica-like, see Fig. 4.1); lichen striatus (fine and adherent, see Fig. 3.52); and lamellar ichthyosis (large and adherent, see Fig. 5.16)
Fissure	Dry or moist, linear, often painful cleavage in the cutaneous surface that results from marked drying and long-standing inflammation, thickening, and loss of elasticity of the integument.	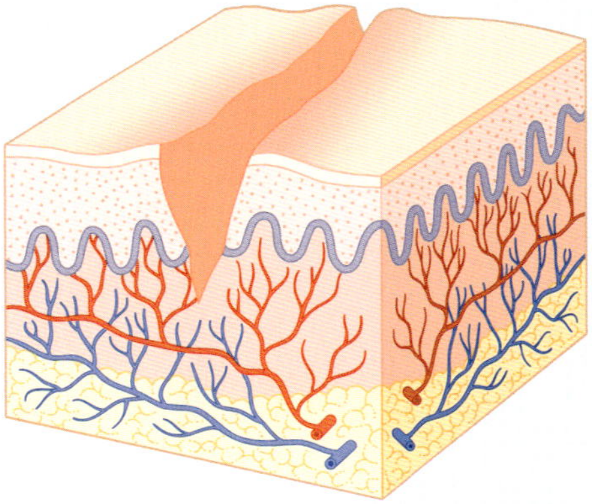	Angular cheilitis (see Fig. 17.46) and dermatitis on the palmar aspect of the fingers (see Fig. 3.58) or the plantar aspect of the foot (see Fig. 3.69)
Erosion	Moist, slightly depressed vesicular or bullous lesions in which part or all of the epidermis has been lost. Because erosions do not extend into the underlying dermis or subcutaneous tissue, healing occurs without subsequent scar formation.	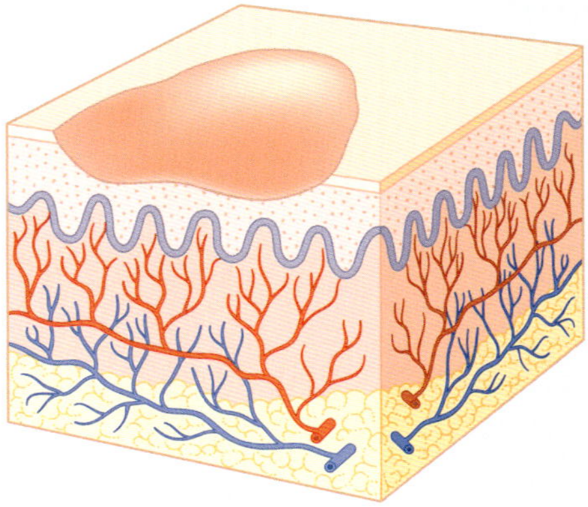	Herpes simplex (see Figs. 3.31 and 15.3); epidermolytic ichthyosis in a neonate (see Fig. 5.6); and superficial forms of epidermolysis bullosa (see Fig. 13.5)

Continued on following page

Table 1.1 Glossary of Dermatologic Terms (Continued)

Lesion	Description	Illustration	Examples
Excoriation	Traumatized or abraded (usually self-induced) superficial loss of skin caused by scratching, rubbing, or scrubbing of the cutaneous surface.	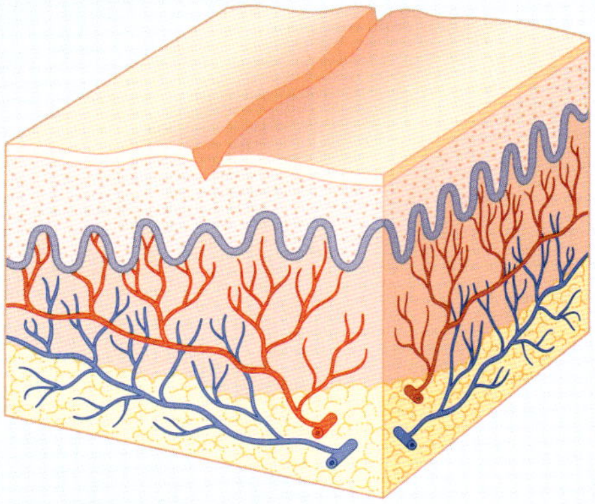	Atopic dermatitis (see Fig. 3.9) and acne excoriée (see Fig. 8.22)
Ulcer	Necrosis of the epidermis and part or all of the dermis and/or the underlying subcutaneous tissue.	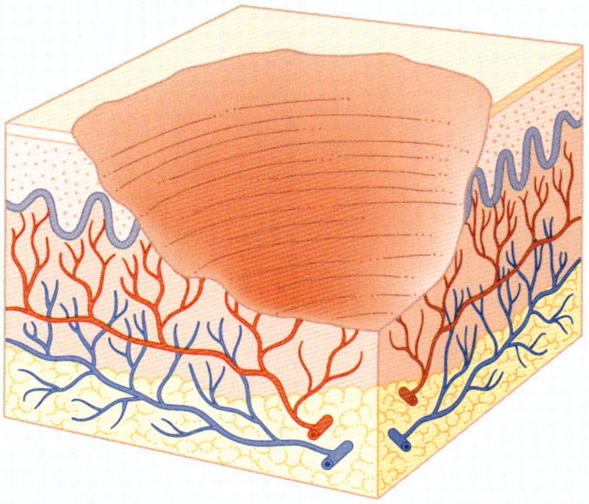	Pyoderma gangrenosum (see Fig. 25.18) and ulcerated hemangioma of infancy (see Figs. 12.15 and 12.26)
Atrophy	Cutaneous changes that result in depression of the epidermis, dermis, or both. Epidermal atrophy is characterized by thin, almost translucent epidermis, a loss of the normal skin markings, and wrinkling when subjected to lateral pressure or pinching of the affected area. In dermal atrophy, the skin is depressed.	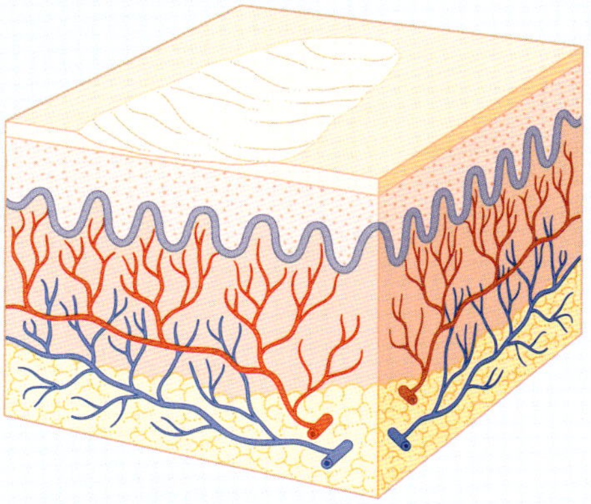	Anetoderma (see Fig. 22.63); morphea (see 22.54 and 22.56); steroid-induced atrophy (see Fig. 3.36); and focal dermal hypoplasia (see Fig. 6.19)
Lichenification	Thickening of the epidermis with associated exaggeration of skin markings. Lichenification results from chronic scratching or rubbing of a pruritic lesion.	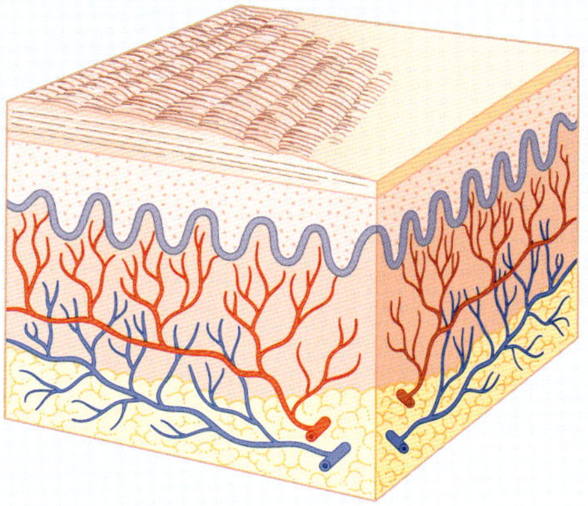	Atopic dermatitis (see Fig. 3.8); chronic contact dermatitis (see Fig. 3.61, *B*); and lichen simplex chronicus (see Fig. 3.43)

Table 1.1 Glossary of Dermatologic Terms (Continued)

Lesion	Description	Illustration	Examples
Scar	A permanent fibrotic skin change that develops after damage to the dermis. Initially pink or violaceous, scars are permanent, white, shiny, and sclerotic as the color fades. Although fresh scars often are hypertrophic, they usually contract during the subsequent 6–12 months and become less apparent. Hypertrophic scars must be differentiated from keloids, which represent an exaggerated response to skin injury. Keloids are pink, smooth, and rubbery and are often traversed by telangiectatic vessels. They tend to increase in size long after healing has taken place and can be differentiated from hypertrophic scars by the fact that the surface of a keloidal scar tends to extend beyond the area of the original wound.	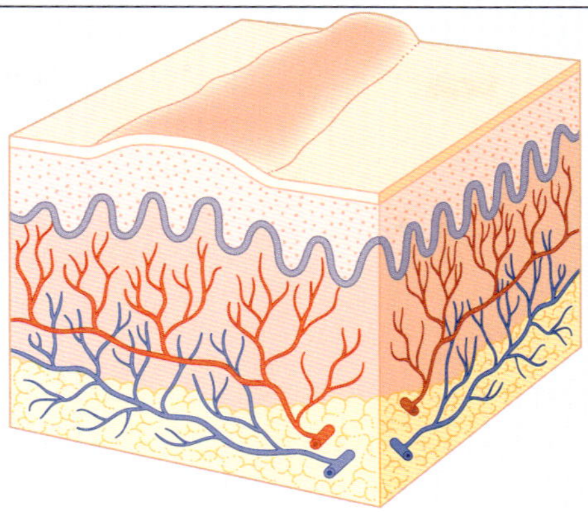	Keloid (see Fig. 9.93); healed areas of recessive dystrophic epidermolysis bullosa (see Fig. 13.26); post-hemangioma scarring (see Fig. 12.21); congenital erosive and vesicular dermatosis with reticulated supple scarring (see Fig. 2.21, *B*); and amniocentesis scars (see Fig. 2.4)

Moniliform refers to a banded or necklace-like appearance. This is seen in monilethrix, a hair deformity characterized by beaded nodularities along the hair shaft.

Multiform refers to disorders in which more than one variety or shape of cutaneous lesions occurs. This configuration is seen in patients with erythema multiforme, urticaria multiforme, early Henoch–Schönlein purpura, and polymorphous light eruption.

Nummular means coin shaped and is usually used to describe nummular dermatitis.

Polycyclic refers to oval lesions containing more than one ring, as commonly is seen in patients with urticaria.

A reticulated or net-like pattern may be seen in erythema ab igne, livedo reticularis, cutis marmorata, cutis marmorata telangiectatica congenita, and lesions of confluent and reticulated papillomatosis.

Serpiginous describes the shape or spread of lesions in a serpentine or snake-like configuration, particularly those of cutaneous larva migrans (creeping eruption) and elastosis perforans serpiginosa.

Umbilicated lesions are centrally depressed or shaped like an umbilicus or navel. Examples include lesions of molluscum contagiosum, varicella, vaccinia, variola, herpes zoster, and Kaposi varicelliform eruption.

Universal (universalis) implies widespread disorders affecting the entire skin, as in alopecia universalis.

Zosteriform describes a linear arrangement along a nerve, as typified by lesions of herpes zoster, although herpes simplex infection can also manifest in a zosteriform distribution.

Distribution and Morphologic Patterns of Common Skin Disorders

The regional distribution and morphologic configuration of cutaneous lesions are often helpful in dermatologic diagnosis.

Acneiform lesions are those having the form of acne, and *an acneiform distribution* refers to lesions primarily seen on the face, neck, chest, upper arms, shoulders, and back (see Figs. 8.3 through 8.8).

Sites of predilection of atopic dermatitis include the face, trunk, and extremities in young children; the antecubital and popliteal fossae are the most common sites in older children and adolescents (see Figs. 3.1 through 3.11).

The lesions of erythema multiforme may be widespread but have a distinct predilection for the hands and feet (particularly the palms and soles) (see Figs. 20.35 through 20.37).

Lesions of herpes simplex may appear anywhere on the body but have a distinct predisposition for the areas about the lips, face, and genitalia (see Figs. 15.1 through 15.14). Herpes zoster generally has a dermatomal or nerve-like distribution and is usually but not necessarily unilateral (see Figs. 15.15 through 15.17). More than 75% of cases occur between the second thoracic and second lumbar vertebrae. The fifth cranial nerve commonly is involved, and only rarely are lesions seen below the elbows or knees.

Lichen planus often affects the limbs (see Figs. 4.54, 4.55, and 4.58). Favorite sites include the lower extremities, the flexor surface of the wrists, the buccal mucosa, the trunk, and the genitalia.

The lesions of lupus erythematosus most commonly localize to the bridge of the nose, malar eminences, scalp, and ears, although they may be widespread (see Figs. 22.3 and 22.4). Patches tend to spread at the border and clear in the center with atrophy, scarring, dyspigmentation, and telangiectases. The malar or butterfly rash is neither specific for nor the most common sign of lupus erythematosus; telangiectasia without the accompanying features of erythema, scaling, or atrophy is never a marker of this disorder other than in neonatal lupus.

Molluscum contagiosum is a common viral disorder characterized by dome-shaped, skin-colored to erythematous papules, often with a central white core or umbilication (see Figs. 15.41 through 15.47). These papules most often localize to the trunk and axillary areas. Although molluscum lesions can be found anywhere, the scalp, palms, and soles are rare sites of involvement.

Photodermatoses are cutaneous disorders caused or precipitated by exposure to light. Areas of predilection include the face, ears, anterior V of the neck and upper chest, dorsal aspect of the forearms and hands, and exposed areas of the legs. The shaded regions of the upper eyelids, subnasal, and submental regions tend to be spared. The major photosensitivity disorders are lupus erythematosus, dermatomyositis, polymorphous light eruption, drug photosensitization, phototoxic reactions, and porphyria (see Chapter 19).

Photosensitive reactions cannot be distinguished on a clinical basis from lesions of photocontact allergic conditions. They may reflect internal as well as external photoallergens and may simulate contact dermatitis from airborne sensitizers. Lupus erythematosus can be differentiated by the presence of atrophy, scarring, hyperpigmentation or hypopigmentation, and periungual telangiectases. Dermatomyositis with swelling and erythema of the cheeks and eyelids should be differentiated from allergic contact dermatitis by the heliotrope hue and other associated changes, particularly those of the fingers (periungual telangiectases and Gottron papules).

Pityriasis rosea begins as a solitary round or oval scaling lesion known as the *herald patch* in 70% to 80% of cases, which may be annular and is often misdiagnosed as tinea corporis (see Fig. 4.49). After an interval of days to 2 weeks, affected individuals develop a generalized symmetric eruption that involves mainly the trunk and proximal limbs. The clue to diagnosis is the distribution of lesions, with the long axis of these oval lesions parallel to the lines of cleavage in what has been termed a *Christmas-tree pattern* (see Figs. 4.50, 4.51, and 4.53). A common variant, inverse pityriasis rosea, often localizes in the inguinal region (see Fig. 4.52), but the parallel nature of the long axis of lesions remains characteristic.

Psoriasis classically consists of round, erythematous, well-marginated plaques with a rich red hue covered by a characteristic grayish or silvery-white mica-like (micaceous) scale that on removal may result in pinpoint bleeding (Auspitz sign) (see Figs. 4.1 through 4.16). Although exceptions occur, lesions generally are seen in a bilaterally symmetric pattern with a predilection for the elbows, knees, scalp, and lumbosacral, perianal, and genital regions. Nail involvement, a valuable diagnostic sign, is characterized by pitting of the nail plate, discoloration, separation of the nail from the nailbed (onycholysis), and an accumulation of subungual scale (subungual hyperkeratosis). A characteristic feature of this disorder is the Koebner or isomorphic response in which new lesions appear at sites of local injury.

Scabies is an itchy disorder in which lesions are characteristically distributed on the wrists and hands (particularly the interdigital webs), forearms, genitalia, areolae, and buttocks in older children and adolescents (see Figs. 18.1 through 18.12). Other family members may be similarly affected or complain of itching. In infants and young children, the diagnosis is often overlooked because the distribution typically involves the palms, soles, and often the head and neck. Obliteration of demonstrable primary lesions (burrows) because of vigorous hygienic measures, excoriation, crusting, eczematization, and secondary infection is particularly common in infants.

Seborrheic dermatitis is an erythematous, scaly or crusting eruption that characteristically occurs on the scalp, face, and postauricular, presternal, and intertriginous areas (see Figs. 3.3, 3.44, and 3.45). The classic lesions are dull, pinkish-yellow, or salmon colored with fairly sharp borders and overlying yellowish greasy scale. Morphologic and topographic variants occur in many combinations and with varying degrees of severity from mild involvement of the scalp with occasional blepharitis to generalized, occasionally severe erythematous scaling eruptions. The differential diagnosis may include atopic dermatitis, psoriasis, various forms of diaper dermatitis, Langerhans cell histiocytosis, scabies, tinea corporis or capitis, pityriasis alba, contact dermatitis, Darier disease, and lupus erythematosus.

Warts are common viral cutaneous lesions characterized by the appearance of skin-colored small papules of several morphologic types (see Figs. 15.19 through 15.37). They may be elevated or flat lesions and tend to appear in areas of trauma, particularly the dorsal surface of the face, hands, periungual areas, elbows, knees, feet, and genital or perianal areas. Close examination may reveal capillaries appearing as punctate dots scattered on the surface.

Changes in Skin Color

The color of skin lesions commonly assists in making the diagnosis (see Chapter 11). Common disorders of brown hyperpigmentation include postinflammatory hyperpigmentation, pigmented and epidermal nevi, café-au-lait spots, lentigines, incontinentia pigmenti, fixed drug eruption, photodermatitis and phytophotodermatitis, melasma, acanthosis nigricans, and Addison disease. Blue coloration is seen in congenital dermal melanocytosis, blue nevi, nevus of Ito and nevus of Ota, and cutaneous neuroblastomas. Cysts, deep hemangiomas, and pilomatricomas often show a subtle blue color, whereas the blue of venous malformations and glomuvenous malformations is often a more intense, dark blue. Yellowish discoloration of the skin is common in infants, related to the presence of carotene derived from excessive ingestion of foods, particularly yellow vegetables containing carotenoid pigments. Jaundice may be distinguished from carotenemia by scleral icterus. Localized yellow lesions may represent juvenile xanthogranulomas, nevus sebaceous, xanthomas, or mastocytomas. Red lesions are usually vascular in origin, such as superficial hemangiomas, spider telangiectases, and nevus flammeus (capillary malformations), or inflammatory, such as the scaling lesions of atopic dermatitis or psoriasis.

Localized lesions with decreased pigmentation may be hypopigmented (decreased pigmentation) or depigmented (totally devoid of pigmentation); Wood lamp examination may help to differentiate depigmented lesions, which fluoresce a bright white, from hypopigmented lesions. Localized depigmented lesions may be seen in vitiligo, Vogt–Koyanagi syndrome, halo nevi, chemical depigmentation, piebaldism, and Waardenburg syndrome. Hypopigmented lesions are more typical of postinflammatory hypopigmentation, pityriasis alba, tinea versicolor, leprosy, nevus achromicus, tuberous sclerosis, and the hypopigmented streaks of pigment mosaicism. A generalized decrease in pigmentation can be seen in patients with albinism, untreated phenylketonuria, and Menkes syndrome. The skin of patients with Chédiak–Higashi and Griscelli syndromes takes on a dull silvery sheen and may show decreased pigmentation.

Racial Variations in the Skin and Hair

The skin of Black and other darker-skinned children varies in several ways from that of lighter-skinned children based on genetic background and customs (see Chapter 11). The erythema of inflamed black skin may be difficult to see and likely accounts for the purportedly decreased incidence of macular viral exanthems such as erythema infectiosum. Erythema in Black children commonly has a purplish tinge that can be confusing to unwary observers. The skin lesions in several inflammatory disorders such as in atopic dermatitis, pityriasis rosea, and syphilis commonly show a follicular pattern in Black children.

Postinflammatory hypopigmentation and hyperpigmentation occur readily and are more obvious in darker-skinned persons, regardless of racial origin. Pityriasis alba and tinea versicolor are more commonly reported in darker skin types, perhaps because of the easy visibility of the hypopigmented lesions in marked contrast to uninvolved surrounding skin. Lichen nitidus is more apparent and reportedly more common in Black individuals; lichen planus is reported to be more severe, leaving dark postinflammatory hyperpigmentation. Vitiligo is particularly distressing to patients with darker skin types, whether Black or Asian, because of the easy visibility in contrast with surrounding skin.

Although darker skin may burn, sunburn and chronic sun-induced diseases of adults such as actinic keratosis and carcinomas of the skin induced by ultraviolet light exposure (e.g., squamous cell carcinoma, keratoacanthoma, basal cell carcinoma, and melanoma) generally have an extremely low incidence in Blacks and Hispanics. Congenital melanocytic nevi also tend to have a lower tendency to transform to malignancy in darker-skinned individuals. Café-au-lait spots are more numerous and seen more often in Blacks, although the presence of six or more should still raise suspicion about neurofibromatosis. Dermatosis papulosa nigra commonly develop in adolescents, especially those who are female, of African descent. Mongolian spots occur more often in persons of African or Asian descent. Physiologic variants in children with darker skin include increased pigmentation of the gums and tongue, pigmented streaks in the nails, and Voigt–Futcher lines, lines of pigmentary demarcation between the posterolateral and lighter anteromedial skin on the extremities.

Qualities of hair may also differ among individuals of different races. Black hair tends to tangle when dry and becomes matted when wet. As a result of its naturally curly or spiral nature, pseudofolliculitis barbae is more common in Blacks than in other groups. Tinea capitis is particularly common in prepubertal Blacks; the tendency to use oils because of hair dryness and poor manageability may obscure the scaling of tinea capitis. Pediculosis capitis, in contrast, is relatively uncommon in this population, possibly related to the diameter and shape of the hair shaft. Prolonged continuous traction on hairs may result in traction alopecia, particularly with the common practice of making tight cornrow braids. The use of other hair grooming techniques such as chemical straighteners, application of hot oils, and hot combs increases the risk of hair breakage and permanent alopecia. Frequent and liberal use of greasy lubricants and pomades produces a comedonal and sometimes papulopustular form of acne (pomade acne).

Keloids form more often in individuals of African descent, often as a complication of a form of inflammatory acne, including nodulocystic acne and acne keloidalis nuchae. Other skin disorders reportedly seen more commonly are transient neonatal pustular melanosis, infantile acropustulosis, impetigo, papular urticaria, sickle cell ulcers, sarcoidosis, and dissecting cellulitis of the scalp. Atopic dermatitis and Kawasaki disease have both been reported most often in children of Asian descent.

Procedures to Aid in Diagnosis

BETTER VISUALIZATION

Although most lesions are diagnosed by clinical inspection, several techniques are used to aid in diagnosis. The Wood lamp (black light) is an ultraviolet A (UVA)-emitting device with a peak emission of 365 nm. With the room completely dark and the light held approximately 10 cm from the skin, the examiner can see (1) more subtle differences in pigmentation and the bright whiteness of vitiligo lesions based on the strong absorbance of the light by melanin, and (2) characteristic fluorescence of organisms such as the pink-orange fluorescence of urine in porphyria (see Chapter 19), the coral red fluorescence of erythrasma, the yellow-orange fluorescence of tinea versicolor, the green fluorescence of ectothrix types of tinea capitis (e.g., *Microsporum*) (see Chapter 17), and sometimes *Pseudomonas* infection. False-positive assessments can result from detection of other fluorescent objects, such as lint, threads, scales, and ointments.

Diascopy involves pressing a glass microscope slide firmly over a lesion and watching for changes in appearance. Purpura, which does not blanch with diascopy because the erythrocytes have leaked into tissue, can be distinguished from erythema caused by vasodilation, which blanches because the pressure from the slides forces the erythrocytes to move out of the compressed vessels. The yellow-brown ("apple jelly") color of granulomatous lesions (e.g., granuloma annulare, sarcoidosis) persists during diascopy, and the constricted blood vessels of nevus anemicus blend in with surrounding skin during diascopy and do not refill when the slide is lifted after diascopy (as do the surrounding normal areas).

Magnification using a lens or lighted devices such as the otoscope, ophthalmoscope, or dermatoscope can be used to more easily visualize lesions such as nailfold capillaries, especially after swabbing the skin with alcohol or applying a drop of oil.[1,2] Indeed, *dermoscopy* (also known as *dermatoscopy* or *epiluminescence microscopy*) refers to examination of the skin with a dermatoscope, a handheld magnifier with an embedded light source. Dermoscopy provides more than just magnification, because it allows the viewer to visualize dermal diagnostic clues. In pediatric patients, dermoscopy can be particularly useful for reassurance regarding the benign nature of pigmented nevi,[3] visualization of vascular lesions, and hair disorders ranging from shaft defects to alopecia areata.[4–8] Reflectance confocal microscopy[9–11] is a noninvasive technology for in vivo imaging of skin at nearly histologic resolution. Although largely used currently to distinguish benign lesions from skin cancer, it has also been used to identify skin accumulation of cysteine for diagnosis of infantile nephropathic cystinosis.[12]

Several diagnostic techniques involve procedures to obtain scales or discharge (by scraping or swabbing) for analysis. Scraping can be performed with a sterile surgical blade, Fomon blade, or even less costly small metal spatula. An endocervical brush (Cytobrush)[13] or moistened swab can be used for obtaining scales and broken hairs for fungal cultures and may be less frightening for young children (see Chapter 17). Vesicular lesions can be scraped for Tzanck smears and obtaining epidermal material for direct fluorescent analysis and viral (primarily herpes) cultures or to show the cellular content such as eosinophils in the vesicular lesions of incontinentia pigmenti. Potential scabies lesions, especially burrows, can be dotted with mineral oil and scraped vigorously for microscopic analysis, which may reveal live mites, eggs, or feces (see Chapter 18). When looking for superficial fungi, both potassium hydroxide (KOH) wet-mount preparations and cultures are often performed, although KOH examination should be performed in a Clinical Laboratory Improvement Amendments (CLIA)-approved setting (see Chapter 17). For skin lesions, the blade or Cytobrush should scrape the active lesional border. For possible tinea capitis, it is important to obtain broken (infected) hairs and scales. The Cytobrush technique has been shown to be more effective than scraping,[13] and vigorously rubbing with a moistened cotton swab (either with tap water or the Culturette transport medium) before inoculation into fungal culture medium is well tolerated, easy, and reliable. Nail scrapings and subungual debris can also be obtained for evaluation; nail clippings can be sent for histopathologic evaluation with special stains to demonstrate fungal elements.

Hair plucks tend to be traumatic for children and often cause hair shaft distortion, but gentle-traction hair pulling yields hair that is appropriate for determining whether alopecia areata is still active (hair-pull test) and for microscopic evaluation of the telogen bulbs of telogen effluvium and the distorted bulb and ruffled cuticle of loose anagen syndrome (see Chapter 7). Cutting the hair shafts may suffice for seeking hair shaft abnormalities via a microscopic trichogram (which may require polarizing light such as to detect trichothiodystrophy) and detecting nits of pediculosis versus hair casts (see Chapter 18).

Patch testing is key to determining or confirming triggers of delayed-type hypersensitivity reactions in children with allergic contact dermatitis (see Chapter 3). Round aluminum (Finn) chambers are taped to the back for 48 hours, and reactions are detected immediately after removal and generally twice thereafter to capture late reactivity. Although a ready-to-apply system is available (TRUE test), many important potential allergens are missing; thus expanded testing is often necessary to comprehensively evaluate possible triggers and is usually best performed by dermatologists who have expertise in patch testing more comprehensively.

Although swabs of mucosae and of purulent skin material are appropriate for microbial cultures, obtaining biopsy material for special stains and cultures of suspected deep fungal or mycobacterial infections is better for pathogen detection (see Therapeutic Procedures section). Biopsies are also important for making a diagnosis based on routine histopathologic, immunofluorescent, and/or immunohistochemical evaluation. For example, immunofluorescent testing is used to delineate the level of cleavage and absent skin proteins in epidermolysis bullosa (see Chapter 13), as well as to define the immune deposits and patterning in immunobullous disorders (see Chapter 13) and Henoch–Schönlein purpura (see Chapter 21); in contrast, immunohistochemistry is important for confirming the diagnosis of Langerhans cells in histiocytosis (see Chapter 10) and a variety of cutaneous lymphoproliferative disorders. Clinicopathologic correlation is important, however, and the pathologic result should be questioned (or repeated) if not consistent with clinical findings.

Therapeutic Procedures

The most common therapeutic procedures in pediatric dermatology are (1) treatment of warts with cryotherapy, (2) treatment of molluscum with cantharidin or curettage, (3) lesional biopsy or excision, and (4) laser therapy. These techniques should only be performed by trained, experienced practitioners. Phototherapy with ultraviolet B (UVB) light, narrow-band UVB, and UVA/UVA1 light is used occasionally in children and is discussed in Chapter 19.

Cryotherapy involves the application of liquid nitrogen to lesional skin, which causes direct injury. It is most commonly used for warts (see Chapter 15) but can be selectively applied to keloids and molluscum contagiosum. Although spray delivery is possible, application with a cotton swab that is adapted with extra cotton to fit the size of the lesion allows better retention of the liquid nitrogen, provides better avoidance of nonlesional skin, and is less frightening for young children. More pedunculated lesions (or filiform warts) can be treated by grasping the lesion with a forceps and freezing the forceps close to the lesion rather than the lesion directly. Generally, freezing is performed until there is a white ring around the lesion, often with two to three freeze-thaw cycles. Cryotherapy is painful and as a result is generally reserved for children 8 years of age and older. Alternative cryotherapy agents that contain dimethyl ether or chlorodifluoromethane achieve temperatures considerably warmer than liquid nitrogen and are not as effective. Potential complications include hypopigmentation and atrophic scarring.

Cantharidin is an extract from the blister beetle, *Cantharis vesicatoria*, that leads to epidermal vesiculation after application to molluscum contagiosum lesions (see Chapter 15). Although traditionally requiring compounding and administration using a wooden applicator, a single-use applicator with cantharidin is in development. Because the extent of blistering cannot be controlled (with some children developing extensive blisters and others virtually none), lesions near the eyes, on mucosae, and near other sensitive areas should not be treated with cantharidin. In addition, lesions should not be occluded. Blistering occurs in 24 to 48 hours, and crusting clears within about a week. Associated discomfort is variable, but application is painless.

Curettage is a scraping technique used most commonly after topical anesthetic application for physical removal of molluscum contagiosum, especially for larger lesions for which cantharidin is less effective. Curettage can also be used after electrodesiccation (with a hyfrecator) to remove the desiccated tissue, most commonly for removal of a pyogenic granuloma (see Chapter 12). Many pediatric dermatologists avoid the use of curettage in younger patients, given the associated discomfort.

Biopsies and excisions are performed in pediatric patients as intervention, not just for diagnosis. The decision to remove a lesion therapeutically should be based on the indication and urgency for removal, the age and maturity of the pediatric patient, the location, and the expected cosmetic result. Careful explanation of the procedure to the parents and child is important to allay concerns and manage expectations. If possible, the area to be biopsied, excised, or injected with anesthesia can be treated initially with a topical anesthetic cream (e.g., 4% lidocaine or 2.5% lidocaine/2.5% prilocaine) under a clear occlusive film (e.g., waterproof transparent dressing [Tegaderm] or Glad Press'n Seal wrap, which adheres more effectively than traditional plastic cling wrap). Buffering the lidocaine with sodium bicarbonate and use of a 30-gauge needle also help to decrease the pain of injection; once buffered, lidocaine with epinephrine must either be kept refrigerated or discarded after a week because of accelerated epinephrine degradation. Regional nerve blocks can be used selectively for larger excisions or cryotherapy. Distraction techniques such as conversation, listening to music, watching a video, or applying vibrations to a contiguous area can also allay fear at almost any age. Punch biopsy is most useful for removing lesions smaller than 6 mm in diameter. For larger lesions and in cosmetically sensitive areas, an elliptical excision is preferred. Elliptical excisions ideally have their long axis following skin lines to minimize tension on the wound and to optimize the ultimate cosmetic appearance of the scar. Shave biopsies are appropriate for the superficial removal of skin tags (acrochordons) and more protuberant small nevi that are cosmetically problematic; however, shave removal can be followed by lesional regrowth and should not be performed if there is any concern about lesional atypia or malignancy. Surgical wounds of 4 mm or larger in diameter should be closed with suture; wounds that are 3 mm or less can be left to heal via secondary intention after hemostasis (including with insertion of Gelfoam), although suturing of any lesion often gives a better cosmetic result. Although octylcyanoacrylates such as Dermabond are appropriate for closure of lacerations, the cosmetic result of their use in elective procedures may be suboptimal and they are generally not recommended. Deep sutures are often required to close the deeper space of larger or deeper wounds (e.g., >6 mm in diameter) using buried absorbable suture materials. Although a variety of methods are available for closing at the surface, interrupted or running subcuticular suturing with nonabsorbable suture material is most often used. Adhesive wound closure strips such as Steri-Strips are often used to further protect the wound from dehiscence.

The most common complications of biopsies and surgical excisions are wound infection, dehiscence, postoperative bleeding, and hematoma (especially on the scalp). Contact dermatitis may also occur, especially in reaction to adhesives or topical antibiotics; many surgeons use petrolatum alone after skin surgery to avoid the risk of contact dermatitis. Parents should be given clear, written postoperative instructions about keeping dressings in place (and the wound completely dry) for the first 48 hours, appropriate wound care thereafter, limitation in physical activity (generally 4 weeks without sports or gym if an excision), managing potential complications, and when to have sutures removed (typically 7 days for the face and 10 to 14 days on the body and extremities).

Light amplifications by stimulated emission of radiation (lasers) produce intense light energy at a specific wavelength that can be emitted as a pulse or continuous wave to target tissue components for destruction. After absorption of the light, heat is generated and the target tissue is selectively destroyed. This process of selective destruction has been called *selective photothermolysis* and carries the benefit of destruction of the target chromophores (substances that absorb specific wavelengths of light) with minimal damage to surrounding tissues.[13]

By far the most common laser used in children is the pulsed-dye laser (PDL; wavelength 585 to 595 nm), which targets hemoglobin and is used for a variety of vascular lesions, including capillary malformations (port wine stains, salmon patches), macular (flat) infantile hemangiomas, ulcerated hemangiomas (in which case it helps speed reepithelialization), spider telangiectasias, and even small pyogenic granulomas. PDL has also been used (with more variable response) for inflammatory linear verrucous epidermal nevus, erythematous striae, warts[14,15], acne,[16] and even some inflammatory dermatoses such as psoriasis and eczema.

The response of a port wine stain to PDL therapy is variable and may depend on the depth of the dermal capillaries, location of the stain (e.g., central facial stains classically respond less to PDL therapy than lesions on the forehead or peripheral face, in part likely related to the more superficial depth of laterally located dilated capillaries),[17] size of the stain, and age at the time treatment is initiated. Sequential treatment sessions are often necessary (generally at 4- to 8-week intervals), and multiple treatments may be necessary to achieve significant improvement.[18] Port wine stains located on the extremities tend to require more treatments than those located elsewhere, and those associated with early-onset hypertrophy have a poorer response and higher complication rate after PDL treatment.[19] Recent studies in adults with facial port wine stains suggest that the effect of the combination of topical rapamycin and PDL may be greater and more persistent than PDL alone.[20]

Other lasers used in pediatric patients include neodymium:yttrium-aluminum-garnet (Nd:YAG; 1064 nm),[21] alexandrite (755 nm),[22] diode (810 nm), Q-switched ruby (694 nm), and intense pulsed light (555 to 950 nm) lasers, which have shown variable benefit in port wine stains, venous malformations, deeper hemangiomas, and pigmented lesions (mongolian spots, nevus of Ota, Becker melanosis).[13,23] The xenon-chloride excimer laser (308 nm) provides a wavelength similar to narrow-band UVB therapy, with the advantage of being able to selectively treat a more targeted area of the skin. It has been demonstrated to be useful in psoriasis, vitiligo, nevus depigmentosus, pityriasis alba, and postinflammatory hypopigmentation.[24–28]

The complete list of 28 references for this chapter is available online at http://expertconsult.inkling.com.

Key References

Haliasos EC, Kerner M, Jaimes-Lopez N, et al. Dermoscopy for the pediatric dermatologist. Part I. Dermoscopy of pediatric infectious and inflammatory skin lesions and hair disorders. Pediatr Dermatol 2013;30:163–71.

Haliasos EC, Kerner M, Jaimes N, et al. Dermoscopy for the pediatric dermatologist. Part II. Dermoscopy of genetic syndromes with cutaneous manifestations and pediatric vascular lesions. Pediatr Dermatol 2013;30:172–81.

Haliasos EC, Kerner M, Jaimes N, et al. Dermoscopy for the pediatric dermatologist. Part III. Dermoscopy of melanocytic lesions. Pediatr Dermatol 2013;30:281–93.

Rudnicka L, Olszewska M, Waskiel A, et al. Trichoscopy in hair shaft disorders. Dermatol Clin 2018;36(4):421–30.

Bonifaz A, Isa-Isa R, Araiza J, et al. Cytobrush-culture method to diagnose tinea capitis. Mycopathologia 2007;163(6):309–13.

Cordisco MR. An update on lasers in children. Curr Opin Pediatr 2009;21:499–504.

Craig LM, Alster TS. Vascular skin lesions in children: a review of laser surgical and medical treatments. Dermatol Surg 2013;39:1137–46.

Dinulos JGH. Cosmetic procedures in children. Curr Opin Pediatr 2011;23:395–8.

Franca K, Chacon A, Ledon J, et al. Lasers for cutaneous congenital vascular lesions: a comprehensive overview and update. Lasers Med Sci 2013;28:1197–204.

2 Cutaneous Disorders of the Newborn

CHAPTER OUTLINE

Neonatal Skin

The skin of the infant differs from that of an adult in that it is thinner (40% to 60%), is less hairy, and has a weaker attachment between the epidermis and dermis.[1] In addition, the body surface area–to–weight ratio of an infant is up to five times that of an adult. The infant is therefore at a significantly increased risk for skin injury, percutaneous absorption, and skin-associated infection. Premature infants born before 32 to 34 weeks' estimated gestational age may have problems associated with an immature stratum corneum (the most superficial cell layer in the epidermis), including an increase in transepidermal water loss (TEWL). This increased TEWL may result in morbidity because of dehydration, electrolyte imbalance, and thermal instability. Interestingly, in the majority of premature infants an acceleration of skin maturation occurs after birth such that most develop intact barrier function by 2 to 3 weeks of life.[2] However, in extremely low-birthweight infants, this process may take up to 4 to 8 weeks.[3] In light of the elevated TEWL levels seen in premature infants, a variety of studies have evaluated the use of occlusive dressings or topical emollients in an effort to improve compromised barrier function.[4–7]

The risk of percutaneous toxicity from topically applied substances is increased in infants, especially those born prematurely.[8,9] Percutaneous absorption is known to occur through two major pathways: (1) through the cells of the stratum corneum and the epidermal malpighian layer (the transepidermal route) and (2) through the hair follicle–sebaceous gland component (the transappendageal route). Increased neonatal percutaneous absorption may be the result of the increased skin surface area–to–weight ratio as well as the stratum corneum immaturity seen in premature neonates. Although transdermal delivery methods may be distinctly advantageous in certain settings, extreme caution must be exercised in the application of topical substances to the skin of infants, given the risk of systemic absorption and potential toxicity. Table 2.1 lists some compounds reported in association with percutaneous toxicity in infants and children.

SKIN CARE OF THE NEWBORN

The skin of the newborn is covered with a grayish-white, greasy material termed *vernix caseosa*. The vernix represents a physiologic protective covering derived partially from secretions of the sebaceous glands and in part as a decomposition product of the infant's epidermis. Vernix contains protein, lipids, and water and provides water-binding free amino acids that facilitate the adaptation from amniotic fluid immersion *in utero* to the dry ambient postnatal state.[10] Although its function is not completely understood, it may act as a natural protectant cream to "waterproof" the fetus *in utero*, where it is submerged in the amniotic fluid.[11] Some studies suggest that vernix be left on as a protective coating for the newborn skin and that it be allowed to come off by itself with successive changes of clothing (generally within the first few weeks of life). It has been suggested that vernix-based topical creams may be effective in augmenting stratum corneum repair and maturation in infants and could play a role in the treatment of epidermal wounds.[12]

The skin acts as a protective organ. Any break in its integrity therefore affords an opportunity for initiation of infection. The importance of skin care in the newborn is compounded by several factors:

1. The infant does not have protective skin flora at birth.
2. The infant has at least one and possibly two open surgical wounds (the umbilicus and circumcision site).
3. The infant is exposed to fomites and personnel that potentially harbor a variety of infectious agents.

Skin care should involve gentle cleansing with a nontoxic, nonabrasive neutral material. During the 1950s, the use of hexachlorophene-containing compounds became routine for the skin care of newborns as prophylaxis against *Staphylococcus aureus* infection. In 1971 and 1972, however, the use of hexachlorophene preparations as skin cleansers for newborns was restricted because of studies demonstrating vacuolization in the central nervous system (CNS) of infants and laboratory animals after prolonged application of these preparations.[13] At the minimum, neonatal skin care should include gentle removal of blood from the face and head, and meconium from the perianal area, by gentle rinsing with water. Ideally, vernix caseosa should be removed from the face only, allowing the remaining vernix to come off by itself. However, the common standard of care is for gentle drying and wiping of the newborn's entire skin surface, which is most desirable from a thermoregulatory standpoint. Recommendations for "first bathing" of the newborn suggest timing it according to local culture, performing it only after the newborn is physiologically stable and able to appropriately thermoregulate, considering the use of water alone or water and an appropriately formulated pH neutral (or acidic) liquid cleanser such as a synthetic detergent (syndet) or liquid baby cleanser, and considering the use of gloves by healthcare workers if performing the initial bath.[14–16]

There is no single method of umbilical-cord care that has been proven to limit bacterial colonization and disease, and cord care practices are quite variable in relation to cultural beliefs and healthcare disparities. Several methods have been reported, including local application of isopropyl alcohol, triple dye (an aqueous solution of brilliant green, proflavine, and gentian violet), and antimicrobial agents such as bacitracin or silver sulfadiazine cream. The routine use of povidone-iodine should be discouraged, given the risk of iodine absorption and transient hypothyroxinemia or hypothyroidism. A safer alternative is a chlorhexidine-containing product.[17] A recent clinical review suggests consideration of application of antimicrobial agents

Table 2.1 Reported Hazards of Percutaneous Absorption in Infants and Children

Compound	Product	Toxicity
Alcohols	Skin antiseptic	Cutaneous hemorrhagic necrosis, elevated blood alcohol levels
Aniline	Dye used as laundry marker	Methemoglobinemia, death
Adhesive remover solvents	Skin preparations to aid in adhesive removal	Epidermal injury, hemorrhage, and necrosis
Benzocaine	Mucosal anesthetic (teething products)	Methemoglobinemia
Boric acid	Baby powder, diaper paste	Vomiting, diarrhea, erythroderma, seizures, death
Calcipotriol	Topical vitamin D_3 analog	Hypercalcemia, hypercalcemic crisis
Chlorhexidine	Topical antiseptic	Systemic absorption but no toxic effects
Corticosteroids	Topical antiinflammatory	Skin atrophy, striae, adrenal suppression
Diphenhydramine	Topical antipruritic	Central anticholinergic syndrome
Lidocaine	Topical anesthetic	Petechiae, seizures
Lindane	Scabicide	Neurotoxicity
Mercuric chloride	Diaper rinses; teething powders	Acrodynia, hypotonia
Methylene blue	Amniotic fluid leak	Methemoglobinemia
N,N-diethyl-*m*-toluamide (DEET)	Insect repellent	Neurotoxicity
Neomycin	Topical antibiotic	Neural deafness
Phenolic compounds (pentachlorophenol, hexachlorophene, resorcinol)	Laundry disinfectant, topical antiseptic	Neurotoxicity, tachycardia, metabolic acidosis, methemoglobinemia, death
Phenylephrine	Ophthalmic drops	Vasoconstriction, periorbital pallor
Povidone-iodine	Topical antiseptic	Hypothyroidism
Prilocaine	Topical anesthetic	Methemoglobinemia
Salicylic acid	Keratolytic emollient	Metabolic acidosis, salicylism
Silver sulfadiazine	Topical antibiotic	Kernicterus (sulfa component), agranulocytosis, argyria (silver component)
Tacrolimus	Topical immunomodulator	Elevated blood levels of immunosuppressive medication
Triple dye (brilliant green, gentian violet, proflavine hemisulfate)	Topical antiseptic for umbilical cord	Ulceration of mucous membranes, skin necrosis, vomiting, diarrhea
Urea	Keratolytic emollient	Uremia

Reprinted with permission from Bree AF, Siegfried EC. Neonatal skin care and toxicology. In: Eichenfield LF, Frieden IJ, Esterly NB, editors. Textbook of neonatal dermatology. 2nd ed. London: Saunders Elsevier; 2008:59–72.

for infants born at home or otherwise outside of birthing centers or hospitals in resource-limited settings but highlights that their use in high-resource countries or the setting of in-hospital delivery has not been found to provide clear benefit.[18]

Physiologic Phenomena of the Newborn

Neonatal dermatology, by definition, encompasses the spectrum of cutaneous disorders that arise during the first 4 weeks of life. Many such conditions are transient, appearing in the first few days to weeks of life only to disappear shortly thereafter. The appreciation of normal phenomena and their differentiation from the more significant cutaneous disorders of the newborn is critical for the general physician, obstetrician, and pediatrician, as well as for the pediatric dermatologist.

At birth, the skin of the full-term infant is normally soft, smooth, and velvety. Desquamation of neonatal skin generally takes place 24 to 36 hours after delivery and may not be complete until the third week of life. Desquamation at birth is an abnormal phenomenon and is indicative of postmaturity, intrauterine anoxia, or congenital ichthyosis.

The skin at birth has a purplish-red color that is most pronounced over the extremities. Except for the hands, feet, and lips, where the transition is gradual, this quickly changes to a pink hue. In many infants, a purplish discoloration of the hands, feet, and lips occurs during periods of crying, breath holding, or chilling. This normal phenomenon, termed *acrocyanosis*, appears to be associated with an increased tone of peripheral arterioles, which in turn creates vasospasm, secondary dilation, and pooling of blood in the venous plexuses, resulting in a cyanotic appearance to the involved areas of the skin. The intensity of cyanosis depends on the degree of oxygen loss and the depth, size, and fullness of the involved venous plexus. Acrocyanosis, a normal physiologic phenomenon, should not be confused with true cyanosis.

CUTIS MARMORATA

Cutis marmorata is a normal reticulated bluish mottling of the skin seen on the trunk and extremities of infants and young children (Fig. 2.1). This phenomenon, a physiologic response to chilling with resultant dilation of capillaries and small venules, usually disappears as the infant is rewarmed. Although a tendency for cutis marmorata may persist for several weeks or months, this disorder bears no medical significance and treatment generally is unnecessary. In some children cutis marmorata may tend to recur until early childhood, and in patients with Down syndrome, trisomy 18, and Cornelia de Lange syndrome, this reticulated marbling pattern may be persistent. When the changes are persistent (even with rewarming) and are deep violaceous in color, cutis marmorata telangiectatica congenita (Fig. 2.2; see also Chapter 12) should be considered. In some infants a white negative pattern of cutis marmorata (cutis marmorata alba)

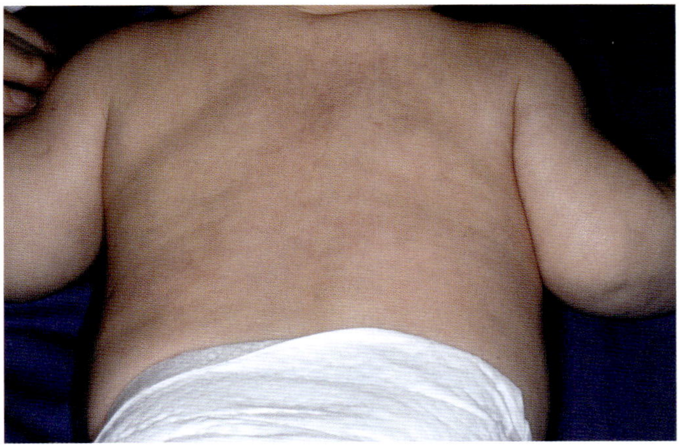

Fig. 2.1 Cutis marmorata. Reticulate bluish mottling that resolves with rewarming.

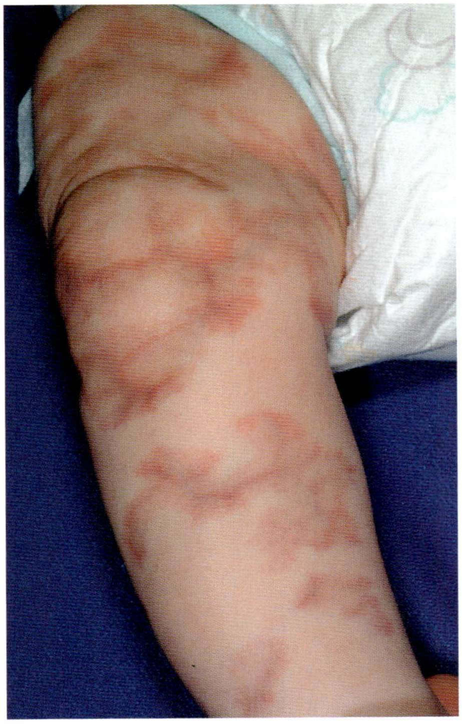

Fig. 2.2 Cutis marmorata telangiectatica congenita. Violaceous, reticulate patches with subtle atrophy. These changes did not resolve with rewarming and were associated with mild ipsilateral limb hypoplasia.

may be created by a transient hypertonia of the deep vasculature. Cutis marmorata alba is also a transitory disorder and appears to have no clinical significance.

HARLEQUIN COLOR CHANGE

Harlequin color change, a form of vascular autonomic dysregulation not to be confused with harlequin ichthyosis (see Chapter 5), is occasionally observed in full-term infants but classically described in premature infants. It occurs when the infant is lying on his or her side and consists of reddening of one-half of the body with simultaneous blanching of the other half. Attacks develop suddenly and may persist for 30 seconds to 20 minutes. The side that lies uppermost is paler, and a clear line of demarcation runs along the midline of the body. At times, this line of demarcation may be incomplete; when attacks are mild, areas of the face and genitalia may not be involved.

This phenomenon appears to be related to immaturity of hypothalamic centers that control the tone of peripheral blood vessels and has been observed in infants with severe intracranial injury as well as in infants who appear to be otherwise perfectly normal. Some medications, including anesthetics and prostaglandin E, may exacerbate the condition.[19] Although the peak frequency of attacks of harlequin color change generally occurs between the second and fifth days of life, attacks may occur anywhere from the first few hours to as late as the second or the third week of life.[20]

INFANTILE TRANSIENT SMOOTH MUSCLE CONTRACTION OF THE SKIN

Believed to be a primitive reflex or autonomic phenomenon, *infantile transient smooth muscle contraction of the skin* refers to a transient rippling of the skin of otherwise-healthy infants, often triggered by cold or blowing air exposure. In a series of nine full-term newborns with this phenomenon, the authors noted several asymptomatic episodes occurring daily for brief periods (usually <1 minute), with completely normal–appearing skin in between episodes. Histologic examination was unremarkable in the skin biopsy specimens from three patients, and the episodes spontaneously resolved over 18 to 24 months. This condition appears to be related to transient arrector pili smooth muscle contraction, without features to suggest smooth muscle hamartoma.[21]

BRONZE BABY SYNDROME

Bronze baby syndrome (BBS) is a term used to describe infants who develop a grayish-brown discoloration of the skin, serum, and urine while undergoing phototherapy for hyperbilirubinemia. Although the exact source of the pigment causing the discoloration is not clear, the syndrome usually begins 1 to 7 days after the initiation of phototherapy, resolves gradually over a period of several weeks after phototherapy is discontinued, and appears to be related to a combination of photoisomers of bilirubin or biliverdin or a photoproduct of copper-porphyrin metabolism.[22–24] Infants who develop BBS usually have modified liver function, particularly cholestasis, of various origins.[25] Although very few babies with cholestasis develop BBS during phototherapy, those who do should be investigated for underlying liver disease.[26] The disorder should be differentiated from neonatal jaundice, cyanosis associated with neonatal pulmonary disorders or congenital heart disease, an unusual progressive hyperpigmentation (universal-acquired melanosis, or "carbon baby" syndrome),[27] and chloramphenicol intoxication ("gray baby" syndrome).[28] Although early recognition of BBS suggests further evaluation for associated disorders, it does not appear to be a contraindication to ongoing phototherapy for hyperbilirubinemia.[29] A distinctive purpuric eruption on exposed skin has also been described in newborns receiving phototherapy and is possibly related to a transient increase in circulating porphyrins.[30] This condition, however, is unlikely to be confused with BBS.

Cephalohematoma

A cephalohematoma is a subperiosteal hematoma overlying the calvarium. These lesions are more common after prolonged labor, instrument-assisted deliveries, and abnormal presentations. They usually develop over the first hours of life and present as subcutaneous swellings in the scalp. They do not cross the midline (Fig. 2.3) because they are limited to one cranial bone, which helps distinguish them from caput succedaneum (see the next section). Occasionally, a cephalohematoma may occur over a linear skull fracture. Other potentially associated complications include calcification (which may persist radiographically for years), osteomyelitis, hyperbilirubinemia, and infection. Signs of an infected cephalohematoma, usually caused by *Staphylococcus aureus* or *Escherichia coli*, include erythema, increasing size, and fluctuance.[31] Although infected lesions (which are rare) may require aspiration,[32] most lesions require no therapy, with spontaneous resorption and resolution occurring over several weeks to months.

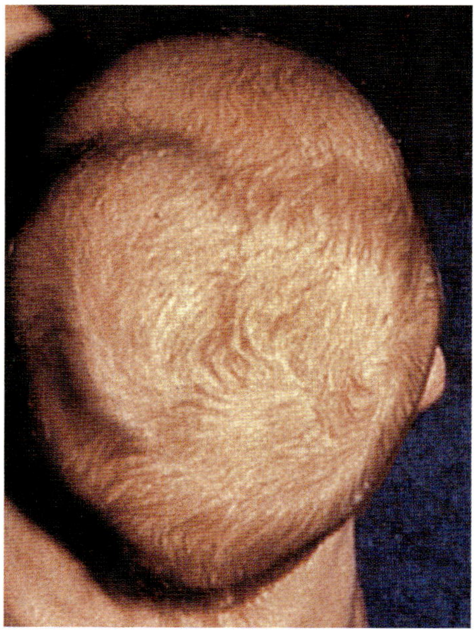

Fig. 2.3 Cephalohematoma. Note the sharp demarcation at the midline.

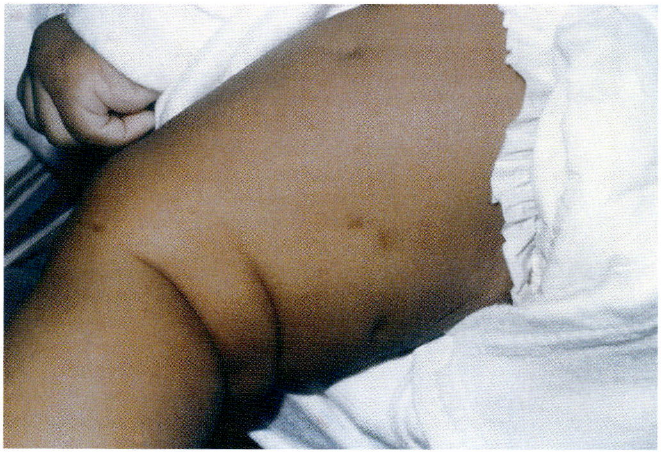

Fig. 2.4 Amniocentesis scars. Multiple depressed scars on the thigh of an infant born to a mother who had an amniocentesis during pregnancy. (Courtesy Lester Schwartz, MD.)

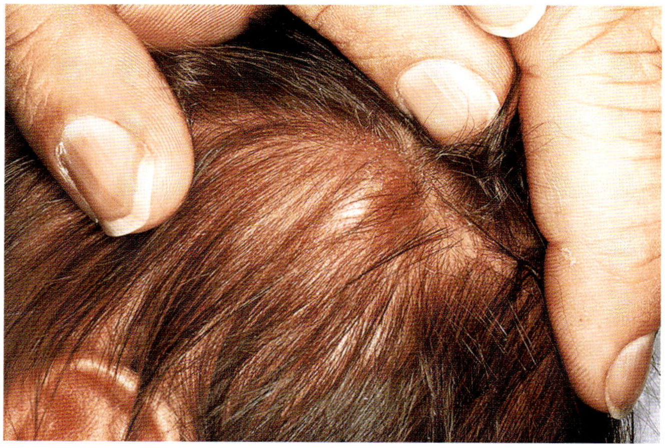

Fig. 2.5 Staphylococcal scalp abscess. Fluctuant, erythematous nodule on the scalp of this 9-day-old infant as a complication of intrauterine fetal monitoring.

Caput Succedaneum

Caput succedaneum is a localized edema of the newborn scalp related to the mechanical forces involved in parturition. It is probably related to venous congestion and edema secondary to cervical and uterine pressure and as such is more common with prolonged parturition and seen most often in primigravidas. Caput succedaneum presents as a boggy scalp mass and may result in varying degrees of bruising and necrosis in addition to the edema, at times with tissue loss. In distinction to cephalohematoma, caput succedaneum lesions often cross the midline. These lesions tend to resolve spontaneously over 48 hours, and treatment is generally unnecessary. One possible complication in cases of severe caput succedaneum is permanent alopecia. *Halo scalp ring* refers to an annular alopecia that presents in a circumferential ring around the scalp in infants with a history of caput.[33] It represents a pressure necrosis phenomenon, and the hair loss may be transient or occasionally permanent.

Complications from Fetal and Neonatal Diagnostic Procedures

Fetal complications associated with invasive prenatal diagnostic procedures include cutaneous puncture marks, scars or lacerations, exsanguination, ocular trauma, blindness, subdural hemorrhage, pneumothorax, cardiac tamponade, splenic laceration, porencephalic cysts, arteriovenous or ileocutaneous fistulas, digital loss (in 1.7% of newborns whose mothers had undergone early chorionic villus sampling), musculoskeletal trauma, disruption of tendons or ligaments, and occasionally gangrene. Cutaneous puncture marks, which occur in 1% to 3% of newborns whose mothers have undergone amniocentesis, may be seen as single or multiple 1- to 6-mm pits, dimples, or round depressed scars on any cutaneous surface of the newborn (Fig. 2.4).[34–36]

Fetal scalp monitoring can result in infection, bleeding, or fontanel puncture, and prenatal vacuum extraction can produce a localized area of edema, ecchymosis, or localized alopecia. The incidence of scalp electrode infection varies from 0.3% to 5%, and although local sterile abscesses account for the majority of adverse sequelae, *S. aureus* or Gram-negative infections, cellulitis, tissue necrosis, subgaleal abscess, osteomyelitis, necrotizing fasciitis, and neonatal herpes simplex infections may also occur as complications of this procedure (Fig. 2.5).[37–39] It is not unusual for new parents to be under the false impression that fetal scalp electrodes are the cause of aplasia cutis congenita (ACC; see later in this chapter).

Scalp injuries sustained during the birth process tend to be minor and include lacerations, erosions, and ecchymoses. Injuries of the scalp and face occur in approximately 16% of vacuum-assisted deliveries and in 17% of forceps-assisted deliveries (Fig. 2.6).[40] In a large series of vacuum-assisted deliveries, occurrence of head injury did not correlate with duration of vacuum application or the number of pop-offs or pulls.[41]

Transcutaneous oxygen monitoring (application of heated electrodes to the skin for continuous detection of tissue oxygenation) and pulse oximetry may also result in erythema, tissue necrosis, and first- or second-degree burns. Although lesions associated with transcutaneous oxygen monitoring generally resolve within 48 to 60 hours, persistent atrophic hyperpigmented craters may at times be seen as a complication. Frequent (every 2 to 4 hours) changing of electrode sites and reduction of the temperature of the electrodes to 43° C, however, can lessen the likelihood of this complication.[42,43]

Anetoderma of prematurity refers to macular depressions or outpouchings of skin associated with loss of dermal elastic tissue seen in premature infants. Reports suggest that these cutaneous lesions may correlate with placement of electrocardiographic or other monitoring electrodes or leads.[44,45]

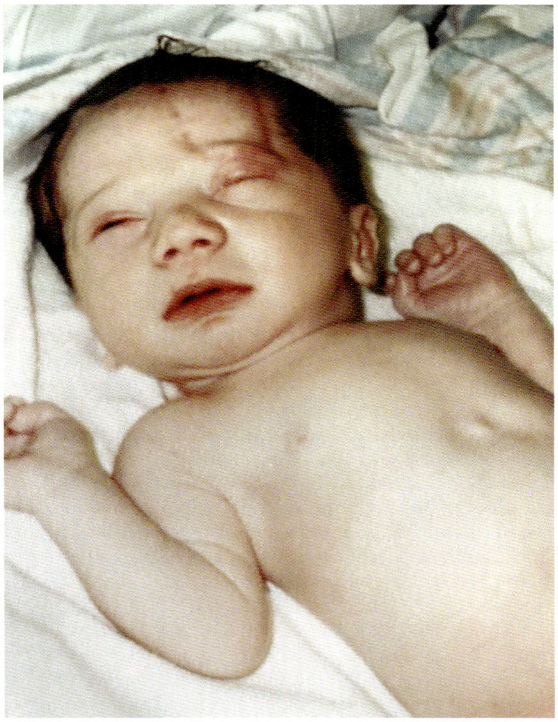

Fig. 2.6 Forceps-induced ecchymoses. This newborn boy was delivered vaginally with forceps assistance and developed this bruising, which conforms to the shape of the forceps blade.

Calcinosis cutis may occur on the scalp or chest of infants or children at sites of electroencephalograph or electrocardiograph electrode placement, as a result of diagnostic heel sticks performed during the neonatal period, or after intramuscular or intravenous administration of calcium chloride or calcium gluconate for the treatment of neonatal hypocalcemia. Seen primarily in high-risk infants who receive repeated heel sticks for blood chemistry determinations, *heel-stick calcinosis* refers to calcified nodules that usually begin as small depressions on the heels. It is considered a form of dystrophic calcinosis cutis (see Chapter 9). With time, generally after 4 to 12 months, tiny yellow or white papules appear (Fig. 2.7, *A*), gradually enlarge to form nodular deposits, migrate to the cutaneous surface, extrude their contents ("transepidermal elimination") (Fig. 2.7, *B*), and generally disappear spontaneously by the time the child reaches 18 to 30 months of age. Although calcified heel nodules are usually asymptomatic, children may at times show signs of discomfort with standing or wearing shoes. In such instances, gentle cryosurgery and curettage can be both diagnostic and therapeutic. Rarely, persistent or symptomatic cases may require surgical excision.[46] Calcinosis cutis after electroencephalography or electrocardiography is more likely to be seen in infants and young children or individuals where the skin has been abraded and usually disappears spontaneously within 2 to 6 months. It can be avoided by the use of an electrode paste that does not contain calcium chloride, and like calcified heel sticks, they may be treated by gentle cryosurgery and curettage.[47,48]

Abnormalities of Subcutaneous Tissue

Skin turgor is generally normal during the first few hours of life. As normal physiologic dehydration occurs during the first 3 or 4 days of life (up to 10% of birthweight), the skin generally becomes loose and wrinkled. Subcutaneous fat is normally quite adequate at birth and increases until about 9 months of age, thus accounting for the traditional chubby appearance of the healthy newborn. A decrease or absence of this normal panniculus is abnormal and suggests the possibility of prematurity, postmaturity, or placental insufficiency.

Sclerema neonatorum and subcutaneous fat necrosis (SCFN) are two disorders that affect the subcutaneous fat of the newborn. Although there is considerable diagnostic confusion between these two entities, there are several distinguishing features that enable a clinical differentiation (Table 2.2). Sclerema neonatorum seems to occur significantly less often than SCFN.

SCLEREMA NEONATORUM

Sclerema neonatorum is a diffuse, rapidly spreading, wax-like hardening of the skin and subcutaneous tissue that occurs in premature or debilitated infants during the first few weeks of life and may rarely present after several months of life.[49] The disorder, usually associated with a serious underlying condition such as sepsis or other infection, congenital heart disease, respiratory distress, intracranial hemorrhage, diarrhea, or dehydration, is characterized by a diffuse nonpitting woody induration of the involved tissues. The process is symmetric, usually starting on the legs and buttocks, and may progress to involve all areas except the palms, soles, and genitalia.[50] As the disorder spreads, the skin becomes cold, yellowish-white, mottled, stony hard, and cadaver-like. The limbs become immobile, and the face acquires a fixed mask-like expression. Infants with this disorder become sluggish, feed poorly, show clinical signs of shock, and, in a large percentage of cases, die.

Although the cause of this disorder is unknown, it appears to represent a nonspecific sign of severe illness rather than a primary

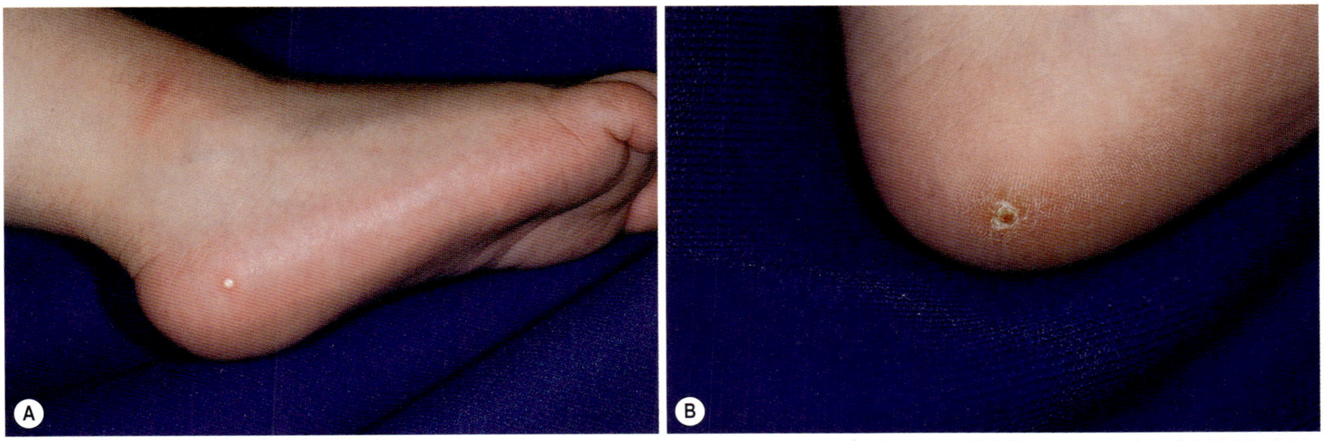

Fig. 2.7 Heel-stick calcinosis. **(A)** Firm, yellow-white papule on the lateral plantar heel of an infant who had multiple heel sticks as a newborn. **(B)** Hyperkeratotic firm papule on the heel of another infant, with early transepidermal elimination before resolution.

Table 2.2 Features of Sclerema Neonatorum and Subcutaneous Fat Necrosis

Sclerema Neonatorum	Subcutaneous Fat Necrosis
Premature infants	Full-term or postmature infants
Serious underlying disease (sepsis, cardiopulmonary disease, diarrhea, or dehydration)	Healthy newborns; may have history of perinatal asphyxia or difficult delivery Also seen in infants with history of therapeutic cooling for HIE
Wax-like hardening of skin and subcutaneous tissue	Circumscribed, indurated, erythematous nodules and plaques
Whole body except palms and soles	Buttocks, thighs, arms, face, shoulders
Poor prognosis; high mortality	Excellent prognosis; treat associated hypercalcemia if present

HIE, Hypoxic-ischemic encephalopathy.

disease. Infants with this disorder are characteristically small or premature, debilitated, weak, cyanotic, and lethargic. In 25% of cases the mothers are ill at the time of delivery. Exposure to cold, hypothermia, peripheral chilling with vascular collapse, and an increase in the ratio of saturated to unsaturated fatty acids in the triglyceride fraction of the subcutaneous tissue (because of a defect in fatty acid mobilization) have been hypothesized as possible causes for this disorder but lack confirmation.[51]

The histopathologic findings of sclerema neonatorum consist of edema and thickening of the connective tissue bands around the fat lobules. Although necrosis and crystallization of the subcutaneous tissue have been described, these findings are more characteristically seen in lesions of SCFN.

The prognosis of infants with sclerema neonatorum is poor, and mortality occurs in 50% to 75% of affected infants. In a series of 51 infants with sclerema neonatorum in a special-care nursery within a Bangladeshi hospital, the fatality rate was 98%.[52] In infants who survive, the cutaneous findings resolve without residual sequelae. There is no specific therapy, although steroids and exchange transfusion have been used.[50]

SUBCUTANEOUS FAT NECROSIS

Subcutaneous fat necrosis (SCFN) is a benign, self-limited disease that affects apparently healthy, full-term newborns and young infants. It is characterized by sharply circumscribed, indurated, and nodular areas of fat necrosis (Fig. 2.8). The cause of this disorder remains unknown but appears to be related to perinatal trauma, asphyxia, hypothermia, and, in some instances, hypercalcemia.[53,54] Although the mechanism of hypercalcemia in SCFN is not known, it has been attributed to aberrations in vitamin D or parathyroid homeostasis. Birth asphyxia and meconium aspiration seem to be commonly associated. In one large series, 10 of 11 infants with SCFN had been delivered via emergency cesarean section for fetal distress, and 9 of the 11 had meconium staining of the amniotic fluid.[55] The relationship among SCFN, maternal diabetes, and cesarean section, if any, is unclear. SCFN after ice-bag application for treatment of supraventricular tachycardia has been reported,[56] and it has also been observed after selective head or generalized cooling for hypoxic-ischemic encephalopathy.[57,58] In a review of neonates with hypoxic-ischemic encephalopathy in Switzerland, 2.8% of all cooled neonates developed SCFN, which occurred independently of the cooling method used and the number of temperature measurements outside the target temperature range.[59]

The onset of SCFN is generally during the first few days to weeks of life. Lesions appear as single or multiple localized, sharply circumscribed, usually painless areas of induration. Occasionally the affected areas may be tender, and infants may be uncomfortable and cry vigorously when they are handled. Lesions vary from small erythematous, indurated nodules to large plaques, and sites of predilection include the cheeks, back, buttocks, arms, and thighs (Fig. 2.9). Many lesions have an uneven lobulated surface with an elevated margin separating it from the surrounding normal tissue. Histologic examination of skin biopsy tissue reveals larger-than-usual fat lobules and an extensive inflammatory infiltrate, needle-shaped clefts within fat cells, necrosis, and calcification. Fine-needle aspiration biopsy has been reported as a useful and less invasive method for diagnosis.[60] Magnetic resonance imaging (MRI), although rarely performed, reveals decreased T1 and increased T2 signal intensity in affected areas.[61]

The prognosis for SCFN is excellent. Although lesions may develop extensive deposits of calcium, which may liquefy, drain, and heal with scarring, most areas undergo spontaneous resolution within several weeks to months. Hypercalcemia is an association observed in up to 56% to 63% of infants in larger series,[62,63] and infants with this finding may require low calcium intake, restriction of vitamin D, and/or systemic corticosteroid therapy. Etidronate therapy has been reported for treatment of recalcitrant SCFN-associated hypercalcemia.[64,65] Infants should be monitored for several months after delivery, because the onset of hypercalcemia can be delayed.[55,66] Other rare systemic complications may include thrombocytopenia, hypoglycemia, and hypertriglyceridemia, all of which tend to be mild or self-limited.

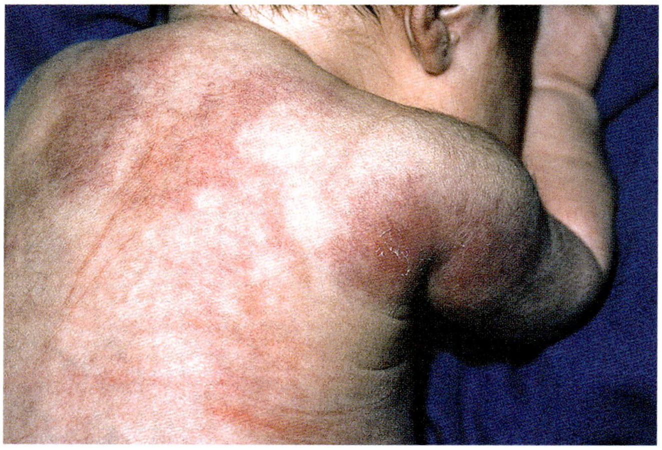

Fig. 2.8 Subcutaneous fat necrosis. Indurated, erythematous plaques on the shoulders and back of this 1-week-old boy.

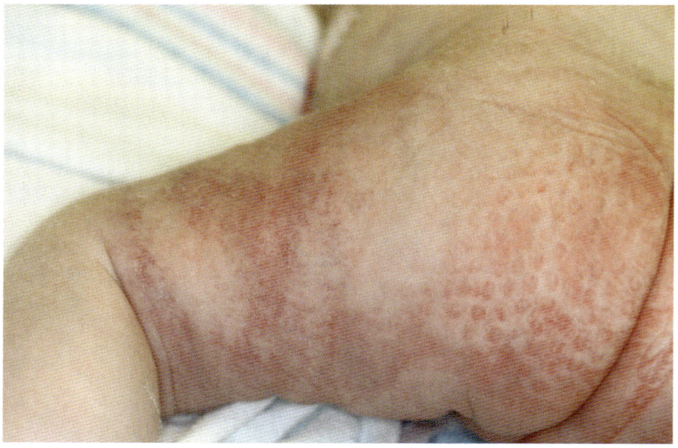

Fig. 2.9 Subcutaneous fat necrosis. This 20-day-old girl presented with firm, indurated erythematous plaques and nodules on the thighs and had been delivered via emergency cesarean section with a history of meconium aspiration, respiratory distress, and hypoglycemia. Her serum ionized calcium was found to be markedly elevated and required therapy with pamidronate.

Miscellaneous Cutaneous Disorders

MILIARIA

Differentiation of the epidermis and its appendages, particularly in the premature infant, is often incomplete at birth. As a result of this immaturity, a high incidence of sweat-retention phenomena may be seen in the newborn. Miliaria, a common neonatal dermatosis caused by sweat retention, is characterized by a vesicular eruption with subsequent maceration and obstruction of the eccrine ducts. The pathophysiologic events that lead to this disorder are keratinous plugging of eccrine ducts and the escape of eccrine sweat into the skin below the level of obstruction (see Chapter 8).

Virtually all infants develop miliaria under appropriate conditions. There are two principal forms of this disorder:

1. Miliaria crystallina (sudamina), which consists of clear superficial pinpoint vesicles without an inflammatory areola (Fig. 2.10)
2. Miliaria rubra (prickly heat), representing a deeper level of sweat gland obstruction and characterized by small discrete erythematous papules, vesicles, or papulovesicles (Fig. 2.11)

The incidence of miliaria is greatest in the first few weeks of life because of the relative immaturity of the eccrine ducts, which favors poral closure and sweat retention. A pustular form of miliaria rubra has been observed in association with pseudohypoaldosteronism during salt-losing crises.[67]

Therapy for miliaria is directed toward avoidance of excessive heat and humidity. Lightweight cotton clothing, cool baths, and air conditioning are helpful in the management and prevention of this disorder. Avoidance of emollient overapplication (e.g., in infants with atopic dermatitis) should also be recommended, especially in warm, humid climates or in the winter when infants are bundled under heavy clothing.

MILIA

Milia, small retention cysts, commonly occur on the face of newborns. Seen in 40% to 50% of infants, they result from retention of keratin within the dermis. They appear as tiny 1- to 2-mm pearly white or yellow papules. Particularly prominent on the cheeks, nose, chin, and forehead, they may be few or numerous (Fig. 2.12) and are often grouped, in which case they have been termed *milia en plaque* (Fig. 2.13). Lesions may occasionally occur on the upper trunk, limbs, penis, or mucous membranes. Although milia of the newborn may persist into the second or third month, they usually disappear spontaneously during the first 3 or 4 weeks of life and accordingly require no therapy. Milia en plaque may occur in a congenital fashion, although they most often occur outside the newborn period, where they may be secondary to skin injury (e.g., abrasions) or blistering disorders.[68] Persistent milia in an unusual or widespread distribution, particularly

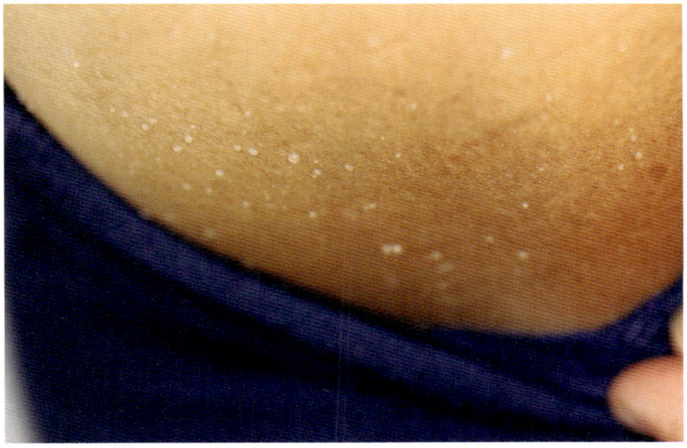

Fig. 2.10 Miliaria crystallina. Note clear, noninflammatory vesicles on the medial thigh of a hospitalized, febrile child.

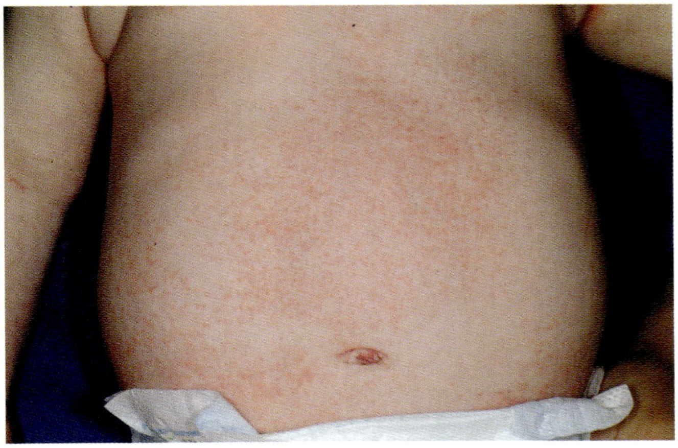

Fig. 2.11 Miliaria rubra. Multiple, erythematous, pinpoint macules and papules in an infant with atopic dermatitis who was being treated with overapplication of greasy emollients.

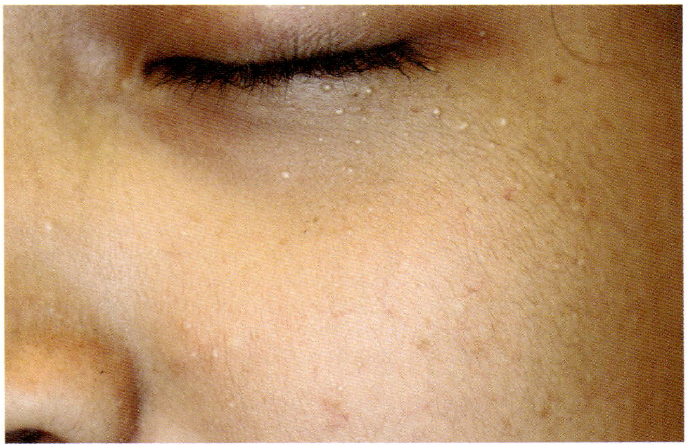

Fig. 2.12 Milia. Multiple small white papules on the cheek of a girl; similar lesions are often noted on the face of healthy newborns.

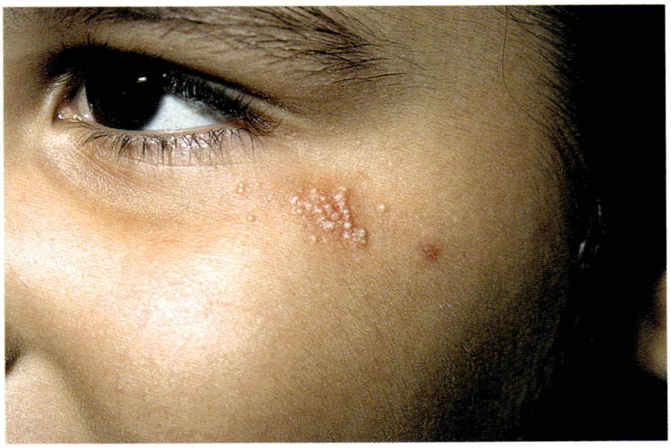

Fig. 2.13 Milia en plaque. Clustered, small, white papules on the lateral cheek.

when seen in association with other defects, may be a manifestation of hereditary trichodysplasia (Marie-Unna hypotrichosis), dystrophic forms of epidermolysis bullosa, Bazex or Rombo syndromes, or type I oral-facial-digital syndrome.

BOHN NODULES AND EPSTEIN PEARLS

Discrete, 2- to 3-mm round, pearly white or yellow, freely movable elevations at the gum margins or midline of the hard palate (termed *Bohn nodules* and *Epstein pearls*, respectively) are seen in up to 85% of newborns. Clinically and histologically the counterpart of facial milia, they disappear spontaneously, usually within a few weeks of life, and require no therapy.

SEBACEOUS GLAND HYPERPLASIA

Sebaceous gland hyperplasia represents a physiologic phenomenon of the newborn manifested as multiple, yellow to flesh-colored tiny papules that occur on the nose, cheeks, and upper lips of full-term infants (Fig. 2.14). A manifestation of maternal androgen stimulation, these papules represent a temporary disorder that resolves spontaneously, generally within the first few weeks of life.

ACNE NEONATORUM

Occasionally infants develop a facial eruption that resembles acne vulgaris as seen in adolescents (Fig. 2.15). Clinical examination typically reveals erythematous papules, pustules, and occasionally comedones (although the latter are more common in infantile acne; see Chapter 8). Although the cause of this disorder is not clearly defined, it appears to develop as a result of hormonal stimulation of sebaceous glands that have not yet involuted to their childhood state of immaturity. In mild cases of acne neonatorum, therapy is often unnecessary; daily cleansing with soap and water may be all that is required. Occasionally, benzoyl peroxide, a topical retinoid, or topical antibiotics may be helpful (see Chapter 8). Unusually severe or recalcitrant cases of acne neonatorum warrant investigation for underlying androgen excess.

A facial acneiform eruption in infants has been associated with the saprophytic *Malassezia* species and has been termed *neonatal cephalic pustulosis* (see Chapter 8). Lesions consist of pinpoint papules, papulopustules, or larger pustules, and they are located on the cheeks, chin, and forehead (Fig. 2.16). A correlation may exist between the clinical severity of lesions and the colonization with this fungal saprophyte.[69,70] In these infants, topical antifungal agents may lead to more rapid resolution of lesions.

ERYTHEMA TOXICUM NEONATORUM

Erythema toxicum neonatorum (ETN), also known as *toxic erythema of the newborn*, is an idiopathic, asymptomatic, benign, self-limiting, cutaneous eruption in full-term newborns. Lesions consist of erythematous macules, papules, and pustules (Fig. 2.17), or a combination

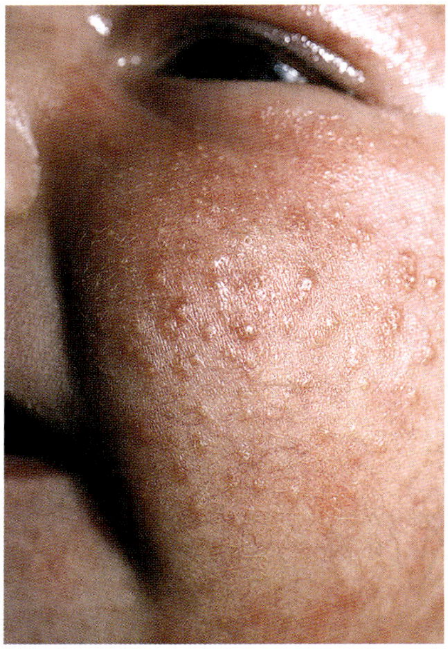

Fig. 2.15 Acne neonatorum. Erythematous papules and papulopustules on the cheek.

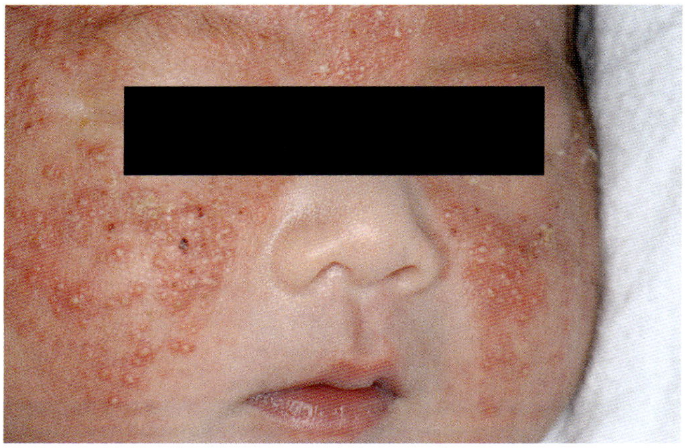

Fig. 2.16 Neonatal cephalic pustulosis. This 2-day-old boy had numerous small and large pustules on the forehead, cheeks, and chin. They cleared rapidly over 1 week with ketoconazole cream.

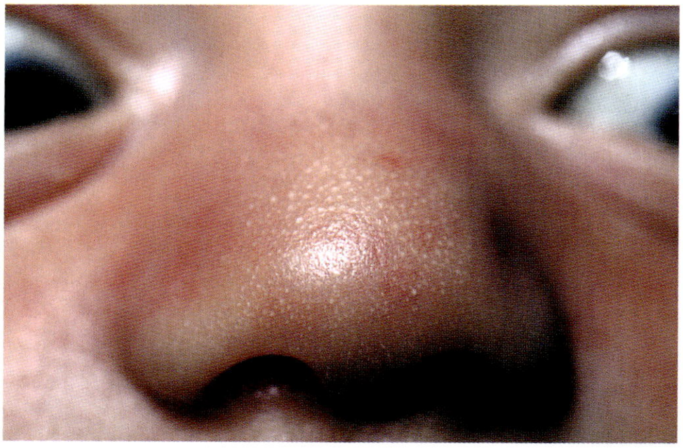

Fig. 2.14 Sebaceous gland hyperplasia. Yellow-white, pinpoint papules on the nasal tip of this 2-day-old boy.

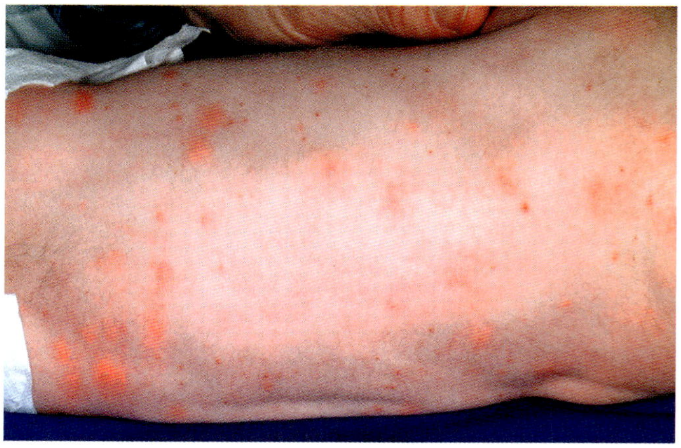

Fig. 2.17 Erythema toxicum neonatorum. Blotchy, erythematous macules and edematous papules.

of these, and may occur anywhere on the body, especially the forehead, face, trunk, and extremities. The fact that these lesions (which histologically reveal follicular-centered eosinophils) often tend to spare the palms and soles may be explained by the absence of pilosebaceous follicles in these areas.

ETN often initially appears as a blotchy, macular erythema that then develops firm, 1- to 3-mm, pale yellow or white papules and pustules. The erythematous macules are irregular or splotchy in appearance, varying from a few millimeters to several centimeters in diameter. They may be seen in sharp contrast to the surrounding unaffected skin, may blend into a surrounding erythema, or may progress to a confluent eruption.

Although ETN appears most commonly during the first 3 to 4 days of life, it has been seen at birth and may be noted as late as 10 days of age.[71] Exacerbations and remissions may occur during the first 2 weeks of life, and the duration of individual lesions varies from a few hours to several days. The cause of ETN remains obscure. One study suggested that it represents an immune response to microbial colonization of the skin at the hair follicle.[72] ETN incidence data are variable. Some authors report an incidence as low as 4.5%; others report incidences varying from 31% to 70% of newborns.[73] Two large prospective series of skin findings in newborns (one in the United States and one in Turkey) found incidences of 7% and 13.1%, respectively.[74,75] In a prospective 1-year multicenter study of more than 2800 neonates in Brazil, the prevalence of ETN was 21.3%, and it was primarily noted in term infants.[76] The incidence of ETN clearly appears to increase with increasing gestational age and birthweight of the infant.[77,76] No sexual or racial predisposition has been noted.

ETN is usually diagnosed clinically. Skin biopsy, which is rarely necessary, reveals a characteristic accumulation of eosinophils within the pilosebaceous apparatus. The diagnosis can be rapidly differentiated from other newborn pustular conditions by cytologic examination of a pustule smear that with Wright or Giemsa staining reveals a predominance of eosinophils. Affected infants may have a peripheral eosinophilia. Although the eosinophilic response has led some observers to attribute the cause of this disorder to a hypersensitivity reaction, specific allergens have never been implicated or confirmed.

Because erythema toxicum is a benign, self-limiting, asymptomatic disorder, no therapy is indicated. Occasionally, however, it may be confused with other pustular eruptions of the neonatal period, including transient neonatal pustular melanosis, milia, miliaria, and congenital infections such as candidiasis, herpes simplex, and bacterial processes. Of these, the congenital infections are the most important diagnostic considerations because of the implications for possible systemic involvement. Table 2.3 lists the differential diagnosis of the newborn with vesicles or pustules.

Table 2.3 Differential Diagnosis of Vesicles or Pustules in the Newborn

Clinical Disorder	Comments
Acrodermatitis enteropathica	Periorificial erosive dermatitis common
Acropustulosis of infancy	Recurrent crops of acral pustules
Behçet syndrome	Oral and genital ulcers; may have cutaneous papules, vesicles, and pustules (Fig. 2.18)
Eosinophilic folliculitis	Scalp and extremities most common sites
Epidermolysis bullosa	Trauma-induced blistering; bullae and erosions
Erythema toxicum neonatorum	Blotchy erythema, evanescent
Incontinentia pigmenti	XLD; linear and whorled patterns; may be vesicles, as well as warty lesions (hypopigmentation and hyperpigmentation occur later)
Infectious	
Bacterial	
Group A or B streptococci	
Staphylococcus aureus	Superficial blisters rupture easily; look for peripheral collarettes (Fig. 2.19)
Listeria monocytogenes	
Pseudomonas aeruginosa	
Other Gram-negative organisms	
Fungal	
Candidiasis	Palms and soles involved; nail changes often present
Viral	
Herpes simplex	Three types: SEM, CNS, disseminated
Varicella-zoster	
Cytomegalovirus	Blueberry muffin lesions more common
Spirochetal	
Syphilis	Red macules, papules; palm and sole scaling
Langerhans cell histiocytosis	Crusting, erosions, palms and soles, LAD
Miliaria	Especially intertriginous, occluded sites; crystallina type presents with clear vesicles without erythema; rubra type presents with red papules and papulopustules
Neonatal cephalic pustulosis	Acneiform disorder, presenting with numerous pustules on the cheeks, forehead, chin; may respond to topical antifungal agents
Pustular psoriasis	
Scabies	Crusting, burrows; palms and soles usually involved
Transient neonatal pustular melanosis	Mainly affects black skin; peripheral collarettes; pigment persists for months
Urticaria pigmentosa	Stroking leads to urtication (Darier sign)
Vesiculopustular eruption of transient myeloproliferative disorder	Vesicles and pustules (face > elsewhere); usually in setting of trisomy 21

CNS, Central nervous system; *LAD,* lymphadenopathy; *SEM,* skin, eyes, and/or mouth; *XLD,* X-linked dominant.

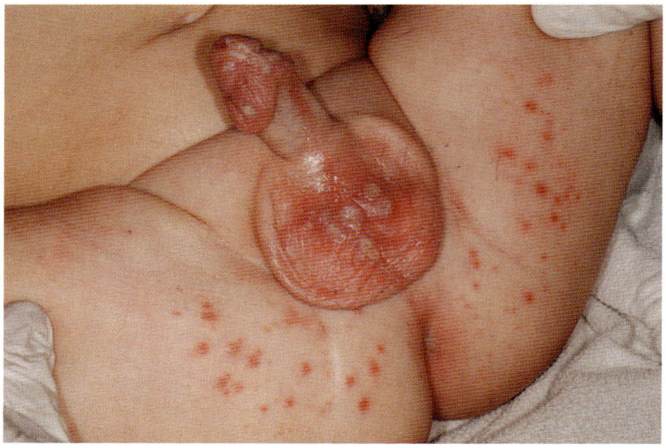

Fig. 2.18 Behçet syndrome. Shallow ulcerations on the scrotum, foreskin, and glans penis of an infant male with oral erosions and the human leukocyte antigen–B51 group genotype. Note the associated papulopustular lesions on the medial thighs and buttocks, another characteristic feature of Behçet syndrome.

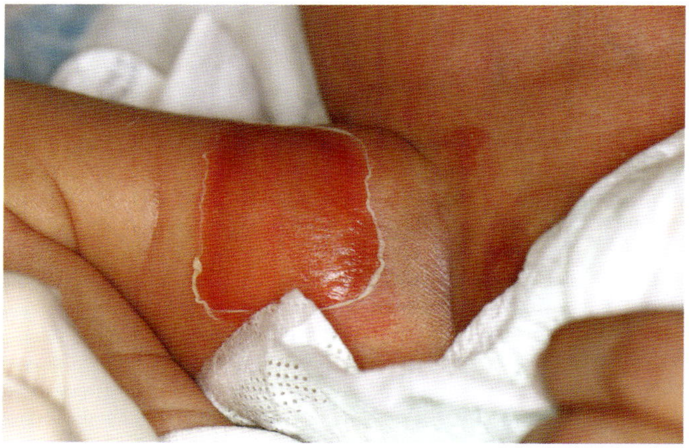

Fig. 2.19 Bullous impetigo. This 11-day-old boy developed flaccid vesicles and bullae that ruptured easily, leaving behind tender red patches with peripheral collarettes as seen here. Staphylococcus aureus grew in culture from the skin swab.

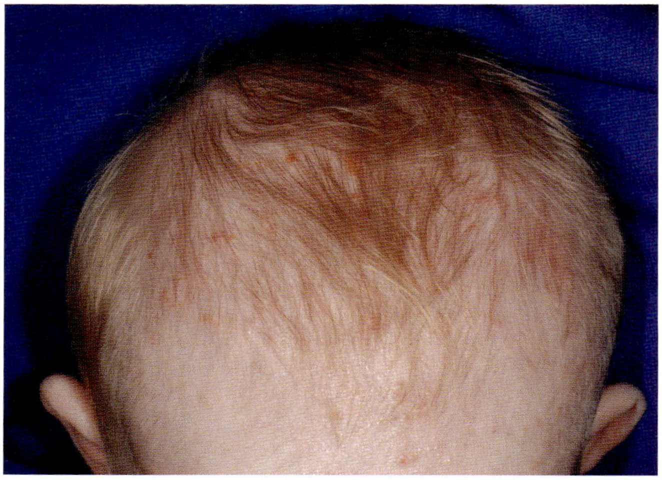

Fig. 2.20 Eosinophilic pustular folliculitis. Erythematous papules and pustules on the scalp of an infant girl, who was subsequently diagnosed with hyperimmunoglobulinemia E syndrome.

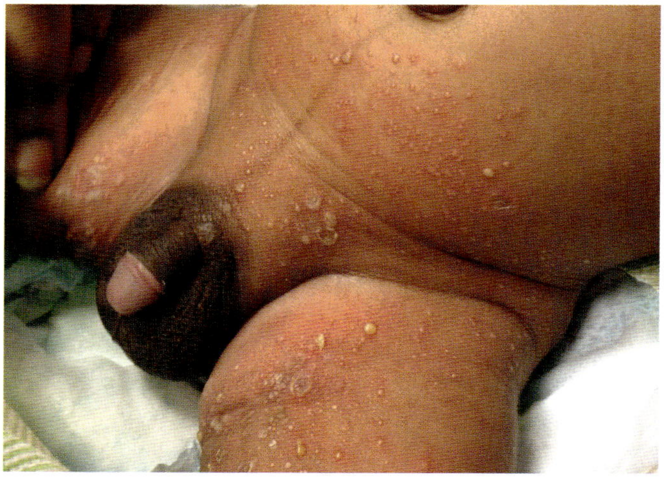

Fig. 2.21 Neonatal *Staphylococcus aureus* pustulosis with multiple pustules in the diaper region. Note some superficial erosions with peripheral collarettes of scale. The culture was positive for *S. aureus*.

EOSINOPHILIC PUSTULAR FOLLICULITIS

Eosinophilic pustular folliculitis (EPF) is an idiopathic dermatosis that occurs in both adults and children (particularly infants). When it occurs in neonates or young infants, it may be clinically confused with other vesiculopustular disorders. Lesions consist of follicular pustules, most commonly occurring on the scalp and the extremities (Fig. 2.20). They tend to recur in crops, in a similar fashion to acropustulosis of infancy (see later), and some suggest that these conditions may be related.[78,79] As opposed to the adult form of EPF, the infancy-associated type does not reveal lesions grouped in an annular arrangement. EPF tends to present before 14 months of age in the majority of patients.[80] Histologic evaluation reveals an eosinophilic, follicular, inflammatory infiltrate, and peripheral eosinophilia may be present. EPF of infancy appears to be distinct from classic (adult) and human immunodeficiency virus (HIV)–associated EPF, although an infant with HIV and EPF has been reported.[81] Importantly, infantile EPF may occasionally be the presenting sign of hyperimmunoglobulinemia E syndrome (HIES) (see Chapter 3). Treatment for EPF is symptomatic, including topical corticosteroids and antihistamines, with eventual spontaneous resolution by 3 years of age in the majority of patients.[80] Topical tacrolimus may be useful in patients who are unresponsive to topical corticosteroids.[82]

IMPETIGO NEONATORUM

Impetigo in newborns may occur as early as the second or third day or as late as the second week of life. It usually presents as a superficial vesicular, pustular, or bullous lesion on an erythematous base. Vesicles and bullae are easily denuded, leaving a red, raw, and moist surface with a peripheral collarette (see Fig. 2.19), usually without crust formation. Blisters are often wrinkled, contain some fluid, and are easily denuded. Lesions tend to occur on moist or opposing surfaces of the skin, as in the diaper area, groin, axillae, and neck folds. *S. aureus* pustulosis (or neonatal pustulosis) is a characteristic manifestation of cutaneous *S. aureus* infection in the neonate or infant. Patients have small pustules on an erythematous base (Fig. 2.21), often distributed in the diaper region. The lesions denude easily on swabbing, and culture is positive for *S. aureus*. Streptococci may occasionally be causative. In term or late preterm neonates with localized involvement and without fever or systemic symptoms, evaluation for serious bacterial illness is generally not required, and treatment in the outpatient setting is often sufficient.[83] However, a complete blood cell count and blood culture are advisable given the rare association with bacteremia.

The term *pemphigus neonatorum* is an archaic misnomer occasionally applied to superficial bullous lesions of severe impetigo widely distributed over the surface of the body. However, a transient neonatal form of pemphigus vulgaris does exist and is caused by transplacental passage of antibodies from a mother with the same disease (see Chapter 13).

SUCKING BLISTERS

Sucking blisters, presumed to be induced by vigorous sucking on the affected part *in utero*, are seen in up to 0.5% of normal newborns as 0.5- to 2-cm oval bullae or erosions on the dorsal aspect of the fingers, thumbs, wrists, lips, or radial aspect of the forearms. These lesions, which must be differentiated from bullous impetigo, epidermolysis bullosa, and herpes neonatorum, resolve rapidly and without sequelae.

TRANSIENT NEONATAL PUSTULAR MELANOSIS

Transient neonatal pustular melanosis (TNPM) is a benign self-limiting disorder of unknown cause characterized by superficial vesiculopustular lesions that rupture easily and evolve into hyperpigmented macules (Fig. 2.22). This disorder is seen in fewer than 1% of newborns[84] and occurs most commonly in infants with black skin. Lesions begin as superficial sterile pustules (Fig. 2.23) that rupture easily to leave a collarette of fine, white scale around a small hyperpigmented macule. Although the distribution may be diffuse, common areas of involvement include the inferior chin, forehead, neck, lower back, and shins. Rarely, vesicles that do not progress to pigmented macules may be detected on the scalp, palms, and soles.

Wright-stained smears of the pustules of TNPM, in contrast to lesions of ETN, demonstrate variable numbers of neutrophils, few or no eosinophils, and cellular debris. Histopathologic evaluation is usually unnecessary.

TNPM is a benign disorder without associated systemic manifestations, and therapy is unnecessary. The pustular lesions usually disappear within 24 to 48 hours, leaving behind hyperpigmented macules that fade gradually, usually over several weeks to months. Occasionally, newborns may have solely the hyperpigmented macules, in which case it is presumed that the pustular phase occurred (and resolved) *in utero*.

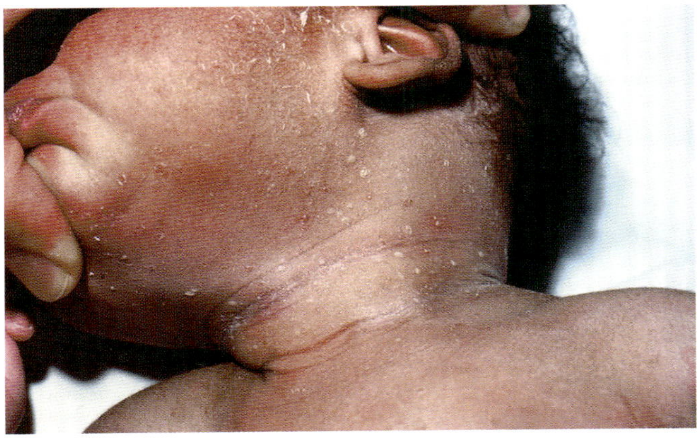

Fig. 2.22 Transient neonatal pustular melanosis. Papules and papulopustules rupture to leave a collarette of fine scales and eventual hyperpigmentation. (Courtesy Nancy B. Esterly, MD.)

ACROPUSTULOSIS OF INFANCY

Acropustulosis of infancy, also known as *infantile acropustulosis (IA)*, is an idiopathic pustular disorder with onset usually between birth and 2 years of age. It is characterized by pruritic, vesiculopustular lesions that recur every few weeks to months. The lesions begin as pinpoint erythematous papules and enlarge into well-circumscribed discrete pustules.[85] They are concentrated on the palms (Fig. 2.24) and soles (Fig. 2.25) and appear in lesser numbers on the dorsal aspect of the hands, feet, wrists, and ankles. Occasional lesions may occur on the face and scalp.

The differential diagnosis of IA includes scabies, dyshidrotic eczema, pustular psoriasis, ETN, TNPM, impetigo, and subcorneal pustular dermatosis. However, the characteristic presentation and course of IA is usually distinctive enough to render a clinical diagnosis. A smear of pustule contents (or histologic evaluation) reveals large numbers of neutrophils and occasionally eosinophils.[85–88] Although the etiology of IA remains unclear, several authors have noted a likely association with preceding scabies infestation.[89–91] IA appears to be common in internationally adopted children.[92]

Patients with IA experience fewer and less intense flares of their lesions with time, and the entire process usually subsides within 2 to 3 years. Pruritus, however, may be severe early in the course, making therapy desirable. Possible associations include irritability, sleeplessness, excoriation, and secondary bacterial infection. Systemic antihistamines, usually in high doses, may relieve pruritus. High-potency topical corticosteroids are quite effective for this condition,[89] and given the limited distribution of lesions, the epidermal thickness at affected (acral) sites, and the periodicity of flares, concerns regarding systemic absorption of these medications should be minimal. Dapsone has long been a recommended therapy for severe cases, but the risk-to-benefit ratio of this agent is not generally justified in patients with IA.

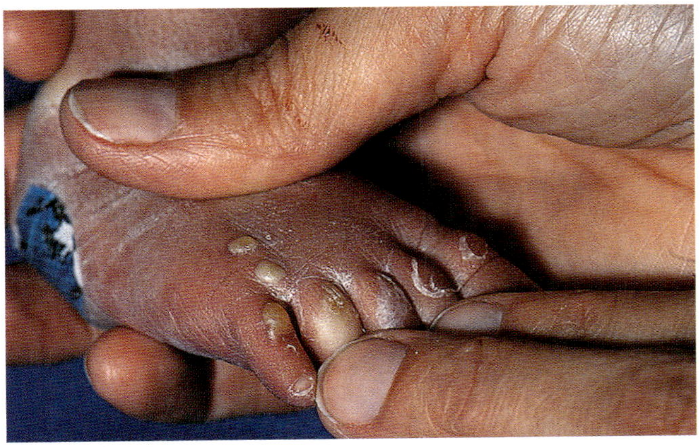

Fig. 2.23 Transient neonatal pustular melanosis. Tense pustules and collarettes of scale at sites of older lesions.

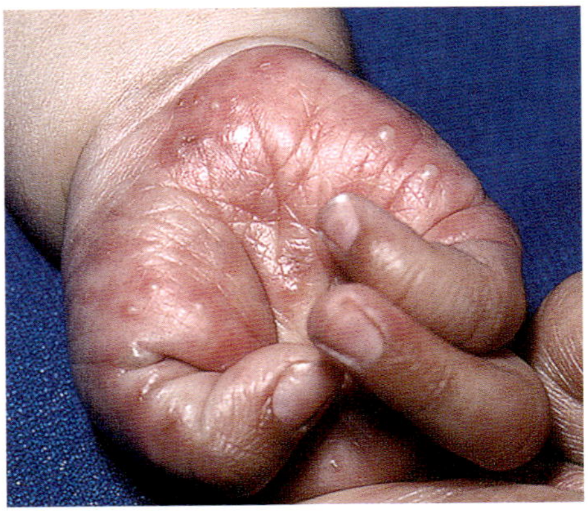

Fig. 2.24 Acropustulosis of infancy. Multiple tense erythematous papules and pustules on the palm of this 4-month-old girl.

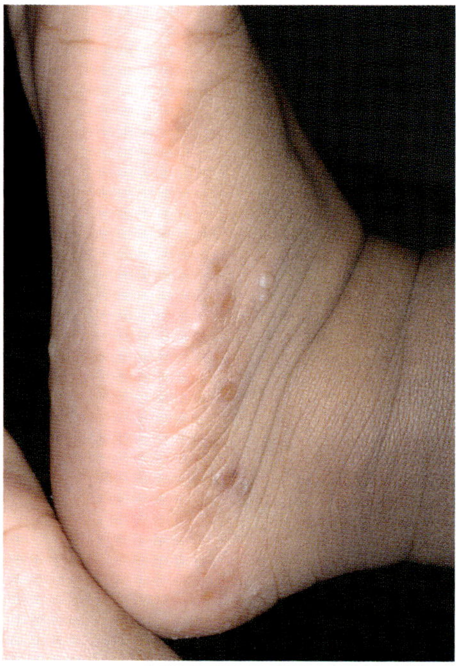

Fig. 2.25 Acropustulosis of infancy. Tense pustules, some of which have ruptured, on the plantar and lateral surfaces of the foot of a 14-month-old girl.

CONGENITAL EROSIVE AND VESICULAR DERMATOSIS

Congenital erosive and vesicular dermatosis (CEVD) healing with reticulated supple scarring is an uncommon disorder characterized by erosive and bullous lesions that, as the name implies, are present at birth and heal with characteristic scarring. Although its cause is unknown, it appears to represent a nonhereditary intrauterine event such as infection or amniotic adhesions, or perhaps an unusual healing defect of immature skin. There are several reports of CEVD occurring in association with neonatal herpes simplex virus infection.[93,94] The disorder generally involves skin of the trunk, extremities, scalp, face, and occasionally the tongue, with sparing of the palms and soles.

CEVD occurs most often in premature infants and presents with extensive cutaneous ulcerations (Fig. 2.26, *A*) and intact vesicles that develop crusting and then heal during the first month of life. Occasionally, blistering may continue to occur beyond infancy.[95,96] Generalized, supple, reticulated scars occur with alternating elevated and depressed areas (see Fig. 2.26, *B*). Up to 75% of the cutaneous surface may be involved, and the skin lesions have been described as having depressed hypopigmented regions alternating with normal to hyperpigmented zones.[97,98] Scars on the trunk and head, which often have a cobblestone-like appearance, may be oriented along the cutaneous lines of cleavage; on the limbs they tend to follow the long axes of the extremities.[98–100] Facial involvement was present in roughly 50% of published cases in one review.[101] Although the eyebrows are usually normal, alopecia may be noted on the scalp. Nails may be absent or hypoplastic, and affected areas on the tongue may manifest scarring and absence of papillae. Dentition is usually normal. Hyperthermia, especially in warm weather or after exertion, is common, and although sweating is absent in scarred areas, compensatory hyperhidrosis in normal-appearing skin may be noted. Chronic conjunctivitis is a major continuing problem for these patients, and corneal scarring may occur.[95,97] Some patients have also been found to have neurologic defects, including mental and motor retardation, hemiparesis, microcephaly, pachygyria, cerebral palsy, and seizures.[97,101]

SEBORRHEIC DERMATITIS

Seborrheic dermatitis is a common, self-limiting condition of the scalp, face, ears, trunk, and intertriginous areas characterized by greasy scaling, redness, fissuring, and occasional weeping. It appears to be related to the sebaceous glands and has a predilection for so-called "seborrheic" areas where the density of these glands is high. It usually presents in infants with a scaly dermatitis of the scalp termed *cradle cap* (Fig. 2.27) and may spread over the face, including the forehead, ears, eyebrows, and nose. Other areas of involvement include the intertriginous zones, umbilicus, and anogenital region (Fig. 2.28). (For a more detailed discussion of seborrheic dermatitis and its therapy, see Chapter 3.)

LEINER DISEASE

The term *Leiner disease*, rarely used in the current era, refers to a shared phenotype for a number of nutritional and immunologic disorders characterized by severe seborrheic dermatitis with exfoliation, failure to thrive, and diarrhea. The disorder may occur during the first week of life but generally starts around 2 to 4 months of age. Patients are particularly at risk for recurrent yeast and Gram-negative infections. Among disorders that may show this phenotype are deficiency or dysfunction of complement, Bruton agammaglobulinemia, severe combined immunodeficiency, and HIES.[102–106]

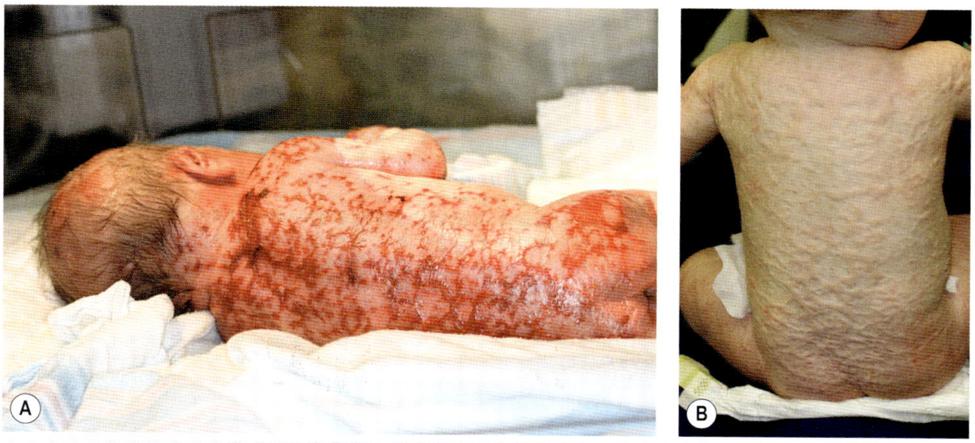

Fig. 2.26 Congenital erosive and vesicular dermatosis healing with reticulated supple scarring. **(A)** Diffuse reticulated erythematous erosions and atrophic plaques involved most of the skin surface in this female infant at 37 weeks' gestational age. **(B)** At age 8 months, prominent generalized reticulate supple scars were distributed on the trunk, face, scalp, and extremities.

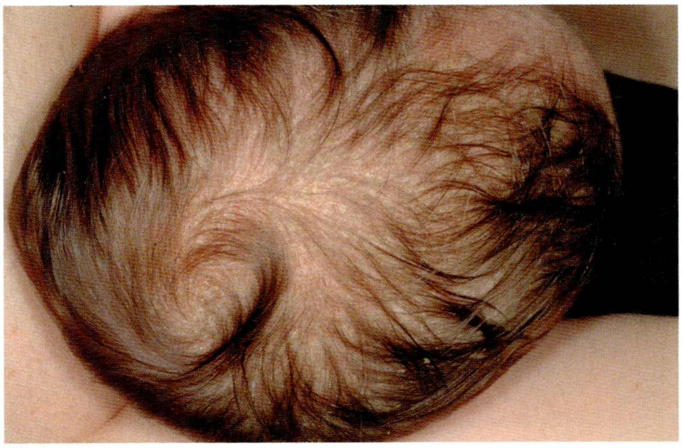

Fig. 2.27 Seborrheic dermatitis of the scalp (cradle cap). Erythema and greasy yellow scales involving the scalp of an infant boy who also had similar changes in the eyebrows.

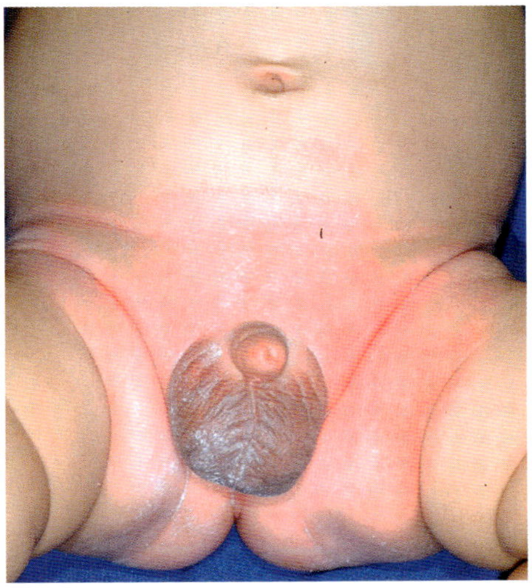

Fig. 2.28 Seborrheic dermatitis. Erythema of the medial thighs, suprapubic region, and buttocks. This presentation can be difficult to distinguish from infantile psoriasis, but the scaling tends to be more mild and the response to topical antiinflammatory therapy more brisk. The whitish debris in this child represents the barrier cream that his parents had applied rather than scaling.

DIAPER DERMATITIS

Diaper dermatitis is perhaps the most common cutaneous disorder of infancy and early childhood. The term is used to describe an acute inflammatory skin reaction in the areas covered by the diaper. The incidence of diaper dermatitis is estimated to be between 7% and 35%, with a peak incidence at 9 to 12 months of age.[107–109] The practice of diapering has evolved through the ages and varies according to local culture, geography, and tradition. Although the earliest materials included beaded cloths, peat moss with animal skin, and dried grass held in place by cloth, technological advancements led to refinement of the cloth diaper and diaper laundry services and eventually development of the disposable diaper in the early 1940s.[110]

The term *diaper rash* is commonly used as a diagnosis, as though the diverse dermatoses that may affect this region constitute a single clinical entity. In actuality, diaper dermatitis is not a specific diagnosis and is best viewed as a variable-symptom complex initiated by a combination of factors, the most significant being prolonged contact with urine and feces, skin maceration, and, in many cases, secondary infection with bacteria or *Candida albicans*. Although diaper dermatitis may often be no more than a minor nuisance, eruptions in this area may not only progress to secondary infection and ulceration but may become complicated by other superimposed cutaneous disorders or represent a manifestation of a more serious disease.

Box 2.1 Differential Diagnosis of Diaper Dermatitis

Chafing dermatitis
Irritant contact dermatitis
Diaper candidiasis
Seborrheic dermatitis
Psoriasis
Intertrigo
Jacquet dermatitis
Perianal pseudoverrucous papules and nodules
Miliaria
Folliculitis
Impetigo
Scabies
Nutritional deficiency (e.g., acrodermatitis enteropathica, cystic fibrosis, biotin deficiency)
Allergic contact dermatitis
Atopic dermatitis
Granuloma gluteale infantum
Langerhans cell histiocytosis
Burns
Child abuse
Epidermolysis bullosa
Congenital syphilis
Varicella/herpes
Tinea cruris
Chronic bullous dermatosis of childhood
Bullous mastocytosis

The three most common types of diaper dermatitis are chafing dermatitis, irritant contact dermatitis, and diaper candidiasis. However, the differential diagnosis of diaper dermatitis is broad (Box 2.1). In patients in whom a response to therapy is slow or absent, alternative diagnoses should be considered and appropriate diagnostic evaluations performed. The following sections contain a brief discussion of several potential causes of diaper dermatitis. Many of these entities are discussed in more detail in other chapters.

Chafing Dermatitis

The most prevalent form of diaper dermatitis is the chafing or frictional dermatitis that affects most infants at some time. Generally present on areas where friction is the most pronounced (the inner surfaces of the thighs, the genitalia, buttocks, and the abdomen), the eruption presents as mild redness and scaling and tends to wax and wane quickly. This form responds quickly to frequent diaper changes and good diaper hygiene.

Irritant Contact Dermatitis

Irritant contact diaper dermatitis usually involves the convex surfaces of the buttocks, the vulva, the perineal area, the lower abdomen, and the proximal thighs, with sparing of the intertriginous creases (Fig. 2.29). The disorder may be attributable to contact with proteolytic enzymes in stool and irritant chemicals such as soaps, detergents, and topical preparations. Other significant factors appear to be excessive heat, moisture, and sweat retention associated with the warm local environment produced by the diaper.

The etiology of irritant contact diaper dermatitis is multifactorial, and past hypotheses have included potential roles for ammonia, bacteria and bacterial products, and urine pH. In 1921 when Cooke demonstrated that an aerobic Gram-positive bacillus (*Bacillus ammoniagenes*) was capable of liberating ammonia from urea, this organism was pinpointed as the causal agent of most diaper dermatoses.[111] More recent studies, however, have refuted the role of urea-splitting bacteria in the etiology of this disorder and incriminate a combination of wetness, frictional damage, impervious diaper coverings, and increase in skin pH. It is suggested that urinary wetness increases the permeability of the skin to irritants as well as the pH of the diaper environment, thus intensifying the activities of the fecal proteases and lipases, the major irritants responsible for this disorder.[112,113]

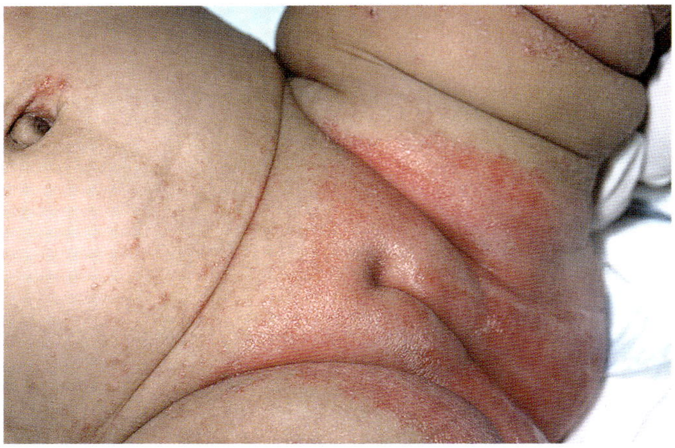

Fig. 2.29 Irritant contact diaper dermatitis. Erythema of the vulva, buttocks, and medial thighs. The inguinal creases were relatively spared.

Several technological innovations in the design of disposable diapers and other diapering products have aimed to reduce moisture and irritancy in this environment, thus decreasing the risk of irritant dermatitis. The introduction of absorbent gelling materials into diaper technology was one such breakthrough and has been shown to result in less diaper dermatitis than conventional cellulose-core disposable diapers.[114] Other innovations have included nonirritating disposable diaper wipes and diapers designed to deliver petrolatum-based formulations to the skin.[115]

A blistering, erosive contact dermatitis has been observed after oral ingestion (either intentional or accidental) of senna-containing laxatives.[116,117] Patients typically have well-demarcated, diamond-shaped eroded plaques with desquamation that in some cases initially could be mistaken for scalding burns. Prolonged contact with stool (e.g., via overnight wearing of the diaper) is often reported. In some countries in the Middle East, such as Jordan and Turkey, where the application of table salt to the skin of infants *(salting)* is a tradition believed to prevent excessive sweating and body odor as an adult, severe erosive dermatitis of the diaper region with ulcerations on the scrotum has been reported, as has associated hypernatremia, which can be fatal.[118,119]

Allergic Contact Dermatitis

Although not traditionally considered a common cause for diaper dermatitis, allergic contact dermatitis has received increasing attention in the literature in recent years (see Chapter 3). Potential associations to consider include chemical constituents of the diaper (rubber additives, rubber accelerator compounds, adhesive resins), topically applied diaper products such as emollients and "butt balms" (emulsifiers), and baby wipes (fragrances and preservatives).[120,121] In a report of six nondiapered children with recalcitrant perianal and buttock dermatitis, all tested positive to methylchloroisothiazolinone/methylisothiazolinone (MCI/MI), a combination preservative found in the wet wipes that were being used for cleansing, with complete clearance on discontinuation of the products.[122] In a review of potential allergens found in diapering products, botanical extracts, α-tocopherol, fragrances, propylene glycol, parabens, and lanolin were among the potential allergens identified.[123] Disperse dyes, which are used to impart color to synthetic fabrics, can also be contact sensitizers and are found in some disposable diapers. When allergic contact dermatitis in the diaper region is suspected in infants, a modified patch testing series (containing fewer allergens than a standard test, given patch test limitations in this population) has been proposed.[124]

Diaper Candidiasis

Candidal (monilial) diaper dermatitis is a commonly overlooked disorder and should be suspected whenever a diaper rash fails to respond to usual therapeutic measures. Cutaneous candidiasis is a possible sequela of systemic antibiotic therapy and should be considered in any diaper dermatitis that develops during or shortly after antibiotic administration.[125]

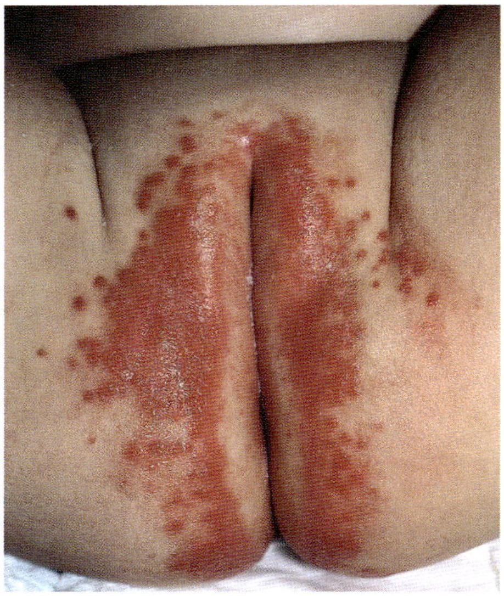

Fig. 2.30 Diaper candidiasis. Beefy-red, erythematous plaques with multiple red satellite papules and papulopustules.

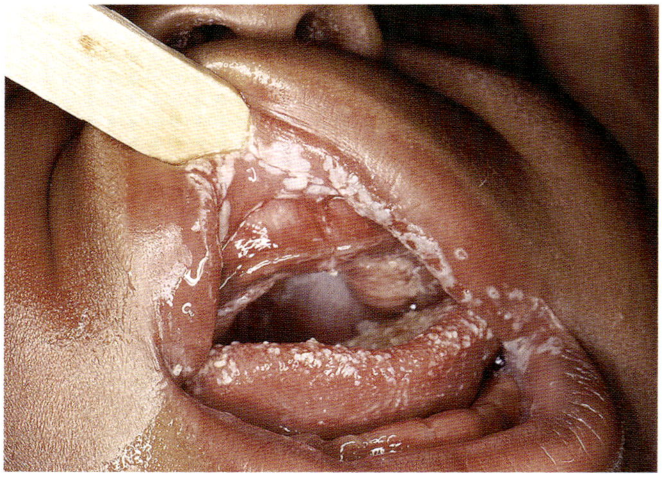

Fig. 2.31 Oral candidiasis (thrush). Gray-white, cheesy patches and plaques of the buccal mucosa, tongue, and gingiva.

Candidal diaper dermatitis presents as a widespread, beefy-red erythema on the buttocks, lower abdomen, and inner aspects of the thighs. Characteristic features include a raised edge, sharp marginalization with white scales at the border, and pinpoint pustulovesicular satellite lesions (the diagnostic hallmark) (Fig. 2.30). Although cutaneous candidiasis commonly occurs in association with oral thrush (Fig. 2.31), the oral mucosa may be uninvolved. Infants harbor *C. albicans* in the lower intestine, and it is from this focus that infected feces present the primary source for candidal diaper eruptions.

If necessary, the diagnosis of candidal diaper dermatitis may be confirmed by microscopic examination of a potassium hydroxide preparation of skin scrapings, which reveals egg-shaped budding yeasts and hyphae or pseudohyphae. Growth of yeast on Sabouraud medium implanted with skin scrapings can also confirm the diagnosis, usually within 48 to 72 hours.

Seborrheic Dermatitis

Seborrheic dermatitis of the diaper area may be recognized by the characteristic salmon-colored, greasy plaques with a yellowish scale

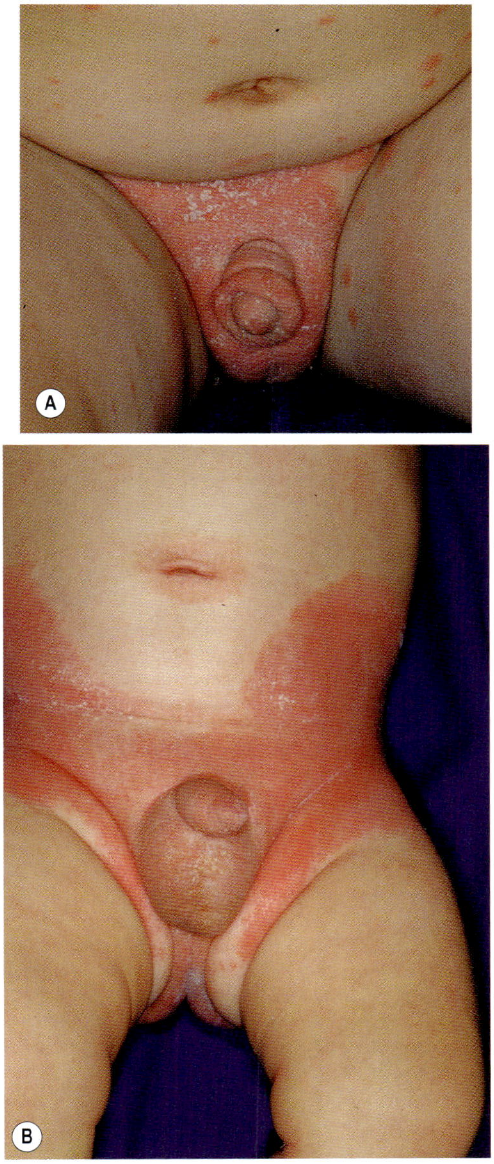

Fig. 2.32 Psoriasis (diaper). **(A)** Sharply demarcated, erythematous, scaly plaques involving the genitals and suprapubic region in this infant boy. **(B)** Thin, scaly, very well demarcated plaques over the diaper area, flanks, and umbilical region of a 3-month-old boy.

and a predilection for intertriginous areas (see earlier). Coincident involvement of the scalp, face, neck, and postauricular and flexural areas helps establish the diagnosis. Seborrheic dermatitis of the diaper region may be difficult to distinguish from psoriasis.

Psoriasis

Psoriasis of the diaper area must also be considered in persistent diaper eruptions that fail to respond to otherwise seemingly adequate therapy (Fig. 2.32). The sharp demarcation of lesions suggests diaper area psoriasis, but the typical scaling of psoriasis may be obscured because of the moisture of the diaper region. The presence of nail changes and red, well-marginated plaques with silvery mica-like scales on the trunk, face, axillae, umbilicus, or scalp may help confirm this diagnosis (see Chapter 4), although affected infants may have involvement limited to the diaper area.

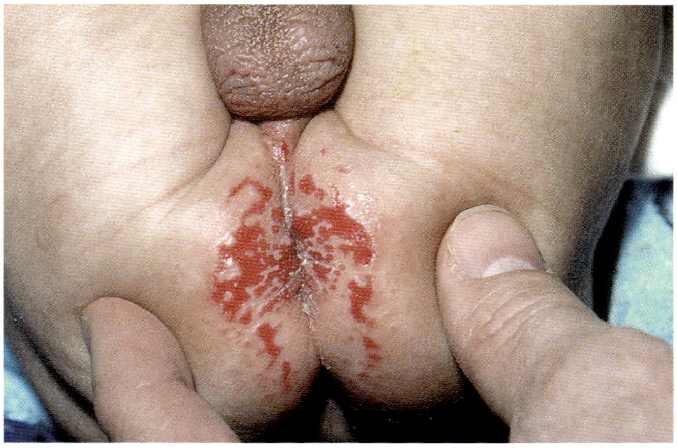

Fig. 2.33 Jacquet dermatitis. Severe diaper area erythema with ulcerated papules and islands of reepithelialization.

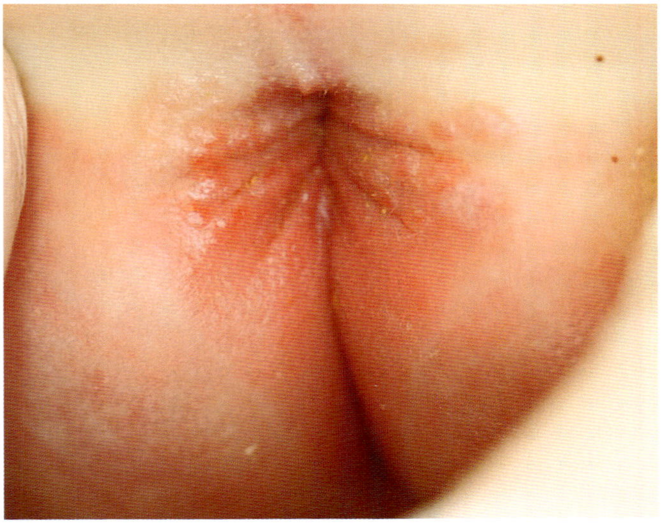

Fig. 2.34 Perianal pseudoverrucous papules and nodules. This 7-week-old boy developed these perianal verrucous papules after a period of severe irritant contact diaper dermatitis/Jacquet dermatitis.

Intertrigo

Intertrigo (see Chapter 17) is a common skin eruption in the diaper area, particularly in hot weather or when infants are overdressed. It usually involves the inguinal creases, the intergluteal area, and the thigh creases (especially in chubby babies) and presents as bright red erythema often with a mild white-yellow exudate. Nondiapered areas of involvement include the anterior neck fold and the axillae.

Jacquet Dermatitis

The term *Jacquet dermatitis* is used to describe a severe erosive diaper eruption with ulcerated papules or nodules (Fig. 2.33). In male infants, erosion and crusting of the glans penis and urinary meatus may result in painful or difficult urination.

Perianal Pseudoverrucous Papules and Nodules

This eruption composed of verrucous (wart-like) papules has been observed to occur in children with incontinence of stool or urine. These patients have verrucous papules (Fig. 2.34) and nodules of the perianal and suprapubic regions, possibly representing a distinct reaction to severe irritant diaper dermatitis. Reported patients had a history of delayed ileoanal anastomosis for Hirschsprung disease, encopresis, or

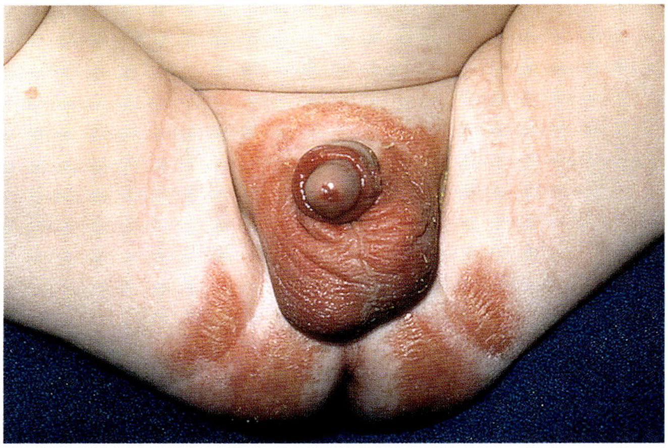

Fig. 2.35 Acrodermatitis enteropathica. Eroded, erythematous patches and plaques in this 4-month-old boy with zinc deficiency. Note the associated balanoposthitis.

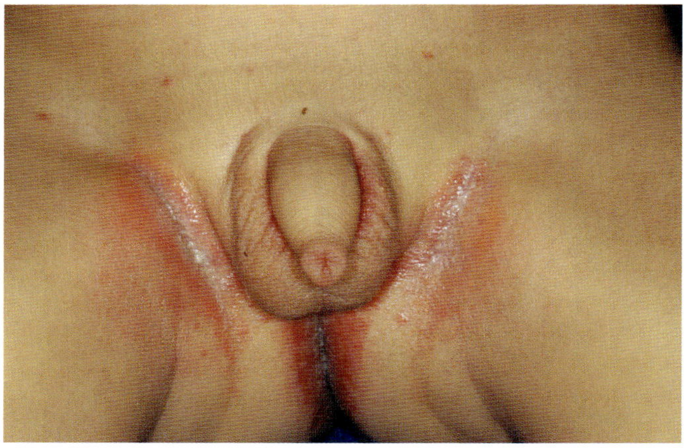

Fig. 2.36 Langerhans cell histiocytosis. Red-brown, eroded plaques in the inguinal creases in an infant male with multiorgan involvement. Note the presence of skin lesions also in the perineum and on the anterior scrotal surface, as well as a few scaly crusted papules on the lower abdomen.

urinary incontinence.[126–128] The importance of this diagnosis lies in differentiating it from condylomata acuminata or other more serious dermatoses.

Acrodermatitis Enteropathica

Acrodermatitis enteropathica, a disorder of zinc deficiency, may mimic a severe irritant contact dermatitis in the diaper area (see Chapter 24). Patients have a periorificial erosive dermatitis that is often most accentuated in the diaper region (Fig. 2.35) but also may involve the perioral face. Erythema and pustules may involve intertriginous or acral sites, and diarrhea, failure to thrive, and alopecia are commonly present.

Langerhans Cell Histiocytosis

Lesions of Langerhans cell histiocytosis (LCH; see Chapter 10) may also have a predilection for the diaper area. This eruption, which often presents in a seborrheic dermatitis–like fashion, classically involves the groin, axillae, and retroauricular scalp. Palms and soles may also be involved. Characteristic lesions consist of yellowish to red-brown papules, often with concomitant erosive (Fig. 2.36) or purpuric qualities. LCH should be considered in any infant with a recalcitrant or hemorrhagic seborrheic dermatitis–like eruption and/or flexural papules with discrete erosions. Lymphadenopathy is common, and multiorgan involvement (especially bones, liver, lung, mucosa, and middle ear) is possible. Skin biopsy with special stains for Langerhans cells is diagnostic.

Treatment of Diaper Dermatitis

Before any consideration for therapy of diaper dermatitis, the appropriate cause must be identified. Educating parents that diaper dermatitis is often recurrent is vital in an effort to prevent perceived management failure. The primary goals in preventing and treating diaper dermatitis include keeping the skin dry, protected, and infection free.[129]

The primary goal in irritant or chafing dermatitis is to keep the area as clean and dry as possible. Frequent diaper changes, gentle cleansing with a moistened soft cloth or fragrance-free diaper wipe (after defecation), exposure to air whenever possible, and the judicious use of topical therapy may be sufficient in most cases. Parents should be educated that minimal to no cleansing is required after urination only. Zinc oxide and petrolatum-based formulations tend to be most effective in forming a barrier to further skin contact with urine and feces; ointments and pastes are generally accepted as the most helpful vehicles. Other useful ingredients may include lanolin, white soft paraffin, and dimethicone. These products should be applied at every diaper change when acute dermatitis is present. Parents should be taught that cleansing the diaper area is necessary only when stool is present, because overwashing in itself can lead to irritation. A low-potency, nonfluorinated topical corticosteroid (e.g., 1% hydrocortisone) applied two to three times daily is appropriate until improvement is noted. Stronger steroids and combination antifungal-corticosteroid preparations should be avoided, given risks of local cutaneous side effects and, more importantly, systemic absorption because of increased skin penetration from occlusion effect.

Secondarily infected (bacterial) dermatitis should be treated with the appropriate systemic antibiotic. Candidal infection requires the use of a topical antifungal agent (e.g., nystatin, clotrimazole, ketoconazole, oxiconazole, econazole, miconazole). It is important to avoid use of topical antifungals such as terbinafine and naftifine, which lack effectiveness against *Candida*.[130] If there is evidence of *Candida* in the mouth (i.e., thrush) as well as the diaper area, topical therapy may be supplemented by oral nystatin. Oral fluconazole, at a dosage of 6 mg/kg per day given once daily for 2 to 4 weeks, is useful for severe cutaneous candidiasis. Although gentian violet has been used for decades for the treatment of oral and diaper candidiasis, reports of bacterial infection and hemorrhagic cystitis in addition to the staining associated with its use suggest that gentian violet be avoided.[131,132] A combination product (0.25% miconazole nitrate, 15% zinc oxide, and 81.35% white petrolatum) is also available, has demonstrated efficacy, and offers the advantage of convenience. Recalcitrant diaper candidiasis may be an initial sign of chronic mucocutaneous candidiasis (see Chapter 17).

GRANULOMA GLUTEALE INFANTUM

Granuloma gluteale infantum is a benign disorder of infancy characterized by purple-red nodules on the skin of the groin, lower abdomen, and inner thighs (Fig. 2.37). Patients have usually received preceding therapy with topical corticosteroids. Although the appearance of these lesions may suggest a malignant process, granuloma gluteale infantum seems to represent a unique response to local inflammation, maceration, and possibly secondary infection (usually *C. albicans*). A similar eruption has been observed in elderly adults.[133] Histologic evaluation of biopsy tissue from granuloma gluteale infantum reveals a nonspecific inflammatory infiltrate, sometimes with giant cells.[134,135]

Lesions of granuloma gluteale infantum resolve completely and spontaneously within a period of several months after treatment of the initiating inflammatory process. Although intralesional corticosteroids or steroid-impregnated tape have been used, such therapy is not recommended.

Developmental Abnormalities of the Newborn

SKIN SIGNS OF OCCULT SPINAL DYSRAPHISM

Spinal dysraphism is a spectrum of disorders defined by absent or incomplete fusion of the midline bony elements and may include

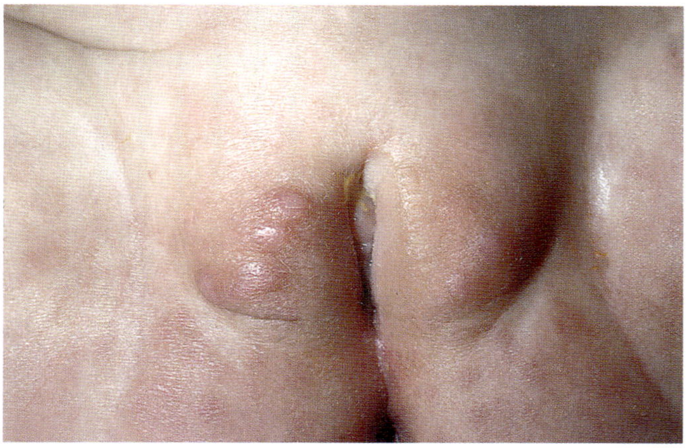

Fig. 2.37 Granuloma gluteale infantum. Erythematous to violaceous papulonodules on the labia majora of this infant with a history of potent topical corticosteroid use in the diaper region.

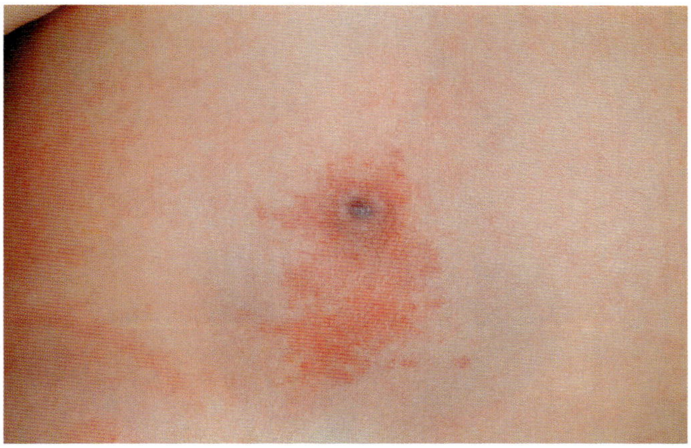

Fig. 2.38 Lumbosacral port wine stain associated with occult spinal dysraphism. Note the associated central depression in this boy who also had an underlying tethered spinal cord.

congenital spinal-cord anomalies.[136] Because occult spinal dysraphism (OSD) can lead to irreversible neurologic complications from tethered cord syndrome, early recognition is desirable. Cutaneous or subcutaneous stigmata may be the presenting sign of OSD, and as such, a working knowledge of potentially associated lesions is vital. Lumbosacral skin lesions that may be associated with OSD and spinal cord defects include hypertrichosis (the classic "faun tail" or finer, lanugo hair), lipomas, vascular lesions (infantile hemangioma, port wine stain; Fig. 2.38), atypical sacral dimples (Fig. 2.39), sinuses, appendages (skin tag, tail), ACC, and melanocytic nevi.[137] Gluteal cleft asymmetry or deviation is another useful finding. The presence of multiple findings increases the risk of OSD.[138,139] In one study, 11 of 18 patients with two or more congenital midline skin lesions had OSD, and the most common midline cutaneous lesions to be associated with OSD were lipomas (either isolated or in combination with other lesions).[140] In a prospective study of infants with lumbosacral infantile hemangiomas, the overall relative risk for spinal anomalies was 640; importantly, 35% of the infants with an isolated lumbosacral hemangioma (and no additional cutaneous findings) had spinal anomalies.[141]

The majority of simple midline dimples are not associated with OSD. Patients with atypical dimples (>5 mm in size, further than 2.5 cm from the anal verge), on the other hand, have a significant risk of associated OSD.[138] The association of nevus simplex (small, dull-pink, vascular malformation, most commonly seen on the occipital scalp, glabella, or eyelids) of the sacrum and OSD is unclear, although

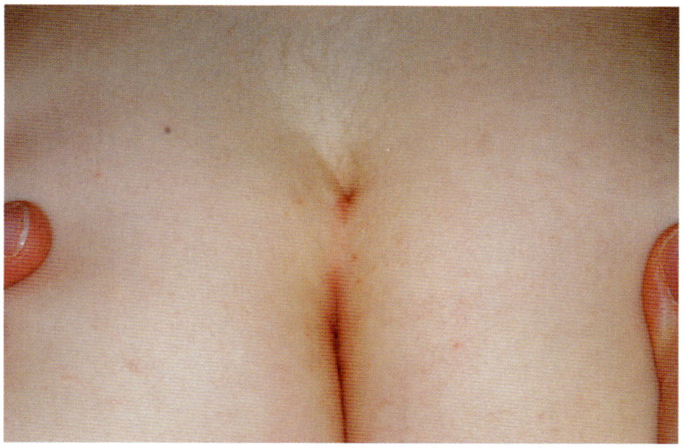

Fig. 2.39 Prominent sacral dimple. This young girl was found to have this prominent dimple superior to the gluteal cleft in association with mild gluteal cleft deviation. Imaging for associated spinal dysraphism was unremarkable.

most agree that these lesions, when occurring alone, do not predict an increased risk of underlying malformations. Cervical OSD is significantly less common, and in those cases associated with cutaneous stigmata, more than one lesion is usually present.[142] It is important to remember that an isolated nevus simplex ("stork bite") of the posterior nuchal or occipital region is *not* an indicator of underlying OSD.

When OSD is being considered, radiographic imaging must be performed. MRI is the diagnostic modality of choice, especially with higher-risk cutaneous findings. Ultrasound screening may be considered in infants younger than 4 months (before ossification of the vertebral bodies is complete), with the advantages being that it is noninvasive and does not require sedation. However, ultrasonography is limited in that small cord lesions (i.e., lipomas or dermal sinus tracts) may be missed,[137] and the overall sensitivity is quite dependent on the experience of the ultrasonographer. In a study of 41 infants with lumbosacral infantile hemangioma, the sensitivity of ultrasound scanning in detecting spinal anomalies was only 50%, with a specificity of 77.8%.[140] Ultrasound may occasionally be associated with false-positive findings, as reported in a study of 439 newborns in whom the study was performed because of cutaneous stigmata. A total of 39 of 439 had abnormal findings, with subsequent MRI revealing unremarkable findings in 17 of them.[143]

In infants with low-risk lesions such as simple dimples or gluteal cleft deviation and without other high-risk findings (e.g., hypertrichosis, skin tags, lipoma, or other mass), the need for imaging is unclear. If it is performed, however, ultrasound may provide a reliable screening when interpreted by an experienced pediatric radiologist.[144] Early neurosurgical referral is indicated if underlying defects are diagnosed.

DRUG-INDUCED FETAL SKIN MALFORMATIONS

There are numerous drugs, including alcohol, hydantoin, valproic acid, warfarin, aminopterin, and isotretinoic acid, that when taken by pregnant women produce an adverse effect on the fetus and newborn. Exposure to these drugs *in utero* may result in a variety of organ malformations, although specific skin malformations are rare. Teratogenic risks as they relate to skin have most commonly focused on antithyroid drugs, especially methimazole (MMI), and their possible role in causing ACC (see later).

CONGENITAL HEMIHYPERTROPHY

Idiopathic congenital hemihypertrophy is a developmental defect in which one side of the body is larger than the other. Although differences in symmetry are often detectable during the newborn period, they usually become more striking with growth of the child. The cutaneous findings most often associated with hemihypertrophy are hyperpigmentation, telangiectasia, abnormal nail growth, and hypertrichosis

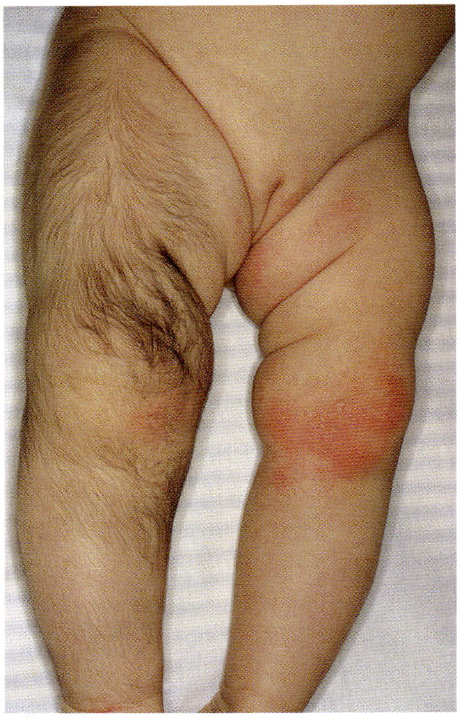

Fig. 2.40 Congenital hemihypertrophy with hypertrichosis. (From Hurwitz S, Klaus SN. Congenital hemihypertrophy with hypertrichosis. Arch Dermatol 1971;103:98–100.

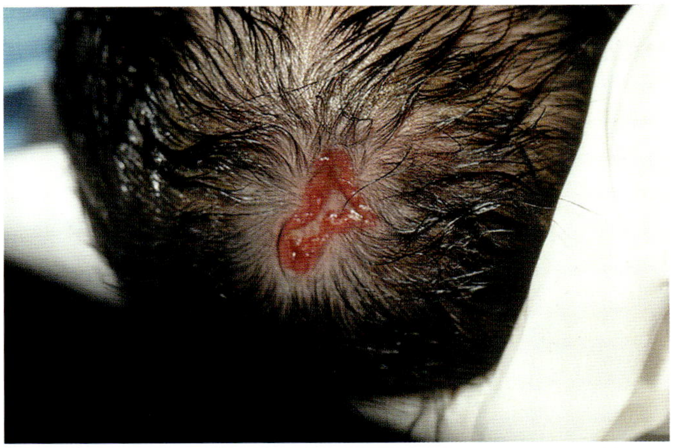

Fig. 2.41 Aplasia cutis congenita. Sharply demarcated ulceration on the scalp of an infant with this disorder.

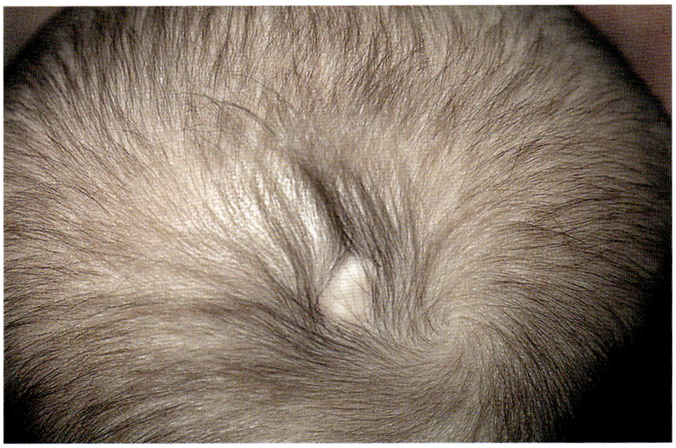

Fig. 2.42 Aplasia cutis congenita. Healed scar with alopecia near the hair whorl in this 8-month-old girl.

(Fig. 2.40). Body temperature and sweating differences have also been reported in patients with this disorder.[145]

Of particular significance is the fact that about 50% of persons with hemihypertrophy may have associated anomalies, including Wilms tumor, aniridia, cataracts, ear deformities, internal hemangiomas, genitourinary tract anomalies, adrenocortical neoplasms, and brain tumors. Therefore patients who exhibit congenital hemihypertrophy should be evaluated for potentially associated conditions. Associated tumors most commonly involve the kidney, adrenal gland, and liver.[146] In patients with hemihypertrophy combined with cutaneous vascular malformations (i.e., port wine stain), the possibility of Klippel–Trénaunay syndrome; Proteus syndrome; congenital lipomatous overgrowth, vascular malformations, epidermal nevi, and scoliosis/skeletal and spinal anomalies (CLOVES) syndrome; or another syndrome comprising a vascular anomaly with hypertrophy should be considered (see Chapter 12).

APLASIA CUTIS CONGENITA

Aplasia cutis congenita is a congenital defect of the skin characterized by localized absence of the epidermis, dermis, and, at times, subcutaneous tissues. Although ACC generally occurs on the scalp, it may also involve the skin of the face, trunk, and extremities. The diagnosis of ACC is usually a clinical one, and the histologic picture varies. Although most cases appear to be sporadic, a variety of potential associations, including teratogens, limb abnormalities, epidermal nevi, underlying embryologic malformations, epidermolysis bullosa, malformation syndromes, and infections, have been proposed.[147]

ACC classically presents as solitary or multiple, sharply demarcated, weeping or granulating, oval to circular, stellate defects ranging from 1 to 3 cm in diameter. Some 70% of scalp lesions are isolated and 20% are double, and in 8% of patients three or more defects may be present.[148] The most common location for ACC is the scalp, and in those cases 80% occur in close proximity to the hair whorl.[149] Although aplasia cutis may also affect the occiput, the postauricular areas, and the face, involvement of these areas appears to be relatively uncommon.

Whereas most scalp defects are small, larger lesions may occur and can extend to the dura or the meninges. Although treatment is generally unnecessary, large scalp lesions (i.e., >4 cm^2) may require surgery with grafting to prevent the potential complications of hemorrhage, venous (sagittal sinus) thrombosis, and meningitis.

At birth, the skin defect may vary from an ulceration with a granulating base (Fig. 2.41) to a superficial erosion or even a well-formed scar. As healing of open lesions occurs, the defect is replaced by smooth, hairless scar tissue (Fig. 2.42), although sometimes the tissue is raised and keloidal. Some lesions may present as a translucent, glistening membrane (membranous aplasia cutis) and when surrounded by a ring of long, dark hair (the "hair collar sign"; Fig. 2.43) may represent a forme fruste of a neural tube defect.[150] This membranous form of ACC may have a recognizable appearance on prenatal sonography as a round hypoechoic defect.[151]

Although most infants with ACC are otherwise well, defects that may occasionally be present include cleft lip and palate, ophthalmologic defects, limb reduction defects, cardiac anomalies, gastrointestinal tract malformations, spinal dysraphism, hydrocephalus, defects of the underlying skull, congenital midline porencephaly, spastic paralysis, seizures, mental retardation, and vascular anomalies.[147] Adams–Oliver syndrome (AOS), a malformation syndrome caused by mutations in the *ARHGAP31*, *DLL4*, *RBPJ*, or *NOTCH1* (autosomal dominant) genes or *DOCK6* or *EOGT* (autosomal recessive) genes, is the association of ACC with transverse terminal limb defects and cardiac and CNS abnormalities.[152–155] The limb defects may include

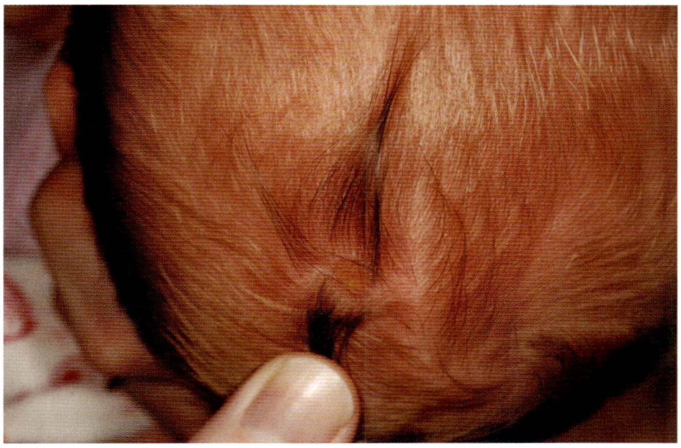

Fig. 2.43 Aplasia cutis congenita, membranous type, with hair collar sign. Note the hairs surrounding the defect in this infant girl, which are longer and darker than her other hair. Magnetic resonance imaging revealed a small tract down to calvarium, without any intracranial or intradural extension.

brachydactyly, syndactyly, loss of terminal phalanges, nail agenesis, or complete absence of the digits, hand, foot, or limb.[156] The cardiac malformations in AOS may include ventricular septal defects, tetralogy of Fallot, left-sided obstructive lesions, and truncus arteriosus.[157] Cutis marmorata telangiectatica congenita (see Chapter 12) is present in nearly 20% of patients with AOS.[158] Up to 50% of patients with trisomy 13 may have scalp ACC, and it may also occur at an increased rate in patients with 4p syndrome. Therefore any patient with signs of scalp ACC and congenital anomalies warrants chromosomal evaluation. Oculocerebrocutaneous (Delleman) syndrome is the association of orbital cysts, cerebral malformations, and focal skin defects including ACC-like lesions and skin tags.[159,160] Other findings in this syndrome include CNS malformations, clefting, and microphthalmia/anophthalmia. ACC in association with fetus papyraceus (vanishing twin syndrome) typically presents with bilateral symmetric buttock and lower extremity involvement as well as truncal lesions.[161] Aplasia cutis of the scalp can also be a feature of scalp-ear-nipple (SEN) syndrome, an autosomal dominant disorder resulting from mutations in *KCTD1*, encoding a protein that affects a transcription factor (AP-2α) that is important in development.[162] Other features of SEN syndrome are minor anomalies of the external ears, digits, nails, and breasts.

The cause of ACC remains unknown. Although most cases are sporadic, familial case reports have suggested autosomal dominant inheritance with reduced penetrance. Incomplete closure of the neural tube or an embryologic arrest of skin development has been suggested as an explanation for midline lesions. This hypothesis, however, fails to account for lesions of the trunk and limbs. In such instances, vascular abnormality of the placenta, with a degenerative rather than an aplastic or traumatic origin, has been postulated as the cause of the cutaneous defects.[163] Antithyroid drugs, most notably MMI, have long been hypothesized as causative teratogens in some cases of ACC. Although causality remains unproven, there are multiple reports of affected infants born to mothers treated with MMI during pregnancy, both as an isolated manifestation and as part of the presentation of "MMI embryopathy," which includes dysmorphism, gastrointestinal tract malformations, and developmental delay.[164] Propylthiouracil has been recommended as the first-line agent in the management of hyperthyroidism during pregnancy, given its equal effectiveness and lack of reports of teratogenic ACC.[165] A heterozygous missense mutation in *BMS1* (which affects ribosomal function) has been identified in autosomal dominant ACC.[166]

Recognition of ACC and differentiation of it from forceps or other birth injury will help prevent possible medicolegal complications occasionally encountered with this disorder. In patients with localized sporadic lesions, aside from cutaneous scarring, the prognosis of ACC is excellent. With conservative therapy to prevent further tissue damage and secondary infection, most small defects of the scalp heal well during the first few weeks to months of life. With aging of the child, most scars become relatively inconspicuous and require no correction. Those that are large and obvious can be treated with plastic surgical reconstruction. Large split-thickness skin grafting has been reported in infants with more extensive defects with good results but can be complicated by hypertrophic scarring and partial skin graft necrosis.[167] Emergency (within the first hours of life) split-thickness skin grafting has been recommended for infants with large ACC defects or defects with large veins or sagittal sinus exposure in an effort to minimize the risks of hemorrhage and infection.[168]

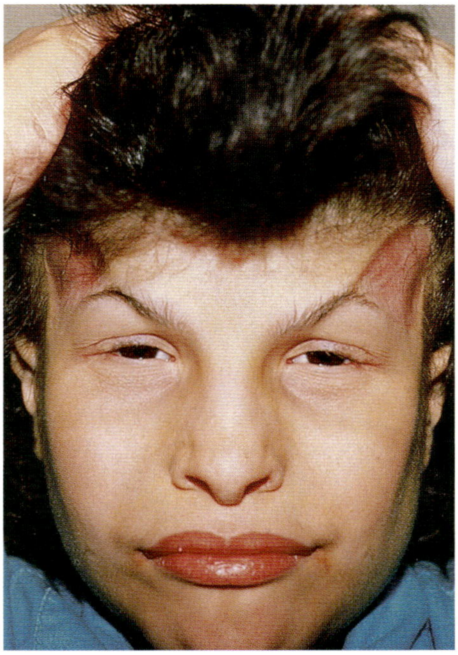

Fig. 2.44 Setleis syndrome. A child with bilateral depressed oval areas on the temples, upwardly slanting eyebrows, narrowed palpebral fissures, and large lips. (Courtesy Seth Orlow, MD.)

Setleis Syndrome

Setleis syndrome was initially described in 1963 by Setleis and colleagues, who described five children of three families, all of Puerto Rican ancestry, who had unique characteristic clinical defects confined to the face.[169] Patients have atrophic skin at the temples (historically likened to forceps marks), coarse facial appearance, absent or duplicated eyelashes of the upper eyelids (distichiasis), eyebrows that slant sharply upward and laterally, and periorbital puffiness (Fig. 2.44; see Chapter 6). Lips may be large with an inverted V contour. Although traditionally believed to have normal intelligence, patients with Setleis syndrome may have associated developmental delay.[170]

Reports of Setleis syndrome have suggested both autosomal recessive and autosomal dominant modes of inheritance,[170,171] and variable expressivity and reduced penetrance may be observed.[172] Setleis syndrome is considered by some to be a form of focal facial dermal dysplasia (see Chapter 6).[173] Homozygous nonsense, missense, and frameshift mutations in *TWIST2* (encoding a basic helix-loop-helix transcription factor) or *de novo* genomic duplication or triplication at 1p36.22p36.21 have been confirmed in some cohorts with the Setleis phenotype.[174–185]

OTHER DEVELOPMENTAL DEFECTS

A congenital dermal sinus or dermoid cyst is a developmental epithelium-lined tract (or cyst) that extends inward from the surface of the skin. Because midline fusion of ectodermal and neuroectodermal tissue occurs at the cephalic and caudal ends of the neural tube, the majority of such defects are seen in the occipital and lumbosacral regions. Dermoids, however, can occur anywhere.

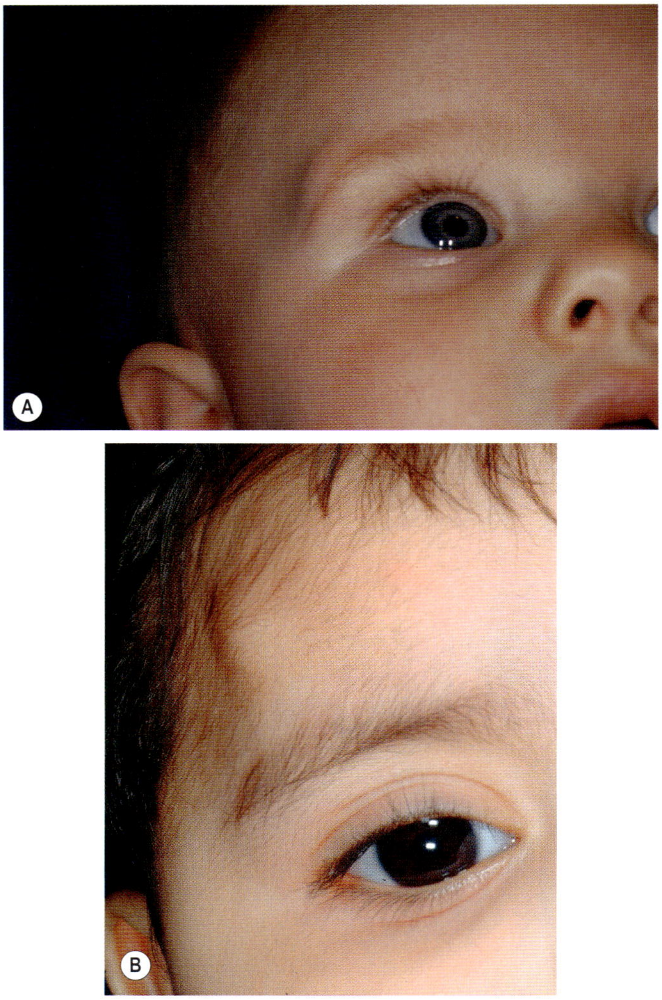

Fig. 2.45 Dermoid cysts. **(A)** A congenital mobile subcutaneous nodule over the lateral eyebrow. **(B)** This mobile, nontender, subcutaneous nodule was present at birth in this 5-month-old girl. The lateral mid-forehead distribution is slightly higher than most dermoids, which present most often in the lateral eyebrow region.

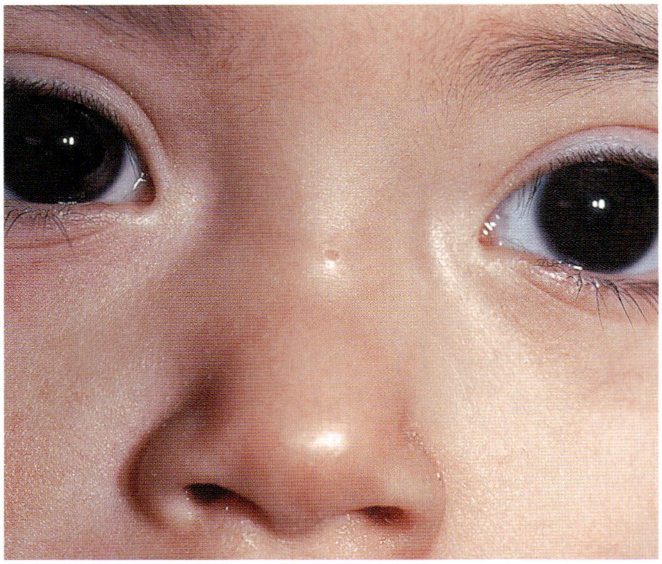

Fig. 2.46 Dermoid sinus. Small sinus ostium at the superior nasal bridge. This patient had no intracranial extension.

Dermal sinus openings may be difficult to visualize, particularly in the occipital scalp region where they may be hidden by hair. A localized thickening of the scalp, hypertrichosis, or dimpling in the midline of the neck or back should alert the physician to the possibility of such an anomaly. These sinuses are of clinical importance as portals for infection that may give rise to abscesses, osteomyelitis, or meningitis.

Dermoid cysts most commonly occur on the orbital ridge, presenting as a nontender, mobile subcutaneous nodule in the eyebrow/orbital ridge region (Fig. 2.45). In this location, there is no association with deep extension. About 3% of dermoids are located in the nasal midline[137] (including glabella, nasal dorsum, and columella), and recognition of these lesions is vital because of the potential for deep extension and CNS communication. Congenital midline nasal masses may represent not only dermoids but also cephaloceles, gliomas, hemangiomas, and a variety of less common neoplasms or malformations. It is vital to consider the diagnostic possibilities carefully when a child's parents seek treatment for a nasal midline mass, given the potential for intracranial connection seen with some of these disorders. Invasive diagnostic procedures should never be performed until radiologic evaluation has been completed.

In midline nasal dermoid cysts or dermal sinuses, an overlying sinus ostium may be present, sometimes with a white discharge or protruding hairs (Fig. 2.46). Presence of such a pit may indicate a higher likelihood of intracranial extension.[176] MRI or computed tomography (CT) of suspicious areas should be performed to evaluate for an underlying tract and CNS connection. Management of dermal sinuses and dermoid cysts consists of surgical excision in an effort to prevent local infection and, in the case of intracranial extension, meningitis and/or abscess formation. Lesions of the lateral forehead or orbital ridge do not require radiographic imaging before surgical excision.

A cephalocele is a herniation of cranial contents through a defect in the skull. Cephaloceles develop as a result of faulty separation of neuroectoderm from surface ectoderm in early gestation and occur most commonly at the occiput, followed by the dorsal nose, orbits, and forehead. These lesions present as a compressible mass that transilluminates with light.[137] Occasionally, an overlying blue hue may be present, which at times can suggest the incorrect diagnosis of deep hemangioma. A useful diagnostic feature is the enlargement of the lesion that may be seen with any maneuver that results in increased intracranial pressure such as crying or straining (called the *Furstenberg sign*). This temporary change is caused by the patent connection between a cephalocele and the CNS. Hypertelorism, facial clefting, and brain malformations may be seen in conjunction with a cephalocele.[177] Surgical resection is the treatment of choice, and multidisciplinary care (plastic surgery, neurosurgery) may be indicated.

A nasal glioma is an ectopic neuroectoderm from early development and may occur in extranasal (60%) or intranasal (30%) locations and less commonly in both extranasal and intranasal sites. This lesion presents as a firm, noncompressible, flesh-colored nodule, sometimes with a blue-red hue, and most often situated at the root of the nose. Hypertelorism may result, and no fluctuation in size is seen, because these lesions have no intracranial connection. An intranasal lesion presents as a protruding mass from the nose, simulating a nasal polyp. *Heterotopic brain tissue* is a term that has been used to similarly describe a rare developmental anomaly that occurs most often on the head and neck, especially in the nasal area, and usually without intracranial communication.[178,179] Surgical excision is the treatment of choice for these lesions.

Congenital fistulas of the lower lip (congenital lip pits) may be unilateral or bilateral and may be seen alone or in association with other anomalies of the face and extremities. They are characterized by single or paired, circular or slit-like depressions on either side of the midline of the lower lip at the edge of the vermilion border. These depressions represent blind sinuses that extend inward through the orbicularis oris muscle to a depth of 0.5 cm or greater. They may occasionally communicate with underlying salivary glands. Excision of lip pits is unnecessary unless mucous gland secretions are problematic.

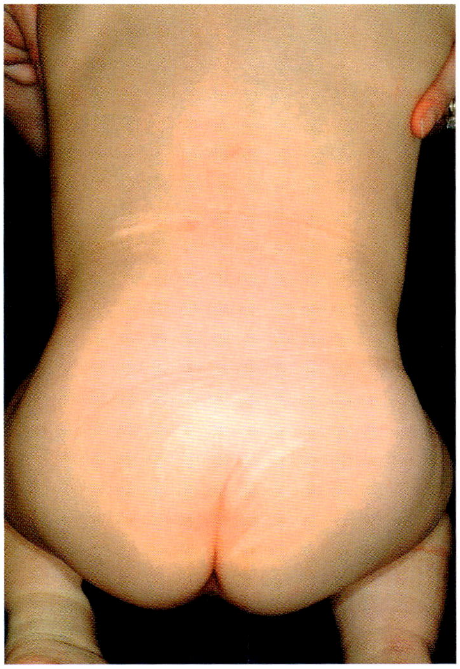

Fig. 2.47 Acquired raised bands of infancy. Numerous linear raised bands on the back of an infant who had similar bands on the extremities. (Courtesy Sarah L. Chamlin, MD.)

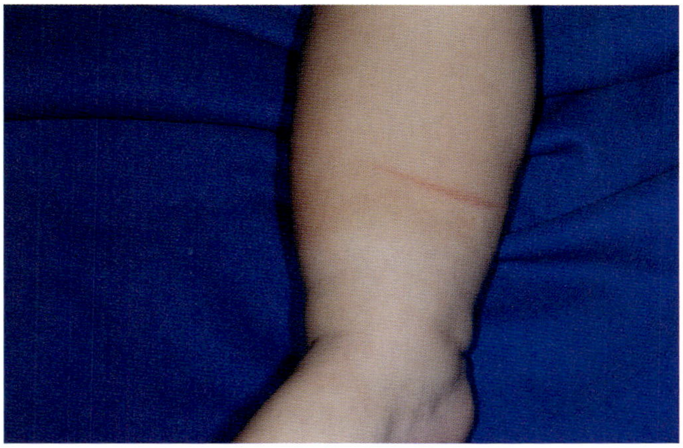

Fig. 2.48 Sock-line hyperpigmentation. Erythematous to hyperpigmented curvilinear streak on the lower leg of a 1-year-old girl whose mother noted the changes shortly after dressing her in tight-fitting socks.

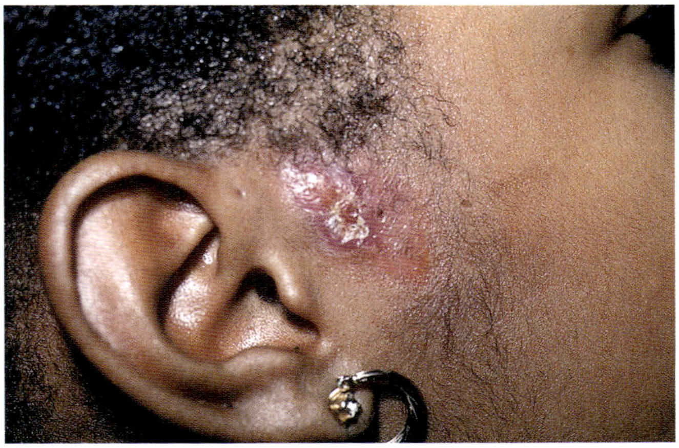

Fig. 2.49 Preauricular sinus with ulceration. This lesion was at risk for recurrent inflammation and infection and ultimately was surgically excised.

Congenital lip pits may be inherited as an autosomal dominant disorder with penetrance estimated at 80%. They may be seen alone or, in 70% of patients, in association with cleft lip or cleft palate. Other associated anomalies include clubfoot, talipes equinovarus, syndactyly, and the popliteal pterygium syndrome (an autosomal dominant disorder with clefting, filiform eyelid adhesions, pterygium, genitourinary anomalies, and congenital heart disease).[180]

Skin dimpling defects (depressions, deep pits, or creases) in the sacral area (see earlier) and over bony prominences may be seen in normal children and infants with diastematomyelia (a fissure or cleft of the spinal cord), congenital rubella or congenital varicella-zoster syndromes, deletion of the long arm of chromosome 18, and Zellweger (cerebrohepatorenal), Bloom, and Freeman–Sheldon (craniocarpotarsal dysplasia, "whistling face") syndromes.

Amniotic constriction bands may produce congenital constriction deformities, and congenital amputation of one or more digits or extremities of otherwise normal infants may occur. The deformities are believed to result from intrauterine rupture of amnion with formation of fibrous bands that encircle fetal parts and produce permanent constriction of the underlying tissue.[181] The most commonly affected areas are the extremities, followed by the umbilical cord, abdomen, and limb–body wall complex.[182] Acquired raised bands of infancy (also known as *raised limb bands*) are linear skin-colored plaques that develop postnatally on the extremities of infants and involve no constrictive defects (Fig. 2.47). They may also occasionally occur on the trunk. Although some argue that these findings are distinct from amniotic constriction bands,[183] coexistence with congenital constriction bands[184] and prenatal ultrasound observation of amniotic bands[185] in reported patients suggests a potential overlap of these two conditions. Sock-line hyperpigmentation (also known as *sock-line bands*) has been described as circumferential, unilateral, or bilateral hyperpigmented streaks on the calf (Fig. 2.48) that are seen in otherwise-healthy children and acquired during infancy and may be related to the wearing of elastic socks or elastic pant legs.[186] It is believed to be distinct from acquired raised bands, must be differentiated from child abuse with a looped cord, and is usually self-limited.[187] These lesions have also been observed on the posterior heel of infants after wearing heel-length socks.[188] Damage to adipose tissue with inflammation and secondary postinflammatory changes have been hypothesized as the cause.

Preauricular pits, cysts, and sinus tracts may develop as a result of imperfect fusion of the tubercles of the first two branchial arches. Unilateral or bilateral, these lesions present as small skin pits that may become infected or result in chronic preauricular ulcerations (Fig. 2.49), retention cysts, or both, necessitating surgical excision. Accessory tragi are fleshy papules, with or without a cartilaginous component, that contain epidermal adnexal structures. Usually seen in the preauricular area, they may also occur on the neck (anterior to the sternocleidomastoid muscle). Accessory tragi may be solitary or localized (Fig. 2.50, *A*) or multifocal, occurring along the embryologic migration line extending from the preauricular cheek to the mouth angle (see Fig. 2.50, *B*). Although generally seen as an isolated congenital defect, they may be associated with other branchial arch syndromes (e.g., oculoauriculovertebral or Goldenhar syndrome). The prevalence of preauricular pits and tags is estimated at around 0.5% to 1.0%.[189,190]

An important consideration with preauricular pits and tags is that of potential associations, the most common concerns being those of hearing or genitourinary defects. Several studies have demonstrated an increased incidence of hearing impairment in the setting of isolated pits or tags, including eustachian tube dysfunction and sensorineural

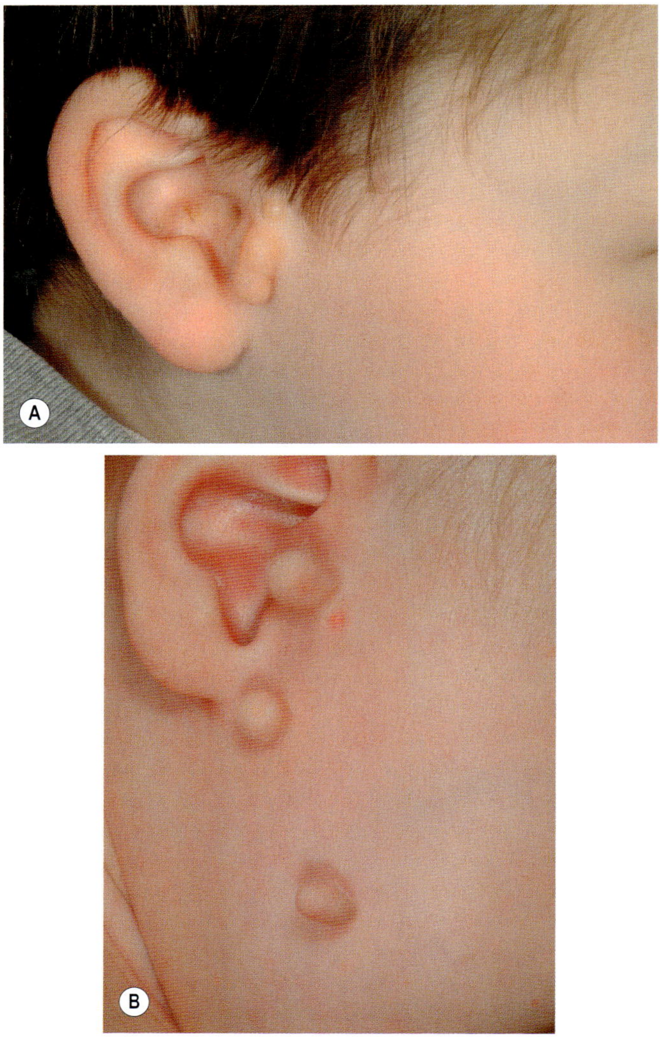

Fig. 2.50 Accessory tragi. These fleshy papules may present in a solitary or localized fashion **(A)** or in a multifocal form, occurring along the embryologic migration line extending from the preauricular cheek to the mouth angle **(B)**.

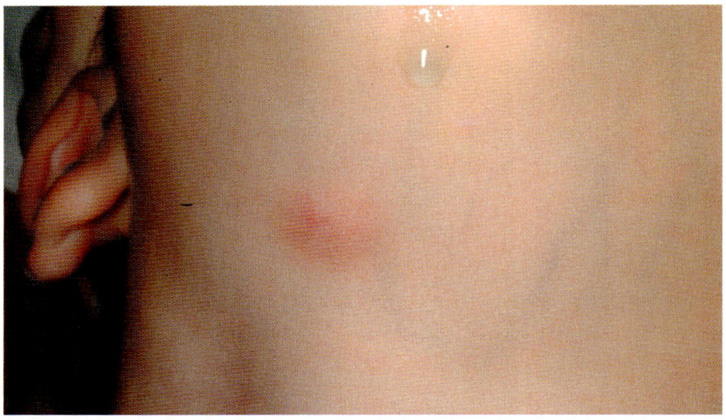

Fig. 2.51 Thyroglossal duct cyst. This congenital nodule of the anterior midline neck was noted to move upward with swallowing.

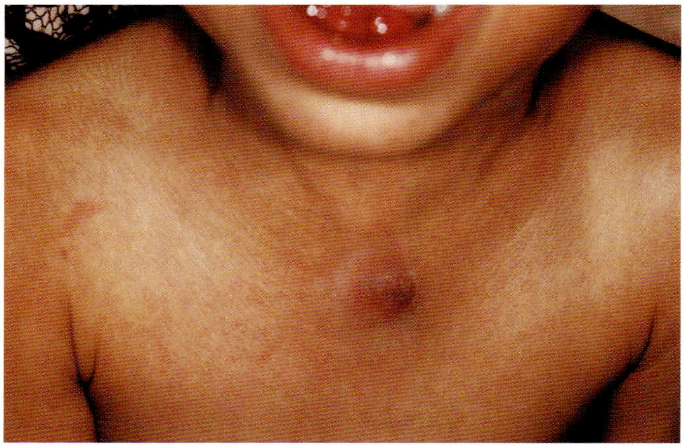

Fig. 2.52 Bronchogenic cyst. This congenital nodule, adjacent to the suprasternal notch, became recurrently inflamed and tender. It was ultimately treated by surgical excision.

hearing loss, suggesting that audiologic evaluation should be performed in these infants.[191–194] The data regarding genitourinary malformations are more controversial, with studies both supporting and refuting an association with preauricular pits or tags.[190,195] It appears that when these preauricular lesions occur in the absence of other dysmorphic or syndromic features, such associations are less likely.

Branchial cleft cysts and sinuses, formed along the course of the first and second branchial clefts as a result of improper closure during embryonic development, are generally located along the lower third of the lateral aspect of the neck near the anterior border of the sternocleidomastoid muscle. Lesions may be unilateral or bilateral and may open onto the cutaneous surface or may drain into the pharynx. Although these lesions may present in childhood, they more commonly come to medical attention during adulthood because of recurrent inflammation. Treatment consists of complete surgical removal or marsupialization (exteriorization, resection of the anterior wall, and suturing of the cut edges of the remaining cyst to the adjacent edges of the skin).

Thyroglossal cysts and sinuses are located on or near the midline of the neck and may open onto the skin surface, extend to the base of the tongue, or drain into the pharynx. Clinically they present as a midline neck cyst that moves with swallowing (Fig. 2.51). These lesions represent persistence of the embryonic structure associated with normal thyroid descent and occasionally may contain ectopic thyroid tissue. Although surgical excision is the treatment of choice, care must be exercised to preserve aberrant thyroid tissue to prevent postoperative hypothyroidism.

Bronchogenic cysts present early, usually at birth, as a nodule (Fig. 2.52) or draining pit, usually over the suprasternal notch. These lesions may develop from ectopic elements of the tracheobronchial tree or may represent ectopic branchial cleft cysts. Surgical excision is the treatment of choice. Fig. 2.53 shows the locations of several types of congenital neck cysts. Small superficial midline neck cysts that appear similar to a giant milium near the sternal notch (Fig. 2.54) have also been observed and appear to be another type of midline developmental anomaly. These lesions have recently been termed *midline anterior neck inclusion cysts (MANICs)*.[196]

Congenital cartilaginous rests of the neck (also known as *wattles*) occur as small fleshy appendages on the anterior neck or over or near the lower half of the sternocleidomastoid muscle. Treatment consists of surgical excision with recognition of the fact that these cutaneous appendages may contain cartilage. Pterygium colli, congenital folds of skin extending from the mastoid region to the acromion on the lateral aspect of the neck, may be seen in individuals with Turner, Noonan, Down, lentigines, electrocardiographic conduction abnormalities, ocular hypertelorism, pulmonic stenosis, abnormal genitalia, retardation of growth, deafness (LEOPARD), and multiple pterygium syndromes; trisomy 18; short-limbed dwarfism; and combined immunodeficiency disease.

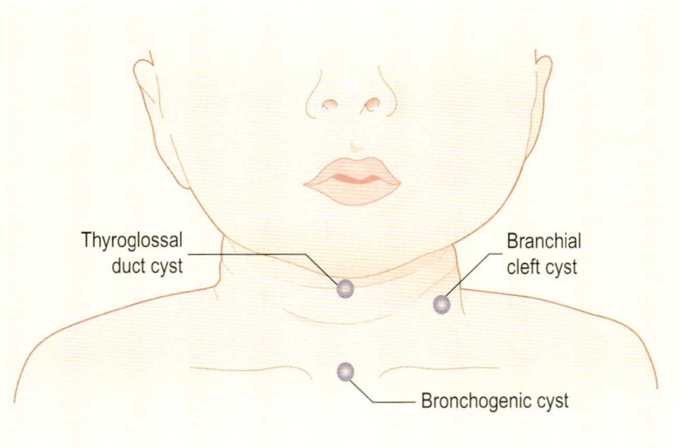

Fig. 2.53 Congenital sinuses of the neck.

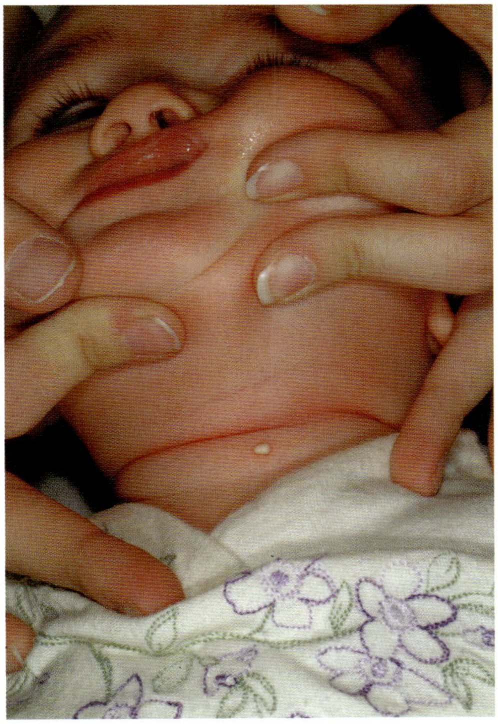

Fig. 2.54 Anterior neck inclusion cyst. This white exophytic cyst was present over the midline anterior neck at birth in this 7-month-old girl.

Supernumerary nipples (polythelia), present at times in males as well as females, are manifested as small brown or pink, concave, umbilicated, or elevated papules along or slightly medial to the embryologic milk line (Fig. 2.55). They are most common on the chest or upper abdomen and occasionally occur at other sites, including the face, neck, shoulder, back, genitals, or thighs. Although much has been written about a relatively high incidence of renal malformation in patients with supernumerary nipples, current studies suggest that this anomaly in an otherwise apparently normal individual does not appear to be a marker of urinary tract malformation.[197–199]

A variety of developmental anomalies may occur in the umbilical region. Urachal cyst or sinus is a lesion that represents persistence of the embryonic urachus, a fibrous cord that develops from the urogenital sinus. A midline nodule near the umbilicus may result, and at times urine drainage may be seen from a fistula connecting the umbilicus to the bladder. Vitelline (omphalomesenteric duct) remnant may present as an umbilical polyp or an umbilicoileal fistula that drains feces onto the skin surface. Complete excision is the treatment of choice for these anomalies.

Congenital Infections of the Newborn

Viral, bacterial, and parasitic infections during pregnancy can be associated with widespread systemic involvement, serious permanent sequelae, and a variety of cutaneous manifestations in the newborn. This section discusses the most significant of these: congenital rubella, congenital varicella-zoster syndrome, neonatal varicella, neonatal herpes, congenital parvovirus B19 infection, congenital syphilis (CS), cytomegalic inclusion disease, congenital Epstein–Barr virus (EBV) syndrome, and congenital toxoplasmosis. Congenital Zika virus infection is briefly discussed, given increasing recognition of its untoward effects on the human fetus.

CONGENITAL RUBELLA

Congenital rubella syndrome (CRS) was initially identified in 1941 by Norman Gregg, an Australian ophthalmologist who observed an unusual form of congenital cataracts in babies of mothers who had had rubella during pregnancy.[200] It occurs after a maternal rubella infection during the first 16 weeks of pregnancy and only rarely when infection is acquired later in gestation. Earlier gestation directly correlates with the likelihood of CRS. Overall, the incidence of CRS in the United States has declined notably in parallel with the decline in rubella cases since licensure of the rubella vaccine in 1969. During 2004 through 2012, 79 cases of rubella and six cases of CRS were reported in the United States and were either import associated or from unknown sources.[201] In 2014 an expert panel reported that since 2004 the incidence of CRS was less than 1 per 5,000,000 births, supporting virtual elimination of the disease from the United States.[202] In 2015 the Pan American Health Organization/World Health Organization declared the Americas region free of endemic transmission of rubella and CRS. Occasional rubella outbreaks, however, have been related to a variety of factors, including occurrence in settings in which unvaccinated adults congregate, in unvaccinated foreign-born adults, and among children and adults in religious communities with low levels of vaccination coverage.[203,204] Studies suggest that young Hispanic women represent a population at elevated risk for delivering an infant affected by CRS, and thus this population needs to be targeted specifically for immunization.[204,205] Importantly, rubella virus continues to circulate in other parts of the world (e.g., Africa, Asia) where rubella vaccination programs are not established and increases the risk of imported rubella in the United States and subsequent CRS.[201,202]

Clinical manifestations of CRS are characterized by the classic triad of congenital cataracts, deafness, and cardiac defects (especially patent ductus arteriosus). *In utero* growth restriction may occur during the last trimester of pregnancy. CNS involvement may result in microcephaly, meningoencephalitis, and mental retardation. Other features include pigmentary retinopathy, hepatosplenomegaly, jaundice, radiolucent bone lesions in metaphyses, and thrombocytopenia.[206] Some infants with CRS may show few manifestations at birth or may be asymptomatic, but findings usually manifest over subsequent months. Occasionally, CRS findings may not become manifest until the second year of life.[207,208]

The most distinct cutaneous feature of CRS is a diffuse eruption composed of blue-red infiltrative papules and nodules and occasionally smaller purpuric macules, measuring 2 to 8 mm in diameter, representing "blueberry muffin" lesions (Fig. 2.56). Blueberry muffin lesions are usually present at birth or within the first 24 hours, and new lesions rarely appear after age 2 days. They may be observed in association with a variety of disorders, usually either infectious or neoplastic (Box 2.2). Histologic evaluation reveals extramedullary hematopoiesis, characteristic of viral infection of the fetus and not unique to infants with CRS but also seen in patients with congenital toxoplasmosis, cytomegalovirus (CMV) infection, erythroblastosis fetalis, congenital leukemia, and twin–twin transfusion syndrome. Other cutaneous manifestations in CRS may include a

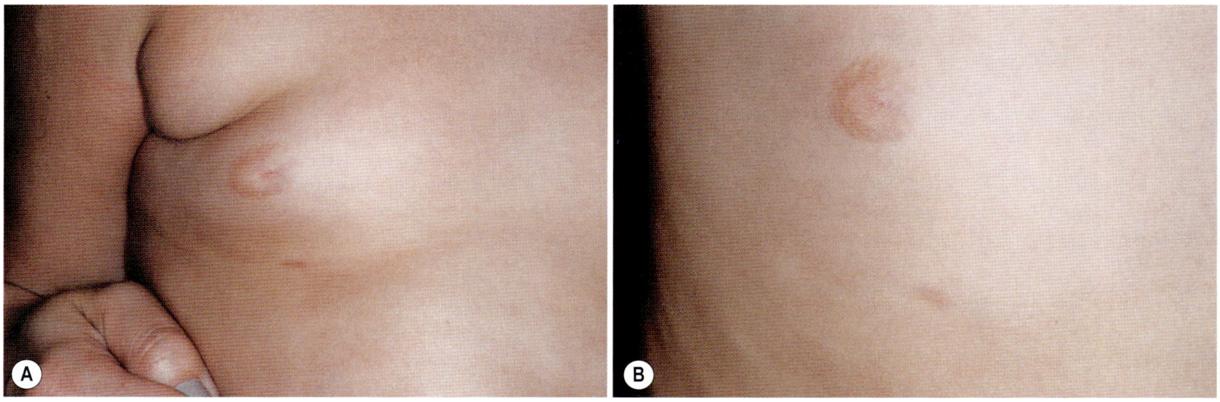

Fig. 2.55 (A) Supernumerary nipple. This papule, inferior and medial to the right breast, was present at birth in this young girl. **(B)** Closer inspection reveals an umbilicated, pink papule representing a well-formed nipple and surrounding areola.

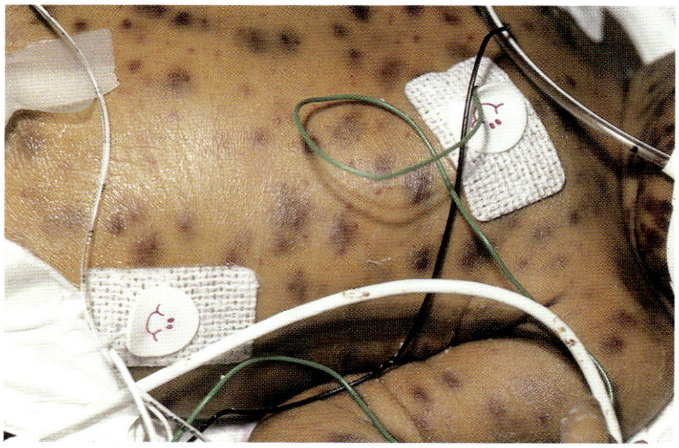

Fig. 2.56 Congenital rubella with blueberry muffin lesions. Multiple violaceous, infiltrative papules and nodules in this newborn with congenital rubella.

Box 2.2 Differential Diagnosis of the Newborn with "Blueberry Muffin" Lesions

Dermal (extramedullary) hematopoiesis
Congenital infection
- Toxoplasmosis
- Rubella
- Cytomegalovirus
- Enterovirus
- Parvovirus B19

Erythroblastosis fetalis
Inherited hemolytic diseases
Twin–twin transfusion
Neoplastic
- Neuroblastoma
- Leukemia
- Histiocytosis
- Alveolar rhabdomyosarcoma

generalized nonspecific maculopapular eruption, reticulated erythema of the face and extremities, hyperpigmentation, and recurrent urticaria. Vasomotor instability, manifested by poor peripheral circulation with generalized mottling and acral cyanosis, may also occur.

The diagnosis of CRS should be suspected in infants with one or more characteristic findings, including congenital cataracts, pigmentary retinopathy, cardiac defects, deafness, thrombocytopenia, hepatosplenomegaly, microcephaly, or blueberry muffin lesions. The diagnosis may be confirmed by isolation of rubella virus from respiratory secretions, urine, cerebrospinal fluid (CSF), or tissue. Neonatal immunoglobulin (Ig) M rubella-specific antibodies or IgG antibodies that persist beyond the time expected for passively transferred immunity are also diagnostic. Real-time reverse transcription polymerase chain reaction (rRT-PCR) can also be performed on throat/nasopharyngeal swabs, serum, and urine. Prenatal diagnosis of congenital infection can be pursued when maternal rubella is diagnosed and is based on detection of rubella virus IgM in fetal blood or detection of viral genome in amniotic fluid, fetal blood, or chorionic villus sampling.[209] Prenatal ultrasound findings most useful in evaluating for CRS include cardiac septal defects, pulmonary artery stenosis, microcephaly, cataracts, microphthalmia, and hepatosplenomegaly.[210]

There is no specific therapy for CRS apart from supportive therapy and recognition of potential disabilities. Because of the high incidence of ophthalmic complications, regular ophthalmologic examinations are indicated. Infants who are congenitally infected may shed virus in urine and the nasopharynx for several months to 1 year and should be considered contagious until that time. The majority of infants who acquire CRS early in gestation will have permanent neurologic and audiologic sequelae, and long-term multidisciplinary care is indicated. A long-term follow-up study of 50 Australian patients with CRS revealed aortic valve disease in 68% and increased incidences of diabetes, thyroid disorders, early menopause, and osteoporosis compared with the general population.[211]

Congenital rubella can be effectively prevented by immunization with live rubella virus vaccine, and universal vaccination is recommended. Efforts focus on immunizing high-risk populations with two doses of rubella vaccine, with a special effort to vaccinate populations at increased risk, including college students, military recruits, and healthcare and daycare workers.[207] Because of the high risk of fetal damage, women known to have contracted maternal rubella during the early months of pregnancy may consider abortion. Although limited data suggest that administration of immunoglobulin to the mother may reduce the amount of viremia and damage when given as early as possible after exposure, it does not appear to prevent congenital infection.

CONGENITAL VARICELLA SYNDROME

Congenital varicella syndrome, also known as *fetal varicella syndrome*, refers to a spectrum of congenital anomalies that may be seen in neonates born to women who contract varicella-zoster virus (VZV) infection during the first 20 weeks of gestation. Overall it is quite rare, probably because primary varicella infection during pregnancy is uncommon given that the majority of women have acquired immunity by childbearing age.[212] The incidence of congenital varicella syndrome after maternal infection is estimated at around 0.4% to 1%, and the highest risk seems to be when infection is acquired between

13 and 20 weeks of gestation.[213,214] Primary VZV infection in a pregnant woman most often results in the birth of a normal newborn, related to either lack of transmission to the fetus or self-limited fetal infection. Although there are rare reports of fetal sequelae in infants born to mothers who develop herpes zoster infection (shingles) during pregnancy, this association is extremely rare.[213,215] Infants born to mothers with a history of maternal varicella during gestation appear to be at increased risk for infantile herpes zoster (shingles). Implementation of universal varicella vaccination programs has been demonstrated to result in reduction of both congenital varicella and neonatal varicella infections.[216]

Congenital varicella syndrome may present with various findings, including low birthweight, ophthalmologic defects (including microphthalmia, Horner syndrome, cataracts, and chorioretinitis), neurologic defects (including mental retardation, seizures, cortical atrophy, encephalomyelitis, and developmental delay), limb hypoplasia with flexion contractures and malformed digits, and gastrointestinal and genitourinary defects.[212] Cutaneous findings include vesicles and/or scarring (often depressed and pigmented) in a dermatomal distribution, although several affected newborns have been reported with cutis aplasia–like absence of skin.

Because the risk of fetal malformation in an infant born to a mother exposed to VZV during pregnancy is so slight, therapeutic abortion is not necessarily indicated. As noted, the majority of women who contract varicella during pregnancy have children with no evidence of the syndrome. Studies to date are inconclusive with regard to the utility of serologic or PCR-based testing of fetal blood or amniotic fluid.[217] Prenatal ultrasound may reveal disseminated organ calcifications.[218] Studies suggest that the use of varicella-zoster immunoglobulin (VariZIG) may clearly modify or prevent disease in the mother who has been exposed and is susceptible. Treatment of mothers with severe varicella with acyclovir or valacyclovir may be considered. Most important is screening of women of childbearing age without a history of varicella for antibody and offering vaccination when indicated. Susceptible women who are already pregnant should be counseled about avoiding contact with individuals who have chickenpox and about the availability of VariZIG should it become necessary.

Neonatal varicella is a varicella infection of the newborn that occurs when a pregnant woman develops chickenpox during the last few weeks of pregnancy or the first few days postpartum. In such instances, the timing of the onset of disease in the mother and her newborn is critical. If the disease onset in the mother is 5 or more days before delivery or in the newborn during the first 4 days of life, the infection tends to be mild. In contrast, if the onset in the mother is within 5 days before delivery to 2 days after delivery or in the newborn between 5 and 10 days of birth, the infant's infection is often severe and disseminated (Fig. 2.57), with pneumonia, hepatitis, or meningoencephalitis and severe coagulopathy and a mortality rate of around 30%. In an effort to prevent neonatal varicella infection, VariZIG (or intravenous immunoglobin [IVIG] if the former is unavailable) should be given as soon as possible after delivery to all infants in whom the mother has the onset of varicella within 5 days before or within 48 hours after delivery, and these infants are also candidates for intravenous acyclovir therapy.[219]

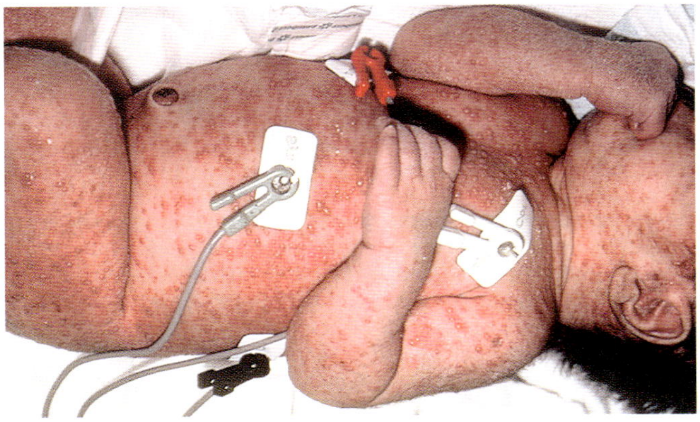

Fig. 2.57 Neonatal varicella. Disseminated, erythematous papules, vesicles, and erosions.

NEONATAL HERPES

Neonatal herpes simplex virus (HSV) infection may range from a mild, self-limited illness to one with devastating neurologic consequences or even death. The overall incidence in the United States is estimated to range between 9.6 and 13.3 cases per 100,000 births.[220,221] Incidence rates likely vary by geographic region and race or ethnicity.[222] Traditionally, up to 70% of neonatal HSV infections were caused by type 2 ("genital") HSV, and the disease was acquired either by ascending *in utero* infection or by spread during delivery through an infected birth canal (perinatal transmission). More recently, type 1 HSV has evolved to be the predominant type causing genital herpes, and neonatal HSV infections in many parts of the world are now caused by HSV-1.[223] Infection of the newborn may also be acquired by intrauterine infection because of maternal viremia with transplacental spread or by postnatal hospital or household contact with other infants or persons with oral HSV infection.[224–226] Of infants with neonatal HSV, 85% acquire their infection during birth (peripartum), 10% postnatally (postpartum), and 5% from *in utero* exposure.[227] Congenital (intrauterine) HSV infection, which is not the focus of this section, is a rare disorder (approximately 5% of all neonatal HSV disease) resulting from intrauterine infection and is characterized by skin vesicles or scarring, chorioretinitis, microphthalmia, microcephaly, and abnormal brain CT findings.[228] Importantly, the majority of infants with cutaneous involvement have lesions at birth or within 12 hours of life (significantly earlier than infants with neonatal herpes).[229]

The risk of neonatal HSV infection in an infant born vaginally to a mother with primary genital infection is high (40% to 57%), whereas the risk to an infant born to a mother with recurrent infection is much lower, around 2% to 5%. The lower rate of transmission with recurrent maternal disease may reflect decreased viral load and partial protection of the fetus by transplacentally acquired antibodies.[230] Most babies with neonatal HSV become infected from mothers who are asymptomatic.

The clinical presentation of neonatal HSV has traditionally been divided into three separate patterns: skin, eyes, and/or mouth (SEM) disease; CNS disease; and disseminated disease. These presentations are summarized in Table 2.4. The exact frequency of the various forms

Table 2.4 Clinical Presentations of Neonatal Herpes

Type	Incidence* (%)	Skin Vesicles (%)	Comment
SEM disease	45	80–85	May progress to more severe infection, especially without early therapy
CNS disease	30	60–70	Clinical overlap with neonatal bacterial sepsis
Disseminated	25	75–80	Multiple organs, including liver, lungs, adrenals, GI tract, and SEM; may progress to respiratory collapse, liver failure, and DIC

Adapted from Kimberlin DW. Herpes simplex virus infections in neonates and early childhood. Semin Pediatr Infect Dis 2005;16:271–81; Kimberlin DW. Herpes simplex virus infections of the newborn. Semin Perinatol 2007;31:19–25; James SH, Kimberlin DW. Neonatal herpes simplex virus infection. Clin Perinatol 2015;42(1):47–59.

CNS, Central nervous system; *DIC*, disseminated intravascular coagulopathy; *GI*, gastrointestinal; *SEM*, skin, eyes, and/or mouth.

*Approximate incidence out of all neonatal herpes patients.

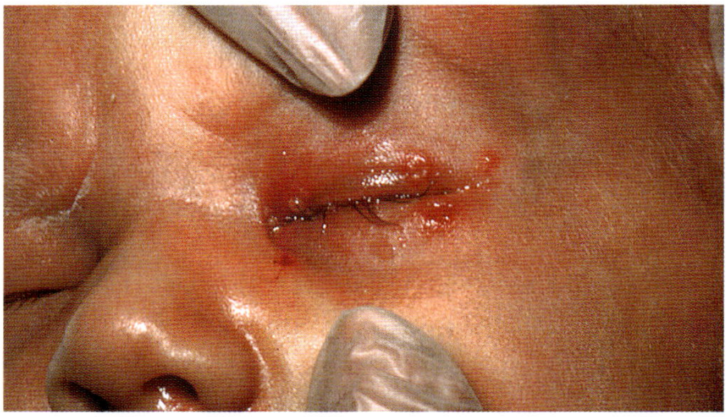

Fig. 2.58 Neonatal herpes simplex infection. Clustered vesicles on an erythematous base in this newborn with congenital herpes simplex infection, skin, eyes, and/or mouth (SEM) type.

Table 2.5 Recommended Evaluation for Suspected Neonatal HSV

Swab specimens from the mouth, nasopharynx, conjunctivae, and anus for HSV culture or PCR assay
Specimens of skin vesicles for HSV culture (if available) or PCR assay
CSF sample for HSV PCR assay
Whole blood sample for HSV PCR assay
Whole blood sample for measuring alanine transaminase (ALT)

From American Academy of Pediatrics. Herpes simplex. In: Kimberlin DW, Brady MT, Jackson MA, Long SS, editors. Red book: 2018 report of the Committee on Infectious Diseases. Elk Grove Village, IL: American Academy of Pediatrics; 2018:437–49.

CSF, Cerebrospinal fluid; *HSV*, herpes simplex virus; *PCR*, polymerase chain reaction.

is unclear, given partial overlap of patterns in some patients and potential delays in the appearance of CNS disease. Most infants affected with neonatal HSV become sick during the first 4 weeks of life; SEM and disseminated disease tend to present earlier (average 9 to 11 days postnatal age) than CNS disease (average 16 to 17 days postnatal age). SEM disease appears to be the least severe and associated with the most favorable prognosis. However, although most infants have SEM disease, 60% to 70% will progress to more diffuse involvement.[231]

Presenting features of neonatal HSV include skin lesions, fever, respiratory distress, and CNS dysfunction. The latter includes seizures, lethargy, poor feeding, irritability, and hypotonia. In a retrospective series of 49 infants with neonatal HSV, 84% presented with seizures, vesicular skin eruption, or critical illness.[232] The skin eruption may vary from erythematous macules to individual or grouped vesicles (Fig. 2.58) or a widespread generalized vesicobullous eruption affecting the skin and buccal mucosa. The vesicles of neonatal HSV may become pustular after 24 to 48 hours and eventually become crusted or ulcerated. Other skin findings may include purpuric, petechial, or zosteriform lesions, as well as large bullae with skin denudation similar to those seen in epidermolysis bullosa.[233] Skin lesions occur most often on the scalp and face, and in breech deliveries they have a predilection for the presenting part. Occasionally, the scalp of the infant may reveal diffuse edematous swelling resembling that seen in caput succedaneum. Rather than resolving spontaneously during the first week, this swelling may become necrotic with resultant drainage and eschar formation and irregularly grouped herpetic vesicles. Fetal scalp monitoring is a risk factor for HSV, because the virus more readily gains entry into the lacerated scalp. Eye involvement, seen only in around 5% of affected infants, may present with conjunctivitis or pathognomonic keratitis.

The disseminated form of neonatal HSV may affect several organs, especially the liver, adrenal glands, lungs, and the CNS. This form is associated with the highest mortality—up to 60%. In the absence of skin lesions or other pathognomonic features, disseminated disease may be difficult to diagnose and should always be considered in the neonate who has risk factors for HSV, possible sepsis (especially if a lack of response to antimicrobial therapy is noted), unexplained pneumonitis (especially in the first week of life), or unexplained nonspecific findings such as thrombocytopenia, coagulopathy, hepatitis, or fever.[231] In addition, infants with an unexplained CSF pleocytosis (usually lymphocytic) merit consideration for the diagnosis of HSV.

The diagnosis of HSV infection in the newborn can be confirmed in a variety of ways. The recommended evaluation from the Committee on Infectious Diseases of the American Academy of Pediatrics is shown in Table 2.5. In the presence of skin lesions, a Tzanck smear can be performed on scrapings from the base of an unroofed vesicle and microscopically reveals multinucleated cells and nuclear inclusions. The Tzanck smear, however, is highly operator dependent and thus may have a relatively low sensitivity; it is also not specific and is rarely if ever performed in the present era. Direct fluorescent antibody study of skin lesion scrapings has a high sensitivity (80% to 90%), excellent specificity,[234] and readily available results. The gold standard for diagnosis of HSV infections remains viral culture, which can be taken from skin (especially vesicular fluid), eyes, mouth, CSF, rectum, urine, or blood.[231] Serologic studies generally are not useful in diagnosing neonatal HSV infection because of the slow serologic response of the newborn and the potential confounding factor of transplacental antibody. PCR studies have been a major advance in the diagnosis of neonatal HSV infection and are especially useful for diagnosing CNS infection, for which they are the diagnostic method of choice. Skin biopsy is rarely indicated, but if it is performed, it reveals characteristic intraepidermal vesicle formation with ballooning degeneration and multinucleation.

Other laboratory findings that may be suggestive of neonatal HSV infection include abnormal coagulation studies, thrombocytopenia, and elevated liver transaminases. Evaluation of CSF in those with CNS or disseminated disease often reveals a lymphocytic pleocytosis and elevated protein, although these findings may be absent in early disease and are not specific for HSV.[235] Electroencephalography and neuroimaging with MRI should also be considered.[235]

The outcome of neonatal HSV infection is quite variable. Prospective data on outcomes were gathered by the Collaborative Antiviral Study Group and revealed that the following were risk factors for mortality: CNS and disseminated disease, decreased level of consciousness at start of therapy, and prematurity. In those with disseminated disease, pneumonitis and disseminated intravascular coagulopathy were important risk factors.[224] Morbidity was greatest in infants with encephalitis, disseminated infection, seizures, or infection with HSV-2 (vs. HSV-1).

Education is vitally important in the prevention of HSV (and therefore neonatal HSV) during pregnancy. Studies have shown that women at greatest risk of acquiring the infection during pregnancy are those who are seronegative and whose partners are HSV positive. It appears that acquisition of infection with seroconversion completed before labor does not affect the outcome of the pregnancy, whereas infection acquired near the time of labor is associated with neonatal HSV and perinatal morbidity.[236] Overall, 70% of infants with neonatal HSV are born to mothers who do not manifest any sign or symptom of genital infection at the time of delivery. Cesarean delivery should be offered to women with active HSV lesions at the time of labor, although not all cases of neonatal HSV can be prevented.[228] The use of acyclovir during pregnancy is controversial, although it may shorten the period of active lesions in the mother. In instances where there is a known history of maternal HSV, use of fetal scalp electrodes should be avoided whenever possible. Viral cultures in mothers with suspected genital HSV during the last few weeks before delivery and routine prophylactic cesarean section for asymptomatic women have not been demonstrated useful and are not routinely recommended.

Newborns with vesicular lesions or suspected HSV should be isolated (contact precautions), evaluated thoroughly for systemic infection, and treated with empiric antiviral therapy. Ophthalmologic evaluation should be performed, and prophylactic topical ophthalmic preparations such as idoxuridine, vidarabine, or trifluorothymidine solution should be initiated. In addition to antiviral therapy, supportive measures are often indicated, including management of seizures, respiratory distress, hemorrhage, and metabolic aberrations. Women with active HSV infection may handle and feed their infants provided they use careful handwashing techniques and wear a disposable surgical mask or dressing to cover the lesions until they have crusted and dried. There is no unequivocal evidence that HSV is transmitted by breast milk or that breastfeeding by a mother with recurrent HSV infection poses a risk to the infant. It therefore appears that if all precautions are used, breastfeeding by a mother with recurrent HSV may be acceptable. After hospital discharge, affected infants should be monitored closely, because 5% to 10% will develop a recurrent infection requiring therapy within the first month of life.[237]

Both vidarabine and acyclovir have been demonstrated effective in the treatment of neonatal HSV. However, because of its safety profile, acyclovir is the treatment of choice.[217] Early studies suggested a dose range of 15 to 30 mg/kg per day for affected infants, but it was subsequently demonstrated that higher dosages are more effective. The survival rate for patients with disseminated HSV treated with high-dose acyclovir (60 mg/kg per day) was significantly higher, with a borderline significant decrease in morbidity.[238] Toxicity was limited to transient neutropenia during therapy, suggesting the importance of monitoring absolute neutrophil counts. In a study of 89 infants with neonatal HSV treated with high-dose acyclovir, the most common clinical adverse events were hypotension and seizure, and the most common laboratory aberration observed was thrombocytopenia, which occurred in 25% of infants.[239] Treatment recommendations are for 14 days for SEM disease and 21 days for CNS and disseminated disease.[235,240] Oral acyclovir suppression for 6 months after acute therapy is recommended for surviving infants with CNS disease, given the demonstrated improved neurodevelopmental outcomes.[241] Algorithmic guidelines on the management of asymptomatic neonates born to women with active genital herpes lesions have been published.[242,243]

CONGENITAL PARVOVIRUS B19 INFECTION

Human parvovirus B19, the same virus that causes erythema infectiosum (fifth disease), may be transmitted by a gravid woman to the fetus and may result in anemia, hydrops fetalis, and even intrauterine fetal demise. The cellular receptor for B19, a virus that lytically infects erythroid precursor cells, is globoside or P-antigen, which is found on erythroblasts and megakaryocytes.[244] Overall, up to 65% of pregnant women are immune to B19 and therefore not at risk,[245] and the majority of infants born to mothers with B19 infection are delivered at term and asymptomatic. The greatest risk appears to be when infection is acquired before 20 weeks' gestation, and the overall incidence of fetal loss is between 1% and 9%.[246–248] The highest risk period for fetal loss is when maternal transmission occurs between 9 and 16 weeks' gestation.[249] Fetal B19 infection may result in severe anemia, high-output cardiac failure, generalized edema, pleural and pericardial effusions, and polyhydramnios. *Hydrops fetalis* refers to fluid accumulation in at least two of the following compartments: subcutaneous, pericardial, pleural, and abdominal.[249] Bony lucencies of long and axial bones noted on plain radiographs have been reported.[250] Although skin findings are not a major feature of congenital B19 infection, blueberry muffin lesions have been described.[251]

In infants who survive congenital B19 infection, there appears to be no increased risk of congenital anomalies or developmental aberrations. Pregnant women exposed to B19 should be reassured regarding the relatively low potential risk and offered serologic testing. Detection of B19 antigens in amniotic fluid or B19 deoxyribonucleic acid (DNA) via PCR are other methods available for diagnostic confirmation.[252] If acute B19 infection is confirmed, serial fetal ultrasonography should be performed to assess for signs of *in utero* infection. Management of severely afflicted fetuses includes fetal digitalization and *in utero* blood transfusions. However, despite management with transfusion in severely anemic or hydropic fetuses with B19 infection, the mortality rate may still approach 25%.[253]

CONGENITAL SYPHILIS

As a result of advances in the detection and treatment of syphilis during the years after the Second World War, the incidence of neonatal syphilis dropped to relatively insignificant levels by the mid-1950s. Since 1959, however, the incidence of primary and secondary syphilis has increased, with a resultant resurgence in the incidence of CS. Surveillance data reported to the Centers for Disease Control and Prevention (CDC) by 50 states and the District of Columbia from 1992 to 1998 revealed 942 deaths among 14,627 cases of CS, resulting primarily from untreated, inadequately treated, or undocumented treatment of syphilis during pregnancy.[254] In the United Kingdom, the number of babies reported with CS increased from 2 in 1996 to 14 in 2005.[255] A review of national surveillance data from 2003 through 2008 revealed an increase in the CS rate from 8.2 cases per 100,000 live births in 2005 to 10.1 cases per 100,000 live births in 2008. This increase paralleled the increase in primary and secondary syphilis among females from 2004 through 2007, and it was noted that the CS rates increased primarily in the South and among infants born to Black mothers.[256] Although the overall rate of CS in the United States decreased during the period from 2008 to 2012, during the years 2012 to 2014 it again increased from 8.4 to 11.6 cases per 100,000 live births.[257] Such data reveal that CS still represents a public health problem and highlight the fact that early prenatal care via early detection and treatment of maternal syphilis is an essential component in CS prevention in neonates.

CS is a disorder in which the fetus becomes infected with the spirochete *Treponema pallidum*, usually after the 16th week of pregnancy. The risk of fetal transmission is estimated to be 70% to 100% for untreated early syphilis.[258] The risk of CS increases with greater maternal spirochetemia and longer duration of maternal primary or secondary syphilis.[259] The widely varied manifestations of CS are determined in part by the stage of maternal syphilis, stage of the pregnancy at the time of infection, rapidity of maternal diagnosis, and treatment and immunologic reaction of the fetus.[260] Of those who die from CS, more than 80% are stillbirths. Among affected live newborns, around 50% are symptom free.[261] Perinatal associations with CS include premature delivery, low birthweight, and small size for gestational age.[262]

The clinical manifestations of CS are divided into lesions of early CS (appearing before 2 years of age) and late CS (occurring after 2 years of age). Skin lesions of early CS are generally infectious, and because there is no primary stage, they may resemble those of acquired secondary syphilis. They differ from those of the second stage of syphilis in that the fetal lesions are generally more widely distributed, more severe, and of longer duration. Lesions of late CS represent either a hypersensitivity reaction on the part of the host or scars and deformities that are direct consequences of infection.

Early Congenital Syphilis

Fetal infection with *T. pallidum* results in multisystem involvement with considerable variation in clinical expression. Although infants with CS commonly exhibit no external signs of disease at the time of birth, many experience clinical manifestations within the first month. Those with florid manifestations at birth appear to be more severely infected, are often premature, and usually have a poor prognosis. Premature infants are more likely to display characteristic features of early CS, including skin findings, hepatosplenomegaly, thrombocytopenia, and radiographic findings in long bones as neonates, compared with full-term infants.[263]

The most common clinical manifestations of early CS are summarized in Table 2.6. Rhinitis (snuffles) is commonly the first sign of CS. Cutaneous lesions of CS are seen in one-third to one-half of affected infants and may be quite varied. Most common is a diffuse papulosquamous eruption that includes the palms and soles, comparable with the rash seen in secondary syphilis in older patients. Vesiculobullous lesions are relatively rare but when they involve the palms and soles are highly diagnostic of CS. The palms and soles are often fissured, erythematous, and indurated, with a dull red, shiny appearance (Fig. 2.59). Concomitant with these changes, desquamation in large, dry flakes may occur over the entire body surface area. Flat, moist, wart-like lesions (condylomata lata) commonly appear in moist areas of skin in infants with CS and are extremely infectious. Intractable diaper dermatitis is occasionally present. Mucous patches, which present as fissures at mucocutaneous junctions, are among the most characteristic and most infectious of the early lesions seen in CS.

Table 2.6 Manifestations of Early Congenital Syphilis

System	Specific Features	Comment
Constitutional	Fever, wasting	
Nasal	Snuffles (nasal discharge)	Commonly the first sign
		2–6 weeks of life
		Ulceration of nasal mucosa
		If deep, may involve cartilage and result in "saddle-nose" deformity
Hematologic	Hemolytic anemia	
	Thrombocytopenia	
Lymphoid	Lymphadenopathy	Epitrochlear nodes highly suggestive
Visceral	Hepatosplenomegaly	50%–75% of patients
		Icterus, jaundice, ascites associated
Mucocutaneous	Papulosquamous lesions	Diffuse eruption
		Palms and soles red, fissured (Fig. 2.59)
		Bright pink-red, fades to coppery brown
		Rare vesiculobullous lesions
		Eventual widespread desquamation
	Condylomata lata	Flat, wart-like lesions in moist areas (especially anogenital, nares, mouth angles)
	Mucous patches	Present in 30%–35% of cases
		Weeping, fissuring at mucocutaneous junctions
		Extend out from lips in radiating fashion
		When deep, may leave scars (rhagades) of perioral region
Osseous	Osteochondritis	15% of patients, especially long bones of extremities; often focal
		Usually asymptomatic, but severe involvement may lead to subepiphyseal fracture and painful pseudoparalysis of Parrot
	Periostitis	Most pronounced at 2–6 months of life
		Usually diffuse
		Calcification and thickening of cortex may lead to permanent deformity (e.g., frontal bossing, anterior bowing of tibia or saber shins)
	Dactylitis	Affects small bones of hands and feet
CNS	CSF abnormalities	Increased protein, mononuclear pleocytosis, positive CSF-VDRL

CNS, Central nervous system; *CSF-VDRL*, cerebrospinal fluid Venereal Disease Research Laboratories test.

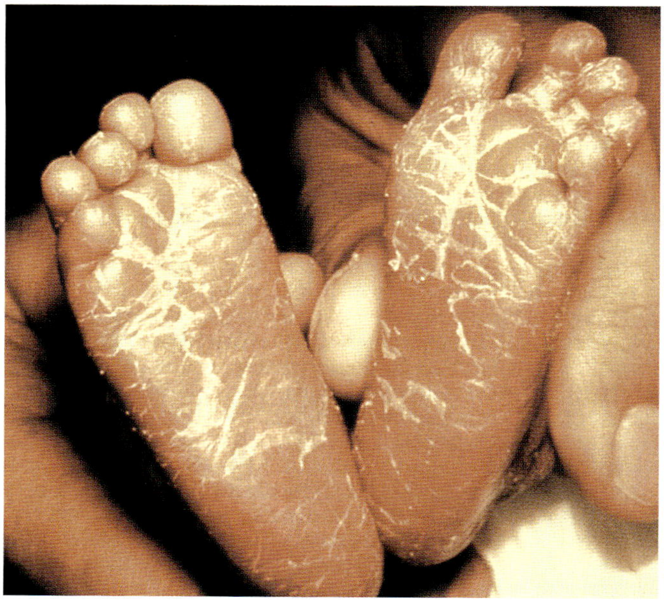

Fig. 2.59 Congenital syphilis. Erythema, scaling, and fissuring of the plantar surfaces in early congenital syphilis.

Necrotizing funisitis, spiral zones of red and blue umbilical cord discoloration interspersed with streaks of chalky white (hence the term *barber-pole umbilical cord*), has been described as a commonly overlooked, early diagnostic feature of CS. The external smooth surface of the umbilical cord without evidence of exudation apparently differentiates necrotizing funisitis from acute bacterial funisitis, an inflammation of the umbilical cord seen in newborns with acute bacterial infection.[264]

Hepatomegaly, when present, is often associated with icterus and occasionally ascites, splenomegaly, and generalized lymphadenopathy. The jaundice, together with anemia, edema, and cutaneous changes, produces a peculiar dirty, whitish brown (café-au-lait) appearance to the skin. Hemolytic anemia and occasional thrombocytopenia are common features of early CS. When occurring with hepatosplenomegaly, jaundice, and large numbers of nucleated erythrocytes in the peripheral circulation, an erroneous diagnosis of erythroblastosis fetalis may be made. Nephrotic syndrome and pneumonitis are occasionally present.

Although only 15% of infants with CS show clinical signs of osteochondritis at birth, 90% show radiologic evidence of osteochondritis and/or periostitis after the first month of life. Syphilitic osteochondritis may occur in any bone but is found most often in the long bones of the extremities. Radiographic findings consist of increased widening of the epiphyseal line with increased density of the shafts, spotty areas of translucency, and a resultant moth-eaten appearance. In most cases, the bony lesions are asymptomatic, but in some infants severe involvement may lead to subepiphyseal fracture with epiphyseal dislocation and extremely painful pseudoparalysis of one or more extremities (so-called "pseudoparalysis of Parrot"). Dactylitis, a rare form of osteochondritis of the small bones of the hands and feet that usually appears between 6 months and 2 years of age, may also occur.

Periosteal lesions are seldom present at birth. Periostitis of the frontal bones of the skull, when severe, may contribute to the flat overhanging forehead that persists as a stigma of children severely infected in infancy. The radiologic changes of periostitis are usually most pronounced between the second and sixth months of life and rarely persist beyond the age of 2 years. Lesions are usually diffuse (in contrast to the localized involvement characteristic of lesions of osteochondritis) and often extend the entire length of the involved bone. First seen as a thin, even line of calcification outside the cortex of the involved bone, the lesions progress and additional layers of opaque tissue are laid down, with the resulting "onion-peel" appearance of advanced periostitis. This eventually produces calcification and thickening of the cortex and, when severe, a permanent deformity. In the tibia, this results in an anterior bowing referred to as *saber shins*. In the skull it is seen (in 30% to 60% of patients) as frontal or parietal bossing.

Even though clinical evidence of CNS involvement is a relatively uncommon finding, CSF abnormalities may be detected in 40% to 50% of infants with CS. IgM immunoblotting and PCR assay on serum or CSF have been shown to be most predictive of CNS infection.[265] Clinical evidence of meningitis with a bulging fontanel, opisthotonos, and convulsions generally portends a poor prognosis. Low-grade syphilitic meningitis may result in a mild degree of hydrocephalus, and children with CNS involvement continuing beyond the period of infancy may go on to demonstrate marked residua with varying degrees of physical and mental retardation.

Late Congenital Syphilis

Late CS refers to findings that persist beyond 2 years of age. It also includes varying signs and stigmata of CS in individuals in whom the diagnosis was overlooked or in those patients who were inadequately treated early in the course of the disease. Signs of late CS are summarized in Box 2.3, and a few are discussed in more detail here.

Perhaps the most pathognomonic signs of late CS are the dental changes. The deciduous teeth are at risk for caries but show no specific abnormalities characteristic of this disorder. The term *Hutchinson incisors* is applied to deformities of the permanent upper central incisors, and the condition is characterized by central notching with tapering of the lateral sides toward the biting edge (so-called "screwdriver teeth"). The simultaneous appearance of interstitial keratitis, Hutchinson incisors, and eighth nerve deafness is called the *Hutchinson triad*. Although described as a time-honored sign of CS because of the relative infrequency of eighth nerve deafness, this triad is actually extremely uncommon and rarely observed. The "mulberry molar" is a malformation of the lower first molars. The mulberry appearance is created by poorly developed cusps crowded together on the crown. Because these teeth are subject to rapid decay, mulberry molars are rarely seen past puberty. When present, however, they are pathognomonic of CS.

Higouménakis sign refers to unilateral thickening of the inner third of the clavicle and is commonly described as a manifestation of late CS. Because fracture of the middle third of the clavicle is the most common fracture occurring at birth, consequent healing and thickening of the involved bone often produces a clinical picture similar to that seen with Higouménakis abnormality. This finding should therefore not be considered a reliable stigma of late CS.

Paroxysmal cold hemoglobinuria is characterized by shaking chills and dark urine within 8 hours of cold exposure, and it may also occur as a manifestation of late CS. It is usually seen in patients with late CS who did not receive treatment, and although it is not pathognomonic, it is highly suggestive of late congenital or untreated acquired syphilis.

Box 2.3 Signs of Late Congenital Syphilis

- Clutton joints (knee effusions)
- Eighth cranial nerve deafness*
- Frontal bossing
- Gummas (skin, subcutaneous, and bone inflammation and ulceration)
- Higouménakis sign (thickening of inner third of clavicle)
- Hutchinson teeth* (peg-shaped upper central incisors)
- Hydrocephalus
- Interstitial keratitis*
- Mental retardation
- Mulberry molars
- Ocular changes (retinitis, optic nerve atrophy)
- Paroxysmal cold hemoglobinuria
- Rhagades (perioral fissuring)
- Saber shins
- Saddle nose
- Short maxillae

*Hutchison triad.

Diagnosis and Treatment of Congenital Syphilis

Determination of the maternal serologic status for syphilis is the standard of care in hospitals, and no newborn infant should be discharged without this information being known.[266] All infants born to mothers who are seropositive require a thorough clinical and laboratory examination, namely a quantitative nontreponemal syphilis test (e.g., Venereal Disease Research Laboratories [VDRL] or rapid plasma reagin [RPR]), and preferably the same as that performed on the mother so that the titers can be compared. In mothers with a reactive RPR or VDRL, important maternal history to consider, which will guide further testing or therapy, includes whether the mother received no therapy, received undocumented therapy, or received therapy less than 1 month before delivery; there is concern of maternal reinfection or relapse (fourfold or greater increase in maternal titers); the mother was treated with a nonpenicillin drug; or the partner was recently diagnosed with syphilis.[266] Confirmation of a reactive nontreponemal test is accomplished with a specific treponemal test, such as the fluorescent treponemal antibody absorption (FTA-ABS) test, the *T. pallidum* particle agglutination (TP-PA), and the microhemagglutination test for *T. pallidum* (MHA-TP). Placental changes may be a useful adjunct in the diagnosis of CS, and include necrotizing funisitis (see earlier in the Early Congenital Syphilis section), villous enlargement, and acute villitis.[267] Diagnosis may be confirmed by positive darkfield examination from the umbilical vein or from moist lesions of the skin or mucous membranes.

Serologic tests in the newborn must be interpreted with caution, because their results may be caused by passive transfer of nontreponemal and treponemal antibodies from the mother and their antibody response may be delayed. A serologic titer in the newborn higher than that of the mother, however, is diagnostic. Additionally, because maternal IgM antibodies do not cross the placenta, detection of IgM in the infant indicates active infection.[255] If no other indications of active infection are evident, with serologic titers equal to or lower than the maternal titer, infants should be monitored closely, with repeated titers taken at appropriate intervals. In cases of passive transfer of antibody, the neonatal titer should not exceed that of the mother and should revert to negative within 4 to 6 months. In cases in which the mother is infected late in pregnancy, both mother and child may be nonreactive at delivery. In such instances, clinical signs and rising titers during the ensuing weeks will confirm the diagnosis.

Evaluation of the infant suspected of having CS should include a thorough physical examination, CSF-VDRL, and cellular/protein analysis and complete blood cell and platelet counts; other tests that may be indicated include ophthalmologic evaluation, long-bone and chest radiographs, neuroimaging, liver function studies, and auditory brainstem response.[266]

Parenteral penicillin G is the treatment of choice for all forms of syphilis. Once the diagnosis of CS is confirmed, treatment should commence immediately with intravenous aqueous crystalline penicillin G at a dosage of 50,000 units/kg every 12 hours for infants aged 1 week or younger, then every 8 hours for infants older than 1 week, for a total of 10 days of therapy. Procaine penicillin G at a dosage of 50,000 units/kg per dose administered intramuscularly once daily for 10 days is an alternative. Treated infants should be monitored closely, with evaluations at ages 2, 4, 6, and 12 months and serologic nontreponemal tests performed every 2 to 3 months until results become nonreactive.[266] Treatment recommendations for infants and children older than age 1 month include higher doses of parenteral penicillin.[266]

Infants with evidence of CNS involvement should receive crystalline penicillin G at a dosage of 200,000 to 300,000 units/kg per day given every 4 to 6 hours for 10 to 14 days. Because studies with benzathine penicillin suggest inadequate penetration of the CNS of newborns when serum penicillin levels are low, its use for CS with CNS involvement is not recommended. However, some experts recommend a single intramuscular dose of benzathine penicillin G at 50,000 units/kg for up to three weekly doses after the course of intravenous aqueous crystalline penicillin.[266]

CYTOMEGALIC INCLUSION DISEASE

Cytomegalic inclusion disease in the newborn is a generalized infection caused by CMV, a DNA virus of the herpesvirus group. It is the most common intrauterine infection in the United States.[268] CMV can be transmitted from person to person via urine, saliva, tears, and genital secretions, as well as via the transplacental route from mother to fetus. Congenital CMV infection occurs in 0.3% to 2.4% of all live births in developed countries,[269] and primary CMV infections are reported in 1% to 4% of seronegative pregnant women. The risk of viral transmission to the fetus is estimated at 30% to 40%.[270] CMV transmission has been reported far less often in association with nonprimary maternal infection.[269] In infants with congenital infection, around 5% to 18% are symptomatic at birth.[271] Although the majority of infected infants are asymptomatic, sequelae of congenital CMV infection in symptomatic patients may range from mild defects to severe or fatal disease. Infants of Native American and African descent have a disproportionately greater risk of mortality from congenital CMV infection compared with Whites, Asians, and Hispanics.[268]

CMV is generally transmitted from a pregnant mother with inapparent infection across the placenta to the fetus late in gestation, although it can also be transmitted by passage through an infected maternal genital tract at the time of delivery or by postnatal CMV-positive blood transfusion. Postnatal transmission may also occur after consumption of infected breast milk, and low birthweight and early postnatal virus transmission are risk factors for symptomatic infection in this setting.[272] In the United States, the CMV seroprevalence is around 50%, leaving many women of reproductive age at risk for maternal infection.[273] Congenital infection is usually suspected based on fetal ultrasound findings, including hydrops, intrauterine growth restriction, microcephaly, ventriculomegaly, and periventricular calcifications. Prematurity occurs in up to 34% of infants with symptomatic congenital CMV infection.[274] Although maternal immunity to CMV was once believed to protect the fetus from infection, it is now known that symptomatic congenital infection can occur after a recurrent maternal infection.[275,276] Because most congenital CMV infections are asymptomatic, diagnosis is most commonly made in infants who manifest several features of the syndrome.

Clinical findings of congenital CMV infection include jaundice, hepatosplenomegaly, anemia, thrombocytopenia, protracted interstitial pneumonia, chorioretinitis, sensorineural hearing loss, microcephaly, hypotonia, and mental retardation. Cerebral calcifications (often paraventricular) may be noted on imaging studies. Cutaneous manifestations include jaundice, petechiae and purpura, a generalized maculopapular eruption, and a generalized blueberry muffin eruption similar to that seen in infants with congenital rubella and toxoplasmosis. Although extremely rare, vesicular lesions have also been reported in infants with this disorder. Most symptomatic cases of congenital CMV infection are fatal within the first 2 months of life. Those who survive often manifest severe neurologic defects, including microcephaly, mental retardation, deafness, spastic diplegia, seizures, chorioretinitis, optic nerve atrophy, and blindness. In infants infected with CMV who do not manifest clinical symptoms at birth, 5% to 15% develop late-onset sequelae such as hearing loss, chorioretinitis, mental retardation, and neurologic defects.[276]

The gold standard for diagnosis of congenital CMV infection remains the detection of virus in saliva, blood, or urine during the first few weeks of life.[269] Viral recovery or a strongly positive serum IgM anti-CMV antibody is considered diagnostic. A variety of serologic assays for CMV antibodies are available, including immunofluorescence, latex agglutination, and enzyme immunoassays. PCR has become increasingly popular in the diagnosis of CMV disease and can be applied to urine, blood, saliva (and other respiratory secretions), amniotic fluid, and CSF. It offers more rapid results and increased sensitivity. Later in infancy, differentiation between intrauterine and perinatal infection is difficult unless signs of intrauterine infection such as chorioretinitis or ventriculitis are present. When the diagnosis remains in doubt, persistent or rising complement-fixation titers may provide confirmatory evidence. Electron microscopic examination for viral particles in urine samples is a rapid diagnostic technique that can also be used, if available. Quantitative PCR examinations on peripheral blood leukocytes can be used to monitor viral load in infected newborns who are infected with CMV.

Prenatal diagnosis is reserved for pregnancies in which ultrasonographic findings suggest suspicion for CMV fetal infection.[271] Available methods include CMV isolation from amniotic fluid and identification of CMV DNA by PCR analysis. Demonstration of IgM anti-CMV antibody in percutaneous umbilical blood samples is also diagnostic, but this test is more difficult and has a lower sensitivity. Diagnosis of primary CMV infection in pregnant women is achieved with sensitive IgM and IgG avidity serologic assays, as well as conventional and molecular detection of virus in blood.[278]

There is no consistently effective therapy for congenital CMV infection, and prognosis for the patient with severe involvement is poor. Ganciclovir has been used, although large-scale studies are lacking, and its use may be associated with toxicity. One phase II collaborative study of ganciclovir treatment in symptomatic congenital CMV revealed hearing improvement or stabilization in 16% of patients but only a temporary decrease in CMV excretion in the urine.[279] Oral valganciclovir (or intravenous ganciclovir in the setting of decreased absorption of oral medications) is recommended as therapy for symptomatic, moderate to severe congenital CMV disease with or without CNS involvement, should be started within the first month of life, and has been associated with improved audiologic and neurodevelopmental outcome at 2 years.[280,281]

CONGENITAL EPSTEIN–BARR VIRUS SYNDROME

Because the majority of young adults are seropositive for EBV, primary infection during pregnancy is uncommon. Although features of congenital EBV infection such as micrognathia, cryptorchidism, cataracts, hypotonia, erythematous skin eruptions, hepatosplenomegaly, lymphadenopathy, and persistent atypical lymphocytosis have been reported, the low rate of EBV infection in pregnancy makes it difficult to assess the full extent of this risk. A prospective study comparing women with serologic evidence of primary, recurrent, or undefined infection with a control group found no differences in pregnancy outcome, birthweights, or incidence of congenital anomalies, suggesting that EBV infection during pregnancy does not represent a significant teratogenic risk.[282]

CONGENITAL TOXOPLASMOSIS

Toxoplasmosis is a parasitic disorder caused by *Toxoplasma gondii*, an obligate intracellular protozoan that may invade multiple tissues including muscle (including the heart), liver, spleen, lymph nodes, and CNS. In humans it can have severe consequences for some populations, including children, fetuses, and those who are immunocompromised. It is estimated that up to 91% of women of childbearing age in the United States are susceptible to *Toxoplasma* infection.[283] This infection in pregnant women may result in serious infantile sequelae if transmitted to the fetus, most notably mental retardation, seizures, and blindness. Toxoplasmosis is transmitted to the fetus transplacentally, and the greatest risk of transmission (60% to 90%) is when acute infection occurs during the third trimester. The severity of fetal infection tends to be greater when infection is acquired during the first trimester. Toxoplasmosis is postnatally transmitted to humans via consumption of, or contact with, raw or inadequately cooked meat (especially pork, lamb, mutton, and wild game) or inadvertent ingestion of oocysts from cat feces in litter or soil.[284] Most pregnant women with acute *T. gondii* infection are asymptomatic without any obvious signs.[285] The highest burdens of congenital toxoplasmosis are found in South America, parts of the Middle East, and some low-income countries in Africa.[286]

Fetal infection with *T. gondii* may result in stillbirth or prematurity. Signs and symptoms of congenital toxoplasmosis may be present immediately at birth or develop during the first few weeks of life and include fever, malaise, vomiting and diarrhea, lymphadenopathy, hepatosplenomegaly, microphthalmia, cataracts, microcephaly, pneumonitis, pericarditis, bleeding diathesis, and seizures. The classic triad of congenital toxoplasmosis consists of chorioretinitis, hydrocephalus, and intracranial calcifications. Up to 80% of patients develop visual or learning disabilities later in life. Hearing impairment, potentially resulting in deafness, may also occur.[287]

Cutaneous findings of congenital toxoplasmosis include a generalized rubella-like maculopapular eruption that generally spares the face, palms, and soles. Blueberry muffin–like lesions (representing extramedullary hematopoiesis) may be present, as may a scarlatiniform eruption or subcutaneous nodules. The skin eruption usually develops during the first weeks of illness, persists for up to 1 week, and may be followed by desquamation or hyperpigmentation.

Laboratory findings in patients with congenital toxoplasmosis are nonspecific and may reveal anemia, eosinophilia, thrombocytopenia, and at times severe leukopenia. Disseminated intravascular coagulation may be present, as may hepatitis. The CSF may be xanthochromic and may contain leukocytes, erythrocytes, and an elevated level of protein. Skull radiographs of affected infants may reveal diffuse, punctate comma-shaped intracranial calcifications.

The diagnosis of congenital toxoplasmosis is made via the combination of clinical findings, serologic studies, DNA-based testing, and occasionally parasite isolation. Measurement of *T. gondii*–specific IgG, IgM, and IgA antibodies in neonatal peripheral blood is recommended, and if there is strong suspicion, peripheral blood, urine, and CSF *Toxoplasma* PCR should also be performed.[288] Much attention has been focused on the prenatal diagnosis of toxoplasmosis, and the recommended testing (published elsewhere) depends on whether the gravid woman is less or more than 16 weeks' gestation.[283]

Most newborns with toxoplasmosis are asymptomatic or have only mild symptoms, although many may have learning disabilities later in life. Because of the serious sequelae that may develop, treatment is recommended even in asymptomatic infants, albeit for a shorter course than those with symptomatic infection. According to most consensus recommendations, infants with symptomatic congenital toxoplasmosis should be treated with a 12-month course of pyrimethamine, sulfadiazine, and leucovorin.[283] In the presence of CSF hyperproteinemia or severe chorioretinitis, systemic steroids are recommended.[288] When *Toxoplasma* infection occurs in pregnant women, treatment with spiramycin is recommended in an effort to prevent mother-to-child transmission; if fetal infection is confirmed or infection is acquired after 18 weeks' gestation, pyrimethamine, sulfadiazine, and leucovorin therapy is recommended.[283,288]

CONGENITAL ZIKA VIRUS INFECTION

In recent years, infection with Zika virus (ZIKV) has been increasingly reported. Outbreaks have been particularly common in South America and have resulted in congenital deformities, most notably microcephaly. This mosquito-borne virus (which may also be transmitted sexually) is a member of the *Flavivirus* genus and typically results in asymptomatic infection or mild, nonspecific clinical features. These may include fever (which tends to be low grade and short lived), macular or maculopapular exanthem, headache, arthralgias, myalgias, conjunctivitis, retroorbital pain, and back pain.[289,290] Although an association between ZIKV infection and neurologic manifestations (primarily Guillain–Barré syndrome) was identified in French Polynesia in 2013, the expanding potential for neurologic sequelae in infants born to infected mothers began to be recognized by 2015, with such abnormalities as microcephaly, cerebellar atrophy, ventriculomegaly, cerebral calcifications, defects in the corpus callosum, cortical malformations, and decreased cerebral artery flow.[291–293] The fetuses of pregnant infected women are also at risk for intrauterine growth restriction and fetal demise. Congenital eye malformations with ZIKV infection may include nonpurulent conjunctivitis, uveitis, chorioretinal atrophy, optic neuritis, colobomata, and retinal hemorrhage. Together the spectrum of congenital neurologic and ophthalmologic features that may be associated with ZIKV infection have been termed *congenital Zika syndrome (CZS)*. The ability of ZIKV to cross the placental barrier is a key factor in causing CZS, although the mechanisms of this transmission are not completely understood.[294] Treatment for ZIKV infection is focused on symptoms, with emphasis on prevention and control measures such as control of mosquito populations; minimizing the risk of mosquito bites, which includes use of repellents and avoidance of unnecessary travel to endemic areas by pregnant women; and avoiding unprotected sexual contact with partners at risk for infection.[290]

The complete list of 295 references for this chapter is available online at http://expertconsult.inkling.com.

Key References

Fortunov RM, Hulten KG, Hammerman WA, et al. Evaluation and treatment of community-acquired Staphylococcus aureus infections in term and late-preterm previously healthy neonates. Pediatrics 2007;120:937–45.
Krafchik B. History of diapers and diapering. Int J Dermatol 2016;55(Suppl. 1):4–6.
Guggisberg D, Hadj-Rabia S, Viney C, et al. Skin markers of occult spinal dysraphism in children. A review of 54 cases. Arch Dermatol 2004;140:1109–15.
Frieden IJ. Aplasia cutis congenita: a clinical review and proposal for classification. J Am Acad Dermatol 1986;14:646–60.
Papania MJ, Wallace GS, Rota PA, et al. Elimination of endemic measles, rubella and congenital rubella syndrome from the Western hemisphere: the US experience. JAMA Pediatr 2014;168(2):148–55.
Smith CK, Arvin AM. Varicella in the fetus and newborn. Semin Fetal Neonatal Med 2009;14(4):209–17.
James SH, Kimberlin DW. Neonatal herpes simplex virus infection. Clin Perinatol 2015;42(1):47–59.
Kimberlin DW, Whitley RJ, Wan W, et al. Oral acyclovir suppression and neurodevelopment after neonatal herpes. N Engl J Med 2011;365(14):1284–92.
Su JR, Brooks LC, Davis DW, et al. Congenital syphilis: trends in mortality and morbidity in the United States, 1999 through 2013. Am J Obstet Gynecol 2016;214(3): 381.e1–9.
Bristow BN, O'Keefe KA, Shafir SC, et al. Congenital cytomegalovirus mortality in the United States, 1990–2006. PLoS Negl Trop Dis 2011;5(4):e1140.
Plosa EJ, Esbenshade C, Fuller MP, et al. Cytomegalovirus infection. Pediatr Rev 2012; 33(4):156–63.
Maldonado YA, Read JS. Diagnosis, treatment and prevention of congenital toxoplasmosis in the United States. Pediatrics 2017;139(2):e20163860.
Mlakar J, Korva M, Tul N, et al. Zika virus associated with microcephaly. N Engl J Med 2016;374:951–8.

3 Eczematous Eruptions in Childhood

CHAPTER OUTLINE

Eczematous eruptions are characterized as inflamed papules and plaques, often in association with pruritus and serous discharge. The specific subtype of eczematous dermatitis is based on the clinical morphology, distribution of lesions, and, in many cases, history of exposure. Biopsy of the skin in these conditions is usually not helpful, except to consider alternative diagnoses with distinct histopathologic features.

Atopic Dermatitis

Atopic dermatitis (AD) is one of the most common skin disorders seen in infants and children, and the most common eczematous disorder. Although the term *eczema* is commonly used, *atopic dermatitis* (or, less commonly, atopic eczema) is a more precise term to describe this subset of dermatitis or inflammation of skin.[1] AD begins during the first 6 months of life in 45% of children, the first year of life in 60% of affected individuals, and before 5 years of age in at least 85% of affected individuals.[2,3] The prevalence of AD in American children is 10% to 13%,[4,5] which is consistent with the prevalence in Scandinavia[6,7] and Japan[8] and represents a marked increase during the past several decades.[9] Of these, 67% have mild disease, 26% have moderate disease, and 7% have severe AD.[5] AD severity is increased in older children, in the eldest child in a family, and in Black and Hispanic children.[5] AD occurs more often in urban areas than in rural areas, in smaller families, and in higher socioeconomic classes, which may suggest that exposure to antigenic pollutants and lack of exposure to infectious agents or other antigenic triggers early in life may play a role in the development of the dermatitis.

The 1-year prevalence of AD in adults is up to 10.2%.[10] Despite its early onset for most patients, a meta-analysis of 7 birth cohort studies with follow-up of up to 26 years revealed no difference in AD prevalence before and after childhood (up to 14.6%),[11] suggesting that the percentage of patients with persistence of AD into adulthood or with relapse after an interval without manifestation is relatively high, although the numbers from studies are variable. In one study, more than 80% of children with mild to moderate AD had recurrent symptoms or required medication use at least into the second decade of life.[12] In another meta-analysis of 45 studies, children with AD of greater severity and that had been persistent already for more than 10 years had the lowest chance for clearance.[13]

PATHOGENESIS OF ATOPIC DERMATITIS

Our improved understanding of the basis for AD has led to new therapeutic interventions (see the Management section). AD involves genetic factors dictating immune response and skin barrier integrity, as well as environmental influences, including one's microbiome.[14] The "inside-out" concept of AD pathogenesis focuses on immune abnormalities as being primary, and the "outside-in" theory considers the epidermal barrier dysfunction (a form of innate immunity) as primary, but it is the interplay of these factors that leads to disease.[14–17]

A role for genetic alterations is suggested by the concordance of 77% in monozygotic twins[18] and the greater probability of having AD if one or, even more so, both parents have AD.[19] By far the most common and influential genetic change is having uniallelic or biallelic loss-of-function mutations in profilaggrin *(FLG)*. *FLG* mutations occur overall in approximately 10% of the population and are the cause of ichthyosis vulgaris, a genetic disorder characterized by climate-dependent dry, scaling skin and hyperlinear palms (see Chapter 5). Mutations in *FLG* occur in 10% to 30% of AD patients.[20–24] In addition to the tight linkage of AD with genes of the epidermal differentiation complex (particularly encoding profilaggrin),[25] genome-wide association (GWA) studies have shown numerous other associated loci, primarily related to epidermal barrier function and innate-adaptive immunity.[26]

Heterozygous loss-of-function mutations in *CARD11* (encoding caspase recruitment domain-containing protein 11) have also been associated[27,28] with moderate to severe AD. Many but not all patients have concurrently been affected by other forms of atopy, pneumonia, bronchiectasis, cutaneous viral infections, oral ulcerations, autoimmunity, neutropenia, hypogammaglobulinemia, or lymphoma. Affected individuals may have reduced T-cell responsiveness *in vitro* with increases in B lymphocytes and abnormal B-cell differentiation.[29] Interestingly, homozygous null mutations in *CARD11* cause a form of severe combined immunodeficiency (SCID), whereas heterozygous gain-of-function mutations lead to a form of B-cell lymphoproliferative disease. Loss-of-function mutations in *CARD14* (vs. the gain-of-function mutations associated with the psoriasis–pityriasis rubra pilaris spectrum) may also underlie a severe variant of AD.[30] Heterozygous gain-of-function mutations in *JAK1* have recently been associated with severe AD with hypereosinophilia but not high levels of immunoglobulin E (IgE).[31] Eosinophilic infiltration of the liver and gastrointestinal tract with hepatosplenomegaly, autoimmune disease, and failure to thrive or short stature are other features, and patients respond to Janus kinase (JAK) inhibition.

In the acute phase of AD, environmental triggers such as irritants, allergens, and microbes and mechanical injury (scratching or rubbing) activate the skin's innate immune system, which includes epidermal Langerhans cells and keratinocytes.[32,33] Expression of cytokines, particularly alarmins interleukin-25 (IL-25), IL-33, and thymic stromal lymphopoietin (TSLP) activate group 2 innate lymphoid cells (ILC2s), leading to T helper 2 (Th2) cell activation.[34] Th2 cells express IL-4, -5, and -13, which promote eosinophilia and IgE production but suppress the expression of epidermal barrier proteins as well as antimicrobial peptides such as β-defensins and cathelicidin. This reduction in antimicrobial peptide production may contribute to the propensity toward development of skin infection in AD patients.[35] TSLP, IL-4/-13, and IL-31 are thought to mediate AD pruritus.[36,37]

Recent studies show that AD T cells also differentiate into Th22 cells, which produce IL-22 and thereby stimulate expression of keratinocyte S100As.[38,39] IL-22 has been implicated in the thickening of skin with lichenification. The role of Th17 cells in AD is not well understood, but increased levels of IL-17 are found in some patients (although not to the extent of Th2 cytokines and IL-22), particularly in young children with recent onset, patients with intrinsic (vs. extrinsic) AD, and people of Asian descent.[40] Although adults with chronic AD also may have increases in Th1 cytokines, Th1 immunity and the Th1/Th2 ratio are very low in children with AD.[41–45] The immune profile of AD is age dependent, with older children and adolescents having an intermediate profile between those of recent-onset AD in young children and in adults.

The intact epidermis itself also plays a role in the skin's innate immune system because it functions as a barrier against water loss (preventing dry skin) and activation of the innate immune system by high-molecular-weight allergens such as dust mite antigens, foods, and microbes. This barrier primarily is composed of tight junction proteins (particularly claudins, middle of the stratum granulosum) and stratum corneum structural proteins and lipids. Filaggrin is the major component of the stratum granulosum of epidermis and binds to keratin.[46,47] Its precursor, profilaggrin, contains 10 to 12 monomers of filaggrin, and fewer monomers within the profilaggrin gene (e.g., 10 vs. 12) have been linked to an increased risk of developing AD,[48] which complements the known increased risk of developing AD with filaggrin insufficiency.[49,50] Filaggrin is also broken down into natural moisturizing factor (NMF), particularly urocanic acid, which promotes skin hydration, providing another explanation for the dry skin of AD and ichthyosis vulgaris. NMF has been shown to be low during the first year of life, especially on the cheeks.[51] AD in association with mutations in *FLG* has been shown to be more severe and more persistent.[12,52]

The stratum corneum lipid matrix predominantly is composed of cholesterol, free fatty acids, and ceramides, densely stacked into a highly ordered, three-dimensional structure of lipid lamellae, which depends on lipid composition. These lipids are secreted by the lamellar bodies into the intercellular space of the stratum corneum. AD skin has a decreased content of very long chain ceramides[53,54] and free fatty acids, related to a deficiency of elongases that synthesize very long-chain fatty acids. The barrier can also be altered by the increased activity of proteases (especially kallikreins 5 and 7), which degrade barrier proteins and are more active at increased pH, as occurs in association with deficiency of filaggrin products (e.g., urocanic acid).

The skin (and perhaps gut) microbiome is another environmental influence on both the barrier and skin immunity.[14] A meta-analysis of 95 studies showed that *Staphylococcus aureus* is found on lesional skin of 70% and nonlesional skin of 39% of patients with AD.[55] Most of the *S. aureus* is methicillin-sensitive *S. aureus* (MSSA), although 7% of patients have methicillin-resistant *S. aureus* (MRSA). Flares of AD are associated with a shift in the microbiome toward a greater percentage of *S. aureus* (and *S. epidermidis*) and reduced bacterial diversity,[56] and the shift is greater in patients with MRSA than MSSA.[57] Commensal organisms are recognized to play a key role in killing *S. aureus* and modulating immune responses. A recent birth cohort suggested that having commensal *Staphylococcus* spp. at day 2 could protect infants against the development of AD.[58] Patients with AD not only have fewer commensals with active disease but also have fewer commensals that are able to kill *S. aureus*.[59] Topical application of commensal organisms (e.g., *Staphylococcus hominis* or *Roseomonas mucosa*)[60] as treatment for AD is a new direction that in early studies appears to reduce AD severity and the use of topical corticosteroid.

Box 3.1 American Academy of Dermatology Clinical Criteria for Atopic Dermatitis

Essential Features

Pruritus (or parental reporting of itching or rubbing) in past 12 months
Eczena (acute, subacute, chronic)
- Typical morphology and age-specific patterns (infants and young children: face, neck, extensors; spares diaper area; any age group: flexural lesions
- Chronic or relapsing history

Important Features (seen in most cases and support diagnosis)

Early age of onset
Personal and/or family history of atopy
IgE reactivity
Xerosis

Associated Features (can help with diagnosis but too nonspecific for diagnosis)

Atypical vascular responses (e.g., delayed blanch response, facial pallor, white dermographism)
Keratosis pilaris/pityriasis alba/hyperlinear palms/ichthyosis
Ocular/periorbital changes
Other regional changes (perioral, periauricular)
Perifollicular accentuation/lichenification/prurigo lesions

Exclusionary Conditions in Children

Contact dermatitis (irritant or allergic; can be concurrent)
Immunodeficiency (and other causes of erythroderma)
Psoriasis
Seborrheic dermatitis
Ichthyoses
Scabies
Cutaneous T-cell lymphoma
Photosensitivity disorders

IgE, Immunoglobulin E.

CLINICAL FEATURES

The cardinal features of AD are pruritus, chronicity, and the age-specific morphology and distribution of lesions (Box 3.1).[61] Extent of involvement may range from mild and limited—for example, to flexural areas—to generalized and severe. The tremendous itch of AD can translate into issues with sleep, especially with wake after sleep onset, but also difficulty in falling asleep, because the pruritus tends to be worst at bedtime. Skin pain[62] can also be a feature.

The morphology of AD and distribution of lesions is often age dependent, although there is considerable overlap (e.g., infants may show the typical distribution of adult AD). Infants with AD typically have intense itching, erythema, papules, vesicles, oozing, and crusting. In infants, AD often begins on the cheeks, forehead, or scalp (Figs. 3.1, 3.2, and 3.3) and then may extend to the trunk (Fig. 3.4) or particularly the extensor aspects of the extremities in scattered, ill-defined, often symmetric patches. Generalized xerosis is common. Exacerbation of facial dermatitis on the medial cheeks and chin is often seen concomitant with teething and initiating foods. This localization likely reflects exposure to irritating saliva and foods, although contact dermatitis or urticaria may contribute. By 8 to 10 months of age the extensor surfaces of the arms and legs often show dermatitis (Fig. 3.5), perhaps because of the role of friction associated with crawling and the exposure of these sites to irritant and allergenic triggers such as those found in carpets. Although dermatitis of the antecubital and popliteal fossae, periorbital areas, and neck are more commonly involved in older children and adolescents, these sites may be affected in infants and young children as well (Fig. 3.6). Typically, lesions of AD spare the groin and diaper area during infancy (Fig. 3.7), which aids in the diagnosis. This sparing likely reflects the combination of increased hydration in the diaper area, protection from triggers by the diaper, and inaccessibility to scratching and rubbing. The "headlight sign" has been used to describe the typical sparing of the nose and medial cheeks in AD, even when there is extensive facial involvement elsewhere (see Fig. 3.1).

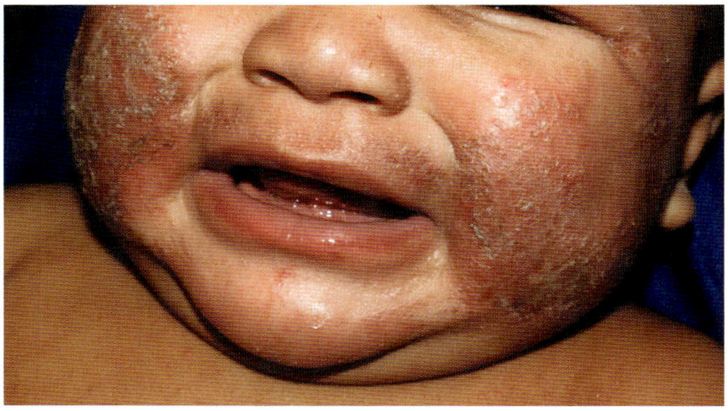

Fig. 3.1 Acute atopic dermatitis (AD) on the cheek of an infant. This boy shows the headlight sign, with relative sparing of the midface and immediate perioral area. The edema and exudation is typical of infantile AD and should not be confused with secondary bacterial infection.

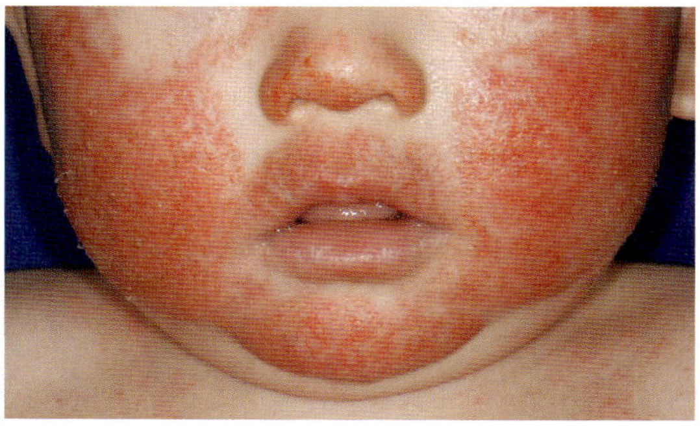

Fig. 3.2 Acute atopic dermatitis in an infant. Despite extensive perioral and nasal tip involvement, the immediate perinasal and infralabial areas are spared.

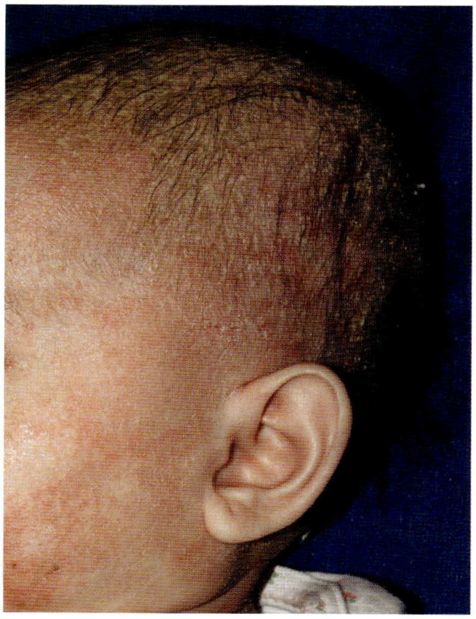

Fig. 3.3 Atopic dermatitis (AD) and seborrheic dermatitis. Seborrheic dermatitis and AD often occur concurrently, especially in infants with early atopic dermatitis. In addition to the presence of AD on the face, head rubbing or excoriations (suggesting scalp pruritus) and recalcitrance to traditional management for seborrheic dermatitis are clues to the combination.

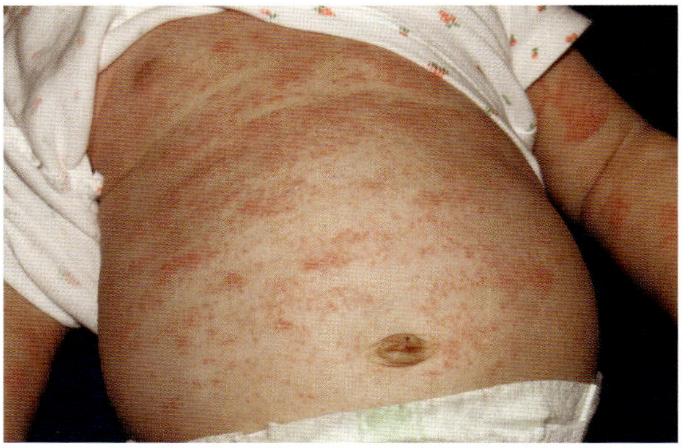

Fig. 3.4 Atopic dermatitis on the trunk and extremities of an infant. In this baby, note the accentuation at the nipple and relative sparing of the antecubital fold.

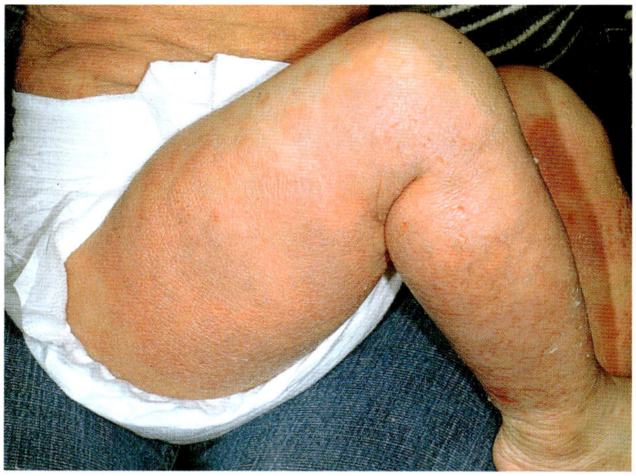

Fig. 3.5 Involvement of the extensor surfaces of the legs and arms is commonly seen during the infantile phase of atopic dermatitis beginning at about 8 months of age, concomitant with crawling and exposure to irritant and allergenic triggers.

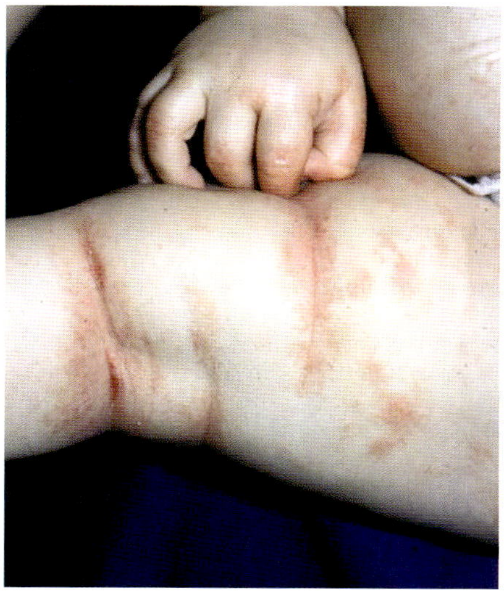

Fig. 3.6 Although antecubital and popliteal fossa involvement is typical of the childhood and adult phases of atopic dermatitis, infants not uncommonly will show involvement at these fold areas. This infant is demonstrating his response to the pruritus.

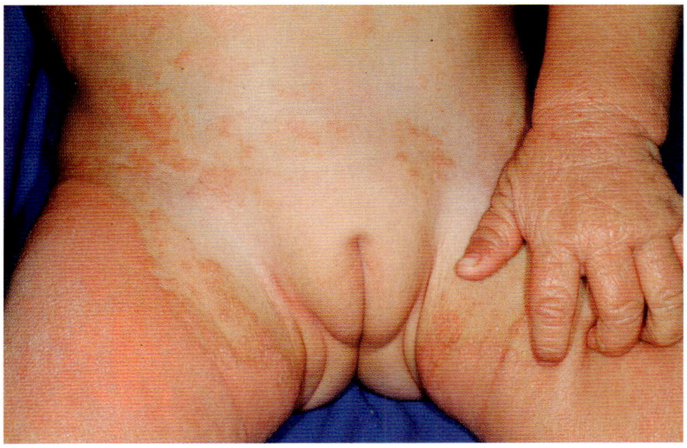

Fig. 3.7 Relative sparing of the diaper area is typical in infants with atopic dermatitis, likely because of the occlusion of this site and protection from scratching and rubbing, as well as from allergenic triggers.

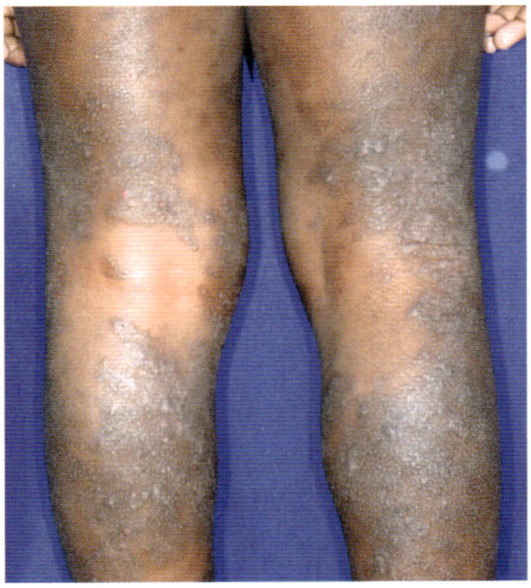

Fig. 3.8 Extensive lichenification on the legs of this affected toddler. Note the follicular accentuation and relative sparing of the popliteal areas.

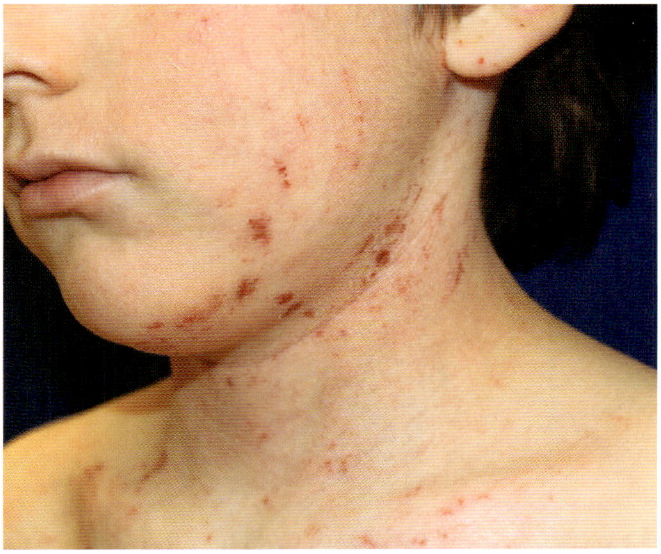

Fig. 3.9 Xerosis with erythema, fissuring, and crusting on the neck and face in this 10-year-old boy.

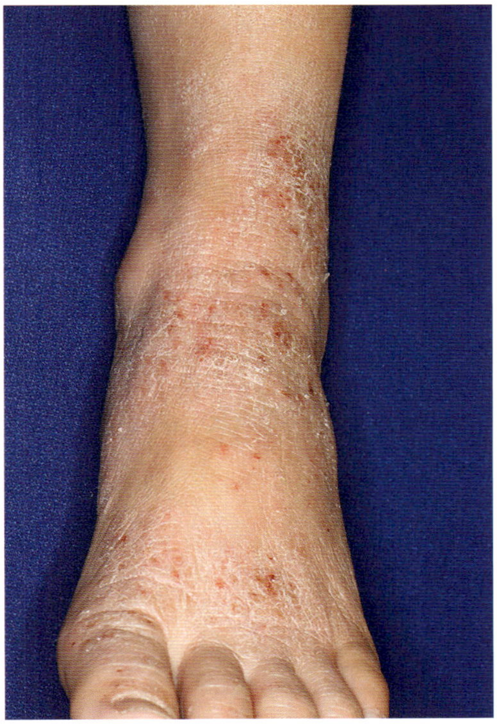

Fig. 3.10 Atopic dermatitis on the ankle and dorsal aspect of the foot. Note the lichenification and crusting.

Not uncommonly, infants initially show signs of seborrheic dermatitis, particularly during the first month or two of life. The associated pruritus and the dry (rather than greasier) scale suggest the combination of both disorders (see Fig. 3.3); the seborrheic component usually clears by 6 to 12 months, whereas the AD features persist. Alopecia may accompany the scalp involvement because of inflammation and chronic rubbing.

By about 2 years of age, children with AD are less likely to have exudative and crusted lesions and have a greater tendency toward chronicity and lichenification (Fig. 3.8). Eruptions are characteristically drier and more papular and often occur as circumscribed scaly patches. The classic areas of involvement in this group are the wrists, ankles, hands, feet, neck, and antecubital and popliteal regions (Figs. 3.9 and 3.10). Facial involvement switches from cheeks and chin to periorbital (Figs. 3.11 and 3.12) and perioral, the latter sometimes manifesting as "lip-licker's dermatitis" (see Fig. 3.56). Dermatitis of the nipples (Fig. 3.13) occurs in some infants and children and can be exacerbated by rubbing on clothing. Pruritus is often severe. Some children with AD show nummular or coin-shaped lesions with sharply defined oval scaly plaques on the face, trunk, and extremities (see Nummular Dermatitis section). In Black children, the lesions of AD are often more papular and follicular (Fig. 3.14). Although localization at flexural areas is more common, some children show an inverse pattern with involvement primarily of extensor areas. Lymphadenopathy may be a prominent feature in affected children (Fig. 3.15), reflecting the role of lymph nodes in handling local infection and inflammation. Nail dystrophy may be seen when fingers are affected, indicating involvement of the nail matrix; children may show secondary staphylococcal or pseudomonal paronychia.

By later childhood and adolescence, predominant areas of involvement include the flexural folds (Fig. 3.16), the face and neck, the

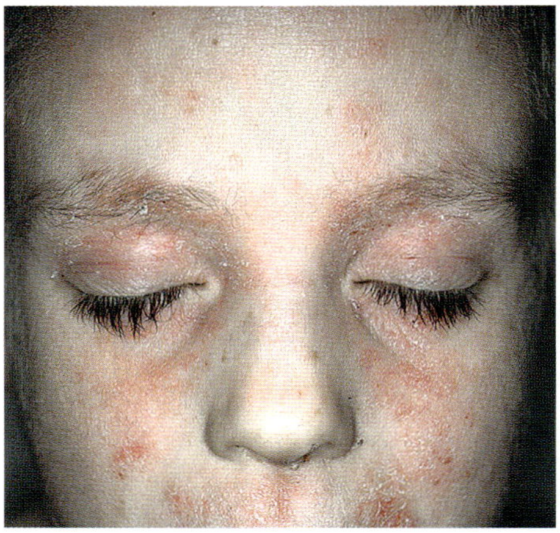

Fig. 3.11 Facial atopic dermatitis in children and adolescents typically affects the periorbital and perioral areas.

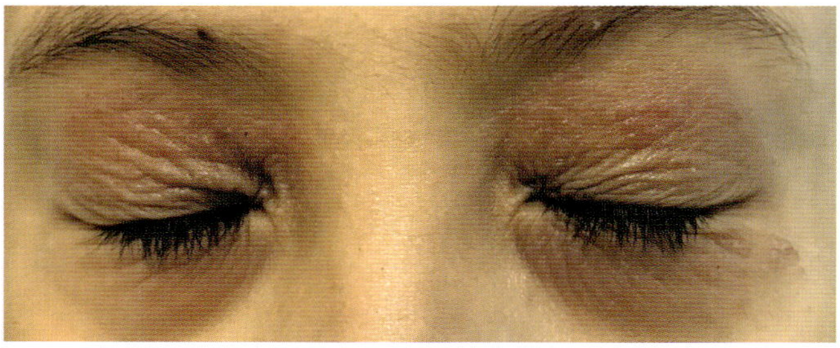

Fig. 3.12 The periorbital areas can be severely lichenified with chronic eyelid dermatitis. Consideration should be given to patch testing with chronic involvement at this site.

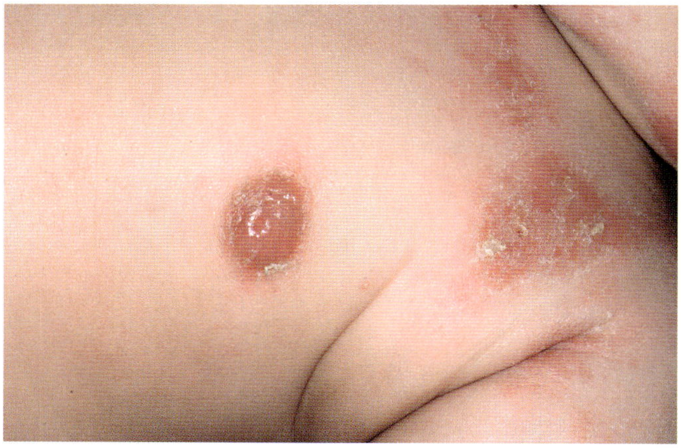

Fig. 3.13 Nipple eczema may occur in infants and children with atopic dermatitis, even without much truncal involvement elsewhere, and is exacerbated by the rubbing of clothes on the affected nipples.

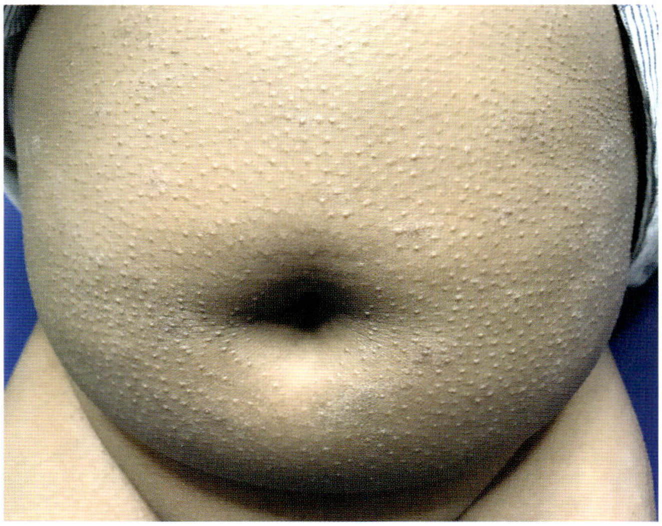

Fig. 3.14 Follicular (or papular) atopic dermatitis (AD) is more commonly seen in Black children with AD and can be difficult to distinguish from lichen nitidus (see Fig. 4.61) and, if on the elbows or knees, juvenile frictional lichenoid dermatosis (see Fig. 3.50).

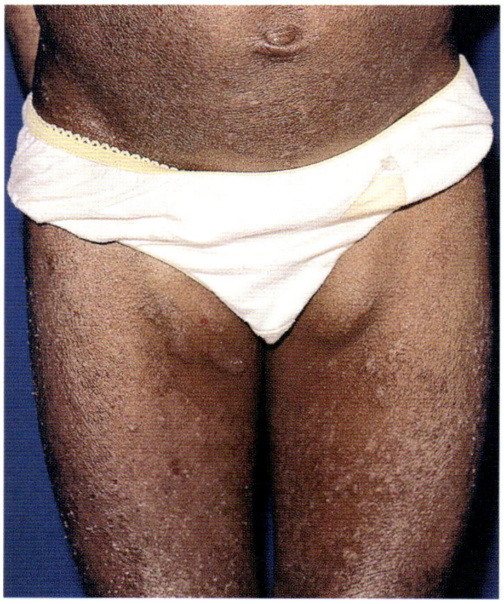

Fig. 3.15 Lymphadenopathy is a common accompanying feature of severe atopic dermatitis (AD), especially when the AD is associated with infection.

upper arms and back, and the dorsal aspect of the hands, feet, fingers, and toes. The eruption is characterized by dry, scaling erythematous papules and plaques and by the formation of large lichenified plaques from lesional chronicity. Weeping, crusting, and exudation may occur from the AD itself but usually is the result of superimposed staphylococcal infection or allergic contact dermatitis. Prurigo nodularis, characterized by well-circumscribed, usually hyperpigmented thickened papules, most commonly on the lower extremities, is most often seen during adolescence (Fig. 3.17).

Postinflammatory reduction of pigmentation may occur at any age, especially in individuals with darker skin. Although postinflammatory hypopigmentation is more common (see Figs. 3.16 and 3.18), pigment reduction may be severe enough to be depigmented, resembling vitiligo (Fig. 3.19), especially on distal extremities. The pigmentary changes are transient and are reversible when the underlying inflammation is controlled; however, 6 months or more may be required for repigmentation (and years if vitiliginous), and sun exposure may accentuate the differences between uninvolved and hypopigmented skin areas. In contrast, hyperpigmentation is predominantly noted at sites of lichenification (Figs. 3.12, 3.15, 3.17, and 3.20.), because the thickened epidermis accumulates epidermal melanin pigment, especially in darker skinned individuals. Children with lichenification show accentuation of skin (Fig. 3.21). Parents may mistake the postinflammatory pigment change seen in some children for scarring or a toxicity of

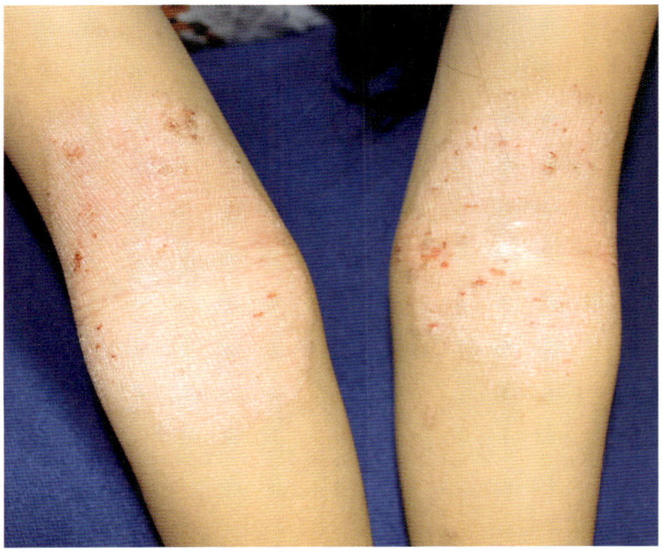

Fig. 3.16 Involvement of antecubital and popliteal areas is characteristic in children and adolescents with atopic dermatitis. Note the associated crusting and postinflammatory hypopigmentation.

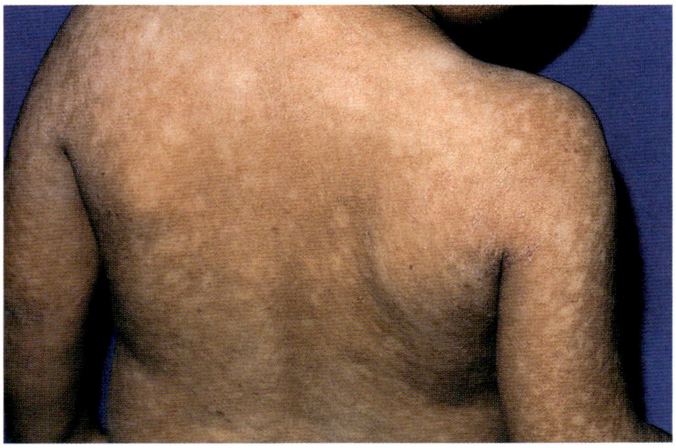

Fig. 3.18 Postinflammatory hypopigmentation of atopic dermatitis (AD). Postinflammatory hypopigmentation is a sequela of AD inflammation, is not related to use of topical steroids, and is not scarring. The postinflammatory hypopigmentation is particularly prominent during summer months, when the surrounding unaffected skin tans after exposure to ultraviolet light, and tends to clear spontaneously after several months if further flares of dermatitis at the site are prevented.

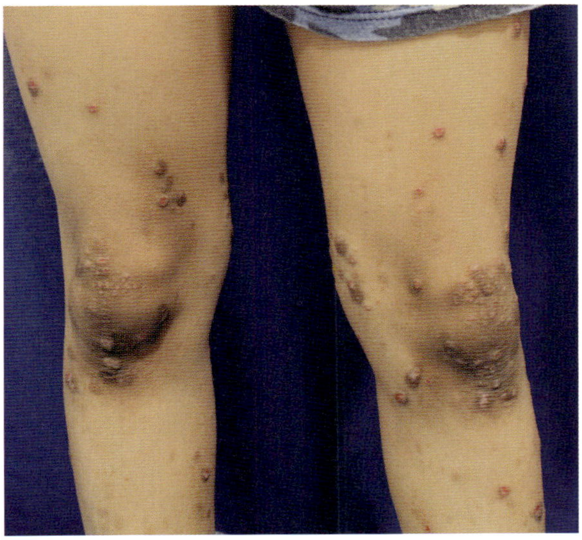

Fig. 3.17 Prurigo nodularis. Well-circumscribed, usually hyperpigmented lichenified papules appear most commonly on the lower extremities. Recurrent gouging of these intensely pruritic papules results in scarring.

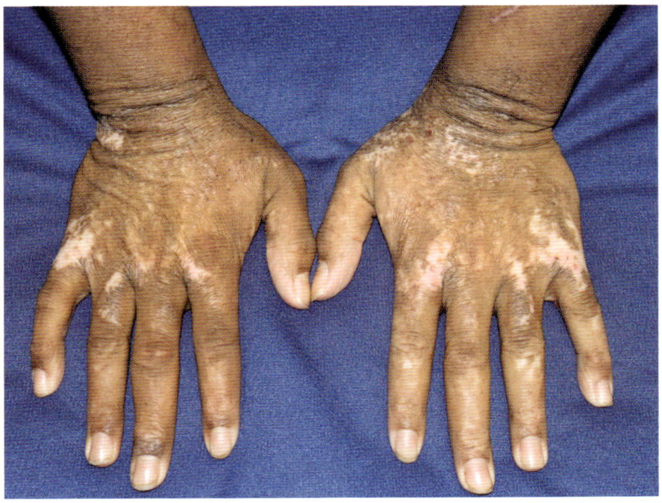

Fig. 3.19 Depigmentation resembling vitiligo occasionally occurs in severely affected children, particularly at sites of chronic atopic dermatitis (AD) on the dorsal aspect of the hands and feet, wrists, and ankles. Repigmentation can occur slowly with improved AD control at these sites.

topically applied medications and need reassurance. AD lesions are not usually scarring, but secondary infection and deep gouging of lesions can leave residual scarring and long-term pigmentary change.

OTHER CLINICAL SIGNS

Several other clinical signs are seen with increased incidence in children with AD, although they may appear in children without AD as well. Dermographism, a manifestation of the triple response of Lewis that occurs in approximately 5% of the normal population, is characterized by a red line, flare, and wheal reaction. A red line develops within 15 seconds at the exact site of stroking, followed within 15 to 45 seconds by an erythematous flare (because of an axon-reflex vasodilation of arterioles). The response finally eventuates in a wheal (because of transudation of fluid from the injured capillaries in the original stroke line) 1 to 3 minutes later. Individuals with AD often demonstrate a paradoxical blanching of the skin termed *white dermographism* (Fig. 3.22). The initial red line is replaced, generally within 10 seconds, by a white line without an associated wheal. Patients with AD may also show circumoral pallor, thought to relate to local edema and vasoconstriction.

Follicular hyperkeratosis, or chicken-skin appearance, particularly on the lateral aspects of the face, buttocks, and outer aspects of the upper arms and thighs, is termed *keratosis pilaris* (see Figs. 7.24 and 7.25).[63] Keratosis pilaris is not seen at birth but is common from early childhood onward and often persists into adulthood. Each lesion represents a large cornified plug in the upper part of the hair follicles, often with surrounding inflammation and vasodilation. Keratosis pilaris is more commonly associated with AD in children who have ichthyosis vulgaris. Moisturizers alone tend to be insufficient as therapy

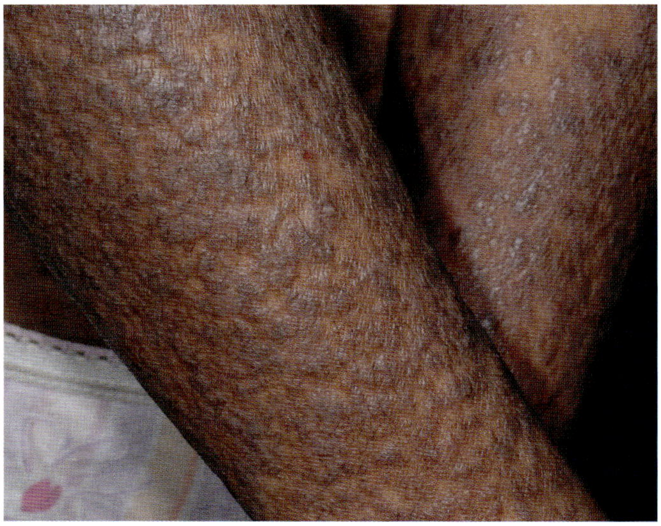

Fig. 3.20 Lichenification. Accentuation of skin markings are notable in thickened, lichenified skin of chronic atopic dermatitis. In darker-skinned individuals, hyperpigmentation tends to be associated with the lichenification.

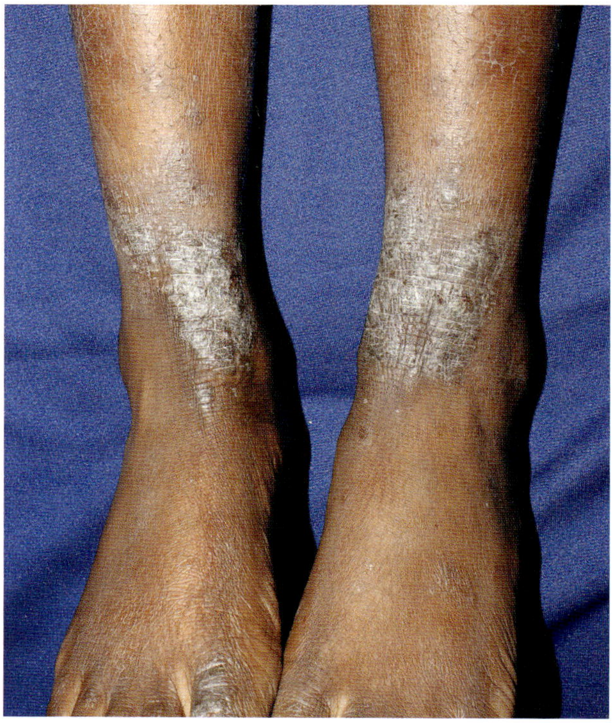

Fig. 3.21 Lichenification appears hyperpigmented in darker skin types (in contrast, see Fig. 3.10 with lichenification at the same site of a child with light skin).

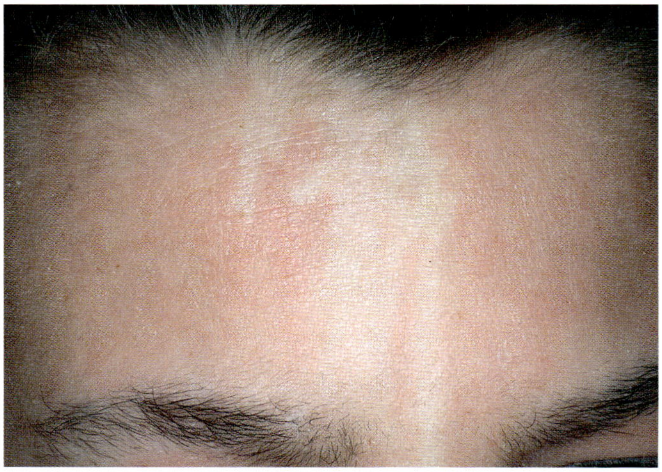

Fig. 3.22 White dermographism is the paradoxical blanching of skin after stroking.

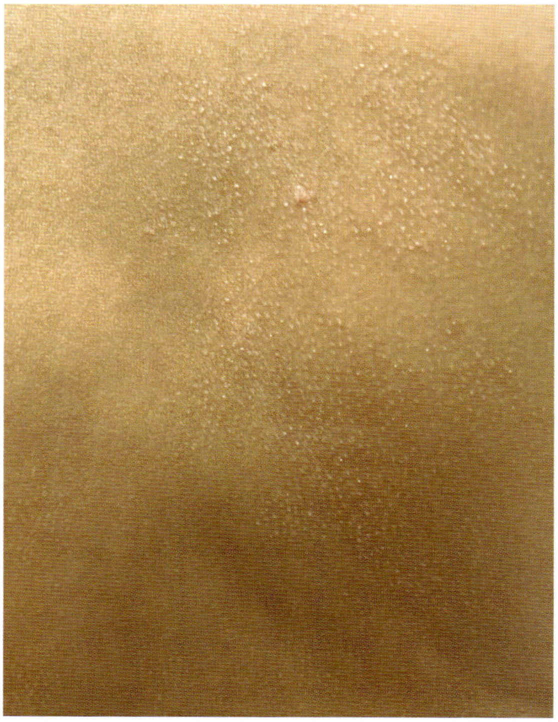

Fig. 3.23 Lichen spinulosus is commonly seen in children with dry skin and sometimes with atopic dermatitis. The characteristic collections of tiny, discrete flat-topped papules are usually asymptomatic.

for keratosis pilaris. Keratolytic agents such as urea or α-hydroxy acids may be helpful. Their use is limited, however, by the increased potential for irritation in children with AD. Treatment should be discouraged unless of significant cosmetic importance, because keratosis pilaris is almost always asymptomatic.

Lichen spinulosus manifests as round collections of numerous tiny, skin-colored to hypopigmented dry spiny papules (Fig. 3.23).[64] More common in Black children, lichen spinulosus usually occurs on the trunk or extremities. Lesions tend to be asymptomatic and may respond to application of emollients and mild topical corticosteroids. Children with AD also show an increased incidence of pityriasis alba, nummular dermatitis, dyshidrotic eczema, and juvenile plantar dermatosis (see related sections).

Individuals with atopic disorders have a distinct tendency toward an extra line or groove of the lower eyelid, the so-called "atopic pleat" (Fig. 3.24). Seen just below the lower lid of both eyes, the atopic pleat may be present at birth or shortly thereafter and is often retained throughout life. This groove (commonly referred to as a *Dennie–Morgan fold*) may result from edema of the lower eyelids and skin thickening; it represents a feature of the atopic diathesis rather than a pathognomonic marker of AD. The atopic pleat has been found with increased incidence in Black children.[65] Slate-gray to violaceous infraorbital discolorations ("allergic shiners"), with or without

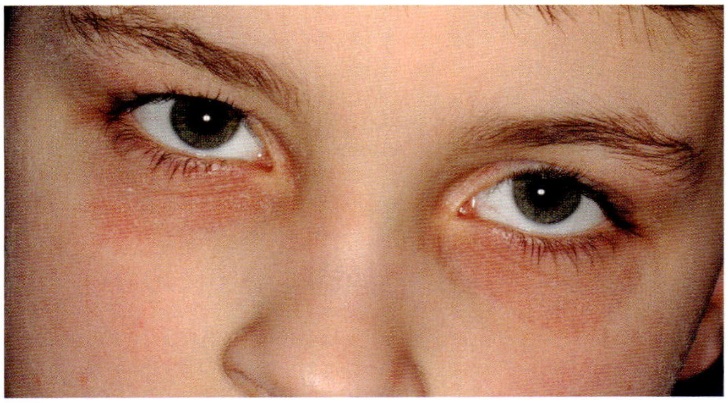

Fig. 3.24 Atopic pleats. Accentuated lines or grooves (Dennie–Morgan folds) are seen below the margin of the lower eyelids. This is a sign of the allergic diathesis and is not specific to atopic dermatitis. Note the mild periorbital dermatitis with hyperpigmentation.

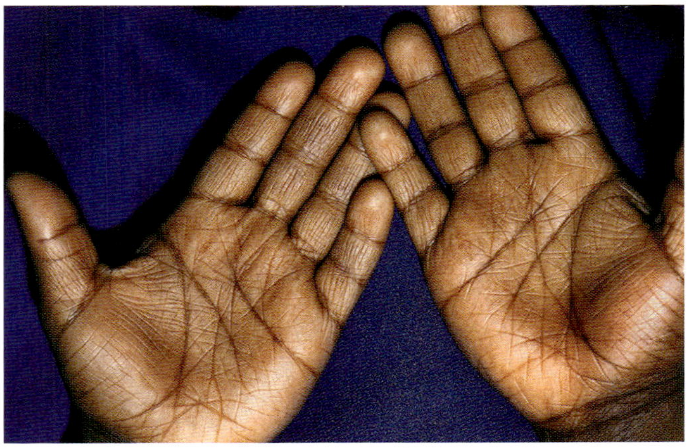

Fig. 3.26 Accentuated palmar creases. Hyperlinearity of the palms is a sign of concurrent ichthyosis vulgaris (see Chapter 5), a genetic disorder of skin associated with an increased risk of atopic dermatitis.

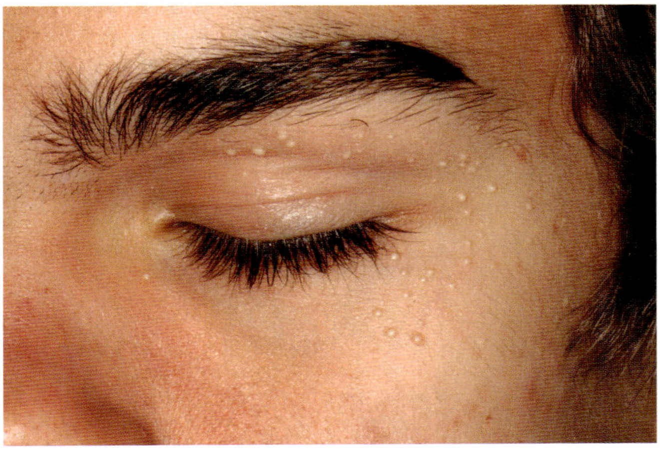

Fig. 3.25 Milia. Note that this child has numerous milia of the periorbital area, small inclusion cysts that are often a sign of chronic rubbing of the skin from periorbital dermatitis and/or allergic conjunctivitis. Milia clear spontaneously but after months to years.

swelling, are also seen in patients with allergies and in patients with AD. Allergic shiners are thought to be a manifestation of vascular stasis induced by pressure on underlying venous plexuses by edema of the nasal and paranasal cavities; the swelling and discoloration become more prominent as a result of repeated rubbing of the eyes and postinflammatory pigment darkening. Another clinical feature, an exaggerated linear nasal crease, is caused by rubbing of the nasal tip (the so-called "allergic salute") and occurs in 7% of schoolchildren.[66] Milia (tiny inclusion cysts; see Chapter 9) of the periorbital area are common in preadolescents (Fig. 3.25), may resemble acne, and are thought to result from the recurrent rubbing. Milia tend to resolve spontaneously, although years may be required; extraction may be performed but is rarely necessary.

Many patients with atopic conditions exhibit an increased number of fine lines and accentuated markings of the palms (Fig. 3.26). These accentuated palmar markings often are a clue to the concurrent diagnosis of ichthyosis vulgaris (see the previous discussion of the pathomechanism and also Chapter 5), a relatively common condition seen with increased incidence in children with AD. Ichthyosis vulgaris is considered a "semi-dominant" disorder because heterozygotes show manifestations (especially in drier, colder climates), but homozygotes tend to have greater severity. Most individuals with ichthyosis vulgaris merely think they have dry skin until the diagnosis is made when they are seen for AD. Diagnosis is based on the accentuated markings on the palms and soles, the characteristic generalized scaling with larger and more severe scaling on the lower extremities, worsening during winter months, and often positive family history.

Allergic keratoconjunctivitis (AKC) is a chronic noninfectious inflammatory condition and is one of the most severe ophthalmic complications associated with atopic dermatitis. AKC has been described in up to 30% of children with AD. It typically begins during late teenage years but has been described as early as 7 years of age.[67] Patients experience chronic itching and pain of the eyes, as well as tearing, redness, and blurred vision. It requires prompt and effective treatment to prevent permanent vision loss; moderate to severe eye irritation, increased redness, discharge, and any visual symptoms are features that require more urgent referral to an ophthalmologist. Complications of AKC include cataracts, keratoconus, infectious keratitis, blepharitis, tear dysfunction, and steroid-induced glaucoma.[68] Treatment options include a combination of mast cell inhibitors, antihistamines, corticosteroids, and calcineurin inhibitors.

Posterior subcapsular cataracts have been described in up to 13% of adult patients with severe AD.[69] Rarely seen in children, these cataracts are usually asymptomatic. Keratoconus (elongation and thinning of the corneal surface) has been reported in about 1% of patients with AD and seems to develop independently of cataracts.[69] Keratoconus is exacerbated by continuous rubbing of the eyes and may require corneal transplantation.

EFFECT ON QUALITY OF LIFE

The quality of life in infants, children, and adolescents with moderate to severe dermatitis is significantly reduced,[70] and having severe AD during childhood can have a great impact on psychosocial development.[71] Infants with AD have been shown to be excessively dependent and fearful. Sleep disturbance affects up to 60% of children with AD overall and 83% of children during flares. Impaired sleep quality occurs in children with mild AD and even inactive AD but is particularly problematic in children with more severe disease,[72] especially wake after sleep onset.[73] Neurocognitive function is impaired in children with sleep problems.[74] Even in clinical remission, children with AD show more sleep disturbance than healthy children,[75] including increased nocturnal wakefulness and a longer latency to rapid-eye-movement (REM) sleep.[75]

Disfigurement associated with moderate to severe AD, coupled with the reduction in sleep, restlessness, and fatigue at school, as well as limitations in participation in sports, isolates the affected child and strains relationships with peers and with teachers.

As a chronic disorder that requires frequent attention, the family of a child with AD carries a high financial burden of parental missed days from work for doctor visits and home care; lost wages owing to interruption of employment; expensive medications; and the costs of special or additional bedding, clothes, and food. The socioeconomic impact of AD in the United States alone is estimated to be $364 million to $3.8 billion annually.[76] The demonstrated average reduction by 1 to 2 hours of parental sleep nightly also translates into increased parental stress[77] and the tendency of affected children to cosleep with parents affects family dynamics.[78] These stressful psychological factors often exacerbate the AD, as may concurrent infectious illness or the stress of assignments at school.

COMORBIDITIES OF ATOPIC DERMATITIS

Allergic Disorders

AD is often associated with other forms of atopy, with 70% to 80% of affected children having an associated increase in IgE levels ("extrinsic" AD). Children with AD overall have a two- to threefold increased risk of developing asthma by 6 years of age and a threefold increased risk of developing allergic rhinitis (AR) compared with children without AD. Greater severity, earlier onset, persistence of the AD, polysensitization, having at least one variant in *FLG*, and parental history of allergic disease further increase the odds of developing these other atopic disorders.[79] Overall, asthma occurs by 6 years of age in approximately 30% of children with AD; AR develops in 43% to 80% of children with AD.[80]

The risk of food allergy is also increased with AD. In one study of almost 1100 infants with predominantly mild to moderate AD who enrolled at 3 to 18 months without a history of food allergy at baseline and were followed prospectively for 36 months, allergy to at least one food developed in 15.9% overall.[81] The most common triggers were peanut (6.6%), cow's milk (4.3%), and egg white (3.9%). The percentage with food allergies increases with greater AD severity, earlier onset, and AD persistence.[82]

Negative predictive values are high for antigen-specific IgE (sIgE), but positive predictive values for sIgE testing tend to be much lower,[81] especially if the cutoff values are low. True food allergy (based on clinical manifestations or food challenge) must be differentiated from the positive sIgE, which is common in infants and children with AD (including in 64% of those with AD beginning before 3 months of age).[83] In one study, 89% of food challenges based on positive sIgE testing were negative, consistent with a false-positive rate for true food allergy.[84] Food allergies to cow's milk and egg usually resolve during childhood, whereas peanut allergy tends to persist.

The approach to prevention of peanut allergy has dramatically changed during the past few years, based on the 2015 Learning Early About Peanut Allergy study, which showed that early introduction (4 to 11 months) of peanut reduced the risk of developing peanut allergy at 60 months of age (1.9%) compared with delayed introduction (13.7%). A panel of the National Institutes of Allergy and Infectious Diseases amended early guidelines[85] to recommend that children with severe AD, egg allergy, or both be exposed to peanut as early as 4 to 6 months of life, but only after evaluation by an allergy specialist (by skin prick testing [SPT], sIgE, or both). Severe AD has been defined as having persistent or frequently recurrent AD with typical morphology and distribution and requiring frequent application of prescription-strength topical antiinflammatory medications despite appropriate use of emollients.[85] Having a low peanut sIgE (<0.35; 6 to 7 g over three or more feedings) or minimal skin prick test reaction (0 to 2 mm) translates into an option to introduce the peanut at home or with supervision in the office setting; having an sIgE of 0.35 or greater should lead to referral to a specialist (given the poor predictive value for a positive sIgE). Having a SPT of 3 to 7 mm allows supervised administration in the office or oral food challenge, whereas having a reaction of more than 8 mm suggests a high likelihood of existent peanut allergy and requires appropriate management with strict peanut avoidance. For those with mild to moderate AD, peanut can be introduced at 4 to 6 months without further assessment (and as desired in those without AD, but ideally well before 1 year of age). Instructions for home feeding, including foods, amounts, subsequent observation, and signs of reaction have been published in the dermatology literature.[86] The expert panel did not recommend a broader panel of food allergen testing, given the poor positive predictive value and in an effort to avoid unnecessary dietary restriction.

The parallel increase in the prevalence of these various atopic disorders, including AD, suggests a shared mechanism or triggers. In fact, AD is often the first atopic feature in children who later develop asthma or AR, although food allergy not uncommonly precedes AD. The *atopic march* refers to the earlier occurrence of AD and later occurrence of one or more of these allergic disorders.[79] Having both AD and allergic sensitization greatly increases the risk of developing asthma and AR.[87]

The concurrence of allergic disorders with AD implicates the AD skin barrier abnormality in increasing the risk through promoting early local and systemic immune reactivity to antigens, with later development of food and environmental allergies, asthma, and allergic rhinitis. The importance of barrier integrity is supported by the association of *FLG* mutations with increased risk of asthma, allergic rhinitis, and food allergies,[88] but only in children with prior development of AD.[89–93] However, latent class analyses have suggested that AD occurs before asthma or AR less often than previously noted,[94] and studies have suggested the concept of multimorbidity with a shared underlying basis (e.g., genetic and/or environmental) driving these disorders.[79]

Biomarker and cluster analyses have begun to further subclassify patients according to phenotype (clinical features) or endotype (biologic/laboratory features[95–96] that are associated with clinical phenotypes). The ability to study biomarkers derived noninvasively through tape strips is likely to help subphenotype pediatric patients in the future,[97–99] allowing prediction of AD course, risk of comorbidities, and therapeutic responses.

INFECTIOUS COMPLICATIONS

In contrast to a prevalence of a carrier state in 5% to 20% of individuals who have no atopic condition, *S. aureus* is recovered in up to 90% of patients from lesions of AD—up to 76% from uninvolved (normal) skin and 50% to 60% from the anterior nares.[100–102] The increased adherence of *S. aureus* to the epidermal cells of individuals with AD[103] and a failure to produce endogenous antimicrobial peptides in the inflamed skin of patients with AD may account for the high rate of *S. aureus* colonization and infection. Although secondary infection in AD is usually from *S. aureus* (72%), 16% of cultures in infected patients with AD yield *S. pyogenes*, and 14% are mixed cultures.[104] Patients infected with group A *Streptococcus* were more likely to be febrile, have facial and periorbital involvement, have bacteremia and cellulitis, and be hospitalized compared with those infected with *S. aureus* alone.[104]

The pyoderma associated with AD is usually manifested by erythema with exudation and crusting (Fig. 3.27, *A* and *B*), particularly at sites of scratching, and occasionally by small pustules at sites of dermatitis (Fig. 3.28). This complication must be considered whenever a flare of chronic AD develops or fails to respond to appropriate therapy. *S. aureus* exacerbates the AD through (1) release of superantigen toxins, which enhance T-cell activation; (2) activation of superantigen-specific and allergen-specific T cells[105]; (3) expression of IgE antistaphylococcal antibodies[106,107]; and (4) increased expression of Th2 cytokines (including IL-31 and TSLP, which are known to cause pruritus directly) and increased expression of IL-22,[108] which is associated with epidermal thickening. Superantigen production also increases the expression of an alternative glucocorticoid receptor that does not bind to topical corticosteroids, leading to resistance.[109] Other factors produced by *S. aureus* are likely to exacerbate AD as well.[110] These observations emphasize the role of *S. aureus* as an important trigger of AD and endorse therapies that decrease the numbers of bacteria on the skin.

Although MRSA colonization and superinfection of AD is increasing, the majority of children with AD harbor MSSA.[100,111] MRSA infection may manifest as pustules (Fig. 3.29, *A*), abscesses (see Fig. 3.29, *B*), or crusting that is indistinguishable clinically from MSSA infection but much more difficult to eradicate; suppression of MRSA often requires that the entire family (including pets, who can harbor MRSA) be treated initially or even on an intermittent basis to reduce colonization, such as with intranasal mupirocin

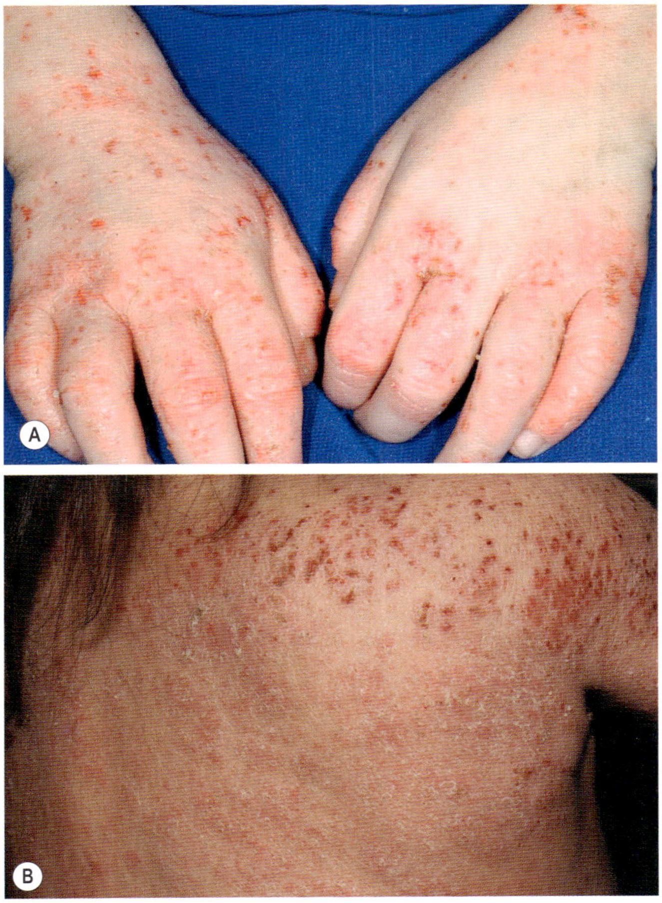

Fig. 3.27 Staphylococcal infection in atopic dermatitis. Sites of excoriation on the dorsal aspects of the hands **(A)** and upper back **(B)** are oozing and crusted. Note the erythema and mild associated edema. The dermatitis and the infection improved with oral administration of cephalexin, and the use of daily baths with sodium hypochlorite helped to maintain control while minimizing crusting.

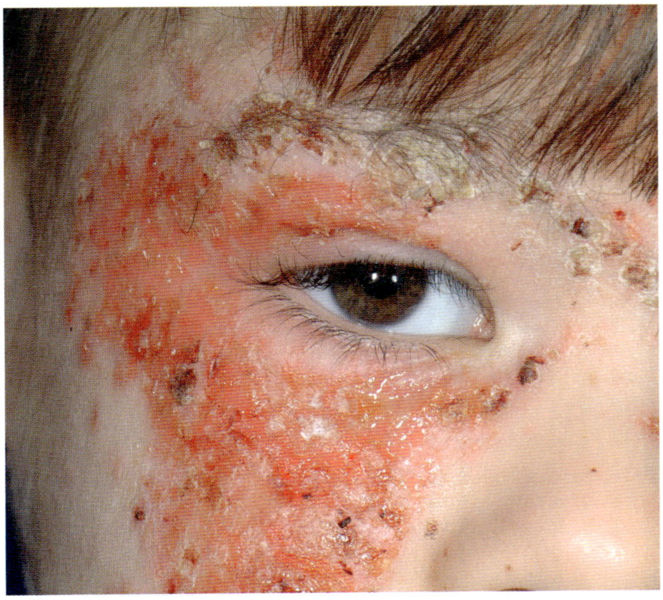

Fig. 3.28 Staphylococcal infection with pustules in atopic dermatitis (AD). Discrete nongrouped pustules and crusting overlying erythema and swelling of the periorbital area of a child with severe AD.

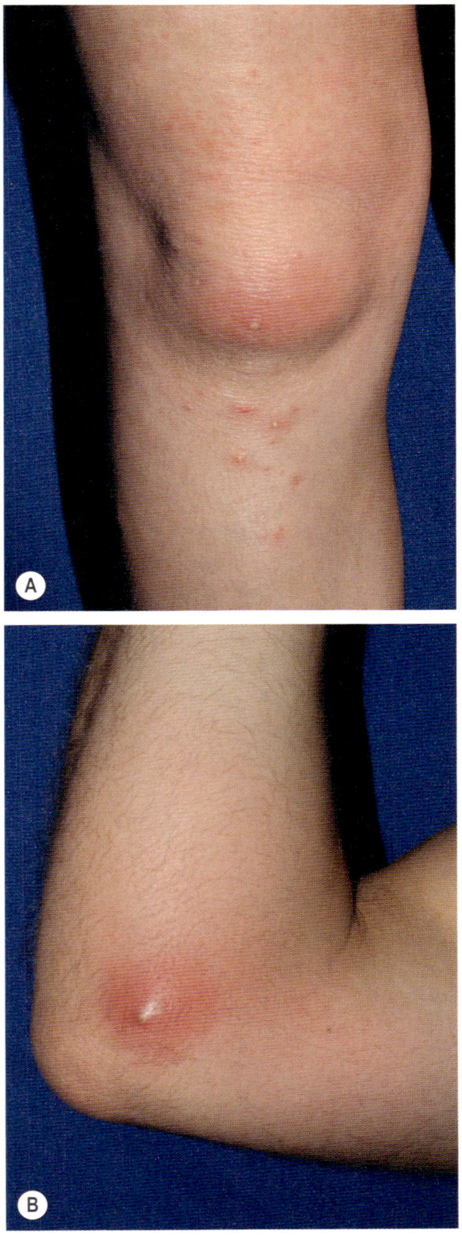

Fig. 3.29 Methicillin-resistant *Staphylococcus aureus* (MRSA) infection in atopic dermatitis (AD). **(A)** Staphylococcal pustulosis on the knees in a girl with severe AD and recurrent MRSA infections. **(B)** Her father has an MRSA abscess on the arm. Decolonization of the entire family is important.

ointment and once to twice weekly bleach baths or use of sodium hypochlorite–containing cleansers.

Greater cutaneous dissemination of certain viral infections has also been noted in children with AD and has been attributed to defects in the generation of antimicrobial peptide and the relative deficiency of Thl cytokine generation and cytotoxic T-cell function. Molluscum contagiosum is a cutaneous viral infection of childhood that most commonly affects the trunk, axillae, antecubital, popliteal fossae, and crural areas (see Chapter 15). Lesions are usually small, dome-shaped papules that often show central umbilication. The often-extensive molluscum lesions tend to be most numerous at sites of active dermatitis and can induce pruritus as well as dermatitis around the molluscum papules ("molluscum dermatitis").

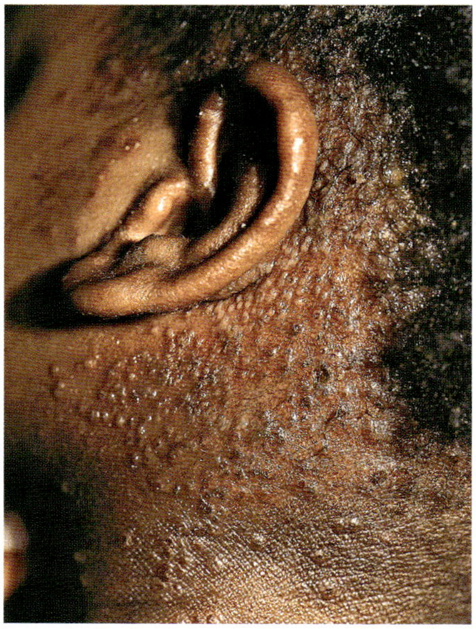

Fig. 3.30 Eczema herpeticum (Kaposi varicelliform eruption). Grouped vesiculopustular lesions on the face, retroauricular, and neck areas. Several of the pustules are beginning to show umbilication. The intense erythema is harder to appreciate in dark skin.

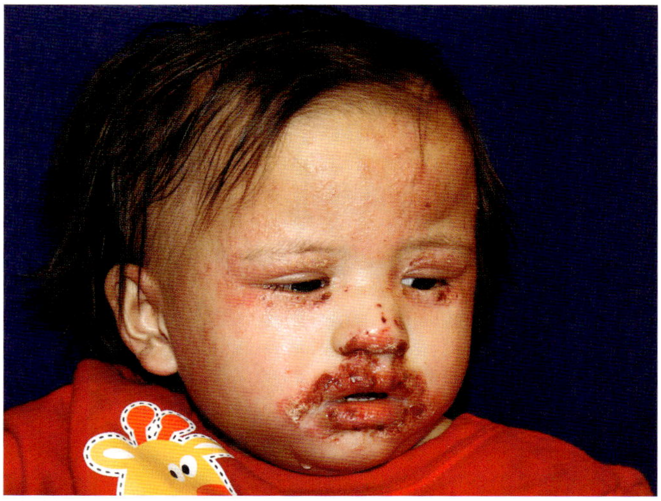

Fig. 3.32 Eczema herpeticum. Infection tends to occur at sites of atopic dermatitis, in this case the periorbital and perioral areas. Although eczema herpeticum with confluence of vesicles and extensive crusting can be confused with bacterial infection, some children also have secondary bacterial infection and need treatment with both acyclovir and antibiotic, such as cephalexin.

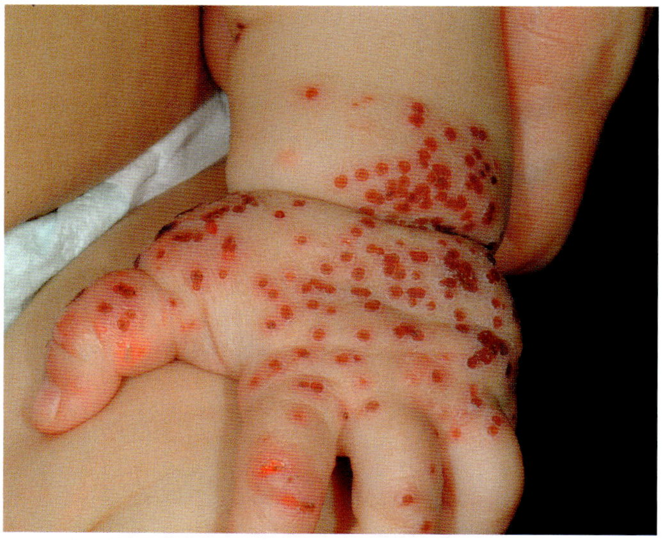

Fig. 3.31 Eczema herpeticum. These small, round umbilicated vesicles and punched out erosions are typical lesions of herpes simplex infection.

Eczema herpeticum (EH, also termed *Kaposi varicelliform eruption*) describes the explosive development of a vesiculopustular eruption caused by herpes simplex virus (HSV) in an individual with an atopic condition. Children with more severe AD and other atopic conditions are at greatest risk.[112] The tendency toward eczema herpeticum is associated with an elevated Th2 and reduced Th1 T-cell immune response to HSV1.[113,114] The clustering and often umbilication of the vesicles is characteristic (Figs. 3.30 and 3.31; see Fig. 8.15), with sites of the dermatitis most commonly affected. Nevertheless, with a confluence of vesicles and crusting, eczema herpeticum can be mistaken for bacterial infection (Fig. 3.32). The diagnosis can be verified by polymerase chain reaction (PCR) and viral culture. If these tests are not available, a Tzanck test can be performed by scraping the floor of vesicles and, after staining the smear with Giemsa or Wright stain, searching for multinuclear virus "giant cells" or balloon cells.

Hospitalization may be necessary, especially in infants younger than 1 year and in association with fever or other systemic symptoms.[115] Early administration of acyclovir has been shown to lead to better outcomes for EH,[116] and use of topical corticosteroids or calcineurin inhibitors has not been associated with poorer outcomes in children hospitalized with EH.[117] Systemic antibiotics should be administered if secondary bacterial infection is strongly suspected but should not be used empirically.[118]

Eczema vaccinatum was a problem when smallpox vaccinations were compulsory, most commonly contracted by accidental contact with a recently vaccinated individual. The global threat of bioterrorism and consideration of smallpox vaccinations has again brought to attention the risk of eczema vaccinatum for patients, particularly children, with AD.[119] Eczema vaccinatum is characterized by the widespread cutaneous dissemination of vaccinia viral lesions that manifest as firm, deep-seated vesicles or pustules that are all in the same stage of development (see Chapter 15). Lesions may become umbilicated or confluent.

Eczema coxsackium (see Chapter 16) is a recently coined term to describe the unusual cutaneous concentration in sites of previous or current AD of vesicles and erosions from coxsackievirus A6 and, less commonly, coxsackievirus A16 infection, which could be confused with EH (Fig. 3.33).[120,121] Fever, oral erosions or ulcerations, and sore throat or mouth are among the most common associated symptoms. Lesions clear spontaneously in an average of 12 days but may persist for a month.

Reactivity to *Malassezia* has been blamed for recalcitrant AD of the head and neck in adolescents. Although there are no documented differences in *Malassezia* species colonization, patients with head and neck AD are more likely to have positive skin prick test results and *Malassezia*-specific IgE compared with healthy control subjects and patients with atopy without head and neck dermatitis. These patients may benefit from a 1- to 2-month course of daily itraconazole or fluconazole followed by long-term weekly treatment.[122]

Other Comorbidities

AD is also associated with several neuropsychiatric disorders, including anxiety, depression, attention-deficit/hyperactivity disorder (ADHD), conduct disorder, and autism.[123–126] In preschool children with AD, there is also a higher risk of enuresis, encopresis, and attachment disorder.[127] The risk of ADHD is highest in children with more severe disease and greater sleep deprivation,[128] reinforcing the impact of these factors on neurocognitive function. One provocative study suggested that use of sedating antihistamines increased the risk of developing ADHD,[129] but further study is needed. Although restlessness and inattention at school, common in sleep-deprived, itchy AD

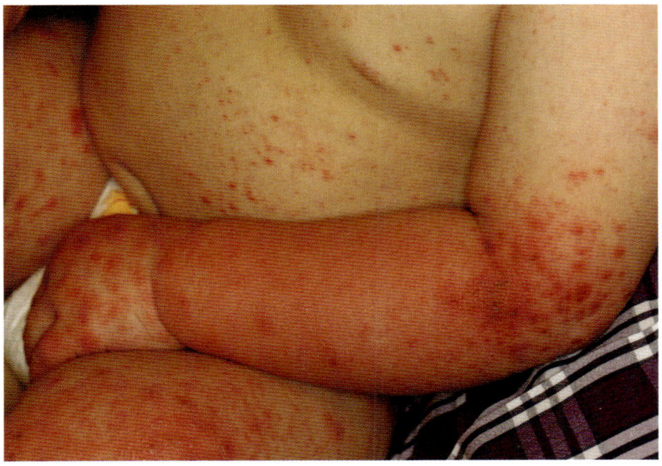

Fig. 3.33 Eczema coxsackium. Children with atopic dermatitis (AD) are at increased risk of widespread cutaneous lesions from coxsackie infection, especially coxsackie A6, which can cluster at sites of AD and be confused with eczema herpeticum.

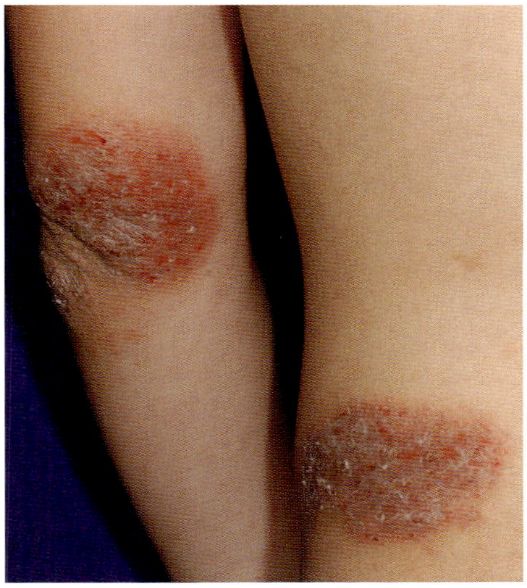

Fig. 3.34 Nummular dermatitis. Characterized by well-defined, round (coin-shaped or nummular) plaques of vesiculopapules overlying erythema and edema. Oozing and secondary infection are common.

children, may be features that resemble those of ADHD, these are not sufficient to meet screening criteria for ADHD for the majority of AD children.[130] Families are also affected, with higher risks of anxiety and depression in caregivers.[131] Children with AD have a higher risk of injury requiring medical attention, related both to comorbid psychiatric and behavioral disorders and their atopy.[132] Additional emerging comorbidities are autoimmune disorders (alopecia areata, vitiligo, rheumatoid arthritis, and inflammatory bowel disease[133]) and obesity,[134] especially during infancy and including central obesity.[135,136]

DIFFERENTIAL DIAGNOSIS

AD is a chronic fluctuating disease. The distribution and morphology of lesions vary with age, but itching is the cardinal symptom of this disorder. Although many skin conditions may occasionally resemble AD, certain characteristics assist in their differentiation. Three common forms of dermatitis that are seen often with AD are contact dermatitis (both irritant and allergic), seborrheic dermatitis, and nummular dermatitis. Each of these disorders is discussed in detail later in the chapters and, as such, is mentioned only briefly here as relevant to AD.

Seborrheic dermatitis is characterized by a greasy yellow or salmon-colored scaly eruption that may involve the scalp, cheeks, trunk, extremities, and diaper area. The major differentiating features include a tendency toward earlier onset, characteristic greasy yellowish or salmon-colored lesions with a predisposition for intertriginous areas, a generally well-circumscribed eruption, and a relative absence of pruritus (see later). Infants may show both atopic and seborrheic dermatitis (see Fig. 3.3), with progression or persistence of the atopic lesions as the seborrheic dermatitis subsides.

Irritant and allergic forms of contact dermatitis are common comorbidities of AD (see related section).[137] Primary irritant dermatitis is commonly seen in infants and young children on the cheeks and the chin (owing in part to the irritation of saliva), the extensor surfaces of the extremities (as a result of harsh soaps, detergents, or rough fabrics), and the diaper area (usually spared in AD; primarily from feces and vigorous cleansing). Irritant dermatitis may also result from bubble baths, personal care products, and handled materials such as modeling clays. Primary irritant dermatitis is generally milder, less pruritic to asymptomatic, and not as eczematous and oozing as the eruptions seen in association with AD. Irritant contact dermatitis to saliva and to exposure to harsh soaps and fabrics occurs more often in children with concomitant AD.

Allergic contact dermatitis (ACD), although relatively uncommon in the first few months of life, can mimic almost any type of eczematous eruption and is characterized by a well-circumscribed pruritic, erythematous, papular, and vesicular eruption. Although such eruptions involute spontaneously on identification and removal of the cause, this disorder often requires a carefully detailed history and

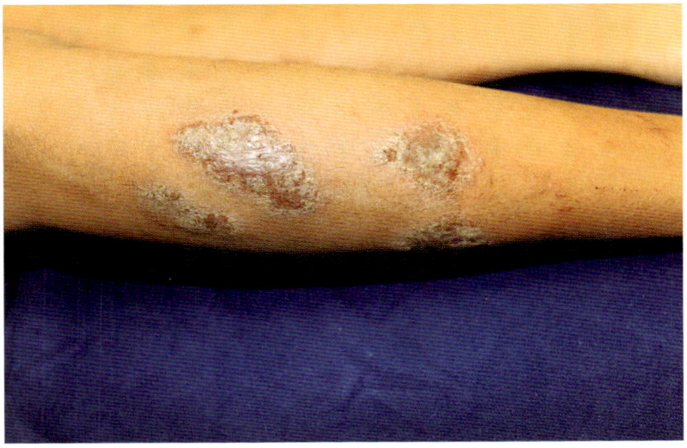

Fig. 3.35 Nummular dermatitis. Some patients show multiple nummular plaques.

prolonged observation before the true causative agent is identified. ACD to nickel occurs often in children with AD[138] and may be misdiagnosed as recalcitrant periumbilical AD. Patients with recalcitrant AD may have concomitant allergic contact reactions, particularly to nickel and less often to topically applied medications and emollients, suggesting the role for patch testing.[139] Positive patch tests for potential allergens other than nickel have been described in up to 45% of children with AD,[138,140,141] and more than half of these are reactions to components in their emollients (lanolin, neomycin, formaldehyde, sesquiterpene lactone mix [including parthenolide], compositae mix, and fragrances) or foaming products (cocamidopropyl betaine).[142] Topical corticosteroids are unusual contact allergens[144–145] but can be tested based on structural class with tixocortol-21-pivalate, budesonide, and hydrocortisone 17-butyrate.[140,146,147]

Nummular dermatitis is a distinctive disorder characterized by coin-shaped lesions. Measuring 1 cm or more in diameter, lesions of nummular dermatitis develop on dry skin and are more often seen during dry winter months. The eruption is characterized by discrete erythematous round plaques formed by the confluence of papules and vesicles (Figs. 3.34 and 3.35). Nummular lesions tend to be secondarily infected and often more recalcitrant to topical therapy. If the combination of medium-strength to potent topical steroid plus topical antibiotic does not suffice, a course of systemic antibiotic may be required. Dilute sodium hypochlorite baths should also be considered.

The lesions of psoriasis, another common skin disease of children, are bright red and topped with loosely adherent silvery micaceous scale (see Chapter 4). Psoriatic lesions usually show a sharply delineated edge and have a predilection for the extensor surfaces (particularly the elbows and knees), the scalp, the buttock, and the genital regions. Approximately 5% of children with psoriasis also show dermatitis, either as typical psoriasis and AD lesions or a psoriasiform dermatitis; these children often have a family history of both atopy and psoriasis.

Scabies in infants and children is commonly complicated by eczematous changes because of scratching and rubbing of involved areas or the application of harsh topical therapeutic agents. The diagnosis of scabies is best made by the history of itching, a characteristic distribution of lesions, the recognition of primary lesions (particularly the pathognomonic burrow when present), positive identification of the mite on microscopic examination of skin scrapings, and the presence of infestation among the patient's family or associates (see Chapter 18).

Langerhans cell histiocytosis (LCH) most commonly occurs before 3 years of age (see Chapter 10). In affected neonates, reddish-brown, purpuric, crusted papules or vesiculopapules are typically present. In infants this skin eruption is often characterized as a scaly, erythematous seborrheic eruption on the scalp, behind the ears, and in the intertriginous regions. On close inspection the presence of reddish-brown, petechial or purpuric lichenoid papules or vesicular or crusted papules in infants is typical. Cutaneous biopsy and identification of $CD1a^+$ Langerhans cells by immunostaining confirms the diagnosis of LCH.

Acrodermatitis enteropathica is an autosomal recessive disorder characterized by vesiculobullous eczematoid lesions of the acral and periorificial areas, failure to thrive, diarrhea, alopecia, nail dystrophy, and frequent secondary bacterial or candidal infection (see Chapters 2 and 24). The characteristic distribution of lesions accompanied by listlessness, diarrhea, failure to thrive, and low serum zinc levels differentiate lesions of acrodermatitis enteropathica from those of AD. Usually a disorder in formula-fed babies with the hereditary form, acrodermatitis enteropathica may also occur in breastfed babies as a result of deficient zinc secretion into maternal breast milk.

Dermatitis during the neonatal or infantile periods is also seen in immune dysregulation, polyendocrinopathy, enteropathy, X-linked (IPEX) syndrome, which manifests with early onset intractable diarrhea and type 1 diabetes mellitus.[148–150] The disorder is often fatal during the first year of life. The cutaneous manifestations are seen in 70% of affected babies and tend to be the first sign.[148] Although an atopic-like dermatitis is most common, the eruption has also been described as psoriasiform or resembling ichthyosiform erythroderma. Lesions are often pruritic, secondarily infected by *S. aureus*, and resistant to treatment with topical corticosteroids. Other common cutaneous manifestations include severe cheilitis, onychodystrophy, and alopecia. Infections of the upper and lower airways and gastrointestinal (GI) tract are common, and affected patients may succumb to sepsis. Food allergies and high levels of IgE and eosinophils are also associated. The autoimmune enteropathy is characterized by persistent, watery, and sometime mucoid or bloody diarrhea during the neonatal period, resulting in malabsorption and failure to thrive. Type 1 diabetes is difficult to control and results from lymphocytic infiltration of the pancreas. Other autoimmune symptoms, such as hypothyroidism, cytopenia, hepatitis, nephropathy, and arthritis can develop in patients who survive the initial acute phase. IPEX syndrome results from mutations in *FOXP3*, leading to absent or dysfunctional regulatory T cells and self-reactive T-cell activation and proliferation. Detection of enterocyte autoantibodies helps make the diagnosis.[151] Treatment generally includes supportive care and systemic immunosuppressive therapy (steroids, methotrexate, tacrolimus), although rapamycin has shown promise. Stem-cell transplantation is the curative treatment[150] if a suitable donor can be found.

Generalized erythroderma in association with atopic features can be seen in other disorders with barrier abnormalities, notably Netherton syndrome (biallelic mutations in *SPINK5*) and SAM syndrome (severe skin dermatitis, multiple *a*llergies and *m*etabolic wasting; biallelic mutations in *DSG1*)[152]; failure to thrive, recurrent infections, and hypotrichosis are associated with both of these ichthyotic disorders (see Chapter 5).

Typical AD may be a feature of several forms of immunodeficiency, most notably in Wiskott–Aldrich syndrome (WAS) and the hyperimmunoglobulinemia E syndrome (HIES) (see related sections). These disorders are distinguished from AD by their recurrent noncutaneous infections and other characteristic features (e.g., thrombocytopenic purpura, bloody diarrhea, and purpuric lesions in WAS and facial and intertriginous staphylococcal abscesses in HIES).

MANAGEMENT

The overall goals of therapy are to reduce itch and maintain sufficient control to minimize any adverse effects of the AD on quality of life. In general, a multistep approach[153] is taken toward management that includes patient and parent education,[154] avoidance of irritants and allergic triggers, good moisturization, normalization of dysbiosis, and use of antiinflammatory medications[155] (Table 3.1). Patient compliance is the main reason for poor outcome and is fueled by concerns about the use of topical corticosteroids and calcineurin inhibitors (see later). Aggressively but safely managing AD flares is important in preventing the exacerbation of disease by delayed or inadequate treatment. The National Eczema Association (NEA) offers a website for education and patient support (www.nationaleczema.org). Age-specific structured educational programs have improved objective and subjective severity scores,[156] and educational videos may improve severity beyond direct education.[157] Written action plans have been shown to improve adherence to therapy.[158,159,161,162] Several guidelines for AD management in children have been published.[163–167]

Preventing the Development of Atopic Dermatitis

Infants in at-risk families (i.e., with at least one parent or sibling who has AD) have a 30% to 50% chance of developing AD by 2 years of age.[168] Limiting the use of skin cleansers is advised. Applying an oil-in-water emollient at least once daily appeared to lower the risk and severity[169–172] of AD, but larger studies have not confirmed this effect.[173,174]

Water hardness has been shown to be associated with an increased prevalence of AD[175,176] and may relate to increased sodium lauryl sulfate residue from washing, leading to greater impairment in barrier function and skin irritation.[177] Although ion-exchange water softeners do not lower the prevalence of AD,[178] they may mitigate the residue deposition seen with hard water.

Table 3.1 Management of Mild, Moderate, and Severe Forms of Atopic Dermatitis

Mild	Moderate	Severe
Bathing and barrier repair* Avoidance of irritant and allergic triggers Intermittent, short-term use of class VI or VII topical steroids (see Table 3.2) ± topical calcineurin inhibitors ± phosphodiesterase 4 (PDE4) inhibitor Treat superinfection	Bathing and barrier repair* Avoidance of irritant and allergic triggers Intermittent, short-term use of class III–V topical steroids (see Table 3.2) ± topical calcineurin inhibitors ± PDE4 inhibitor Treat superinfection Oral antihistamines for sleep	Bathing and barrier repair* Avoidance of irritant and allergic triggers Class II topical steroids for flares (see Table 3.2); class III–V topical steroids ± tacrolimus ointment for maintenance Treat superinfection Oral antihistamines for sleep Consider systemic immunosuppressants, immunomodulatory biologics (e.g., dupilumab), ultraviolet light therapy

*Barrier repair may be accomplished by application of effective emollients and/or barrier-repair agents.

Despite the fact that maternal dietary antigens are known to cross the placenta, most studies have provided no evidence that avoidance of maternal dietary antigens during pregnancy or lactation has a protective effect during the first 18 months of life on the development of AD or on food sensitization by 7 years of age.[179–181] In fact, there is increasing evidence that early exposure to food antigens may reduce the risk of developing food allergies. As a result, breastfeeding without restricting maternal diet as a strategy to prevent food allergy is recommended until 4 to 6 months unless contraindicated for medical reasons. Although there is no evidence that breastfeeding protects against the development of pediatric AD at any age,[182,183] peanut, milk, and wheat intake during pregnancy may be associated with reduced allergy and asthma in children.[184,185] As a result, if available and affordable, hydrolyzed infant formulas, rather than cow's-milk or soy-milk formulas, can be given to at-risk infants who are not exclusively breastfed, although they may not affect the risk of AD. Solid foods, including potentially allergenic foods, should not be delayed beyond 4 to 6 months of age in at-risk infants.[186,187]

Probiotics have recently received considerable attention as a means of prevention of AD. Evidence that reduced diversity in the gut microbiota is a risk factor in the development of AD[188–191] provides further rationale for probiotic use. Although there is some evidence of benefit prenatally in prevention (for reviews[192–195]) there is insufficient evidence to recommend probiotics as part of standard management of infantile AD.[195,196] Of note, however, mixtures of probiotics appear to be more helpful than use of a single probiotic, and a recent trial of a mixture of different probiotic strains led to a significantly greater reduction in SCORAD during 12 weeks of therapy than placebo, with a greater use of topical steroids in the placebo arm.[197]

Although early studies suggest some benefit of prebiotics (fiber compounds that stimulate the growth of advantageous organisms) and fatty acids (such as the γ-linolenic acid alone or in combination with omega-3 fatty acids),[195] there is insufficient evidence to recommend these approaches for either reducing the risk of developing AD or treating AD.

Avoidance of Irritant Triggers

Certain climatic factors, such as temperature, air pollution/urban environment, and psychological stress, are linked to AD and difficult to control.[198] Many patients have problems with eccrine sweating and sweat retention during the summer months, leading to increased pruritus, especially in the face of lichenification. The increased vasodilation of already inflamed skin from increased summer heat further contributes to pruritus and cutaneous erythema. Nevertheless, children with AD should be encouraged to participate as actively in sports as possible. Swimming is an excellent sport for children with AD if exposure to chlorinated pool water is tolerated. Children should be coated with an emollient (after sunscreen application) as a protectant against pool chemicals; rinsing immediately after swimming followed by application of emollient may decrease the risk of irritation. Children should also be kept cool after application of the thick emollient, or, if sweating is anticipated, a less occlusive moisturizer should be applied. Air-conditioning is important during hot weather to decrease pruritus. The pruritus and erythematous papules of miliaria rubra, which can develop when sweating and using an occlusive moisturizer, can be confused by parents with exacerbation of the dermatitis, setting up a cycle of worsening involvement from repeated application of the occlusive emollient. Recognition and education in decreasing the frequency of emollient application are vital in this situation.

Overdressing children during winter months should also be avoided to prevent overheating. The low humidity of winter months and use of indoor heating also increases skin xerosis and may promote dermatitis; humidifiers may be useful but may increase the exposure to mold allergens if they are not cleaned often. Saliva is a major irritant for infants with AD, and exposure to large amounts of saliva with teething and eating, including saliva mixed with food, exacerbates the facial dermatitis. Protecting the face before meals or naptime with a thick, protective emollient may be helpful. Similarly, older children with AD are at risk for lip-licker's dermatitis because of the irritant effects of saliva.

Attention to clothing is also important. Soft cotton clothing is recommended over traditional wool or other harsh materials, which tend to precipitate itching and scratching, and in one study fabric softener decreased skin dryness.[199] There is only low-quality evidence regarding AD improvement or decrease in bacterial colonization from use of special textiles, particularly silk and silver-coated cotton.[200–201] Affected children should avoid use of harsh soaps and detergents, fabric softener sheets, products with fragrance, and bubble baths. Cigarette smoking in homes of children with AD should be avoided, because it can lead to an increase in irritation and pruritus and may also increase the tendency toward subsequent development of asthma.[203]

Avoidance of Triggering Allergens

It may be possible to identify potential allergen triggers by taking a careful history and doing selective allergy tests.[204] However, triggers that can easily be avoided are difficult to find for most affected individuals, and without a documented or proven food allergy, avoiding potentially allergenic foods as a means of managing AD is not recommended. Food allergy leading to dermatitis is unusual. Testing for allergy to milk, egg, peanut, wheat, and soy is only recommended in children younger than 5 years of age with moderate to severe AD who have persistent AD despite optimized management with topical therapy or who have a reliable history of an immediate reaction after ingestion of a specific food.[205,206] Food antigen–specific IgE levels correlate better than a radioallergosorbent test and prick tests,[207] but the level of sIgE is not clinically useful for predicting the development of clinically relevant food allergy. Negative skin prick tests or serum allergen-specific IgE levels are highly predictive at eliminating potential allergens. However, at 6 months of age, 83% of patients with severe AD show IgE food sensitization to milk, eggs, and/or peanuts, and 65% of these children retain food sensitivity by 12 months of age. In comparison, 5% of 6-month-old infants and 11% of 12-month-old infants without atopy show IgE food sensitization.[208] Fewer than 40% of children with moderate to severe AD with food sensitization show reactivity during food challenges,[209] and many of these eruptions are urticarial. In a longitudinal study, 16% of more than 1000 infants with AD (all severities) developed food allergies, particularly to peanut (7%), milk (4%), and egg (4%), with the highest risk in infants with greater AD severity.[81,209] Foods may also induce extracutaneous manifestations in pediatric patients with AD, particularly involving the GI tract. Foods may also act as irritants, especially citrus foods, and reactions to chemicals in foods, such as tartrazine or other colorings, may occur. For children in whom food allergies are suspected to be relevant, comanagement with a pediatric allergist is recommended.

The most common food allergens often contaminate other foods and are difficult to avoid entirely. Restrictions in diet should not worsen the quality of the patient's and family's life more than the AD itself. Challenges of agents that may trigger IgE reactivity are best conducted under medical observation, because anaphylaxis has occasionally been reported. It should be remembered that excessively restrictive diets in atopic children may lead to weight loss, calcium deficiency, hypovitaminosis, and kwashiorkor.[210] Proper nutritional counseling and supplementation should be included in management, including warning against the use of protein-poor rice and almond milk for cow's milk, hydrolyzed, and elemental formulas. After the first few years of life, the risk of significant reactivity to food diminishes (particularly with eggs, milk, soy, and wheat). Unless a careful dietary history suggests food sensitivity as a trigger, improvement through dietary manipulation in children older than 5 years is rarely noted.

In contrast to potential reactivity to foods, reactivity of children and adolescents with AD to aeroallergens increases with age. The most common aeroallergen triggers are house-dust mites *(Dermatophagoides pteronyssinus)*, grass pollens, animal dander, and molds, particularly *Alternaria*. Plant pollens, particularly ragweed, also contain an oleoresin capable of producing sensitization and eczematous contact dermatitis. Airborne dermatitis may involve the exposed surfaces of the face, neck, arms, legs, and V area of the chest but can be distinguished from photosensitivity, which results in sharper lines of demarcation between normal skin and eczematous skin. Exacerbation of facial dermatitis during pollen season or after children contact a pet should alert parents to the possibility of allergy to an aeroallergen or contact allergen (see Allergic Contact Dermatitis section). Cat exposure during infancy can increase the risk of developing AD,[211] especially in infants with an *FLG* mutation.[212] Cat exposure in children with AD has been shown to increase the risk of developing asthma, although dog exposure may be protective.[213] Epicutaneous application of aeroallergens by atopy patch test on unaffected atopic skin shows reactivity as an eczematoid patch in 30% to 50% of patients with AD but tends to be negative in patients with only respiratory allergy to these triggers or in healthy volunteers. However, patch tests have not been standardized, and their performance and interpretation vary widely.

The value toward AD control of mite-allergen avoidance measures (encasing mattresses and pillows, washing bedding in hot water weekly, vacuuming living areas and bedrooms frequently, keeping only soft nonfurry toys, cleaning carpets regularly or removing them, and eliminating pets) is controversial, and a meta-analysis found no value in encasing mattresses to prevent allergic diseases or symptoms.[214] Immunotherapy for food allergies or aeroallergens has long been controversial as treatment for AD, unlike its efficacy for treating AR and extrinsic asthma; recent double-blind, placebo-controlled studies, however, suggest some value of specific oral and sublingual immunotherapy, including to peanuts.[215,216]

Use of Bathing and Emollients

Although water exposure can increase xerosis through evaporative loss, daily baths hydrate the skin, especially if the water loss is prevented by emollient application within a few minutes after bathing. Baths are also fun for infants and children, contribute to parent–child bonding, and remove surface bacteria and desquamated scale. Whether to limit the duration of bathing is controversial, but many recommend limiting the bath to approximately 10 minutes. Older children and adolescents should be instructed to avoid excessively warm baths and showers. Only mild soaps with lower pH to suppress protease activation (such as Dove or Basis) or soapless cleansers (such as Cetaphil, CeraVe, or Aquanil) should be used if a cleanser is felt to be needed. Bubble baths can be irritating and are contraindicated in moderate to severe AD. Bath oils[217] have not been found beneficial and can be hazardous if they make the tub slippery.

The addition of dilute sodium hypochlorite (bleach) to the bath (¼ cup per half-tub of water with full-strength 5% to 6% commercial bleach [range commercially is 3% to 8%] or 1 mL/L for local soaks or compresses) or use of a sodium hypochlorite wash is helpful in controlling the dermatitis, especially for children with a history of skin infection when used as maintenance therapy (see Topical Antiinflammatory Medications section).[100] Although the antibacterial effect has been implicated in AD improvement, there is growing evidence that dilute sodium hypochlorite has direct antiinflammatory and barrier-promoting effects on skin[218] (see Treatment of Secondary Cutaneous Infections section), rather than being antibacterial, given its low concentration.[219] Children may complain about sitting in a tub bath because of stinging, particularly during acute exacerbations with raw skin and crusting. In such instances, the addition of 1 cup of salt or baking soda may make the bath more tolerable until more aggressive therapy with topical steroids and treatment of secondary infection with oral antibiotics leads to improvement.

In general, dryness is worse during cold months when it is aggravated by heat in the house and low humidity. Key to maintaining hydration is the application of a good emollient, particularly within minutes after bathing. In general, the thicker and greasier the emollient, the higher the content of oil relative to water and the more effective the emollient (e.g., ointment is better than cream, which is better than lotion). Petrolatum itself has been shown to upregulate gene expression of filaggrin and antimicrobial peptides, increase stratum corneum thickness, and reduce cutaneous inflammation. Pure petrolatum is rarely a cause of contact dermatitis.[220] Nevertheless, nonointment emollients, particularly emollient creams, can be substituted when use of a greasy ointment is objectionable and may have inherent antiinflammatory properties. Some patients, especially those with sensory issues and poor tolerance of ointments and creams, find oils to be helpful, although in general oils do not penetrate the skin as well as oil–water mixtures. Purified sunflower seed and safflower seed oils improve the AD skin barrier, whereas olive oil and mustard seed oil are detrimental to skin barrier recovery and can cause erythema,[221–223] emphasizing that oils are not interchangeable. Similarly, virgin coconut oil is superior to mineral oil in reducing AD severity[224] and to olive oil in decreasing *S. aureus*,[225] although potential concern about contact sensitization have been raised. "Barrier repair" agents, with additives such as N-palmitoylethanolamine,[226] ceramide,[227] and glycyrrhetinic acid,[228] also show mild antiinflammatory properties and may be beneficial for children with mild to moderate AD but are much more costly than emollients.

Wet wraps of plain water can be applied at night after bathing and emollition or after application of the topical antiinflammatory agent to decrease pruritus and the sensation of burning at night.[229–231] Short-term use (up to 14 days) of wet wraps over topical corticosteroids is more efficacious than wraps over bland emollients alone but can be associated with transiently increased steroid absorption. Although wet gauze bandage wraps (such as Kerlix or Kling) are often used in a hospital setting, dressing the young child at home in moist pajamas and socks that cling to the skin and are topped by a dry layer to avoid excessive cooling can be very soothing and promote sleep. Unna boots can also be loosely applied to the legs or arms at night (under self-adherent wraps) to decrease pruritus and protect from scratching.

Open wet compresses may be useful in children with weeping, oozing, or crusted lesions. Aluminum acetate (as in Burow solution, 1:20 or 1:40) is germicidal and suppresses the weeping and oozing of acutely inflamed lesions. Burow solution 1:40 is prepared by dissolving one packet or effervescent tablet (Domeboro) in a pint of cool or tepid tap water. These compresses are applied with a gauze or a soft cloth (e.g., a man's handkerchief or strips of bed-sheeting) two to three times daily for 10 to 15 minutes for up to 5 days. Washcloths and heavy toweling interfere with evaporation and therefore are not as effective. Compresses should be lukewarm, moderately wet (not dripping), and remoistened at intervals. After the compress, the topical antiinflammatory agent may be applied.

Topical Antiinflammatory Medications

Topical corticosteroids have been the mainstay of treatment for AD (see Table 3.1) and are available in a wide range of potencies from the weakest class VII corticosteroids (e.g., hydrocortisone acetate) to the ultrapotent class I steroids (Table 3.2). The use of more potent topical corticosteroids when applied to large surface areas, under occlusion, or for long periods may lead to adverse effects (Box 3.2), most commonly local atropy. The face and intertriginous areas are the most susceptible sites and may show local effects, even when weaker steroids are used for prolonged periods. Because of their increased body surface area-to-weight ratio, small children have the greatest risk of systemic absorption of topically applied steroids.

The potency of a topical corticosteroid is largely determined by vasoconstrictor assay and is related to its vehicle as well as to its chemical formulation. The concentration of each topical corticosteroid is only significant with respect to potency relative to other corticosteroids of the same chemical formulation. Accordingly, hydrocortisone acetate 2.5% is much weaker than triamcinolone acetonide 0.1%, which in turn is weaker than clobetasol propionate 0.05%, even though the concentrations would suggest the opposite. It also should be recognized that hydrocortisone acetate differs chemically from hydrocortisone butyrate, hydrocortisone probutate, and hydrocortisone valerate, which as midpotency steroids are stronger than hydrocortisone acetate. Similarly betamethasone dipropionate is stronger than betamethasone valerate. Halogenated steroids are usually stronger than nonhalogenated steroids.

Ointments are the most commonly chosen vehicle for treating AD. Corticosteroid ointments afford the advantage of occlusion, more effective penetration, and in general greater efficacy than equivalent cream or lotion formulations. Ointments are particularly effective in the management of dry, lichenified, or plaque-like areas of dermatitis. Ointment formulations, however, may occlude eccrine ducts, inducing sweat retention and pruritus, and hair follicles, leading to folliculitis. As with emollients, formulations in ointments may not be as well tolerated during the summer months of increased heat, perspiration, and high humidity. Creams and lotions are more cosmetically elegant and afford the advantages of greater convenience and acceptability

Table 3.2 Relative Potencies of Topical Corticosteroids (from Most Potent to Weakest)

Class	Drug	Dosage Form(s)	Strength (%)
I. VERY HIGH POTENCY			
	Augmented betamethasone dipropionate	Ointment	0.05
	Clobetasol propionate	Cream, ointment, foam	0.05
	Diflorasone diacetate	Ointment	0.05
	Halobetasol propionate	Cream, ointment	0.05
II. HIGH POTENCY			
	Amcinonide	Cream, lotion, ointment	0.1
	Augmented betamethasone dipropionate	Cream	0.05
	Betamethasone dipropionate	Cream, ointment, foam, solution	0.05
	Desoximetasone	Cream, ointment	0.25
	Desoximetasone	Gel	0.05
	Diflorasone diacetate	Cream	0.05
	Fluocinonide	Cream, ointment, gel, solution	0.05
	Halcinonide	Cream, ointment	0.1
	Mometasone furoate	Ointment	0.1
	Triamcinolone acetonide	Cream, ointment	0.5
III–IV. MEDIUM POTENCY			
	Betamethasone valerate	Cream, ointment, lotion, foam	0.1
	Clocortolone pivalate	Cream	0.1
	Desoximetasone	Cream	0.05
	Fluocinolone acetonide	Cream, ointment	0.025
	Flurandrenolide	Cream, ointment	0.05
	Fluticasone propionate	Cream	0.05
	Fluticasone propionate	Ointment	0.005
	Mometasone furoate	Cream	0.1
	Triamcinolone acetonide	Cream, ointment	0.1
V. LOWER-MEDIUM POTENCY			
	Hydrocortisone butyrate	Cream, ointment, solution	0.1
	Hydrocortisone probutate	Cream	0.1
	Hydrocortisone valerate	Cream, ointment	0.2
	Prednicarbate	Cream	0.1
VI. LOW POTENCY			
	Alclometasone dipropionate	Cream, ointment	0.05
	Desonide	Cream, gel, foam, ointment	0.05
	Fluocinolone acetonide	Cream, solution, oil	0.01
VII. LOWEST POTENCY			
	Dexamethasone	Cream	0.1
	Hydrocortisone	Creams, ointments, lotions, solutions	0.25, 0.5, 1
	Hydrocortisone acetate	Creams, ointments	0.5–1

during hot weather and in intertriginous areas but often contain additives that may be irritating or sensitizing. Traditional gels and foams are not well tolerated in individuals with AD, but they may be most effective in the management of acute weeping or vesicular lesions. Topical corticosteroids in emollient-based foam formulations and hydrocolloid gels (in contrast to the alcohol-containing foams and gels) are particularly useful for hairy areas, to avoid occlusion, and for cosmesis. Oil preparations are most commonly used for scalp dermatitis. Best applied to a wet scalp, oil formulations can be shampooed out after exposure for at least 1 hour to overnight. Fluocinolone acetonide oil, however, spreads easily and has been shown to be helpful after the bath for children with extensive AD.[232]

Occlusion of treated areas with polyethylene film such as Saran wrap or the use of flurandrenolide-impregnated polyethylene tape enhances the penetration of corticosteroids up to 100-fold. This mode of therapy is particularly effective for short periods (8 to 12 hours a

Box 3.2 Potential Side Effects of Topical Corticosteroids

Local Cutaneous Side Effects

Atrophy
Striae
Periorificial granulomatous dermatitis
Acne
Telangiectasia
Erythema
Hypopigmentation
Ocular effects
Cataracts
Glaucoma

Systemic Side Effects

Hypothalamic–pituitary–adrenal axis suppression

day on successive days) for patients with chronic lichenified or recalcitrant plaques of dermatitic skin. Occlusive techniques, however, are contraindicated for prolonged periods and are not recommended in infected or intertriginous areas. Given that the diaper is an occlusive dressing, application of steroids in the diaper area of infants should be avoided or limited to short-term use of low-strength topical steroids.

Concern about the use of topical steroids has led to "steroid phobia" among families and even physicians[233–235] internationally.[236] As a result, compliance may be decreased and weak topical steroids insufficient for adequate control may be used. In a recent study, 81% of parents or adult patients with AD had fears about the use of topical steroids, and 36% admitted nonadherence as a result.[237] Considering the widespread use of topical corticosteroids, few local adverse reactions occur when topical steroids are carefully chosen and used appropriately based on site of application and severity of the dermatitis (Fig. 3.36).[238] Recently, topical steroid addiction has been cited as an adverse effect of topical corticosteroids, but it is virtually never seen in children with AD who use topical steroids and should not discourage the use of topical steroids in pediatric patients. In older patients with AD, this disorder is characterized by a burning or stinging, sharply delineated erythematous eruption, primarily on the face and genital region, occurring days to weeks after discontinuation of prolonged, inappropriate, and frequent use of moderate- to high-potency topical corticosteroids.[239]

In general, group I corticosteroids are not recommended for patients younger than the age of 12 years, should not be used in

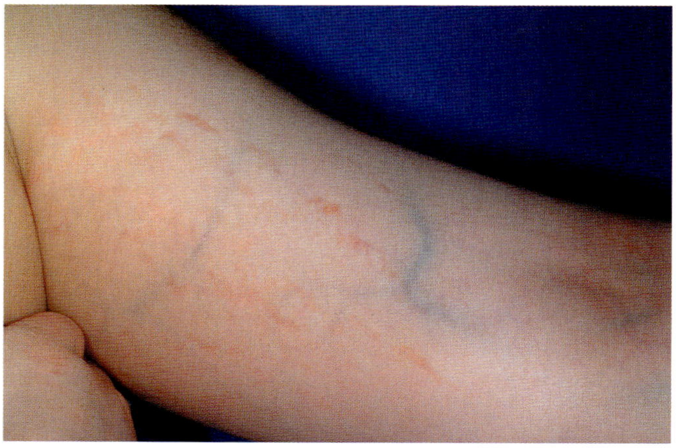

Fig. 3.36 Steroid-induced atrophy. Although unusual, steroid-induced atrophy in this patient with atopic dermatitis resulted from the twice-daily application of a class III–IV topical steroid over 1 year. Note the excellent control of the dermatitis but the obvious striae and prominence of veins because of atrophy of overlying skin.

intertriginous areas or under occlusion, and require a rest period after 14 days of use. Use of this group of ultrapotent steroids is usually reserved for lichenified plaques and recalcitrant dermatitis of the hands and feet and should be limited. Potent topical corticosteroids (class II) may safely be used once or twice daily for up to 2 weeks, except in sensitive areas, and are often applied at the first sign of flare to rapidly reverse the itch and inflammation.

A variety of steroid-free topical antiinflammatory agents have been introduced to allow patients to decrease their application of topical steroids and thus associated risks. Topical calcineurin inhibitors (TCIs; tacrolimus ointment 0.03% and pimecrolimus cream 1%) have been approved as alternative therapy for AD in children older than 2 years.[240,241] Several studies and anecdotal reports have suggested good efficacy and safety for tacrolimus ointment 0.1% (in children older than 2 years) and for tacrolimus 0.03% ointment and pimecrolimus cream in infants younger than 2 years, but their use is off-label.[242,243] Tacrolimus and pimecrolimus prevent the formation of a complex that includes calcineurin, a phosphatase.[244] Without this complex, the phosphate group from the nuclear factor of activated T cells (NF-AT) cannot be cleaved, the NF-AT transcription factor cannot be transported to the nucleus, and production of cytokines associated with T-cell activation is inhibited. Tacrolimus and pimecrolimus also inhibit mediator release from mast cells and basophils and decrease IgE receptor expression on cutaneous Langerhans cells.[245]

Tacrolimus ointment has good efficacy in children with moderate to severe AD.[246] The efficacy of the 0.1% ointment is comparable to a mid-potency topical corticosteroid,[247] and that of the 0.03% ointment to a low-potency steroid. Pimecrolimus cream is also comparable to a low-potency steroid and is indicated for pediatric patients with mild to moderate AD.[248,249] Assays of systemic absorption of tacrolimus and pimecrolimus have shown transient low levels in the blood, if at all, and no adverse effects on systemic immunity have been demonstrated.[246,250]

In 2006 the US Food and Drug Administration (FDA) placed a boxed warning on the class of calcineurin inhibitors based on the theoretical potential for TCIs to cause skin carcinogenesis and lymphoma. This theoretical risk was based on the known risk of malignancy (posttransplant lymphoproliferative disease and nonmelanoma skin cancer) in transplant patients who are profoundly immunosuppressed by systemically administered tacrolimus and in animal studies when treated with 26 to 47 times the maximum recommended dosage. Although a meta-analysis identified an increased risk of lymphoma in patients with severe AD, the number of malignancies and lymphomas is very low in AD children in postmarketing registries.[251–256] In addition, task forces of the American College of Allergy, Asthma, and Immunology; the American Academy of Allergy, Asthma, and Immunology; and the American Academy of Dermatology found no evidence to support the issuance of a black box warning.[257–260] Although preliminary data from a European cohort study suggested a borderline association of the use of tacrolimus in AD children and pediatric lymphoma, data did not account for disease severity.[261] There was also no evidence for an association of pimecrolimus with lymphoma. No lymphoma or nonmelanoma skin cancer occurred in a 10-year cohort study with almost 45,000 person-years of use of tacrolimus ointment.[262] Regardless of the limited evidence for risk, the boxed warning remains and patients need to be advised of potential risks and to practice sun protection during use.

To date, the only confirmed safety issue associated with the use of calcineurin inhibitors in children is burning or pruritus with application, described in the minority of affected children, particularly those with active inflammation. This sensation has been shown to result from stimulation of TRPV1 receptors in skin with depletion of substance P.[263] Calcineurin inhibitors do not have the atrophogenic potential of the corticosteroids and can be safely used on the head, neck, and intertriginous areas. Furthermore, no adverse effects on the eyes have been found, allowing safe application in periorbital areas. No increase in cutaneous infections has been noted in children.[264] Given that the potential local effect of TCI has been described more often when skin is inflamed, many practitioners recommend calming the inflammation with a short course of topical corticosteroids, then continuing with TCI to maintain control.

In 2016 the first topical phosphodiesterase 4 (PDE4) inhibitor (crisaborole) became commercially available for treating mild to moderate AD in children 2 years and older,[265,266] and subsequently 3 months of age. PDE4 activity is increased in AD and promotes degradation of cyclic adenosine monophosphate (cAMP). As a result, the cyclic AMP response is reduced and production of proinflammatory cytokines is increased in AD skin. Crisaborole has a good safety profile, although burning and stinging on application can occur in up to 50% of patients, particularly when applied to the face.[267]

The choice of topical steroid, TCI, or crisaborole depends on the severity and localization of the dermatitis, the age of the pediatric patient, and the history of use of topical antiinflammatory agents. For children with mild AD, intermittent use of a low-strength topical steroid with emollient application to maintain clearance usually suffices. However, children with moderate to severe disease often show a cycle of rapid recurrent flaring when topical antiinflammatory suppression is discontinued. A commonly used regimen to maintain control in these children while minimizing the risk of chronic steroid application is to apply mid- to high-potency topical steroids for acute flares (e.g., for a few days to up to 2 weeks twice daily), followed by a maintenance regimen. Alternative options for maintenance are "dialing down" to a low-strength topical corticosteroid, switching to a nonsteroidal topical agent (e.g., TCI or PDE4 inhibitor), or "proactive therapy" to retain control.[268–270] The typical regimen for proactive therapy is to taper use from twice daily (in response to a flare) to once daily for a week or two, and then two to three times a week on areas that are now clear or almost clear but recurrently flare without continued local immunosuppression.

For sites of severely lichenified dermatitis, salicylic acid can be compounded into preparations with steroids to improve penetration. Tar (liquor carbonis detergens or crude coal tar) can be also be used as an adjunctive therapy in patients with chronic dermatitis in the form of tar baths (e.g., Cutar) or compounded with topical corticosteroids (e.g., compounding triamcinolone 0.1% with 6% salicylic acid and 5% to 10% liquor carbonis detergens in Aquaphor ointment). The objectionable odor, staining properties, potential for irritation, risk of causing folliculitis, and low potential risk of later carcinogenesis make tar a choice only for only selected patients.

Several new nonsteroidal antiinflammatory medications are currently under development for AD and have shown promise in phase 2 trials. The topical aryl hydrocarbon receptor modulating agent (TAMA)[271] tapinarof was found to be superior to vehicle in patients with primarily moderate AD, approximately 30% of whom were adolescents. Several cytokines, including type 2 cytokines, require activation of the JAK/STAT signaling pathway. Topical formulations of JAK inhibitors (ruxolitinib and delgocitinib) have improved AD severity and reduced itch significantly more than vehicle[272,273] and numerically more than active comparators.

Role of Antihistamines

Reduction of the pruritus of AD is best achieved by reducing AD severity, generally through application of topical antiinflammatory medications. Sedating antihistamines (targeting the histamine 1 receptor), such as hydroxyzine, diphenhydramine, and doxepin, may help itchy children fall asleep, although they have little direct effect on the pruritus itself. Nonsedating antihistamines may be valuable as treatment for other atopic conditions such as AR and have been shown to decrease the risk of urticaria, but they have limited value in decreasing pruritus because they do not tend to be sedating.[274] Long-term use in young children has not led to behavioral, cognitive, or psychomotor developmental abnormalities.[275]

The histamine 4 receptor (H4R) is a recently discovered receptor subtype that has been shown to mediate the proinflammatory function of T cells, mast cells, eosinophils, and inflammatory dendritic epidermal cells. An oral antihistamine antagonist of H4R, adriforant, did not reduce the severity of adult moderate to severe AD when compared with placebo in a phase 2b trial.[276] Leukotriene antagonists such as montelukast, which are used extensively in asthma prophylaxis, have largely been ineffective.[277]

Treatment of Secondary Cutaneous Infections

Antistaphylococcal antibiotics are important in the management of patients with heavy *S. aureus* colonization or infection because of the role of *S. aureus* overgrowth in triggering dermatitis. Topical antibiotics, such as mupirocin or fusidic acid (the latter is not currently available in the United States), can be used for localized impetiginized lesions, but systemic antibiotics are required for more extensive involvement. Despite the increase in community-acquired (CA) MRSA nationally, most atopics still harbor MSSA.[100,105] As a result, cephalexin is still used most commonly (and successfully) to empirically treat secondarily infected dermatitis and will cover both staphylococcal and streptococcal organisms.[104] The chronic administration of antistaphylococcal therapy for AD should be avoided in an effort to minimize the risk of development of MRSA and *S. aureus* resistant to topical antibiotics.[278]

Dilute sodium hypochlorite (bleach) baths are now the standard of care as a maintenance measure for decreasing flares in moderate to severe AD. The addition of ½ cup of 5% to 6% sodium hydroxide per full tub of water (1 mL/L or 4 mL/gallon) markedly reduces the severity and extent of the dermatitis in children with a history of staphylococcal infections, although likely not because of any anti-bacterial properties, given its low concentration of sodium hypochlorite.[100,279,280] Even daily maintenance dilute sodium hypochlorite baths are generally well tolerated and may be needed for more severe AD. A washcloth can be used to distribute the bleach-bath water to the head and neck, avoiding the eyes and mouth. If skin erosions from secondary infection make bathing uncomfortable, postponing bleach baths until after the first few days of treatment may be necessary. If a bath is not possible, a 5- to 10-minute wet compress with bleach solution or a shower using a sodium hypochlorite–containing wash (such as CLn), or soaks of hands or feet can be used.[281] Application of mupirocin ointment to the nares and hands of patients and caregivers twice daily for 5 sequential days each month, and use of gentle antibacterial soaps[282] may also decrease colonization.

Antiviral treatment of cutaneous herpes simplex infections is important in preventing widespread dissemination, which rarely is life threatening. Administration of oral acyclovir (100 mg tid to qid for children younger than 6 years; 200 mg qid for older children; or for adolescents 500 mg valacyclovir twice daily) for a week usually controls the infection. More extensive involvement may require hospitalization and intravenous acyclovir treatment, especially in younger children. For children with recurrent EH, a course of prophylactic administration of oral acyclovir or valacyclovir once daily for 6 months or longer effectively suppresses the recurrences. Adjunctive therapies include topical compresses and concurrent administration of topical or systemic antibiotics if bacterial infection is also suspected. In general, topical corticosteroids can be continued during the course of systemic acyclovir therapy without affecting clearance of the viral infection if the dermatitis is problematic. Molluscum infections (see Chapter 15) can be managed by curettage after application of topical anesthetics[283] or by cantharidin application.[284] Children with molluscum and AD (but not nonatopic children) may show improvement in both their dermatitis and the molluscum lesions by treatment with high doses of oral cimetidine (40 mg/kg per day divided twice daily) for a 3-month course.[285,286] Imiquimod has not been found beneficial in double-blind, randomized trials.

Other Considerations for Atopic Dermatitis that Fails to Respond: Adherence and Alternative Diagnoses

Moderate to severe AD may be recalcitrant to topical antiinflammatory therapy. Although secondary staphylococcal infection is a common reason for recalcitrance, several other factors should be considered before initiating systemic immunosuppressive therapy or phototherapy.[287] Poor adherence is a major reason for failure to respond. In one study with electronic-cap monitoring to detect opening of tubes, mean adherence of patients with mild to moderate AD was 32%, increasing on or near office visit days.[288] Shortening the time between prescription of the medication and the follow-up office visit[289]; prescribing once-a-day treatment; using sticker charts to engage children[290]; providing adequate education about the disease, the use of treatment, and why it is needed; and adapting instruction on medication use to existing elements of the family routine (e.g., linking to bathing or brushing the teeth)[291] may be helpful.

Chronic, unresponsive dermatitis, especially involving the face, hands, or feet, may result from ACD,[292] and comprehensive patch testing should be undertaken (see Contact Dermatitis section). Several other alternative diagnoses that may require different intervention are described (see Differential Diagnosis section).

Management of Children with Severe Atopic Dermatitis Requiring Systemic Immunosuppressive Therapy

Systemic immunosuppressive therapy[293,294] and ultraviolet light treatment have long been considered the alternatives for children and adolescents with recalcitrant moderate to severe disease. Narrow-band ultraviolet B light therapy, which avoids intervention with systemic immunosuppressive therapy, has been reported to cause at least moderate improvement in 89% of children and complete clearance in 40% during a median of 3 months.[295] Significant reductions in severity can be seen in as little as 3 weeks after initiation.[296] Nevertheless, the requirement for frequent treatments in a medical office (two to three times weekly) and holding still in a hot, enclosed box while wearing protective goggles, as well as the unknown risk of long-term cutaneous damage from ultraviolet light, complicate the use of this form of therapy for most pediatric patients. Home-based therapy may be an option, but phototherapy units are costly.

Systemic immunosuppressants have more often been the choice as intervention, and have been used by approximately 1% of AD patients overall[296–298] (despite 7% with AD having severe disease). Pediatric AD guidelines for the two most commonly used immunosuppressants, cyclosporine and methotrexate, are similar to those for pediatric psoriasis.[299] Their use has been limited by the potential risks of immunosuppressant therapy and requirement for laboratory monitoring. Dupilumab, the first targeted AD therapy, inhibits the shared receptor for IL-4 and IL-14 (IL-4R). Dupilumab was FDA approved for adolescents in 2019 and for children ages 6 to 11 years in 2020.

Systemic Immunosuppressant Therapy

Systemic corticosteroid therapy is effective for most patients with AD, but the rapid rebound after discontinuation of therapy and high risk of potential side effects make its use impractical for patients with AD and contraindicated for most pediatric patients.[300] Systemic administration of nonsteroidal antiinflammatory medications to children with AD has largely replaced the use of systemic corticosteroids by pediatric dermatologists in the management of more recalcitrant severe AD, but systemic steroids are still the most commonly used systemic medication overall for pediatric AD.[298]

Cyclosporine has the most rapid onset of action and greatest efficacy among the nontargeted systemic agents, but also the highest risk of potential side effects.[301] Therapy is initiated with 3 to 5 mg/kg per day (microemulsion for preferred). Response may be seen within 1 to 3 months, but medication should be tapered once significant improvement is achieved; trough levels can be determined in patients without a sufficient response to determine if a higher dosage can be administered. Discontinuation of treatment usually leads to relapse flares, but low-dose continuing treatment or intermittent courses in children can be effective.[302–304] In one study that predated the availability of dupilumab, cyclosporine was the most common first-line agent for treating pediatric AD severe enough to require medication.[305] Several experts now recommend initial treatment with cyclosporine to rapidly suppress the severe AD (e.g., for 3 months) followed by continued treatment with an alternative, safer immunosuppressant, such as methotrexate or mycophenolate mofetil, or with ultraviolet light, should immunomodulatory agents be inavailable or ineffective. Renal and hepatic function and blood pressure must be carefully monitored during cyclosporine therapy.

Methotrexate is a safer alternative to cyclosporine as first-line or maintenance therapy after cyclosporine-induced improvement.[306–308] Its major limitation is the delay in onset of action compared with cyclosporine, a limitation that is shared with mycophenolate mofetil and azathioprine. Continued improvement in severity and quality of life can occur beyond 10 months after initiation.[306] However, methotrexate can be effective or very effective in 75% of children with severe AD. In general, treatment is well tolerated (in one study, 14% experienced minor nausea and 14% had slight elevation in hepatic transaminases) and serious adverse events are quite rare. Low-dose therapy (0.3 to 0.5 mg/kg per week)[309] is administered with folic supplementation. Although not studied in AD, for pediatric psoriasis a 6- to 7-day per week regimen of folic acid was found to be more effective in limiting gastrointestinal toxicity than weekly folic acid administration. The need for a small test dose of methotrexate has not been demonstrated. Complete blood cell counts and hepatic transaminates should be monitored at least monthly during the first 6 months and then quarterly.

Mycophenolate mofetil has been found to cause at least 60% improvement in 91% of treated children with a dosage of 40 to 50 mg/kg per day for children and 30 to 40 mg/kg per day for adolescents with maximal effects at 8 to 12 weeks.[310] Complete blood cell counts and liver function testing should be performed.

Azathioprine (2.5 to 3.5 mg/kg per day) has effectively suppressed severe, recalcitrant AD in 58% to 92% of children during a 3-month trial.[311–313] Pretreatment determination of thiopurine methyltransferase level can predict the risk of developing myelosuppression, and hepatic functions should also be monitored. In one study the thiopurine methyltransferase (TPMT) levels changed unpredictably during treatment in 25% of patients, suggesting that periodic assessment of TPMT levels is warranted to optimize clinical response.[313] Azathioprine should be used with caution, given its recent link with hepatosplenic T-cell lymphoma.

Interferon-γ downregulates Th2 lymphocyte function, and treatment with recombinant interferon-γ (50 μg/m² daily or every other day) has led to improvement in some patients, including pediatric patients.[314–316] Flu-like symptoms are particularly common early in the treatment course. The high price and benefit for only a subset of individuals also limit the use of interferon-γ in children who are severely affected with AD.

Targeted Immunomodulatory Agents

The increased understanding of the pathogenesis of AD, including in children, has led to an extensive pipeline of new therapeutics in trial for AD[317] and generation of biologics that specifically target Th2 pathway components. As noted, dupilumab inhibits activation of the shared receptor (IL4Rα) of key type 2 cytokines IL-4 and IL-13. For all dosing, a loading dose double the treatment dose is given. The pivotal double-blind, randomized controlled trial in 251 adolescents with moderate to severe AD showed achievement of the co-primary endpoints of Investigator Global Assessment (IGA), clear (0) to almost clear (1) (24% on dupilumab every 2 weeks vs. 2% on placebo), and at least a 75% reduction from baseline on the Eczema Area and Severity Index (EASI-75) in 42% using dupilumab every 2 weeks vs. 8% placebo.[318,319] In general, administration every 2 weeks was superior to every 4 weeks. In *post hoc* analyses, 80% of adolescents taking dupilumab every 2 weeks (versus 24% on placebo) who did not achieve IGA 0/1 at week 16 achieved meaningful improvement from baseline ($p < .0001$).[319] Dosing is weight based at 200 mg every other week for those less than 60 kg and 300 mg every other week for those 60 kg and more; a loading dose of twice the standard dose is given initially. In the phase 3 trial for 6- to 11-year-olds, approximately 30% achieved IGA 0/1 and approximately 70% EASI-75, regardless of whether given every 2 or every 4 weeks, versus 11% and 27% on placebo, respectively.[319,320] However, dosing of 300 mg every 4 weeks for children <30 kg and 200 mg every 2 weeks gave superior blood levels and efficacy, resulting in these on-label dosing recommendations. At the time of writing, trials were ongoing for pediatric patients as young as 6 months.

The side effect profile of dupilumab in pediatric patients shows the risk of injection site reactions, as with other biologics. Conjunctivitis has been seen at about twice the frequency in those on dupilumab versus placebo in trials, but rarely leads to discontinuation (Fig. 3.37). In the adolescent trial the occurrence of bacterial infection was reduced and dupilumab improved comorbid asthma and allergic rhinitis, reducing IgE concentrations for food and aeroallergens.[319] Dupilumab has not been found to suppress vaccine-induced immunity[321] in adults.

Increased facial erythema, despite improved severity elsewhere, is not an uncommon experience with dupilumab and may be related to unmasking of contact dermatitis[322–324] (see Contact Dermatitis section). In fact, recall dermatitis at the site of previous positive patch tests has been shown to occur after injection of dupilumab[325] and patch testing may still be possible although sometimes suppressed.[323] Other possible causes of increased facial erythema include *Malassezia* reactivity, Demodex, or the need for higher dosing. Psoriasis-like

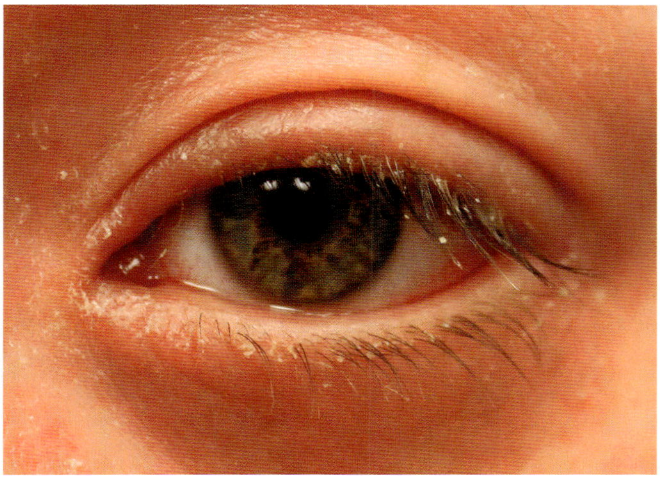

Fig. 3.37 Conjunctivitis, blepharitis, and concomitant periorbital dermatitis (edema, erythema, and scaling) that developed while using dupilumab therapy. Inflammation of the bulbar conjunctiva is occasionally seen with use of dupilumab, but the eyelids and periorbital area are a common site of allergic contact dermatitis.

lesions have been reported in a minority of patients given dupilumab after clearance or near-clearance of the dermatitis. In addition, although alopecia areata has been reported to reverse with treatment in those with concomitant AD and alopecia areata,[326–330] dupilumab-induced alopecia during dupilumab therapy with reversal after drug discontinuation has also been described.[331,332]

Several additional targeted systemic approaches to improving AD are currently being studied and appear promising in early trials. Most advanced are the IL-13 inhibitors (lebrikizumab[333] and tralokinumab),[334] based on the predominance of the type 2 cytokine IL-13 in AD skin, and JAK inhibitors (baricitinib,[335] abrocitinib [primarily JAK1],[336] and upadacitinib[337] [primarily JAK1]), based on the concept that signaling in AD is primarily through JAK1. Nemolizumab targets the "itch-specific" cytokine IL-31 and strongly suppresses the itch but has little antiinflammatory effect.[338–340]

Use of Complementary Treatment Approaches

The impact of vitamin D_3 levels and potential value of vitamin D_3 supplementation remain controversial. Low levels of vitamin D_3, including in cord blood,[341] have been associated with childhood AD,[342,343] and AD severity may be greater with lower vitamin D levels.[344] Oral vitamin D_3 has been shown to upregulate the expression of cathelicidin, including in the skin of individuals with AD. However, topically applied vitamin D_3 analogue irritates AD skin and has been used to generate a mouse model of AD. Although one small open-label study of oral vitamin D_3 supplementation in children with AD who were vitamin D deficient showed clinical improvement,[345] small double-blind trials show improved serum levels of vitamin D_3 with supplementation but no clinical improvement in AD.[344,346] At this time there is insufficient evidence to recommend vitamin D_3 supplementation for AD.[347]

Alternative medicine, particularly herbal remedies and homeopathy, is used in 42.5% to 63.5% of patients with AD.[348,349] More than half reported no improvement but tried the therapies based on recommendation from nonphysicians, concern about the potential risks of topical steroids, and dissatisfaction with conventional treatment. Of concern is that these complementary approaches have potential side effects, have not been adequately tested for safety and efficacy, and require time and effort that might otherwise be directed toward use of physician-prescribed treatment. The benefit from administration of traditional Chinese herbal therapy has been variable.[350–352] Regardless, the demonstration of hepatic toxicity, cardiac adverse events, and idiosyncratic reactions from this therapy has raised concerns; furthermore, the discovery of glucocorticoid contamination in some preparations warns that these alternative agents be used with caution.[353]

Massage therapy has been advocated as a means to improve the clinical signs of AD in young children, in addition to improving the psychological well-being of the patients and family members.[354] Psychological counseling, behavioral modification, hypnotherapy, and biofeedback can also be helpful in decreasing scratching.[157] Psychological intervention for families can also be beneficial, because increased parental stress and depression correlate with higher levels of biologic markers of inflammation.[355]

Pityriasis Alba

Pityriasis alba is a common cutaneous disorder, especially in children with darker skin, characterized by asymptomatic hypopigmented patches, usually on the face, neck, upper trunk, and proximal extremities (Figs. 3.38 and 3.39).[356,357] Individual lesions vary from 1 cm or more in diameter and may show a fine scale. This disorder is thought to represent a nonspecific dermatitis with residual postinflammatory hypopigmentation and occurs more often in individuals with darker skin types.[358] Histologic evaluation shows normal numbers of melanocytes but decreased epidermal melanosomes and melanocyte degeneration.[359] Most cases appear after sun exposure because

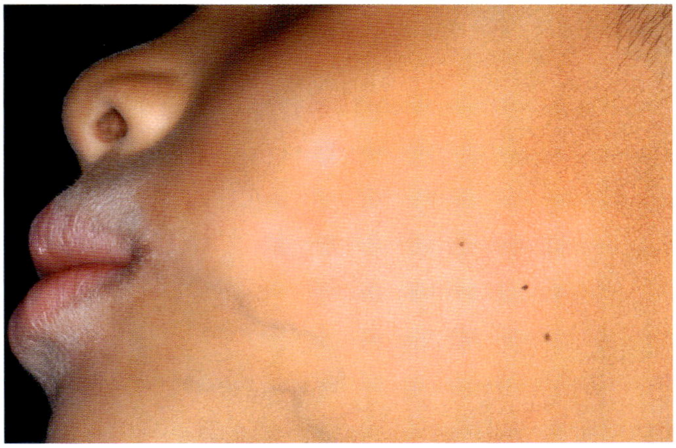

Fig. 3.38 Pityriasis alba. Circumscribed scaly hypopigmented lesions on the cheek. These patches are thought to represent postinflammatory hypopigmentation and are most easily visible in children with darker skin. Note the concomitant lip-licker's dermatitis.

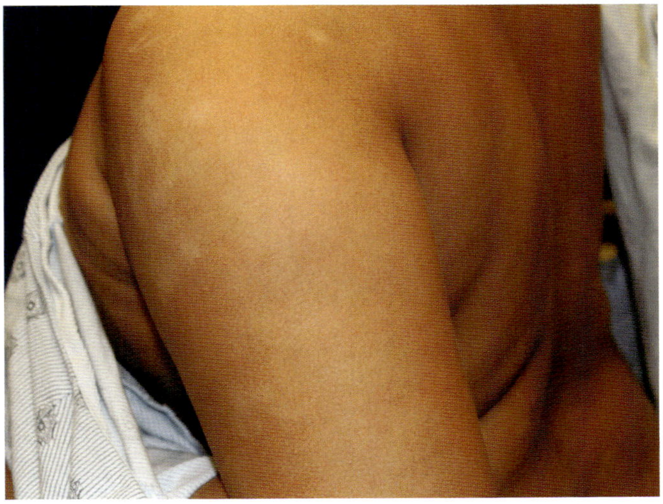

Fig. 3.39 Pityriasis alba. The upper arm is another common site.

of the contrast that results between areas that can show a pigmentary response to ultraviolet light and the pityriasis alba areas that do not.

The differential diagnosis of the hypopigmented macules of pityriasis alba includes tinea versicolor, vitiligo, and the white macules seen in association with tuberous sclerosis; nevus depigmentosus; cutaneous T-cell lymphoma; leprosy; postinflammatory hypopigmentation secondary to atopic dermatitis, psoriasis, tinea corporis, or pityriasis rosea; and, in light-skinned individuals, nevus anemicus. Application of mild topical corticosteroids or calcineurin inhibitors for a few weeks followed by frequent moisturization and protection of the sites and surrounding area from sun exposure allows repigmentation of involved areas. Patients and parents should be warned that, as with any form of postinflammatory hypopigmentation, repigmentation may take several months to years. Effective moisturization during drier months may help prevent recurrence of the pityriasis alba in subsequent summers.

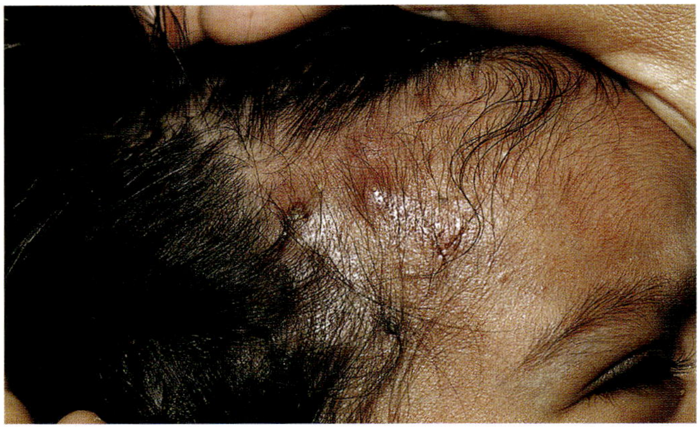

Fig. 3.41 Hyperimmunoglobulinemia E syndrome (HIES). In addition to atopic dermatitis, most infants and children with HIES show erythematous, slightly purulent cold abscesses, shown here on the forehead and scalp. (Reprinted with permission from Bolognia JL, Jorizzo JL, Rapini RP. *Dermatology*. St. Louis, MO: Elsevier; 2003.)

Hyperimmunoglobulinemia E Syndrome

HIES[360–364] is a rare immunodeficiency disorder characterized by very high levels of IgE in association with AD and recurrent cutaneous and sinopulmonary infections.[365–367] The AD is seen in 100% of patients, usually within the first 6 months, and is of variable severity (Fig. 3.40). Most patients have an autosomal dominant form (AD-HIES), a subset of which has been called *Job syndrome*. AD-HIES results from mutations in the gene encoding signal transducer and activator of transcription 3 *(STAT3)*.[368,369]

Many neonates or infants with AD-HIES have pruritic papulopustules, especially on the face, which show eosinophilic folliculitis or eosinophilic dermatitis by biopsy of lesional skin.[370] Infections often begin during the first 3 months of life. Cutaneous candidiasis may also be an early clinical feature (83%). Cutaneous *S. aureus* infections may take the form of excoriated crusted plaques, pustules, furuncles, cellulitis, paronychia, lymphangitis, or abscesses, especially on the neck, scalp, periorbital areas, axillae, and groin (Fig. 3.41). The abscesses are slightly erythematous and tender but not nearly to the degree expected for a normal individual. Although some patients demonstrate cutaneous manifestations only,[371] patients with HIES usually have recurrent bronchitis and pneumonias with resultant empyema, bronchiectasis, and in 77% of patients, pneumatocele formation. The pneumatoceles tend to persist and become the site of further infections with bacteria *(Pseudomonas)* or fungi *(Aspergillus, Scedosporium)*. Rarely, massive hemoptysis ensues. Other common sites of infection include the ears, oral mucosae, sinuses, and eyes. Visceral infections other than pneumonia are unusual.

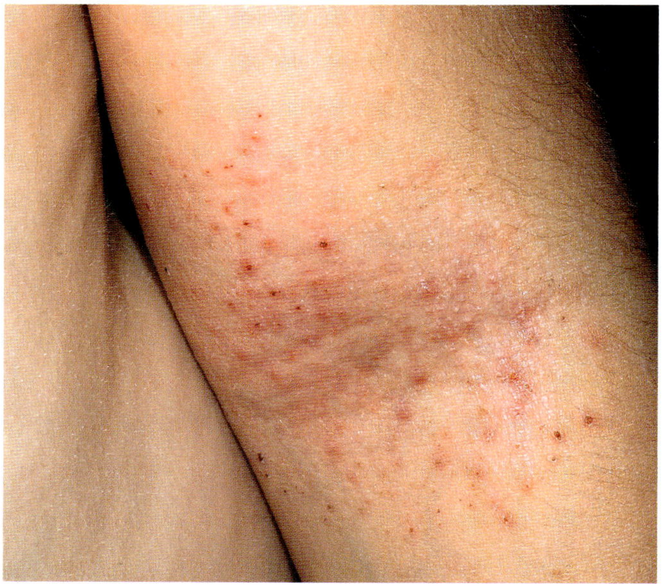

Fig. 3.40 Hyperimmunoglobulinemia E syndrome with atopic dermatitis of the antecubital area.

By late childhood and adolescence, patients with HIES begin to develop characteristic facial features with thickened, doughy skin, prominent forehead, broad nose, deep-set eyes, pitted scars, and prominent follicular ostia,[365] perhaps reflecting bony abnormalities and recurrent facial abscesses. Osteopenia is usually detected by adolescence or early adulthood, and patients have an increased risk of bone fractures, often because of unrecognized or minor trauma.[372] Scoliosis occurs in 64% of patients 16 years of age or older, and hyperextensibility of joints has been reported in 70% of patients. Dental abnormalities associated with HIES syndrome include retention of primary teeth, lack of eruption of secondary teeth, and delayed resorption of the roots of primary teeth.[373] Focal brain hyperintensities and an increased incidence of lymphoma are other features. Patients with HIES of intermediate phenotypes that include staphylococcal and mucocutaneous candidal infections may have *STAT3* mosaicism.[374]

The abnormalities in *STAT3* signaling impair Th17-cell development, leading to insufficient expression of IL-17 and IL-22, which drive expression of antimicrobial peptides, thus promoting *S. aureus* and candidal infections.[375]

The diagnosis of HIES is largely based on clinical findings and the presence of very high levels of IgE. There are no specific tests to confirm the diagnosis other than the finding of HIES-related mutations. Patients have markedly elevated levels of polyclonal IgE. Although levels of more than 2000 IU/mL are needed to consider the diagnosis in older children and adults, the normal levels of IgE in infants (0 to 50 IU/mL) are considerably lower than those in older children. A 10-fold increase in IgE levels above normal levels for age should trigger consideration of HIES, although these levels of IgE are more common in AD without HIES.[376] Affected individuals tend to have IgE antibodies directed against *S. aureus* and candida. Levels of IgE are not related to clinical course and may decrease to normal in affected adults. Approximately 93% of patients have eosinophilia of the blood and sputum. Abnormal polymorphonuclear leukocyte and monocyte chemotaxis has been noted but is intermittent and not correlated with infection. Cell-mediated immunity (Th1 driven) is often abnormal as well and may manifest as anergy to skin testing, altered responses in mixed leukocyte culture, and impaired blastogenic responses to specific antigens such as *Candida* and tetanus. The decrease in memory ($CD27^+$) B cells is noted in 80% of patients, in contrast to individuals with AD and high levels of IgE.[377]

Autosomal recessive HIES (AR-HIES)[367,378,379] is much less common than AD-HIES. In 78% of cases, it results from loss-of-function mutations in *DOCK8* (dedicator of cytokinesis 8), which is highly expressed in lymphocytes and regulates the actin cytoskeleton.[379] In a large series of 64 DOCK8-deficient patients, 62% had low IgM levels, less than 50% were able to mount recall immune responses, and 20% had lymphopenia, in addition to the typical hyper IgE and eosinophilia.[379] Early AD was a feature in 97% of patients, with almost 70% having severe AD. The neonatal eosinophilic skin eruption was only described in 35%. Abscesses occur in 60% but tend to be more inflamed than the cold abscesses of AD-HIES. Upper respiratory infections and allergies (>70%) are also shared features with AD-HIES. Cardinal features that are not part of the *STAT3*-deficient form include severe viral infections (extensive warts and molluscum, herpes, and life-threatening cytomegalovirus infections), early malignancy (cutaneous and mucosal squamous cell carcinomas in 8%[380]) neurologic changes (primarily aneurysms and strokes; 36%), and an increased risk of autoimmune issues (anemia, thrombocytopenia, and vasculitis).[381,382] In contrast to STAT3 deficiency, pneumatoceles and parenchymal lung abnormalities are unusual, and patients fail to show the bone fractures and retention of primary teeth of the dominant form. DOCK8 deficiency leads to impaired migration of dendritic cells to lymph nodes and defective CD4 T-cell priming. In B cells, DOCK8 also serves as an adaptor protein upstream of STAT3, which likely accounts for some of the overlap with AD-HIES. The T-cell lymphopenia and low interferon-γ production contribute to the high risk of viral infections.

The majority of patients AR-HIES without *DOCK8* mutations have biallelic mutations in *PGM3*,[383] the gene encoding phosphoglucomutase 3, leading to impaired synthesis of UDP-GlcNAc (uridine diphosphate N-acetylglucosamine), which is an important precursor for protein glycosylation. Although *PGM3* mutations may lead to SCID, patients with milder disease have high levels of IgE, atopy, and frequent sinopulmonary infections with bronchiectasis, as well as neurocognitive impairment. Autoimmune disorders and increases in Th17 cells are distinguishing features. Joint hyperextensibility and scoliosis have been described. AR-HIES can also result from homozygous mutations in *TYK2* (which activates STAT3), although *TYK2* mutations are usually associated with more profound immunodeficiency. Nontuberculous mycobacterial infections are a characteristic feature of patients with *TYK2* mutations.[384,385]

HIES must be distinguished from a number of other disorders in which IgE levels may be elevated. Most common is AD (including *CARD11* heterozygous loss-of-function mutations), which shows similar inflammatory cutaneous features and often very high levels of IgE, especially if severe[376]; the concurrent presence of abscesses, coarse facies, noncutaneous infections, and dental and bony abnormalities in HIES may enable differentiation. WAS can be distinguished by thrombocytopenia with cutaneous petechiae and hemorrhagic episodes. Eosinophilia and elevations of IgE levels with dermatitis can also be seen in patients with DiGeorge syndrome, the Omenn syndrome type of SCID, graft-versus-host disease (GVHD), and selective IgA deficiency. Loss-of-function mutations in *ERBB2IP*, including ERBIN, leads to a phenotype with hyper IgE, eosinophilic esophagitis, and allergic manifestations of AD-HIES but without mucosal *Candida* infections and with the addition of hypermobility and vascular abnormalities.[386] Homozygous mutations in *IL6ST*, encoding the GP130 cytokine receptor subunit required for cytokine signaling (e.g., IL-6, oncostain M; all through JAK-STAT signaling), lead to hyper IgE, eosinophilia, AD, recurrent infections, bronchiectasis, and scoliosis, as well as craniosynostosis.[387]

The mainstay of therapy for HIES is antistaphylococcal antibiotics, and patients are usually treated prophylactically with trimethoprim-sulfamethoxazole. When other bacterial or fungal infections develop, infections must be treated with appropriate alternative antibiotics. Recombinant interferon-γ has shown inconsistent efficacy. The cutaneous and pulmonary abscesses often require incision and drainage. The pneumatoceles should be removed surgically, especially if present for longer than 6 months, to prevent microbial superinfection. Therapy for AD as discussed in previous sections is also useful for HIES; omalizumab has improved the severe dermatitis of a recalcitrant patient with a relatively low level of IgE.[388] Alendronate sodium may alleviate the osteopenia.[372]

Early stem cell transplantation is an important intervention for patients with AR-HIES from *DOCK8* mutations,[389] which has a 34% mortality rate.[379] Hematopoietic stem cell transplantation is not a treatment of choice for AD-HIES unless there are severe complications, such as lymphoproliferative disease.

Wiskott–Aldrich Syndrome

WAS is a rare X-linked recessive disorder that in its classic form consists of dermatitis that meets criteria for AD, bleeding from microthrombocytopenia and platelet dysfunction, and recurrent severe pyogenic infections.[390–392] Bleeding is the most common manifestation, but the presence of mild to severe AD distinguishes WAS from X-linked thrombocytopenia and X-linked neutropenia with myelodysplasia, which are both allelic. The majority of patients are male, but full expression has been reported in girls.[393]

The dermatitis usually develops during the first few months of life and fulfils criteria for AD (Fig. 3.42). Excoriated areas commonly have serosanguineous crust and often show petechiae or purpura. IgE-mediated allergic problems such as urticaria, food allergies, and asthma are also seen with increased frequency.

The hemorrhagic diathesis results from both quantitative and qualitative defects in platelets. Platelets from patients with WAS are small and structurally abnormal with a reduced half-life, although megakaryocyte numbers are normal. Epistaxis and bloody diarrhea are often the initial manifestations. Mucocutaneous petechiae and ecchymoses (Fig. 3.42), spontaneous bleeding from the oral cavity, hematemesis, melena, and hematuria are common, but the severity varies.

Recurrent bacterial infections begin in infancy as placentally transmitted maternal antibody levels diminish and include staphylococcal impetigo, furunculosis, otitis externa and media, pneumonia, pansinusitis, conjunctivitis, meningitis, and septicemia. Infections with encapsulated bacteria such as pneumococcus, *Haemophilus influenzae*, and *Neisseria meningitidis* predominate. With advancing age, T-cell function progressively deteriorates and patients become increasingly susceptible to infections caused by herpes and other viruses and to *Pneumocystis jiroveci*.

Additional clinical features may be hepatosplenomegaly, lymphadenopathy, and autoimmune complications. The most common autoimmune complication is hemolytic anemia, occurring in 36% of patients and usually before 5 years of age.[394] Other autoimmune disorders that clearly seem linked to WAS are autoimmune neutropenia (25%),

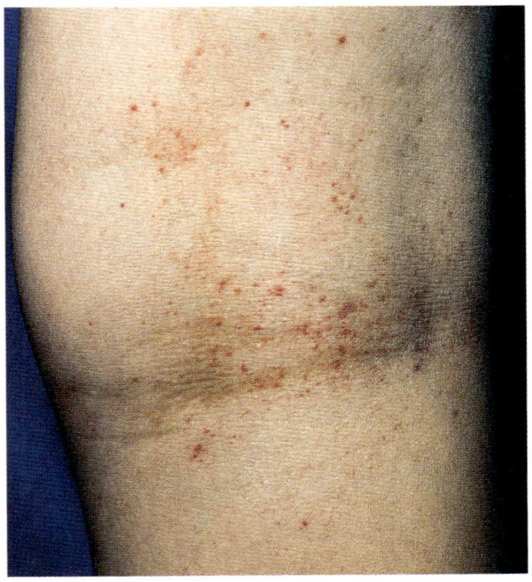

Fig. 3.42 A bleeding diathesis as a result of thrombocytopenia and platelet dysfunction, the most common manifestation in patients with Wiskott–Aldrich syndrome (WAS), may appear as petechiae, ecchymoses, and purpuric patches. The dermatitis of patients with WAS is indistinguishable from atopic dermatitis.

arthritis (29%), IgA nephropathy, and central nervous system vasculitis and painful cutaneous small-vessel vasculitis (22%), which can appear as purplish induration of skin and soft tissues.

The clinical course of WAS is progressive, usually resulting in death by adolescence without transplantation. Overall, 40% of patients die of infection, 21% of hemorrhage (usually intracranial), and 25% of malignant neoplasia. Lymphoreticular malignancies occur overall in 13% to 22% of patients,[395] with an average age of onset of 9.5 years. Non-Hodgkin lymphoma[395,396] is the most common malignancy and is often linked to Epstein–Barr (EBV) infection, and extranodal and brain involvement predominate. Fewer than 5% who develop lymphoma survive more than 2 years.

Individuals with WAS have mutations in the gene that encodes WAS protein (WASp), and the extent of WASp depletion correlates with disease severity. WASp, through complexing with other proteins, activates Arp2/3 and ultimately polymerizes the actin cytoskeleton to enable cell movement, formation of dendrites and of immune synapses, T-cell activation, and B-cell homeostasis. Platelet abnormalities result from defective migration in proplatelet formation, inherent platelet defects increasing fragility, and autoimmunity against platelets. T-regulatory cell dysfunction has been blamed for the increased risk of autoimmune complications. The mechanism for the AD is not defined but could relate to T-cell activation defects and the abnormal interactions of WAS Langerhans cells with T cells after antigenic stimulation.

Laboratory studies show thrombocytopenia in 100% of patients, with platelets usually less than 80,000/mm^3 and often less than 20,000/mm^3. Platelets tend to be small, and aggregation is sometimes defective. Eosinophilia is common, but lymphopenia is not usually seen until after 6 to 8 years of age. Total serum γ-globulin is usually normal, but levels of IgM are often low, with variable IgG levels and increased levels of IgA, IgE, and IgD. The number of T lymphocytes and response *in vitro* to mitogens may be normal in early life but often decreases with advancing age. Delayed hypersensitivity skin-test reactions are usually absent, and antibody responses to polysaccharide antigens are markedly diminished.

Several conditions may be confused with WAS. Many other immunodeficiencies are characterized by dermatitis, increased susceptibility to infections, and the development of malignancy but do not share the bleeding diathesis. The clinical findings of hemorrhage, petechiae, and recurrent sinopulmonary infections in WAS help to differentiate WAS from AD.

Bone marrow transplantation with human leukocyte antigen (HLA)-identical marrow is the treatment of choice. Full engraftment results in normal platelet numbers and functions, immunologic status, and, if T lymphocytes engraft, clearance of the dermatitis.[397] Optimal survival occurs with matched sibling donors and allogeneic transplantation before age 5 years (87%). Despite the good result of matched unrelated donors in young children (71%), there is a higher risk of acute GVHD after transplant (56%) versus matched siblings (16%).[398] Mixed chimerism (i.e., engraftment of T cells but not myeloid or B cells) increases greatly the risk of chronic GVHD. If a matched donor is unavailable, infusion of autologous stem cells modified *ex vivo* by gene therapy is an alternative approach.[399]

Appropriate antibiotics and transfusions of platelets and plasma decrease the risk of fatal infections and hemorrhage. Intravenous infusions of γ-globulin are also useful in patients. Topical corticosteroids may improve the dermatitis, and chronic administration of oral acyclovir is appropriate for patients with EH. Splenectomy has been used selectively for patients with severe platelet abnormalities; however, splenectomy increases the risk of infection by encapsulated organisms, markedly increasing the risk of mortality after transplantation. Children with WAS are unable to mount immune responses after administration of vaccines against encapsulated organisms. Rituximab has been used successfully in some children with EBV-induced lymphoma to prolong survival.[400]

Lichen Simplex Chronicus

Lichen simplex chronicus (circumscribed neurodermatitis) is a localized, chronic pruritic disorder characterized by patches of dermatitis that result from repeated itching, scratching, and rubbing of the involved area. The pruritus may begin in an area of normal-appearing skin or may be initiated in a preexisting lesion of atopic, seborrheic, or contact dermatitis, lichen planus, or psoriasis.

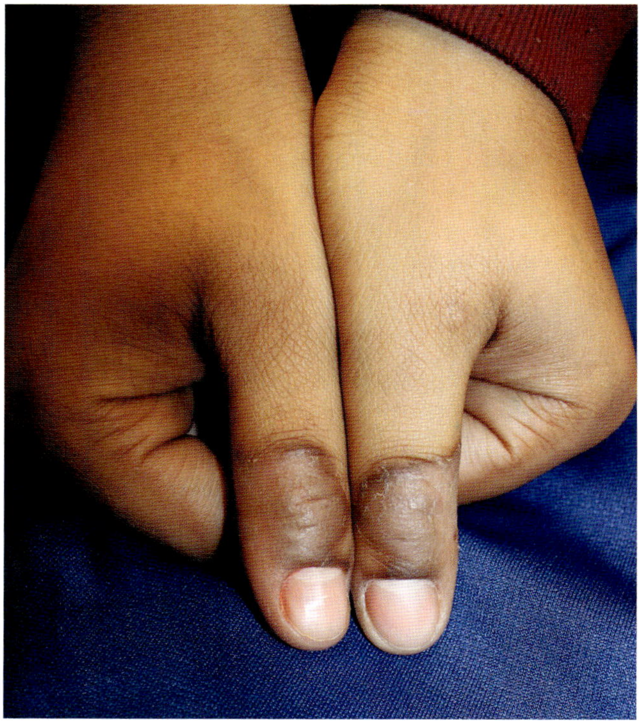

Fig. 3.43. Lichen simplex chronicus. Localized plaques of dermatitis result from repeated rubbing or scratching of the involved area.

Lesions of lichen simplex chronicus generally occur in adolescents or adults but may be seen in younger children. The disorder may develop at any location on the body, but the most common areas of involvement are those that are easily reached and may be scratched unobtrusively (particularly during periods of tension and concentration). These include the nape or sides of the neck, wrists, ankles, hands, and pretibial areas. Other common sites of involvement include the inner aspects of the thighs, vulva, scrotum, and perianal areas.

The clinical features of lichen simplex chronicus include single or multiple oval plaques with a long axis that usually measure up to 15 cm in diameter (Fig. 3.43). During the early stages, the skin is reddened and slightly edematous with exaggerated skin markings. Older, more typical lesions are characterized by well-circumscribed, dry, thickened, scaling, pruritic, often hyperpigmented plaques.

The diagnosis of lichen simplex chronicus is dependent on the presence of pruritic lichenified plaques in the characteristic sites of predilection. Lesions of tinea corporis may be differentiated by a lack of lichenification, by the presence of a scaly border (often with clearing in the center), by demonstration of hyphae on microscopic examination of skin scrapings, and by fungal culture. Psoriatic plaques generally may be differentiated by a characteristic thick, adherent white or silvery scale, their underlying deep red hue, and characteristic areas of involvement. Lesions of AD may be differentiated by history, more poorly demarcated lesions, the presence of atopic stigmata, and a tendency toward involvement in antecubital and popliteal areas.

The successful management of lichen simplex chronicus depends on an appreciation of the itch-scratch-itch cycle and the associated scratching and rubbing that accompany and perpetuate this disorder. Topical application of potent corticosteroids, under occlusion if necessary, and the administration of systemic antihistamines (such as diphenhydramine or hydroxyzine) usually induces remission of the pruritus and the eruption within a period of several weeks. Use of tap water compresses before application of the topical corticosteroid or compounding topical steroid with salicylic acid (e.g., 6% salicylic acid and 0.1% triamcinolone powder in hydrophilic ointment) may increase penetration of the topical antiinflammatory agent. Other techniques include application overnight of flurandrenolide-impregnated tape, protection from scratching and rubbing by occluding with adherent dressings, and injection of intralesional triamcinolone acetonide (e.g., 5 to 10 mg/mL) in tolerant adolescents.

Seborrheic Dermatitis

Seborrheic dermatitis refers to a self-limiting erythematous, scaly, or crusting eruption that occurs primarily in the so-called "seborrheic areas" (those with the highest concentration of sebaceous glands), namely the scalp, face, and postauricular, presternal, and intertriginous areas. Seborrheic dermatitis in the pediatric population is most commonly seen in infants and adolescents. The cause of seborrheic dermatitis is not well understood. Its predilection for areas of high sebaceous gland density and the correlation of activity with increased hormonal levels during the first year of life[401] and adolescence suggests a relation to sebum and sebaceous glands. Seborrheic dermatitis of adolescence and adulthood has been attributed to *Pityrosporum ovale (Malassezia ovalis)*, a lipophilic yeast normally found in abundance on the human scalp.[402] However, the relationship between seborrheic dermatitis in infants and that of adolescents and adults is controversial. It is unclear if this organism plays a causal role in disease in infants.[403,404] Many infantile cases improve with topical ketoconazole, suggesting that overgrowth of yeast may, at least in some instances, play a role in the pathogenesis of this disorder.

Seborrheic dermatitis appears in infancy between the second and tenth week of life (usually the third or fourth) and peaks in incidence at 3 months of age.[405] Infantile seborrheic dermatitis often begins with a noneczematous, erythematous, scaly dermatitis of the scalp (termed *cradle cap*) or the diaper area and is manifested by thin dry scales or sharply defined round or oval patches covered by thick, yellowish brown, greasy crusts. Although the condition is limited to the scalp in most affected infants, it may progress to the forehead, ears, eyebrows, nose, and back of the head (see Figs. 3.3 and 2.27). Erythematous greasy, salmon-colored, sharply marginated scaly patches may also involve the intertriginous and flexural areas of the body, the postauricular areas, the trunk, umbilicus, anogenital areas, and groin (Fig. 3.44). Pruritus is slight or absent, and the lesions usually lack the dry, fine scaling character associated with AD. Overlap of seborrheic dermatitis and AD, however, may occur with the features of AD becoming more prominent as the seborrheic dermatitis subsides. In one study, 49% of infants with AD had a history of infantile seborrheic dermatitis, in contrast to 17% of controls.[406]

The differential diagnosis of seborrheic dermatitis during infancy includes AD, psoriasis, LCH, and immunodeficiency. Lesions of AD are almost always pruritic, are poorly defined, and have dry, fine scaling. In addition, the occluded diaper area is usually spared in AD, in contrast to the common diaper area involvement of seborrheic dermatitis. Psoriasis can be quite difficult to differentiate because it can present in infants in a fashion very similar to that of seborrheic dermatitis, with sharply marginated, brightly erythematous scaling patches. Psoriasis tends to show a slower response to topical corticosteroid therapy and can be distinguished, if necessary, by skin biopsy. Although LCH can at times be mistaken for seborrheic dermatitis, the presence of discrete 1- to 3-mm yellowish to red-brown crusted or eroded papules, purpuric lesions, hepatosplenomegaly, or lymphadenopathy supports the diagnosis of LCH; histopathologic and immunohistochemical examination of cutaneous lesions confirms the diagnosis of LCH. When the erythema and scaling of infantile seborrheic dermatitis becomes severe, generalized, and exfoliative, the diagnosis of immunodeficiency must be considered. The lack of constitutional findings (diarrhea, fever, weight loss), alopecia, associated infections, and the spontaneous clearance or rapid response to therapy of seborrheic dermatitis help to distinguish the conditions. Severe generalized seborrhea-like dermatitis in association with failure to thrive, recurrent skin and other infections, and chronic diarrhea (once called *Leiner syndrome*) can be seen in several immunodeficiency disorders, including C3 and C5 complement deficiencies, C5 dysfunction, hypergammaglobulinemia E syndrome, SCID (especially Omenn syndrome), and X-linked agammaglobulinemia.[407]

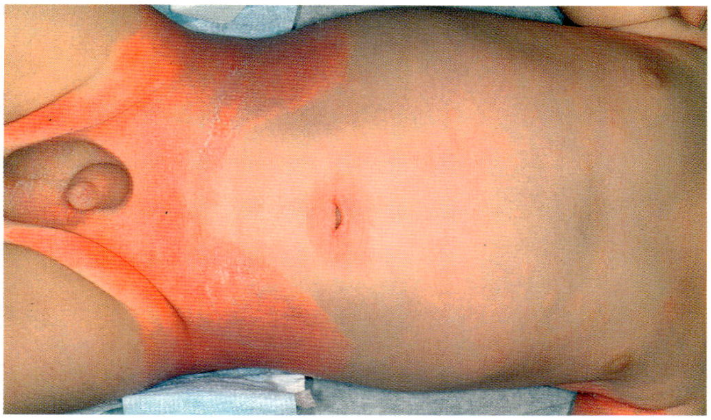

Fig. 3.44 Seborrheic dermatitis. A cause of diaper rash in young infants, seborrheic dermatitis is difficult to distinguish clinically from infantile psoriasis but tends to be less erythematous, to have thinner scaling, and to respond more quickly to topical antiinflammatory medications.

Between puberty and middle age, seborrheic dermatitis may appear on the scalp as a dry, fine, flaky desquamation, commonly known as *dandruff*. This seborrhea is an extreme form of normal desquamation in which scales of the scalp become abundant and visible, often overlying inflammation. Erythema and scaling of various degrees may also involve the supraorbital areas between the eyebrows and above the bridge of the nose, nasolabial crease (Fig. 3.45), lips, pinnae, retroauricular areas, and aural canals. Blepharitis is a form of seborrheic dermatitis in which the eyelid margins are red and covered with small, white scales. Seborrheic dermatitis may also involve the sideburns, beard, and mustache areas, with diffuse redness, greasy scaling, and pustulation. The severity and course of seborrheic eruptions of the eyelids and bearded areas are variable and have a tendency to chronicity and recurrence.

Occasionally an adolescent patient may have an eruption that has clinical features of both seborrheic dermatitis and psoriasis. Such eruptions may be termed *sebopsoriasis*. Lesions of seborrheic dermatitis can be differentiated from those of psoriasis by a lack of the characteristic vivid red hue or micaceous scale, a predisposition toward flexural rather than extensor aspects of the extremities, and the fact that lesions of seborrhea generally tend to remain within the confines of the hairline. Lesions of psoriasis (or sebopsoriasis) commonly extend beyond the hairline and in general are more resistant to standard antiseborrheic therapy.

The prognosis of infantile seborrheic dermatitis is excellent. In some patients, the disorder clears within 3 to 4 weeks, even without treatment, and most cases clear spontaneously by 8 to 12 months of age. The condition generally does not recur until the onset of puberty, although mild scaling of the scalp, particularly at the vertex, can be seen in some affected children through preschool years. Treatment of infantile scalp seborrheic dermatitis is best managed by frequent shampooing.[408] Although antiseborrheic shampoos, including ketoconazole shampoo,[409] may be useful, in infants or young children, these products may be drying or irritating to the eyes. A gentle "no-tears" shampoo usually suffices. If the scales are thick and adherent, removal can be facilitated by the thin application of mineral or baby oil followed by gentle scalp massage with a soft toothbrush and then shampooing. Antiseborrheic shampoos are alternatives if therapy with no-tears shampoo is not effective. If there is a significant inflammatory component, a topical corticosteroid lotion, oil, or solution, with or without 3% to 5% salicylic acid, may be applied once to twice daily. For involvement other than the scalp, a low-strength topical corticosteroid or topical antifungal agent is usually effective when applied once to twice daily.

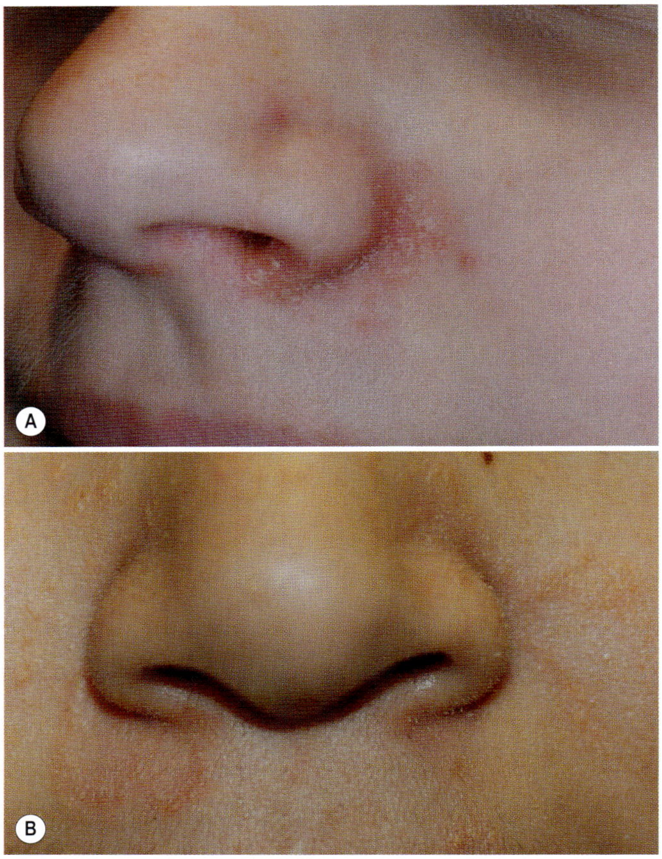

Fig. 3.45 Seborrheic dermatitis. **(A)** Facial seborrheic dermatitis in adolescents typically involves nasolabial folds and may result from overgrowth of lipophilic yeasts of the normal flora. In **(B)** tinea faciei was considered, but the distribution and bilaterality are atypical for tinea.

Adolescents with seborrhea of the scalp may try a variety of antiseborrheic shampoos, tar shampoo, ketoconazole shampoo, or 5% tea tree oil shampoo.[408,410] Antiseborrheic shampoos may contain selenium sulfide (e.g., Sebulex, Exsel, and Selsun), salicylic acid (e.g., T-Sal), or zinc pyrithione (e.g., Head and Shoulders or DHS Zinc). If the scale is extremely thick and adherent, it can be loosened by warmed mineral oil massaged into the scalp or by the use of P&S Liquid (Baker Cummins), ideally left on overnight. Scales are then loosened by scrubbing gently with the fingers or a soft brush, and the scalp is shampooed. For patients with associated erythema or pruritus, topical corticosteroid lotions, gels, oils, or foams may be used. Seborrheic dermatitis of the face or intertriginous areas in adolescents usually responds quickly to the application of a mild corticosteroid, calcineurin inhibitor, or antifungal medication. If these are too greasy, a foam preparation of ketoconazole is available.[411]

Blepharitis may be managed by warm-water compresses, gentle cleansing with a dilute solution of a nonirritating or baby shampoo, and mechanical removal of scales when necessary. Topical corticosteroids on the eyelids or eyelid margins should be used with caution, although calcineurin inhibitors (e.g., tacrolimus or pimecrolimus) or PDE4 inhibitors (e.g., crisaborole) may be used safely in this area.

Seborrheic dermatitis of the intertriginous or diaper areas occasionally may be complicated by secondary candidal or bacterial infection. Candidal infection is usually seen in the diaper areas as discrete erythematous scaling papules and sometimes pustules, especially at the periphery of the affected area. Secondary bacterial infection is more commonly seen as oozing at the neck fold and other intertriginous sites. In such instances, topical anticandidal or antibacterial agents are generally helpful. For patients with disease refractory to topical treatment or for those with significant secondary bacterial infection, bacterial cultures and appropriate systemic antibiotics are necessary.

Intertrigo

Intertrigo is a superficial inflammatory dermatitis that occurs in areas where the skin is in apposition (Fig. 3.46; see also Fig. 17.43). As a result of friction, heat, and moisture, the affected areas become intensely erythematous in a well-demarcated pattern, macerated, and often secondarily infected by bacteria or *Candida* or, in adolescents, by dermatophytes (see Chapter 17). Intertrigo with secondary streptococcal infection often presents with oozing and can be associated with bacteremia.[412,413] Treatment is directed toward elimination of the macerated skin. Open wet compresses, dusting powders (such as Zeasorb), topical corticosteroid lotions, and, when indicated, appropriate antibiotics or fungicidal agents may be used.

Dyshidrotic Eczema

Dyshidrotic eczema (pompholyx) is an acute recurrent or chronic eczematous eruption of the palms, soles, and lateral aspects of the fingers, characterized by deep-seated, variably inflamed lesions that range from tapioca-like vesicles to large, tense bullae (Figs. 3.47

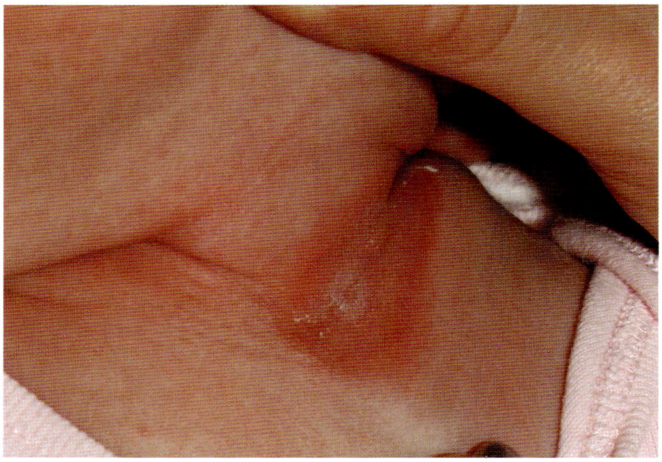

Fig. 3.46 Intertrigo of the neck fold. Intertrigo is a superficial inflammatory dermatitis that occurs at sites of skin apposition, most commonly involving the neck, inguinal, and antecubital and popliteal folds. Secondary bacterial or yeast infection is common.

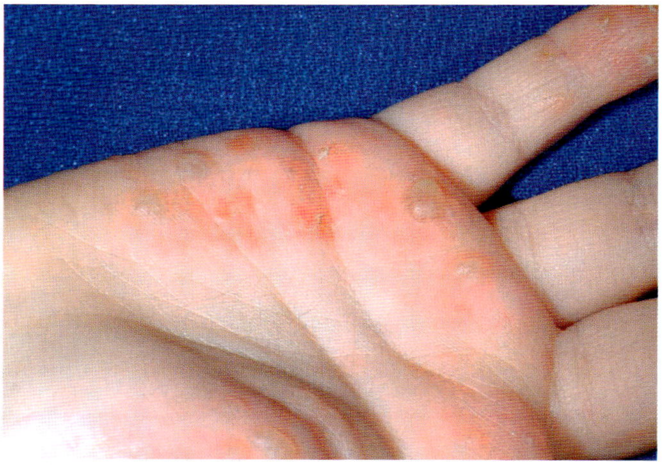

Fig. 3.47 Pompholyx, or dyshidrotic eczema. An acute recurrent or chronic eruption of the palms, soles, and lateral aspects of the fingers with deep-seated tapioca-like vesicles to large, tense bullae.

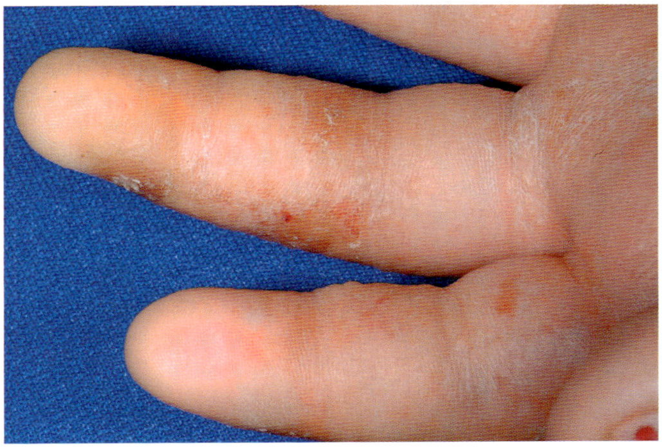

Fig. 3.48 Pompholyx, or dyshidrotic eczema. Superficial crusting and desquamation often replace the ruptured tiny vesicles of dyshidrotic eczema.

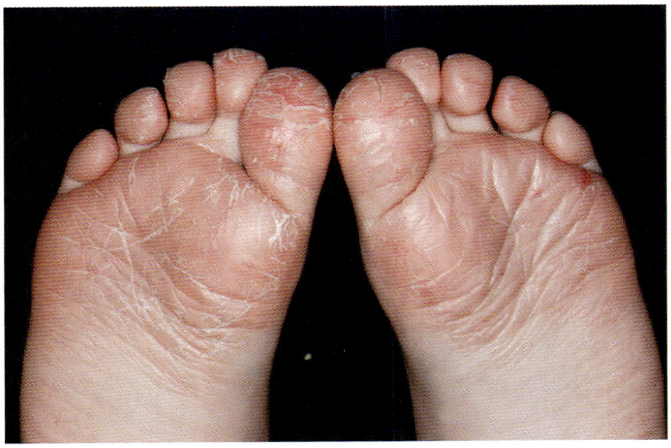

Fig. 3.49 Juvenile plantar dermatosis. Scaling, lichenification, and fissuring in chronic juvenile plantar dermatitis. Note the sparing of toe regions without contact. This patient also has ichthyosis vulgaris, which explains the hyperlinear soles.

and 3.48).[414] The distribution of lesions generally is bilateral and somewhat symmetric. Patients complain of considerable pruritus and/or burning. Hyperhidrosis is often associated. Attacks usually last a few weeks, but relapses are frequent, often several times per year.

Dyshidrotic eczema may be confused with contact dermatitis or tinea, disorders commonly unilateral or more localized. ACD (see Allergic Contact Dermatitis section) on the feet or hands most commonly results from exposure to potassium dichromate (for tanning leather) or rubber but occasionally is caused by paraphenylenediamine (PPD; in hair dyes and as an additive to henna), nickel, fragrance mix, and colophony (in glues and also in violin rosin).[415] Fungal culture and patch testing can be performed to distinguish these disorders from tinea and contact dermatitis, respectively. Id reactions and pustular psoriasis must also be considered in the differential diagnosis of this disorder and are most commonly bilateral. Juvenile plantar dermatosis is limited to the feet and tends to be bilateral (Fig. 3.49). A reaction on the palms and soles resembling dyshidrotic eczema has also been described after intravenous immunoglobulin (IVIG), most commonly after the first IVIG treatment in adults with neurologic disorders.[416,417] In a minority of these cases, eczematous lesions may be extensive. Severe dyshidrotic eczema may also occur after IVIG therapy for Kawasaki disease[418] or Stevens–Johnson syndrome.[416]

The natural course of dyshidrotic eczema is one of frequent recurrence. Open wet compresses tend to open the vesicles, and application of moderate to potent topical corticosteroids, although not curative, helps relieve the manifestations of this disorder. Topical tacrolimus 0.1% ointment has been used successfully as an alternative that allows rotational therapy.[419] When infection is present, antibiotics may be administered topically or systemically. Although not a disorder of eccrine glands *per se*, the use of topical aluminum chloride in concentrations of 12% (e.g., Certain Dri) to 20% (e.g., Drysol) or topical glycopyrronium may decrease the associated hyperhidrosis and help to control the disorder if not too irritating. Hyperhidrosis can also be controlled by oral administration of glycopyrrolate if topical application of drying agents is ineffective or too ineffective. For adolescents with recalcitrant hyperhidrosis, intradermal injections of botulinum toxin might be considered.[420] Phototherapy with either narrow-band ultraviolet B light or high doses of ultraviolet A1 light[421] and even short courses of oral corticosteroids with gradual tapering have been used.

Juvenile Plantar Dermatosis

Juvenile plantar dermatosis (dermatitis plantaris sicca or "sweaty-sock dermatitis") is a common dermatosis of infancy and childhood, most commonly localized to the distal aspect of the soles and toes, particularly the great toes, but sparing the interdigital spaces. Associated with hyperhidrosis and thought to represent a frictional irritant dermatitis, the disorder is manifested acutely by a symmetric, smooth, red, glazed, and fine scaling but can become lichenified with chronicity (see Fig. 3.49). Similar changes have also been reported on the fingertips in up to 5% of patients with excessive perspiration. Untreated juvenile plantar dermatosis generally tends to persist for several years, and although there is no seasonal pattern, some patients report slight worsening of the condition during the summer and in cold weather.

The differential diagnosis of juvenile plantar dermatosis includes tinea pedis, palmoplantar psoriasis, pityriasis rubra pilaris, and shoe-related contact dermatitis. Tinea pedis can manifest as scaling and erythema of the plantar foot but is more likely to involve the interdigital spaces. Associated pustulation of tinea may be mistaken for secondary staphylococcal infection. Potassium hydroxide scrapings and culture may be required to distinguish tinea pedis and juvenile plantar dermatosis. The plaques of psoriasis are often thicker and more erythematous. Pityriasis rubra pilaris may closely resemble psoriasis but often shows a salmon-orange coloration on the palms and soles. Both psoriasis and pityriasis rubra pilaris usually show lesions elsewhere. Contact dermatitis owing to a component of shoes is more commonly on the dorsum of the foot, but the plantar foot is occasionally involved (see Shoe Dermatitis section).

Although treatment is not always completely successful, children with hyperhidrosis of the feet should wear all-cotton socks and avoid occlusive footwear whenever possible, remove their shoes when indoors, change their socks whenever they are damp, dust an absorbent powder into shoes and socks (to help lessen perspiration), and use an emollient cream as soon as the shoes and socks are removed. Patients do not usually tolerate topical agents for hyperhidrosis, but oral glycopyrrolate tends to be very effective and may reduce the severity of the dermatitis; dosing is 1 to 5 mg per day, and the most common complications are dry mouth and eyes. Use of a medium-strength to potent topical steroid is usually effective in diminishing the pruritus and inflammation associated with juvenile plantar dermatitis. Low-strength topical steroids are often not effective, given the thick overlying stratum corneum of the plantar surface. Topical or systemically administered antistaphylococcal antibiotics may be needed if patients show crusting or pustulation suggesting secondary infection. Careful application of a cyanoacrylate (e.g., Super Glue) to fissured areas often provides relief from the associated discomfort.

Frictional Lichenoid Dermatitis

Frictional lichenoid dermatitis (frictional lichenoid eruption, juvenile papular dermatitis, recurrent summertime pityriasis of the elbows

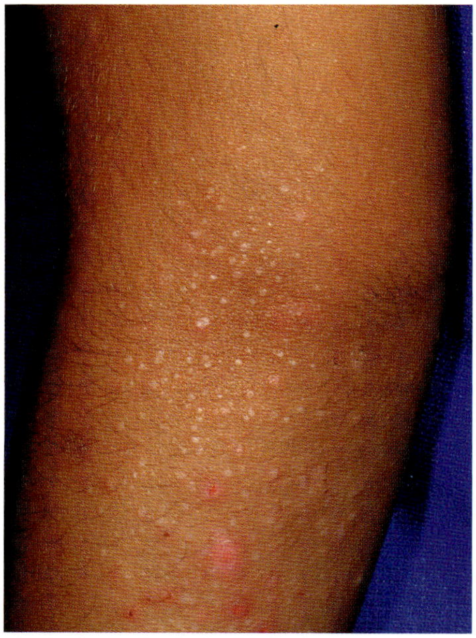

Fig. 3.50 Frictional lichenoid dermatosis. Aggregates of lichenoid papules occur primarily on the elbows, knees, knuckles, and backs of the hands of children. Although many of the papules are monomorphic and tiny, suggesting lichen nitidus (see Chapter 4), the associated pruritus, localization, and concurrent presence of lichenoid papules of various sizes on the elbows allow the diagnosis to be made clinically.

and knees) is a recurring cutaneous disorder affecting children, especially boys, between 4 and 12 years of age.[422] Most cases are seen in the spring and summer when outdoor activities are common, and many cases have been associated with playing in sandboxes (sandbox dermatitis) or on grass. Approximately half of the affected children have AD, allergic rhinitis, or asthma.[423] The eruption is characterized by aggregates of discrete lichenoid papules, 1 or 2 mm in diameter, which occur primarily on the elbows, knees, and backs of the hands of children in whom such areas are subject to minor frictional trauma without protection of clothing (Fig. 3.50). Lesions may be hypopigmented, and associated pruritus is often severe but may be absent. It tends to occur in children with a predisposition to atopy.

The differential diagnosis of this disorder includes psoriasis, AD, molluscum, flat warts, lichen nitidus, and the papulovesicular acrolocated syndrome (Gianotti–Crosti syndrome; see Chapter 16). The management of frictional lichenoid dermatitis includes avoidance of frictional trauma to the involved areas (as might occur with leaning on elbows and knees) and application of topical corticosteroids and emollient, especially to ease any associated pruritus.

Nummular Dermatitis

Nummular dermatitis (also called *nonmular eczema*) is characterized by discoid or coin-shaped plaques. The name is derived from the Latin word *nummulus* ("coin-like"), because of the shape and size of the lesions. The plaques of nummular dermatitis are composed of minute papules and vesicles, which enlarge by peripheral extension to form discrete, usually round or oval, erythematous, often lichenified and hyperpigmented plaques that measure 1 cm or more in diameter (see Figs. 3.34 and 3.35). They usually occur on the extensor surfaces of the hands, arms, and legs as single or multiple lesions on dry or asteatotic skin. Pruritus is usually associated and may be intense. Occasionally the face and trunk may be involved. The surrounding skin may be xerotic, particularly in children with AD and nummular dermatitis, but in many patients is normal. Secondary staphylococcal infection is common and manifests as crusting and exudation.

Nummular dermatitis must be differentiated from ACD, AD (which may be seen concurrently), psoriasis, and superficial dermatophyte infections of the skin. History of exposure, patch testing if appropriate, fungal culture, and biopsy of lesional skin can help to distinguish these conditions.

Effective therapy requires application of class II to IV topical corticosteroids, preferably in an ointment base or under occlusion. The combination of a refined tar preparation (liquor carbonis detergens 5% to 10%) in a strong corticosteroid used twice daily is an alternative means of treatment. Secondary staphylococcal infection should always be considered, especially in recalcitrant lesions, and commonly requires systemic administration of antibiotic (such as cephalexin) in addition to a potent topical steroid. Although in general the use of topical antibiotic with topical steroid is discouraged for AD beyond for mild secondary infection, nummular dermatitis often responds better to concurrently applying topical steroid and topical mupirocin. For severe cases that are recalcitrant to topical medication, methotrexate is the treatment of choice.[424]

Winter Eczema

Winter eczema, also known as *asteatotic eczema, eczema craquelé*, or *xerotic eczema*, is a subacute eczematous dermatitis characterized by pruritic scaly erythematous patches, usually associated with dryness and dehydration (asteatosis) of the epidermis. Generally seen on the extremities and occasionally on the trunk, these changes are most common during winter when the humidity is low, particularly in adults and adolescents who bathe or shower often with harsh or drying soaps. Frequent bathing with incomplete drying and resultant evaporation of moisture causes dehydration of the epidermis, with redness, scaling, and fine cracking that may resemble cracked porcelain (hence the term *eczema craquelé*). Treatment of winter eczema is centered in the maintenance of proper hydration of the stratum corneum and is dependent on the routine use of emollients, limiting the time and temperature of showers, use of mild soaps, and topical therapy with corticosteroids (preferably those in an ointment base) for individual lesions.

Lichen Striatus

Lichen striatus is a self-limiting inflammatory dermatosis that follows Blaschko lines, the path of ectodermal embryologic development of skin.[425,426] Although not considered contagious or inherited, lichen striatus has been described in more than one family member.[427,428] It has followed viral infections, vaccination (e.g., hepatitis B virus), and trauma, but its cause is unknown. The inflammatory infiltrate of lichen striatus shows plasmacytoid dendrocytes and, similar to other lichenoid disorders, a type I interferon signature.[429] The mean age of onset is 4 years of age, although older children may be affected. Girls appear to be affected two to three times more often than boys. In a large series, 60 of 115 affected children were atopic.[426]

The eruption is usually asymptomatic (but sometimes is pruritic) and reaches its maximum extent within a few weeks to months. Only 6% of affected children show more than one band. Lesions begin as 2- to 4-mm erythematous to hypopigmented, slightly scaling, flat-topped papules that rapidly coalesce to form the curvilinear band. The line of involvement tends to be narrow but can range from several millimeters to 1 or 2 cm in width. Most commonly lichen striatus affects an extremity but occasionally the face (Fig. 3.51),[430] neck, trunk, or buttocks is affected. Nail involvement is seen, typically by extension of an extremity lesion.[431,432] In dark-skinned or tanned individuals the eruption may appear as slightly scaly (Fig. 3.52) or as a band-like area of hypopigmentation (Fig. 3.53). Although the band is usually continuous, it may occasionally be interrupted by or interspersed with coalescent plaques several centimeters in diameter along a line of Blaschko.

The differential diagnosis of lichen striatus most commonly includes inflammatory linear verrucous epidermal nevus (ILVEN), which tends to be more psoriasiform (Fig. 3.54; see also Chapter 9 and Fig. 9.40) and blaschkitis[433] (more eczematous) (Fig. 3.55). In contrast to lichen striatus, blaschkitis is usually papulovesicular, pruritic,

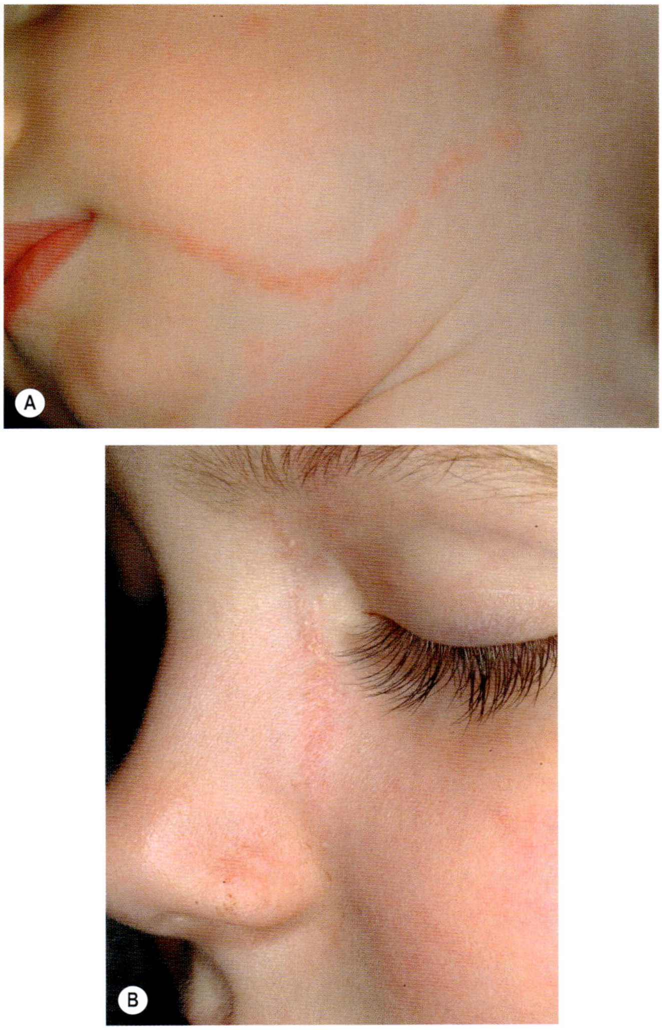

Fig. 3.51 (A and B) Lichen striatus. A self-limiting, usually unilateral linear or curvilinear collection of small, erythematous, flat-topped papules that follows one of the Blaschko lines, lines of the embryologic development of skin. Lines on the face tend to be particularly thin.

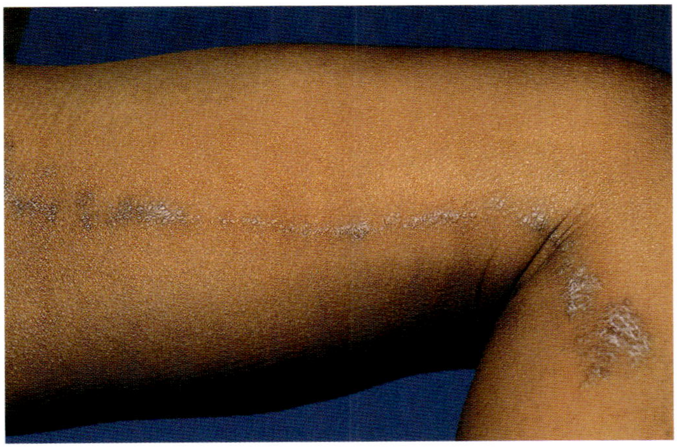

Fig. 3.52 Lichen striatus. Linear collection of papules of lichen striatus, most commonly seen on the extremities. The erythema is more difficult to appreciate on darker skin, but the mild scaling may be more apparent.

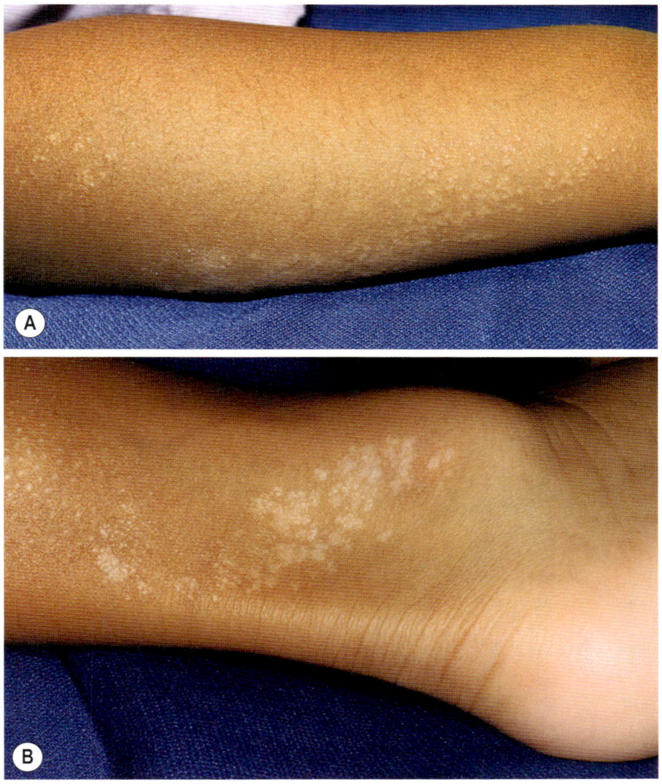

Fig. 3.53 (A and B) Lichen striatus. The linear and curvilinear streaks of lichen striatus may be collections of hypopigmented papules or macules from the onset, particularly in children with darker skin types.

involves multiple bands, tends to last for about a month, recurs often, and tends to respond to topical antiinflammatory medication. Biopsy of blaschkitis shows pure spongiosis without a lichenoid infiltrate. Other acquired inflammatory lesions distributed along lines of Blaschko can include linear forms of lichen planus, linear lichen nitidus, lichenoid drug eruptions,[434] lichenoid chronic GVHD, lupus erythematosus, AD, and linearly arranged ("koebnerized") lesions of verruca plana. When the diagnosis remains in doubt, histopathologic examination of a cutaneous biopsy specimen will help exclude other possible linear eruptions.

Lichen striatus usually resolves spontaneously within 3 to 24 months (mean duration, 6 months)[426] but occasionally lasts longer (up to 3.5 years)[435] and often leaves an area of hypopigmentation that subsequently disappears. Recurrences occur in 2% of children. Therapy is generally unnecessary, and topical corticosteroids do not tend to hasten resolution but can reduce pruritus if present. However, facial lesions have responded to tacrolimus,[436] and combination of a topical tazarotene and topical steroid has been associated with lesional clearing.[437]

Contact Dermatitis

Contact dermatitis may be defined as an eczematous eruption produced either by local exposure to a primary irritating substance (irritant contact dermatitis) or by an acquired allergic response to a clinically relevant sensitizing substance (allergic contact dermatitis [ACD].[147] A contact allergen can sensitize but does not cause a reaction on first exposure. With continued or repeated exposure, the allergen may trigger a contact dermatitis based on a type IV allergic reaction. An irritant, on the other hand, may be defined as a substance that produces an eczematous response on the basis of irritation rather than by immunologic means and can occur in anyone; allergens only

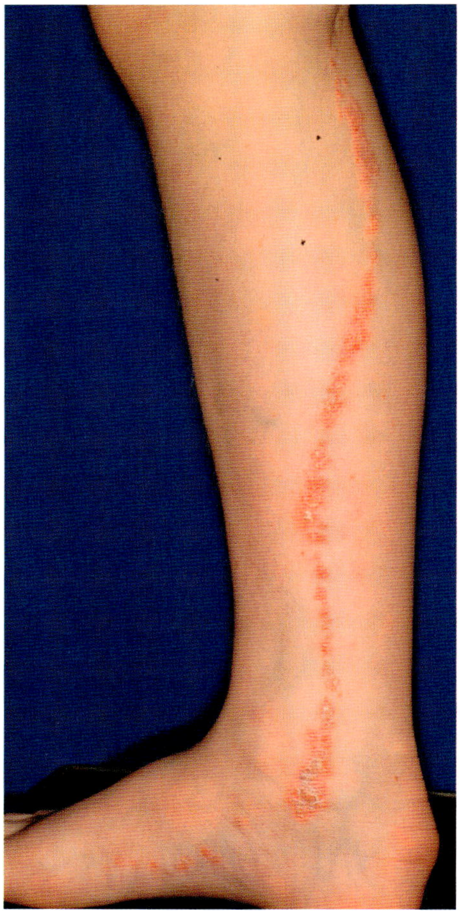

Fig. 3.54 Inflammatory linear verrucous epidermal nevus (ILVEN). Lichen striatus must be differentiated from ILVEN, a persistent mosaic lesion that follows the lines of Blaschko (see Chapter 9). The papules of ILVEN tend to be more erythematous, less discrete, more scaly, and more pruritic than those of lichen striatus, but biopsy or observation over 2 to 3 years may be necessary to determine the diagnosis.

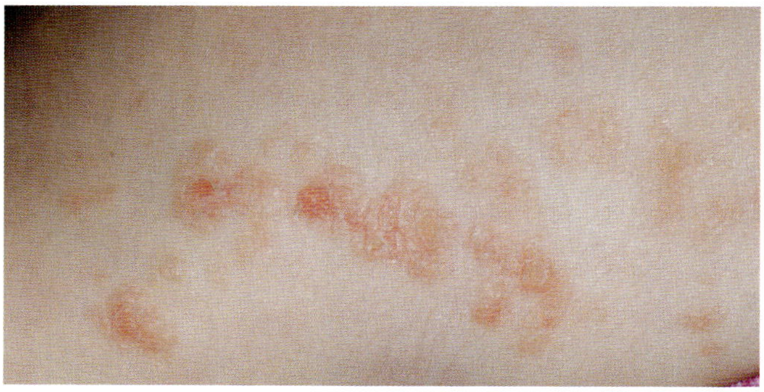

Fig. 3.55 Blaschkitis. Although distributed along a Blaschko line, lesions of blaschkitis are eczematous, are often multiple, and last for just a few weeks, in contrast to those of lichen striatus or ILVEN.

can trigger contact dermatitis in susceptible individuals. Photocontact reactions (see Chapter 19) such as phytophotodermatitis after contact with the juice or rinds of certain lemons and limes (and several other plant-based products) occur only when the skin is exposed to ultraviolet light. ACD should be distinguished from contact urticaria, which can be diagnosed by the morphology of the lesions (urticarial) and is best treated with antihistamines.[438,439]

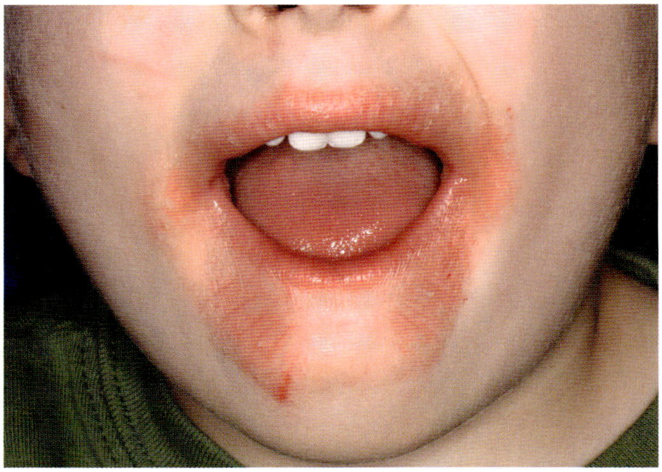

Fig. 3.56 Lip-licker's dermatitis. Chronic contact dermatitis with lichenification and hyperpigmentation in the shape of licking from the tongue and sometimes beyond.

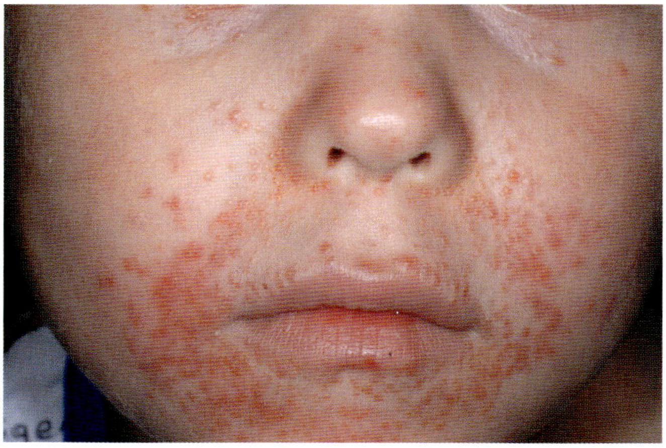

Fig. 3.57 Periorificial granulomatous dermatitis. The discrete, tiny, noneczematous papules are usually seen in a perioral distribution but may be perinasal and/or infraorbital. The morphology and distribution help to distinguish periorificial granulomatous dermatitis from perioral irritant or allergic contact dermatitis.

PRIMARY IRRITANT DERMATITIS

Common substances that produce primary irritant dermatitis include harsh soaps, bleaches, detergents, solvents, acids, alkalis, bubble baths, certain foods, saliva, urine, feces, and intestinal secretions. The severity of the dermatitis varies from person to person or from time to time in the same person as a result of the condition of the skin at the time of exposure, the strength of the irritant, the location of the eruption, the cumulative effect of repeated exposures to the irritating substance, and local factors such as perspiration, maceration, and occlusion.

In children, the lips and adjacent skin commonly become dry and, as a result of a licking habit, inflamed and scaly (lip-licker's dermatitis) (Fig. 3.56). If extensive, lip-licker's dermatitis must be distinguished from ACD, especially that caused by mango (see Fig. 3.63), and perioral granulomatous dermatitis (Fig. 3.57), which is characterized by small erythematous papules of the perioral and often suborbital areas and is exacerbated by application of topical corticosteroids (see Chapter 8). Saliva also commonly becomes trapped between the thumb and mouth of thumb suckers, and a similar reaction is commonly seen in toddlers who continue to use pacifiers for long periods. In infants with AD, saliva is a significant irritant associated with the extensive drooling from teething and contributes to the dermatitis on the cheeks and chin. In the infant and young child, circumoral erythema may also represent a contact dermatitis in response to foods such as citrus foods, carrots, shrimp, and spinach. The dermatitis is caused by direct contact with the skin, not from ingestion of the offending food substances, although exposure is aggravated by regurgitation of food particles, dribbling of saliva, and rubbing of the involved areas.

Diaper dermatitis is the most common form of irritant contact dermatitis in infancy (see Chapter 2), with a peak age of incidence of 9 to 12 months of age. ACD in the diaper area is rare. Irritant diaper dermatitis typically affects the exposed convex surfaces and spares the folds, which are protected. Toddlers and younger children who use pull-up diapers at night and children with enuresis not uncommonly show an irritant dermatitis of the buttocks region related to exposure to urine and limited absorbency of the pull-up. Perianal dermatitis is often irritant related as a result of exposure to stool but must be distinguished from perianal psoriasis (see Chapter 4) and perianal streptococcal cellulitis (see Chapter 14).

Juvenile plantar dermatosis has been linked to exposure to sweat and is more commonly seen in children with plantar hyperhidrosis (see previous discussion). Excessive handwashing, especially during winter months and in compulsive handwashers, is the most common cause of dermatitis on the dorsum of the hands. The increased attention to handwashing as a means to decrease the spread of infectious disease has markedly increased the risk of developing irritant hand dermatitis in school-aged children. "Slime," a concoction often made at home with boric acid salt, glue, and water, is a growing cause of irritant hand dermatitis, particularly on the palm[440–442] and palmar aspects of the fingers (Fig. 3.58). Although most commonly an irritant dermatitis, ingredients in the detergents, shaving cream, shampoos, or contact lens solution that are used as the source of the boric acid or the glue may trigger ACD because they contain fragrance, methylchloroisothiazolinone/methylisothiazolinone (MCI/MI), isothiazolinones, and other potential allergens (see Allergic Contact Dermatitis).

Soccer and hockey shin guards typically trap sweat and cause friction, leading to an irritant contact dermatitis on the anterior aspect of the lower legs of school-aged children that can become lichenified if chronic. Strategies to reduce friction, such as wearing a cotton sock under the guard and coating the area with absorbent powder or petrolatum before using the guards, together with topical antiinflammatory therapy for the dermatitis as needed, have been helpful.[444] Should the dermatitis persist or worsen, ACD should also be considered, particularly as related to the rubber compounds and neoprene components in sporting equipment (Table 3.3). Irritant dermatitis can develop under tight rings or watches because of the trapping of sweat, detergents, or other irritants (Fig. 3.59). Irritant reactions may also occur from exposure to fiberglass particles attached to clothes after exposure to fiberglass insulation panels or drapes.[445] Because clothes washed in a washing machine in which fiberglass materials have been washed are also capable of inducing this cutaneous reaction, children whose parents have been exposed may also be affected. Fiberglass dermatitis presents as a pruritic, patchy folliculitis or subacute dermatitis. Microscopic examination of skin scrapings from involved areas or suspected articles of clothing may reveal pale, greenish, granular rod-like fibers one to two times the width of a hair. The use of methylphenidate transdermal patches in children with ADHD often leads to irritant reactions confined to the site of patch application; ACD to the patch is rare.[446]

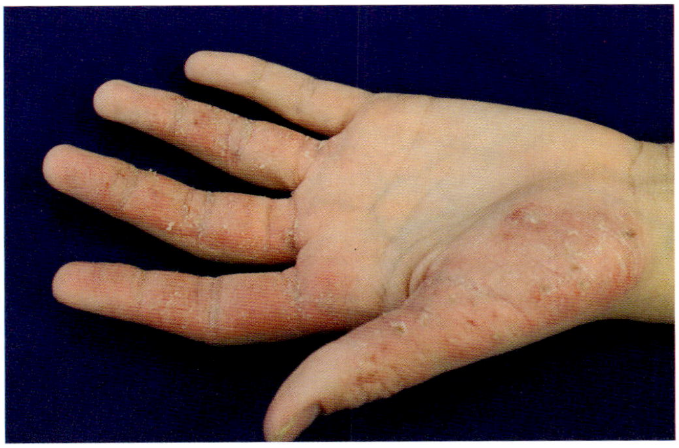

Fig. 3.58 Hand dermatitis. Slime, made at home from boric acid salt, glue, and water, is a cause of irritant (and sometimes allergic) contact dermatitis on the palms.

Avoidance of the irritant is key to improvement. Low-potency topical corticosteroids or calcineurin inhibitors are used to treat the dermatitis of face and intertriginous areas; medium-strength topical steroids, or even potent topical steroids for hands and feet, may be required. Moisturizing creams or ointments lubricate and protect the affected areas. The treatment of irritant diaper dermatitis is discussed in Chapter 2.

ALLERGIC CONTACT DERMATITIS

ACD may account for up to 20% of all dermatitis in childhood and is likely to be underdiagnosed.[146,147,447] Key areas of involvement are the eyelids, neck, hands, axillae, anogenital area, and lower extremities. ACD represents a type IV immunologic (delayed hypersensitivity or cell-mediated) reaction in which antigenic contact with cutaneous Langerhans cells and T-lymphocyte activation are key. Despite their clinical similarity, nickel sensitization involves Th1/Th17 and Th22 lymphocytes, but fragrance allergy and, to a lesser extent, rubber allergy largely involve Th2 lymphocyte activation.[448,449] After sensitization to the offending allergen, ACD will develop on reexposure to the sensitizing substance. Sensitization may occur after only a few exposures to the offending substance, or allergy may occur after years of contact. Once the area has become sensitized, however, reexposure to the offending allergen may result in an acute dermatitis within a relatively brief period (generally 8 to 12 hours after exposure to the sensitizing allergen).

Reactions to *Rhus* family of contact allergens (e.g., poison ivy) are the most common triggers in children. Other major sources of clinically relevant ACD in children are metals (especially nickel, chromates, cobalt, and occasionally gold), fragrances and Balsam of Peru, lanolin/wool alcohols, cocamidopropyl betaine (CAPB; foaming product in "no-tears" shampoos and cleansers),[450] topical antibiotics (neomycin and bacitracin), formaldehyde, and rubber products[146,147,451] (see Table 3.3). Other triggers to consider in children are PPD contaminating temporary henna tattoos,[452] disperse dyes in clothing,[453] and the preservatives MCI and MI, which are sometimes in wet wipes. Girls are at greater risk for developing contact allergy, especially during adolescence and on the face, because of their greater exposure to ear piercing (nickel), cosmetics (preservatives and fragrances), and hair products. Initial sensitization to common allergens and occasionally ACD itself may occur during infancy.[454] Of tested children, 23% to 49% have AD, although it is unclear whether this high number represents a referral bias or truly increased risk[139,455–457]; the greatest relevant reactivity in this group is to allergens in the emollients.[140]

In a recent study of baby and child products, the most prevalent allergen found in commercially available products was fragrance (48%) to give the "fresh baby" smell.[458] Betaines were found in 18% of products, especially cocamidopropyl betaine, derived from coconut oil or fatty acids. Lanolin was still in 10% of products, and propylene glycol was found in 9%. Propylene glycol is not only in topical products but is also used in food products, tablets, and liquid medications (including hydroxyzine syrup), increasing the risk of systemic contact dermatitis.[459] At this time, only 3% of products each had MCI/MI and formaldehyde releasers, which is much lower than the frequency of use less than 10 years ago (10% of products), suggesting response to concerns about sensitization risk. A second study from the United Kingdom similarly evaluated 438 "baby products" and found that 88% had at least one potential contact allergen (especially parabens, fragrances, cetyl/stearyl alcohol, methylisothiazolinone, sodium lauryl sulfate, and lanolin). Interestingly, branded products and those marked as "sensitive," "gentle," "organic," or "fragrance-free" had more reference allergens than those without this marketing.[460]

Table 3.3 Most Common and Relevant Sensitizers in Children and Their Sources*

Group	Allergen	Sources	Typical Distribution	Other Comments
Plant	Urushiol	Poison ivy, sumac, oak	Extremities in linear streaks; face, genitals	If aerosolized, can be extensive and on face resemble angioedema
Metal	Nickel	Jewelry, snaps, buckles, eyeglasses, keys, coins, cell phones, tablets, laptop computers, orthodontics	Subumbilical, face, eyelids, earlobes, neck, wrists	Detect with glyoxime on objects
Topical antibiotic	Neomycin	Antibiotic-containing ointments	Face, eyelids	Bacitracin can also sensitize
Fragrance and balsam of Peru	Fragrance mix Balsam of Peru *(Myroxylon pereirae)*	Cosmetics, perfumes, sunscreens, toothpaste, flavoring agents in food and drink, lozenges, lip balms, topical healing agents, insect repellents	Face, eyelids, mouth, lips, neck, hands	Cross reacts with eugenol/isoeugenol (essential oils from several spices, such as cloves and cinnamon); vanilla, tiger balm, benzoin, propolis, colophony, citrus peel
Preservative	Thimerosal	Creams, lotions, mascara, vaccines	Torso, face	Largely removed
Metal	Cobalt	Buttons, snaps, jewelry, cement, ceramics, vitamin B_{12}	Umbilical, earlobes, neck, hands	Contaminant with nickel
Metal	Chromate	Leather (tanned), cement, paints, matches, green felt	Umbilical, hands, soles	
Metal	Gold	Jewelry, occupational exposure to jewelry, medicinal use; rarely dental gold	Face, eyelids, earlobes, neck wrists, fingers; rarely mucosal	Long-lasting patch reaction
Rubber accelerant	Thiuram	Elastic (waistband, socks), gloves, shoes (soles and insoles), pesticides	Waistline, feet, hands	Washing clothes with bleach causes release
Emollient	Lanolin/wool alcohols	Emollients, lip balms, soaps, aftershave, baby and bath oil, hand sanitizers	Hands, body	Sheep wool products
Emulsifier	Propylene glycol	Skin care products and cosmetics, topical medications, foods, coated oral medications	Face; can be generalized or scattered	More often causes an irritant dermatitis
Preservative	Formaldehyde/formaldehyde releasing	Lotions, cosmetics, shampoo, newsprint, wrinkle-resistant clothes	Hands, face, ears, trunk (sparing axillae)	
Oxidative chemical	Paraphenylenediamine	Hair dyes, printer ink, contaminant in henna tattoos (black)	Hairline, ears, hands, sites of tattoos	
Preservative	Methylchloroisothiazolinone/ methylisothiazolinone (MCI/MI)	Many infant products, such as wet wipes, protective creams, liquid soaps, shampoos, household cleaners, paints	Especially hands; can be head and neck, feet, diaper region, generalized	
Surfactant	Cocamidopropyl betaine (CAPB)	Cleansing products for children (such as tear-free formulations)	Face, hands	
Dye	Disperse dyes	Diaper material, colored synthetic garments (school and athletic uniforms)	Areas of high friction (e.g., around the axillae sparing the vault, anterior thighs)	
Rubber accelerant and antioxidant	Mixed dialkyl thiourea	Neoprene in computer mouse pads, wetsuits, shoes, athletic braces, shin guards, protective pads	Areas of friction and sweating under athletic equipment	
Adhesives	p-tert-butylphenol formaldehyde	Glues, surface coating and adhesives in shoes, ECG pads, leather goods, upholstery, hobbies	Hands, feet	

ECG, Electrocardiogram.
*For additional information, see http://www.truetest.com and choose the specific antigen.

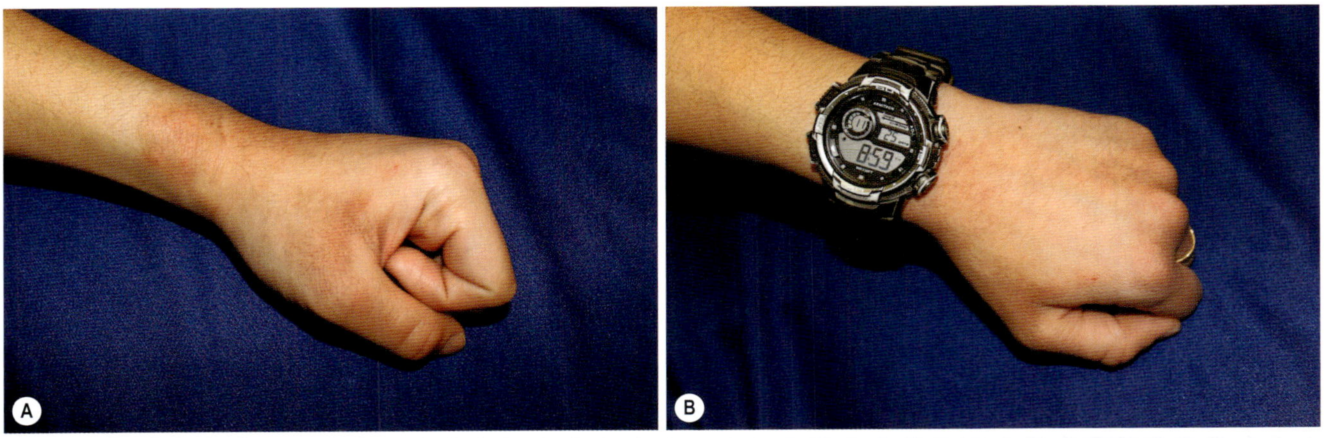

Fig. 3.59 Irritant contact dermatitis. **(A)** Tight watches or rings can trap sweat or water with detergent to cause irritation. **(B)** Allergic contact dermatitis might also be considered, but watch backs are largely stainless steel and do not contain releasable nickel or other components that can trigger allergic reactions.

The diagnosis of ACD is based on the appearance and distribution of skin lesions and aided when possible by a history of contact with an appropriate allergen (Table 3.4; see Table 3.3). Appearance on exposed areas only, linearity, and sharp edges are also clues to a reaction to a contactant, although ACD usually expands beyond the contact area in contrast to irritant contact dermatitis. For example, linearly distributed vesicles and bullae overlying erythema are typical of poison-ivy reactions. Dermatitis can appear at a distant site because of allergen transfer from one body site to another or by "recall reactions," which are flares at sites of prior allergen exposure. Contact dermatitis can also occur from exposure of a child to a contact allergen from a family member *(connubial dermatitis)*. Particularly common are fragrances, hair products, and henna contaminated by paraphenyldiamine (PPD).[461–463]

Dermatitis on the eyelids, hands, feet, and legs is most commonly associated with positive reactions on patch testing. Eyelid dermatitis often results from preservatives in cosmetics, fragrances, or emollients applied to the hands. Shoe dermatitis occurs more often on the dorsal aspect of the feet; in children, the most common allergens are potassium dichromate, thimerosal, cobalt chloride, mercapto mix, colophonium, mercury, and nickel.[464] Subumbilical or earlobe dermatitis is typical of nickel contact allergy, and axillary-vault dermatitis should lead to investigation of sensitivity to deodorant or fragrances, whereas axillary dermatitis sparing the vault may relate to clothing dyes. Toilet seat dermatitis (buttock and posterior thighs) could result from ACD to essential oils, lacquer, or paint in a wooden toilet seat but now more commonly is irritant contact dermatitis from detergents or ACD to a cleansing component (Fig. 3.60) and responds well to treatment of the dermatitis followed by prevention with the use of toilet seat covers.[465] Occasionally, oral lichenoid reactions occur after ingestion of allergens. The histopathologic picture of ACD usually does not allow differentiation from primary irritant dermatitis or AD.

The acute lesions of ACD are characterized by intense erythema accompanied by edema, papules, vesiculation (sometimes bullae), oozing, and a sharp line of demarcation between involved and normal skin. In the subacute phase, vesiculation is less pronounced and is mixed with crusting, scaling, and thickening of the skin. Chronic lesions, conversely, are characterized by lichenification, fissuring, scaling, and little or no vesiculation.

Autosensitization Dermatitis or Id Reaction

Id reaction (autosensitization dermatitis, autoeczematization) describes a hypersensitivity disorder characterized by the acute onset of small edematous papules or papulovesicles. Id reactions to nickel are

Table 3.4 Distribution of Dermatitis and Possible Triggers

Localization	Triggers
Eyelids	Cosmetics, emollients (hands), fragrances, hair dyes, metals, nail products
Hairline, postauricular, ear helix	Hair dyes, hair products
Earlobes, neck	Fragrance, metal jewelry
Periaxillary	Textile dyes, formaldehyde and formaldehyde releasers
Axillary vault	Deodorants
Subumbilical	Metal (snaps, belt buckles)
Extremities, linear streaks	Poison ivy and oak, phytophotodermatitis
Plantar aspect of feet	Adhesive, rubber in shoes
Dorsal aspect of feet	Leather (chromates, dyes), rubber, adhesive

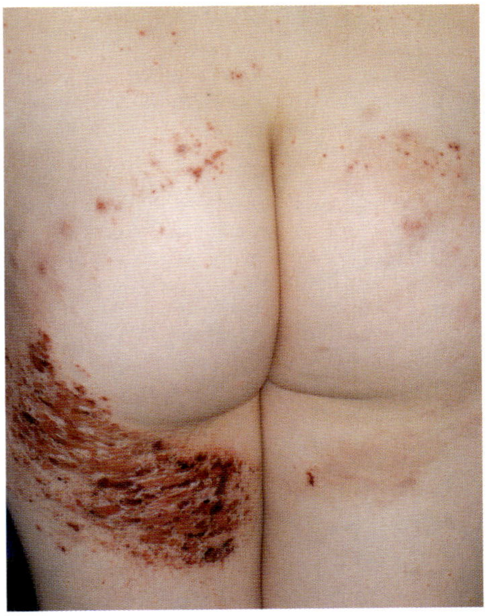

Fig. 3.60 Toilet seat dermatitis. This boy's mother used wipes with iodopropynyl butylcarbamates and fragrance to clean the seat. The dermatitis cleared after a switch to dilute bleach water.

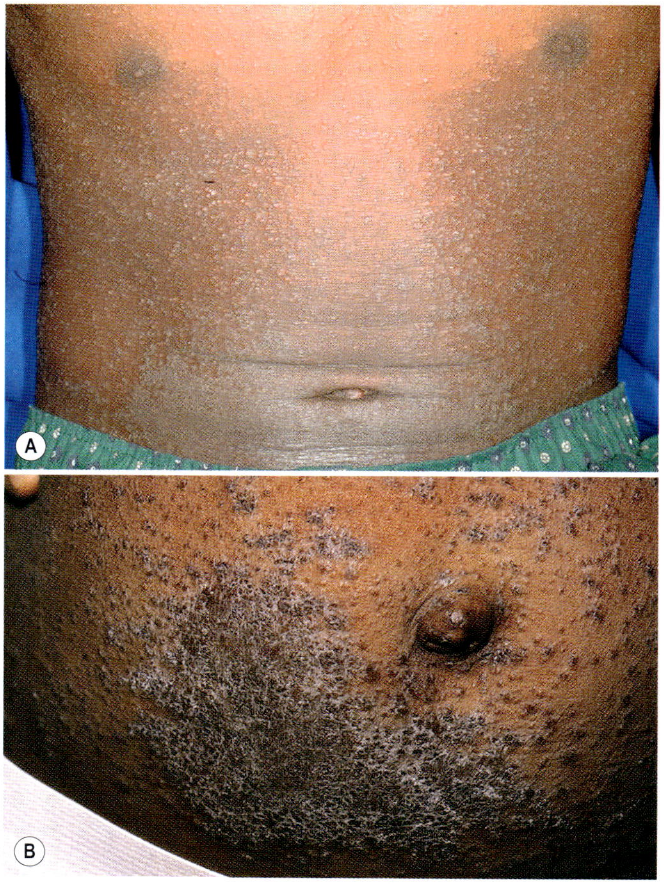

Fig. 3.61 Nickel contact dermatitis with id reaction. **(A)** Note the characteristic subumbilical (or periumbilical) hyperpigmented plaque of dermatitis in this patient with nickel contact dermatitis. **(B)** The lichenification and hyperpigmentation indicate a chronic dermatitis. The tiny discrete papules seen around the plaque extend across the entire trunk and represent an id reaction to the dermatitis.

found in up to 50% of patients[466] and may appear on the trunk (Fig. 3.61), forearms, flexor aspects of the upper arms, and extensor aspects of the upper arms and thighs and, less commonly, the face. The eruption is nearly always symmetric but may demonstrate light sensitivity or an isomorphic response (the Koebner phenomenon), in which trauma elicits new lesions. Lesions are generally associated with moderate to severe pruritus. The disorder usually appears acutely over a few days and nearly always is preceded by an exacerbation of the preexisting dermatitis by infection, rubbing, or inappropriate therapy. The acute eruption may subside spontaneously in a few weeks if the primary dermatitis is controlled. Relapses, however, are common, particularly when the initial local lesion flares and is followed by a further disseminated eruption.

The diagnosis of id reaction is made clinically on the basis of a generalized papulovesicular eruption that develops in the wake of preexisting eczematoid dermatitis. Treatment depends on the use of open wet compresses, antihistamines, and topical corticosteroid preparations. Control of the primary lesion is critical to prevent further or recurrent antigenic stimulation. Although seldom indicated, a 2- to 3-week course of systemic corticosteroids may at times be necessary in cases unresponsive to more conservative therapy.

Id reactions may also be seen in response to infectious agents, particularly in bacterial and dermatophyte infections. The tiny papules of the id reaction associated with tinea capitis most commonly are localized to the head and neck. Often, the id reaction of tinea capitis occurs after initiation of treatment with oral antifungal agents and is erroneously considered to be a drug reaction. Recognition of the underlying infection and continuing the antimicrobial treatment is critical for clearance.

Table 3.5 Allergen Components in the Commercially Available T.R.U.E. Test Kit

Panel 1.2	Panel 2.2	Panel 3.2
Nickel sulfate	p-tert-butylphenol formaldehyde resin	Diazolidinyl urea
Wool alcohol (lanolin)	Epoxy resin	Quinoline mix
Neomycin sulfate	Carba mix	Tixocortol-21-pivalate
Potassium dichromate	Black rubber mix	Gold sodium thiosulfate
Caine mix	Cl^+ Me^- isothiazolinone (MCI/MI)	Imidazolidinyl urea
Fragrance mix	Quaternium-15	Budesonide
Colophony	Methyldibromo glutaronitrile	Hydrocortisone 17-butyrate
Paraben mix	p-phenylenediamine	Mercaptobenzothiazole
Negative control	Formaldehyde	Bacitracin
Balsam of Peru	Mercapto mix	Parthenolide
Ethylenediamine dihydrochloride	Thimerosal	Disperse blue 106
Cobalt dichloride	Thiuram mix	Bronopol

T.R.U.E., Thin-Layer Rapid Use Epicutaneous.

Patch Testing

Patch tests may be used to confirm the diagnosis of ACD if a specific agent is suspected, even in young children.[467] Different panels of antigens for patch testing are available in Europe, the United States, and Japan, which has led to efforts to standardize testing internationally. In the United States, the Thin-Layer Rapid Use Epicutaneous (T.R.U.E.) patch test kit (Allerderm; http://www.truetest.com) is commercially available and has been expanded to 36 allergens (Table 3.5). These test kits have allergens for reactivity against the most common contact allergens measured and preloaded onto hypoallergenic tape for easy use; however, the potential allergens are not inclusive and lack flexibility. Of the most relevant allergens in children,[468] dialkyl thioureas and CAPB are not found in the latest T.R.U.E. test kits. Also, although MCI/MI is in this kit, MI alone is not but is often positive (and thus missed).[469] A Pediatric Dermatology Workgroup of the American Contact Dermatitis Society designated the 38 most important allergens for testing in children 6 to 17 years of age (FDA-approved ages for patch testing), noting that a typical back of a child can hold 40 to 60 patches.[470] Of these 38, 15 are not included (or are only partially represented) in the T.R.U.E. test kits at this time.[471] The North American Contact Dermatitis Group (NACDG) and American Contact Dermatitis Society screening allergen series are more extensive sets of test substances.[472] Among these 38, the ones most likely to cause ACD per the Pediatric Contact Dermatitis Registry are nickel (13.0%), fragrance (9.4%), Balsam of Peru (6.5%), propylene glycol (5.0%), bacitracin and CAPB (both 4.6%), and neomycin and formaldehyde (both 4.4%). A list of 21 key allergens for testing in preschool children has also been published.[473]

When patch testing is performed, patches should be placed on grossly normal, nonhairy skin such as the back or volar forearm.[474] Distraction techniques such as having the child watch a video are very useful, particularly for testing smaller children.[475] Patch testing should be deferred in the presence of extensive active dermatitis; false-positive reactions may be obtained, and a strongly positive patch-test reaction may cause acute exacerbation of the dermatitis. Antihistamines affect type I reactions and not type IV reactions; thus their administration is not a contraindication to patch testing. Systemic corticosteroid and immunosuppressive therapy might mask patch-test responses, and it is preferable that oral steroids be discontinued at least 3 weeks before patch testing. Potent topical steroids have also

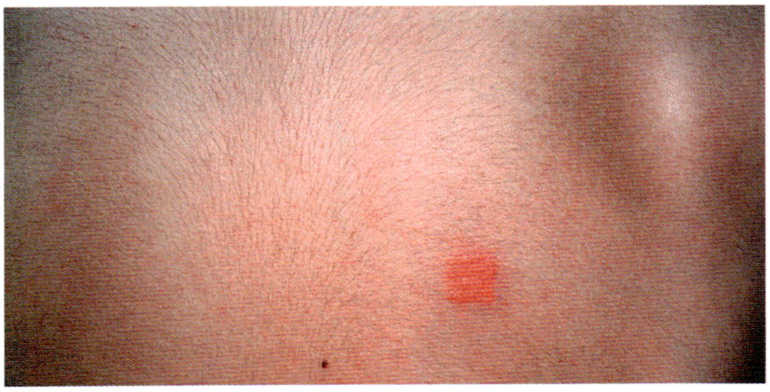

Fig. 3.62 Patch testing. Positive patch test reaction to p-tert-butylphenol formaldehyde resin in a patient with shoe dermatitis because of reactivity to the glue (see Fig. 3.71).

been shown to suppress patch-test reactivity[476] and should be avoided at the site of testing for 1 week before patch testing.

Patch tests generally should be kept in place for 48 hours, and a reading can be made after an interval of 20 to 60 minutes after removal of the patch to allow the skin to recover from the effects of pressure and occlusion (Fig. 3.62). The patch or its removal may produce mild transient erythema or a temporary blanching effect, resulting in false reactions.

Reactions are graded based on redness, induration, and presence of blistering. Unless testing for weak sensitizers (such as fabrics or cosmetics), a doubtful reaction (faint macular erythema only) is usually of no significance. A 1 plus (1+) reaction is characterized by erythema, infiltration, and possibly papules. The addition of vesicles to this response indicates a 2 plus (2+) reaction, and a bullous reaction is read as 3 plus (3+). A second reading of the patches should be performed at 72 to 96 hours after the patches are placed. This reading distinguishes irritant from allergic reactions, because irritant reactions often resolve after patches are removed, whereas allergic reactions increase in time. Delayed reading at 5 days or beyond may be needed for certain allergens (metals such as nickel, cobalt, potassium dichromate, and gold; topical antibiotics such as neomycin and bacitracin; topical corticosteroids; PPD). In one study 66% of children had a positive reaction at 48 hours, 84% at 72 hours, and 50% between days 7 and 9; 13% only had delayed reactions to offending agents, stressing the need to include the late observation.[477]

Based on the results, families can learn more about specific allergens at https://www.truetest.com/global/patientinfo.htm. The Contact Allergen Management Program (CAMP) of the American Contact Dermatitis Society provides detailed lists of products that patients are able to use through a website (https://www.contactderm.org/resources/acds-camp) and free app (https://www.contactderm.org/files/CAMP_App_User_Guide.pdf). It may also be advisable for patients to test a product on a limited area on the upper inner arm twice a day for 1 week (the repeat open application test [ROAT]).

Occasionally, positive reactions may have no clinical significance. In that case the reaction is termed *contact allergy* rather than ACD. Similarly, the offending material may not give rise to a positive reaction at the site of the test but may show a positive test if carried out on an area of skin closer to the point of the previously existing dermatitis. The value of patch tests is corroborative, and they should be used only as a guide in an attempt to confirm a suspected allergen. Scratch and intracutaneous tests are not useful in contact allergic dermatitis.

Poison Ivy (Rhus) Dermatitis

In the United States, poison ivy, poison oak, and poison sumac produce more cases of ACD than all other contactants combined.[478] The plants causing poison ivy dermatitis are included under the botanical term *Rhus* and are *Toxicodendron* species. Poison ivy and poison oak are the principal causes of *Rhus* dermatitis in the United States. Regardless of the specific *Rhus* plant, the clinical appearance of the dermatitis may be identical. The *Rhus* group belongs to the family of plants known as Anacardiaceae, and cross reactions may occur. These include furniture lacquer derived from the Japanese lacquer tree, oil from the shell of the cashew or Brazil nut, the fruit pulp of the gingko tree, and the marking nut tree of India, from which a black "ink" used to mark apparel is produced. The ACD to this ink is termed *dhobi itch*. The rind of the mango also cross reacts, and the possibility of contact dermatitis to *Rhus* should be considered in children with perioral dermatitis after eating mango or on the hands of mango pickers[479] (Fig. 3.63).

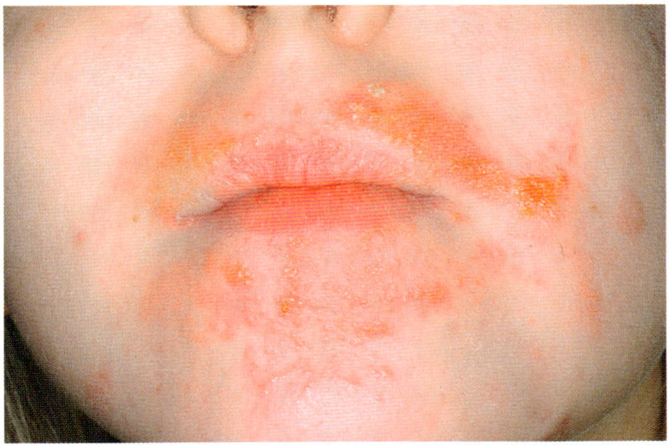

Fig. 3.63 Mango dermatitis. Individuals who react to *Rhus* family plants may demonstrate a perioral dermatitis after eating mango but only when in contact with the mango rind, not from the fruit itself.

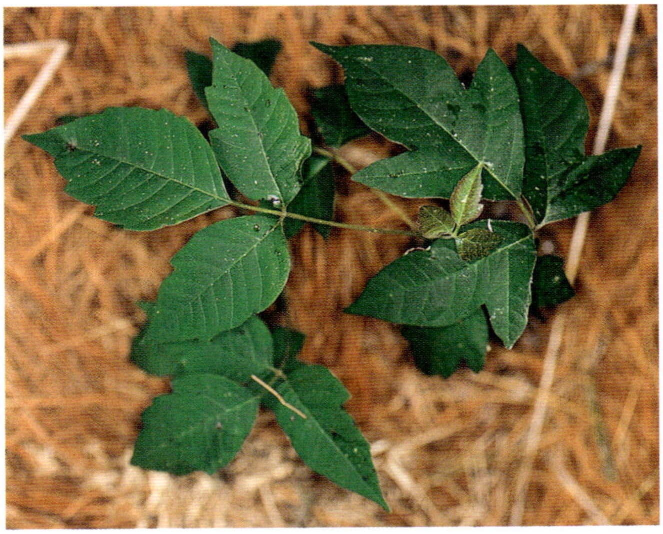

Fig. 3.64 Poison ivy plant. A member of the *Rhus* family, showing three notched leaflets. (Courtesy Dr. Jon Dyer.)

The poison ivy plant (Fig. 3.64) characteristically shows three leaflets notched at the edge. It grows luxuriantly as a tall shrub or woody rope-like vine in vacant lots, among grasses, and on trees or fences throughout all sections of the United States except the extreme southwest. Poison sumac grows as a shrub or tree, never as a vine. It has 7 to 13 leaflets (arranged in pairs along a central stem), with a single leaflet at the end, is relatively uncommon, grows less abundantly, and is found only in woody or swampy areas primarily east of the Mississippi River. Poison oak, conversely, grows as an upright shrub, is most prominent on the West Coast, and is not a problem in the eastern United States. Although *Rhus* dermatitis is more common in the summer, the eruption may occur at any time of year by direct contact with the sensitizing allergen from the leaves, roots, or twigs of the plants.

The eruption produced by poison ivy and related plants is a delayed contact hypersensitivity reaction to an oleoresin (urushiol) of which the active sensitizing ingredient is a pentadecylcatechol. It is characterized by itching, redness, papules, vesicles, and bullae (Fig. 3.65).

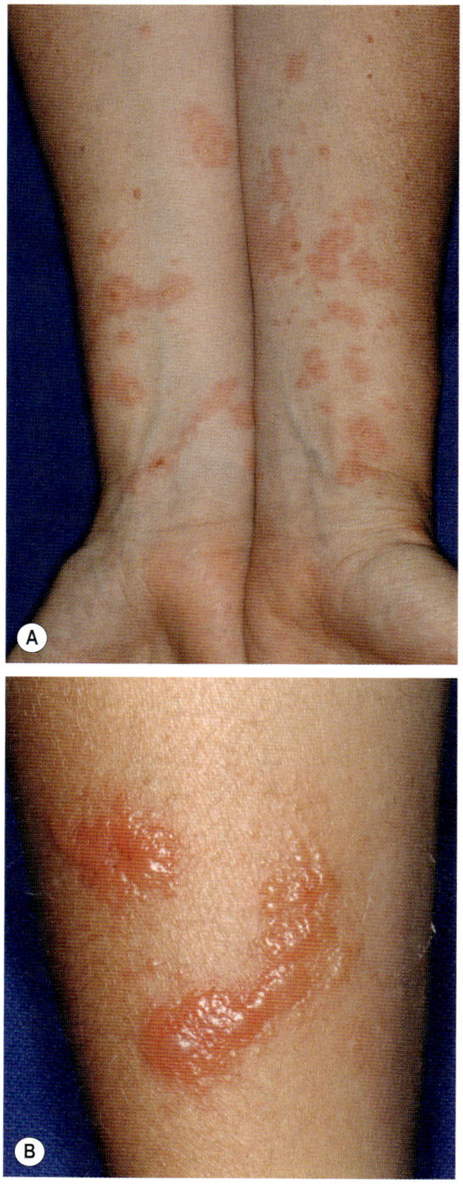

Fig. 3.65 **(A)** *Rhus* dermatitis with Koebner phenomenon. **(B)** A characteristic linear vesicular eruption on the forearms with poison ivy *(Rhus)* dermatitis.

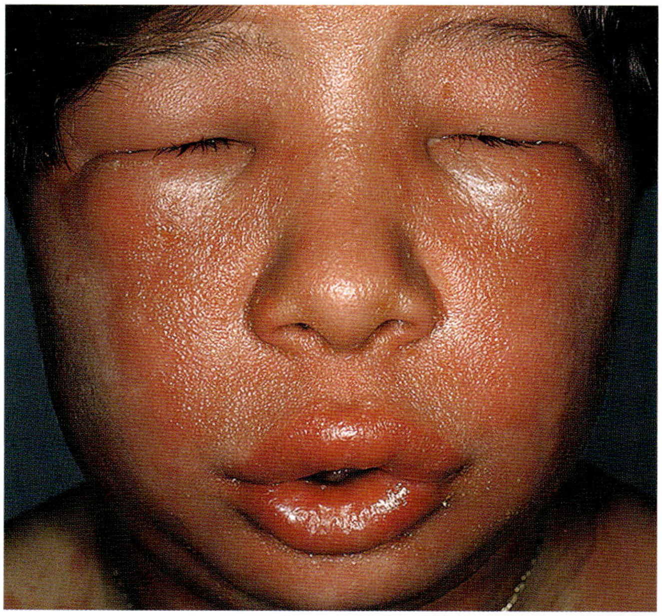

Fig. 3.66 *Rhus* dermatitis. The entire face may become swollen with *Rhus* dermatitis, especially if the patient was exposed through aerosolization. The fine vesiculation distinguishes contact dermatitis from angioedema.

Although often irregular and spotty, a linear distribution is highly characteristic because of scratching and transfer of the urushiol oleoresin (Koebner phenomenon). When contact is indirect, such as from a pet that has the oleoresin on its fur, the dermatitis is often diffuse, thus making the diagnosis more difficult unless the true nature of exposure is suspected. In the fall, when brush and leaves are burned, it must be remembered that the sensitizing oil may be vaporized and transmitted by smoke to exposed cutaneous surfaces, often presenting as a diffuse facial dermatitis with periorbital swelling (Fig. 3.66).

Rhus dermatitis usually first appears in susceptible, sensitized individuals within 1 to 3 days after contact with the sensitizing oleoresin; in highly sensitive individuals it may occur within 8 hours of exposure. Such temporal differences are probably the result of the degree of exposure, individual susceptibility, and variation in cutaneous reactivity of different body regions.

About 70% of the population of the United States would acquire *Rhus* dermatitis if exposed to the plants or the sensitizing oleoresin contained in its leaves, stems, and roots. The result is an acute eczematous eruption that, barring complications or reexposure to the offending allergen, persists for 1 to 3 weeks. Because the undiluted sap from plants of the *Toxicodendron* species turns black when exposed to dry surfaces and skin, dramatic black lacquer- or enamel-like deposits on the skin ("black spot poison ivy") and clothing of individuals exposed to poison ivy or other urushiol-containing plants may rarely be seen.[480,481] These spots typically cannot be removed with soap and water and may precede the development of typical dermatitis.

The best prophylaxis, as with any type of ACD, is complete avoidance of the offending allergen. Patients should be instructed in how to recognize and avoid members of the poison *Rhus* group. When poison ivy is present in the garden or in children's play areas, chemical destruction or physical removal is indicated. Heavy-duty vinyl gloves should be used if the plants are uprooted, because the urushiol is soluble in rubber and can penetrate latex gloves.[482] No topical measure is totally effective in the prevention of poison ivy dermatitis, but certain commercially available barrier preparations with quaternium-18 bentonite (organoclay) have been shown to diminish reactivity significantly (IvyBlock, StokoGard, Hollister Moisture Barrier, Hydropel).[483] Desensitization to the oleoresin of poison ivy by systemic administration of *Rhus* antigen is unreliable and should be reserved only for extremely sensitive individuals who cannot avoid repeated exposure to the antigen. Systemic reactions are not uncommon with the use of hyposensitization procedures.

In an effort to minimize the degree of dermatitis, individuals with known exposure should wash thoroughly with soap and water as rapidly as possible so that removal of the oil is accomplished, preferably within 5 to 10 minutes of exposure. If the oleoresin is not carefully removed shortly after exposure, the allergen may be transmitted by the fingers to other parts of the body (particularly the face, forearms, or male genitalia) (Fig. 3.67). However, the fluid content of vesicles and bullae is not contagious and does not produce new lesions. Thus unless the sensitizing antigen is still on the skin, the disorder is neither able to be spread on an individual nor contagious from one person to another.

Complete change of clothing is advisable, and whenever possible, contaminated shoes and clothing should be washed with soap and water or cold water mixed with alcohol to remove the urushiol. Harsh soaps and vigorous scrubbing offer no advantage over simple soaking and cool water. Thorough washing may not prevent a severe dermatitis

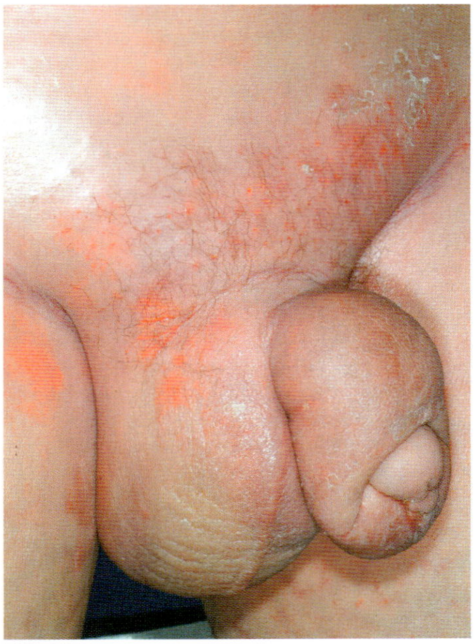

Fig. 3.67 *Rhus* dermatitis. The oleoresin may be transmitted by the fingers to other parts of the body, including the male genitalia.

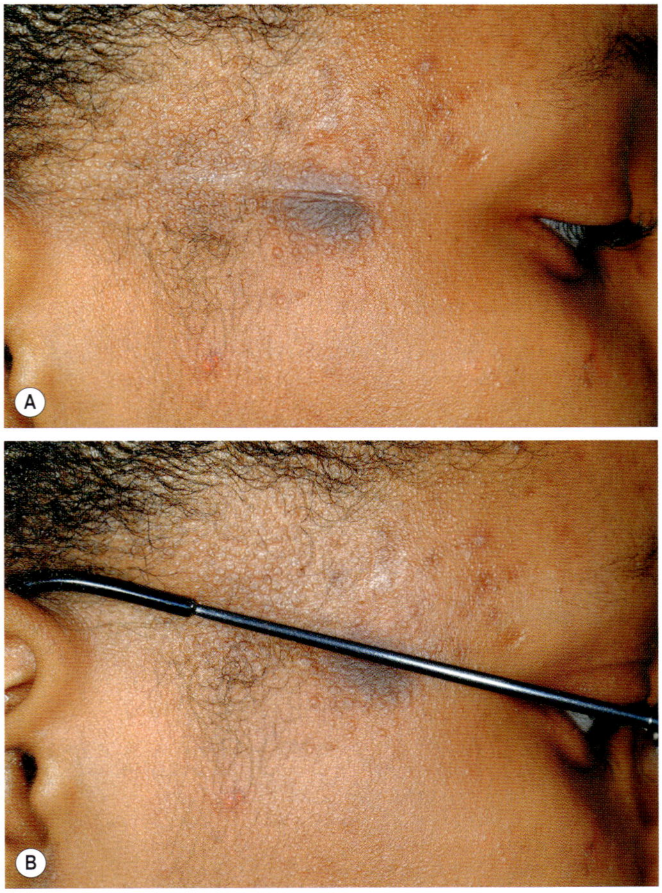

Fig. 3.68 Nickel contact dermatitis. This dermatitis **(A)** represents a reaction to nickel-containing eyeglass frames **(B)**.

in highly sensitive persons. It may, however, reduce the reaction and prevent spread of the oleoresin. When early washing is not feasible, it is worthwhile to wash at the first opportunity in an effort to remove any oleoresin remaining on the skin or clothing and thus prevent its transfer to other parts of the body.

In the management of mild *Rhus* dermatitis, treatment with an antipruritic "shake" lotion such as calamine lotion is helpful. Topical preparations containing potential sensitizers such as diphenhydramine or benzocaine should be avoided. As in other acute eczematous eruptions, cool compresses with plain tap water or Burow solution are soothing, help remove crusts, and relieve pruritus. Administration of potent topical corticosteroids and systemic use of antihistamines and antipruritic agents are helpful. Because the acutely involved areas tend to be vesicular and weeping, creams and lotion forms of topical steroids are more commonly used than occlusive ointments.

In severe, more generalized cases of *Rhus* dermatitis, short-term systemic corticosteroid treatment may be indicated. Systemic corticosteroid therapy may be initiated with dosages of 1 mg/kg per day of prednisone or its equivalent. Steroids should be tapered gradually over 2 to 3 weeks. Premature termination of systemic corticosteroids may result in a rapid rebound, with return of the dermatitis to its original intensity.

Metal and Metal Salt Dermatitis

Nickel dermatitis, the most common ACD to metal, is also by far the most common cause of contact allergy in children undergoing patch testing, with a prevalence of 10.3% to 40% in tested children worldwide.[455,468,484] Nickel may be added to other metals to increase metal strength (in chromium or cobalt) or as plating to increase attractiveness and durability (a variety of metals, including gold).

Earlobe dermatitis is a cardinal sign of nickel dermatitis. Ear piercing has repeatedly been shown to be a strong risk factor for both females[485] and males.[486] The current trend toward piercing of additional body areas in both males and females has increased the numbers of nickel-sensitive individuals. A positive family history of nickel ACD appears to be a risk factor.[466] Several studies have shown an increased risk of nickel sensitivity in girls (perhaps because of piercing).[487] Because piercing of ears or other sites is responsible for an increased tendency of sensitization to nickel and nickel products, piercing should be done with a stainless steel needle. Persons undergoing piercing should be advised to wear only stainless steel earrings or titanium earrings until the earlobes (or other sites) are completely healed, usually about 3 weeks. Although stainless steel contains up to 20% nickel, the nickel is bound tightly and usually causes no problems.

Prominent pruritic periumbilical and subumbilical papules should also trigger consideration of contact allergy to nickel from the nickel-containing buttons on pants and belt buckles and may present as recalcitrant lichenified plaques in children with AD.[488] Circular erythematous scaling patches on the midline trunk of infants may signal reactivity to the metal snaps in baby clothes, and at least 6% of the fasteners in children's clothing have been shown to release nickel ion.[489] Other potential triggers are zippers, clothing hooks, the dorsal eyelets on shoes, nickel-containing eyeglass rims (Fig. 3.68), shoe buckles, musical instruments,[490] razors,[491] gaming systems,[492] laptops,[493] tablets,[494] and cell phones and cell phone accessories.[495,496] Although the concentration of nickel in orthodontic appliances is low and has not been found to sensitize against nickel, patients who are already nickel sensitive, usually from exposure through ear piercing, rarely may show gingival reactions induced by the appliance[497]; the prevalence of reactions to orthodontic appliances is approximately 0.03%.[498] Students should be aware of the presence of nickel in seats with metal studs, which may lead to patches on the posterior thighs,[499] and metal ballet balance bars may lead to hand dermatitis. Hand dermatitis may also be associated with nickel allergy, because nickel may be present in the metal handles of scissors, keys, doorknobs, and the wheels of skateboards. Nickel coins in the United States no longer contain nickel, but small amounts are present in coins from other countries, and reactions to coin rolling or after coin ingestion by young children have been described.[500] Patch testing for nickel sensitivity can be performed, but false negatives are not uncommon, and repeated testing may be helpful. If a substance is suspected of containing free nickel, application of a test solution of dimethylglox-ime in a 10% aqueous solution of ammonia (Allerderm Ni kit) to the suspected item will usually cause the suspected metal to turn pink.

Once the presence of hypersensitivity to nickel has been established, the hypersensitivity usually lasts for years. Patients must therefore be taught how to avoid contact with nickel objects through the use of proper substitutes. If possible, wearing clothes with nickel should be avoided, and substitution of pants with elasticized waists for jeans with metal snaps and leather for metal belt buckles should be considered. Periodic coating of the offending metal with clear nail polish (including after each washing if laundered) may prevent loss of nickel, but sewing cloth over the nickel snap is not effective because sweating encourages nickel to leach through the fabric into contact with skin. In general, watches with stainless steel backs should be worn; application of an adhesive moleskin on the back of a watch may be helpful. Sterling silver or platinum jewelry is usually tolerated. Nickel-free eyeglass frames are available. The majority of inexpensive earrings contain some nickel,[501] so that individuals with the allergy should wear only surgical stainless steel earrings, "hypoallergenic" earrings with titanium (which looks like platinum), or earrings with plastic casings (Blomdahl, Simply Whispers). Vinyl gloves can be worn by patients who are sensitive to nickel to avoid hand contact with nickel. Mid- to high-potency topical steroids can be used to treat a reaction, but avoidance of nickel is required for full efficacy. Dietary avoidance of nickel is difficult but has been recommended by some authors in patients with severe nickel-induced hand ACD and those with systemic contact dermatitis who do not respond to avoidance. Foods with high nickel content include canned foods, chocolate, cocoa, soybeans, cashews, almonds, oatmeal, legumes, and several types of fish and shellfish.

Chromates are an ingredient in the manufacture of many products such as cement, mortar, leather, paints, and anticorrosives. They are used in the dye of the green felt fabric used for pool tables and the yellow-green pigment of tattoos and cosmetics. Dichromates are used to toughen the collagen in leather and allow it to resist wear, water, and changes because of heat. Most contact reactions in children that are caused by chromates manifest as shoe dermatitis (see Shoe Dermatitis section).

Cobalt blue pigment is found in glass and pottery and used in the blue and green of watercolor paints and crayons. It is inextricably linked to nickel in metal-plated objects and costume jewelry, and it can be found in cosmetics, joint replacements, and cement. Oral administration of vitamin B_{12}, which also contains cobalt, can cause intractable hand eczema, and injection may lead to dermatitis at the injection site in individuals who are sensitive to cobalt.

Allergic reactions to aluminum (Al) are probably not rare and develop most often from vaccination with Al-adsorbed vaccines, including those for diphtheria, tetanus, and pertussis; *Haemophilus influenza*; pneumococcus; hepatitis A and B; and human papillomavirus.[502,503] Children most commonly present with intensely itchy subcutaneous nodules or indurations localized to the site on the anterolateral thigh from 3 weeks to 4 years after the vaccination. Exacerbation of the itching may occur with intercurrent upper respiratory or GI tract infections, sometimes as a prodromal sign. These itchy indurated areas persist for a median duration of 4.6 years. In one study patch testing with aluminum showed reactivity in 95% of those affected, and almost 20% of these reported ACD after exposure to Al-containing deodorants, cosmetics, sunscreens, emollients, and buttons.[503] Other contactants that contain aluminum are Al-precipitated pollen extracts used for allergen-specific immunotherapy, ear drops, and pigments used in tattooing. More than 90% of children with these reactive lesions had milder reactions after vaccines beyond infancy, suggesting that the value of continued vaccination outweighs the risk of avoidance of Al-adsorbed vaccines.

Shoe Dermatitis

Shoe dermatitis is an extremely common form of contact dermatitis in childhood that usually results from rubber products, especially given the increasing trend for athletic shoes. It is commonly misdiagnosed as tinea pedis, a disorder that occurs uncommonly in children before puberty. In one study, more than 50% of children with foot dermatitis showed reactivity to suspected contact allergens.[504]

Shoe dermatitis usually begins on the dorsal surface of the base of the great toe. It may remain localized or spread to involve the dorsal surfaces of the feet and other toes. The thick skin of the plantar surfaces is generally more resistant but may demonstrate dermatitis over the sole, ventral surface of the toes, instep, or even the entire plantar surface that may be confused with juvenile plantar dermatosis or psoriasis. Erythema, lichenification, and, in severe cases, weeping and crusting are typical, but the interdigital spaces usually are spared. In contrast, maceration, scaling, and occasional vesiculation of the interdigital webs, particularly between the fourth and fifth toes, are usually seen with tinea pedis. Irritant dermatitis from friction and ill-fitting shoes may also sharply localize to the dorsal aspects of the toes.

Rubber components are the principal allergens[505]; these include accelerators (most commonly mercaptobenzothiazole but also thiuram, carbamate, and diphenylguanidine) and rubber antioxidants. Rubber accelerators facilitate the transformation of liquid rubber to solid. Several components of the approved patch-test kit in the United States test for rubber, including the carba mix, the black rubber mix, mercaptobenzothiazole, mercapto mix, and the thiuram mix (see Table 3.5); however, additional testing should be performed if shoe dermatitis is suspected but an agent is not found in this standard kit, because it is not fully inclusive. Rubber is a common component of the insoles of shoes and particularly of box toes. Rubber cement may be used in joining shoe uppers, outer leather, and linings.

Individuals with rubber sensitivity may also react to exposure to pacifiers (perioral); wearing latex gloves or handling rubber bands or balloons (hand dermatitis); wearing underwear, swimwear, and socks with elastic (especially if clothes are bleached; waist and inguinal areas); handling rubber handle grips (sweaty hands)[505]; wearing swim goggles (periorbital); using cosmetic applicators (face); and wearing adhesive bandages. In adolescent boys and men, penile contact dermatitis may result from wearing rubber condoms.

Neoprene is a form of rubber in which dialkyl thioureas are used to speed up vulcanization, making it tougher and more pliable for shaping. It is now widely used in sporting equipment, mouse pads and computer cases, wetsuits, athletic shoes, shin guards and other protective pads, orthopedic braces, leggings, and Halloween masks. Components of neoprene-containing items that cause ACD are diethyl thiourea (a dialkyl thiourea that is not in the T.R.U.E. test) and p-tertiary (tert)–butylphenol formaldehyde resin in adhesive.[507]

Less commonly, chromates in leather and adhesives (colophony and p-tert-butylphenol formaldehyde resin) can cause foot dermatitis (Fig. 3.69). p-tert-butylphenol formaldehyde resin has also recently been implicated in ACD from the foam padding of a bra.[508] The nickel in eyelets and arch supports should also be considered. Iatrogenic ACD

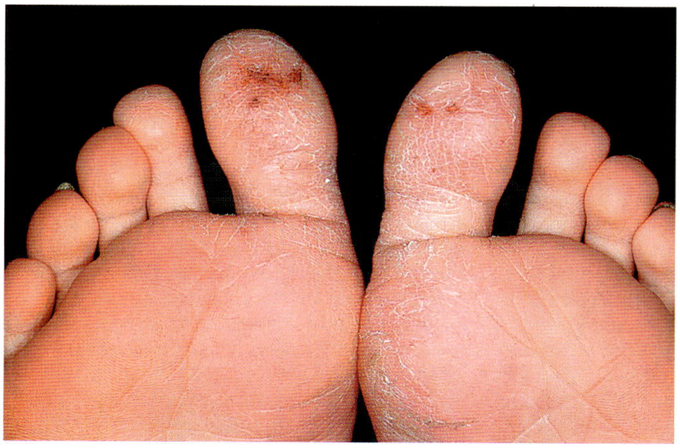

Fig. 3.69 Shoe dermatitis. The recalcitrance of this patient's dermatitis to potent topical steroids led to patch testing, which showed reactivity to p-tert-butylphenol formaldehyde resin (see Fig. 3.64), a component of the glue used in shoes. More commonly, shoe dermatitis is seen on the dorsal aspect of the feet and results from rubber products in shoes or chromates used to tan the leather.

also often occurs on the foot, particularly because of neomycin or bacitracin in topical antibiotics.[509] Hyperhidrosis and wearing of occlusive hosiery and shoes contribute to shoe-contact allergy by leaching out allergens and increasing their percutaneous penetration.

Patients with shoe sensitivity should avoid the offending allergen and control associated hyperhidrosis. Use of shoe substitutes depends on whether the reactivity is to rubber, chromates, or adhesives. Vegetable-tanned footwear is a substitute if reactivity is to chromates. Open sandals, unlined sewn leather moccasins (such as from L.L. Bean), wooden clogs, or plastic “jelly” sandals are other alternatives. In addition, polyvinyl shoes, although they increase the tendency to perspiration, commonly lack many of the potential sensitizers seen in regular shoes; Bass Weejuns loafers and vinyl tennis shoes may also be acceptable substitutes. Because the inner sole is a common source of contact sensitization, removal and replacement with cork insoles, Dr. Scholl’s Air Foam pads, or Johnson’s Odor-Eaters held in place with a nonrubber adhesive such as Elmer’s glue are often helpful.

The management of active shoe dermatitis, as in other eczematous disorders, is aided by use of open wet compresses, topical corticosteroids, and antipruritic agents. Because hyperhidrosis is usually responsible for the “leaching” out of potential sensitizing agents, use of measures that minimize excessive perspiration of the feet is advisable. Athletic equipment can be lined with water-repellent canvas as an adjunct to the use of a protective sock or sleeve. The topical use of aluminum chloride, available as Drysol or Certain Dri, or tannic acid soaks (two teabags in 1 quart of water) once or twice weekly, often assist in the control of hyperhidrosis. Noncaking agents such as Zeasorb powder dusted freely into shoes and hosiery not only tend to lessen perspiration but also may act as a mechanical barrier, thus limiting contact with potential allergens and irritants. When painful fissures are present, soaking the foot in water for 20 minutes at bedtime followed by the careful application of superglue or liquid adhesive into the fissured areas, the use of topical corticosteroids and emollient creams, and occlusion at night with plastic wrap or small plastic bags will hasten resolution and lessen discomfort. Barrier socks (Microair), which have three layers of fabric that provide a physical barrier and are breathable, have been helpful in decreasing reactions if exposure cannot be avoided.[510] Individuals with rubber allergy should wear vinyl rather than rubber gloves and avoid bleaching clothes with elastic and using rubber swim goggles, rubber headphones, and latex condoms.

Dermatitis to Cosmetics and Topical Medications

The most common cosmetic agents causing ACD are lipsticks, antiperspirants, hair dyes with PPD, substances in commercial and home permanent wave formulations, lanolins, acrylics, nail lacquers, benzalkonium and ascorbic acid in contact-lens solutions, fragrances (perfumes), sunscreen components (particularly benzophenone and increasingly octocrylene), and a number of preservatives used in cosmetics and shampoos. These allergens are the most common triggers of ACD of the hands.[511] Because early use of cosmetics abets this problem, it is recommended that cosmetics be avoided in young children. Even “toy” cosmetics contain fragrance, particularly cinnamic aldehyde.[512] In many instances the eyelids are affected not by cosmetics applied to the lids and lashes but by preparations applied to the scalp, face, and nails. Exposure to peppermint oil most commonly leads to perioral dermatitis.[513] Peppermint oil is found in cosmeceuticals, personal hygiene products (mouthwashes, toothpastes, and bath preparation), topical medications (cooling sensation), and food.

ACD is increasingly blamed on preservatives and vehicle components.[514] MCI/MI (Kathon CG)[515] and MI alone[515] are used as preservatives in baby shampoos, soaps, wet wipes, and protective creams. The dermatitis usually manifests on the face, perianal/buttock area, or hands and resists topical and oral antibiotics and corticosteroids. One study found that MCI/MI ranked third in positive patch-testing results in pediatric patients.[516,517] Lesions from MCI/MI on the buttock may be confused with baboon syndrome, which is characterized by well-defined symmetric erythema on the buttocks and sometimes on the upper thighs and axillae and usually is related to oral drug ingestion.[518] Recent studies found that testing to higher concentrations of MCI/MI as well as to MI alone is necessary to detect ACD to MCI or MI.[519] However, the T.R.U.E. test identifies only the MCI/MI mix at lower concentration.

Another common cause of fingertip and facial dermatitis is CAPB, a surfactant contained in many no-tears shampoos and soaps, contact-lens solutions, and moist baby and facial wipes. CAPB reactivity has been found in 11.3% children who have undergone patch testing.[468,520]

Formaldehyde and formaldehyde releasers (such as quaternium-15, diazolidinyl or imidazolidinyl urea, bromonitropropanediol/bronopol, and dimethylol dimethyl hydantoin)[514] are other preservatives that may trigger contact allergy. A reaction to tosylamide/formaldehyde resin in nail polish is seen largely in female patients who paint their nails[521] but has been described in boys, including from application to the nails as a deterrent to nail biting.[522] Dermatitis tends to occur on the eyelids, cheeks, lips, chin, and neck, rather than on the nails themselves. Although the incidence of lanolin sensitivity from emollients is low, lanolin and its derivatives may be present under many different names (e.g., wool wax, wool grease, and wool fat). Lanolin sensitivity should be suspected in children with AD who tolerate application of petrolatum but not the application of lanolin-containing emollients, such as Aquaphor or Eucerin.

In the United States, parabens (compounds containing p-hydroxybenzoic acid) are often added in low concentrations to creams, lotions, and cosmetics in an attempt to retard microbial growth; although possible allergens, they are much weaker than other preservatives such as MCI/MI, CAPB, and formaldehyde/formaldehyde releasers and, in fact, were named the nonallergen of the year in 2019 by the American Contact Dermatitis Society.[523] Thimerosal is an organic mercurial compound used as a preservative. It has largely been removed from vaccines but can be found in cosmetics, eye drops, and contact-lens solutions. Although positive patch testing to thimerosal may occur, reactivity is unlikely to be clinically relevant, and rates of sensitization will likely decline with the removal of thimerosal from many vaccines.[524] Although still in the T.R.U.E. test kit, the NACDG has removed thimerosal from their standard testing trays because of its low clinical relevance.

More than 5000 different fragrances are in use today, and the ingredient “fragrance” on a label represents a mixture of many. Reactivity to fragrance has been shown to increase with age.[525] Use of perfumes in adolescent girls has been associated with the “atomizer sign,” the presence of primary dermatitis at the Adam’s apple where the perfume is sprayed.[526] Deodorants can be triggers for ACD in the axillary vault and generally cause an eczematous dermatitis (see Metal and Metal Salt Dermatitis section); inclusion of sandalwood and ylang ylang oils in some deodorants encourages sensitization through shaved axillae. Antiperspirants containing zirconium may produce allergic granulomatous reactions. If near the axillary area but not in the vault, disperse dye in clothing is the most likely cause of the reactivity (see Clothing Dermatitis section). Even baby washes and shampoos have fragrance as a component. “Unscented” or “fragrance-free” means that the product has no perceptible odor but does not necessarily mean devoid of fragrance chemicals; it may just reflect the addition of masking agents. Furthermore, manufacturers are not required in the United States to list specific fragrances and often do not list essential oils and fragrances used for reasons other than aroma (e.g., preservatives, bisabolol, citrus oil). Testing to both fragrance mix and balsam of Peru captures 70% to 80% of fragrance allergies. True fragrance-free products are available.[527]

The most common allergy-containing fragrances are cinnamic alcohol and cinnamic aldehyde, which are among the eight components of the fragrance mix used in contact allergy testing. Cinnamic alcohol and cinnamic aldehyde are components of chewing gums, toothpaste, mouthwash, flavored lip balms, chewable vitamins,[528] detergents, soaps, and deodorants.[529] Other fragrances are used in perfumes, aftershaves, colognes, and even food flavorings. Reactions to fragrance mix were noted in 18% of 500 children in a study in the United Kingdom.[456]

Balsam of Peru (*Myroxylon pereirae* tree extract) is an oleoresin that may contain some of the fragrances in the fragrance mix as well as a range of other components (such as citrus peel, tea tree oil, benzoic acid, and others). Individuals who react to balsam of Peru may react to beeswax, colophony, various spices, turpentine, and coumarin. Balsam of Peru is found in many body washes, shampoos, and diaper area topical products. Balsam of Peru cross reacts with other balsam derivatives, such as balsam of pine, which is found in fluocinolone oil.[530] Its presence as a flavoring in citrus peel and spices (e.g., cinnamon, cloves, vanilla, nutmeg, paprika, and curry) has led to systemic contact dermatitis reactions to citrus products, spices, pickles, chocolate,

Table 3.6 Classification of Topical Corticosteroids Based on Chemical Structure and Cross Reactivity

Group A	Group B	Group C	Group D1	Group D2
Hydrocortisone acetate	Amcinonide	Desoximethasone	Alclometasone	Difluprednate
Methylprednisolone	Budesonide*	Dexamethasone	Beclomethasone	Hydrocortisone 17-butyrate*
Prednisolone	Desonide	Diflucortolone	Betamethasone dipropionate	Prednicarbate
Tixocortol-21-pivalate*	Fluocinolone	Fluocortolone	Betamethasone 17-valerate	
	Fluocinonide	Halometasone	Clobetasol	
	Halcinonide		Diflorasone	
	Triamcinolone		Fluticasone	
			Mometasone	

*Used to test reactivity.

wine, and colas[531]; avoidance of ketchup in affected children can lead to marked clearance of widespread, recalcitrant dermatitis.[532] Balsam of Peru also cross reacts with a chemical in Mastisol, often used to increase adhesive adherence

A variety of topical prescription and over-the-counter formulations are capable of producing contact and (at times) systemic contact reactions. Of these, ethylenediamine, benzocaine and its derivatives, topical antibiotics, and topical preparations with diphenhydramine are the most common. Topical application of diphenhydramine (such as in Caladryl) is generally frowned on because it reportedly could cause sensitization and lead to a generalized reaction after systemic administration of diphenhydramine, but occurrence is exceedingly rare. In addition, application of over-the-counter topical antibiotics may cause contact dermatitis and may lead to worsening of cutaneous inflammation despite appropriate use. Neomycin sulfate has long been considered the most allergenic of the topical antibiotics, but bacitracin allergy now exceeds it in prevalence in some studies, and anaphylactic reactions to topical application of bacitracin have been described[533]; both are ingredients in "triple antibiotic" formulations. Although neomycin and bacitracin are not chemically related, both bacitracin and neomycin cosensitization may occur concurrently when topical antibiotics with both are applied. Fusidic acid is an antibiotic used topically outside the United States that can cause both ACD and anaphylaxis after topical application.[534] Recently, ACD to potassium peroxymonosulfate, used as a chemical shock treatment for hot tubs and swimming pools to clear the water, has been described.[535]

Ethylenediamine, a compound stabilizer seen in various topical creams, including with nystatin cream, cross reacts with certain antihistamines, among them hydroxyzine and promethazine hydrochloride. Ingestion of a cross-reacting oral antihistamine in an ethylenediamine-sensitive individual can cause generalized dermatitis[536]; systemic contact dermatitis may also occur from administration of hydroxyzine but without reactivity to ethylenediamine.

The trend in adolescents of hair streaking and dyeing and henna tattoos has increased exposure to dyes containing PPD. In addition to typical contact allergic dermatitis, these reactions to PPD may resemble erythema multiforme or vesicular erythema multiforme.[537] Because of the tendency to use PPD in the mixture to darken and increase the precision of design of the temporary henna tattoo, children may show ACD to PPD at any site of henna tattooing.[452,538] Henna itself is rarely a sensitizer. Concentrations of PPD as high as 17.5% have been found in henna-tattoo preparations despite the limit of 6% PPD allowed in hair dyes. Once sensitized to PPD after a henna tattoo, children not only have a lifelong potential reactivity to permanent oxidative hair dye[539] but also may show systemic contact dermatitis to components that cross react with PPD such as hydrochlorothiazide, sulfonamide medications, and ester anesthetics such as benzocaine.[540] PPD may be a component of fur dyes, dark-colored cosmetics, inks, rubber products, and photographic supplies. PPD reactions in children may also occur because of "connubial dermatitis," in which a child is sensitized through contact with the product on a parent.[463]

ACD from topical corticosteroids has been increasing in incidence and should be considered when patients with dermatitis are worsening despite the application of topical steroids.[541] Sensitization can also occur from ophthalmic solutions and aerosolized inhaled corticosteroids.[542] Reactions to topical steroids can be anywhere, but typically those from ophthalmic solutions involve the conjunctivae, eyelids, and periorbital areas, whereas ACD to inhaled steroids is usually on the face, sometimes with extension. Generalized eruptions may occur after systemic exposure to a cross-reacting steroid. Five groups of corticosteroids have been classified based on their chemical structures (A, B, C, D1, and D2) (Table 3.6). Sensitization to group A steroids (in over-the-counter hydrocortisone and oral prednisone) is highest (overall 5.72%).[543] Topical steroids can be screened by ROAT on the forearm. Tixocortol pivalate, budesonide, and hydrocortisone 17-butyrate are used to test for allergy to topical corticosteroids, although the combination of tixocortol pivalate and budesonide detect almost 90% of the patients with corticosteroid allergies. Positive reactions to topical steroids may not be detectable until 5 days or more after patching. The majority of individuals who test positive to topical steroids have other positive patch tests as well, and it should be remembered that ACD may result from the excipient (e.g., preservative or penetration enhancer) or even the nickel from the tube, rather than the steroid itself.

Adhesive Tape Dermatitis

Although most cutaneous reactions related to the wearing of adhesive tape are of a mechanical rather than contact sensitivity type, allergic reactions may be caused by the rubber compounds (rubber accelerators or antioxidants) that have been incorporated into the adhesive or the vinyl backing of the adhesive (Fig. 3.70). Dermicel (Johnson &

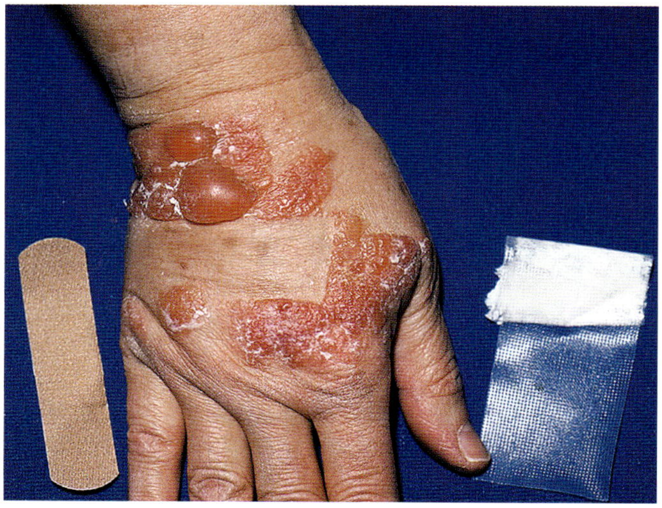

Fig. 3.70 Tape contact dermatitis. Note that this patient did not react to the cloth Band-Aid *(left)* but rather to the larger tape *(right)*.

Johnson), Steri-Strips, or Micropore surgical tape (3M Company), nonrubber acrylate, and spray-on bandages are helpful for those individuals allergic to or irritated by ordinary adhesive tapes. Nevertheless, acrylates in plastics are increasingly becoming an emerging allergen and can reach the skin without direct contact.

Clothing Dermatitis

Although nonspecific irritation from fabrics, rubber, dyes, and cleaning solutions is not uncommon, ACD caused by true sensitization to fabrics is occasionally seen in childhood. Permanent press and crease-resistant fabrics have been responsible for many cases of contact dermatitis because of the use of formaldehydes and formaldehyde-releasing preservatives. Of textiles, blended cottons, corduroy, silk, and rayon have the highest concentrations of formaldehyde, whereas polyester has the least. In a recent survey of 65 children suspected of having contact dermatitis, 7.5% reacted to formaldehyde and 3.8% to each of the listed formaldehyde-releasing preservatives.[468] This type of dermatitis is more likely to occur in individuals whose clothes are tight fitting and close to the skin. The inner thighs, axillary lines, and popliteal fossae are particularly susceptible.

Dermatitis attributable to dyes in wearing apparel such as school and athletic uniforms is increased from clothing dyed black or dark blue (because the concentration of dyes in dark clothing is much higher than that of dyes in light-colored clothing, and dark colors tend to bleed more readily than dyes of lighter hue). Disperse dyes may be used in patch testing, but the garment can also be directly applied for patch testing. Children may also react to the epoxy resin in the adhesive holding a knee patch onto jeans and elastic or rubber waist bands in underwear in which the rubber components are leached out after exposure to bleach.

Compositae Dermatitis

Compositae is one of the largest plant families (10% of the world's flowering plants) and includes among its members chrysanthemum, ragweed, artichoke, sunflower, lettuce, spinach, chamomile, gingko, feverfew, parthenium, and dandelions. Contact allergy to compositae is well recognized in florists, gardeners, and farmers but only occasionally occurs in children.[544] Bisabolol, a compositae derivative, is a component of moisturizers and has been implicated in pediatric ACD.[545]

The complete list of 545 references for this chapter is available online at http://expertconsult.inkling.com.

Key References

Weidinger S, Beck LA, Bieber T, et al. Atopic dermatitis. Nat Rev Dis Primers 2018;4(1):1.

Paller AS, Kong HH, Seed P, et al. The microbiome in patients with atopic dermatitis. J Allergy Clin Immunol 2019;143(1):26–35.

Palmer CN, Irvine AD, Terron-Kwiatkowski A, et al. Common loss-of-function variants of the epidermal barrier protein filaggrin are a major predisposing factor for AD. Nat Genet 2006;38:441–6.

Paller AS, Spergel JM, Mina-Osorio P, et al. The atopic march and atopic multimorbidity: many trajectories, many pathways. J Allergy Clin Immunol 2019;143(1): 46–55.

Borok J, Matiz C, Goldenberg A, et al. Contact dermatitis in atopic dermatitis children-past, present, and future. Clin Rev Allergy Immunol 2019;56(1):86–98.

Jacob SE, McGowan M, Silverberg NB, et al. Pediatric contact dermatitis registry data on contact allergy in children with atopic dermatitis. JAMA Dermatol 2017: 153(8):765–70.

Boguniewicz M, Fonacier L, Guttman-Yassky E, et al. Atopic dermatitis yardstick: practical recommendations for an evolving therapeutic landscape. Ann Allergy Asthma Immunol 2018;120(1):10–22.e2.

Eichenfield LF, Tom WL, Berger TG, et al. Guidelines of care for the management of atopic dermatitis. Section 2. Management and treatment of atopic dermatitis with topical therapies. J Am Acad Dermatol 2014;71(1):116–32.

Sidbury R, Davis DM, Cohen DE, et al. Guidelines of care for the management of atopic dermatitis. Section 3. Management and treatment with phototherapy and systemic agents. J Am Acad Dermatol 2014;71(2):327–49.

Work Group, Sidbury R, Tom WL, et al. Guidelines of care for the management of atopic dermatitis. Section 4. Prevention of disease flares and use of adjunctive therapies and approaches. J Am Acad Dermatol 2014;71(6):1218–33.

Simpson EL, Paller AS, Siegfried EC, et al. Dupilumab in adolescents with uncontrolled atopic dermatitis: a randomized, double-blinded, placebo-controlled, parallel-group, phase 3 clinical trial. JAMA Dermatol 2019;156(1):44–56.

Paller AS, Siegfried EC, Thaçi D, et al. Efficacy and safety of dupilumab with concomitant topical corticosteroids in children 6 to 11 years old with severe atopic dermatitis: a randomized, double-blinded, placebo-controlled phase 3 trial. J Am Acad Dermatol 2020:S0190–9622(20)31152-X.

Jacob SE, Brankov N, Kerr A. Diagnosis and management of allergic contact dermatitis in children: common allergens that can be easily missed. Curr Opin Pediatr 2017:29(4):443–7.

4 Papulosquamous and Related Disorders

CHAPTER OUTLINE

Childhood Psoriasis

Psoriasis is a relatively common immune-mediated disorder, which occurs overall in 0.5% to 0.8% of pediatric patients, with a linear increase in prevalence by age from 0.2% at 2 years to 1.2% at 18 years.[1–5] Psoriasis rarely is present at birth.[6,7] Approximately one-third of adults with psoriasis noted the onset of disease during the first 2 decades of life. As in the adult population, psoriasis occurs most often in white children.[7] The severity of the condition may vary from a life-threatening neonatal pustular or exfoliative dermatosis to a mild, localized disorder that causes no distress. Psoriasis usually follows an irregularly chronic course marked by remissions and exacerbations of unpredictable onset and duration. It negatively affects the quality of life of both the pediatric patient and the parents.[8,9]

Both complex genetic and environmental factors contribute to the risk of psoriasis. An immediate family history has been reported in 30% to 49% of pediatric patients,[6,10] and the risk of occurrence in monozygotic twins is two to three times that of dizygotic twins.[11] The major genetic determinant is *PSOR1* (35% to 50% of patients), which is within the major histocompatibility complex on chromosome 6.[12] Early-onset psoriasis has been linked to human leukocyte antigen (HLA) antigen Cw6, and 73.7% of patients with guttate psoriasis show HLA Cw6 antigen, in contrast to a rate of 7.4% in the general population. Autosomal dominant mutations in caspase recruitment domain family member 14 (*CARD14*; *PSOR2*) also lead to a psoriatic[13] (or pityriasis rubra pilaris [PRP]) phenotype. Deficiency of IL-36 receptor antagonist (DITRA) from variants in *IL36RN* is the major cause of generalized pustular psoriasis (GPP) in patients without plaque psoriasis.[14–16] At least 64 susceptibility loci for psoriasis have now been identified, including genes regulating T-cell function, especially interleukin (IL)-23 function, tumor necrosis factor (TNF) activation, nuclear factor (NF)-κB signaling, T-helper (Th) 2 cytokines, interferon (IFN)-mediated antiviral responses, and macrophage activation.[17–19]

Evidence that psoriasis is a Th17/IL-23 pathway–mediated disorder is also based on the success of targeted therapy, such as cyclosporine and inhibitors of TNF, IL-23p40 and IL-23p19, and IL-17/ IL-17 receptor. The majority of T cells in psoriatic plaques are CD45RO+ memory-effector T cells that migrate into skin exposed to an antigenic trigger. The innate immune system plays a key role in psoriasis, initiating a cascade that involves toll-like receptor-mediated[20] activation of plasmacytoid dendritic cells, included by complexes that contain antimicrobial peptides.[20,21] The activated dendritic cells express IL-12 and IL-23, leading to Th1 and Th17 cell expression of TNF-α/IFN-γ and IL-17/IL-22, respectively. These cytokines stimulate the keratinocytes to produce more IL-1β and IL-6, TNF-α, chemokines, and antimicrobial peptides, further contributing to immune activation and cutaneous inflammation.[22]

Skin injury and streptococcal infections[23,24] are well-known environmental triggers for psoriasis. Additionally, the occurrence of psoriasis has been linked to *Staphylococcus aureus* infection[25] and Kawasaki disease,[26] suggesting a role for superantigens. Psoriasis has been triggered by administration of growth hormone therapy, IFN (e.g., for chronic hepatitis), and other drugs (particularly, lithium, β-blockers, antimalarials, and sodium valproate).[27] Flares of psoriasis have also clearly been linked to psychological and physical stress.

CLINICAL MANIFESTATIONS

Classic lesions of psoriasis consist of round, brightly erythematous, well-marginated plaques covered by a characteristic grayish or silvery-white (mica-like, or "micaceous") scale, attached primarily at the center rather than the periphery of lesions.[28–30] Psoriatic papules coalesce to form plaques that measure 1 cm or more in diameter. The disorder may present as solitary lesions or countless plaques in a generalized distribution (Fig. 4.1). Follicular-based scaling occurs in psoriasis (Figs. 4.2 and 4.3), generally in the presence of more typical lesions, and must be differentiated from PRP.[31] Lesions are usually bilaterally symmetric with a distinct predilection for the scalp (Fig. 4.4) and hairline (Fig. 4.5), elbows, knees and legs (Figs. 4.6 and 4.7), and lumbosacral and anogenital regions. However, lesions may also be found on the trunk or in a flexural distribution with involvement of the axillae (Fig. 4.8 groin (Figs. 4.9, 4.10 and 4.11), and umbilical region. *Inverse psoriasis* reflects lesions in these flexural regions, which is seen without any extensor surface involvement in 2.8% to 6.0% of patients or in association with only regional involvement in 30% of patients. Lesions may also be limited to the palms (Fig. 4.12, *A*) and soles (Fig. 4.12, *B*).[32] A linear variant that courses along the Blaschko lines rarely occurs (Fig. 4.13)[33] and may be associated with more extensive psoriasis (usually with later onset) and/or juvenile psoriatic arthritis (JPsA).[34]

Removal of psoriatic scale results in fine punctate bleeding points. This phenomenon (termed the *Auspitz sign*) is highly characteristic and relates to the rupture of capillaries high in the papillary dermis of lesions. The Koebner phenomenon (an isomorphic response) is commonly seen in psoriasis (Fig. 4.14) but also in verrucae, *Rhus* dermatitis, lichen planus, lichen nitidus, Darier disease, and PRP. This valuable diagnostic sign of psoriasis describes the occurrence of skin lesions at sites of local injury, such as after irritation (a scratch or sunburn) (Fig. 4.15), a surgical scar, or a preexisting disease such as seborrheic or atopic dermatitis. The Koebner phenomenon likely is responsible for psoriasis of the diaper region and around enteral feeding tubes.[35] A peripheral white ring is often the first sign of involution of a psoriatic plaque (termed a *Woronoff ring*). However, when the central portions of the plaques resolve, the involuting lesions may appear nummular (small circles), annular (with central clearing) (Fig. 4.16), gyrate, or arcuate (semicircular).

Facial Psoriasis

Facial psoriasis is more common in children than in adults and occurs without other involvement in 4% to 5% of patients. Involvement of the periorbital area is most typical (Fig. 4.17), and lesions may be subtle, leading to confusion with atopic dermatitis (Fig. 4.18). The plaques of psoriasis tend to be more clearly delineated than patches of atopic dermatitis, are less pruritic, and may show an annular configuration. It should be noted, however, that at least 5% of pediatric patients show an eczema/psoriasis overlap, either showing typical

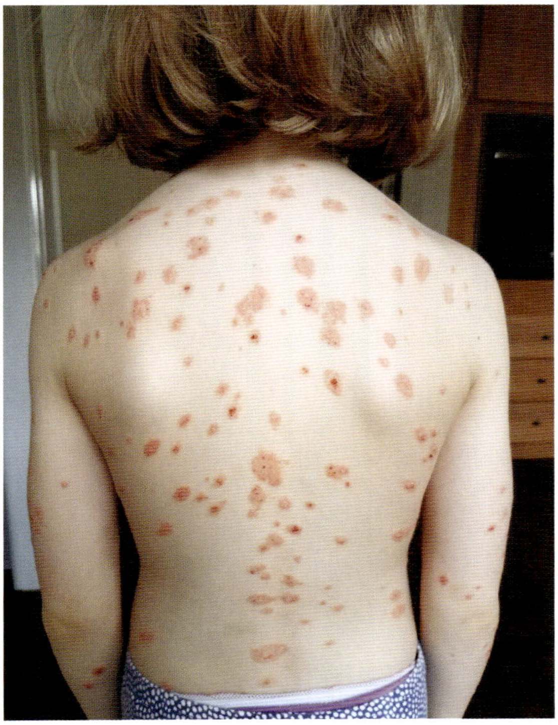

Fig. 4.1 Psoriasis. Typical small plaques on the back and arm in this girl with generalized involvement.

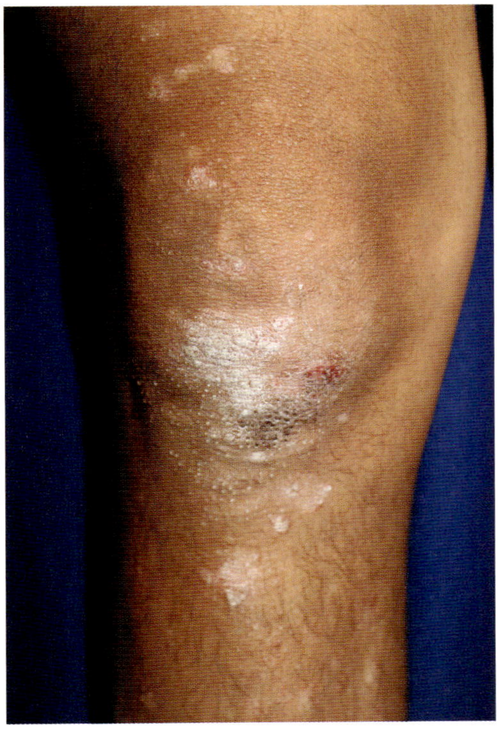

Fig. 4.2 Follicular psoriasis. Scaling follicular-based papules, especially on the knees or elbows, may be a feature of psoriasis but are generally accompanied by more typical or larger plaques that enable the diagnosis and distinguish it from pityriasis rubra pilaris.

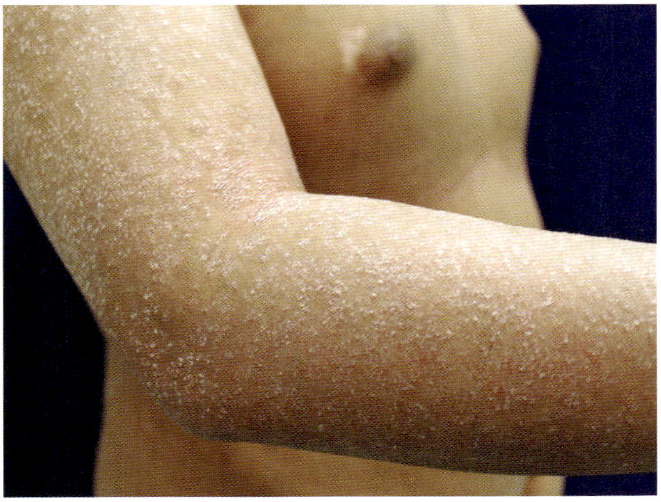

Fig. 4.3 Follicular psoriasis. The extremities were studded with follicular-based erythematous papules but the patient also had typical psoriatic lesions.

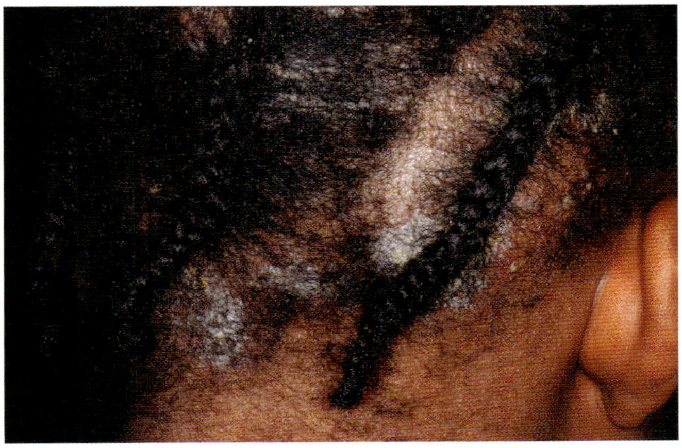

Fig. 4.4 Scalp psoriasis. Discrete plaques of scale overlying erythema. Oiling of the scalp may observe the scaling and make diagnosis more challenging. If concomitant alopecia or lymphadenopathy is present, tinea capitis needs to be considered, especially if psoriasis is confined to the scalp.

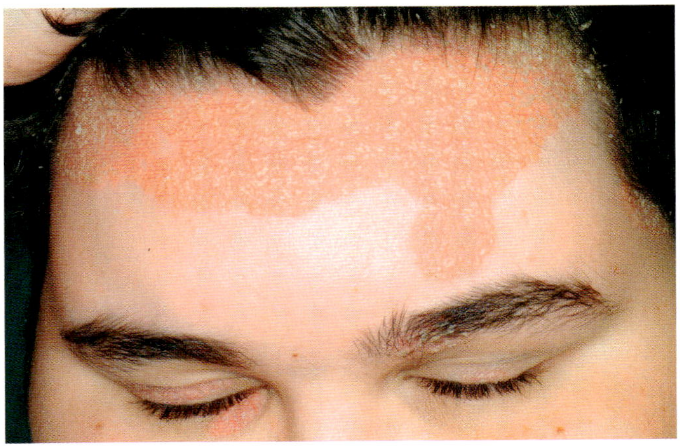

Fig. 4.5 Psoriasis. Psoriasis often involves the forehead, particularly contiguous to the scalp. Note the eyelid and brow involvement. Given the yellowish scaling, this has been called *sebopsoriasis*.

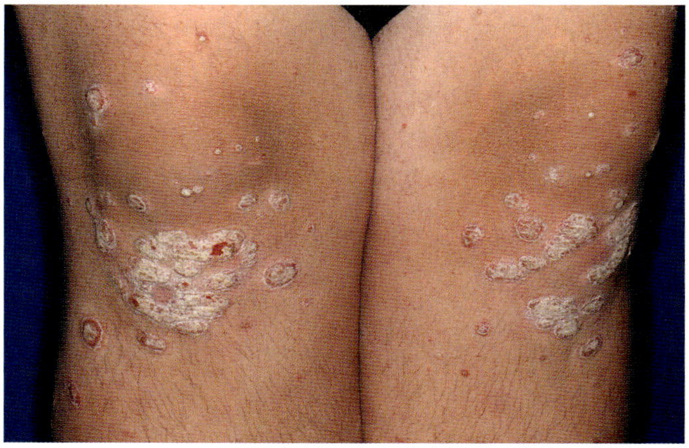

Fig. 4.6 Psoriasis. Typical plaques of psoriasis with thick, micaceous scale overlying erythema on the knees.

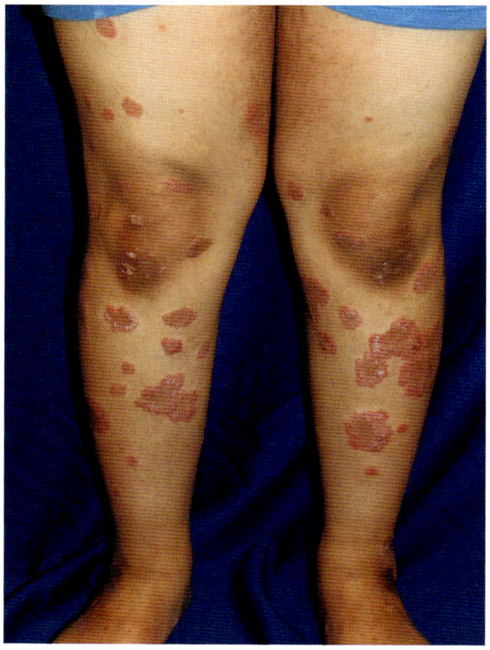

Fig. 4.7 Well-demarcated, erythematous, scaling plaques cover much of the anterior aspect of the legs.

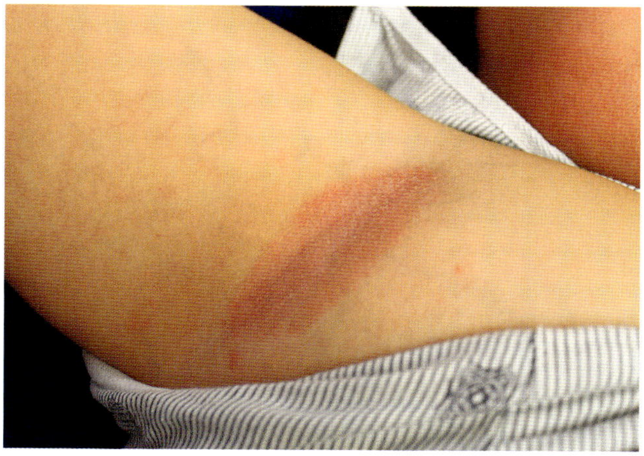

Fig. 4.8 The axilla may be involved in psoriasis but may not show the classic scale because the area is occluded and moist.

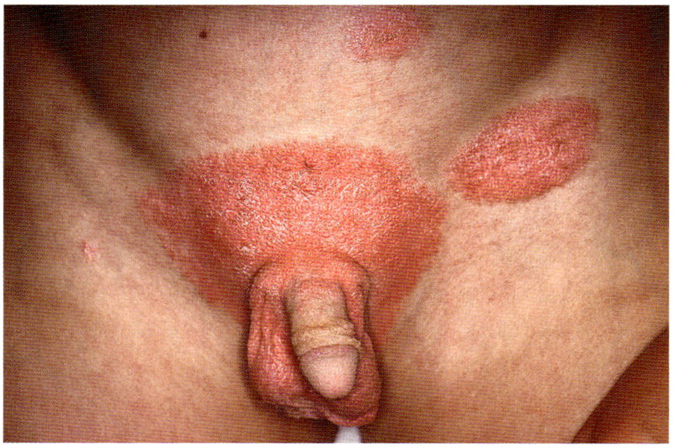

Fig. 4.9 Psoriasis. Discrete, brightly erythematous plaques of inverse psoriasis in a 3-year-old boy. Note that the scaling tends to be thinner in an intertriginous area.

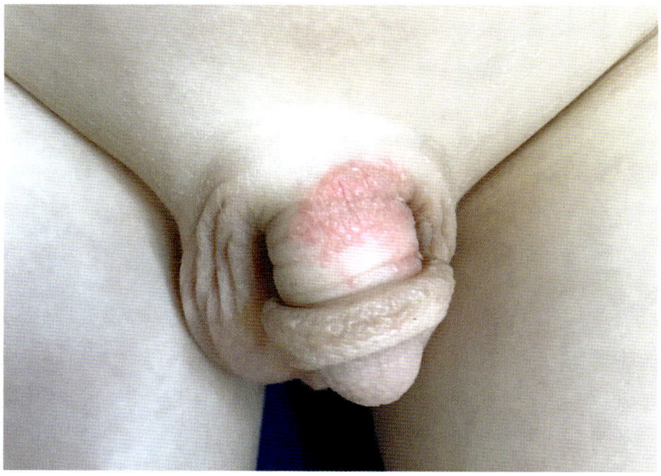

Fig. 4.10 Psoriasis. Discrete pink scaling plaque on the penile shaft. This boy was also found to have perianal streptococcal cellulitis (Fig. 4.19) and responded to the combination of oral antistreptococcal antibiotic and topical tacrolimus ointment.

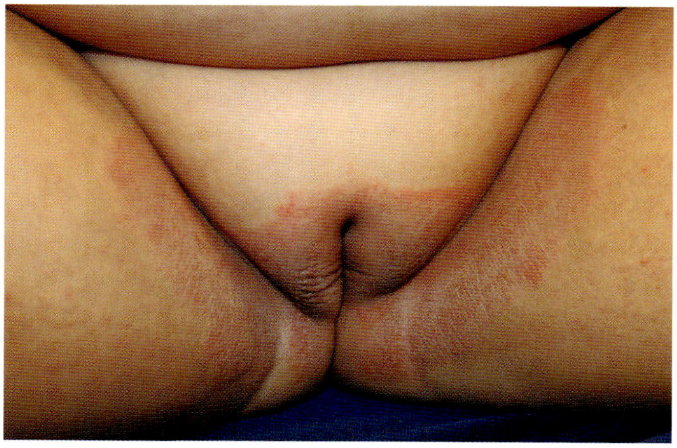

Fig. 4.11 Psoriasis. Well-demarcated, erythematous plaques of the external labia and inguinal areas.

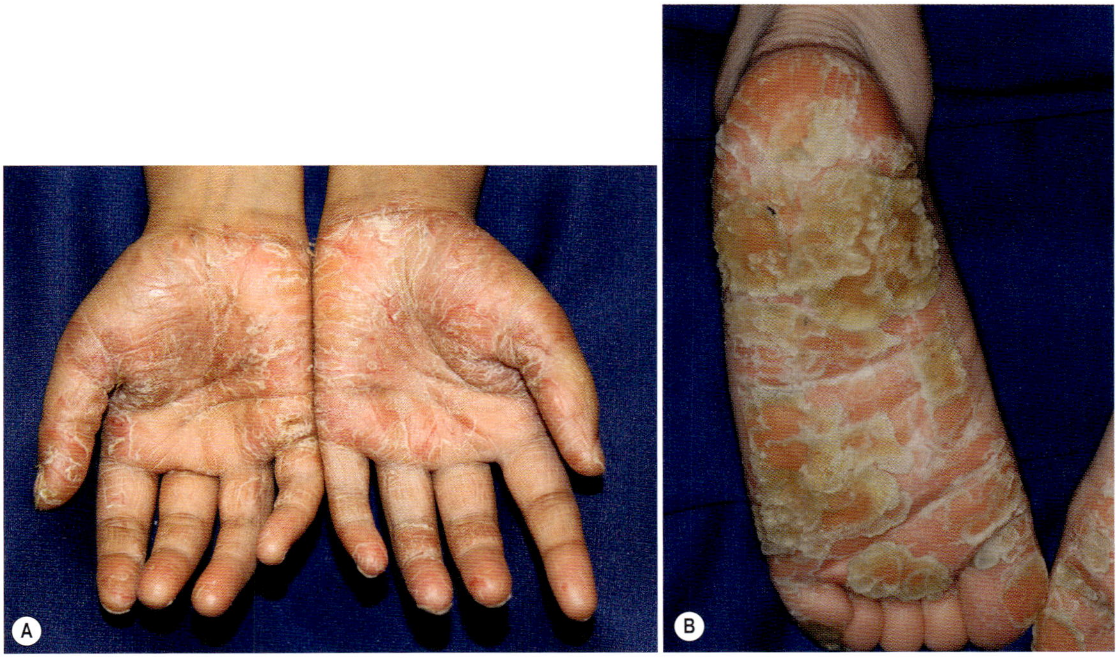

Fig. 4.12 Psoriasis. Involvement of the psoriasis on the palms **(A)** and soles **(B)**.

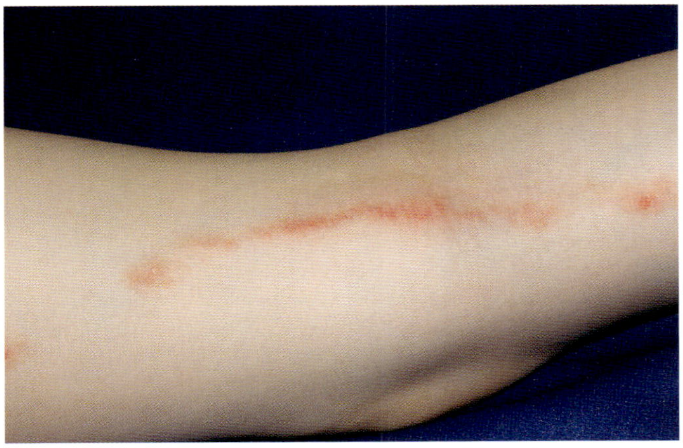

Fig. 4.13 Linear psoriasis. This patient first developed this streak of erythema and mild scaling at 5 years of age. Generalized psoriasis had its onset after a streptococcal infection 18 months later. Later treatment with ustekinumab led to clearance of both the linear psoriasis and the generalized plaques of psoriasis (shown in Fig. 4.1).

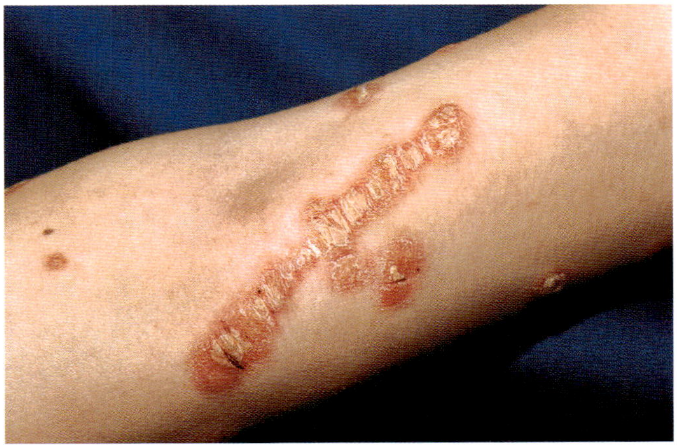

Fig. 4.14 Psoriasis. This patient shows the Koebner phenomenon, with development of a linear plaque of psoriasis after trauma to the arm.

lesions of both atopic dermatitis and psoriasis or lesions that are intermediate (e.g., nummular and psoriasiform).[36] Almost all patients with the overlap have a family history of both atopic disease and psoriasis. Although mucosae do not tend to be affected in psoriasis, geographic tongue is a frequently unrecognized feature of psoriasis in many children (Fig. 4.19). Geographic tongue, with or without GPP, has been associated with mutations in *IL36RN* or, if without a variant in *IL36RN*, with a reduction in the ratio of expression of IL-36 receptor to IL-36γ in tongue mucosa.[37]

Guttate Psoriasis

Seen in up to 44% of pediatric patients, guttate psoriasis generally occurs in children and young adults and is often the first manifestation of psoriasis.[11] Lesions are drop-like (guttate), round or oval, measure from 2 to 6 mm in diameter (Fig. 4.20), and generally occur in a symmetric distribution over the trunk and proximal aspects of the extremities (occasionally the face, scalp, ears, and distal aspects of the extremities). Guttate psoriasis is often, but not necessarily, triggered by group A streptococcal infection of the oropharynx or perianal area[29,38] Two-thirds of patients with guttate psoriasis give a history of an upper respiratory tract infection 1 to 3 weeks before the onset of an acute flare of the disorder.[39] Although guttate psoriasis may clear spontaneously (Fig. 4.21), 40% of affected children progress to the plaque type,[40] which may ultimately be more severe psoriasis than in children with plaque disease initially.[29]

Scalp Psoriasis

The scalp is commonly the initial site of psoriatic involvement (20% to 40%), and scalp psoriasis occurs more often in affected girls than boys,[29] perhaps due to the Koebner phenomenon associated with combing, brushing, and vigorous shampooing. Most typical are well-demarcated, erythematous plaques with thick, adherent silvery scales similar in appearance to those on other parts of the body (Fig. 4.22). However, psoriatic lesions of the scalp, eyebrows, and ears (the superior and postauricular folds and external auditory meatus) may instead be greasy and more salmon-colored, suggesting a diagnosis of seborrheic dermatitis. In this variant, often termed *sebopsoriasis*, lesions may present with features of both seborrhea and psoriasis.

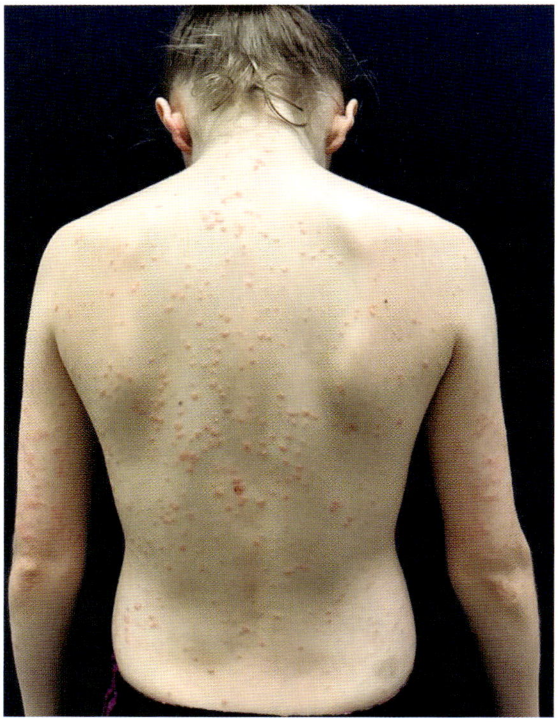

Fig. 4.15 Psoriasis. Sunburn on the upper chest and neck led to a flare in an adolescent previously in excellent control.

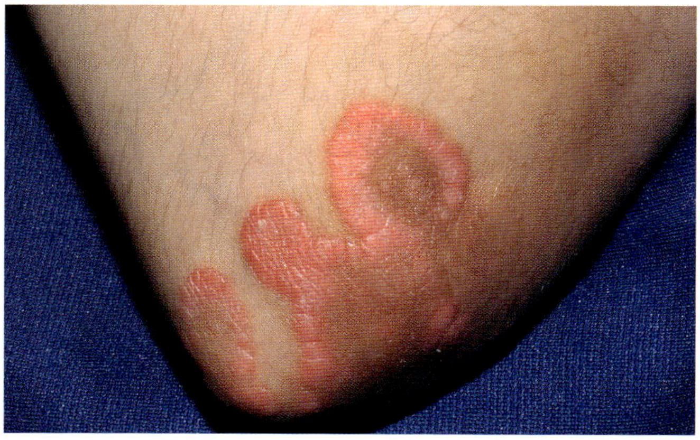

Fig. 4.16 Psoriasis. Annular plaques on the elbow. Note the central clearing, leaving hyperpigmentation.

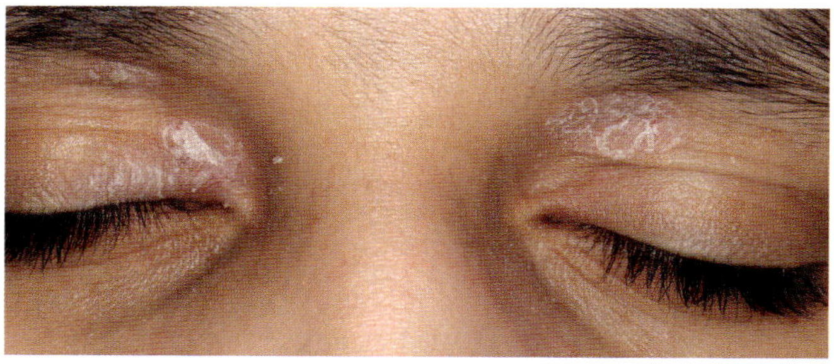

Fig. 4.17 Psoriasis. Eyelid involvement is often mistaken for atopic or contact dermatitis.

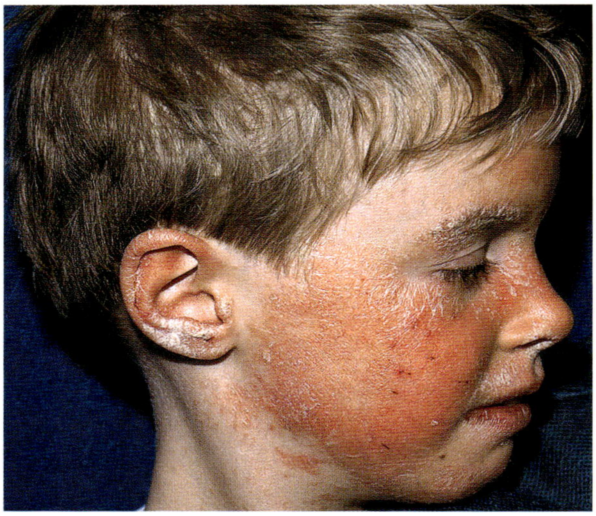

Fig. 4.18 Psoriasis. Facial psoriasis most commonly involves the periorbital area, but more extensive facial involvement can occur.

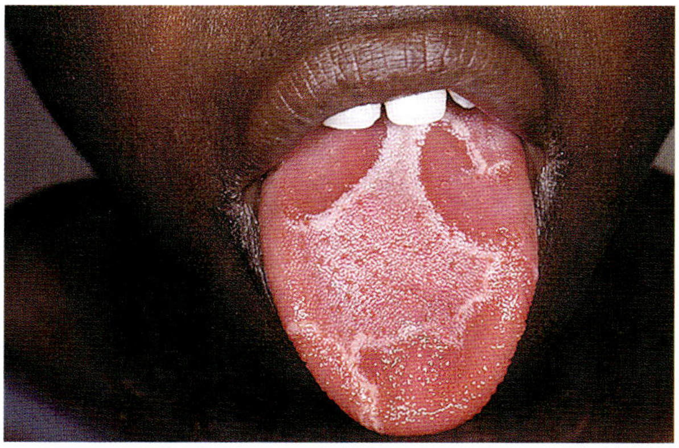

Fig. 4.19 Psoriasis. Geographic tongue can be seen as the most common mucosal manifestation of patients with psoriasis.

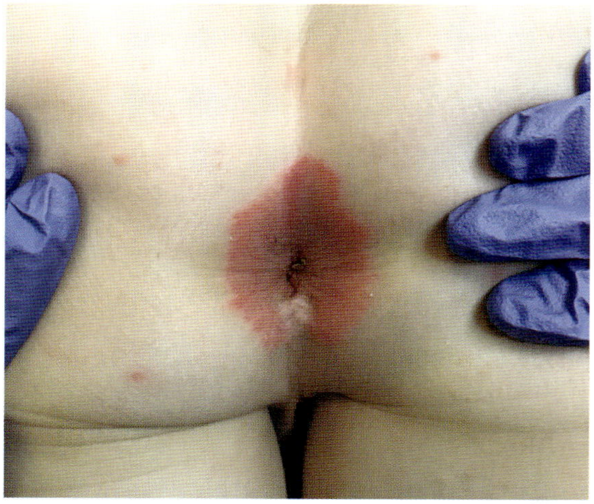

Fig. 4.20 Guttate psoriasis. Guttate (teardrop) lesions appeared after a streptococcal infection. Guttate lesions are 0.2 to 0.6 mm in diameter. This girl's guttate psoriasis lesions persisted, were recalcitrant to topical intervention, and cleared quickly with initiation of adalimumab injections.

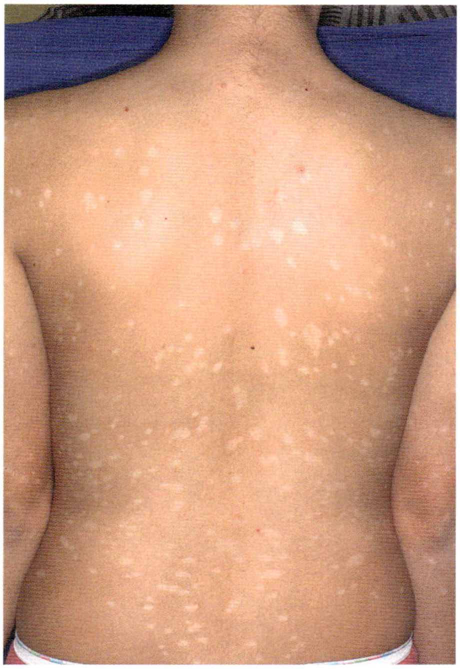

Fig. 4.21 Guttate psoriasis. These small hypopigmented macules are the postinflammatory residual lesions of guttate psoriasis.

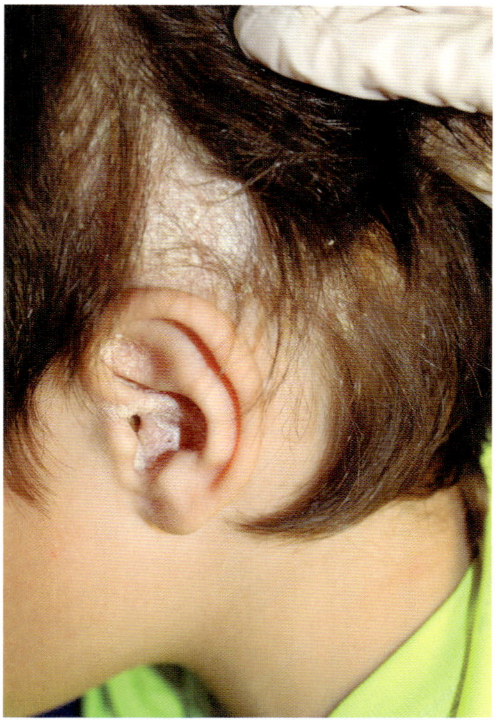

Fig. 4.23 Scalp psoriasis. Scaling on the scalp and within the antihelix of the ear.

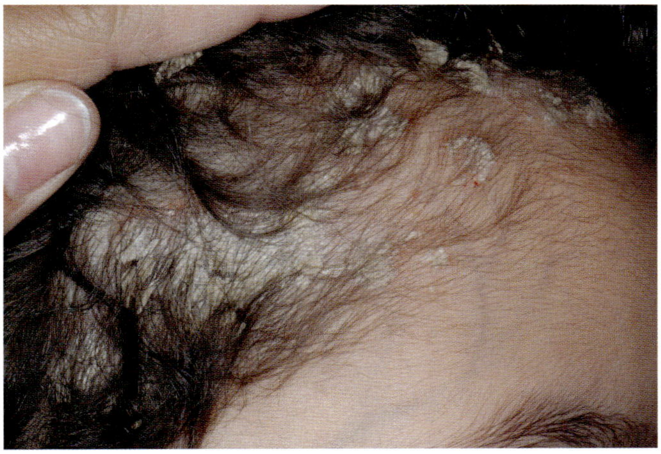

Fig. 4.22 Scalp psoriasis. Thick, discrete scaling overlying erythema on the scalp.

Whereas lesions of seborrheic dermatitis generally remain within the hairline, lesions of psoriasis often extend beyond the confines of the hairline onto the forehead (see Fig. 4.5), preauricular, postauricular, ear (Fig. 4.23), and nuchal regions. Lesions of the postauricular area commonly fissure (Fig. 4.24). Rapid response to therapy further distinguishes seborrhea from psoriasis. Another scaling disorder of the scalp that may be a variant of psoriasis is pityriasis amiantacea (asbestos-like) (Fig. 4.25)[41]; the alternative term, *tinea amiantacea*, should be abandoned, because the disorder is unrelated to dermatophyte infection. Pityriasis amiantacea usually begins in school-aged children and adolescents as large plates of scale firmly adherent to the hair and scalp. Focal hair loss and secondary infection may be associated. Most patients have no other signs of psoriasis, and later development of more typical psoriasis only occurs in 2% to 15% of patients. Pretreatment of affected scalp areas with fluocinolone 0.01% oil daily for at least an hour and then shampooing with a keratolytic shampoo is usually effective.

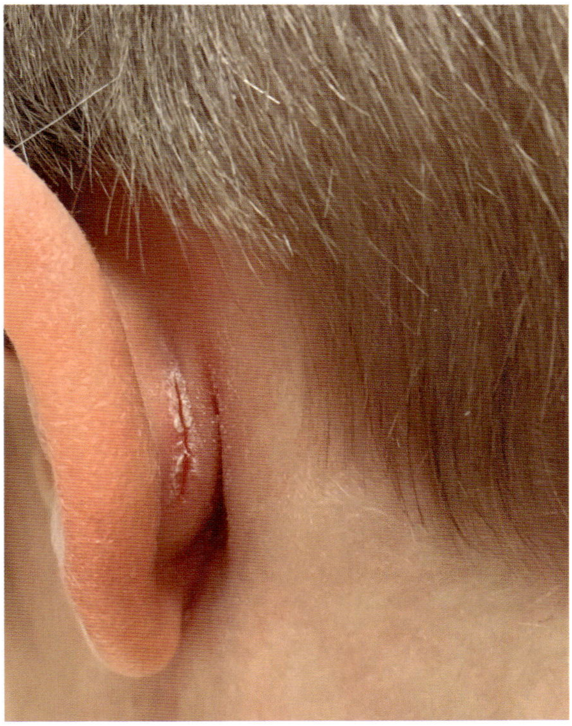

Fig. 4.24 Psoriasis. Fissures of the postauricular area from psoriasis.

Diaper-Area Psoriasis

Psoriatic diaper rash (see Fig. 2.32) with or without dissemination is the presenting manifestation in 13% and 4% of patients, respectively.[36] This form of psoriasis must be differentiated from infantile seborrheic dermatitis (see Chapter 3) and, when localized to the diaper area, other forms of diaper dermatitis (see Chapter 2). The sharply

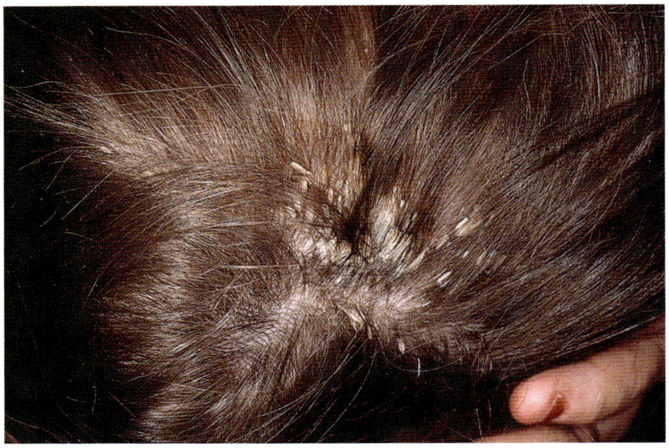

Fig. 4.25 Pityriasis (tinea) amiantacea. In this severe form of psoriasis of the scalp, the scales are strongly adherent (asbestos-like).

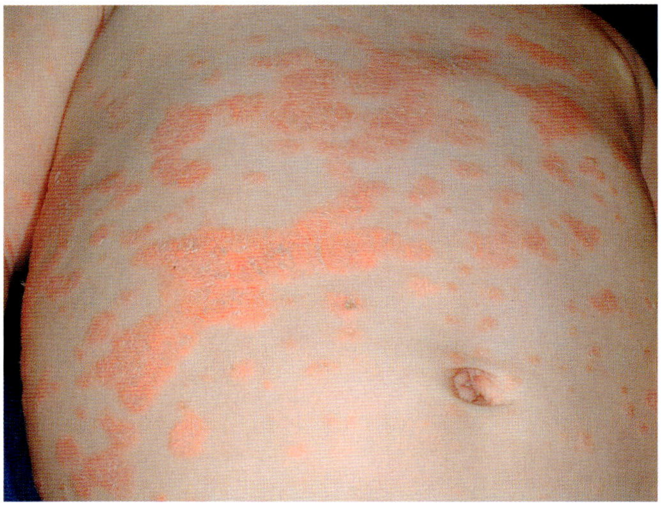

Fig. 4.26 Psoriasis in an infant. In addition to diaper-area involvement, this infant showed disseminated plaques of typical psoriasis.

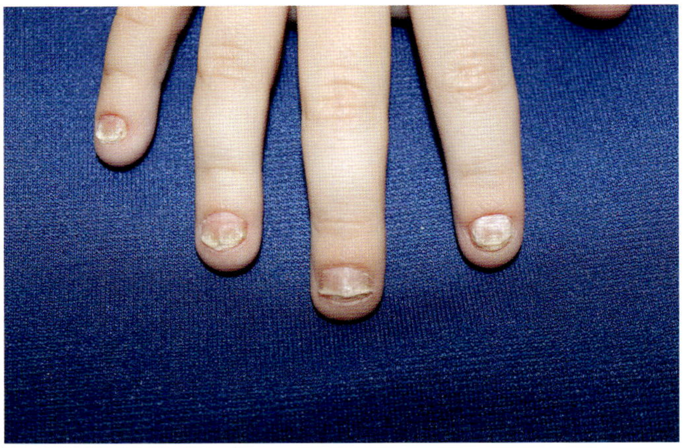

Fig. 4.27 Nail psoriasis. Several fingers show severe onycholysis with oil spots and nail pitting.

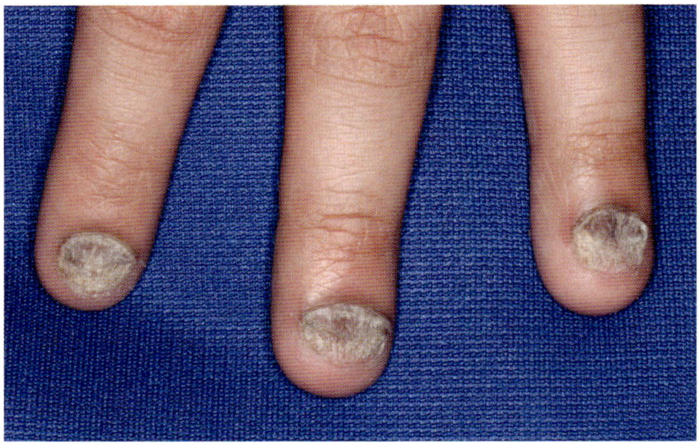

Fig. 4.28 Nail psoriasis. Note the trachyonychia or rough, ridged longitudinal striations, sometimes called *sandpapered* nails (see Chapter 7).

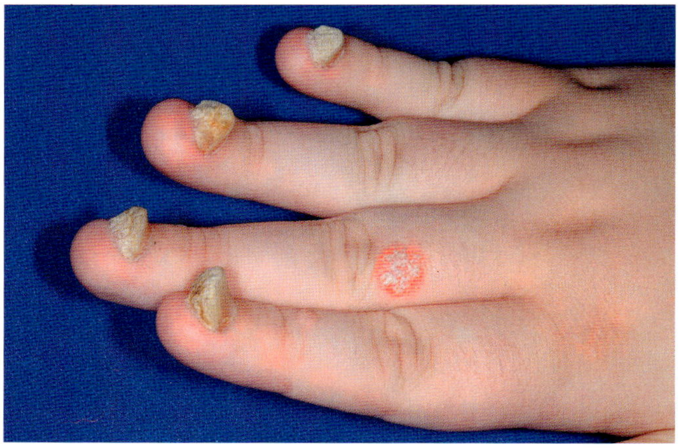

Fig. 4.29 Nail psoriasis. Extensive subungual hyperkeratosis in a teenager. Note the isolated small plaque on one finger.

defined plaques, bright-red coloration, shininess, and larger, drier scales of psoriasis help to differentiate it from seborrheic dermatitis. Many infants with diaper-area psoriasis also show psoriasiform lesions elsewhere (Fig. 4.26). Because of the increased moisture of the occluded diaper region, scale may not be visible clinically but can be revealed by scraping the area gently. The incidence of psoriasis in the diaper area during infancy probably reflects the Koebner phenomenon, triggered by trauma from exposure to stool and urine, and resolves when toilet trained. Nevertheless, boys and girls out of diapers may also show genital area involvement. Of prepubertal girls with a genital region complaint, 17% had psoriasis[42] particularly involving the vulva, perineum, and natal cleft.

Nail Involvement

Although statistics vary, the nails appear to be affected in 25% to 50% of pediatric patients with psoriasis, more commonly during the second decade of life and in males[29] (Figs. 4.27, 4.28, and 4.29). Nail involvement has also been associated with more severe disease, palmoplantar psoriasis, and psoriatic arthritis.[43] Pitting is most common[44] (69% to 92% with nail involvement), manifesting as small, irregularly spaced depressions measuring less than 1 mm in diameter.[44] Larger depressions or punched-out areas of the nail plate may also be noted. These pits are thought to represent small intermittent psoriatic lesions in the nail matrix region that forms the superficial layers of the nail plate. Psoriatic pitting may be indistinguishable from the nail pitting seen in alopecia areata (see Chapter 7) and atopic dermatitis (see Chapter 3), although other features assist in differentiating these disorders. Discoloration (especially leukonychia in 73% with nail changes), longitudinal ridges, onycholysis (separation of the distal and lateral nail plate edges), and subungual hyperkeratosis (lifting of the nail plate with nail thickening) (see Fig. 4.29) are also commonly seen. Secondary bacterial, candidal, and occasionally dermatophyte infections occur with increased incidence.

Other Forms of Psoriasis

Pustular psoriasis and erythrodermic (exfoliative) psoriasis are the most severe variants of childhood psoriasis,[45,46] but occur in only approximately 1% of pediatric patients with the disease.[11] Pustular psoriasis has been described as early as the first week of life.[47,48] Although much less common than plaque and guttate psoriasis, pustular psoriasis is more commonly the first manifestation of psoriasis in affected infants and children than in adults.

The erythema of pustular psoriasis develops and rapidly becomes studded with superficial, pinpoint-sized up to 2- or 3-mm pustules (Fig. 4.30). The lesions of GPP in children show an annular morphology in 60% of patients (Fig. 4.31).[47,49] Sheets of erythema and pustulation can involve the flexures, genital regions, webs of the fingers, and periungual areas.[50] The cutaneous inflammation typically progresses in an explosive manner from discrete sterile pustules to crusts and ultimately to generalized exfoliative dermatitis. More than 90% of the skin shows intense erythema, massive exfoliation, and associated abnormalities of temperature and cardiovascular regulation. The nails often become thickened or separated by subungual lakes of pus. Mucous membrane lesions in the mouth and tongue are not uncommon. Fever, malaise, and anorexia are typically associated with GPP. Affected children may show failure to thrive. The predominant histologic feature on biopsy is the large intraepidermal unilocular pustule containing polymorphonuclear leukocytes (the spongiform pustules of Kogoj) with little, if any, surrounding spongiosis or inflammation. Although staphylococcal infection may at times occur as a secondary complication, lesions are usually sterile.

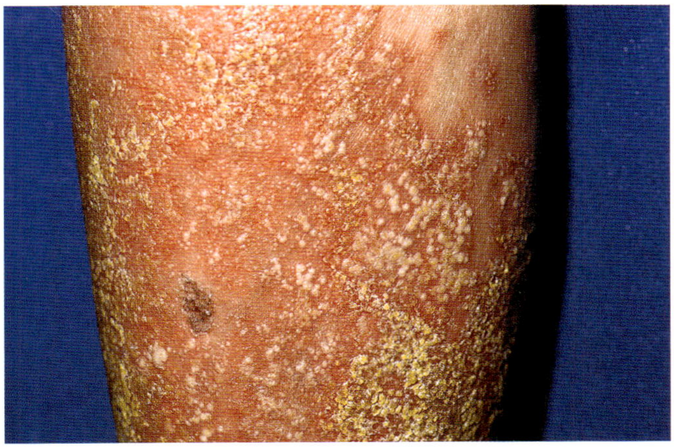

Fig. 4.30 Pustular psoriasis. Collections of small pustules, some with an annular configuration, overlying bright erythema.

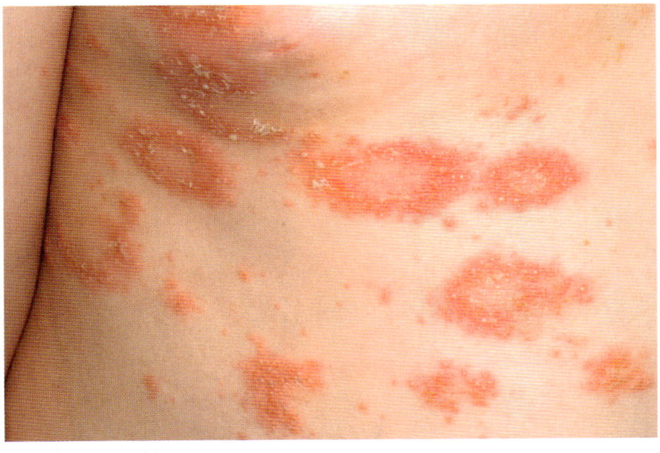

Fig. 4.31 Pustular psoriasis. Note the annular configuration of the pustules.

Deficiency of IL-36 receptor antagonist (encoded by *IL36RN*) or DITRA is an important cause of GPP in patients without plaque psoriasis.[14–16] Early age of onset is a feature of individuals with homozygous or compound heterozygous *IL36RN* variants. DITRA in babies is often characterized by irritability, tender skin, diarrhea, dysphagia, and failure to thrive in association with their pustular psoriasis and/or exfoliative erythroderma. In one study of 66 children with pediatric-onset GPP without plaque psoriasis, other signs of DITRA included severe cutaneous inflammation, confluent areas of purulence, and perianal and flexural erosions.[51] Neutrophilia and thrombocytosis are common, but other organs are not involved.[52] Poor response to standard therapy and early recurrence after discontinuation of medication are other clues to diagnosis. The discovery of IL-36 pathway activation in DITRA has led to the recognition that IL-36 is important in driving both pustular and plaque psoriasis. Given that individuals with knockout mutations in the IL-36 receptor have normal immune function, inhibition of IL-36 has emerged as a new potential therapeutic approach.[53]

Although pustular psoriasis is most often generalized, it can be limited to the palms and soles (pustulosis palmaris et plantaris) or to fold areas.[54] Pustulosis palmaris et plantaris is a bilaterally symmetric, chronic pustular eruption on the palms and soles characterized by deep-seated 2- to 4-mm sterile pustules that develop within areas of erythema and scaling. Plaque or pustular psoriasis may be seen elsewhere on the body. Within several days the pustules resolve and leave a yellow-brown scale that is generally shed within 1 or 2 weeks. Phases of quiescence and exacerbation are characteristic, and exfoliating crusted lesions may be seen concurrently with newly developing pustules. Pustular psoriasis localized to the neck fold tends to have its onset during infancy.[54] The disorder is often misdiagnosed as dermatitis caused by bacterial or candidal infection (Fig. 4.32). Biopsy facilitates making the diagnosis, particularly given that many lesions clinically appear more papular than pustular. Other fold areas may be affected, and dissemination to GPP is not uncommon.

Psoriasis-like pustules during the neonatal period or in infancy, often in association with sterile multifocal osteomyelitis or periostitis, should also raise the possibility of inappropriate activation of IL-1 from biallelic variants in the IL-1 receptor antagonist (deficiency of IL-1 receptor antagonist [DIRA]). Pustules may be widespread or grouped and more localized. DIRA also may feature joint swelling and pain, oral stomatitis, and pyoderma gangrenosum, especially during childhood.[50,55,56] Most neonates with DIRA are born prematurely.

Pustular psoriasis may also present after infancy in association with sterile lytic lesions of bone (sometimes called *chronic recurrent multifocal osteomyelitis* [*CRMO*]) as part of several syndromes.[57] CRMO in association with congenital dyserythropoietic anemia and neutrophilic dermatoses comprises Majeed syndrome, an autosomal recessive disorder caused by mutations in *LPIN2*.[58] Synovitis, acne, pustulosis, hyperostosis, osteitis (SAPHO) syndrome (see Chapter 8)

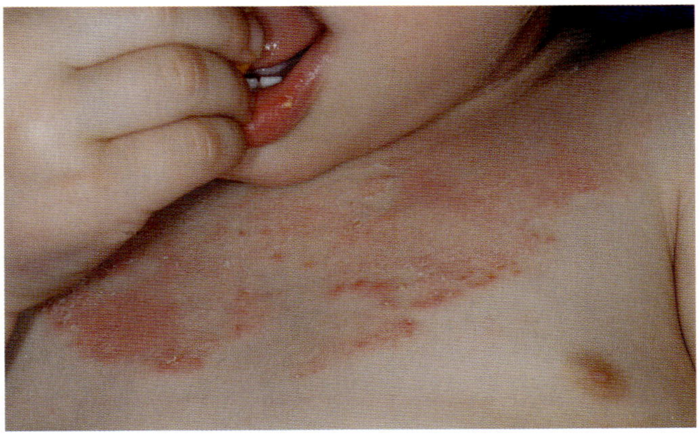

Fig. 4.32 Localized pustular psoriasis in an infant. In infants, pustular psoriasis may be localized to intertriginous areas, particularly the neck fold, and be confused with dermatitis or infection. This form is difficult to treat and may eventuate in generalized pustular psoriasis.

describes the constellation of synovitis, acne, palmoplantar pustulosis and psoriasis, hyperostosis, and osteitis and usually affects the bones of the lower limb, pelvis, and clavicle.[59,60] The bone and joint lesions can severely affect quality of life but may respond to immunosuppressive medications such as methotrexate and aggressive intervention for acne with isotretinoin.[61]

Pustules overlying erythroderma can also be an occasional feature of patients with variants in *CARD14*,[62] which typically has its onset during infancy or early childhood. More commonly, however, patients with *CARD14* alterations often show signs of recalcitrant plaque-type psoriasis or PRP (see Pityriasis Rubra Pilaris section, later) and respond most rapidly to ustekinumab.[63]

Patients with extensive pustular or erythrodermic psoriasis usually require hospitalization, and courses are not uncommonly complicated by cutaneous infection and bacterial septicemia. The disease is cyclic and associated with complete clearance of the pustular phase and unexplained exacerbations that span decades. Relapses are common and become progressively more severe, often with a poor prognosis. Unless localized and mild, management of pustular psoriasis usually requires systemic medications (e.g., retinoids, cyclosporine, methotrexate, and biologics; see Systemic Medications). Children with DITRA have been shown to have a higher recurrence rate after discontinuation of systemic retinoids than children with GPP without the IL36RN variant.[51] Pediatric patients with DIRA often respond rapidly to subcutaneous administrations of anakinra 2 to 4 mg/kg per day.

Comorbidities

Many of the comorbidities experienced by adults with psoriasis also occur in children. As such, affected children should receive routine screening in collaboration with pediatricians, with referral to rheumatologists, gastroenterologists, endocrinologists, and cardiologists as appropriate[64] (see Table 4.3).[64] Pediatric patients with moderate to severe plaque psoriasis have demonstrated impaired physical, emotional, social, and school functioning in comparison to healthy children,[65] on par with children who have arthritis or asthma, and to a greater extent than children with diabetes.[66] In one study, 65% of children with psoriasis experienced stigmatization and 43% complained about fatigue.[67] Indeed, pediatric patients with psoriasis have a higher risk of developing psychiatric disorders,[68] especially depression[69] and anxiety.[68,70] The risk of these neuropsychiatric issues is further compounded by the increased risk of having other medical issues, particularly the most common comorbidity, obesity.[71–74]

Obesity (defined as having a body mass index [BMI] at the 95th percentile or higher) occurs in 38.5% of children with moderate to severe psoriasis[71] and tends to precede the onset of psoriasis by at least 2 years in more than 90% of affected children.[75–77] In one study, the odds ratio (OR) of being obese at the time of psoriasis onset was 2.58 (confidence interval [CI], 1.48 to 4.52).[77,78] Being[78] overweight ("excess adiposity," 85th to <95th percentile BMI) or obese occurs in pediatric psoriasis with an OR of 2.65 (95% CI, 1.70 to 4.15) globally; in the United States, the OR is 4.22 (CI, 2.05 to 8.67).[10] Although obesity is linked to greater severity, excess adiposity is not dependent on psoriasis severity. Although the association is not as high as with psoriasis, a study of 320 children with JPsA[79] demonstrated that almost 20% were obese and 36.3% overweight. Waist circumference percentile and waist-to-height ratio, which are both better indicators of metabolic risk than BMI percentile, are only increased in children with moderate to severe psoriasis.[10] Early evidence suggests that aggressive therapy for psoriasis does not lead to reductions in weight or waist circumference.[10]

In a study of 20 US children with psoriasis, metabolic syndrome (as defined by having at least three of the following: elevated triglycerides, high-density lipoprotein cholesterol, fasting blood glucose, waist circumference percentile, and blood pressure) occurred in 30% of those with psoriasis but 5% of the control group ($p < 0.05$).[80,81] Although some studies have shown no association, others have suggested a 1.5- to 3-fold increased OR of having hyperlipidemia, hypertension, diabetes, metabolic syndrome, polycystic ovarian syndrome, nonalcoholic liver disease, and elevated hepatic transaminases.[78,82] These odds largely reflect the increase in obesity, and in one study the risk for these comorbidities was 42% to 64% higher among obese children with psoriasis than nonobese children without psoriasis.[78] Although a longitudinal study is needed, these data suggest that early intervention with lifestyle modification may decrease the long-term metabolic risk for these children.

Inquiry about pain, joint swelling, or limping, as well as examination of the joints for arthritis, should be part of the routine evaluation. Joint pain has been described in approximately 10% of US children with moderate to severe psoriasis, although only 1% to 4% in European countries.[10,71] JPsA comprises about 7.5% of juvenile idiopathic arthritis,[83] and criteria have been established by the International League of Associations for Rheumatology (ILAR).[84–87] These include arthritis with psoriasis or arthritis and (1) a family history of confirmed psoriasis in a parent or sibling, (2) dactylitis,[88] or (3) nail pitting or onycholysis.[88] The diagnosis is excluded if the patient has a positive rheumatoid factor titer or signs of systemic disease (daily fever, evanescent erythematous eruption, generalized adenopathy, hepatomegaly or splenomegaly, or serositis).

The occurrence of JPsA is biphasic. Younger children affected by psoriatic arthritis tend to be female with dactylitis and small-joint involvement that is more likely to progress and persist. The swelling often includes the juxtaarticular tissue, resulting in a blunt, "sausage-shaped" appearance of the involved fingers or toes. Progression to polyarthritis occurs in 30%, leading to flexure deformities and severe bone destruction (osteoporosis, shortening and tapering of the involved distal phalanx) with long-standing disease. On radiologic examination, this resembles a sharpened pencil (the so-called "pencil-in-cup" or "pencil-and-goblet" deformity) at the metatarsophalangeal and metacarpophalangeal joints. However, 72% have their onset when older than 4 years, with a male predominance and high prevalence of enthesitis[83] and axial joint disease.[84] Psoriatic skin lesions occur in approximately 60% of children with psoriatic arthritis, are identical to those seen in patients who do not manifest joint disease, and are not related in severity to that of the joint disease. Either skin disease or arthritis may develop initially, and in most patients flares of joint and skin disease do not correlate. Rheumatoid arthritis is also seen with increased frequency in children with psoriasis; in one cross-sectional register study in Denmark, the OR of having JPsA was 10.08 (95% CI, 7.97 to 12.74) and of rheumatoid arthritis 6.61 (95% CI, 2.75 to 15.87).[83,89]

The risk of developing Crohn's disease has been found to be higher in pediatric psoriasis,[73] but the possibility of increased risk of ulcerative colitis is controversial. Asymmetric anterior uveitis has been described in 14% to 17% of children with JPsA. The cutaneous lesions of psoriasis may develop several years after the onset of persisting uveitis.[90] Vitiligo[89] and asthma[91,92] have recently been linked to pediatric psoriasis.

DIAGNOSIS OF PSORIASIS

The diagnosis of psoriasis can usually be made clinically, although biopsy can be performed if the diagnosis is in question. Biopsy sections show epidermal thickening (acanthosis with elongation of the rete ridges), retention of nuclei in the stratum corneum (parakeratosis), and a mononuclear infiltrate. Focal collections of neutrophils in the stratum corneum or subcorneal layer (Munro microabscesses) are an additional feature in biopsies from patients with pustular psoriasis. Skin biopsies in DIRA and DITRA show features similar to those seen in pustular psoriasis.[42]

COURSE

Most patients have long-term mild to moderate disease, often with plaques confined to areas of frictional trauma such as the elbows, knees, buttocks, and scalp. The course of psoriasis, however, is unpredictable, ranging from spontaneous remissions to frequent exacerbations without an evident trigger. Although sunlight generally is beneficial and often leads to improvement during the summer, sunburns can elicit the Koebner phenomenon and lead to exacerbation. With appropriate therapy, satisfactory control of the disease is possible.

DIFFERENTIAL DIAGNOSIS

Guttate psoriasis and plaque psoriasis are most commonly confused with dermatitis and other papulosquamous disorders described in this chapter, especially pityriasis rosea or pityriasis lichenoides chronica (PLC) (Box 4.1). PRP is the hardest to differentiate, especially when involved areas are largely the palms, soles,

Box 4.1 Differential Diagnosis of Psoriasis

Guttate and Plaque Psoriasis

Pityriasis rubra pilaris
Pityriasis rosea
Pityriasis lichenoides chronica
Psoriasiform dermatitis
Lichen planus
Drug eruptions
Widespread dermatophytosis

Facial Psoriasis

Discoid lupus erythematosus
Seborrheic dermatitis

Scalp Psoriasis

Tinea capitis
Seborrheic dermatitis

Nail Psoriasis

Trauma
Onychomycosis
Lichen planus

Diaper Area Psoriasis

Seborrheic dermatitis
Irritant dermatitis
Candidal diaper dermatitis

Pustular Psoriasis

Staphylococcal pustulosis
Candidal pustulosis
Herpes simplex infection
Acute generalized exanthematous pustulosis (viral, drug)
Extensive eosinophilic folliculitis
Interleukin-1 receptor antagonist deficiency
Palmoplantar pustular psoriasis
Candidiasis
Infantile acropustulosis

Erythrodermic Psoriasis

Extensive pityriasis rubra pilaris
Congenital ichthyosiform erythroderma
Erythrokeratodermia variabilis

elbows, and knees. Although follicular accentuation is classically seen in PRP, this finding may occasionally be present in psoriasis as well. Focal areas of sparing and sometimes more salmon coloration of PRP can help to distinguish the conditions clinically; biopsy sections of PRP may show perifollicular inflammation and alternating parakeratosis and orthokeratosis (stratum corneum without nuclei). Children with variants in *CARD14* may present with plaque psoriasis (or sometimes erythrodermic/pustular types), PRP, or a phenotype that has characteristics of both psoriasis and PRP[63,65]; facial erythema is often prominent. A plaque-type psoriasiform eruption and, less often, a generalized or annular pustular psoriatic eruption may follow Kawasaki disease (see Chapter 21).[93–95] Psoriasiform dermatitis with a distribution that is often atypical for psoriasis and shows a Th1 (IFNγ) immunophenotype[96] is a common occurrence in children taking TNF inhibitors, especially for Crohn's disease (see later). Generalized and localized forms of pustular psoriasis can be differentiated from infectious causes of pustulosis by cultures and from noninfectious conditions, such as eosinophilic folliculitis or infantile acropustulosis, by biopsy. Psoriasiform dermatitis may also be seen in boys with immune dysregulation, polyendocrinopathy, enteropathy, or X-linked (IPEX) syndrome (see Chapter 3). Atypical cases of psoriatic arthritis must be differentiated from other types of juvenile idiopathic arthritis or systemic lupus erythematosus.

THERAPY OF PEDIATRIC PSORIASIS

Education is a key component of psoriasis therapy. Patients and parents must understand the chronicity of the disorder and the tendency in 38% of pediatric patients for spontaneous remissions lasting for variable periods.[97] Most patients respond well to available therapies, but the response is slower than with dermatitis.[98–104] The therapeutic approach should be simplified and tailored to the individual patient to optimize compliance, because therapy is time consuming. Patients and family members of the patient should understand the rationale for treatment and any potential risks. Older children and adolescents should be empowered to maintain their own therapeutic routine with parental guidance. The concept that injury to skin may exacerbate psoriasis (Koebner phenomenon or isomorphic response) should also be explained (Table 4.2). Removal of potential trigger factors, including medications, and rapid intervention for streptococcal infection should be explored.

Table 4.1 Monitoring for Comorbidities in Children with Psoriasis*

Comorbidity	When to Screen	Recommendation for Screening
Obesity and overweight	Yearly monitoring starting at 2 years of age	Body mass index (BMI) percentile
Diabetes	Every 3 years if overweight (if risk factors) or obese, starting at 10 years or onset of puberty	Fasting serum glucose
Hyperlipidemia	9–11 years old; 17–21 years old More often if cardiovascular risk factors	Fasting lipid panel
Hypertension	Yearly starting at 3 years of age	Blood pressure measurement
Nonalcoholic fatty liver disease (NAFLD)	If overweight (and other risk factors) or obese starting 9–11 years of age; earlier if very obese or family history of NAFLD	Alanine aminotransferase level
Arthritis	Any age	By history and examination
Inflammatory bowel disease	At any age	By history of gastrointestinal problems or unexplained weight loss
Psychiatric issues	Yearly screening, regardless of age, but consider substance abuse starting at 11 years of age	Screen with questions about feeling anxious, worrying, depressed or hopeless; interest or pleasure in activities*

*Modified from Osier E, Wang AS, Tollefson MM, et al. Pediatric psoriasis comorbidity screening guidelines. JAMA Dermatol. 2017;153(7):698–704.

Table 4.2 Prevention of Psoriasis in Pediatric Patients

Site of Potential Psoriasis	Preventive Behavior
Creases and folds	Minimize friction by maintaining appropriate weight Avoid irritating underarm deodorants
Face	Avoid irritating soaps and burning from exposure to ultraviolet light
Genital and perianal regions	Avoid irritation from tight garments and exposure to accumulated feces and urine
Hands and feet	Minimize excessive sweating and exposure to irritants such as harsh soaps Avoid tight shoes
Nails	Avoid long fingernails or toenails, trauma to nails in play situations, excessive use of nail polish and remover, and wearing tight shoes Hydrate nails before trimming and avoid manipulation of cuticles
Scalp	Avoid vigorous brushing, combing, or scratching of scalp

Topical Therapy

The topical therapies most commonly used in children include topical corticosteroids, topical calcineurin inhibitors, and vitamin D_3 analogues (calcipotriene and calcitriol). Use of topical retinoids, keratolytics, tar preparations, and anthralin (also called *dithranol*) is less common (Table 4.3). Most topical interventions are off-label. Emollients are important adjunctive measures to decrease associated scaling and dryness, but do not replace medications that treat inflammation.

The mainstay of treatment for plaque psoriasis remains topical corticosteroids (see Chapter 3, Table 3.2), which often produce dramatic resolution of lesions as monotherapy. As with atopic dermatitis, parents of children with psoriasis may have “steroid phobia,” and time must be taken to reassure about safety when used correctly.[105] Application up to twice daily of class II to IV (potent to midpotent) topical steroids is required to improve lesions on the trunk and extremities. Ointments tend to penetrate the psoriatic scale better and are preferred. If individual thick plaques fail to respond, a short course of an ultrapotent topical steroid ointment (such as clobetasol, halobetasol, or augmented betamethasone dipropionate) can be initiated.

Vitamin D_3 analogues are steroid-sparing alternatives that are best applied twice daily, but their onset of action is slow (often 6 to 8 weeks). Calcipotriene[106] (cream, ointment, or solution) and calcitriol (ointment) are most effective when combined with potent topical steroids, either directly (i.e., commercially available as betamethasone propionate [0.064%] and calcipotriene [0.005%] ointment) or mixed 1:1 before application (e.g., with halobetasol or augmented betamethasone dipropionate).[107] However, once- to twice-daily application of these potent topical steroids, with or without a vitamin D_3 analogue, should be restricted to 2 to 4 weeks because of the risk for developing local atrophy, including striae (especially in the preadolescent/adolescent population), with continued use. After this limited treatment period, one can initiate a “weekend therapy” regimen that combines class I steroids (used on weekend days only) and topical calcipotriene/calcitriol weekdays; this regimen is best administered by a dermatologist familiar with the use of these regimens.[108] Vitamin D_3 analogue monotherapy may also be efficacious in children.[109,110] Irritant dermatitis, particularly on the face and intertriginous areas, occurs in up to 20% of patients treated with these analogues. Once the acute lesions are under control, treatment can be tapered to lower-potency steroids and/or emollients.

Use of halogenated midpotent-to-potent steroids should be avoided in the diaper area, intertriginous areas, and on the face. In contrast, calcineurin inhibitors, particularly tacrolimus ointment 0.1%, are useful with twice-daily application for 1 to 2 months, especially for facial and intertriginous psoriasis.[111]

The topical retinoid tazarotene is available in 0.05% and 0.1% strength creams and gels. Tazarotene is best applied once a day in combination with once-daily application of a mid- to high-potency topical steroid; however, even with the topical steroid, tazarotene is often too irritating for use in childhood psoriasis.

Keratolytic agents to enhance penetration, such as 6% salicylic acid, are often compounded into a steroid ointment with or without tar. Keratolytic agents, occlusion, or steroid-impregnated tapes are alternative treatments for more hyperkeratotic, resistant lesions. Tar, which is both antiinflammatory and antiproliferative, is available over the counter for addition to the bath, as a single agent, or compounded (in the form of 1% to 10% crude coal tar or 5% to 10% liquor carbonis detergens) into a prescription with topical steroids and/or salicylic acid. However, tar preparations stain skin and clothing, have an odor that is often objectionable to children and adolescents, and increase the risk of developing folliculitis.

An alternative to tar therapy is short-contact anthralin therapy, formulated in a temperature-sensitive vehicle that releases the active medication at skin-surface temperature.[112,113] Anthralin, also called dithranol, is applied for 5 minutes initially, with gradually increasing times of exposure as tolerated and needed for efficacy. Discoloration of skin or clothing is significantly less than that with tar. Contact with the face, eyes, and mucous membranes should be avoided.

Treatment of Scalp Lesions

Psoriatic scalp lesions can be difficult to treat and not uncommonly are recalcitrant to even systemic therapy. Topical corticosteroids may be applied in the form of oils, solutions, or foams, and calcipotriene solution may be steroid-sparing. Combination betamethasone

Table 4.3 Topical Treatments for Psoriasis in Children

Medication	Use in Children	Potential Side Effects and Comments
Emollients	Useful in mild disease; adjunct	None
Topical steroids	First-line therapy	Local side effects: atrophy, striae Systemic side effects: impaired growth, adrenal suppression, cataracts, tachyphylaxis
Calcitriol or calcipotriene	Usually adjunct with steroids	Irritation
Tacrolimus/pimecrolimus	Face, intertriginous areas	Burning with initial applications
Tazarotene	Usually adjunct with steroids	Irritation
Tar	Thicker plaques	Irritation, staining, folliculitis
Anthralin	Short contact application	Irritation; less staining than tar
Salicylic acid	Thicker plaques; usually compounded with steroids ± tar	Irritation

propionate (0.064%) and calcipotriene (0.005%) ointment in a suspension is approved by the US Food and Drug Administration (FDA) for scalp psoriasis for children 12 years and above.[114] Clobetasol and fluocinolone shampoos are also available. Removal of scales can be facilitated by softening scales through application of oil-based medications. For example, fluocinolone 0.01% oil under shower cap occlusion can be applied for 1 hour to overnight to the wet, affected scalp and should be followed by washing with shampoos containing keratolytic agents (e.g., salicylic acid), tar, a steroid (0.01% fluocinolone or clobetasol), or zinc. Alternatively, plain mineral oil or a phenol and saline (Baker Cummins P&S) solution can be applied overnight with a shower cap for occlusion. In the morning, the patient can shampoo, use a conditioner after shampooing, and then apply a steroid foam or solution if needed.

Treatment of Nail Psoriasis

Psoriatic nails are extremely distressing to the patient, respond slowly to therapy, and are difficult to treat topically because of the failure of topical agents to penetrate the nail plate. Instillation of class I steroid solutions into the subproximal nailfold area can be successful, especially applied under occlusive tape at night, but application nightly of flurandrenolide-impregnated tape to the base of the nail for approximately 6 months tends to yield better results. Injections of triamcinolone suspension (10 mg/mL) into the nailfold of the abnormal nail with a 30-gauge needle every 4 to 6 weeks is painful, even with the use of topical anesthetic creams, and should be reserved for the motivated older child or adolescent who fails to respond to topical application. Nightly application of tazarotene 0.05% or 0.1% gel under occlusion, if tolerated, has been shown to cause improvement.[115] Use of topical indigo naturalis oil extract has been described.[116] Disfiguring nail psoriasis that is unresponsive to topical measures may respond to systemic intervention (generally methotrexate or a biologic medication), but the decision to start a systemic medication must be carefully weighed.

Compresses for Pustular Psoriasis

Local applications of wet dressings with Burow solution 1:40 or potassium permanganate 1:5000 (one crushed 65-mg tablet into 250 mL of water) often help relieve acute flares of the pustular aspect of palmoplantar or generalized pustular psoriasis.

Ultraviolet Light

Most patients with psoriasis benefit from exposure to sunlight and accordingly are often better during the summer months. However, sunburn precautions must be taken through the use of sunscreens, avoidance during hours of most intense sunlight, and sun-protective clothing, because sudden overexposure may result in sufficient epidermal injury to cause exacerbation of the disorder. For those who can arrange exposure to sunlight on a regular basis, this can be an important aspect of therapy alone or in combination with topical therapies. Although natural sunlight is easier for children and less aggressive than artificial ultraviolet therapy, ultraviolet treatments under professional supervision may also be used as therapy,[117–122] especially when psoriasis involves more than 10% to 20% body surface area, involves the palms and soles, and/or is recalcitrant to topical therapy.[119] Response to phototherapy is enhanced by preexposure application of oil or ointment,[118] so that the use or lack of use of an emollient before phototherapy should be consistent throughout the phototherapy treatment course. Narrowband ultraviolet B (nbUVB) (≈311 nm) has a higher ratio of therapeutic-to-toxic wavelengths than broadband UVB light (290 to 320 nm) and is considered as efficacious. More than 90% of children treated with nbUVB improve by more than 75%[123–125] and more than 75% become clear/almost clear[126] with reduction in use of topical steroids.[126]

The nbUVB light is best initiated in a light box at a dermatology office as outpatient therapy. Once patients and parents know how to increase the doses of ultraviolet light gradually, judge the effects of the daily treatment, and practice preventive eye care, home light-box therapy can be initiated. Home light boxes are ultimately less invasive to the mainstream activities of a family and may be more cost-effective than in-office therapy, although careful monitoring is required. In general, ultraviolet light therapy is started at 70% to 75% of the minimal erythema dose and increased by about 10% to 20% with each treatment as tolerated. A minimum of three treatments per week is required to clear psoriasis. Although rarely used in young children, phototherapy may be administered to young children who are accompanied by parents in the light unit. Tricks such as use of singing together or listening to music can be used to distract the child during treatment. Acutely, nbUVB therapy is associated with skin darkening, a chance of skin burning, and sometimes early pruritus. Although long-term data are lacking in children with psoriasis, recurrent exposure to nbUVB light could theoretically increase the long-term risk of the development of skin cancer and premature aging.

The excimer laser (≈308 nm) is fiber-optically targeted UVB light that can treat localized plaques of psoriasis without exposing normal skin to unnecessary radiation. Although its use in children has been limited,[119,127] it is painless and offers safety advantages over nbUVB therapy.[128] Psoralens and ultraviolet A (PUVA) light (320 to 400 nm) is used rarely in children because of the ocular toxicity, generalized photosensitivity, and risk of later development of actinic changes and cutaneous carcinomas[129]; topical application of the psoralens with UVA is a safer alternative but rarely needed. Protective eyewear must be worn for 24 hours after each PUVA exposure because of the risk of cataract development. The use of topical PUVA light in a hand/foot box has proven effective in adolescents and older children with psoriasis of the hands and feet.

Systemic Therapy[130–132]

Oral medications are reserved for children with erythrodermic and pustular forms of psoriasis or for those with plaque psoriasis recalcitrant to topical therapies that is moderate to severe, highly visible, and/or affecting function (e.g., palmoplantar).[130,132–134] In general, systemic corticosteroids should be avoided. Although occasionally effective, steroids are often ineffective or lead to flares of psoriasis when withdrawn, including triggering of pustular psoriasis. Especially in guttate psoriasis, examination for the possibility of pharyngitis or perianal cellulitis should be performed, and culture for β-hemolytic streptococci obtained as appropriate. Antibiotics should be prescribed if the culture is positive, although recurrent positive cultures may signal a carrier state. Although important for treating streptococcal infections, trials of antibiotic therapy are usually not helpful.[135] Some pediatric patients with refractory psoriasis have been shown to improve after tonsillectomy for the treatment of chronic and recurring streptococcal infection.[24,136–138] One study showed that 86% of adult patients who underwent tonsillectomy showed sustained improvement (30% to 90%) 2 years after the procedure in contrast to the unchanged status of control patients. Clinical improvement correlated with reduction in circulating keratin peptide–reactive skin-homing (CLA+) T cells (which also recognize cross-reacting streptococcal M proteins), suggesting that the tonsils generate the T cells recognizing these determinants.[24]

The various systemic medications that are available for treating moderate to severe psoriasis are shown in Table 4.4. Methotrexate is the most commonly used systemic agent in children[130] and is indicated for severe unresponsive psoriasis, exfoliative erythrodermas, pustular psoriasis,[119,139] and psoriatic arthritis. It is occasionally used for nail psoriasis if nonsystemic agents are ineffective. Methotrexate has antimitotic, antichemotactic, and antiinflammatory activities. After appropriate screening tests (blood counts; hepatic testing; and, if deemed appropriate by the physician based on clinical situation and individual risk factors, renal functions, tuberculosis screening, and pregnancy testing in female patients of childbearing age),[1] oral methotrexate is initiated at an oral dosage of 0.2 to 0.5 mg/kg per week and can be increased to 0.7 mg/kg per week if needed for efficacy.[133,140,141] The upper limit in children is usually 20 to 25 mg per week. If methotrexate is not efficacious orally, a trial of subcutaneous weekly administration can be undertaken, especially in obese children requiring higher dosing. Methotrexate assays can be performed to determine if a dosage increase is needed in children who respond inadequately after 12 weeks.[142]

The most common side effects are nausea, abdominal discomfort, fatigue, headaches, and anorexia. The most significant side effect is bone marrow suppression. Administration of folic acid diminishes the risk of nausea, mucosal ulcerations, and macrocytic anemia.[143] The

Table 4.4 Treatment of Pediatric Psoriasis with Phototherapy and Systemic Agents

Intervention	Baseline Laboratory Tests	Dosing	Follow-up Tests	Potential Side Effects and Comments*
Methotrexate	CBC, LFTs; Renal function and TB testing at physician discretion	0.3–0.6 mg/kg/wk	Monthly CBCs, LFTs for first 3 months and then every 3–6 mo; annual TB testing if at risk	GI toxicity, fatigue most common; bone marrow suppression and hepatotoxicity
Cyclosporine	BP; CBC, LFTs, BUN, Cr, Mg^{++}; TB and HIV testing if at risk Some recommend fasting lipids, potassium, and uric acid	2–5 mg/kg/d; can go higher based on drug trough levels	BP checks weekly in first month then at follow-up visits; monthly CBCs, LFTs for first 6 mo and then every 3 mo; annual TB testing if at risk	Renal and hepatic toxicity, hypertension, hypertrichosis, immunosuppression, UVB-induced skin cancer
Acitretin	CBC, LFTs, fasting lipids, pregnancy testing if fertile female	0.5–1 mg/kg/d	LFTs, fasting lipid levels after 1 mo and with dose increases, then every 3 mo; pregnancy testing as appropriate	Cheilitis, hyperlipidemia, musculoskeletal pain, hair loss, skin fragility, bone toxicity if used long-term, teratogenicity
PDE4 inhibitor: Apremilast	Generally not needed	30 mg twice daily is adult dose; also available in 10 and 20 mg	None	Diarrhea, nausea, vomiting, headache, upper respiratory infection, mood change, weight loss
TNF inhibitor: etanercept	TB testing required; optional CBC, LFTs	0.8 mg/kg sc injection weekly (max 50 mg)	Annual TB testing	Increased risk of mycobacterial infection and possibly lymphoma
TNF inhibitor: adalimumab	TB testing required; optional CBC, LFTs	24 mg/m^2 sc every 2 wk	Annual TB testing	Increased risk of mycobacterial infection and possibly lymphoma
TNF inhibitor: infliximab	TB testing required; LFTs; optional CBC	3.3–5 mg/kg IV at 0, 2, 6, then every 7–8 wk	Annual TB testing; LFTs every 3 mo	Increased risk of mycobacterial infection and possibly lymphoma; rarely used for psoriasis unless need very rapid intervention
Interleukin 12/23 inhibitor: ustekinumab	TB testing required; optional CBC, LFTs	0.75 mg/kg if $\leq$60 kg, 4 wk, every 12 wk; 45 mg if 60–100 kg or 90 mg if $>$100 kg	Annual TB testing based on risk factors	Increased risk of mycobacterial/*Salmonella* infection and possibly lymphoma

BP, Blood pressure; *BUN,* blood urea nitrogen; *CBC,* complete blood count; *Cr,* creatinine; *GI,* gastrointestinal; *HIV,* human immunodeficiency virus; *IV,* intravenous; *LFTs,* liver function tests; *Mg,* magnesium; *MMR,* measles, mumps, and rubella; *sc,* subcutaneous; *TB,* tuberculosis; *PDE4,* phosphodiesterase-4; *TNF,* tumor necrosis factor-alpha; *UVB,* ultraviolet B.

*All interventions other than phototherapy, acitretin, and apremilast are immunosuppressive. If suggested by history or examination, undertake baseline hepatitis A, B, and C and/or HIV testing. Before starting any immunosuppressive agent, vaccinations should be up-to-date. Live and live attenuated vaccines should be avoided; among common ones are varicella, MMR, and intranasal influenza. See text for more details.

dosage is 1 mg/day (may skip the day of methotrexate administration). For young children, two chewable multivitamins (each containing 400 μg folic acid) can be given. Although weekly dosing of folic acid on the day after methotrexate administration (same total weekly dose) has commonly been used in Europe, a recent study showed a significant increase in the occurrence of gastrointestinal side effects with weekly dosing (five- to sixfold that of six to seven times weekly).[130] Switching to subcutaneous administration of methotrexate also reduces gastrointestinal complaints. Liver and bone marrow function should be monitored by blood testing, but testing should not be in the 72 hours after methotrexate administration, when transaminases may be transiently elevated. Obese children may have hepatic steatosis and a higher risk of transaminase abnormalities. Liver biopsy is unnecessary in children, and overall hepatic toxicity is rare. Live vaccines such as measles, mumps, and rubella (MMR); poliovirus; and intranasal influenza vaccines may not be given to a child taking weekly methotrexate. Sulfa drugs, including trimethoprim/sulfamethoxazole (Bactrim), should be avoided while taking methotrexate. Improvement is sometimes seen by as little as 3 weeks after initiation of treatment but more commonly requires 10 weeks. Once clearing is achieved, the methotrexate should be gradually lowered (e.g., 2.5 mg/month) during the subsequent months.

Cyclosporine has been used in young patients with severe unresponsive psoriasis, exfoliative erythrodermas, or pustular psoriasis.[133,144] Its mechanism of action involves inhibition of cytokine production by T lymphocytes. Cyclosporine is usually initiated orally at a dosage of 4 to 5 mg/kg per day (and 3 mg/kg per day if microemulsion) and maintained for 3 to 4 months until marked improvement occurs, followed by gradual downward titration and discontinuation within a year of initiation (generally with transition to an alternative, safer therapy). The dosing can be increased if trough cyclosporine levels prove to be low. The potential complications are hypertension, renal and hepatic toxicity, and hypertrichosis; however, concerns about future leukemias, lymphomas, cutaneous carcinomas, and other oncogenic risks are heightened with childhood use. Live vaccines (e.g., MMR and poliovirus) cannot be used in patients receiving cyclosporine therapy. Patients must also avoid macrolide-family medications (e.g., azithromycin) because they can markedly increase cyclosporine levels.

Retinoids tend to be less effective than methotrexate or cyclosporine as a single agent for treating plaque-type psoriasis;[145] in one study, 44% achieved a Psoriasis Area and Severity Index [PASI] score of 75 (at least 75% improvement from baseline in the PASI). However, retinoids are more effective for exfoliative erythrodermas and for pustular psoriasis that does not respond to compresses and topical corticosteroids alone.[146,147] Oral retinoids are often used more successfully in combination with topical ointments, ultraviolet light treatment, methotrexate, or cyclosporine. Acitretin normalizes epidermal differentiation and has an antiinflammatory effect. The usual regimen is oral administration at a dosage of 0.5 to 1 mg/kg per day, although the dosage can be titrated depending on patient response and laboratory results (maintenance dosing is usually 0.2 to 0.4 mg/kg per day).[108] Complications related to retinoid usage are most commonly dryness of the skin and mucous membranes and elevation of serum triglyceride levels. The potential for skeletal toxicity (premature epiphyseal closure and hyperostosis), although rare, must be monitored clinically and, if appropriate, radiographically during infancy, childhood, and puberty in patients who receive retinoids long term. Screening tests include blood counts, fasting lipid profiles, and hepatic studies. Retinoids cause severe teratogenicity and should be used with caution in adolescent girls. Isotretinoin may be an alternative retinoid for female adolescents with pustular psoriasis because of its much more rapid clearance, but generally it is not as effective as acitretin.

Apremilast is an oral phosphodiesterase 4 (PDE4) inhibitor approved for use in adult moderate to severe psoriasis. Gastrointestinal adverse events, particularly diarrhea, nausea, and abdominal discomfort, are not infrequent but tend to be self-limited and do not often lead to treatment discontinuation. Laboratory monitoring is not needed. Although off-label and in phase 3 trials at the time of writing, pK studies suggest dosing of 20 mg twice daily for children ≥15 to <35 kg and ≥6 years of age and 30 mg twice daily for children ≥12 years and ≥35 kg.[148]

Dimethylfumarate, a fumaric acid ester, is an immunosuppressant available outside of the United States for treating moderate to severe psoriasis. In a retrospective study of 14 pediatric patients (median age at onset, 15 years), only 36% of patients were nonresponders and 36% showed complete clearance.[149] Severe diarrhea and flushing were the causes of discontinuation in two patients, although transient mild elevation in liver function testing or leukopenia was noted in 36% of the children.

Biologic[150] agents target specific components of the immune system that have been shown to be increased in psoriasis[151] and have been found to have an earlier onset of response and higher efficacy than nonbiologic agents[152] (Figs. 4.33, A and B).[150,151] Currently available biologic agents inhibit either TNF-α (adalimumab, etanercept, infliximab) or IL-12 /IL-23 (ustekinumab),[153] although additional TNF, IL-17, IL17Ra, and IL-23p19 inhibitors are commercially available for adults with plaque psoriasis and in phase 3 trials in pediatric patients at this time. During 2010–2014, biologics comprised 9.6% of all prescribed medications for psoriasis (pediatric and adult) but accounted for 86% of their cost.[154] All biologics are administered subcutaneously with the exception of intravenous infliximab and have been associated with injection site reactions in the minority of patients. Infection, especially mycobacterial infection for the TNF inhibitors, is the only other risk that has been seen in trials with children. TNF inhibitors, especially etanercept, are the most commonly used biologic agents for pediatric psoriasis to date.[155–159] In a trial of 211 pediatric patients with moderate to severe plaque-type psoriasis, 57% achieved PASI 75 by 12 weeks of once-weekly therapy with 0.8 mg/kg etanercept; only 11% of patients treated with the vehicle control achieved this degree of improvement.[71,160] In the 5-year open-label extension, etanercept retained its efficacy and showed no long-term unexpected side effects, mycobacterial infection, or malignancy.[161]

Use of adalimumab, a TNF inhibitor administered every other week, has been described in several anecdotal reports, but has only been tested in pediatric patients in one double-blind, randomized trial. Papp et al. compared full-dose (0.8 mg/kg every other week) and half-dose (0.4 mg/kg every other week) subcutaneously administered adalimumab with oral methotrexate (0.1 to 0.4 mg/kg given weekly) in children 4 years old and above in a 16-week study.[162] PASI 75 was achieved in 58% of those on full-dose adalimumab, 44% of those on half-dose adalimumab, and 32% of those taking methotrexate, although the mean dosage of methotrexate (0.15 mg/kg per week) was below the standard given by pediatric dermatologists (0.3 to 0.5 mg/kg per week). There was no significant difference in the occurrence of adverse events, including infections, between the adalimumab and methotrexate groups. Adalimumab is currently approved in Europe for children 4 years of age and above, but not yet in the United States.

Two other TNF inhibitors deserve mention. Intravenously administered infliximab is generally reserved for severe flares of pustular or erythrodermic psoriasis that demand rapid response. Certolizumab is a TNF inhibitor that is biochemically distinct (pegylated), achieved higher PASI 75 scores than adalimumab and etanercept in adults, and is currently FDA approved for psoriasis in adults; it is given subcutaneously every 2 weeks and, in contrast to other biologics, fails to traverse the placenta, making it safe for use during pregnancy.

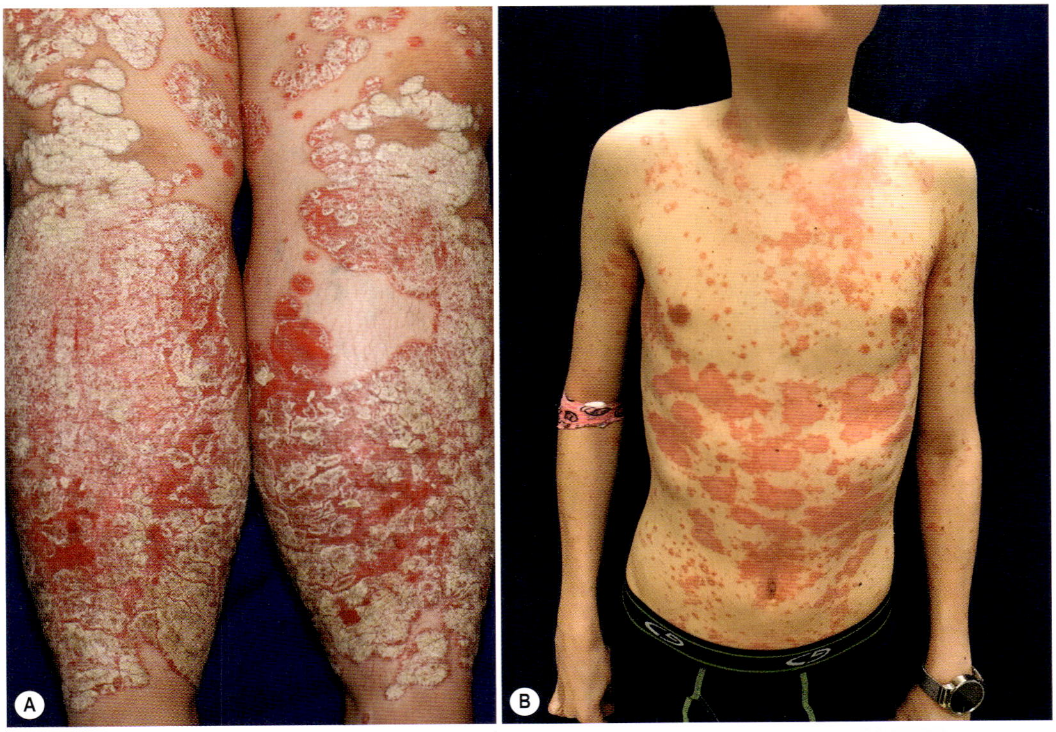

Fig. 4.33 Psoriasis. **(A)** Severe psoriasis in an obese adolescent that cleared almost entirely with adalimumab therapy. **(B)** Severe psoriasis that cleared entirely with ustekinumab therapy.

Ustekinumab administration has been reported anecdotally to improve moderate to severe psoriasis in children as young as 2 years of age.[163–165] Landells et al. compared[166] 12 weeks of standard-dose ustekinumab (0.75 mg/kg for <60 kg; 45 mg for >60 to <100 kg, and 90 mg for >100 kg) with half-standard dosing and placebo for adolescents 12 years and above with moderate to severe plaque psoriasis.[166] PASI 75 was achieved in approximately 80% of children with both ustekinumab doses compared with 11% on placebo; PASI 90 was reached in about 60% taking ustekinumab compared with 5% taking placebo. Ustekinumab and other drugs that inhibit Th17/IL-23 pathway activation may be the optimal therapy for *CARD14*-related psoriasis and PRP.[63] Ustekinumab is approved in the United States and Europe for treating plaque psoriasis in adolescents 12 years and older. Inhibitors of IL-17A (ixekizumab and secukinumab), the IL-17A receptor (brodalumab), and IL-23p19 (guselkumab, tildrakizumab, and risankizumab) are currently approved for use in adults but not in children. Nevertheless, there are anecdotal reports suggesting efficacy, such as the use of secukinumab for DITRA.[167] Interestingly, however, Cordoro et al. have shown predominantly IL-22-expressing T cells in lesional skin of pediatric psoriasis, in contrast to the predominantly IL-17A-expressing cells in adult psoriasis,[168] raising the question of whether inhibition of IL-17A will be as effective in children as in adults.[168]

Multiple factors need to be considered in making the choice of systemic agent, including patient preference, cost, tolerance, adverse effects, dosing schedule, and mode of administration. Of importance, biologic agents are also considerably more costly than methotrexate,[169] which is a major deterrent to their use when access is an issue.

Although primarily used for plaque psoriasis, TNF inhibitors have led to improvement for recalcitrant palmoplantar pustular[170] and erythrodermic[171] psoriasis. TNF inhibitors can show loss of efficacy with time; in adults, the 4-year drug survival for etanercept or adalimumab is approximately 40%.[172] Should a TNF inhibitor lose its efficacy, switching to an alternative TNF inhibitor (or a different class of medication) can significantly improve psoriasis severity.[173]

The long-term risks of biologic therapy in children are unknown, although to date serious acute adverse events are rare. Patients may be at risk for mycobacterial and *Salmonella* infections,[174] and baseline intermediate-strength purified protein derivative (PPD) or QuantiFERON gold with annual reevaluation is recommended; the need to obtain baseline and follow-up levels of other laboratory tests (e.g., blood counts and liver function tests) in children is controversial. Adverse effects on the development of the immune system in young children and an increased risk of lymphoma are theoretical concerns. Assessment of a recent claims database that included 9045 biologics-naïve pediatric psoriasis patients showed a significantly increased lymphoma rate (not of cancer overall) compared with the US Surveillance, Epidemiology, and End Results (SEER) database, but not relative to the >77,000 child comparator cohort.[175]

Development of Psoriasis and Psoriasiform Dermatitis During Administration of Tumor Necrosis Factor Inhibitors

Children taking TNF inhibitors, especially those with Crohn's disease that is well controlled, may develop new-onset psoriasiform dermatitis.[175–179] This seemingly paradoxical inflammatory cutaneous response has also been described in children with juvenile idiopathic arthritis, hidradenitis suppurativa, or Behçet syndrome. The psoriasis from TNF inhibitors favors the scalp, periorificial skin, nails, dorsal aspect of hands and feet (Fig. 4.34), and often the palms and soles, where it can be pustular. Lesions are not uncommonly secondarily infected with *S. aureus*. The eruptions are described after a wide range of duration of treatment, ranging from one dose to up to 63 months. Its occurrence in no way affects the response to the biologic agent for the original indication, and the risk of occurrence is not reduced by concurrent administration of methotrexate. The mechanism for the development of psoriasis despite suppression by TNF inhibition remains unclear. Cytokine imbalance with increased expression of IFN, known to increase the risk of psoriasis in chronic active hepatitis, has been proposed.[180] Patients with Crohn's disease who developed psoriasis on infliximab were more likely to have homozygous *IL-23R* polymorphisms, suggesting a genetic tendency.[177] An infectious trigger, particularly streptococcal or staphylococcal infection, has been suggested as well.

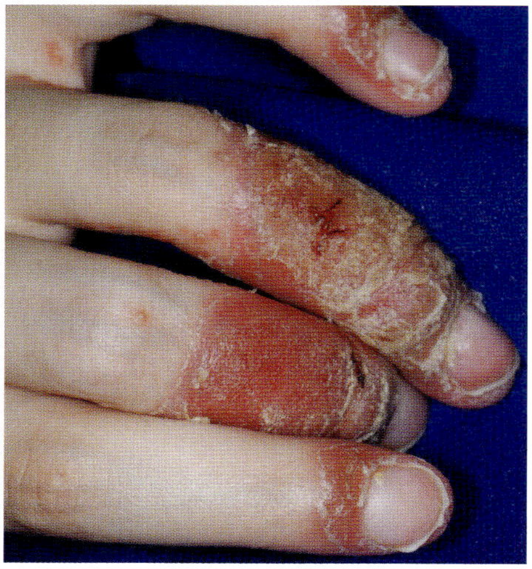

Fig. 4.34 Psoriasiform eruption induced by tumor necrosis factor (TNF) inhibitor on the dorsal aspect of the hands.

Approximately half of affected children require a change in their initial anti-TNF agent, and about one-third discontinue TNF inhibitors entirely.[176] Trying topical therapy alone is warranted before considering an alternative systemic regimen. Initiation of methotrexate[181] or ustekinumab[182] are other therapeutic options.

THERAPY FOR PSORIATIC ARTHRITIS

Many patients with psoriatic arthritis require only nonsteroidal antiinflammatory drugs, maintenance of joint position, functional splinting, and physiotherapy. The combination of methotrexate and a biologic agent is now most commonly used for more recalcitrant cases. Occasionally arthroscopic synovectomy or joint replacement is required.

PSYCHOSOCIAL AND EDUCATIONAL SUPPORT

Psoriasis affects the family as well as the child. Caregivers of the children often experience anxiety and/or depression related to the child's psoriasis.[183] The National Psoriasis Foundation (www.psoriasis.org) is available as a support group for patients and families of patients and provides superb educational material about psoriasis.

Reactive Arthritis

Reactive arthritis (formerly called *Reiter syndrome*) most commonly occurs in young men between 20 and 40 years of age,[184] but has been described in children as young as 9 months of age. It has been reported in almost 100 children, usually boys.[185] In affected adults, reactive arthritis usually occurs after sexually transmitted infection, particularly *Chlamydia*, or gastrointestinal infection and has been associated with human immunodeficiency virus (HIV) infection.[184] In children, it usually develops after an acute enteric infection, particularly one caused by *Shigella flexneri*, *Salmonella typhimurium*, *Campylobacter*, or *Yersinia*. Diarrhea and other symptoms of gastrointestinal disease are often gone by the time of arthritis onset, so history is important. Fever, anorexia, weight loss, and malaise may be other early signs. Several weeks may pass between the onset of fever and diarrhea and the clinical findings of reactive arthritis.

The classic triad of reactive arthritis includes nonbacterial conjunctivitis, urethritis, and arthritis. However, the complete triad is rarely seen at onset, may take several weeks to develop, and is incomplete in the majority of affected children. Conjunctivitis is the most common ocular manifestation and occurs overall in 50% of children. It tends to be bilateral, is self-limited with clearance in weeks, and ranges in severity from mild injection to mucopurulent inflammation. Acute, painful anterior uveitis; iritis; keratitis; corneal ulceration; and optic neuritis have rarely been described. The arthritis typically is asymmetric and involves more than one joint, most commonly large weight-bearing joints, such as the hip, knee, and ankle. However, other large or small joints can be affected, and involvement occasionally is symmetric. In contrast to the pattern in affected adults, the sacroiliac joint is rarely involved in pediatric cases. Many children also show enthesitis, a typical feature of reactive arthritis characterized by focal tenderness at sites where ligament and tendon insert into bone. The arthritis and enthesitis tend to resolve after a few months but occasionally persist or recur. The urethritis in children is usually asymptomatic, and detection of sterile pyuria may be the only evidence of urethral inflammation. Less commonly, inflammation of the meatus may be clinically detectable or urethral discharge may be noted.

The cutaneous manifestations of reactive arthritis may develop either in association with or independently of the other features of the disorder. Most classic are the circinate balanitis/vulvitis and keratoderma blennorrhagica. The circinate balanitis/vulvitis occurs in 15% to 75% of affected children[186,187] and presents as well-defined erosions on the glans penis in uncircumcised males and on the vulva in females; circumcised male patients often show inflamed hyperkeratotic plaques on the shaft and scrotum. The keratoderma blennorrhagica occurs in 8% to 25% of children[185,186] and appears as psoriasiform scaling, inflammatory papules, pustules, and plaques on pressure or weight-bearing areas of the palms and soles (Fig. 4.35).

Psoriasiform papules and plaques have also been described on the extensor surfaces of the extremities and the dorsal aspects of the feet and hands. Oral lesions consist of painless erythema, shallow erosions, and small pustules that may occur on the buccal mucosa, gums, lips, palate, and tongue. Oral lesions generally resolve spontaneously after a period of several days. Lesions on the tongue, particularly when thickly coated, may simulate a geographic tongue. Nail changes resembling psoriasis have also been seen.[188]

Diagnosis of the disorder is made based on the constellation of clinical features and is supported by nonspecific laboratory findings. Rheumatoid factor is negative, but most affected children show HLA-B27 antigen. Sterile pyuria and significant elevation of erythrocyte sedimentation rate are usually found. Mild anemia with leukocytosis may be present as well. If performed early, stool cultures may yield the triggering bacterial organism. Although biopsy of the skin lesions may be helpful, it does not distinguish the cutaneous lesions of reactive arthritis from those of psoriasis. Reactive arthritis must be differentiated from other seronegative arthropathies, including psoriatic arthritis,[189] juvenile idiopathic arthritis, infectious arthropathies (especially gonococcal and Lyme disease), Kawasaki disease,[190] Behçet syndrome, and rheumatic fever.

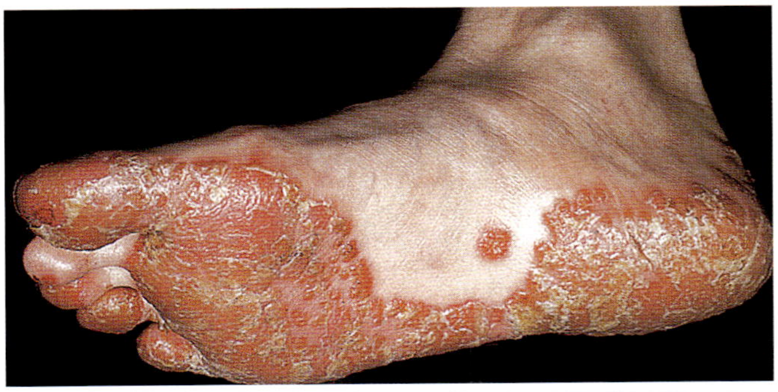

Fig. 4.35 Keratoderma blennorrhagicum, showing thickened, psoriasiform papules and plaques on the foot of a patient with reactive arthritis. (Reprinted with permission from Schachner LA, Hansen RC, eds. Pediatric dermatology. Edinburgh, Scotland: Mosby; 2003: Fig. 15.16.)

Reactive arthritis is almost always self-limiting in children and clears without sequelae.[186] A minority of children show recurrent or chronic arthritis. Treatment consists primarily of bed rest and administration of nonsteroidal antiinflammatory drugs. The cutaneous lesions may respond to topical corticosteroids. Ophthalmologic consultation is appropriate for patients with ocular manifestations. Occasionally, intraarticular injection of corticosteroids or administration of systemic medication is required. Sulfasalazine, methotrexate, acitretin, cyclosporine, and infliximab[191] have been used for patients with severe, unresponsive disease.

Pityriasis Rubra Pilaris[192]

PRP is a chronic skin disorder characterized by small follicular papules, disseminated yellowish-pink scaly plaques surrounding islands of normal skin, and hyperkeratosis of the palms and soles (Figs. 4.36 through 4.42.).[192] Although most pediatric cases are acquired without

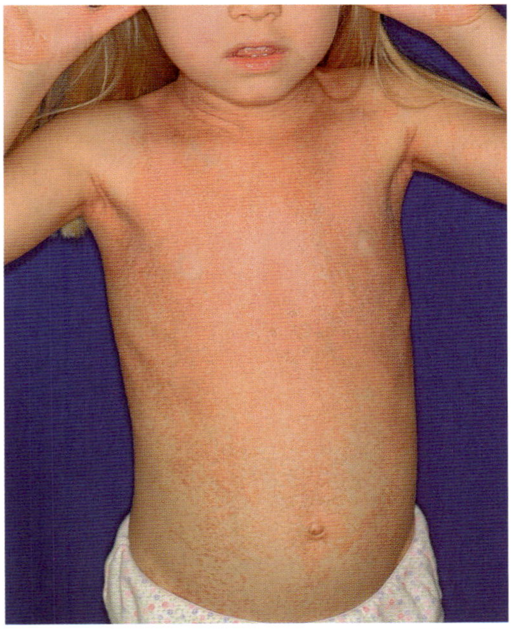

Fig. 4.36 Pityriasis rubra pilaris. Symmetric, diffuse, well-circumscribed, salmon-colored plaques representing the coalescence of erythematous papules. The discrete papules can be seen at the borders.

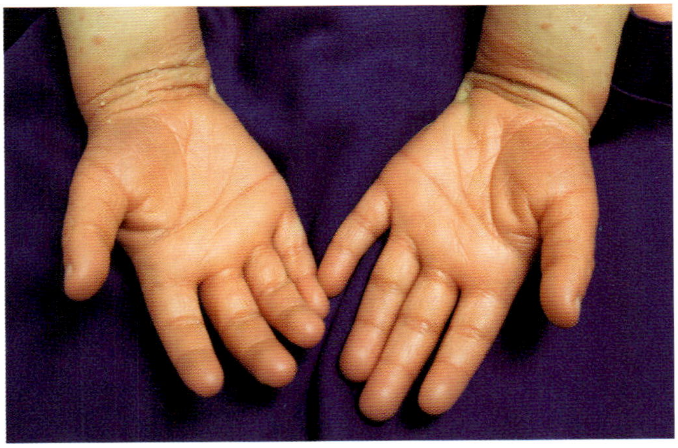

Fig. 4.37 Pityriasis rubra pilaris. Note the well-circumscribed palmar erythema and keratoderma.

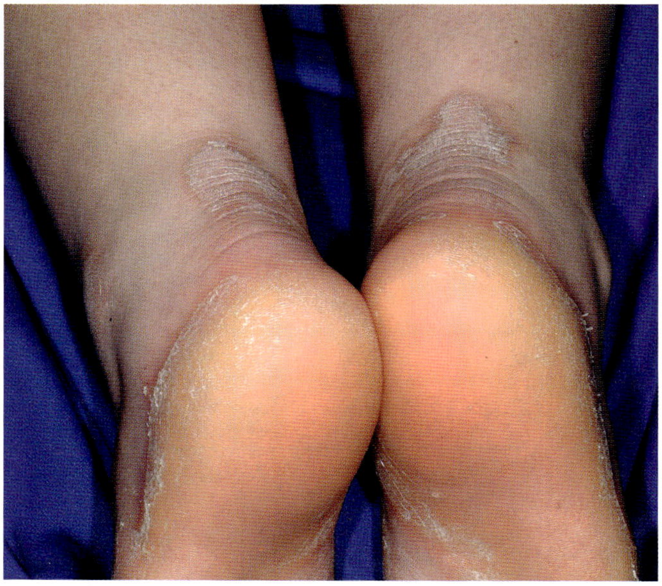

Fig. 4.38 The keratodermic sandal of a patient with type IV pityriasis rubra pilaris.

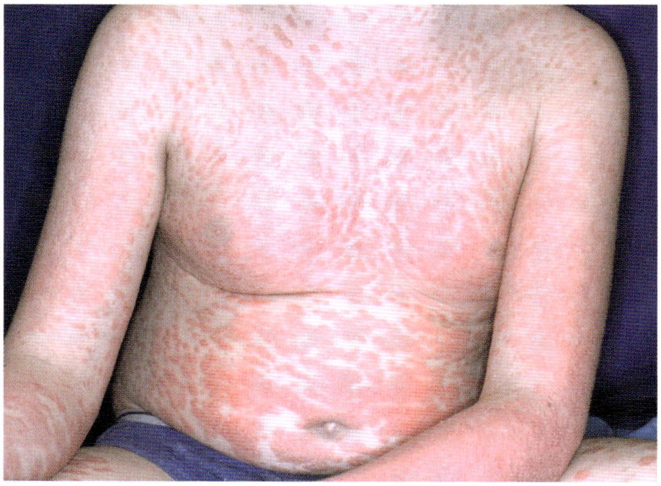

Fig. 4.40 Individuals with mutations in *CARD14* may show changes of pityriasis rubra pilaris, sometimes with unusual patterning on the trunk.

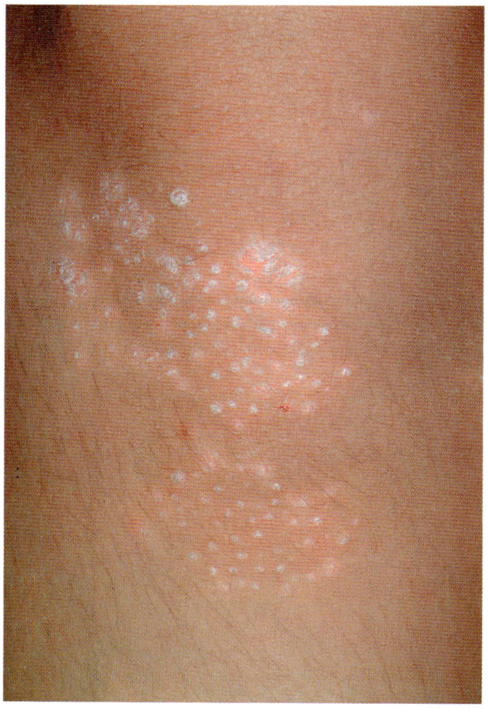

Fig. 4.39 Pityriasis rubra pilaris. Follicular scaling papules on the knee, a common site.

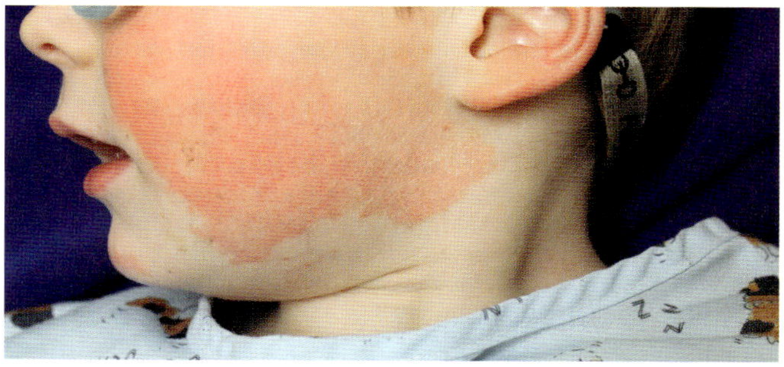

Fig. 4.41 Facial characteristics of PRP can include bright erythema of the cheeks and ears. This boy had no variant in *CARD14*.

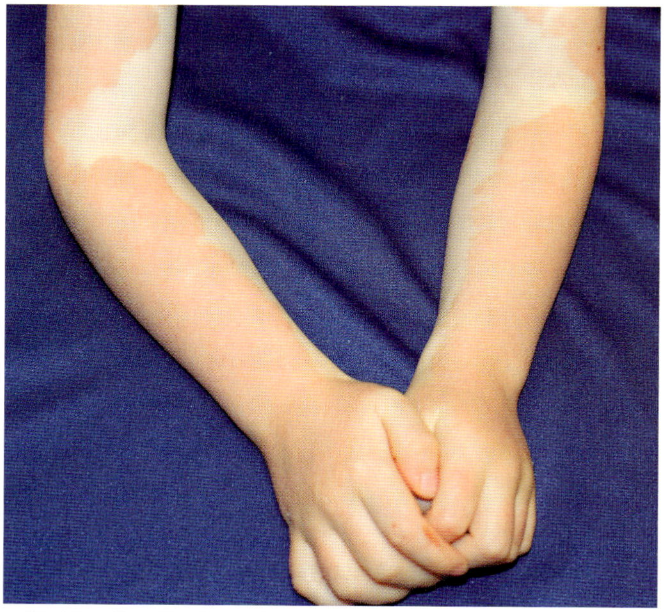

Fig. 4.42 Well-demarcated salmon-colored plaques of PRP.

a family history of the disorder,[193] autosomal dominant PRP has been described in families[194] and is now known to result from activating mutations in *CARD14* (*PSORS2*), which encodes the caspase recruitment domain family member 14.[195,196] *CARD14* is expressed by keratinocytes and activates NF-κB signaling.[197] Individuals with these *CARD14* mutations may present with cutaneous manifestations that resemble forms of psoriasis (see earlier) or PRP. Some of the distinguishing features of PRP resulting from *CARD14* mutations (which has been called *CARD14-related papulosquamous eruption* [CAPE]) are early age of onset, prominent involvement of the cheeks and sometimes chin and ears, patterning of lesions and "skip" areas on the trunk (see Fig. 4.40), a family history of psoriasis or PRP, and poor response to topical agents and isotretinoin.[63] Nevertheless, sporadic forms of PRP can show early onset, molecular evidence of *CARD14* activation without gene variants,[198] and may be indistinguishable clinically and histologically from the hereditary form (see Fig. 4.41).

Keratoderma of the palms and soles develops in the majority of children with PRP and can be present before or after the appearance of other features.[199] When seen on the soles, this has been referred to as a *keratodermic sandal* (see Fig. 4.38). The keratoderma shows a sharply demarcated border, sometimes extending to involve the dorsum of the hands and feet. The salmon color and sometimes edema help to distinguish the keratoderma from psoriasis, ichthyosis, hereditary palmoplantar keratoderma, and erythrokeratodermias (see Chapter 5). PRP-like manifestations, especially the palmoplantar keratoderma, are a rare manifestation of dermatomyositis.[200] Thickening of the elbows, knees (see Fig. 4.39), ankles, and Achilles tendon (see Fig. 4.38) is seen in most affected children.[201] Lesions can cover large body surface areas, but typically show the salmon color and sharp demarcation (see Fig. 4.42). Although not always present, the most characteristic clinical feature is the 1-mm follicular-based papule with a central keratotic plug that is often surrounded by salmon-colored erythema (see edges of coalescent scale, Fig. 4.36). Initially discrete, the papules usually coalesce into well-demarcated hyperkeratotic plaques with a coarse texture similar to the surface of a nutmeg grater. The plaques are generally symmetric and diffuse and contrast sharply with islands of normal skin that occur within the affected areas. Despite their frequency in affected adults, the distinct follicular-based papules on the dorsal aspect of the fingers are found in a minority of affected children.[199]

More than 40% of pediatric patients show cephalic involvement (see Fig. 4.41), often extending from the face to the neck and onto the upper trunk in a cape-like configuration with sharp borders (see Fig. 4.36). Scalp scaling may be extensive, with large, adhesive scales and underlying salmon-colored erythema. Although perioral and periorbital areas may show the keratotic papules and erythema, the mucosae are spared. Ectropion has been described in children with extensive PRP, including resulting from *CARD14* variants; arthritis and contractures of the fingers may also be a feature of severe *CARD141*-related PRP (Fig. 4.43).

The nails are dystrophic in 13% of patients and can show thickening, onycholysis, transverse striations, and subungual debris (see Fig. 4.44). The characteristic pitting of nails seen in psoriasis, however, is not a feature. The Koebner phenomenon, a hallmark of psoriasis, has been described in approximately 10% of children with PRP. Pruritus is only occasionally a feature but may occur in children with diffuse disease.

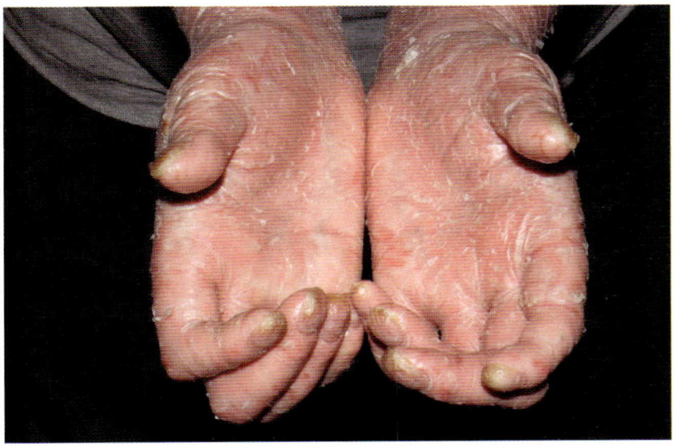

Fig. 4.43 Severe PRP resulting from *CARD14* mutation with associated ectropion and severe keratoderma of the hand with contractures.

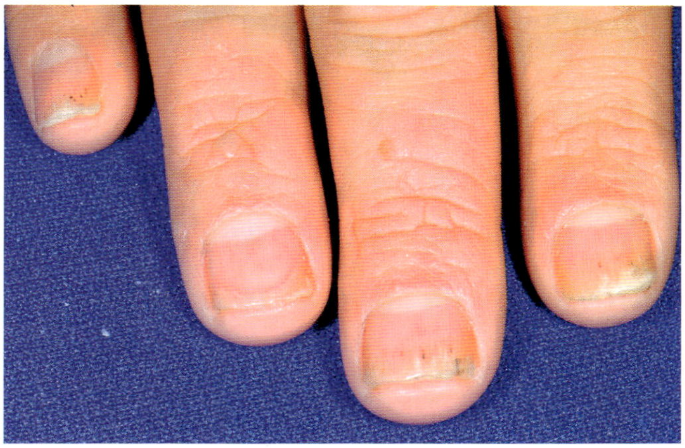

Fig. 4.44 Unusual nail changes in a girl with extensive pityriasis rubra pilaris (PRP). Note the onycholysis and splinter hemorrhages. Her skin disease was more typical of PRP than psoriasis and cleared with oral retinoids.

The onset of PRP in children may be acute, as is more typical of adults, appearing and spreading during a few days. Alternatively, the eruption may begin on the scalp and forehead and extend gradually. Exfoliative, rapidly progressive dermatitis with associated malaise, chills, and fever is rarely described in children. Biopsy of a follicular-based papule can aid in diagnosis if it shows the characteristic follicular keratosis, as well as epidermal parakeratosis and dermal mononuclear infiltrates, particularly surrounding the hair follicle.

The disorder has been classified into five types[202] based on the age of onset, lesion distribution, and disease course in six types: types I and II in adults; types III (classical juvenile), IV (circumscribed juvenile), and V (atypical juvenile) in children; and a type VI in patients with HIV infection, which has been reported in a child[203] (Table 4.5). Of these, type IV PRP is the most common in pediatric patients.[204] However, many pediatric cases cannot easily be fit into any of these classifications. In addition, children may originally exhibit characteristics of one type that then evolve into another type. An alternative system of classification of five types has been proposed based on the presentation and courses in 104 children. This newer classification adds a new type I that shows only palmoplantar keratoderma without follicular plugging (20% of children) but combines Griffiths types I and III into a single classification that includes all ages.[199]

The clinical course of PRP is variable. In a review of 29 pediatric cases, 52% showed clearance within 6 months (mean 2.7 months), and an additional 11% were symptom free by 1 year after onset.[204] In another study of 30 children, 43% showed 90% to 100% clearing, an additional 23% showed at least 30% clearing, and 17% showed a poor outcome.[205] However, in a more recent study of 28 patients, two-thirds of patients with type III and IV juvenile PRP (i.e., most of the patients) had a protracted course lasting longer than 3 years.[206] The prognosis does not correlate with acute versus gradual onset or extent of involvement. The course at times is characterized by spontaneous remissions and exacerbations; some children have disease that evolves into a phenotype more typical of psoriasis than PRP.

Patients with milder, more localized PRP may respond to emollients, topical corticosteroids, tazarotene,[207] calcipotriol, and/or keratolytic agents (e.g., formulations containing urea, salicylic acids, or α-hydroxy acid). Calcineurin inhibitor therapy may clear facial lesions.[208]

Unless known to have a mutation in *CARD14*, nonresponders with more extensive disease are best treated with systemic retinoid therapy (e.g., isotretinoin, acitretin, alitretinoin[209,210]), which has been shown to be more effective in children than UVB light. Alternatives are methotrexate,[211–213] cyclosporine, azathioprine, and apremilast.[205,214,215] Adequate therapeutic trials of retinoids require at least 4 to 6 months and careful monitoring. Extensive extraspinal

Table 4.5 Classification of Pityriasis Rubra Pilaris in Adults and Children*

Type		Incidence	Clinical Features
I	Classic adult	Most adults	Follicular keratotic papules, first on face and extending caudally; progresses to generalized keratoderma with islands of sparing; palms and soles usually involved; generally clears within 3 years
II	Atypical adult	Rare	More ichthyosiform scaling; coarse palmoplantar keratoderma; long duration
III	Classic juvenile	14% to 35% of children	Same as type I
IV	Circumscribed juvenile	Most common type in children	Thick plaques on knees, elbows; palms, and soles involved
V	Atypical juvenile	Rare, familial; onset in first years of life	"Sclerodermatous" changes on palms and soles; follicular hyperkeratosis
VI	PRP in association with human immunodeficiency virus	Only described in 1 4 year old child	Classified as type IV based on distribution

Griffiths WA. Pityriasis rubra pilaris. Clin Exp Dermatol. 1980;5(1):105–12.
Menni S, Brancaleone W, Grimalt R. Pityriasis rubra pilaris in a child seropositive for human immunodeficiency virus. J Am Acad Dermatol. 1992;27:1009.

hyperostosis has been described in a child with PRP after long-term administration of oral retinoid therapy.[216] Given the self-limited nature of the disorder in many affected children, retinoids should be tapered and discontinued as tolerated after several months of continuous therapy. TNF inhibitors with or without retinoids have also been helpful in many patients.[217–222] Treatment with Th17/IL-23 inhibitors, especially ustekinumab, has also proven effective for several patients with recalcitrant PRP,[221,223,224] including with *CARD14* variants, which is consistent with the role of IL-23 as an intermediate in the *CARD14*-induced NF-κB signaling pathway.[63,224]

Pityriasis Lichenoides[225,226]

Pityriasis lichenoides (formerly called *parapsoriasis*) is a spectrum of cutaneous eruptions that has been subdivided into two forms[226,227]: (1) an acute form, pityriasis lichenoides et varioliformis acuta (PLEVA, Mucha–Habermann disease), and (2) a chronic form, PLC.[225,226] Overall, 19% to 38% of cases occur in pediatric patients,[228,229] occasionally during the first decade of life and even at birth.[230] In a recent study of 75 children (median age, 8) in which 40 had long-term follow-up, 67% had PLC, 29% had PLEVA, and 4% were mixed,[225] but other studies have shown approximately equal frequencies.[226] Some children show clinical and/or histologic features of both the acute and chronic forms, suggesting considerable overlap and confirming the concept that these groups represent a spectrum of disease. As a result, a newer classification is based on distribution into diffuse, central (neck, trunk, and extremities), and peripheral (acral) forms, rather than the morphology of lesions.[231] Acral involvement, including of the face, is more common in children than in adults, and the disorder persists longer before spontaneous remission in children as well.[232]

PLEVA is a polymorphous eruption that usually begins as asymptomatic to pruritic, symmetric 2- to 3-mm, oval or round, reddish-brown macules and papules. The papules occur in successive crops and rapidly evolve into vesicular, necrotic, and sometimes purpuric lesions (Figs. 4.45 and 4.46). These develop a fine crust and gradually resolve with or without a varioliform scar. Lesions may involve the entire body but are often most pronounced on the trunk, proximal thighs, and upper arms, especially the flexor surfaces. The face, scalp, mucous membranes, palms, and soles are often spared or may be involved to a lesser degree. Transient hypopigmentation or hyperpigmentation may result. The course usually lasts for periods of a few weeks to several months. Patients occasionally have associated fever and constitutional symptoms. A rare variant, the febrile ulceronecrotic form, is characterized by large, coalescing, ulceronecrotic

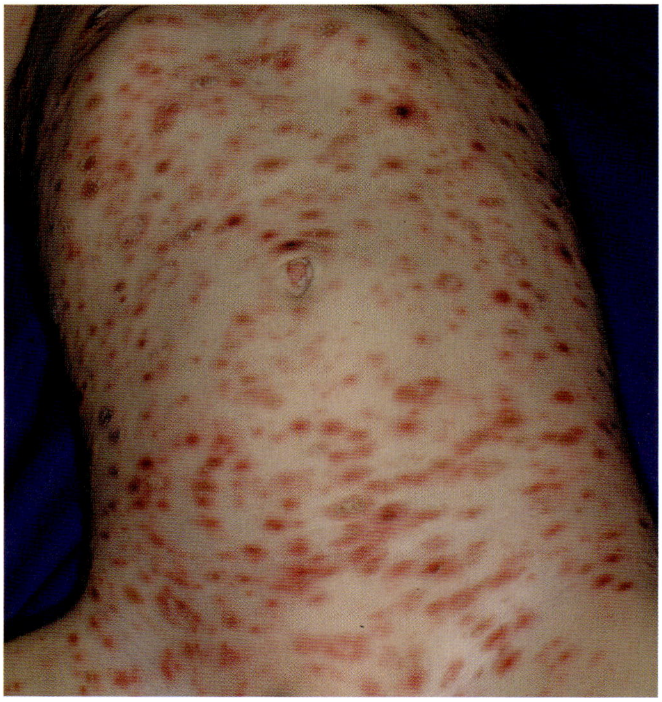

Fig. 4.45 Pityriasis lichenoides et varioliformis acuta. Symmetric oval and round, reddish-brown macular, papular, necrotic, and crusted lesions on the chest and abdomen of a 3-year-old boy.

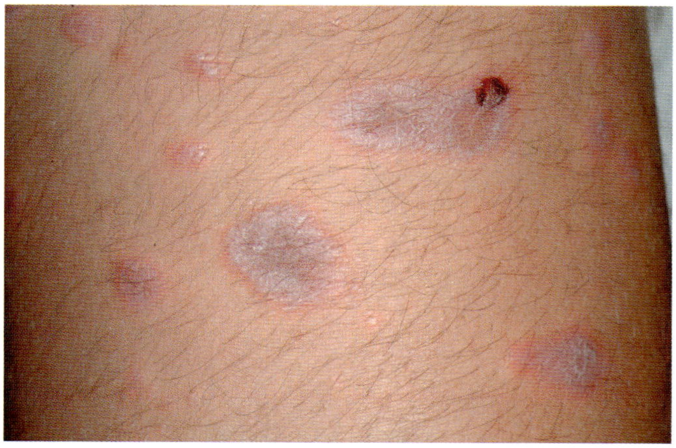

Fig. 4.46 Pityriasis lichenoides et varioliformis acuta. Symmetric oval and round, scaling papules and plaques. In skin of color, the red to purpuric hue of the lesions may be more subtle.

nodules and plaques associated with high fever and arthralgias[233–238]; 50% of reported cases have been in children.[239] Febrile ulceronecrotic PLEVA may be associated with gastrointestinal, pulmonary,[240] and central nervous system[241] involvement.

PLC may begin *de novo* or may evolve from PLEVA. Lesions characteristically appear as scaling papules and plaques (Figs. 4.47 and 4.48) that resolve with dyspigmentation but no scarring.

In the early stages, pityriasis lichenoides may be mistaken for chickenpox, arthropod bites, impetigo, vesicular pityriasis rosea, vasculitis, or scabies; chronic forms may be confused with psoriasis, lichen planus, pityriasis rosea, and secondary syphilis. The duration of the eruption (often in crops); the presence of macules and papules interspersed with vesicular, crusted, or hemorrhagic lesions with or without varioliform scarring; and subsequent hypopigmentation or hyperpigmentation help to differentiate pityriasis lichenoides from other conditions. When the diagnosis remains in doubt, histopathologic examination of a skin biopsy specimen will often substantiate the proper diagnosis, showing heavy mononuclear cell perivascular infiltration and, in more acute lesions, erythrocyte extravasation into the dermis, intraepidermal vesicle formation, and epidermal necrosis.

The cause of pityriasis lichenoides is unknown. However, studies demonstrating T-cell clonality[242,243] and a predominant plasmacytoid dendritic eruption with high expression of type 1 cytokines[244]/IFN−γ[171α] suggest that pityriasis lichenoides is a benign lymphoproliferative process in which a vigorous host immune reaction prevents the condition from evolving into lymphoma. The common temporal association of preceding exposure to viral infection, especially to parvovirus or human herpesvirus (HHV)-8,[238,245,246] or immunization, especially to MMR,[247] implicates an abnormal immune response to a viral antigenic trigger. These results are consistent with rare reports of cutaneous T-cell lymphoma (CTCL) occurring in patients with clinical manifestations or a history of PLEVA or PLC.[248–250] CD30+ T cells in the biopsy specimens of a few patients with pityriasis lichenoides[251] show overlap with lymphomatoid papulosis (see later)[245] and suggests a spectrum of lymphoproliferative disorders from benign (PLEVA, PLC), to lymphomatoid papulosis, to CTCL. Indeed, approximately 5% of children develop CTCL (see Chapter 10), especially mycosis fungoides presenting as nodules, hypopigmentation, or poikiloderma, after several years of pityriasis lichenoides.[252,253]

A recent long-term study found that children with PLEVA had a mean disease duration of 35 months, whereas those with PLC had a mean duration of at least 78 months.[225,253] Residual postinflammatory pigmentary alterations can last for several years. Narrowband ultraviolet light is the most effective therapy,[254] and most children show clearance in sun-exposed areas.[255] The improvement from exposure to ultraviolet light may also explain the common onset during autumn or winter months.[256–258] Systemic antibiotics,[228] particularly erythromycin, azithromycin,[259,260] or a tetracycline, are first-line therapy because of their ease compared with phototherapy, but require a 2- to 3-month trial. If successful, antibiotics can be tapered, but continued administration at low to full dosage may be required for sustained clearance. Tetracyclines should not be administered to children younger than 8 years of age (depending on the status of eruption of secondary teeth) or to pregnant adolescents. Methotrexate,[261] cyclosporine,[262] cyclophosphamide,[241] and TNF inhibitors[236] are appropriate to consider for severely affected children, such as those with the febrile ulceronecrotic form. Topical corticosteroids and/or oral antihistamines may be helpful for pruritus and insomnia, but do not hasten resolution.

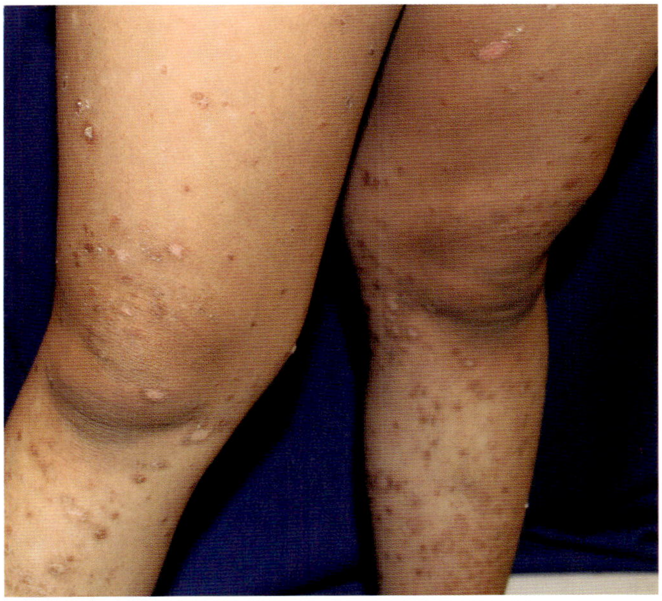

Fig. 4.47 Pityriasis lichenoides chronica. Small, dusky erythematous scaling papules with numerous residual macules of postinflammatory hyperpigmentation and hypopigmentation.

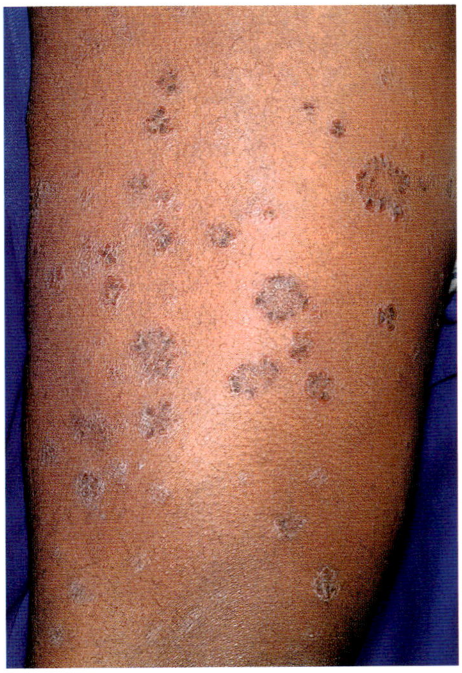

Fig. 4.48 Pityriasis lichenoides chronica. Annular scaling plaques with associated hyperpigmentation in an Black patient.

Pityriasis Rosea

Pityriasis rosea is an acute, benign, self-limiting disorder that affects male and female patients equally.[263,264] Approximately 50% of cases occur before adulthood, with only 4% of cases before 4 years of age. Most patients are otherwise well; however, a prodrome of headache, malaise, pharyngitis, lymphadenopathy, and mild constitutional symptoms is present in approximately 5% of affected patients, particularly in association with more florid involvement. The etiology of pityriasis rosea remains controversial. A viral disorder is suggested by the occasional presence of prodromal symptoms, the course of the disease, epidemics with seasonal cluster, occasional reports of simultaneous occurrence in closely associated individuals, and a tendency to lifelong immunity in 98% of cases. There is evidence both to support and refute the idea that pityriasis rosea is a reaction to HHV-6 and/or -7.[265] High circulating levels of Th17/IL-22 cytokines have been described, as in psoriasis.[266,267]

Some 70% of cases start with a single isolated lesion, the so-called "herald patch" (Fig. 4.49), which is found most commonly on the trunk, upper arm, neck, or thigh. This characteristic initial lesion presents as a sharply defined oval area of scaly dermatitis (typically

2 to 5 cm in diameter, but rarely large enough to encircle the trunk)[268] with a finely scaled, slightly elevated border that gradually expands. After an interval of 2 to 21 days, a secondary generalized eruption of smaller papules (0.2 to 1 cm) appears in crops, characteristically sparing the face (in 85% of individuals), scalp, and distal extremities. In about 25% of cases itching, particularly of secondary lesions, may be noted. The orientation of the long axis of these lesions is most characteristic (Fig. 4.50). The typically ovoid lesions run parallel to the lines of skin cleavage, leading to a pattern resembling a "Christmas tree" on the back, wrapping around the trunk horizontally at the axillary area and suprapubic areas, and following inguinal folds. The smaller lesions also show a "collarette of scale" that surrounds the lesions (Figs. 4.49 and 4.51). Although the truncal distribution is most common, some patients, particularly children, show an inverse distribution of lesions on the face, axillae, and groin (Fig. 4.52). This atypical form of pityriasis rosea may be particularly difficult to diagnose if there is no history of a herald patch and if the characteristic morphology of lesions goes unrecognized. The face and neck are more often involved in children than in adults, particularly in Black children. Black children with pityriasis rosea may also have more extensive eruptions, which are more papular (34%) and resolve with residual dyspigmentation.[269] Papular lesions in pityriasis rosea are more common in young children[270] (Fig. 4.53).

Vesicular, pustular, follicular, urticarial, erythema multiforme–like, and hemorrhagic variants,[270] as well as lesions in a unilateral or blaschkoid distribution, have also been described. The herald patch occasionally is the only manifestation. Involvement of the oral mucous membranes occurs in up to 16% of patients, most often as asymptomatic erythematous patches that rarely appear erosive, hemorrhagic, or bullous.[271,272]

The secondary eruption peaks within a few days to a week. Clearance usually occurs within 6 weeks, initially in the lesions that appeared earliest, but may require as long as 5 months. The disorder is rarely recurrent.[265] Postinflammatory hypopigmentation or

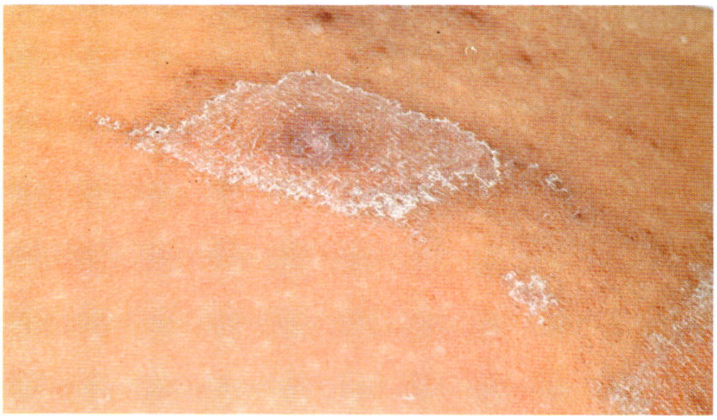

Fig. 4.49 Herald patch (pityriasis rosea). Oval lesion with finely scaled elevated border, occasionally misdiagnosed as tinea corporis.

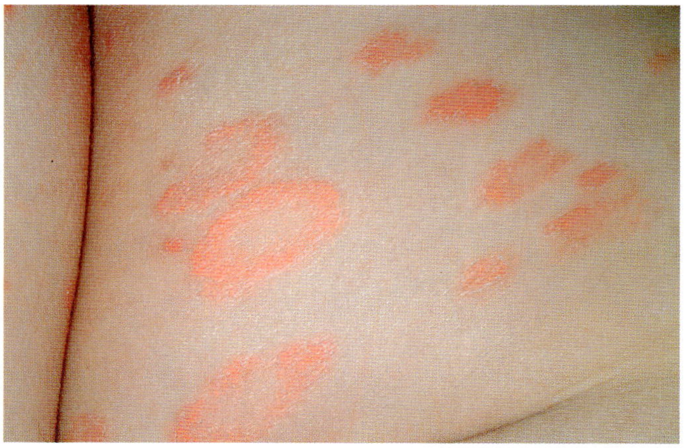

Fig. 4.51 Pityriasis rosea. The collarette of scale can be subtle.

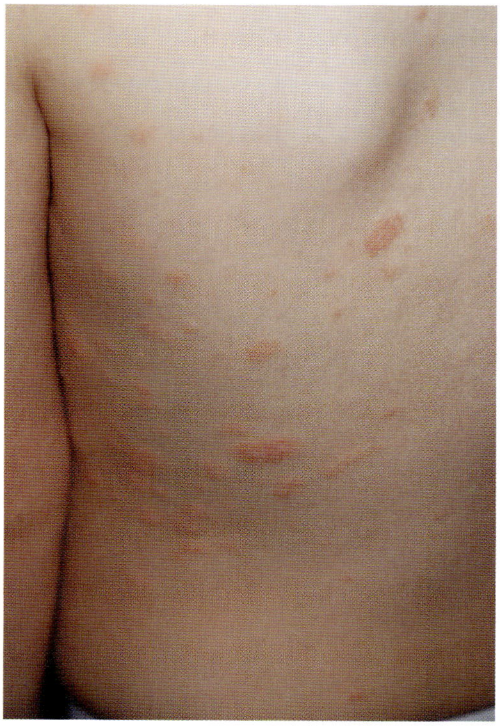

Fig. 4.50 Pityriasis rosea. The lesions of pityriasis rosea typically follow skin lines, which are easiest to appreciate on the trunk.

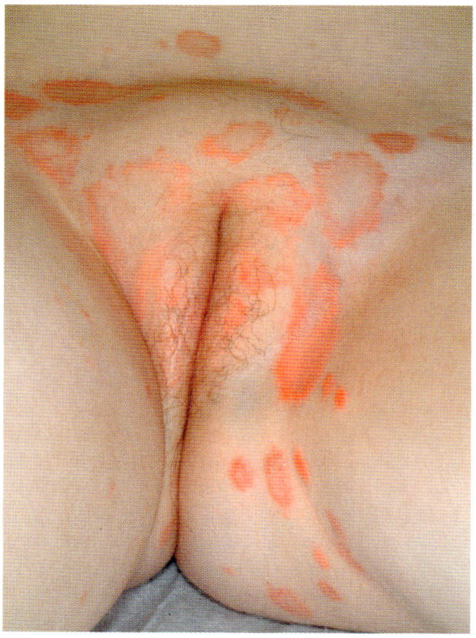

Fig. 4.52 Pityriasis rosea. Inverse pattern showing the distribution along skin lines. Scaling may be more difficult to appreciate in intertriginous areas.

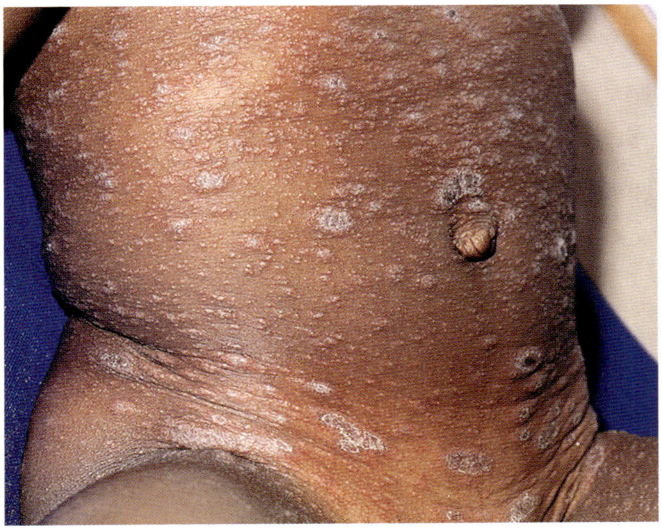

Fig. 4.53 Pityriasis rosea. Truncal involvement with larger plaques and predominantly round papular lesions, most commonly see in young children and Blacks. Note the peripheral scale and distribution along skin lines.

hyperpigmentation may commonly be noted, particularly in dark-skinned individuals, and may persist for weeks to months after clearance of the pityriasis rosea.

The diagnosis of pityriasis rosea depends on recognition of the distribution of lesions and the characteristic appearance of the oval lesions with their fine peripheral or collarette scales. The histologic features of pityriasis rosea are not diagnostic and resemble those of a subacute or chronic dermatitis. The herald patch may be mistaken for tinea corporis, and the full-blown eruption must be differentiated from widespread tinea infection, drug eruption, PLEVA, seborrheic dermatitis, nummular eczema, psoriasis (particularly the guttate variety), and, importantly, secondary syphilis. The latter must be considered in sexually active individuals who show involvement of the palms and soles, an unusual (but occasional) site for lesions of pityriasis rosea. The hemorrhagic form of pityriasis rosea must also be distinguished from vasculitis, including Henoch–Schönlein purpura, and viral disorders with thrombocytopenia.

Most patients require no treatment beyond reassurance as to the nature and prognosis of the disorder. Pruritus, if present, usually responds to topical antipruritics (calamine lotion, lotions containing menthol and/or camphor, lotions with pramoxine), oral antihistamines, colloidal starch or oatmeal baths, and mild topical corticosteroid formulations. Exposure to ultraviolet light or sunshine tends to hasten resolution of lesions, and in the summertime it is not uncommon to see patients with pityriasis rosea under covered areas with little to no evidence of the eruption on sun-exposed regions.[273] The value in speeding clearance of systemic steroids, erythromycin, and acyclovir is controversial.

Lichen Planus

Lichen planus is a disorder primarily of adults, but 2% to 11% of reported cases occur in children and adolescents,[274,275] including as those young as 3 weeks of age. The etiology of lichen planus is unknown, but evidence suggests a cytotoxic Th1-cell and plasmacytoid dendritic cell–mediated immune response, as seen with cutaneous lupus erythematosus.[276] Familial cases are rare[277] but have an earlier age at onset; increased severity; greater likelihood of chronicity; and an increased incidence of erosive, linear, ulcerative, and hypertrophic forms. Several cases in children have been described after hepatitis B vaccination.[278–280] The association of lichen planus with hepatitis C, as seen in adults,[281] has not been noted in children.[278,282] Lesions resembling lichen planus are a common manifestation of chronic graft-versus-host disease (see Chapter 25).

The primary lesion is a small, shiny, flat-topped polygonal, reddish or violaceous papule (Figs. 4.54 and 4.55).[283] Individual papules vary from 2 mm to 1 cm or more and may be closely aggregated or widely dispersed. Lichen planus is generally mildly to intensely pruritic in adults but is not uncommonly asymptomatic in affected children.[274] The disorder is usually limited to a few areas, with the lower legs the most common site[278]; lichen planus also often affects the flexural surfaces of the ankles and wrists, the genitalia (Fig. 4.56), and the lower back. Involvement of the face (Fig. 4.57), palms, and soles is unusual.[284] Lichen planus pigmentosus inversus is a rare variant with involvement in the skin folds.[285]

At times, one may detect characteristic small grayish puncta or streaks that form a network over the surface of papules. These delicate white lines, termed *Wickham striae*, become more visible under magnification with a hand lens or by wetting the lesion with an alcohol swab or a drop of oil, which renders the horny layers of lesions more transparent. Occasionally, lesions may coalesce to form plaques or a linear configuration (the Koebner phenomenon) at sites of minor trauma, such as scratch marks (Fig. 4.58).

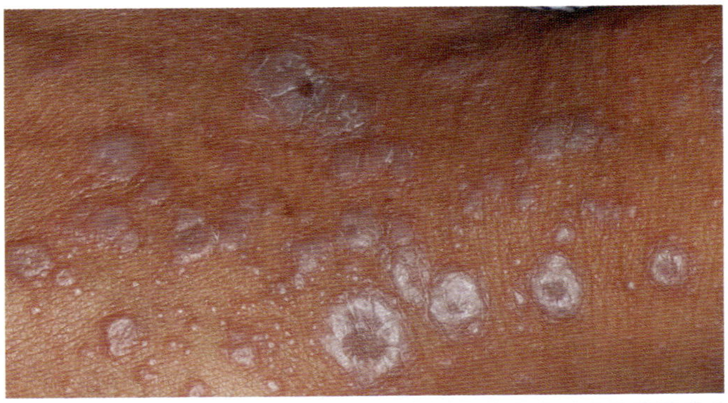

Fig. 4.54 Lichen planus. The shiny, flat-topped polygonal violaceous papules of lichen planus. Note the Wickham striae (linear whitish-gray streaks) on the surface.

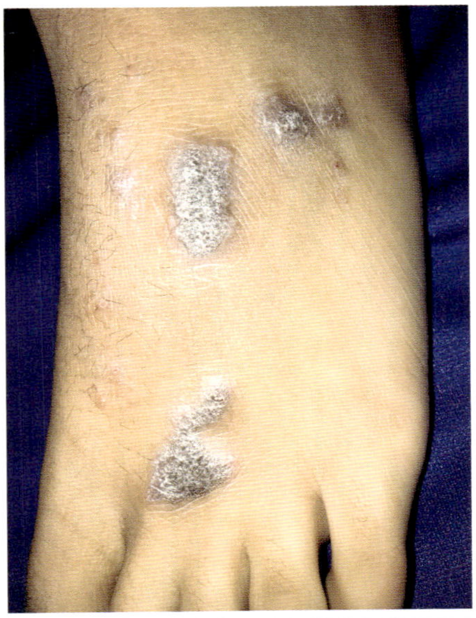

Fig. 4.55 Lichen planus. The shiny, flat-topped polygonal violaceous papules and plaques of lichen planus. Note the white, lacy Wickham striae and the intense residual hyperpigmentation.

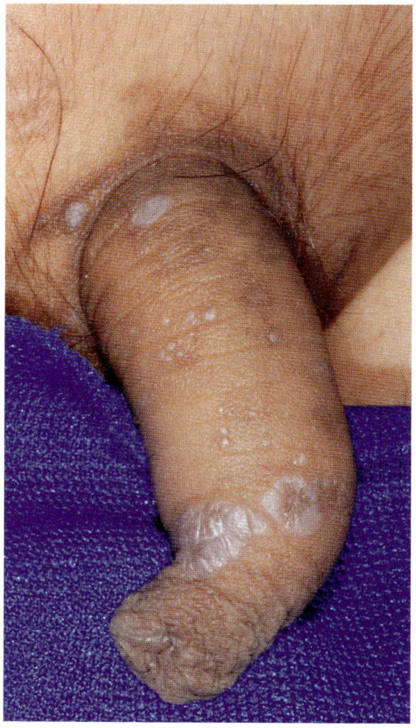

Fig. 4.56 Lichen planus. Typical violaceous lesions of lichen planus on the penile shaft, a common site.

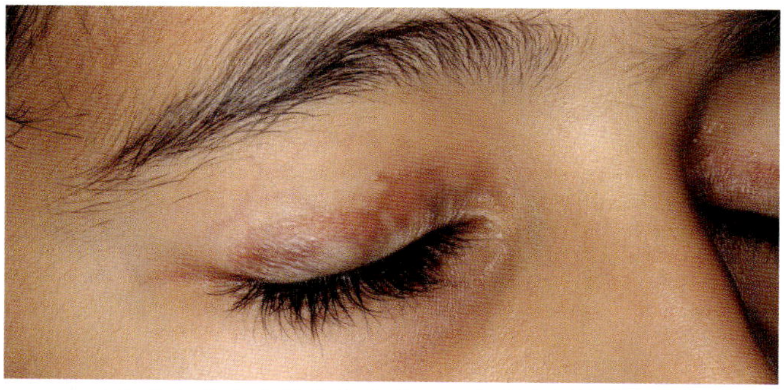

Fig. 4.57 Lichen planus. Mildly pruritic violaceous lesions on the eyelids with postinflammatory intense hyperpigmentation; biopsy confirmed lichen planus.

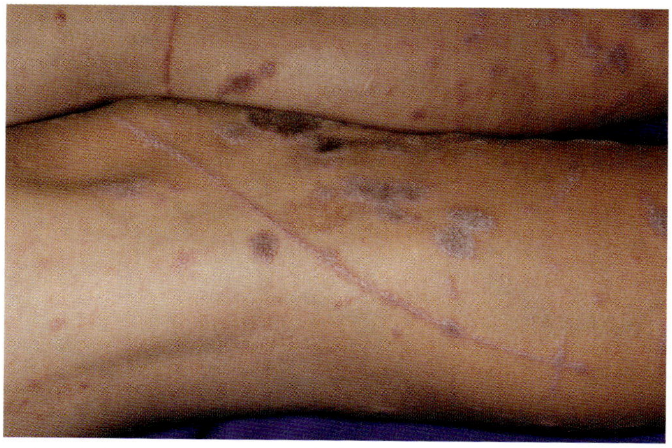

Fig. 4.58 Lichen planus. Note the linearity of lesions from scratching and the Koebner phenomenon.

Mucous membrane involvement is seen in up to 40% of pediatric patients[286] and is much less common than in adult patients (50% to 70% of adult patients).[274,279] When present, lesions usually appear as pinhead-sized white papules forming annular or linear lace-like patterns on the mucosal aspects of the cheeks (Fig. 4.59).[287,288] Lesions on the palate, lips, and tongue are less characteristic and except for their reticulated appearance may easily be mistaken for areas of leukoplakia. In one pediatric series of oral lichen planus, the tongue was the most commonly affected site (75% of cases).[289] On the lips the papules are more often annular, sometimes with adherent scaling reminiscent of that seen in lupus erythematosus. Although the typical reticulated mucosal lesions of lichen planus are asymptomatic, painful ulcerative lesions have been found on the tongue; oral mucous membranes; and mucosal surfaces of the pharynx, esophagus, gastrointestinal tract, vulva, and vagina. Oral lichen planus has been described in a girl with autoimmune polyendocrinopathy-candidiasis-ectodermal dystrophy.[289] Ocular lichen planus is rare in children, but presents as dry eyes with persistent conjunctival hyperemia and progressive symblepharon.[290]

Up to 10% of adult patients with lichen planus demonstrate involvement of one to all nails, but nail involvement appears to be less common in affected children; one study, however, noted nail involvement in 19% of 100 children.[274,278] Violaceous lines or papules in the nailbed may occasionally be seen through the nail plate. The nail dystrophy consists of loss of luster, thinning of the nail plate, longitudinal ridging or striation, splitting or nicking of the nail margin, atrophy, overlapping skin folds (pterygia), marked subungual hyperkeratosis, lifting of the distal nail plate, red or brown discoloration, and at times complete and permanent loss of the nail (Fig. 4.60).[291] Some children with 20-nail dystrophy (trachyonychia, see Chapter 7) may have lichen planus, but biopsy of the nail matrix would be needed to confirm the diagnosis in the absence of cutaneous changes.[292]

Although lichen planus is considered to be papulosquamous, many variations in morphology and configuration may be noted. These variations include vesicular, bullous, actinic, annular, hypertrophic (Fig. 4.61), atrophic, linear,[293] erythematous, and follicular forms (Table 4.6).[293–295] Lichen planus pemphigoides is a rare autoimmune blistering disease in which the typical lichen planus lesions evolve into bullous lesions with a mean lag time of 8 weeks (see Chapter 13).[294] The extremities are most commonly involved, and approximately half of the affected children show palmoplantar lesions. Direct and indirect immunofluorescence shows the presence of circulating antibodies.[296]

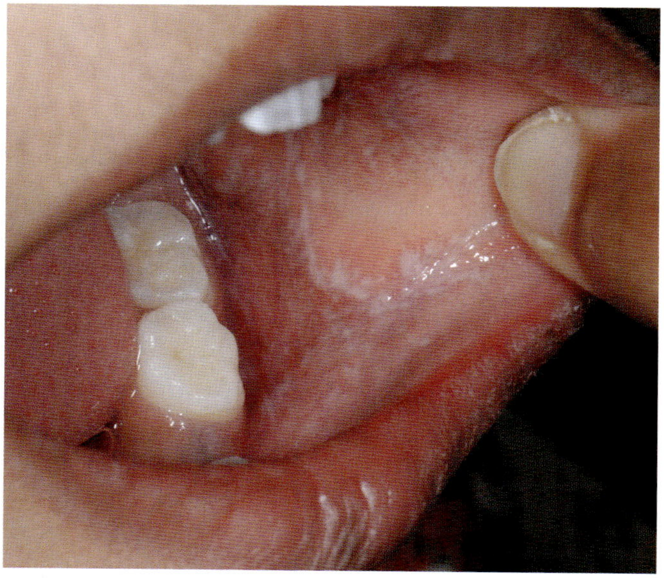

Fig. 4.59 Oral lichen planus. Wickham striae on the buccal mucosa.

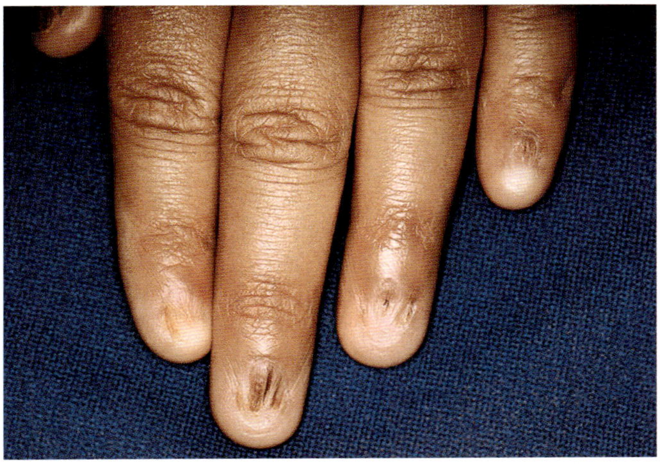

Fig. 4.60 Lichen planus of the nails. Anonychia and pterygium formation.

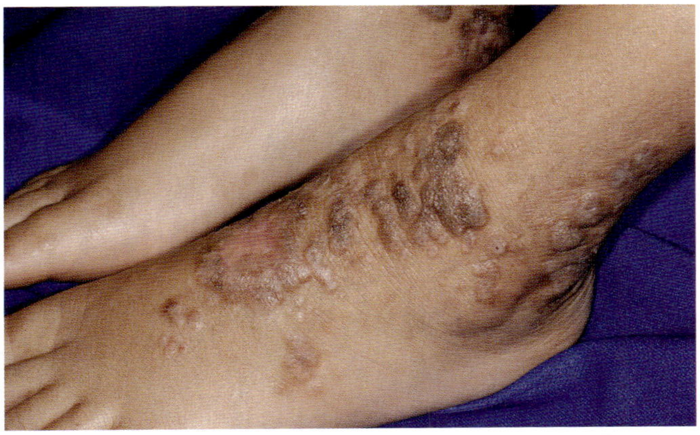

Fig. 4.61 Lichen planus. The plaques of lichen planus may be hypertrophic but show the characteristic violaceous coloration and intense hyperpigmentation.

Many drugs may produce an eruption that resembles lichen planus (lichenoid drug eruption). Most commonly implicated are antihypertensives (captopril, enalapril, labetalol, and propranolol), diuretics (especially hydrochlorothiazide), antimalarials (especially hydroxychloroquine and quinidine), metals (especially gold salts), and penicillamine. Among other agents rarely implicated but used often in children and adolescents are griseofulvin, tetracycline, carbamazepine, phenytoin, and nonsteroidal antiinflammatory drugs. Leflunomide,[296,297] human growth hormone,[297] and even papillomavirus vaccination[298] have recently been implicated. In contrast to other drug eruptions, in which the latent period between introduction of the drug and the reaction is within 1 month, the latent period with lichenoid drug eruptions is typically several months to years after initiation of a medication. Similarly, the time to clearance after discontinuation of the medication is also prolonged and can take several weeks to months. The lichenoid lesions of lichenoid drug eruptions tend to be more eczematous, psoriasiform, or pityriasis rosea–like than the typical papules of lichen planus. Lesions occur much less commonly on oral mucosae than on skin.[299] In addition, they uncommonly show Wickham striae and are often photodistributed, particularly on the extensor forearms. Nail changes may be a late development, even after discontinuation of the offending medication.[296] The histologic picture resembles lichen planus, but shows more eosinophils.

The diagnosis of lichen planus depends on the recognition of the typical purple, polygonal, pruritic papules and plaques. When the diagnosis is in doubt, histopathologic examination of a cutaneous lesion can confirm the proper diagnosis. Characteristic changes are destruction of the basal cell layer (liquefactive degeneration), sawtoothing of the rete pegs, and a band-like lymphocytic infiltrate that hugs and invades the lower epidermis. Although cases of lichen planus occasionally clear in a few weeks, two-thirds of affected individuals with acute forms display spontaneous resolution within 8 to 15 months. In most patients, the lesions tend to flatten but are often replaced by an area of intense hyperpigmentation that tends to persist for several months to years (Fig. 4.62). Occasionally, lichen planus itself may persist for years, and 10% to 20% of patients suffer one or more recurrences of their disorder.

The standard therapy for lichen planus in pediatric patients involves administration of class I to IV topical steroids and oral antihistamines to reduce the pruritus and eventually flatten and clear lesions.[278] Topical tacrolimus has been effective in cases recalcitrant to topical steroids.[300] For more extensive or recalcitrant cases, the addition of a 2- to 6-week course of systemic corticosteroids (1 mg/kg per day) is usually helpful in ameliorating the associated pruritus and hastening

Table 4.6 Variants of Lichen Planus

Variant Type	Characteristics
Bullous	Bullae develop on existent LP lesions
LP pemphigoides	LP + bullous pemphigoid with autoimmune reactivity, usually against type XVII collagen (bullous pemphigoid 180 antigen)
Actinic	Onset during spring, summer; primarily sun-exposed surfaces (face, neck, dorsum of arms and hands); often annular configuration; most commonly in children and young adults
Annular	Occur in 10% of patients, often scattered amid typical lesions of LP
Hypertrophic	Pruritic, thick, hyperkeratotic plaques, especially on the legs and dorsal regions of the feet; persistent
Atrophic	May represent a resolving phase in which larger plaques become centrally depressed with residual hyperpigmentation
Hemorrhagic/purpuric	Shows nonblanching component on diascopy
Linear	LP occurring spontaneously along the lines of Blaschko; presumably reflects somatic mosaicism
Erosive/ulcerative	Intensely painful ulcerations on the palms and soles; chronic lesions may evolve into squamous cell carcinoma; erosive lesions may occur on mucosal surfaces
LP/lupus erythematosus	Overlapping features of lupus and LP; lesions are usually acral and patients may show high titers of ANA
Lichen planopilaris	Follicular LP; keratotic plugs surrounded by violaceous erythema, especially on scalp but can affect any hair-bearing area; usually results in cicatricial alopecia

ANA, Antinuclear antibodies; *LP*, lichen planus.

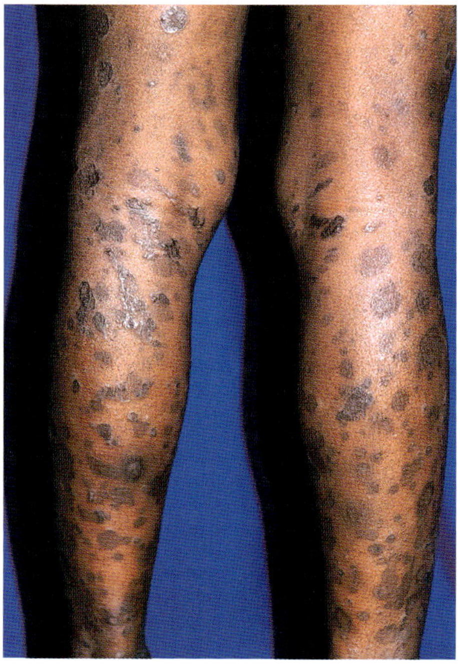

Fig. 4.62 Lichen planus. Intense residual postinflammatory hyperpigmentation.

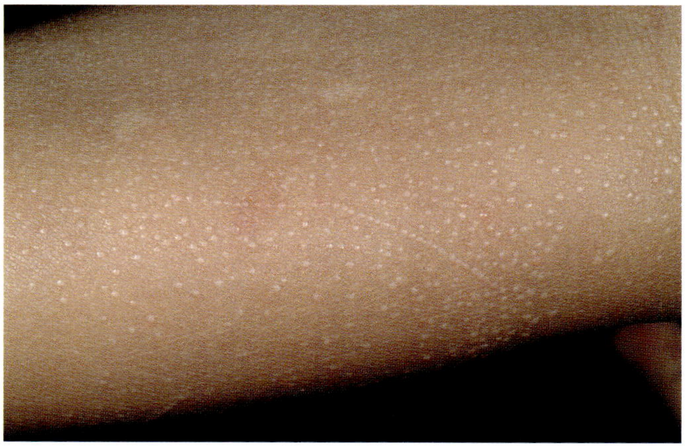

Fig. 4.63 Lichen nitidus. Sharply demarcated, pinpoint- to pinhead-sized monomorphic, round, usually flesh-colored lesions. Lesions may be distributed in a linear configuration after trauma to the site (Koebner phenomenon).

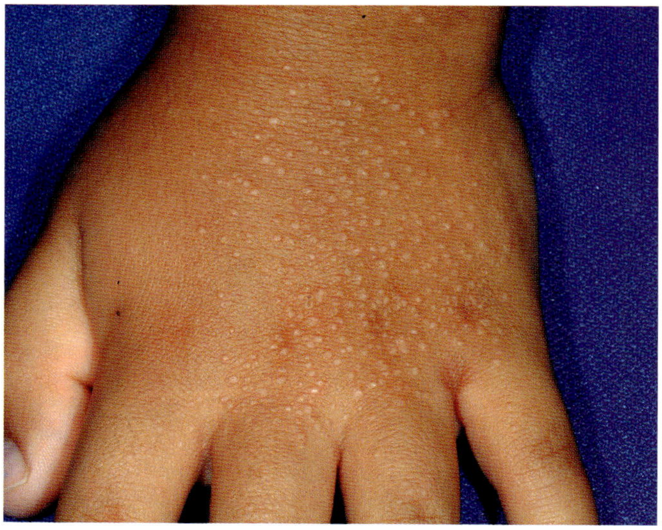

Fig. 4.64 Lichen nitidus. Note the even distribution of these pinpoint- to pinhead-sized round lesions on the dorsal aspect of the hand.

clearance.[301] Acitretin has also been effective for lichen planus, especially if hypertrophic.[302] Hypertrophic lichen planus lesions may also respond to application of class I topical steroids under occlusion, flurandrenolide-impregnated tape, or intralesional injections of triamcinolone. When traditional forms of therapy fail, metronidazole,[303] griseofulvin,[304] dapsone,[274] PUVA or nbUVB light therapy,[274] oral retinoids,[301] cyclosporine,[305] mycophenolate mofetil, and thalidomide[306] have been shown to be effective in selected cases. Patients with lichen planus pemphigoides often respond to topical corticosteroid and oral dapsone therapy, but a systemically administered steroid may be required.

If drug-induced lichen planus is considered, medications should be discontinued whenever possible. Mucous membrane lesions should be treated if symptomatic, eroded, or ulcerated. Topical anesthetics such as diphenhydramine elixir, viscous lidocaine, topical corticosteroids (such as Kenalog in Orabase), or topical tacrolimus ointment[307] may be beneficial. Because erosive forms of oral lichen planus may have an increased risk of malignant transformation, patients with oral lesions should avoid carcinogenic factors (such as tobacco) and receive periodic follow-up examinations and biopsy of suspicious lesions.[308] Nails may respond to administration of systemic corticosteroids, methotrexate, and/or intralesional steroids, but local application of potent steroids under occlusion or flurandrenolide-impregnated tape at the nail base can be used if the disorder is largely limited to the nail.[291]

Lichen Nitidus

Lichen nitidus is an uncommon benign dermatosis that affects individuals of all ages but is most commonly seen in preschool and school-aged children. Although the etiology remains unknown, association with lichen planus has been reported,[309] and some authorities consider lichen nitidus to be a variant of lichen planus. Familial cases have rarely been described.[310,311] Lichen nitidus has been seen in association with Down syndrome,[312] Niemann–Pick disease,[313] and Russell–Silver syndrome.[314]

The individual papules of lichen nitidus are sharply demarcated, pinpoint to pinhead sized, round or polygonal, and usually flesh-colored (Figs. 4.63 and 4.64). The surface of each lesion is flat, shiny, and slightly elevated, sometimes with a central depression in perforating lichen nitidus.[315] The eruption is arranged in groups, primarily located on the trunk, genitalia, abdomen, and forearms of affected individuals but may be generalized.[316] Linear lesions in lines of trauma (Koebner reaction) are common. Minute, grayish, flat papules on the buccal mucous membrane and nail changes (thickening, ridging, pitting, onycholysis)[317] have occasionally been noted, even before the appearance of cutaneous papules.[318] A rare variant is spinous follicular lichen nitidus, which may be localized or generalized and is often associated with perifollicular granulomas.[319] Lichen nitidus occasionally clears spontaneously after a period of several weeks to months but more often lasts much longer (occasionally years) with little or no response to treatment. As with lichen planus, significant postinflammatory pigmentary changes may persist.

Biopsy can confirm the diagnosis and characteristically shows claw-like projections of the rete ridges encircling an inflammatory infiltrate of lymphocytes, histiocytes, and occasionally giant cells, resembling a hand clutching a ball. Topical corticosteroids or calcineurin inhibitors occasionally clear the lesions but more often are not effective. nbUVB phototherapy has cleared generalized lichen nitidus.[320] Because lichen nitidus is usually asymptomatic and tends to resolve spontaneously, intervention is elective.

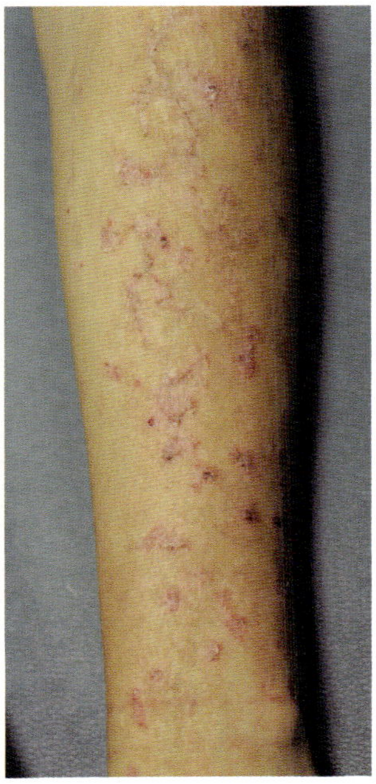

Fig. 4.65 The lichenoid papules and plaques of keratosis lichenoides chronica often have a reticulated or linear patterning and are most commonly found on the limbs and face.

Keratosis Lichenoides Chronica

Keratosis lichenoides chronica is a rare, chronic, progressive dermatosis that is much more common in adults than in pediatric patients.[321–323] Lesions may be present from birth or appear during infancy and are sometimes pruritic in children.[324] Familial occurrence (probably autosomal recessive) is more common in pediatric cases than in adults. The characteristic pink-red to violaceous lichenoid papules and scaling verrucous lesions show a linear or reticulated pattern (Fig. 4.65). The eruption tends to be symmetric, particularly on the limbs and, less commonly, the abdomen and buttock. Pediatric patients often have facial involvement, with well-defined, scaling, erythematous papules that may appear purpuric or resemble seborrheic dermatitis. Alopecia of the anterior scalp (receding frontal hairline), eyebrows, and eyelashes may be noted. The palms and soles may show keratoderma, and nails may be discolored with thickening and longitudinal ridging. Occasionally, mucosae are affected: painful ulcerations or keratoses of the oropharyngeal or genital mucosae, hoarseness, and keratoconjunctivitis have been described. Biopsy sections resemble those of lichen planus but show focal areas of parakeratosis.

Keratosis lichenoides chronica may persist for decades and is unresponsive to topical corticosteroid therapy, although one reported patient improved with the application of topical tacrolimus ointment.[325] Ultraviolet light exposure, PUVA therapy, methotrexate, and oral administration of retinoids,[326] alone or in combination, may be beneficial. Keratosis lichenoides chronica in two siblings has been associated with gain-of-function mutations in *NLRP1*, resulting in inflammasome activation and increased IL-1 signaling.[327]

The complete list of 327 references for this chapter is available online at http://expertconsult.inkling.com.

Key References

Menter A, Cordoro KM, Davis DMR, et al. From the academy joint AAD-NPF guidelines of care for the management and treatment of psoriasis in pediatric patients. J Am Acad Dermatol 2019, in press.

Eichenfield LF, Paller AS, Tom WL, et al. Pediatric psoriasis: Evolving perspectives. Pediatr Dermatol 2018;35(2):170-81.

Relvas M, Torres T. Pediatric psoriasis. Am J Clin Dermatol 2017;18(6):797-811.

Tangtatco JA, Lara-Corrales I. Update in the management of pediatric psoriasis. Curr Opin Pediatr 2017 Aug;29(4):434-442.

Paller AS, Mercy K, Kwasny MJ, et al. Association of pediatric psoriasis severity with excess and central adiposity: an international cross-sectional study. JAMA Dermatol 2013;149(2):166-76.

Mercy K, Kwasny M, Cordoro KM, et al. Clinical manifestations of pediatric psoriasis: results of a multicenter study in the United States. Pediatr Dermatol 2013;30(4):424-8.

Craiglow BG, Boyden LM, Hu R, et al. CARD14-associated papulosquamous eruption: a spectrum including features of psoriasis and pityriasis rubra pilaris. J Am Acad Dermatol. 2018;79(3):487-94..

Osier E, Wang AS, Tollefson MM, et al. Pediatric psoriasis comorbidity screening guidelines. JAMA Dermatol 2017;153(7):698-704.

Becker L, Tom WL, Eshagh K, et al. Excess adiposity preceding pediatric psoriasis. JAMA Dermatol 2014;150(5):573-4.

Cordoro KM. Topical therapy for the management of childhood psoriasis: part I. Skin Therapy Lett 2008;13(3):1-3.

Ersoy-Evans S, Altaykan A, Sahin S, et al. Phototherapy in childhood. Pediatr Dermatol 2008;25(6):599-605.

Roenneberg S, Biedermann T. Pityriasis rubra pilaris: algorithms for diagnosis and treatment. J Eur Acad Dermatol Venereol. 2018;32(6):889-98.

Yang CC, Shih IH, Lin WL, et al. Juvenile pityriasis rubra pilaris: report of 28 cases in Taiwan. J Am Acad Dermatol 2008;59(6):943-8.

Geller L, Antonov NK, Lauren CT, et al. Pityriasis lichenoides in childhood: review of clinical presentation and treatment options. Pediatr Dermatol 2015;32(5):579-92.

Bowers S, Warshaw EM. Pityriasis lichenoides and its subtypes. J Am Acad Dermatol 2006;55(4):557–72, quiz 573–6.

Ersoy-Evans S, Greco MF, Mancini AJ, et al. Pityriasis lichenoides in childhood: a retrospective review of 124 patients. J Am Acad Dermatol 2007;56(2):205-10.

Browning JC. An update on pityriasis rosea and other similar childhood exanthems. Curr Opin Pediatr 2009;21(4):481-5.

Kanwar AJ, De D. Lichen planus in childhood: report of 100 cases. Clin Exp Dermatol 2010;35(3):257-62.

5 Hereditary Disorders of Cornification (the Ichthyoses and Palmoplantar Keratodermas)

The hereditary disorders of cornification, or the ichthyoses, are a group of disorders characterized by scaling, skin thickening, and usually underlying inflammation,[1,2] leading to a significant impact on quality of life.[3] In many patients, itch is also an issue.[4] Ichthyoses are largely distinguished by their clinical and, in some cases, histologic and ultrastructural features. During the past 2 decades, next-generation sequencing has facilitated the discovery of the underlying molecular basis of most of the forms of ichthyosis, further refining classification[2,5] and facilitating our understanding of the role and interactions among epidermal proteins and lipids[6] in normal epidermal function. Most variants have been identified in exomes by whole-exome sequencing, but pathogenic variants have been discovered in intronic regions[7] and require more comprehensive investigations, including whole-genome sequencing.

Desquamation is the end result of proteolytic degradation of corneodesmosomes (the intercellular junctions within the stratum corneum) and is abetted by friction and cell hydration. Desquamation requires normal epidermal differentiation and depends on a gradient of pH, the presence of protease inhibitors, and the generation of hygroscopic molecules within the stratum corneum cells. Abnormalities in desquamation and differentiation usually result from abnormal corneocyte shedding (retention hyperkeratosis) or from increased epidermal cell proliferation (epidermal hyperplasia).

In addition to the stratum granulosum–based tight junction, the stratum corneum plays an important role in the epidermal barrier. The stratum corneum is composed of stacked corneocytes and surrounding highly hydrophobic lipid layers (lamellae) formed by the secretion of lamellar body contents at the interface of the stratum granulosum and the stratum corneum. Most of the mutations that lead to ichthyosis affect lipid metabolism or epidermal proteins, leading to barrier dysfunction and resulting in increased transepidermal water loss and decreased water-holding capacity.[8,9] Many of the features of ichthyosis are thought to be continuous compensatory attempts to restore the barrier (e.g., upregulated epidermal lipid synthesis, epidermal hyperproliferation, and inflammation with increased expression of Th17 cytokines).[10–13] This homeostatic response likely allows survival of affected individuals but may also contribute to the ichthyosis phenotype.

Nonsyndromic Forms of Ichthyosis

Four major forms of nonsyndromic ichthyosis[14–16] have been delineated, based largely on clinical and genetic characteristics:

1. Ichthyosis vulgaris, the most common ichthyosis, transmitted as an autosomal semi-dominant trait (meaning it can manifest when one allele is abnormal and to a greater extent when both alleles have a pathogenic gene variant)
2. Recessive X-linked ichthyosis (RXLI), expressed only in males and transmitted as an X-linked recessive trait
3. Keratinopathic ichthyosis, an autosomal dominant trait (most commonly epidermolytic ichthyosis [EI])
4. Autosomal recessive congenital ichthyosis (ARCI) (most collodion babies; exhibits a spectrum of characteristics from lamellar ichthyosis [LI] to congenital ichthyosiform erythroderma [CIE]).

ICHTHYOSIS VULGARIS

Ichthyosis vulgaris is by far the most common genetic form of ichthyosis, and the majority of individuals affected by the disorder are undiagnosed (Table 5.1), either because of the minimal clinical manifestations (which are affected by climate) or because the condition is dismissed as dry skin. This disorder, which is not present at birth, may be noted after the first 2 to 3 months of life and often not until later in childhood. Ichthyosis vulgaris generally improves with age, in summer, and in warm moist environments. Scales are most prominent on the extensor surfaces of the extremities and are most severe in cold and dry weather. Scales on the pretibial and lateral aspects of the lower leg are large and plate-like, resembling fish scales (Fig. 5.1, *A*); the flexural areas are characteristically spared. In other areas, small, white, bran-like scales may be seen. Scales tend to be darker on dark-skinned individuals. Scaling of the forehead and cheeks, common during childhood, generally diminishes and clears with age, but hyperlinearity and mild to moderate thickening of the palms and soles are characteristic (Fig. 5.1, *B*). Discrete hyperkeratosis may occur on the elbows, knees, and ankles.

A reduced or absent granular layer in skin sections may help to differentiate ichthyosis vulgaris from other forms of ichthyosis. Given that filaggrin is the major protein of the granular layer, it is not surprising that mutations in *FLG*, the gene encoding for profilaggrin, the precursor of filaggrin, are responsible.[17] In fact, *FLG* mutations are observed in 7.7% of Europeans and 3.0% of Asians, although not all manifest with ichthyosis vulgaris, given the dependence of its phenotype on environmental factors.[17–19] Ichthyosis vulgaris is now known to be a semi-dominant condition, in contrast to the previous assumption of dominant inheritance, i.e., manifestations are seen with a mutation on one allele in 1:12 Europeans but are worse if null mutations are on both alleles (probability, 1:576). The cleaved product of profilaggrin, filaggrin, plays an important role in linking a protein (involucrin) and lipids (ceramides) in the corneocyte envelope (see Chapter 3). In addition, filaggrin breaks down to amino acid metabolites that increase skin hydration (a natural moisturizing factor). Without filaggrin, the epidermis cannot provide normal barrier function; transepidermal water loss is increased, leading to xerosis; and the ingress of foreign

Table 5.1 Comparison of the Most Common Types of Ichthyosis

	Ichthyosis Vulgaris	X-Linked Recessive Ichthyosis	Keratinopathic Ichthyosis: Epidermolytic Ichthyosis	ARCI: Classic Lamellar Ichthyosis	ARCI: Classic Congenital Ichthyosiform Erythroderma
Prevalence	1:30 (1:12 with mutation)	1:1500 males	1:300,000	1:300,000	1:300,000
Inheritance	Autosomal semi-dominant	X-linked recessive	Usually autosomal dominant	Usually autosomal recessive	Autosomal recessive
Onset	2 months and beyond	17% at birth; 83% by 1 year	Birth, with superficial blistering	Birth, as collodion baby	Birth, as collodion baby
Character of scales	Fine, white to larger scales, esp. on legs	Large, brown	Verrucous scale, superficial blisters	Large, plate-like scales	Fine white scaling overlying erythema
Localization	Can be generalized; relative sparing of flexures; hyperlinear palms	Accentuation at neck and behind ears; relative sparing of flexures	Generalized; especially at flexures and overlying joints	Generalized; ectropion, occasional alopecia, nail dystrophy	Generalized; ectropion; occasional alopecia
Distinct histologic features	Often shows decreased granular layer	None	Epidermolytic hyperkeratosis	Massive orthokeratosis; moderate acanthosis	More acanthosis
Molecular basis	Mutations in profilaggin *(FLG)*; worse if both alleles	Deletions in *ARSC1* (arylsulfatase C)	Mutations in *KRT1* and *KRT10*; superficial form with mutations in *KRT2*	Most commonly mutations in *TGM1*; rarely other types (see CIE)	Mutations in *TGM1; ALOXE3; ALOX12B; NIPAL4; ABCA12; CYP4F22; PNPLA1; LIPN; CerS3; SDR9C7; SLC27A4*
Comments	Increased risk of atopic dermatitis and keratosis pilaris	Accumulation of cholesterol sulfate; FISH analysis to detect deletion; genital abnormalities rare; asymptomatic corneal opacities; contiguous gene deletion: with anosomia, retardation (Kallmann syndrome), and/or chondrodysplasia punctata	Superficial form shows more superficial blistering and much less thickening; secondary *Staphylococcus aureus* infection; palm/sole thickening predominantly with *KRT1* mutation	Transglutaminase activity can be measured in skin samples	May be associated with neurologic abnormalities

ARCI, Autosomal recessive congenital ichthyosis; *CIE*, congenital ichthyosiform erythroderma; *FISH*, fluorescent *in situ* hybridization analysis.

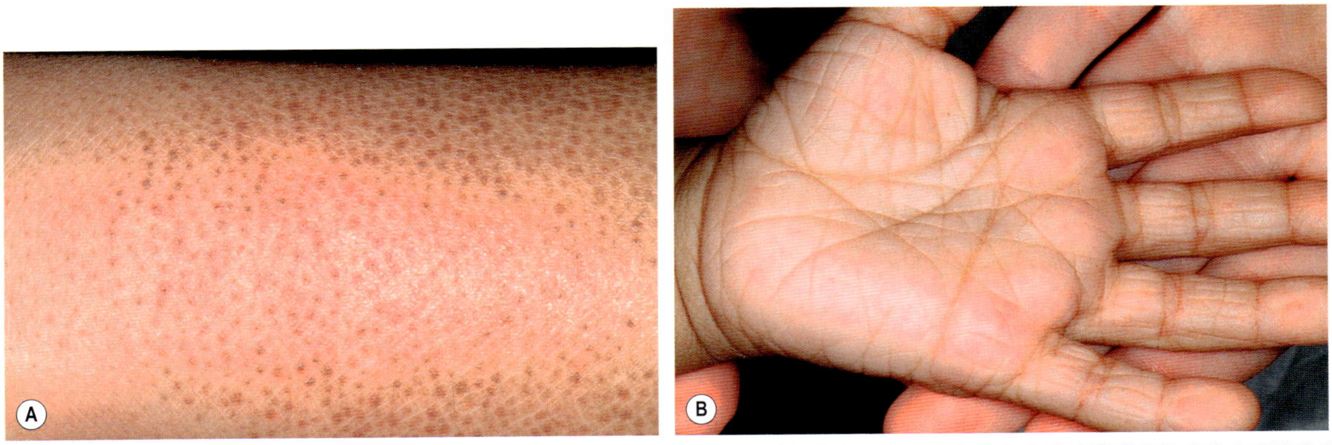

Fig. 5.1 Ichthyosis vulgaris. **(A)** Scales are most prominent on the extensor surfaces of the extremities, especially the lower extremities. **(B)** The palms and soles are thickened with increased palmar markings.

substances (such as allergens and pathogens) occurs more readily, thereby increasing the risk of exposure to triggers of atopy.

Patients with ichthyosis vulgaris often have an atopic background with a tendency toward atopic dermatitis (AD) (see Chapter 3).[20,21] The risk is highest in individuals with two mutated alleles. Overall, up to 30% of patients of a Northern European background with AD and more than 20% of Japanese with AD[22,23] have *FLG* mutations. *FLG* mutations are uncommon in darker-skinned populations, even with ichthyosis vulgaris,[24] although *FLG2* variants have been correlated with more persistent AD in Blacks.[25] Filaggrin-2 is expressed in the stratum granulosum and is essential for proper epidermal cornification[26] (see Peeling Skin Syndrome later). Signs of

AD may be seen before other clinical signs of ichthyosis vulgaris, and most individuals with the condition never show evidence of AD. Individuals with AD and a *FLG* mutation tend to have more severe and more persistent AD, particularly if *FLG* mutations occur on both alleles. The occurrence of other forms of atopy (asthma, allergic rhinitis) typically follows the onset of AD in children with *FLG* mutations, suggesting that the barrier defect of ichthyosis and the occurrence of AD are a driving force toward the development of other atopic conditions. Mechanistic studies have shown increased penetration of allergens and chemicals in filaggrin-deficient skin, and epidemiologic studies have found higher levels of hand eczema, irritant contact dermatitis, and nickel sensitization in association with *FLG* variants.

The diagnosis of ichthyosis vulgaris should be considered in patients with AD who show large scales, particularly on the extensor aspects of the extremities; examination of the palms and soles shows the hyperlinearity. Keratosis pilaris, which is commonly associated with ichthyosis vulgaris and atopy[18] (see Chapter 3 and Chapter 7, Figs. 7.25 and 7.26), is most predominant on the upper arms, buttocks, and thighs.

An autosomal recessive form of ichthyosis vulgaris can result from biallelic mutations in *CASP14*, which encodes caspase 14, the enzyme that degrades filaggrin monomers in the stratum corneum to hygroscopic amino acids. In addition, mutations in *ASPRV1*, which encodes skin aspartic protease (SASPase), lead to a severe ichthyosis vulgaris–like disorder with large, plate-like scales (Fig. 5.2, *A*) and hyperlinear thickened palms (Fig. 5.2, *B*) that has recently been described in humans.[27] SASPase enables profilaggrin-to-filaggrin processing, and the described missense mutations reduce this processing.

Emollients may improve dry skin but do not normalize the epidermal gene expression profile of filaggrin.[28] Excessive exposure to factors that decrease skin barrier functions and increase the risk of AD should be avoided. Individuals with ichthyosis vulgaris should be protected against neonatal exposure to cats to prevent AD and should abstain from smoking to prevent asthma.[19]

Although rare in children, "acquired" ichthyotic scaling has been described in patients with nutritional disorders such as hypovitaminosis or hypervitaminosis A, hypothyroidism, sarcoidosis, dermatomyositis, leprosy, tuberculosis, human immunodeficiency virus (HIV) infection, and neoplastic disorders, particularly lymphomas. It should be noted that these forms were described before the availability of testing for *FLG*/profilaggrin mutations; given the many undiagnosed patients, it is possible that the underlying condition increased the risk of manifesting the ichthyosis in an individual with a *FLG* mutation. Pityriasis rotunda, a rare variant of acquired ichthyosis, is characterized by asymptomatic, circular or oval, brown scaly patches on the trunk or extremities. Seen primarily in individuals of Japanese, African, and West Indian origin, its occurrence in Whites is extremely rare. The condition may at times be associated with an underlying disorder, may follow pregnancy, or may be familial. In contrast to ichthyosis vulgaris, pityriasis rotunda is chronic, is resistant to treatment, and tends to improve only when the underlying disorder is treated.

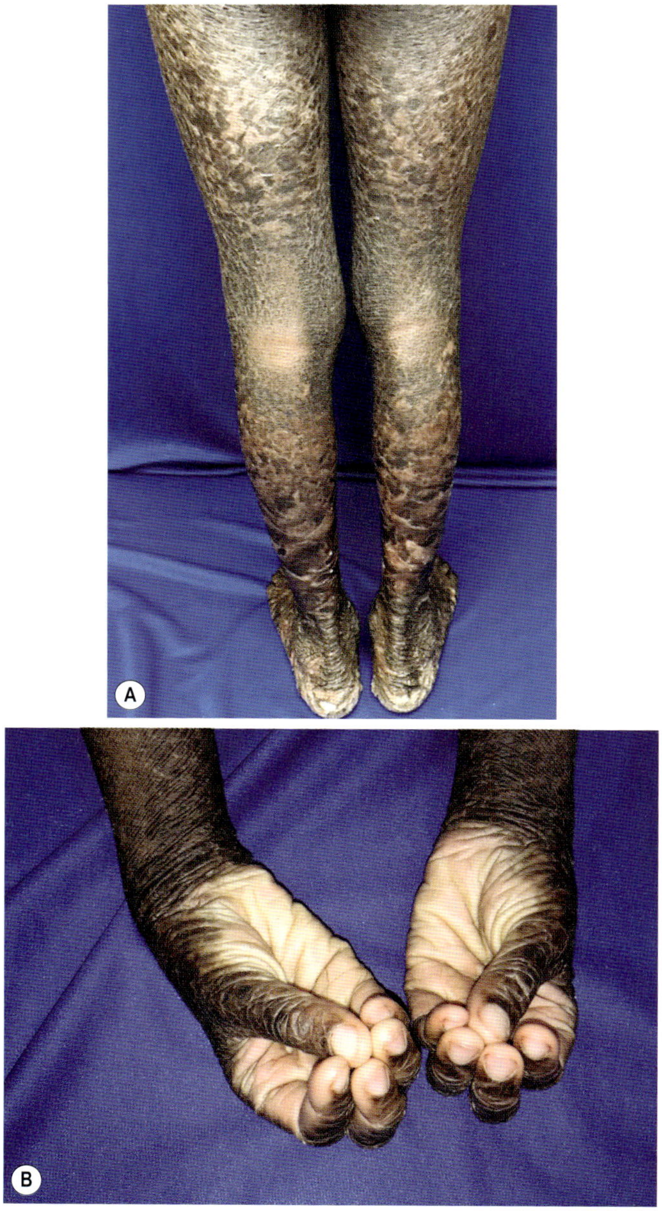

Fig. 5.2 *ASPRV1* deficiency. Generalized scaling **(A)** and palmoplantar hyperlinearity **(B)** can be confused with ichthyosis vulgaris, but tend to be more severe and the scaling more lamellar in character.

RECESSIVE X-LINKED ICHTHYOSIS

RXLI occurs in 1:1500 males and results from a mutation (deletion of the entire gene in 90%) in the *ARSC1* gene that encodes steroid sulfatase (STS), also known as *arylsulfatase C* (see Table 5.1). The disorder has rarely been described in females who have Turner syndrome or carry the mutation on both alleles. Female carriers do not tend to show ichthyosis because the affected gene is located at the distal tip of the X chromosome, a location that escapes X-inactivation. Thus rather than having random inactivation of one of the X chromosomes, as dictated by the Lyon hypothesis, both of the alleles are expressed in every cell, providing sufficient enzyme. STS normally is concentrated in lamellar bodies and secreted into the spaces between stratum corneum cells. It degrades cholesterol sulfate, generating cholesterol for the epidermal barrier. Cholesterol sulfate itself is an epidermal protease inhibitor, so STS deficiency prevents normal degradation of the stratum corneum desmosomes and leads to corneocyte retention.[29,30]

Low placental production of estrogens and elevated sulfated steroid levels have been described in the urine of mothers of boys with RXLI, associated with a difficult or prolonged labor and failure to have cervical dilation.[31] Deletion of both *ARSC1* and a contiguous gene (up to 10% of patients) results in both ichthyosis and Kallmann syndrome (associated with mental retardation, hypogonadism, and anosmia; deletion of *KALI* gene), X-linked recessive chondrodysplasia punctata (bone dysplasia with stippled epiphyses; deletion of arylsulfatase E/*ARSE*), and/or retardation with autism (neuroligin 4/*NLGN4*).[32,33] RXLI is commonly predicted prenatally by chromosomal microarrays, which have a high sensitivity for the detection of microdeletions. The presentation can be highly variable, and in one study, most patients had "dry" skin or "eczema" rather than recognized ichthyosis.[34] Fluorescent *in situ* hybridization (FISH) analysis for the STS gene is another way to show the gene deletion. RXLI can be confirmed by reduced arylsulfatase C activity in leukocytes or by elevated blood levels of cholesterol sulfate and increased mobility of β-lipoproteins.[35]

RXLI typically manifests within the first 3 months of life. Approximately 17% of affected individuals show scaling at birth,

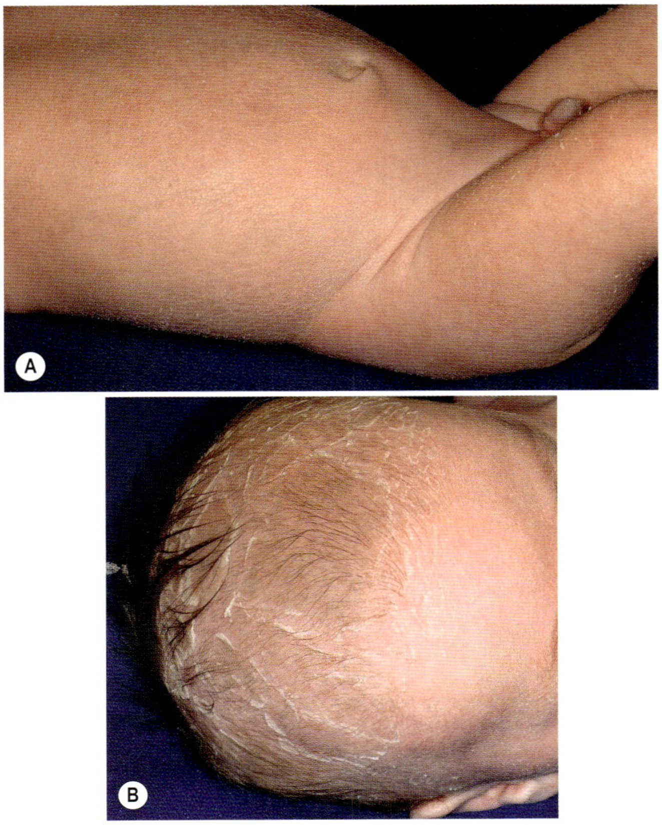

Fig. 5.3 Recessive X-linked ichthyosis. Scaling may be subtle, particularly in younger infants. This 6-month-old boy was diagnosed *in utero* by increased maternal estradiol levels and then FISH analysis of chorionic villus samples. Note the fine scaling on the trunk **(A)** and the large scales on the scalp **(B)**.

often in the form of a mild collodion-like membrane. Most develop scaling during the first 6 months of life (Fig. 5.3). The severity of the scaling can range from mild to severe. This form of ichthyosis generally involves the entire body, with accentuation on the scalp, neck, abdomen, back, front of the legs, and feet but spares the palms, soles, central face, and flexural areas (Fig. 5.4, *A*). Scales may be small to large and tend to be brown in coloration and darker in darker-skinned patients. The sides of the neck often appear dark and unwashed (Fig. 5.4, *B*). Patients may shed or molt their scales episodically, particularly in the spring and fall. RXLI can be difficult to distinguish from ichthyosis vulgaris and may occur concurrently; RXLI is more severe with concomitant FLG mutation, and palmar hyperlinearity is a diagnostic clue.[36]

Boys with X-linked ichthyosis rarely have hypogonadism and/or cryptorchidism; testicular cancer has been described in one patient.[37] Deep corneal opacities may be found in approximately 50% of affected adult males and less often in female carriers of this disorder. The opacities, easily detectable by slit-lamp examination, are discrete and diffusely located near the Descemet membrane or deep in the corneal stroma. Although they are a marker for the disorder in older patients, these opacities do not affect vision.

The features of RXLI may be seen in patients with autosomal recessive multiple sulfatase deficiency (Fig. 5.5), a syndromic form of ichthyosis characterized by features of mucopolysaccharidoses, metachromatic leukodystrophy, X-linked recessive chondrodysplasia punctata, and RXLI. The disorder results from mutations in sulfatase-modifying factor 1 *(SUMF1)*, which encodes the α-formylglycine–generating enzyme required for posttranslation modification of sulfatases.[38,39] Progressive neurologic deterioration, a feature of the metachromatic leukodystrophy, usually leads to death during infancy.

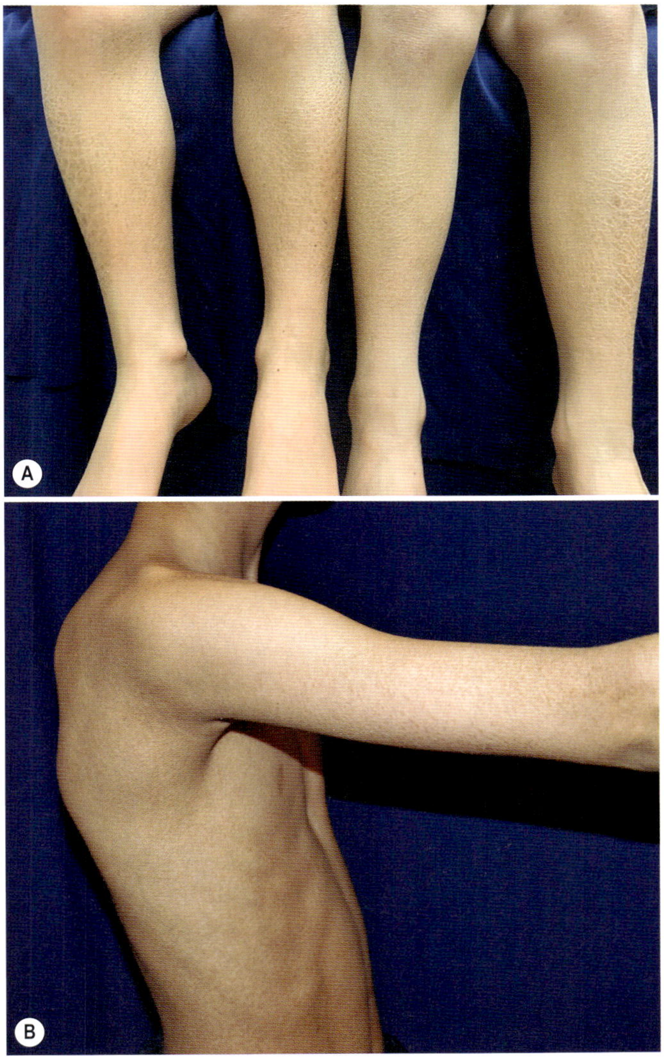

Fig. 5.4 Recessive X-linked ichthyosis. **(A)** Scales tend to be polygonal and hyperpigmented, as seen in these two affected brothers. **(B)** Polygonal, hyperpigmented scaling on the neck, trunk, and arm.

KERATINOPATHIC ICHTHYOSES

Keratinopathic ichthyosis includes the epidermolytic forms of ichthyosis associated with keratin gene mutations. The major subgroups are EI (formerly called *bullous CIE, Brocq type*)[40] and superficial EI (formerly called *ichthyosis bullosa of Siemens*). The designation *epidermolytic hyperkeratosis* is a histologic description that is not specific to this group of disorders, although it traditionally referred to EI.

Mutations are usually point mutations that lead to an abnormal, but full-length keratin that incorporates into the keratin filament. The resultant keratin network functions poorly, leading to skin cell collapse and clinical blistering, especially in response to trauma. The thickening of skin is thought to be compensatory to protect against blistering, but has also been linked to abnormal lamellar-body secretion.[41] Virtually all forms are inherited in an autosomal dominant manner, although EI may rarely be autosomal recessive.[42–44] EI results from mutations in *KRT1* or its partner in intermediate filament formation, *KRT10*; both are expressed throughout the suprabasal layers of epidermis. Superficial EI is caused by mutations in *KRT2*, which is only expressed in more superficial epidermis and also partners with keratin 10.[45–47]

EI affects approximately 1 in 300,000 individuals, and 50% of patients have new mutations. The skin is red and may be tender at

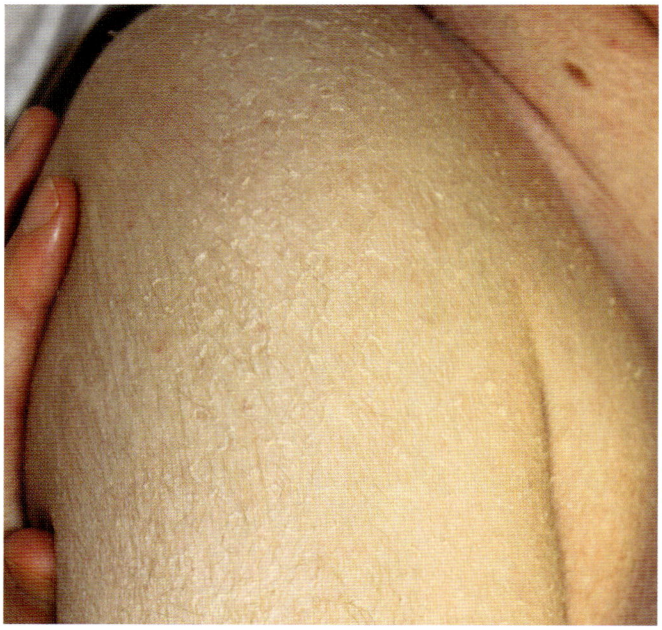

Fig. 5.5 Multiple sulfatase deficiency. Scaling with failure to desquamate in a neurologically impaired boy.

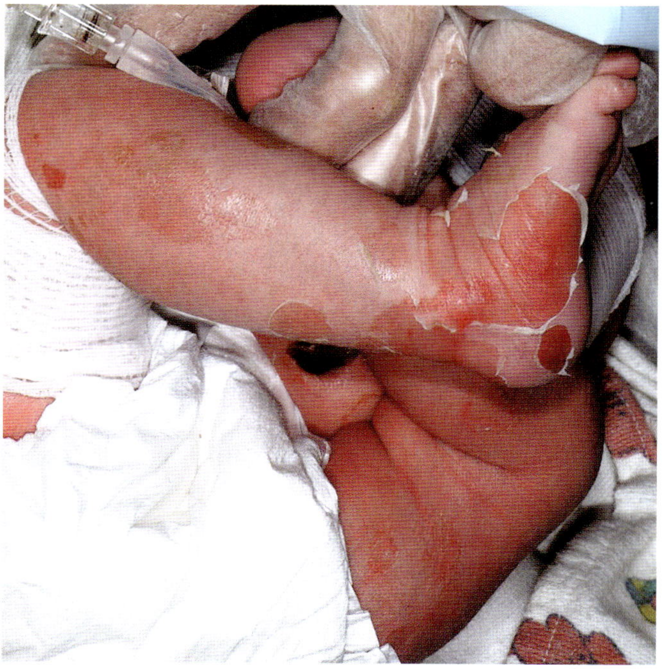

Fig. 5.6 Epidermolytic ichthyosis. In the neonate, superficial blisters predominate and may be mistaken for epidermolysis bullosa.

birth. Superficial bullae generally appear within the first week of life (often within a few hours after delivery; Fig. 5.6) and may be confused with those of epidermolysis bullosa (see Chapter 13) or with staphylococcal scalded skin syndrome (see Chapter 14). Skin thickening may be present at birth, sometimes even with the typical scale of EI, but often appears during the months after birth (Fig. 5.7) with only subtle thickening during the neonatal period, especially on the elbows and knees. The blisters are primarily seen in areas of trauma and can

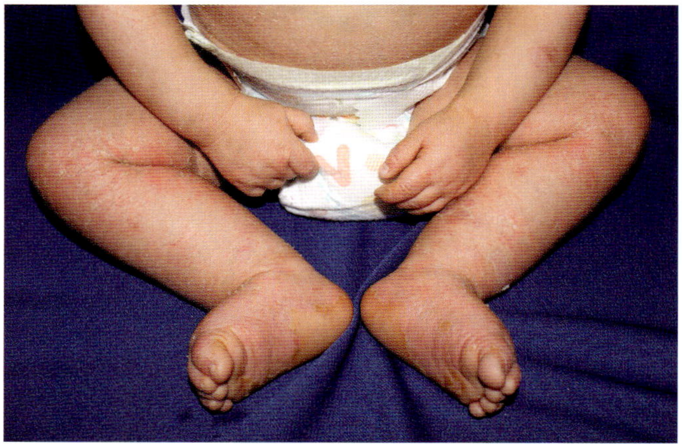

Fig. 5.7 Epidermolytic ichthyosis. Within the first several months, blistering tends to be reduced, but scaling becomes apparent, as seen in this 8-month-old with a variant in *KRT10*.

occur in crops. They vary from 0.5 cm to several centimeters in diameter. They tend to heal quickly, consistent with their superficial location. When ruptured, they discharge clear fluid and leave raw denuded areas. Secondary bacterial infection, especially with *Staphylococcus aureus*, is commonly associated with this disorder.

Verruciform grayish-brown scales eventually cover most of the skin surface; the flexural creases and intertriginous areas show particularly marked involvement (Figs. 5.8 and 5.9).[48] Palms and soles have varying degrees of thickening and scaling (Fig. 5.10), but much more marked involvement often occurs in individuals with mutations in *KRT1*, because keratin 9 expression in the palms and soles can compensate for abnormal keratin 10 expression, but expression of *KRT1* (which is the partner for both keratins 9 and 10) remains critical.[48] Facial involvement may occur, but ectropion does not. Although scalp involvement may result in nit-like encasement of hair shafts, the hair, eyes, teeth, and nails are normal. A disagreeable body odor is commonly associated with severe forms of this disorder due to the thick, macerated scale and overgrowth of bacteria and, less often, candida. Skin biopsy specimens show marked hyperkeratosis with lysis of the epidermal cells above the basal cell layer (epidermolytic hyperkeratosis) leading to the bullae.[49] Keratolytic agents are often poorly tolerated in keratinopathic forms of ichthyosis and can increase skin fragility.

The epidermolytic hyperkeratotic form of epidermal nevus shows a histologic appearance identical to that of epidermolytic ichthyosis, but is not associated with skin fragility or a blistering tendency (see Chapter 9). This form of nevus represents a mosaic condition in which the affected skin, but not the normal intervening skin, carries a mutation in *KRT1* or *KRT10* (Fig. 5.10).[50] Individuals with more extensive forms of the epidermolytic hyperkeratotic form of epidermal nevus can have offspring with generalized epidermolytic ichthyosis, reflecting a germline mutation. Prenatal diagnosis can be performed in at-risk families.[51]

Mutations in regions of *KRT1* and *KRT10* that are less critical than the α-helical rod domain can lead to milder forms of EI with thickening limited to the fold areas. Mutations in *KRT1* and *KRT10* can also cause an annular variant (annular EI),[52,53] in which annular erythematous polycyclic scaling plaques on the trunk and extremities slowly enlarge, resolve, and later recur.

Ichthyosis Curth–Macklin (formerly called *ichthyosis hystrix*) has its onset of manifestations during early childhood as progressively worsening diffuse or striate palmoplantar keratoderma (PPK) that can be associated with deep fissuring, flexural contracture, and digital constriction. Affected individuals develop characteristic "porcupine quill–like" verrucous yellow-brown scaling, especially on the hands and feet and overlying the large joints (Fig. 5.11). Binuclear cells and pathognomonic concentric perinuclear "shells" of aberrant keratin are characteristic ultrastructural findings.[54] *KRT1* mutations have been described in some,[55,56] but not all, affected patients.

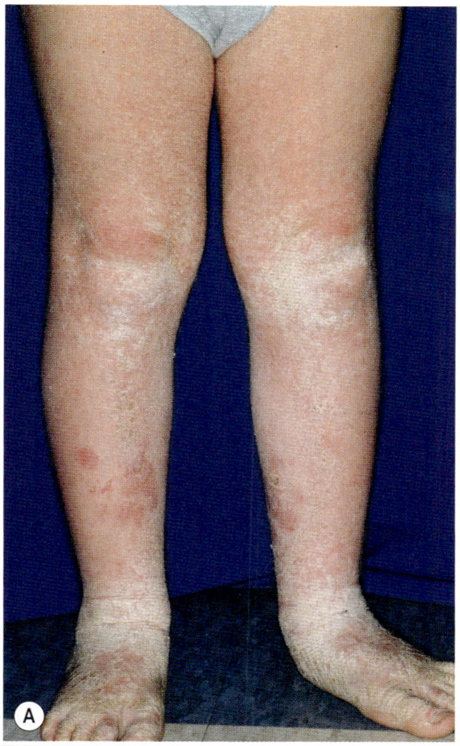

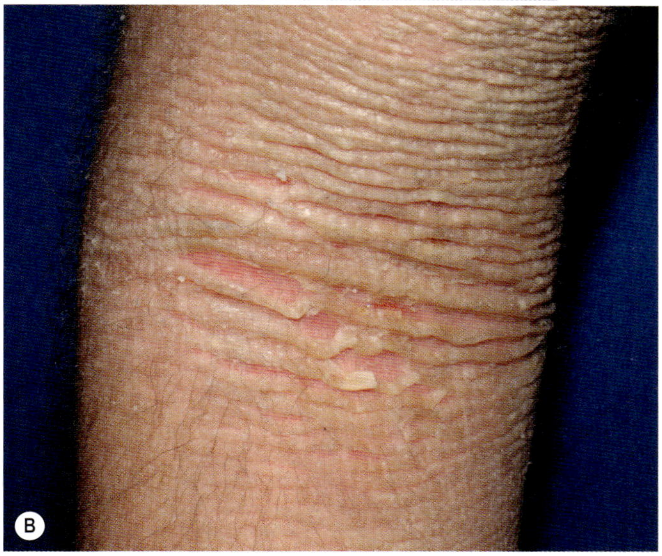

Fig. 5.8 Epidermolytic ichthyosis. **(A)** Thick verrucous scale on the legs of a 6-year-old boy. Note the intensification of scaling over the knees and ankles and the areas of blistering on the legs. **(B)** The scaling can take on a corrugated appearance.

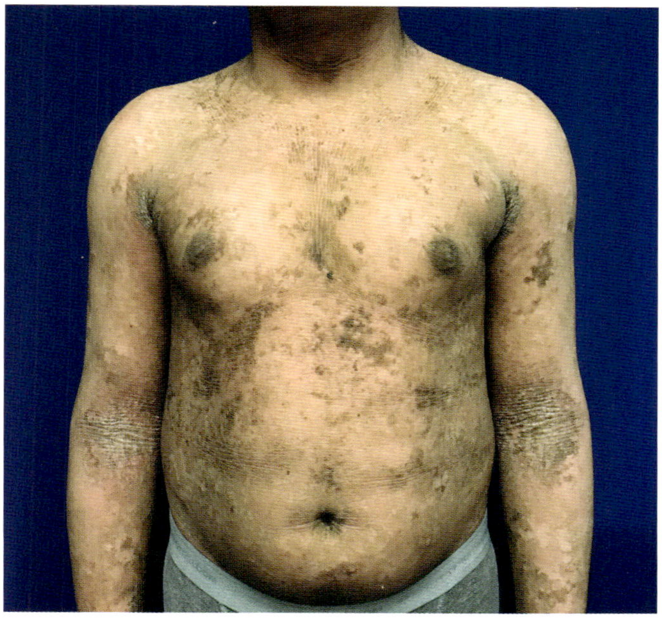

Fig. 5.9 Extensive corrugated scale of epidermolytic ichthyosis with accentuation in the fold areas.

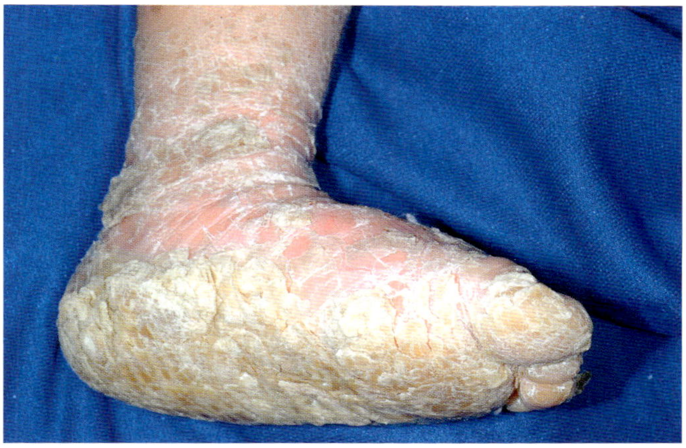

Fig. 5.10 Epidermolytic ichthyosis. The marked hyperkeratotic sole in this child virtually ensures that the underlying gene defect involves *KRT1*.

Superficial EI shows milder thickening and more superficial blistering. The palms and soles are minimally thickened, if at all. Although large, tense bullae can occur (Fig. 5.12, *A*), in general, the appearance of blisters has been likened to molting (mauserung phenomenon) and can appear as subtle peeling skin, especially by adolescence and adulthood (Fig. 5.12, *B*), because of the superficial location of the cleavage plane. Accordingly, less hyperkeratosis is seen in sections of skin biopsies, and the lysed areas of epidermis only begin halfway up the stratum spinosum. Affected individuals may be misdiagnosed as mild EI clinically, but the limited localization of the epidermolysis histologically and the finding of mutations in *KRT2* by molecular genetic testing can distinguish the disorders.[57,58]

Ichthyosis with confetti (IWC), also called *congenital reticular ichthyosiform erythroderma* or *ichthyosis variegata*, is an autosomal dominant keratinopathy characterized by generalized erythroderma and lack of blistering, and this is often mistaken for CIE. IWC is distinguished by its progressive reversion of affected areas to normal-appearing skin in a "confetti" pattern of macules.[59–63] These specific mutations, typically frameshift mutations in exon 6 or 7 of *KRT1* or KRT10, predispose to postzygotic translocations that allow protein expression of the mutated allele and correct the phenotype.[64] In general, *KRT1* mutations are associated with the "confetti" first appearing during infancy,[59] whereas *KRT10* mutations tend to manifest the cleared areas beginning during childhood or even young adulthood (Fig. 5.13, *A* and *B*).[65] Other major features include malformation of ears, hypoplasia of mammillae, and[66] dorsal acral hypertrichosis.[67] Severe cases of pityriasis rubra pilaris from *CARD14* mutations may resemble IWC because of the extensive erythroderma with areas of sparing[68] (see Chapter 4); severe manifestations of *CARD14* mutations can include ectropion and PPK, requiring differentiation from CIE (see later).

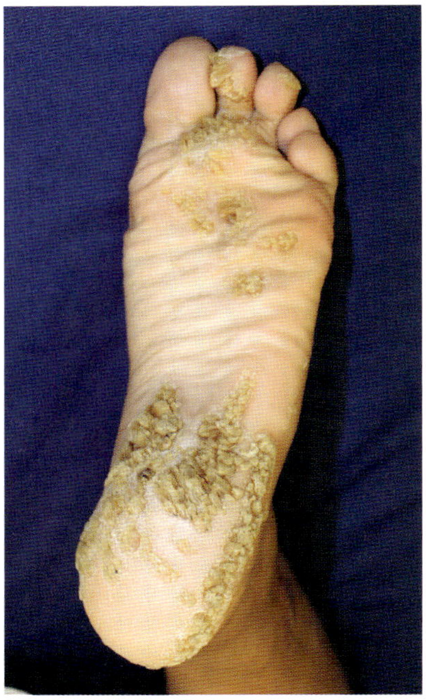

Fig. 5.11 Ichthyosis hystrix. Verrucous plaques on the plantar surface. This girl had undergone grafting of the palms to increase hand function.

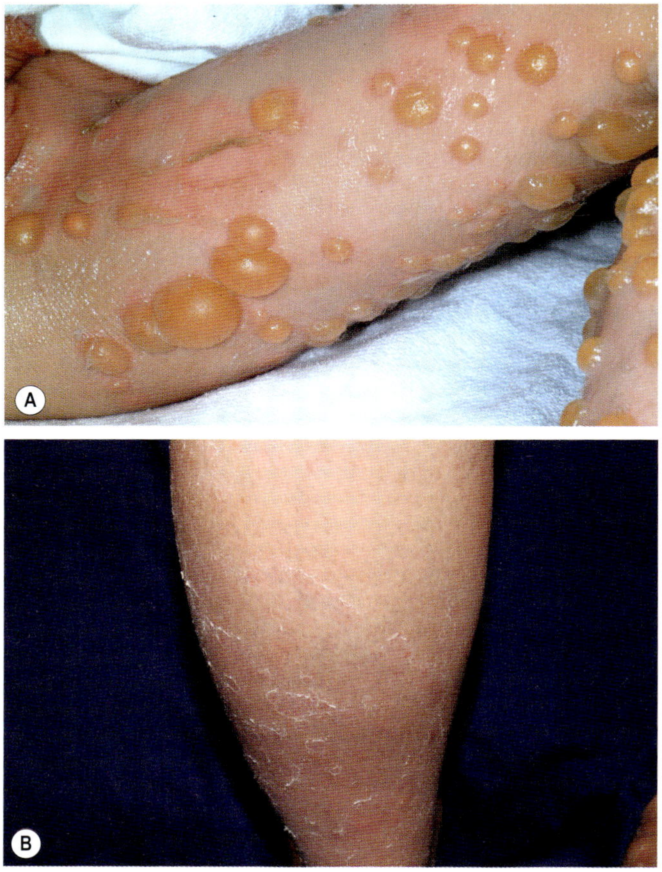

Fig. 5.12 Superficial epidermolytic ichthyosis. **(A)** Occasionally, affected individuals may show tense bullae that resemble bullous pemphigoid (see Chapter 13). The bullae on this patient arose when he developed a viral exanthema. **(B)** More typically, there is mild kyperkeratosis and a "molting" appearance with desquamation of superficial scale.

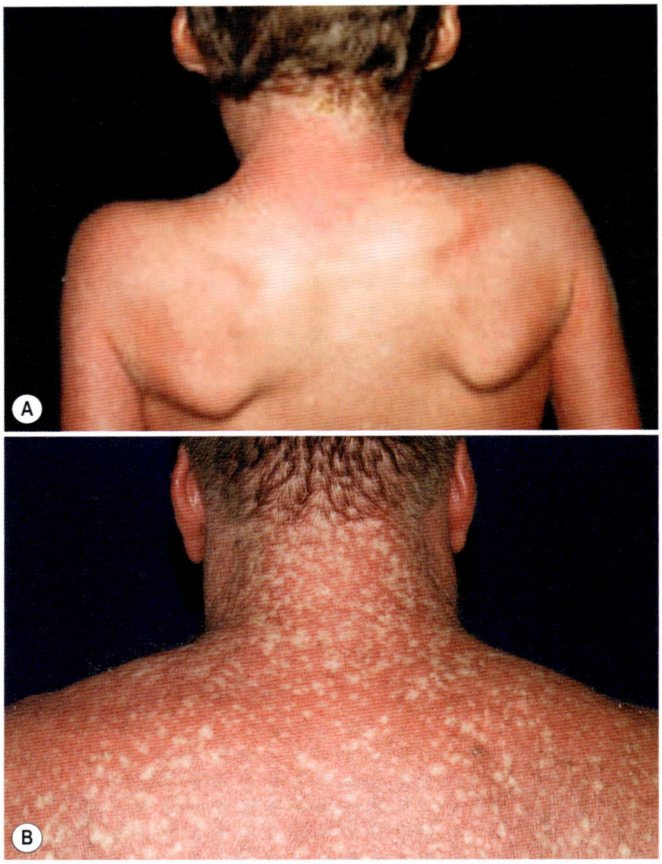

Fig. 5.13 Ichthyosis en confetti. At 5 years of age, this boy with IWC and a *KRT10* variant has a few white areas **(A)**. In this 50-year-old man with IWC and a *KRT10* variant, the entire neck and trunk are studded with white areas of clearance **(B)**.

COLLODION BABY

Collodion baby is a descriptive term for an infant who is born with a membrane-like covering resembling collodion (Fig. 5.14).[69,70] The collodion baby is not a specific disease entity, but rather a phenotype common to several forms of ichthyosis. At least 65% of collodion babies have ARCI (see Autosomal Recessive Congenital Ichthyosis), a group of genetically distinct forms of ichthyosis with overlapping clinical features[71]; some infants in this group (5% to 6%) shed their collodion membranes and show apparently normal skin (self-healing collodion baby [SHCB]).[72,73] Having a collodion membrane at birth, however, is not a necessary feature for ARCI.[74] Less often, collodion babies shed their membranes and show features of syndromic forms of ichthyosis (Conradi–Hünermann–Happle [CHH] syndrome, trichothiodystrophy [see Chapter 7], or RXLI). There is one case of a collodion membrane associated with medication use in a mother who received infliximab before and throughout the course of the pregnancy; although the collodion membrane shed and the skin appeared normal 1 year after birth, no genotype analysis was performed to consider a mild variant of ichthyosis rather than resulting from medication use during pregnancy.[75]

At birth, collodion babies are completely covered by a cellophane- or oiled parchment–like "membrane" that, due to its tautness, may distort the facial features and extremities. Thus peripheral edema with digital constriction, flattened ears, and bilateral eversion of the eyelids, lips, and at times the vulva often cause affected infants to resemble one another during the first few days of life. Among the problems facing these infants are an inability to suck properly, respiratory difficulty because of restriction of chest expansion by the thick membrane, cutaneous and systemic infection, and aspiration pneumonia. Despite the thickening of

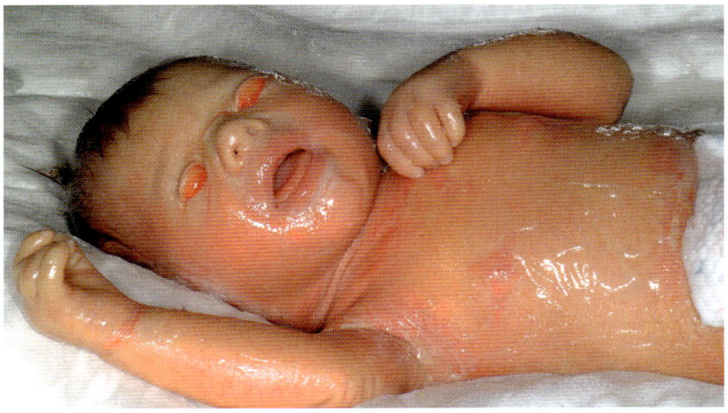

Fig. 5.14 Collodion baby. Note the shiny thickened skin, mild ectropion, mild eclabium, and ear deformity. In this 5-day-old baby, the "membrane" is starting to crack and desquamate.

the stratum corneum, this membrane is a poor barrier, leading to excessive transcutaneous fluid and electrolyte loss,[76] hypernatremic dehydration, increased metabolic requirements, and temperature instability.

Collodion babies are often born prematurely. Patients born as collodion babies may develop neurologic abnormalities. These should be interpreted in the context of history. Although most likely related to premature birth, syndromic disorders should also be considered. For example, patients with Sjögren–Larsson syndrome are very occasionally born with a collodion membrane and may resemble LI during childhood but tend to progressively develop neurologic features.

Supportive care is of primary importance in the management of collodion babies.[77,78] They are traditionally managed in a humidified incubator with special attention given to the prevention of temperature instability, sepsis, and fluid and electrolyte imbalance. Systemic antibiotic therapy should be initiated if infection is detected, but not prophylactically. Desquamation is encouraged by the application of emollients rather than manual debridement; given the poor cutaneous barrier and potential toxicity, use of keratolytic agents should be avoided during the first several months of life.

AUTOSOMAL RECESSIVE CONGENITAL ICHTHYOSIS

ARCI encompasses a wide range of clinical phenotypes that range from classic harlequin ichthyosis (HI) and nonbullous CIE to classic LI.[79] The same individual may show a range of overlapping clinical features; for example, retinoid treatment may decrease the lamellar scaling but increase visible erythroderma.[80] Failure to thrive may be a feature of ARCI, especially if severe, and short stature may ensue.[81] Overall, ARCI occurs in approximately 1 in 100,000 to 300,000 live births. The diagnosis is based on clinical findings; biopsy is not helpful unless needed to exclude alternative diagnoses. The features of the ARCI group of disorders usually persist throughout the affected individual's lifetime. Many affected individuals complain of associated pruritus. Severely affected patients tend to experience hypohidrosis, which may lead to heat intolerance, with hyperpyrexia and heat exhaustion during periods of hot, humid weather and vigorous physical exercise. Although the hypohidrosis may reflect obstruction of eccrine glands by hyperkeratosis, persistence with ameliorative retinoid therapy suggests an eccrine gland/duct developmental abnormality in many affected with ichthyosis. Squamous cell carcinomas have been reported at a younger age, but are rare.[82]

Mutations in 12 known genes have been shown to result in the ARCI phenotype, and most of these mutated genes have been related to the CIE phenotype (see Table 5.1). A few cases of autosomal dominant LI have been described.[83] The discovery of the underlying genetic basis in families with ARCI has facilitated the prenatal diagnosis based on genotyping rather than the riskier diagnosis by fetal skin biopsy.[84]

Overall, 34% to 55% of individuals with ARCI have mutations in the gene encoding transglutaminase 1 *(TGM1)*, and these patients typically feature the LI phenotype.[85] *TGM1* crosslinks several proteins to form the cornified envelope surrounding corneocytes. In patients missing transglutaminase, transglutaminase activity is undetectable in frozen skin specimens.[86]

The 11 genes linked to ARCI are largely involved in synthesis and metabolism of the intracellular lipids of the stratum corneum, including the critical epidermal ω-O-acylceramides from N-acyl fatty acids[87–89] (Table 5.2). HI is the most severe form of CIE and has been shown to result from nonsense mutations in the gene encoding the ABCA12 transporter.[90,91] Missense mutations in *ABCA12* cause a milder CIE phenotype than null type mutations.[92] A deficiency of ABCA12 perturbs lipid transport, formation of lamellar bodies, keratinocyte terminal differentiation, and transfer of proteolytic enzymes required for normal desquamation.[93–95] In addition, genes encoding lipoxygenases,[96] *ALOX12B* (encoding 12(R)-lipoxygenase) and *ALOXE3* (encoding lipoxygenase-3),[97,98] are often mutated. Other genes with biallelic mutations leading to ARCI are *LIPN*,[99] *CYP4F22*,[100] *PNPLA1*,[101,102] *SLC27A4*,[103] *NIPAL4*,[104–106] and *CERS3*[87,107–109] Studies[110] in PNPLA1-deficient mice and keratinocytes suggest that topical application of ω-O-acylceramides could be a replacement therapy for these forms of CIE.[110] Other genes found to be mutated in ARCI include *SDR9C7*[111,112] and *SULTB1*[113] (see Table 5.2). Although biallelic mutations in *CAPN12*[114] (encoding calpain 12) and *CASP14*[115] (encoding caspase 14) also are autosomal recessive and congenital, these disorders are not associated with collodion membranes and more closely resemble exfoliative ichthyosis (superficial exfoliation overlying intense erythroderma) and ichthyosis vulgaris (fine, white scaling without erythroderma), respectively, and thus are not included here as part of ARCI.

The clinical features of the classic LI phenotype may range from very mild to severe. Individuals who show the greatest severity of LI have large, lamellar, plate-like scales with relatively mild underlying erythroderma; ectropion (eversion of an edge or margin of the eyelid resulting in exposure of the palpebral conjunctiva) (Fig. 5.15); and mild eclabium (eversion of the lips) (see Table 5.1). Lamellar scales are large, quadrangular, yellow to brown-black, often thick, and centrally adherent with raised edges resembling armor plates (hence the term *lamellar*) (Fig. 5.16). Scales are most prominent over the face, trunk, and extremities, with a predilection for the flexor areas. Cheeks are often red, taut, and shiny; more scales appear on the forehead than on the lower portion of the face. The palms and soles are almost always affected in LI; severity varies from increased palmar markings to a thick keratoderma with fissuring. Digital involvement may lead to pseudoainhum (constricting bands of the digits) and autoamputation.[116] The scalp is scaly (Fig. 5.17) with variable alopecia, which can be extensive and scarring. Involvement of the nails is variable. They may be stippled, pitted, ridged, or thickened, often with marked subungual hyperkeratosis.

Variant forms of LI from mutations in *TGM1* manifest in a more limited distribution of lesional skin. Patients with bathing suit ichthyosis (BSI) are born with a full collodion membrane and transition to LI, but within the first months of life, the scaling on the extremities clears[117] (Fig. 5.18). The residual LI on warmer skin areas (e.g., axillae, trunk, scalp, and neck) has been linked to temperature-sensitive mutations in *TGM1*.[118] Mutations in *TGM1* that encode proteins sensitive to hydrostatic pressure can result in SHCB. Affected neonates show either a generalized or acral[119] collodion membrane at birth that clears entirely as the baby transitions to the dry environment postnatally.[72] The *TGM1* mutations in both BSI and SHCB phenotypes are missense mutations that are predominantly in the catalytic core domains.[120] *ALOX12B* and *ALOX3B* mutations have also been described with SHCB.[73,121]

Mutations in *SDR9C7* lead to early keratoderma of the extensor elbows and knees with PPK. Affected individuals usually are not born with a collodion membrane and tend to have generalized scaling with variable erythema.[122] Patients with biallelic mutations in *SULT2B1* either are collodion babies or have dry, scaling, erythematous skin at birth and thereafter have larger, dark scales that resemble RXLI[123] or LI (although scales are not as large). The skin is erythematous and thickened, with accentuation overlying the joints.

Classic nonbullous CIE is characterized by a much more prominent erythrodermic component that may first become apparent as the collodion membrane (or HI scale) is shed; some patients show CIE at birth without a classic collodion membrane. Affected individuals show fine,

Table 5.2 Role of Genes Mutated in Congenital Ichthyosiform Erythroderma

Gene (% affected)	Gene Product	Function	Comments
ABCA12 (9%)	ABCA12 transporter	Lipid transport for formation of lamellar bodies and provision of intracellular lipids of the stratum corneum; deficiency also leads to premature terminal differentiation and normal transfer of proteolytic enzymes for desquamation	Nonsense mutations: harlequin ichthyosis; missense mutations: more severe CIE
ALOX12B (7%)	12(R)-lipoxygenase	Oxidizes acylglucosylceramide (to be a substrate for ω-O-acylceramide)	
NIPAL4 (6%)	Ichthyin	Needed to convert ω-O-free fatty acids to ω-O-fatty acid-CoA in the formation of ω-O-acylceramides from N-acyl fatty acids	
ALOXE3 (3%)	Lipoxygenase-3	Oxidizes acylglucosylceramide (to be a substrate for ω-O-acylceramide)	
PNPLA1 (3%)	Patatin-like phospholipase domain containing 1	Esterification of ω-hydroxyceramides to acylceramides	Some patients with PNPLA1 mutations have a phenotype that could be confused with EKV and is not generalized
CYP4F22 (2%)	Cytochrome P450 family 4 subfamily F member 22	Epidermal ω-hydroxylase that converts longer chain (C28-C34) N-acyl fatty acids to ω-hydroxy-free fatty acids	
LIPN (<1%)	Lipase N	Adds a ω-hydroxyl group to oxidized acylglucosylceramide to make ω-acylglucosylceramide	Ichthyotic changes may begin during early childhood
SLC27A4 (<1%)	Fatty acid transport protein 4/FATP4	Fatty acid transporter that associates with ichthyin (for triglyceride and ω-hydroxy-fatty acid-CoA synthesis)	Prematurity, polyhydramnios, perinatal respiratory distress, and thick white vernix-like scaling at birth that can be confused with KID syndrome; atopy diathesis
CERS3 (<1%)	Ceramide synthase 3	Synthesis of ω-hydroxy-ceramide from ω-hydroxy-fatty acid-CoA	
SDR9C7 (<1%)	Short chain dehydrogenase/reductase family 9C member 7	Converts retinal to retinol; affects vitamin A metabolism and terminal differentiation	Usually are not born with collodion membrane
SULTB1 (<1%)	Sulfotransferase family 2B member 1	Cytosolic sulfotransferase important for making cholesterol sulfate from cholesterol	

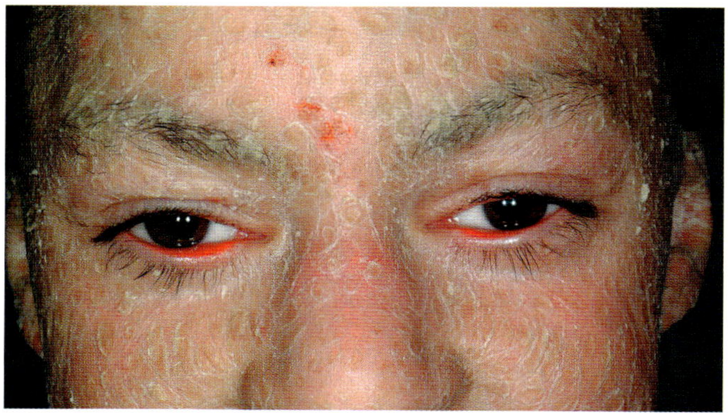

Fig. 5.15 Lamellar ichthyosis. Lamellar ichthyosis phenotype of autosomal recessive congenital ichthyosis (ARCI). Large plate-like scaling on the forehead and cheeks. This patient shows moderate ectropion.

white scales on the face, scalp, and trunk, although scaling may consist of more plate-like scales on the extensor surfaces of the legs (Fig. 5.19). The degree of ectropion is variable but often milder than with LI and there is less PPK. Cicatricial alopecia is possible (but not as frequent as in severe LI), and nails may show thickening and ridging. Some patients with CIE show intrauterine growth retardation and/or failure to thrive, although nutritional deficiency and gastrointestinal abnormalities are uncommon.[124] In general, phenotypes of CIE

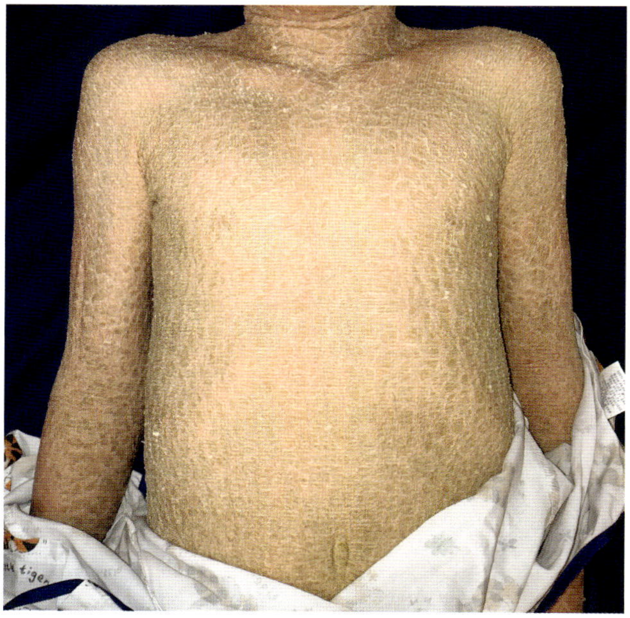

Fig. 5.16 Lamellar ichthyosis. Lamellar ichthyosis phenotype of autosomal recessive congenital ichthyosis (ARCI). Large plate-like scaling on the trunk and arms.

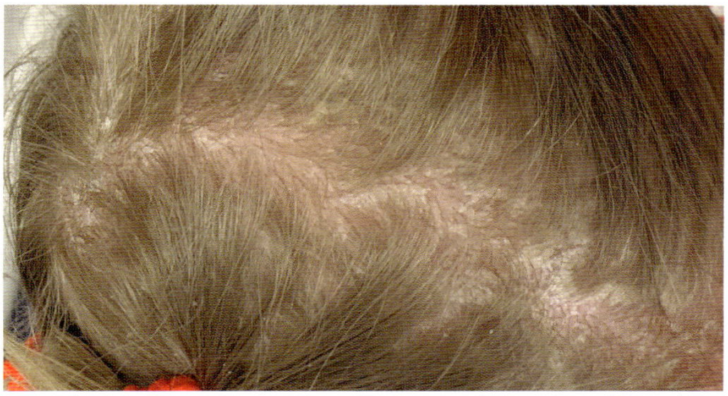

Fig. 5.17 Lamellar ichthyosis. Thick scaling on the scalp. This girl has minimal alopecia, but some have severe alopecia that becomes cicatricial.

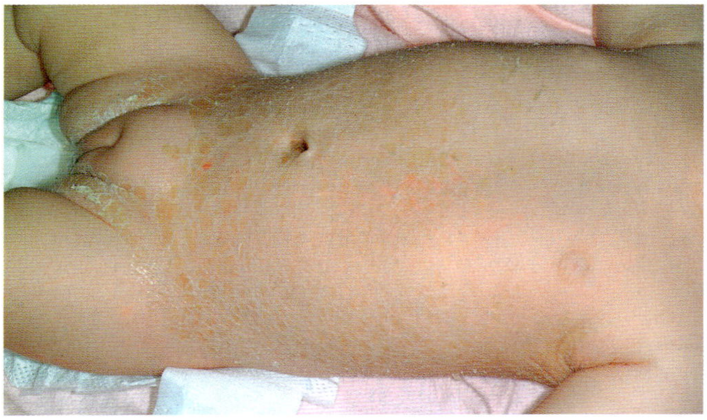

Fig. 5.18 Lamellar ichthyosis, temperature sensitive. Bathing suit distribution, lamellar ichthyosis phenotype of autosomal recessive congenital ichthyosis (ARCI). This distribution of the ichthyosis, largely involving the trunk and intertriginous areas with sparing of the face and limbs, signals a temperature-sensitive mutation in *TGM1*, encoding transglutaminase 1. This baby was born with a full collodion membrane.

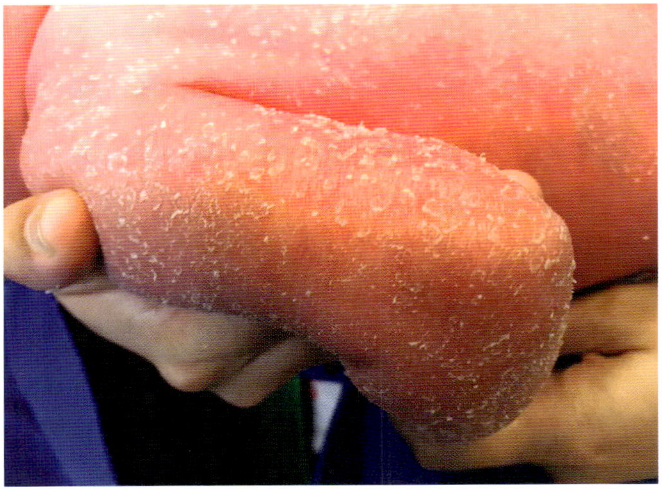

Fig. 5.19 Congenital ichthyosiform erythroderma. CIE phenotype of autosomal recessive congenital ichthyosis (ARCI). The severity of the erythema and scaling can be highly variable. This infant has biallelic missense variants in *ABCA12*, which resulted in a collodion membrane at birth rather than harlequin ichthyosis and evolution to severe erythroderma and scaling.

among the various gene-linked subsets are not specific enough to pinpoint a particular gene without genotyping, although *LIPN* mutations have been reported to have a later onset (early childhood).[125] "Skip areas" without scaling, resembling erythrokeratodermia variabilis, have been described in association with variants in *PNPLA1*[101] (Fig. 5.20).

Among the many different subtypes of CIE, HI is the most distinctive and severe form of ARCI. HI manifests at birth as profoundly thickened, armor-like skin that is fissured into polygonal, triangular, or diamond-shaped plaques that simulate the traditional costume of a harlequin (Fig. 5.21).[126] Rigidity of the skin results in marked ectropion; everted O-shaped lips with a gaping fish-mouth deformity; and a distorted, flattened, and undeveloped appearance to the nose and ears. The skin rigidity can restrict respiratory movements, sucking, and swallowing. The hands and feet are ischemic, hard, and waxy, often with poorly developed digits and an associated rigid and claw-like appearance. Flexion deformity of the limb joints is common, and the nails may be hypoplastic or absent. Restrictive dermopathy (see Chapter 6) shows congenital contractures, tight skin, ectropion, and intrauterine growth retardation and can thus sometimes be confused with HI, but it shows no hyperkeratosis or scaling.

Death is usually associated with prematurity, pulmonary infection (in part associated with hypoventilation caused by thoracic rigidity), poor feeding, excessive fluid loss, poor temperature regulation, or

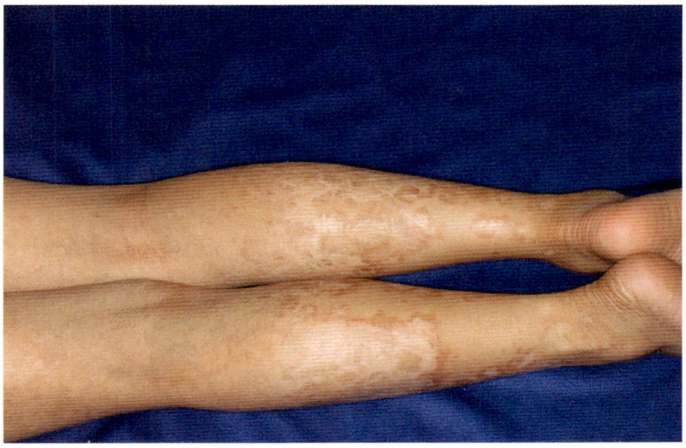

Fig. 5.20 Congenital ichthyosiform erythroderma. This girl has a *PNPLA1* variant, leading to ARCI. However, she had symmetric areas of less involvement, which brought erythrokeratodermia variabilis into the differential.

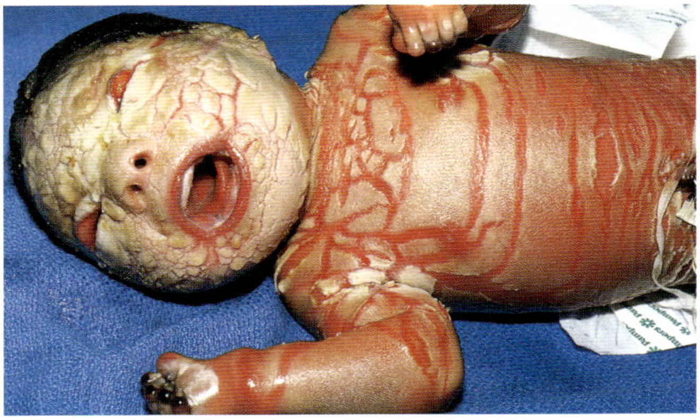

Fig. 5.21 Harlequin ichthyosis. Profoundly thickened, armor-like skin with fissuring, leading to the polygonal, triangular, or diamond-shaped plaques that simulate the costume of a harlequin. Note the severe ectropion, eclabium, and digital infarction. (Courtesy Sylvia Suarez, MD.)

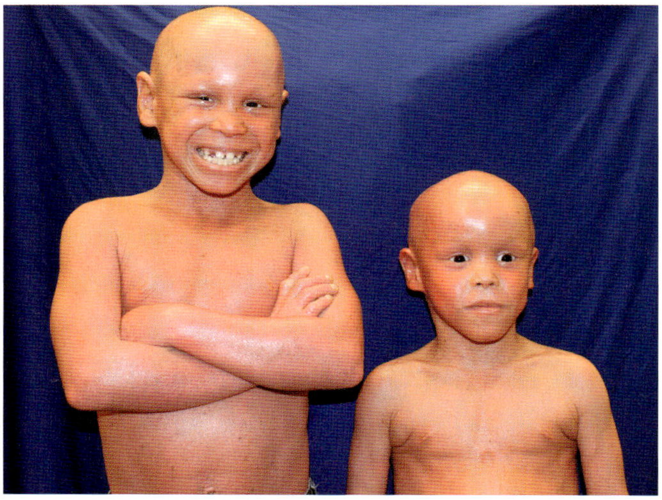

Fig. 5.22 Harlequin ichthyosis. These two brothers with *ABCA12* variants survived the neonatal period without retinoid intervention. With application of moisturizer multiple times daily, they are thriving, but have recurrent methicillin-resistant *Staphylococcus aureus* (MRSA) infections, and one suffers from early-onset synovitis. Note the severe erythroderma and total alopecia.

sepsis as a result of cutaneous infection. The severity may be variable, however, and prolonged survival has been achieved by intensive supportive measures, emollients, and in some cases, oral administration of systemic retinoids.[127–130] Initiation of aggressive intervention for babies with HI is controversial. Even with administration of systemic retinoids or spontaneous clearance of the armor-like scaling, the optimal outcome resembles that of severe CIE (Fig. 5.22). Physicians often reserve initiation for babies who survive the first few weeks, because most infants are stillborn or die during the neonatal period (usually during the first few hours or days of life); however, it is unclear whether the use of systemic retinoids leads to a better outcome than excellent supportive care, especially during the neonatal period of therapy.[131] In addition to initiation of systemic retinoids, topical application of tazarotene or surgical lysis has been used to quickly reduce the encasing bands in HI, which can lead to digital and limb constriction.[132]

HI babies who survive the neonatal period have an increased risk of developing arthritis during childhood, perhaps associated with the high frequency of T cells expressing interleukin-17A or interleukin-22 (IL-17A/IL-22), which is highest in HI among the forms of CIE.[11] Pulmonary issues can be ongoing in infants and young children. Prenatal diagnosis of HI has been suspected based on ultrasound-based discovery of distal arthrogryposis[133] and can be performed definitively by molecular analysis.[134]

Another form of ARCI, *ichthyosis prematurity syndrome (IPS)*, is distinctive in its neonatal appearance and course. Resulting from biallelic mutations in *SLC27A4/FATP4*, affected babies are characteristically born more than 6 weeks premature in association with polyhydramnios and opaque amniotic fluid because of the extensive shedding of epidermal cells.[135,136] Affected neonates have generalized thick, spongy white, desquamating skin that resembles vernix caseosa, accentuated on the scalp and eyebrows, which can be confused with the neonatal thick, white scaling at birth in keratitis-ichthyosis-deafness (KID) syndrome.[137,138] Neonates often have perinatal respiratory distress and sometimes life-threatening neonatal asphyxia of amniotic keratin debris. During the neonatal period, the scaling may evolve to resemble cobblestones overlying moderate erythroderma. Although the marked thickening clears within weeks, xerosis with follicular keratosis and pruritus persist, and patients often show AD, dermographism, asthma, and eosinophilia (which tends to classify IPS as a syndromic form). More than 70% develop respiratory and/or food allergy.[139]

OTHER FORMS OF NONSYNDROMIC ICHTHYOSIS

Loricrin Keratoderma

Loricrin keratoderma (also called *Camisa disease*, a variant of Vohwinkel keratoderma) is an autosomal dominant disorder with ichthyosis and PPK.[140–142] Mutations occur in the gene encoding loricrin, a protein that is linked by transglutaminase-1 to involucrin and other proteins of the corneocyte envelope, thereby participating in barrier function and normal epidermal maturation.[143,144] Affected individuals may be born with a collodion membrane and later show a mild, minimally erythrodermic, generalized ichthyosis with flexural accentuation. The PPK is initially noted during the first weeks of age, is often transgrediens, and usually shows a honeycomb pattern that resembles that of Vohwinkel syndrome (connexin defect). Pseudoainhum may occur but usually not until adolescence or even adulthood; the starfish-shaped keratoses of Vohwinkel syndrome are not seen with loricrin keratoderma. Alopecia and knuckle pads are occasionally seen, but not other ectodermal abnormalities or hearing impairment. Parakeratosis on routine skin biopsy is a characteristic histologic feature, but termination mutations in the C-terminus have been linked to milder PPK without pseudoainhum and without parakeratosis on affected skin biopsy.[145]

Erythrokeratodermias

Erythrokeratodermias are a group of predominantly autosomal dominant ichthyoses. Erythrokeratodermia variabilis (EKV) is characterized by two distinct types of lesions: (1) sharply marginated, pruritic, or burning areas of erythema with finer scaling that are often figurate in configuration and undergo changes in size, shape, and distribution during a period of days to weeks (Fig. 5.23); and (2) hyperkeratotic plaques with thick, yellow-brown scales that usually overlie erythema (Fig. 5.24). Lesions are most often symmetrically distributed on the limbs, trunk, and buttock with relative sparing of the face, scalp, and flexures. In contrast to the chronic but remitting appearance of these plaques and figurate lesions, plaques on the knees, elbows, Achilles tendons, and soles of the feet are often persistent. PPK has been described in 50% of affected families.

Although lesions are usually noted at birth or shortly thereafter during the first year of life, in a few individuals the onset has been noted during late childhood or early adulthood. The disorder may partially regress at puberty and tends to improve in summer. Patients usually tend to respond well to systemically administered retinoids.[146] EKV has been known to result from mutations in genes that both map

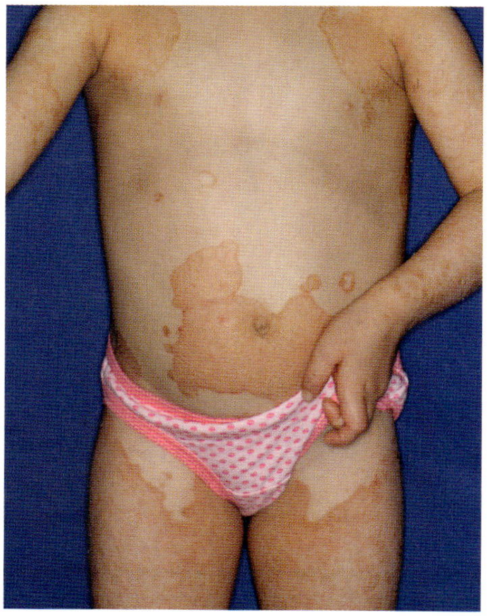

Fig. 5.23 Erythrokeratodermia variabilis (EKV). This girl shows well-demarcated plaques that sometimes are migratory.

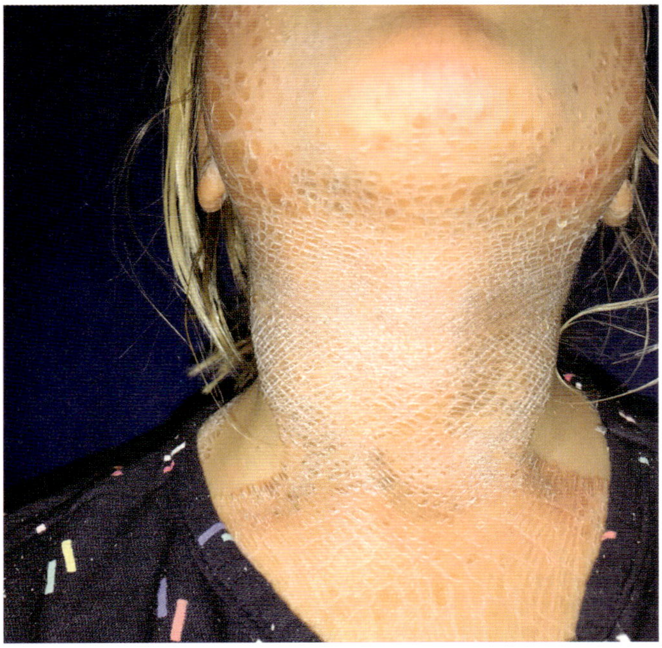

Fig. 5.24. Erythrokeratoderma variabilis (EKV). This girl shows fixed, well-demarcated plaques. Note the symmetric sparing on the clavicular areas.

to chromosome 1p35.1 and encode interacting connexins: the *GJB3* encoding connexin 31[147] and *GJB4* gene encoding connexin 30.3.[148–150] Well-demarcated plaques of mild erythema, thickening, and scaling, rather than generalized CIE-like involvement, have been described with mutations in *PNPLA1*[101] (see CIE). Migrating plaques have also been described in neutral lipid storage disease (Chanarin–Dorfman syndrome) from variants in *ABHD5*.

Mutations in *GJA1*, encoding connexin 43, are associated with plaques of progressive erythrokeratoderma that often begin during infancy with areas of hyperpigmentation, particularly periorally and over the joints. Associated features are PPK, leukonychia, and often profound hyperpigmentation, even in light-skinned individuals (Fig. 5.25).[151,152]

Erythrokeratodermia with cardiomyopathy (EKC) is an autosomal dominant disorder characterized by erythrokeratodermia that tends to begin during infancy, early failure to thrive, woolly hair with alopecia, and nail and variable dental abnormalities[153] (Fig. 5.26). Signs of cardiomyopathy tend to develop by the end of the first decade and may require transplantation. The disorder results from missense mutations, all leading to proline substitution and clustered within the same region-terminal region. Two children with *DSP* mutations and a similar phenotype responded dramatically to treatment with ustekinumab[12] after failure to respond to broader immunosuppressants or retinoids, one of whom was demonstrated to have high expression of Th1/Th17 pathway genes in the skin and increases in IL-17-/IL-22-expressing cells in the blood before initiating therapy.

Individuals with symmetrical EKV lesions during early infancy that clear by 25 years of age may develop progressive spinocerebellar ataxia in adulthood in association with heterozygous mutations in *ELOVL4*.[154] Patients with biallelic *ELOVL4* mutations[155] or heterozygous mutations in *ELOVL1*[156] have ichthyosis in association with spastic diplegia and severe neurodevelopmental delay and must be distinguished from Sjögren–Larsson syndrome (SLS; see Sjögren–Larsson Syndrome). Mutations in *ELOVL1* also lead to sensorineural deafness. *ELOVL1* and *ELOVL4* encode elongases needed for synthesis of very long-chain fatty acids in skin, eyes, and the neurologic system.

Progressive symmetric erythrokeratodermia (PSEK; Darier–Gottron syndrome) tends to have its onset during infancy, stabilizes after 1 or 2 years, and may partially regress at puberty. PSEK has been distinguished from EKV by the absence of the migrating red patches; the

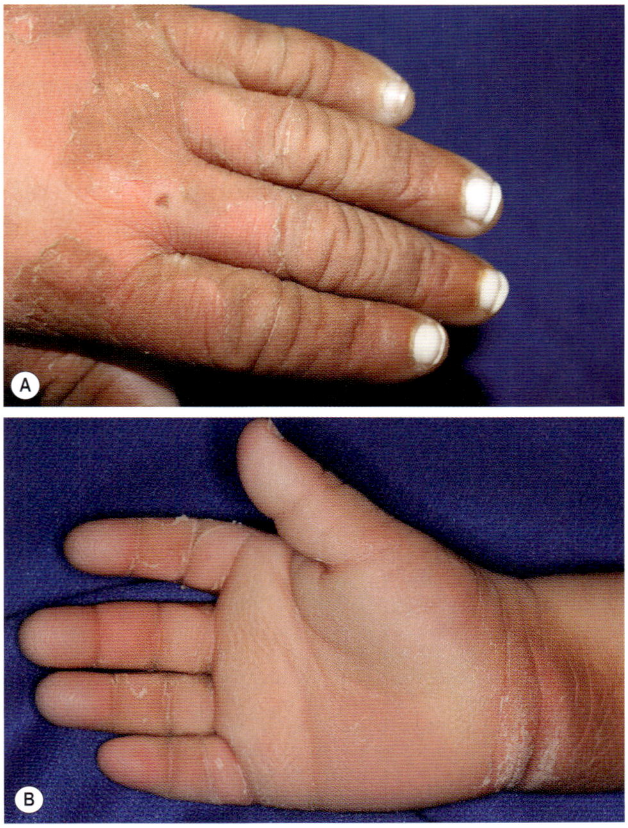

Fig. 5.25 Erythrokeratodermia variabilis (EKV). Variants in *GJA1*, encoding connexin 43, cause a form of EKV with distinguishing clinical features**.** **(A)** Note the white nails and hyperpigmented, thickened skin that peels to reveal underlying erythema. **(B)** The palms have keratoderma with the "honeycombing" pattern that is often seen with connexin defects.

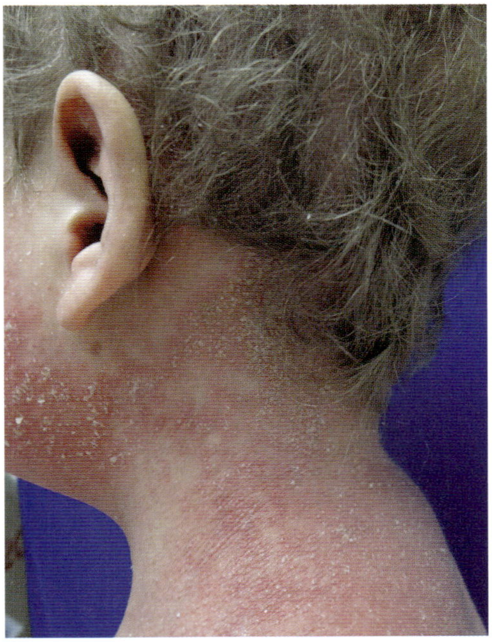

Fig. 5.26 Erythrokeratodermia with cardiomyopathy (EKC). Features of erythroderma and scaling can resemble psoriasis and sparse, woolly hair can be the early signs of this deficiency of desmoplakin and high risk of developing cardiomyopathy in childhood.

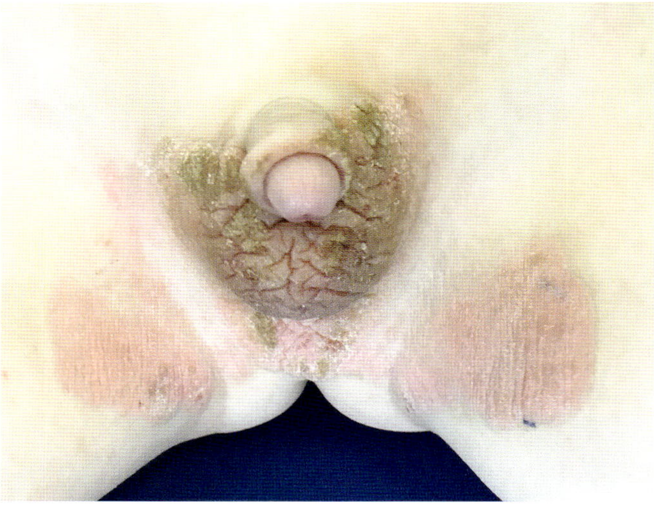

Fig. 5.27 Progressive symmetric erythrokeratodermia (PSEK). Thick psoriasiform plaques with hyperpigmented verrucous scaling of the genital and perioral areas are characteristic of PSEK, which results from variants in *KDSR*, encoding an enzyme needed for ceramide synthesis.

typical sparing of the chest and abdomen with scaling, often verrucous plaques limited to the extremities, genitals/buttocks (Fig. 5.27), and face; and a higher incidence of PPK (≈ 50% of cases). PSEK has recently been shown to result from biallelic mutations in *KDSR*, encoding 3-ketodihydrosphingosine reductase, an enzyme required for ceramide synthesis. Affected individuals tend to respond well to retinoids, perhaps because retinoids can induce an alternative pathway for ceramide generation.[157] Some cases have associated thrombocytopenia.[158] Biallelic mutations in *KRT83* (a gene linked with monilethrix with heterozygous mutations) have also been found to cause a form of PSEK without hair or nail abnormalities.[159] Transgrediens PPK with nail dystrophy and extension onto the extremities, periorificial (cheilitis, perianal, groin up to the abdomen, buttocks) keratotic plaques, and associated woolly hair and scant eyebrows have been described in patients with heterozygous or biallelic mutations in *PERP*, encoding a p53/p63 tetraspan membrane component of desmosomes.[160] Signs begin during the first months of life and may be confused with Olmsted syndrome.

Peeling Skin Syndrome

Peeling skin syndrome (PSS; also called *exfoliative ichthyosis* or *keratolysis exfoliativa congenita*) encompasses a group of unusual autosomal recessive diseases characterized by lifelong, spontaneous superficial peeling of the skin that may be persistent or periodic.[161–163] The Nikolsky sign tends to be positive. Seasonal variation with worsening during summer months has been described. PSS must be distinguished from other causes of peeling skin, such as staphylococcal scalded skin syndrome in infants (generalized) or localized epidermolysis bullosa simplex (acral forms). In general, proteases are activated in these peeling skin disorders.[164]

Generalized PSS may be noninflammatory (type A) or inflammatory (type B).[165] Mutations in *CHST8*, which encodes a Golgi transmembrane N-acetylgalactosamine-4-O-sulfotransferase (GalNAc4-ST1), cause exfoliative ichthyosis (PSS3), an asymptomatic form of noninflammatory generalized peeling skin that usually begins by 6 years of age, but may be congenital.[166] Skin biopsy shows a thickened stratum corneum with an intracorneal or subcorneal separation.

Superficial peeling skin without inflammation has also been described in association with moderate diffuse PPK (which is easily removed without pain) in families with biallelic loss-of-function mutations in *SERPINB8*,[167] encoding the protease inhibitor SERPIN8, and leading to disadhesion of keratinocytes in the basal and suprabasal epidermal layers. In contrast to mutations in *SERPIN7* (Nagashima-type PPK),[168] water exposure does not alter the appearance of the keratoderma. Homozygous mutations in *FLG2*, encoding filaggrin 2, have been found to cause generalized PSS (PSS6). Superficial trauma leads to focal areas of denudement in association with chronic hyperkeratotic plaques on joint areas. The condition characteristically improves with advancing age. Generalized peeling in association with leukonychia, acral punctate keratosis, cheilitis, and knuckle pads are the features of PLACK syndrome, a form of PSS due to loss-of-function mutations in *CAST*, the gene encoding calpastatin, inhibitor of the protease calpain.[169] In addition, biallelic deleterious mutations in *CAPN12*, encoding calpain 12, have led to intense erythroderma and exfoliative scaling in association with hypotrichosis and severe nail dystrophy[114] in an infant who also had biallelic mutations in *ABCA12* but no features of HI (e.g., harlequin scaling at birth, total alopecia) other than the intense erythroderma. Calpain 12 is a protease that plays an important role in epidermal differentiation and hair follicle cycling.

Inflammatory generalized skin peeling results from mutations in *CDSN* and loss of corneodesmin,[170] found in the stratum corneum and hair follicle (PSS1). This form always begins at birth. Patients show erythematous migratory peeling patches and complain of associated pruritus or burning. Short stature and easily removable anagen hairs may be associated.[161] Biopsy specimens reveal psoriasiform thickening of the epidermis and a subcorneal or intracorneal split. The differential diagnosis includes Netherton syndrome (NS) and SAM syndrome. SAM syndrome is characterized by severe dermatitis, multiple allergies, and metabolic wasting due to biallelic mutations in *DSG1* (encoding desmoglein 1[171]) (Fig. 5.28). However, there is wide phenotypic variability, ranging from dermatitis and PPK without systemic manifestations to the food allergies with limited skin involvement.[171] Parents may demonstrate PPK.

An acral or localized form of hereditary PSS is characterized by lifelong painless peeling of predominantly the dorsal aspect of the hands and feet in superficial sheets[172] and exacerbation during summer months with increased sweating.[166,173] A facial variant has been described.[174] This form is caused by mutations in *TGM5* encoding transglutaminase-5,[175,176] which crosslinks epidermal proteins (PSS2),[177] or *CSTA*, encoding cystatin A, a protease of the cornified cell envelope.[178,179]

Keratosis Linearis–Ichthyosis Congenital–Keratoderma

Keratosis linearis–ichthyosis congenital–keratoderma (KLICK) is a rare, autosomal recessive disorder characterized by distinctive striate hyperkeratosis in the flexures (perpendicular to the fold) and PPK.[180,181] It results from a single-nucleotide deletion in the 5′ untranslated regions (UTRs) of the proteasome maturation protein (*POMP*) gene, which reduces levels of *POMP* and leads to proteasome insufficiency, increased endoplasmic reticulum (ER) stress, and perturbed processing of profilaggrin in differentiating keratinocytes.[182,183]

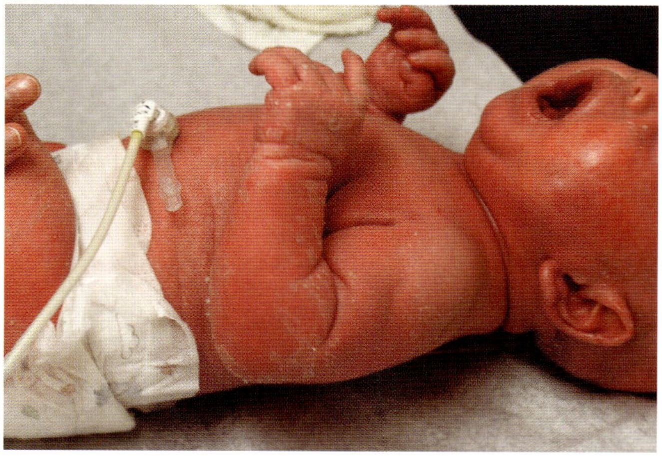

Fig. 5.28 SAM syndrome. SAM syndrome (severe dermatitis, multiple allergies, and metabolic wasting syndrome) presents as generalized erythroderma and failure to thrive. Note the superficial desquamation due to deficiency of the desmosomal protein desmoglein 1.

Syndromic Forms of Ichthyosis

Syndromic forms of ichthyosis[184] may be associated with a variety of extracutaneous abnormalities, most commonly involving the hair (e.g., Netherton; ichthyosis follicularis, alopecia, and photophobia [IFAP] and ichthyosis, hypotrichosis, and sclerosing cholangitis [IHSC] syndromes and ichthyosis with hypotrichosis; trichothiodystrophy) and neurologic system (e.g., Sjögren–Larsson; Refsum; cerebral dysgenesis, neuropathy, ichthyosis, and palmoplantar keratoderma [CEDNIK]; and mental retardation, enteropathy, deafness, neuropathy, ichthyosis, and keratoderma [MEDNIK] syndromes). Some syndromic disorders are often lethal in the neonate (e.g., Neu–Laxova syndrome), infant (e.g., Gaucher disease type 2; arthrogryposis, renal dysfunction, and cholestasis [ARC] syndrome; multiple sulfatase deficiency), or child (e.g., CEDNIK syndrome).

NEUTRAL LIPID STORAGE DISEASE WITH ICHTHYOSIS

Neutral lipid storage disease with ichthyosis, or Chanarin–Dorfman syndrome, is a rare autosomal recessive disorder seen primarily in individuals of Middle Eastern or Mediterranean descent.[185–187] The clinical phenotype can variably include liver steatosis with hepatomegaly, muscle weakness/myopathy, ataxia, neurosensory hearing loss, subcapsular cataracts, nystagmus, strabismus, mental retardation, and nephritic syndrome,[188] but ichthyosis of the CIE phenotype is an almost constant finding. Patients are often born as collodion babies, occasionally with ectropion and eclabium. Skin biopsies show skin thickening with foamy keratinocyte cytoplasm due to prominent neutral lipid droplets in the basal cells and eccrine glands seen best on oil-red O-stained frozen sections. Serum lipids are normal, although the triglyceride content of lymphocytes, macrophages, and fibroblasts in culture is 2 to 20 times that of normal cells. Muscle and liver enzymes may be elevated twofold to threefold. The diagnosis is confirmed by a peripheral blood smear, which shows lipid droplets in granulocytes (Jordan anomaly) that are also seen in the leukocytes of heterozygous carriers of Chanarin–Dorfman syndrome. Mutations have been identified in *ABHD5* or *CGI-58*,[189] a gene encoding an enzyme expressed during differentiation in lipid-transporting lamellar granules of epidermis[190] and required for triglyceride degradation and normal barrier function.[191,192] A diet of moderate amounts of carbohydrates and medium-chain triglycerides, together with oral acitretin 0.5 mg/kg per day, has been shown to improve both the CIE and liver function tests.[193]

CHIME SYNDROME

Individuals with CHIME syndrome (also called *Zunich neuroectodermal syndrome*) show a combination of coloboma, heart defects, ichthyosiform dermatosis, mental retardation, and ear anomalies, including conductive hearing loss.[194,195] The autosomal recessive disorder is caused by mutations in *PIGL*,[196–198] a de-N-acetylase required to make glycosylphosphatidylinositol (GPI), which is a membrane glycolipid that anchors the C-terminus of proteins (receptors, enzymes, adhesion molecules) during posttranslational modification.[199] The skin is notably thickened and dry at birth, with pruritus often developing during the first months of life (Fig. 5.29). The colobomas are usually retinal, although choroidal colobomas have been described. Several heart defects, including pulmonic stenosis, ventricular septal defect, transposition of the great vessels, and tetralogy of Fallot, have been associated. Patients show a typical facies with hypertelorism; a broad, flat nasal root; upslanting palpebral fissures; epicanthic folds; a long columella but short philtrum; macrostomia; full lips; and cupped ears with rolled helices. All patients show brachydactyly. The hair may be fine and sparse, and trichorrhexis nodosa has occasionally been described. Some patients have renal or urologic anomalies, and cleft palate has been described.

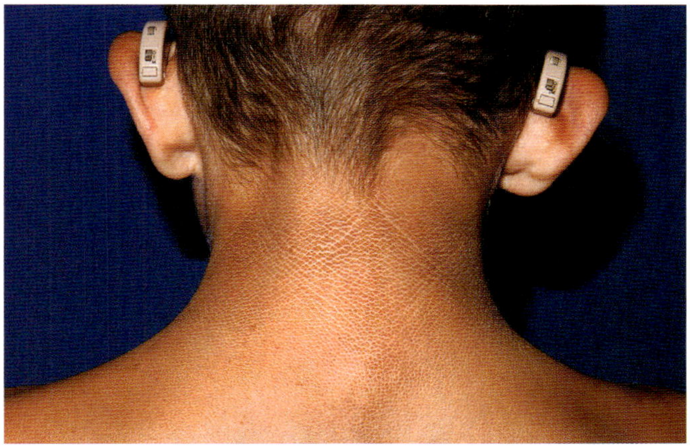

Fig. 5.29 CHIME syndrome. Thickened skin on the back of the neck. Note the hearing aids because of conductive hearing loss.

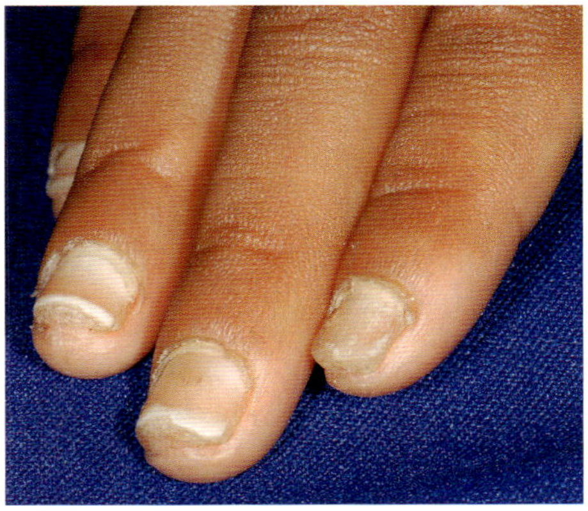

Fig. 5.30 KID syndrome. Note the fine, stippled papules studding the dorsal aspect of the fingers and the subungual hyperkeratosis.

KID SYNDROME

KID syndrome is a rare autosomal dominant disorder characterized by keratitis, congenital ichthyosis, and neurosensory deafness.[200,201] Patients are usually born with erythematous skin that progressively becomes thickened and leathery during the first months of life. Generalized tiny stippled papules are characteristic (Fig. 5.30), and 90% of patients develop well-defined verrucous plaques, especially on the face and limbs. Alopecia may be congenital (25%) and ranges from sparse hair to total alopecia (Fig. 5.31); a thick yellow scale may cover the scalp at birth. Most patients show PPK with a stippled or leathery pattern. Nails tend to be dystrophic and may show leukonychia,[202] and sweating may be diminished.

The hearing loss is congenital, neurosensory, and nonprogressive; it can be detected by brainstem auditory-evoked potential testing. In contrast, ocular features are rarely seen at birth but progress and become evident by childhood or early adolescence. Photophobia may be the earliest sign, and the characteristic corneal vascularization and keratoconjunctivitis sicca lead to pannus formation and marked reduction in visual acuity.[203] KID syndrome must be distinguished from IFAP syndrome (see Chapter 7), an ichthyotic condition in which patients have total alopecia, thickened skin with spiny projections, PPK, and photophobia with decreased visual acuity. Neonates with IPS can resemble babies with KID syndrome,[138] given the alopecia and thick white, confluent scaling on the scalp, upper face, and extremities.

Almost half of patients with KID syndrome have recurrent bacterial and candidal infections of the skin, eyes, and ear canals.[200,204] Some patients have demonstrated abnormal chemotaxis and impaired lymphocyte proliferative responses to *Candida albicans*. The follicular occlusion syndrome (including hidradenitis suppurativa) has been described in some patients, may lead to scarring alopecia, and may require surgical intervention.[205] More than 10% of patients develop squamous cell carcinoma of the skin, especially acral (Fig. 5.32), or

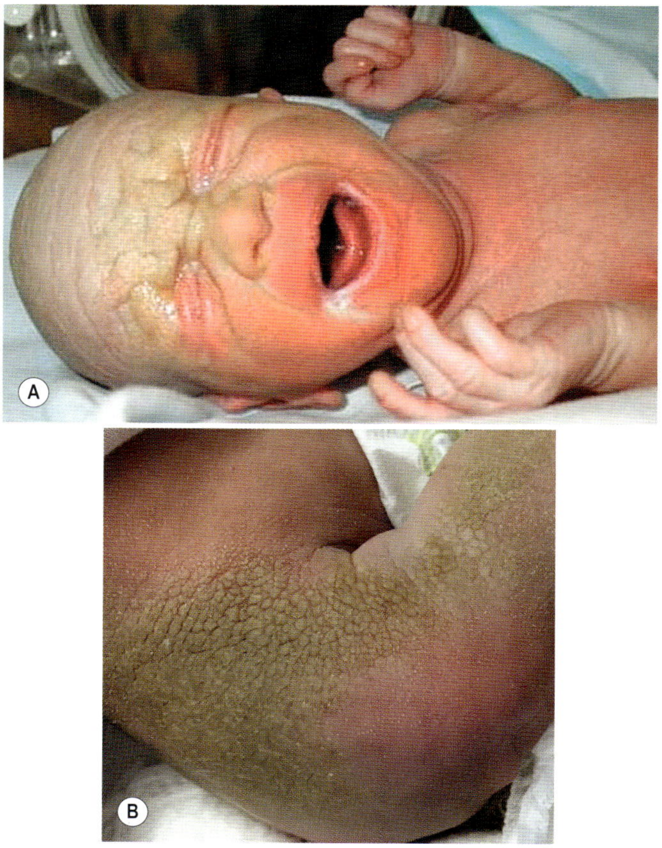

Fig. 5.31 (A) KID syndrome. Markedly thickened skin with fine stippling on the cheeks and perioral skin. Note the total alopecia in this patient, who was found to have a mutation in *GJB2*, which encodes connexin 26. **(B)** Note the fine projections, including between the thick scales, in this newborn. (**A** Courtesy Amy Theos, MD. **B** Courtesy Sapna Vaghani, MD, and Daniela Russi, MD.)

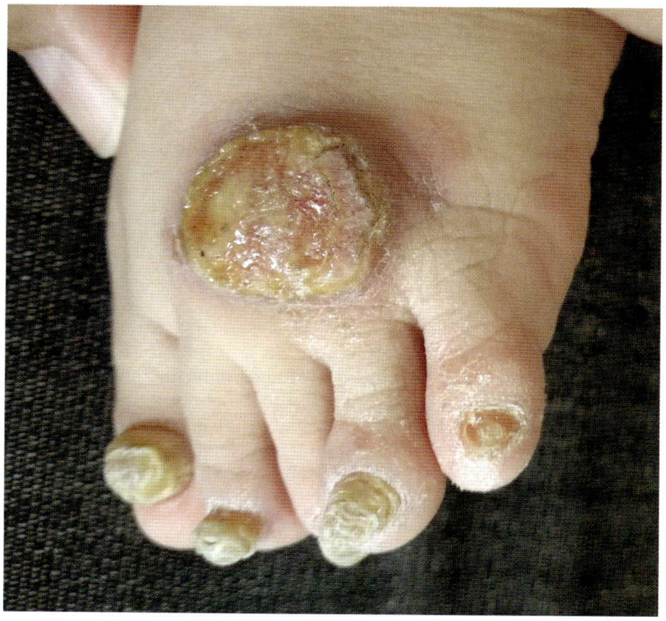

Fig. 5.32 KID syndrome. This 3-year-old girl with KID syndrome developed a squamous cell carcinoma. Note the nail abnormalities and skin thickening.

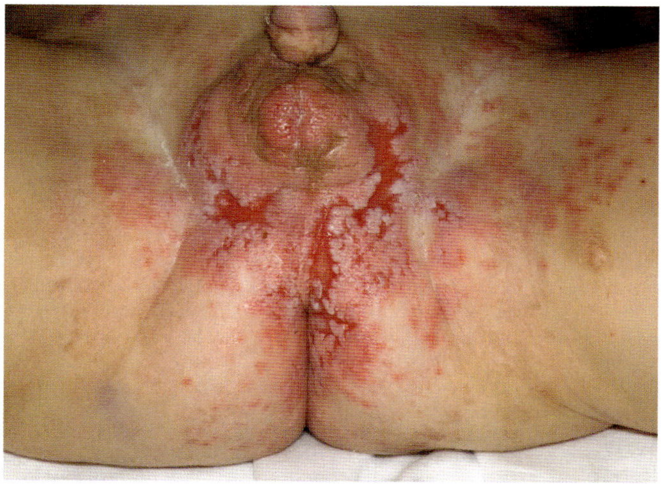

Fig. 5.33 Mosaicism for *GJA2* mutation. This baby had symmetric acantholytic plaques of the genital and perianal region as the presenting sign. During the next 10 years, blaschkoid verrucous plaques with erosions, resembling the verrucous lesions of KID syndrome, developed in numerous locations.

tongue,[200,206] including during childhood. Trichilemmal tumors[207–210] and Dandy–Walker malformation[211] have been described.

The disorder results from mutations in *GJB2*[212] or, occasionally, *GJB6*, genes encoding connexins 26[213] and 30,[214] respectively. The latter connexin is also mutated in patients with Clouston syndrome, which shares the alopecia, nail dystrophy, PPK, and sometimes photophobia of KID syndrome (see Chapter 7). Connexins are critical for the formation of gap junction hemichannels at cell–cell contact sites, which enable intercellular communication. The hyperactive (open) hemichannels increase intracellular calcium levels,[215,216] which likely contribute to the ichthyotic features.

A baby with KID syndrome from a connexin 26 mutation has recently been described whose unaffected mother had the same point mutation but had an additional, more distal, null mutation in the same allele that protected her from having phenotypic manifestations; the second mutation leading to reversion was lost in the baby, presumably by prezygotic reversion during meiosis of the maternal gamete.[217] Revertant mosaicism can also develop in patients with KID, as evidenced by progressively enlarging patches of normal-appearing skin beginning at 20 years of age in a young woman with KID syndrome.[202] Mosaic alterations in *GJB2* have been associated with porokeratotic eccrine nevus[218–220] and a progressive, hyperkeratotic disorder with acantholysis resembling Darier or Hailey–Hailey disease (Fig 5.33).

Therapy for KID syndrome is largely supportive. Chronic administration of fluconazole has improved the verrucous plaques of cutaneous candidiasis.[221,222] Cochlear implants[223] and corneal transplants have been used to correct the sensorineural hearing loss and corneal vascularization, respectively.[203,224–226] Oral retinoids may improve ichthyotic lesions, but only occasionally help with the vision or hearing abnormalities.[227] Mefloquine, a US Food and Drug Administration (FDA)–approved antimalarial drug, inhibits the aberrant connexin 26 hemichannels in keratinocytes from a mouse model of KID syndrome and may be a future intervention.[228]

NETHERTON SYNDROME

Netherton syndrome (NS) is an autosomal recessive condition that combines ichthyosis, atopy, and hair shaft deformities. It presents during the neonatal or early infantile period with generalized scaling erythroderma but not a true collodion baby phenotype. Neonates with NS are usually born prematurely and develop the eruption *in utero* or during the first weeks of life. Failure to thrive is often profound, requiring hospitalization for nutritional support and correction of the associated hypernatremic dehydration.[229]

Patients may have diarrhea associated with intestinal villus atrophy, and the majority experience sepsis, upper and lower respiratory infections, and cutaneous *S. aureus* infection.[230] Adults with NS are also at risk for extensive papillomavirus infection,[231] usually involving the genital region, and may develop squamous cell carcinoma.[82,232–234] A variety of immunologic abnormalities have been described, suggesting that NS should be considered a primary immunodeficiency disorder.[235] These include reduced memory B cells, defective response to vaccination, impaired antibody amplification and class switching, decreased natural killer (NK)–cell cytotoxicity, a skewed T-helper (Th) 1 phenotype, and increased proinflammatory cytokine levels.[230,236] Treatment with intravenous immunoglobulin may cause an increase in NK-cell cytotoxicity and clinical improvement.[230,236]

Ichthyosis linearis circumflexa, the characteristic skin change associated with NS, is characterized by migratory, polycyclic scaly lesions with a peripheral double-edged scale (Fig. 5.34). Although most commonly seen in association with NS, patients may show only the ichthyosis linearis circumflexa without the hair shaft abnormalities or other features of NS. Ichthyosis linearis circumflexa is not generally seen before 2 years of age and occurs eventually in only 70% of patients. The ichthyosiform erythroderma that is the typical manifestation in the neonatal and infantile periods tends to improve with increasing age. Partial remissions have been noted, and spontaneous fluctuation is common, but there is little tendency to spontaneous resolution.

The classic hair shaft abnormality, trichorrhexis invaginata ("bamboo hairs," "ball-and-socket deformity"), is thought to result from a

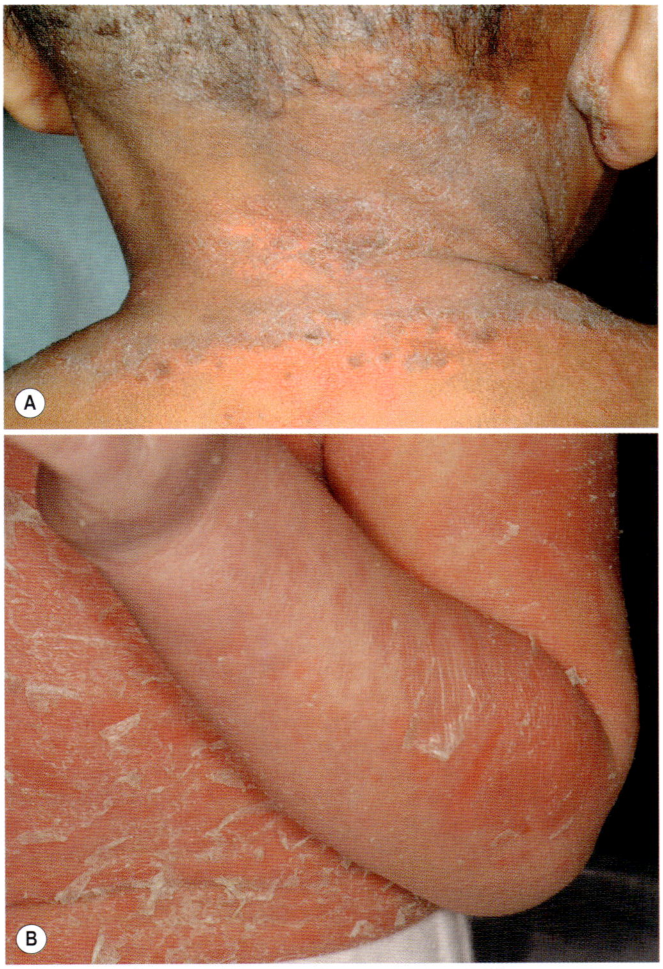

Fig. 5.34 Netherton syndrome. Polycyclic scaling lesions, many showing the scale edge. **(A)** Note the underlying erythroderma, scalp involvement, and short hair. **(B)** Sometimes there is more global erythroderma and larger desquamative scaling.

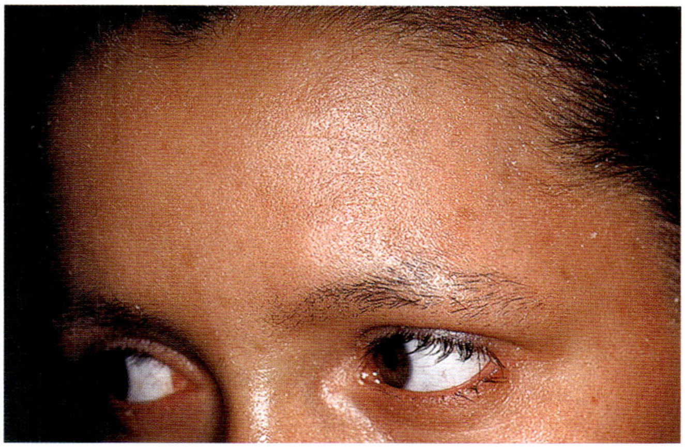

Fig. 5.35 Netherton syndrome. Dry, lusterless hair that breaks and thus remains short and unmanageable. Note the eyebrow alopecia and facial erythroderma.

defect in keratinization of the internal root sheath. The hair defect results in easy hair breakage and hair that is poorly manageable, dry, and lusterless (Fig. 5.35) (see Chapter 7, Fig. 7.6). Multiple hairs from different areas should be examined, because only 20% to 50% of hairs may be affected. Examination of hairs from the eyebrow region often is most fruitful, and dermoscopy facilitates visualization of the "matchstick" hair defect.[237,238] Finding the hair shaft disorder is particularly difficult in the affected neonate.

NS results from loss-of-function mutations in *SPINK5*, which encodes lymphoepithelial Kazal-type-related inhibitor *(LEKTI)*, a serine protease inhibitor.[239] The increase in serine protease activity (kallikreins 5 and 7) leads to decreases in desmosomal proteins (desmoglein 1 and desmocollin 1) with premature degradation of corneocyte desmosomes and excessive desquamation.[240–242] Routine histologic examination of skin-biopsy sections is of limited value, but immunohistochemical studies show absent or reduced expression of *LEKTI*,[243–245] and electron microscopic studies have revealed features that are specific to NS.[246,247]

Approximately two-thirds of patients show pruritic atopic-like dermatitis, food allergies, urticaria, angioedema, asthma, eosinophilic esophagitis, and/or anaphylaxis. In addition, most patients have increased levels of circulating eosinophils and immunoglobulin E (IgE). These atopic manifestations likely result from the unregulated kallikrein 5 activity, which activates *PAR2* and *TSLP* (as in AD; see Chapter 3), as well as other cytokines,[248] and contributes to both the very poor skin barrier and the cutaneous inflammation.

NS can be confused with AD, given the pruritic, erythematous scaling skin and propensity toward atopy.[249] NS should also be distinguished from other forms of ichthyosis, especially with abnormal hair, profound barrier defects, and early failure to thrive (Table 5.3). These include SAM syndrome,[250] epidermal growth factor receptor (EGFR) deficiency,[251,252] ADAM17 deficiency,[253–260] and erythrokeratodermia-cardiomyopathy.[12] In some patients, numerous pustules are present before the classic double-edged scale becomes obvious, raising the possible diagnosis of pustular psoriasis.[261,262] Alopecia with ichthyosis is also a feature of trichothiodystrophy[253] (see Chapter 7), ichthyosis hypotrichosis syndrome,[256–259,263] and IHSC syndrome[254,255] (see Table 5.3).

Treatment of NS is largely supportive. The marked impairment in barrier function, highest among the various orphan forms of ichthyosis, can lead to significant absorption of topically applied medication, necessitating careful monitoring of serum levels or adrenal suppression. Patients often respond to application of topical calcineurin inhibitors, but in some of these patients (not all), there is significant absorption,[264] risking systemic immunosuppression.[265,266] Particular care must be taken with topical corticosteroids. Application of hydrocortisone 1% ointment caused Cushing syndrome in an 11-year-old boy. In one case report, a premature neonate with NS experienced reversal of metabolic abnormalities, reduction in skin exfoliation, and subsequent weight gain

Table 5.3 Differential Diagnosis of Netherton Syndrome: Genetic Disorders with Ichthyosis and Alopecia

Disorder	Inheritance	Gene	Features Resembling Netherton Syndrome	Differentiation from Netherton Syndrome
SAM syndrome	AR Loss-of-function mutations	*DSG1** *SAM-like syndrome can also result from a *DSP* mutation	CIE with PPK, no collodion membrane; failure to thrive; hypernatremia; barrier defect; dermatitis; high IgE; malabsorption; eosinophilic esophagitis; multiple food allergies; recurrent infections; hypotrichosis; hypoalbuminemia	May have microcephaly, growth hormone deficiency, developmental delay, cardiac defects; psoriasiform dermatitis with acantholysis in skin sections; absence of desmoglein
Erythrokeratodermia-cardiomyopathy	AD Missense mutation	*DSP* in single spectrin repeat	Erythroderma; sparse, abnormal hair (ultimately woolly); early failure to thrive; sometimes allergies	Later development of cardiomyopathy
ADAM17 deficiency	AR Loss-of-function mutations	*ADAM17*	Psoriasiform erythroderma/widespread pustules; failure to thrive; malabsorption; short, broken hair; recurrent infections	Bloody diarrhea; cardiomyopathy/ cardiomyositis
EGFR deficiency	AR Loss-of-function mutations	*EGFR*	Erythema, scaling, and widespread pustules; alopecia; failure to thrive, watery diarrhea, high IgE and eosinophils, hypernatremia, hypoalbuminemia; recurrent bronchiolitis	Cardiovascular issues
Trichothiodystrophy	AR Loss-of-function mutations	*ERCC2, ERCC3, GTF2H5, C7Orf11* (see Chapter 7)	CIE-like ichthyosis; short, brittle hair; "tiger tail" hair shaft defect under polarized microscopy	May have impaired intelligence, decreased fertility, short stature, and photosensitivity
IHS (also called autosomal recessive ichthyosis with hypotrichosis [ARIH] syndrome)	AR Loss-of-function mutations	*ST14* (encodes matriptase); abnormal filaggrin processing	Generalized, congenital ichthyosis with sparing of face, palms, and soles; diffuse nonscarring alopecia of scalp, eyelashes, and eyebrows from birth, but improves to sparse, unruly hair during adolescence and merely recession of the frontal hair line by adulthood	May have patchy follicular atrophoderma and hypohidrosis; photophobia from corneal abnormalities; blepharitis; dental abnormalities; hair microscopy may show pili torti or pili bifurcati
IHSC (or NISCH) syndrome	AR Loss-of-function mutations	*CLDN1* (encodes claudin 1, structural protein of tight junctions)	Congenital generalized scaling, predominantly on the limbs and abdomen and sparing skin folds, palms and soles; coarse, curly hair with frontotemporal cicatricial alopecia	Congenital paucity of bile ducts or sclerosing cholangitis leads to neonatal jaundice with hepatomegaly; oligodontia, and enamel dysplasia; blood smears show small eosinophils and keratinocyte vacuoles without lipid contents

AR, Autosomal recessive; *CIE,* congenital ichthyosiform erythroderma; *Ig,* immunoglobulin; *IHS,* ichthyosis hypotrichosis syndrome; *IHSC,* ichthyosis-hypotrichosis-sclerosing cholangitis; *NISCH,* neonatal ichthyosis sclerosing cholangitis; *PPK,* palmoplantar keratoderma; *SAM,* severe dermatitis, multiple allergies, and metabolic wasting.

*Netherton syndrome must also be distinguished from severe atopic dermatitis and immunodeficiency disorders.

when treated four times daily with a topical ointment that contained zinc oxide, cod liver oil, lanolin, and sodium bicarbonate.[267]

Anecdotal reports suggest that suppression of the cutaneous immune activation may be beneficial. Administration of infliximab (with resultant decreased thymic stromal lymphopoietin levels[268,269]) and narrow-band ultraviolet B (UVB) light[270–273] have led to marked cutaneous improvement within a few months. Based on the finding of increased Th17/IL-23 expression in the skin of patients with Netherton syndrome, targeted monoclonal antibodies ustekinumab and secukinumab have been used with remarkable success in treating NS.[10–13,274,275] Inhibition of kallikrein[276,277] or the combination of kallikreins 5 and 7 has been proposed as a therapeutic option: in mouse models of NS, either kallikrein 5 itself[278] or only inhibition of both kallikreins simultaneously rescued the epidermal barrier and the postnatal lethality.[278] An early-phase gene therapy trial is underway in Europe, with the normal *SPINK5* gene introduced by lentivirus into the grafted patient keratinocytes.[245]

REFSUM DISEASE

Refsum disease is an autosomal recessive neurocutaneous disorder caused by a deficiency in oxidation of phytanic acid, a branched, long-chain fatty acid derived from dietary chlorophyll.[279–282] The clinical features usually develop in late childhood or early adult life and progress slowly during months to several years. Neurologic manifestations are most prominent and include sensorineural deafness; anosmia; failing vision; night blindness due to retinitis pigmentosa; and a progressive weakness, foot drop, and loss of balance caused by a mixed sensorimotor neuropathy and cerebellar involvement. Delayed diagnosis may result in severe neurologic impairment, wasting, and depression. The associated ichthyosis, which can either coincide with or postdate the neurologic features, resembles ichthyosis vulgaris or, in severe untreated cases, LI. Accentuated palmoplantar markings, stubby thumbs with digital asymmetry, and cardiac arrhythmias may be associated features.

Refsum disease results from mutations in one of two genes, either *PHYH* (also named *PAHX*), which encodes the peroxisomal enzyme phytanoyl-CoA hydroxylase, or *PEX7*, which encodes the PTS2 (peroxisomal targeting signal 2) receptor.[283] Phytanic acid cannot be synthesized by humans and is mainly derived from plant chlorophyll. Normally serum levels are undetectably low, but in Refsum disease may account for up to 30% of serum lipids. The accumulation of phytanic acid disturbs the cholesterol balance and may alter lipid degradation.[284] Histology shows variably sized vacuoles in the epidermal basal and suprabasal cells, corresponding to the lipid accumulation seen with lipid stains of frozen sections. The diagnosis is based on the demonstration of increased levels of phytanic acid in the patient's serum, tissue, or urine. Therapy consists of a chlorophyll-free diet and avoidance of phytanic acid–containing foods.

SJÖGREN–LARSSON SYNDROME

The ichthyosis of the autosomal recessive disorder SLS usually manifests in the neonatal period as fine, white scaling, accentuated in flexural areas.[285] Erythema is occasionally present at birth but clears within months. Presentation as a collodion baby occurs only occasionally. By 1 year of age, the ichthyosis of SLS is not erythrodermic but shows generalized velvety thickening (often with a yellowish hue), particularly on the trunk and neck, with minimal desquamation (Fig. 5.36), PPK, and relative sparing of the face.[286,287] The skin is characteristically pruritic, and most patients are hypohidrotic. The degree of scaling varies from mild to more severe (Fig. 5.37) and does not change with increasing age.[288,289] Hair and nails are normal. The neurologic disease usually presents within the first year with failure to reach normal developmental milestones and the onset of spasticity. Phenotypic variability is seen,[290] and some patients have been described with mild neurologic features of SLS without associated skin disease.[291] Spasticity and muscle paresis is most pronounced in the legs,[288] and most affected persons become dependent on a wheelchair for mobility. Most patients have a learning disability to a variable degree and a speech disorder, and some show seizures, short stature, kyphosis, and enamel hypoplasia. The pathognomonic retinal "glistening dots" are not present in all patients, but photophobia is common.

SLS results from inactivating mutations in the fatty aldehyde dehydrogenase gene (*FALDH* or *ALDH3A2*), leading to abnormal metabolism of long-chain aldehydes[292] and alcohols. Epidermal cells in affected individuals show abnormal lamellar bodies and lipid droplets, consistent with defective lipid metabolism.[293] A prenatal diagnosis of SLS is possible by measurement of fatty acid oxidation (FAO) activity in cultured amniocytes or chorionic cells, histologic analysis, and/or analysis of fetal deoxyribonucleic acid (DNA) if the gene defect is known. The ichthyosis is treated with topical keratolytic agents and retinoids[288]; oral acitretin (0.5 mg/kg per day initially with 0.25 mg/kg per day maintenance) decreased the severity of ichthyosis and increased quality of life in eight affected children, with 57% of those with pruritus per parental report.[294] Dietary supplementation with medium-chain fatty acids is generally not helpful.[286] The leukotriene inhibitor zileuton was only reported to decrease the associated pruritus in 1 of 10 patients in one trial[295,296] and had no ameliorative effect on the progressive neurologic deterioration.[297] Clinical research is testing the efficacy of aldehyde dehydrogenase–specific activator drugs and peroxisome proliferator-activated receptor alpha (PPAR-α) agonists to increase mutant *FALDH* activity, dietary lipid modification, and gene therapy.[292] Ichthyosis with more severe neurologic changes than SLS (spastic diplegia, seizures, and intellectual disability) can also result from biallelic mutations in *ELOVL4*, a fatty acid elongase that catalyzes the first and rate-limiting step in very long-chain fatty acid synthesis (see Erythrokeratodermia Variabilis and Progressive Symmetric Erythrokeratodermia section).[155]

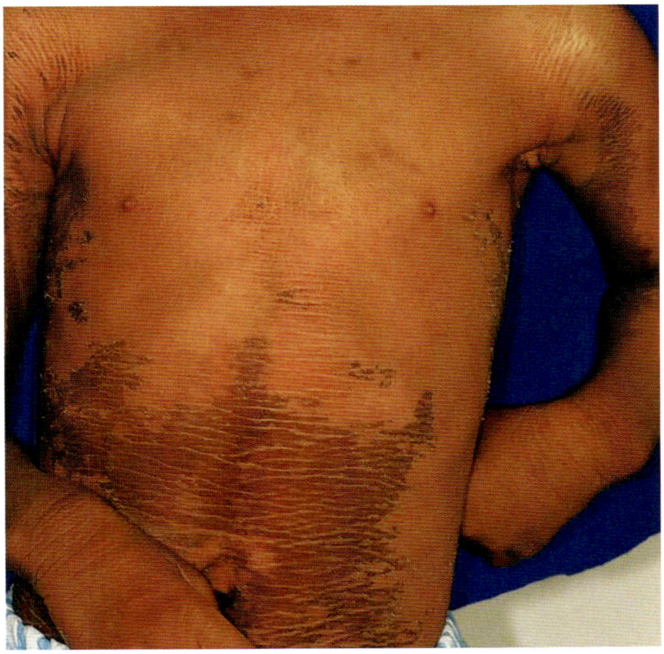

Fig. 5.37 Sjögren–Larsson syndrome. Thick, lamellar scaling in a girl with neurologic issues, particularly spasticity.

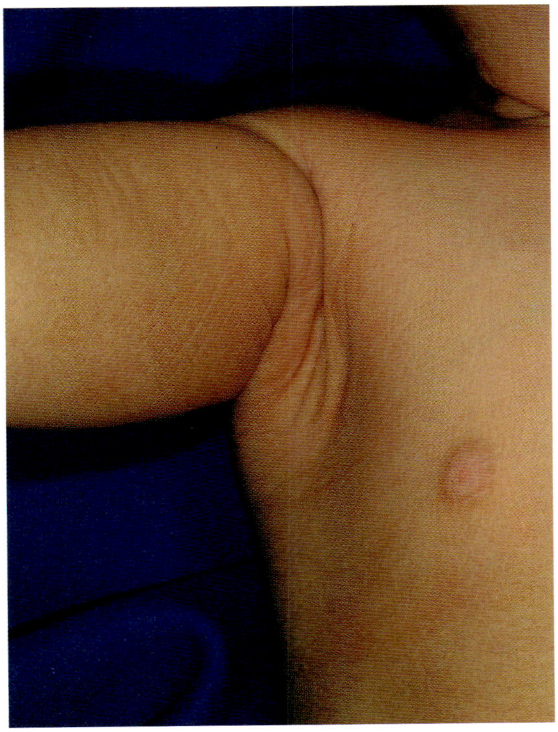

Fig. 5.36 Sjögren–Larsson syndrome. The skin shows velvety thickening with a yellowish hue and minimal desquamation.

NEU–LAXOVA SYNDROME

Neu–Laxova syndrome is an autosomal recessive form of congenital ichthyosis associated with a high risk of early death. Affected babies have severe intrauterine growth retardation, an edematous appearance, lung hypoplasia, microcephaly, and abnormal brain development with lissencephaly and agenesis of the corpus callosum.[298–301] The ichthyosis tends to be present at birth but ranges in severity from mild to a harlequin appearance. Patients tend to show typical facies, including protuberant eyes with a flattened nose, slanted forehead, micrognathia, deformed ears, and a short neck. Some affected neonates show microphthalmia or cleft palate. Syndactyly, limb or digital hypoplasia, and limb contractures are common, and X-rays often show poor bone mineralization. Mutations occur in one of three genes of the L-serine biosynthesis pathway: phosphoglycerate dehydrogenase (*PHGDH*),[302,303] phosphoserine aminotransferase (*PSAT1*), or phosphoserine phosphatase (*PSPH*).[304] Ceramide expression is reduced.[305] Neu–Laxova represents the severe end of the spectrum of disorders caused by mutations in these genes (others have variable neurologic manifestations). Craniofacial and limb defects have been seen in a variety of syndromes with reduced intrauterine movement (fetal akinesia/hypokinesis sequence).

GAUCHER SYNDROME TYPE 2

Gaucher syndrome type 2 results from an absence of lysosomal β-glucocerebrosidase, which hydrolyzes glucosylceramide to ceramide. The neonate with Gaucher syndrome type 2 (acute infantile cerebral form) may be a collodion baby[306,307] with the onset during infancy of neurologic signs and hepatosplenomegaly.[308] Other neonatal features may be hydrops, arthrogryposis, cholestasis, and cytopenias.[309] Blueberry muffin lesions have been reported in one neonate, possibly reflecting dermal erythropoiesis.[310] Glucosylceramide and ceramide are critical components of the intercellular bilayers of the stratum corneum and play a role in epidermal barrier function.[9] The absence of glucocerebrosidase leads to abnormal skin thickening and increased transepidermal water loss. Even when the skin appears normal clinically in affected patients, ultrastructural abnormalities in lamellar membranes may be seen.[311–315] Enzyme replacement therapy can improve the visceromegaly and hematologic abnormalities, but does not cross the blood–brain barrier to alter neurologic manifestations of Gaucher disease.[309,312] Mutations in the gene encoding UDP–glucose ceramide glucosyltransferase (UGUG or glucosylceramide synthase/GCS), which transfers glucose to ceramide to synthesize glucosylceramide, have been reported to cause ichthyosis with a collodion membrane at birth and lethality during the neonatal period.[313]

CEDNIK SYNDROME

CEDNIK syndrome first manifests between 5 and 11 months of age with progressive neurologic deterioration.[314,315] Affected infants show a generalized mild LI phenotype with sparing of skin folds but palmoplantar thickening. The hair tends to be fine and sparse. Microcephaly, neuropathy, cerebral dysgenesis, sensorineural deafness, optic nerve atrophy, neurogenic muscle atrophy, and cachexia are associated, and affected individuals usually die within the first decade of life. Patients with CEDNIK syndrome have mutations in *SNAP29*, a component of the secretory (SNARE [soluble NSF attachment protein receptor]) pathway that is important for vesicle fusion and lamellar granule maturation and secretion. In mouse models, keratinocyte-specific SNAP29 deficiency leads to abnormal skin differentiation, increased proliferation, and poor barrier formation.[316] In CEDNIK syndrome, glucosylceramide- and kallikrein-containing granules are abnormally retained in the stratum corneum, leading to retention hyperkeratosis and an abnormal epidermal barrier.

MEDNIK SYNDROME

MEDNIK syndrome is an autosomal recessive disorder that shows manifestations at birth or within the first weeks of life.[317–319] Among the ichthyoses, it most closely resembles EKV and, in fact, has also been called *EKV3*. Nail thickening and mucosal involvement may be associated. Patients show congenital sensorineural deafness, psychomotor and growth retardation, mental retardation, and peripheral neuropathy. The severe, congenital, chronic diarrhea is life-threatening. MEDNIK syndrome results from mutations in *AP1S1*, encoding a subunit (1A) of an adapter protein complex (AP-1) that is involved in the organization and transport of proteins during skin and spinal cord development.[320]

DEAFNESS–DYSTONIA SYNDROME

Another ichthyotic disorder with deafness and neurologic abnormalities is deafness–dystonia syndrome. This autosomal recessive disorder results from mutations in *FITM2* (fat storage-inducing transmembrane 2), which affects neutral lipid storage and metabolism.[321] The ichthyotic scaling is most prominent on the shins and is associated with scarring alopecia. The first manifestation is typically deafness beginning around 6 months, with progression during the first decade. Other features are global developmental delay, dystonic movements, sensory neuropathy, and low body mass index.

ARC SYNDROME

The distinguishing features are the associated arthrogryposis (contractures of the limbs, particularly of the knee, hip, and wrist; rocker bottom feet; talipes equinovarus), renal tubular degeneration with metabolic acidosis, and intrahepatic bile duct hypoplasia with cholestasis. "Arthrogryposis"; "Renal"; and "Cholestasis (ARC) syndrome usually presents with lamellar scaling within the first days to year of life but not at birth.[322–325] The extent of involvement ranges from mild involvement, particularly over fold and joint areas, with PPK to severe generalized scaling. Ectropion and mild scarring alopecia may be present. Patients may also show cerebral malformations with microcephaly and intellectual impairment, hypothyroidism, deafness, dysmorphic features, hip dislocation, osteopenia, exocrine pancreatic insufficiency, and large, dysfunctional platelets with bleeding diathesis. Death ensues during the first year of life. ARC syndrome results from mutations in *VPS33B* (vacuolar protein sorting 33B) and, less often, *VIPAS39*, which regulate SNARE protein-mediated fusion of membrane vesicles required for lamellar body secretion.[326] Incomplete ARC syndrome has been described without the arthrogryposis.[327] Mutations in *VPS33B* have also been described in patients with autosomal recessive keratoderma-ichthyosis-deafness (ARKID) syndrome, an autosomal recessive disorder characterized by diffuse PPK (sometimes leading to autoamputation), sensorineural deafness, and fine generalized scaling without other features of ARC syndrome.[328]

CONRADI–HÜNERMANN–HAPPLE SYNDROME

The key clinical features of CHH syndrome (also called *X-linked dominant chondrodysplasia punctata type II*) are linear ichthyosis, chondrodysplasia punctata, cataracts, and short stature.[329] Neonates tend to show severe ichthyosiform erythroderma with patterned, yellowish, markedly hyperkeratotic plaques (Fig. 5.38, *A*). However, some cases are so mild that the diagnosis is only made by detection of blashkoid streaks of ichthyosis and/or follicular atrophoderma later in life.[330] After the first 3 to 6 months of life, the erythroderma and scaling resolve, leaving erythema and later follicular atrophoderma in a distribution that follows Blaschko lines, hypopigmentation and hyperpigmented streaks, particularly on the trunk (Fig. 5.38, *B* and *C*), and circumscribed cicatricial alopecia of the scalp and eyebrows (Fig. 5.39). Patients may show persistent psoriasiform lesions in intertriginous areas (ptychotropism) (Fig. 5.40). Skin biopsy sections may show intracorneal calcifications and keratin-filled follicular ostia.[331] In addition to the cutaneous findings, patients with CHH show asymmetric skeletal involvement with punctate calcification of the epiphyseal regions that usually results in an asymmetric shortening of the long bones (especially the humeri and femora) and sometimes in severe kyphoscoliosis, facial dysplasia, and hip dislocation. Unilateral or bilateral sectorial cataracts, patchy, coarse, lusterless hair, nasal bone dysplasia with saddle-nose deformity (see Fig. 5.39), and a high-arched palate further characterize the disease. The bony abnormalities, but not the skin lesions, of CHH syndrome have been described in association with teratogenic exposures to medications and infections and maternal autoimmune diseases.[332]

X-chromosomal inactivation explains the distribution of skin lesions along Blaschko lines, the sectorial cataracts, and the asymmetric skeletal abnormalities. Abnormal cholesterol synthesis/metabolism has been detected in patients with CHH, and mutations have been identified in emopamil-binding protein (EBP), which encodes 3β-hydroxysteroid-Δ8,Δ7-isomerase, a key component in cholesterol biosynthesis. Abnormal lamellar granules and malformed intercellular lipid layers have been detected ultrastructurally,[333] and plasma sterol analysis shows markedly elevated levels of 8(9)-cholesterol and 8-dehydrocholesterol.[334]

CHILD SYNDROME

CHILD syndrome is a congenital disorder characterized by congenital hemidysplasia, ichthyosiform erythroderma, and limb defects.[335] Also known as *unilateral CIE*, the hallmark of the disorder is the sharp midline demarcation and its largely unilateral cutaneous and skeletal features (Fig. 5.41). This X-linked dominant condition occurs almost exclusively in girls and is presumed to be lethal in affected males. The only case in a boy is thought to represent early postzygotic mosaicism.[336] The inflammatory ichthyosiform skin lesions of CHILD syndrome may be present at birth or develop during the first few months of life. They are characterized by yellow and waxy scaling and/or streaks of inflammation and scaling that is often patchy but may follow

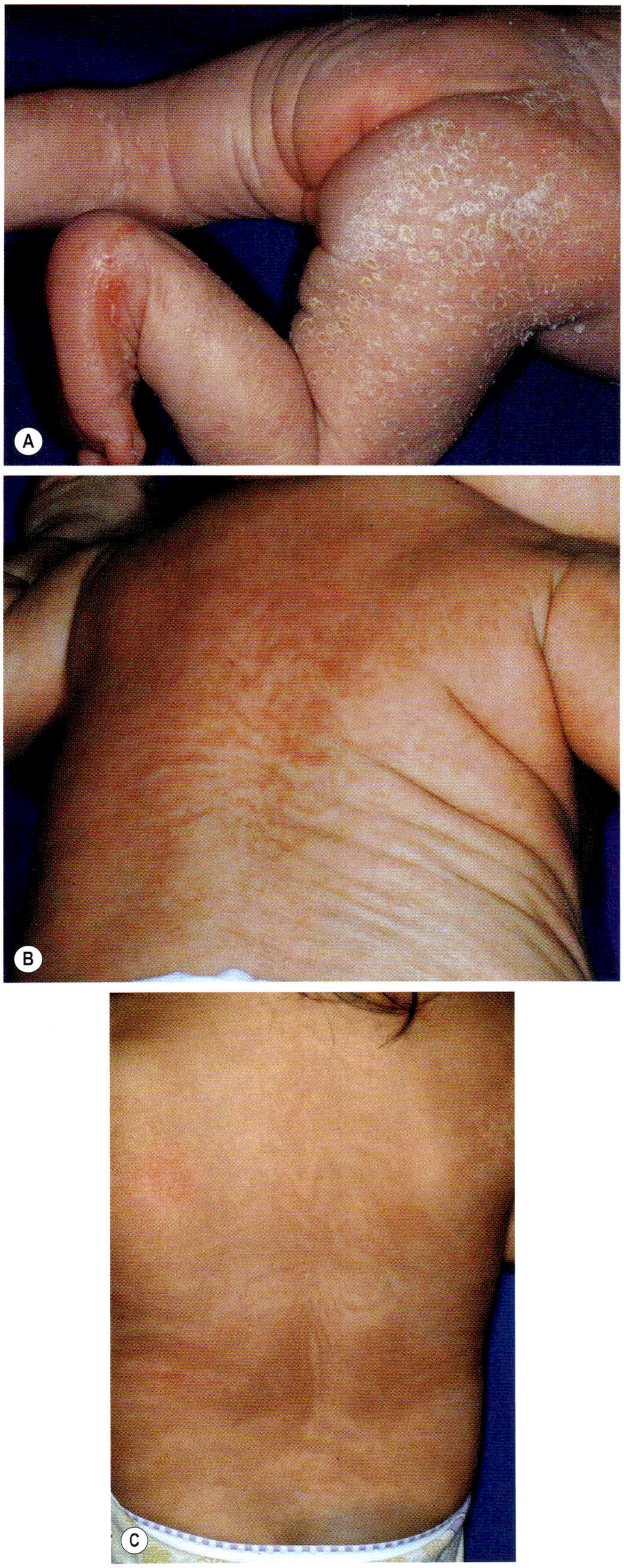

Fig. 5.38 Conradi–Hünermann–Happle syndrome. Congenital scaling **(A)** and residual hyperpigmentation during infancy after scale clearance **(B)** and later during childhood **(C)** in a distribution that follows Blaschko lines.

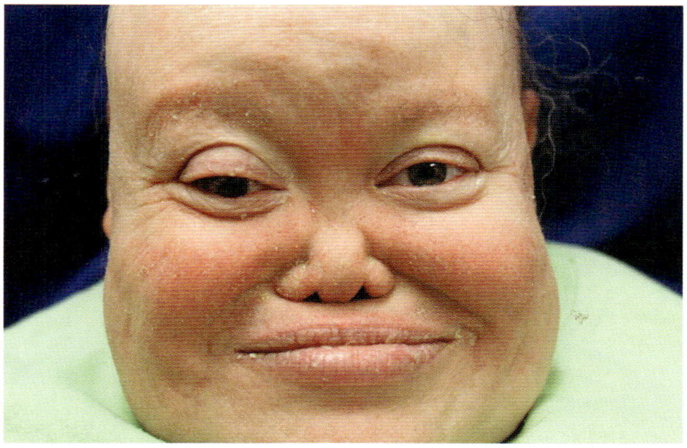

Fig. 5.39 Conradi–Hünermann–Happle syndrome. Cicatricial alopecia of the eyebrows. Approximately half of this patient's scalp hair was replaced by cicatricial alopecia as well. Note the saddle deformity of the nose.

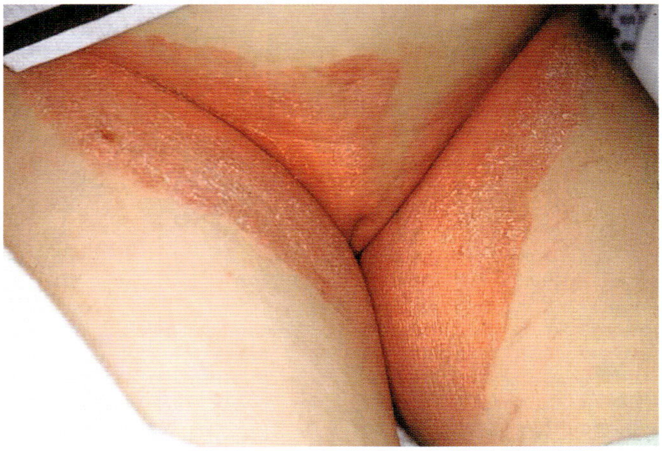

Fig. 5.40 Conradi–Hünermann–Happle syndrome. Bilateral ptychotropism with psoriasiform plaques.

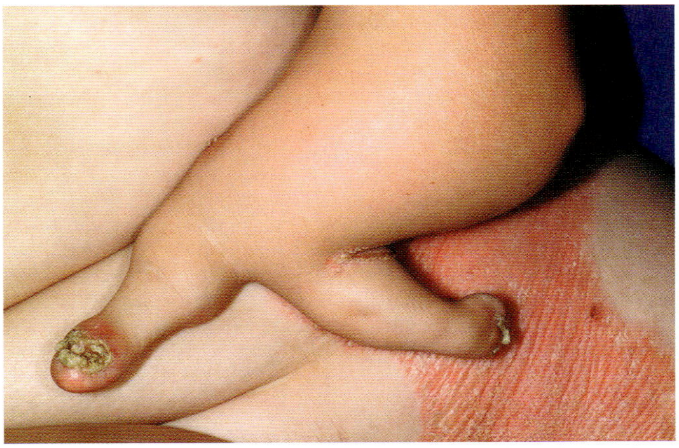

Fig. 5.41 CHILD syndrome. Unilateral congenital ichthyosiform erythroderma with marked deformity of the arm. This girl's ipsilateral leg was also markedly shortened and required amputation.

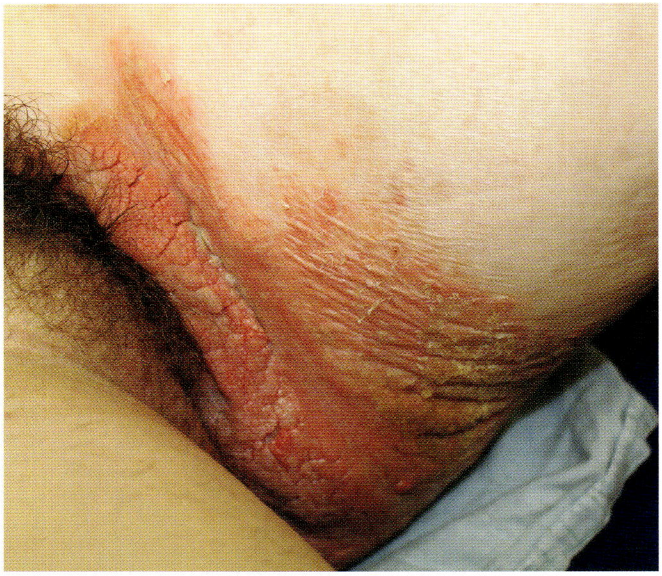

Fig. 5.42 CHILD syndrome. This teenager shows a ptychotropic plaque and verrucous xanthoma of the left vulva.

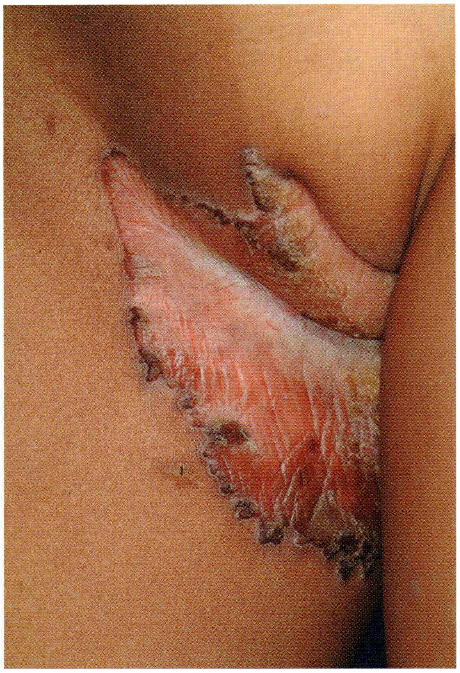

Fig. 5.43 CHILD nevus. The ptychotropism of a sharply demarcated, thickened plaque of the inguinal area that ends abruptly at the midline. This girl showed mild thickening and hyperpigmentation involving only the right side of her body but no limb deformities or hemidysplasia.

Blaschko lines. Similarly, streaks of normal skin may be interspersed within the area of the CHILD nevus, and affected individuals may have minimal limb abnormalities.[337] Biopsy of skin lesions shows epidermal thickening with characteristic infiltration of the papillary dermis of histiocytes showing foamy cytoplasm (verruciform xanthoma). Exuberant verrucous overgrowth, including of mucosal areas (Fig. 5.42), has been described.

Unilateral alopecia and severe nail dystrophy with claw-like nails have been described. The face is typically spared. With increasing age, lesions may improve or even clear spontaneously, but lesions in intertriginous areas (ptychotropism) tend to persist and be the most severely affected sites.[338] Rarely, a localized hyperkeratotic plaque with a sharp demarcation at the midline is the sole manifestation of CHILD syndrome (CHILD nevus) (Fig. 5.43). A mild form of CHILD syndrome has been described in three generations,[339] suggesting genetic control of the skewing of X inactivation.[340]

Ipsilateral skeletal hypoplasia, ranging in severity from hypoplasia of the fingers to complete agenesis of an extremity, is an important feature of CHILD syndrome. As with the skin changes, unilaterality is not absolute, and slight changes may be present on the contralateral side. The molecular basis for the unilaterality is not understood, but the epidermal changes correlate with mutant gene expression in the epidermis; leukocytes show skewing of X-chromosome inactivation, and virtually all circulating cells express the normal gene.[341] Punctate epiphyseal calcifications may be demonstrable by radiography but tend to disappear after the first few years of life. Cardiovascular and renal abnormalities are the major visceral manifestations of CHILD syndrome, although anomalies of other viscera have been described. Inactivating mutations have been identified in the *NSDHL* gene encoding a 3β-hydroxysteroid dehydrogenase,[342] which functions upstream of EBP in the cholesterol synthesis pathway. Treatment with keratolytic agents and retinoids is poorly tolerated, but topical application of compounded 2% lovastatin/2% cholesterol leads to dramatic improvement.[341,343] Use of alternative statins, such as simvastatin, and addition of glycolic acid compounded with the cholesterol also have been beneficial.[343,344]

Treatment of Nonsyndromic and Syndromic Ichthyoses

Treatment of patients with most forms of ichthyosis involves topical application of keratolytic agents and topical or systemic administration of retinoids.[1,345–347] The Foundation for Ichthyosis and Related Skin Types (FIRST; www.firstskinfoundation.org) is a support group for patients and families with disorders of cornification. In additional to educational materials, FIRST provides information about commercially available treatment options. Several other foundations worldwide support families with ichthyosis and have educational websites as well (e.g., www.ichthyosis.org.uk and www.ictiosis.org).

The management of all types of ichthyosis consists of retardation of water loss, rehydration and softening of the stratum corneum, and alleviation of scaliness and associated pruritus. Daily to twice-daily baths using a superfatted soap or a soapless cleanser followed immediately by application of the emollient to moist skin can be helpful for all forms. Shorter baths are preferred for patients with ichthyosis vulgaris, especially with associated AD. However, many patients with LI or EI have found long baths to be particularly helpful. Ichthyosis vulgaris and RXLI can be managed quite well by topical application of emollients and the use of keratolytic agents to facilitate removal of scales from the skin surface.

α-Hydroxy acid preparations such as lactic and glycolic acids are the most commonly used as agents to desquamate excessive scale and increase hydration.[345,348] Urea in concentrations of 10% to 20% has a softening and moisturizing effect in addition to a keratolytic effect on the stratum corneum and is helpful in the control of dry skin and pruritus. Urea 40% is available for thicker skin areas, such as palms and soles. Salicylic acid is another effective keratolytic agent and can be compounded into petrolatum at concentrations between 3% and 6% to promote shedding of scales and softening of the stratum corneum. When it is used to cover large surface areas for prolonged periods, however, patients should be monitored for salicylate toxicity, most commonly complaints of tinnitus. The combination of 6% salicylic acid in propylene glycol may be particularly helpful for keratoderma of the palms and soles, especially when used under occlusive wraps. The LI phenotype of ARCI generally requires more potent keratolytic agents; individuals with milder forms of LI often respond well to the topical application of tazarotene (Fig. 5.44).[349,350] As the skin normalizes, the risk of irritation from tazarotene increases, sometimes leading to dermatitis and then requiring therapy to be intermittent.

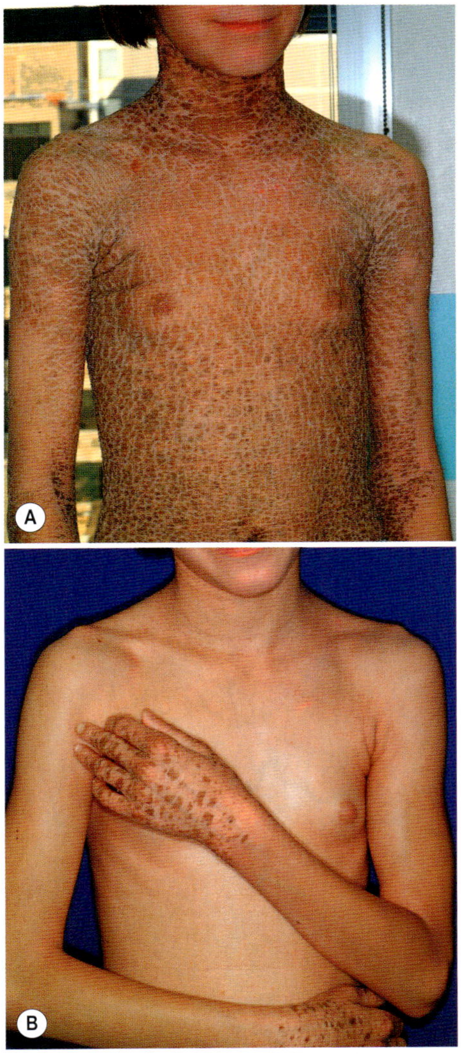

Fig. 5.44 **(A)** and **(B)** Clearance of the lamellar phenotype of ichthyosis with topically applied tazarotene. After 2 months of nightly application of tazarotene 0.1% cream, this girl experienced remarkable improvement in her ichthyosis.

Topical N-acetylcysteine (NAC) with or without urea (e.g., 10% N-acetylcysteine in 5% urea) has also been used for ichthyoses, most often for LI.[351–353] NAC requires compounding, can be irritating, and may have an associated sulfuric odor that can be masked somewhat by the addition of rosemary oil or other intense scents. Topical vitamin D analogues may be beneficial for some patients. For infants in the first 6 to 12 months of life, treatment should be limited to bathing and emollients, with the introduction of keratolytic agents after this time.

The skin of EI is quite fragile, and patients generally will tolerate only intermittent, short-term use of keratolytic agents, if at all. Similarly, individuals with NS and CHILD syndrome tolerate topically applied keratolytic agents poorly. It should be remembered that individuals with ichthyosis usually have a barrier abnormality that can lead to increased percutaneous absorption. Although topical antiinflammatory medications may be used for associated dermatitis or to decrease intense pruritus, the risk of detectable levels of corticosteroids or calcineurin inhibitors must be kept in mind. For example, topical tacrolimus ointment has been found to be helpful for individuals with NS, but toxic levels have sometimes been detected,[264] emphasizing the need for careful monitoring.[266]

Oral retinoids (isotretinoin, acitretin) have led to dramatic improvement in some pediatric patients with the ichthyoses but should be used with caution because of their many potential side effects that limit long-term therapy, particularly bone toxicity.[354,355] Alitretinoin may be more effective at reducing erythema than acitretin but is less effective at reducing scaling[356] and is only available in Europe (not FDA approved).

Oral retinoids are generally reserved for use in adolescents and adults with more severe ichthyotic disorders that do not show a satisfactory response to topical agents. Because of the teratogenicity of retinoids, isotretinoin, with its much shorter half-life than acitretin, has often been used preferentially for fertile females with ichthyosis as an additional precaution to birth control. In general, oral retinoids are most effective for patients with a prominent scaling phenotype, particularly LI, and are not indicated for more erythrodermic forms, particularly NS.

Understanding the role of cutaneous inflammation in causing the phenotypic manifestations of ichthyosis has led to new directions in therapy. Anecdotal reports of improvement in NS with infliximab[268,269] and in a mouse model of HI from *in utero* overexpression of the anti-inflammatory cytokine interleukin 37b suggest that targeted anti-inflammatory therapy may be a new approach.[357] Transcriptional analysis of the skin (and blood) of patients with psoriasis has shown a shared Th17 signature, resembling that of psoriasis and implying that targeted biologics for psoriasis might ameliorate the skin disease in ichthyosis.[10,11,13] Two children with variants in *DSP*, the gene encoding desmoplakin, and erythrokeratodermia demonstrated marked improvement in both inflammation and scaling when administered the IL-12/IL-23 inhibitor ustekinumab.[12] Recombinant transglutaminase-1 enzyme encapsulated in liposomes reversed the ichthyosis phenotype and barrier function in a skin-humanized mouse model of LI,[358] but has not yet advanced to human trials.

Patients with the ichthyoses tend to be more susceptible to cutaneous infection, particularly dermatophyte and staphylococcal infections. Secondary infection should be considered when patients with ichthyosis (particularly ARCI and EI) develop a new eruption. The accumulation of scale predisposes to overgrowth of bacteria and an odor, which in addition to the significant cosmetic ramifications of these disorders, may lead to additional problems in social acceptance by peers. Patients with thick scale may benefit from use of mild antibacterial soaps (e.g., Lever 2000 or Cetaphil antibacterial soap) or use of antibacterial washes if not too irritating. Many patients benefit from the addition of bleach (4 mL per gallon or 1 mL per L; ½ cup per full standard tub) or baking soda (1 cup) into the bath water. Dermatophyte infections often require administration of systemic antifungal medications.[359]

Sweating is often inadequate in patients with ichthyosis due to the occlusion of eccrine ducts. Affected individuals should be guarded against overheating during winter months and kept in air conditioning during warmer months, with frequent wetting of the skin or even cooling suits (see Chapter 7) during sports activities.

The ectropion of patients with ARCI exposes the conjunctivae and cornea, resulting in irritation.[360] Bland moisturizing drops can be administered several times daily to provide protective moisture, and patients may benefit from wearing eye patches at night if the eyes cannot close entirely. Systemic treatment with retinoids may improve the ectropion,[361] and apremilast being used for concomitant psoriasis in a man with LI led to improved ectropion.[362]

Some physicians recommend plastic surgery to correct the ectropion,[363] because damage to the cornea may impair vision; however, this surgery is complex and often unsuccessful. Periorbital application of tazarotene (0.05% to 1.0% cream)[364,365] and N-acetylcysteine have decreased ectropion when used sparingly. Injection of small aliquots of hyaluronic acid into each eyelid has also been used to promote eyelid closure and reduce exposure keratopathy.[366]

Ichthyosis of the ear canal can lead to accumulation of skin debris and conductive hearing loss. In a recent survey, 80% with ichthyosis reported ear pruritus, 66% had trouble hearing, and 29% reported ear pain.[367] Regular professional ear cleaning and use of ear softeners can decrease the risk of hearing loss and recurrent ear infections.

In countries without significant dietary supplementation with vitamin D_3, ichthyosis, particularly the epidermolytic and lamellar forms (Fig. 5.45), has been associated with an increased risk of the development of rickets, which may be exacerbated by retinoid

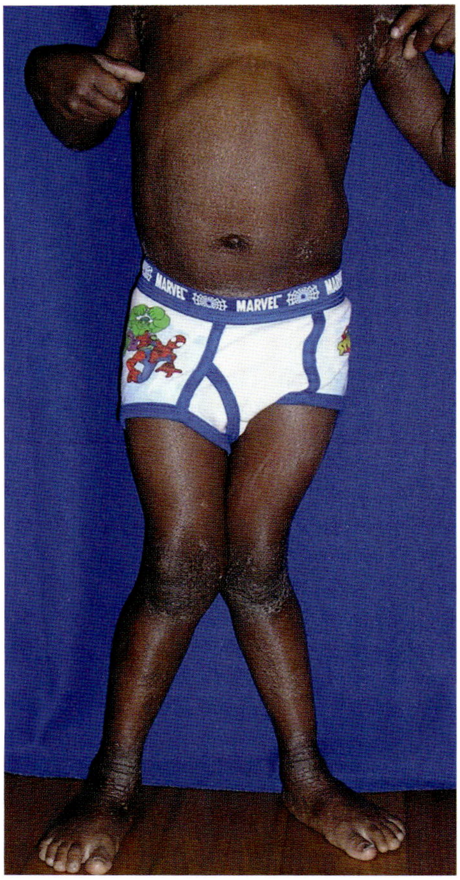

Fig. 5.45 Patients with ichthyosis are at increased risk for the development of rickets, as shown in this boy from Nigeria.

therapy.[368] Serum levels of parathyroid hormone at 75 pg/mL or more and 25(OH)D_3 at 8 ng/mL or less significantly increase the risk of developing rickets,[369] and a high level of alkaline phosphatase is another marker of rickets development.[370–373] The increased risk may relate to decreased ultraviolet light exposure, failure of UVB light to penetrate the thickened scale, and/or an abnormality in processing of vitamin D_3 in response to UVB light. Nevertheless, vitamin D_3 supplementation should be considered.

Other Disorders of Differentiation

DARIER DISEASE

Darier disease (keratosis follicularis, Darier–White disease; acral form, acrokeratosis verruciformis of Hopf) is an autosomal dominant disorder that most commonly first manifests between 8 and 15 years of age as flesh-colored papules that become covered with a yellow, waxy scaling crust (Figs. 5.46 to 5.48).[374] Lesions often coalesce to form thickened, warty plaques that are malodorous. Sites most often affected include the forehead, temples, ears, nasolabial folds, scalp, upper chest, and back in the so-called "seborrheic" distribution. Isolated scalp involvement has been reported and may be the presenting sign.[375] Linear streaks of Darier disease along Blaschko lines have been attributed to gene mosaicism.[376] Localized congenital Darier disease has been described and may represent type 2 mosaicism.[377] Lesions of Darier disease are often worsened by exposure to ultraviolet radiation, heat,[378] friction, and other forms of trauma. Secondary bacterial or herpes simplex virus infection is common.[379] *S. aureus* has been isolated from almost 70% of lesional skin areas, and colonization is correlated with more severe disease.[380]

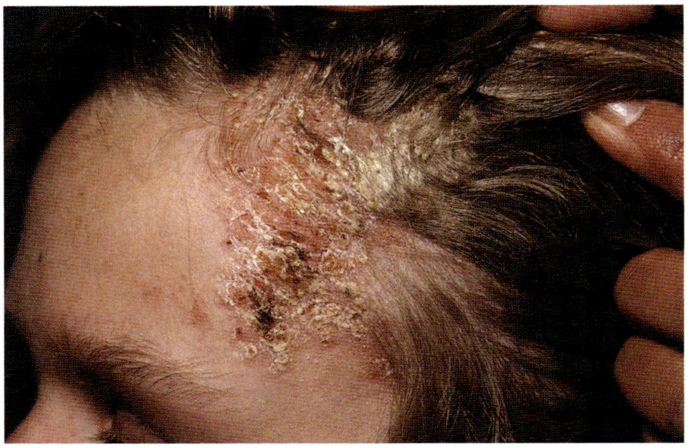

Fig. 5.46 Darier disease. Thickened, warty plaques on the forehead and temples are characteristic and tend to be symmetrically distributed.

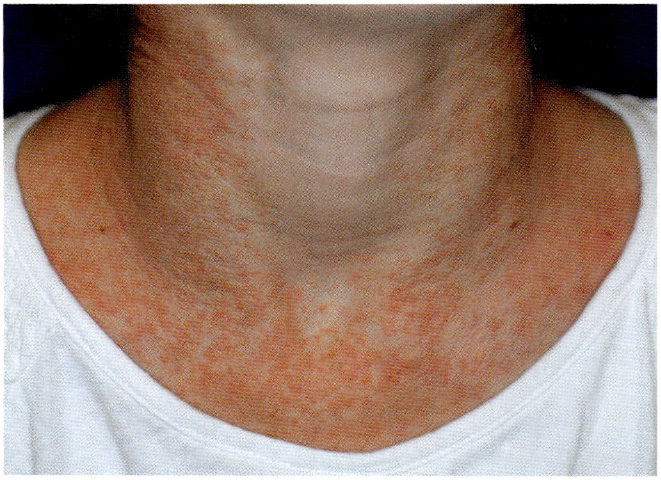

Fig. 5.47 Darier disease. The discrete keratotic papules of Darier disease have led to the alternative name *keratosis follicularis*.

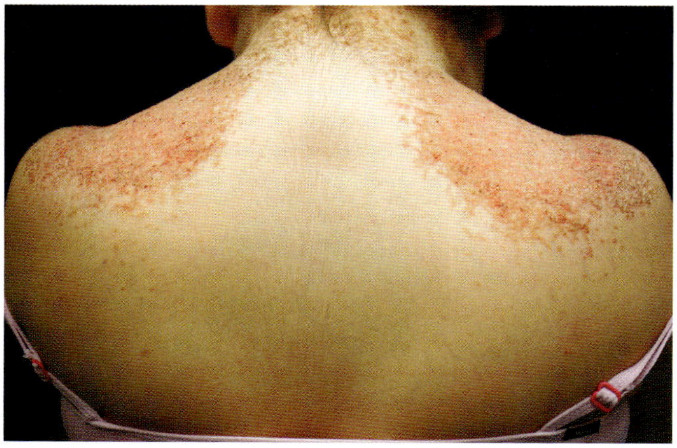

Fig. 5.48 Darier disease. Characteristic patterning of keratotic erythematous papules on the shoulders.

Punctate keratoses on the palms and soles, either raised or with a central pit, occur in most patients. Keratoses resembling flat warts may be found on the dorsal aspects of the hands (acrokeratosis verruciformis), which dermoscopically show[381] the papules as irregular and white with cobblestoning. In some patients, these acral keratotic lesions are the only manifestation; these cases have all been linked to p.Pro602Leu mutations in *ATP2A2*.[382] Guttate leukoderma has been described in a few patients with darker skin.[383,384] The nails are easily broken and often show a characteristic V-shaped scalloping of the free edge (see Chapter 7). Subungual thickening with streaks of discoloration and subungual hemorrhage may be seen (see Fig. 7.72). White, centrally depressed papules or verrucous white plaques simulating leukoplakia are often seen on the mucosae of the cheeks, palate, and gums[385] and may involve the rectum and vulva. Neuropsychiatric problems, including learning disability (in more than 40% of patients),[386] schizophrenia, bipolar disorder, and/or seizures, are seen in approximately 5% of patients,[387] and bone cysts may be associated with Darier disease as well.[388]

The characteristic histopathologic changes of Darier disease include intraepidermal suprabasal clefts or lacunae and the formation of acantholytic "corps ronds" (cells with a basophilic nucleus surrounded by a clear halo) and "grains" (small, dark cells with a pyknotic nucleus) in the stratum corneum. Mutations responsible for Darier disease involve *ATP2A2*, which encodes the sarcoplasmic/endoplasmic reticulum calcium ATPase type 2 (SERCA2).[389] Epidermal differentiation requires elevations in calcium levels for intercellular junction assembly, and the affected enzyme participates in the calcium pump system.[390–396] Although 12% to 40% of patients with Darier disease have no identifiable *ATP2A2* mutation, no other gene has been associated.[397]

Systemic[398,399] administration of retinoids has resulted in significant improvement in most affected individuals.[400] Infection control is of paramount importance for some individuals. Topical application of 5-fluorouracil,[401,402] tacrolimus ointment,[403] and diclofenac gel[404] have been reported to be helpful. Doxycycline has been helpful in a few patients.[405,406] Recalcitrant areas have been treated successfully with carbon dioxide, erbium:yttrium-aluminum-garnet (YAG), and pulsed-dye lasers.[407–410] Miglustat, a commercially available inhibitor of sphingolipid synthesis, corrects the defect in differentiation and adhesion of Darier keratinocytes *in vitro* and may be a future systemic treatment.[395] Cyclooxygenase-2 (COX-2) inhibition has been shown to restore the UVB-induced downregulation of SERCA2 expression in keratinocytes, suggesting the possibility that celecoxib could be another therapeutic modality for Darier disease.[411]

HAILEY–HAILEY DISEASE (FAMILIAL BENIGN PEMPHIGUS)

Hailey–Hailey disease is an autosomal dominant genodermatosis characterized by recurrent vesicles and erosions that most commonly appear on the sides and back of the neck, in the axillae, in the groin, and in the perianal regions (Fig. 5.49).[412] The disorder usually has its onset in the late teens or early twenties but has been reported in a 5-month-old infant.[413] Most cases have a fairly constant course. The primary lesions are small vesicles that occur in groups on normal or erythematous skin. The vesicles may enlarge to form bullae and rupture easily, leaving an eroded base; they exude serum and develop crusts resembling impetigo. The Nikolsky sign may be present. Lesions tend to spread peripherally with an active, often serpiginous, border, and central resolution with peripheral extension often results in circinate lesions. In the intertriginous area, lesions tend to form erythematous plaques with dry crusting and soft, flat, and moist granular vegetations. Burning or pruritus is common, and particularly in the intertriginous areas lesions tend to become irritating, painful, and exceedingly uncomfortable. Mucosal involvement is uncommon, but papular lesions of the oral mucosa, esophagus, vagina, and conjunctivae have been described. As with Darier disease, mosaic forms of Hailey–Hailey disease have been described and course along lines of Blaschko[414]; streaks of Hailey–Hailey disease may present during childhood in individuals with genomic *ATP2C1* mutations who develop a second mutation in the normal allele (type 2 mosaicism).[415]

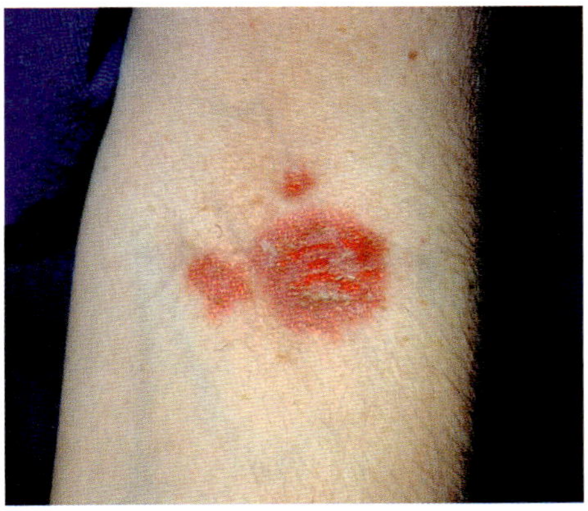

Fig. 5.49 Hailey–Hailey disease. Crusted, erosive plaques that are symmetrically distributed, especially at fold areas.

Skin sections from the advancing border of a lesion show a suprabasal vesicle with acantholysis of epidermal cells that resembles a dilapidated brick wall. Mutations have been identified in *ATP2C1*, encoding a secretory calcium (Ca^{++})/manganese (Mn^{++})–adenosine triphosphatase (ATPase) pump of the Golgi apparatus.[416]

The cutaneous lesions of Hailey–Hailey disease are induced by several external stimuli, particularly heat, humidity, friction from ill-fitting clothing, exposure to ultraviolet light, and bacterial or candidal infection. Intervention includes avoidance of these precipitating factors through wearing lightweight clothing, avoidance of friction and overheating, and treatment with topical or systemic antimicrobials as required for colonization or infection. Patients may experience spontaneous improvement with exacerbations and remissions.

Topical application of corticosteroids or calcineurin inhibitors[417] has been the mainstay of treatment for most patients; topical calcitriol has led to improvement as well.[418] Topical application of gentamicin led to lesional clearance in a patient with an *ATP2C1* premature stop mutation, attributed both to the antibacterial effect and to the ability of aminoglycoside therapy to induce readthrough of a pathogenic nonsense mutation[419]; oral antibiotics are used for recurrent secondary infections. Because of the role of sweating as an exacerbation, botulinum toxin type A injections have been useful for selected patients.[420] Naltrexone has led to improvement in several patients,[421–424] and the use of minocycline and doxycycline[425,426] has been described. In persistent and disabling cases, oral retinoids,[427] photodynamic therapy,[428,429] ablative laser therapy, narrowband UVB,[430] dermabrasion, or excision of involved regions followed by split-thickness skin grafts have been used.

Porokeratoses

The porokeratoses are a group of hyperkeratotic disorders characterized by a thread-like, raised hyperkeratotic border that shows a typical thin column of parakeratosis, or cornoid lamella, on histologic examination of lesional tissue.[431,432] The cornoid lamella can be more easily seen clinically by dermoscopy.[433]

Porokeratosis is thought to be a disorder of dysregulated keratinization with epidermal cell hyperproliferation and premature apoptosis of keratinocytes.[434] The porokeratoses may appear in several classic forms: (1) classic porokeratosis of Mibelli, (2) linear porokeratosis, (3) punctate porokeratosis and porokeratosis palmaris et plantaris disseminata (PPPD), and (4) disseminated superficial actinic porokeratosis (DSAP)/disseminated superficial porokeratosis. Several other unusual variants have been described, and many disorders can occasionally show cornoid lamellation and be confused histologically (not clinically) with porokeratosis (e.g., psoriasis, Fox–Fordyce disease).[435]

Porokeratosis of Mibelli may manifest as one, a few, or many annular lesions that usually appear during childhood, enlarge over years, and persist indefinitely (Figs. 5.50 and 5.51).[436] Boys are affected more commonly than girls. The disorder has a predilection for the face, neck, forearms, and hands but also may affect the feet,

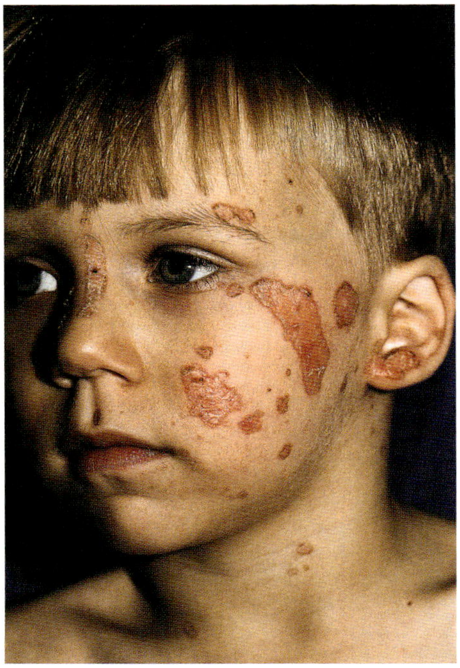

Fig. 5.50 Porokeratosis. Multiple erythematous annular lesions surrounded by a wall-like ridge of scaling.

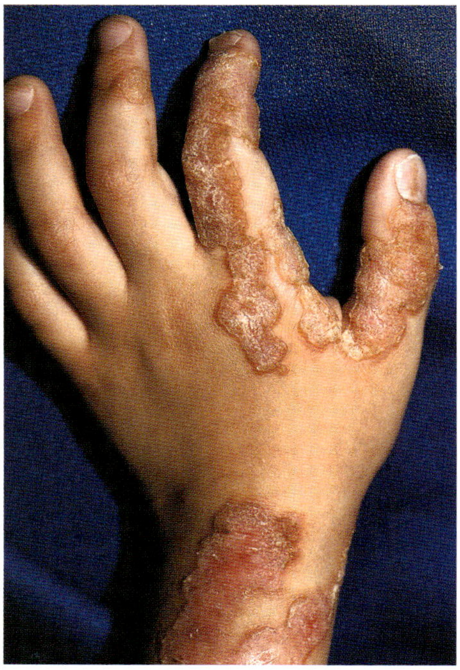

Fig. 5.51 Porokeratosis. Annular lesions with a hyperkeratotic, peripheral, wall-like ridge.

ankles, buccal mucosa, and glans penis. Porokeratosis on the scalp may be associated with alopecia. The initial lesion begins as a crateriform hyperkeratotic papule that gradually expands to a plaque of circinate or irregular contour measuring from a few millimeters to several centimeters in diameter. If several lesions are present, they are usually unilateral. The diagnostic feature of this disorder is the raised hyperkeratotic peripheral ridge, which has been compared with the Great Wall of China. A useful technique to accentuate the scaling is to stain the edges with gentian violet (surgical marking pen), wipe off the ink with an alcohol pad, and then view the ring to see the characteristic collarette of scale.[437] Lesions are commonly mistaken for tinea corporis, warts, or granuloma annulare.

Linear porokeratosis presents in infancy or childhood as one to several collections of porokeratotic lesions that resemble porokeratosis of Mibelli but follow the lines of Blaschko, similar to epidermal nevi.[438,439] Although unusual, linear porokeratosis may be indistinguishable clinically from inflammatory linear verrucous epidermal nevi (ILVEN; Fig 5.52). Ulcerated forms of linear porokeratosis have been described.[440]

Porokeratotic eccrine ostial and dermal duct nevus (PEODDN) is a form of linear porokeratosis that involves the adnexal structures, specifically the eccrine ostia and ducts and hair follicles.[441–443] PEODDN includes the previously termed *porokeratotic eccrine and hair follicle nevus* and *porokeratotic adnexal ostial nevus*. The nevus may be present at birth, but if not, usually appears during the first years of life and occasionally during adulthood. Lesions present as multiple asymptomatic, hyperkeratotic, sometimes spiny papules and plaques and punctate pits, often filled with a comedo-like keratin plug (Fig. 5.53).[444,445]

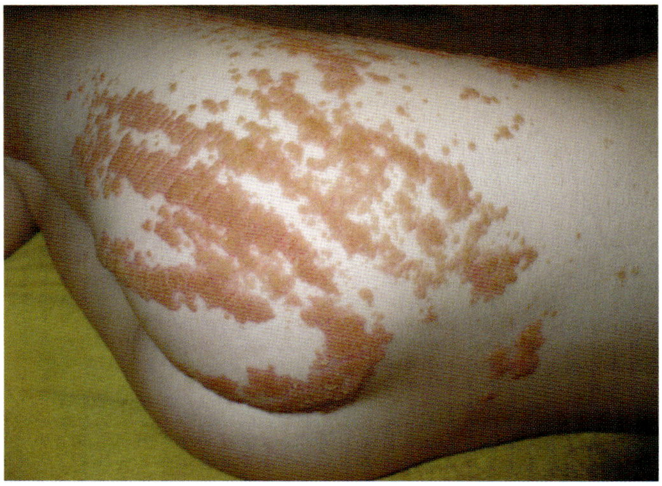

Fig. 5.52 Linear porokeratosis. Blaschkoid plaques of erythema and scaling that resemble inflammatory linear verrucous epidermal nevi (ILVEN) but resulted from a genomic and a somatic mutation in *PMVK*, leading to blockade of cholesterol biosynthesis. Topical treatment with compounded 2% lovastatin/2% cholesterol led to virtual disappearance.

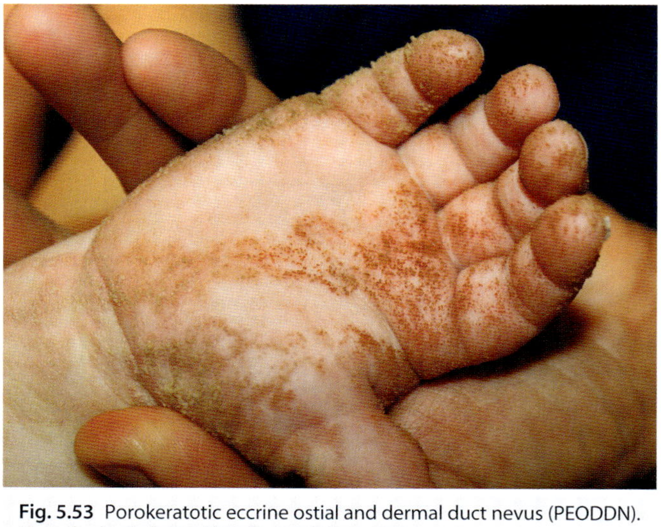

Fig. 5.53 Porokeratotic eccrine ostial and dermal duct nevus (PEODDN). Note the hyperkeratotic spiny papules.

The collections of papules tend to be distributed along Blaschko lines, particularly on the distal extremities, although lesions have been described on the face, proximal extremities, and trunk, including associated with unilateral breast hypoplasia. Lesions may be erythematous and eroded, especially during the neonatal period. Biopsy sections show a dilated eccrine acrosyringium and, in some cases, hair follicle with an overlying cornoid lamella. In most patients, the lesions are static, but progressive extension has been described. Spontaneous improvement of lesions on the extremities has been noted, whereas lesions on the palms and soles tend to persist.

Punctate porokeratosis presents as 1- to 2-mm punctate papules of the palms and soles during adolescence or adulthood. The peripheral raised rim may be difficult to appreciate, and differentiation from keratoderma punctata, Darier disease, and Cowden disease may require biopsy. PPPD is an autosomal dominant variant of punctuate porokeratosis that occurs more often in males. Small "seed-like" keratotic papules with a slightly elevated peripheral rim first develop during childhood or adolescence on the palms and soles. Lesions subsequently disseminate to other areas of the body, including parts not exposed to sunlight and the mucous membranes. Lesions may be asymptomatic to pruritic.

DSAP is the most common form of porokeratosis but rarely presents in its disseminated form during childhood[446–448] and only occasionally during late adolescence. Women are more often affected than men. An autosomal dominant disorder, most cases are sporadic and first show manifestations during the third or fourth decade of life. Lesions appear on sun-exposed areas of the skin, particularly on the lower legs and forearms, and are usually multiple, with most patients having more than 50 lesions. Most lesions measure 0.5 to 1 cm, with a range from 0.1 to 4.5 cm in diameter, and are asymptomatic to mildly pruritic. In contrast to the borders of the lesions of porokeratosis of Mibelli, the ridges are only slightly elevated above the cutaneous surface. Several individuals have been described with both DSAP and linear porokeratosis. Linear porokeratosis may be present during childhood in patients with DSAP as type 2 mosaicism with mutation in the normal allele (loss of heterozygosity), leading to an earlier and more severe lesion distributed along a line of Blaschko with DSAP appearing later, especially after ultraviolet light exposure.[446,448–450] Involvement with type 2 mosaicism may be extensive (see Fig. 5.52). Disseminated superficial porokeratosis is also autosomal dominant and has its onset during the third or fourth decade of life. Lesions primarily occur on the extremities and are bilaterally symmetric but do not spare sun-protected areas, as occurs in DSAP. Immunosuppression (e.g., HIV infection or organ transplantation[447]) can also trigger the appearance of disseminated porokeratotic lesions.[451]

Porokeratosis usually results from mutations in genes encoding components of the cholesterol/isoprenoid biosynthesis pathway. Most of these mutations to date have been linked with DSAP, which is genetically heterogenous. Most commonly, heterozygous gene alterations are found in *MVD*, which encodes mevalonate diphosphodecarboxylase, or *MVK*, which encodes mevalonate kinase.[452] However, variants in these same genes are most often found to cause porokeratosis in children.[452] These gene products play a role in regulating calcium-induced keratinocyte differentiation and could protect keratinocytes from apoptosis induced by UV light, a known trigger.[453] Other genes of the same pathway[452] that are occasionally linked to porokeratosis are *PMVK* (phosphomevalonate kinase),[454] *FDPS* (farnesyl diphosphate synthase), and *SLC17A9* (solute carrier family 17, member 9),[455] with other candidate genes also suggested.[456,457] Somatic mutations in *GJB2* (encoding connexin 26, the gene implicated in KID syndrome with genomic mutations) are thought to be responsible[218] for the PEODDN form of linear porokeratosis[458]; the spiky hyperkeratotic papules of PEODDN have been associated with deafness[459] and KID syndrome.[460]

Porokeratosis is a feature of CDAGS syndrome, an autosomal recessive disorder characterized by craniosynostosis and clavicular hypoplasia, delayed closure of the fontanel and deafness, imperforate or anteriorly displaced anus, genitourinary malformations (especially hypospadias and urethrorectal fistula), and the porokeratotic skin eruption.[461–463] Other features include hearing loss and nonscarring alopecia.[462] The lesions typically affect the face (especially cheeks and chin) and extremities (elbows, knees, dorsal aspect of hands). The disorder has been mapped to chromosome 22q12-13,[464] but the underlying molecular defect is unknown.

Lesions of porokeratosis are slowly progressive and relatively asymptomatic but may require intervention for cosmesis. The development of squamous cell carcinoma or Bowen disease within lesions has occasionally been reported with all forms except the punctuate form, but the risk is highest with long-standing lesions.

A variety of therapies have been used, including keratolytics, diclofenac gel,[465–468] topical and oral retinoids,[469,470] topical imiquimod,[471] topical 5-fluorouracil, topical ingenol mebutate,[472] cantharidin,[473] cryotherapy, electrodesiccation, laser ablation,[474–476] photodynamic therapy with methyl aminolevulinate cream,[477–480] dermabrasion, curettage, and excision. Children with linear forms of porokeratosis associated with biallelic mutations in *PMVK* or *MVD* (i.e., with marked reduction in enzyme activity) may benefit from topical application of the combination of a statin and cholesterol, as has been helpful for CHILD syndrome and consistent with the cascade of mutations in genes associated with the cholesterol/isoprenoid biosynthesis pathway.[481] This observation suggests that topical application of compounded statin/cholesterol may be beneficial for other forms of porokeratosis from genetic alterations that disrupt cholesterol biosynthesis.

Palmoplantar Keratodermas

PPK (palmar and plantar hyperkeratosis, keratoderma of the palms and soles) describes a diffuse or localized thickening of the palms and soles that may occur as part of a genetic disorder or as an inflammatory disorder such as pityriasis rubra pilaris, psoriasis, or reactive arthritis (see Chapter 4).[482–484] Genetic forms of PPK may be nonsyndromic,[485,486] appearing alone or in association with other cutaneous/adnexal features (such as with LI, EI, pachyonychia congenita [see Chapter 7], hidrotic ectodermal dysplasia [see Chapter 7], or epidermolysis bullosa simplex [see Chapter 13]). Alternatively, PPK may be syndromic, as in Carvajal syndrome (cardiac arrythmia) or Vohwinkel syndrome (deafness).

Several classification systems have been proposed for the inherited forms of PPK, the simplest of which is striate, focal, diffuse, or punctate PPK. The identification of the underlying molecular defect allows further classification. In some cases, mutations in a particular gene can cause more than one pattern. For example, mutations in *DSG1* can cause focal and diffuse PPKs, although striate PPK is the more typical outcome.[487] Finally, a classification by functional subgroup has also been proposed and includes abnormalities in structural proteins (keratins), cornified envelopes (loricrin), cell–cell communication (connexins), cohesion (desmoplakin 1, desmoglein 1, plakophilin), and transmembrane signaling (cathepsin C).[488] Hereditary forms of PPK often first manifest when the affected child starts to walk and are usually symmetrical. Diffuse forms may initially appear focal, but the more extensive involvement is notable within the first few years of life.

In general, the treatment of all forms of hyperkeratosis of the palms and soles is palliative and consists of application of keratolytic formulations, such as 10% to 20% salicylic acid in a thick emollient cream (under occlusion at night if tolerated); intermittent use of Keralyt gel or 40% salicylic acid (Mediplast) plasters; periodic soaking of the affected area in water; and gentle removal of excessive keratinous material by a pumice stone, scalpel, or single-edged razor blade. Painful fissures can be treated by a formulation of 30% tincture of benzoin in zinc oxide or cyanoacrylate (Superglue) before the application of a keratolytic formulation. Patients should wear comfortable shoes and avoid pressure or friction to affected areas. Although oral retinoids are helpful, they are recommended only for short-term use for the temporary relief of individuals with significant disability; topical retinoids may be helpful for more limited keratoderma. Surgical excision and grafting have been used with variable results.[489] Specific therapeutic recommendations are noted later for certain forms of PPK.

STRIATE PPK

Striate PPK is characterized by focal keratoderma on the soles that often develops during infancy. Focal or characteristic streaks of keratoderma may develop on the palmar surface, especially if traumatized. Plantar involvement is nummular, not linear. The condition usually results from heterozygous mutations in the gene encoding either desmoplakin or desmoglein-1[490–494] and affects the ability of keratin filaments to attach to the cell membrane. Striate PPK can be a feature of mild homozygous mutations in *DSG1*[495] (vs. the more typical resulting SAM syndrome) and heterozygous mutations in the end domains of *KRT1*.[496] Carvajal syndrome and children with Costello syndrome (see Fig. 6.13) both feature striate PPK and curly hair,[497] although the PPK is often more extensive on the plantar aspects.

FOCAL KERATODERMAS

Pachyonychia congenita (PC) describes a group of autosomal dominant conditions characterized most prominently by a characteristic nail dystrophy in association with painful plantar keratoderma (see Fig. 5.54) that has a great impact on quality of life (see Chapter 7; Figs. 7.67 and 7.68). Mutations occur in one of five keratins: *KRT6a*, *KRT6b*, *KRT6c*, *KRT16*, or *KRT17*.[498,499] Presentation with focal PPK alone with minimal or no nail changes occasionally is caused by mutations in *KRT16* but is typical with mutations in *KRT6c*.[500] High-frequency ultrasound has shown bullae underlying the plantar keratoderma, which likely contribute to the pain.[501] Treatment is difficult, and only mechanical treatments, topical retinoids, and topical steroids have shown significant therapeutic efficacy.[502]

PPK and deafness due to mutations in the mitochondrial genome occur in the mitochondrial transfer RNA (tRNA) encoding the *MTTS1* gene. The focal PPK is typically first seen at 5 to 15 years of age.[503] Most prevalent over the plantar surface, keratotic plaques may also develop on the palm and at other pressure sites, including the knees and elbows, Achilles tendons, and the dorsal surface of the toes. Palmar involvement is most pronounced in adults who are manual workers. Hearing loss occurs in approximately 60% of patients, and the PPK occurs in approximately 30%.

Richner–Hanhart syndrome (tyrosinemia type II) is an autosomal recessive disorder caused by a deficiency of hepatic tyrosine aminotransferase (mutations in the *TAT* gene)[504] and resulting in accumulation of tyrosine.[505,506] The early cutaneous lesions may be seen during childhood as sharply demarcated, yellowish keratotic papules of the palmar and plantar surfaces and sometimes occur during the late teenage years. The lesions become more erythematous, erosive, and painful with time. Nail dystrophy may be associated. Photophobia and bilateral tearing commonly occur within the first 3 months of life and progress to corneal erosions; herpetic ulceration is often erroneously diagnosed. Mildly affected individuals have been described and may have just focal PPK with mild or no ocular manifestations.[507,508] The treatment of choice is dietary restriction of tyrosine with a low-phenylalanine, low-tyrosine diet.

Howel–Evans syndrome (tylosis with esophageal cancer) is a late-onset form of autosomal dominant focal PPK associated with the development of mucosal squamous cell carcinoma in 95% of affected patients by the age of 65 years, particularly of the esophageal mucosa (38-fold increased risk).[509] The PPK is most prominent on pressure areas on the soles and is usually fully penetrant, with the onset between 6 and 12 years of age. Palmar involvement is most prominent in manual laborers. Frictional hyperkeratosis may occur at other areas of trauma such as the elbows and knees, and oral leukokeratosis is often seen. Follicular hyperkeratoses are common and may be the initial manifestation in younger patients. The condition results from mutations in *RHBDF2*, which encodes the inactive rhomboid protease iRhom2 and results in dysregulation of EGFR signaling.[510]

DIFFUSE KERATODERMAS

Epidermolytic PPK (EPPK; Vörner type) is an autosomal dominant disorder characterized by sharply circumscribed congenital thickening of the palms and soles (Fig. 5.55). Most patients have hyperhidrosis, which may lead to maceration and fissuring. The waxy hyperkeratosis, limited to the palms and soles, is surrounded by an erythematous border. Transgrediens (to the dorsal surface) may be seen, and some patients show thickened skin over the joints (knuckle pads).[511,512] Mild thickening over the elbows and knees may occur. An associated odor suggests secondary bacterial or fungal infection. Biopsy sections often show epidermolytic hyperkeratosis similar to that seen in EI, although more than one sample may be required to demonstrate the epidermolysis. Blistering, however, is not usually seen except the increased fragility that can occur with retinoid therapy. The disorder results from mutations in keratin 9, a form of keratin protein expressed only in the palms and soles.[513] Personalized ribonucleic acid interference (RNAi)–based therapy has been developed in a *KRT9*-mutated mouse model of EPPK.[514]

Diffuse nonepidermolytic PPK (NEPPK; Unna type) is an autosomal dominant genodermatosis that clinically is indistinguishable from EPPK other than tending to be milder, but it does not show epidermolysis in biopsy sections. This form of PPK has been attributed largely to mutations in noncritical regions of the gene that encodes keratin 1 and to mutations in *KRT6a* or *16* (without the nail changes of PC, also caused by mutations in these genes).[515] Greither syndrome, with transgrediens involvement in a glove-and-sock distribution, is considered a more severe form of diffuse NEPPK, and mutations have been found in *KRT1*.[516] Diffuse NEPPK is a component of Naegeli–Franceschetti–Jadassohn syndrome and dermatopathia pigmentosa reticularis, allelic disorders resulting from mutations in *KRT14* that are also characterized by abnormal sweating, reticulate hyperpigmentation, absence of dermatoglyphics, and other ectodermal anomalies (see Chapter 7).[517,518]

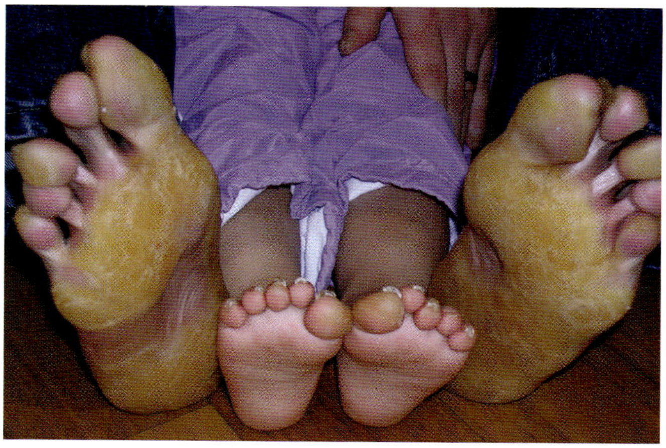

Fig. 5.54 Pachyonychia congenita. Focal palmoplantar keratoderma at sites of pressure. Note the autosomal dominant inheritance, mild plantar keratoderma at this age, and abnormal nails in the 2-year-old daughter.

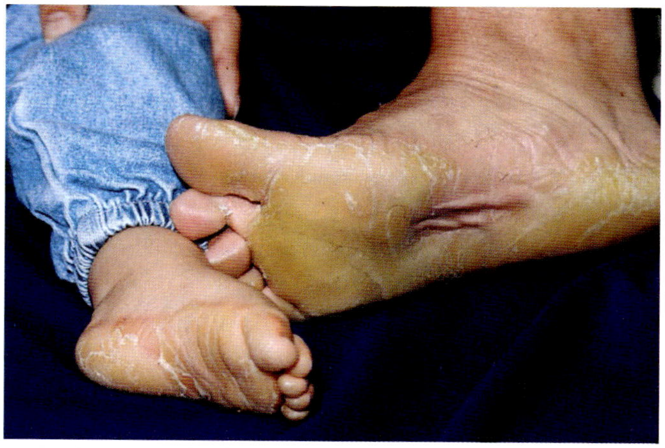

Fig. 5.55 Epidermolytic palmoplantar keratoderma. Waxy thickening is limited to the palms and soles and is usually surrounded by an erythematous border. This is an autosomal dominant disorder, as shown in mother and daughter.

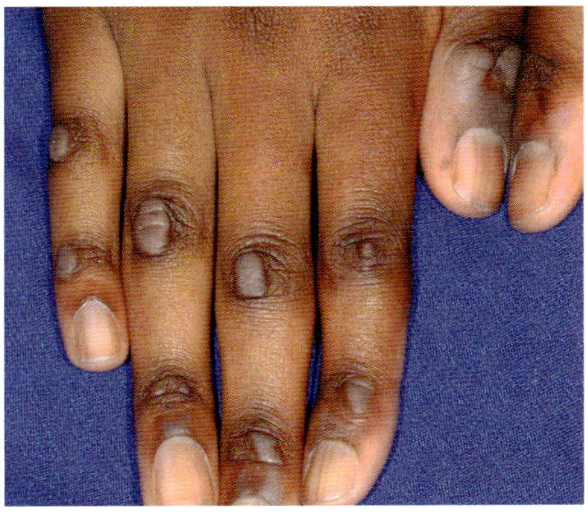

Fig. 5.56 Knuckle pads. These hyperkeratotic plaques can be seen as an isolated entity but may be associated with palmoplantar keratoderma.

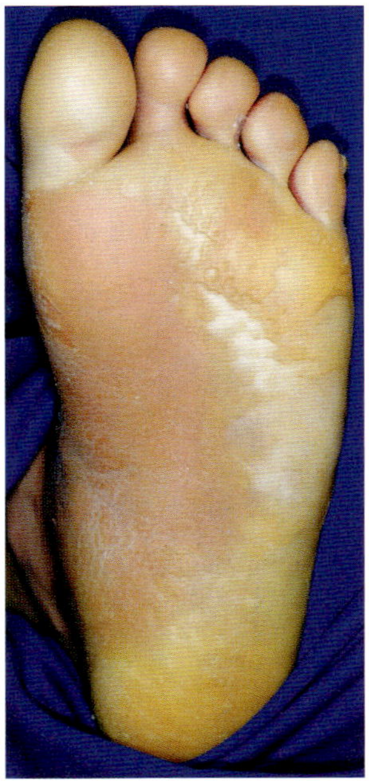

Fig. 5.57 Mal de Meleda palmoplantar keratoderma. Diffuse plantar keratoderma overlying erythema that extends to the dorsal aspects of the feet and hands. The Mal de Meleda type is one of the few autosomal recessive forms of hereditary palmoplantar keratoderma.

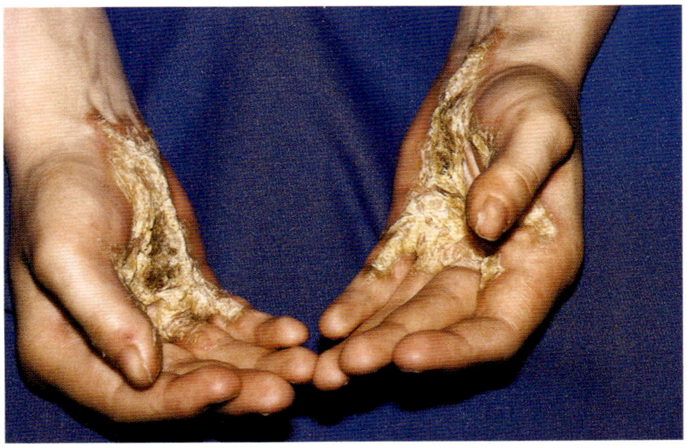

Fig. 5.58 Olmsted syndrome. Mutilating, painful plaques of keratoderma on the palms and soles begin during infancy to early childhood.

PPK associated with hearing loss occurs in individuals with Vohwinkel syndrome, an autosomal dominant mutilating keratoderma characterized by extensive PPK with a distinct "honeycomb" pattern and constrictions (pseudoainhum) that may lead to amputation of distal digits.[519] In some cases, distinctive hyperkeratotic starfish-like plaques are present over the elbows, knees, and sometimes the knuckles. Sensorineural deafness is a common accompanying feature. Mutations in the *GJB2* gene encoding connexin 26 underlie Vohwinkel syndrome; nonmutilating PPK with deafness, knuckle pads, and leukonychia (Bart–Pumphrey syndrome) and, as if mosaic, PEODDN.[520,521] Knuckle pads can also be a feature of other forms of PPK[488,511,522] and occur as an isolated entity (Fig. 5.56).[523] Knuckle pads should not be confused with calluses (usually more lateral) and pachydermodactyly, a form of soft tissue fibromatosis that affects the second to fourth fingers and has been linked to the repetitive friction and trauma of gaming in adolescents. The ichthyotic variant of Vohwinkel syndrome also shows PPK with a honeycomb appearance and pseudoainhum but has associated ichthyosis and no deafness (see Loricrin Keratoderma section earlier).

Clouston syndrome (hidrotic ectodermal dysplasia) is an autosomal dominant condition that results from mutations in the *GJB6* gene encoding connexin 30 (see Chapter 7).[524] Keratoderma (hyperkeratosis) of the palms and soles is common and may be diffuse or focal. It occasionally extends to involve the sides and dorsal aspects of affected hands and feet. Nails grow slowly and may appear thickened or thinned, striated, discolored, brittle, or hypoplastic. The tips of the digits show pseudoclubbing (see Chapter 7, Fig. 7.23), and hyperpigmentation may overlie digital joints. Paronychial infections are common and may result in partial to complete destruction of the nail matrix. Body hair may be sparse, eyebrows and eyelashes may be thinned or absent, and the skin has a smooth texture. Scalp hair, generally normal during infancy and childhood, may become thin, fragile, or sparse to absent after puberty. Diffuse PPK with dystrophic, leukodermic nails and exuberant, bushy scalp hair has been linked to biallelic mutations in *FAM83G*, which is likely a repressor of Wnt signaling and proliferation.[525]

Mal de Meleda (keratosis palmoplantaris transgrediens) is an autosomal recessive form of diffuse PPK associated with inflammatory keratotic plaques that extend to the dorsal aspects of the hands and feet and may overlie joints (Fig. 5.57).[526] Hyperhidrosis, superinfection, and occasionally perioral erythema, brachydactyly, and nail abnormalities may be associated. Female carriers may show mild PPK with interdigital fissures and keratotic papules.[527] Flexion contractures and spontaneous amputation of the digits occur in severe cases. Mal de Meleda is the result of mutations in *ARS* component B, which encodes *SLURP-1*.[528,529] The role of *SLURP-1* in epidermal homeostasis and tumor necrosis factor (TNF) α inhibition explains the hyperproliferative and inflammatory phenotype.

Olmsted syndrome (mutilating PPK with periorificial plaques) is a rare autosomal dominant disorder characterized by the progressive development of mutilating, painful plaques of keratoderma on the palms and soles that begins during infancy to early childhood (Fig. 5.58).[530,531] The borders of the keratoderma tend to be erythematous, and hyperkeratotic plaques may affect intertriginous folds. Contractures and autoamputation from progressive constriction of the digits are common. Periorificial areas become thickened and fissured to varying degrees. Patients often show alopecia, corneal defects, and nail dystrophy and may have oral leukokeratosis. The risk of cutaneous squamous cell carcinoma is increased. Olmsted syndrome results from mutations in *TRPV3* (transient receptor potential cation channel, subfamily V, member 3),[532,533] which encodes a cation channel in the skin and brain that senses temperature and regulates vasoconstriction. This channel also plays a role in regulation of calcium ion transport and hair cycling, which may explain the PPK and alopecia of Olmsted syndrome, and in cutaneous inflammation,[534] which may explain the associated erythema and contribute to the pain.

X-linked Olmsted syndrome has been linked to mutations in *MBTPS2* and is allelic with ichthyosis follicular, atrichia, and photophobia/IFAP and keratosis follicularis spinulosa decalvans (KFSD) syndromes[535] (see Chapter 7).[536] Patients show the alopecia, periorificial keratoderma, and severe palmoplantar keratoderma. Recent studies have shown that the TRPV3 regulatory region is a target for MBTPS2, which may contribute to the overlapping features.[537]

Oral retinoids can be helpful in decreasing the keratoderma and the intense associated discomfort,[538] and low-dose retinoid with topical combination calcipotriol/betamethasone dipropionate has also been successful in patients with associated pruritus.[539] In addition to oral retinoids, EGFR inhibitors have been shown to improve the PPK.[540] Full-thickness excision of plaques with skin grafting has been successful in several patients.[541]

Alopecia and mutilating keratoderma can also be seen in PPK–congenital alopecia syndrome, which can be autosomal dominant and milder or autosomal recessive and associated with pseudoainhum, sclerodactyly (which must be distinguished from Huriez syndrome, see next paragraph), contractures, and sometimes cataracts; the underlying cause is unclear.[542]

Sclerotylosis (Huriez syndrome, PPK with scleroatrophy) is an autosomal dominant PPK that presents at birth with a diffuse, symmetric keratoderma of the palms and soles. The fingers have a pseudosclerodermatous appearance with scleroatrophy, adermatoglyphia, and often hypohidrosis of the palms and soles (Fig. 5.59).[543] Contractures of the digits are often seen, and reticulate erythema is sometimes seen on the dorsal surface. Raynaud phenomenon is not a feature, which can distinguish further from scleroderma. Nail abnormalities, including longitudinal ridging, hypoplasia, and clubbing, have been reported. Patients show an increased risk of developing highly metastatic squamous cell carcinoma of the palms or soles during the third and fourth decades,[544] and bowel cancer has been described. The disorder results from variants at a specific splice site in *SMARCAD1*, which is a chromatin remodeler that is involved in ultraviolet light–induced DNA repair.[545] Autosomal dominant adermatoglyphia[546] and Basan syndrome, which lacks the sclerodermatous changes and tendency for squamous cell carcinoma but has been associated with facial milia and acral bullae, are allelic variants.[547]

Sclerodactyly and PPK with an increased risk of squamous cell carcinoma are also features of Micali syndrome,[548,549] an autosomal recessive disorder that results from mutations in *RSPO1*, mapped to 1q34 and encoding R-spondin 1.[550–552] Variable features include chronic periodontal disease with early loss of teeth, bilateral cataracts and optic nerve coloboma, and hypertriglyceridemia. Deficiency of R-spondin 1 in men results in PPK and the risk of squamous cell carcinoma alone, but in female individuals with 46,XX leads to sex reversal with the development of ambiguous genitalia, hypospadias, hypoplastic testes, and low testosterone levels.

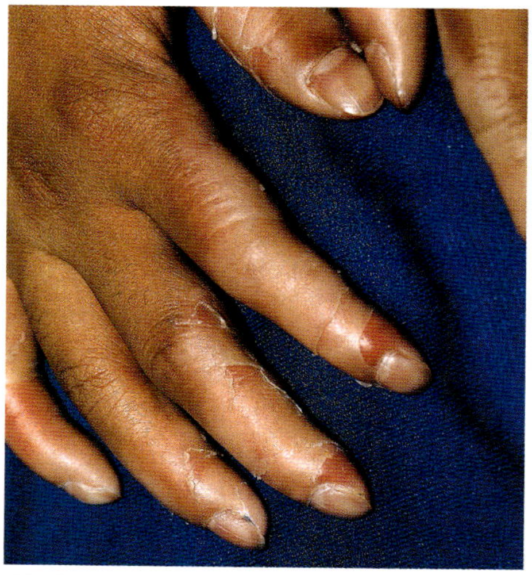

Fig. 5.59 Huriez syndrome. Palmoplantar keratoderma is associated with sclerodactyly. Affected individuals have a high risk of developing local squamous cell carcinoma.

Naxos disease and Carvajal syndrome (PPK with arrhythmogenic cardiomyopathy) are autosomal recessive forms of PPK associated with an early risk of sudden death from cardiac arrhythmia.[553–557] The keratoderma, which develops during infancy, tends to be more diffuse in Naxos disease and more striate in Carvajal syndrome. Patients with Carvajal syndrome also progressively develop striated lichenoid keratoses of the flexural areas and follicular keratoses of the knees and elbows. Both are associated with woolly hair from birth. The prominent cardiac abnormalities, including electrocardiograph (ECG) changes, ventricular arrhythmias, and ventricular structural alterations, may not become clinically apparent until the middle of the second decade of life. In general, right ventriculopathy has been associated with Naxos disease and left ventriculopathy with Carvajal syndrome, but some patients have abnormalities of both ventricles.[555,558] The disorders result from mutations in *JUP*, which encodes the desmosomal component plakoglobin,[559] or in *DSP*, which encodes desmoplakin. Keratoderma and woolly hair, but not cardiomyopathy, can occur in individuals with mutations in *KANK2*, which encodes a nondesmosomal protein that controls activation of steroid receptors, including the vitamin D receptor.[560] Sparse, woolly hair and dilated cardiomyopathy are seen in erythrokeratodermia with cardiomyopathy (also *DSP* mutations) and infants with mutations in *PPP1R13L*, leading to the absence of iASPP, a transcriptional regulator of innate immunity.[561] Cardiomyopathy is present during infancy with *PPP1R13L* mutations, but has its onset later during childhood with *DSP/JUP* mutations. Skin manifestations also tend to be milder with *PPP1R13L* mutations.

The Papillon–Lefévre syndrome and its variant, Haim–Munk syndrome, are autosomal recessive disorders that usually first show erythema and diffuse to localized psoriasiform hyperkeratosis of the palms (Fig. 5.60, *A*) and especially the soles during infancy or early childhood, coinciding with the timing of eruption of the primary teeth.[562–564] The keratoderma often extends to the dorsal aspects of the hands and feet (Fig. 5.60, *B*). Psoriasiform lesions occur on the knees and elbows. Rapidly progressive periodontitis and periosteal changes of the alveolar bone result in loss of both deciduous and permanent teeth (Fig. 5.60, *C*). Gingival involvement may manifest as early as 1 year of age and tends to be present by 5 years of age. Patients are usually edentulous by 15 years. Late-onset periodontitis after several years of PPK has also been described.[565] Although an increased risk of acral lentiginous melanoma has been suggested, the reports are primarily in the Japanese population, which has a high incidence of this melanoma.[566] Haim–Munk syndrome (originally described in individuals descended from Cochin, India) has the additional features of arachnodactyly, acroosteolysis, and onychogryphosis but not the calcification of the falx cerebri or susceptibility for bacterial infection described in some patients with Papillon–Lefévre syndrome.[567] Nevertheless, the same gene mutation can cause either disorder.[568]

Both disorders result from mutations in the *CTSC* gene, encoding cathepsin C, leading to impaired innate immune responses,[569] cell autophagy,[570] and desquamation from activation of serine proteases.[571,572] Diffuse NEPPK and chronic periodontal disease with loss of teeth are also a feature of Micali syndrome (see later). Papillon–Lefévre syndrome responds well to topical tazarotene 0.1% cream or low-dose acitretin therapy.[573] Gingivitis in association with palmar linearity, plantar keratoderma, and mild ichthyosis (predominantly axillary) is also a feature of the HELIX syndrome (hypohidrosis, electrolyte imbalance, lacrimal gland dysfunction, ichthyosis, and xerostomia), which results from biallelic mutations in *CLDN10B*, encoding the tight-junction protein claudin-10b. The severe deficiency in saliva secretion increases the risk of the gingival inflammation and dental enamel issues.[574]

PUNCTATE PPK

Punctate PPK (also called *keratosis punctata palmaris et plantaris*; PPKP) is characterized by discrete keratoses of the palms and soles, usually has its onset during early adolescence or beyond, and has been classified into three autosomal dominant subdisorders.[575–577] Punctate papules of the palms and soles are also a feature of porokeratosis punctata palmaris et plantaris, Cole disease (in association with guttate hypopigmentation),[578,579] keratosis punctata of the palmar creases, Darier disease, and Cowden syndrome (see Chapter 9).[580] Oral retinoids have been used as treatment.[581]

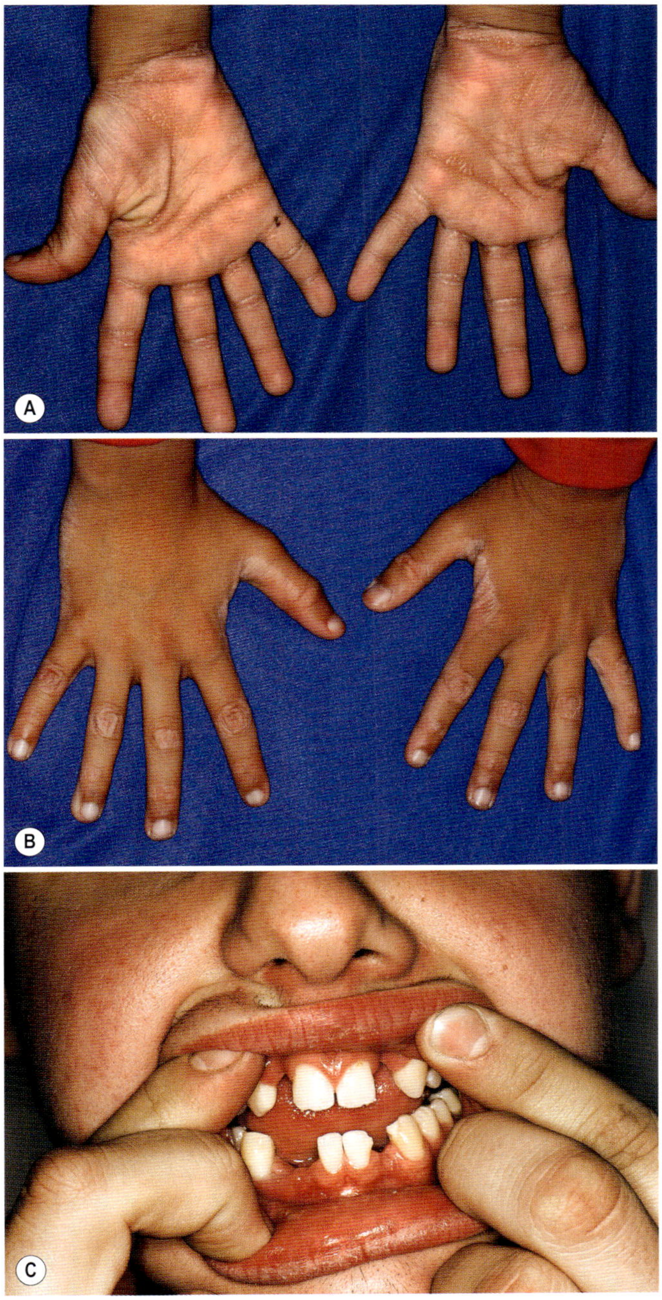

Fig. 5.60 Papillon–Lefévre syndrome. Focal plaques of palmoplantar keratoderma **(A)** with transgrediens extension **(B)** are associated with the progressive periodontitis **(C)** and periosteal changes of the alveolar bone that begins during infancy or early childhood and result in loss of both deciduous and permanent teeth.

PPKP1A (also known as *Buschke–Fischer–Brauer disorder*) features multiple tiny punctate keratoses, typically confined to the palmoplantar creases and volar aspects of the digits. The central keratinous plug may be lost or can be picked out, leaving a shallow depressed pit with a keratotic base. Lesions can be particularly painful when walking or from pressure on the hands in persons who perform manual labor. The disorder results from heterozygous mutations in one of two genes: *AAGAB*,[582,583] which encodes a protein that participates in membrane trafficking of EGFR and other proteins, and *COL14A1*, which encodes collagen 14.[584]

PPKP2 has tiny hyperkeratotic spiny papules, sometimes also involving the volar aspect of the hands.[585] Cornoid lamellae have been associated in some cases. Facial sebaceous hyperplasia[586] may be associated.

PPKP3 (also called *hereditary acrokeratoelastoidosis [of Costa]*) is characterized by persistent, asymptomatic, whitish papules and plaques that are most prevalent at the margins of the hands (especially thenar and hypothenar areas) and pressure areas on the palms and soles (border of ventral and dorsal areas).[587] Lesions are sometimes found on the knuckles and nailfolds. Biopsy shows hyperkeratosis, acanthosis, and decreased numbers of coarsely fragmented elastic fibers. Aquagenic PPK can be seen.[588] Although the condition is generally bilateral, unilateral involvement has been described.[589] The underlying genetic basis is unknown. A unique homozygous mutation in *SLURP1* (the gene altered in the Mal de Meleda form of PPK) has been reported to cause the acrokeratoelastoidosis phenotype in one family.[590]

AQUAGENIC PPK

Aquagenic wrinkling of the palms (also called *acquired aquagenic PPK*, *aquagenic syringeal acrokeratoderma*, and *transient aquagenic palmar hyperwrinkling*) is a transient and recurrent keratoderma of the palms and lateral fingers induced by exposure to water.[591–593] Rarely, papules are also noted on the dorsal aspect. In one study, the mean age of onset was 9 years (range, 20 months to 15 years).[594] Exposure to water elicits a whitening of the wet palm within a few minutes and visible thickening ("hand in the bucket sign"), often associated with a tight, tingling, pruritic, or even painful sensation (Fig. 5.61). The cause is thought to be an increase in the stratum corneum's water-binding capacity because of the increased electrolyte concentration in sweat. Although biopsy is generally unnecessary, it often shows dilation of the eccrine acrosyringia and hyperplastic eccrine sweat glands.

Aquagenic wrinkling of the palms was originally described in patients with cystic fibrosis,[595,596] with a prevalence of 40% to 84% among affected individuals.[597] It is most obvious in patients with the DeltaF508 mutation in the *CFTR* gene (encoding cystic fibrosis transmembrane conductance regulator)[598] and may be a cutaneous sign of carriers or patients with cystic fibrosis.[597,599,600] Aquagenic wrinkling can also be seen in individuals with increased sweat chloride levels but without cystic fibrosis.[601] Nevertheless, a sweat chloride test should be performed for children diagnosed with aquagenic wrinkling with further investigation if positive. Unilateral involvement has been described in a child.[602] Tobramycin can induce aquagenic wrinkling without exposure to water,[603] and COX-2 inhibitors have also been associated.[604–606] Topical aluminum chloride[607] and palmar injection of botulinum toxin have been used for symptomatic patients.[608]

The lesions must be distinguished from hereditary papulotranslucent acrokeratoderma, an autosomal dominant disorder with onset during childhood with persistent palmar papules,[609] although exposure to water may lead to worsening. This condition also often begins at puberty and is often accompanied by palmar hyperhidrosis.

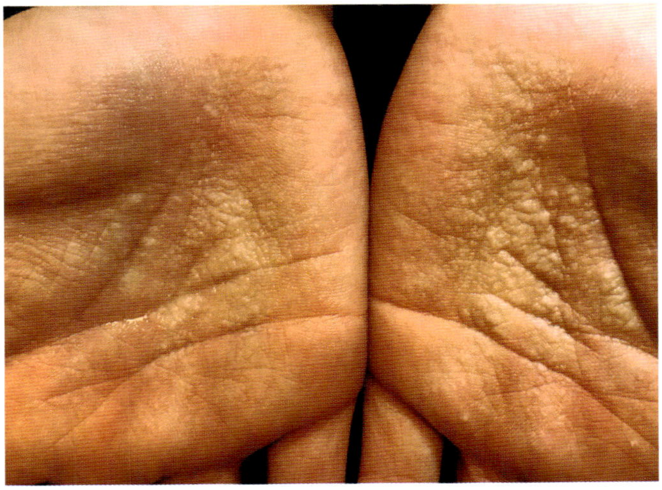

Fig. 5.61 Aquagenic wrinkling of the palms. The palm becomes whitened and thickened within a few minutes after exposure to water.

Exposure to water can also lead to a white, spongy appearance in autosomal dominant diffuse nonepidermolytic PPK in individuals with mutations in *AQP5*, encoding water-channel protein aquaporin-5.[610] This white, spongy reactivity to water exposure is also seen in "Nagashima-type" PPK, an autosomal recessive diffuse PPK in individuals of Japanese and Chinese descent.[611] The PPK is well demarcated and erythematous with transgrediens extension to the dorsal surfaces of the hands and feet and the Achilles tendon but is mild and nonprogressive, in contrast with Mal de Meleda PPK. Nagashima-type PPK results from loss-of-function mutations in *SERPINB7*, which encodes a serine protease inhibitor, suggesting that the enhanced water permeation is caused by activation of proteases.[612–614]

The complete list of 614 references for this chapter is available online at http://expertconsult.inkling.com.

Key References

Oji V, Tadini G, Akiyama M, et al. Revised nomenclature and classification of inherited ichthyoses: results of the first ichthyosis consensus conference in Soreze 2009. J Am Acad Dermatol 2010;63(4):607–41.

Traupe H, Fischer J, Oji V. Nonsyndromic types of ichthyoses: an update. J Dtsch Dermatol Ges 2014;12(2):109–21.

Arin MJ. The molecular basis of human keratin disorders. Hum Genet 2009; 125(4):355–73.

Vahlquist A, Fischer J, Torma H. Inherited nonsyndromic ichthyoses: an update on pathophysiology, diagnosis and treatment. Am J Clin Dermatol 2018;19(1): 51–66.

Takeichi T, Akiyama M. Inherited ichthyosis: non-syndromic forms. J Dermatol 2016;43(3):242–51.

Prado R, Ellis LZ, Gamble R, et al. Collodion baby: an update with a focus on practical management. J Am Acad Dermatol 2012;67(6):1362–74.

Fleckman P, Newell BD, van Steensel MA, et al. Topical treatment of ichthyoses. Dermatol Ther 2013;26(1):16–25.

Hernández-Martin A, Aranegui B, Martin-Santiago A, et al. A systematic review of clinical trials of treatments for the congenital ichthyoses, excluding ichthyosis vulgaris. J Am Acad Dermatol 2013;69(4):544–549.e8.

Mazereeuw-Hautier J, Vahlquist A, Traupe H, et al. Management of congenital ichthyoses: European guidelines of care, part one. Br J Dermatol 2019;180(2): 272–81.

Mazereeuw-Hautier J, Hernandez-Martin A, O'Toole EA, et al. Management of congenital ichthyoses: European guidelines of care, part two. Br J Dermatol 2019; 180(3):484–95.

Sakiyama T, Kubo A. Hereditary palmoplantar keratoderma "clinical and genetic differential diagnosis." J Dermatol 2016;43(3):264–74.

Guerra L, Castori M, Didona B, et al. Hereditary palmoplantar keratodermas. Part I. Non-syndromic palmoplantar keratodermas: classification, clinical and genetic features. J Eur Acad Dermatol Venereol 2018;32(5):704–19.

Guerra L, Castori M, Didona B, et al. Hereditary palmoplantar keratodermas. Part II: syndromic palmoplantar keratodermas - diagnostic algorithm and principles of therapy. J Eur Acad Dermatol Venereol 2018;32(6):899–925.

Petrof G, Mellerio JE, McGrath JA. Desmosomal genodermatoses. Br J Dermatol 2012;166(1):36–45.

6 Hereditary Disorders of the Dermis

Several hereditary disorders of the skin primarily manifest as disorders of the dermis. Clinical manifestations range from laxity of skin to infiltrated papules and from rigidity to thinning of the dermis. Disorders of mucopolysaccharides are reviewed in Chapter 24.

Ehlers–Danlos Syndrome

Ehlers–Danlos syndrome (EDS) consists of a group of six inherited disorders of collagen characterized by increased cutaneous elasticity, hyperextensibility of the joints, and fragility of the skin, sometimes with the formation of pseudotumors and large gaping scars. The 1997 Villefranche classification[1] was refined in the 2017 International Classification (Table 6.1).[2] For all subtypes other than the hypermobile type, confirmation of subtype relies on molecular genetic analysis.

Most forms of EDS are linked to mutations in genes encoding fibrillar collagens, enzymes involved in posttranslational modification of these proteins, or extracellular matrix proteins. Mutations in type V and type III collagen cause classic and vascular EDS, respectively, whereas mutations involving the processing of type I collagen are involved in the arthrochalasis and dermatosparaxis types and of collagen crosslinking in the kyphoscoliotic type of EDS. In addition to the clinical classification of EDS, a grouping according to pathogenetic mechanism has also been proposed (Table 6.2).[3] The underlying cause for most individuals with the hypermobile type remains unknown.

The prevalence of EDS, including the mild forms, may be as high as 1:5000 individuals. The spectrum of severity of EDS ranges from almost imperceptible findings to severe, debilitating disease. The most common type with skin manifestations is the classical type (Box 6.1). The vascular type tends to be most devastating. The kyphoscoliosis, arthrochalasis, and dermatosparaxis types are considerably less common than other forms. The effect on quality of life can be considerable, and three-quarters of affected individuals report fatigue[4] that may be affected by pain, sleep disturbance, difficulty with concentration, and diminished social functioning.[5]

The skin of individuals with the **classical** type (cEDS) is velvety, soft, and has a doughy consistency. After being stretched, it returns to its normal position as soon as released, in contrast to the lax skin of cutis laxa. Skin hyperextensibility (Fig. 6.1) should be tested at a site not subjected to mechanical forces or scarring, such as the volar surface of the forearm. In contrast to 10% of apparently normal individuals, approximately 50% of patients with EDS can touch the tip of their nose with their tongue (Gorlin sign) (Fig. 6.2). In addition, the skin of the hands, feet, and at times the elbows tends to be lax and redundant, thus resulting in a loose-fitting glove- or moccasin-like appearance. A number of patients have pressure-induced herniation of subcutaneous fat on the wrists or on the medial or lateral aspect of the heels, evident when the patient is standing (piezogenic pedal papules) (Fig. 6.3).[6] In addition to abnormal elasticity, the skin of patients with the classical (but not the hypermobile) form of EDS is extremely fragile, and minor trauma may produce gaping "fishmouth" wounds (Fig. 6.4). It has poor tensile strength and cannot hold sutures properly. This leads to dehiscence, poor healing, and the formation of wide, papyraceous, wrinkled hernia-like scars, particularly over areas of trauma (such as the knees, forehead, pretibial areas, and elbows). Blood vessels are fragile, resulting in hematomas and a chronic bruise-like appearance, particularly on the anterior aspect of the lower extremities (Fig. 6.5). The resolution of hematomas is accompanied by fibrosis, which produces soft subcutaneous nodules (molluscoid pseudotumors, especially over joints such as the elbows and fingers) and small calcified subcutaneous nodules, especially on the shins and forearms (spheroids). Facial dysmorphism of the midface and orbital areas and infraorbital creases (epicanthal folds) are common, especially in children.[7]

Hyperextensible joints may result in "double-jointed" fingers or subluxation of larger joints (Fig. 6.6). This may occur spontaneously or follow slight trauma. Generalized hypermobility is determined by a score of 5 or higher in the 9-point scale established by Beighton and colleagues[1] (Fig. 6.8; Table 6.3). Sprains, dislocations or subluxations, and pes planus occur as complications, and patients complain of chronic joint and limb pain despite normal skeletal radiographs.[8,9] Muscle hypotonia and delayed gross motor development have been described. Hiatal hernia, postoperative hernias, and anal prolapse have been noted as manifestations of the tissue hyperextensibility and fragility.[10] Anomalies of the heart and dissecting aortic aneurysms have rarely been described in the classical form,[11,12] in contrast to the arterial form. Mitral valve prolapse is a common manifestation, but aortic root dilatation is uncommon; both can be assessed by echocardiography, computed tomography (CT), or magnetic resonance imaging (MRI) examinations.[10]

The diagnosis of classical EDS is primarily clinical. Routine histopathologic examination of skin from patients with EDS is usually normal but may show loose collagen and irregular fibroblasts[13]; electron microscopy demonstrates disorganized collagen fibers and fibrils with variable cross-sectional diameters. Studies of platelet function and coagulation are usually normal despite a tendency for bruising and increased bleeding, further implicating the defective structural integrity of skin and blood vessels.

The underlying molecular defect for 93% of patients with the classical form of EDS is mutations in the α1 *(COL5A1)* or α2 *(COL5A2)*

Table 6.1 2017 International Classification of Ehlers–Danlos Syndrome

Type	Mutations (Protein Products)	Skin Findings	Joint Changes	Inheritance	Other Comments
1. **Classical*** (cEDS)	*COL5A1, COL5A2* (type V collagen)	Hyperextensibility, bruising, velvety skin, widened atrophic scars, molluscoid pseudotumors, spheroids	Hypermobility and its complications, joint dislocations	AD (usually)	Mitral valve prolapse Hernias
CLASSICAL VARIANT					
EDS/OI overlap	*COL1A1* (type I collagen)	Classic EDS features		AD	Blue sclerae, short stature, osteopenia/fractures May have late arterial rupture
2. **Classic-like** (clEDS)	*TNXB* (tenascin X)	Hyperextensibility, marked hypermobility, severe bruising, velvety skin, no scarring tendency	Hypermobility	AR	Parents (especially mothers) with one TNXB mutation can have joint hypermobility
3. **Cardiac-valvular** (cvEDS)	*COL1A2* (type I collagen alpha 2 chain)	Classic EDS features		AR	Severe cardiac valve issues as adult
4. **Vascular*** (vEDS)	*COL3A1* (type III collagen)	Thin, translucent skin; bruising; early varicosities; acrogeria	Small joint hypermobility	AD	Abnormal type III collagen secretion; rupture of bowel, uterus, arteries; typical facies; pneumothorax
5. **Hypermobile*** (hEDS)	Unknown; some may have *COL5A1* mutations	Mild hyperextensibility, scarring, textural change	Hypermobility, chronic joint pain, recurrent dislocations	AD	Sometimes confused with joint hypermobility syndrome
6. **Arthrochalasis*** (aEDS)	Exon 6 deletion of *COL1A1* or *COL1A2*	Hyperextensible, soft skin with or without abnormal scarring	Marked hypermobility with recurrent subluxations	AD	Congenital hip dislocation Arthrochalasis multiplex congenita Short stature
7. **Dermatosparaxis*** (dEDS)	*ADAMTS2* (type I collagen N-peptidase)	Severe fragility Sagging, redundant skin		AR	Severe bruising Also occurs in cattle
8. **Kyphoscoliosis*** (kEDS)	*PLOD1* (lysyl hydroxylase) *FKBP14* (FKBP prolyl isomerase 14 or FKBP22)	Soft, hyperextensible, bruising, atrophic scars	Hypermobility	AR	Severe muscle hypotonia, congenital kyphoscoliosis, scleral fragility and rupture, marfanoid habitus, osteopenia; sensorineural hearing loss with FKBP14 deficiency
9. **Brittle cornea syndrome** (BCS)	*ZNF469* (zinc finger protein 469) *PRDM5* (PR domain zinc finger protein 5)	Skin hypermobility	Joint hypermobility	AR	Kyphoscoliosis Characteristic thin, brittle cornea, ocular fragility, blue sclera, and keratoconus
10. **Spondylocheirodysplastic form** (spEDS) (includes former progeroid form)	SLC39A13 (ZIP13 zinc transporter) *β4GALT7* or *β3GalT6* (galactosyltransferase I or II, key enzymes in glycosaminoglycan synthesis)	Soft, hyperextensible, bruising, atrophic scars	Hypermobility	AR	Bone abnormalities but without congenital hypotonia and progressive kyphoscoliosis Moderate short stature, wrinkled palms with thenar and hypothenar atrophy, blue sclerae; progeroid subtype has loose facial skin, curly hair, alopecia, developmental delay, spondyloepimetaphyseal dysplasia with bone fragility, and severe kyphoscoliosis
11. **Musculocontractural** (mcEDS)	*CHST14* (dermatan 4-O-sulfotransferase) or *DSE* (dermatan sulfate epimerase)	Fragile, hyperextensible skin with atrophic scars and delayed wound healing	Hypermobility	AR	Progressive kyphoscoliosis, adducted thumbs in infancy, clubfoot, arachnodactyly, contractures, characteristic facial features, hemorrhagic diathesis
12. **Myopathic** (mEDS)	*COL12A1* (type 12 collagen alpha 1 chain)			AD or AR	Muscle weakness in infancy/childhood with large joint contractures and distal joint hypermobility; may have hypertrophic scarring
13. **Periodontal** (pEDS)	*C1R* or C1S (complement components C1r and C1s)	Can have classic EDS features	Can have hypermobility	AD	Periodontitis Marfanoid habitus Prominent eyes Short philtrum

AD, Autosomal dominant; *AR*, autosomal recessive; *EDS*, Ehlers–Danlos syndrome; *OI*, osteogenesis imperfecta.
*In original Villefranche classification.

Table 6.2 Classification of Ehlers–Danlos Syndrome by Pathogenesis

Group A: Disorders of Collagen Primary Structure and Collagen Processing
Classical type: *COL5A1, COL5A2*, rarely COL1A1 (selected genotypes) Cardiac-valvular type: *COL1A2* Vascular type: *COL3A1*, rarely *COL1A1* (selected genotypes) Arthrochalasia type: *COL1A1, COL1A2* Dermatosparaxis type: *ADAMTS2*
Group B: Disorders of Collagen Folding and Crosslinking
Kyphoscoliotic type: *PLOD1, FKBP14*
Group C: Disorders of Structure and Function of the Interface Between the ECM and Muscle ("Myomatrix")
Classic-like type: *TNXB* Myopathic type: *COL12A1*
Group D: Disorders of Glycosaminoglycan Biosynthesis
Spondylodysplastic type: *B4GALT7, B3GALT6* Musculocontractural type: *CHST14, DSE*
Group E: Disorders of Complement Pathway
Periodontal type: *C1R, C1S*
Group F: Disorders of Intracellular Processes
Spondylodysplastic type: *SLC39A13* Brittle cornea syndrome: *ZNF469, PRDM5*

Box 6.1 **Major and Minor Criteria for Classical Ehlers–Danlos Syndrome**

- Major criteria
  1. Skin hyperextensibility and atrophic scarring
  2. Generalized joint hypermobility
- Minor criteria
  1. Soft, doughy skin
  2. Easy bruisability
  3. Skin fragility with trauma
  4. Molluscoid pseudotumors
  5. Subcutaneous spheroids
  6. Hernia
  7. Epicanthal folds (especially during childhood)
  8. Complications of joint hypermobility (pain, flexible pes planus, sprains, luxation/subluxation
  9. Family history of a first-degree relative with Ehlers–Danlos syndrome (EDS) per clinical criteria
- Minimal criteria to suggest classical EDS: Skin hyperextensibility and atrophic scarring plus either the other major criterion (joint hypermobility) or at least three minor criteria
- Molecular testing is necessary to confirm the diagnosis

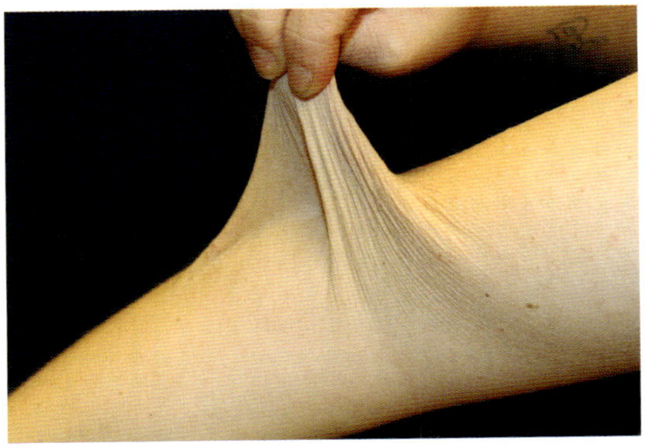

Fig. 6.1 Ehlers–Danlos syndrome. Skin hyperextensibility on the arm.

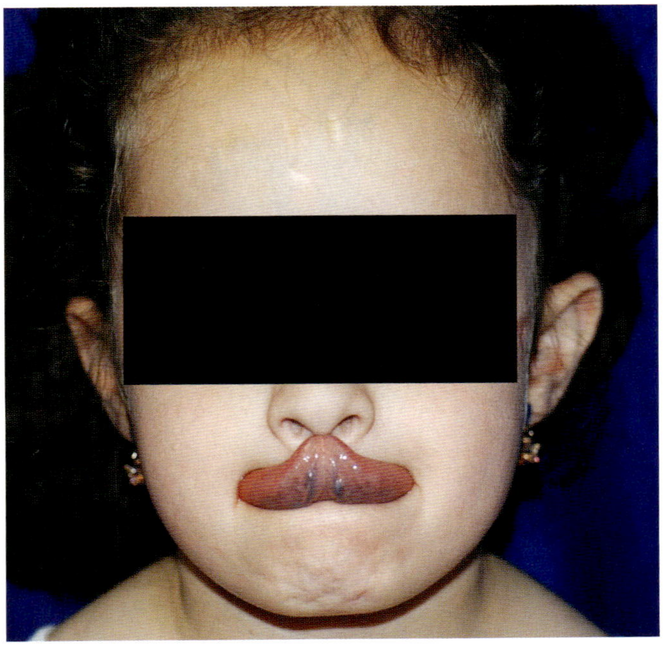

Fig. 6.2 Ehlers–Danlos syndrome (EDS). Gorlin sign is five times more common in EDS than in normal individuals. Note the scars on the forehead.

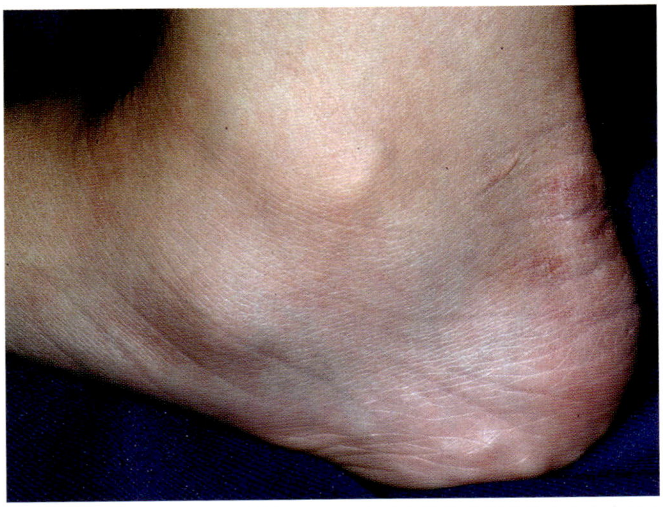

Fig. 6.3 Ehlers–Danlos syndrome. Piezogenic pedal papules are caused by pressure-induced herniation of subcutaneous fat, seen here on the lateral aspect of the heel.

chain of type V collagen, a minor fibrillar collagen that regulates collagen fibril diameter. These mutations typically lead to haploinsufficiency for *COL5A1* and are dominant negative for *COL5A2*.[7,14,15] Autosomal recessive type I EDS has been described from homozygous variants in exon 64b of *COL5A1*, an alternatively spliced isoform that accounts for only 30% of *COLA5A1*.[16] Patients with mutations in *COL1A1* at a nonglycine site (mutations at glycine sites lead to osteogenesis imperfecta [OI]) may exhibit features of classic EDS alone or with subtle features of OI (blue sclera, relatively short stature, osteopenia, or fractures).[17] Some children with nonglycine substitutions in type I collagen have classic EDS but develop spontaneous arterial rupture during adulthood.[18]

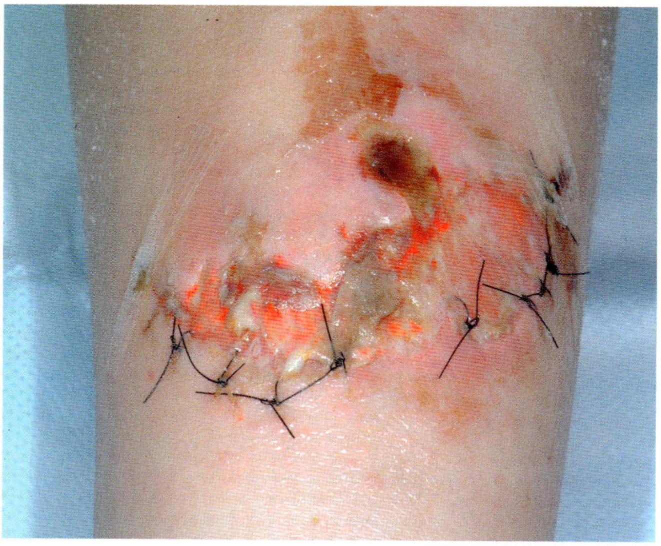

Fig. 6.4 Ehlers–Danlos syndrome. Minor trauma results in a large wound on the shin. The wound dehisced despite placement of several sutures.

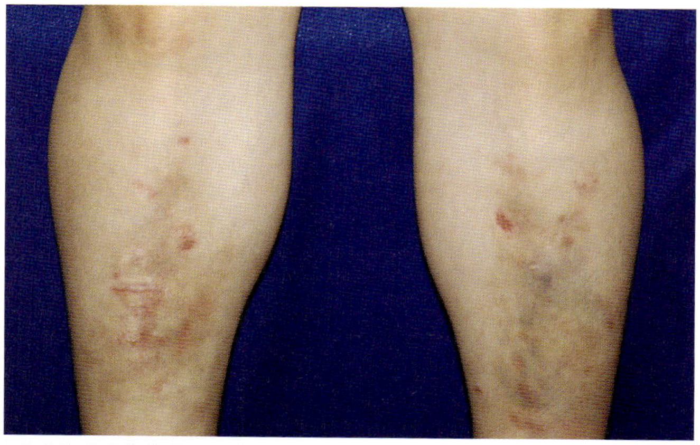

Fig. 6.5 Ehlers–Danlos syndrome. Poor wound healing and persistent discoloration with active ecchymosis of the anterior aspect of the lower extremities of this adolescent girl.

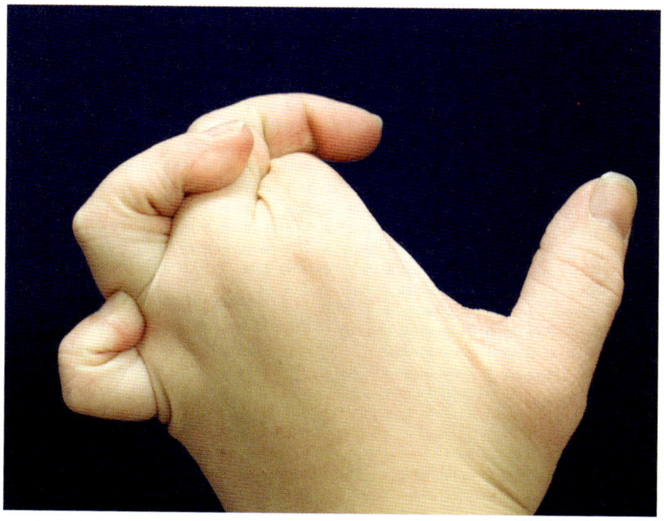

Fig. 6.6 Ehlers–Danlos syndrome. Hyperextensible joints may result in double-jointed fingers, as seen in this girl.

Table 6.3 Beighton Scale for Generalized Joint Hypermobility (≥5/9 Meets Criteria*)

Finding	Negative	One Side	Both Sides
Passive flexion of thumb to forearm	0	1	2
Passive dorsiflexion of fifth finger >90 degrees	0	1	2
Hyperextension of elbows >10 degrees	0	1	2
Hyperextension of knees† >10 degrees	0	1	2
Hyperextension of knees is done by being able to touch the floor with palms It is 0 if no It is 1 if yes	0	1	2

*Present = 1.
†Touching the floor with palms open and knees fully extended.

The **"classic-like"** autosomal recessive form of EDS (clEDS), caused by a deficiency of the extracellular matrix protein tenascin-X, shows typical EDS (hyperextensibility, bruising) but normal wound healing and without atrophic scarring.[19–21] Serum levels of tenascin-X are undetectable. Heterozygous carriers may exhibit only joint hypermobility. A contiguous gene syndrome caused by a 6p deletion can present with tenascin-X deficiency, as well as congenital adrenal hyperplasia (deletion in *CYP21A2*) with or without ovarian failure (deletion in *MSH5*).[22,23]

The **cardiac-valvular** type (cvEDS) results from a total absence of the proα2-chain of type I collagen. Severe progressive cardiac valve issues (especially aortic and mitral) predominate in adults, but may not be present in the first decade. The typical features of cEDS are commonly seen.

The **vascular** type of EDS (vEDS) is characterized by extensive bruising and often thin, translucent skin that is not hyperextensible.[10,24–26] Joint hypermobility is usually limited to the digits, and only 17% of patients meet Beighton criteria.[27] The facial appearance is often typical, with sunken eyes, a thin upper lip, and decreased facial fat. Spontaneous rupture of arteries, particularly midsized arteries, may occur during childhood, although its peak age of incidence is the third or fourth decade of life[28,29]; the diagnosis of vascular EDS may be missed until a devastating vascular complication occurs. Arterial or intestinal rupture often presents as acute abdominal or flank pain (including from gastrointestinal [GI] bleeding or bowel perforation), and intracranial aneurysms may be associated with cerebrovascular accidents.[30] Arterial rupture is the most common cause of death. Pregnancies may be complicated by prepartum and postpartum arterial bleeding and by intrapartum uterine rupture. Vaginal and perineal tears from the delivery heal poorly, and pneumothorax occurs in 11% of affected individuals. In one series, 94% of patients with vEDS showed blue sclerae.[27] Given the autosomal dominant nature of vEDS, the diagnosis should be considered if there is a family history of arterial dissection or rupture under 40 years of age, or if spontaneous pneumothorax or unexplained sigmoid colon rupture with other vEDS features exists.[2]

The vascular form of EDS has been associated with mutations in type III collagen (*COL3A1*), resulting in a reduced amount of type III collagen in dermis, vessels, and viscera. The mean lifespan is reduced to 51 years of age. However, the prognosis is related to the underlying *COL3A1* mutation, with individuals with null mutations having a better prognosis than those with missense or exon-skipping mutations.[31]

vEDS may be confused with periodontal EDS and Loeys–Dietz syndrome (LDS). The latter is an autosomal dominant disorder characterized by joint hypermobility with dislocations; soft, velvety skin; arterial tortuosity; widespread vascular aneurysm and dissection[32]; and an increased risk of atopy.[33] The disorder has been divided into LDS type 1 and type 2. Patients with type 1 disease have a marfanoid habitus (but do not fulfill Ghent criteria for Marfan syndrome [MFS] including lack of ectopia lentis), craniofacial abnormalities, and mutations in *TGFBR1* (transforming growth factor [TGF]-β1 receptor), whereas patients with type 2 have mutations in *TGFB2R* and no craniofacial or skeletal anomalies.[32]

The most common form of EDS, the **hypermobile** type (hEDS), is associated with extensive joint hypermobility and dislocations, particularly of the shoulder, patella, and temporomandibular joints. The skin is often soft and velvety but heals well and only occasionally shows hyperextensibility. Children often receive a diagnosis of chronic pain syndrome because no specific underlying cause is identified.[34] Up to 40% of school-aged children may show a score of 5 or higher using the 9-point Beighton criteria, leading to overdiagnosis and making diagnosis of hEDS difficult.[35] It is also hard to distinguish from benign joint hypermobility syndrome,[36] and the term *joint hypermobility syndrome* has been suggested to encompass any child with symptomatic joint hypermobility,[35,37] including those with hypermobility-type EDS. The autonomic burden of hypermobility-type EDS is as high as in fibromyalgia and is primarily characterized by orthostatic issues (dizziness or even transient loss of consciousness with postural change or standing), palpitations, shortness of breath, and GI complaints.[38] Involvement during infancy may present as unexplained fractures, with parents accused of child abuse and neglect, and an affected parent unaware of the EDS diagnosis.[39]

Patients with the **arthrochalasis** type (aEDS) show generalized joint hypermobility with severe recurrent subluxations and congenital bilateral hip dislocation. The skin may be hyperextensible, fragile, and easy to bruise. Early and significant muscle hypotonia, kyphoscoliosis, and mild osteopenia have been described. Mutations in *COLA1A1* or *COL1A2* that result in skipping of exon 6 lead to defective collagen synthesis.[40]

The **dermatosparaxis** form of EDS (dEDS) is characterized by severe skin fragility with sagging, redundant skin[41]; wound healing leads to wide atrophic scars, especially past infancy.[42] The skin may be soft and doughy in texture with easy bruisability. Characteristic facies, gingival hyperplasia, large umbilical and inguinal hernias, delayed closure of the fontanels, postnatal growth failure, and premature rupture of the fetal membranes may be seen. Electrophoretic demonstration of procollagen $\alpha 1(I)$ or $\alpha 2(I)$ chains from collagen or cultured fibroblasts is seen with the arthrochalasis and dermatosparaxis forms.

The **kyphoscoliotic** type of EDS (kEDS) is characterized by generalized joint laxity with severe muscle hypotonia at birth, which leads to gross motor delay and congenital progressive scoliosis.[43] Severe hypotonia is predominant during infancy, and patients are thought to have congenital muscular dystrophy or myopathies. By the second or third decade of life, patients tend to lose the ability to ambulate. The skin may be fragile and heals with atrophic scars. Easy bruisability and arterial rupture have been described.[44] Patients often show a marfanoid habitus, osteopenia, and scleral fragility with rupture of the ocular globe. Because of *PLOD1* mutations, this form shows a deficiency of collagen lysyl hydroxylase. The diagnosis can be confirmed by finding a high ratio of lysyl pyridinoline (LP) to hydroxylysyl pyridinoline (HP) crosslinks (LP/HP) in the urine by high-performance liquid chromatography (HPLC).[43,45] Mutations in *FKBP14*,[46,47] which catalyzes the folding of type III collagen, are an unusual cause of kEDS[46] and are associated with sensorineural healing loss and a higher risk of serious vascular abnormalities in adulthood than with *PLOD1* mutations.

The **brittle cornea syndrome** (BCS), an autosomal recessive condition caused by mutations in either *ZNF469* or *PRDM5*, is characterized by thin, brittle cornea; ocular fragility; blue sclera; and keratoconus, as well as associated skin and joint hypermobility and kyphoscoliosis.[48–50]

The **spondylocheirodysplastic** form of EDS (spEDS) resembles the kyphoscoliotic form but lacks the severe muscular hypotonia from birth and progressive kyphoscoliosis. spEDS shows moderate and progressive short stature, variable hypotonia, and bowing of the limbs, with osteopenia and pes planus; delayed motor and cognitive development; and translucent, doughy, hyperextensible skin.[51] Biallelic mutations in *SLC39A13*, which encodes the zinc transporter protein ZIP13, important for intracellular zinc homeostasis, are causative.[52,53]

The progeroid forms of EDS are now classified as subsets of spondylodysplastic EDS. They are caused by biallelic mutations in either galactosyltransferase I *(B4GALT7)* or II *(B3GalT6)*, key enzymes in initiating glycosaminoglycan (GAG) synthesis.[54–56] In addition to the typical features of spEDS from *SLC39A13* mutations, both have joint hypermobility and blue sclerae. Each has its own gene-specific minor criteria for diagnosis, including gene-specific craniofacial features. For example, spEDS from *B4GALT7* mutations is also characterized by craniofacial features, elbow contractures, clouded cornea, and characteristic radiographic features, whereas spEDS from *B4GALT6* mutations is associated with joint contractures (typically of the hands), peculiar fingers, talipes equinovarus, and dental issues.[54,57]

Musculocontractural EDS (mcEDS) is a variant with characteristic facial features, multiple contractures, a hemorrhagic diathesis with large subcutaneous hematomas, and several other systemic complications; this variant has been linked to dysfunction of dermatan sulfate from mutations in both alleles of genes encoding dermatan 4-O-sulfotransferase *(CHST14)*[58,59] or dermatan sulfate epimerase (DSE).[60]

The **myopathic** form (mEDS) can be autosomal dominant or recessive, but the congenital muscle hypotonia or atrophy, proximal joint contractures, and distal joint hypermobility are major criteria. Many patients have soft, doughy skin and atrophic scarring.The **periodontal** type (pEDS; formerly type VIII EDS) is a dominant form of EDS and shows variable interfamilial and intrafamilial clinical manifestations (including patients without skin or joint abnormalities).[61] The periodontal type is associated with early gingival regression and periodontitis, joint hypermobility, mild skin findings, and often a marfanoid body habitus, as well as prominent eyes, a short philtrum, pretibial hyperpigmentation, and hoarseness (Fig. 6.7).[62–64] Acrogeria and prominent vasculature are often associated. It results from heterozygous variants in C1R and C1S, encoding complement subcomponents C1r and C1s.

MANAGEMENT OF EHLERS–DANLOS SYNDROME

Management is mainly supportive, but cardiovascular workup, physiotherapy, pain management, and psychological and genetic counseling are important. Wearing a medical bracelet warning of EDS and carrying information for teachers and healthcare workers can be helpful. The Ehlers–Danlos National Foundation (www.ednf.org) is a national support group. Children with skin fragility should use protective pads on the shins, knees, and forehead to decrease the risk of laceration and bruising. Low-impact sports (such as swimming) are preferable to contact sports and weight training in patients with hypermobility. Physical and occupational therapists or rheumatologists can suggest devices (such as splints and braces) to make movement more comfortable. Children with significant hypotonia or motor developmental delay should be referred for appropriate physical therapy to improve muscular strength and coordination. Pain medication should be tailored to individual needs. Psychological counseling to help develop coping strategies and treat depression can be important, especially in patients with hypermobility and chronic pain.

A baseline echocardiogram should be performed in all patients with EDS to evaluate aortic root diameter and cardiac valves. Echocardiograms should be repeated in children and adolescents

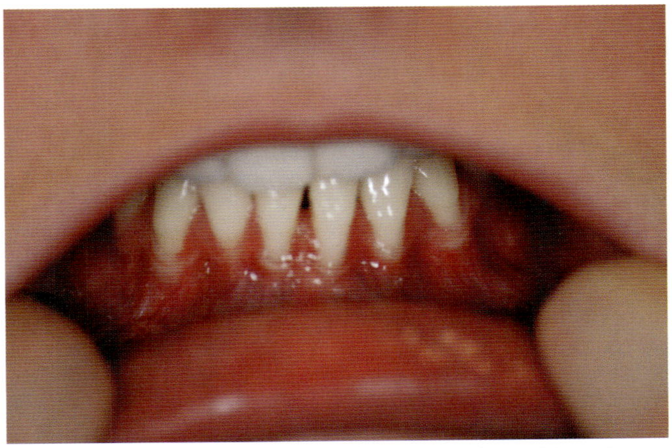

Fig. 6.7 Periodontitis in a girl with periodontal Ehlers–Danlos syndrome.

approximately every 3 years if the results are normal and annually if results are abnormal. Patients who have mitral valve prolapse and regurgitation should be given prophylactic antibiotics to prevent bacterial endocarditis.

Surgical procedures present problems, because tissues are friable and difficult to suture.[65] Therefore edges of wounds should be approximated without tension by closely spaced sutures in two layers (absorbable and retained); adhesive reinforcement (e.g., Steri-Strips) to minimize scar spread; and pressure bandages to aid healing, diminish scarring, and lower the risk of hematoma and pseudotumor formation. Sutures should be kept in place for at least twice as long as for normal skin, and use of absorbable suture material that does not get removed has been proposed. Prophylactic antibiotics after injury and close monitoring for postoperative infection are important to minimize postoperative complications.

Ascorbate is a cofactor that stimulates prolyl hydroxylase and lysyl hydroxylase, enzymes that catalyze the formation of hydroxyproline and hydroxylysine to promote collagen deposition. Doses of 2 to 4 g/day have been administered to patients with the kyphoscoliosis type to improve wound healing and decrease the bleeding tendency.[66] Ascorbic acid sometimes decreases the bleeding tendency in other types. Antiinflammatory drugs may improve the musculoskeletal pain associated with EDS, but those interfering with platelet function and prolonging bleeding (acetylsalicylic acids, nonsteroidal antiinflammatory drugs [NSAIDs] other than celecoxib family) should be avoided in patients with significant bruising. Dental procedures require extra precautions as well, because of increased bleeding.[67] More than half of patients who undergo posterior spinal fusion for scoliosis develop various complications.[68]

In patients with the vascular type of EDS, blood pressure should be maintained in the normal range, and annual surveillance of the aortic vasculature is important.[26] Invasive vascular procedures (such as arteriography and catheterization) increase the risk of vascular rupture and should be replaced by Doppler ultrasound and/or magnetic resonance angiography (MRA).[26] Surgery should be avoided if possible but may be required for arterial or bowel complications.[69] Manipulation of vascular and other tissues should be minimized if surgery is required. Celiprolol, a long-acting β_1 antagonist and partial β_2 agonist, decreased by threefold the incidence of arterial rupture or dissection in patients with vascular EDS[70]; no other β-blockers have been rigorously tested. Pregnancy for women with EDS is considered high risk, but particularly with the vascular type of EDS (up to 12% die from uterine rupture or peripartum arterial rupture). Planned caesarean section may be preferable to vaginal delivery.[71] Infants with EDS are prone to premature birth because of early rupture of membranes.[72] Preterm delivery occurs in 40% of pregnancies with affected neonates and 21% of pregnancies of affected mothers.[73–76]

Marfan Syndrome

MFS is an autosomal dominant disorder that occurs in approximately 1:5000 persons[77] and affects primarily the skeletal, ocular, and cardiovascular systems.[78–84] Mutations primarily occur in the *FBN1* gene that encodes fibrillin-1 (66% to 91%) and rarely in *TGFBR1* or *TGFBR2*, the genes also associated with LDS (see Ehlers–Danlos Syndrome section). Fibrillin-1 is secreted into the extracellular matrix and polymerizes to form microfibrils of the zonular fibers of the lens, which are associated with elastic fibers in the aorta and skin.[85,86] The microfibrils stabilize latent TGF-β-binding proteins (LTBPs), which bind to and maintain TGF-β in an inactive state.[80] Deficiency of fibrillin-1 thus leads to abnormal TGF-β signaling. About 27% of cases occur by spontaneous mutation; recurrence as a result of parental germline mosaicism has been described.[87,88]

Diagnosis is best made by clinical examination (including careful cardiac evaluation and measurement of body proportions) (Box 6.2), echocardiography, slit-lamp ophthalmologic examination, and radiographs or imaging as needed to find criteria. Cardiac examinations should be repeated every year until adulthood.[79,84] Early diagnosis is critical because of the potentially fatal complications, but the clinical features evolve with advancing age, and diagnosis is difficult. Family history is also important, but manifestations may not be evident until adolescence, and expressivity is variable, so generations appear to be skipped. The Ghent diagnostic criteria (Box 6.3) were simplified in 2010, eliminating major and minor criteria and giving more weight to ectopia lentis and aortic root aneurysm/dissection.[89] Other organ involvement contributes to a systemic score to guide diagnosis if aortic disease, but not ectopia lentis, is present. A more important role

Box 6.2 Most Common Features of Marfan Syndrome

- Autosomal dominant disorder
- Present in ≥75% of individuals with Marfan syndrome (MFS):
  - Positive wrist and thumb sign
- Present in ≥50% and <75% of individuals with MFS:
  - Dolichostenomelia
  - Pes planus
  - Joint hypermobility
  - Aortic root dilatation
  - Mitral valve prolapse
  - High arched palate with crowded dentition
  - Typical facial features
  - Lens displacement (ectopia lentis)
- Present in ≥25% and <50% of individuals with MFS:
  - Pectus excavatum or carinatum requiring surgery
  - Myopia
  - Scoliosis
  - Striae

**Dolichostenomelia* refers to a habitus in which the limbs are unusually long, as is typical of MFS (*dolichos*, long; *steno*, narrow or close; *melia*, of the limbs).

Box 6.3 Revised Ghent Criteria for Marfan Syndrome

Without a family history of Marfan syndrome (MFS), any of these combinations allow diagnosis:

1. Aortic diameter (Z score* ≥2) AND ectopia lentis
2. Aortic diameter (Z ≥2) AND fibrillin-1 *(FBN1)* mutation
3. Aortic diameter (Z ≥2) AND systemic criteria (≥7 points; see criteria later)
4. Ectopia lentis AND fibrillin-1 *(FBN1)* mutation with known aortic diameter (Z ≥2)

With a positive family history, these features allow the diagnosis:

1. Ectopia lentis
2. Systemic criteria (≥7 points) (see criteria later)
3. Aortic diameter (Z ≥2 above 20 years old, ≥3 below 20 years old)

Alternative diagnoses (no family history of MFS):
Ectopia lentis syndrome: ectopia lentis with or without systemic criteria AND: (1) with an *FBN1* mutation but one not known to be associated with aortic diameter (Z ≥2) OR (2) no *FBN1* mutation
MASS: aortic diameter (Z <2) AND systemic criteria (≥5 with at least one skeletal feature) but without ectopia lentis
MVP syndrome: MVP AND aortic diameter (Z <2) AND systemic criteria (<5) without ectopia lentis

Systemic criteria (maximum total: 20 points; score .7 indicates systemic involvement):
Wrist AND thumb sign = 3 (wrist OR thumb sign = 1)
Pectus carinatum deformity = 2 (pectus excavatum or chest asymmetry = 1)
Hindfoot deformity = 2 (plain pes planus = 1)
Pneumothorax = 2
Dural ectasia = 2
Protrusio acetabuli = 2
Reduced US/LS AND increased arm/height AND no severe scoliosis = 1
Scoliosis or thoracolumbar kyphosis = 1
Reduced elbow extension = 1
Facial features (3/5) = 1 (dolichocephaly, enophthalmos, downslanting palpebral fissures, malar hypoplasia, retrognathia)
Skin striae = 1
Myopia >3 diopters = 1
MVP (all types) = 1

MASS, Mitral valve prolapsed and myopia, mild and nonprogressive aortic root dilatation, marfanoid skeletal changes, and skin features (especially striae); *MVP*, mitral valve prolapse; *US/LS*, upper segment/lower segment ratio.
*Z score is the standard deviation from normal means of the inner to inner-edge diameter of the aortic root at the sinus of Valsalva, normalized for the subject's body surface area and age.

is assigned to genotyping *FBN1* and other relevant genes. Criteria now enable diagnosis of ectopia lentis and distinction from MASS syndrome (mitral valve prolapse and myopia, mild and nonprogressive aortic root dilatation, marfanoid skeletal changes, and skin features, especially striae) and mitral valve prolapse syndrome. Criteria are still less reliable in children, especially because several of the more specific features are age dependent (e.g., aortic dilatation, ectopia lentis, dural ectasia, protrusion acetabuli),[78,79,90] and care should still be made to avoid branding children unnecessarily with MFS, given the potential stigma and lifestyle restrictions.

Patients are often tall with long extremities ("marfanoid habitus"; see Fig. 6.8). The arm span characteristically is greater than the height and, after puberty, the upper segment (vertex to pubis)–to–lower segment (pubis to sole) ratio is less than 0.86. Arachnodactyly, kyphoscoliosis, pectus carinatum or excavatum, and a hindfoot deformity or flat feet are commonly seen in patients with this disorder. Joint laxity from capsular, ligamentous, and tendinous involvement may cause hyperextensibility and/or dislocation. Patellar dislocation is not uncommon; dislocation of the hip, often detected during the newborn period, may be the first sign of MFS. The thumb sign (thumb extends well beyond the ulnar border of the hand when overlapped by fingers) and wrist sign (thumb overlaps the fifth finger as they grasp the opposite wrist) are screening tests for the joint hypermobility of MFS.[91] Dural ectasia is occasionally seen in children, and imaging is performed largely to consider an additional Ghent criterion for diagnosis, but its presence is nonspecific. Specific facial features and pneumothorax are additional criteria (see Box 6.3).

Lack of subcutaneous fat and the presence of striae, most prominent on the upper chest, arms, thighs, and abdomen, are the most common cutaneous manifestations of MFS. In addition, elastosis perforans serpiginosa (EPS; see Elastosis Perforans Serpiginosa section) occurs with increased incidence in patients with MFS.

The most common ocular abnormalities are lens displacement (ectopia lentis; the hallmark of ocular involvement, seen in at least 55% of affected children and usually bilateral) and myopia (almost half of children). Retinal detachment, cataracts, or glaucoma may impair vision and cause blindness.[92]

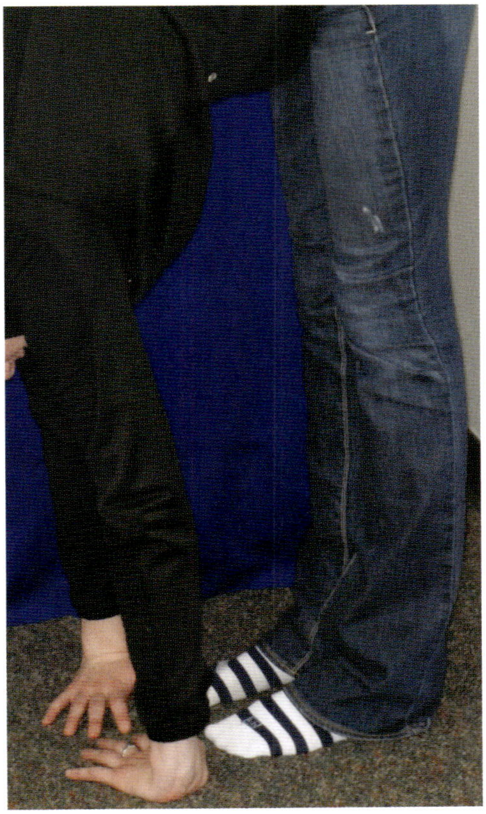

Fig. 6.8 Marfan syndrome (MFS). The long arm span and decreased upper-to-lower body ratio are characteristic of the "marfanoid habitus."

Cardiovascular abnormalities occur in almost 70% of children with MFS. Dilatation of the aorta is the most common defect and is generally greatest at the sinuses of Valsalva, diffuse dilatation of the proximal segment of the ascending aorta with aortic regurgitation often occurs, and dilatation of the pulmonary artery has been detected in 8% of affected children.[93] Mitral valve prolapse occurs in approximately 60% of affected children and adolescents.[94] Left ventricular dilatation may predispose patients to alterations of repolarization and fatal ventricular arrhythmias.[95] The most severely affected children, those with neonatal MFS, almost always have aortic dilatation and severely impaired valves, leading to congestive heart failure, pulmonary hypertension, and a risk of early death.[88] In a child diagnosed with MFS, serial echocardiography at 6- to 12-month intervals is recommended, with the frequency depending on the aortic diameter in relation to the body surface area and the rate of increase. Pregnancy has been associated with significant cardiac complications (aortic dissection, arrhythmia), postpartum hemorrhage, thromboembolism, premature babies, and babies who are small for gestational age.[96–98]

Conditions most often considered when patients have cutaneous and other system concerns are vEDS (aortic root dilatation or dissection) (see Ehlers–Danlos Syndrome and Table 6.1), the MASS phenotype, LDS (aortic root dilatation or dissection), Shprintzen–Goldberg syndrome, homocystinuria, and methylmalonic aciduria with homocystinuria (Table 6.4).[99] Patients with MFS do not have the translucent and velvety skin or easy bruising of EDS or LDS.[80] Patients with homocystinuria have ectopia lentis and a marfanoid habitus, but mental retardation is a distinguishing feature. Individuals with an inherited deficiency in processing cobalamin C/vitamin B_{12} similarly may have marfanoid features in addition to macrocytic anemia and neurodevelopmental issues.[100] Perhaps hardest to distinguish is MASS, a marfanoid disorder caused by *FBN1* mutations but with a better prognosis. Striae are a prominent feature, and atrophic skin patches with abnormal elastic fibers may be present.[101] Pectus excavatum and marfanoid skeletal features are most common.[102] Among the distinguishing features are a stable and mild aortic root dilatation and lack of ectopia lentis, but distinguishing MASS from MFS can be difficult in children and adolescents.

The prognosis of MFS depends on the extent and severity of cardiovascular defects. Death usually occurs in adulthood, but occasionally during childhood, as a result of cardiovascular sequelae, especially due to complications related to dilatation of the aortic root.[103,104] A rare neonatal form of MFS features the marfanoid body disproportion, lax skin, emphysema, ocular abnormalities, joint contractures, kyphoscoliosis, adducted thumbs, crumpled ears, micrognathia, muscle hypoplasia, and deficient subcutaneous fat over joints.[105] Severe cardiac valve insufficiency and aortic dilatation result in death during the first 2 years of life. A neonatal progeroid variant of MFS with prematurity, congenital lipodystrophy, and frameshift mutations at the 3′ end of *FBN1* has been described. In the differential diagnosis of progeria, the marfanoid habitus with accelerated linear growth, severe myopia, and dilatation of the aortic bulb allow correct diagnosis.[106,107]

Children with MFS but without serious cardiac issues can participation in some sports but should avoid potentially harmful exertion, particularly contact sports (to protect the aorta and lens), sports with bursts of activity (such as sprinting), and isometric exercises (such as weightlifting), which might lead to further aortic root dilatation, aortic rupture, or congestive heart failure.[84] Scuba diving should be avoided because of the risk of pneumothorax.

Systemic pharmacologic therapy has been directed at limiting aortic root dilatation.[108,109] The largest study in children, the Pediatric Heart Network trial, showed that atenolol, a β-blocker, and losartan, an angiotensin receptor blocker that reduced TGF-β pathway aberrant signaling, each reduced the rate of aortic dilatation.[108,109] When atenolol is used, the dose should be individualized and uptitrated on the basis of hemodynamic response to achieve maximal β-blockade. Doses of 1.4 mg/kg per day losartan (100 to 150 mg per day in adult-sized adolescents) are recommended. For patients with severe or progressive aortic root dilatation, the combination of β-blocker and angiotensin receptor blocker therapy should be considered. Given that the

Table 6.4 Genetic Basis for Marfan Syndrome and Related Disorders

Disorder	Subtype	Gene	Distinguishing Features
Marfan syndrome (MFS)	—	FBN1	—
MASS syndrome	—	FBN1	MASS = Mitral valve prolapse/Myopia, Aortic root dilatation, Striae/skin features, and Skeletal features of Marfan syndrome No ectopia lentis Arterial disease is milder and not progressive
Loeys–Dietz syndrome (LDS)	LDS1 LDS2 LDS3 LDS4 LDS5 Other	TGFBR1 TGFBR2 SMAD3 TGFB2 TGFB3 SMAD2	No myopia or ectopia lentis; includes craniosynostosis, hypertelorism, bifid uvula Has translucent, velvety skin and bruising of EDS
Shprintzen–Goldberg syndrome (SGS)	—	SKI	Skeletal, skin, and cardiovascular features of MFS and LDS Milder vascular issues (limited to risk of aneurysm or dissection of aortic root) Craniosynostosis, hypotonia, learning difficulties
Homocystinuria		CBS	Marfanoid habitus Ectopia lentis, but downward displacement Widened epiphyses and metaphyses with early osteoporosis Mental retardation and seizures Thromboses and early atheroma formation Malar flush
Cobalamin C (CblC) defect		MMACHC	Marfanoid features, arachnodactyly, joint laxity, and scoliosis, macrocytic anemia, developmental delay, behavioral issues

FBN1 encodes fibrillin-1; *TGFBR1* and *TGFBR2* encode the TGF-β receptors 1 and 2; *TGFB2* and *3* encode TGF-β2 and TGF-β3; *SMAD2* and *SMAD3* encode proteins that are critical signal transducers for TGF-β receptors; *SKI* encodes the SKI proto-oncogene, which represses TGF-β activity; *CBS* encodes cystathionine beta-synthase; *MMACHC* (Methylmalonic aciduria CblcC type with Homocystinuria) is critical for the conversion of cobalamin/vitamin B12 into adenosylcobalamin (required for methylmalonyl CoA mutase) and methylcobalamin (cofactor for methionine synthase, which converts homocysteine to methionine).

greatest improvement was noted in younger children, medical therapy should be prescribed even in young children with evidence of early aortic root dilatation. There is limited evidence to support the routine use of angiotensin-converting enzyme inhibitors or calcium channel blockers for prophylactic treatment of aortic enlargement. Not all patients respond, and those who experience progressive aortic root dilatation with its ongoing risk for aortic dissection should be considered for prophylactic aortic root surgery. In one study, striae together with elevated TGF-β and matrix metalloproteinase (MMP)-3 serum levels correlated with a higher risk of aortic dissection.[110] Aneurysmal and valvular heart defects may require prosthetic replacement, but this should be postponed as long as possible to avoid recurrent prosthesis replacement, particularly in growing children.

Early and regular ophthalmologic examinations are required to detect correctable amblyopia and retinal detachment. Ectopia lentis and even complete luxation may be tolerated for decades, but lens extraction may be required to treat diplopia, glaucoma, cataracts, or retinal detachment. Repair of the pectus excavatum is indicated if cardiopulmonary compromise occurs, but should be delayed until skeletal maturation is nearly complete to prevent recurrence and should employ internal stabilization. Scoliosis may be lessened in adolescent girls by estrogen therapy, but this therapy may also produce an overall decrease in height. Bracing, physical therapy, and vertebral fusion may all be necessary to prevent severe scoliosis. The website for the National Marfan Foundation is www.marfan.org.

Osteogenesis Imperfecta

OI refers to a group of inherited disorders of bone fragility in which the skin may be thin, atrophic, and somewhat translucent.[111–113] The easy bruisability and bone fractures may raise the possibility of child abuse. Wound healing may be normal, but scars are commonly atrophic or hypertrophic. Patients often show hyperlaxity of ligaments and hypermobility of joints, but joint dislocation does not occur. Blue sclerae are distinctive features in approximately 90% of patients but can also be seen in MFS and EDS; increased electron-dense granular material between scleral fibers permits scattering of light by normal pigment within the orbit. Otosclerosis with hearing loss may begin during adolescence (50% of the common type I by adulthood), and fragile, discolored teeth are particularly common in the more unusual forms (dentinogenesis imperfecta [DI]). Patients may show mitral and aortic valve dilatation and regurgitation and cystic medionecrosis of the aorta.

More than one classification scheme has recently been proposed; the newer Sillence classification[113] includes types 1 through 5 and the more-newly recognized, less common, and largely autosomal recessive forms based on clinical features. The classification described by Marini et al.[114] separates types of OI based on genetics and extends the five Sillence classification subtypes to 12 subtypes (I through XII) and an unclassified/other category (Table 6.5). OI has also been classified by severity of clinical features (mild to extremely severe), fracture frequency, bone densitometry, and level of mobility.[113] Changes in 16 genes may be classified under OI,[113] presenting variable clinical features, severity, and prognosis.[114] More than 85% of affected individuals have an autosomal dominant form of OI (AD OI), of which most are type I OI, the mildest form.

Patients with AD OI almost all have mutations in type I collagen, which is composed of two α1 *(COLIA1)* and one α2 *(COLIA2)* polypeptide chains, forming a triple helical structure. Dominant OI can also result from mutations in *IFITM5*, leading to abnormalities in matrix mineralization. Overall, 10% to 15% of cases are autosomal recessive and result from a mutation in one of at least 11 genes involved in posttranslational processing of type I collagen and bone formation (see Table 6.4). Some of these encode proteins involved in a complex required for proline (P986) hydroxylation of type I collagen *(CRTAP, P3H1, CYPB)*.[115–117] Others are involved in collagen mineralization *(BRIL* and *PEDF)*, collagen crosslinking, folding and chaperoning *(FKBP65* and *HSP47)*, and osteoblast development (osterix, *OASIS, TRICB*, and *WNT1*) (see Table 6.4).

Table 6.5 Classification of Osteogenesis Imperfecta

Type	Frequency/ Inheritance	Gene; Protein	Clinical Features	Effect of Gene Alteration
I	AD (>50%)	*COL1A1, COL1A2*; type I collagen	Also called *nondeforming OI with blue sclerae* Fractures (90% to 95%), blue sclerae (100%), hearing loss (begins in adolescence and is in >50% by 40 years), vertigo, normal stature, rarely DI	Collagen I quantity
II	AD*	*COL1A1, COL1A2* glycine substitutions; type I collagen	Also called *perinatal lethal OI* Multiple fractures, severe rib (beading) and long bone (crumped, accordion-like) deformities, frog leg positioning, blue-gray sclerae, small for gestational age 20% stillborn and 40% die by 1 month	Collagen I structure
III	AD	*COL1A1, COL1A2* glycine substitutions; type I collagen	Also called *progressive deforming OI* Severe deformities; multiple fractures with progressive deformities, short stature (less than third percentile) with severe progressive scoliosis, marked osteopenia, nonambulatory Triangular face, hearing loss in adults, may have DI Progressive whitening of sclerae Majority now survive into adulthood and have normal growth velocity/decreased fractures with cyclic IV bisphosphonates	Collagen I structure
IV	AD	*COL1A1, COL1A2* glycine substitutions; type I collagen	Also called *common variable OI*; milder than OI III Moderately short, mild to moderate scoliosis, recurrent fractures with variable deformity, osteoporosis Typically ambulatory DI common, adult-onset hearing loss, usually normal sclerae	Collagen I structure
V	AD (4% to 5%)	*IFITM5*; BRIL	Also called *OI with calcification in interosseous membranes* Mild to moderate fractures (especially forearms, legs affected) and short stature, dislocation of radial head White sclerae, no DI Rarely, painful hyperplastic callus	Matrix mineralization
VI	AR	*SERPINF1*; PEDF	Similar to type III, moderately short, scoliosis, white sclerae, no DI Abnormal bone mineralization	Matrix mineralization
VII	AR	*CRTAP*; cartilage-associated protein	Moderately deforming Clinically types II and III, but milder forms documented Rhizomelic shortening of humerus and femur, coxa vara, "popcorn epiphyses" White sclerae, no DI	3-hydroxylation of collagen
VIII	AR	*LEPRE1*; prolyl-3-hydroxylase-1/P3H1	Moderately deforming Clinically types II and III, but milder forms documented Rhizomelic shortening of humerus and femur, coxa vara, "popcorn epiphyses" White sclerae, no DI	3-hydroxylation of collagen
IX	AR	*PPIB*; peptidyl-prolyl isomerase B/CyPB	Clinically types II and IV Fractures with generalized osteopenia, wide anterior fontanel Moderate growth deficiency, gross motor delay No rhizomelia or DI, white sclerae	3-hydroxylation of collagen
X	AR	*SERPINH1*; HSP47	Clinically type III	Collagen chaperone
XI	AR	*FKBP10*; FKBP10 (also called FKBP65)	Clinically type III Can have joint contractures	Telopeptide hydroxylation for crosslinking
XII	AR	*BMP1*; BMP1/mTLD	Clinically type III	Collagen processing (cleaves C-propeptidase)
OTHERS				
	AR	*CREB3L1*; OASIS	Clinically type III	Osteoblast development
	AR	*SP7/OSX*; SP7/osterix	Clinically type II	Osteoblast development
	AR	*TMEM38B*; TRICB	Clinically type III	Osteoblast development
	AD/AR	*WNT1*; WNT1	Clinically type II (AD) or type III (AR)	Osteoblast development
	AR	*PLOD2*; PLOD2	Clinically type III; can have congenital joint contractures	Telopeptide hydroxylation
	XLR	*PLS3*; plastin 3	Clinically closest to type IV; no features beyond childhood fractures; manifests in hemizygous males and variable in heterozygote females	Bone formation and remodeling

AD, Autosomal dominant; *AR*, autosomal recessive; *DI*, dentinogenesis imperfecta; *OI*, osteogenesis imperfecta; *XLR*, X-linked recessive.
*Usually new mutation; parental germline mosaicism in 2% to 6% of cases.

Supportive orthopedic therapy includes physical therapy to prevent contractures and immobility-induced bone loss, orthoses to protect the lower limbs,[118] and, in more severe cases, bisphosphonates.[119] Cyclical treatment with intravenous bisphosphonates is the mainstay of medical therapy for children with moderate to severe OI and has been shown to increase bone mass density, improve muscle strength and mobility, and decrease fractures and bone pain.[111,120]

Cutis Laxa

Cutis laxa (generalized elastolysis) results from mutations in one of 14 genes that disrupt the elastic tissue network in skin[86,121–126] (Box 6.4; Table 6.6). In general, the products of these genes are either (1) proteins involved in the assembly of elastic fibers and upregulation of TGF-β signaling (e.g., *ELN, FBLN4, FBLN5,* and *LTBP4*); (2) Golgi proteins that facilitate secretion of elastic network components (e.g., *ATP6VOA2, RIN2,* and *GORAB*); or (3) mitochondrial proteins (e.g., *PYCR1, ALDH18A1,* and *SLC2A10*).[122] Some affect protein glycosylation (*ATP6VOA2, ATP6V1E1,* and *ATP6V1A*).[126,127]

Cutis laxa can be acquired or congenital, with the genetic forms inherited as either autosomal dominant or autosomal recessive forms, the latter usually being more severe. An X-linked form (X-linked cutis laxa, or occipital horn syndrome; formerly Ehlers–Danlos syndrome type IX) is now classified as a copper transport disease caused by a mutation in the copper transporting adenosine triphosphatase (ATPase), α-polypeptide *ATP7A*.

Patients with cutis laxa present a striking picture of loose, inelastic, redundant skin that sags and hangs in pendulous folds, as if it were too large for the body. The drooping and ectropion of the eyelids, together with the sagging facial skin and accentuation of the nasal, labial, and other facial folds, help produce the "bloodhound" or aged appearance (Fig. 6.9).

Most dominant cases result from heterozygous frameshift mutations in the gene encoding elastin.[128] The autosomal dominant form may appear at any age and presents as a cosmetic problem with few systemic changes.[129] The skin in cutis laxa is extensible but, in contrast to that of EDS, does not spring back to place on release of tension. Special stains for elastic tissue (Verhoeff–van Gieson stain) of skin biopsy specimens demonstrate significantly decreased or absent dermal elastic fibers.

Systemic manifestations caused by weakened supportive tissue include aortic root dilatation (55%), hernias (51%; ventral, hiatal, or inguinal), pulmonary emphysema (37%), pulmonary artery stenosis, diverticulae of the GI tract or urinary bladder, and uterine or rectal prolapse.[128] In patients with the severe autosomal recessively inherited disease, the disorder is gradually progressive, and death from pulmonary complications related to emphysema may occur early in infancy or in many instances in the second to fourth decades of life.

Box 6.4 Most Common Features of Cutis Laxa

- Autosomal dominant or autosomal recessive forms
- Autosomal recessive forms subdivided into those with cardiovascular features (ARCL-1); those with developmental delay (ARCL-2); and those with developmental delay, athetosis, and corneal clouding (ARCL-3). A variety of underlying molecular bases for each group have been discovered (see Table 6.5)
- Skin
  - Loose, inelastic skin
- Most common other features:
  - Facial dysmorphism
  - Aortic dilatation
  - Pulmonary artery stenosis
  - Pulmonary emphysema
  - Diverticulae: gastrointestinal, genitourinary
  - Uterine or rectal prolapse
  - Ventral, hiatal, inguinal hernias

ARCL, Autosomal recessive cutis laxa.

The autosomal recessive forms have traditionally been divided into three subgroups based on clinical characteristics: autosomal recessive cutis laxa (ARCL)-1, -2, and -3 (see Table 6.6).[130–142] Most genes mutated in ARCL have been identified, and the group is quite heterogeneous. All patients tend to have cutis laxa and facial dysmorphism. Hernias (umbilical, inguinal, diaphragmatic) are common. ARCL-1 is characterized by severe cardiopulmonary lesions, including infantile emphysema and cardiac defects, and bladder diverticulae.[143] Fibulin-5 deficiency has been associated with supravalvular aortic stenosis. Fibulin-4 deficiency (mutations in *FBLN4*, also called *EFEMP2*) may be associated with mild to moderate cutis laxa and has been linked to arachnodactyly, tortuous vessels with aneurysm, joint laxity, microcephaly, bone fractures, and pulmonary artery occlusion[144] (Fig. 6.10). Fibulins-4 and -5 are critical in elastic fiber assembly in the skin and other elastic tissues. More recently, *LTBP4* mutations (ARCL type 1C) have been found in patients with emphysema and severe GI and genitourinary (GU) tract involvement but no vascular abnormalities.

Patients with ARCL-2 (which includes "wrinkly skin syndrome") have mild cutis laxa with growth, distinct facial features, hip dysplasia, and often developmental delay without prominent vascular lesions or emphysema, in contrast to ARCL-1. Patients with ARCL-2A may show pretibial pseudoecchymotic skin lesions that resemble those found in EDS,[145] and ARCL-2B is associated with osteoporosis and fractures. The most recently described ARCL-2C and D are characterized by generalized skin wrinkling with sparse subcutaneous fat and often large skin folds with abnormal fat distribution; some have congenital heart defects and/or seizures.[127] ARCL-3, or De Barsy syndrome,[139] can be distinguished from ARCL-2 by athetoid movements and corneal opacities, but otherwise there is overlap between ARCL-2 and ARCL-3.[139,140,146,147] Gerodermia osteodysplastica, resulting from mutations in *GORAB*, shows features of ARCL-2A, ARCL-2B, and ARCL-3 (De Barsy syndrome) but has no associated corneal opacities or athetoid movement and characteristically has osteopenia with fractures (as in ARCL-2B). In fact, more severe cases of ARCL-2B show juvenile cataract and dystonic movement, as in ARCL-3.[148] Cutis laxa is a major component for children with Lenz–Majewski syndrome in association with generalized hyperostosis, proximal symphalangism, syndactyly, brachydactyly, mental retardation, hypertelorism, and enamel hypoplasia.[149] Lenz–Majewski syndrome has recently been linked to gain-of-function mutations in phosphatidylserine synthase 1 (*PTDSS1*), which affect phospholipid synthesis.[150] Neonatal brachydactyly with later severe dwarfism, intellectual disability, and hyperostotic skeletal dysplasia are distinguishing features.[151]

Cutis laxa is also a component of several additional syndromes[150–160] (Box 6.5). Cutis laxa is a component of macrocephaly, alopecia, cutis laxa, and scoliosis (MACS) syndrome, an autosomal recessive disorder that results from deficiency of *RIN2*, leading to decreased fibulin-5 and microfibrils.[157] Arterial tortuosity syndrome (ATS) features facial dysmorphism, vessel tortuosity, and joint laxity with scoliosis. Costello syndrome is an autosomal dominant disorder characterized by soft, loose skin of the neck, hands, and feet with excessive wrinkling and deep creases resembling cutis laxa.[152,158,159] The digits tend to be hyperextensible, with loose skin and characteristic ulnar deviation at the wrist (Fig. 6.11). Affected children develop papillomatous plaques (Fig. 6.12, *A*) and/or papules (Fig. 6.12, *B*) around the nares, mouth, and anal areas; acanthosis nigricans; and sometimes striate palmoplantar keratoderma (Fig. 6.13). Although prenatal overgrowth and polyhydramnios occur, patients tend to have postnatal failure to thrive and a distinctive appearance with craniofacial findings that resemble those of lysosomal storage disorders. The facies are coarse with thick lips, macroglossia, and relative macrocephaly. Severe short stature, mental retardation, curly hair, palmoplantar keratoderma (sometimes striate), and hypertrophic cardiomyopathy are other associated manifestations. Costello syndrome results from activating mutations in *HRAS*[161–163] and is associated with a 15% lifetime risk for malignancy, most commonly rhabdomyosarcoma.[164] Deficiency of transaldolase (TALDO) presents with hepatosplenomegaly, liver failure, and cirrhosis in association with dysmorphic features, hypertrichosis, cutis laxa, congenital heart disease, hemolytic anemia, thrombocytopenia, and GU malformations[160,165]; patients may die *in utero* with hydrops fetalis.

Table 6.6 Cutis Laxa and Related Disorders

Disorder	ADCL	ARCL-1A	ARCL-1B	ARCL1C/ URDS	ARCL-2A	ARCL-2B	ARCL-2C	ARCL-2D	ARCL-3/ De Barsy	GO	XLCL	MACS	ATS	Lens-Majewski
Gene	*ELN*	*FBLN4/ EFEMP2*	*FBLN5*	*LTBP4*	*ATP6V0A2*	*PYCR1*	*ATP6V1E1*	*ATP6V1A*	*ALDH18A1; PYCR1*	*GORAB*	*ATP7A*	*RIN2*	*SLC2A10*	*PTDSS1*
Protein	Elastin	Fibulin-4	Fibulin-5	LTBP4	ATP6V0A2	PYCR1	ATP6V1E1	ATP6V1A	P5CS; PYCR1	GORAB	ATP7A	RIN2	GLUT10	PSS1
Lax skin	+++*	++	+++	+++	+++	+++	+++	+++	+++	++	+++	++	+++	++
Facial features												—		
Prominent ears	+++	+	+++	+	—	—	+	+	—	—	++		+	++
Hypertelorism	—	+++	—	+++	—	—	++	++	—	—	—		++	++
Retrognathia	—	+++	—	+++	+++	+++	++	++	—	—	—		+++	+++
Other dysmorphism	—	++	—	++	—	++	++	++	++	+++	++		++	+++
Emphysema	++	++	+++	+++	—	—	—	—	—	—	—	—	—	—
Supravalvular aortic stenosis	—	—	+++	—	—	—	—	—	—	—	—	—	—	—
Aortic aneurysm	++	+++	—	—	+	—	+	+	—	—	—	—	++	—
Arterial tortuosity	—	+++	+	—	—	—	—	—	++	—	++	—	+++	—
Hernias	++	+++	+++	+++	+++	++	+	+	++	++	+++	+	++	—
Bladder diverticula	—	—	+	+++	+	—	—	—	—	—	+++	—	—	—
Delayed motor development	—	+	+	—	+++	—	—	+	+++	+++	+++	—	—	—
Mental retardation	—	—	—	—	+++	+++	—	—	+++	++	+++	—	—	++
Growth delay	—	++	+	+++	+++	+++	—	—	+++	+++	+	—	—	++
IUGR	—	—	—	+	+++	+++	—	—	+++	+++	—	—	—	
Lax joints	—	+	—	++	+++	+++	+	+	++	+++	++	+++	+++	++
Hypotonia	—	+	—	+++	+++	—	++	++	++	++	++	—	—	—
Congenital hip dislocation	—	+	—	—	+	+++	+	+	++	++	—	—	—	++
Patent anterior fontanel	—	—	—	++	+++	—	—	—	++	++	++	—	—	++
Occipital horns	—	—	—	—	—	—	—	—	—	—	+++	—	—	—
Osteoporosis	—	—	—	—	—	++	—	—	—	+++	++	+	—	—
Scoliosis	—	—	—	—	++	+	++	—	++	+++	++	+++	++	+++
Macrocephaly	—	—	—	—	—	—	—	—	—	—	—	+++	—	—
Microcephaly	—	—	—	—	—	+	—	—	++	++	—	—	—	—
Gingival hyperplasia	—	—	—	—	—	—	—	—	—	—	—	+++	—	—
Corneal opacity	—	—	—	—	—	+	—	—	+++	—	—	—	—	—
Athetoid motion	—	—	—	—	—	+	—	—	+++	—	—	—	—	—
Alopecia	—	—	—	—	—	—	—	—	—		—	+++	—	+

ADCL, Autosomal dominant cutis laxa; *ARCL*, autosomal recessive cutis laxa; *ATS*, arterial tortuosity syndrome; *GO*, gerodermia osteodysplastica; *GORAB*, golgin, RAB6-interacting; *IUGR*, intrauterine growth retardation; *LTBP4*, latent transforming growth factor β-binding protein 4; *MACS*, macrocephaly alopecia cutis laxa scoliosis syndrome; *P5CS*, Δ^1-pyrroline-5-carboxylate synthase; *URCS*, Urban–Rifkin–Davis syndrome; *URDS*, Urban–Rifkin–Davis syndrome; *XLCL*, X-linked cutis laxa.

*Incidence of finding range: —, *not reported* to +++, *common*. Of note, some of these disorders have been reported in a very small number of patients, and thus the incidence range may be inaccurate at this time.

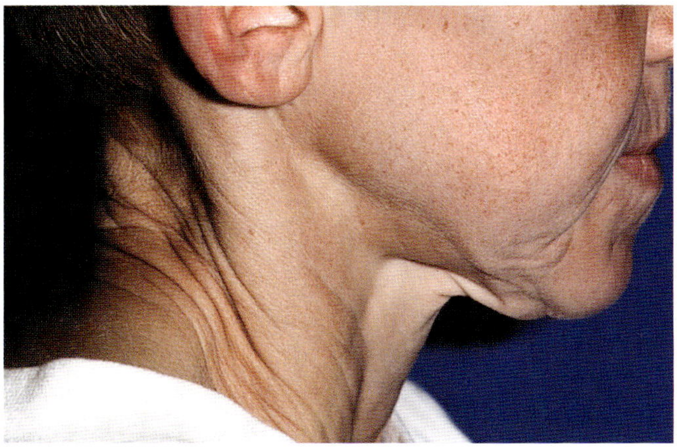

Fig. 6.9 Cutis laxa. Sagging skin in an affected 8-year-old child.

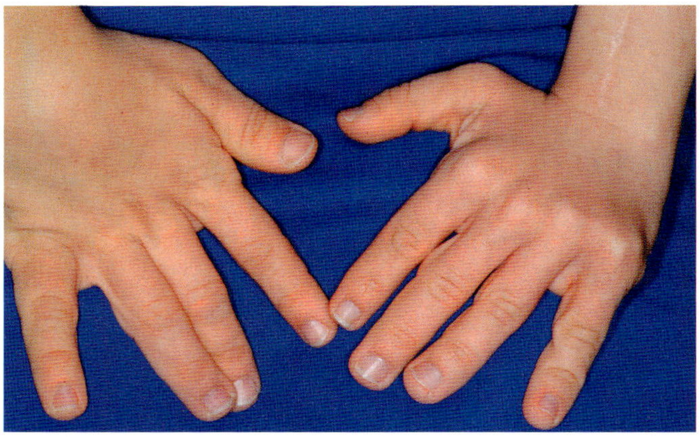

Fig. 6.11 Costello syndrome. Note the loose, hyperextensible skin of the digits.

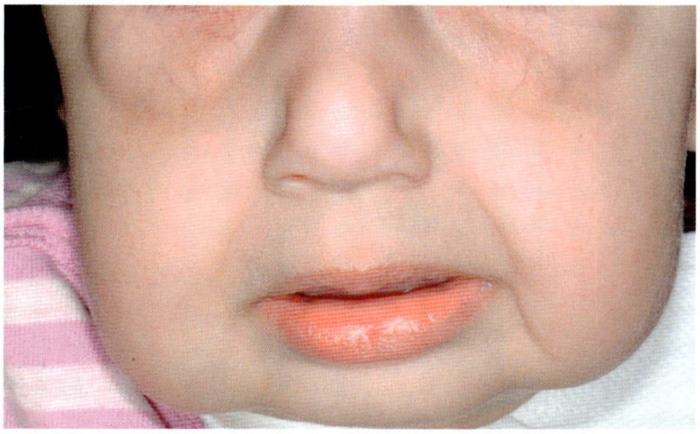

Fig. 6.10 Cutis laxa. This 2-year-old girl with fibulin-4 deficiency shows the sagging infraorbital and cheek skin of cutis laxa.

Box 6.5 **Other Rare Genetic Disorders with Wrinkled or Lax Skin (not in Table 6.5)**

- Ablepharon–macrostomia syndrome
- Barber–Say syndrome
- Cantú syndrome
- Costello syndrome
- GAPO syndrome
- Kabuki makeup syndrome
- Menkes syndrome
- Progeria
- Patterson pseudoleprechanism
- SCARF syndrome
- Transaldolase deficiency
- Williams syndrome

GAPO, Growth retardation, alopecia, pseudoanodontia, and optic atrophy; *SCARF,* skeletal abnormalities, cutis laxa, craniostenosis, psychomotor retardation, and facial abnormalities.

Cutis laxa has also been described in a child with typical Kabuki makeup syndrome.[156]

Cutis laxa can be an acquired condition (Box 6.6), although it occurs less commonly in children than in adults.[166] It can be localized, but in its generalized form ill-defined areas of loose skin appear insidiously but progressively, usually first on the face and then progressing in a cephalocaudal direction. The development of cutis laxa is often preceded by an urticarial eruption. Emphysema, aortic aneurysms with subsequent rupture, and GI and GU diverticulae have been associated. Although most affected children have not had systemic evidence of acquired cutis laxa, aortic dilatation, emphysema, and severe tracheobronchomegaly have led to the demise of children with acquired cutis laxa. Children may develop cutis laxa after drug

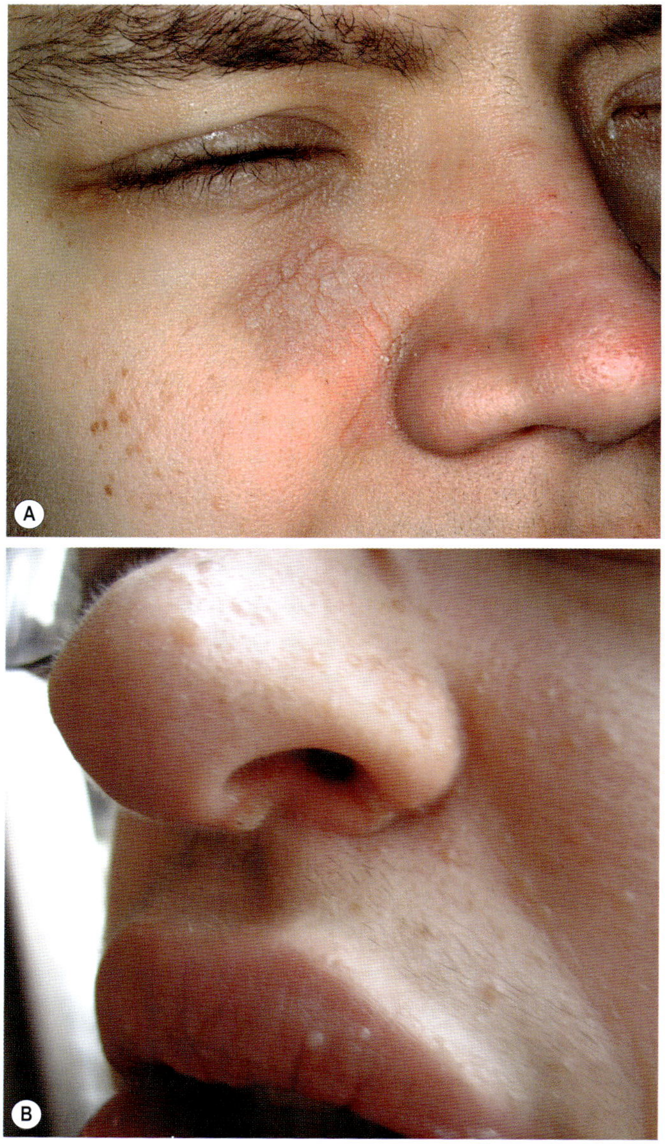

Fig. 6.12 Costello syndrome. Papillomata on the face can be confluent verrucous plaques **(A)** or small papules **(B)** and tend to occur on the midface. Note the coarse, curled eyelashes **(A)**.

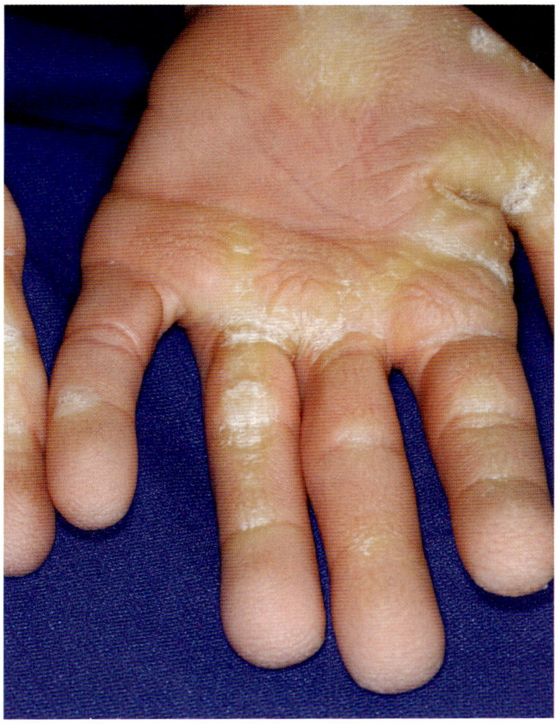

Fig. 6.13 Costello syndrome. Striate keratoderma on the palmar aspect of the fingers is sometimes seen, in addition to keratotic plaques on the palms.

Box 6.6 Associations with Acquired Cutis Laxa

Infections: *Toxocara canis* (cat scratch); *Treponema pallidum* (syphilis); *Borrelia burgdorferi* (Lyme disease); *Onchocerca volvulus* (onchocerciasis)
Medications: isoniazid; penicillins; D-penicillamine
Inflammatory diseases: celiac disease; sarcoidosis; dermatitis herpetiformis, Sweet syndrome
Rheumatic disorders: systemic lupus erythematosus; rheumatoid arthritis
Others: α1-antitrypsin deficiency; mastocytosis; nephrotic syndrome; amyloidosis; malignancy

exposure to penicillin, D-penicillamine,[167] or isoniazid. EPS may be related[168] (see Elastosis Perforans Serpiginosa section). Marshall syndrome (also called *type II acquired cutis laxa*) is a postinflammatory elastolysis characterized by well-demarcated, nonpruritic erythematous plaques that appear in crops during a period of days to weeks, often in association with fever, malaise, and peripheral eosinophilia.[169] Several children have developed cutis laxa after Sweet syndrome,[170] especially at sites of previous inflammation.[171] Acquired cutis laxa has been described in a child with extensive cutaneous mastocytosis.[172] Systemic involvement is rare, but fatal aortitis has been described. Interestingly, a child with acquired cutis laxa after *Toxocara* infestation was found to have compound heterozygous mutations in elastin and a fibulin-5 mutation on one allele, suggesting that environmental factors may trigger acquired cutis laxa in genetically predisposed individual.[173]

Therapy for cutis laxa is limited. Surgery can correct diverticulae, rectal prolapse, or hernias, and plastic surgery can make a dramatic improvement in patients, inevitably with important psychological benefit.[174] Unlike patients with EDS, patients with cutis laxa have no vascular fragility and heal well, enabling repeated facelift procedures. Pulmonary function studies may aid in the early detection of emphysema.

Pseudoxanthoma Elasticum

Pseudoxanthoma elasticum (PXE) is a genetic disorder of the elastic tissue that involves the skin, eyes, and cardiovascular system (Box 6.7).[175] Approximately 1:60,000 individuals are affected.[176] PXE is now recognized to be a metabolic disease rather than a primary disease of elastic tissue.[177,178] It has been linked to mutations in the adenosine triphosphate (ATP)–binding cassette (ABC) subfamily C member 6 *(ABCC6)* gene, which encodes a transmembrane ABC transporter that promotes release of nucleotide triphosphates.[179–181] Although *ABCC6* is expressed primarily in the liver and kidneys, its low levels of expression in other tissues is sufficient to prevent calcification; its absence at these sites leads to ectopic calcification.[182] Nucleoside triphosphates are the precursors of inorganic pyrophosphate (PPi), the circulating factor that inhibits mineralization and thus prevents PXE.[183] Deficiency of ABCC6 also increases tissue-nonspecific alkaline phosphatase (TNAP), which degrades PPi, and an inhibitor of TNAP has been shown to prevent calcifications in mouse models of PXE.[182] The chemical chaperone 4-phenylbutyrate,[184] which has been used for urea cycle disorders, thalassemia, and hepatic cholestasis, corrects defects that involve transport to the membrane, as in PXE, and has been shown in a humanized mouse PXE model to rescue the cardiac calcification defect.

Most of the demonstrated gene mutations would be predicted to lead to autosomal recessive inheritance patterns, although pseudodominant inheritance due to familial consanguinity has been described. PXE demonstrates marked phenotypic heterogeneity even among patients from the same family,[185] suggesting an important role for genetic and environmental factors.[186]

Lesions often develop prepubertally, especially on the lateral aspects of the neck, but may be overlooked because they are small and asymptomatic.[187–189] Most commonly, the diagnosis becomes apparent when the patient reaches the second or third decade of life. The severity may range from extensive flexural cutaneous elastic tissue involvement with severe retinal and cardiovascular complications, often resulting in early blindness and coronary artery disease, to primarily skin changes, milder eye findings, and, rarely, vascular disease. Earlier onset of cutaneous signs has not been associated with a worse prognosis. The cutaneous lesions are characterized by soft, yellowish (xanthoma-like) papules and polygonal plaques on the neck (Fig. 6.14); below the clavicles; in the axillae; and on antecubital fossae, periumbilical areas, and the perineum and thighs. They vary from several papules to linear plaques resembling plucked chicken skin, morocco leather, or orange skin *(peau d'orange)*. Dermoscopic evaluation under polarized light shows irregular yellowish streaks alternating with superficial linear blood vessels.[190] The skin becomes more redundant with advancing age and tends to show progressive calcification at affected sites. Oral, anal, and vaginal mucosal lesions may occur, most commonly infiltration of the lip mucosa. Skin lesions that are similar clinically and ultrastructurally to PXE have been described in patients with β-thalassemia[191] or sickle cell anemia[192,193] or as a complication of D-penicillamine use,[194] but these are rare in children.

Box 6.7 Most Common Features of Pseudoxanthoma Elasticum

- Autosomal recessive
- Skin
  - Yellow papules and plaques (*peau d'orange*, "plucked chicken skin")
- Ocular
  - Angioid streaks
  - Retinal epithelial mottling *(peau d'orange)*
  - Loss of central vision
- Vascular calcifications, hemorrhage
  - Gastrointestinal bleeding
  - Hypertension
  - Cerebrovascular accidents
  - Claudication, myocardial infarction

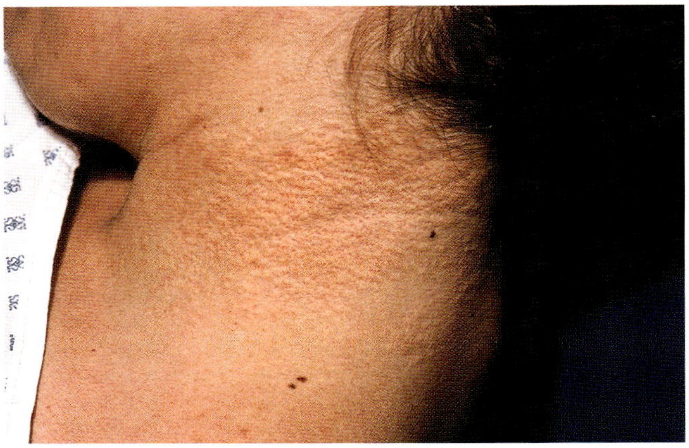

Fig. 6.14 Pseudoxanthoma elasticum. Xanthoma-like papules and plaques on the neck have been likened to plucked chicken skin.

The characteristic angioid streaks are slate-gray to reddish-brown linear bands, resembling vasculature radiating from the optic papilla. Seen ultimately in 94% of patients,[195] angioid streaks represent visualization of the choroid through tears in the calcified and brittle elastic lamina of the Bruch membrane.[196] Angioid streaks usually do not appear until the third decade of life but have been described in children as young as 10 years of age. Characteristic irregular retinal epithelial mottling *(peau d'orange)*, resulting from degenerated elastic tissue, is commonly detected in children with PXE and usually precedes angioid streaks.[188] Loss of central vision (because of retinal hemorrhage and choroidal neovascularization with scarring, not the angioid streaks per se) is the most common disability and may develop in more than 70% of patients with this complication.[197] These retinal changes are not pathognomonic, because they may also be found in patients with thalassemia,[198] sickle cell anemia, Paget disease of the bone, idiopathic thrombocytopenic purpura, acromegaly, EDS, and lead poisoning.[199] Carriers uncommonly may experience ophthalmologic complications.[200]

Calcification of degenerated elastic tissue of the internal lamina of blood vessels with subsequent hemorrhage is a common and potentially serious complication of PXE. The midsized arteries of the extremities, GI tract, and renal vasculature are sites of early manifestations of this degenerative damage. Both hypertension from resultant renal artery stenosis and GI bleeding may occur during adolescence. Late vascular sequelae in PXE include cerebrovascular accidents, intermittent claudication, and myocardial infarction. Severe coronary artery disease has been noted in adolescents with PXE and may respond to bypass surgery, and cardiovascular manifestations may be present during the first decade of life.[201] In addition, an infant with *ABCC6* mutations and a brother with typical manifestations of PXE since adolescence died of generalized arterial calcification, leading to extensive arterial stenosis and myocardial ischemia.[202] Early evidence suggests that carriers of *ABCC6* loss-of-function mutations have an increased risk of coronary artery disease, so parents should be counseled about preventive intervention.[203] Recent studies in mice suggest that statins can prevent, but not reverse, aberrant mineralization in mouse models of PXE.[204]

The diagnosis of PXE is based on the clinical findings and on histopathologic evidence of calcification in elastic tissue and basophilic degeneration of the elastic tissue in the middle and deeper zones of the dermis. Elastic tissue degeneration also affects connective tissue elements of the aorta and medium-sized muscular arteries in the heart, kidneys, GI tract, and other organs.

ABCC6 is thought to distribute to the dermis a reduced form of vitamin K. The form of vitamin K is a cofactor of matrix Gla-protein, an inhibitor of ectopic calcification, suggesting a reason for the dermal calcification.[176] A recessive disorder that resembles severe PXE clinically and histologically, PXE-like disorder with multiple coagulation factor deficiency,[205] usually starts during adolescence and results from deficiency of an enzyme that activates matrix Gla-protein. This matrix Gla-protein activator (γ-glutamyl carboxylase or GGCX) is also important for vitamin K–dependent clotting, leading to cerebral aneurysms and a bleeding diathesis in addition to PXE-like changes.[206–210] In addition to the yellowish, often coalescent papules of PXE in fold areas, PXE-like with multiple coagulation factor deficiency has generalized cutis laxa, especially at the skin folds, as well as facial dysmorphism, but has less vascular and ocular involvement (only subclinical atherosclerotic plaques and ocular angioid streaks). Generalized arterial calcification of infancy (GACI) with extensive tissue mineralization can also result from the same variants in *ABCC6* as PXE, and siblings with GACI without PXE or typical PXE with skin lesions and angioid streaks have been described.[211,212] GACI is more commonly caused by mutations in *ENPP1*,[213] which can also variably be associated with these features of PXE.

Because of the risk of progressive visual loss, patients under 40 years of age are advised to have fundal examination every other year and self-monitor visual acuity with the Amsler grid.[195] Because of the potential risk to eyes and calcified vessels when traumatized, contact sports and high-intensity cardiovascular exercise should be prohibited for persons with PXE to minimize the risk of future visual loss. Intravitreal injection of vascular endothelial growth-factor antagonists prevent neovascularization and thereby reduce the loss of visual acuity,[214] with or without laser and photodynamic therapeutic options.[196,210,215,216] Avoidance of high-cholesterol foods and smoking, control of blood pressure, and safe aerobic exercises are appropriate because of the vascular risks. Serial cardiac evaluation (careful auscultation and echocardiographic monitoring) to detect mitral valve prolapse is also important. Ultrasound studies have also shown impaired left ventricular function, impaired aortic elastic properties, and a high prevalence of peripheral artery disease. Because carriers also showed cardiovascular issues, albeit milder, carriers of PXE should be identified and monitored.[217]

Early studies suggested that patients who extensively ingested dairy products rich in calcium and phosphate have more severe later disease. In addition, clinical and histologic improvement in skin lesions has been described in 50% of patients treated systemically with aluminum hydroxide, which binds phosphate.[218] The demonstration in a mouse model of PXE that increased dietary intake of magnesium prevents connective tissue mineralization led to a 2-year trial in affected patients, but results are not yet available.[219,220] The first-generation bisphosphonate, etidronate, was tested in a 1-year randomized, double-blind trial of 74 adults for its reduction of ectopic calcification with mixed results; etidronate lowered arterial calcification and subretinal neovascularization events, but did not reduce lower extremity calcification—the primary endpoint—without adverse events. Warfarin has been shown to accelerate the ectopic mineralization[221] and should be avoided if possible. Plastic surgery may improve the appearance of sagging skin, although extrusion of calcium particles through the surgical wound may result in delayed healing and unsightly scars.[222] Nonablatic fractional laser resurfacing has also been used with good results.[223] GI bleeding can usually be managed conservatively. Two support groups, the National Association for Pseudoxanthoma Elasticum (http://www.napeusa.com/) and PXE International (www.pxe.org), are available.

Elastosis Perforans Serpiginosa

EPS (also termed *perforating elastoma*) is a perforating disorder of elastic tissue characterized by an annular, arciform, or linear arrangement of keratotic papules.[224,225] The individual papules measure 2 to 4 mm in diameter, but collectively can lead to lesions as long as 15 to 20 cm in overall length. The papules are generally capped by a distinctive keratotic plug, which when forcibly dislodged reveals a bleeding crateriform lesion. Biopsy shows elongated tortuous channels within the epidermis that are perforated by abnormal and degenerated elastic tissue extruded from the dermis. Lesions show a predilection for distribution on the posterolateral aspects of the neck (Fig. 6.15) and occasionally the chin, cheeks, mandibular areas of the face, antecubital fossae, elbows, and knees.[226]

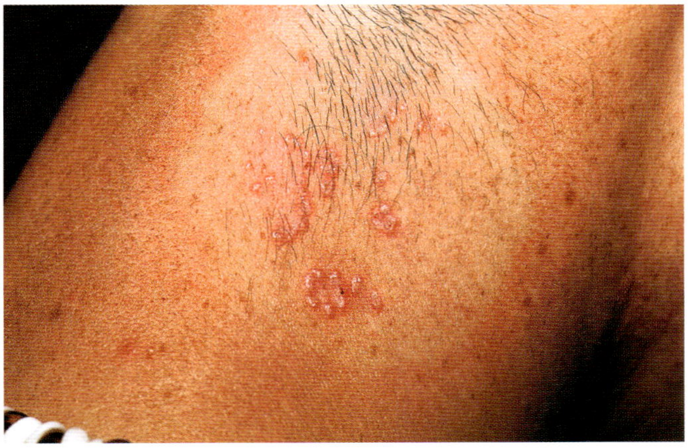

Fig. 6.15 Elastosis perforans serpiginosa. Annular, arcuate, and linear arrangement of erythematous keratotic papules on the posterolateral aspects of the neck. (Courtesy Annette Wagner, MD.)

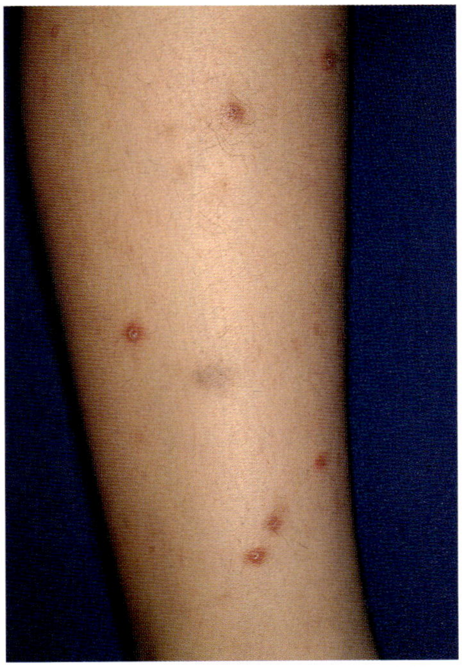

Fig. 6.16 Reactive perforating collagenosis. Pruritic papules with keratotic plugs stud the legs of this otherwise normal girl; biopsy is helpful in distinguishing among the perforating disorders.

This cutaneous disorder primarily affects young persons, especially those in the second decade of life, and generally disappears spontaneously within 5 to 10 years. Up to 44% of reported cases have been seen in association with Down syndrome, OI, EDS, PXE, cutis laxa, Rothmund–Thomson syndrome, acrogeria, morphea, or MFS or as a complication of penicillamine therapy.[227–230] Thorough history and physical examination should suffice to consider underlying causes.[230] Treatment with stripping of the surface keratinous material by repeated application of Scotch tape, cryosurgery, keratolytic agents, imiquimod,[231–233] laser, or photodynamic therapy (PDT)[232,233] may result in improvement of some lesions, but recurrences are common even if therapy is effective.

EPS must be distinguished from three other perforating disorders of the skin that feature transepidermal elimination of altered dermal substances: reactive perforating collagenosis (Fig. 6.16), perforating folliculitis, and Kyrle disease. These perforating disorders occur more commonly in adults, especially in association with chronic renal disease and diabetes,[234] but can occur in children, including siblings. The underlying basis for the perforation and extrusion of dermal material is poorly understood, but skin biopsy can distinguish among them. As with EPS, treatment can be difficult. Topical retinoids and topical and intralesional corticosteroids often provide no relief; narrowband ultraviolet B (UVB) light has been shown to decrease the pruritus and promote resolution of reactive perforating collagenosis.[235]

Focal Dermal Hypoplasia

Focal dermal hypoplasia (Goltz syndrome) is characterized by linear streaks of dermal hypoplasia (Box 6.8). The condition is X-linked dominant and thought to be lethal in homozygous males; 90% of patients are female. The disorder results from mutations in *PORCN*, which encodes a protein that is critical for the secretion of Wnt, an important protein for skin and bone development.[236–238] Although the disorder in male individuals usually reflects postzygotic mosaicism of the mutated *PORCN* gene[239,240] (see Fig. 6.17), classic features of Goltz syndrome have also been described in a male with Klinefelter syndrome.[241]

Many of the cutaneous manifestations of focal dermal hypoplasia are present from birth.[242,243] These include the widely distributed linear areas of hypoplasia of the skin, often with associated telangiectasia (Figs. 6.17 and 6.18); soft, yellow, reddish-yellow, or yellow-brown nodular outpouchings, often in a linear distribution (caused by herniation of the subcutaneous fat through the thinned dermis); and sometimes erosions or ulcers from the cutaneous hypoplasia that gradually heal with atrophy. Patients often show streaky hyperpigmentation or hypopigmentation or depigmentation (Fig. 6.19), sometimes with hyperpigmented freckles in the hypopigmented areas.[244] Erythematous papillomas of the affected skin or mucosae of the oral, anal, or genital region may develop and progress.[245] Nail changes occur in 89% of affected individuals[246] (micronychia, atrophy, V-nicking, and longitudinal ridging).[246,247] Patchy or diffuse sparseness of hair and hypodontia with enamel hypoplasia[247] have also been described. Skeletal abnormalities are most commonly digital abnormalities (syndactyly [68%] and ectrodactyly/"lobster claw" deformities [68%]) and leg-length discrepancy (57%)[245,246,248] (Fig. 6.20). Increased risk of fracture and osteoporosis have recently been suggested.[245] Associated ocular abnormalities include colobomas (chorioretinal in 61% and iris in 50%), microphthalmia (44%), nystagmus (33%), strabismus (22%), anophthalmia (11%), cataracts (11%), and papillomas of the conjunctivae and eyelids (5%).[248] Eye, hair, teeth, and limb abnormalities may occur without cutaneous features.[249] Nutritional and GI problems are common and include underweight (77%), short stature (65%), oral motor dysfunction (41%), constipation (35%), gastroparesis (35%), and gastroesophageal reflux (24%).[250,251] Obstructive sleep apnea may require tonsillectomy.[251] Other associated abnormalities may

Box 6.8 Most Prominent Features of Focal Dermal Hypoplasia (Goltz Syndrome)

- X-linked dominant, 10% of patients are male
- Linear or reticular patterns of:
  - Thinned dermis
  - Focal fat herniation
  - Hyperpigmentation or hypopigmentation
  - Papillomas
  - Ulcerations
- Ectodermal abnormalities
  - Sparse hair
  - Thin nails
  - Hypodontia, enamel hypoplasia
- Skeletal abnormalities, especially digital anomalies
- Ocular colobomas, strabismus, microphthalmia
- Diagnosis
  - Clinical features
  - Osteopathia striata (plain radiography)

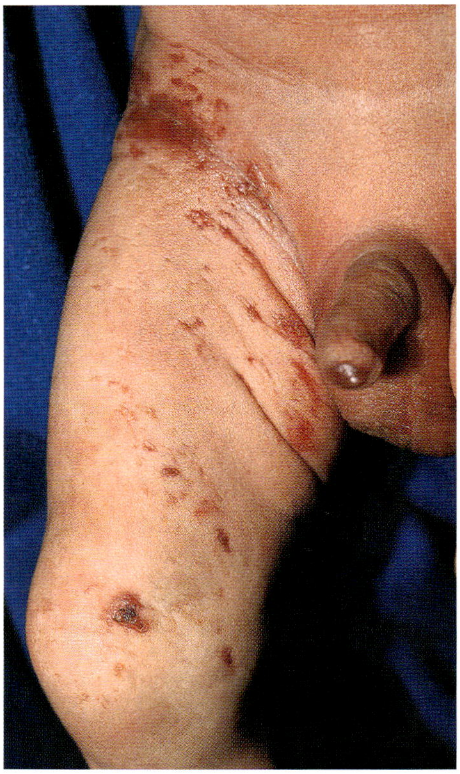

Fig. 6.17 Focal dermal hypoplasia (Goltz syndrome). Linear streaks of dermal hypoplasia with visible telangiectasia in an affected boy. The condition is presumed to be lethal in male individuals, suggesting that this boy's manifestation reflects postzygotic mosaicism.

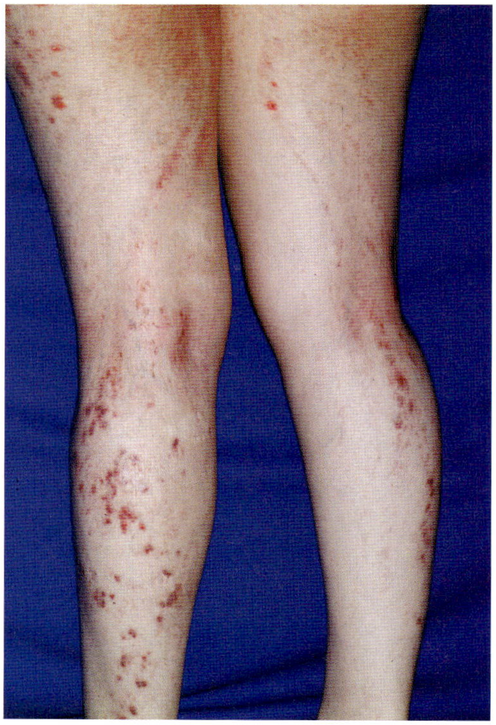

Fig. 6.18 Focal dermal hypoplasia. Streaks of dermal hypoplasia with visible telangiectasia that follow Blaschko lines. This girl underwent a series of pulsed-dye laser treatments, which reduced the visibility of telangiectasia and improved cosmesis on her face, arms, and legs.

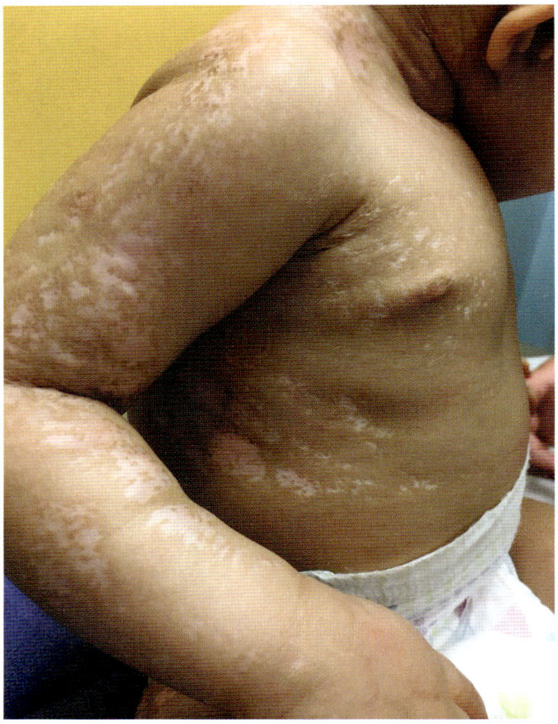

Fig. 6.19 Focal dermal hypoplasia. Depigmented streaks along Blaschko lines in this girl with Goltz syndrome.

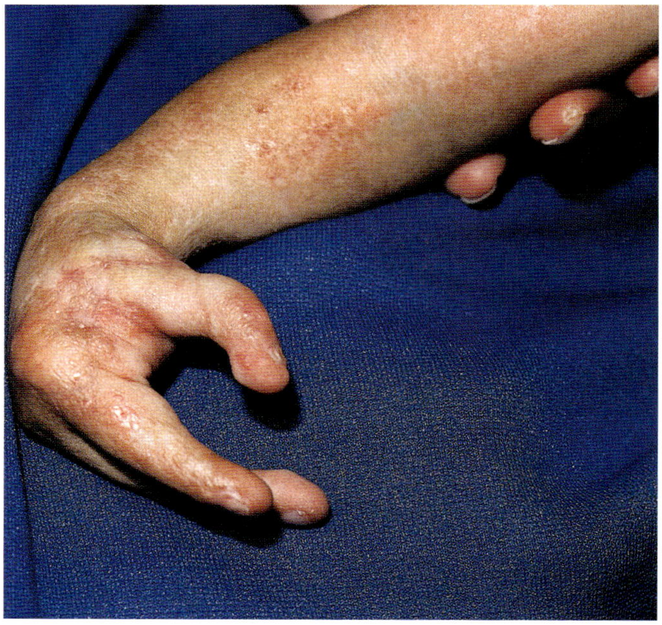

Fig. 6.20 Focal dermal hypoplasia. Skeletal deformities are common, especially involving the hand.

include umbilical or inguinal hernia, cleft lip and/or cleft palate, central nervous system abnormalities (microcephaly, mental retardation, myelomeningocele, and hydrocephalus[252]), giant cell tumor of bone,[253] and multiple basal cell carcinomas.[254]

Virtually all cases of focal dermal hypoplasia reveal fine parallel linear striations in the metaphyses of long bones at or near epiphyseal junctions on radiographs. Although striations can be seen with other bony abnormalities, this linear change in the metaphyseal regions of the long bones (termed *osteopathia striata*) is a useful diagnostic sign of this disorder. Although rarely necessary to confirm the diagnosis, biopsy of an affected area of skin can be performed and shows hypoplasia of dermal connective tissue with upward extension of the subcutaneous fat tissue almost to the normal epidermis.[255,256] Even mildly affected females (from mosaicism[256] or skewed X-inactivation) or males (mosaicism) require genetic counseling because of the risk of having severely affected offspring.[242,257–259] Surgical intervention can ameliorate the developmental defects such as syndactyly or polydactyly and remove papillomas of the skin or mucous membranes. Pulsed-dye laser therapy can reduce telangiectasia, and ablative fractional laser resurfacing can induce dermal thickening.[260] Dental care can dramatically improve the hypodontia and enamel dysplasia.[261] Families can find support resources internationally through the National Foundation for Ectodermal Dysplasias (www.nfed.org).

Focal dermal hypoplasia should not be confused with focal facial dermal dysplasia (FFDD), which is characterized by bitemporal, round, scar-like lesions that resemble forceps marks (Fig. 6.21).[262] Thought to result from incomplete fusion of the ectodermal groove between the maxillary and mandibular prominences,[263] FFDD is currently classified into four subtypes. Patients with type I FFDD (autosomal dominant Brauer syndrome) have additional facial characteristics (flattened nasal tip, sparse lateral eyebrows, distichiasis [double row of eyelashes]) that are mild. FFDD type II (autosomal dominant Brauer–Setleis syndrome) is characterized by the addition of thin and puckered periorbital skin, absent eyelashes and/or distichiasis, upslanting palpebral fissures, a broad nasal tip and flat nasal bridge, and large lips.[129,264] Individuals with type III FFDD (autosomal recessive Setleis syndrome; see also Chapter 2) show the bitemporal lesions of focal facial dermal hypoplasia in association with a coarse facial appearance, anomalies of the eyelashes and lateral eyebrows,[265,266] dysplastic low-set ears, and a characteristic mouth with large lips and an inverted V contour with downturned corners. Setleis syndrome results from mutations in *TWIST2*, a transcription factor important for development.[267] Heterozygotes for *TWIST2* mutations may show partial features such as distichiasis and partial absence of the lower eyelashes.[268] Patients with type IV FFDD (autosomal recessive) typically have preauricular hypoplasia, which may resemble membranous aplasia cutis congenita,[269] but no other associated anomalies; however, buccal mucosal polyps have been described.[270,271] Type IV FFDD results from homozygous loss-of-function mutations in *CYP26C1*, a retinoic acid–degrading enzyme.[270]

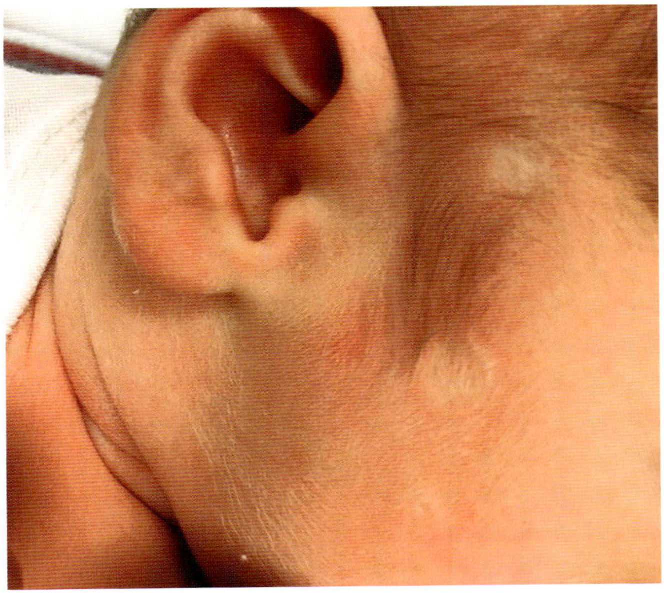

Fig. 6.21 Focal facial dermal hypoplasia. Bitemporal, round, scar-like lesions that resemble forceps marks, but represent a developmental defect.

Focal dermal hypoplasia must also be distinguished from microphthalmia with linear skin defects (MLS) syndrome (also called *MIDAS* for *microphthalmia, dermal aplasia, and sclerocornea syndrome*).[272] This X-linked-dominant developmental defect is characterized by microphthalmia and other eye abnormalities in association with linear, jagged skin defects typically involving the face, scalp, neck, and occasionally the upper trunk.[273] Other features can include short stature, developmental delay, structural brain abnormalities,[274] seizures, diaphragmatic hernia, congenital heart defects, and even pseudotail,[275] although there is wide phenotypic variability. Mutations in mitochondrial holocytochrome C-type synthase *(HCCS)* at chromosome Xp22.2 are responsible.[276] *HCCS* encodes an enzyme involved in mitochondrial oxidative activity.

Laminopathies

Four laminopathies are included among disorders of premature aging: progeria, atypical progeroid syndrome, restrictive dermopathy, and atypical Werner syndrome (see end of Werner Syndrome, later). They result from mutations either in *LMNA*, encoding the nuclear lamina protein lamin A, or *ZMPSTE24*, encoding a critical zinc metalloproteinase in lamin A processing.[277] Recently, a study of 87 patients with metabolic syndrome showed nuclear shape abnormalities and abnormal lamin A/C nuclear distribution in 11%; novel missense mutations in *LMNA* or *ZMPSTE24* were found in 3 of these patients, suggesting that some patients with metabolic syndrome have a laminopathy.[278] This possibility was further confirmed by the report of an additional dominant negative mutation in *ZMPSTE24* in a man with truncal and abdominal fat accumulation, partial lipodystrophy, metabolic syndrome with acanthosis nigricans, obesity, type 2 diabetes and hyperlipidemia, and dilated cardiomyopathy.[279]

Progeria (Hutchinson–Gilford syndrome [HGPS]) is a rare disease that results from a specific mutation (1824C→; G608G) on one allele of *LMNA* in >90% of cases.[277,280 283] Although this common mutation does not even change an amino acid, it does activate a cryptic splice site in exon 11, so mutant lamin A precursor, or progerin, lacks a series of 50 missing amino acids and is thus permanently modified by lipid farnesylation. Farnesylation of progerin prevents its proper insertion into the nuclear lamina and leads to progressive deformities in the nuclei of patients with HGPS. It is unclear if nonfarnesylated progerin also has toxicity.[284] Interestingly, progerin has also been shown to accumulate with aging in normal cells[285] and is induced in adult cells exposed to ultraviolet A (UVA) but not UVB light.[286] Although the mutations in HGPS are dominant negative, an autosomal recessive form with homozygous *LMNA* mutations (R527C) has been described.[287] Affected children show features of HGPS but have additional GI and skeletal abnormalities, and carrier parents are asymptomatic.

HGPS first manifests by 24 months of age with cutaneous alterations (mean age is <12 months) and often failure to thrive.[288] The most commonly reported early skin feature is sclerodermoid change, which most commonly involves the abdomen and thighs, generally present by 3 years old.[288] Other early changes are perioral and nasolabial cyanosis, prominent superficial veins of the scalp and body (Fig. 6.22), hypopigmentation and hyperpigmentation at sites of sclerodermatous change, and scalp alopecia, which progresses in a predictable pattern with midscalp and vertex area loss after other areas.[288 290] Patients progressively develop additional signs of premature aging, including early skin wrinkling, osteopenia with fractures, and atherosclerosis.[291] Other characteristics are reduced birthweight with postnatal growth retardation[292]; profound midfacial hypoplasia and micrognathia, but the appearance of hydrocephalus because upper head size is minimally reduced; generalized atrophy of muscle and subcutaneous tissue with a beaked nose and a bird-like appearance; and ocular surface disease.[293] The teeth become crowded, irregular in form, or deficient in number, and deciduous dentition is often retained.[294] Speech becomes high-pitched and squeaky, and intelligence is generally normal. The chest becomes narrow and the abdomen protuberant; due to a mild flexion of the knees, a "horse-riding" stance becomes apparent. Menarche is achieved in more than half of affected girls, despite little to no sign of pubertal development and minimal body fat.[295]

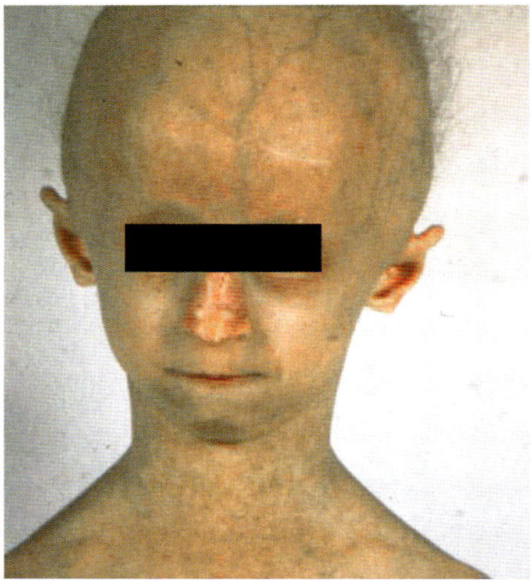

Fig. 6.22 Progeria. Alopecia, subcutaneous atrophy, prominent scalp veins, and bird-like facies. (Courtesy Schachner LA, Hansen RC, eds. Pediatric dermatology. 3rd ed. New York, NY: Elsevier; 2003.)

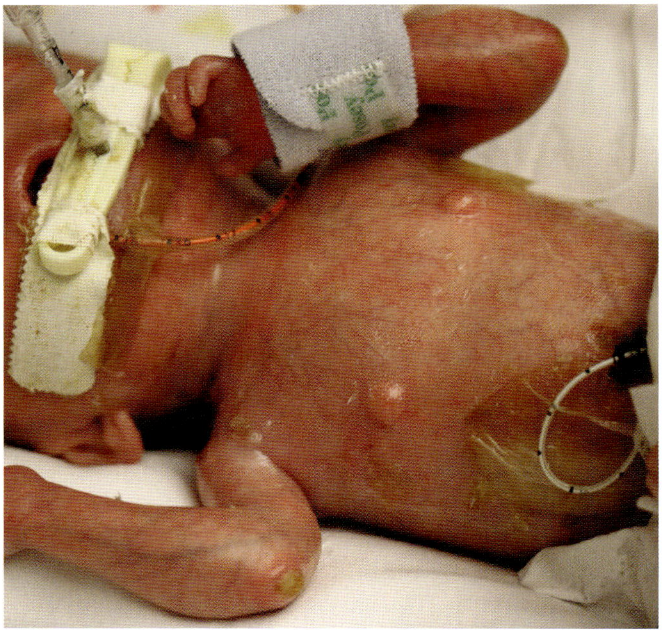

Fig. 6.23 Restrictive dermopathy. Note the translucent skin, protuberant nipples, and ulcers topped with thick keratotic crust.

Cardiac murmurs commonly occur after the age of 5 years and are soon followed by atherosclerosis-induced hypertension, cardiomegaly, angina, myocardial infarction, and congestive heart failure. Without intervention, death usually occurs at a mean age of 14.6 years, usually due to the coronary artery disease.[296] Progeria should be distinguished from scleroderma and from atypical Werner, Hallermann–Streiff, Cockayne, Bloom, and Rothmund–Thomson syndromes.

In preclinical models, treatment with three medications has been found to reverse the nuclear distortion in progeric cells: farnesyltransferase inhibitors, the combination of a bisphosphonate and a statin, and rapamycin (or its analog temsirolimus),[297] although all three have different effects on the many abnormalities in progeric cells.[298,299] Farnesyltransferase inhibitor treatment for at least 2 years has led to some type of improvement in all treated patients involving weight, cardiovascular flexibility, bone structure, and/or sensorineural hearing.[300] Farnesyltransferase inhibitor therapy also increased mean survival by 1.6 years[301,302] and decreased the rate of clinical strokes, headaches, and seizures.[303,304] Combination therapy with the farnesyltransferase inhibitor lonafarnib, a statin (pravastatin), and a bisphosphonate (zoledronic acid) improved bone mineral density, but added no cardiovascular benefit.[305] Growth hormone treatment increases weight by approximately 50% and linear growth by only about 10%. **Atypical progeroid syndromes** are progeroid disorders caused by missense *LMNA* mutations other than G608G that lead to nuclear abnormalities but are not rescued by farnesyltransferase inhibitors.[306] They have a variable presentation, ranging from a neonatally lethal restrictive dermopathy-like tight skin disorder (see later) to HGPS-like disorders with growth retardation, skin atrophy, partial alopecia, and diabetes.

Restrictive Dermopathy

Restrictive dermopathy is a rare, fatal autosomal recessive disorder characterized by taut, translucent, thin skin with fissures and erosions underlying sometimes dramatic hyperkeratosis (Fig. 6.23).[307–310] The intrauterine course is characterized by polyhydramnios with reduced fetal movements beginning at about 31 weeks' gestational age.[311,312] Clavicular hypoplasia is a consistent *in utero* characteristic.[313] Affected neonates show a dysmorphic facies (fixed, round open mouth with micrognathia; a small pinched nose; hypertelorism; enlarged fontanels; and widened sutures) and flexion contractures. Death usually occurs shortly after birth[314,315] due to pulmonary atelectasis, but affected babies have survived as long as months with respiratory and nutritional support. Biopsy sections show a flat epidermal junction and a thin dermis with compact collagen fibers, sparse elastic fibers, and rudimentary skin appendages. Restrictive dermopathy most commonly results from loss-of-function mutations in both alleles of *ZMPSTE24 (FACE1)* and occasionally from dominant negative mutations in *LMNA*.[316–320] In the face of *ZMPSTE24* deficiency, prelamin A accumulates, although the mechanism for the dermopathy is unclear.[321]

Werner Syndrome

Werner syndrome (progeria of the adult) is a rare autosomal recessive disorder that results from mutations in the *WRN* gene, which encodes Werner protein, a deoxyribonucleic acid (DNA) helicase enzyme that maintains genomic stability.[322–325] Patients usually develop and appear normal until adolescence, when they lack the pubertal growth spurt. Premature graying of hair at the temples may be seen then, and patients develop progressive alopecia, short stature, bird-like facies, and an apparent aged appearance. Cutaneous features include sclerodermoid changes of the skin of the extremities and, to a lesser degree, the face and neck; telangiectasias; mottled or diffuse pigmentation; keratoses; and indolent ulcers over pressure points, particularly on the soles and ankles.

Patients with Werner syndrome develop severe, often generalized, vascular disease; diabetes mellitus (71%); hypogonadism (80%); osteoporosis (91%); cataracts (100%); loss of subcutaneous tissue and severe muscle wasting in the legs, arms, feet, and hands with large abdominal fat deposits (leading to a body habitus of a stocky trunk with spindly extremities)[326]; soft tissue calcification; a high-pitched voice or hoarseness; and a predisposition to neoplastic disease (hepatoma, thyroid adenocarcinoma, ovarian carcinoma, melanoma, meningioma, leukemia, fibrosarcoma, osteogenic sarcoma, and carcinoma of the breast).[327,328] Patients may be thought to have insulin resistance with lipodystrophy[326] or scleroderma.[329] The mean age of death is 54 years. Therapy for Werner syndrome is supportive, but a study in a mouse model suggests that vitamin C supplementation may reverse aging abnormalities and lengthen the lifespan.[330] Bosentan, an endothelin receptor antagonist, has been shown to accelerate healing of the ulcerations.[331]

Atypical Werner syndrome affects about 15% of patients clinically diagnosed with Werner syndrome (see later) but results from mutations in *LMNA* rather than *WRN*.[332] Affected individuals start to show aging as young adults but at an accelerated rate compared with patients who have Werner syndrome and usually have no diabetes or cataracts. Mutations in a variety of other genes involved in DNA damage repair and response have led to phenotypes confused with Werner syndrome, supporting the concept that genomic instability plays a key role in accelerated aging. These have included mutations in *POLD1, CTC1, SPRTN, ERCC4, MDM2*, and *SAMHD1*.[333–338]

Stiff Skin Syndrome

Stiff skin syndrome (SSS) is a heterogeneous condition with scleroderma-like changes and associated contractures. Congenital fascial dystrophy is considered a subset in which the involvement exclusively involves the fascia. SSS results from heterozygous mutations in specific domains of *FBN1*, the gene encoding fibrillin-1 that is also altered in MFS.[339] However, these mutations causing SSS do not prevent fibrillin-1 secretion or assembly into microfibrils, which is the issue with MFS.[340] In SSS there is excessive microfibrillar deposition with impaired elastogenesis and increased TGF-β signaling in the dermis.[339]

Characterized by well-demarcated cutaneous and subcutaneous induration without inflammation that first develops between the neonatal period and early childhood, SSS is most severe on the legs, thighs, buttocks, and overlying joints.[341–346] Segmental SSS has been described,[347,348] in which the distribution is limited. Segmental involvement accounts for 35% of cases and has an average age of onset of 4.1 years (vs. 1.6 years for widespread SSS,[347] although onset may be in the first weeks regardless of distribution). Patients with segmental SSS do not tend to progress beyond the first months of onset and share a similar percentage of familial involvement (24% and 22%, respectively, in one series),[347] although somatic mosaicism for the *FBN1* mutation should also be considered. Contractures primarily involve the lower extremities with characteristic demarcation at the inguinal canal, although the shoulder girdle may also be affected.[349] Joint stiffness begins during early childhood, can significantly limit movement, and can be progressive, although the skin induration is relatively stable. Although limited joint mobility is a characteristic feature of those with widespread involvement, it has also been described in 44% with segmental SSS. Hypertrichosis may be associated (primarily of the lumbar area). Viscera are not affected, and patients lack immunologic abnormalities.

Biopsies show a characteristic lattice-like array of thick collagen, although the site is variable (e.g., may involve dermis and subcutaneous tissue or fascia or both). Adipocyte entrapment is a characteristic feature, but inflammation and mucin deposition are absent.[350,351] The condition needs to be distinguished from scleroderma neonatorum, subcutaneous fat necrosis, morphea, connective tissue nevi, and other scleroderma-like conditions, including progeria.[352] Management is through physical therapy, which should be initiated as early as possible.[353] Systemic administration of corticosteroids and other immunosuppressive agents has resulted in no improvement, although two cases of segmental SSS reportedly improved with the combination of mycophenolate mofetil and physical therapy.[354] Losartan led to improvement in a patient with segmental involvement.[348]

Winchester Syndrome

This autosomal recessive disorder has been described in fewer than a dozen patients.[355,356] Other names are multicentric osteolysis, nodulosis, and arthropathy (MONA); nodulosis, arthropathy, and osteolysis (NAO); and Torg syndromes.[357,358] It is characterized by short stature, coarse facies, corneal opacities, thickened leathery and hypertrichotic skin, hypertrophic lips and gingivae, generalized osteolysis, and progressive painful arthropathy with joint stiffness and contractures of distal phalanges.[359] Osteolysis may first be detectable after 1 year of age and can be progressive. Symmetric restrictive banding has been reported to develop in early adulthood.[360] The disorder has been attributed to mutations in both alleles of *MMP2*.[357,361]

Buschke–Ollendorff Syndrome

Buschke–Ollendorff syndrome is an autosomal dominant disorder that, when fully expressed, manifests as connective tissue nevi (with increased elastic fibers [68%], collagen [14%], or both [18%])[362] and osteopoikilosis.[363–367] The estimated incidence is estimated at 1:20,000.[368] It results from loss-of-function mutations in the *LEMD3* gene (encoding MAN1), which lead to enhanced TGF-β signaling and upregulation of TGF-β and bone morphogenetic protein (BMP) gene targets.[369,370] Although more than 50% of affected individuals have both skin and bone alterations,[362] dermal lesions are absent in 19% and bony lesions in 24%, with variability in presentation among family members.

The connective tissue nevi appear as collections of subtle, 3-mm, skin-colored to yellow papules or plaques (dermatofibrosis lenticularis disseminata), most often on the buttocks, proximal trunk, and limbs. Most connective tissue nevi are asymmetrically distributed and grouped, and individual lesions may coalesce into plaques. They occasionally occur on the scalp and are associated with alopecia.[371] Most patients first develop skin lesions in early childhood with advancement in number and size with age, although smaller lesions may also resolve during adulthood.[372–374] The bony lesions (osteopoikilosis) often appear after 15 years of age but are present in 46% under 8 years of age.[362] The osteopoikilosis is characterized by discrete spherical areas of increased radiodensity, most often noted in the epiphyses and metaphyses of long bone, pelvis, scapulae, and carpal and tarsal bones (Fig. 6.24). Although it causes no clinical problems, in the absence of cutaneous changes, osteopoikilosis may be misdiagnosed as bony metastases. Melorheostosis, which presents with an appearance of dripping wax along the outer bone, is much less common (5%), but can be associated with pain and can hinder growth. Other skeletal abnormalities, including short stature (5%), otosclerosis, spinal stenosis (2%),[364] supernumerary vertebrae and ribs, syndactyly,[375] and ossifying fibromas,[376] have been described, all in association with the osteopoikilosis. Limited anterior–posterior X-rays of the hands, wrists, ankles, knees, and pelvis rather than a full skeletal survey have been recommended.[377] In one cohort of six patients, 50% had cognitive delay,[362] although reported in only 5% in the literature.

Other connective tissue nevi (isolated or in association with tuberous sclerosis or Proteus syndrome,[377,378] papular elastorrhexis,[329]

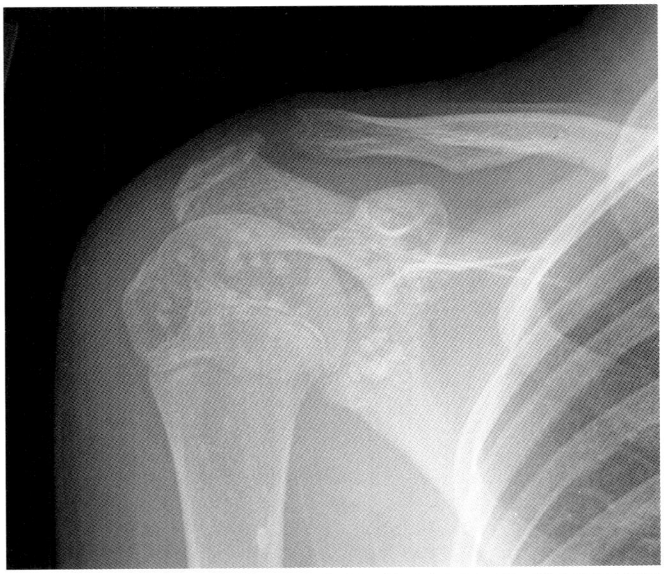

Fig. 6.24 Buschke–Ollendorff syndrome. An oncology consultation was recommended because the small round radiodensities on X-rays of this boy with Buschke–Ollendorff syndrome were not recognized to be osteopoikilosis.

morphea, and PXE) are the most common disorders considered in the differential diagnosis. The lesions of papular elastorrhexis resemble dermatofibrosis lenticularis disseminata but show decreased, fragmented elastic fibers rather than elastomas. Although usually sporadic, papular elastorrhexis has been described as familial with an autosomal dominant mode of inheritance.[380] No therapy is available or necessary.

Lipoid Proteinosis

Lipoid proteinosis (hyalinosis cutis et mucosae) is an autosomal recessive disorder characterized by hoarseness beginning in infancy and the later appearance of yellowish, beaded papules and nodules in the skin.[381–383] Both the hoarseness and the cutaneous lesions result from the abnormal deposition of hyaline material at the dermal–epidermal and microvascular basement membranes and papillary dermis.[384] The underlying molecular basis of lipoid proteinosis is mutations in extracellular matrix protein 1 *(ECM1)*, a secreted protein that may play roles in skin adhesion and protein interactions near the basement membrane.[385,386] There is considerable phenotypic heterogeneity, however, even with the same mutation.[387] The largest group of patients with lipoid proteinosis is in South Africa, where an *ECM1* c.826C>T founder mutation has been detected.

Hoarseness secondary to vocal cord involvement is a clinical feature in virtually every case, and adolescents and adults with this disorder can be recognized instantly because of their husky voice and thickened eyelids. The voice may be hoarse from birth or become so within the first few years of life and becomes progressively worse during early childhood.

Vesicles or small bullae develop during infancy or early childhood in about 50% of children, but rapidly erode with hemorrhagic crusting.[388,389] Ultrastructural analysis of these lesions and cultured keratinocytes shows "free-floating" intact desmosomes, consistent with the role of *ECM1* in cell–cell adhesion.[390] Distinctive linear or discrete varioliform scars subsequently develop, particularly on the face, trunk, and upper extremities (Fig. 6.25). Herpes simplex infection, impetigo, or epidermolysis bullosa may be considered as alternative diagnoses.

Patients first develop the typical discrete or confluent 2- to 3-mm yellowish-white to yellowish-brown papules in later childhood. These papules are found most commonly on the face, eyelids, neck, and hands. In about 50% of individuals, a string of bead-like papules, often followed by a loss of cilia, appears on the free eyelid margins. The flexural areas often show a yellow, waxy appearance with diffuse thickening of the skin. Many patients with lipoid proteinosis have hyperkeratotic plaques on the elbows, knees, and palms, with infiltrative plaques at sites of trauma. In one review of 17 patients from 10 families, individuals with verrucous elbow plaques during the first years of life were those with the mildest involvement on the face and buttocks.[391]

Also characteristic in patients with extensive manifestations are eversion of the lips (with their surfaces studded with tiny yellow papules and ulcerations), hypertrophic or vegetative lesions at the corners of the mouth, round papules just below the lip on the midline of the chin, and radiating fissures at the corners of the mouth. Partial alopecia of the scalp, eyebrows, eyelashes, or bearded area is common by later childhood. Other features that have been described are hypohidrosis, hypertrichosis, hypoplasia or aplasia of permanent teeth, parotid pain and recurrent parotid swelling as a result of obstruction of the Stensen duct, and impaired nail growth.

Because of hyaline deposition, the tongue becomes involved in 68%. It is characteristically thick, firm, and woody; is bound to the floor of the mouth; has lateral indentations; and is difficult to extrude.[392] The soft palate, tonsils, uvula, and undersurface of the tongue show extensive irregular yellow-white infiltrations and ulceration. Dysphagia caused by pharyngeal infiltration and respiratory obstruction as a result of severe laryngeal involvement can complicate the disorder. Central nervous system involvement is usually restricted to asymptomatic calcification (seen in 70% of patients older than 10 years of age), which can be seen on radiographic examination as bilateral bean-shaped opacities above the sella turcica. However, lipoid proteinosis is associated with attacks of rage and seizures; in one series, the most common seizure was focal with motionless staring, originating from the mesial temporal areas[393] with severity variable but unrelated to the extent of calcification.

Diagnosis is aided by a history of hoarseness from early childhood; thickening, stiffening, and difficulty in extrusion of the tongue; an impaired ability to swallow; characteristic involvement of the skin and mucous membranes; and histopathologic examination of involved tissue. Histologic features consist of thick homogeneous bands of eosinophilic, periodic acid–Schiff-positive, hyaline-like amorphous material in the upper dermis, with an associated patchy distribution surrounding blood vessels, sweat glands, and arrector pili muscles.

Lipoid proteinosis has a chronic but relatively benign course. Treatment is chiefly symptomatic and consists of surgical or laser removal of laryngeal nodules or tracheostomy for laryngeal obstruction and cosmetic measures such as laser resurfacing or dermabrasion for unappealing cutaneous lesions on the face or other exposed surfaces. Acitretin can improve the hoarseness[394,395] and, in some patients, the skin lesions.[389,396]

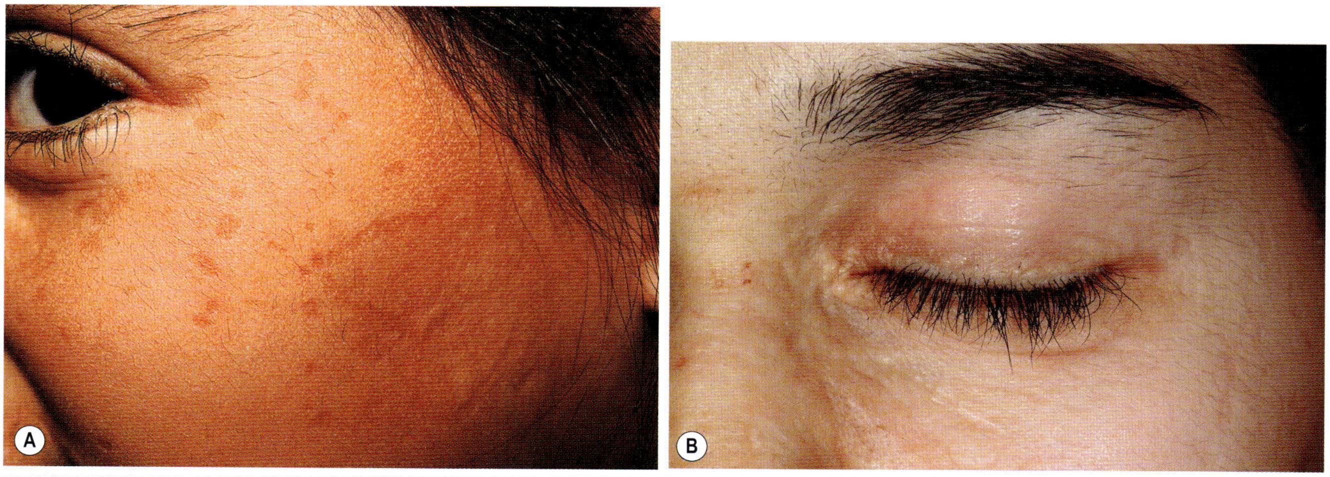

Fig. 6.25 Lipoid proteinosis. **(A)** Linear or varioliform scars develop after clearance of the vesicular, crusted lesions of childhood. **(B)** Confluent bead-like papules line the upper eyelid in about 50% of individuals with lipoid proteinosis but tend to first appear later in childhood. Note the waxy skin of the infraocular area.

Infantile Systemic Hyalinosis and Juvenile Hyaline Fibromatosis

Infantile systemic hyalinosis (ISH) and juvenile hyaline fibromatosis (JHF) are similar autosomal recessive conditions that represent allelic variants, with ISH of earlier onset and greater severity. ISH and JHF result from mutations in the gene that encodes capillary morphogenesis gene 2 (*CMG2*; also called *anthrax toxin receptor 2* or *ANTXR2*).[397–399] The term *hyaline fibromatosis syndrome* has been proposed to encompass both.[400] *CMG2/ANTXR2* is thought to play a role in basement membrane matrix assembly and endothelial cell morphogenesis (in addition to being the receptor for anthrax).[401] In general, milder phenotypes are associated with in-frame and missense mutations within the cytoplasmic domain, but modifier genes and/or environmental effects are thought to account for exceptions.[397]

The histologic and ultrastructural features of ISH and JHF are similar, and a unified classification based on severity has been suggested.[402] The deposition of hyaline material, characterized as an acellular proteinaceous material that appears pink and glassy in routine sections, occurs in multiple organ systems.

ISH[400] presents within the first few weeks of life, although intrauterine growth restriction and reduced fetal movements have been described. The predominant cutaneous findings of ISH are diffusely thickened skin; small nodules of the perianal region, ears, and lips; and a reddish-blue to hyperpigmented discoloration overlying bony prominences.[403,405] The joint contractures and osteopenia lead to the frog-leg position and virtual immobility that are typical of affected infants.[406] Patients with ISH also develop malabsorption and a protein-losing enteropathy, leading to diarrhea and failure to thrive. Oral manifestations include thickening of the oral mucosa, extensive overgrowth of the gingival tissue, marked curvature of the dental roots, and replacement of the periodontal ligament by hyaline fibrous material. These oral findings may cause difficulty in feeding and compound the nutritional deficiency resulting from malabsorption. Thyroid dysfunction has also been described.[407] The condition is usually fatal by 2 years of age because of recurrent pulmonary infections and diarrhea.

JHF, also known as *juvenile systemic hyalinosis*, encompasses mild to moderate disease within the spectrum of *CMG2* mutations.[408] JHF has a later onset than ISH, and patients survive into adulthood; the oldest reported patient was 58 years old.[409] JHF is characterized by joint contractures (especially of the small joints of the hands and feet), gingival hypertrophy, generalized osteopenia, and papular and nodular skin lesions, typically on the scalp, perianal and perinasal areas (Fig. 6.26), palms, and trunk.[410,411] Some children experience rectal bleeding because of the anal lesions.[412]

The differential diagnosis of these hyaline fibromatoses includes infantile myofibromatosis, Winchester syndrome, Farber lipogranulomatosis, and mucopolysaccharidoses. A progeroid syndrome with hard, painless, keloid-like nodules is Penttinen syndrome, characterized by a premature aged appearance with typical facies starting in early childhood, lipodystrophy, contractures, acro-osteolysis with brachydactyly, corneal clouding, and progressive sensorineural hearing deficit.[413,414] Penttinen and Penttinen-like syndromes result from mutations in *PDGFRB* (platelet-derived growth factor receptor-beta), the same gene mutated in infantile myofibromatosis. Imatinib treatment may improve the features of these disorders.

There is no satisfactory treatment at this time for ISH/JHF, although administration of interferon α-2b led to remarkable improvement in skin nodules, gingival hypertrophy, and joint mobility in a girl with JHF.[415] Early dental intervention with good hygiene is important, and gingivectomy may be required[416] with careful anesthetic management.[417,418] Lesions can be partially excised if ulcerated or disfiguring, but tend to recur.[419]

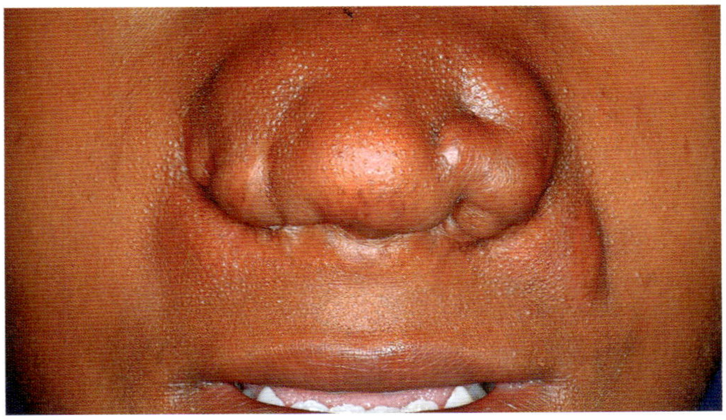

Fig. 6.26 Juvenile hyaline fibromatosis. Note the nodules on the nose and the gingival hypertrophy. Fine papules can be seen on the nose and perinasal area; the patient had dozens of visible 1- to 2-mm papules on the chin as well.

The complete list of 419 references for this chapter is available online at http://expertconsult.inkling.com.

Key References

Malfait F, Francomano C, Byers P, et al. The 2017 international classification of the Ehlers-Danlos syndromes. Am J Med Genet C Semin Med Genet 2017;175(1):8–26.

Brady AF, Demirdas S, Fournel-Gigleux S, et al. The Ehlers-Danlos syndromes, rare types. Am J Med Genet C Semin Med Genet 2017;175(1):70–115.

Colombi M, Dordoni C, Venturini M, et al. Spectrum of mucocutaneous, ocular and facial features and delineation of novel presentations in 62 classical Ehlers-Danlos syndrome patients. Clin Genet 2017;92(6):624–31.

Tinkle BT, Saal HM. Committee on Genetics: health supervision for children with Marfan syndrome. Pediatrics 2013;132(4):e1059–72.

Loeys BL, Dietz HC, Braverman AC, et al. The revised Ghent nosology for the Marfan syndrome. J Med Genet 2010;47:476–85.

Singh MN, Lacro RV. Recent clinical drug trials evidence in Marfan syndrome and clinical implications. Can J Cardiol 2016;32(1):66–77.

Berk DR, Bentley DD, Bayliss SJ, et al. Cutis laxa: a review. J Am Acad Dermatol 2012;66(5):842, e1–17.

Naouri M, Boisseau C, Bonicel P, et al. Manifestations of pseudoxanthoma elasticum in childhood. Br J Dermatol 2009;161(3):635–9.

Maas SM, Lombardi MP, van Essen AJ, et al. Phenotype and genotype in 17 patients with Goltz-Gorlin syndrome. J Med Genet 2009;46(10):716–20.

Bree AF, Grange DK, Hicks MJ, et al. Dermatologic findings of focal dermal hypoplasia (Goltz syndrome). Am J Med Genet C Semin Med Genet 2016;172c(1):44–51.

Merideth MA, Gordon LB, Clauss S, et al. Phenotype and course of Hutchinson-Gilford progeria syndrome. N Engl J Med 2008;358(6):592–604.

Saussine A, Marrou K, Delanoe P, et al. Connective tissue nevi: an entity revisited. J Am Acad Dermatol 2012;67(2):233–9.

7 Disorders of Hair and Nails

Hair

Hair is a protein by-product of follicles distributed everywhere on the body surface except the palms, soles, vermilion portion of the lips, glans penis, penile shaft, nail beds, and sides of the fingers and toes. Although hair is of minimal functional benefit to humans, the psychologic effects of disturbances of hair growth are commonly a source of great concern to children, adolescents, and their parents.

In the human fetus, groups of cells appear in the epidermis at about the eighth week of gestation. These differentiate to form the hair follicles, and hair begins to develop between the eighth and twelfth weeks of fetal life. This growth continues throughout fetal development. Although there are indications that some hair is lost during gestation and at the time of birth, the majority of hairs on the newborn are 5 to 6 months old.

Lanugo hairs are fine, soft, unmedullated, and poorly pigmented hairs seen only in fetal and neonatal life, except in the rare hereditary syndrome hypertrichosis lanuginosa. They appear as a fine, dense growth over the entire cutaneous surface of the fetus. Lanugo hair is normally shed *in utero* in the seventh or eighth month of gestation, but may cover the entire cutaneous surface of the premature newborn infant. Postnatal hair may be divided into vellus and terminal types. Vellus hairs are the fine, lightly pigmented hairs seen on the arms and faces of children. Terminal hairs are the mature, thick, darker hairs on the scalp, eyebrows, eyelashes, and areas of secondary-sexual hair distribution. The number and distribution of individual hair follicles are genetically determined and constant from birth. As the infant's skin grows, however, the density of hair follicles reduces from 1135 per cm^2 at birth to 615 per cm^2 by adulthood.

The average human scalp contains 100,000 hairs. The average growth rate of terminal hair is approximately 2.5 mm/week (1 cm/month). The hair shaft represents the equivalent of the stratum corneum of skin, with the follicular keratinocytes dictating the characteristics of the shaft. The hair root is characterized by three definable cyclic stages of growth: anagen (Fig. 7.1, *A*), catagen, and telogen (Fig. 7.1, *B*; Box 7.1). The human hair follicle has a long phase of regular growth (the anagen phase) that lasts 2 to 6 years, with an average of 3 years. The hairs then undergo a period of partial degeneration (the catagen phase), lasting up to 3 weeks, followed by a resting (telogen or club) phase. The telogen phase of the follicle lasts for about 3 months. At the end of this time, new growth is initiated. As new hairs grow, they push out the old telogen hairs that have remained in the resting follicles. In healthy individuals, 85% to 90% of the scalp is in the actively growing anagen stage and 1% is in the brief transitional (catagen) stage; 10% to 15% is in the resting or telogen stage, with an average of 50 to 100 hairs shed and simultaneously replaced each day. Although scalp hair has a long anagen phase, eyelash and extremity hair have a lower anagen/telogen ratio and thus tend to be shorter.

Neonatal Hair

The first crop of terminal scalp hair is in the actively growing anagen phase at birth, but within the first few days of life there is a physiologic conversion to the telogen phase. Consequently, a high proportion of neonatal scalp hairs are shed during the first 4 months of life (Fig. 7.2). This telogen shedding (telogen effluvium of the newborn) usually is gradual hair loss, particularly between 2 and 4 months and most noticeable at the occipital area. Rarely the hair loss occurs in the first 4 weeks of life in a frontal-temporal pattern.[1] This physiologic hair shedding at the occipital area is not related to the baby's sleeping position (i.e., friction).[2] Replacement of the first terminal hairs is generally completed before the first 6 months of life. The neonatal hairline commonly extends along the forehead and temples to the lateral margin of the eyebrows. These terminal hairs gradually convert to vellus hairs during the first year of life. Premature infants are often covered by lanugo hairs, which are more densely distributed on the face, limbs, and trunk. This retention of lanugo hair is probably related to the cyclic activity *in utero* and the normal shedding of telogen vellus hairs in the fetus during the last few weeks of gestation.

Tools for Diagnosis of Hair Loss Disorders

Evaluation of hair disorders starts with taking a good history and performing a careful physical examination, including of the hair and the entire scalp. Careful attention must be paid to the timing of the hair loss, whether there is shedding, whether any contacts have hair loss, recent illness and exposures, medication history, nutrition, and signs or symptoms of other illness, such as thyroid or other autoimmune disease. Examination of the scalp should be focused on determining if the hair loss is nonscarring vs. scarring, hair characteristics, and if there is any patterning (Box 7.2). Several tools are available to help with differentiation among possible diagnoses[3,4] (Box 7.3). The hair tug test involves holding the hair between the index finger and the thumb near the root and tugging with the other hand at the distal part; if the hair fractures, fragility is suggested. The hair pull test, in contrast, involves gently pulling at a batch of hairs between the index finger and the thumb. The test is performed at multiple locations on the scalp and is positive if more than 10% of hairs are released. In general, telogen hairs are released, and their identity can be visualized by light microscopy or trichoscopy; however, the hair pull test is positive for alopecia areata (AA), with microscopic evidence of the typical tapered hairs. Trichoscopy is a technique that often allows direct visualization of hairs, rather than pulling of hairs for microscopic evaluation.[5] Loss of follicular ostia identified scarring or cicatricial alopecia, whereas preserved ostia assures of a nonscarring process. One can also visualize scalp erythema, dyspigmentation, pustules, and edema more easily through trichoscopy. Yellow and black dots, as well as exclamation point hairs, are typical of AA. In contrast, comma-shaped hairs and corkscrew hairs are features of tinea capitis. Hair shaft disorders can

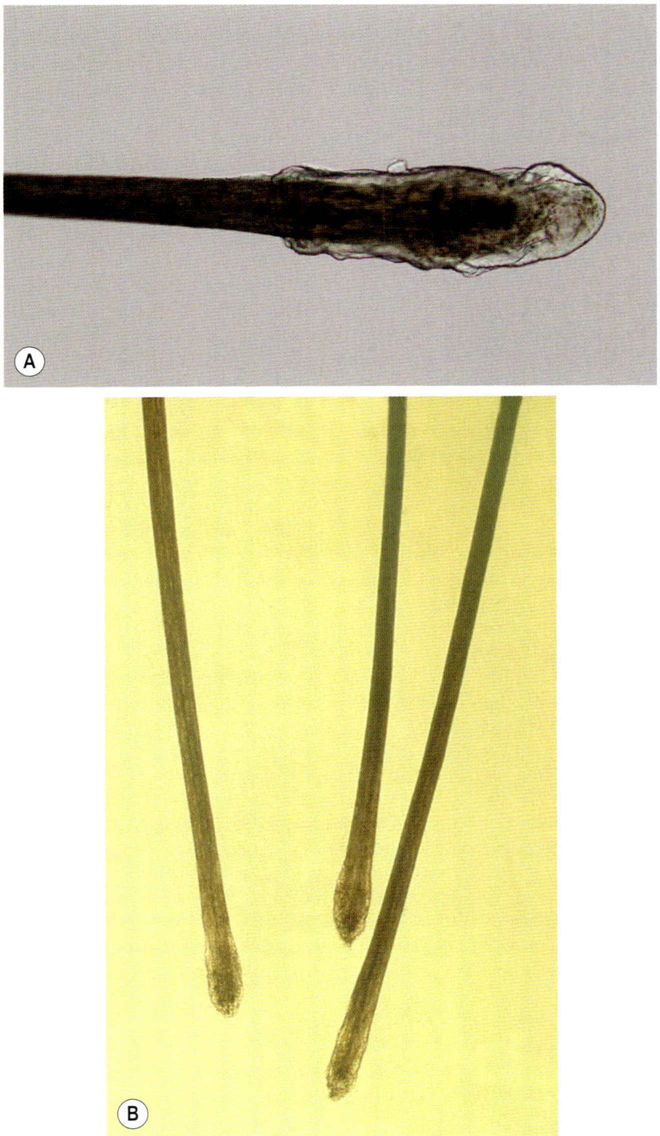

Fig. 7.1 Stages of growth of the hair root. **(A)** Anagen hairs are the growing hairs that comprise 90% of hair at any time and persist for several years. Anagen hairs are pigmented and have a translucent sheath. **(B)** Telogen hairs are in a resting phase that persists for 3 months. Note the small bulb and lack of sheath.

Box 7.1 Cyclic Stages of Human Hair Growth

1. Anagen phase (active growth phase) lasts 2 to 6 years (average 3 years)
2. Catagen phase (stage of partial degeneration) lasts 10 to 14 days
3. Telogen phase (resting stage) lasts 3 to 4 months

Box 7.2 Clinical Examination of Alopecia

1. Overall characteristics: pattern of loss, extent, color, texture, length, breakage
2. Scalp features: scarring vs. nonscarring, inflammation, trichoscopy (follicular openings), pigmentary change, scaling, crusts, pustules
3. Hair beyond scalp: eyebrows, lashes, extremity hair, secondary sexual hair if adolescent
4. Special tests: trichoscopy of shaft, hair pull, hair tug, hair mount (see Box 7.3)

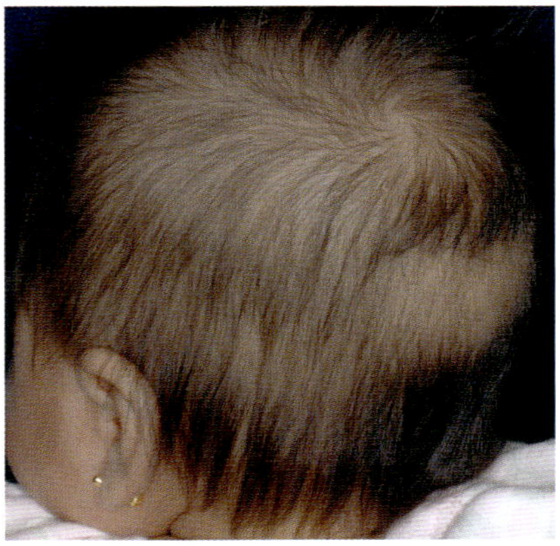

Fig. 7.2 Telogen shedding of the newborn. This 4-month-old girl shows generalized thinning of scalp hair, reflecting telogen effluvium.

Box 7.3 Special Tests of Hair and Scalp

Hair pull: Grasp about 50 hairs between first three fingers and pull gently but firmly away from scalp at four scalp regions (i.e., frontal, occipital, temporal bilaterally); positive pull test means more than 10% of hairs pull out easily (are in telogen) and is seen with active alopecia areata.
Hair tug: Hold a group of hairs with one hand and use other hand to pull away at distal end, looking for hair breakage (which can then be analyzed microscopically in a hair mount). This can be helpful with fragile hair syndromes such as monilethrix.
Hair mount: Hairs are separated, oriented side by side on a glass slide, covered with mounting medium (such as Permount), and covered with a coverslip without air bubbles. This technique allows one to distinguish anagen from telogen bulbs based on shape and pigmentation, distorted bulbs and cuticles (as in loose anagen syndrome), and hair shaft abnormalities.
Trichoscopy: Can replace hair mounts and microscopy when examining shaft. Disease-specific findings such as for alopecia areata (follicular openings showing yellow dots; "exclamation-point" hairs), tinea capitis (comma or corkscrew hairs), and trichotillomania (coiled or flame hairs); black dots at follicular opening suggest broken hairs and can be seen with alopecia areata, tinea, and trichotillomania.

also be visualized by dermoscopy; one can see uniform elliptical nodes and constrictions (monilethrix), shaft telescoping (trichorrhexis invaginata), twists along the long axis (pili torti), alternating light and dark areas (pili anulati), waves at short intervals (woolly hair), splitting into fibers (trichorrhexis nodosa), or, using polarized light, alternating light and dark bands (trichothiodystrophy).[5]

Alopecias

Clinical examination allows hair loss disorders to be divided into nonscarring (noncicatricial) or scarring (cicatricial) types (see Box 7.2).[6–8] Causes of nonscarring alopecia include alteration of the hair growth cycle, inflammatory cutaneous disease, and structural abnormalities of the hair.[9,10] Some traumatic disorders, such as traction alopecia, pressure alopecia, or trichotillomania, can scar if severe but often resolve without clinical evidence of scarring. Evaluation typically involves gentle traction on the hair (hair-pull test) to determine if hair comes out easily (as in loose anagen syndrome [LAS], AA, or telogen effluvium) and microscopic or trichoscopic evaluation of hair shafts to seek hair shaft abnormalities (see Box 7.3).

NONSCARRING ALOPECIAS WITH HAIR SHAFT ABNORMALITIES

Hair Shaft Abnormalities with Increased Fragility

Variations in the structure of the hair shaft are a common occurrence and at times may provide clues to other pathologic abnormalities[11,12] (Box 7.4). Because each hair shaft anomaly has a distinctive morphology,

Box 7.4 Structural Hair Shaft Defects with Fragility (and Associated Disorders)

Trichorrhexis Nodosa

- Trauma (most common)
- Argininosuccinic aciduria
- Citrullinemia
- Oculodentodigital dysplasia
- Trichothiodystrophy
- Trichohepatoenteric syndrome

Monilethrix

- Hair keratin mutations (KRT81, KRT83, KRT86)
- Desmoglein 4 mutations

Trichorrhexis Invaginata

- Netherton syndrome

Pili Torti

- Menkes syndrome
- Crandall syndrome
- Björnstad syndrome
- Bazek–Dupré–Christol syndrome
- Rombo syndrome
- Hypotrichosis with juvenile macular degeneration
- Mitochondrial enzyme defects

Trichothiodystrophy

- Group I: mutations in *XPD, XPB, p8*
- Group II: mutations in *TTDN1*
- Group III: Pollitt syndrome, Sabinas syndrome (genes unknown)

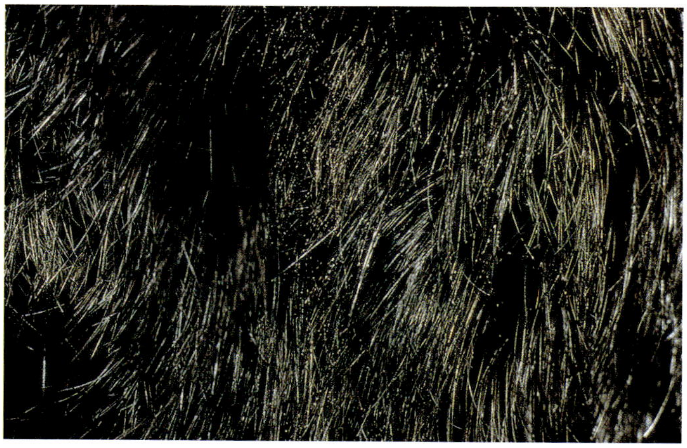

Fig. 7.3 Trichorrhexis nodosa. Grayish-white nodules, which resemble two interlocking brushes or brooms microscopically, may be seen on the hair.

the diagnosis often can be established in the office by trichoscopy (using a dermatoscope)[13] (see Box 7.3)[8] or by microscopic examination of snipped hairs.[9] Other than reduction of trauma to reduce breakage, there is no effective treatment for this group of disorders.

Trichorrhexis Nodosa. Trichorrhexis nodosa, the most common hair shaft anomaly, is a distinctive disorder manifested by increased fragility.[9,14] Grayish-white nodules may be seen on the hair (Fig. 7.3), which under trichoscopy or light microscopy have the appearance of two interlocking brushes or brooms, the result of segmental longitudinal splitting of fibers without complete fracture. The disorder features dry, lusterless, short hair that is easily fractured.

Usually "acquired" in adolescents without other issues, trichorrhexis nodosa most commonly results from trauma to the hair. The injury may result from the use of hot combs, excessively hot hairdryers, hair straighteners, and other chemical treatments or the cumulative cuticular damage from vigorous combing and brushing, repeated salt-water bathing, prolonged sun exposure, and frequent shampooing. Cream rinses and protein conditioners are helpful. If hair-straightening procedures, vigorous grooming habits, and thermal and chemical trauma to the hair are discontinued, the acquired form of trichorrhexis nodosa generally improves within 2 to 4 years.

Less commonly trichorrhexis nodosa is genetic and manifests during infancy. Infants with the autosomal dominant form show normal hair at birth, but the hair that regrows within a few months is abnormal; the hair defect tends to improve with advancing age. Trichorrhexis nodosa may also be a manifestation of children with the late-onset form of argininosuccinic aciduria, a condition that results from lack of argininosuccinase. In this condition, the hair is usually normal at birth and first becomes fragile at 1 to 2 years of age with a dull, matted appearance, especially at the occipital area. The hair defects are associated with psychomotor retardation, cerebellar ataxia, and a marked increase of argininosuccinic acid in the blood, urine, and cerebrospinal fluid.[15,16] Dietary treatment of the metabolic abnormality leads to normalization of the appearance and integrity of the hair. Similar clinical manifestations are found in infants with citrullinemia, caused by a deficiency of argininosuccinic acid synthetase. Trichorrhexis nodosa is the most common hair shaft abnormality, but pili torti has been described and hair bulbs may be atrophic. Some patients show an eruption that resembles acrodermatitis enteropathica. Trichorrhexis nodosa has also been described in oculodentodigital dysplasia,[17,18] trichothiodystrophy (TTD), and trichohepatoenteric syndrome, characterized by facial dysmorphism, liver disease, immune defects, and severe diarrhea requiring intravenous nutrition.[19]

Monilethrix. *Monilethrix* (beaded hair) is an autosomal dominant disorder characterized by partial alopecia from breakage and variation in hair shaft thickness with small node-like deformities that produce a beaded appearance and internodal fragility. The nodal pattern can be seen by trichoscopy (Fig. 7.4) but can be subtle.[20,21] In individuals with this disorder, normal neonatal lanugo hairs are shed during the first few weeks of life. The regrown hair, which generally appears at about the second month of life, is dry, lusterless, and brittle and fails to grow to any appreciable length because of breakage (Fig. 7.5, *A*). In severe cases, the infant may remain bald or the scalp hair may be sparse, easily fractured, and stubble-like with follicular prominence from keratosis. Although generally a disorder of scalp hair, body hairs may also be affected. The clinical findings are limited to the occiput and nape in more

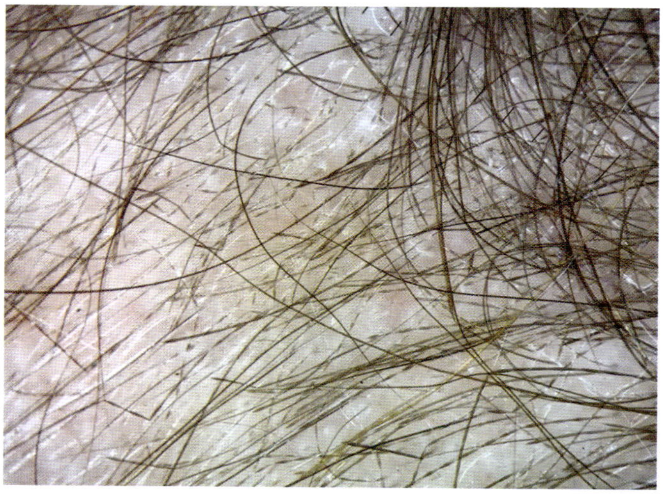

Fig. 7.4 Monilethrix. The distinct beading of monilethrix can be appreciated under trichoscopy (using the dermatoscope).

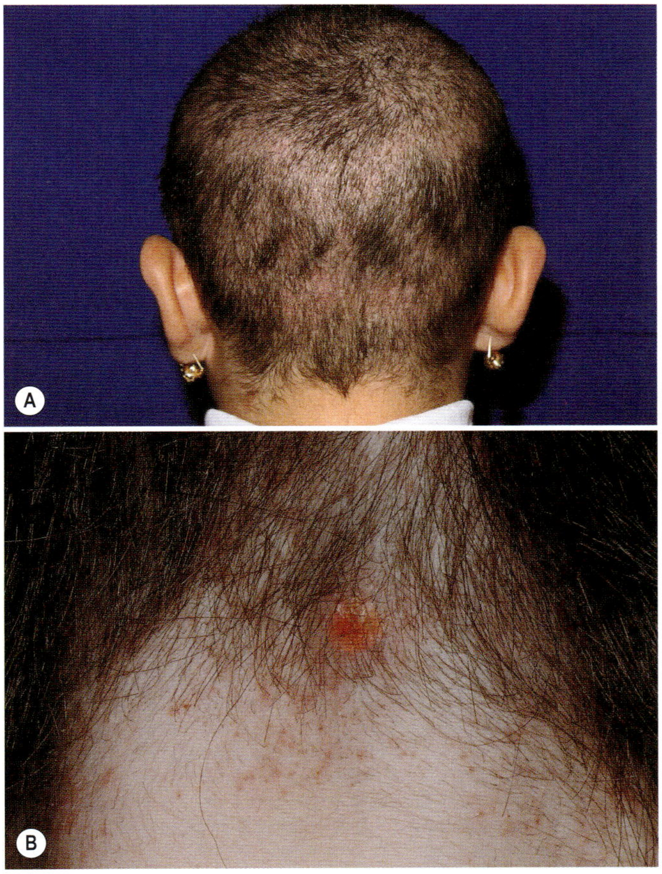

Fig. 7.5 Monilethrix. **(A)** The hair is dry, lusterless, brittle, and fails to grow to any appreciable length. The occipital area is most commonly and most severely affected in most cases. **(B)** The follicles are prominent and often hyperkeratotic. This girl was scratching at her occipital area, which led to further breakage and an erosion.

limited cases (Fig. 7.5, *B*). Occasionally this disorder is not apparent during infancy but becomes apparent later in childhood or during adult life. Follicular keratosis is associated in some pedigrees and may affect the face, scalp, and extremities. Some patients show koilonychia. Spontaneous improvement or remission may occur at puberty or during pregnancy, suggesting a hormonal influence,[22] but the condition may persist unchanged throughout adulthood. Administration of oral retinoids,[23] topical minoxidil,[24] and low-dose oral minoxidil[25] have been reported to improve the alopecia.

Monilethrix most commonly is autosomal dominant and results from mutations in hair (or trichocyte) keratins. These hair keratins have a high cysteine content, making them "hard" keratins with a high degree of crosslinking. Of the 26 known hair follicle–specific keratins, three have been associated with monilethrix and all are type II keratins.[26] Mutations in *KRT81* and *KRT86* are most common.[27] Mutations in *KRT83* also lead to monilethrix,[27,28] but homozygous deletion variants in *KRT83* result in generalized ichthyosis with palmoplantar keratoderma and no hair defects.[29] Because keratins provide structural integrity to hair, abnormalities in these keratins lead to hair fragility, with breakage occurring at the internodal sites. Mutations in hair keratins have also been linked to pure hair and nail ectodermal dysplasia (PHNED) (*KRT85*), woolly hair with hypotrichosis (*KRT71* and *KRT74*), and pseudofolliculitis barbae (*KRT75*). The majority of the hair keratins remain unlinked to human phenotypes but may impart variants in hair strength, texture, or curliness.[30]

Autosomal recessive monilethrix has been linked to mutations in *DSG4*, which encodes desmoglein 4, a transmembranous cell-adhesion molecule of the cadherin family that is predominantly expressed in the hair cortex and upper cuticle.[31–33] Desmoglein 4 is thought to integrate keratin filaments into desmosomes.[34] Desmoglein 4 mutations may also manifest as autosomal recessive hypotrichosis, which resembles monilethrix but lacks the characteristic beaded appearance of the hair shaft under light microscopy.[35]

Pseudomonilethrix. *Pseudomonilethrix* was originally described as an autosomal dominant developmental defect of fragile hair with irregularly shaped nodes.[10,36] In fact, the hair changes are artifactual and related to overlapping hairs under the pressure of an overlying glass slide.[37] Pseudomonilethrix is seen more commonly when fine hairs are handled by forceps.

Trichorrhexis Invaginata. *Trichorrhexis invaginata* (bamboo hair) is characterized clinically by dry, lusterless, easily fractured, sparse, and short hair. Under light microscopy, the hairs show a peculiar intussusception or telescope-like invagination along the hair shaft, which microscopically resembles the ball-and-cup joints of bamboo.[9,38] Variations in trichorrhexis invaginata occur, most commonly "golf-tee hair," presenting the expanded proximal end of an invaginate node,[39] which is easily seen by trichoscopy.[40] The hair defect in trichorrhexis invaginata is thought to be abnormal keratinization of the hair shaft, which results in softening of the hair cortex and promotes intussusception of the distal portion of the hair shaft into the softer proximal portion.

Although trichorrhexis invaginata may occur as an isolated finding, this hair shaft abnormality is characteristic of Netherton syndrome (see Fig. 7.6), an autosomal recessive genodermatosis that has been linked to mutations in *SPINK5* (see Chapter 5).[41] Neonates with this disorder characteristically show generalized exfoliative erythroderma and failure to thrive, often associated with hypernatremic dehydration, recurrent infections, and sepsis. Severely affected neonates may show extremely sparse and even absent hair, making the diagnosis based on hair shaft examination difficult. However, the eyebrows are almost always short and broken (Fig. 7.6, *A* and 5.35); eyebrow hairs should be

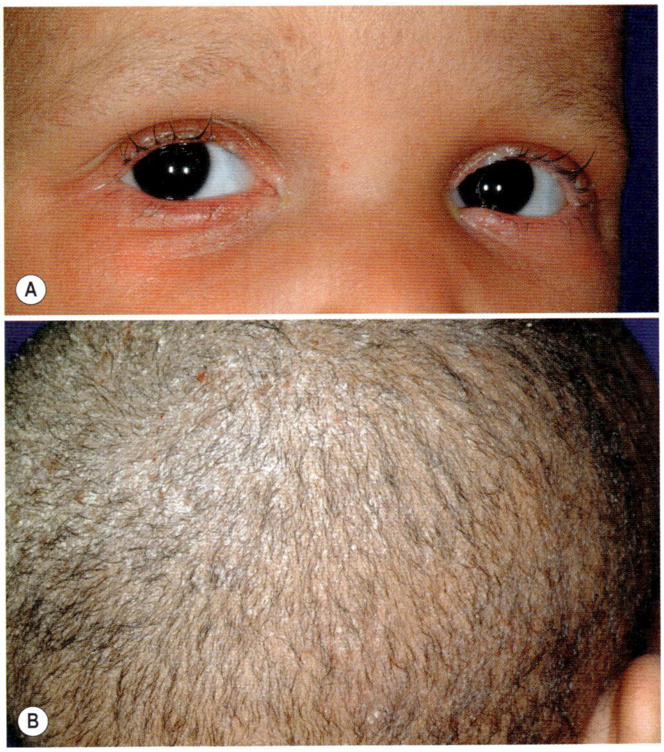

Fig. 7.6 Netherton syndrome. **(A)** The characteristic microscopic features of Netherton hair (trichorrhexis invaginata) are often found in eyebrow hairs. Note the sparse, broken brows and lashes in this young girl who also shows the periorbital dermatitis. **(B)** Short, broken hair throughout the scalp. Note the desquamative scaling and excoriations.

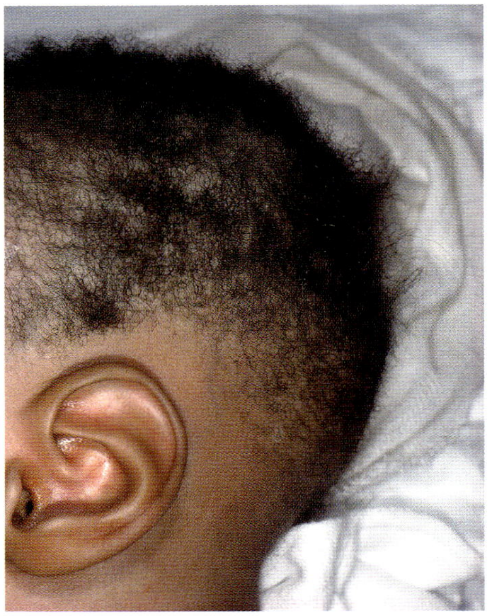

Fig. 7.7 Menkes syndrome. The hair is fine, dull, hypopigmented compared with other family members, and stands on end. It looks and feels like steel wool.

examined in cases in which the abnormality cannot be demonstrated from scalp hair, and trichoscopy (dermoscopy) can be helpful.[8,42–45]

Beyond infancy, many affected individuals show the characteristic skin finding of ichthyosis linearis circumflexa, with walls of scale surrounding red patches, in addition to their dry, lusterless hair that breaks easily (see Fig. 7.6, *B* and Fig. 5.34*A*). Atopic conditions usually accompany the ichthyosis. Although spontaneous remission of the hair defect has been described (generally between 6 and 15 years of age), the vast majority show persistence.

Pili Torti. *Pili torti* hairs show three or four regularly spaced twists that occur at irregular intervals along the hair shaft.[9,46] The hair shaft appears flattened at the site of the twist, which is almost always through 180 degrees. The dry, fragile hair is often lighter in color than expected and shimmers in reflected light with a "spangled" appearance because of the hair twisting. The hair tends to be short, especially in areas subject to trauma, and may extend out from the scalp. Pili torti must be distinguished from twisted hair, which has been described in association with anorexia nervosa.[47]

Pili torti may occur as an isolated phenomenon with onset at birth or early infancy.[48] This genetic disorder shows both autosomal dominant and autosomal recessive inheritance patterns. The appearance of the hair in patients with pili torti may become more normal with time, although twisted hairs can still be found in the adult scalp; those who still manifest the disorder at puberty, however, are unlikely to show significant improvement with age. A late-onset autosomal dominant form has also been described, in which brittle hair and patchy alopecia develop after puberty. Mental retardation has been noted in some pedigrees. Pili torti has been associated with several mitochondrial disorders (see Pili Torti section).

Menkes syndrome (trichopoliodystrophy) is an X-linked recessive neurodegenerative disorder that affects male infants. Classic Menkes syndrome affects 90% to 95% of patients, with a less common mild form associated with long survival and occipital horn syndrome (previously called X-linked cutis laxa or Ehlers–Danlos syndrome type IX) showing largely connective tissue manifestations. Carrier females may exhibit pili torti. Classical Menkes syndrome is characterized by coarse facies; pili torti; temperature instability; seizures; psychomotor retardation; arterial intimal changes; soft, doughy skin that may resemble localized areas of cutis laxa[49]; joint laxity; low or absent plasma copper and ceruloplasmin levels; growth failure; increased susceptibility to infection; and death, generally by age 3 or 4 years.[50,51] Clinical features often include premature birth, hypothermia, and relatively normal development until 2 to 6 months of age, when drowsiness and lethargy are noted, intractable seizures begin, and growth and development cease. Rarely neonates demonstrate erythroderma as an early sign.[52]

Usually the hair is fine, dull, sparse, and poorly pigmented in infancy; it stands on end and looks and feels like steel wool (Fig. 7.7). Additional features include tortuosity of cerebral and other medium-sized arteries; osteoporosis; frequent subdural hematomas; widening of the metaphyses with spurring; and frequent fractures, at times simulating the radiologic findings characteristic of patients with battered child syndrome.[53] Although pili torti is generally a prominent feature of this disorder, other less commonly reported hair abnormalities include monilethrix and trichorrhexis nodosa.

Menkes syndrome results from mutations in *ATP7A*,[54] which encodes a copper-transporting adenosine triphosphatase (ATPase) that incorporates copper into copper-dependent enzymes and maintains copper levels by removing excessive copper from the cytosol.[55] The combination of clinical features, bone abnormalities, and low plasma copper and ceruloplasmin levels establishes the correct diagnosis. Parenteral administration of copper histidine occasionally prevents neurologic degeneration and pigmentation if initiated in the neonatal or infantile period[56] but often is ineffective.[57]

Crandall syndrome, an X-linked recessive disorder, consists of pili torti with alopecia, sensorineural deafness, and hypopituitarism.[58] *Björnstad* syndrome is characterized by sensorineural deafness, pili torti, and occasionally mental retardation. The syndrome is autosomal recessive, but families with an autosomal dominant pattern have been described.[59] The recessive form has more recently been linked to mutations in *BCS1L*, which encodes an ATPase needed to assemble complex III in the mitochondria. More severe defects in *BCS1L* markedly increase reactive oxygen species and are lethal to neonatal infants with multisystemic involvement (complex II deficiency and growth retardation, aminoaciduria, cholestasis, iron overload, lactic acidosis, and early death [GRACILE] syndrome).[60]

Bazex–Dupré–Christol and *Rombo* syndromes are X-linked dominant traits characterized by congenital hypotrichosis with pili torti, numerous facial milia, trichoepitheliomas, vellus hair cysts, and an increased risk of the early development of basal cell carcinomas.[38,61–64] Distinguishing features are follicular atrophoderma, hypohidrosis, comedones and facial and neck pigmentation in Bazex–Dupré–Christol syndrome, and atrophoderma vermiculatum and photosensitivity in Rombo syndrome. Females often do not show the hypotrichosis, with normal and pili torti hairs intermingled.[65]

Hypotrichosis with juvenile macular dystrophy (HJMD) is characterized by the development of sparse, short hair from birth or in the first months of life. Fusiform beading and pili torti may be seen by microscopy. Macular degeneration first develops in the first or second decade, leading to blindness by early adulthood. Patients suspected of having HJMD should have annual ophthalmologic evaluations, because early retinal pigmentation and atrophy precede the decrease in visual acuity. The disorder is autosomal recessive and caused by mutations in *CDH3*, which encodes P-cadherin.[66,67] *CDH3* mutations also cause ectodermal dysplasia, ectrodactyly, and macular dystrophy (Table 7.1).

Individuals with mitochondrial enzyme abnormalities have shown a wide variety of abnormalities, predominantly failure to thrive and neuromuscular changes; however, skin or hair abnormalities have been described in 10% of affected children.[68] Hair abnormalities range from alopecia to dry, thick, brittle hair to hypertrichosis, especially on the back. Syndromic disorders with hair abnormalities may also affect mitochondrial function (e.g., Björnstad syndrome and cartilage–hair hypoplasia). Light-microscopy examination of affected hair has shown a variety of hair shaft defects associated with increased fragility, including pili torti, TTD, trichorrhexis nodosa, and diffuse longitudinal grooving with flattened hair shafts.[68,69] Patchy erythematous lesions have been described, and many of the patients with skin manifestations have shown mottled pigmentation.

Pili Bifurcati. *Pili bifurcati* is an uncommon anomaly of hair growth characterized by intermittent bifurcation of the hair shaft in which affected hairs divide into two separate shafts that subsequently become rejoined along the hair shaft.[70,71] This bifurcation is repeated at

Table 7.1 Classification for Ectodermal Dysplasias*

Disorder†	Inheritance	Gene	Protein	Function
GROUP 1				
EDA/NF-kB Pathway				
Hypohidrotic ectodermal dysplasia	XLR	*EDA1*	Ectodysplasin (EDA)	Membrane ligand
Hypohidrotic ectodermal dysplasia	AD	*EDAR*	EDA receptor (EDAR)	Receptor of EDA
		EDARADD	EDAR-associated death domain	Adaptor molecule
Hypohidrotic ectodermal dysplasia	AR	*EDAR*	EDAR	Receptor of EDA
		EDARADD	EDAR-associated death domain	Adaptor molecule
		TRAF6	TNF receptor associated factor 6	Activates IKK
Hypohidrotic ectodermal dysplasia with immune deficiency (males) ± osteopetrosis (males) ± lymphedema	XLR	*NEMO/ IKBKG*	NF-kB essential modulator	NF-kB activation
Incontinentia pigmenti (females)	XLD	*NEMO/IKKγ*	NF-κB essential modulator	NF-κB activation
Hypohidrotic ectodermal dysplasia with immune deficiency	AR	*IkBα*	IkBα	NF-kB activation
p63 Pathway				
Ectrodactyly-ectodermal dysplasia-clefting syndrome	AD	*p63*	p63	Transcription factor
Rapp–Hodgkin syndrome	AD	*p63*	p63	Transcription factor
Ankyloblepharon-ectodermal dysplasia-clefting syndrome (AEC)	AD	*p63*	p63	Transcription factor
Acrodermatoungual-lacrimal-tooth (ADULT)	AD	*p63*	p63	Transcription factor
Limb-mammary syndrome	AD	*p63*	p63	Transcription factor
Curly hair, ankyloblepharon, and nail dystrophy (CHAND) syndrome	AR	*RIPK4*	RIPK4	Serine/threonine protein kinase
Popliteal pterygium syndromes (spectrum) Popliteal pterygium Bartsocas-Papas Cocoon	AR, AD AR AR	IRF6 *RIPK4* CHUK	IRF6 RIPK4 CHUK	Transcription factor Kinase Kinase
Ectodermal dysplasia	AD	*KDF1*	KDF1	Keratinocyte differentiation factor
Trichodentoosseous syndrome (TDO)	AD	*DLX3*	DLX3	Transcription factor
Clefting-ectodermal dysplasia	AR	*PVRL1*	Nectin 1	Interacts with cadherins, esp. at adherens junctions
Ectodermal dysplasia-syndactyly syndrome	AR	*PVRL4*	Nectin 4	Interacts with cadherins, especially at adherens junctions
Hypotrichosis with juvenile macular dystrophy ± ectrodactyly/ other ectodermal defects	AR	*CDH3*	Cadherin 3/ P-cadherin	Adhesion molecule for cell–cell binding
WNT Pathway				
Witkop syndrome	AD	*MSX1*	MSX1	Transcription factor
Focal dermal hypoplasia	X-linked dominant	*PORCN*	PORCN	Regulates Wnt signaling
Oculodentodigital dysplasia (ODDD)	AD	*WNT10A*	Wnt10A	Wnt pathway
Hypohidrotic ectodermal dysplasia	AR, AD	*WNT10A*	Wnt10A	β-catenin-mediated signaling
Schöpf–Schulz–Passarge syndrome	AR	*WNT10A*	Wnt10A	β-catenin-mediated signaling
Ectodermal dysplasia	AR	*KREMEN1*	KREMEN1	Receptor involved in Wnt regulation
Structural Element				
Clouston syndrome	AD	*GJB6*	Connexin 30	Intercellular junctions
Ectodermal dysplasia	AR	*GRHL2*	Grainyhead-like 2	Transcription factor
Oculodentodigital dysplasia (ODDD)	AR	*GJA1*	Connexin 43	Intercellular junctions
Ellis van Creveld syndrome	AR	*EVC, EVC2*	EVC, EVC2	Ciliopathy
Ectodermal dysplasia 4, hair/nail type (ECTD4)	AR	*KRT85*	KRT85	Keratin

Continued

Table 7.1 Classification for Ectodermal Dysplasias—cont'd

Disorder†	Inheritance	Gene	Protein	Function
Keratitis-ichthyosis-deafness syndrome, autosomal dominant (KID) (see Chapter 5)	AR	*GJB2*	Connexin 26	Intercellular junctions
Ectodermal dysplasia: skin fragility syndrome (see Chapter 13)	AR	*PKP1*	Plakophilin 1	Desmosomal plaque/ stability
Naegeli- Franceschetti- Jadassohn syndrome (see Chapter 11)	AD	*KRT14*	KRT14	Keratin
Pachyonychia congenita	AD	*KRT 6a, 6b, 6c, 16, 17*	KRT 6a, 6b, 6c, 16, 17	Keratin

*Many forms of ectodermal dysplasia remain unclassified.
†Some more recently described forms of ectodermal dysplasia are not yet named.
AD, Autosomal dominant; *AR*, autosomal recessive; *IKK*, inhibitor of kappa light polypeptide gene enhancer in B-cell kinase; *TNF*, tumor necrosis factor; *TNFR*, tumor necrosis factor receptor; *XLD*, X-linked dominant; *XLR*, X-linked recessive.

intervals, and the anomaly appears to be transitory, with only a small percentage of hairs exhibiting the bifurcation. This disorder should not be confused with pili multigemini, a disorder in which multiple hairs project from a single hair follicle.

Trichothiodystrophy. *TTD* is a heterogeneous group of autosomal recessive disorders in which patients have dry, brittle, cysteine-deficient hair as an isolated finding or in association with often-multisystemic disease.[72] To date, four genes have been linked to autosomal recessive TTD: *ERCC2 (XPD)*, *ERCC3 (XPB)*, *p8* or *GTF2H5 (TTDA)*, and *C7Orf11/ MPLKIP (TTDN1)*. The function of *TTDN1* is not well understood, but it likely regulates cell cycling and transcription efficiency.[73] The other three genes encode subunits of transcription/repair factor IIH (TFIIH), a multiprotein complex involved in transcription and nucleotide excision repair.[74,75] A recently described form of autosomal recessive TTD results from mutations in *GTF2E2*, which encodes a subunit of the basal transcription factor II E (TFIIEβ) and is associated with proficient nucleotide excision repair.[76]

Light microscopy of TTD hairs shows a wavy, irregular outline and a flattened shaft that twists like a folded ribbon. Two types of fracture may be seen: trichoschisis (clean transverse fracture) or an atypical trichorrhexis nodosa with only slight splaying of the cortical cells. Trichoscopy using polarized light or polarizing microscopy shows the characteristic alternating light and dark bands, the "tiger-tail" appearance.[77–79] Although the severity of hair shaft defects is inversely proportional to the hair sulfur content, there is no association between the extent of systemic disease and percentage of abnormal hairs.[79] Sparse hair is often associated with the shaft defect. Some patients have described cyclic hair loss with fever, which may reflect a mutation leading to thermosensitive *XPD*.

A review of 112 published cases of TTD described the abnormalities beyond hair defects.[80] Ichthyosis has been noted in 65% and clinical evidence of photosensitivity in 24% of these patients. The ichthyosis may resemble autosomal recessive congenital ichthyosis (ARCI) or ichthyosis vulgaris (see Chapter 5), and some patients show marked depletion of the granular layer in skin biopsy sections.[81] Of the patients who have TTD with ichthyosis, 37% show a collodion phenotype at birth.[80] Patients may also show xerosis, palmoplantar keratoderma, atopic dermatitis, and/or follicular keratosis.[81] Nail abnormalities have been described in 63% of patients overall, especially dystrophy with thickening or yellow discoloration.

Among the most common noncutaneous features are developmental delay/intellectual impairment (86%), short stature and low weight (73%),[82] and ocular abnormalities (51%, especially cataracts). Facial dysmorphism is seen in 66% of patients, especially microcephaly, large or protruding ears, and micrognathia. An outgoing personality is a characteristic feature. Bone abnormalities are seen radiographically in 38%, particularly osteosclerosis and delayed bone age. Gonadal abnormalities were noted in 14% overall, most commonly hypogonadism and cryptorchidism. Recurrent infections have been noted in 46%, particularly involving the respiratory and gastrointestinal tracts and the inner ear, but were uncommonly associated with immunodeficiency or neutropenia.[83,84] Overall, mortality in the first decade of life is increased 20-fold. Not only is there the increased risk of infection, but children with TTD are at high risk for poor outcomes after routine procedures. Complications during pregnancy are noted in 26% of patients, most commonly intrauterine growth retardation, but also preterm delivery; preeclampsia; hemolysis, elevated liver enzymes, and low platelets (HELLP) syndrome; and prematurity.[85,86] The newly described form *(GTF2E2)* is a nonphotosensitive form and is characterized by ichthyosis, failure to thrive, and delayed motor and cognitive development. Unlike xeroderma pigmentosum, TTD is not prone to cancer, although squamous cell carcinoma has been described.[87,88]

Subgroups of TTD have been classified based on clinical characteristics (brittle hair, intellectual impairment, decreased fertility, and short stature [BIDS]; ichthyosis, brittle hair, infertility, developmental delay, short stature [IBIDS]/Tay syndrome; photosensitivity, ichthyosis, brittle hair, infertility, developmental delay, short stature [PIBIDS]). However, a new classification has been proposed that divides patients based on their mutations as group I (mutations in genes encoding subunits of TFIIH: *XPD/ERCC2*, *XPB/ERCC3*, *TTDA*, or *p8/GTF2H5*), II (*TTDN1/ MPLKIP* and *GTF2E2*), and III (no known molecular basis).[81] Group I includes patients with photosensitivity (either clinical or *in vitro*) and is the most common subtype. Most individuals in group II are not photosensitive and show an increased risk of developmental delay, delayed bone age, seizures, and autistic behavior.[89] Currently unclassified but nonphotosensitive patients (such as those with Pollitt and Sabinas syndromes, which have been linked to gene defects)[90] are in group III. Using this classification, ichthyosis and the collodion-baby phenotype are most highly correlated with group I, whereas hypogonadism has been found more in groups II and III.

An X-linked form of nonphotosensitive TTD has been described, characterized by the typical sparse, brittle hair; severe intellectual impairment with microcephaly; and short stature, but also facial dysmorphism and an aged appearance, hypogammaglobulinemia, seizures, endocrine abnormalities, and brain malformations.[91] Ichthyosis and photosensitivity are not features. The disorder results from mutations in *RNF113A*, which encodes a protein of unknown function.

Marie Unna Hypotrichosis. *Marie Unna hypotrichosis* is an autosomal dominant disorder manifested by almost complete congenital absence of scalp hair, eyebrows, and eyelashes.[92–94] The hair regrows to normal density but is coarse, flattened, and twisted. Beginning at puberty the hair becomes progressively sparser, particularly on the vertex and scalp margins, resulting in a high frontal (Fig. 7.8) and nuchal hairline. By adulthood, only a sparse fringe of hair at the scalp margin may remain, and eyelashes, eyebrows, and body hair, including secondary-sexual hair, tend to be sparse. Scattered follicular horny plugs may be associated but no scarring. Trichoscopy/light microscopy of the shaft shows variations in shaft diameter and twisting or bending at odd angles. Other ectodermal structures are unaffected, except that 50% of affected individuals show exceptionally widely spaced upper incisor teeth. Mutations that cause Marie Unna hypotrichosis affect *U2HR*, an open-reading frame upstream of the hairless gene that inhibits hairless expression; as a result, hairless expression and Wnt signaling are increased.[95,96]

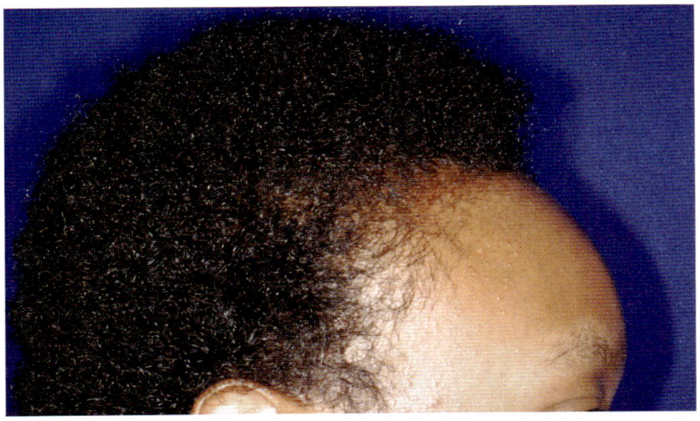

Fig. 7.8 Marie Unna hypotrichosis. Note the loss of hair at the frontal hairline and the sparse, coarse eyebrows. Progressive alopecia will leave him largely alopecic as an adult.

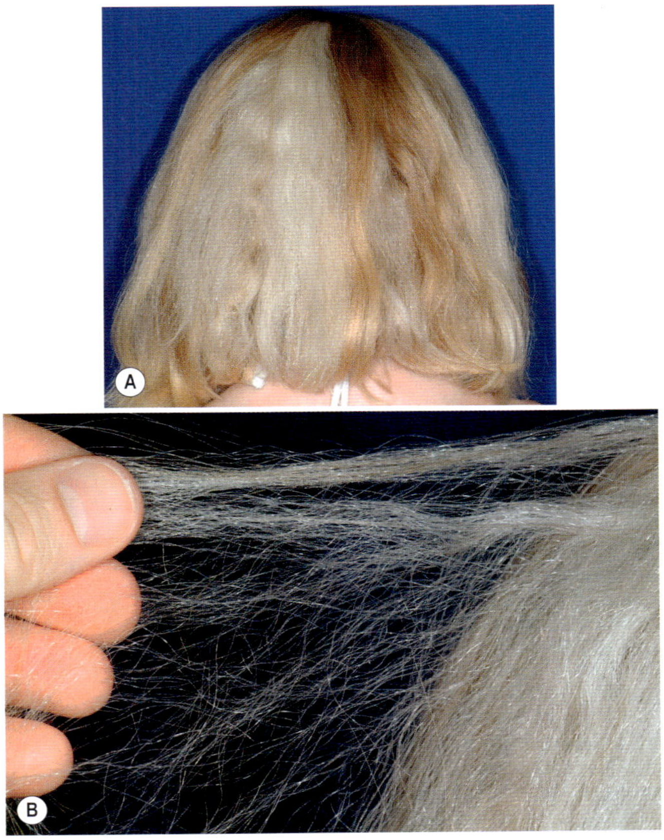

Fig. 7.9 Woolly hair nevus. The affected hair is lighter **(A)**, sometimes sparser, and more "woolly" in consistency from the normal surrounding scalp hair **(B)**.

Hair Shaft Abnormalities Without Increased Fragility

Pili Annulati. *Pili annulati* (ringed hair) is an autosomal dominant condition with onset shortly after birth. The hair looks shiny with attractive highlights but has alternating bright and dark bands on close inspection. The bright areas are the result of light scattering from clusters of air-filled cavities within the cortex that appear as dark areas under light microscopy, especially in more proximal hair regions.[97] Pili annulati may increase the risk of developing AA[98] and has been reported to markedly improve or clear after the occurrence of alopecia totalis.[99] The gene mutated in pili annulati has been linked to chromosome 12q24.33, but no mutations in candidate genes have been found.[100]

Pseudopili annulati is an unusual variant of normal hair in which bright bands are seen at intervals along the hair shaft. Secondary to periodic twisting or curling of the hair shaft, this banding is conspicuous only in blond hairs and represents an attractive optical effect caused by reflection and refraction of light by flattened and twisted hair surfaces.

Woolly Hair

Woolly hair describes a tight, curly hair that is usually present from birth and shows abnormalities under light microscopy.[9] The individual scalp hairs are fine and dry, light-colored, and corrugated at intervals, resembling the wool of sheep. Recognition of woolly hair is important because of the many associated abnormalities. Disorders characterized by generalized woolly hair, keratoderma, and dilated cardiomyopathy have been linked to mutations in indesmosomal proteins (desmoplakin,[101,102] plakoglobin,[103] and desmocollin-2[104] for *Naxos* disease and *Carvajal* syndrome; desmoplakin for erythrokeratodermia with cardiomyopathy/EKC, see Chapter 5); keratoderma and woolly hair without cardiomyopathy may also result from mutations in *KANK2* (see Chapter 5). Diffuse woolly hair has also been associated with ocular abnormalities, keratosis pilaris atrophicans, and/or ulerythema ophryogenes, keratosis follicularis spinulosa decalvans (KFSD),[105] giant axonal neuropathy (GAN) syndrome, and primary osteoma cutis.

Woolly hair without associated systemic manifestations can be inherited as either an autosomal dominant or autosomal recessive trait, both of which result from abnormalities of the inner-root sheath of the hair follicles. The entire scalp tends to be affected from birth, but nonscalp hair is normal. The hair grows slowly, is hypopigmented, and shows varying degrees of hypotrichosis. Plucked hair shows a dystrophic bulb and sometimes nonspecific shaft defects. The dominant form results from mutations in *KRT25*, *KRT71*, or *KRT74*, encoding type 1 hair keratin 25, or its parners, type 2 keratins 71 and 74, respectively.[106–108]

The recessive forms have now been explained by mutations in two interacting genes, *LPAR6* (encoding the lipophosphatidic acid [LPA] receptor 6/*P2RY5*)[111,112] and *LIPH* (encoding lipase H).[109,110] Lipase H reduces phosphatidic acid to LPA,[113] which is involved in lipid and energy metabolism. Biallelic missense mutations in KRT25 have also been reported to cause an autosomal recessive form of woolly hair.[114,115] Topical minoxidil has been reported to increase hair thickness and numbers in patients with *LIPH* deficiency.[116] Woolly (often yellow) hair has also been a feature associated with mutations in *PERP*, encoding a desmosomal component; the disorder may manifest as an autosomal dominant disorder characterized by palmoplantar keratoderma, cheilitis, and periorificial involvement, resembling Olmsted syndrome, or as an autosomal recessive disorder with more generalized erythrokeratoderma.[117]

The woolly hair nevus is a sporadic condition characterized by the development of one or more patches of hair different in color, shape, and consistency from the normal surrounding scalp hair (Fig. 7.9). The hairs on the affected area are usually smaller in diameter, lighter in color, and sparser than those on the rest of the scalp.[118] When examined under a dissecting microscope, the individual hairs are noted to twist about their long axis. The majority of reported cases of woolly hair nevus have been recognized during the first few months of life, but some have appeared in young adulthood.[119,120] In about 50% of cases, woolly hair nevus coexists with a linear epidermal nevus in the same area or elsewhere.[121,122] Ocular involvement has been described as an associated feature. Epidermal nevi with woolly hair are linked to mutations in *HRAS*.[123,124] Hairs within the woolly hair patch show follicular miniaturization with increased vellus hairs.[125]

Acquired Progressive Kinking of the Hair. *Acquired progressive kinking* of the hair is a rare disorder of scalp hair, with onset in adolescence or in young adulthood.[126] The condition is characterized by a rapid onset of extreme curliness of the hair (mainly on the frontoparietal region of the scalp and vertex), often in association with an increased coarse texture, diminished luster, and striking unruliness. The disorder is more common in males than in females. Hair may become

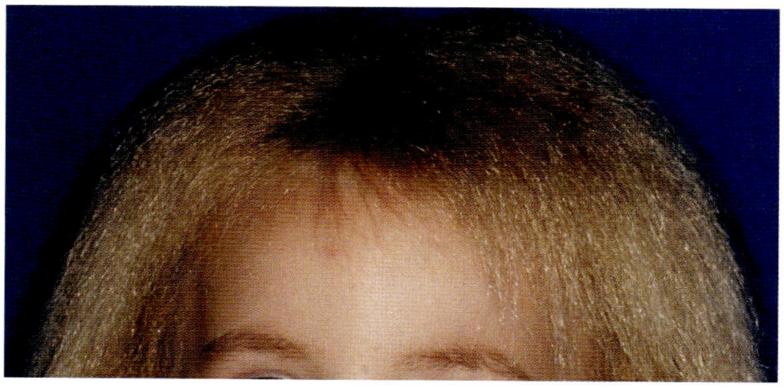

Fig. 7.10 Uncombable hair syndrome. Blond hair that is dry and frizzy and does not lie flat on the scalp, thus making combing impossible. (Courtesy Sarah Chamlin, MD.)

darker or remain unaltered in color, and the rate of growth may be decreased or unchanged.[127] Examination of abnormal hairs by light microscopy reveals alterations in hair shaft diameter and partial twisting of the hair on its longitudinal axis.

Although the etiology of this disorder is unknown, it may follow treatment with systemic retinoids, including isotretinoin. The localization of hair kinking, family history of androgenetic alopecia (AGA), pathologic features of the affected scalp, and tendency to evolve into AGA suggest acquired kinking as a harbinger of AGA.[128] No therapy is effective, and application of topical minoxidil has not affected the progressive thinning of hair in the areas of kinking.[128] Spontaneous reversion to normal hair has been reported.[129] Coarse hair, but not woolly hair, is also a feature of Hajdu–Cheney syndrome, resulting from mutations in *NOTCH2*. Other features include craniofacial abnormalities, short stature, acroosteolysis with broad nails and digits, synophrys, coarse skin, and premature tooth loss with periodontitis.[130]

Uncombable Hair Syndrome. The *uncombable hair syndrome* (pili trianguli canaliculi, spun-glass hair syndrome) is a unique hair disorder characterized by very pale, silvery, blond, or straw-colored hair. The hair is dry, frizzy, and unruly, and it does not lie flat on the scalp, thus making combing impossible (Fig. 7.10).[131,132] The syndrome is autosomal recessive and results from mutations in one of three genes: *PADI3* (encoding peptidylarginine deiminase 3), *TGM3* (encoding transglutaminase 3), or *TCHH* (encoding trichohyalin[133]). PADI and TGM3 are enzymes responsible for posttranslational modifications in trichohyalin, a hair shaft protein.

The onset is usually during infancy or early childhood, and eyebrows, lashes, and body hair are normal. Affected children may have minor nail abnormalities,[134] and some show both uncombable hair and loose anagen hair (see Loose Anagen Syndrome section).[135] However, more significant nail abnormalities or other features beyond the hair issue should prompt a search for a second disorder; one child with uncombable hair and congenital anonychia was found to have homozygous mutations in both *PADI3* and *RSPO4*, encoding R-spondin 4 (see nails).[136] The characteristic structural defect of uncombable hair—the presence of canalicular depressions along the hair shaft—can be demonstrated by scanning electron microscopy[137] or by routine microscopy of the hair in cross-section.[138] Cross-sectional microscopy shows a variety of shapes, including triangular, quadrangular, and reniform. The longitudinal grooving and abnormal shape in cross-section, however, are not specific for uncombable hair syndrome and have been described in several other syndromes, among them Marie Unna hypotrichosis, the ectodermal dysplasias with clefting, hypohidrotic ectodermal dysplasia (HED), oral-facial-digital syndrome type I (OFD1), and progeria. The clinical appearance of the spun-glass hair requires a sizable proportion of abnormal hairs, and at least 50% of hairs are abnormal by scanning electron microscopy. The hair tends to become progressively more manageable by adolescence, and some patients have responded to biotin administration.[134]

Uncombable hair syndrome must be distinguished from extremely unruly hair, which is seen in 2% of individuals. Extremely unruly hair that tends to stand up from the area of the posterior parietal whorl toward the frontal hairline may be associated with microcephaly and is a potential indicator of abnormal brain growth and morphogenesis, similar to upsweep of anterior scalp hair and aberrant parietal whorl position.

Loose Anagen Syndrome

LAS occurs in 10% of all children who have alopecia[139] and is characterized by actively growing anagen hairs that are loosely anchored and can be easily and painlessly pulled from the scalp.[140] Although considered an autosomal dominant disorder, 70% of cases are sporadic, and in one series, 95% were girls.[141] A mutation in a hair keratin (*KRT75*, formerly called *K6HF*) has been found in some families, but its relevance is unclear because it does not reliably segregate with the loose anagen phenotype.[26] The mean age of onset in girls is 30 months of age, but of diagnosis is 5 years of age.[141] Most patients are white, and although many patients are blonde, about half of the reported cases have brown hair. Affected children generally have sparse, short, scalp hairs that seldom require cutting (Fig. 7.11, *A*). Examination shows patchy or subtle diffuse thinning with hairs of uneven length (Fig. 7.11, *B*). The hair often appears to be limp, and a matted texture with a "bed head" appearance is sometimes noted at the occiput. Of the actively growing anagen hairs, the majority show ruffled cuticles (resembling floppy socks) and pigmented misshapen anagen bulbs (resembling hockey sticks) (Fig. 7.11, *C* and *D*). Gentle pulling tends to yield several hairs, allowing the diagnosis to be made by light-microscopic examination of the hair; forceful extraction of hairs may lead to misshaping of normal anagen hairs and thus should be avoided. Shedding of the hair is cyclic, and the inability to extract large amounts of hair by a gentle pull test does not definitively rule out the diagnosis.

LAS has been classified into three phenotypes. Type A is characterized by sparse hair that cannot grow long. Type B features unruly hair that is diffuse or patchy. Type C has normal-appearing hair, but excessive shedding of the loose anagen hairs. Types A and B almost exclusively affect children. Although no treatment is available for this disorder, it is reassuring for patients and their families to know that other abnormalities are not associated with this disorder, and children with this condition tend to improve with time. Gentle hair care and volumizing shampoos/conditioners have been recommended. There is no good evidence to date that oral biotin administration or application of topical minoxidil is helpful.

Loose anagen hair is also a feature of an autosomal recessive Noonan-like syndrome (Noonan-like syndrome with loose anagen hair)[142] that has been linked to mutations in *SHOC2*[143] or *PPP1CB*,[144] encoding a subunit of protein phosphatase 1, which forms a complex with *SHOC2*. In addition to the fine, sparse, unruly hair, affected children show the Noonan syndrome facies and broad neck; macrocephaly; reduced growth with delayed bone age (often from growth hormone deficiency); variable cognitive defects; hyperactivity; hypernasal voice; darkly pigmented, thickened skin with dermatitis; and cardiac defects. LAS has also been described in hypohidrotic ectodermal dysplasia.[145]

NONSCARRING ALOPECIAS WITHOUT HAIR SHAFT ABNORMALITIES[146]

Congenital/Genetic Disorders

Congenital Triangular Alopecia. *Congenital triangular alopecia* is characterized by an area of alopecia that, although sometimes notable at birth in babies with abundant scalp hair, is usually detected at 2 or 3 years of age (Fig. 7.12). It is often earlier in boys than girls because of the shorter hair.[147–149] An initial appearance during adulthood has been described.[150] The area is triangular and overlies the frontotemporal suture, with the base of the triangle directed forward. The triangular patch may extend to the hairline, but often a fringe of hair may separate it from the forehead. Generally measuring 3 to 5 cm from base to apex, the area may be completely bald or partially covered by vellus hairs and remains unchanged throughout life. The differential diagnosis includes AA, trichotillomania, and traction alopecia. Dermoscopy of the affected area shows normal follicular openings with vellus hairs,[149] whereas dermoscopy of AA shows dystrophic and exclamation-point hairs.[151] Although unilateral in 80% to 90% of affected individuals, it may be bilaterally symmetric, and on rare occasions, similar triangular patches may be noted on the temporoparietal area, occipital scalp, or nape.[152]

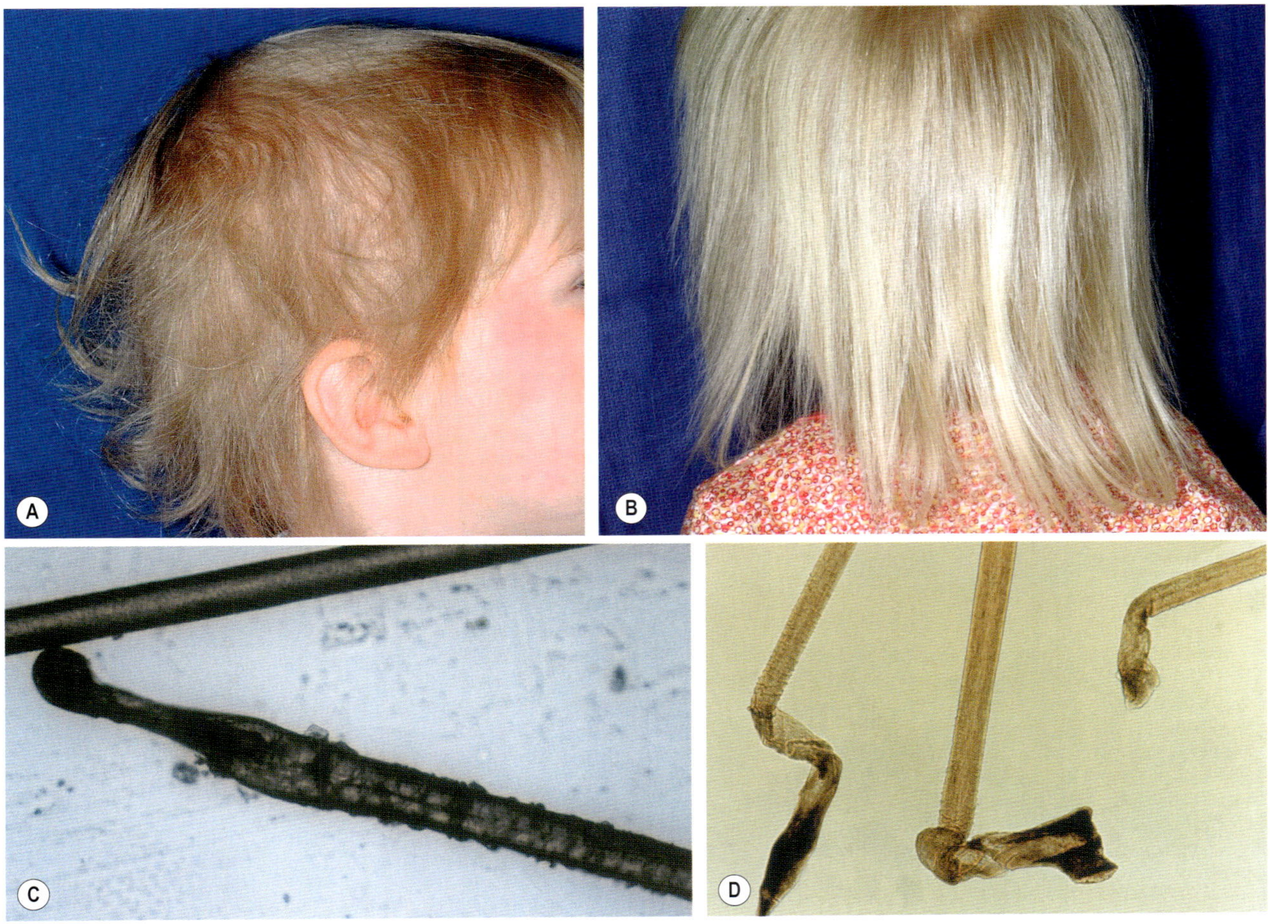

Fig. 7.11 Loose anagen syndrome. **(A, B)** The typical patient is a blonde preschool girl whose hair comes out easily and has become lusterless, fine, sparse, and uneven. When viewed under light microscope, the hairs that are easily able to be removed without plucking show a ruffled cuticle **(C)** and distorted bulb **(D)**.

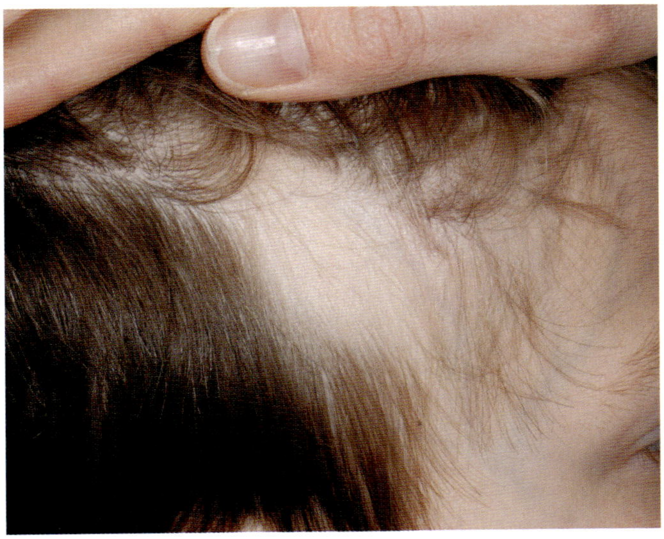

Fig. 7.12 Congenital triangular alopecia. This triangular patch of alopecia may not appear until 2 to 3 years of age or even later but then persists unchanged.

The condition is almost always sporadic, although the association with developmental delay and seizures has been described in a mother and daughter.[153] Congenital triangular alopecia has been described in a patient each with phakomatosis pigmentovascularis, Down syndrome, and Dandy–Walker malformation.[148] Hair transplants have been used to repopulate the area of triangular alopecia.[154] Bilateral congenital localized patches of alopecia of the parietal area that resemble the alopecia of congenital triangular alopecia have been seen in patients with Gomez–Lopez–Hernandez syndrome (cerebellotrigeminal–dermal dysplasia). Although the alopecia classically affects the parietal area, other sites have been reported to show symmetric alopecia.[155] Other features are skull defects (craniosynostosis with brachycephaly, midfacial hypoplasia), neurologic abnormalities, short stature, hypertelorism, and corneal opacities.[156]

Atrichia with Papular Lesions

Individuals who initially have hair but lose it all, with the first hair shedding shortly after birth, likely have *atrichia with papular lesions* (APL; resulting from mutations in the hairless gene) or, alternatively, *vitamin D–dependent rickets type IIA* (caused by mutations in the vitamin D receptor).[157,158] Affected individuals never regrow scalp hair and tend to be nearly totally devoid of eyebrows, lashes, and axillary and pubic hair (Fig. 7.13). Follicular cysts and milia-like lesions may appear on the skin later in life (hence the nomenclature of "with papular lesions"). Scalp biopsies show disintegration of the lower two-thirds of the hair follicle, which is often replaced by cysts. Patients with vitamin D–resistant rickets are clinically and histologically identical to patients with APL[159] but show the additional manifestations of early-onset

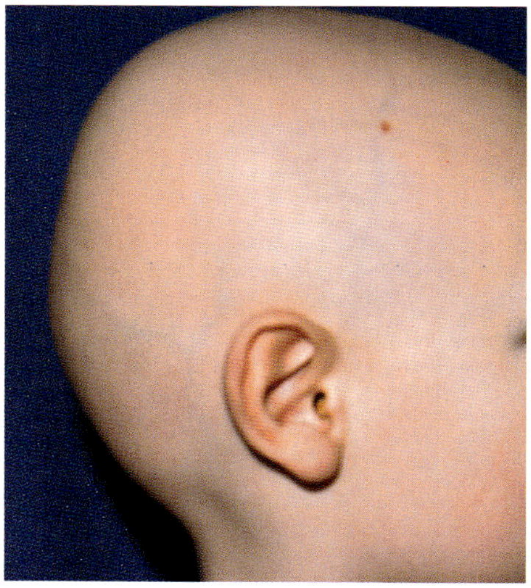

Fig. 7.13 Congenital atrichia. This boy lost his hair during the first year of life and has never regrown it. A mutation in the hairless gene was demonstrated.

rickets, hypocalcemia, secondary hyperparathyroidism, and elevated 1,25-dihydroxyvitamin D_3.[160] The similarity in phenotype reflects the direct regulatory effect of the vitamin D receptor and hairless gene on each other via a transcriptional mechanism.[161,162] This group of patients is often misdiagnosed as having alopecia universalis, and they must be also be distinguished from patients with PHNED, an autosomal recessive disorder resulting from mutations in *KRT85*, *KRT74*, or the *HOXC13* homeobox gene,[163] which usually presents with congenital complete alopecia and uniformly small, dystrophic nails.[164–168] Sometimes, lacrimal duct obstruction[169] and very short, sparse, fragile hair may be present in PHNED and is easily visualized by trichoscopy.[170]

Hypotrichosis Simplex

Hypotrichosis simplex is a group of rare autosomal dominant and autosomal recessive nonscarring alopecias in which patients are usually born with normal hair. Hair loss can begin in the first months or even as late as the first decade (Fig. 7.14) and can progress to almost complete loss of scalp hair by adulthood. Graying has been reported to coincide with hair loss. Some individuals show sparse, fine, short hairs, especially at the crown, but hair on sites other than the scalp is normal. The disorder has considerable genetic heterogeneity. Autosomal dominant forms result from mutations in genes encoding corneodesmin, a

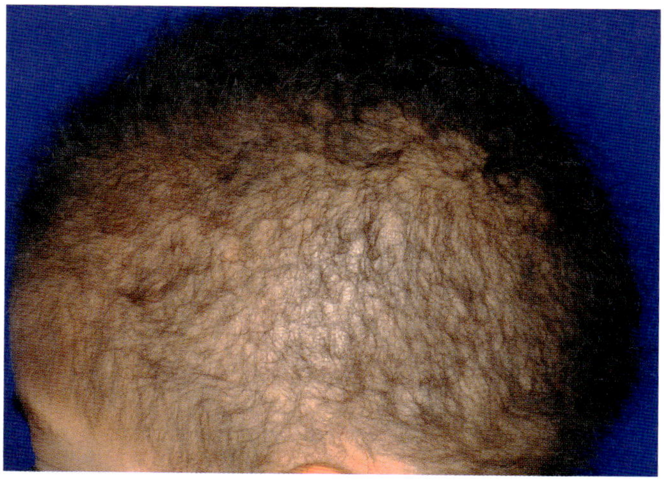

Fig. 7.14 Hypotrichosis simplex. This girl with localized autosomal recessive hypotrichosis began to lose hair in the first months of life and was found to have homozygous variants in *C3ORF52*. She had no other medical issues.

protein of the corneocyte desmosomes and inner hair sheath (see Peeling Skin Syndrome section, Chapter 5)[171,172]; a protein of the pre–messenger ribonucleic acid (mRNA) processing spliceosome *(SNRPE)*[173]; and *APCDD1*, an inhibitor of Wnt pathway signaling.[174] Localized autosomal recessive hypotrichosis most often results from variants in the lipase pathway (see Woolly Hair section). Homozygous variants in the gene encoding C3ORF52, which is co-expressed and interacts with lipase H in the inner root sheath of the hair follicle, reduced lipase H-mediated lipophosphatidic acid biosynthesis and leads to hypotrichosis without woolly hair.[175] Localized autosomal recessive hypotrichosis can also be associated with scalp follicular keratosis, which can be confused with monilethrix.

Hallermann–Streiff; Sensenbrenner; Coffin–Siris; Nicolaides-Baraitser; and growth retardation, alopecia, pseudoanodontia, and optic atrophy (GAPO) syndromes all show hypotrichosis in association with facial dysmorphism and other physical signs (see Online only). In *Hallermann–Streiff* syndrome (oculomandibulodyscephaly), hypotrichosis of the scalp, eyebrows, and eyelids is associated with dwarfism, beaked nose, and brachycephaly. The alopecia is most prominent at the frontal and parietal areas and is especially marked along suture lines. Axillary and pubic hair may also be scant, and cutaneous atrophy, largely limited to the scalp and nose, may appear as thin, taut skin and prominent underlying blood vessels. Other features include frontal and parietal bossing, mandibular hypoplasia, microphthalmia, low-set ears, thin and small lips, high-arched palate, atrophy of the skin of the face, congenital cataracts, blue sclerae, motor and occasionally mental retardation, and dental abnormalities.

Sensenbrenner syndrome, or cranioectodermal dysplasia, is a rare autosomal recessive disorder manifested by small stature, dolichocephaly, an unusual facies, and tubulointerstitial nephritis leading to early end-stage renal failure.[176] The typical facies show frontal bossing, hypertelorism, prominent epicanthal folds, antimongoloid palpebral fissures, eversion of the lip, and full-rounded cheeks. Patients have small, gray, widely spaced teeth; short, fine, hair; and hypohidrosis.[177] Sensenbrenner syndrome is a ciliopathy that results from mutations in *IFT122*,[178] *WDR35*,[179] or *IFT43*.[180]

Patients with *Coffin–Siris syndrome* most commonly show a constellation of severe mental retardation; a characteristic coarse-appearing facies; scalp hypotrichosis with hypertrichosis of the eyebrows, eyelashes, face, and back; hypotonia; hypoplastic to absent fifth fingernails and distal phalanges; and feeding problems with postnatal growth deficiency.[181] Coffin–Siris syndrome is autosomal dominant and results from mutations in one of several components of the SWItch/sucrose nonfermenting (SWI/SNF; also called *BAF*) adenosine triphosphate (ATP)–dependent chromatin-remodeling complex.[182,183] Of these, mutations in *ARID1B* are most common (76% in one series).[184,185] A related disorder is *Nicolaides–Baraitser* syndrome, which results from mutations in *SMARCA2*, which encodes one of two subunits of this BAF chromatic remodeling complex. Nicolaides–Baraitser syndrome is an autosomal dominant disorder with cardinal features that include intellectual disability of varying extents, short stature, microcephaly, typical facies, and sparse scalp hair in association with brachydactyly, seizures, and behavioral problems.[186]

As mentioned, *GAPO* is an acronym for *growth retardation, alopecia, pseudoanodontia, and optic atrophy*.[187] Distinctive craniofacial features include an aged appearance with frontal bossing, high forehead, midfacial hypoplasia, hypertelorism, and thickened eyelids and lips. GAPO syndrome is autosomal recessive and results from mutations in *ANTXR1*, which encodes anthrax toxin receptor 1.[188] Although the alopecia usually affects the entire scalp and starts shortly after birth, it occasionally starts as late as 2 years of age and can be partial at first (occipital[189] or in a pattern resembling androgenetic alopecia).[190] Eyebrows and lashes are also sparse.

Cartilage–hair hypoplasia syndrome is an autosomal recessive disorder that occurs primarily in inbred Amish or Finnish populations.[191,192] Patients have short limbs and sparse, fine scalp and body hair. Several patients with hyperextensible digits and soft, doughy skin, reflecting degenerated elastic tissue, have been described.[193] Defective cell-mediated immunity is seen in most patients and results in relative anergy, altered T-cell responses, and increased susceptibility to severe viral infections, particularly varicella.[194] Patients may have infantile neutropenia, Diamond–Blackfan anemia, severe combined immunodeficiency, celiac syndrome, and/or toxic megacolon. Mild to

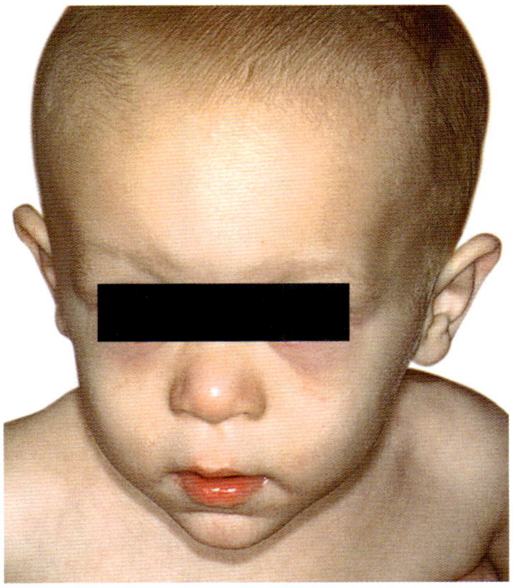

Fig. 7.15 Trichorhinophalangeal syndrome, type I. This 9-month-old boy shows the distinctive facies, including the pear-shaped nose and elongated philtrum, the thin upper lip, and the receding chin, as well as the sparse hair. He had hip dysplasia as well.

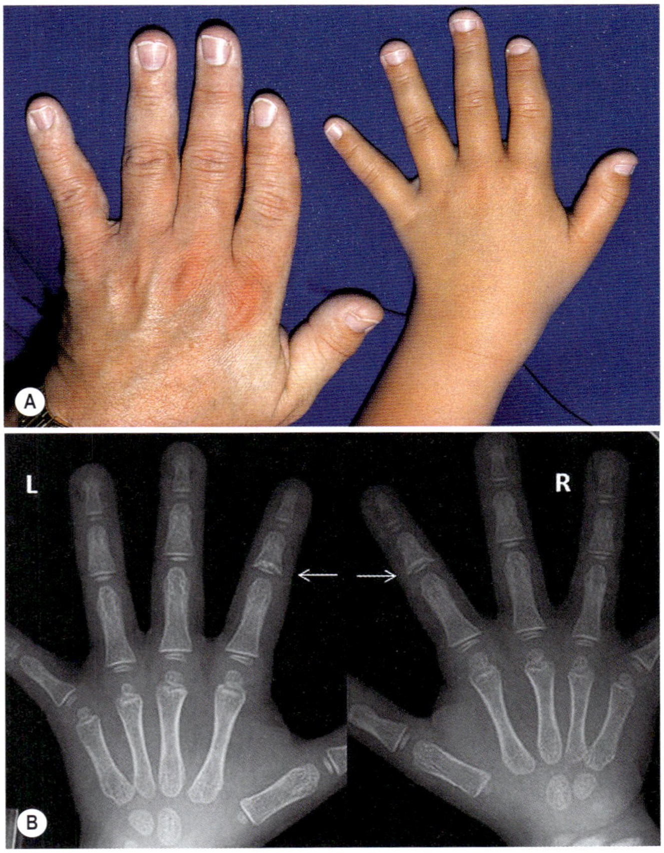

Fig. 7.16 Trichorhinophalangeal syndrome, type I. **(A)** Brachydactyly in an affected father and daughter with short stature and typical facies. Note the deviation of the middle phalanges. **(B)** Cone-shaped epiphyses of the second finger of this child's left and right hands.

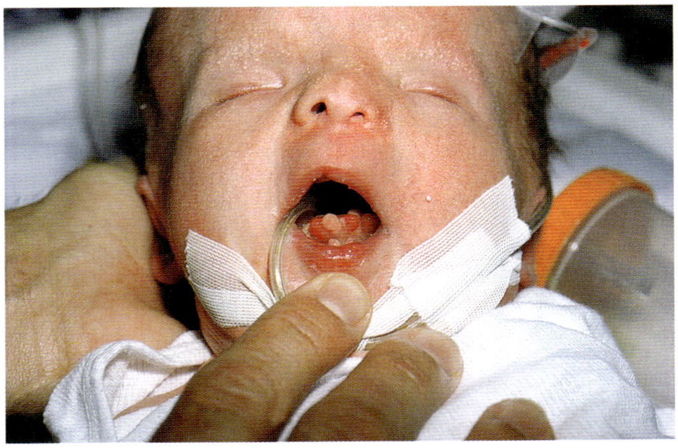

Fig. 7.17 Oral-facial-digital syndrome, type I. This infant girl shows the asymmetric hypoplasia of nasal cartilages and lobulated cleft tongue. Note the many facial milia on the cheek and eyelids. The hair continues to be sparse and dry.

severe bronchiectasis has been noted in more than 50% of patients.[195] Approximately 10% develop malignancy, especially lymphoreticular; an increased prevalence of early basal cell carcinomas has also been described.[196] The disorder results from mutations in ribonuclease (RNase) *MRP,* which cleaves RNA in mitochondrial deoxyribonucleic acid (DNA) synthesis and preribosomal RNA in the nucleolus.[197] Alopecia is seen with macrocephaly, cutis laxa, and scoliosis in macrocephaly, alopecia, cutis laxa, and scoliosis (MACS) syndrome (see Chapter 6).

Trichorhinophalangeal syndrome (TRPS) type I is an autosomal dominant disorder characterized by a distinctive facies with pear-shaped nose, elongated philtrum, thin upper lip, supernumerary incisors, and receding chin (Fig. 7.15) and skeletal abnormalities, including brachydactyly, deviation of the middle phalanges (Fig. 7.16, *A*), hip malformation, and short stature.[198–200] Most patients show fine, sparse, slow-growing hair, but almost-normal hair to complete baldness have been described. The underlying molecular basis is a mutation in *TRPS1,* which encodes a transcription factor. The diagnosis is made by the demonstration of cone-shaped epiphyses of the fingers seen on plain radiography (Fig. 7.16, *B*). These findings may not be detectable until 3 years of age or older. The type II form of TRPS (Langer–Giedion syndrome) is a contiguous gene syndrome, with contiguous deletion of *TRPS1, RAD21,* and *EXT1,* which gives patients the associated multiple exostoses. These exostoses are typically first seen on the scapulae, elbows, and knees during infancy or preschool years. Type III TRPS results from mutations in *TRPS1,* but manifests with much more severe short stature and generalized shortening of all phalanges and metacarpals than TRPS type I.[201] Good retention of frontal scalp hair has been shown after transplantation in a patient in whom minoxidil was not helpful.[202]

Oral-facial-digital syndrome, type 1 (OFD1) is an X-linked dominant ciliopathy largely limited to girls. Typically, the disorder is thought to be lethal in boys, although surviving boys with in-frame or missense mutations have been described.[203,204] The disorder results from mutations in *OFD1,* which encodes a centrosomal protein of primary cilia. Facial features occur in almost 70% of patients and include hypoplasia of nasal cartilage and hypertelorism with lateral displacement of the inner canthi (dystopia canthorum)[205] (Fig. 7.17). Among the oral anomalies described are tongue hamartomas, lobulated cleft tongue, cleft lip and palate, maldeveloped frenula, asymmetry of the lips and tongue, and maxillary gingival swelling.[206] Associated hand malformations are common and include brachydactyly, syndactyly, clinodactyly, and polydactyly. Almost half of affected individuals show central nervous system (CNS) involvement, most commonly retardation or selective cognitive impairment. Cutaneous abnormalities occur in the minority of patients but include numerous milia at birth[207] and sparse fine or coarse, dry, and lusterless hair to frank alopecia. Polycystic kidney disease with renal insufficiency is occasionally seen in children but more often occurs with advancing age (>50% after age 36 years).[208] Other "ciliopathies" share the CNS, skeletal, and cystic renal abnormalities of OFD1. An autosomal recessive form of OFD syndrome has been described, resulting from homozygous variants of the helicase gene

DDX59.[209] Features include lobulated or bifid tongues with hamartomas, developmental delay with microcephaly, and variable polydactyly.

Ectodermal Dysplasias

Ectodermal dysplasias are a complex group of approximately 200 developmental disorders that were traditionally classified based on their sites of abnormalities (hair, teeth, nails, and/or eccrine glands) and other ectodermal and nonectodermal features.[210] Newer classifications focus on the molecular basis of these disorders (now known in almost 100 ectodermal dysplasias),[211,212] the function of the affected proteins, and the clinical features.[213] The newest classification, developed by a National Institutes of Health international advisory board, divides ectodermal dysplasias based on major developmental pathway (EDA, TP63, WNT) or component of a complex molecular structure (e.g., keratins, connexins, cadherins) (see Table 7.1). This group also proposed a definition of ectodermal dysplasia as a genetic condition affecting the development and/or homeostasis of two or more ectodermal derivatives, including hair, teeth, nails, and certain glands. If a disorder affects only one ectodermal derivative (an attenuated phenotype) but involves a gene known to be associated with ectodermal dysplasia, the disorder is grouped as a nonsyndromic trait of the causative gene.

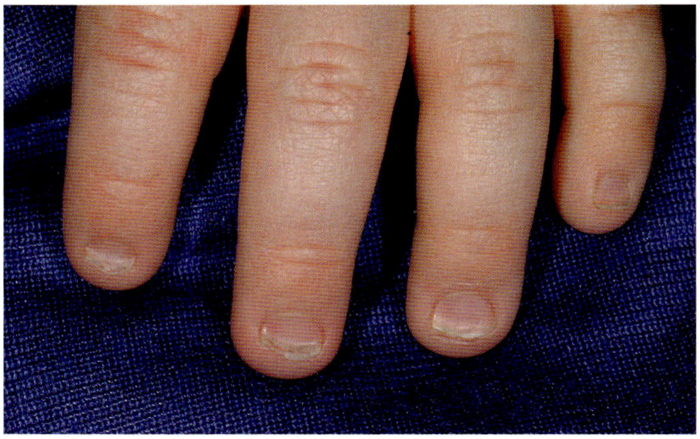

Fig. 7.18 Trichodental syndrome (Witkop syndrome). Slow-growing, small, spoon-shaped nails are a characteristic feature in addition to the slow-growing lusterless hair, sparse outer eyebrows, and small, sometimes absent teeth.

EDA and Wnt Signaling Pathways.

HYPOHIDROTIC ECTODERMAL DYSPLASIA. *HED* is characterized by the triad of reduced sweating, hypotrichosis, and defective dentition[214] resulting from variants in genes of the EDA and WNT pathways (see Table 7.1).[215] The majority of affected individuals are male, and overall 92% have a mutation in one of four genes (see Table 7.1): ectodysplasin-A1 (*EDA1* on the X-chromosome) in 58%; its ectodysplasin receptor (*EDAR*) in 16%; Wnt10A (*WNT10A*) in 16% (classified as a WNT-related disorder); and EDAR-associated death domain (*EDARADD*) in 2%.[216] HED may also result from a heterozygous mutation in *TRAF6*, which is upstream of *NEMO* and promotes nuclear factor-κB (NFκB) activity,[217] and in X-chromosome located *XEDAR*, encoding the receptor for EDA2, a different EDA isoform that binds to Traf6.[218] Female carriers with an *EDA1* mutation show random inactivation of the abnormal gene and can show manifestations ranging from none to extensive dental defects, alopecia, and patchy hypohidrosis following the lines of Blaschko, which are lines of embryologic development of skin. Mutations in the receptor *(EDAR)*, the death domain *(EDARADD)*, or WNT10A *(WNT10A)* may be inherited in a recessive or dominant pattern.[213] The phenotype with recessive mutations closely resembles those in X-linked recessive HED, whereas dominant mutations tend to be less severe with respect to sweating and hair loss.[219]

Mutations in *WNT10A* can lead to a spectrum of ectodermal defects that can include isolated oligodontia, mild manifestations of HED,[220,221] oculoonychodermal dysplasia (OODD), or Schöpf–Schulz–Passarge syndrome. The nail changes of OODD (fragility, longitudinal ridging, splitting, koilonychias, onycholysis, and pterygium) begin in early childhood and are associated with palmoplantar keratoderma, agenesis of the permanent teeth, and sometimes facial erythema and atrophic tongue papillae. Schöpf–Schulz–Passarge syndrome may manifest solely with bilateral eyelid cysts and palmoplantar keratoderma, but often includes nail, hair, and/or dental abnormalities.[222,223]

Trichodental syndrome, also known as *Witkop syndrome* or the tooth-and-nail syndrome, is an autosomal dominant disorder characterized by fine, dry, slow-growing lusterless hair; sparseness or absence of the lateral halves of the eyebrows; congenitally missing and small teeth; and slow-growing, small, spoon-shaped nails (especially toenails) (see Fig. 7.18).[224,225] Mutations have been described in *MSX1*, which directs the formation of teeth and nails.[226] Oligodontia of primary or permanent teeth in association with a low frontal hairline, a low and broad nasal bridge, thick lips, and sparse hair are seen in patients with biallelic mutations in *KREMEN1*.[227,228] KREMEN1 is the receptor for Dickkopf-1, which forms a complex to potently inhibit Wnt (including Wnt10A) signaling.

Hypohidrotic ectodermal dysplasia with immunodeficiency (HED-ID) affects 1:250,000 births[229] and is usually caused by hypomorphic mutations in *NEMO*,[230] an X-linked gene. Autosomal dominant HED-ID results from hypermorphic (gain-of-function) point mutations or N-terminal truncations in *IKBA/NFKBIA*, which impair its phosphorylation and degradation, and thus reduce activation of the NF-kB pathway.[231] *NEMO* mutations tend to cause incontinentia pigmenti in girls (see Chapter 11) and amorphic mutations (i.e., there is effectively no gene product) tend to be lethal in males. Features of HED have been described in 77% of boys with immunodeficiency and *NEMO* mutations; osteopetrosis and lymphedema have been noted in 8% with HED-ID.[232] Boys with HED-ID occasionally show the clinical vesiculopapules and histologic features of incontinentia pigmenti, but the distribution is not blaschkoid.[233] Most mutations in *NEMO* that lead to HED-ID occur in exon 10 and affect the C-terminal zinc finger domain, which is critical for normal dendritic cell immune stimulation,[234] but mutations leading to HED-ID can be scattered throughout the *NEMO* gene.[235] Rarely, girls can have delayed skewing of the mutant *NEMO* allele, leading to both the typical pigmented streaks of incontinentia pigmenti and immunodeficiency, especially defective tumor necrosis factor alpha (TNF-α) production and mycobacterial infection.[236]

FEATURES OF ECTODERMAL DYSPLASIA IN HED. Affected children often appear more like each other than like their own unaffected siblings[237]; classic features are usually obvious by later infancy. Most have a distinctive pathognomonic facies: a square forehead with frontal bossing, large conspicuous nostrils, wide cheekbones with flat malar ridges, a thick everted lower lip, and a prominent chin. Ears may be small, satyr-like (pointed), low-lying, and anteriorly placed (Fig. 7.19, *A* and *B*, Fig. 7.20). Artificial intelligence technology, trained to recognize the classic features of X-linked HED, distinguishes affected males and, to a lesser extent, carrier females, suggesting its use as a screening tool.[238] Many of the features are more prominent in children than in adults, particularly the broad forehead, prominent eyes, and short philtrum.

Alopecia is often the first feature to attract attention but is seldom complete; overall 80% of males with the X-linked type have sparse hair.[239] The hair also tends to be lightly pigmented and short. The skin is soft, thin, and light-colored but shows fine wrinkling and sometimes darkening of the periorbital areas. Many affected neonates are born with red, peeling skin, but collodion-like thickening has occasionally been described.[240,241] Atopic dermatitis and other atopic conditions occur with increased incidence, and periorbital dermatitis is particularly common. The paucity of nail changes helps distinguish HED from other ectodermal dysplasias, although nail changes were described in up to 50% of male and female carriers in a recent self-reported survey.[239]

The decreased capacity for perspiration occurs in virtually all affected males and has a profound effect on life quality.[242] Hypohidrosis often results in hyperthermia, and patients manifest with intermittent fevers, especially during hot weather or after exercise or meals. These recurrent fevers of unknown origin may be the presenting manifestation in affected infants. Hypoplastic lacrimal and mucous glands can lead to decreased tearing or epiphora, chronic nasal discharge, and an increased risk of otitis media and respiratory tract infections.[243] Although sebaceous glands may be hypoplastic, exuberant sebaceous hyperplasia has been reported.[244] Females and female carriers may have breast hypoplasia. Dentition is generally delayed, and dental anomalies vary from complete to partial absence of teeth with peg-shaped or conical incisors (see Fig. 7.19, *B*).

FEATURES OF IMMUNODEFICIENCY IN HED-ID. Boys with HED-ID usually have recurrent infections. Serious pyogenic infections occur in 86% of

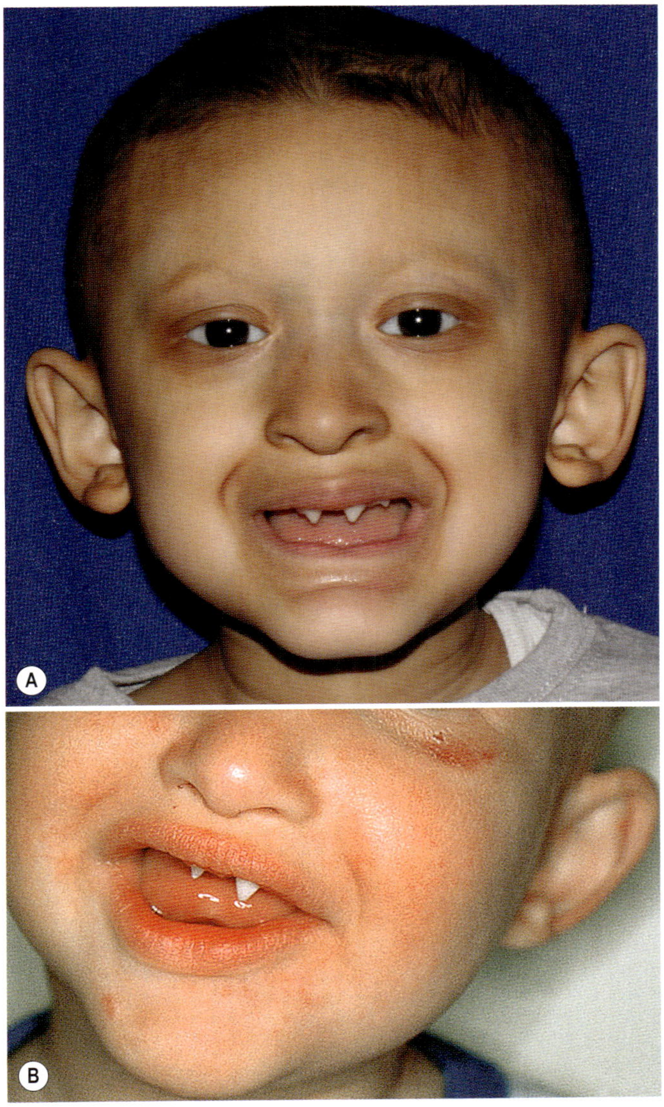

Fig. 7.19 Hypohidrotic ectodermal dysplasia (HED). **(A)** This boy shows the short, sparse hair; large conspicuous nostrils; wide cheekbones with flat malar ridges; periorbital wrinkling; a thick everted lower lip; prominent chin; and low-lying, anteriorly placed, pointed ears. **(B)** Conical incisors in a toddler with HED. Note the periorbital wrinkling, flat malar ridges, and prominent ears.

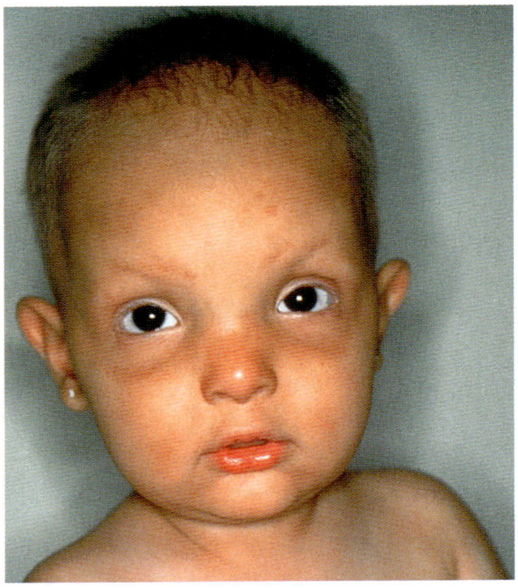

Fig. 7.20 Hypohidrotic ectodermal dysplasia (HED). This girl is a carrier for a mutation in ectodysplasin but shows all of the characteristic facies features. Girls with HED may also have a mutation in a gene encoding the receptor for ectodysplasin, inherited as an autosomal disorder.

affected individuals, and mycobacterial infections (especially atypical *Mycobacterium avium*) in 44%.[237,245,246] Pneumocystis and viral and candidal infections occur less often. Bacteremia or sepsis is common,[237,247] and the most common sites of infection are the lungs, sometimes leading to bronchiectasis, and the skin, sometimes with abscesses. Inflammatory colitis affects 21% of boys and presents as intractable diarrhea and/or failure to thrive. Some patients develop autoimmune hemolytic anemia. Natural killer-cell dysfunction has been described in all patients, but otherwise a range of immune defects have been described, largely reflecting the functional impairment in CD40, interleukin (IL)-1, TNF-α, and toll receptor signaling.[237,248] Almost 60% of affected boys show hypogammaglobulinemia, with high levels of immunoglobulin (Ig) M in 15%. Hyper-IgM syndrome much more commonly results from mutations in *CD40* ligand *(CD40L)*[249] and may manifest with CD40L deficiency as oral aphthae and warts.[250] Individuals with HED-ID are at high risk for early death from infections without transplantation.[251–254] Global survival after transplantation is 74% within a mean of the first 5 years.[255] Preexisting mycobacterial infection or colitis is associated with a poor outcome.

Therapy for patients with all forms of HED is directed toward temperature regulation: cool baths and drenching with water, air conditioning, light clothing, and cooling suits. Reduction of activities that cause normal perspiration may be beneficial.[256] Lubricating eye drops and nasal irrigation can compensate for the decreased glandular secretion. Topical or oral minoxidil may promote some hair growth with long-term use.[257] Dental intervention should begin by 2 years of age and can include dental prostheses, with implants in older adolescents and adults, to improve mastication, encourage normal speech development, and reduce cosmetic disfigurement.

In mouse and dog models of X-linked HED, the prenatal or perinatal administration of recombinant Fc-EDA protein or ligand replacement using an EDAR-agonist antibody can improve dentition, lacrimation, sweating, and bronchopulmonary gland function.[258–260] Intraamniotic administration at 26 and 31 weeks' gestational age of recombinant EDA protein with an Fc domain, which helps with fetal gastrointestinal absorption after ingestion of amniotic fluid, led to the development of normal sweat glands and evidence of the presence of tooth buds and salivary and Meibomian glands in treated twins with EDA deficiency.[261] Prenatal diagnosis has been made noninvasively by tooth-germ ultrasound.[262] The National Foundation for Ectodermal Dysplasias (NFED) provides excellent education materials on management of the hypohidrosis and dental abnormalities (www.nfed.org); support groups are also available outside the United States (www.ectodermaldysplasia.org; www.displasiaectodermica.org; www.ektodermale-dysplasie.de).

P63-RELATED FORMS OF ECTODERMAL DYSPLASIA. *TP63* encodes p63, which plays a critical role in the maturation of ectodermal, orofacial, and limb development. Mutations in *TP63* lead to a group of autosomal dominant disorders with ectodermal dysplasia, orofacial clefting, and limb malformations as key characteristics. These clinical manifestations have traditionally been used to classify subtypes, but significant clinical and genotypic overlap and intrafamiliar variability in phenotype are recognized.[263–266] Included are *Rapp–Hodgkin* syndrome (clefts of the lip, palate, and/or uvula; small, narrow, dysplastic nails; hypodontia with small conical teeth; and maxillary hypoplasia)[267]; *ankyloblepharon–ectodermal dysplasia–clefting* (AEC or Hay–Wells syndrome; ankyloblepharon or congenital fusion of the eyelids in association with facial clefting and midfacial hypoplasia)[268,269]; *ectrodactyly, ectodermal dysplasia, and cleft lip/palate* (EEC) syndrome; *limb-mammary* syndrome (ectrodactyly, cleft palate, and mammary gland abnormalities); *acrodermatoungual-lacrimal-tooth* (ADULT) syndrome[270]; and nonsyndromic split hand/foot malformation.

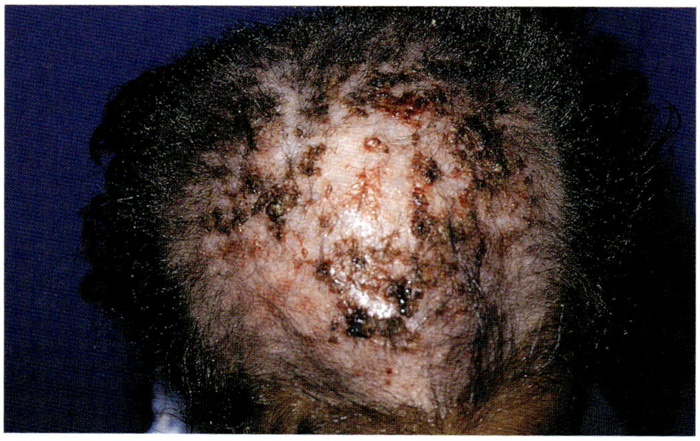

Fig. 7.21 Ankyloblepharon-ectodermal dysplasia-clefting syndrome. Scalp dermatitis with secondary staphylococcal infection is a chronic problem and leads to cicatricial alopecia.

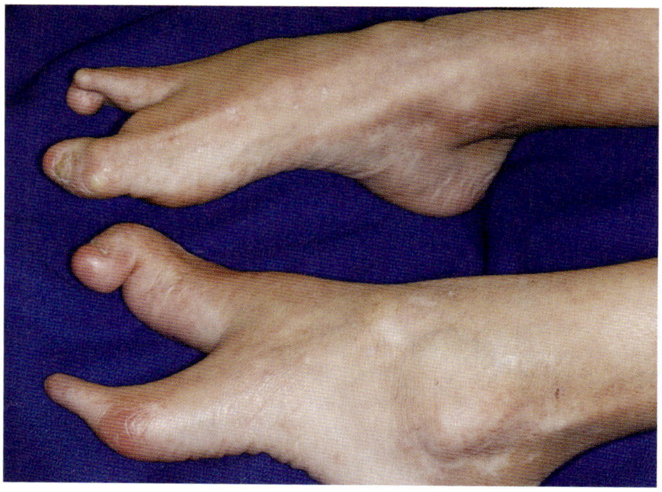

Fig. 7.22 Epidermal dysplasia-ectrodactyly-clefting (EEC) syndrome. This spectrum of developmental abnormalities results from mutations in the gene encoding p63.

The skin, hair, teeth, nails, and glands (eccrine, sebaceous, lacrimal, mammary) are abnormally developed.[271] The skin tends to be dry, itchy, and hypopigmented. Extensive erosions have been described in 80% of neonates with the AEC phenotype. The hair is often sparse and wiry, and nails tend to be dystrophic. Scalp dermatitis and erosions with secondary chronic staphylococcal infection may be recurrent in the first few years of life and lead to cicatricial alopecia, especially of the vertex and frontal scalp (Fig. 7.21). Teeth are often decreased in number with malformations and enamel hypoplasia.[272] Hypohidrosis may be present,[273] tearing is often decreased, and nipple hypoplasia has been described. Patients may show split hand/foot malformations (lobster claw deformity; ectrodactyly) (Fig. 7.22) and/or syndactyly.[274] Short stature, poor weight gain, and hypospadias are other commonly described characteristics.[275] Ectodermal dysplasia with clefting and/or ectrodactyly/syndactyly can be caused by mutations in a variety of other genes, that is, other disorders (see Table 7.1).

Disorders with p63 mutations also should be distinguished from the phenotype resembling AEC/EEC, but with hypogammaglobulinemia, which results from heterozygous variants in *CHUK* (*IKKA*; conserved helix-loop-helix ubiquitous kinase).[276,277] CHUK is a direct target of p63 and a component of the IKK complex, which participates in NF-kB pathway activation. *CHAND syndrome*,[278] characterized by curly hair from birth, ankyloblepharon, and nail dystrophy,[279,280] results from biallelic variants in *RIPK4*, which encodes a serine/threonine protein kinase. Heterozygous or biallelic mutations in *IRF6* (encoding interferon regulatory factor 6, a transcription factor) cause popliteal pterygium syndrome, a milder phenotype within the popliteal pterygia spectrum, characterized by cutaneous webbing across one or more joints, cleft lip and/or palate, nail dystrophy, syndactyly, and genital malformations. Biallelic mutations in *RIPK4*, *CHUK*, and *IRF6* also result in severe disorders within this spectrum (*Bartsocas-Papas* and *Cocoon syndrome*).[281] A constellation of ectodermal defects also results from a heterozygous variant in *KDF1*, encoding a recently described keratinocyte differentiation factor that acts upstream of p63[282–284] Features include lusterless scalp hair with thinning of the lateral eyebrows, a broad nasal root and sometimes everted nostrils, hypohidrosis, lost (and in one case natal) teeth, nail dystrophy, hyperlinear palms, keratosis pilaris, and hidradenitis suppurativa. Ectrodactyly with cutis aplasia, including with scalp erosion and inflammation that could easily be confused with p63 mutation, is a feature of mutations in *UBA2*, encoding a protein that regulates protein modification by sumoylation.[285–287]

The *trichodentoosseous syndrome* is an autosomal dominant disorder characterized by kinky, curly hair at birth that tends to become straighter during childhood; small, widely spaced, pitted, eroded, and discolored teeth with early caries as a result of defective enamel; thickness and splitting of the nails; dolichocephaly, frontal bossing, and a square jaw, giving affected persons a distinctive facies; normal physical development; and increased bone density, especially of the cranial bones. The condition results from mutations in *DLX3*, a crucial regulator of hair follicle differentiation and cycling.[288]

Cleft lip/palate–ectodermal dysplasia features spoon-shaped, slow-growing fingernails and toenails, short brittle hair with pili torti, palmoplantar keratoderma, mental retardation, malformed ears, and partial syndactyly. It results from mutations in nectin 1, encoded by *PVRL1*.[289,290] Mutations in nectin 4, encoded by *PVRL4*, lead to ectodermal dysplasia–syndactyly syndrome (EDSS), characterized by slowly progressive scalp alopecia with twisted hair on trichoscopy, dental abnormalities (widely spaced, peg-shaped, conical), and syndactyly.[291–294]

Ectodermal Dysplasia Related to Abnormalities in Structural Proteins.

CLOUSTON SYNDROME (HIDROTIC ECTODERMAL DYSPLASIA). The most common hidrotic type of ectodermal dysplasia is *Clouston syndrome*, an autosomal dominant disorder characterized by nail dystrophy, hyperkeratosis of the palms and soles, and hair defects.[295] Most cases have been reported in French-Canadian families. Unlike HED, individuals with the hidrotic form have a normal facies and show no abnormality of sweating, although eccrine syringofibroadenomas have been described.[296] The teeth develop normally but are prone to caries. The predominant feature is congenital nail dystrophy, which may be the only manifestation in about one-third of affected individuals.[297] The nails are thickened, thinner or shortened, striated, and often discolored (Fig. 7.23). They may resemble the nails of pachyonychia congenita (PC) and are difficult to distinguish without genotyping until other features develop, such as the painful character of the plantar keratoderma of PC, which is often present by 5 years of age, and the alopecia of HED. The nails grow slowly and commonly show chronic paronychial infections, which may lead to partial to complete destruction of the nail matrix. Typically the skin and soft tissue surrounding the nail and at the finger pad appear thickened and swollen, leading to the term *drumstick fingers*. The palmoplantar keratoderma can extend to the dorsal aspects of the hands and feet. Hair may be normal during infancy and childhood but thereafter often becomes sparse, fine, and brittle and may eventuate in total alopecia (Fig. 7.24). Body hair may be sparse; eyebrows and eyelashes may be thinned or absent. The skin may show a mottled hyperpigmentation with thickening and hyperpigmentation over the knees, elbows, and knuckles. Ocular abnormalities may include strabismus, conjunctivitis, and premature cataracts.

Clouston syndrome has been attributed to mutations in *GJB6*,[298] encoding connexin 30, a structural component of the intercellular gap junction. One patient with Clouston syndrome and bigenic mutations (one of each allele) of *GJB6* and *GJA1* (encoding connexin 43) has been described.[299] Mutations in *GJB6* have also been noted in patients with keratitis, congenital ichthyosis, and neurosensory deafness (KID) syndrome (see Chapter 5), who share the palmoplantar keratoderma

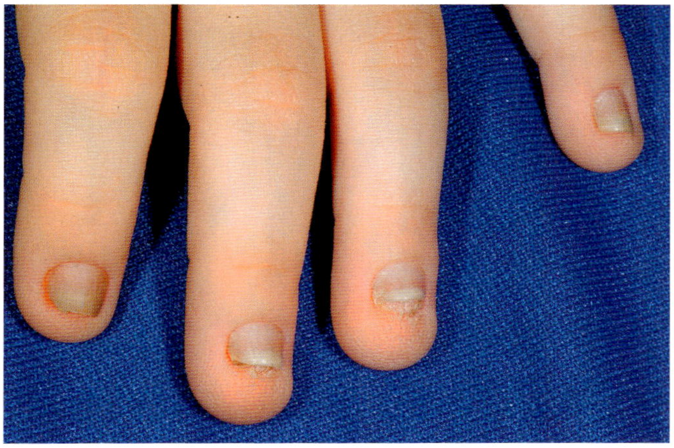

Fig. 7.23 Hidrotic ectodermal dysplasia (Clouston syndrome). Nail dystrophy, accentuation of ridging on the digital tips, and bulbous swelling of the soft tissue surrounding the nail and at the finger pad are the most typical manifestations of this syndrome. The nails can be confused with pachyonychia congenita, but the hair changes of hidrotic ectodermal dysplasia and the characteristic discomfort of the plantar keratoderma of pachyonychia congenita help to distinguish the disorders.

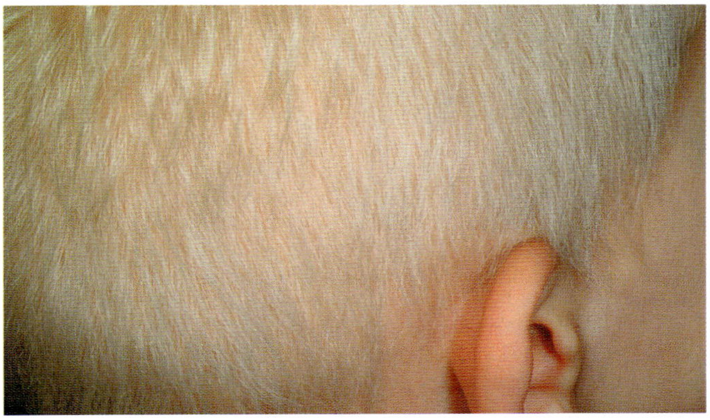

Fig. 7.24 Hidrotic ectodermal dysplasia. This child shows the fine, sparse, brittle hair of Clouston hidrotic ectodermal dysplasia. Not uncommonly, the hair abnormality does not develop until after puberty.

and sometimes early alopecia with thickening of the scalp. Clouston syndrome should also be distinguished from an autosomal recessive disorder that results from mutations in encoding grainyhead-like 2 *(GRHL2)*; in addition to nail dystrophy or loss and marginal palmoplantar keratoderma, patients show hypodontia and enamel hypoplasia, oral hyperpigmentation, dysphagia, and sometimes deafness or asthma.[300] The combination of tretinoin and minoxidil has caused hair growth in Clouston syndrome.[301]

Oculodentodigital dysplasia (ODDD), an autosomal dominant disorder, results from mutations in *GJA1*, which encodes connexin 43[17,18]. In addition to abnormalities of the eyes, teeth, and digits, patients with ODDD show curly hair (sometimes with trichorrhexis nodosa); focal keratoderma; a characteristic facies with hypoplastic ala nasi; and neurologic, cardiac, and hearing defects. Mutations in *GJA1* have also been linked to erythrokeratodermia variabilis with leukonychia and skin hyperpigmentation (see Chapter 5).

Ellis van Creveld syndrome is an autosomal recessive disorder that features nail dysplasia in association with chondrodysplasia, polydactyly, orofacial abnormalities, and sometimes cardiovascular malformations.[302] The mutated genes, *EVC* and *EVC2*, localize to cilia and are thought to be involved in hedgehog signaling.[303]

DISORDERS OF FOLLICULAR PLUGGING

Keratosis Pilaris

Keratosis pilaris is a common skin condition characterized by keratinous plugs in the follicular orifices surrounded by a variable degree of erythema (see Chapter 3).[304] These small follicular-based papules are most commonly distributed on the cheeks (Fig. 7.25), extensor areas of the upper arms, and anterior and lateral thighs (Fig. 7.26) but may be widespread. Occasionally, facial keratosis pilaris overlies intense erythema (keratosis pilaris rubra)[305] and may also be pigmented (erythromelanosis follicularis faciei et colli).[306–308]

Children with keratosis pilaris tend to have xerosis and sometimes atopic dermatitis; 35% have variants in *FLG* (filaggrin deficiency[309]) and may manifest ichthyosis vulgaris. Histopathologic sections show follicular plugs, hair abnormalities, and an absence of sebaceous glands.[309] Keratosis pilaris does not tend to be symptomatic but may be cosmetically distressing, especially if quite inflammatory or extensive.

Treatment is difficult but usually requires application of keratolytic agents such as creams or lotions containing lactic acid, glycolic acid, salicylic acid, or urea and gentle exfoliation by a pumice stone, washcloth, loofah sponge, or Buf-Puf. Responsive patients must maintain therapy to achieve continued remission or improvement. Fractional carbon dioxide laser has been effective in reducing the keratotic papules and hyperpigmentation, but not the erythema.[310] The intense erythema of keratosis pilaris rubra may be lessened by pulsed-dye laser therapy[311,312] or photopneumatic (vacuum-assisted pulsed-light)

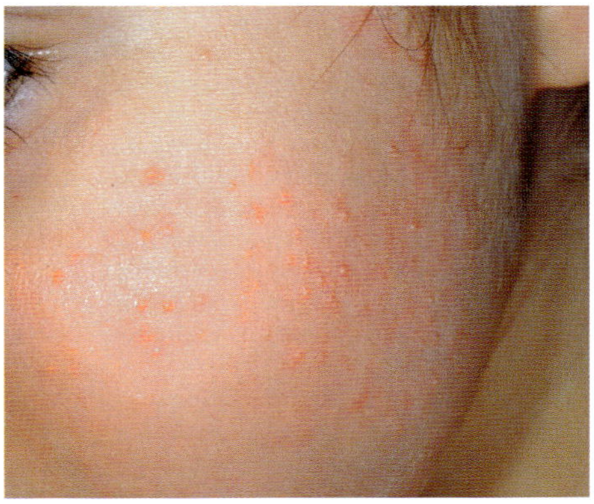

Fig. 7.25 Keratosis pilaris. Keratotic, follicular-based plugs with variable associated erythema are common on the lateral cheeks of young children.

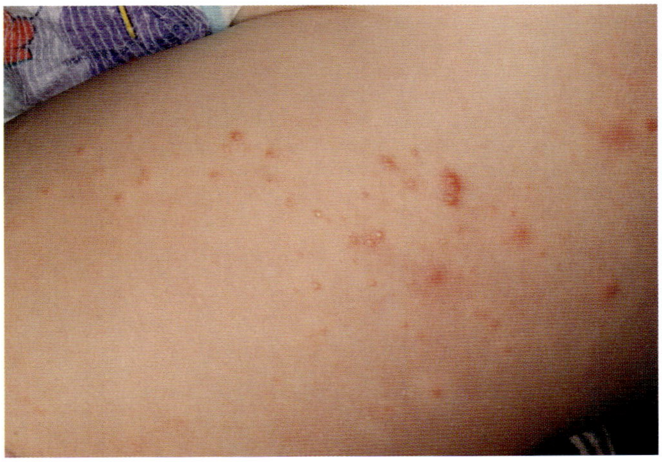

Fig. 7.26 Keratosis pilaris. The lateral thighs are a common site. The follicular lesions can be inflamed papules or even pustules, resembling bacterial folliculitis.

Table 7.2 Classification of Keratosis Pilaris Atrophicans

	Atrophoderma Vermiculata	Ulerythema Ophryogenes	Keratosis Follicularis Spinulosa Decalvans
Skin lesions	Erythematous papules, follicular plugs, horn cysts, atrophic	Follicular papules, plugging, scarring	Milia, thorn-like follicular projections, atrophic scars
Sites	Cheeks, neck, limbs	Lateral eyebrows, extending medially	Scalp, eyebrows, eyelashes, cheeks, nose, neck, dorsal hands, fingers
Alopecia	Absent	Minimal eyebrows	Scarring alopecia of the scalp
Photophobia	Absent	Absent	Marked, corneal opacities
Inheritance	Sporadic or autosomal dominant	Sporadic or autosomal dominant	X-linked recessive or autosomal dominant

Reprinted with permission from Schachner LA, Hansen RC, eds. *Pediatric Dermatology*. 4th ed. Edinburgh, Scotland: Mosby; 2011.

therapy.[313] The erythema is sometimes decreased by treatment with low-strength topical steroids or calcineurin inhibitors.[314]

Keratosis Pilaris Atrophicans

Numerous terms have been used to describe a group of interrelated syndromes characterized by inflammatory keratotic follicular papules and later by atrophy. Commonly described as atrophic variants of keratosis pilaris, these include ulerythema ophryogenes, atrophoderma vermiculata, and keratosis follicularis spinulosa decalvans[315,316] (Table 7.2).[317] This group of disorders has been attributed to abnormal keratinization of the follicular infundibulum, resulting in obstruction of the growing hair shaft, chronic inflammation, and scarring. No therapy is terribly effective,[318] although topical keratolytic and antiinflammatory agents (topical corticosteroids and calcineurin inhibitors) may reduce the keratotic and inflammatory components, respectively. In general, systemic retinoids have not been helpful. Durable eyebrow reconstruction using individual hair follicle micrografts in an adult with quiescent disease has been reported.[319]

Ulerythema ophryogenes (keratosis pilaris atrophicans faciei) is characterized by persistent reticular erythema, small horny papules, atrophy, and scarring of the outer half of the eyebrows (Fig. 7.27).[320] The disorder is more common in boys and usually starts in the first months of life. Occasionally the disorder extends to include the adjacent skin, adjacent scalp, and cheeks.

Ulerythema ophryogenes and keratosis pilaris have been described in patients with two similar but distinct "*RAS*opathies" of the *RAS-MAPK* signaling pathway, the *cardiofaciocutaneous* (CFC) syndrome[321] and *Noonan* syndrome. Patients with CFC syndrome often show widespread keratosis pilaris–like lesions of the face, ears, scalp, and extensor surfaces of the extremities (82% of patients) in association with scarcity or absence of the eyebrows (73%).[322,323] Similarly, Noonan syndrome is associated with keratosis pilaris–like lesions and sparse eyebrows; both are characterized by curly/wavy hair. The atrophy and scarring of ulerythema ophryogenes are absent in CFC and Noonan syndromes.

Both CFC and Noonan syndromes share features of short stature, congenital cardiac abnormalities (particularly pulmonary valve stenosis), retardation, macrocephaly, hypertelorism, a high forehead, pectus carinatum, and many pigmented nevi.[324,325] Lymphedema and a low posterior hairline are more typical features of Noonan syndrome. Patients with CFC syndrome often show hypoplastic supraorbital ridges, bitemporal constriction, and an antimongoloid slant, features not described in Noonan syndrome.[322]

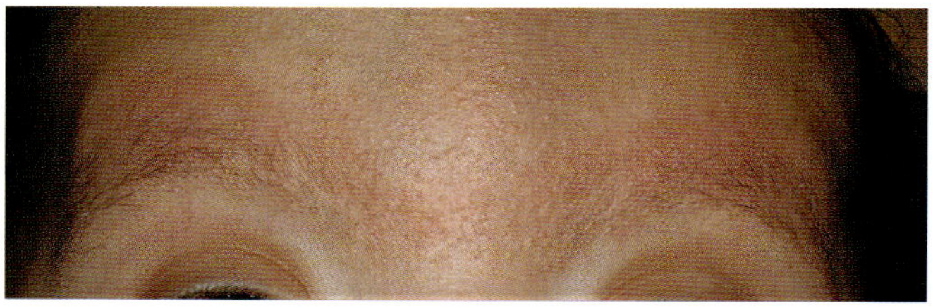

Fig. 7.27 Ulerythema ophryogenes. Extensive keratosis pilaris with alopecia and scarring of the eyebrows in this boy with Noonan syndrome.

As with clinical features, there is overlap in genes that are mutated in Noonan and CFC syndromes (*BRAF, KRAS, MAPK1* [encoding MEK1], and *MAPK2* [encoding MEK2]).[326–329] However, the genes most commonly altered in Noonan syndrome are *PTPN11* (50%) and *SOS1* (10% to 13%).[327] Individuals with Noonan syndrome associated with LAS have a unique mutation in *SHOC2*, a scaffold protein required for the *RAS-MAPK* signaling cascade.[330] A recent study noted genotype–phenotype correlation during the first year of life, with thin hair linked to mutations in *SHOC2* and *BRAF*, whereas keratosis pilaris was associated with mutations in *SOS1, BRAF*, and *SHOC2*.[331] Other *RAS*opathies with skin features are lentigines, electrocardiographic abnormalities, ocular hypertelorism, pulmonic stenosis, abnormal genitalia, retardation of growth, and sensorineural deafness (LEOPARD) syndrome; neurofibromatosis; neurofibromatosis–Noonan syndrome; Legius syndrome; the newly described *CBL*-mutation-associated syndrome (café-au-lait spots, see Chapter 11); and Costello syndrome (see Chapter 6). Ulerythema ophryogenes has also been associated with Cornelia de Lange[332] and Rubenstein–Taybi[333] syndromes, as well as with woolly hair.[334]

Atrophoderma vermiculata (folliculitis ulerythema reticulata, atrophoderma vermicularis) usually has its onset between 5 and 12 years of age.[315] This disorder is characterized by the formation of numerous tiny symmetric, atrophic, and at times erythematous pits on the cheeks, periauricular areas, and occasionally the forehead and eyebrows. These cribriform lesions generally measure 1 to 2 mm across and 1 mm deep and are separated from each other by narrow ridges of normal-appearing skin. Laser and dermabrasion have been advocated to improve the cosmetic appearance of affected individuals when the condition is stable, usually after puberty. Low-dose isotretinoin (0.5 mg/kg per day) for two 6-month courses has been reported to cause cosmetic improvement.[335]

Keratosis follicularis spinulosa decalvans (KFSD) is characterized by atrophic keratotic follicular papules of the scalp, eyebrows, and eyelashes that eventuate in scarring alopecia (Fig. 7.28). Associated

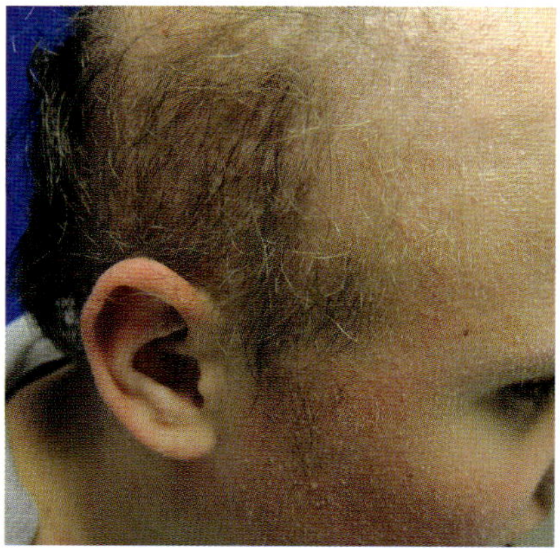

Fig. 7.28 Keratosis follicularis spinulosus decalvans. This patient showed widespread spiny, follicular-based keratoses, photophobia, and abnormal hair with cicatricial alopecia.

features are palmoplantar keratoderma, corneal dystrophy, photophobia, and atopy.[336] KFSD is usually an X-linked recessive disorder, and female carriers may show milder manifestations.[337] The initial signs are photophobia with tearing, ophthalmitis, and conjunctival and corneal inflammation, which occur in the first weeks or months of life; congenital glaucoma and cataracts have been noted in association. Extensive keratosis pilaris of the face, extremities, and trunk tends to begin during early childhood, often in association with facial erythema. Cicatricial alopecia of the scalp begins around puberty and slowly progresses in association with follicular inflammation and fibrosis; eyebrows also tend to be affected. Some patients show palmoplantar keratoderma and marked xerosis. Acne keloidalis nuchae (see Acne Keloidalis section) and tufted hair folliculitis has been described in several patients.[338] *Ichthyosis follicularis, congenital atrichia, and photophobia* (IFAP) is another X-linked condition in which affected neonates show keratotic follicular papules with a sandpapery feel to the skin, atrichia or severe hypotrichosis, and photophobia from birth (Fig. 7.29).[339–341] In contrast to KSFD, the alopecia of patients with IFAP does not scar. Mental retardation and developmental delay have been described in both KSFD and IFAP syndromes. Other features are gingival hyperplasia and angular stomatitis, psoriasiform plaques, palmoplantar erythema with thickening, short stature, and seizures. One boy with IFAP syndrome developed Hodgkin lymphoma,[342] but association with the syndrome was unclear.

IFAP and KFSD are allelic and result from mutations in a zinc metalloprotease *(MBTPS2)* that is important for cholesterol homeostasis, handling endoplasmic reticulum stress, and cell differentiation.[343,344] Mutations in *MBTPS2* also cause *X-linked Olmsted* syndrome (see Chapter 5) and *BRESEK/BRESHECK* syndrome. The latter disorder is characterized by brain anomalies, retardation (intellectual, associated with microcephaly), ectodermal dysplasias (atrichia and photophobia, but not ichthyosis follicularis), skeletal deformities (especially vertebral and hand anomalies), Hirschsprung disease, eye or ear anomalies, cleft lip/palate or cryptorchidism, and kidney anomalies.[345] The most common features are included in the BRESEK acronym. Female carriers can show mild phenotypes (e.g., hypotrichosis, hyperkeratosis, nail dystrophy, ichthyotic changes, typically along the lines of Blaschko).[346–348]

KFSD may also be autosomal dominant in inheritance,[63,349] although the underlying molecular defect is unclear.[350] Marked facial erythema, extensive folliculitis, onychodystrophy, and multiple caries have been described in these patients.

Ichthyosis in association with hair abnormalities may also be seen in ichthyosis hypotrichosis syndrome, ichthyosis–hypotrichosis–sclerosing cholangitis syndrome, Netherton syndrome (see Chapter 5), and TTD. Another disorder with nonscarring partial alopecia that must be distinguished is hereditary mucoepithelial dysplasia.[351] In addition to extensive keratosis pilaris and psoriasiform plaques, affected individuals show fiery red mucosal inflammation (hard palate, gingival, tongue, perianal, and perineal), and ocular photophobia with keratitis, cataracts, and corneal opacities.

The follicular scarring of these disorders should be distinguished from disorders of follicular atrophoderma without keratotic plugs. These include perifollicular atrophoderma of acne scarring (see Chapter 8), Conradi–Hünermann syndrome (see Chapter 5), Rombo syndrome, and Bazex syndrome. Treatment of these disorders of follicular plugging is challenging, with most patients refractory to systemic and topical steroids, systemic antibiotics, dapsone, and methotrexate. Some patients with IFAP/KSFD show improvement with systemic retinoids.[340,349,352,353]

CENTRAL CENTRIFUGAL CICATRICIAL ALOPECIA

Central centrifugal cicatricial alopecia (CCCA) is a disorder characterized by hair breakage and thinning, primarily involving the vertex with progression centrifugally.[354] Tender papules and sometimes pustules and pruritus may be associated. Dermoscopy reveals a perifollicular grayish halo. It occurs predominantly in female patients of African ancestry and has been described in adolescents; in many cases, a mother is affected. Hair grooming habits (such as relaxers and hot combs) have been linked, but the condition may occur without any history of a hair treatment. Although usually without inflammation clinically, biopsies show varying degrees of lymphocytic inflammation

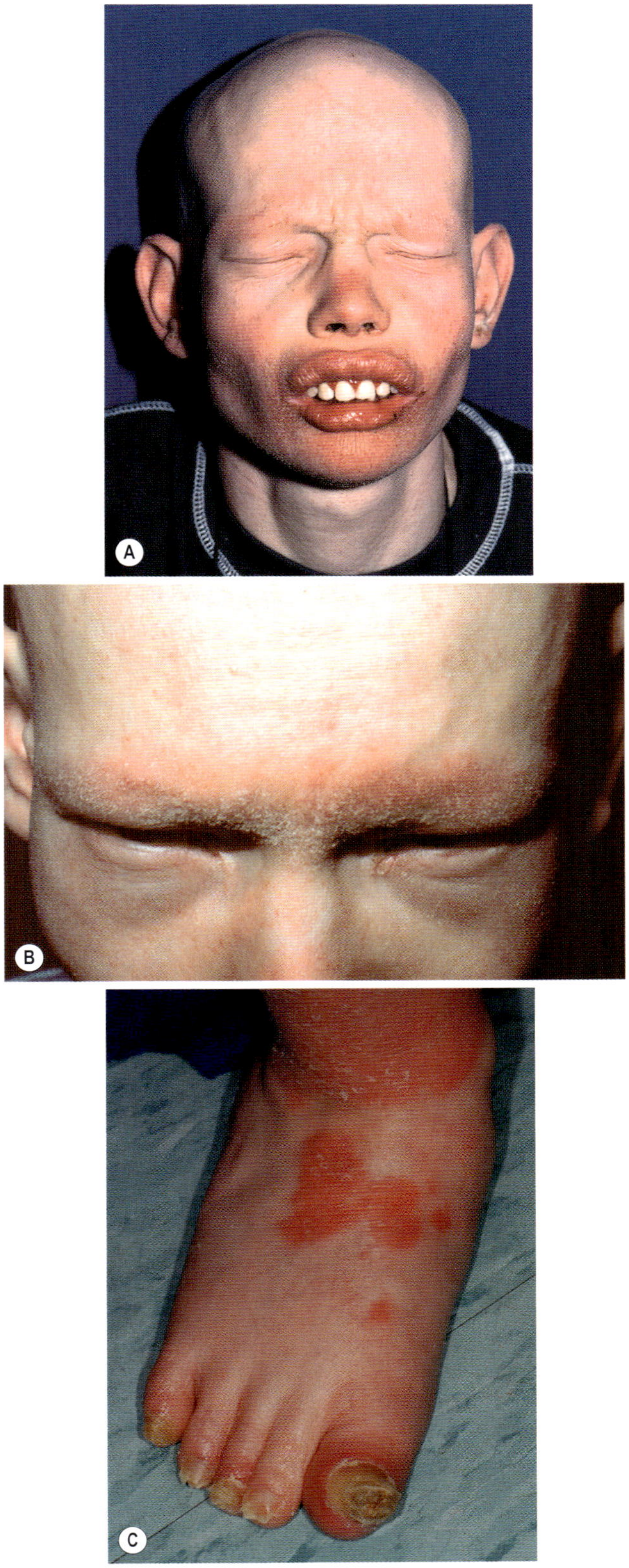

Fig. 7.29 Ichthyosis follicularis, congenital atrichia, and photophobia syndrome. **(A)** Note the total alopecia and the erythematous, scaling skin. **(B)** Note the spiny, keratotic follicular papules of the eyebrows and lashes and the atrichia. The patient's photophobia prevents him from looking at the camera and has led to tearing. **(C)** Periungual erythema and marked nail yellowing and thickening; note the psoriasiform plaques at the ankle and on the dorsal aspect of the foot.

in association with reduced follicular density, degeneration of follicles, and fibrosis. Tinea capitis is the most common differential diagnosis, but folliculitis, including folliculitis decalvans, is a consideration that can be ruled out by biopsy. Heterozygous loss-of-function mutations in *PADI3*, encoding peptidyl arginine deiminase, type 3 (PADI3), have recently been implicated.[355] PADI3 is an enzyme that posttranslationally modifies proteins, such as trichohyalin, which are involved in hair shaft formation. Biallelic *PADI3* mutations have been noted in children with uncombable hair syndrome.[133] Treatment is challenging, but primarily is directed at decreasing inflammation through topical and intralesional steroids and antiinflammatory antibiotics such as doxycycline. Surgery to remove scarred areas should be deferred until inflammation has abated for 9 to 12 months.

OTHER SCARRING ALOPECIAS

Scarring or cicatricial alopecia is the end result of a wide number of inflammatory processes in and around the pilosebaceous units, resulting in irreversible destruction of tissue and consequent permanent scarring alopecia.[146,356] If scarring is not easy to determine clinically, histologic analysis of a biopsy is helpful.[357,358] The scarring may be the result of a developmental defect (aplasia cutis) (see Figs. 2.41 and 2.42); inflammatory changes due to severe bacterial, viral, or fungal infection; physical trauma (halo alopecia from caput succedaneum[359] [see Chapter 2], irradiation, long-term trichotillomania, thermal or caustic burns); neoplastic or infiltrative disorders (including severe alopecia mucinosa); various dermatoses (lichen planus, lupus erythematosus, localized or systemic scleroderma [see Chapter 22]); keratosis pilaris atrophicans, a group of disorders of hair plugging; or various dermatologic syndromes such as folliculitis decalvans, dissecting cellulitis of the scalp, acne keloidalis, and pseudopelade.

Follicular Mucinosis

Follicular mucinosis (alopecia mucinosa) is an inflammatory disorder characterized by sharply defined follicular papules or infiltrated plaques with scaling, loss of hair, and accumulation of mucin in sebaceous glands and the outer root sheaths of affected hair follicles.[360–362] A relatively uncommon condition affecting children as well as adults, the disorder is characterized by often pruritic, grouped follicular papules that often coalesce into scaling plaques or nodular, boggy infiltrated plaques with overlying erythema and scaling (Fig. 7.30). Lesions usually measure 2 to 5 cm in diameter. Distributed primarily on the face, scalp, neck, and shoulders (occasionally the trunk and extremities), lesions are usually devoid of hair. Except in the scalp or eyebrows, the alopecia is generally not conspicuous.

The cause of follicular mucinosis is unknown, although cases have been linked with administration of infliximab.[363] In the majority of cases (in those <40 years of age), it is a benign idiopathic condition.[364] In older adults, however, the presence of boggy infiltrated plaques of alopecia mucinosa may be the first sign of cutaneous T-cell lymphoma.[365,366] Cutaneous T-cell lymphoma has rarely been described in children with follicular mucinosis,[367] so affected children must be monitored carefully.[368–370]

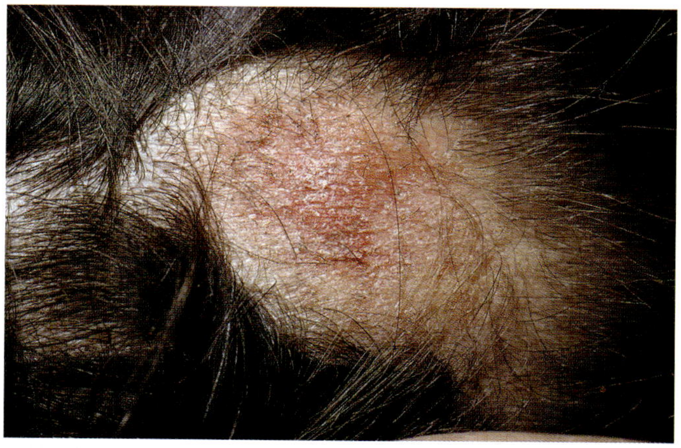

Fig. 7.30 Alopecia mucinosa. An erythematous, mildly scaling, infiltrated hairless plaque. Biopsy shows mucin in the follicular area. Alopecia mucinosa tends to be a benign condition in children but has been associated with cutaneous T-cell lymphoma in adults.

Follicular mucinosis must be differentiated from lichen spinulosus,[371] pityriasis rubra pilaris, tinea infection, pityriasis alba, granulomatous diseases, and the papulosquamous group of disorders. When the diagnosis remains in doubt, cutaneous biopsy of an affected area is generally confirmatory, showing accumulation of mucin within the hair and sebaceous glands.

Solitary or few lesions usually clear spontaneously within 2 years. More numerous and widely distributed plaques tend to be more chronic. Destruction of follicles may give rise to permanent alopecia, and the disorder may persist with new lesions continuing to appear over years. Although some cases appear to benefit from topical or intralesional corticosteroids, such claims are difficult to evaluate because spontaneous healing is the rule.

Folliculitis Decalvans

Folliculitis decalvans is characterized by successive crops of patchy, painful folliculitis leading to progressive hair loss and scarring.[372] The disorder must be distinguished by culture from bacterial folliculitis caused by *Staphylococcus aureus*, although the two forms often coexist, leading to the hypothesis that folliculitis decalvans results from an abnormal host response to staphylococcal toxins.[373] Folliculitis decalvans may begin during adolescence in male patients but is rarely seen in female patients before 30 years of age. Although the scalp is the most commonly affected site, hair-bearing areas of the trunk, axillae, and pubic region may be affected. Typical lesions show round to irregular bald, atrophic patches, each surrounded by crops of follicular pustules. Tufted folliculitis is a variant in which tufts of hair tunnel beneath the surface and emerge from dilated follicular openings amid areas of scarring.[373]

Treatment of folliculitis decalvans is difficult. Systemic antibiotics that penetrate the follicle well (tetracyclines, clindamycin, erythromycin) with or without rifampicin often prevent disease extension, but continued administration is required to prevent relapse.[374] Isotretinoin monotherapy ≥0.4 mg/kg per day, given for ≥3 months, led to considerable improvement with a low risk of relapse in a retrospective series.[375] Several reports have also found photodynamic light therapy[376–378] to be helpful in some patients.

Dissecting Cellulitis of the Scalp

Dissecting cellulitis of the scalp, also termed *perifolliculitis capitis abscedens et suffodiens*, is characterized by painful fluctuant nodules and abscesses of the scalp connected by tortuous ridges or deep sinus tracts with cicatricial alopecia.[8] The connection can often be demonstrated by applying pressure to one nodule and observing purulent drainage emerging from another. Lesions are usually first noted at the occipital area or vertex but may progress to involve the entire scalp. The disorder occurs most commonly in Black male teenagers and young adults.[379,380] The response in some patients to antiandrogen therapy and occurrence after anabolic steroids[381] suggests a role for androgenic stimulation. An association with acne conglobata and hidradenitis suppurativa has also been described ("follicular occlusion triad"), suggesting an inflammatory reaction to *Propionibacterium acnes*. Other purulent disorders of the scalp, including bacterial folliculitis and inflammatory tinea capitis (kerion), must be considered.[382,383] Features of dissecting cellulitis have also been described as a manifestation of Crohn's disease.[384]

The disorder has a chronic, relapsing course. Although use of oral tetracyclines or erythromycin with or without surgical drainage of lesions may be effective, many studies suggest systemic administration of isotretinoin to be the treatment of choice, although the disease recurs with discontinuation, as with other approaches.[380,385,386] Response to TNF inhibitors is variable, but some have experienced improvement.[387] Laser ablation has also been advocated.[388]

Acne Keloidalis

Acne keloidalis (folliculitis keloidalis) is a chronic scarring folliculitis and perifolliculitis of the nape and occipital scalp.[389–391] Initial lesions

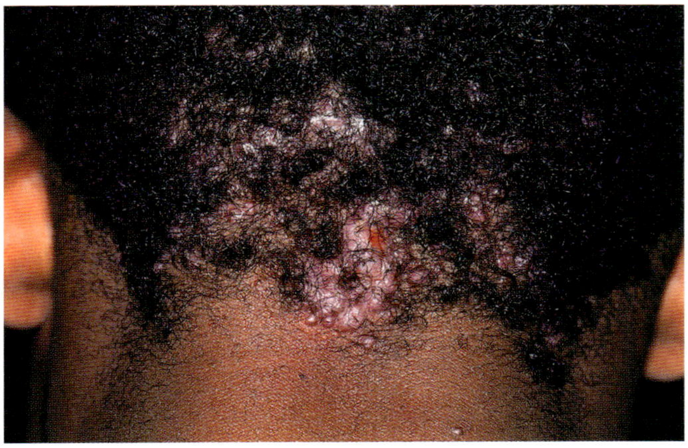

Fig. 7.31 Acne keloidalis. Scarring folliculitis with keloidal scarring at the nape and occipital scalp in this 17-year-old Black adolescent.

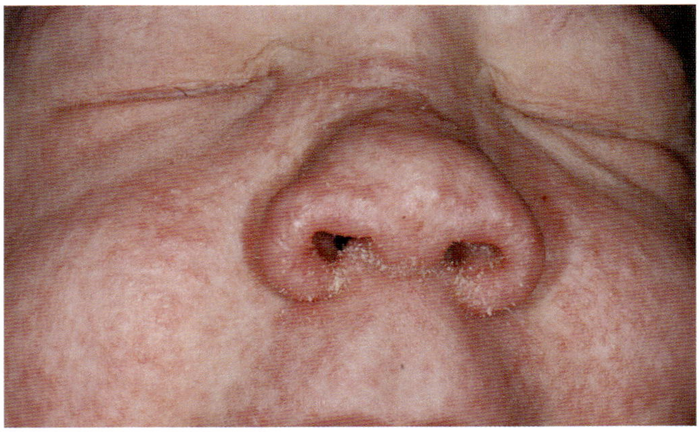

Fig. 7.32 Trichodysplasia spinulosa. Note the keratotic spines and follicular-based erythematous papules on the face in this boy who had received a transplant and was receiving immunosuppressive medications.

tend to be inflammatory papules and occasionally pustules, which evolve into firm keloidal, often coalescent papules and plaques (Fig. 7.31). Severe cases may show abscesses and sinus formation. Patients may complain of pruritus and discomfort. The disorder is seen most commonly in postpubertal males, especially Blacks between the ages of 14 and 25 years, but is occasionally described in females.[392] Chronic scalp folliculitis and components of the metabolic syndrome or hypertension are associations.[393]

Acute inflammation of the follicle is thought to be the primary pathologic process, followed by a granulomatous foreign body reaction to released hair and subsequent fibrosis; a variety of triggers have been proposed, among them irritation from shirt collars or helmets, bacterial folliculitis, or ingrown hairs after a short haircut. Treatment of this disorder is difficult and consists of long-term systemic antibiotics and intralesional corticosteroids. Patients should avoid close "clipper" haircuts and scratching of the area. Excision with second-intention healing has been helpful for selected patients, especially with fibrotic nodules.[394,395] Lasers, particularly the 810-nm diode, erbium:yttrium-aluminum-garnet (YAG), and long-pulsed neodymium:YAG.[396–398] Targeted ultraviolet B (UVB) light therapy has shown promise.[399]

Pseudofolliculitis Barbae

Pseudofolliculitis barbae, commonly called *razor bumps* or *ingrown hair*, is an inflammatory condition of hair follicles of the beard area that is particularly common in adolescent males of African ancestry with curly, coarse hair (see Chapter 14).[390,391,394,400,401] The condition can affect adolescent girls with tightly curled hair, however, especially if shaving occurs on the face because of hirsutism or because of hair removal elsewhere (waxing, plucking, or shaving of the axillae or pubic area). Erythematous, 2- to 4-mm, flesh-colored or often hyperpigmented, follicular-based papules are characteristic. The shape of the hair follicle, hair cuticle, and direction of hair growth predispose the patient to the inflammatory response when hair is shaved or plucked.[402] A single-nucleotide polymorphism (SNP) in *KRT75*, encoding hair keratin 75, has been linked with a much greater tendency to develop pseudofolliculitis barbae, especially in individuals with curly hair.[403] It is theorized that the pressure and traction exerted by close and regular shaving destabilizes the hair keratin.[403]

Pseudofolliculitis barbae is thought to represent a foreign-body reaction around an ingrown hair. Optimal therapy has been controversial, as there are few double-blind trials. Some advocate temporarily discontinuing shaving or other forms of hair removal and then instituting alternative techniques that decrease the closeness of the shave, such as use of an electric razor (avoiding the "closest" shave setting), the Bumpfighter razor (American Safety Razor Company, Staunton, VA),[404] or chemical depilatories. Others have found that use of a good regimen with copious shaving cream or gel to condition the hair, shaving with a multiblade razor daily, and postshave moisturization is well tolerated.[405] Shaving should always be in the direction of hair growth, and pretreatment with an antibacterial soap or benzoyl peroxide wash may decrease the potential inflammation from bacterial overgrowth. Adjunctive topical agents are retinoids, low-potency topical steroids, topical antibiotics, and depigmenting agents. Nonlaser epilation is not recommended and may exacerbate pseudofolliculitis barbae; however, the neodymium:yttrium-aluminum-garnet (Nd:YAG) 1064-nm and diode (800 to 810 nm) lasers have been used to epilate the curly hairs and can cause significant improvement.[406–408] Eflornithine cream, which inhibits hair growth, may also be helpful but may be associated with the development of local irritation.

Pseudopelade

Pseudopelade is a nonspecific scarring form of slowly progressive alopecia of the scalp generally seen in adults, although it has been described rarely in children. It may represent the end result of discoid lupus erythematosus (see Chapter 22) or lichen planopilaris (see Chapter 4). It is characterized by multiple small, round, oval, or irregularly shaped hairless cicatricial patches of varying sizes. Affected areas are shiny, ivory white or slightly pink, and atrophic. Lesions commonly coalesce to form finger-like projections and have been compared with footprints in the snow. Lesions generally appear at the vertex of the scalp. A few hair-containing dilated follicles may be interspersed between the patches. The condition tends to resolve spontaneously after several years, leaving the alopecia. Therapy is often unsuccessful, although intralesional injections of triamcinolone have temporarily benefited some patients. Cosmetic improvement has also been achieved by the multiple-punch autograft technique of hair transplantation.

Trichodysplasia Spinulosa

Trichodysplasia spinulosa is an uncommon alopecic disorder that classically presents as usually asymptomatic, small, comedo-like, follicular-based papules with central keratotic spines on the alae nasi, cheeks, eyebrows, and ears[409,410] (Fig. 7.32). However, the disorder may involve the trunk and upper extremities or even may be generalized.[411] Sometimes the face skin is thickened, creating a leonine facies. The disorder typically occurs in patients immunocompromised from use of immunosuppressive drugs. Dermoscopy is a helpful tool to identify the multiple vellus hairs projecting from the dilated follicular openings. Histology shows distended anagen hair follicles with dilated infundibula, plugged with numerous (up to 50) keratinous material and often poorly formed vellus hairs.

Polymerase chain reaction (PCR) and sequencing from skin scrapings detect the trichodysplasia spinulosa–associated polyomavirus (TSPyV) infection, which specifically targets inner root sheath keratinocytes.[412] TSPyV is seroprevalent in the normal population, with infection commonly occurring during early childhood, probably

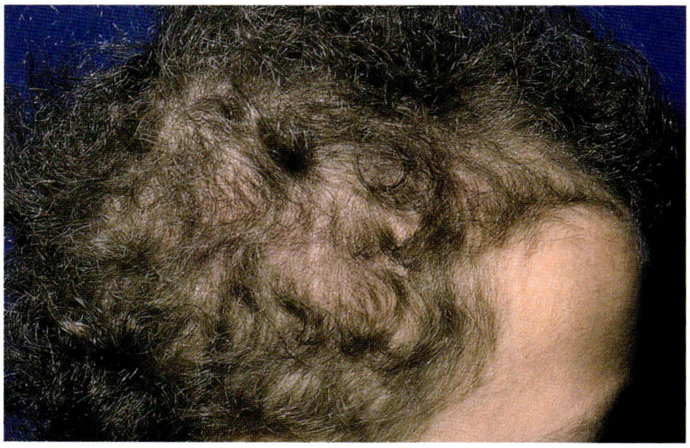

Fig. 7.33 Telogen effluvium. Hair shedding is increased and, if a significant amount, a detectable increase in sparsity of hair may be noted. The loss is diffuse across the scalp but tends to stabilize after a few months and usually returns to normal within about 6 months.

Box 7.5 **Potential Triggers of Telogen Effluvium**

Emotional stress
Fever (high)
Medications (see Box 7.6)
Nutritional disorders
- Biotin deficiency
- Crash dieting; anorexia; picky eater
- Essential fatty acid deficiency
- Iron deficiency

Hypervitaminosis A
Pica and associated lead poisoning
- Physiologic telogen effluvium of the newborn
- Parturition
- Severe chronic illness
- Severe infection
- Surgery
- Thyroid disease (hyperthyroidism or hypothyroidism)

Box 7.6 **Pediatric Medications That May Be Associated with Telogen Effluvium**

Albendazole
Amphetamines
Angiotensin-converting enzyme inhibitors (e.g., captopril, enalapril)
Anticoagulants (e.g., heparin, warfarin)
Anticonvulsants (e.g., valproic acid, carbamazepine)
β-blockers (e.g., propranolol)
Cimetidine
Danazol
Interferon-α
Lithium
Oral contraception (during use or with discontinuation)
Retinoids (e.g., isotretinoin)

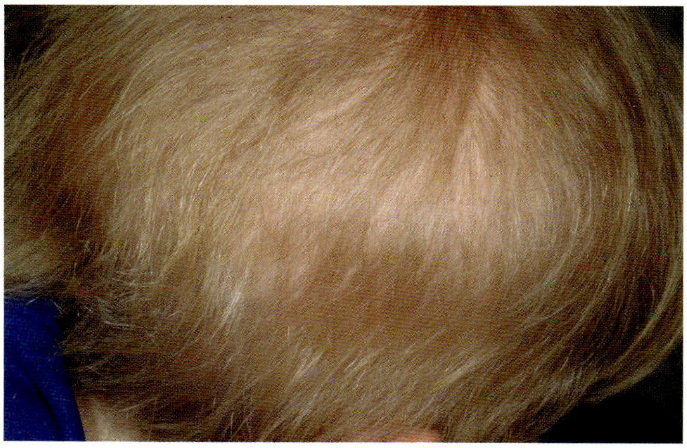

Fig. 7.34 Short anagen syndrome. Anagen hairs cycle more rapidly, leading to finer hair that never needs a haircut.

spread through respiratory droplets[413]; 63% to 90% of adults are infected. Topical cidofovir (1% to 3%) or oral valganciclovir with tapering of the immmunosuppression[414] and physical extraction of the keratin spicules[415] have led to improvement.

Telogen Effluvium

The normal cyclic pattern of anagen and telogen hair phases may be interrupted by a variety of different stimuli, resulting in *telogen effluvium*. Telogen effluvium represents the most common type of alopecia in children and is characterized by excess hair shedding with diffuse thinning of scalp hair to varying degrees (Fig. 7.33).[7] The average individual who shampoos at least every other day loses 50 to 100 telogen hairs per day, but 25% of scalp hair (25,000 hairs) must be shed before unmistakable thinning becomes apparent.[416–418]

Several stimuli are capable of producing an interruption in the anagen phase of the hair follicles (Box 7.5). Telogen effluvium may be suggested by a history of a stressful event preceding the onset of alopecia by 6 to 16 weeks that shifts more hairs into telogen phase. Most common are acute illnesses, especially with fever and infection, major trauma, surgery, or childbirth. Initiation of medications (Box 7.6) or discontinuation of medications, particularly oral contraceptives, isotretinoin, anticonvulsants, cimetidine, and terbinafine, has also been implicated.[419,420] More chronic telogen effluvium has been associated with chronic illness, thyroid abnormalities, iron-deficiency anemia, malabsorption (e.g., celiac disease), malnutrition (e.g., anorexia nervosa, but sometimes poor eating habits in children),[47] inflammatory bowel disease,[421] systemic lupus erythematosus,[422] lead poisoning (in contrast to anagen effluvium in thallium poisoning), and zinc deficiency. The proportion of follicles affected and the severity of the subsequent alopecia depend on the duration and severity of the trigger and individual variations in susceptibility.

The diagnosis may be confirmed by both counting the number of hairs shed each day and determining the percentage of telogen hairs in the scalp. Telogen hair represents approximately 15% and anagen 85% of scalp hair. If 25% or more of gently pulled hairs are telogen, telogen effluvium can be diagnosed. Parents often bring in a bag full of hairs (or can send a bag of hairs for assessment after the visit). Anagen hair roots can be recognized by their intact outer and inner hair sheaths, with or without a portion of the dermal papilla adherent to the tip of the root (see Fig. 7.1, *A*). Telogen hair roots have uniform shaft diameters, contain no pigment, and are club shaped (see Fig. 7.1, *B*), much like the tip of a cotton-tipped applicator.

Increased telogen hair loss can also be seen in children with *short anagen* syndrome, in which the short, fine hair is present from birth,[423] is shed excessively, and does not require haircuts (Fig. 7.34). The pull test tends to be positive, but hairs are <6 cm in length and are tapered (i.e., uncut). The shortening of the anagen phase (4 to 10 months), despite a normal rate of growth, leads to the decrease in the maximal hair length and an increase in the number of hairs in telogen. Topical minoxidil may increase hair density but not hair length; its use is generally unnecessary. The disorder tends to resolve spontaneously during puberty and adulthood.[424]

Elongation of the anagen phase has also recently been described as a result of mutations that deplete fibroblast growth factor 5 (FGF5), a regulator of hair length.[425] Because anagen hairs are already the majority of scalp hair but represent the minority of hairs of the eyelashes and extremities, trichomegaly (very long eyelashes) and longer extremity hair are the clinical manifestations in this recessive disorder that is homologous to the "angora" mutation in several species.

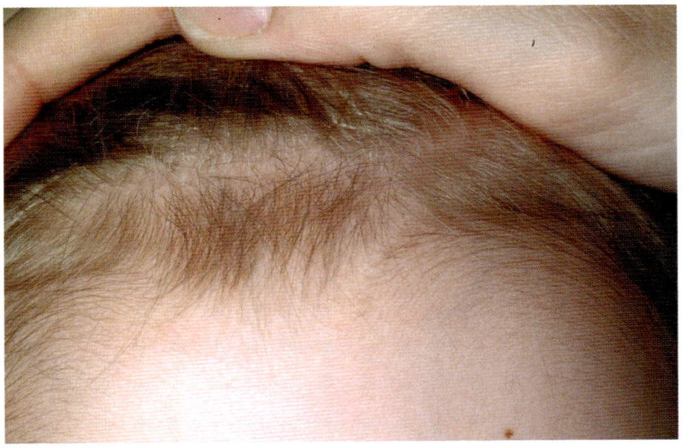

Fig. 7.35 Telogen effluvium. A rim of short hair (fringe-like) can be seen at the scalp borders in patients with telogen effluvium with hair regrowth.

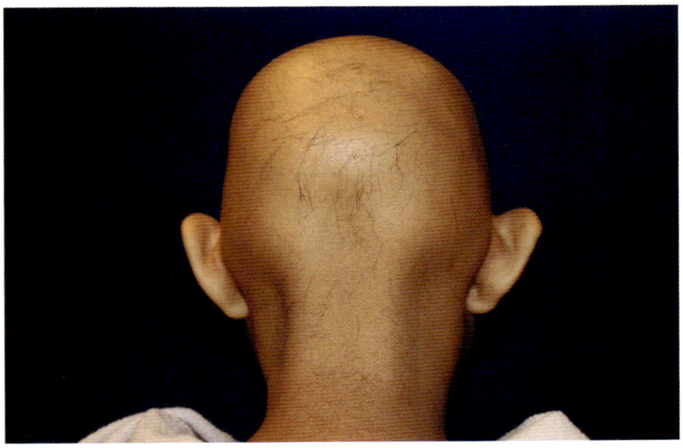

Fig. 7.36 Chemotherapy-induced alopecia. One year after receiving chemotherapy, this young girl still had virtually no hair. Topical minoxidil was not helpful, but oral minoxidil led to better regrowth.

There is no effective treatment for telogen effluvium, but complete regrowth almost invariably occurs within months unless the stressful event is repeated or the underlying trigger is sustained. A fringe of hair at the scalp margin can be shown as evidence of early hair regrowth (Fig. 7.35). Daily application of minoxidil may reduce shedding[426] in patients with chronic effluvium.

Careful explanation of the cause of this disorder and its favorable prognosis, with careful instructions to the patient to avoid unnecessary manipulation, tends to suffice. Blood tests for underlying disorders should be performed based on personal and family history and on examination, especially if no trigger is obvious. Adolescents predisposed to AGA may show incomplete regrowth after telogen effluvium with a residual pattern of hair loss consistent with AGA. Rarely, prolonged illness with high fevers destroys some follicles completely and only partial recovery ensues. Telogen effluvium occasionally occurs more than once in an individual, suggesting a predisposition to more significant hair loss with stress.

Anagen Effluvium

In *anagen effluvium*, hair shaft production is markedly reduced, leading to tapering of the shaft and shedding.[427] Given that more than 80% of scalp hair is in anagen phase, hair loss is usually profound. Anagen effluvium usually occurs in patients administered radiation or chemotherapy for malignancy. Most commonly implicated are cyclophosphamide, methotrexate, 6-mercaptopurine, and doxorubicin.[419,420] The alopecia tends to begin at a mean of 1.5 months after chemotherapy with regrowth starting about 2.6 months after cessation of chemotherapy, although the time course is quite variable.[428] Scalp cooling has been associated with reduction in hair loss in women with breast cancer, but no information is available in pediatric cancer patients.[429] In addition, anagen effluvium may be associated with exposure to high levels of colchicine[430] and toxic levels of boric acid, lead, thallium, arsenic, bismuth, and warfarin.[419,431] Anagen effluvium has also been reported in a young boy who required extracorporeal membrane oxygenation for cardiorespiratory failure, presumably related to hair matrix apoptosis from the shift of hypotension with hypoxia to reperfusion.[432]

The clinical features of anagen effluvium depend on the degree of toxicity created by the causative agent. With lower doses of the toxic agent, only segmental thinning or narrowing may occur without actual fracture of the hair shaft. Gentle hair pulls yield "pencil point" dystrophic hairs with proximal tips tapered to a point.[417] With extensive anagen effluvium, the remaining hairs are telogen, and the hair plucks late in the course may show as many as 100% telogen hairs. A careful history, documented evidence of hair loss, microscopic examination of spontaneously shed and manually epilated hairs, and appropriate physical and toxicologic examinations help to establish the correct diagnosis. Cessation of the responsible drug or toxin generally results in regrowth of hair.

A cicatricial form of alopecia may also occur after administration of chemotherapy, leading to permanent hair loss, defined as incomplete hair growth lasting longer than 6 months after stopping chemotherapy. In one study, permanent chemotherapy-induced alopecia occurred in 12% of children[428] (Fig. 7.36). Response to topical minoxidil is limited at best, although significant improvement was described in an adult with oral minoxidil.[433]

Alopecia Areata

AA is one of the most common hair loss disorders with a prevalence of 0.1% to 0.2% of the population; 18% of patients with AA seen by dermatologists are under 18 years of age.[434] Within the spectrum are alopecia totalis (AT; loss of all scalp hair), alopecia universalis (AU; loss of all body hair) (these collectively develop in approximately 5% of pediatric cases), and the ophiasis pattern (wrapping around the sides and back of the scalp). However, it has been suggested that these imprecise terms be abandoned and that the extent be defined based on the Severity of Alopecia Tool (SALT) score (with ≥50% reflecting severe AA), plus whether there is any body hair.[435] The pediatric SALT has been adjusted slightly[436] to reflect[436] differences by age, and a computer imaging algorithm has been developed to quantify SALT from photographs.[437] As an additional tool, the distal thumb (thumbprint area) is approximately 1% of the scalp, helping to delineate extent in those with milder involvement.[438]

The cumulative lifetime risk of developing AA is 2.1%, with the peak incidence occurring during young adulthood.[439] Prepubertal onset occurs less often than onset during adolescence, is associated with a family history of AA, and has a poorer prognosis. Occurrence in young infants is unusual, and the disorder is very rare in neonates.[440] Many families describe seasonality to flares (increased hair loss), with fall and early winter the peak months (and April to August relatively stable).[441]

There is a strong association between AA and atopic dermatitis, which is greatest among prepubertal children and in individuals with alopecia totalis and alopecia universalis.[442–445] Loss-of-function mutations in *FLG* (encoding filaggrin) have been associated with a more severe course and associated atopy but not a higher risk.[446] In a National Alopecia Areata registry of pediatric AA that was heavily skewed towards AT/AU (46%), 33% had atopic dermatitis, 21% asthma, 20% allergic rhinitis, 14% "allergy," and 5% urticaria.[447] In contrast, ≤3% of the patients reported another immune disorder (most often vitiligo [3%], psoriasis [2%], or Hashimoto thyroiditis [<1%]).[448] There is no sexual predilection for the disorder. Familial occurrence is reported in 8% to 52% of children, with an estimated lifetime risk of 7.1% in siblings, 7.8% in parents, and 5.7% in offspring.[449] Occurrence in both identical twins is 55%, emphasizing the importance of genetic as well as environmental factors.

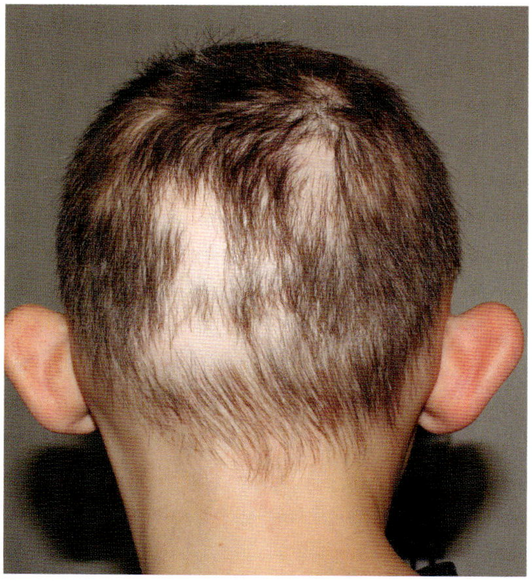

Fig. 7.37 Alopecia areata. Individuals with this common hair disorder suddenly develop one or more round or oval, well-circumscribed, clearly defined patches of hair loss.

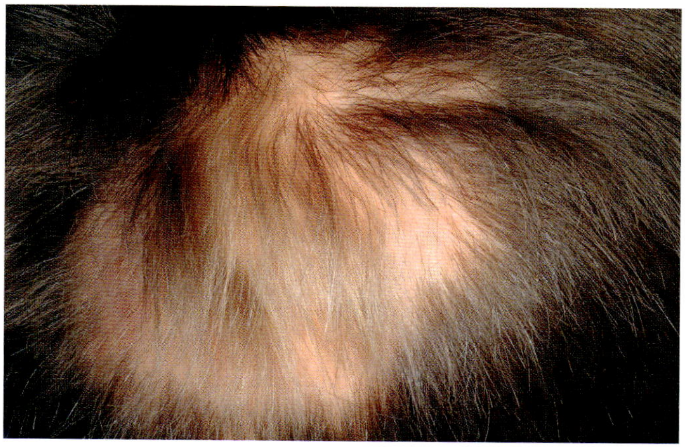

Fig. 7.38 Alopecia areata. Regrowing hair may be vellus hair or appear hypopigmented but is eventually replaced by normally pigmented terminal hair.

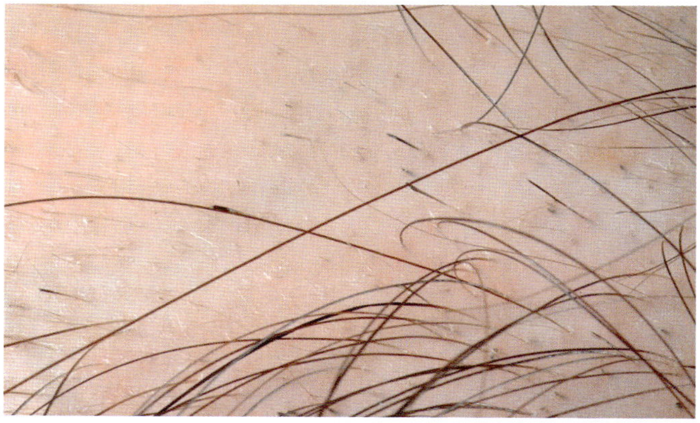

Fig. 7.39 Alopecia areata. "Exclamation-point hairs" in a girl with an ophiasis pattern of hair loss. Under the microscope, these hairs demonstrate a tapered shaft to an attenuated bulb (the "dot" of the exclamation point).

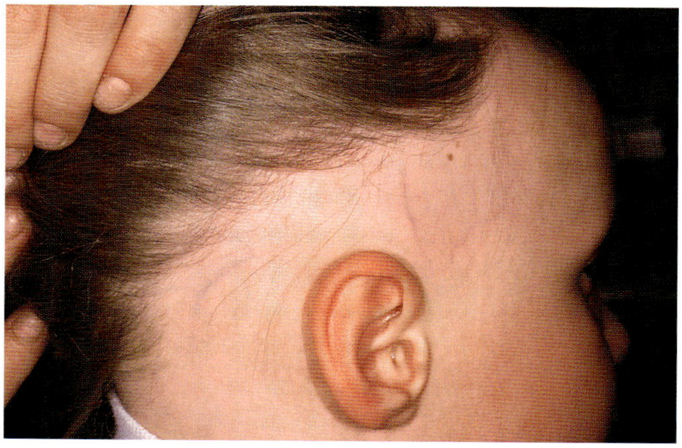

Fig. 7.40 Alopecia areata. The ophiasis pattern involves hair loss in a band extending from the occiput bilaterally along the hair margin toward the region above the ear and sometimes circling to the anterior scalp.

The typical clinical picture of AA generally consists of a sudden (overnight or several days) appearance of one or more round or oval, well-circumscribed, clearly defined patches of hair loss (Fig. 7.37).[450–452] Overall 83% of children have this patchy loss involving less than 50% of the scalp. Occasionally the initial patches may lack a regular outline and at times may demonstrate scattered long hairs within the bald areas. In other instances the initial loss may be diffuse, with discrete patches of alopecia being apparent only after 1 or 2 weeks, if at all. The primary patch may appear on any hairy cutaneous surface but usually occurs on the scalp. The skin is smooth, soft, and almost totally devoid of hair. Rarely, slight erythema or edema may be found at an early stage. Depigmented or hypopigmented hair shafts, simulating poliosis, may be seen (Fig. 7.38). Discrete islands of hair loss sometimes are separated by completely uninvolved or partially involved scalp. Around the margins of patches of alopecia, pathognomonic "exclamation-mark" hairs may be detected (Fig. 7.39). These loose hairs, with attenuated bulbs and short stumps, are easily plucked out of the scalp. Examination of such hairs under a low-power microscope reveals an irregularity in diameter and a poorly pigmented hair shaft that tapers to an attenuated bulb. The hair bulb represents the dot of the exclamation point. Dermoscopic evaluation of the affected scalp can be very helpful, showing the tapered hairs and sometimes yellow perifollicular dots, demarcating the hyperkeratotic follicular plugs.[453,454]

The ophiasis pattern of hair loss begins as a bald spot on the posterior occiput and extends anteriorly and bilaterally in a 1- to 2-inch-wide band encircling the posterior scalp, usually extending above the ear but occasionally to the anterior aspect of the scalp (Fig. 7.40). The ophiasis pattern is generally associated with a poor prognosis.[455] Progression to the totalis or universalis forms (Fig. 7.41) occurs more slowly but more often in children than in adults. Alopecia may involve any hair; eyebrows and eyelashes may be lost with or without patches of hair loss on the scalp (Fig. 7.42).

Nail defects are seen in 10% to 20% of cases. Although more extensive disease is associated with more nail involvement, some patients may have extensive nail dystrophy with little hair change. The most characteristic nail abnormality is a fine, grid-like stippling, regularly arranged in horizontal and/or vertical rows with smaller and shallower pits than those seen in patients with psoriasis (Fig. 7.43, *A*). Pitting overall is described in 20% and longitudinal ridging (trachyonychia) in 8%.[456] Proximal shedding (onychomadesis), opacification, and serration of the free edges may also be seen (Fig. 7.43, *B*). Nail dystrophy tends to occur more often and be more severe in patients with AT and AU.

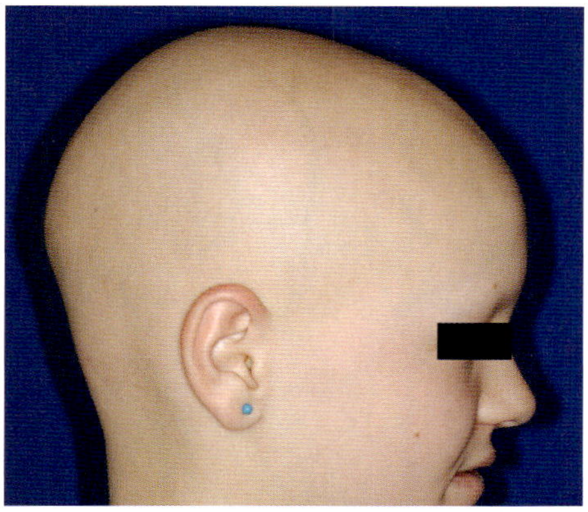

Fig. 7.41 Alopecia universalis. All hair is lost on the scalp and elsewhere. This is associated with a much poorer prognosis for hair regrowth.

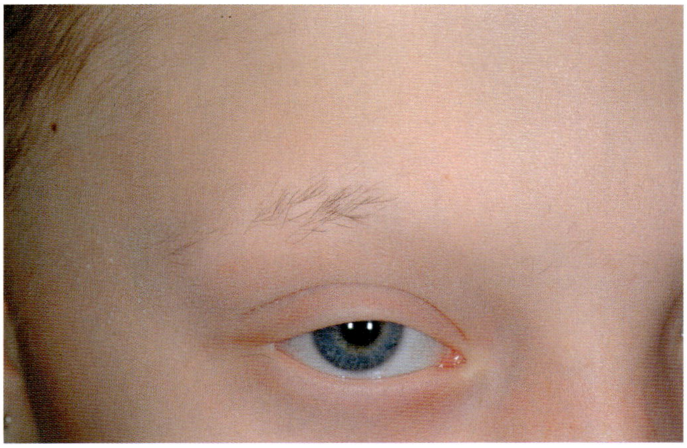

Fig. 7.42 Alopecia areata. The alopecia may involve the eyebrows and eyelashes, even without hair loss on the scalp; in this situation, trichotillomania must also be considered.

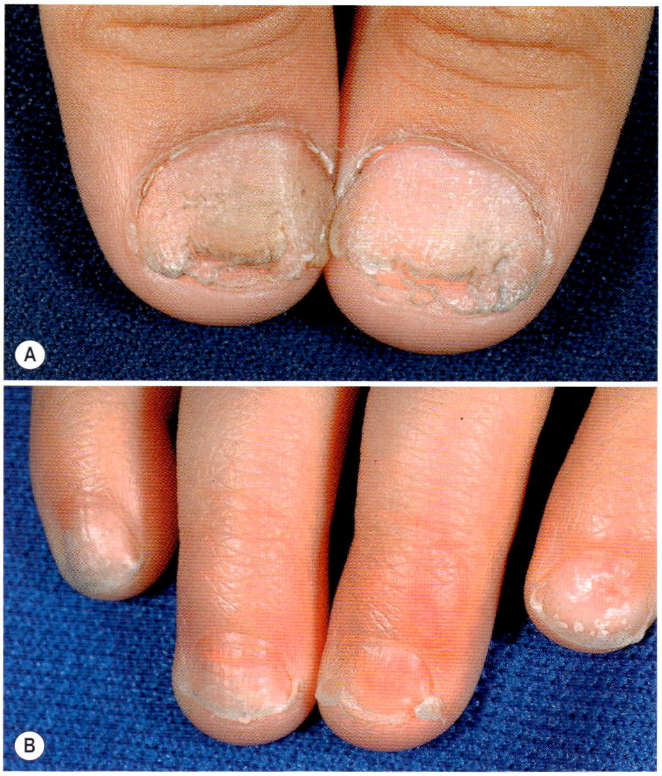

Fig. 7.43 Alopecia areata with nail changes. **(A)** The nails in this boy with alopecia areata are covered with shallow pits resulting from alteration in the proximal matrix. **(B)** Punctate opacification, proximal shedding (onychomadesis), Beau lines (horizontal dells), and serration of the free edges are all seen in the nails of this young girl with alopecia universalis.

The diagnosis of AA is based on its clinical picture. The sudden appearance and circumscribed nonscarring, patterned nature of hair loss distinguish it from other disorders of alopecia. Trichotillomania is typically associated with bizarre, irregular patches of hair loss with areas of broken hairs of different lengths. The absence of signs of inflammation and scaling will generally help distinguish this disorder from that of tinea capitis. When the diagnosis is in doubt, dermoscopic or microscopic examination of hairs, potassium hydroxide mounts, fungal cultures, and cutaneous punch biopsy will generally establish the proper diagnosis. AU beginning in infants must be distinguished from congenital alopecias such as atrichia with papules.[457] The AA spectrum can be a feature in 33% of children with autoimmune polyendocrinopathy–candidiasis–ectodermal dystrophy (APECED) syndrome, resulting from mutations in *AIRE* (see Chapter 23).[458]

Although associated autoimmune disorders in affected children are quite rare, a family history of other autoimmune disorders, especially thyroiditis, is common, and autoantibodies may be detected in patient sera.[459] An increased incidence has also been noted in patients with trisomy 21. No guidelines for laboratory testing are available. However, the minority of patients have evidence of hypothyroidism (Hashimoto's disease in 50%)[460], hyperthyroidism (Graves' disease in 25%), or subclinical (asymptomatic thyroid dysfunction (15%), suggesting that laboratory testing for thyroid disease could be restricted to patients with a family history of the condition, clinical findings of potential thyroid dysfunction, or a history of trisomy 21. Severity, duration of disease, and age at diagnosis do not appear to alter the risk[460] of having thyroid dysfunction.

The risk of celiac disease in association with AA is small and does not appear higher than in the general population.[461] The National Alopecia Areata Registry cited a 0.31% self-reported prevalence of celiac disease in children younger than 13 years with AA,[447] and the alopecia in patients with AA and celiac disease may improve on a gluten-free diet. A proposed recommendation is screening only if there are signs and symptoms of celiac disease with a low threshold for testing or in patients with a first-degree relative with celiac disease or a concurrent immune (e.g., trisomy 21, IgA deficiency) or autoimmune (e.g., dermatitis herpetiformis, thyroiditis) disorder.[461]

The course of AA is variable and difficult to predict.[462] New patches of hair loss may appear for 4 to 6 weeks and occasionally for several months. Spontaneous regrowth may occur. In general, when the process is limited to a few patches, the prognosis is good, with complete regrowth occurring within 1 year in 60% to 80% of patients; progression to total loss of scalp hair is unusual (<10%) and portends a considerably worse prognosis. About 30% of patients with patchy AA will have future episodes once regrown. In general, the earlier the onset, the poorer the prognosis. Elevated serum levels of IL-15 have been described in patients with AA, with levels higher with more severe involvement[463]; it is unclear if levels can be followed to predict the course. Other prognostic indicators of a worse outcome are family history of autoimmune disease, personal history of atopy, and nail abnormalities.

Therapy for AA at best controls the condition but does not cure it or prevent development of new areas.[464–466] Because of the chronic nature of the condition and the slow growth of hair, any trial of a treatment modality requires at least 4 months. The sudden hair loss, cosmetic ramification, and unpredictable course make AA a frightening disorder for affected patients and families[467]; psychological support and counseling are required for all patients and parents. Adequate camouflage of alopecic areas may be achieved by hats, headbands, or hairstyle changes. In children with severe involvement, wigs can be helpful. Locks of Love is an organization that provides hair prostheses to financially disadvantaged children under the age of 18 years (locksoflove.org).[468] The National Alopecia Areata Foundation (naaf.org) is a national support group for affected children and their families. Given the high percentage of children with patchy AA who show spontaneous remission within a year, physicians may prescribe no therapy. In general, patients with more extensive AA or with limited involvement unresponsive to topical corticosteroids should be referred to a dermatologist.

The most commonly used therapy for more limited AA in children is class I to III topical corticosteroids, with or without occlusion (such as may be achieved under a wig, bathing cap, or Saran Wrap). Because the regrowth rate without medications is high, it has been hard to demonstrate clear evidence of the efficacy of steroids. In one study, clobetasol cream was more effective than 1% hydrocortisone in decreasing the extent of hair loss by 12 weeks of twice-daily use when used for 6 weeks on and 6 weeks off for a total of 24 weeks.[469] If a class I (ultrapotent) steroid is employed, its use should be limited to intermittent-pulse therapy; longer use may result in significant local atrophy and systemic absorption.

Intradermal corticosteroid injections commonly result in regrowth in tufts at injection sites within 4 to 6 weeks but are too uncomfortable for most children, even with the use of topical anesthetic creams. When an intralesional corticosteroid is used, a syringe with a 30-gauge needle or jet injection is best. Triamcinolone acetonide is injected in concentrations of 2.5 mg/mL (eyebrow area) to 10 mg/mL (scalp). Dosage should be limited to 0.1 mL per site, spaced at least 1 cm apart, with injections at intervals of at least 4 to 6 weeks.[451] Transient local atrophy may occur. Efficacy appears to be greatest in those who have less than 75% hair loss and with a relatively short duration of hair loss.

Minoxidil has been shown to stimulate follicular DNA synthesis. Although largely used for AGA, 2% to 5% topical minoxidil solution or 5% foam has been shown to cause cosmetically acceptable hair regrowth in approximately 20% to 45% of patients when used twice daily for 2 months.[470–472] The best results occur in patients with limited hair loss and when used concurrently with topical corticosteroids or anthralin. Cutaneous side effects may include local irritation, allergic contact dermatitis, and hypertrichosis, especially on the forehead (Fig. 7.44). Although quite rare, three children treated with topical minoxidil developed tachycardia, palpitations, and dizziness.[473] Prostaglandin F2a analogues (e.g., latanoprost, bimatoprost, travoprost) have not been helpful for alopecia of the eyelashes or brows[474]and have been linked to periorbital hyperpigmentation.[475] However, there are anecdotal reports of improvement after use for scalp AA.[476,477]

Anthralin cream is an alternative therapy that seems to elicit hair growth by nonspecific immunostimulation.[478] The 1% cream is usually applied as short-contact therapy, initially for 30 minutes with a gradual increase in exposure as tolerated to a maximum of 2 hours before shampooing of the scalp. A mild dermatitis is often required for regrowth, so concurrent use of topical corticosteroids is not recommended. New hair growth is usually seen in 3 months, but 6 months or more may be required for an acceptable response. Scalp irritation, folliculitis, and staining of the skin or clothes are potential adverse effects.

Two studies have demonstrated low levels of vitamin D in individuals with AA,[479–481] and a boy with AA responded to topical calcipotriol,[482] but no causal relationship with vitamin D deficiency has been confirmed. In a retrospective analysis of almost 100 children with AA and documented levels of 25-OH-vitamin D when not on supplementation, the frequency of deficiency was similar to that in a larger pediatric population (both 22%). The level of serum vitamin D and SALT scores were weakly positively correlated ($r = 0.35$, $p = 0.009$)[483] in one study, but a meta-regression analysis of several studies found no significant association.[484]

Treatment of more extensive AA (>50%), AT, and AU is very difficult. Topical application of corticosteroids is generally not helpful, but anthralin has shown greater responses. Topical immunotherapy is considered the treatment of choice for chronic, severe AA[452] and has been shown to decrease the T-cell infiltration.[485] Squaric acid dibutyl ester (SADBE) and diphenylcyclopropenone (DCP) are used most commonly because they are effective but not mutagenic or carcinogenic. Patients are initially sensitized on the arm to the contact allergen (e.g., SADBE 2%); then increasing concentrations of the allergen, beginning at 0.001% to 0.01%, are applied to the scalp until mild erythema and scaling develop. Contact dermatitis at the sensitization site (about 20% of treated children)[486] or treatment site and regional lymphadenopathy are the risks of this therapy but only occasionally lead to discontinuation.[487,488] Immunotherapy may be performed weekly by the physician or administered with careful monitoring by responsible parents at home on a daily basis, gradually increasing the frequency of application and dosing. In a recent meta-analysis of 45 studies that included children (>2000 patients), 75% of those with patchy alopecia and 55% with AT/AU had some hair regrowth, although only 25% and 32% of these, respectively, experienced complete regrowth.[489] A poorer response has been associated with disease extent ≥50%, having an atopic history, and having nail involvement. Recurrence rates were 38% with maintenance treatment and 49% without.[490,491] Responses to SADBE and DCP were similar, suggesting that they are alternative approaches, including in patients with anergy or adverse effects from one or the other. Combination DCP and anthralin gave superior results than DCP alone in one retrospective analysis of 47 patients.[492] In patients who are atopic with extensive AA, the addition of oral fexofenadine to the contact allergen treatment may increase the response.[493] Although photochemotherapy with systemic psoralen followed by ultraviolet A (PUVA) light and cyclosporine therapy have been successful in some adults with this disorder, their efficacy and potential toxicity probably do not justify their use in children.

Although not recommended for general use, systemic corticosteroids may be considered for carefully selected patients with severe involvement and rapidly progressive hair loss who are psychologically

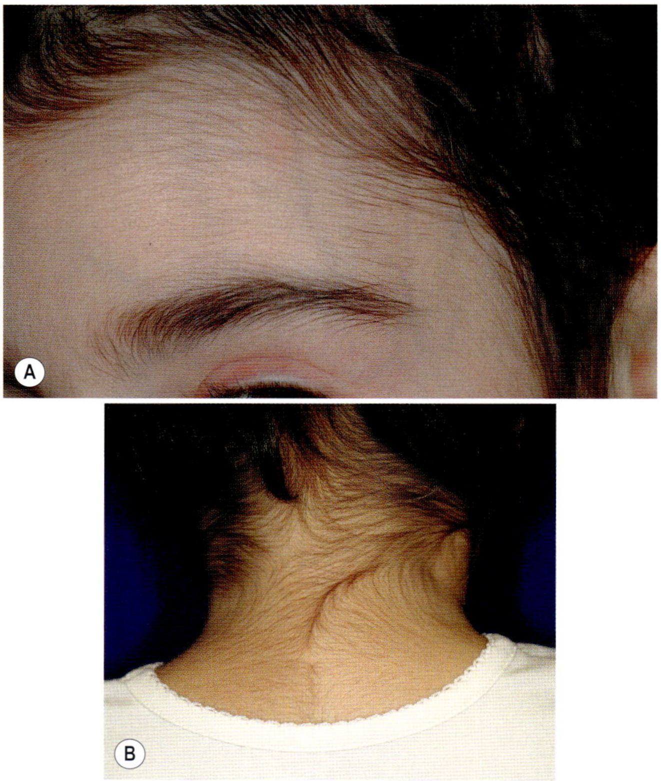

Fig. 7.44 Hypertrichosis induced from topical medications. Children who apply both topical corticosteroids and minoxidil are at particularly high risk for developing localized hypertrichosis, especially on the forehead **(A)** and nape **(B)**.

handicapped by their disorder. In such instances, prednisone may be administered in dosages of 0.5 to 1 mg/kg per day for 4 weeks until hair loss ceases and then tapered to alternate-day therapy for a few months. It must be emphasized that close follow-up evaluation is indicated in such cases and that the potential side effects associated with systemic corticosteroid therapy must be explained to the patient and parents. Pulse therapy with intravenous methylprednisolone has also been administered at a dosage of 250 mg twice daily for three sequential days with cessation of hair loss,[494] but the long-term outcome after corticosteroid therapy is poor.[495,496] In one retrospective study of 24 children with multifocal disease to AU, five to six monthly treatments on 3 consecutive days of 8 mg/kg intravenous methylprednisolone led to a complete response in 38% and no response in 33%, but 81% relapsed within a mean of 9.5 months after therapy.[497] Not surprisingly, patients with duration of less than 6 months and an onset at younger than 10 years of age and multifocal vs. diffuse disease responded better. Continuing application of topical minoxidil after a steroid taper has been shown to decrease hair loss.

Methotrexate (0.3 to 0.6 mg/kg per week) led to greater than 50% hair regrowth in children with recalcitrant AA in whom it was used for more than 2 months; the mean time to regrowth in one study was 4.4 months, and all responders experienced improvement within 6 months.[498,499] However, achieving long-term control is unusual, with relapse in most cases when stopped.[500] Sulfasalazine has shown cosmetically acceptable improvement in about 25% of treated adults[501] when used at a dosage of 1.5 g twice daily (but starting with 0.5 g/dose and then 1 g/dose for the first and second month, respectively). Trials with TNF inhibitors have been disappointing,[502] and AA has developed during TNF inhibitor therapy.[503] Hydroxychloroquine showed dramatic improvement in four children with 92% to 100% hair loss treated for 8 to 24 months in a retrospective review of nine patients.[504]

Light therapy is another approach for AA.[505,506] Most trials have used the 308-nm excimer laser or light, although 904-nm pulsed infrared diode laser and fractional lasers have also been used. The frequency of light therapy ranges from twice weekly to every other week. The proposed mechanism is light-induced inhibition of the T cells involved in the perifollicular inflammation. Excimer laser therapy twice weekly is painless and caused hair regrowth in 60% of recalcitrant patches of AA in children in less than 3 months; only 22% of responders relapsed after 6 months.[507]

Recent studies, including a genome-wide association study (GWAS) of more than 1000 affected individuals,[508] have shed light on the underlying pathomechanism of AA.[508–516] Whereas most of the linked genes involve the immune system, a receptor for stress-induced proteins *(NKG2D)* is also strongly linked, which is of interest because a stressful event precedes the onset of AA in 9.5% to 58% of patients.[517,518] These mechanistic studies have led to the discovery that systemic administration of Janus kinase (JAK) inhibitors (ruxolitinib, tofacitinib) prevent the development of AA in the *C3H/HeJ*-grafted mouse model and in pilot studies led to almost complete hair regrowth after up to 5 months of 20 mg ruxolitinib twice a day orally in adults with severe AA.[519,520] A meta-analysis of 30 reports of use of JAK inhibitors (tofacitinib, ruxolitinib, baricitinib) for AA (four cohort studies; 26 case reports) suggested good responses in 46% and partial responses in an additional 21%,[521] with better responses in pediatric vs. adult patients (although most reports involved adults). The mean time to initial hair growth was 2.2 months and to complete hair growth 6.7 months. Recurrences after discontinuation were common.

At the time of writing, no double-blind, randomized trials of the use of oral or topical JAK inhibitors in pediatric patients had been reported, although anecdotal results have been described. In one retrospective assessment of 13 adolescents, the mean percentage reduction in SALT score was 61% with a median of 93% after an average of 6.5 months[522] (range, 2 to 16 months) of 5 mg twice daily of tofacitinib; in another, eight adolescents with AU responded to 5 mg twice daily tofacitinib with >50% scalp regrowth within 5 months and significant improvement in SALT scores; the most rapid growth was after 3 months.[523] In one study of four preadolescent children (8 to 10 years old) with AT, 5 mg twice daily led to full hair regrowth in 50% (after 3 and 6 months' duration).[524] In another study with three 4- to 5-year-olds with total AA, 2.5 mg tofacitinib (primarily once daily) led to at least 50% hair regrowth within 6 to 21 months.[525] Regrowth of scalp hair tends to be better in those with a duration of AA for <10 years, although eyebrow and eyelash hair may respond to treatment without a scalp hair response. In general, evidence of scalp hair regrowth is faster than eyebrow, which tends to be faster than eyelash growth (in one study, 3.1 vs. 4.3 vs. 5.5 months, respectively).[526] Because of concerns regarding safety, baseline and repeated monitoring of blood counts (cytopenias), metabolic panel (increased transaminases and creatinine), and serum lipids (increased high-density lipoprotein [HDL] and low-density lipoprotein [LDL]) is important. Varicella zoster infection has been a common adverse event (primarily adults), but other infections and nonmelanoma skin cancer are rarely described.[527] Oral JAK inhibitors have been linked to serious infections in 2% to 6% of patients, and the long-term risks of use in pediatric patients are unknown.[528]

Results with topical JAK inhibitors, although presumably safer, have been less promising than with oral treatment. After topical application of a compounded liposomal base preparation of 2% tofacitinib twice daily in 11 children under 16 years of age, 91% of whom had 70% hair loss or more, only 3 had cosmetically acceptable hair regrowth after a treatment duration of 25 to 72 weeks of therapy.[529] Eyebrow regrowth from the use of ruxolitinib 0.6% cream has been described in an adolescent after 12 weeks of treatment.[530] In a study of six children and teenagers, only two had cosmetically acceptable regrowth of scalp hair (both on 2% tofacitinib in a liposomal base for 9 to 12 months).

With the growing use of dupilumab for atopic dermatitis, the relationship between atopic dermatitis and AU has received more attention. In adults, AA has also been associated with activation in skin and blood of Th1 and Th2 immune axes, as well as with the IL-23 (but not Th17) cytokine pathways.[531–533] In fact, several patients with AA and atopic dermatitis have had hair regrowth when administered dupilumab.[534–537] However, others with atopic dermatitis and no alopecia have experienced AA when taking dupilumab,[538,539] suggesting the need for further evaluation to understand the mechanism for these different responses.

Androgenetic Alopecia

AGA occurs in both males (common balding or male-pattern baldness) and females (preferentially called *female-pattern hair loss*[540] [FPHL]) and can begin during adolescence[541,542] or even as young as 7 years[543,544]; in general, the earlier the onset, the more profound the subsequent alopecia. Both AGA and FPHL are characterized by patterned, progressive hair loss from the scalp, although the patterning is different in females vs. males. Dihydrotestosterone (DHT) is the primary androgen implicated, converted from testosterone by the enzyme 5-a-reductase. There is increased expression of androgen receptors and/or an exaggeration formation of DHT in the scalp. These androgens gradually decrease the size of scalp hair follicles, resulting in miniaturized hairs. In addition, the anagen growth phase is shortened, leading to more hairs in the telogen phase. The conditions are inherited as polygenic traits influenced by both maternal and paternal genes[545]; in one study, 83% of adolescents with AGA had an affected first-degree relative.[541] Chronic low-grade inflammation in the scalp may also favor hair loss.

Most patients with AGA note thinning of scalp hair rather than shedding, although shedding may occur early in the course and be confused with telogen effluvium or diffuse AA. AGA during adolescence occurs twice as often in males as patterned hair loss in females and is generally more severe. The mildest and often earliest form of AGA in males is thinning at the vertex, often in conjunction with symmetric bitemporal triangular recession of the hairline (Fig. 7.45). In FPHL, there are two typical patterns: (1) centrifugal expansion of thinning from the midscalp (but not accentuation at the vertex as in males) and (2) frontal accentuation or Christmas tree pattern. In girls, the frontal hairline is relatively unaffected, but widening of the central hair part is often seen, leading to scalp visibility (Fig. 7.46). This female pattern of more diffuse hair loss is observed in 20% to 33% of adolescent males.[541,544]

Given the patterning of the scalp hair loss, comparing the density of hair at the frontal to vertex region vs. the occiput (which is not under

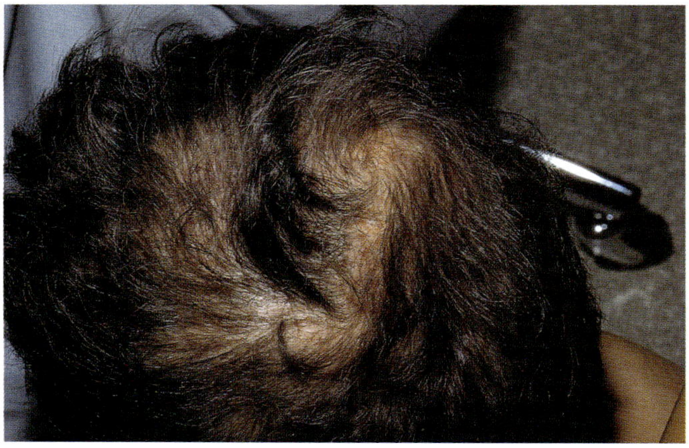

Fig. 7.45 Androgenetic alopecia. The scalp hair is thinned progressively but most notably between the frontal region of the scalp and the vertex.

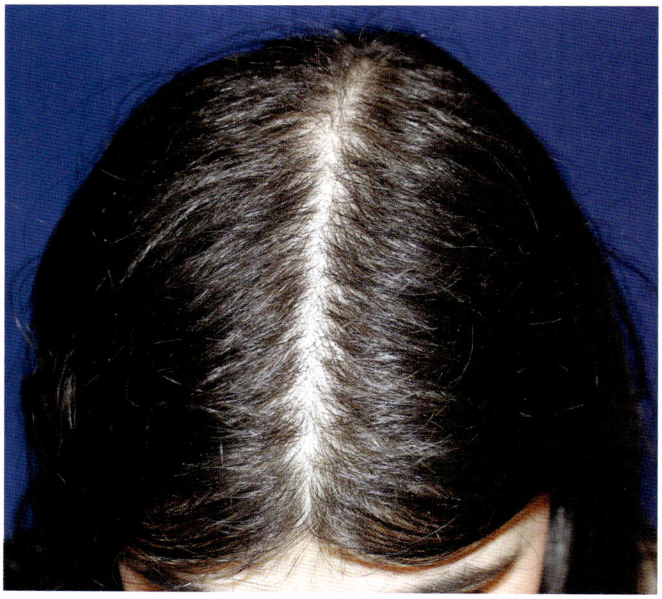

Fig. 7.46 Androgenetic alopecia. Widening of the central hair part is often seen, leading to scalp visibility.

androgenic control) can be of value. In FPHL, a piece of black (if light-colored hair) or white (if dark) fabric or paper can be placed behind the hair to more easily visualize the hairs clinically. Dermoscopy is a useful adjunctive measure to visualize the miniaturized hairs in affected areas.[8] The presence of follicular ostia should be sought, because loss of ostia suggests a scarring process and should lead to an alternative diagnosis, such as CCCA or frontal fibrosing alopecia. Other forms of alopecia in the differential diagnosis are chronic telogen effluvium, frontal trichotillomania, and a more generalized form of AA. With chronic telogen effluvium, hair pull is positive from multiple areas of the scalp, including the occiput. If confirmation is required, scalp biopsy can be performed, particularly with horizontal sectioning to determine the ratio of terminal to vellus hairs (>7:1 is normal; <4:1 is diagnostic; in contrast, the terminal:vellus hair ratio in chronic telogen effluvium is generally 9:1, showing lack of miniaturization). Other supporting histologic features are the perifollicular inflammation and some fibrosis.

Hormonal evaluation and endocrinologic consultation for female patients should be considered, although hyperandrogenism is unusual without other signs (menstrual irregularities, moderate to severe acne, and/or hirsutism). Laboratory evaluation should include testing for free and total testosterone; dehydroepiandrosterone sulfate (DHEA-S); 17-OH-progesterone (to consider late-onset congenital adrenal hyperplasia); and, if appropriate, levels of prolactin, vitamin D, thyroid hormones, and serum ferritin (for iron deficiency). In one study 37.5% of 19 affected adolescent girls had increased levels of androgens and 47% showed at least one additional clinical feature of hyperandrogenism. Laboratory testing should also be considered in boys who have diffuse thinning (more of a female pattern) or abnormal pubertal development.

The occurrence of AGA and FPHL during teenage years can be quite disturbing to the affected young men and women. Careful examination and repeated reassurance are required to discourage expensive and ineffective therapeutic regimens. Without treatment, the course tends to be progressive; the aim of treatment is to retard the further thinning of the hair and to promote hair growth.

Topical minoxidil and oral finasteride are US Food and Drug Administration (FDA)–approved treatments (minoxidil is over-the-counter) but are only approved for use in patients over the age of 18 years. Guidelines of use are available.[546] Minoxidil solution or foam promotes hair growth and decreases hair loss in approximately 60% of male and female patients when applied twice daily.[547–549] Administration of oral minoxidil has minimally greater efficacy than topical, but is associated with a high risk of hypertrichosis and the occasional occurrence of edema and electrocardiogram (EKG) abnormalities. The mechanism of action of topical minoxidil most likely involves its stimulation of follicular proliferation and vascularization of the follicle. Although 2% has been approved for women and 5% for men, the 5% strength has been found to be more effective and can be initiated off-label, with 2% as an alternative should any issue arise. One mL of minoxidil solution or a half-cap of foam is spread evenly on the dry scalp once daily (girls) to twice daily (boys). Evidence of hair growth requires at least 3 to 6 months, and treatment response should not be assessed before 6 months. A transient increase in telogen hair shedding is common during the 2 to 8 weeks after initiation (telogen shedding in preparation for anagen hair growth), and patients should be warned to avoid becoming discouraged. Application of minoxidil must be continued to maintain hair growth, and hair loss resumes 4 to 6 months after discontinuation. The addition of weekly microneedling, which stimulates hair follicle stem cells but may also improve minoxidil penetration, markedly increased the hair count and improved the patient evaluation during a 12-week period in comparison with minoxidil alone.[550]

The most common side effect of topical minoxidil is hypertrichosis on nonscalp sites, possibly from transfer of the solution.[551] Irritation can occur, usually from the propylene glycol in the solution (higher in 5% vs. 2%), and may lead to scalp pruritus and scaling; allergic contact dermatitis is less common and requires patch testing for diagnosis. Orthostatic hypotension has rarely been described. Topical minoxidil should not be used in pregnant or lactating adolescents.

Oral finasteride (1 mg daily) is often combined with minoxidil for treatment in males, given their different mechanisms of action. As with topical minoxidil, improvement is slow, and follow-up initially at 6 months is appropriate, with a trial of at least a year unless an issue arises. Finasteride specifically inhibits type II 5-a-reductase, leading to a reduction in both serum and scalp levels of dihydrotestosterone. Sexual dysfunction (decreased libido, erectile or ejaculatory dysfunction) has been described in 1% to 2% of patients. Other risks are gynecomastia, testicular pain, depression or mood alteration, and hypersensitivity reactions. Postmarketing reports suggest that these adverse effects sometimes persist more than 3 months after discontinuation ("postfinasteride syndrome"), but a causal relationship has not been demonstrated. Finasteride is known to cause feminization of the male fetus and should not be used for adolescent girls.[552] Oral dutasteride 0.5%, which inhibits both type I and type II 5-a-reductase and is available outside of the United States, has been shown to be more effective than finasteride with the same side effect profile.[553]

Spironolactone has shown some benefit in girls with AGA at doses of 50 to 200 mg/day[554]; similarly, cyproterone acetate in doses of 50 to 100 mg/day in combination with ethinyl estradiol has been successful in inducing hair regrowth and preventing progression but is not currently available in the United States. Spironolactone can be combined with topical minoxidil for FPHL; patients with FPHL and hirsutism or acne have a better response to spironolactone than with FPHL alone.[555] Food supplements with plant extracts, including of *Serenoa repens*, a treatment of benign prostatic hyperplasia, have been proposed as a "natural" alternative for treating male AGA.[556] A report of hot flashes in an 11-year-old girl linked to oral ingestion of *S. repens* for telogen effluvium warns of their danger in pediatric patients.[557]

In male AGA, ketoconazole shampoo has been shown to increase hair density, size, and percentage in anagen,[558] but there is no evidence in women with FPHL. Randomized, double-blind, controlled office- or home-based studies have suggested modest efficacy of office-based low-level laser therapy, either as monotherapy or with other interventions.[559–561] Wavelengths between 600 and 1550 nm (red/infrared spectrum) are usually used. Surgical procedures, such as scalp reduction with or without tissue expansion, scalp flaps, and multiple-punch autografting hair transplantation, may also be considered in patients with advanced AGA but are inappropriate for use in adolescents, given that the course of the AGA is unpredictable.[562]

Traumatic Alopecias: Traction Alopecia and Trichotillomania

Traumatic alopecia results from the forceful extraction of hair or the breaking of hair shafts by friction, pressure, traction, or other physical trauma. The usual causes are cosmetic practices and trichotillomania. Other causes of traumatic alopecia include pressure, such as occurs in neonates who develop caput succedaneum with a scalp ring from birth trauma or use of suction at delivery[359] (see Chapter 2), and as is seen in association with the habit of head banging; prolonged bed rest in one position, such as may be seen in chronically ill patients; postoperative alopecia (as a result of pressure-induced ischemia during long surgical procedures); thermal or electric burns; repeated vigorous massage; a severe blow to the scalp; occipitoparietal alopecia, such as may be induced by spinning on the crown of the head during break dancing; pressure from orthodontic headgear[563]; or prolonged use of wide-strapped, heavy headphones, such as those commonly used by individuals while jogging. Prolonged or forceful trauma may cause scarring alopecia.

Alopecia from cosmetic practices most often results from traction but has been described as resulting from pulling, frequent brushing with nylon bristles, the use of hot combs and oils, and hair-straightening practices such as teasing. *Traction alopecia* is characterized by oval or linear areas of hair loss at the margins of the hair line, along the part, or scattered through the scalp, depending on the type of traction or trauma.[564–566] Peripheral scalp hair loss may occur in individuals who wear their hair in ponytails or braids or use hair extensions[567] or barrettes (Fig. 7.47). Overall, 17.1% of school-aged Black girls showed traction alopecia, with the percentage increasing toward the end of high school and with a history of braids on relaxed hair.[568] In one study, traction alopecia occurred three times more often in girls with cornrows compared with either ponytails or braids.[569] Hair loss from hair rollers is usually most conspicuous in the frontocentral area or around the margins of the scalp. With persistence, scarring can occur.

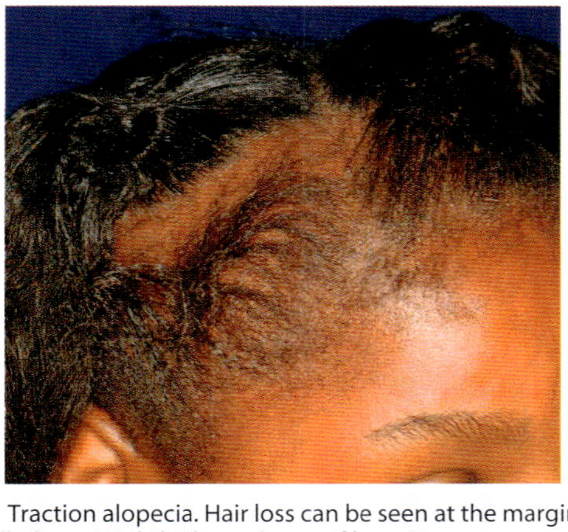

Fig. 7.47 Traction alopecia. Hair loss can be seen at the margins where hair is pulled most tightly through use of barrettes.

Traction alopecia must be distinguished from CCCA, seen primarily in Black individuals and generally starting at the vertex of the scalp. In severe chronic forms, however, the entire scalp may be involved. Traction folliculitis may present as perifollicular erythema and pustules at sites of traction.[570]

Trichotillomania is a self-limiting, self-induced form of traction alopecia produced either consciously or by habitually plucking, pulling, or cutting the hair in a bizarre manner.[571–573] Trichotillomania-by-proxy has also been described, in which a parent with trichotillomania pulls the hair of a child as part of the overwhelming urge to depilate.[574] Seen in both sexes, it more commonly occurs in adolescents and females, although 20% experience trichotillomania before 12 years of age,[575] and the condition may occur in preschool children. The scalp is the most common site of involvement, but the eyebrows, eyelashes, and even pubic hair may also be affected as the patient plucks, twirls, or rubs hair-bearing areas, resulting in the epilation or breakage of hair shafts (Fig. 7.48).

The habit is usually practiced in bed before the child falls asleep (when the parent does not notice the habit). In young individuals, the condition is commonly associated with a habit of finger or thumb sucking (Fig. 7.49). In a study of children 10 to 17 years of age with

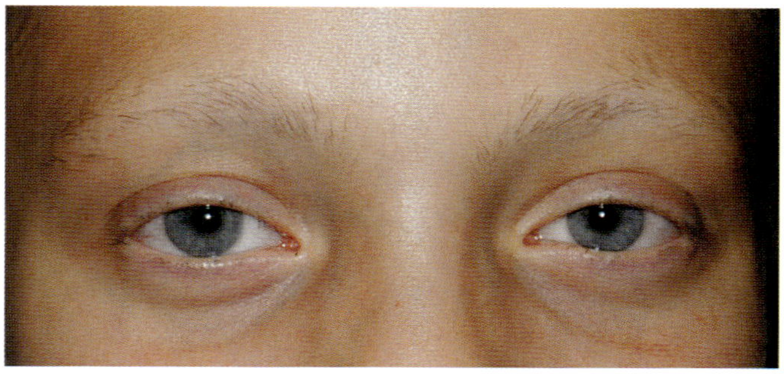

Fig. 7.48 Trichotillomania. The eyebrows and eyelashes may be pulled out or broken by repetitive plucking, twirling, or rubbing.

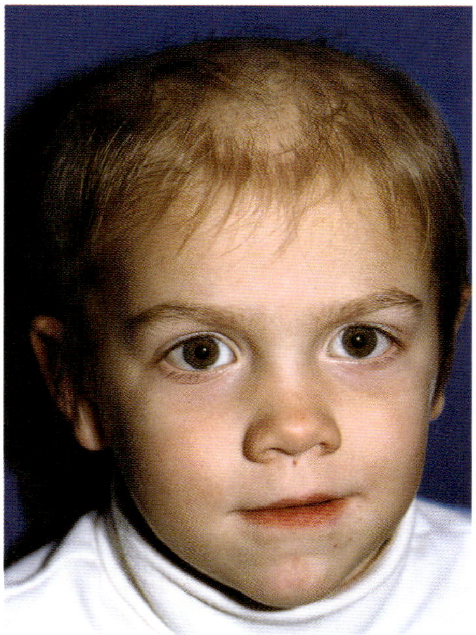

Fig. 7.49 Trichotillomania. In younger children trichotillomania is often a habit of twirling or plucking associated with finger or thumb sucking and does not reflect significant psychologic disturbance.

trichotillomania, hair pulling most often occurred when doing homework, working on the computer, watching television, or sitting on the toilet, with most isolating themselves during hair pulling.[576] Eyebrow and eyelash pulling occurred in addition to the scalp hair. In these older children, other compulsive behaviors, such as nail biting (onychophagia), skin and lip picking, picking at acne (acne excoriée), nose picking, lip biting, and cheek chewing, are often seen. In 2013 the American Psychiatric Association changed trichotillomania in its *Diagnostic and Statistical Manual of Mental Disorders (DSM)* 5 classification tool from an impulse-control disorder not elsewhere classified to an obsessive-compulsive disorder. Depression, attention-deficit/hyperactivity disorder (ADHD), and tics are the most common comorbid psychiatric disorders.

Trichotillomania usually begins insidiously as an irregular linear or rectangular area of partial hair loss. Affected areas are generally single; often frontal, frontotemporal, or frontoparietal; and commonly appear on the contralateral side of right- or left-handed individuals. The affected patches have irregularly shaped angular outlines and are never completely bald (Fig. 7.50). Within the involved regions, the hair is short or stubbly and broken off at varying lengths (Fig. 7.51).

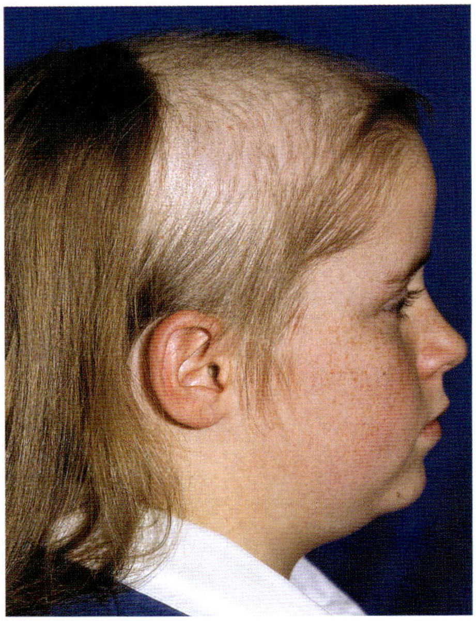

Fig. 7.50 Trichotillomania. The affected areas have irregularly-shaped, angular outlines and are never completely bald. They tend to be sites that are easy to reach.

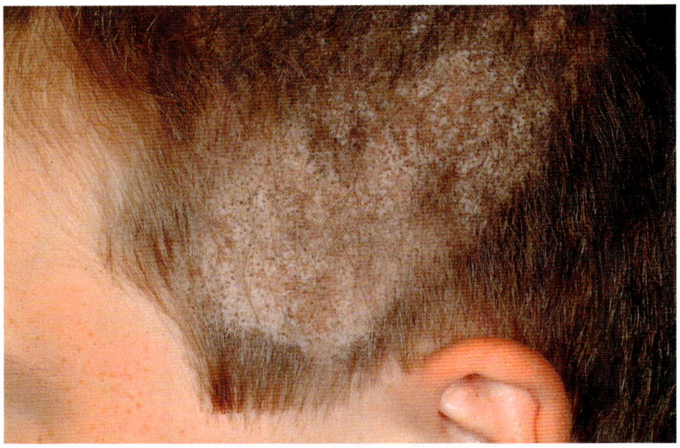

Fig. 7.51 Trichotillomania. This boy tried to cover a patch of trichotillomania with eyebrow pencil but continued to pluck hairs.

If one maintains a high index of suspicion, trichotillomania can generally be distinguished from other forms of hair loss by its characteristic configuration and distribution. Trichoscopy can be helpful, showing the irregularly broken hairs, as well as a variety of other specific signs (such as the V sign, flame hairs, coiled hairs, and follicular microhemorrhage).[577,578] Occasionally the diagnosis can be confirmed by the finding of wads of hair under the pillow or bed or by observation of the habit by a parent, teacher, or physician. When the diagnosis is suspected, regrowth of hair in a carefully shaved or occluded patch of scalp in the involved area (to prevent manipulation) may confirm the correct diagnosis. The possibility of associated trichophagia and trichobezoar should be considered[579]; Rapunzel syndrome is a rare form of trichobezoar in which the swallowed hair extends from the stomach into the small bowel, resulting in intestinal occlusion and requiring surgical removal.[580]

Trichotillomania should be distinguished from AA, although both have been described in the same individuals, often with the AA as the trigger to the trichotillomania.[581] Clinical differentiation from AA is usually based on the bizarre configuration, irregular outline, and presence of short, stub-like, broken hairs. Differentiation from tinea capitis may require microscopic examination of plucked hairs with potassium hydroxide and fungal culture (see Chapter 17). Of particular significance is the fact that the broken hairs of trichotillomania, unlike those of certain forms of tinea capitis, remain firmly rooted in the scalp, and the cutaneous surface is normal and stubbled rather than erythematous or scaly. If the diagnosis remains in doubt, biopsy of the involved area may be helpful.

The management of trichotillomania is often difficult and requires a strong relationship among the doctor, patient, and parents. Although patients occasionally will admit to touching the affected areas, they commonly will deny plucking, rubbing, or excessive manipulation. Blunt accusation is often detrimental, but gentle suggestion of the cause may lead to dialog that is important for reversal. Psychopathologic changes are reported to be present in some 50% to 75% of affected individuals. These changes are usually mild, but severe psychologic disturbance occurs in approximately 5% of patients with trichotillomania, most commonly in older children and teenagers. In general, the disorder is limited in preschool-aged children and may be more episodic in children than in affected teenagers.

If patients are reassured, given an opportunity to express their emotional needs, and offered a reasonable therapeutic regimen such as a mild shampoo, mild topical steroid (e.g., hydrocortisone 1%) lotion, and behavioral modification techniques, the habit will sometimes disappear, especially in young children. For those individuals with persistent or severe obsessive-compulsive or emotional problems, however, psychiatric intervention should be considered. Cognitive behavioral therapy with relapse prevention can reduce trichotillomania severity by 64% at 6-month follow-up evaluation.[582,583] For habitual trichotillomania in young children, substitution therapy (such as with a soft tag to stroke or a long-haired doll) and provision of rewards can be helpful.[584] Olanzapine, clomipramine, or a highly selective serotoninergic reuptake inhibitor (SSRI) (e.g., fluvoxamine, fluoxetine, paroxetine, sertraline, or citalopram) may be of benefit. Despite the value of oral N-acetylcysteine in a large trial of adults with trichotillomania and case reports in children with 1200 to 1800 mg/day[585,586] (with or without an SSRI), a recent trial of 39 children ages 8 to 17 years did not show benefit during 12 weeks of treatment.[587] A trichotillomania support group, the Trichotillomania Learning Center, is available at www.trich.org.

Eruptive Vellus Hair Cysts

Eruptive vellus hair cysts are characterized by 1- to 3-mm, skin-colored to hyperpigmented follicular papules, most commonly on the anterior chest (Fig. 7.52).[588] Lesions usually are not grouped and tend to be smooth-surfaced with a round or domed shape. Vellus hair cysts have less commonly been described on the upper and lower extremities, face, neck, abdomen, axillae, posterior trunk, and/or buttocks. If darker blue in color and on the face, they have been confused with nevus of Ota.[589] Although usually seen in children between 4 and 18 years of age, these cysts can occur at any age.

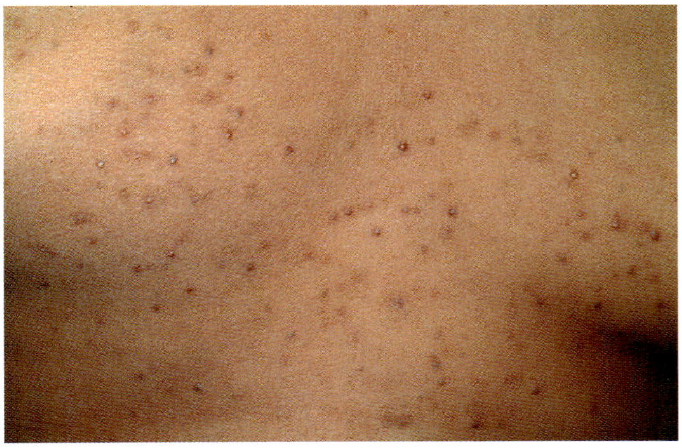

Fig. 7.52 Vellus hair cysts. One- to 3-mm, skin-colored to hyperpigmented follicular papules on the anterior chest.

The histologic picture of an eruptive vellus hair cyst is a small, mid-to-upper dermal keratinizing cyst filled with lamellar keratin and small-diameter nonpigmented or lightly pigmented hair shafts. Vellus hair cysts can be distinguished from steatocystoma multiplex by the inclusion of sebaceous glands in the cyst wall of steatocystoma multiplex.[590] However, lesions with features of both types of cysts have been described; both types of lesions have been seen in the same individuals, and kindreds with the autosomal dominant inheritance of both vellus hair cysts and steatocystoma multiplex have been reported with keratin 17 mutations, suggesting a common causation for the two types of cystic lesions.[591,592] An alternative diagnostic technique to biopsy is to perform a tiny incision at the top and examine the expressed contents microscopically for vellus hairs.[593] The co-occurrence of[594] eruptive vellus hair cysts with steatocystoma multiplex (and trichofolliculomas) has been described. Multiple eruptive vellus hair cysts have been described in association with preauricular pits, lipomas, joint hypermobility, and cardiac defects in a multigeneration family with autosomal dominant inheritance.[595]

Vellus hair cysts are most commonly confused with comedonal acne, milia, molluscum contagiosum, syringomas, folliculitis, keratosis pilaris, steatocystoma multiplex, and other adnexal tumors; dermoscopic evaluation can be helpful in making the diagnosis.[596] The cysts may resolve spontaneously during a few months to years by transepidermal elimination. Patients desiring therapy can be treated by incision of individual cysts and expression of their contents followed by gentle curettage, light electrodesiccation with expression of contents,[597] therapy with topical vitamin A acid (tretinoin), lactic acid (12% lotion), or laser.[598]

Hypertrichosis and Hirsutism

Excessive hairiness may be localized or diffuse, congenital or acquired, and normal or pathologic.[422] Hair in the pubic area of infants may be benign and often resolves spontaneously by 1 year of age, especially if on the scrotum in boys and labia majora or mons in girls without other evidence of virilization or sexual development.[599] The terms *hypertrichosis* and *hirsutism* are commonly and inappropriately used synonymously to describe excessive hair on the body.[600,601] *Hirsutism* implies an excessive growth of body hair in women or children (mostly girls) in an androgen-induced hair pattern (upper lip, chin, sideburn areas, neck, anterior chest, breasts, linea alba, abdomen, upper inner thighs, and legs).[602] Hirsutism most commonly represents a physiologic variant of hair growth, often seen in several family members, which comes to medical attention only because of societal pressure to remove excessive hair (Fig. 7.53). *Hypertrichosis*, conversely, refers to a generalized or localized pattern of non-androgen-dependent excessive hair growth in a male or female without evidence of masculinism or menstrual abnormality.

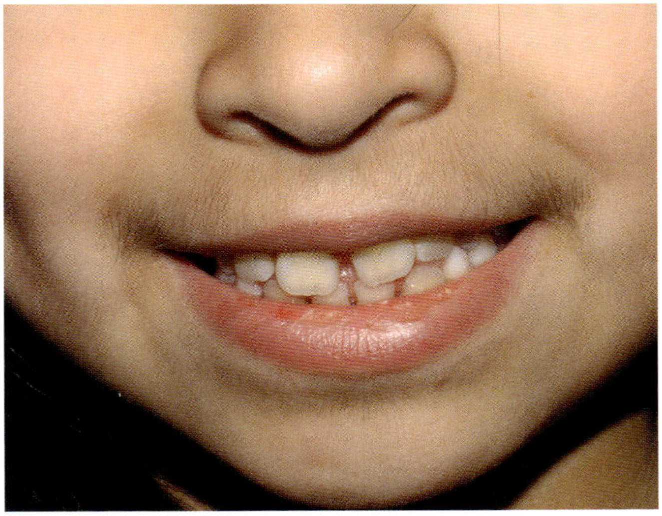

Fig. 7.53 Familial hirsutism. This 6-year-old girl has excessive terminal hair on the upper lip, which led to embarrassment. Her mother and maternal grandmother experienced the same increase in mustache hair.

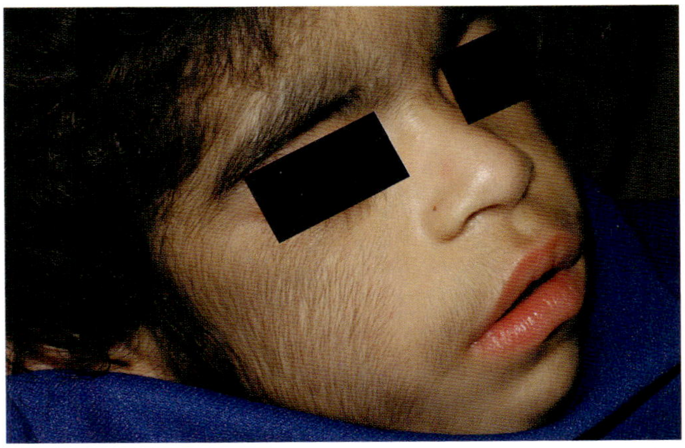

Fig. 7.54 Drug-induced hypertrichosis. This toddler developed hypertrichosis from administration of diazoxide for hyperinsulinemia.

ACQUIRED GENERALIZED HYPERTRICHOSIS

Generalized hypertrichosis may be associated with neurologic disorders (postencephalitic hypertrichosis, multiple sclerosis), anorexia nervosa, acrodynia, hypothyroidism, porphyria, dermatomyositis, gross malnutrition, and various forms of drug-induced hypertrichosis.

Although congenital adrenal hyperplasia (resulting from biallelic variants in *CYP21*) is more often associated with hirsutism (especially early pubic hair), limb hypertrichosis without hirsutism has rarely been reported in affected children.[603] Drug-induced hypertrichosis (Fig. 7.54) is most commonly seen in children who are administered phenytoin or cyclosporine, usually after 2 or 3 months of treatment, but other medications have been implicated as well[604] (Box 7.7; see Fig. 22.21). Localized hypertrichosis can be acquired from topical application of minoxidil (see Fig. 7.44) and topical corticosteroids (Fig. 7.55). Reversible generalized hypertrichosis has also been described in an infant exposed to topical minoxidil from her caregiver grandfather who held her extensively on his shoulders.[605] In adults, but not in children, acquired forms of hypertrichosis lanuginosa are strongly associated with internal malignancy, especially adenocarcinoma.

Box 7.7 Medications That May Cause Hypertrichosis

Adrenocorticotropic hormone (ACTH)
Corticosteroids
Cyclosporine
Danazol
Diazoxide
Glucocorticosteroids
Hexachlorobenzene (drug-induced porphyria cutanea tarda)
Minoxidil
Omeprazole
Penicillamine
Phenytoin
Psoralens and ultraviolet light exposure
Streptomycin
Testosterone
Valproic acid

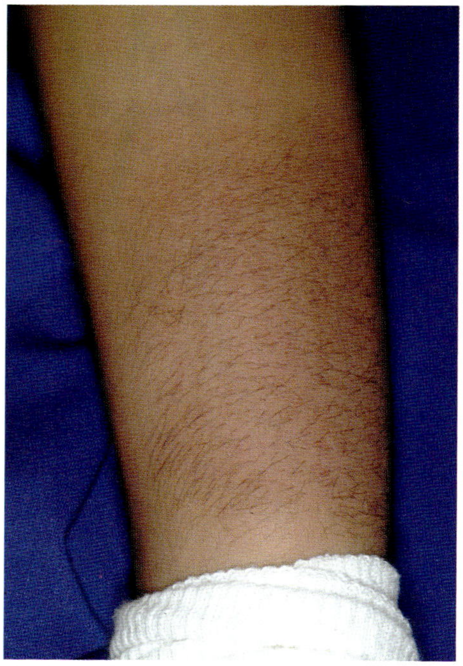

Fig. 7.55 Drug-induced hypertrichosis. Overgrowth of terminal hair was noted strictly at the site at which this boy's parents continued to apply a medium-strength topical corticosteroid for many months after clearance of his nummular dermatitis.

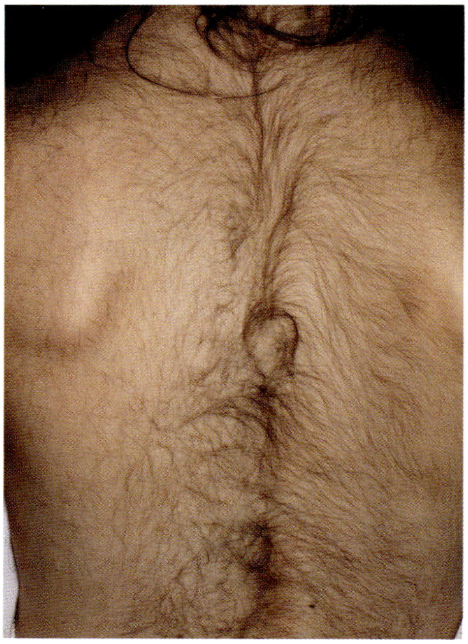

Fig. 7.56 Hypertrichosis. Generalized terminal hair growth in this girl with gingival hyperplasia.

CONGENITAL HYPERTRICHOSIS

The original fine, soft, unmedullated, and usually unpigmented lanugo hairs are shed *in utero* during the seventh or eighth month of gestation. Premature infants, however, commonly display this fine coat of lanugo hair, particularly on the face, limbs, and trunk. In these infants the fine lanugo hairs are shed during the first 3 months of life and replaced by normal terminal hair growth, generally before the first 6 months. Congenital generalized hypertrichosis can present as an isolated finding or may be associated with other anomalies.[606]

Hypertrichosis lanuginosa is a rare inherited disorder in which lanugo hairs persist or are overproduced throughout life.[607,608] Affected infants may be unusually hairy at birth or may develop hypertrichosis during early childhood. In some children, the hair will be spontaneously lost during childhood; in others, it will remain into adulthood. Generalized hypertrichosis can be very disfiguring. Affected children have been called *monkey-men, dog-face,* and *human Skye terriers.* Sporadic, autosomal recessive, and autosomal dominant cases have been described. Congenital[609] glaucoma, skeletal abnormalities, and missing teeth have been described in association.

Ambras syndrome is a generalized condition of hypertrichosis in which the hair appears to be vellus rather than lanugo hair.[610–612] The hypertrichosis is most evident on the face, ears, and shoulders and persists throughout life. Dysmorphic facial features have been associated. Ambras syndrome has been linked to a rearrangement in chromosome 8q that downregulates the expression of *TRPS1* (also mutated in trichorhinophalangeal syndrome).[613]

Hypertrichosis with gingival hyperplasia is a distinct autosomal dominant disorder in which affected individuals have excessive terminal body and facial hair in an identical distribution to that of hypertrichosis lanuginosa, as well as gingival hyperplasia (Fig. 7.56). Although the hypertrichosis is most commonly present at birth or in infancy, the hypertrichosis begins at puberty in some cases. The gingival hyperplasia is usually noted with delayed tooth eruption and has been described as pink, firm, and pebbly. The disorder is complicated by interference with chewing, respiration, and speech, and periodontal abscesses have been described because of difficulty in dental eruption. Gingival debulking may be required. A large deletion on 17q24.2-q24.3 has been found to be responsible for congenital generalized hypertrichosis, with or without gingival hyperplasia.[614] Whole-exome sequencing in a girl with congenital generalized hypertrichosis and gingival hyperplasia showed a homozygous intronic mutation in the ABC lipid transporter gene *ABCA5*, which is within the deleted region on chromosome 17; the mutation caused aberrant splicing of the transcript and decreased follicular protein levels.[615] Generalized hypertrichosis can also be a manifestation of a "potassium channelopathy," usually resulting from heterozygous activating mutations in *ABCC9*, which encodes the sulfonylurea receptor *SUR2*. In addition to the hypertrichosis, affected individuals have a spectrum of features ranging from acromegalic facies (with or without gingival hypertrophy)[616,617] to Cantú syndrome with its neonatal macrosomia, coarse facial features, osteochondrodysplasia, and cardiomegaly.[618] *SUR2* is expressed in the dermal papilla and is stimulated by minoxidil in inducing hair growth.[619] Isolated congenital hypertrichosis has also been linked to duplication in 17q11.2, a region that includes *FOXN1*, which plays a role in follicular keratinocyte differentiation. Nonsense mutations in *FOXN1* are associated with congenital alopecia, nail dystrophy and T-cell immunodeficiency.[620]

Box 7.8 Congenital Syndromes Associated with Generalized Hypertrichosis

Acromegaloid facial appearance syndrome (affected genes: *PGM1; GLO1; IGHG3; HP*)
Barber–Say syndrome *(KMT2A)*
Cantú syndrome (hypertrichosis with osteochondrodysplasia) *(ABCC9; KCNJ8)*
Coffin–Siris syndrome (BAF complex genes)
Cornelia de Lange (Brachmann–de Lange) syndrome *(NIPBL; SMC1A; SMC3; RAD21; HDAC8)*
Craniofacial dysostosis
Eye disorders
- With amaurosis congenital, cone-rod type
- With congenital lamellar cataracts and mental retardation
- With pigmentary retinopathy

Gorlin–Chaudhry–Moss (oculo-facio-cardio-dental) syndrome *(BCOR)*
Gingival hyperplasia
- Congenital generalized hypertrichosis with gingival hyperplasia
- Zimmerman–Laband syndrome

Hemimaxillofacial dysplasia
Lipodystrophies
- Berardinelli–Seip syndrome *(BSCL)*
- Donohue syndrome (leprechaunism) *(INSR)*

Mitochondrial encephalopathy, lactic acidosis, and stroke-like episodes (MELAS) syndrome
Mucopolysaccharidoses
- Hunter syndrome
- Hurler syndrome
- Sanfilippo syndrome

Porphyrias (see Chapter 19)
- Erythropoietic porphyria (Gunther disease)
- Familial porphyria cutanea tarda
- Hepatoerythropoietic porphyria

Rubinstein–Taybi syndrome *(CREBBP; EP300)*
Schinzel–Giedion syndrome *(SETBP1)*[MAJ359]
Stiff skin syndrome
Toxin exposure
- Fetal alcohol syndrome
- Fetal hydantoin syndrome

Weidemann–Steiner syndrome *(KMT2A)*
Winchester (Torg–Winchester) syndrome (see Chapter 6) *(MMP2)*

X-linked dominant hypertrichosis has been described in a Mexican pedigree. Affected males show excessive generalized terminal hair growth, especially on the face and upper torso; female individuals are less severely affected and can show asymmetric hairiness thought to represent random inactivation (lyonization) of the affected chromosome. This condition sometimes improves after puberty.[621] In another Mexican kindred, congenital universal hypertrichosis was associated with deafness and dental anomalies as an X-linked recessive disorder.[622]

Generalized hypertrichosis is also a feature of several syndromes (Box 7.8), among them congenital erythropoietic porphyria (see Chapter 19) and, most commonly, *Cornelia de Lange* syndrome.[623] This congenital, genetically heterogeneous disorder features marked hypertrichosis; cutis marmorata; hypoplastic genitalia, nipples, and umbilicus; prenatal and postnatal growth retardation; malformation of the limbs, gastrointestinal tract, diaphragm, heart, and genitourinary systems; mental retardation; and a characteristic low-pitched and growling cry. The face of affected individuals is characterized by overgrowth of the eyebrows; long eyelashes; high upper lip; saddle-nose; and a cyanotic hue about the eyes, nose, and mouth. Children with this disorder often have recurrent respiratory tract infections and gastrointestinal reflux; seizures have been observed in about 20% of reported cases, and most patients die before the age of 6 years. To date, heterozygous mutations in five genes have been described, most commonly *NIPBL* (60%).[623] These genes all encode structural or regulatory proteins involved in cohesin, a protein complex that regulates the separation of sister chromatids during cell division.[624]

LOCALIZED FORMS OF HYPERTRICHOSIS

Nevoid Hypertrichosis

Growth of hair abnormal in length, shaft diameter, or color may occur in association with other nevoid abnormalities or as isolated circumscribed developmental defects (Fig. 7.57).[625,626] Abnormal tufts of hair in the lumbosacral and, at times, the posterior cervical or thoracic areas (the faun-tail nevus,[627] Fig. 7.58) may be associated with an underlying kyphoscoliosis, duplication of a portion of the spinal cord (diastematomyelia), or tethered cord. Although neurologic signs of this disorder generally appear during early childhood, they may be delayed until the affected person's teenage or adult years. Early detection by imaging allows neurosurgical intervention and prevents the potential neurologic sequelae. Symmetric localized hypertrichosis has also been described at the elbows (hypertrichosis cubiti)[628,629] and anterior cervical area (anterior cervical hypertrichosis) (Fig. 7.59). *Hypertrichosis cubiti* and *anterior cervical hypertrichosis* are usually isolated disorders. However, anterior cervical hypertrichosis has been described as an autosomal recessive disorder in association with developmental delay; peripheral neuropathy with or without retinal

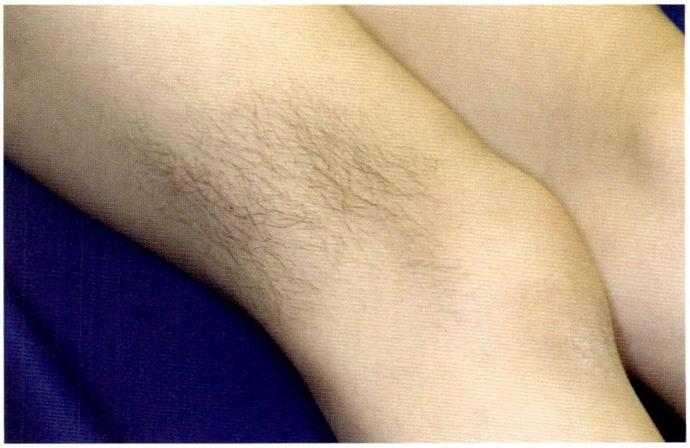

Fig. 7.57 Nevoid hypertrichosis. Isolated patch of hypertrichosis on the leg. (Courtesy Dr. Brandi Kenner-Bell.)

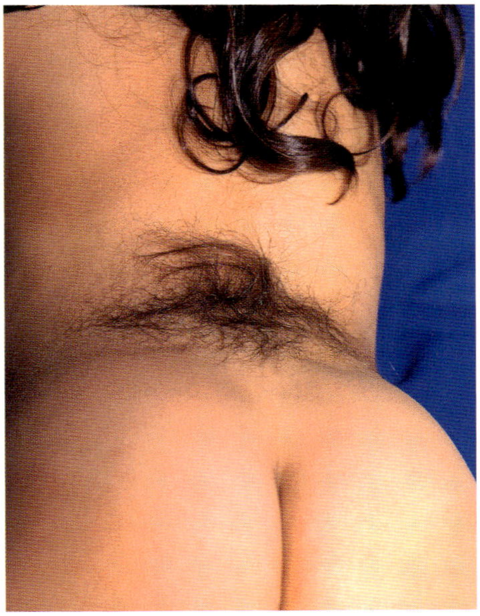

Fig. 7.58 Faun-tail deformity. Abnormal tufts of hair in the lumbosacral area suggest an underlying tethered cord or diastematomyelia.

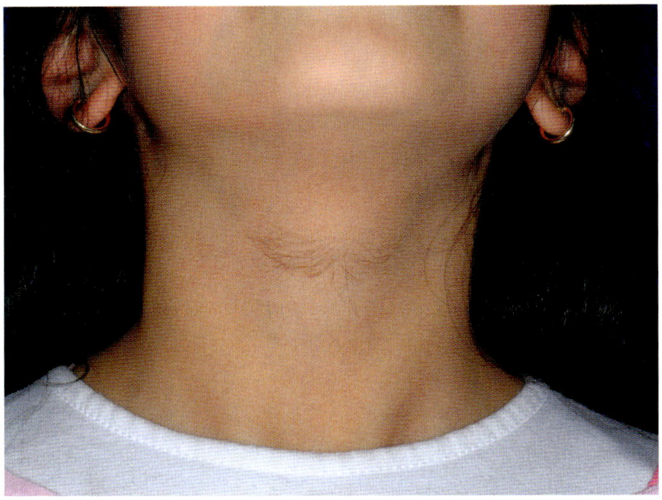

Fig. 7.59 Anterior cervical hypertrichosis. A form of nevoid hypertrichosis, this patch of hair at the anterior aspect of the neck is usually not associated with other pathology.

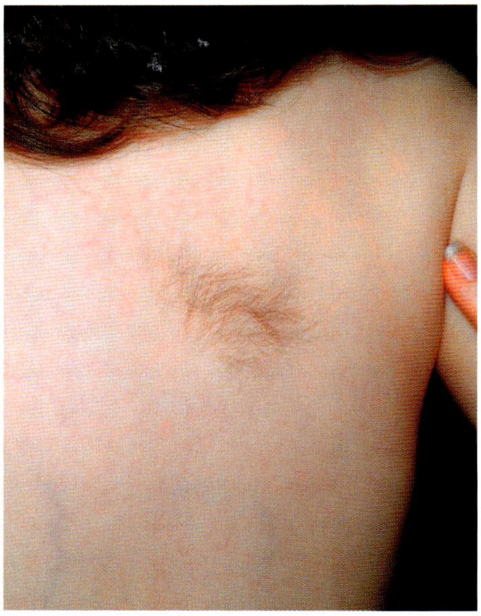

Fig. 7.60 Nevoid circumscribed hypertrichosis. This hair follicle hamartoma shows congenital growth of thicker, darker, and longer hairs without associated hyperpigmentation or associated follicular prominence.

abnormalities[630]; and hypertrichosis cubiti with short stature, facial asymmetry, intrauterine growth retardation, developmental and speech delay, and infantile spasms.[631]

Hypertrichosis is often a characteristic of melanocytic nevi, smooth muscle hamartomas and Becker nevus, plexiform neurofibromas, and linear epidermal nevus. Nevoid circumscribed hypertrichosis (Fig. 7.60), a hair follicle nevus, presents as an isolated patch of hypertrichosis. Increased local hair growth may be seen after wearing a cast or at sites of thrombophlebitis, stasis dermatitis, X-ray or ultraviolet light irradiation, chemical irritation, or local hormonal stimulation. Extensive congenital smooth muscle hamartomas may show hypertrichotic and skin-colored to lightly hyperpigmented patches in association with excessive skin folds and follicular dimpling (sometimes called *Michelin baby syndrome*).[632] Multiple patches of congenital hypertrichosis in association with blaschkoid streaks of hypopigmentation have spontaneously cleared shortly after birth.[633]

Symmetric, large, hypertrichotic, indurated hyperpigmented patches on the middle and lower body first appear during the first or second decade in autosomal recessive *H syndrome*.[634] In addition to hyperpigmentation and hypertrichosis, patients show hepatosplenomegaly, heart anomalies, hearing loss, hypogonadism, hallux valgus, low height, camptodactyly, and occasionally hyperglycemia. Mutations have been found in the nucleoside transporter hENT3, encoded by *SLC29A3*.[635]

Idiopathic Hirsutism

Idiopathic hirsutism describes the presence in girls of excessive body hair in a male sexual pattern (the face, particularly the upper lip; chest; abdomen; arms; and legs) in the absence of clinical evidence of disturbed endocrine or metabolic function (see Fig. 23.16).[636,637] Idiopathic hirsutism is assumed to relate to increased stimulation of the hair follicles of genetically predisposed girls by normal levels of androgenic hormones. Hirsutism is quantified by the Ferriman–Gallwey scale, with scores of 6 to 8 considered mildly hirsute, 8 to 15 serious, and greater than 15 overt hirsutism. Other signs of hyperandrogenism are acne, oligomenorrhea or amenorrhea, and AGA/FPHL.

The incidence of hirsutism in any population is difficult to assess, because the range of normal is quite wide and subject to individual acceptance and includes that which is not always socially acceptable in a particular culture. Hispanic, Jewish, and Welsh women in general have more hair than their counterparts of Northern European, Japanese, and Indian heritage. The physician should be cognizant of what is normal and acceptable to some individuals, yet unacceptable and a source of anguish to others. Performing a history and physical examination (including body mass index [BMI] and waist circumference) will determine the need for full endocrinologic investigation. When hirsutism is observed in a postpubertal girl without other signs of masculinity (receding hairline, deepening of the voice, or evidence of menstrual disturbance), endocrine disease is unlikely. When the disorder does not appear to be physiologic and particularly if associated with other signs of androgen excess or premature puberty (sexual hair before 8 years of age in girls), abnormalities of the pituitary, adrenals, and ovaries must be ruled out. These include "exaggerated adrenarche," late-onset congenital adrenal hyperplasia, virilizing tumors,[638,639] Cushing syndrome, hyperprolactinemia, acromegaly, Achard–Thiers (diabetes, hypertension, and hirsutism) syndrome, and *polycystic ovary syndrome* (PCOS)[640] (see Chapters 8 and 23).[641,642] Of these, PCOS is by far the most common and is increasing in prevalence in parallel to the increasing trend toward obesity in teenagers (3% of unselected adolescents in one study).[643]

In addition to signs of hyperandrogenism,[644] the presence of oligomenorrhea or amenorrhea and acanthosis nigricans are a clue to PCOS (see Chapter 23).[645] Oligomenorrhea is defined as menstrual cycles of more than 35 days, with fewer than eight menstrual cycles per year defined as chronic anovulation. It is harder to diagnose oligomenorrhea in adolescents, but persistent irregularity more than 2 years after the onset of menses should be considered abnormal. Obesity is a significant risk factor for PCOS, and 40% to 60% of women with PCOS are overweight or obese, especially with abdominal adiposity. PCOS commonly runs in families, and several genetic loci have been identified in GWAS studies,[646] including variants in *DENND1A*, which encodes connecdenn 1, a protein that regulates human ovarian androgen biosynthesis.[647]

If an endocrine abnormality is suspected, minimal laboratory testing for excessive androgen production should include levels of 17-ketosteroids (for mild adrenal hyperplasia), free plasma testosterone, dehydroepiandrosterone sulfate levels, and morning and evening cortisol; luteinizing hormone (LH) and follicle-stimulating hormone (FSH) ratios and transabdominal ultrasound (to rule out small ovarian cysts) may be useful. Hormonal evaluations are best carried out in the morning during the third to fifth day of menstruation. Criteria for diagnosis and testing for PCOS are reviewed in Chapter 23.

Treatment of Hypertrichosis and Hirsutism

The appearance of excessive hair may be modified in several ways.[636] Cutting with scissors or clipping close to the skin with hair trimmers, although occasionally not psychologically acceptable to the patient, are the simplest methods and least likely to irritate the skin. These techniques do not stimulate faster or thicker growth.[600] Bleaching with hydrogen peroxide may make excessive hair less conspicuous for up to 4 weeks and works best for light-skinned children, because yellow bleached hair may be emphasized when viewed against darkly pigmented skin. Plucking and wax epilation (essentially a form of widespread plucking) by application of a warm wax preparation to the affected areas are too painful for children but may be an option for older adolescents. Chemical depilatories that contain sulfides, thioglycolates, or enzymatic depilatory agents destroy the projecting hair shafts, causing minimal damage to underlying skin. Of these, the sulfide-containing preparations are more effective but more irritating and produce a disagreeable hydrogen sulfide odor. The thioglycolate-containing agents are less irritating but slower in action and less effective on coarse hairs. Enzymatic agents are less offensive but not as effective as other types. Children with extensive hypertrichosis must limit treatment with chemical depilatories to localized sites because of the risk of systemic absorption and toxic reactions. Eflornithine cream 15% is a prescription medication for twice-daily application that inhibits ornithine decarboxylase, a hair follicle enzyme that participates in hair growth. As a result, eflornithine may decrease further growth, although it does not minimize existing hair. Local irritation may occur.

Electrolysis and laser are more permanent hair removal techniques that are uncomfortable, and thus their use may be limited for prepubertal children. In electrolysis, an electric current is delivered to the hair follicle, destroying it. In contrast, laser and intense pulsed light remove unwanted hair through the selective photothermolysis of the melanin-rich hair follicles with minimal absorption by surrounding tissues.[648,649] Laser systems used for the treatment of hypertrichosis/hirsutism include the ruby laser (694 nm), the long-pulsed diode laser[650] (800 or 810 nm), the alexandrite laser (755 nm), and the Nd:YAG laser (1084 nm); broad-spectrum intense pulsed light (570 to 1200 nm) has also been used.[651] In one study comparing six treatments given at 1-month intervals of Nd:YAG laser vs. the intense pulsed light (755 nm), Nd:YAG was more effective and safer (less erythema and residual hyperpigmentation) than the intense pulsed light.[652] The diode, alexandrite, and Nd:YAG laser are safest for treatment of hirsutism in dark-skinned patients.[653,654] Application of topical anesthesia may be required. Treatment may require years for cosmetically acceptable results if hypertrichosis is generalized.

If an adolescent has hirsutism and hyperandrogenemia, therapy should be specific to the underlying trigger under the guidance of a gynecologist or endocrinologist. For example, dexamethasone 0.25 to 0.5 mg at night generally reverses the hyperandrogenic signs of adrenal hyperplasia.[655] For PCOS in adolescents, the most important intervention is lifestyle modification with increasing exercise and controlling dietary intake. In PCOS, loss of at least 10% of initial body weight improves menstrual function and metabolic abnormalities.[656] The administration of metformin or other insulin sensitizers is adjunctive to lifestyle changes but can improve insulin resistance, adiposity, oligomenorrhea, and serum androgen levels, as well as hirsutism.[657,658]

Antiandrogens and oral contraceptives are the traditional treatment for management of hirsutism. The combination of ethinyl estradiol and drospirenone, for example, reduces the Ferriman–Gallwey score in adolescents by approximately 50% over a 12-month period.[659] Spironolactone in doses of 50 to 200 mg/day; cyproterone acetate, 50 to 100 mg/day (available in Europe); and cimetidine have antiandrogenic activity. Intermittent low-dose finasteride (2.5 mg every 3 days) for 6 months has been shown to be effective in reducing the hirsutism score in teenaged girls with idiopathic or PCOS-related hirsutism.[660]

Pigmentary Changes of Hair

PREMATURE GRAYING

Graying of human hair is caused by a reduction in the activity of melanocytes within hair follicles. Premature graying of hair, termed *canities*, refers to a loss of color, especially of scalp hair, at an age earlier than that generally accepted as physiologic (before the age of 20 in whites and 30 in Blacks). It most commonly occurs in children with vitiligo or AA. Canities have also been described in children with pernicious anemia, hyperthyroidism and other thyroid disorders, progeria, Werner syndrome, ataxia-telangiectasia, Rothmund–Thomson syndrome, tuberous sclerosis, neurofibromatosis, and Waardenburg and Vogt–Koyanagi syndromes. There is a familial tendency toward developing premature graying in children who are otherwise healthy. Premature graying may be readily masked, if desired, by chemical rinses and dyes. Chloroquine interferes with pheomelanin synthesis and may lead to hair lightening with a silvery discoloration in blonde and red-haired persons.[661]

GREEN DISCOLORATION

The spontaneous appearance of green discoloration in the hair of light-haired individuals may occur as a result of exposure to copper used as an algae retardant in swimming pools or household tap water containing excessive amounts of copper.[662,663] The introduction of fluoride into a town water supply may acidify water and cause copper to be leached from the plumbing system. Sometimes a ground wire connects a faulty electric apparatus to the copper water pipes, thus diverting sufficient flow of electric current through the water system to dissolve copper.

If resulting from swimming, the use of a copper-based algicide should be discontinued. In cases related to household tap water, electric grounding of household plumbing and adjustment of the pH of the tap water will help prevent recurrences. Copper-induced discoloration of the hair can be treated in several ways: bleaching with 3% hydrogen peroxide for 2 to 3 hours, washing with the chelating agent edetic acid (EDTA-Metalex) for 30 minutes, use of a penicillamine-containing shampoo, or application of 1.5% 1-hydroxethyl diphosphonic acid.

Nails

The nails are convex horny structures originating from a matrix that develops from a groove formed by epidermal invagination on the dorsum of the distal phalanges at 9 weeks' gestation. At 10 weeks' gestation, a smooth, shiny quadrangular area can be recognized on the distal dorsal surface of each digit, and formation is completed by 20 weeks' gestation. The nail apparatus consists of a nail matrix of proliferating epidermal cells (Fig. 7.61), largely located under the proximal nailfold. In the thumbs and in a variable number of digits, a white crescent-shaped lunula is usually seen projecting from under the proximal nailfolds and represents the distal portion of the matrix. The cells of the lunula form the lower surface of the nail plate, whereas the more proximal matrix forms the exposed surface of the nail plate. Although the nail plate is translucent and essentially colorless, most of the exposed nail appears pink as the result of transmission of color from the adherent richly vascular underlying nail bed. The lateral borders of the nail plate lie under the edge of the lateral nailfolds. The hyponychium is the area of skin where the distal border of the nail plate becomes detached from the nail bed.

Unlike hair, nails grow continuously throughout life and normally are not shed. Although the nails of individual fingers grow at different rates, the normal rate of fingernail growth varies between 0.5 and 1.2 mm per week; the rate of toenail growth is slower than that of the fingernails. Nails grow more quickly in children than in adults.

Many nail disorders occur in children.[664] Dermatoses that characteristically involve the skin and hair may also affect the nails. Among these are atopic dermatitis, psoriasis, lichen planus, Darier disease, AA, onychomycosis, dyskeratosis congenita (DC) and other ectodermal dysplasias, and certain forms of epidermolysis bullosa.[665] Some nail deformities require surgical correction for cosmetic or functional improvement.[666]

MEDIAN NAIL DYSTROPHY AND HABIT-TIC DYSTROPHY

Median nail dystrophy (also termed *solenonychia* or *dystrophia unguium mediana canaliformis*) and *habit-tic dystrophy* (also termed *onychotillomania* or *habit-tic deformity*) are uncommon disorders that usually

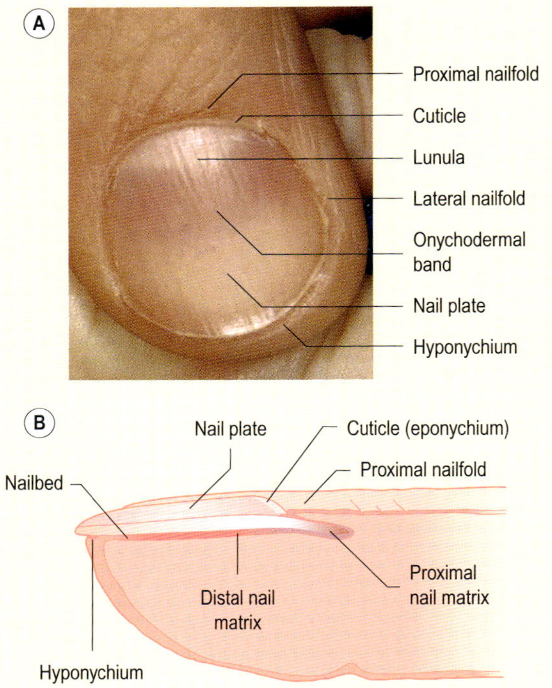

Fig. 7.61 **(A)** Visible structures of the nail. **(B)** Anatomic structure of the nail apparatus.

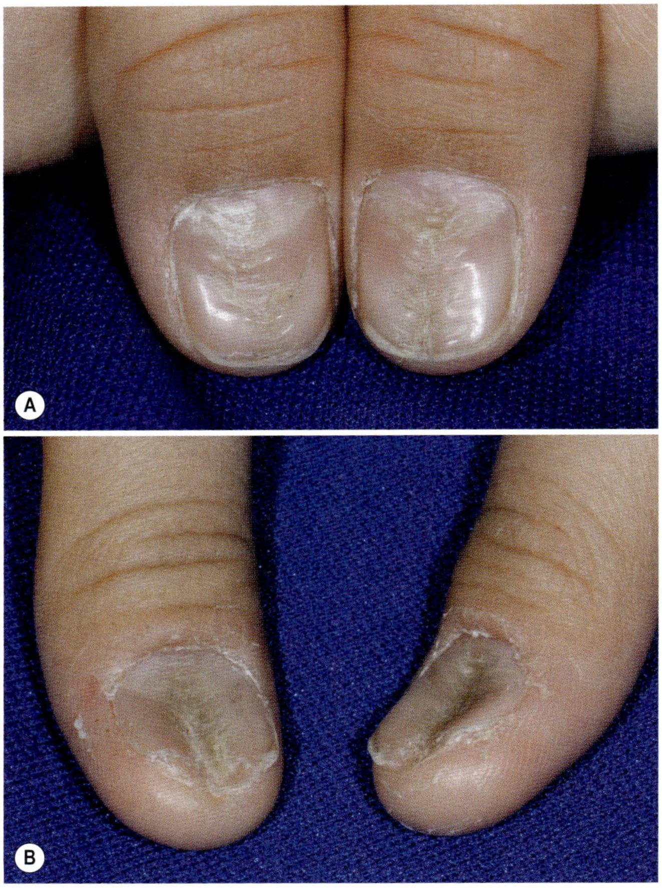

Fig. 7.62 Median nail dystrophy/habit-tic dystrophy. **(A)** and **(B)** Central depression to varying degrees and fir tree–like or irregularly spaced horizontal splits extending toward the lateral margins. Neither boy admitted to any trauma to the nail, although scaling and swelling of the periungual area can be seen in **(B)**.

affect the thumbs. Both disorders have a central canal-like depression or split of varying severity with cracks or lines extending from the central longitudinal lesion toward the lateral nail edges (Fig. 7.62). In median nail dystrophy the lines are typically described as feathery cracks resembling a Christmas tree, and in habit-tic dystrophy they are described as more horizontally arrayed and irregularly spaced; however, the two disorders can look identical, leading to their grouping by some experts as one disorder. A temporary defect in the matrix that interferes with nail formation is thought to be the cause, leading to the depression or split initially appearing at the cuticle and proceeding outward as the nail grows. Median nail dystrophy has been described during administration of isotretinoin,[667,668] during use of cryotherapy,[669] and with habitual use of smartphones and tablets,[670] whereas habit-tic dystrophy is commonly linked to continuous picking of the nail cuticle of the affected digit and has been described in association with guitar playing.[671] The disorder may improve spontaneously after years, especially after the causative trauma ceases. Other than avoidance of trauma, there is no effective treatment, although 4 months of tacrolimus 0.1% ointment led to significant improvement in a 19-year-old man with median nail dystrophy,[672] and 10 sessions of 1064-nm Nd:YAG laser caused improvement in an adult.[673] Injected triamcinolone acetonide and tazarotene have also been used with some success.

ONYCHOSCHIZIA

Lamellar splitting of the nail plate at its distal free edge, or *onychoschizia*, is a common complaint of girls and women. The condition usually results from repeated trauma, frequent exposure to nail polish, or excessive immersion in water with detergents. The defect is aggravated by excessive manicuring and the frequent use of solvents to remove nail polish, which further dehydrates the nail. The regular use of an emollient hand cream to the nail and its cuticles, the avoidance of excessive manipulation, the use of several layers of nail polish in an effort to splint the nail, and avoidance of all but oily polish removers are beneficial.

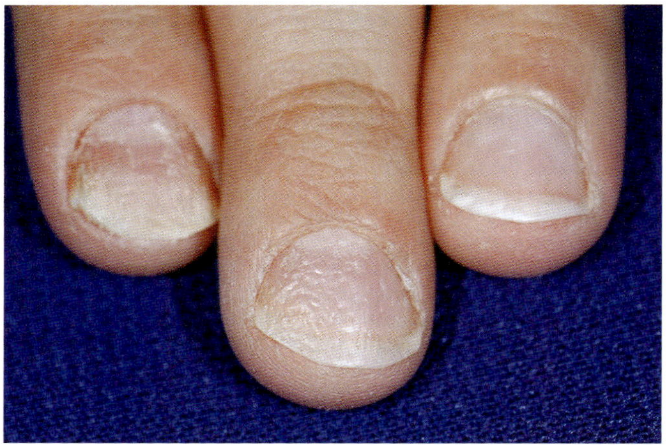

Fig. 7.63 Pitting. Nail pitting associated with psoriasis.

NAIL PITTING

Pitting of the nails is a common problem of children and most commonly is associated with the nail involvement of psoriasis (Fig. 7.63),[674] atopic dermatitis, or AA. Less common associations are lichen planus, vitiligo, reactive arthritis, and chronic renal failure. The punctate depressions result from alterations in the proximal matrix and may vary

Table 7.3 Associations with Nail Matrix Arrest

Conditions	Infection	Medications	Trauma
Acrodermatitis enteropathica	Coxsackie virus*	Antibiotics	Perinatal, often superimposed candida
Alopecia areata	Streptococcus	Antiseizure	Periungual
Amelogenesis imperfect	Syphilis	Chemotherapy	
Epidermolysis bullosa	*Trichophyton tonsurans*	Retinoids	
Febrile illness	Varicella	Nutritional deficiency	
Hypoparathyroidism	Kawasaki disease	Pemphigus vulgaris	
		Pemphigus vulgaris	
		Radiation therapy	
		Stevens–Johnson syndrome	
		Systemic lupus erythematosus	

*Most common cause.

from small to large and deep. One nail or several may be affected. Clustered pits may be seen in children who have experienced localized trauma, whereas shallow, randomly distributed pits are usually seen in children with psoriasis or atopic dermatitis. Transverse rows of regularly spaced pits have been described in children with AA (see Fig. 7.43, *A*). The pathomechanism for nail pits likely involves pinpoint areas of aberrant epidermis and inflammation of the nail matrix.

NAIL MATRIX ARREST (BEAU LINES AND ONYCHOMADESIS)

Nail matrix arrest develops as a nonspecific reaction to any stress that temporarily interrupts nail formation and becomes visible on the surface of the nail plate several weeks or more after onset of the disease that caused the condition. *Beau lines* are transverse grooves or furrows that originate under the proximal nailfold (Table 7.3). They first appear at the cuticle and move forward with the growth of the nail. Because normal nails grow at a rate of approximately 1 mm per week, the duration and time of the illness often can be estimated by the width of the furrow and its distance from the cuticle. *Onychomadesis* (proximal complete separation of the nail) results from full but temporary arrest of growth of the nail matrix (Fig. 7.64).[675,676] Triggers are similar for Beau lines and onychomadesis and involve stressful events (see Table 7.3) such as birth trauma,[677,678] chemotherapy and other drugs,[679,680] infections and febrile illnesses,[675,681,682] and prolonged intensive-care hospitalization.[683] Of these, nail matrix arrest after hand-foot-and-mouth disease (HFMD) from Coxsackie infection is most common in children.[675,684,685] Nail changes are typically seen 1 to 2 months after onset of the HFMD and lasts for approximately 4 weeks (range, 1 to 8 weeks).[684,686] Changes occur more often on fingernails than toenails and, if both are involved, tend to occur spontaneously. However, involvement of all toenails and fingernails is unusual. Onychomadesis has been described at birth. In all cases, the nail changes resolve spontaneously.[687]

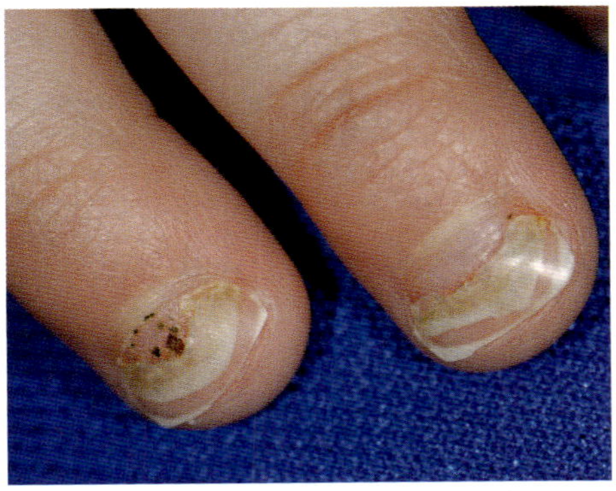

Fig. 7.64 Onychomadesis. Nails showed this deep transverse groove and nail separation.

SPOON NAIL

Spoon nail (*koilonychia*) is a common deformity in which the normal contour of the nail is lost. The nail is thin, depressed, and concave from side to side, with turned-up distal and lateral edges. Although the diagnosis is usually apparent, liquid will pool on the nail plate because of the concavity, leading to a positive "water drop" test.[688] Koilonychia of the hallucal nails is common in newborns and young infants and resolves spontaneously during childhood.

The condition may be a secondary feature of several dermatologic disorders. It occurs in association with nail thickening in psoriasis, onychomycosis, iron and other nutritional deficiencies, some cases of pachyonychia congenita (in which subungual thickening from the hyponychium changes the direction of nail growth), and trauma.[689] Koilonychia can also be seen in disorders with nail thinning or ridging, such as in lichen planus, trachyonychia, and focal dermal hypoplasia. Cases have been described in association with severe iron-deficiency anemia, although the pathomechanism is unclear. Koilonychia may also be inherited as an isolated autosomal dominant trait. Koilonychia can be confused with platyonychia, or flattened nails, which have been described primarily in patients with cirrhosis, and with pincer nails, characterized by excessive curvature at the lateral aspects of the nail plate, leading to an appearance of ingrown nails. Pincer nails are usually a congenital deformity but can be acquired in individuals with epidermolysis bullosa, digital epidermoid cysts, and distal phalangeal exostosis. Because they can be quite painful, pincer nails are often corrected surgically.

RACKET NAIL

Racket nails, or *brachyonychia*, are short, wide nails that show loss of curvature. Most commonly found on the thumb and halluces, racket nails are associated with short, stubby phalanges, presumably reflecting an arrest in distal phalangeal formation. This disorder may be inherited in an autosomal dominant mode as an isolated entity, but has been described in association with several pediatric syndromes such as acrodysostosis, acroosteolysis, cartilage–hair hypoplasia syndrome, Larsen syndrome, pyknodysostosis, and Rubinstein–Taybi syndrome.

Racket nails may be confused with *nail clubbing* or acropachy (Table 7.4), which results from overgrowth of the fibrovascular support stroma of the distal phalanx. Increased flexibility of the distal nail plate because of edematous tissue is an early sign of clubbing. Also typical is the angle greater than 180 degrees (Lovibond angle) formed by the proximal nailfold and nail plate when viewed from a lateral position. Clubbing in children is usually a sign of internal disease, but can be a component of a syndrome. An example is pachydermoperiostosis (also called *primary hypertrophic osteoarthropathy* [PHO]), an autosomal dominant or recessive disorder characterized by digital clubbing, periostosis, arthropathy, pachydermia, coarsening of facial features, hyperhidrosis, acne, seborrhea, and folliculitis (see Chapter 23). PHO results from mutations in either *HPGD*[690] or *SLCO2A1*.[691] These genes encode for a 15-hydroxyprostaglandin dehydrogenase and a prostaglandin transporter protein, respectively, and are responsible for degradation of

Table 7.4 Clubbing in Children

History	System	Disease
ACQUIRED		
Generalized	Pulmonary	Cystic fibrosis
		Bronchiectasis
		Tuberculosis, aspergillosis
		Asthma complicated by lung infections
		Sarcoidosis
		Pulmonary fibrosis
		Tumors
	Cardiovascular	Cyanotic congenital heart disease
		Subacute bacterial endocarditis
		Myxomas
	Gastrointestinal	Inflammatory bowel disease
		Gardner syndrome
		Parasitosis
		Cirrhosis
		Chronic active hepatitis
	Endocrine	Diamond syndrome (myxedema, exophthalmos, and clubbing)
		Hypervitaminosis A
		Malnutrition
Limited to one or more digits		Aortic/subclavian artery aneurism
		Brachial plexus injury
		Trauma
		Maffucci syndrome
		Gout
		Sarcoidosis
		Severe herpetic whitlow
Hereditary		Pachydermoperiostosis
		Familial, isolated
Pseudoclubbing*		Apert syndrome
		Pfeiffer syndrome
		Rubinstein–Taybi syndrome

Modified from Baran R, Dawber PR. *Diseases of the Nails and Their Management*. London, UK: Blackwell Scientific; 2001. Reprinted with permission from Schachner LA, Hansen RC, eds. *Pediatric Dermatology*. 4th ed. Edinburgh, Scotland: Mosby; 2011.

*Broad distal phalanges with normally shaped nails.

prostaglandin E2. Clubbing may also be the sole manifestation of mutations in *HPGD* (autosomal dominant) or *SLCO2A1* (autosomal recessive).[692]

TRACHYONYCHIA

Trachyonychia is characterized by excessive ridging, longitudinal grooves and striations, opalescent discoloration, a rough sandpaper-like quality of the nails, a tendency toward breakage and fragmentation (onychorrhexis), and splitting at the free margins[693,694] (Fig. 7.65). The condition was called *20-nail dystrophy* with involvement of all nails, but this term has fallen out of favor because not all trachyonychia[695] involves 20 nails (and because occasionally all 20 nails are affected by other dystrophic nail disorders). Trachyonychia has been described more in boys than girls,[696] with a peak age of occurrence between 3 and 12 years of age.

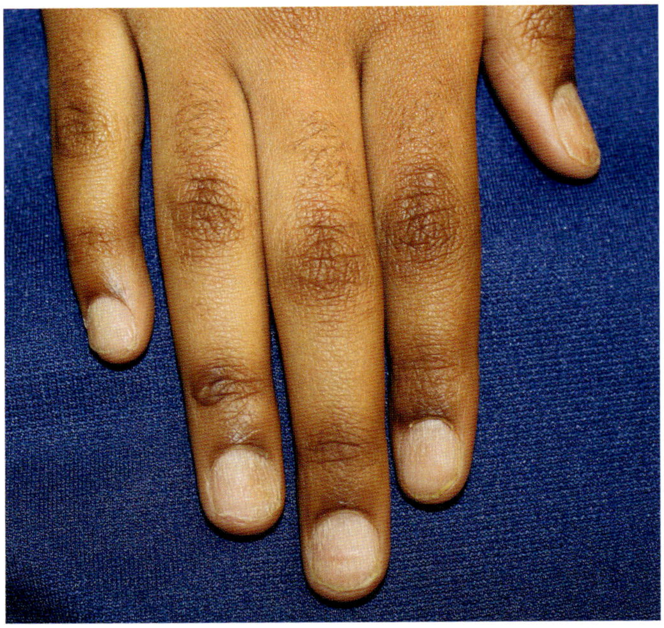

Fig. 7.65 Twenty-nail dystrophy (trachyonychia). Excessive ridging, longitudinal striations, and a rough texture of all 20 nails in an adolescent. Note the rough edges associated with the longitudinal striations.

Trachyonychia has been divided based on clinical appearance into two types: (1) opaque trachyonychia, the more severe type, which appears as nails that have been roughened by sandpaper, and (2) shiny trachyonychia, which is characterized by opalescent, shiny nails with numerous pits. Trachyonychia is usually an isolated entity but has been described commonly and primarily in association with psoriasis, atopic dermatitis, AA, and lichen planus. In fact, trachyonychia may occur months to years before other signs of cutaneous disease. The course of trachyonychia is variable, but spontaneous improvement may occur in months to years; in one study 82% showed total resolution or marked improvement in a mean period of 66 months,[697] suggesting that observation is an appropriate intervention.[698] Application of potent topical corticosteroids to the base of the nail, particularly in the form of flurandrenolide tape, may reverse the changes of trachyonychia after several months of nightly usage. Tazarotene gel application and betamethasone dipropionate ointment, applied for 3 to 6 months[699] to the nail base, have also been used. Filing the nails and application of clear nail polish may reduce the tendency toward snagging and tearing of the nail plates.

ONYCHOGRYPHOSIS

Onychogryphosis is a hypertrophic nail deformity most commonly seen in the toenails. Some cases of nail hypertrophy are developmental. The nails become thick and circular in cross-section instead of flat (thus resembling a claw). The disorder is most commonly seen in elderly individuals but may occur in children with poor hygiene. Management requires regular paring or trimming and, when severe, treatment by a podiatrist using files, nail clippers, or mechanical burrs. Onychogryphosis is commonly associated with secondary onychomycosis but may be seen in a variety of forms of ichthyosis, such as Haim–Munk syndrome (see Chapter 5) and in severe epidermolysis bullosa simplex (see Chapter 13).

CONGENITAL MALALIGNMENT OF THE GREAT TOENAILS

Congenital malalignment of the great toenails is a disorder in which lateral rotation of the nail matrix leads to lateral deviation of the great toenail from the longitudinal axis of the distal phalanx and, at times,

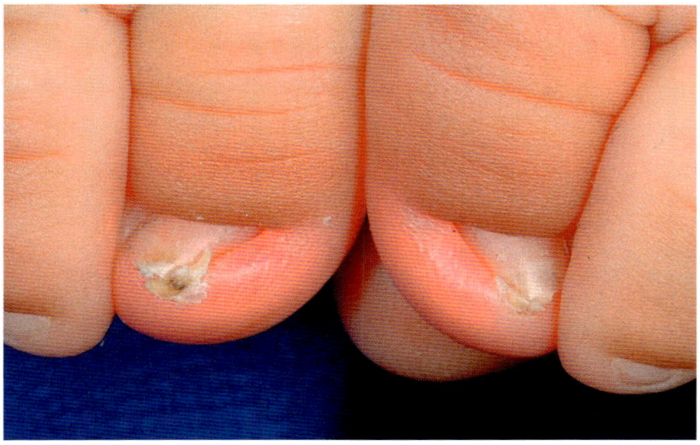

Fig. 7.66 Congenital malalignment of the great toenails. Lateral rotation of the nail matrix leads to lateral deviation of the great toenail from the longitudinal axis of the distal phalanx and, at times, thickening, discoloration, and shortening of the nail plate. Note the secondary severely ingrown toenails and overgrowth of the medial nailfold.

thickening, discoloration, and shortening of the nail plate (Fig. 7.66).[700,701] Resultant onychodystrophy may lead to onychogryphosis and chronic ingrown toenails. Paronychia can be associated.[702] The disorder may be inherited as an autosomal dominant disorder[703] and often improves spontaneously.[704] Usually a condition present in infancy and early childhood, later onset in teenage years has been described.[705] If improvement is not seen during the first year and the deviation is severe, surgical realignment of the nail with local anesthesia can be performed, preferably before age 2 years.[666]

INGROWN NAILS

Ingrown toenail *(onychocryptosis)* is a common disorder in which the lateral edge of the nail is curved inward and penetrates the underlying tissue with resulting erythema, edema, pain, and in chronic forms, the formation of granulation tissue. Generally seen on the great toes of affected individuals, the main cause of the deformity is compression of the toe from side to side by ill-fitting footwear and improper cutting of the nail (in a half-circle rather than straight across). The pseudo-ingrown toenail, also seen as a transient deformity in newborns, is a common phenomenon (2.4% of infants)[706] and generally self-corrects by the time the child reaches the age of 12 months. Treatment, if required, consists of wearing properly fitting footwear, allowing the nail to grow out beyond the free edge, control of acute infection by compresses, topical and at times systemic antibiotics, and, in many instances (once the infection has subsided), surgical treatment. The traditional therapy for recurring cases has been excision of the lateral aspect of the nail (wedge resection) with the use of local anesthesia followed by curettage or chemical destruction of the nail matrix to prevent regrowth of the offending portion of the nail.[707–709] Although phenol and sodium hydroxide have traditionally been used for chemical destruction, these techniques tend to lead to extensive tissue destruction with delayed healing. Partial avulsion with 90% bichloroacetic acid has been suggested as an effective but safer technique.[710] An alternative technique using a flexible tube secured with a suture (FTSS) was associated with a lower recurrence rate than matricectomy and faster recovery.[711] However, two simpler techniques are particularly useful in children. Excellent cosmesis has been achieved with few to no recurrences[712] by simply excising the nailfold itself rather than the matrix.[713] In addition, the slit tape–strap procedure can be used as adjunctive or monotherapy, in which the slit in an elastic tape is fitted around the nail, lifting the nail edges. Pain was reduced in an average of 5 days, with cure in approximately 21 weeks and recurrence in less than 10% after treatment.[714]

Retronychia refers to inflammation of the proximal nailfold and occurs when the new nail growing from the matrix pushes the old nail upwards, interrupting the longitudinal nail and embedding the nail plate into the proximal nailfold. It usually results from trauma and can be treated initially in children with clobetasol ointment nightly for a few months. Alternative therapy for recalcitrant or recurrent retronychia is complete nail-plate avulsion, although permanent nail dystrophy results in approximately one-third of treated patients.[715,716]

NAIL ATROPHY

Atrophic nails range from complete absence of the nail (anonychia) to nails that are poorly or partially developed (micronychia). Congenital anonychia is an autosomal recessive disorder characterized by isolated congenital anonychia or hypoplasia, usually of all the fingernails and toenails. The disorder results from mutations in the R-spondin 4 (*RSPO4*) gene, which is only expressed in the mesenchymal tissue underlying the digit tip epithelium and activates Wnt/β-catenin signaling.[717,718] Anonychia can be associated with junctional epidermolysis bullosa, trauma, infectious paronychia, and inflammation (e.g., Stevens–Johnson syndrome, chronic graft-versus-host disease, and lichen planus). Micronychia has been described in patients with ectodermal dysplasias, teratogen exposure (e.g., fetal hydantoin syndrome), and chromosomal abnormalities (e.g., Turner syndrome; Noonan syndrome; and trisomies of chromosomes 3, 8, 13, and 18). Micronychia is a prominent feature of nail–patella syndrome and congenital onychodysplasia of the index fingers (COIF).

NAIL–PATELLA SYNDROME

Nail–patella syndrome, also termed *osteoonychodysplasia*, is an autosomal dominant disorder that results from mutations in *LMX1B*.[719–721] *LMX1B* encodes a transcription factor (LIM homeobox) that regulates dorsoventral polarity in the developing limb (including nail development), as well as bone, eye, and glomerular basement-membrane development.[722,723] Genetic heterogeneity has been suspected, given that some families do not have linkage or mutations in *LMX1B*.[724]

Nail changes are seen in 98% of affected individuals.[725,726] They vary from a triangular lunula (most consistent feature), especially of the thumbs and index fingers, to severe dysplasia and micronychia, to absence of the medial and distal aspects of the index and thumb nails.[727] Median nail defects can be seen, especially with more severe nail involvement; these can range from a longitudinal crease or fracture to pseudopterygium.[728] Nail involvement is symmetric and often shows progression from the index to fifth fingernails. Occasionally the toes are affected. Softening, spooning, discoloration, central grooving, splitting and cracking, narrowing, and less commonly, thickening of nails have been described.

The knees have a flattened profile with a small or absent patella, and the elbows show radial head dysplasia. Both are subject to recurrent dislocation, flexion contractures, and arthritis. The pathognomonic iliac horns extend from the center of the iliac bones. Renal involvement occurs in 30% to 60% of patients and presents with (often asymptomatic) proteinuria and/or microscopic hematuria, edema, and hypertension. Progression to nephrotic syndrome occurs in less than 20% of patients, and renal failure requiring dialysis or transplantation occurs in 10%.[729] Affected patients also risk the development of glaucoma and dystrophic dental enamel. An increased risk of ADHD and depression has been described, perhaps related to the role of *LMX1B* in the development of mesencephalic dopaminergic neurons and the serotonergic system.[730] Support groups are available at www.npsw.org and www.npsuk.org.

CONGENITAL ONYCHODYSPLASIA OF THE INDEX FINGERS

COIF, also known as *Iso and Kikuchi syndrome*, is characterized by asymmetric, ulnar-deviated micronychia of the index fingers. Involvement may be unilateral or bilateral, and polyonychia may be associated. X-rays of the underlying phalangeal bone show a characteristic Y-shaped bifurcation or a sharp distal phalangeal tip. Deformities of other fingers are rarely present.[731] Usually a sporadic condition, autosomal dominant inheritance and occurrence in twins have been described.[732]

PACHYONYCHIA CONGENITA

PC describes a group of autosomal dominant conditions characterized by characteristic nail dystrophy in association with painful plantar keratoderma (see Chapter 5).[733] Mutations occur in one of five keratins: *KRT6a, KRT6b, KRT6c, KRT16*, and *KRT17*,[734–738] and classification is based on the underlying affected gene (i.e., PC-6a, PC-6b, PC-6c, PC-16, and PC-17). Of these, PC-6a (41%) and PC-16 (31%) are the most common. The historical terms *PC-1* (Jadassohn–Lewandowsky syndrome) and *PC-2* (Jackson–Lawlor syndrome) are no longer used, given their overlapping features and lack of concordance with underlying gene changes. At this time, genotyping is being performed free of charge through the Pachyonychia Congenita Project (www.pachyonychia.org). Recent studies have focused on dysregulated inflammation and oxidative stress as key mechanisms underlying the associated keratolysis and plantar pain.

At birth, fingernail and toenail changes are present in almost 70% and 60% of patients, respectively (Fig. 7.67), but the plantar keratoderma is in only 7% (see Chapter 5, Fig. 5.36, C). By 5 years of age, however, more than 75% of patients have toenail and fingernail dystrophy, as well as plantar keratoderma. Ultimately, 98% of affected individuals show toenail dystrophy, and fingernail dystrophy occurs in 76%. A late-onset form is unusual,[739] and most previously reported cases have not had genotyping to confirm the diagnosis.

Typical nails have marked subungual hyperkeratosis with a pinched V-shape, but premature nail termination is common. Most individuals have dystrophic changes of all 10 toenails, but the hallucal nails are most often affected (Fig. 7.68). Periungual infection (especially staphylococcal and candidal) is reported by most affected individuals, and nails may be shed. The keratoderma tends to be predominantly at pressure points, but can be exquisitely painful with a profound impact on quality of life and functioning (see Chapter 5, Fig. 5.36, C). The pain in part results from underlying bullae.[740] Hyperhidrosis of the palms and soles may be associated.

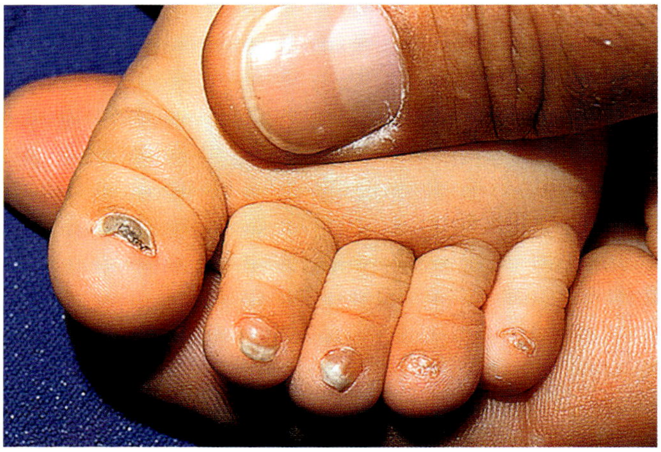

Fig. 7.67 Pachyonychia congenita. The nails may be thickened or discolored at birth but often show changes first on the toenails and during infancy.

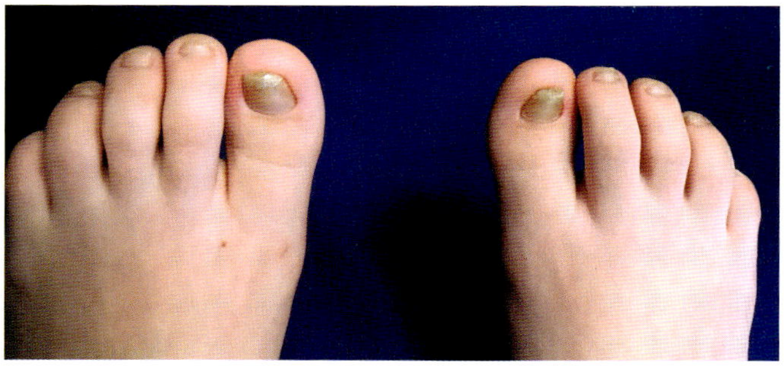

Fig. 7.68 Pachyonychia congenita. Only the hallucal nails were involved in this 4-year-old without fingernail changes but with extensive small cysts on the face and trunk.

Additional clinical manifestations include cysts, follicular keratoses, hoarseness, and oral leukoplakia. The steatocysts and pilosebaceous cysts, formerly thought to be specific to PC-6b and PC-17, are now known to be common in PC-6a as well. These cysts usually first manifest at early puberty, particularly on the head, neck, upper chest, and upper arms. Pinhead-sized follicular papules may appear in areas of trauma on the extensor surfaces of the extremities, popliteal fossae, lumbar region, buttocks, and less commonly, on the face and scalp. Early oral lesions are often present in the form of opaque white plaques (leukokeratosis) on the dorsum of the tongue or the buccal mucosa at the interdental line and are often confused with thrush (candidal infection) in the infant. Less common associated findings include cheilitis, scrotal tongue, corneal dystrophy, and hoarseness, the latter specific for PC-6a.

Differences that distinguish PC subtypes include (1) later onset and less frequent occurrence of nail dystrophy and keratoderma in PC-K6b, PC-K6c, and PC-K16; (2) concurrent fingernail and toenail thickening in PC-K6a and PC-K17; (3) more palmar (vs. plantar) keratoderma in PC-K16; (4) cysts primarily in PC-K17 and follicular hyperkeratoses primarily in PC-K6a; (5) hoarseness and/or oral leukokeratoses in the first year of life, most often in PC-K6a; and (6) natal teeth exclusively in PC-K17. Among pediatric patients, PC affects the social interactions and function of adolescents more profoundly than younger children, related to the highly visible nail changes and painful plantar thickening.

In the young child, PC must be distinguished from HED (Clouston syndrome), which can show similar nail alterations at birth and painful keratoderma.[741] The presence of hypotrichosis can distinguish HED. Indeed, alopecia is not a feature of PC except in the rare situation in which biallelic mutations in *KRT17* are inherited.[742] Hypertrophic nail dystrophy at birth is also a feature of biallelic mutations in *FZD6*, encoding frizzled 6, a Wnt-signaling pathway receptor in the nail matrix.[743,744]

The subungual hyperkeratosis persists for life, and treatment is directed toward relief of the painful hyperkeratosis of the soles and the nail dystrophy.[745] Mechanical nail treatment (filing, grinding, and trimming) is particularly effective after soaking the nails.[746] Mechanical intervention can also improve the keratoderma, but topical agents (retinoids, steroids, keratolytics, emollients) are not very helpful, and pain control management is key. Administration of systemic retinoids has been successful for some, but not all, patients and is rarely appropriate in pediatric patients.[747] As a last resort, surgical avulsion and matrix destruction followed by scarification of the nail bed to prevent regrowth can be performed. Toenail regrowth is less than fingernails, but in one study of 81 toenails with known fate removed using a variety of techniques from individuals with PC, including children, 43% never regrew and 34% partially regrew.[748] Plantar sweating has been shown to increase the painful blistering at hyperkeratotic sites and can be controlled by oral administration of glycopyrrolate or injections of botulinum toxin.[749]

The pain of PC feet is the most debilitating issue and can profoundly affect quality of life. The pain is chronic and has been described as throbbing and stabbing, especially during weight bearing. The majority of patients have hyperalgesia, static allodynia, and tingling[750] at sites of pain, suggesting the medications used for neuropathic pain may be of value. *K16* small interfering ribonucleic acid (siRNA) injections into the palmoplantar keratoderma have resulted in clearance, but are too painful to sustain.[751] Oral rapamycin decreased painful plantar thromboses and keratoses in patients with *K6a* mutations (based on suppression of *K6a* expression), but led to unacceptable gastrointestinal and mucocutaneous adverse events.[752] A pilot study of topical rapamycin for plantar surfaces was promising,[753] and a larger trial is ongoing. Interestingly, chemotherapy in an adult with lifelong painful plantar keratoderma led to complete resolution.[754] A support group is available for affected families (www.pachyonychia.org).

DYSKERATOSIS CONGENITA

Dyskeratosis congenita (DKC) may be inherited as X-linked recessive, autosomal dominant, or autosomal recessive, and pathogenic variants

Table 7.5 The 11 Genes Mutated in Dyskeratosis Congenita

Gene	Protein	Inheritance	Frequency (%)
DKC1	Dyskerin	XLR	17–36
TINF2	TIN2: TRF1-interacting nuclear factor 2	AD*	11–24
TERC/hTR	TERC: telomerase RNA component	AD	6–13
TERT	TERT: telomerase	AD, AR	1–17
ACD	Adrenocortical dysplasia protein homolog	AD, AR	<1
RTEL1	Replication of telomere	AD, AR	<1
CTC1	CTS telomere replication complex component 1	AR	<1
NHP2	NOLA2: nuclear protein family A, member 2	AR	<1
NOP10	NOLA3: nuclear protein family member A, 3	AR	<1
WRAP53/ TCAB1	WD repeat-containing protein encoding RNA antisense to p53	AR	<1
PARN	Poly(A)-specific ribonuclease	AR	<1

AD, Autosomal dominant; *AR*, autosomal recessive; *RNA*, ribonucleic acid; *XLR*, X-linked recessive.
*DKC associated with *TINF2* variants has been reported to occur as AD or *de novo*.

have been described in 11 genes altogether to date, accounting for 70% of studied individuals with DKC (Table 7.5).[755–757] The protein products of these genes affect the maintenance of telomeres, which are repetitive base pairs at the ends of chromosomes. Telomeres "cap" and protect the ends of chromosomes to prevent the DNA damage checkpoint machinery from recognizing chromosome ends as double-stranded DNA breaks (DSBs) that require recombination. The risk of telomere shortening and failure to protect is unstable chromosomes, increased cell cycle arrest and apoptosis, and the development of cancer. The enzyme telomerase synthesizes new telomere repeat DNA onto existing ends and includes the catalytic subunit TERT, the RNA template component TERC, and other factors. Of note, however, telomere abnormalities can occur in tissues without telomerase, such as in Werner syndrome (see Chapter 6), in which loss of a DNA helicase causes abnormalities in mesenchymal tissues (dermis, adipose tissue, bone) with little or no telomerase.

Prevention of senescence and apoptosis is particularly important in rapidly dividing cells. DKC is considered a "telomeropathy" because most patients show severe shortening of telomeres. Mutations causing these diseases are in genes encoding factors that support the ability of telomerase to extend telomere ends (*DKC1, TINF2, TERT, TERC/hTR, NOP10* encoding NOLA3, *NHP2* encoding NOLA2, *WRAP53/TCAB1, PARN, ACD,* and *POT1*), as well as encoding factors that may play more complicated roles in telomere replication (*CTC1, STN1,* and *RTEL1*). The most common cause of DKC is mutations in *DKC1* (a gene on the X chromosome that encodes dyskerin, a nucleolar protein that stabilizes telomerase). Although DKC is sometimes classified among disorders of aging, patients do not appear old and have no increased risk of atherosclerosis.

DKC is characterized most commonly by nail dystrophy (75%), reticular pigmentation (55%), and oral leukoplakia (55%)[757] (Table 7.6). However, in a study of 60 patients, all three features of the triad were only seen in 37% of patients, and 10% (all of whom had milder autosomal dominant forms) had none of the features of this triad.[758] The thin, dystrophic nails usually appear first between the ages of 5 and 13 years. Mildly affected nails show ridging and longitudinal grooving; severely affected nails are shortened and show pterygium formation, resembling the nails of lichen planus or graft-versus-host disease (Fig. 7.69). Cutaneous changes usually develop after the onset of nail changes, most commonly during late childhood to teenage years. A fine reticulated grayish-brown hyperpigmentation, sometimes surrounding hypopigmented, atrophic, telangiectatic patches on the face, neck, shoulders, upper back, and thighs, is characteristic (Fig. 7.70). The poikilodermatous change is sometimes confused with Rothmund–Thomson syndrome (*RECQL4* mutations), epidermolysis bullosa simplex with mottled pigmentation (usually *KRT5* mutation), Naegeli–Franceschetti–Jadassohn syndrome/dermatopathia pigmentosa reticularis (*KRT14* mutation), or Clericuzio-type poikiloderma with neutropenia (another *C16orf57* mutation).[759] Mucous membrane changes consist of leukoplakia and, rarely, blisters and erosions of the oral (Fig. 7.71) and anal mucosae, esophagus, and urethra. Similar changes of the tarsal conjunctiva may result in atresia of the lacrimal ducts, excessive lacrimation, chronic blepharitis, conjunctivitis, and ectropion. The teeth tend to be defective and subject to early decay. Periodontitis may develop, and affected persons have an increased incidence of cutaneous malignancy, predominantly squamous cell carcinoma in the areas of leukoplakia.

Other mucocutaneous changes may include epiphora (>30%), dermatoglyphic changes, early graying of the hair, palmoplantar hyperkeratosis, and hyperhidrosis. The hair of the scalp, eyebrows, and eyelashes is often sparse and lusterless. Unusual changes are bullae of the palms and soles; wrinkled atrophic skin over the elbows, knees, and penis; and a diffuse atrophic, transparent, and shiny appearance on the dorsal aspects of the hands and feet. Patients commonly have atrophy of the muscles and bones of the feet and hands, giving a "cupped" appearance to the palms.[760–762]

Most cases have been in males, consistent with an X-linked disorder, but carrier females may show mild to complete clinical features. The median age of diagnosis is 15 years, because many patients first seek treatment as teens or young adults.Overall, approximately 90% of patients develop life-threatening bone marrow failure characterized by severe aplastic anemia with neutropenia, splenomegaly, and a hemorrhagic diathesis. The risk of developing bone marrow failure correlates with having more of the triad features[758] and more mucocutaneous features overall. However, a 3-year-old presented with bone marrow failure and only nail dystrophy.[763] Acute myeloid leukemia and myelodysplastic syndrome have also been described. Pulmonary fibrosis and hepatic cirrhosis are other life-threatening complications. Epithelial tumors often first develop by the mid-teens, commonly in areas of mucosa with leukoplakia. Squamous cell carcinoma of the tongue is most common, but cutaneous squamous cell carcinoma, acute myeloid leukemia, and myelodysplastic syndrome are not uncommon.

Variants of DKC include Hoyeraal–Hreidarsson syndrome, which is DKC with cerebellar hypoplasia, developmental delay, and intrauterine growth retardation,[764] and Revesz syndrome with bilateral exudative retinopathy, cerebellar hypoplasia, and growth retardation.[765] Multiple features of DKC, including nail dystrophy and abnormal skin pigmentation, are seen in patients with poikiloderma with neutropenia (primarily mutations in *USB1*) and ectodermal dysplasia/short stature syndrome[766] (*GRHL2*). The genes affected in these disorders encode products that are also implicated in telomere maintenance and DNA repair pathways. Absent dermatoglyphics with nail dystrophy can be a feature of SMARCAD syndrome (SMARCAD1-associated congenital facial milia, adermatoglyphia, reduced sweating, contractures, acral bullae and dystrophy of nails), an autosomal dominant disorder that includes a spectrum from the group formerly designated as Basan syndrome (most typically with the adermatoglyphia, milia, and neonatal acral bullae) to autosomal dominant adermatophyphia with hypohidrosis.[767]

Screening for DKC is best performed by flow cytometry and fluorescence *in situ* hybridization (flow-FISH) of leukocyte subsets[763] to detect telomere shortening. The average life expectancy is 44 years. Patients

Table 7.6 Findings, Complications of Dyskeratosis Congenita and Suggested Monitoring

System	Findings	Potential Complications	Monitoring/Treatment
Skin	Nail dystrophy* Reticulated pigmentation* Hyperhidrosis Early graying or sparse hair Telangiectasia Acrocyanosis Cutaneous atrophy Palmoplantar keratoderma Absent dermatoglyphics	Cutaneous SCCs	Annual skin examination Sun protection
Oral	Leukoplakia* Erythematous patches Dyspigmentation Taurodontism Tooth decay and loss	Oral cancer	Biannual dental examinations
Growth and development	Short stature Developmental delay		
Head and neck		SCC	Annual otolaryngology examinations
Eyes	Epiphora Ectropion, entropion Trichiasis, sparse lashes	Corneal abrasion Infections	Annual eye examinations
Gastrointestinal	Esophageal stenosis Hepatic fibrosis	Dysphagia	Esophageal dilatation Annual liver function tests Liver ultrasounds
Genitourinary	Urethral stenosis Epithelial malignancy		
Lungs	Pulmonary fibrosis	High risk with transplant	Annual PFTs
Bones	Osteoporosis Avascular necrosis hips, shoulder	Fractures	Ca^{++}, vitamin D_3
Hematologic	Low blood counts*	Bone marrow failure* Myelodysplastic syndrome Leukemia	Biannual blood counts Baseline bone marrow Chemotherapy as appropriate

Ca^{++}, Calcium; *PFT*, pulmonary function test; *SCC*, squamous cell carcinoma.
*Present in more than 75% of patients.

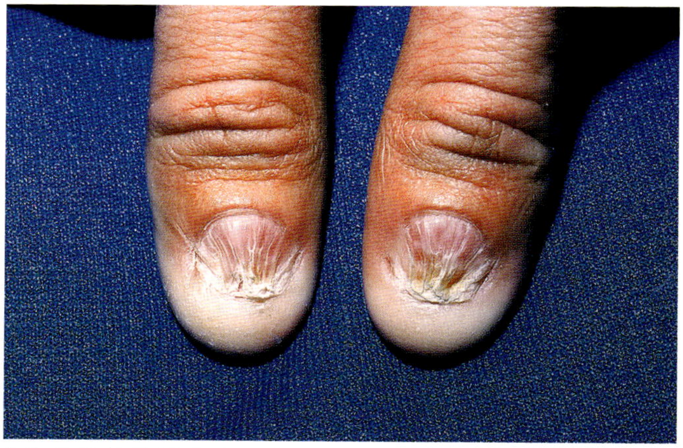

Fig. 7.69 Dyskeratosis congenita. Shortened nails with pterygium formation.

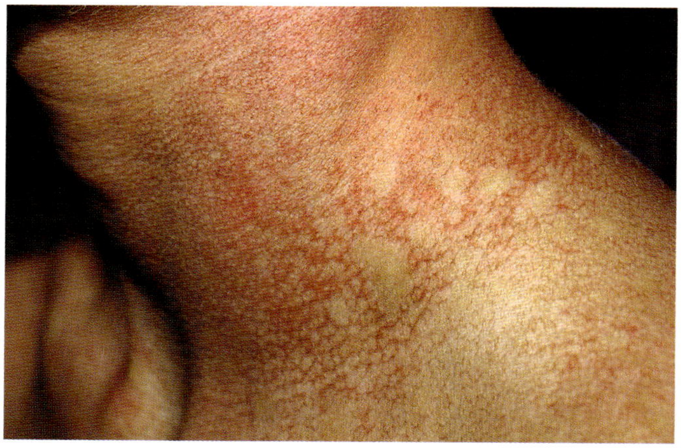

Fig. 7.70 Dyskeratosis congenita. Reticulated hyperpigmentation surrounding hypopigmented, atrophic, telangiectatic patches.

usually die of bone marrow failure (≈60% to 70%), pulmonary disease (≈10% to 15%), or malignancy (≈10%). Recommended disease surveillance includes biannual blood counts, bone marrow evaluations annually, hepatic ultrasounds, annual pulmonary functional tests, and skin cancer screening. Treatment of bone marrow failure is recommended with a hemoglobin persistently below 8 g/dL, platelets less than 30,000/mm^3, and neutrophils less than 1000/mm^3. If a matched donor without genetic and clinical evidence of DKC is available, stem cell transplantation should be considered but carries substantial risk. The 10-year survival rate probability is 30%, with mortality generally attributed to pulmonary or hepatic fibrotic or vascular complications related to disease progression or toxicity related to myeloablative regimens, even reduced-intensity conditioning.[768,769] Long-term survival after transplantation has been poor.

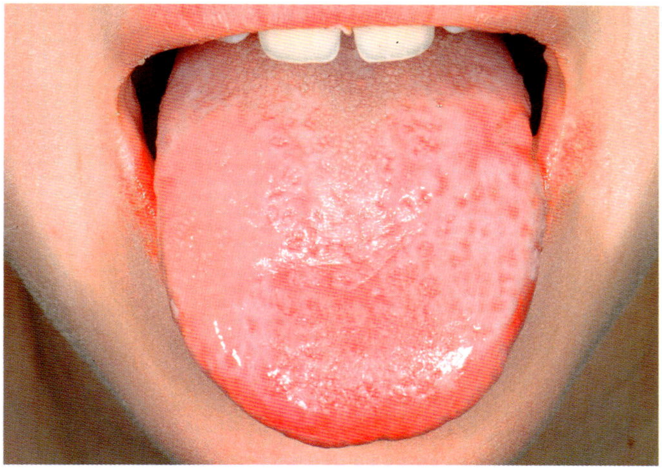

Fig. 7.71 Dyskeratosis congenita. Leukoplakia of the oral mucosa.

Lung transplantation should be considered for those with pulmonary fibrosis. A trial of androgens such as oxymetholone may be considered before transplantation from an unrelated donor and has improved blood counts in 60% of treated patients[770]; however, androgens may cause hepatic tumors, and the combination of androgen and granulocyte colony–stimulating factor (G-CSF) has led to splenic rupture. Management of patients otherwise consists of bougienage for esophageal stenosis; fulguration, curettage, and surgical excision of leukokeratosis of the buccal and anal mucosae; and lifelong, regular supervision for early detection of mucosal or cutaneous carcinomas.

DISORDERS OF THE NAIL BED

Onycholysis refers to separation of the nail plate from the underlying hyponychium and can occur for a wide variety of reasons (Box 7.9).[771,772] Vigorous cleaning of the subungual debris that tends to accumulate exacerbates this condition. Onycholysis may result from exposure to sunlight (photoonycholysis)[773] in individuals administered tetracyclines, especially doxycycline (see Fig. 8.16),[774] griseofulvin,[775] thiazides, or voriconazole.[776]

Abnormalities of the nail bed may be seen through the transparent nail plate. Onycholysis that occurs proximal to the hyponychium may resemble a yellow-brown oil spot, a nail change that is considered pathognomonic of psoriasis but is rarely seen in children. Notching of the distal nail plate may be seen in Darier disease in association with longitudinal red and white streaks (Fig. 7.72) (see Disorders of Nail Coloration section and Chapter 5). Nail bed hemorrhages are usually the result of trauma. As the hemorrhage ages, it changes color from red to purple to brown and moves more distally. Larger hematomas may resemble melanocytic nevi, although more commonly melanocytic nevi of the nail bed manifest as longitudinal pigmented streaks of the nail.

Injuries to fingers or toes may result in nail avulsion, painful subungual hematoma, or nail bed laceration, which are often managed in the emergency room. Nail bed removal results in scarring and deformity and is generally not necessary when the nail plate is intact and well adherent, especially with just a minimally displaced underlying distal phalanx fracture.[777] Hematomas should be decompressed through trephining, in which a hole is created in the nail plate by electrocautery or rotating a hot paperclip to drain the blood, thereby reducing pain and pressure.[778] Nail bed lacerations are repaired with 6-0 sutures or octyl-2-cyanoacrylate.[779,780]

PARONYCHIA

Paronychia refers to inflammation surrounding the nail, generally after breakdown in the barrier between the nail plate and the adjacent nailfold.[781,782] At times, the cuticle is obscured, and the nailfold is replaced by granulation tissue. Acute paronychia, characterized by painful, erythematous, indurated swelling of the proximal or lateral nailfolds, often with purulent draining, is usually caused by *S. aureus* infection; bacterial cultures can be performed to consider a bacterial etiology (see Chapter 14). Abscesses associated with acute staphylococcal infections may spontaneously decompress or may require drainage and local wound care along with a course of appropriate antibiotics. Chronic paronychia with nail dystrophy presenting with nonpurulent erythema of the periungual areas, nail ridging, and cuticle loss is more commonly due to candidal infection. Candidal

Box 7.9 Underlying Causes of Onycholysis

Chemical Irritants

Cosmetics, especially with formaldehyde
Depilatories
Detergents
Nail polish removers
Organic solvents

Inflammatory Disorders

Alopecia areata
Atopic dermatitis
Contact dermatitis
Lichen planus
Psoriasis

Infectious Disorders

Bacterial paronychia
Candidiasis
Herpes simplex (whitlow)
Onychomycosis
Verrucae

Medications

Anticonvulsants (valproic acid)
Chemotherapeutic agents (especially taxanes)
Griseofulvin
Retinoids (isotretinoin)
Tetracyclines (photoonycholysis)
Thiazides (photoonycholysis)

Systemic Disorders

Iron-deficiency anemia
Rheumatic disease
Thyroid disease (hyperthyroidism or hypothyroidism)

Trauma

Compulsive subungual cleaning
Sportsman toe

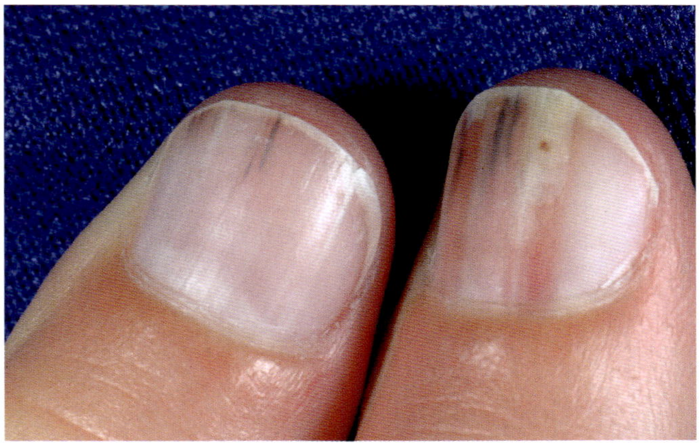

Fig. 7.72 Darier disease. Longitudinal reddish-purple and white streaks of the nail.

paronychia is often associated with repeated exposure of the fingers to wetness (see Figs. 17.47 and 17.51). Toddlers who suck their fingers or thumb usually have candidal paronychia, but a more acute process with purulence and crusting overlying the erythema and swelling may also reflect a herpetic whitlow of the finger or toe. Infants with sucking blisters show blisters filled with clear fluid. Potassium hydroxide scrapings to detect the pseudohyphae of *Candida albicans* (see Chapter 17) and direct fluorescence assays and cultures to consider herpes simplex infection (see Chapter 15) should be performed to distinguish these disorders. Even pediatric leishmaniasis may present as paronychia[783] and should be considered from exposure in endemic areas. Treatment of paronychia should be directed toward clearance of the infecting organism. In individuals beyond the age of infancy, efforts to keep the fingers dry, including avoidance of sucking and wet work, are critical for clearance. Paronychia is rarely seen with tinea unguium (see Chapter 17).

Periungual inflammation may also result from noninfectious causes. These include psoriasis and acropustulosis (see Chapter 4), chemical irritants including nail cosmetics,[784] and medications (particularly isotretinoin[772], indinavir[785], and small-molecule inhibitors of the epidermal growth factor receptor[786,787]/EGFR, and mitogen-activated protein kinase[788] [MAPK/MEK]). Soaks with dilute bleach[788] or 2% povidone-iodine[789] have improved the condition. EGFR inhibitors often cause pseudopyoderma granuloma as well, which has been successfully treated in some patients with topical timolol under occlusion.

DISORDERS OF NAIL COLORATION

A longitudinal streak of brown pigmentation of the nail *(melanonychia striata)*, which may extend to involve the entire nail (Fig. 7.73), usually is benign in children[790] (see Chapter 9), as opposed to the new onset of melanonychia striata in an adult, which raises the possibility of melanoma. Multiple streaks of melanonychia striata are not uncommon in those with phototypes IV to VI skin[791] and may begin during childhood. Melanonychia can also be horizontally arrayed (transverse melanonychia) or involve the entire nail. Abnormal nail pigmentation may be seen in systemic diseases[792] or in association with the ingestion of various chemicals or medications. Brown pigmentation of multiple nails may be associated with the ingestion of phenolphthalein as a reaction to antimalarials, minocycline, gold therapy, cancer chemotherapy, or zidovudine in pediatric human immunodeficiency virus (HIV) infection.[793] Brown-black pigmentation of the nailfold and nail matrix can be a sign of melanoma of the nail bed (Hutchinson sign), Peutz–Jeghers syndrome, and Laugier–Hunziker syndrome (see Chapter 11). Brown nail pigmentation has also been described as a manifestation of Addison disease or Graves disease.[794] Orange-brown chromonychia of the distal nails has been observed in Kawasaki disease,[795] including in 72% of 40 pediatric patients in one series.[796] The transverse discoloration of the acral nail begins 5 to 8 days after the onset of fever and clears entirely within several weeks. In argyria, the lunulae show a distinctive slate blue discoloration, and in hepatolenticular degeneration (Wilson disease), the lunulae may present an azure blue discoloration. Blue discoloration of the nails has also been described from administration of azidothymidine (AZT)[772] and imatinib.[797] Lithium carbonate can cause brownish-black transverse bands at the margins of the lunulae, and pigmentation in the form of transverse bands has been reported in patients receiving zidovudine,[797,798] bleomycin, and doxorubicin. Gray or blue-gray nails can occur in individuals with ochronosis or argyria, as a reaction to quinacrine or phenolphthalein, or with macrocytic anemia and vitamin B_{12} deficiency.[799] When a green discoloration is seen in association with onycholysis, *Pseudomonas aeruginosa* infection must be considered (Fig. 7.74).

Longitudinal erythronychia is characterized by one or more linear pink-red, usually asymptomatic, bands on the nail plate that originate at the proximal nailfold, cross the lunula, and extend to the free edge of the nail plate.[800] With time, the lesion may become brown, especially if hemorrhage is associated. One or more digits may be involved. Localized cases in children can be associated with a wart, vascular or glomus tumor, epidermal nevus, onychopapilloma (benign nail unit tumor that occasionally occurs in adolescents),[801] or postsurgical scar, whereas multiple nails are often affected in Darier disease (see Chapter 5) and lichen planus (see Chapter 4).[802] Nail fragility with splitting or V-shaped nicks, onycholysis, splinter hemorrhage, and/or subungual keratosis may be associated. *Red lunulae*[803] can be seen in patients with AA, lupus erythematosus, dermatomyositis, congestive heart failure, reticulosarcoma, psoriasis, carbon monoxide poisoning, lymphogranuloma venereum, and after stem cell transplantation. When the distal 1- to 2-mm portion of the nail has a normal pink color and the rest of the nail has a white appearance, the disorder has been termed *Terry nails*[804] (Fig. 7.75). Seen in patients with cirrhosis; chronic congestive heart failure; adult-onset diabetes; and polyneuropathy, organomegaly, endocrinopathy, M component, and skin changes (POEMS) syndrome, Terry nails may also be seen in normal children younger than 4 years of age, in the very elderly, and at times in normal individuals without evidence of cirrhosis or other systemic disease.

The term *leukonychia* (white nails) is used to describe a disorder in which at least a portion of the nail becomes white. The white color

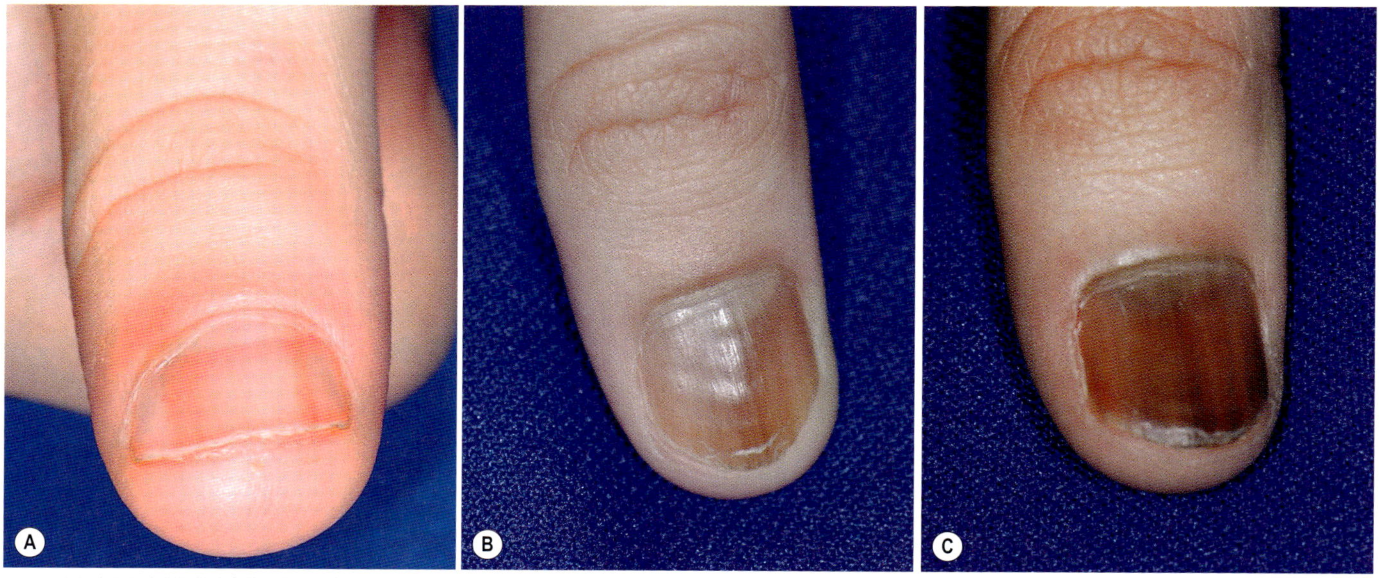

Fig. 7.73 Melanonychia. Nail pigmentation can progress, as occurred in this girl over 12 years. This benign nail pigmentation began as discrete longitudinal streaks **(A)** and progressively covered half **(B)** and then all **(C)** of the nail. Although no biopsy was performed, this most likely represents a benign pigmented nevus of the nail matrix.

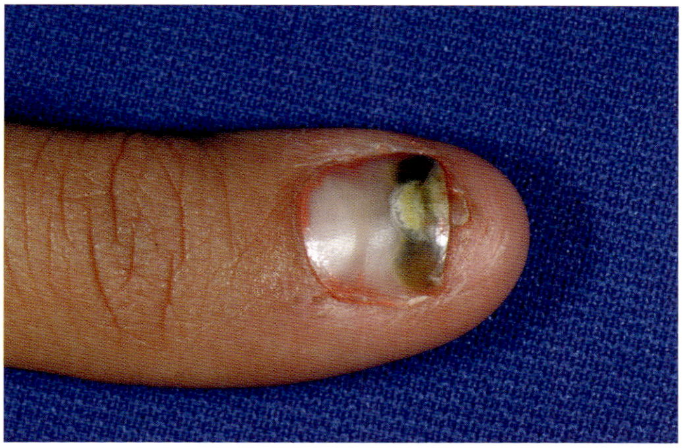

Fig. 7.74 Pseudomonas paronychia. Note the green discoloration.

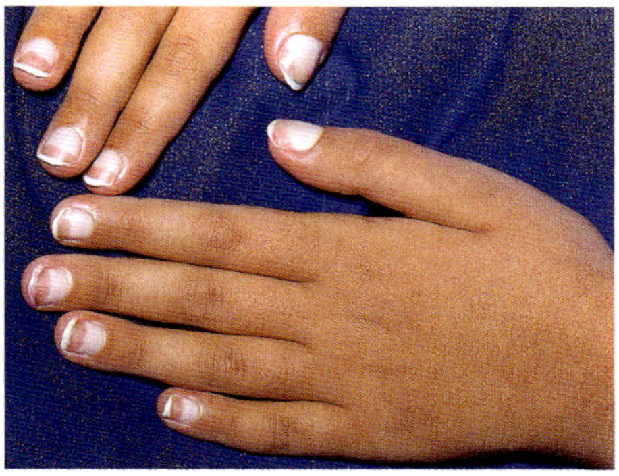

Fig. 7.75 Terry nails. The distal 1 to 2 mm of the nail have a normal pink color, and the rest of the nail has a white appearance. This girl had hepatic cirrhosis.

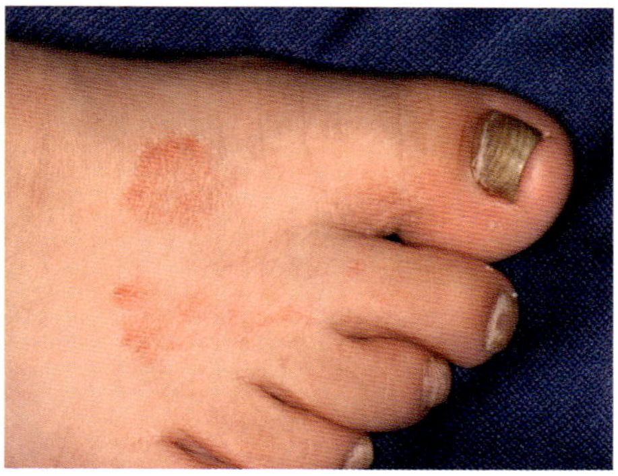

Fig. 7.76 Nail discoloration from onychomycosis. Horizontal striations were colored yellow on the hallucal nail but white on other nails. Note the annular, scaling, erythematous lesion on the top of the foot and the erythema and scaling interdigitally, both signs of tinea pedis.

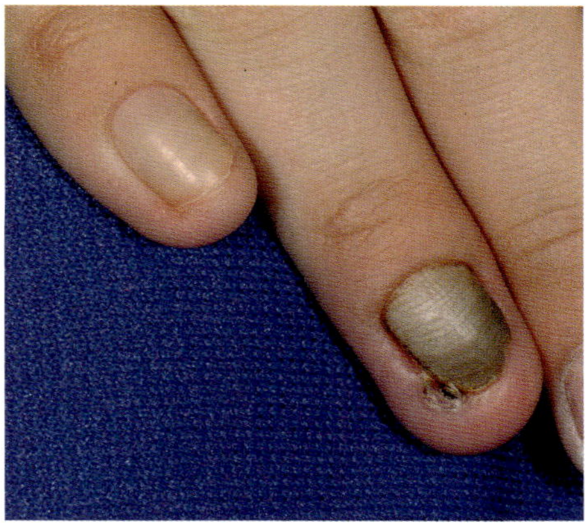

Fig. 7.77 Yellow nail syndrome. Yellowish discoloration of the nails is associated with slow growth, thickening, excessive curvature, and an absence of lunulae in some of the nails of this 8-year-old boy who had congenital chylothorax. The toenails were also affected.

may be seen as punctuate, striate, or encompassing much or all of the nail. Several forms of leukonychia striata have been described. The most common are variably sized white areas, sometimes multiple, that result from local manipulation. They tend to be horizontal in orientation (rather than following the shape of the nailfold or lunula), do not extend across the entire nail, are not depressed (vs. Beau lines from nail matrix arrest), and grow out with the nail. *Mees bands* are transverse 1- to 2-mm white bands that follow the lunula, tend to extend to the margins, and move distally as the nail grows out; they have been described in arsenic or heavy metal poisoning, septicemia, dissecting aortic aneurysm, and renal failure. The white transverse bands in *Muehrcke nails* affect the vascular bed under the nail plate and do not move as the nail grows out; they have been associated with hypoalbuminemia, such as from nephrotic syndrome, cirrhosis, or cytostatic chemotherapy agents. The *half-and-half* nail results from renal disease and azotemia and shows whitening of the proximal nail bed with red, pink, or brown coloration of the distal half. Similar changes have been described in association with isoniazid treatment.[805] The toenail may also be white because of superficial onychomycosis or proximal subungual onychomycosis (see Chapter 17); however, these forms of onychomycosis are uncommon in children in comparison with the more typical distal lateral subungual onychomycosis, in which the nail plate is yellow with subungual debris, thickening, and onycholysis (Fig. 7.76). Leukonychia is associated with palmoplantar keratoderma, knuckle pads, and hearing loss in Bart–Pumphrey syndrome, caused by mutations in *GJB2*, encoding connexin 26, and with erythrokeratodermia variabilis from mutations in connexin 43 (see Chapter 5). Congenital porcelain-like whitening of all (leukonychia totalis) or part (leukonychia partialis) of the 20 nails can be inherited as an autosomal recessive or autosomal dominant disorder without other manifestations as a result of mutations in *PLCD1*, encoding a phospholipase of the nail matrix that controls nail growth.[806] Leukonychia has been linked to selenium deficiency in a boy with Hirschsprung disease and responded to selenium supplementation.[807]

Yellow nail syndrome is a disorder associated with severe long-term lymphedema and, most commonly, respiratory disease, especially chronic bronchitis, bronchiectasis, interstitial pneumonitis, and pleural effusion.[808] Other associations include persistent hypoalbuminemia, thyroid disease, immunologic deficiencies (IgA), lymphoreticular malignancy, rheumatoid arthritis, lupus erythematosus, Hodgkin disease, and nephrotic syndrome. Yellow nails have been linked to exposure to titanium in candy or children's toothpastes (not sunscreens), but these children have had recurrent respiratory infections[809]; high levels of titanium were detected in nail clipping, and the condition improved when exposure to titanium was reduced. Most often a phenomenon of middle-aged individuals but also described in neonates (often with the lymphedema of fetal hydrops) and young children, the nails show a pale yellow or greenish-yellow to brown discoloration of the nails (Fig. 7.77) associated with slow growth; thickening; excessive curvature from side to side (on its long axis); increased hardness, onycholysis, or spontaneous shedding of the nails; absence of lunulae; and swelling of the periungual tissues, as might be seen in patients with chronic paronychia. The nail changes improve spontaneously in 30% of patients, but administration of oral and topical vitamin E, including in combination with triazole antifungals,[810] has been reported to be effective in some individuals.[811–813] Yellowing of the nail can be seen in adolescents from use of nail polish remover or administration of isotretinoin.[814]

The complete list of 814 references for this chapter is available online at http://expertconsult.inkling.com.

Key References

Rudnicka L, Olszewska M, Waskiel A, et al. Trichoscopy in hair shaft disorders. Dermatol Clin 2018;36(4):421–30.

Castelo-Soccio L. Diagnosis and management of alopecia in children. Pediatr Clin North Am 2014;61(2):427–42.

Singh G, Miteva M. Prognosis and management of congenital hair shaft disorders with fragility-part I. Pediatr Dermatol 2016;33(5):473–80.

Singh G, Miteva M. Prognosis and management of congenital hair shaft disorders without fragility-part II. Pediatr Dermatol 2016;33(5):481–7.

Cantatore-Francis JL, Orlow SJ. Practical guidelines for evaluation of loose anagen hair syndrome. Arch Dermatol 2009;145:1123–8.

Wright JT, Fete M, Schneider H, et al. Ectodermal dysplasias: classification and organization by phenotype, genotype and molecular pathway. Am J Med Genet A 2019;179(3):442–7.

Gilhar A, Etzioni A, Paus R. Alopecia areata. N Engl J Med 2012;366(16):1515–25.

Carmina E, Azziz R, Bergfeld W, et al. Female pattern hair loss and androgen excess: a report from the multidisciplinary androgen excess and PCOS committee. J Clin Endocrinol Metab 2019;104(7):2875–2891.

Gonzalez ME, Cantatore-Francis J, Orlow SJ. Androgenetic alopecia in the paediatric population: a retrospective review of 57 patients. Br J Dermatol 2010;163(2):378–85.

Chu DH, Rubin AI. Diagnosis and management of nail disorders in children. Pediatr Clin North Am 2014;61(2):293–308.

Chernoff KA, Scher RK. Nail disorders: Kids are not just little people. Clin Dermatol 2016;34(6):736–41.

Savage SA. Dyskeratosis Congenita. In: Adam MP, Ardinger HH, Pagon RA, et al., editors. GeneReviews®. Seattle (WA): University of Washington, Seattle 1993–2020. 2009 Nov 12 [updated 2019 Nov 21].

8 Acne Vulgaris and Other Disorders of the Sebaceous and Sweat Glands

CHAPTER OUTLINE

Disorders of the Sebaceous Glands

ACNE VULGARIS

Acne vulgaris is the most common skin problem in the United States, affecting nearly 80% to 85% of individuals at some point between 11 and 30 years of age.[1,2] Although not a serious disease, acne may be the source of permanent scarring and, even more importantly, psychosocial morbidity and decreased emotional well-being. Withdrawal from society, depression, and decreased self-esteem may occur in individuals with more significant disease. Girls and boys with acne have more feelings of uselessness and lower body satisfaction compared with those without acne, and these features are compounded by the fact that acne typically presents in adolescents, who tend to be psychologically vulnerable and sensitive to modification in their physical appearance.[3] Acne severity has been shown to be directly correlated with extent of embarrassment and lack of enjoyment of or participation in social activities.[4] Patients with even mild to moderate acne have demonstrated high scores on the Carroll Rating Scale for Depression and an increased prevalence of suicidal ideation (SI).[5] In addition, patients with severe acne may have poorer academic performance[6] and higher unemployment rates.[7] Issues such as these highlight that the potential benefits of acne therapy extend far beyond the simple cosmetics of the disease.

Pediatric acne is the terminology applied to acne occurring from birth through 11 years of age; *adolescent acne* describes patients from age 12 to adulthood.[8] The contemporary classification of pediatric acne based on age of onset of the disease is shown in Fig. 8.1.

Acne vulgaris is seen routinely by primary care physicians, and so familiarity with the treatment of this condition is vital. The majority of acne patients with mild to moderate disease respond well to traditional therapies; patients with severe or recalcitrant disease may merit treatment with agents most appropriately prescribed by dermatologists. Although the underlying cause of acne vulgaris remains unknown, considerable data concerning its pathogenesis have accumulated in recent decades to allow a rational and therapeutically successful approach to its management. There is no single "gold standard" therapy for acne, and treatment regimens must be individualized and occasionally fine-tuned to achieve the optimal response.

The tendency to develop acne is often familial and is felt by some to be inherited as an autosomal dominant trait. However, because of the high prevalence, the genetics of the disease remain unclear. Adolescent acne usually begins around the time of onset of puberty, occurring earlier in girls than boys. However, the onset of acne may occur significantly earlier, and it may be the first sign of pubertal maturation in girls, correlating with increasing levels of dehydroepiandrosterone (DHEA), an adrenal androgen.[9] Natural history studies show that in 80% of patients the incidence and severity of acne decline by the early 20s, although as many as 50% of adults older than 25 years are affected and a minority may have persistence into middle age.[10,11] An important consideration is the timing of onset of puberty, which has followed a downward trend for many years. Studies from the mid-twentieth century onward suggest that breast and pubic hair development in American girls is occurring at younger ages, with Black girls disproportionately represented.[12] As a result the regional definitions of precocious puberty have been revised such that puberty is currently considered precocious if it occurs before 8 years of age in European girls, before 7 years of age in American White girls, and before 6 years of age in Black girls. A similar trend has not been identified in boys, in whom the cut-off age for precocious puberty continues to be 9 years.[13,14]

An understanding of acne pathogenesis helps the practitioner conceptualize and formulate the therapeutic plan. Four interrelated processes, including hyperkeratinization, androgen stimulation, bacterial infection, and inflammation, are traditionally believed to be involved in this multifactorial disease. A pictorial representation of acne pathogenesis is shown in Fig. 8.2.[15] Individual acne lesions usually begin with obstruction of the pilosebaceous unit (composed of the hair follicle and the sebaceous gland). These units are localized primarily to the face and trunk, and these "follicular plugs" (or microcomedones) are caused by excessive numbers of desquamated epithelial cells from the wall of the follicle in combination with excessive amounts of sebum, the oily, lipid-rich substance produced by the sebaceous glands. Sebum production is stimulated by adrenal and gonadal androgens and rises to maximum levels during late adolescence. These microcomedones enlarge into *comedones*, which may be open (blackheads) or closed (whiteheads). The reason for the black appearance of open comedones is unclear; one hypothesis suggests compaction and oxidation of the keratinous material at the follicular opening results in this finding. Melanin pigment may also play a role.[16,17]

Propagation of acne lesions occurs when *Cutibacterium acnes* (formerly *Propionibacterium acnes*), a resident anaerobic organism, proliferates in this environment of sebum and follicular cells with the production of chemotactic factors and proinflammatory mediators, which contribute to inflammation.[18] Hypersensitivity to this organism may also play a part in the more severe forms of acne.[19] Observations regarding the potential mechanisms of *C. acnes* induced inflammation have suggested activation of toll-like receptor signaling, stimulation of antimicrobial peptide activity, induction of matrix metalloproteinase production, and inflammasome activation.[20–22] The clinical counterpart to these infectious and inflammatory events are papules and pustules. With continued inflammation and macrophage recruitment, larger lesions (cysts and nodules) may result. Finally, sequelae of active acne lesions include dyspigmentation (usually hyperpigmentation or, occasionally, hypopigmentation) and scarring. Box 8.1 summarizes the various types of acne lesions.

Although the pathway in Fig. 8.2 has traditionally been used to explain acne pathogenesis, ongoing research continues to shed light on these processes. Subclinical inflammation, even before the formation of the microcomedone, may be present in acne as demonstrated by upregulated levels of inflammatory cytokines and cells in uninvolved skin from acne patients.[23] Another study supporting this hypothesis used digital photographic images to follow the evolution of acne lesions and showed that nearly 30% of inflammatory lesions arose from normal-appearing skin (as opposed to comedones).[24] Further elucidation of the mechanisms that give rise to acne lesions will enable better targeting of acne therapies.

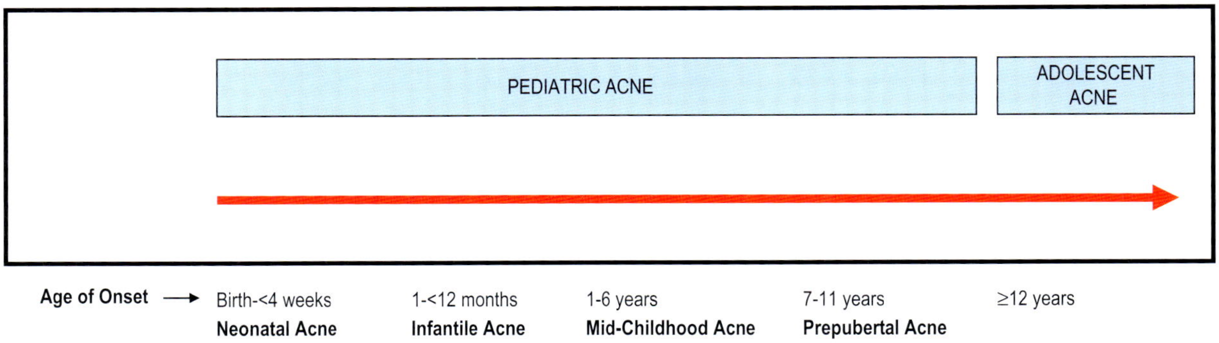

Fig. 8.1 Contemporary classification of acne vulgaris in childhood and adolescence. (Modified from references 51, 70, and 267.)

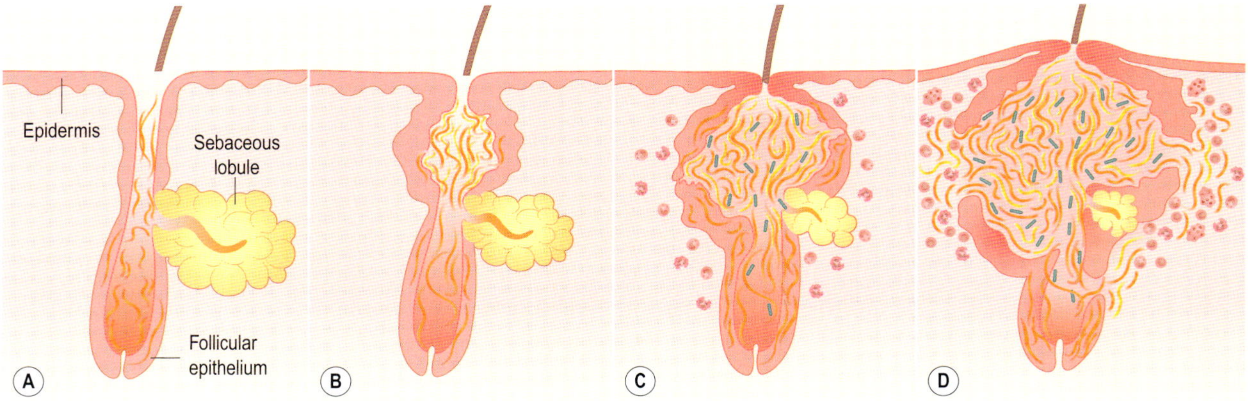

Fig. 8.2 Traditional view of acne pathogenesis. **(A)** Early comedone, with mild follicular plugging. **(B)** Later comedone. **(C)** Inflammatory papule/pustule. **(D)** Nodule/cyst. It should be noted that emerging studies suggest that subclinical inflammation may occur earlier in the pathogenesis, even before follicular plugging **(A)**. (Reprinted with permission from Zaenglein AL, Thiboutot DM. Acne vulgaris. In: Bolognia JL, Jorizzo JL, Rapini RP, editors. Dermatology. Edinburgh: Mosby; 2003.)

Box 8.1 Types of Acne Lesions

- Active lesions (increasing severity)
  - Microcomedone (may not be clinically apparent)
  - Open comedone (blackhead)
  - Closed comedone (whitehead)
  - Papule
  - Pustule
  - Nodule
  - Cyst-like nodule
- Sequelae
  - Dyspigmentation (usually hyperpigmentation)
  - Scarring (sometimes keloidal)

In addition to the established pathogenic factors discussed previously, there may be other triggers or exacerbating conditions that contribute to acne vulgaris. These other factors are less well understood and in some cases controversial. Stress appears to be a common trigger for acne, possibly via increased activation of the hypothalamic–pituitary–adrenal axis and the resultant increase in androgen production. Acute worsening of acne has been documented in college students during examination periods and correlated with an increased perceived stress score.[25] Mechanical factors such as skin occlusion from sports gear (i.e., helmets, chin straps, shoulder pads) may exacerbate the condition. Applications topically applied to hair and skin, especially pomades and greasy ointments, may contribute to physical obstruction of the pilosebaceous unit and worsen the disease. Several medications may worsen acne, including anabolic steroids, progestins, lithium, isoniazid, hydantoin, and gold.[26] Pathologic androgen excess is often associated with acne (see later), and although endocrinologic evaluation is not indicated for the majority of patients, it should be considered in patients who have additional signs as listed in Box 8.2.[27] Individuals with moderate to severe keratosis pilaris appear to have lower prevalence and severity of facial acne vulgaris.[28]

Box 8.2 Potential Signs of Androgen Excess in Acne Patients

Young Children

- Body odor
- Axillary hair
- Pubic hair
- Clitoromegaly

Adult Women

- Recalcitrant/late-onset acne
- Menstrual irregularity
- Hirsutism
- Male- or female-pattern alopecia
- Infertility
- Acanthosis nigricans
- Truncal obesity

Modified from Strauss JS, Krowchuk DP, Leyden JJ, et al. Guidelines of care for acne vulgaris management. J Am Acad Dermatol 2007;56:651–63.

The role of diet in the pathogenesis of acne vulgaris remains controversial, and controlled studies have refuted the value of dietary restrictions. For many years the elimination of various foods such as chocolate, soft drinks, milk, ice cream, fatty foods, shellfish, and iodides was recommended. The misconception that iodine is injurious to patients with acne vulgaris originated with the concept that iodides administered orally as a medication occasionally initiate a papulopustular acneiform eruption. The concept that chocolate exerts an adverse effect on acne has been challenged, and one controlled double-blind study found that it failed to affect either the course of the disease or the production and composition of sebum.[29] However, the possibility that diet plays a role in the pathogenesis or exacerbation of acne continues to be addressed. A review of two non-Westernized populations (one in Papua New Guinea and the other in Paraguay) revealed an astonishing difference in acne prevalence compared with individuals in Westernized societies.[30] One potential explanation asserted for these differences is the diets of these populations, which are composed mainly of minimally processed plant and animal foods and are nearly devoid of the carbohydrates typical in Western diets, which may result in high insulin levels. Hyperinsulinemia, in turn, may promote the development of acne by its ability to increase androgen production.[30] It remains unclear whether adhering to a diet with a low glycemic load (LGL) can effect a change in acne, although several studies seem to suggest an association.[31–34] Studies have suggested increased sex hormone–binding globulin, reduced androgen levels, and reduced acne lesion development in young men who ate an LGL diet, although the associated weight loss in this cohort and the lower saturated fat content and higher fiber level in the LGL diet are considered by some as potential confounders.[35,36] In a cross-sectional study of 50 nonobese adults with acne vulgaris, high glycemic index and high glycemic load diet was positively associated with acne vulgaris, and an inverse correlation between glycemic index and adiponectin (a hormone derived from subcutaneous fat that exhibits antiinflammatory effects) was noted.[37] The association between milk consumption and development of acne has been explored, with several studies (some of which were limited by their retrospective and/or questionnaire-based design) suggesting a positive association, possibly related to a combination of exogenous hormones and growth factors and stimulation of endogenous hormones.[38–42] Interestingly, skim milk was consistently associated with acne in most (but not all) of these studies, suggesting that fat content alone may not explain the acne-causing ability of milk in the studied cohorts.[35,41] Other dietary factors that have been studied with regard to acne pathogenesis include omega-3 fatty acids, antioxidants, zinc, vitamin A, and dietary fiber.[36,43] Acne presents with a combination of the various lesion types previously discussed: comedones, papules, pustules, cysts, nodules, scarring, and dyspigmentation. The earliest lesion type is usually the comedone, and mild acne may be limited to these lesions (Figs. 8.3 and 8.4). With increasing severity, patients develop inflammatory lesions, including papules and pustules (Figs. 8.5 and 8.6). Nodules and cyst-like nodules may be present in patients with moderate to severe disease (Figs. 8.7 and 8.8) and may result in permanent acne scarring (Figs. 8.9 and 8.10). Dyspigmentation is a common sequela, especially in patients with darker complexions (Figs. 8.11 and 8.12). The primary sites for acne lesions correlate with the areas most concentrated with sebaceous glands: the face, chest, back, and shoulders. In patients with regressing acne lesions, macular erythema (Fig. 8.13) and hyperpigmentation are commonly seen. Although patients commonly regard these as active lesions and "scars," they usually imply effectiveness of the therapy, and their temporary nature should be explained to the patient. The scarring that occurs in patients with the more severe papulopustular and nodulocystic forms of acne develops because of fibrous contraction after the inflammatory phase. In addition to sharply punched-out pits and craters, hypertrophic or keloidal scars may also develop. The severity of the scarring depends on the depth and degree of the inflammation and on the patient's individual susceptibility.

Acne fulminans is a rare and severe form of acne vulgaris, occurring primarily in boys and young men. Patients present with an acute onset of painful, pustular, nodular, and occasionally ulcerative acne lesions concentrated on the chest (Fig. 8.14), shoulders, back, and face. Fever, leukocytosis, polyarthralgia, and elevation in inflammatory markers may also be present, and the skin lesions usually result in permanent scarring. Osteolytic bone lesions may be present, especially in the clavicle, sternum, and long bones.[44] Ironically, acne fulminans has most often been ascribed to treatment with oral isotretinoin. Systemic corticosteroids are the mainstay of therapy, with the addition of isotretinoin after the acute inflammatory stage has subsided. A recent acne fulminans consensus treatment guideline recommends temporary discontinuation of isotretinoin while oral corticosteroids are started, with reintroduction at a very low dose (0.1 mg/kg per day) once lesions begin to heal over, with very gradual isotretinoin dose escalation.[45] Other reported therapies include etanercept, infliximab, anakinra, cyclosporine, and dapsone.[45–47]

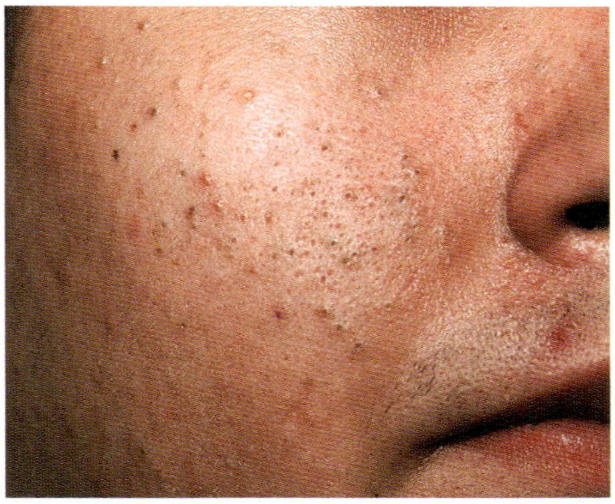

Fig. 8.3 Acne vulgaris: comedonal. Open comedones present as blackheads.

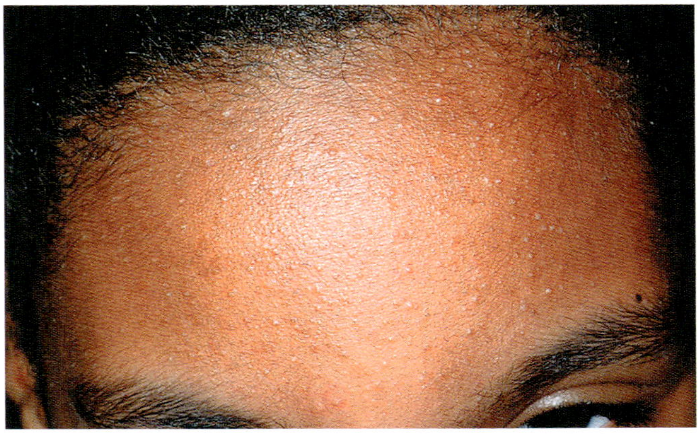

Fig. 8.4 Acne vulgaris: comedonal. Closed comedones present as whiteheads.

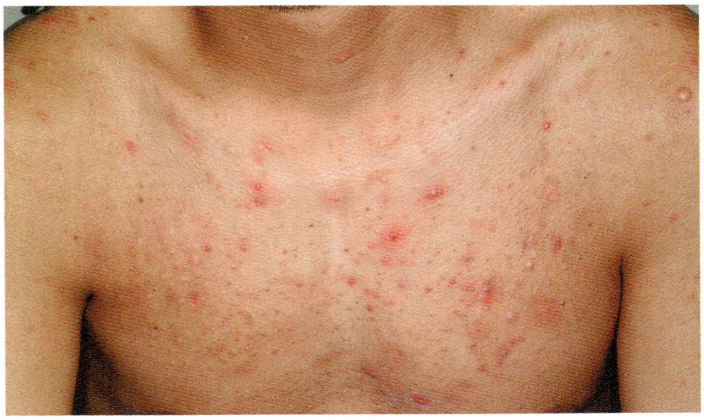

Fig. 8.5 Acne vulgaris: inflammatory. Note the erythematous papules and pustules, as well as open and closed comedones.

Acne Therapy

Before any attempt is made to treat acne, patient education is vital. Important considerations include explaining the nature and natural

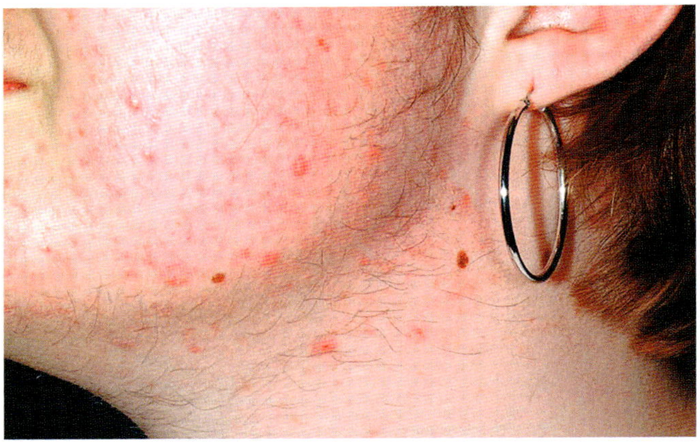

Fig. 8.6 Acne vulgaris: inflammatory. This adolescent girl has inflammatory papules and papulopustules, as well as hirsutism.

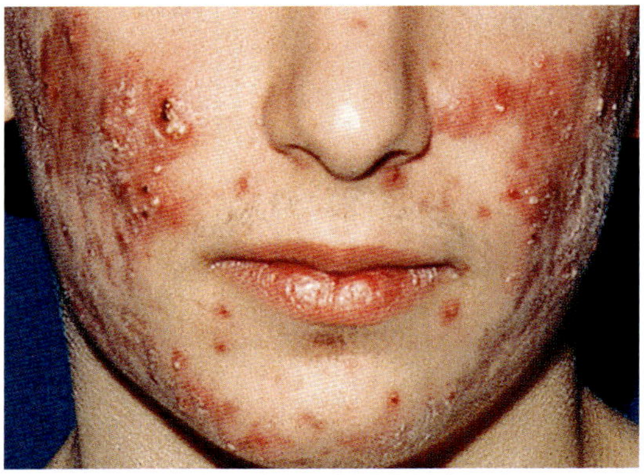

Fig. 8.7 Acne vulgaris: nodulocystic.

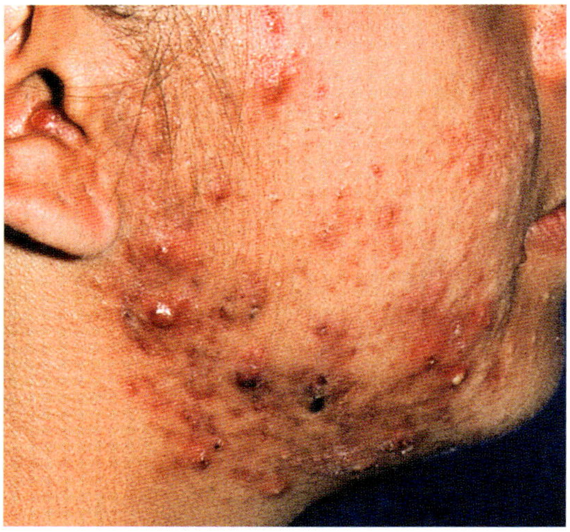

Fig. 8.8 Acne vulgaris: nodulocystic.

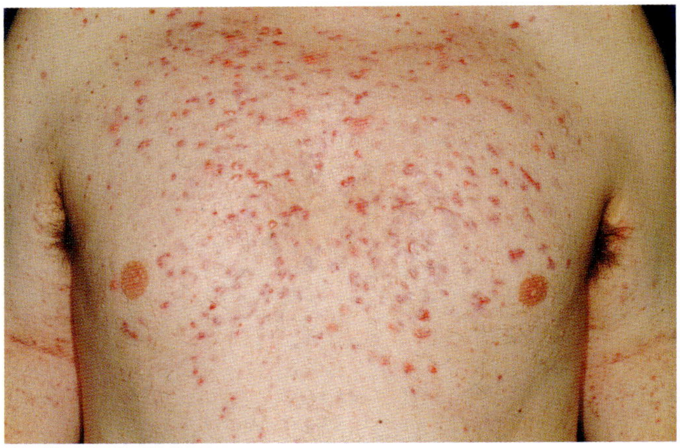

Fig. 8.9 Acne scarring. This patient has severe nodular acne vulgaris with scarring involving the trunk.

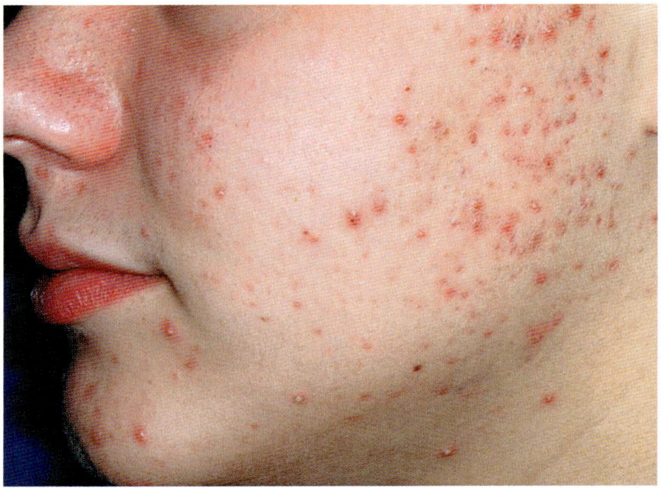

Fig. 8.10 Acne scarring.

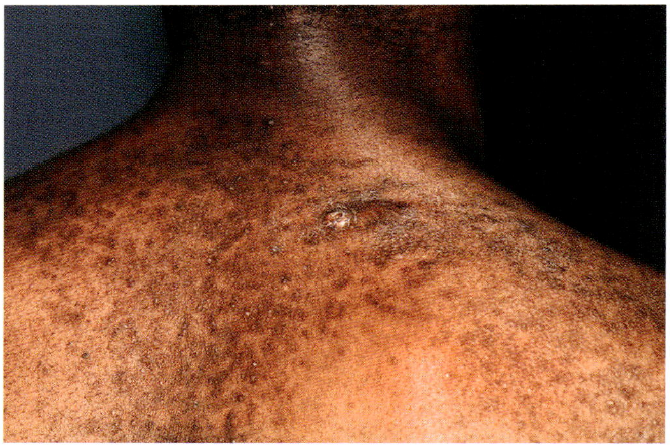

Fig. 8.11 Acne-induced dyspigmentation.

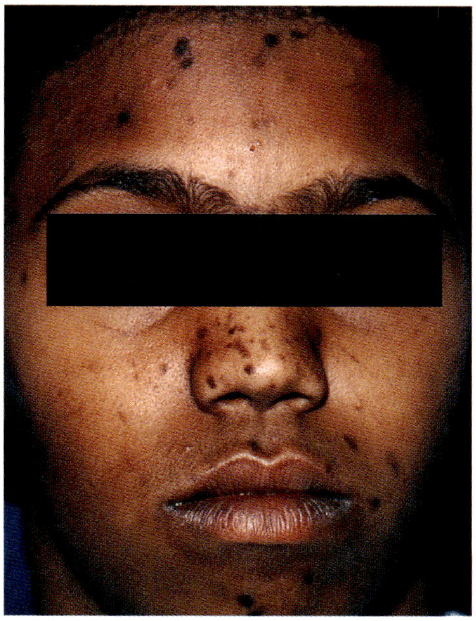

Fig. 8.12 Acne-induced dyspigmentation. Note the "T-zone" distribution corresponding to prior acne lesions.

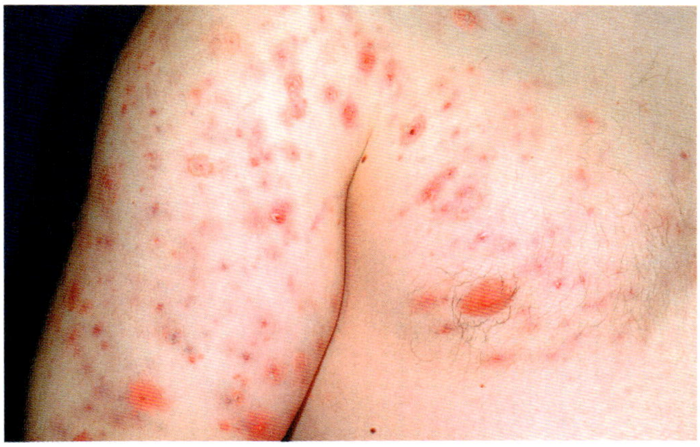

Fig. 8.13 Residual postacne erythema. Note erythematous macules at sites of prior lesions.

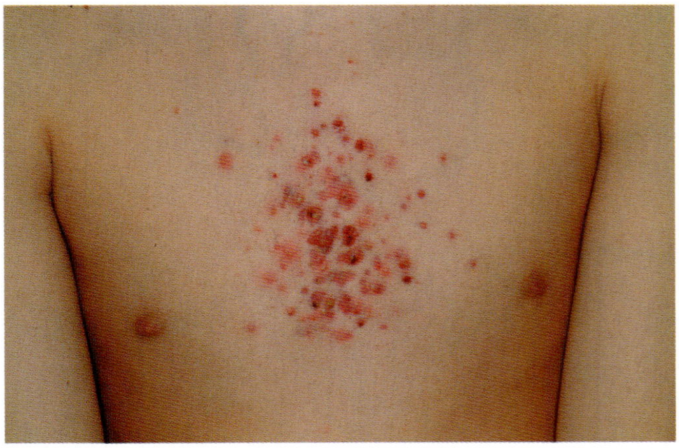

Fig. 8.14 Acne fulminans. This patient developed acute worsening of his acne lesions on starting isotretinoin therapy and required systemic corticosteroids.

Box 8.3 **Pearls for Increasing Adherence in Acne Therapy**

- Use written action plans for topical and systemic medication use.
- Keep the treatment regimen as simplified as possible; use of fixed-dose combination agents (when possible) may facilitate this goal.
- Consider the vehicles of prescribed agents and tolerability by the individual patient.
- Take time to educate the patient regarding expectations (length of time to see improvement, likelihood of mild irritation early in the course of therapy, potential side effects).
- Review appropriate application of topical medications.
- Reinforce the importance of ongoing use (maintenance therapy), once improved.
- Consider psychologic comorbidities and encourage open discussion regarding acne-associated stressors.

Modified from Eichenfield LF, Krakowski AC, Piggott C, et al. Evidence-based recommendations for the diagnosis and treatment of pediatric acne. Pediatrics 2013;131(3):S163–86; Eichenfield LF, Mancini AJ. PedAcne resource guide: a comprehensive overview of pediatric acne & companion to the online self-assessment exam. New York: Educational Testing and Assessment Systems; 2013; and Yan AC, Baldwin HE, Eichenfield, et al. Approach to pediatric acne treatment: an update. Semin Cutan Med Surg 2011;30:S16–21.

history of acne vulgaris, dispelling acne myths regarding causes and treatments, highlighting the need for adherence with therapy and appropriate follow-up care with the physician, reviewing the correct usage of medications and the potential side effects, and emphasizing the expected gradual improvement in symptoms with therapy. Patient education materials are very useful to this end and will help increase adherence with treatment. Such materials can be created and personalized by the physician or purchased from national organizations such as the American Academy of Dermatology (www.aad.org) or the American Academy of Pediatrics (www.aap.org). Box 8.3 lists some clinical pearls for increased adherence in acne therapy.

Acne treatment in the past was hindered by mythical concepts regarding its causes, a more limited armamentarium of treatment options, and a lack of appreciation for the dire psychosocial consequences that can result for the acne patient. With the current level of understanding of acne pathogenesis, the ever-expanding array of therapeutic approaches, and recognition of both the physical and emotional benefits of successful therapy, every patient with acne who desires treatment should be able to benefit from physician intervention. The primary care provider is optimally situated to offer therapy to patients with mild and moderate disease, and case-based education has been shown to significantly increase pediatric provider knowledge on treating acne in accordance with published evidence-based recommendations.[48] For those with recalcitrant or severe involvement, referral to a dermatologist is often necessary. Although acne therapy is a combination of art and science, a solid understanding of the various classes of medication and their proper use in both monotherapy and combination therapy provides the foundation for designing treatment plans. A conceptual framework is shown in Table 8.1 for an acne treatment algorithm. Contemporary treatment algorithms are also available in the published literature.[49–53]

Topical therapies are first-line treatment for patients with mild acne and are very useful as part of a combination therapy regimen for patients with moderate or severe acne. Prescription-strength topical agents are summarized in Table 8.2. Benzoyl peroxide (BP) and topical retinoids (vitamin A acids), although potential irritants, appear to be the most effective topical agents. Based on current understanding of acne pathogenesis, these two products offer a highly effective therapeutic approach that can be tailored to each patient. Although success in the management of acne vulgaris can be achieved by the use of these agents alone, the therapeutic effect can be increased substantially by their use in combination, despite the fact that they are applied at separate times.

Daily facial cleansing, preferably in the morning and at bedtime, is a useful step in acne management. The goal of cleansing is to remove excess oil, dirt, and makeup. Use of a gentle, soap-free, pH-balanced cleanser or acne wash is recommended.[51] It is important that the acne patient be appropriately educated that harsh scrubbing and use of abrasive devices or sponges may increase inflammation and actually worsen acne or increase the risk of scarring.

Table 8.1 Acne Treatment Algorithm

	SEVERITY (LESION TYPE)				
Therapy	**Mild (Comedonal)**	**Mild (Inflammatory/Mixed)**	**Moderate (Inflammatory/Mixed)**	**Severe (Inflammatory/Mixed)**	**Severe (Nodular/Scarring)**
Initial therapy options[*,†]	Topical retinoid BP Salicylic acid cleanser	BP/retinoid combo BP/antibiotic combo Antibiotic/retinoid combo + BP	BP/retinoid combo BP/antibiotic combo ± topical retinoid Antibiotic/retinoid combo + BP ± oral antibiotic	BP/retinoid combo + oral antibiotic BP/antibiotic combo + topical retinoid + oral antibiotic Antibiotic/retinoid combo + BP + oral antibiotic	Isotretinoin
Alternative therapy options[*,†,‡]	Add BP or retinoid if not already prescribed BP/antibiotic combo BP/retinoid combo Antibiotic/retinoid combo	Substitute another combo product Add missing component (e.g., topical retinoid, BP, topical antibiotic) Change type, strength or formulation of topical retinoid	Substitute another combo product Add missing component (i.e., topical retinoid, BP, topical antibiotic, oral antibiotic) Change type, strength or formulation of topical retinoid Consider hormonal therapy[§] for female patients Consider oral isotretinoin	Consider changing oral antibiotic Consider isotretinoin Consider hormonal therapy[§] for female patients	Consider hormonal therapy[§] for female patients
Maintenance therapy	Topical retinoid or BP/retinoid combo	Topical retinoid or BP/retinoid combo	Topical retinoid or BP/retinoid combo	Topical retinoid or BP/retinoid combo	Topical retinoid or BP/retinoid combo

Adapted from Zaenglein AL, Thiboutot DM. Expert committee recommendations for acne management. Pediatrics 2006;118(3):1188–99; Thiboutot D, Gollnick H, Bettoli V, et al. New insights into the management of acne: an update from the Global Alliance to Improve Outcomes in Acne Group. J Am Acad Dermatol 2009;60:S1–50; Eichenfield LF, Krakowski AC, Piggott C, et al. Evidence-based recommendations for the diagnosis and treatment of pediatric acne. Pediatrics 2013;131(3):S163–86; Thiboutot DM, Gollnick HP. Treatment considerations for inflammatory acne: clinical evidence for adapalene 0.1% in combination therapies. J Drugs Dermatol 2006;5(8):785–94; Gollnick H, Cunliffe W, Berson D, et al. Management of acne: a report from a Global Alliance to Improve Outcomes in Acne. J Am Acad Dermatol 2003;49(Suppl. 1):S1–37; and Zaenglein AL, Pathy AL, Schlosser BJ, et al. Guidelines of care for the management of acne vulgaris. J Am Acad Dermatol 2016;74:945–73.

BP, Benzoyl peroxide.

*If combination products not available to patient, consider substitution of individual components as separate prescriptions.

†Topical dapsone may be considered in place of topical antibiotic.

‡If needed as determined by physician assessment and patient satisfaction.

§Combined oral contraceptive or oral spironolactone.

BP and salicylic acid are the active ingredients in most over-the-counter (OTC) acne products. In fact most BP acne products are now limited to OTC status, excepting some prescription combination products. Salicylic acid helps reduce sebum and decrease comedones and is found in various concentrations as a gel, lotion, wash, or cream. It may be an alternative comedonal therapy for those who cannot tolerate topical retinoids (now considered the mainstay of comedonal acne therapy). Glycolic acid, one of the α-hydroxy acids, is found naturally in fruits and yogurt and may be useful in decreasing hyperkeratosis associated with acne.

BP is traditionally the most commonly used topical preparation for acne vulgaris and, as noted earlier, is available as an OTC product and in some select prescription (primarily fixed-dose combination) products. It is a powerful antimicrobial, useful for reducing colonization of *C. acnes*, and also has some comedolytic and antiinflammatory effects. BP is available in a variety of strengths and comes as a gel, wash, cream, lotion, and even shaving cream. It is usually used once or twice daily. BP products may bleach colored clothing or linens, and patients should be warned of this possibility. Combination products of BP with topical antibiotics (erythromycin or clindamycin) are readily available, and these agents appear to be more effective than either ingredient used alone.[54–56] Combination BP/topical retinoid products are also available. These agents are discussed in more detail in the paragraphs that follow.

Potential side effects of BP include irritant contact dermatitis and rarely allergic contact dermatitis.[26,57] Irritant dermatitis is particularly problematic when the product is used excessively or in association with abrasive soaps or astringents or both. Therapy must be individualized and initiated gradually, particularly in fair-skinned or atopic individuals. BP should be applied as a thin film and rubbed in gently, gradually increasing the frequency and strength of the preparation as tolerance is developed (generally over several weeks). As with most topical agents, a small portion of the product is generally sufficient for application to the entire face. If irritation or excessive dryness develops, the preparation may be discontinued for several days and then restarted more sparingly, and/or noncomedogenic facial emollients may be used (in small amounts).

Topical retinoids (see Table 8.2) are a very effective class of medication used in the treatment of acne. These drugs normalize the keratinization process within the follicles, which reduces obstruction and therefore the formation of microcomedones and comedones. Some topical retinoids may also have antiinflammatory activity. These agents are thus both comedolytic and anticomedogenic and, as such, function to help prevent new acne and treat existing lesions. They have also been shown to have a beneficial effect on secondary lesions, such as scarring and pigmentation.[58] The prototype drug in this class is tretinoin, an acid of vitamin A. Newer-generation agents include adapalene and tazarotene. Tazarotene was used initially in the treatment of psoriasis and subsequently received approval for the treatment of acne vulgaris. Although success in the management of acne can often be achieved by the use of topical retinoids alone, the therapeutic effect can be substantially increased by their use in combination with BP or a topical antibiotic. A tretinoin/clindamycin combination (Table 8.3; see Table 8.2) has been found to improve both comedonal and inflammatory acne, and an adapalene/BP combination product was found to be more effective than either agent alone and placebo.[59]

Topical retinoids are generally applied once nightly and should be applied sparingly. A useful analogy for the patient is to use a "pea-sized" or "chocolate chip–sized" amount of product for a full-face application. The traditional recommendation was for retinoids to be applied to a dry face, with 30 to 45 minutes of "air drying" allowed after washing and before applying the product. However, this appears to be unnecessary with the newer formulations of tretinoin, adapalene, and tazarotene. The primary side effect of topical retinoids is irritation, which can be minimized by appropriate application and use. In general the cream forms are less drying than the gels, solutions, or

Table 8.2 Prescription Topical Therapies for Acne Vulgaris

Drug	Brand*	Formulation
ANTIMICROBIALS		
Clindamycin	Cleocin T	1% solution, gel, pledgets, lotion
	ClindaMax	1% lotion
	Clindets	1% pledgets
	Clindagel	1% gel
	Evoclin	1% foam
Clindamycin/BP†	BenzaClin	1% (5% BP) gel
	Duac	1% (5% BP) gel
	Acanya	1.2% (2.5% BP) gel
	Onexton	1.2% (3.75% BP) gel
Dapsone	Aczone	5%, 7.5% gel
Erythromycin	Emgel, Erygel, A/T/S	2% gel
	Eryderm, Erymax, T-Stat, A/T/S	2% solution 1.5% solution
	Staticin	2% ointment
	Akne-Mycin	2% solution + ZA
	Theramycin Z	2% swab
	Emcin Clear, Erycette	
Erythromycin/BP†	Benzamycin, Benzapak, Actipak	3% (5% BP) gel
Minocycline	Amzeek	4% foam
Sulfacetamide	Klaron	10% lotion
	Plexion	10% (5% sulfur) cloths, wash
	Clenia	
	Rosula	10% (5% sulfur) cream, wash
	Avar, Avar LS	10% (4% sulfur) wash 10% (5% sulfur; 2% in LS) wash, foam
Azelaic acid	Azelex	20% cream
RETINOIDS		
Adapalene	Differin‡	0.1% cream, lotion 0.3% gel
Adapalene/BP†	Epiduo	0.1% (2.5% BP) gel
	Epiduo Forte	0.3% (2.5% BP) gel
Tazarotene	Tazorac	0.05, 0.1% cream 0.05, 0.1% gel
	Fabior	0.1% foam
Tretinoin	Retin-A	0.025, 0.05, 0.1% cream 0.01, 0.025% gel
	Retin-A Micro	0.04, 0.06, 0.08, 0.1% gel
	Avita	0.025% cream, gel
	Atralin	0.05% gel
Tretinoin/clindamycin†	Ziana	0.025% (1.2% clindamycin) gel
	Veltin	0.025% (1.2% clindamycin) gel

BP, Benzoyl peroxide; *ZA*, zinc acetate.
*Listed are examples; this list is not exhaustive. Many of these preparations are available in generic form as well.
†Combination therapy product.
‡Note that 0.1% gel is available without a prescription.

Table 8.3 Fixed-Dose Combination Acne Therapies

Active Agents	Brand(s)	Formulation
Clindamycin/BP	BenzaClin	1%/5% gel
	Duac	1%/5% gel
	Acanya	1.2%/2.5% gel
	Onexton	1.2%/3.75% gel
Erythromycin/BP	Benzamycin	3%/5% gel
	Benzapak	3%/5% gel
	Actipak	3%/5% gel
Adapalene/BP	Epiduo	0.1%/2.5% gel
	Epiduo Forte	0.3%/2.5% gel
Clindamycin/tretinoin	Ziana	1.2%/0.025% gel
	Veltin	1.2%/0.025% gel

BP, Benzoyl peroxide.

pledgets, although again, newer formulations have minimized this effect, even with the gel vehicle. In patients with sensitive skin, good initial choices for retinoid therapy are tretinoin cream (in a lower strength), adapalene cream, or one of the micro preparations. If the product is tolerated well and more effect is desired, the patient can then be advanced to higher strengths, a gel or pledget formulation, or tazarotene. Another popular strategy used to decrease the incidence of irritation is to have the patient begin therapy 3 nights weekly, increasing as tolerated over a few weeks to nightly application.[60] Because retinoids may degrade significantly when mixed with BP, such combination therapy should be used only in the form of preformulated combination products (see Tables 8.2 and 8.3) or, if used as individual agents, they should be applied at different times.[61]

Increased sun sensitivity is another potential side effect of topical retinoids, and patients should be counseled regarding the appropriate use of a sunscreen with a sun protection factor of 30 or higher, especially if they are also using a photosensitizing oral agent. The risk of teratogenicity with use of the topical retinoids is controversial but remains a concern given the well-established teratogenic potential of the oral retinoid, isotretinoin. There are sporadic reports of congenital malformations in infants born to women who used topical tretinoin during pregnancy, but controlled human studies are lacking for this drug, which is classified as a pregnancy category C (studies in animals have revealed adverse effects on the fetus and there are no controlled studies in women or studies in women and animals are not available), as is adapalene (tazarotene, however, is classified as pregnancy category X). The limited transdermal uptake, lack of alteration of plasma retinoid levels, epidemiologic data, and margin of safety when compared with known teratogens all suggest the unlikelihood of tretinoin being a human developmental toxicant.[62–65] However, until a formal consensus exists, the potential risks of topical retinoids should be discussed in detail with women of childbearing potential, and their use should probably be avoided during pregnancy.

Topical antibiotics (see Table 8.2) exert their effect primarily by decreasing the population of *C. acnes*, and they may also have antiinflammatory effects. The most commonly used topical antibiotics for acne are clindamycin, erythromycin, and sulfacetamide. These agents are most useful for inflammatory acne, and in patients with mixed inflammatory and comedonal disease they should be used in combination with another agent that has comedolytic properties (e.g., BP or retinoid). These agents are usually well tolerated and are applied once or twice daily. As with other topical agents, lotions and creams are less drying than solutions, pledgets, and gels. Monotherapy with topical antibiotics should be discouraged, given the greater development of bacterial resistance, which can be lessened by the concomitant use of a preparation containing BP (see later).

Topical erythromycin has been used for decades in the treatment of acne and is usually well tolerated. The addition of zinc to erythromycin may increase its therapeutic efficacy.[66] Topical erythromycin has fallen out of favor with many acne experts given its reduced efficacy compared with clindamycin, secondary to resistance of cutaneous organisms.[53] Topical clindamycin is another well-tolerated antibiotic preparation for acne. Although pseudomembranous colitis is usually associated with oral clindamycin, there are rare reports of this complication with topical application of this agent.[67,68] Therefore if a patient using topical clindamycin develops persistent diarrhea, this rare complication should be considered. Topical sulfonamide preparations (mainly sulfacetamide) are also available by prescription and may be particularly useful in patients who also show evidence of rosacea. These medications are often well accepted, although some patients may find their odor offensive. Patients with allergies to oral sulfa drugs should not use topical sulfonamides. Topical dapsone, a newer arrival in the acne antibiotic market, appears to be most effective against inflammatory lesions, although its mechanism may not be related to *C. acnes* reduction. Topical dapsone may result in clinically insignificant mild hemolysis in patients with glucose 6-phosphate dehydrogenase deficiency.[69] More recently, minocycline foam has been approved as another topical option.

The landscape of topical acne therapy has evolved significantly in recent decades, with the increasing availability of fixed-dose combination therapies (see Table 8.3). These agents are approved for mild to moderate acne vulgaris, and they offer the advantages of improved adherence and complementary mechanisms of action of the individual active ingredients.[70] Available fixed-dose combination products include those combining BP and clindamycin, BP and adapalene, clindamycin and tretinoin, and BP and erythromycin. Each of these products, to receive US Food and Drug Administration (FDA) approval, was demonstrated to have superior efficacy over placebo as well as the individual active ingredients ("monads") in large, multicenter clinical trials.

With increasing use of topical antibiotics for the treatment of acne vulgaris, the development of resistant strains of *C. acnes* is being observed. Cross-resistance of *C. acnes* to erythromycin and clindamycin is now widespread.[71] In one study, erythromycin-resistant organisms were isolated from 51% of patients treated with oral erythromycin but also from 42% of patients treated with topical clindamycin.[72] Antibiotic-resistant propionibacteria may be transmissible between acne-prone individuals as well as between patients and their physicians.[73] Data suggest that the concomitant use of BP with topical (as well as oral) erythromycin or clindamycin diminishes the emergence of resistant bacterial strains.[27,49,74]

Azelaic acid is a naturally occurring dicarboxylic acid produced by the fungal organism *Pityrosporum ovale*. It has antibacterial and anticomedonal properties and is felt by some to be equal in efficacy to BP or tretinoin. The effectiveness of azelaic acid may be increased by using it in combination with other topical medications such as retinoids, antibiotics, or BP.[75] Another benefit of this agent is its ability to decrease hyperpigmentation caused by acne. Azelaic acid is marketed as a 20% cream and is applied twice daily. Side effects are rare but include burning, tingling, mild erythema, and pruritus.

Physicians are commonly consulted regarding the safety of acne treatment in women who are pregnant, may become pregnant, or are breastfeeding an infant. Although there are no long-term studies on the use of topical antibiotics during pregnancy, erythromycin seems to be safe. Because it is estimated that approximately 8% of topically applied clindamycin can be absorbed,[62] this drug is probably best avoided for women who are breastfeeding, are pregnant, or are contemplating pregnancy. Although approximately 5% of topically applied BP is absorbed through the skin, it is rapidly metabolized to benzoic acid, enters the dermal blood vessels as benzoate, and is then transported to the kidneys and excreted in the urine. Thus BP appears to be safe during pregnancy, although controlled studies are lacking. The use of tretinoin is discussed earlier in this section.

Oral antibiotics (Table 8.4) are the most common form of systemic therapy used in the treatment of acne vulgaris, despite the fact that the only agent with FDA-approval for this indication is extended-release minocycline. These agents are quite effective and are best reserved for patients with moderate or severe inflammatory acne. They are useful in decreasing *C. acnes*, free fatty acids found in sebum, and inflammation (via their inhibitory effect on neutrophil chemotaxis). Oral antibiotics generally require 4 to 8 weeks to achieve their maximum effect, and it is usually necessary to continue therapy for several months, with gradual tapering as tolerated once the disease activity has diminished. The most commonly used antibiotics for treating acne are the tetracycline-class drugs (tetracycline, minocycline, doxycycline, and, more recently approved, sarecycline) and erythromycin. Less commonly, clindamycin, trimethoprim-sulfamethoxazole, azithromycin, and cephalexin are used. These medications are usually given on a twice-daily basis.

The safety of long-term antibiotic therapy for acne has been a concern of patients, parents, and physicians. Although the risk-to-benefit ratio of the most commonly used medications is favorable, each agent carries its own inherent potential toxicities, some of greater concern than others. The development of *C. acnes* resistance has been demonstrated for most of the agents used in this setting, especially erythromycin and clindamycin, in which case cross-resistance patterns may emerge.[76,77] General guidelines for oral antibiotic use in acne include avoiding the oral agent if topical agents will suffice, continuing treatment for no longer than is necessary, reusing the same drug when possible (if restarting oral therapy is required), and avoidance of concomitant oral and topical treatment with dissimilar antibiotics.[77] In addition, it is recommended that treatment be limited

Table 8.4 Oral Antibiotics for Acne Vulgaris

Drug	Usual Dosage*	Comments/Side Effects
COMMONLY USED		
Tetracycline	250–500 mg	Dental staining <9 years Dairy products decrease absorption GI upset, photosensitivity, teratogenic, PTC, VVC, IBD
Minocycline	50–100 mg 55, 65, 80, 105, 115 mg ER (1 mg/kg once daily)	Dental staining <9 years Dairy products decrease absorption Vertigo (lower incidence with ER), GI upset, blue-gray skin pigmentation, severe drug reactions with hepatitis/pneumonitis, lupus-like reactions, SJS, teratogenic, hepatitis, PTC, VVC, IBD
Doxycycline	50–100 mg 75, 100, 150 mg ER, once daily 20 mg ("subantimicrobial dose")	Dental staining <9 years Dairy products decrease absorption Photosensitivity, photoonycholysis, GI upset (rare), teratogenic, PTC, VVC, IBD
Erythromycin	250–500 mg	GI upset (common), VVC, drug–drug interactions, prolongation of the QT interval; no longer recommended by most experts given increased resistance
LESS COMMONLY USED		
Trimethoprim-sulfamethoxazole	80/400 mg, 160/800 mg	Severe drug reactions, SJS, bone marrow suppression, hepatitis, GI upset, VVC, fixed drug eruption; routine use for acne strongly discouraged
Azithromycin	Varied; often pulse dosing	GI upset, occasional drug reactions
Clindamycin	75–150 mg	Pseudomembranous colitis, GI upset, drug reactions, VVC
Cephalexin	250–500 mg	GI upset, drug reactions, VVC

ER, Extended release formulation; *GI*, gastrointestinal; *IBD*, inflammatory bowel disease; *PTC*, pseudotumor cerebri; *SJS*, Stevens–Johnson syndrome; *VVC*, vulvovaginal candidiasis.
*Usually given twice daily for acne unless otherwise noted in table.

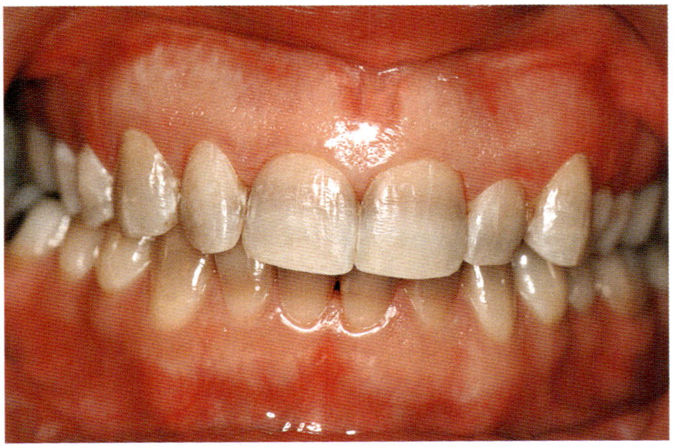

Fig. 8.15 Dental staining from tetracycline. (Courtesy Maria Simon, DDS.)

to the shortest possible duration, with reevaluation in 3 to 4 months, in an attempt to minimize bacterial resistance and that concomitant therapy with BP and/or a retinoid be used and continued for maintenance after completion of systemic therapy.[53,78] In patients who do not respond to oral antibiotics, the possibility of resistant strains should be considered. Overall, the commonly used oral antibiotics for acne are well tolerated, side effects are uncommon, and routine laboratory testing is unnecessary. Concomitant use of antibiotics and oral contraceptive agents may result in decreased efficacy of the latter, and this possibility should be discussed with female patients.

Tetracycline-class antibiotics (especially doxycycline and minocycline) are the gold standard of oral antibiotic therapy for acne. These agents have a long track record of safety and efficacy, although side effects are possible. The possibility of dental staining (Fig. 8.15) in children younger than 9 years of age precludes their use in this population, who only occasionally have moderate to severe acne. Tetracycline-class antibiotics should also not be used in pregnant women, given the deposition of the drug in developing teeth as a result of its chelating properties and the formation of a tetracycline–calcium orthophosphate complex.

The most common side effects of the tetracyclines are photosensitivity and gastrointestinal upset. The risk of phototoxicity is greatest with tetracycline and doxycycline and extremely rare with minocycline. Pseudotumor cerebri is a rare side effect, the risk being greatest when isotretinoin and a tetracycline are taken concomitantly. Tetracyclines cannot be taken with dairy products or antacids, which impair absorption. In addition, tetracycline (but not doxycycline or minocycline) absorption is impaired in the presence of food, and thus the medication must be taken 1 hour before or 2 hours after a meal. This feature may result in decreased adherence among active teenagers. Tetracyclines should be used with caution in patients with renal disease.

Doxycycline has the benefit of sustained absorption in the presence of food but may result in severe photosensitivity reactions. One such type of reaction is "photoonycholysis," which presents with erythema and separation of the nail plate from the nailbed (Fig. 8.16). These patients usually also have an associated photosensitivity rash on exposed areas of skin. Pill esophagitis is another potential side effect of oral doxycycline and can usually be prevented by taking the medication with a full glass of water and avoiding recumbency for at least 1 hour after dosing. In a retrospective cohort study of patients with acne who were treated with oral tetracycline-class antibiotics, the hazard ratio (HR) for developing inflammatory bowel disease (IBD) was increased for all agents in this class but most notably for doxycycline (HR of 1.63).[79] However, a definitive causal link between tetracycline-class antibiotics and development of IBD remains to be proven. Off-label use of subantimicrobial-dose doxycycline hyclate (20-mg tablets taken twice daily) has been reported in acne vulgaris and has been shown to significantly reduce the number of lesions without any detectable antimicrobial effect on skin flora or alteration of resistance patterns.[80] An extended-release formulation of doxycycline is available and can be administered once daily.

Minocycline is the most widely prescribed systemic antibiotic for the management of acne in the United States, Canada, and the United Kingdom, and it is estimated that 65% of prescriptions for this drug are for acne.[81] It is particularly effective against *C. acnes* and also has antiinflammatory properties. Similar to doxycycline, an extended-release formulation of minocycline is available and may improve adherence as well as decrease the incidence of vestibular side effects. Although the side effect profile is somewhat similar to that of other tetracyclines, minocycline rarely causes photosensitivity. Other side effects more specific to minocycline are headache, dizziness, vertigo, and a blue-gray pigmentation of mucosae (see Fig. 11.64*A*) or at sites of previous inflammation such as acne scars.

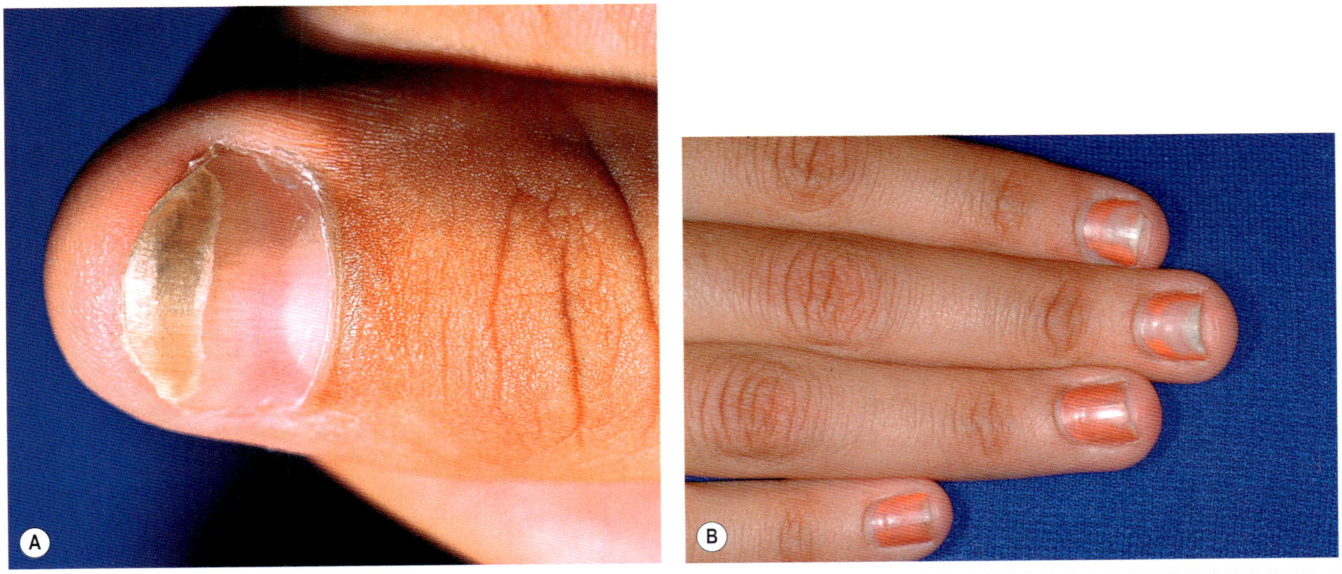

Fig. 8.16 Doxycycline-induced photoonycholysis in two patients. Note distal nail plate separation with new nail growing in proximally **(A)** and separation of nail plate from underlying nailbed in the index and middle fingers **(B)**.

Occasional yet potentially serious toxicities may be associated with minocycline, including autoimmune hepatitis, drug-induced lupus (DIL), serum sickness–like reaction (SSLR), and drug reaction with eosinophilia and systemic symptoms (DRESS).[81–83] DRESS (see Chapter 20) is characterized by a diffuse erythematous rash, facial (especially periorbital) edema, lymphadenopathy, fever, and internal organ involvement (most commonly the liver). It tends to occur within 6 to 8 weeks of starting the drug and is similar to the hypersensitivity reaction occasionally seen with the aromatic anticonvulsants (phenytoin, carbamazepine, phenobarbital, lamotrigine). SSLR (see Chapter 20) presents with fever, urticarial rash, periarticular swelling with arthralgia, and occasional nephritis and lymphadenopathy. A comparative study reviewing adverse events of tetracycline, minocycline, and doxycycline revealed that these reaction patterns (DIL, SSLR, and DRESS, also known as *drug hypersensitivity reaction* or *drug hypersensitivity syndrome*) are all more common with minocycline than with the other two medications.[84] Also of note is the fact that SSLR and DRESS usually occur within 2 months of beginning treatment, whereas DIL may be delayed for up to 2 years.[84] Like doxycycline, minocycline use has been linked to a possible increased risk of IBD, but this link remains definitively unproven.

Autoimmune hepatitis, DIL, arthritis, vasculitis, and development of autoantibodies have been unified under the moniker of minocycline-induced autoimmunity (MIA). A study of 27 children with MIA revealed a mean duration of treatment of 13 months before the diagnosis. The majority of patients had polyarthralgia or polyarthritis, mostly of the hands and feet. Other features included constitutional symptoms, livedo reticularis, Raynaud phenomenon, elevation of liver enzymes, and elevated antinuclear antibody titers. Importantly, 26% of patients had chronic autoimmunity, manifested mostly as persistent arthritis.[85] Many patients with minocycline-associated DIL have no skin eruption. Polyarteritis nodosa has been reported, and positivity for antinuclear antibody and perinuclear antineutrophil cytoplasmic antibody supports the diagnosis.[51,86] Antihistone antibodies, traditionally considered pathognomonic for DIL, are often negative in patients with minocycline-associated disease. In a study of a cohort of patients with minocycline-induced liver injury, 80% of whom were female with a median age of 19 years, a markedly increased carrier frequency (compared with population controls) for human leukocyte antigen (HLA)–B*35:02 was found, suggesting increased risk in those carrying this HLA allele.[87]

Although these major types of tetracycline class drug reactions are rare overall, their possibility should be discussed with the patient, especially when minocycline is being considered. Many experts consider doxycycline to be a safer alternative, even in patients who have a history of MIA.

Erythromycin was traditionally a useful antibiotic for acne vulgaris, but its use is often limited by the fairly high incidence of gastrointestinal disturbance, even with the enteric-coated preparations. Otherwise it has few side effects and carries the distinct benefit of no phototoxicity. However, the high prevalence of erythromycin-resistant *C. acnes* organisms further limits its clinical utility. Other antibiotics occasionally used for acne include clindamycin, trimethoprim-sulfamethoxazole, azithromycin, and cephalexin. Prolonged use of oral clindamycin is not desirable because of the risk of pseudomembranous colitis caused by the toxin liberated by *Clostridium difficile*, which is able to grow in large numbers in the intestinal tract of some patients who receive this drug. Trimethoprim-sulfamethoxazole can be very effective for acne, but it is not recommended as a first-line agent given the severe and potentially life-threatening reactions (i.e., DRESS, Stevens–Johnson syndrome, and toxic epidermal necrolysis) and bone marrow suppression that may occur.

The most common complication of antibiotic therapy in adult female patients is vaginal candidiasis, but it rarely occurs in teenagers. This complication is proportionately more common in women who take combined oral contraceptives (COCs) concomitantly with their systemic antibiotics. Another concern in patients who are also taking COCs is the possibility of the oral antibiotic diminishing the effectiveness of the contraceptive. Although this possibility remains controversial, it should be discussed with patients and alternative forms of birth control considered during the period of treatment. Patients on long-term antibiotic therapy may rarely develop a condition termed *Gram-negative folliculitis*, caused by superinfection of the pilosebaceous units with Gram-negative organisms. This condition should be considered in the acne patient presenting with a pustular eruption and who has a history of antibiotic treatment for 3 to 6 months. It is manifested by a pustular folliculitis (often with lesions situated around the nose and mouth) or deep nodulocystic lesions topped by pustules and recalcitrant to the acne regimen. The organisms causing Gram-negative folliculitis include *Escherichia coli*, *Pseudomonas aeruginosa*, *Serratia marcescens*, *Klebsiella* spp., and *Proteus mirabilis*.[88] It may be related to impaired host responses in cell-mediated or humoral immunity.[89] Gram-negative folliculitis may respond to a change in antibiotics to reduce Gram-negative organisms, but it responds more consistently to isotretinoin.[88,90]

Hormonal therapies are another option for the treatment of acne in female patients. The primary goal of these therapies is to oppose the effects of androgens on the sebaceous glands.[91] Hormonally driven acne may have some distinguishing clinical features, including larger and deep-seated inflammatory nodules in the mandibular and anterolateral neck regions, menses-associated flares, and associated signs of hyperandrogenism such as hirsutism and menstrual irregularities. If polycystic ovary syndrome (PCOS) is suspected, initial laboratory testing should include serum total and free testosterone, DHEA sulfate, and luteinizing hormone and follicle-stimulating hormone levels, as well as the 17-hydroxyprogesterone level if late-onset congenital adrenal hyperplasia is suspected. Abnormal findings should prompt referral to an endocrinologist.

Hormonal acne therapies include androgen receptor blockers, adrenal androgen production blockers, ovarian androgen production blockers, and enzyme inhibitors, and they may be prescribed in consultation with a gynecologist or endocrinologist. This group of medications may have other beneficial effects on the hirsutism, androgenetic alopecia, and menstrual irregularities in some female patients.[26] COCs contain both an estrogen and a progestin, and those with a lower intrinsic androgenic activity type of progestin (desogestrel, norgestimate, and drospirenone) are most desirable for acne therapy. Drospirenone, a novel progestin, has both antiandrogenic and antimineralocorticoid activity and is reportedly better tolerated in terms of weight gain and mood changes.[92] Norgestimate and ethinyl estradiol (Ortho Tri-Cyclen); norethindrone, ethinyl estradiol, and ferrous fumarate (Estrostep Fe); drospirenone and ethinyl estradiol (Yaz); and drospirenone, ethinyl estradiol, and levomefolate calcium (Beyaz) are FDA-approved for use in the treatment of acne vulgaris. COCs may be the first-line treatment in female patients with skin manifestations of hyperandrogenemia.[93] Risks of COCs include venous thromboembolism, myocardial infarction, and ischemic or hemorrhagic stroke, although these risks seem to be more clinically significant in patients with other risk factors such as tobacco use, diabetes mellitus, and hypertension.[94] Box 8.4 lists contraindications to treatment with COCs. Antiandrogenic agents include spironolactone, flutamide, cyproterone acetate, gonadotropin-releasing hormone antagonists, and 5-α-reductase inhibitors. Spironolactone, which is used primarily as a diuretic in the treatment of hypertension, competes for androgen receptors on target cells and inhibits 5-α-reductase. It is usually started at 25 to 50 mg/day, and maintenance doses, which vary by the individual, range from 25 to 200 mg/day.[93] Potential side effects of spironolactone therapy include menstrual irregularities (in as many as half of treated women), nausea, dizziness, polyuria, and hyperkalemia, although the latter has been shown to be rare in otherwise healthy women.[95,96] In a study of 27 women with severe acne who were treated with spironolactone and a combined contraceptive (drospirenone and ethinylestradiol), this combination was demonstrated to be effective and safe, without hyperkalemia or other serious side effects.[97]

Isotretinoin (13-*cis* retinoic acid; Absorica, Amnesteem, Claravis, Myorisan, Sotret, Zenatane) is a derivative of vitamin A that is highly effective for recalcitrant nodulocystic acne, and the availability of this agent revolutionized the treatment of severe disease. Although the precise mechanism of action is unknown, its effects appear to be related to marked inhibition of sebum synthesis, lowering of *C. acnes* concentration, inhibition of neutrophil chemotaxis, and comedolytic and antiinflammatory effects. Isotretinoin therapy often, but not always, results in complete and permanent remission of acne vulgaris.[98] Preteens and young teenagers seem to have the highest rate of relapse. In patients who experience a recurrence of disease,

Box 8.4 Contraindications to Treatment with Combined Oral Contraceptive Agents

Pregnancy
Breast cancer (current or past)
Breastfeeding (<6 months postpartum)
History of the following:

- Diabetes with end organ damage or if <35 years of age
- Deep vein thrombosis or pulmonary embolism
- Hypertension (uncontrolled)
- Major surgery with prolonged immobilization
- CVA
- Ischemic heart disease
- Valvular heart disease with high risk
- Hypercholesterolemia
- Migraine headache and >35 years of age (or <35 years of age and focal neurologic symptoms)
- Liver disease (hepatitis, cirrhosis, liver tumor)
- Smoking and >35 years of age
- Known thrombogenic mutations
- Systemic lupus with antiphospholipid antibodies

Adapted from Zaenglein AL, Pathy AL, Schlosser BJ, et al. Guidelines for the management of acne vulgaris. J Am Acad Dermatol 2016;74(5):945–73; Harper JC. Use of oral contraceptives for management of acne vulgaris. Practical considerations in real world practice. Dermatol Clin 2016;34: 159–65; and Nguyen HL, Tollefson MM. Endocrine disorders and hormonal for adolescent acne. Curr Opin Pediatr 2017;29:455–65.
CVA, Cerebrovascular accident.

however, the flares may be milder and more responsive to therapies used before isotretinoin therapy. Repeat courses may occasionally be necessary. Although approved by the FDA for treatment of severe acne, in recent guidelines for management of acne vulgaris, the expert working group agreed that indications for isotretinoin therapy include moderate acne that is either treatment resistant or that produces physical scarring or significant psychosocial distress.[53]

Patients usually start by taking 0.5 mg/kg per day of isotretinoin, increasing the dosage to 1 mg/kg per day, usually for around 16 to 24 weeks. A lower starting dosage is often used in patients with severe acne to prevent exacerbation. Cumulative dosing goals, ranging from 120 to 150 mg/kg for the entire course of treatment, have been advocated because they may decrease the rate of relapse.[99,100] Early in the course of isotretinoin therapy, there may be a temporary flare of lesions, and patient education regarding this possibility is vital. Although isotretinoin is truly a miracle drug for severe forms of acne, it has several potential side effects and should only be prescribed by physicians experienced in its use.

Potential adverse effects of isotretinoin are numerous and are summarized in Table 8.5. Laboratory monitoring during therapy is typically limited to fasting serum lipid profiles and hepatic function studies (in addition to monthly pregnancy tests for female patients of childbearing potential). Recent studies have suggested that monitoring of lipid and hepatic panels may be indicated less frequently, especially if findings are normal when tested 2 months into therapy.[101,102] A risk management program, iPLEDGE (www.ipledgeprogram.com), was approved by the FDA and drug manufacturers and implemented in March 2006. This mandatory distribution program, which requires prescribers, patients, pharmacies, drug wholesalers, and manufacturers in the United States to register and comply, was created in an effort to prevent the use of isotretinoin during pregnancy because of its teratogenic effects (see later). Under this system, prescribers must record two negative pregnancy tests before a female patient can commence therapy with isotretinoin. The iPLEDGE program represents the most rigorous risk management program in history for such a widely prescribed drug.[103] Overall the risk of major side effects from isotretinoin (assuming pregnancy is avoided) is quite low. Unfortunately, a retrospective cohort study found no significant decrease in fetal exposure in female patients of childbearing age compared with the prior risk management program (System to Manage Accutane-Related Teratogenicity [SMART]).[104]

Table 8.5 Potential Isotretinoin-Associated Adverse Effects

Side Effect	Comment
Dry skin and nasal membranes	Occasional epistaxis
Dry eyes	Most problematic for contact-lens wearers; may develop conjunctivitis, chalazion, hordeolum
Cheilitis	May be quite severe
Photosensitivity	
Decreased night vision	
Corneal opacities	
Alopecia	Diffuse thinning; generally reversible but can be the start of androgenetic alopecia
Headache	
Pseudotumor cerebri	Most common with concomitant use of tetracycline-class antibiotic
Musculoskeletal pain	
Hyperostosis	Mainly seen with prolonged use
Elevated triglycerides, cholesterol	Rare pancreatitis
Hepatitis	
Inflammatory bowel disease	Controversial; current evidence insufficient to prove an association or causal relationship
Rhabdomyolysis	
Teratogenicity	See text for discussion
Depression, suicidal ideation	See text for discussion

Isotretinoin is a known human teratogen and is a pregnancy category X drug. Major fetal malformations have been observed in exposed infants, including abnormalities of the skull, ear, eye, central nervous system, and heart. As little as one pill can have devastating consequences on the developing fetus.[26] To qualify for therapy, females of childbearing potential must have two negative serum or urine pregnancy tests and commit to either abstinence or use of two forms of contraception, one of which must be a primary form (COC, intrauterine device, injectable or implantable hormonal birth control product, partner's vasectomy, or tubal ligation), for at least 1 month before initiation of therapy and for 1 month after discontinuing therapy. Abstinence is most desirable for female patients on isotretinoin therapy. A signed patient consent form is required. Unfortunately, even with dedicated pregnancy prevention programs and education regarding isotretinoin-associated teratogenicity, inadequate birth control efforts continue to be practiced by some female patients being treated with isotretinoin. Ongoing fetal exposure to isotretinoin has been demonstrated to be an international problem, highlighting the need for more effective strategies that incorporate considerations for cultural differences.[105]

The risks of isotretinoin-related depression and SI have come to the forefront in recent years. The exact association, if any, remains controversial, and arguments both supporting and refuting the potential for mood disturbance have been made. Epidemiologic data have demonstrated a lower suicide rate in 12- to 18-year-old isotretinoin users compared with the annual rate of suicide for that population in the United States. Critical literature reviews have failed to confirm an association, and although retinoid receptors are widely distributed in the brain, there is no known pharmacologic mechanism to account for isotretinoin-induced psychiatric symptoms.[106–108] In one systematic literature review it was noted that studies comparing depression before and after treatment did not show a significant increase and that, surprisingly, some revealed a trend toward fewer or less severe depressive symptoms after isotretinoin therapy.[108] A meta-analysis of the literature confirmed these observations, finding a lower prevalence of depression after isotretinoin treatment of acne, with decrease in mean depression scores.[109] In a cross-sectional questionnaire-based study exploring the relationship of SI, mental health problems, and social functioning to acne severity among adolescents, SI was reported two to three times more often in those with increasingly severe acne compared with those with little to no acne. Mental health problems and poorer school functioning were also associated with substantial acne, and the authors concluded that adverse events such as depression and SI that have been ascribed to acne therapies may actually reflect the burden of the disease rather than a medication effect.[110] Given these observations and others, it is recommended that isotretinoin patients (a population at greater risk for psychiatric comorbidity) be appropriately screened and monitored for symptoms of depression and SI, with prompt referral to a mental health professional if concerns arise.[111]

The potential association between isotretinoin use and IBD, which was first suggested in the mid-1980s, continues to be debated. A case-control study of more than 8000 cases of IBD compared with nearly 22,000 controls revealed a strong association between previous isotretinoin exposure and ulcerative colitis, but not Crohn's disease, with the risk increasing in a dose-dependent manner.[112] In another case-control study and meta-analysis, there was no increased risk ratio for IBD in patients who had been treated with isotretinoin.[113] In a retrospective population-based cohort study in Canada, no significant association between isotretinoin use and IBD was found, although in a secondary analysis of individuals limited to ages 12 through 19 years, a weak IBD association was noted for both isotretinoin and topical acne medications.[114] In two other studies, including a meta-analysis and a large single-center retrospective study, there was no increased risk of IBD identified with isotretinoin exposure.[115,116] Hence, as supported by the position statement of the American Academy of Dermatology, current evidence is insufficient to prove either an association or a causal relationship between isotretinoin use and IBD in the general population.[117] Until more is known, however, it is prudent to mention this possible association to patients and parents and to monitor patients appropriately during therapy.

It is a common notion that skin surgery or other procedures should be delayed after isotretinoin therapy, given the traditional belief that the agent impairs normal wound healing or may result in abnormal scarring. However, in a systematic review of the literature over a 35-year period, there was insufficient evidence to support delaying skin surgery, fractional ablative or nonablative laser procedures, or a variety of cosmetic procedures (manual dermabrasion, superficial chemical peels, laser hair removal) in patients either receiving or having recently completed isotretinoin treatment.[118]

There are a variety of miscellaneous treatments for acne vulgaris, and these are listed in Table 8.6.[26,119–121] Box 8.5 lists examples of therapeutic approaches based on acne type and severity.

NEONATAL ACNE

Although acne is usually a disorder of adolescents and young adults, neonates and infants are occasionally affected. Neonatal acne has its onset within the first weeks of life and may be congenital in up to 20% of newborns.[122] Infantile acne (see Infantile Acne section), on the other hand, usually presents between 1 and 12 months of life and tends to be more severe and more persistent.[123] Both types occur more often in boys than in girls.

Neonatal acne typically presents with mildly erythematous papules involving the face and scalp and less commonly the chest and back (Fig. 8.17). Comedones occasionally may be present, although these tend to be more characteristic of infantile acne. Neonates presenting with more pustular lesions may have a variant referred to as *neonatal cephalic pustulosis* (see below). Neonatal acne should be distinguished from other potentially papulopustular disorders of the neonate, including infection (bacterial, candidal, or viral), erythema toxicum neonatorum, miliaria (prickly heat), eosinophilic folliculitis, and milia (typically noninflamed white papules rather than pustules).

The cause of neonatal acne is believed to relate to increased production of DHEA by the fetal adrenal glands. Another factor may be androgens, both delivered transplacentally and manufactured by the neonatal testicles. Testicular androgen production serves as a stimulus to primed adrenal glands, which may partially explain the

Table 8.6 Alternative Treatments for Acne Vulgaris

Treatment	Comment
Comedone extraction	Performed with comedone extractor
Injections	Intralesional triamcinolone injected into large cysts or nodules
Light therapy	Blue light (may photoinactivate *C. acnes*) Red light (may have antiinflammatory effect) Combination blue-red light Intensed pulse light (IPL) Photodynamic therapy (PDT) Photopneumatic therapy
Laser therapy	KTP, pulsed dye laser (rarely used) Resurfacing laser (including both nonablative and ablative resurfacing lasers); useful for acne scarring
Dermabrasion/dermasanding	Useful for acne scarring
Collagen injection	Useful for acne scarring
Chemical peels	Useful for acne scarring and hyperpigmentation
Punch grafts/tissue augmentation	Useful for acne scarring
Trichloroacetic acid	Useful for atrophic acne scars
Radiation therapy	Outdated modality
Topical tea tree oil	Other herbal agents including oral barberry extract, oral ayurvedic compounds, gluconolactone solution

Adapted from Rothman KF. Acne update. Dermatol Ther 1997;2:98–110; Zaenglein AL, Pathy AL, Schlosser BJ, et al. Guidelines of care for the management of acne vulgaris. J Am Acad Dermatol 2016;74(5):945–73; Elman M, Slatkine M, Harth Y. The effective treatment of acne vulgaris by a high-intensity, narrow band 405–420 nm light source. J Cosmet Laser Ther 2003;5(2):11–17; Goodman GJ. Management of post-acne scarring: what are the options for treatment. Am J Clin Dermatol 2000;1(1):3–17; and Lee JB, Chung WG, Kwahck H, et al. Focal treatment of acne scars with trichloroacetic acid: chemical reconstruction of skin scars method. Dermatol Surg 2002;28(11):1017–21.
KTP, Potassium titanyl phosphate.

Box 8.5 Acne Treatment Vignettes*

Mild Comedonal Acne

Topical retinoid once daily, *or*
Topical retinoid/BP combination product once daily, *or*
BP wash once daily

Mild–Moderate Combined Acne (Inflammatory and Comedonal Lesions)

BP cleanser daily and topical retinoid once daily, *or*
BP/topical antibiotic combination product in AM and topical retinoid in PM, *or*
BP cleanser daily and topical retinoid/topical antibiotic combination product once daily

Moderate–Severe Combined Acne (Inflammatory and Comedonal Lesions)

Oral antibiotic and topical retinoid once daily, *or*
Oral antibiotic and topical retinoid/BP combination product once daily, *or*
Oral antibiotic, BP wash, spironolactone and topical retinoid once daily (female patient), *or*
COC, oral antibiotic and topical retinoid/BP combination product once daily (female patient)

Severe or Scarring Acne

Isotretinoin

BP, Benzoyl peroxide; *COC*, combined oral contraceptive.
*These vignettes are therapeutic examples only and not intended to be specific recommendations; acne therapy should always be tailored to the specific patient and severity of involvement.

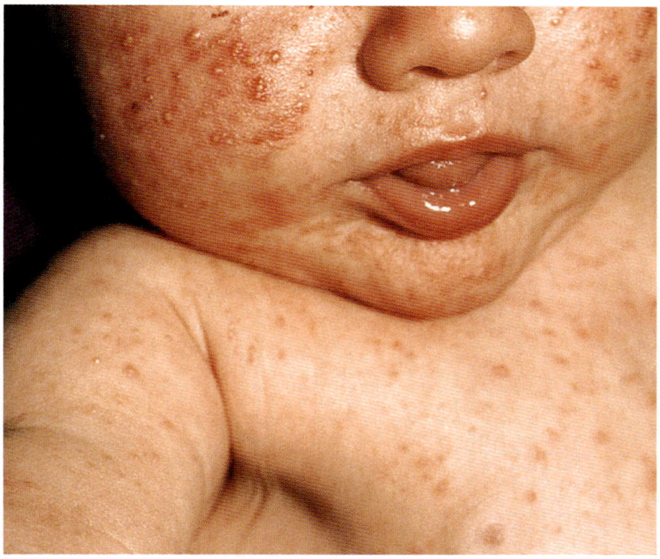

Fig. 8.17 Neonatal acne. This newborn had typical papules and pustules with rapid resolution over 1 month.

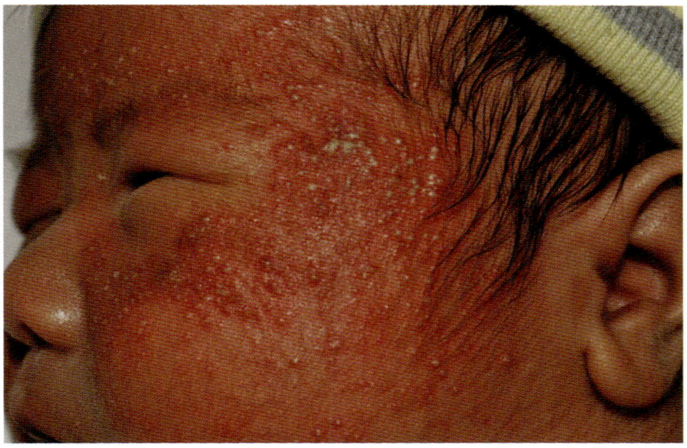

Fig. 8.18 Neonatal cephalic pustulosis. This 2-day-old male neonate (also shown in Fig. 2.16) presented with numerous inflammatory papules and pustules on the face; ketoconazole cream applied twice daily led to rapid resolution over 1 week.

increased incidence of neonatal acne in male babies.[98] In babies with neonatal acne, a family history of acne may or may not be present.[124]

In recent years a neonatal pustular eruption that presents in a similar fashion to neonatal acne has been described and has been termed *neonatal cephalic pustulosis.* This disorder presents with multiple facial papules and pustules (Fig. 8.18), and direct examination of pustule smears may reveal yeasts of *Malassezia furfur* or *Malassezia sympodialis.*[125,126] In a 1996 series of 13 neonates with such a pustular eruption, smears were notable for *M. furfur* in 8 of the patients, all of whose conditions cleared rapidly after application of ketoconazole cream.[125] Colonization of neonates with *Malassezia* begins at birth and increases over the first few weeks of life.[127] However, the exact role of *Malassezia* in this setting is poorly understood, with inconsistent findings in subsequent reports.[128] The association between neonatal cephalic pustulosis and neonatal acne remains unclear.[129]

Neonatal acne usually regresses spontaneously over 3 to 6 months, only occasionally persisting longer. In mild cases, therapy is generally unnecessary; daily cleansing with a gentle soap and water may be all that is required. Exogenous oil such as baby oils, creams, ointments, and lotions may aggravate the condition and should be avoided. For infants with more inflammatory or persistent disease, a low-strength

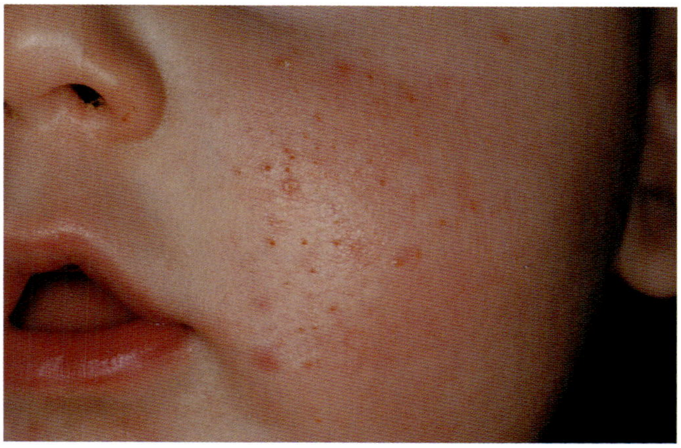

Fig. 8.19 Infantile acne. This child with infantile acne presented with primarily open and closed comedones.

(2.5% to 5%) BP gel or a topical antibiotic (e.g., erythromycin gel) are reasonable treatment options. In the otherwise-well neonate with a significantly pustular facial eruption (i.e., more suggestive of neonatal cephalic pustulosis), topical antifungal therapy can be considered. If there is a significant comedonal component or nodules are present, the infant more likely has infantile acne (see Infantile Acne section), and other therapeutic options may be necessary, including oral antibiotics.

INFANTILE ACNE

Infantile acne presents between 1 and 12 months of life. Clinically the infant most often has open and closed comedones (Fig. 8.19), but inflammatory papules and pustules occasionally occur (Fig. 8.20). They may also develop larger papules and nodules with the potential for scarring (Fig. 8.21), even without comedonal lesions. Lesions occur most commonly on the face, but the neck, back, and chest may also be involved. Most experts consider treatment of infantile acne vital to prevent scarring and permanent facial disfigurement.

The patient with infantile acne should have a concomitant growth assessment (with charting of height and weight) and examination for any features of precocious puberty or androgen excess, including axillary odor, clitoromegaly, presence of axillary or genital hair, breast development, and increased muscle mass. Left-hand radiography for bone age may be a useful screening test.[130] If any concerns are noted, an evaluation for hyperandrogenism should be performed (Box 8.6).

Treatment for infantile acne depends on the severity of the clinical lesions. Mild to moderate disease is usually treated with a combination of BP, topical antibiotics, and/or topical retinoids. The latter should always be included in patients with more comedonal disease. For disease that does not respond to topical measures, oral erythromycin is an excellent first-line antibiotic therapy, and the ethylsuccinate form is generally well tolerated. Refractory involvement or the presence of nodules or scarring suggests the need to consider oral isotretinoin therapy.[131] Intralesional steroids have also been used to treat larger nodules.

MID-CHILDHOOD ACNE

Mid-childhood acne is defined as acne that has its onset between 1 and 7 years of age. This is an important diagnosis to render because acne that begins during this age range is generally considered abnormal. This is related to the fact that children of these ages do not produce significant levels of either adrenal or gonadal androgens. Mid-childhood acne is the most likely type to be associated with an underlying endocrinologic disorder. Diagnoses such as late-onset congenital adrenal hyperplasia, androgen-secreting tumors of the adrenal glands or gonads (benign or malignant), and true precocious puberty can all present with early acne.[70,132] A hyperandrogenism evaluation (see Box 8.6) or referral to a pediatric endocrinologist is strongly recommended in this setting. Treatment for mid-childhood acne is similar to that outlined in the previous section for infantile acne.

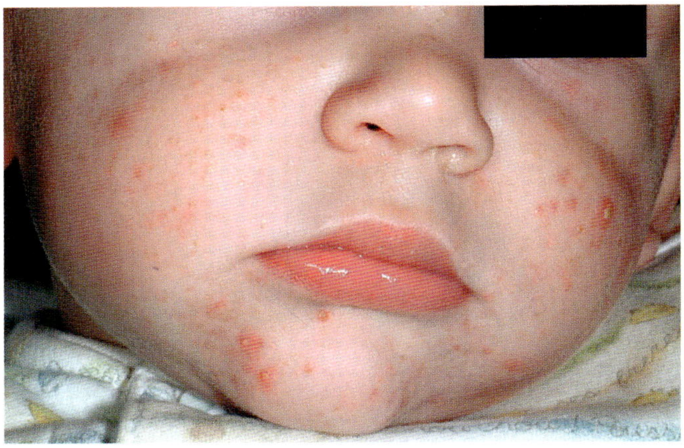

Fig. 8.20 Infantile acne. This infant had more persistent involvement with larger lesions such as the deep papulopustule on the left cheek.

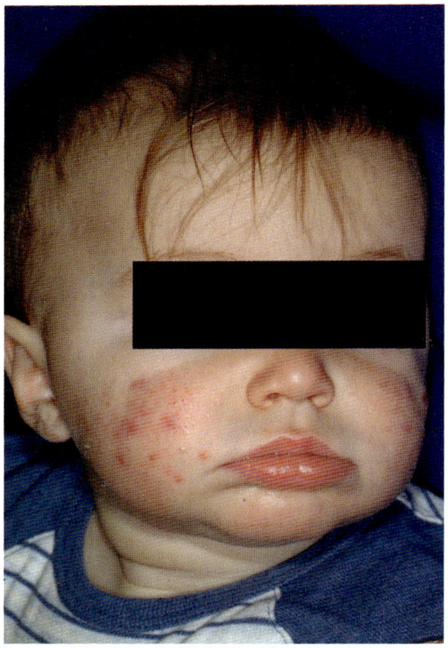

Fig. 8.21 Infantile acne. This infant had many inflammatory papules and nodules, which resulted in some permanent scarring.

Box 8.6 Recommended Laboratory Evaluation for the Child with Acne and Suspected Hyperandrogenism

- Serum testosterone (free and total)
- Luteinizing hormone (LH)
- Follicle-stimulating hormone (FSH)
- Dehydroepiandrosterone sulfate (DHEAS)
- 17-Hydroxyprogesterone (17-OHP)
- Prolactin
- Radiographic bone age

An important consideration for any infant or young child with acne is the possibility of virilization related to exogenous androgen exposure. Topical androgens (primarily in the form of testosterone gel or cream) are being increasingly used by male patients with hypogonadism, in addition to use as an off-label therapy for increased libido and enhanced manhood.[133,134] Inadvertent exposure of young children through contact with the treated individual has been increasingly reported and may result in clitoromegaly, appearance of secondary sexual hair, penile or testicular enlargement, frequent erections, growth acceleration, increased muscle mass, greasy hair, and acne.[134,135] This resultant pseudo-precocious puberty (PPP) highlights the need to obtain a thorough family history and inventory of medications being used by close contacts.

Table 8.7 Common Clinical Features of Polycystic Ovary Syndrome (PCOS)

Feature	Comment
Oligo- or anovulation*	Chronic anovulation may predispose to infertility and endometrial cancer
Hyperandrogenism*	Associated skin findings include hirsutism,[†,‡] acne,[§] hair loss (androgenetic alopecia)
Polycystic ovaries*	Defined as ovary volume >10 mL or cysts (2–9 mm) count ≥12 per ovary; however, criteria may be less specific in adolescents
Hyperinsulinemia	Associated with insulin resistance; often associated with acanthosis nigricans[‡] (see Chapter 23)
Overweight/obesity	
Other	Cardiovascular disease, obstructive sleep apnea, nonalcoholic steatohepatitis, psychiatric disorders

Adapted from Nguyen HL, Tollefson MM. Endocrine disorders and hormonal therapy for adolescent acne. Curr Opin Pediatr 2017;29:455–65; Schmidt TH, Khanijow K, Cedars MI, et al. Cutaneous findings and systemic associations in women with polycystic ovary syndrome. JAMA Dermatol 2016;152(4):391–8; and Housman E, Reynolds RV. Polycystic ovary syndrome: a review for dermatologists. J Am Acad Dermatol 2014;71:847.e1–10.

*Considered the hallmark clinical features of PCOS; two out of these three criteria required to confirm diagnosis per 2003 Rotterdam criteria.

†Defined as excessive sexual hair (a male-like distribution); distinguished from *hypertrichosis*, which is generalized excessive hair growth.

‡These two features appear to be the most reliable cutaneous markers for PCOS.

§Acne in these patients may be more severe, with nodulocystic lesions and accentuation on the chin, jawlines, and back.

ANDROGEN EXCESS AND ACNE

It is well recognized that androgens precipitate acne in both men and women, in addition to the potential effects of hyperandrogenemia in younger children as discussed in the previous sections. Acne may be produced or aggravated by increased adrenal gland production in response to stress, adrenal tumors, gonadal dysgenesis, Cushing syndrome, and ovarian androgen excess, such as that occurring in patients with PCOS (see Chapter 23). Clinical manifestations of PCOS are summarized in Table 8.7. This condition seems to be quite common. In one study of women with acne (but lacking menstrual disorders, obesity, or hirsutism), polycystic ovaries were found in 45%, compared with 17% of age-matched controls.[136] Adolescent girls with severe, persistent, or recalcitrant forms of acne, especially in the setting of other signs of androgen excess (e.g., menstrual irregularity and hirsutism) should be screened for this disorder with laboratory examinations (as discussed earlier) and transabdominal ovarian ultrasound. In patients with acne who show rapid development of virilizing signs such as voice deepening, increased muscle mass, or androgenetic alopecia, the evaluation should focus more on a search for a tumor rather than polycystic ovaries.[137] *Metabolic syndrome* (previously referred to as *syndrome X*) describes the clinical presentation of severe insulin resistance, obesity, hypertension, dyslipidemias, and microvascular angina. Occasionally, ovarian hyperandrogenism and polycystic ovaries may occur in this setting.[138] Treatment for PCOS typically consists of hormonal agents and antiandrogens such as spironolactone.

ACNE ROSACEA

Acne rosacea (also known simply as *rosacea*) is a chronic vascular inflammatory disorder usually limited to the face and characterized by erythema, telangiectasia, papules and pustules, and occasionally hyperplasia of the sebaceous glands and the soft tissues of the nose (rhinophyma). Rosacea is primarily a disease of adults between the ages of 30 and 50 but may also appear as early as the second decade of life, at times coexisting with acne vulgaris. Rosacea most often manifests as erythema and telangiectasia of the cheeks. A variety of ocular lesions may occur in the setting of rosacea. This association is termed *ocular rosacea* and is characterized by blepharitis, conjunctivitis, episcleritis, iritis, keratitis, and occasionally corneal ulceration and subsequent opacity. Several aberrant responses have been identified in rosacea, including altered toll-like receptor 2 (*TLR2*) expression, enhanced vasodilation triggered by cathelicidin, and greater lesional skin activity of reactive oxygen species.[139]

There are several potential exacerbating factors in rosacea, including sun exposure, stress, cold weather, hot beverages, alcohol consumption, and certain foods.[140] Avoidance of these factors may help prevent flares in certain individuals. Although the causes of rosacea and ocular rosacea are not well understood, a primary genetic predisposition is suggested because single genes may control mediators involved in rosacea pathways, namely enzymes, neuroendocrine transmitters, and cytokines.[141] Complete clearing of rosacea is rarely achieved, but satisfactory control can usually be accomplished by the use of topical or oral agents. Systemic therapy options include metronidazole, doxycycline, minocycline, tetracycline, and clarithromycin, and the most useful topical therapy appears to be metronidazole.[142] Topical sulfonamide preparations, azelaic acid, and sulfa-based washes may also be useful. Patients with rosacea tend to tolerate topical retinoids and BP poorly. Oral isotretinoin has been effective in patients with severe rosacea, predominantly of the granulomatous type. The telangiectasias may improve after pulsed-dye laser therapy or photodynamic therapy with red light. Two topical α-adrenergic receptor agonists have been approved for the facial erythema of rosacea: brimonidine gel and oxymetazoline hydrochloride cream. A subset of individuals treated with brimonidine gel, however, may experience worsening of facial erythema or rebound erythema, which in some cases has been worse than the baseline changes.[143,144] Rhinophyma, if it develops, is a difficult finding to treat and usually requires aggressive dermatologic surgical procedures with or without laser surgery.

Although clinically classic acne rosacea does not typically occur in young children, two entities that do classically occur in childhood may be related: periorificial dermatitis and idiopathic facial aseptic granuloma (IFAG). These are discussed in more detail later in this chapter.

POMADE ACNE

A variety of external agents can induce acne-like eruptions on repeated exposure to the skin of susceptible persons. These include greasy or oily sunscreen preparations, heavy makeup bases, and grooming agents. An acneiform eruption induced by various grooming substances used on the scalp has been termed *pomade acne*. It is usually seen on the forehead and temples and consists of numerous, closely set, closed comedones. The cheek and chin may also be involved if the agent has been applied over the entire face. Pomade acne may in fact represent true acne vulgaris potentiated by the use of occlusive products. It usually responds to standard acne therapy along with discontinuation of the offending comedogenic preparation.

ACNE COSMETICA

Acne cosmetica is a variant of acne described in women, usually women who are older than 20 years of age, that is attributed to the frequent or heavy use of cosmetics,[145] particularly those containing lanolin, petrolatum, certain vegetable oils, butyl stearate, isopropyl myristate, sodium lauryl sulfate, lauryl alcohol, or oleic acid. The lesions are predominantly small, scattered, closed comedones on the face. Although common in women without a history of acne, those with a history of adolescent acne seem to be the most susceptible. A prominent feature is a coarse facial appearance associated with prominent dark follicles that is often more distressing to the patient than the actual acne lesions themselves. The most extensive eruptions are seen in women who attempt to mask the lesions under a heavy coating of cosmetics. Fortunately most cosmetic companies today are aware of the problem of comedogenicity, and many cosmetics are now marketed as "noncomedogenic." A variant of acne cosmetica, consisting of deep-seated nodules and closed comedones that heal very slowly with hyperpigmentation, may occur after facial beauty treatments.[146]

ACNE EXCORIÉE

Acne excoriée (also known as acne excoriée des jeunes filles, acne excoriée of Brocq, skin picking disorder, and excoriation disorder) is a form of acne most commonly seen in adolescent girls. It is a self-inflicted skin condition in which the patient feels compelled to pick real or imagined acneiform lesions, which then propagates the disorder.[147] In the *Diagnostic and Statistical Manual of Mental Disorders*, fifth edition (DSM-5), this disorder is included under obsessive-compulsive disorder (OCD), along with other body-focused repetitive behavior disorders.[148–150] Associated comorbidities may include not only OCD but also anxiety, body dysmorphic disorder, substance use disorders, eating disorders, trichotillomania, kleptomania, compulsive buying, and borderline personality disorder.[151] Patients usually spontaneously admit the self-inflicted nature of the condition (although some may be unaware of their behavior), unlike most artifactual dermatoses[147,152] (see Chapter 26). Acne excoriée is often precipitated by emotional stress. Excoriation or squeezing of acne lesions may vary from mild to moderate irritation (Fig. 8.22) to severe scarring and occasional gross mutilation. Therapeutic options include cognitive behavior therapy, habit reversal training, and pharmacologic therapies, including selective serotonin reuptake inhibitors, doxepin, clomipramine, pimozide, and olanzapine.[151,153] It has been noted that many dermatologists focus on treatment of the acne component in this disorder, whereas a combined approach that includes appropriate referral for mental health services is optimal.[154]

ACNE CONGLOBATA

Acne conglobata is a severe suppurative form of acne vulgaris that is usually chronic and seen in men (especially Blacks) between 18 and 30 years of age. It is characterized by cysts, abscesses, and sinus tracts and often heals with cosmetically disfiguring keloidal scars. Axial and/or peripheral arthritis may be associated, and the latter tends to involve large joints in an oligoarticular pattern.[155] Treatment is challenging and may include nonsteroidal antiinflammatory drugs (NSAIDs), prednisone, methotrexate, penicillamine, and isotretinoin. Adalimumab and other tumor necrosis factor (TNF) antagonists may also be useful.[156]

Synovitis, acne, pustulosis, hyperostosis, and osteitis (SAPHO) syndrome is an association of musculoskeletal disorders (synovitis, arthritis, hyperostosis, osteitis) with skin conditions, including palmoplantar pustulosis and acne conglobata.[157,158] Sacroiliitis may also occur,

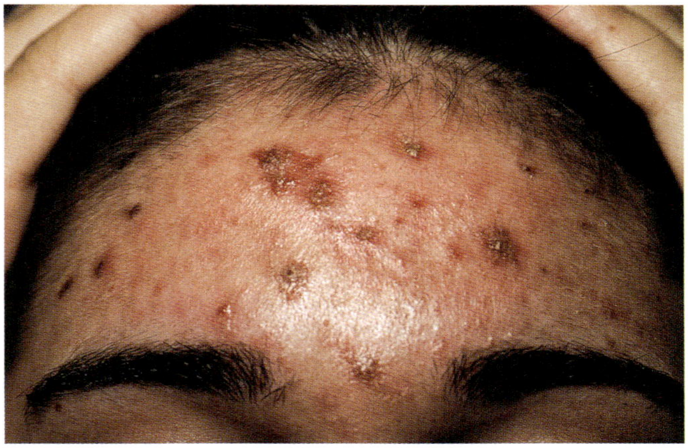

Fig. 8.22 Acne excoriée. Note the numerous excoriated and crusted papules of the forehead.

with or without hidradenitis suppurativa (HS) (see later) or a peripheral arthropathy.[159,160] Skin involvement is very common in SAPHO syndrome and may occur before or after the onset of bone and joint symptoms. Palmoplantar pustulosis appears to be the most common associated skin finding,[161] but the diagnosis is based on the typical oligoarticular findings (including erosions and joint space narrowing) in the absence of infectious or other etiologies, and skin findings are not necessarily required for the diagnosis.[161] Acne occurs in around 25% of patients. Bone lesions are present in the majority of patients, and articular lesions in around half of patients.[162] The most common skeletal site of involvement in adults is the anterior chest wall, whereas in pediatric patients, involvement of the long bones is most commonly noted.[163] Reported treatment options for SAPHO syndrome include NSAIDs, steroids, joint injections, antibiotics, methotrexate, colchicine, bisphosphonates, TNF inhibitors (including infliximab and etanercept), anakinra, ustekinumab, apremilast, and surgical interventions.[155,164–168]

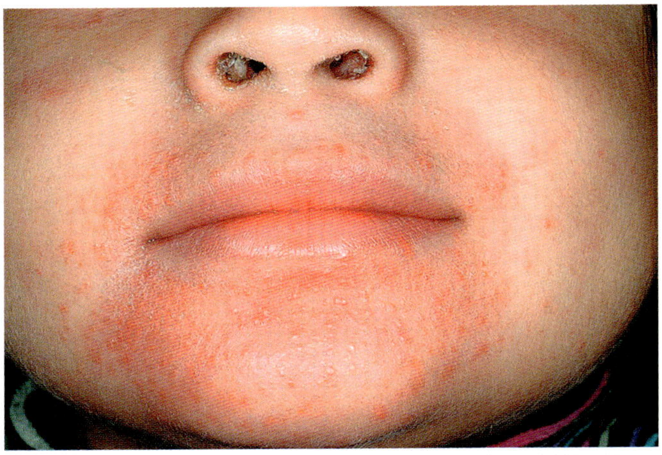

Fig. 8.23 Periorificial dermatitis. Numerous erythematous papules in a perioral distribution.

ACNE WITH FACIAL EDEMA/SOLID FACIAL EDEMA

Acne vulgaris (or acne rosacea) may at times be associated with an inflammatory edema of the middle face (cheeks, forehead, periorbital areas, base of the nose, and glabella), which has been termed *solid facial edema* or *Morbihan disease*. Although its pathogenesis is unknown, it is believed to be a manifestation of chronic cutaneous inflammation and edema, analogous to that occurring in the legs of patients with recurrent cellulitis and venous insufficiency. Occasionally it may be the only presenting symptom of these acneiform disorders.[169] Solid facial edema is challenging to treat and is often unresponsive to oral antibiotics or topical therapies, with variable responses to oral corticosteroids and isotretinoin.[170,171] Carbon dioxide laser blepharoplasty and surgical debulking have been reported for eyelid involvement.[172,173]

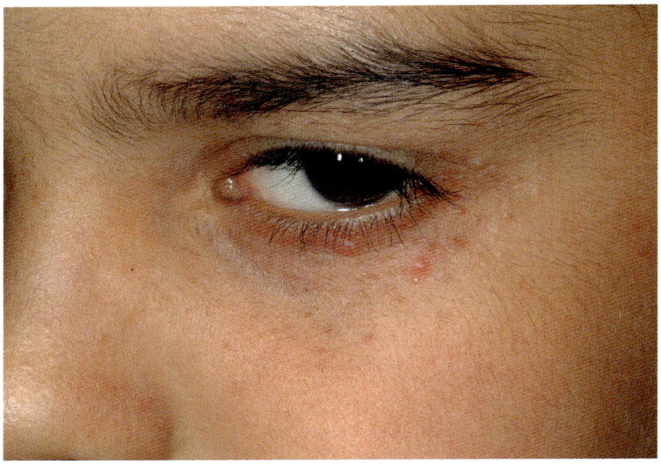

Fig. 8.24 Periorificial dermatitis. Erythematous papules and papulopustules and hyperpigmented macules of the inferior eyelid and periorbital region.

PERIORIFICIAL DERMATITIS

Periorificial dermatitis (known traditionally as *perioral dermatitis*) is a fairly common acneiform condition in children as well as young women, in whom it was originally described. Patients exhibit erythematous discrete papules and papulopustules distributed in perioral (Fig. 8.23), nasolabial, and periocular (Fig. 8.24) locations. Occasionally, flesh-colored papules or nodules may be present.[174] As the papules resolve, they may be replaced by a diffuse redness or erythematous scale. In a retrospective review of 222 children with periorificial dermatitis, the condition was most likely in White girls, with an average age at presentation of 6.6 years.[175]

Some consider periorificial dermatitis to be a juvenile form of acne rosacea and in particular the subtype of ocular rosacea, in part related to the overlapping histologic features in these conditions. The cause of periorificial dermatitis is unknown, but in many patients, use of mid- to high-potency topical corticosteroids seems to be related to the pathogenesis.[176,177] In one retrospective study of 79 children with the disorder, 72% had a history of previous topical, inhaled, or systemic steroid exposure.[178] However, periorificial dermatitis also occurs in children who have no preceding history of corticosteroid therapy. Blepharitis, conjunctivitis, chalazion, and hordeolum (stye) (Fig. 8.25) may occur in children with periorificial dermatitis and account for the significant clinical overlap with ocular rosacea.[179]

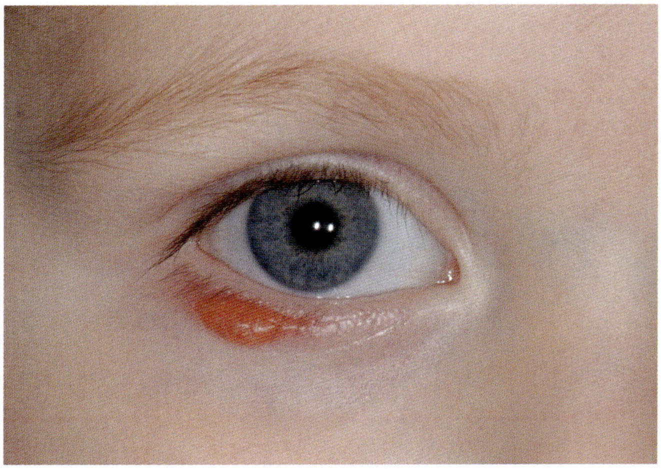

Fig. 8.25 Hordeolum (stye) in a patient with periorificial dermatitis. This male toddler had a history of recurrent perioral and periorbital papules and pustules, as well as recurrent styes.

Granulomatous periorificial dermatitis is a less common variant of periorificial dermatitis and is characterized by discrete yellow-brown papules (Fig. 8.26), less prominent erythema, and a granulomatous infiltrate on histologic examination. In addition to facial involvement, patients with this disorder may have extrafacial lesions clinically and histologically identical to the facial ones.[180] Ocular features such as those previously listed may also be present. Most reported cases of granulomatous periorificial dermatitis have been in prepubertal children, especially in those with a preceding history of topical corticosteroid application to the affected areas. Some patients have been initially misdiagnosed as having sarcoidosis, based primarily on histopathologic findings. Nonetheless, sarcoidosis and Blau syndrome (see Chapter 25), an entity that may be difficult to distinguish from sarcoidosis, may be in the differential diagnosis in patients with more extensive periorificial dermatitis (and with more generalized involvement).

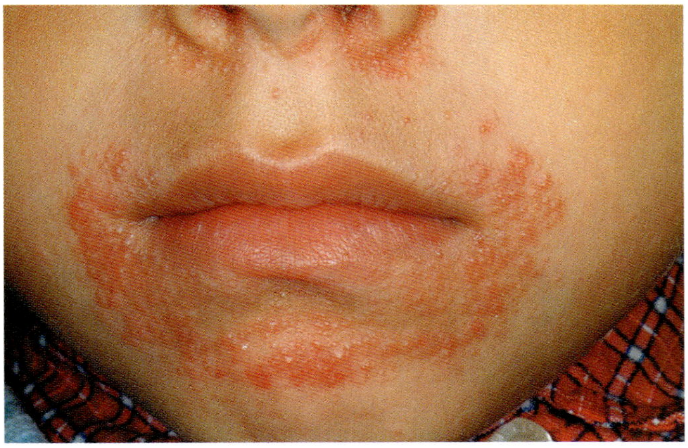

Fig. 8.26 Granulomatous periorificial dermatitis. Note the translucent quality of the erythematous papules and the nasolabial fold involvement.

Periorificial dermatitis is generally self-limited, although resolution may take months to years, and the lesions may occasionally heal with scarring. Treatment options include topical antibiotics (the most effective being metronidazole, erythromycin, or sulfur-based products) and, in more severe cases, oral erythromycin or tetracyclines (in patients older than 8 years). The authors have also used pimecrolimus cream either as monotherapy or in conjunction with another topical or oral agent with good efficacy and tolerability. In patients treated with oral antibiotics, treatment should be continued for a minimum of 6 to 8 weeks, with gradual tapering, in an effort to avoid the rapid rebounding that is commonly seen with shorter courses of therapy. If erythromycin is used (i.e., in younger children), enteric-coated preparations are recommended and generally well tolerated. Oral metronidazole has been reported with good response.[181] Ivermectin, given as a single dose orally or applied once daily topically, has been reported as another effective treatment option.[182]

IDIOPATHIC FACIAL ASEPTIC GRANULOMA

Idiopathic facial aseptic granuloma (IFAG) was initially described in the French literature as *pyodermite froide du visage* and believed to be a pyoderma.[183] More recently it has been viewed as a possible manifestation of granulomatous rosacea in childhood.[183–185] The possible link of IFAG to rosacea is based on its association with relapsing chalazia, facial telangiectasias, erythema and flushing, conjunctivitis, and conjunctival hyperemia, as well as its response to therapies traditionally used in rosacea.[185–187] IFAG presents as a large inflammatory nodule, often solitary, on the face (usually the cheek) of a child (Fig. 8.27). Some have suggested that the most common localization for these nodules is within a triangular-shaped area of the cheek, delimited by the lateral canthus, mouth angle, and earlobe.[188] The differential diagnosis is broad and may include pilomatricoma, cyst, infection, pyogenic granuloma, Spitz nevus, xanthogranuloma, and vascular lesion.[189] IFAG lesions on the eyelids may share overlapping features with hordeola and chalazia.[190] Histologic evaluation (when performed) reveals follicular and perifollicular inflammation with granulomas, a similar picture to that of granulomatous rosacea. Lesions of IFAG may resolve spontaneously in some patients but typically require treatment to speed healing. Reported therapies for the condition have included oral antibiotics (erythromycin, clarithromycin, or tetracycline-class antibiotics), oral metronidazole, and topical azelaic acid or metronidazole. Fortunately most lesions resolve without scarring.

FORDYCE SPOTS

Fordyce spots are a relatively common benign condition characterized by minute yellow to yellow-white macules and globoid papules distributed on the vermilion region of the lips and the buccal mucosa. Other less common locations include the glans penis (Fig. 8.28) or labia minora. Fordyce spots are composed of "free" (i.e., not associated with hair follicles) sebaceous glands, and they probably represent a normal anatomic variant. They may present or become more prominent during puberty. Fordyce spots are asymptomatic, and treatment is unnecessary.

Disorders of the Apocrine Glands

Apocrine sweat glands are found in only a few areas: the axillae, anogenital region, and areolae of the breasts. They are poorly developed in childhood but begin to enlarge with the approach of puberty, triggered by androgen production. Apocrine secretion is sterile and odorless when it initially appears on the cutaneous surface. Associated odor develops as a result of bacterial decomposition of the secreted substances.

FOX–FORDYCE DISEASE

Fox–Fordyce disease (also known as *apocrine miliaria*) is a chronic papular eruption of apocrine gland–bearing areas, principally the axillae, the breast areolae, and the pubic and perineal regions. It is seen primarily in young women and is a disorder of unknown etiology. It appears to be related to apocrine sweat retention associated with obstruction and rupture of the intraepidermal portions of the affected apocrine glands. Fox–Fordyce disease is usually seen in postpubescent girls and women and is quite rare in prepubertal children as a result of quiescence of the apocrine glands.

This disorder presents with dome-shaped, flesh-colored to erythematous follicular papules (Fig. 8.29) in the affected areas. Pruritus may be severe, is often paroxysmal, and is aggravated by emotional stress. Treatment is notoriously difficult and may include topical or intralesional corticosteroids, topical antibiotics, topical retinoids, topical calcineurin inhibitors, botulinum toxin type A, and fractional CO_2 or

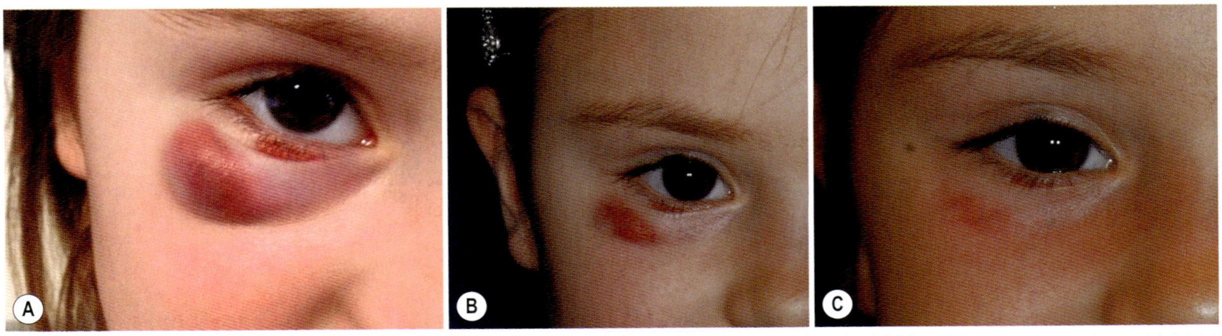

Fig. 8.27 Idiopathic facial aseptic granuloma. **(A)** This 7-year-old girl presented with a large, fluctuant nodule on the right inferior periorbital cheek. Note the associated hordeolum of the inferior eyelid margin. After 6 weeks of treatment with oral erythromycin and metronidazole gel, the nodule was markedly improved **(B)** and the erythema continued to fade with continued therapy for several months **(C)**.

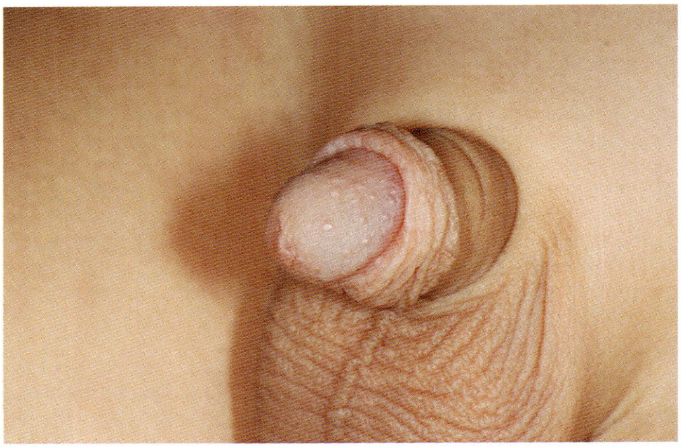

Fig. 8.28 Fordyce spots. Asymptomatic, pink to yellow papules on the glans penis of a 3-year-old boy.

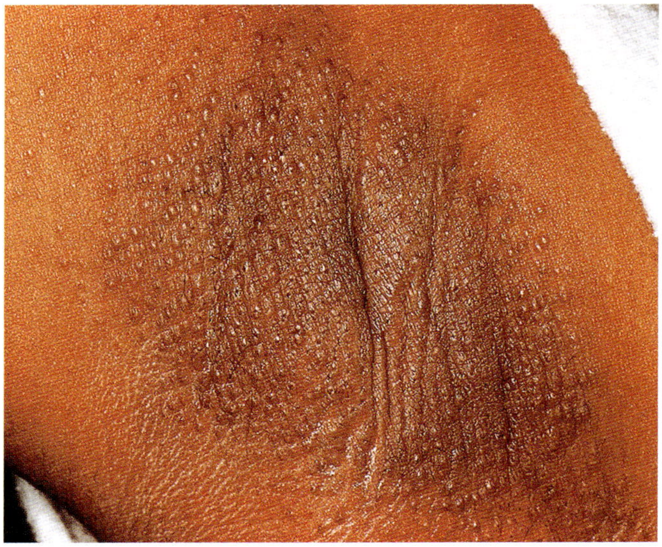

Fig. 8.29 Fox–Fordyce disease (apocrine miliaria). Small, round, follicular papules in the axilla of an adolescent girl.

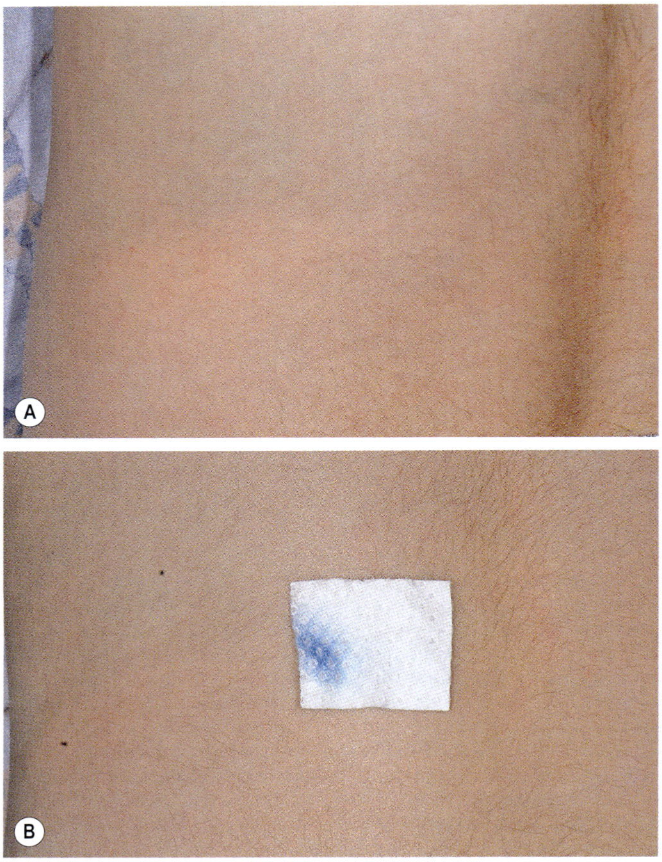

Fig. 8.30 Chromhidrosis. This 9-year-old boy had diffuse cutaneous pigmentation that improved after showering but rapidly reaccumulated. Note the blue hue to the skin, highlighted by the normal-colored stripe seen after rubbing **(A)** and the accumulation of blue pigment on the alcohol pad used to rub **(B)**. Surface cultures for bacteria and fungi were negative, but some improvement was noted after antifungal therapy.

erbium glass laser therapy.[191–194] Surgical excision of the affected areas is occasionally necessary in severely afflicted patients.

CHROMHIDROSIS

Chromhidrosis is a rare disorder in which the sweat appears colored. It typically involves the apocrine glands (apocrine chromhidrosis), although eccrine chromhidrosis may also occur, albeit less often. The cause of chromhidrosis is unclear, although it may be associated with drug ingestion (especially quinine, clofazimine, and rifampicin) in some patients. Eccrine chromhidrosis has been reported in association with hyperbilirubinemia, primarily in men, but also in an adolescent with sickle cell disease.[195] The reported colors in chromhidrosis include yellow, blue (Fig. 8.30), green, red, and black. *Pseudochromhidrosis* refers to chromhidrosis occurring as the result of an extrinsic factor, such as skin surface chemicals found in dyes (e.g., from clothing) and other colored chemicals or from chromogenic organisms, including *corynebacteriae* (which may result in red pseudochromhidrosis), *Pseudomonas aeruginosa* (which may color the sweat green), *Bacillus* spp., and *M. furfur* (the latter two associated with blue pseudochromhidrosis).[196–198] Treatment for chromhidrosis is difficult, aimed at reducing perspiration, and may include topical antiperspirants, capsaicin, and botulinum toxin type A.[199–203]

HIDRADENITIS SUPPURATIVA

Hidradenitis suppurativa (HS) is a chronic suppurative and scarring disease that primarily involves apocrine gland-bearing skin in the axillary, inguinal, and anogenital regions. The breasts (primarily inframammary regions) and scalp are less commonly involved. HS affects Blacks and females more often than Whites or males, usually develops after puberty, and has traditionally been ascribed to plugging of the apocrine duct and associated bacterial infection. Prepubertal individuals may occasionally be affected, but this is primarily a disorder with onset well after puberty.[204] It is most common in obese individuals. Some studies have suggested that the primary event may be a folliculitis with secondary involvement of the apocrine glands.[205,206] Some authors have thus suggested an alternative name, *acne inversa*.

The cause of HS is poorly understood. Genetic factors, hormonal influences, obesity, smoking, and tight-fitting clothing have each been hypothesized to play a role.[206,207] Dysregulation of the immune response may be implicated and is supported by the beneficial effect of biologic agents in some patients, studies demonstrating upregulation of some immune components such as *TLR2*, and the observed potential association with other inflammatory conditions such as Crohn's disease.[208] Familial HS has been shown to segregate in an autosomal dominant manner and may be associated with mutations in the γ-secretase genes, which include *NCSTN*, *PSENEN*, and *PSEN1*.[209–212]

These observations offer insight that may facilitate the development of new therapies.

Several severity classifications have been developed for HS, the most classic of which is the Hurley staging system, which is a three-stage classification of severity. Hurley stage 1 is characterized by abscess formation without sinus tracts and scarring. Hurley stage 2 reveals single or multiple separated areas of recurrent abscesses with sinus tracts and scarring. Hurley stage 3 reveals multiple interconnected sinus tracts and abscesses that cover the entire affected anatomic region. Limitations of the Hurley score include the lack of incorporation of inflammatory features, the inability to revert from stage 3 back down to a lower stage (given inclusion of scarring, which is irreversible, in both stages 2 and 3) even if in complete remission, and lack of precision for disease monitoring in clinical trials given the existence of only three stages.[213] Refinement of this system to better allow for severity ratings in the early stages has been proposed.[214] A newer scoring system, the Severity Assessment of Hidradenitis Suppurative score, differentiates only between fistulas and inflammatory lesions other than fistulas (rather than the various inflammatory lesions of HS), and correlates significantly with the Hurley staging and the modified Hidradenitis Suppurative Score.[215]

The earliest clinical finding in HS is a painful, inflammatory abscess-like swelling, usually 0.5 to 1.5 cm in diameter, in the affected apocrine areas. Over time the abscess enlarges and may rupture, resulting in purulent, foul-smelling drainage. With further development and enlargement of abscesses, sinus tracts form (Fig. 8.31) and eventually scarring ensues with the development of deep fibrosis and dermal contractures. Hypertrophic scarring may be seen, as may open comedones (Fig. 8.32). HS may be extremely debilitating in severely afflicted patients, with chronic pain, drainage, and secondary infection. Bacteriologic study of early lesions often reveals coagulase-positive staphylococci or streptococci, probably representing secondary infection. Occasionally *Escherichia coli, Pseudomonas aeruginosa*, or other Gram-negative organisms contaminate lesions. HS has a significant impact on quality of life and has been shown to result in more impairment than found with several other dermatologic conditions, including chronic urticaria, psoriasis, and atopic dermatitis.[216] Various quality-of-life measures have confirmed that HS has a significant impact on physical, social, and emotional well-being.[217]

Therapy for HS is often challenging. Management must be individualized based on the severity of disease, with correction of any associated metabolic disorders (including assessment for precocious puberty), attention to weight control, symptom management, and medical therapy.[218] Initial measures include antibiotics (topical clindamycin may suffice for mild disease; when more moderate to severe, oral agents are often recommended, especially tetracycline-class antibiotics and clindamycin) and local wound care. Intralesional steroid injections, oral cyclosporine, and combination oral clindamycin-rifampin therapy have been reported as useful.[208,219,220] Incision and drainage may be useful in certain instances, but for more severe cases surgical modalities are generally necessary. These include local excision, unroofing of lesions with marsupialization, punch debridement (mini-unroofing), incision and drainage, and wide excision with primary or secondary closure, skin grafting, or flaps.[221–223] Carbon dioxide and Nd:YAG laser therapies are other options that seem to be quite effective.[220,224] Low efficacy and a high risk-to-benefit ratio have been suggested as possible limitations for isotretinoin and the TNF-α inhibitors (e.g., etanercept and infliximab) in this setting,[225–227] although these agents have been found to be helpful in some studies.[220,228,229] Adalimumab, another TNF-α antagonist, has gained increasing acceptance as an effective agent for HS when dosed on a weekly basis and is now FDA approved for use in affected adults.[230–233] Other biologic agents that have shown potential include ustekinumab and anakinra.

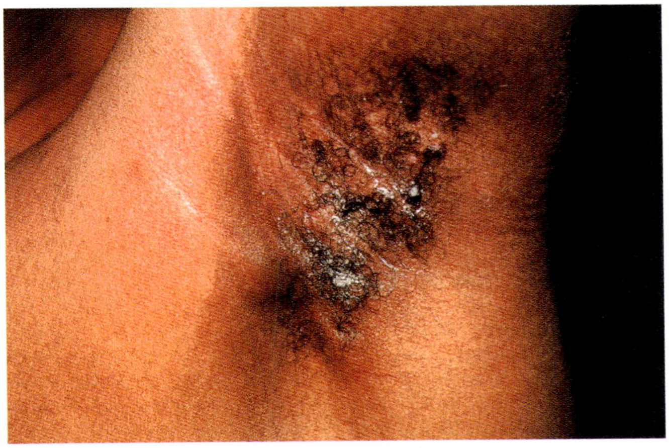

Fig. 8.31 Hidradenitis suppurativa. Erythematous papules, cysts, nodules, and sinus tracts are seen in the axilla of this adolescent boy.

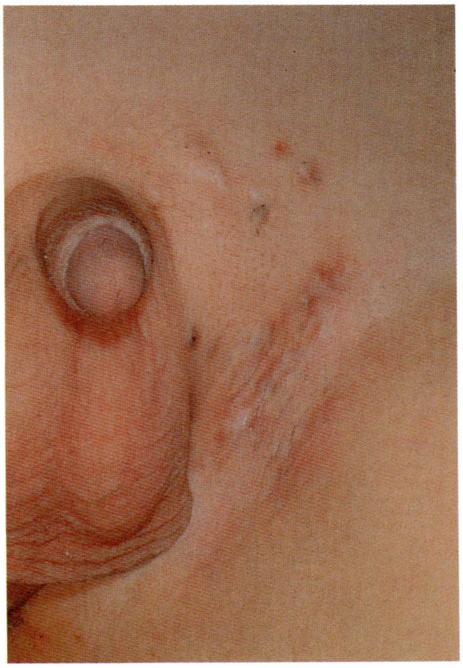

Fig. 8.32 Hidradenitis suppurativa. Sinus tracts with chronic scarring and cyst-like papules in the inguinal region of a young boy with chronic disease. Note the associated open comedones.

Several disorders have been described in which HS is present in conjunction with other inflammatory processes. These presentations seem to fall under the umbrella of autoinflammatory disorders (see Chapter 25). The association of pyoderma gangrenosum, acne, and HS (PASH) was described as a syndrome sharing some clinical overlap with pyogenic sterile arthritis, pyoderma gangrenosum, and acne (PAPA) syndrome (see Chapter 25) but lacking the joint inflammation and with the added feature of suppurative hidradenitis in skin folds.[234] Whereas PAPA syndrome is related to mutations in the *PSTPIP1* gene, no mutations (aside from some microsatellite repeats of unclear significance in the promoter region) were found in this original cohort with PASH syndrome, nor were there mutations found in other genes linked to several other autoinflammatory disorders. Subsequently, however, mutations in nicastrin *(NCSTN)* and *PSTPIP1* have been identified in some patients with PASH syndrome,[235,236] but the lack of identified mutations in other PASH patients highlights the genetic heterogeneity of the disorder.[237] The association of pyogenic arthritis with pyoderma gangrenosum, acne, and hidradenitis suppurativa (PAPASH) has significant clinical overlap with PASH, and in the originally reported patient a missense mutation in the *PSTPIP1* gene was noted and felt to be related to the clinical presentation.[238] A patient has also been reported with the findings of pyoderma gangrenosum, acne, suppurative hidradenitis, and axial spondylarthritis, for which the author proposed the term *PASS*.[239] The clinical overlap in these described associations highlights the need for continued study of the clinical presentations and molecular bases.

Disorders of the Eccrine Glands

The eccrine sweat glands are distributed over the entire skin surface and found in greatest abundance on the palms and soles and in the axillae. They represent the principal means of maintaining homeostatic balance by evaporation of water. Their secretion depends on their sympathetic nerve supply, which is controlled by various stimuli, including thermal and emotional types. By these mechanisms the quantity and quality of sweat may be varied. Ectodermal dysplasias associated with decreased eccrine sweating are discussed in Chapter 7.

HYPERHIDROSIS

Hyperhidrosis (idiopathic hyperhidrosis or primary pediatric hyperhidrosis) is a disorder characterized by the excessive production of sweat in response to heat or emotional stimuli and not related to an underlying disease or drug toxicity; it is defined as the production of sweat beyond what is physiologically necessary to maintain thermal homeostasis.[240] Hyperhidrosis is a poorly understood disorder, and the clinical spectrum ranges from a mild increase over the normal level of physiologic sweating to an extreme, debilitating expression of the disease. Such extreme sweating may be socially embarrassing and occupationally disabling and may negatively affect the patient's psychological well-being.[241,242] Hyperhidrosis may be palmoplantar and/or axillary and, in rare instances, generalized. In patients with these forms of idiopathic hyperhidrosis, neurovascular or metabolic abnormalities are absent. Idiopathic localized unilateral hyperhidrosis is a rare form of hyperhidrosis localized to a sharply demarcated area on the face or upper extremities of an otherwise healthy individual.[243,244] Auriculotemporal nerve (Frey) syndrome is the constellation of facial flushing and hyperhidrosis in response to gustatory stimuli and is discussed in Chapter 12. The International Hyperhidrosis Society offers a website (www.sweathelp.org) that provides patient education and support services.

There are a variety of treatment options for idiopathic hyperhidrosis (Table 8.8). The first-line therapies are topical and consist of both OTC and prescription-strength antiperspirant preparations. The active ingredient in many of these is either aluminum chloride or formaldehyde. These products are best applied to dry skin at bedtime, and their effect may be potentiated when they are used along with plastic wrap occlusion overnight (when practical). However, for some patients occlusion results in more irritation. Topical glycopyrrolate, an anticholinergic agent that has become available in the United States as glycopyrronium cloths and is approved for axillary hyperhidrosis in patients 9 years of age and older, has also been demonstrated to be effective in those with craniofacial hyperhidrosis.[245–247] The systemic anticholinergic side effects reported in some patients with use of this topical agent for hyperhidrosis suggest some systemic absorption.

Systemic anticholinergic agents such as glycopyrrolate or propantheline bromide are often useful but may occasionally be limited by their side effect profiles, which include dry eyes, dry mouth, dizziness, constipation, and urinary hesitancy. Oral glycopyrrolate appears to be very effective and well tolerated in children with hyperhidrosis. It is usually started at a dose of 1 mg taken once to twice daily and may be titrated to a maximal dose of 6 mg daily (usually divided into twice or three times daily dosing). In a series of 31 pediatric patients (between 9 and 18 years of age) treated with oral glycopyrrolate, 90% reported improvement and nearly three-quarters reported no side effects, with dry mouth and dry eyes reported by 26% and 10% of patients.[248] The α-adrenergic receptor agonist clonidine has also been used for hyperhidrosis, and in one series of 13 patients receiving this therapy, the response rate was 46%.[249] Sedative agents such as diazepam may be useful before an anxiety-provoking event, but their continual use is not recommended.

Iontophoresis is a successful therapy for some patients. This therapy involves a small device that delivers a direct current using tap water (with or without anticholinergic agents) as the conductive medium. Its proposed mechanism of action is the development of keratotic plugs in the eccrine sweat ducts, and its effect may last up to 6 weeks between treatments. This treatment appears to be quite safe, with side effects limited to dryness, burning, tingling, and fissuring of treated sites. Iontophoresis units are available without a prescription via the internet at several sites, including www.drionic.com, www.hidrexusa.com, and www.rafischer.com.

Botulinum toxin type A, injected either intradermally or "intracutaneously" (more superficial injections), has been demonstrated to be quite effective in the treatment of axillary or palmoplantar hyperhidrosis.[244,250,251] This agent works by blocking presynaptic acetylcholine release. Studies have revealed improved quality of life and an excellent safety profile with this modality.[251–253] The effects of botulinum toxin type A injections last for 4 to 9 months, but the need for repeat injections and variable patient tolerability of the procedure may be limiting. Botulinum toxin type B has also been efficacious for this condition but may be more limited by injection site pain and autonomic side effects. Microwave thermolysis is another treatment that has been reported in adults with hyperhidrosis.[254]

In patients with severe and recalcitrant idiopathic hyperhidrosis, surgical therapy may be indicated. Thoracoscopic sympathectomy (or endoscopic thoracic sympathectomy) is the traditionally used procedure, although postoperative compensatory and gustatory sweating may be a problem.[255–258] Up to 20% of patients may have such severe disabling compensatory sweating that they regret having had the procedure.[259] Other reported complications include Horner syndrome, intrathoracic bleeding, and pneumothorax.[260] However, in a series of 28 patients between 6 and 21 years of age who had failed at least one form of medical therapy for primary focal hyperhidrosis of the palms, all achieved postoperative resolution,

Table 8.8 Therapeutic Options for Primary Hyperhidrosis

Treatment Class	Comment
Topical antiperspirants	Aluminum chloride, formaldehyde, others Both OTC and prescription strengths Usually applied at bedtime
Topical anticholinergics	Glycopyrronium cloths
Oral anticholinergics	Glycopyrrolate, propantheline bromide, oxybutynin May be limited by side effects (dry eyes, dry mouth, bowel/bladder dysfunction) Clinical experience greatest with glycopyrrolate
Other systemic agents	Clonidine, calcium channel blockers, benzodiazepines
Iontophoresis	Safe and well tolerated Tap water used, with or without anticholinergic agents Efficacy variable
Botulinum toxin types A or B	Injected intradermally or intracutaneously Effective, but painful Often requires repeat injections at 3- to 6-month intervals
Thoracic sympathectomy	Reserved for patients with severe or recalcitrant disease Postoperative compensatory sweating may occur Video-assisted surgery: quicker and fewer complications

Modified from Stolman LP. Treatment of hyperhidrosis. Dermatol Clin 1998;16(4):863–9; Gelbard CM, Epstein H, Hebert A. Primary pediatric hyperhidrosis: a review of current treatment options. Pediatr Dermatol 2008;25(6):591–8. © 2008 by John Wiley & Sons, Inc. Reprinted by permission of John Wiley & Sons, Inc. Brown AL, Gordon J, Hill S. Hyperhidrosis: review of recent advances and new therapeutic options for primary hyperhidrosis. Curr Opin Pediatr 2014;26:460–5; Grabell DA, Hebert AA. Current and emerging medical therapies for primary hyperhidrosis. Dermatol Ther 2017;7:25–36; and Qbrexza [package insert]. Menlo Park, CA: Dermira, Inc.; 2019.
OTC, Over the counter.

which was sustained for a median of 17 months with improved quality-of-life scores and temporary compensatory sweating seen in only one patient.[261]

DYSHIDROSIS

Dyshidrosis (dyshidrotic eczema or pompholyx) is the term applied to a condition of recurring vesiculation of the palms, soles, and lateral aspects of the fingers in which hyperhidrosis is often associated. It is not a primary disorder of eccrine glands but rather a type of eczematous eruption. It is discussed in more detail in Chapter 3.

ANHIDROSIS

Anhidrosis is the abnormal absence of (or in the case of hypohidrosis, decrease in) perspiration from the surface of the skin in the presence of appropriate stimuli, which may result in hyperthermia. This condition may be caused by a deficiency or abnormality of the sweat glands (as in hypohidrotic ectodermal dysplasia; see Chapter 7) or of the nervous pathways from the peripheral or central nervous system leading to the sweat glands (as in syringomyelia, leprosy, anticholinergic drug therapy, or sympathectomy). Cool baths, air conditioning, light clothing, and reduction of the causes of normal perspiration help to relieve symptoms.

In congenital insensitivity to pain with anhidrosis (CIPA), also known as *hereditary sensory and autonomic neuropathy type IV*, patients have recurrent episodes of fever, anhidrosis, absence of reaction to noxious stimuli, self-mutilating behavior, and mental retardation. These patients commonly show evidence of oral self-mutilation, including biting injuries and scarring of soft tissues of the mouth and oral mucosa.[262] They are at risk for infections of the skin and skeleton, most often caused by *S. aureus*.[263] Immunologic dysfunction, including cell-mediated and humoral immune defects as well as abnormalities in the innate immune response, have been reported.[264] This autosomal recessive condition has been ascribed to mutations in the *NTRK1 (TRKA)* gene as well as the *SCN9A* gene. Defects in the *NTRK1* gene, which encodes the receptor tyrosine kinase for nerve growth factor, impair intracellular signal transduction in response to nerve growth factor.[265] The *SCN9A* gene is one of the nine genes encoding voltage-gated sodium channels, which play a crucial role in converting mechanical or chemical stimuli into electrical signals within excited cells. Nav1.7 is the sodium channel encoded by the *SCN9A* gene, and mutations have also been linked to primary erythromelalgia (PE) (see Chapter 12) and paroxysmal extreme pain disorder (PEPD).[266]

BROMHIDROSIS

Bromhidrosis is an embarrassing malodorous condition in which an excessive and usually offensive odor emanates from the skin. It may be of two types: (1) apocrine, resulting from bacterial degradation of apocrine sweat; or (2) eccrine, from the microbiologic degradation of stratum corneum softened by excessive eccrine sweat.

The term *apocrine bromhidrosis* refers to an exaggeration of the axillary odor normally noted by all postpubertal individuals. *Eccrine bromhidrosis* refers to the excessive odor produced by bacterial action on the stratum corneum when it becomes macerated by eccrine sweat. This disorder occurs primarily on the plantar surfaces of the feet and intertriginous areas, particularly the inguinal region. Eccrine bromhidrosis may also occur in association with metabolic disorders including phenylketonuria, maple syrup urine disease, and isovaleric acidemia.

Bromhidrosis is best managed by regular thorough cleansing (preferably with an antibacterial soap), the use of commercial deodorants and antiperspirants, the application of topical antibiotics as necessary, and frequent changes of clothing. Plantar bromhidrosis may be associated with pitted keratolysis (see Chapter 14).

MILIARIA

Miliaria (see Chapter 2) is a common dermatosis caused by sweat retention and is characterized by a papulovesicular eruption secondary to prolonged sweating with obstruction of the eccrine ducts. The pathophysiologic events that lead to this disorder are keratinous plugging of eccrine ducts followed by disruption of the normal escape of eccrine sweat into the skin. The clinical findings vary depending on the depth of obstruction of the eccrine duct within the skin. The three forms of miliaria are miliaria crystallina (sudamina), miliaria rubra (prickly heat), and miliaria profunda. The incidence of miliaria is greatest in the first few weeks of life because of a relative immaturity of the eccrine ducts that favors poral closure and sweat retention. In addition, older infants and children may develop miliaria in any situation predisposing them to increased sweating or skin obstruction (e.g., warm summer climates, swaddling with several layers of clothing during winter months, febrile illnesses).

Miliaria crystallina is characterized by clear, thin-walled, noninflammatory vesicles, 1 to 2 mm in diameter, occurring in crops on otherwise normal-appearing skin (see Chapter 2, Fig. 2.10). The vesicles are asymptomatic and occur most often in intertriginous areas, particularly on the neck and axillae, or on parts of the trunk covered by clothing. Lesions of miliaria crystallina are highly characteristic and easily differentiated from other vesicular diseases. When the diagnosis is in doubt, rupture of vesicles with a fine needle results in release of the clear, entrapped sweat. The obstruction in miliaria crystallina is quite superficial, either within or just beneath the stratum corneum. Miliaria rubra (prickly heat) is the most common form of miliaria. These lesions have a predilection for occluded areas of skin, especially the upper trunk, back, volar aspects of the arms, and body folds. The face may also be involved. Clinically there are discrete but closely aggregated, small erythematous papules (Fig. 8.33) or papulovesicles. The lesions of miliaria rubra are always nonfollicular, which helps differentiate this disorder from folliculitis. Viral exanthems and drug reactions may sometimes be in the clinical differential diagnosis, but the distribution of lesions combined with the history and physical examination usually allow for distinction. Miliaria pustulosa is a variant of miliaria rubra consisting of distinct superficial pustules that are also not associated with hair follicles. Lesions tend to occur in areas of skin that have had previous inflammation and often appear coexistent with lesions of miliaria rubra.

Miliaria profunda is a more pronounced form of miliaria quite uncommon outside of the tropics. This disorder usually follows repeated episodes of miliaria rubra and is characterized by firm, white, 1- to 3-mm papules. This papular presentation is related to the deep level of obstruction. Lesions are most prominent on the trunk and proximal extremities, and this form of miliaria is extremely rare in infants and children.

The key to the management of miliaria is prevention by avoidance of excessive heat and humidity. In infants, all that is generally required is parental reassurance and advice on proper clothing and temperature regulation. The lesions of miliaria are self-limited, but simple strategies such as cool baths, light clothing, and use of air conditioning can make the patient more comfortable while awaiting

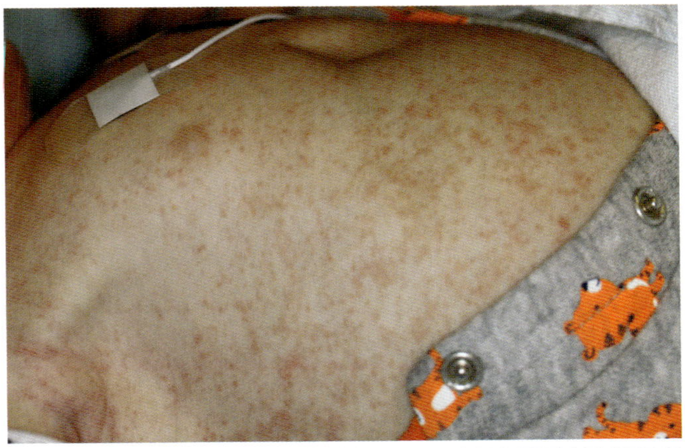

Fig. 8.33 Miliaria rubra. Erythematous macules and papules diffusely distributed on the trunk of a hospitalized febrile infant.

resolution. Topical preparations are of little value and in fact may further propagate the condition by compounding eccrine duct obstruction.

The complete list of 274 references for this chapter is available online at http://expertconsult.inkling.com.

Key References

Thiboutot D, Gollnick H, Bettoli V, et al. New insights into the management of acne: an update from the Global Alliance to Improve Outcomes in Acne Group. J Am Acad Dermatol 2009;60:S1–50.

Eichenfield LF, Krakowski AC, Piggott C, et al. Evidence-based recommendations for the diagnosis and treatment of pediatric acne. Pediatrics 2013;131(3): S163–86.

El-Hallak M, Giani T, Yeniay BS, et al. Chronic minocycline-induced autoimmunity in children. J Pediatr 2008;153(3):314–19.

Halvorsen JA, Stern RS, Dalgard F, et al. Suicidal ideation, mental health problems, and social impairment are increased in adolescents with acne: a population-based study. J Invest Dermatol 2011;131(2):363–70.

Greywal T, Zaenglein AL, Baldwin HE, et al. Evidence-based recommendations for the management of acne fulminans and its variants. J Am Acad Dermatol 2017;77: 109–17.

Zaenglein AL, Pathy AL, Schlosser BJ, et al. Guidelines of care for the management of acne vulgaris. J Am Acad Dermatol 2016;74(5):945–73.

Barros B, Thiboutot D. Hormonal therapies for acne. Clin Dermatol 2017;35: 168–72.

Lee YH, Scharnitz TP, Muscat J, et al.. Laboratory monitoring during isotretinoin therapy for acne: A systematic review and meta-analysis. JAMA Dermatol 2016;152(1):35–44.

Van der Zee HH, Jemec GBE. New insights into the diagnosis of hidradenitis suppurativa: clinical presentations and phenotypes. J Am Acad Dermatol 2015;73:S23–6.

Grabell DA, Hebert AA. Current and emerging medical therapies for primary hyperhidrosis. Dermatol Ther 2017;7:25–36.

9 Cutaneous Tumors and Tumor Syndromes

CHAPTER OUTLINE

Because of the increasing public awareness and incidence of skin cancer, physicians are often consulted regarding tumors of the skin. In children, the vast majority of cutaneous tumors are benign, and their importance lies predominantly in the cosmetic defect they may create or in their occasional association with systemic disease. Malignant skin lesions, however, despite their relative rarity in children, cannot be completely disregarded or ignored. Each lesion in children, as in adults, must be assessed individually with a consideration of its cosmetic effect, its possible association with systemic manifestations, and its capacity for malignant degeneration.

Cutaneous tumors can be differentiated into those arising from epidermal (or mucosal) cells, from melanocytes, from the epidermal appendages, or from dermal or subcutaneous cells or tissues. The latter category includes tumors of fibrous, neural, vascular, fatty, muscular, and osseous tissues. Skin tumors can also be divided into benign (the vast majority of lesions in children) and malignant. The term *nevus* (plural *nevi*) has a broad meaning in dermatology. Strictly defined, this term refers to a circumscribed congenital abnormality of the skin. When this term is used, therefore, it is appropriate to include a qualifying adjective (e.g., epidermal nevus, melanocytic nevus, or vascular nevus), thus specifying the cell of origin. In commonplace practice, however, the term *nevus* is usually used to imply a benign tumor of pigment cells (melanocytes). Hence to many practitioners a nevus is the same as a "mole."

In this chapter we will discuss several cutaneous tumors (and corresponding tumor syndromes where applicable). Pigmented lesions are discussed as a separate entity apart from the previously described classification, given their high incidence.

Pigmented Lesions

Pigmented lesions, especially melanocytic nevi (moles), are the most common neoplasms found in humans. In this section we will discuss melanocytic nevi (both congenital and acquired) and several variants, including dysplastic, Spitz, and halo types. Nevus spilus and Becker nevus, two distinct pigmented lesions, will also be discussed, as will malignant melanoma (MM), which, although rare in childhood, does occasionally occur.

Melanocytic Nevi

Melanocytic nevi are extremely common skin neoplasms composed of "nevocytes" or nevus cells that are believed to be slightly altered melanocytes. The melanocyte is a dendritic cell that produces melanin and transfers it to keratinocytes (epidermal cells) and hair cells, thus supplying the normal brown pigment to skin and hair. Both melanocytes and nevus cells are of neural origin. Melanocytes originate in the neural crest and early in fetal life migrate from there to the skin. After birth some melanocytes occasionally remain in the dermis of certain races (Asians, Native Americans, Blacks, and individuals from the Mediterranean region), where they may appear as congenital dermal melanocytosis (formerly Mongolian spots; see Chapter 11). Blue nevi and the nevi of Ota and Ito (see Chapter 11) also represent examples of arrested melanocytic migration in which the melanoblasts remain in the dermis.

Melanocytic nevi can be either congenital (described in more detail later) or acquired. Acquired nevi usually appear after infancy, increase in size and number during early childhood, and peak during the third or fourth decade, with slow involution as aging progresses. The predisposition of an individual to the development of acquired melanocytic nevi seems to be related to several factors, including skin type, race, genetic predisposition, and ultraviolet light exposure. These lesions tend to be few in childhood, increasing in number with age to a peak in the third decade. Sun exposure, sunburns, and fair skin pigmentation seem to be associated with their development in childhood.[1] In one large cross-sectional study, nevus counts were found to steadily increase with age from a median of 3 at age 2 years to 19 at age 7 years.[1] High numbers of nevi were associated with moderate sun exposure and outdoor activities. In another study, 5- and 6-year-old children with a history of sunburns or an increased number of holidays in foreign countries with a sunny climate had significantly higher nevus counts than controls without these characteristics.[2] Higher numbers of childhood nevi have been demonstrated in areas of skin chronically exposed to the sun and in children with lighter skin, blond hair, and blue eyes.[3] Higher nevus counts are noted in children who reside in sunny climates (e.g., Australia) compared with age- and race-matched control children. Melanocytic nevi may also occur in higher numbers in children with a history of leukemia and/or a history of chemotherapy, and in these settings the lesions may occur with greater incidence on acral areas such as the palms and soles.[4–6] Children who have received allogeneic hematopoietic stem cell transplantation (HSCT) may have higher nevus counts, larger nevi, and a propensity toward development of atypical nevi; factors associated with increase nevus counts in this population include malignant indication for the HSCT, pretransplant chemotherapy, history of total body irradiation, and myeloablative conditioning.[7]

The primary importance of melanocytic nevi lies in their possible transformation into MM. These lesions are felt to be both markers of an increased risk of cutaneous melanoma and, in some cases, direct precursor lesions.[8] The annual transformation rate of a single mole into melanoma seems extremely low, with an estimate of 0.0005% or lower for individuals younger than 40 years.[8] Nonetheless, melanocytic nevus cells were seen histologically in proximity to MM in 51% of cases in one study.[9] Genetic analyses of nevi and melanoma reveal nonrandom patterns of genetic alteration (loss of heterozygosity), confirming the notion that the former are precursor lesions for the latter.[10] These findings highlight the relevance of close monitoring of melanocytic nevi for atypical features as well as the importance of sun protection education. The Study of Nevi in Children project is a population-based study cohort documenting the clinical and dermoscopic (magnified light; also known as dermatoscopy) evolution of nevi in childhood and adolescence over time. Study investigators have reported age-related, anatomic site–related, and native skin pigment phenotype–related dermoscopic findings in pediatric nevi.[11] This cohort also highlighted that although nevi counts tend to increase during childhood, existing nevi may decrease in size, fade, or completely disappear and that these changes are not typically concerning in this patient population.[11]

Melanocytic nevi are subdivided into types and clinically described based on the microscopic location of the nevus cells. Accordingly they are classified as junctional, intradermal, or compound lesions. Junctional nevi have proliferation of nevocytes at the dermal–epidermal junction, compound nevi reveal cells at the junction and in the dermis, and intradermal nevi reveal loss of the epidermal component with nests of cells limited to the dermis. Interestingly, these histologic subtypes progress in parallel to the natural history of nevus maturation (junctional nevi early in life, then compound nevi, and finally intradermal nevi with eventual atrophy of the dermal component during later adulthood).[12] Melanocytic nevi have a wide range of clinical appearances. They may occur anywhere on the cutaneous or mucocutaneous surface and may be flat, slightly elevated, dome-shaped, nodular, verrucous, polypoid, cerebriform, or papillomatous.

Junctional Nevi

Junctional nevi usually occur as hairless, light to dark brown or black macules (Fig. 9.1). They range from 1 mm to 1 cm in diameter, with a smooth and flat (nonpalpable) surface and preservation of skin furrows. Although most junctional nevi are round, elliptical, or oval and show a relatively uniform pigmentation, some may be slightly irregular in configuration and color. Most junctional nevi represent a transient phase in the development of compound nevi and are found only in children. An exception to this rule, however, is seen on the palms, soles, and genitalia where the lesions often retain their junctional appearance.

Compound Nevi

Compound nevi are more common in older children and adults but may also be present in younger children. They may appear similar to junctional nevi but tend to be more elevated and accordingly vary from a slightly raised papule to a larger, papillomatous papule or plaque. They are flesh colored to brown (Fig. 9.2), may have a smooth or verrucous surface, and may have dark coarse hairs within them (Fig. 9.3), especially when occurring on the face. During later childhood and adolescence, compound nevi tend to increase in thickness and depth of pigmentation. It is at this stage that many children are brought to the physician for evaluation.

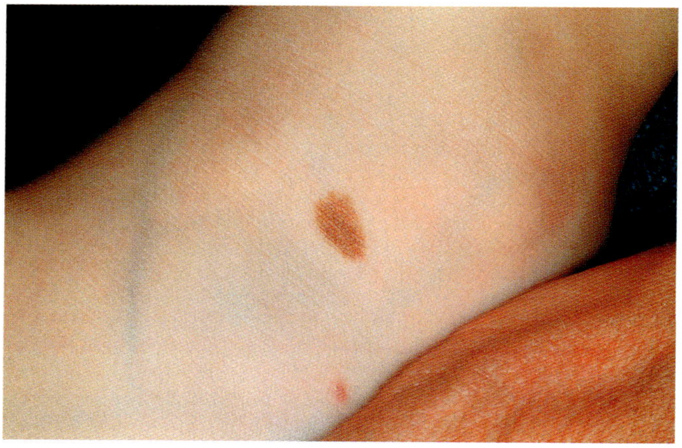

Fig. 9.1 Junctional melanocytic nevus. A well-demarcated, tan macule.

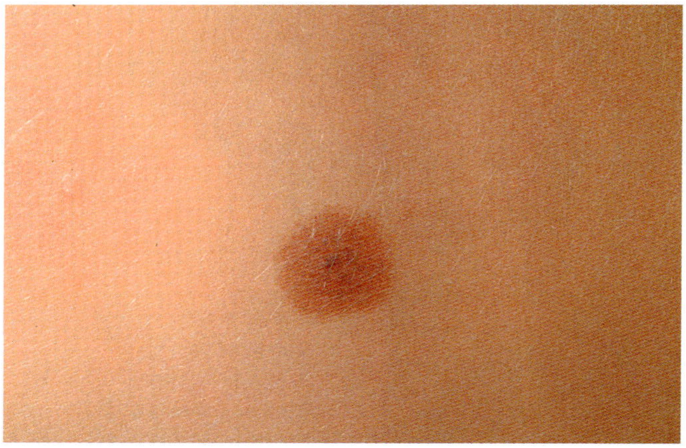

Fig. 9.2 Compound melanocytic nevus. A well-demarcated, tan papule with some darker speckling centrally.

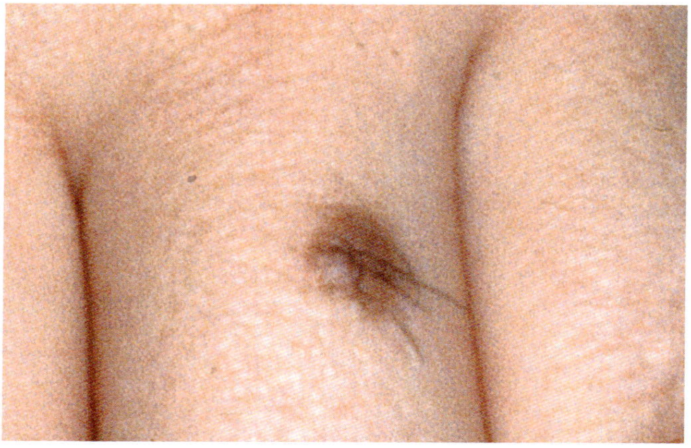

Fig. 9.3 Compound melanocytic nevus. Note the coarse, terminal hairs within the nevus.

Intradermal Nevi

Intradermal nevi are seen most commonly in adults. They are usually dome-shaped, soft, "fleshy" papules (Fig. 9.4). They may be sessile (attached by a broad base) or more pedunculated (attached by a more narrow base) and range from a few millimeters to 1 cm or more in diameter. Intradermal nevi may be clinically indistinguishable from compound nevi, and their color varies from nonpigmented (flesh-colored) lesions to those of varying shades of brown. They may occur anywhere on the skin surface and are often found on the head and neck; coarse hairs often are present. After the third decade of life, as nevus maturation continues, there is destruction and replacement of nevus cells by fibrous or fatty tissue, and by 70 years of age most individuals have few remaining nevi. In fact, nevi that persist into old age appear to have an increased risk of malignant degeneration.[8]

Treatment decisions regarding melanocytic nevi are usually related to their cosmetic appearance, repeated irritation of the lesion, or fear of potential malignant transformation. The majority of melanocytic lesions require no treatment; by careful clinical evaluation the patient can often be reassured as to their benign nature. Removal of nevi, when indicated, is best achieved by punch biopsy or complete surgical excision. Any nevus being removed because of concern for malignant degeneration should be removed with a full-depth excision, because microscopic tumor depth is the primary prognostic indicator in MM. Every excised nevus should be subjected to histopathologic examination.

Many authors advocate for the routine excision of pigmented lesions in certain anatomic locations (e.g., palms, soles, scalp, and genitalia) because of the belief that the likelihood of malignant

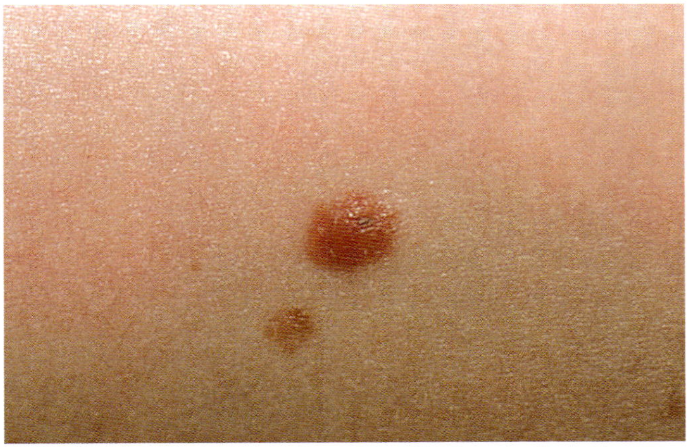

Fig. 9.4 Intradermal melanocytic nevus. A tan, fleshy papule with adjacent intradermal nevus.

transformation is greater in these areas. It seems that prophylactic excision of all nevi in these locations is unwarranted. However, lesions in acral sites may reveal atypical clinical and histologic features,[13,14] possibly in relation to repetitive trauma. Recognition of these histologic variations is vital to avoid the misdiagnosis of the "acral lentiginous" subtype of MM, which occurs primarily after the seventh decade of life. Benign acral melanocytic neoplasms (including nevi and lentigines) often reveal their long axes to be parallel to the dermatoglyphic lines on palms and soles and when on the feet in children are most often distributed over the forefoot.[15] Scalp nevi in children (and particularly adolescents) may also commonly reveal mild clinical atypia, both clinically and histologically, although the vast majority behave in a biologically benign fashion (see more later).[16] Scalp nevi that reveal significant atypia and/or that may be difficult to monitor clinically, however, may merit excision.

Occasionally, pigmented nevi show recurrence after excision, which may be a significant source of anxiety for the patient, the parent, and at times the physician. Recurrent lesions (which have been called *pseudomelanoma* by some) present as circumscribed pigmentation within the surgical scar (Fig. 9.5). This finding is usually not an indication of malignancy but instead represents proliferation of nevus cells from the peripheral epidermis, sweat ducts, or hair follicles. Options for management include close clinical follow-up care (assuming the original pathologic examination revealed no atypical findings) or repeat excision.

Meyerson Nevus

The term *Meyerson nevus* (also known as *Meyerson phenomenon* or *halo dermatitis*) refers to a localized eczematous eruption that occurs in the region of a melanocytic nevus and was originally described by Meyerson in 1971.[17] The inflammatory reaction does not appear to be a marker for atypia within the nevus, although there are reports of the phenomenon in association with dysplastic lesions.[18] The Meyerson phenomenon may be associated with acquired or congenital melanocytic nevi (CMN).[19] It has also been described in association with nonmelanocytic lesions including nevus sebaceus, dermatofibroma, and smooth muscle hamartoma.[20–22] The Meyerson nevus presents clinically as a scaly erythematous plaque overlying a pigmented nevus (which may or may not be clinically noted at time of initial evaluation). The overlying dermatitis may be treated with a topical corticosteroid, which often leads to complete resolution, enabling closer inspection of the underlying nevus (Fig. 9.6). If left untreated, the dermatitis often resolves spontaneously over time.[23]

MELANONYCHIA STRIATA

Melanonychia striata (also known as *longitudinal melanonychia*) is most commonly seen in individuals with darker skin complexions, especially Blacks, of whom up to 90% may have at least one such

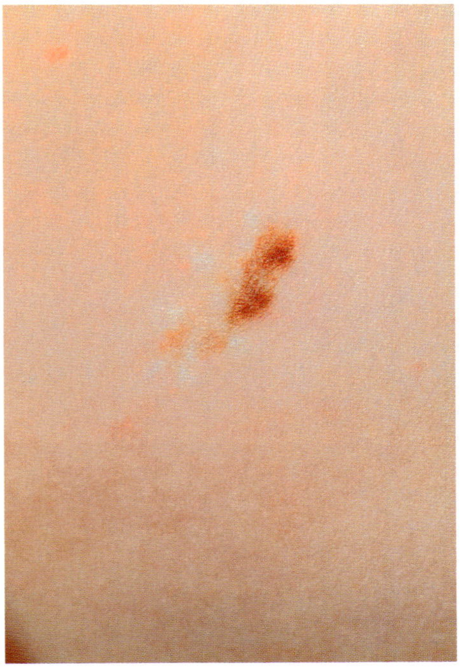

Fig. 9.5 Recurrent melanocytic nevus (within a surgical scar). The initial nevus had been incompletely excised.

streak. It is significantly less common in children with white skin. Melanonychia striata presents as a brown linear band of pigmentation on a fingernail (Fig. 9.7) or toenail. The pigmentation extends from the proximal nailfold to the distal margin of the digit, and the width may vary from less than 1 mm to several millimeters. Drugs, pregnancy, trauma, and human immunodeficiency virus (HIV) infection may all be associated with melanonychia striata, although the majority of patients have no underlying association.

Melanonychia striata may represent benign melanocytic hyperplasia (i.e., melanocytic nevus or lentigo) or a nail matrix melanoma. In children, the majority of cases seem to be related to benign lesions,[24,25] although the possibility of melanoma must always be entertained. The presence of multiple bands, as occasionally seen in people with darker skin, is reassuring and mitigates against malignancy. Worrisome features may include very dark or nonhomogeneous bands, changing pigmentation or shape (especially when rapidly evolving), blurred lateral borders, associated nail dystrophy, extension of the pigmentation onto the proximal or lateral nailfolds (Hutchinson sign; Fig. 9.8),[26] and broad bands (Fig. 9.9). However, the last two features may also occur in benign pediatric nail matrix nevi and should not be presumed to confirm the diagnosis of melanoma.[27] In a series of 30 childhood cases of melanonychia striata, histopathologic diagnoses included subungual lentigo (20 patients), subungual nevus (5 patients), and atypical melanocytic hyperplasia (5 patients), with no diagnosed melanomas or evidence of aggressive clinical behavior.[28] Dermatoscopic evaluation may be useful for monitoring in the hands of clinicians experienced in its use, but the patterns and accuracy remain to be confirmed in this setting, and patterns observed in adults with nail apparatus melanoma may be observed in the setting of benign pediatric cases.[29–31] In patients with melanonychia striata and significantly atypical or concerning features, nail matrix biopsy for histologic evaluation should be strongly considered. Although this procedure may result in permanent nail plate dystrophy, this risk is justified when concerns for possible melanoma exist.

CONGENITAL MELANOCYTIC NEVI

CMN represent a special group of melanocytic lesions with an increased risk of transformation to MM. By strict definition, these

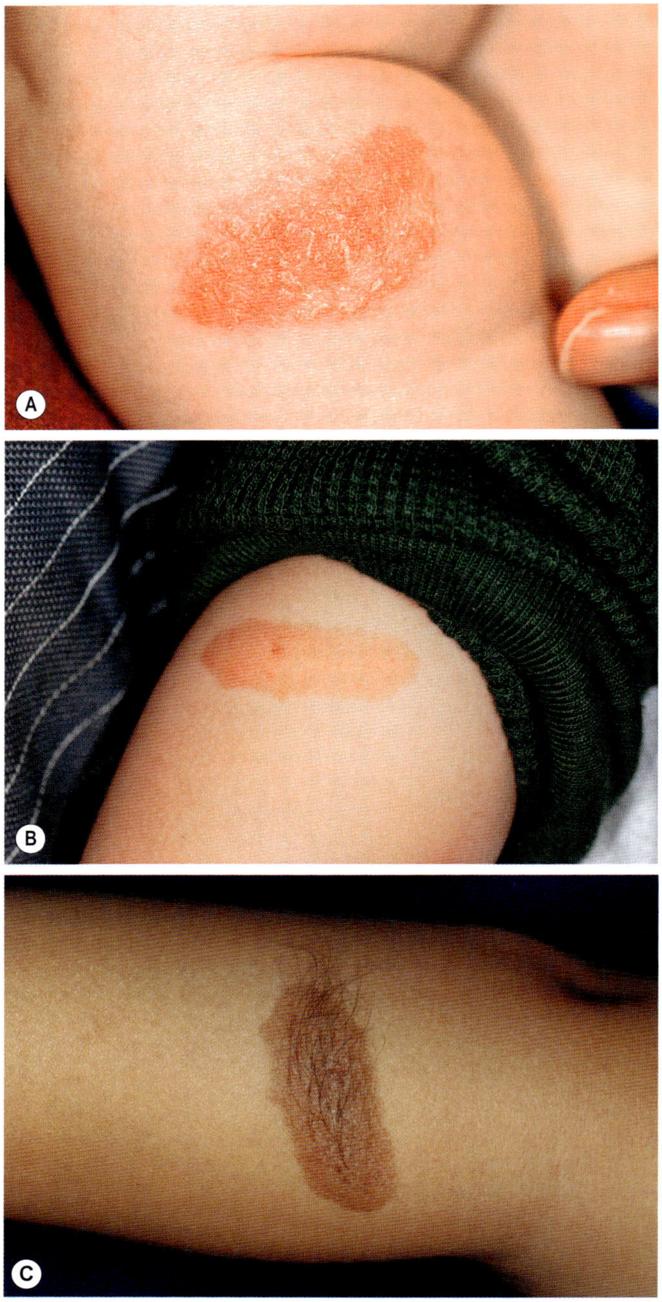

Fig. 9.6 Meyerson nevus. **(A)** This 9-month-old boy sought treatment for this scaly plaque on the proximal forearm (note the faint outline of the underlying pigmented nevus). **(B)** At the follow-up examination, the congenital melanocytic nevus can be clearly appreciated after 2 weeks of treatment with a topical corticosteroid. **(C)** At 4 years of age, the congenital nevus has darkened and developed coarse terminal hair growth.

lesions are present at birth. However, in some patients with small and medium-sized lesions, they may be initially noted sometime during the first year of life rather than immediately at birth. Congenital nevi have been classified traditionally according to their greatest diameter in adulthood. According to this nomenclature, they have been traditionally defined as *small* (<1.5 cm in greatest diameter), *medium-sized* (1.5 to 19.9 cm), or *large* (≥20 cm) congenital nevi. An interdisciplinary group of experts in the field developed a consensus-based

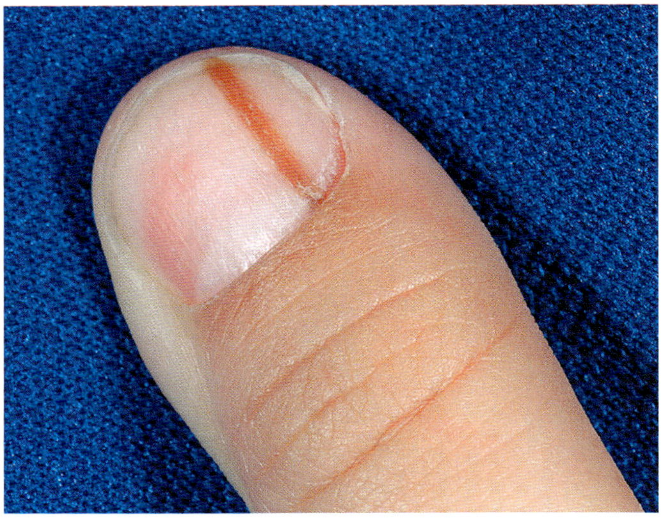

Fig. 9.7 Melanonychia striata. A 2-mm, evenly pigmented band. Note the absence of pigmentation of the proximal nailfold (negative Hutchinson sign).

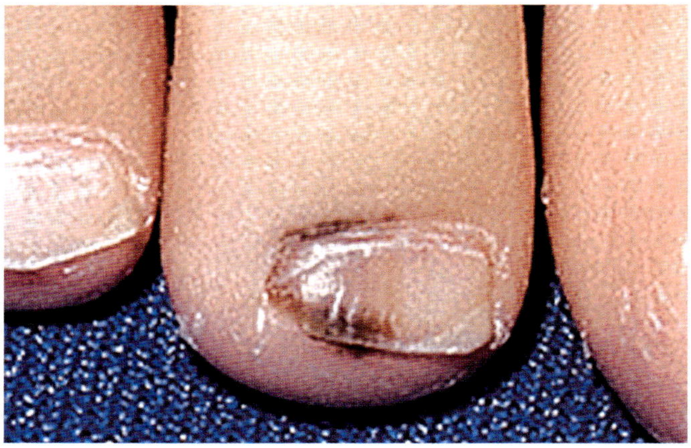

Fig. 9.8 Melanonychia striata with Hutchinson sign. Note pigmentation involving both the proximal nailfold and the distal nailfold regions. This patient underwent nail matrix biopsy; the lesion was a compound nevus without atypia.

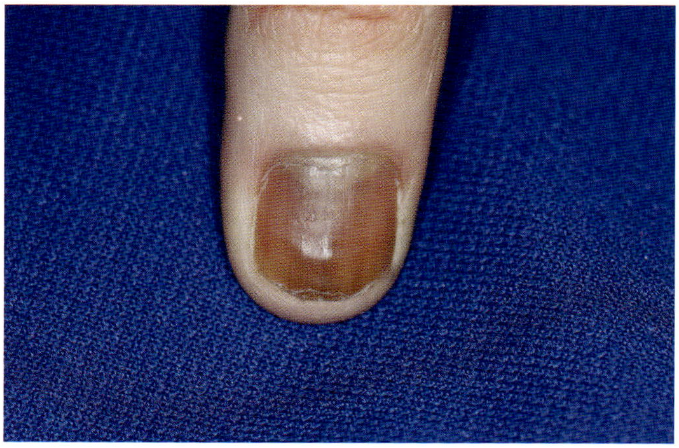

Fig. 9.9 Melanonychia striata. This teenaged girl had changes that began at 3 years of age, with gradual broadening of the band and eventual involvement of the entire nail unit. Nail matrix biopsy revealed junctional nevus with benign features.

categorization scheme for CMN that includes modified size categories (again, based on projected adult size) as follows: *small* (<1.5 cm), *medium* (M1: 1.5 to 10 cm; M2: >10 to 20 cm), *large* (L1: >20 to 30 cm; L2: >30 to 40 cm), and *giant* (G1: >40 to 60 cm; G2: >60 cm).[32] This classification includes other descriptors of CMN, including number of satellite nevi, anatomic localization, color heterogeneity, surface rugosity, hypertrichosis, and presence of dermal or subcutaneous nodules. Such a standardized classification scheme hopefully helps facilitate collaborative international studies and database development for the study of large and giant CMN.[32]

It is estimated that approximately 1% of newborns have a small congenital nevus (with some more recent studies suggesting an incidence of up to 3% of neonates), and large lesions occur in around 1 in 20,000 newborns.[33–36] Giant melanocytic nevi occur in 1 in 500,000 newborns.[37] Nevus spilus, or speckled lentiginous nevus (see later), may represent a distinct subtype of congenital melanocytic nevus that presents early in life as a café-au-lait macule, with the development of the more characteristic nevi a bit later in life.[38] Whereas malignant potential may be a primary concern with CMN, the potential psychosocial consequences, especially with large or giant lesions, are significant and may include social difficulties, psychological morbidities, behavioral and emotional impairment, and predisposition to taunting or bullying.[39]

Congenital nevi have some characteristic histopathologic features, including extension of nevus cells into the deeper dermis and subcutis, between the collagen bundles (as single cells), and in association with appendages, nerves, and vessels.[40,41] These features may be useful when histologic confirmation of a congenital lesion is desired, but such findings may not be noted in every congenital nevus. This pattern of deep extension is important to keep in mind when surgical intervention of such a lesion is being considered. Activating mutations in genes of the mitogen-activated protein kinase (MAPK) signal transduction pathway may be associated with nevi (see also later), including congenital nevi. The most notable of these are the *NRAS* and *BRAF* genes. A mutation in *BRAF (V600E)* has been noted in the majority of small congenital (and acquired) nevi, whereas medium, large, and giant CMN are often associated with mutations in *NRAS*.[42–44] In a series of large and giant CMN, *NRAS* mutations were noted in nearly 95% of cases, whereas in small- and medium-sized CMN, 70% bore *NRAS* mutations and 30% revealed *BRAF* mutations.[45] In a series of patients with multiple CMN and neurocutaneous melanosis (NCM) (see later), both the cutaneous and neural lesions contained missense mutations in codon 61 of *NRAS*, whereas unaffected tissues and blood were negative for this mutation, suggesting postzygotic mutation in a progenitor cell within the neuroectoderm.[46] Other reported gene mutations in molecular pathways for pediatric nevogenesis include *HRAS* (some Spitz nevi, atypical Spitz nevi, speckled lentiginous nevi), *BRAF with loss of BAP1* (some atypical Spitz nevi), and *GNAQ/GNA11* (some blue nevi).[47]

Small and medium-sized CMN usually present as flat, light- to dark-brown or pink macules (Fig. 9.10) or papules or as brown to dark brown, well-circumscribed patches or plaques. They may reveal some pigment variation, and the surface may have hair (Fig. 9.11). With time they tend to become more elevated, and coarse dark brown hairs may become more prominent. When an extremity is circumferentially involved with a medium- or large-sized congenital nevus, limb underdevelopment may occur (Fig. 9.12).[12]

Large CMN are uniformly present at birth and present as dark brown to black plaques, often with a verrucous or cobblestoned surface and hypertrichosis (Fig. 9.13). Color variation is common in these lesions and may make clinical examination for concerning features more challenging. Giant CMN often occur on the posterior trunk and may occupy a significant portion of the skin surface. They may have a dermatomal distribution and may involve an entire upper or lower extremity or the scalp. These lesions have been variably named *coat-sleeve, stocking, bathing trunk,* or *giant hairy* nevi, depending on their sites of involvement. As with large CMN, giant nevi present as large, brown to black plaques with varying degrees of nodularity, color variation, and hypertrichosis (Fig. 9.14). Erosions or ulcerations in these giant lesions may occur (Fig. 9.15), and although once believed to be consistently ominous findings, they are often benign and usually not indicative of MM.[48] Large and giant congenital nevi may be

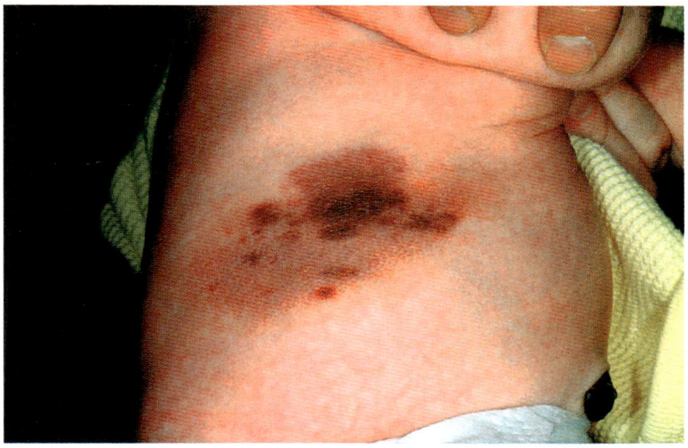

Fig. 9.10 Early congenital melanocytic nevus. Note the various shades of brown and red in this 2-week-old infant boy.

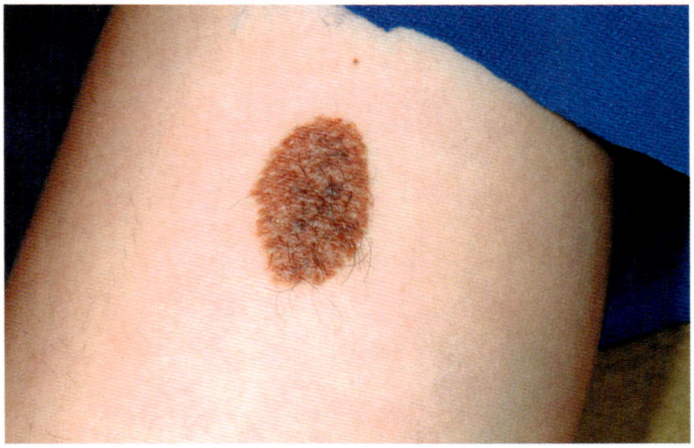

Fig. 9.11 Congenital melanocytic nevus. A well-demarcated, brown plaque with some pigment variation and hypertrichosis.

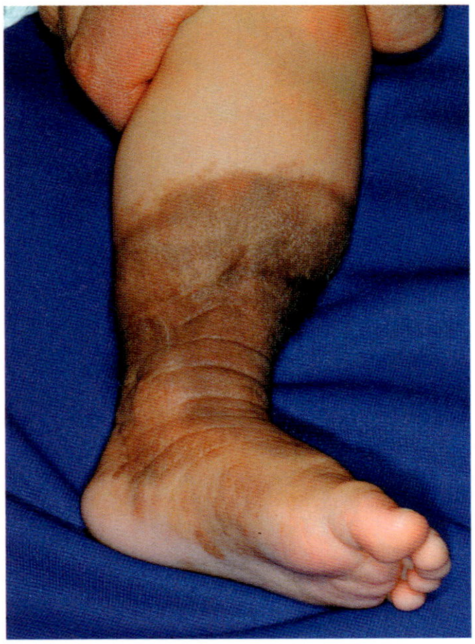

Fig. 9.12 Congenital nevus of the lower extremity. Note the limb hypoplasia in the ankle region associated with this circumferential lesion.

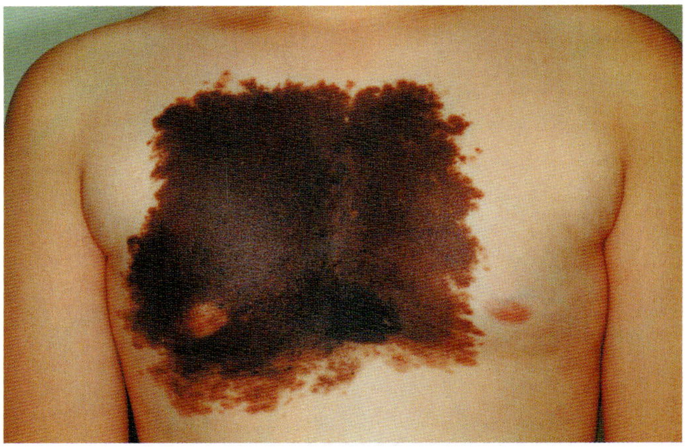

Fig. 9.13 Large congenital melanocytic nevus.

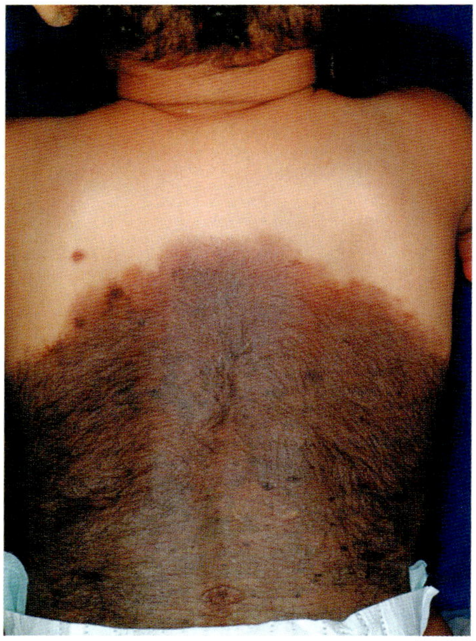

Fig. 9.14 Giant congenital melanocytic nevus. Note the marked hypertrichosis and adjacent satellite lesions.

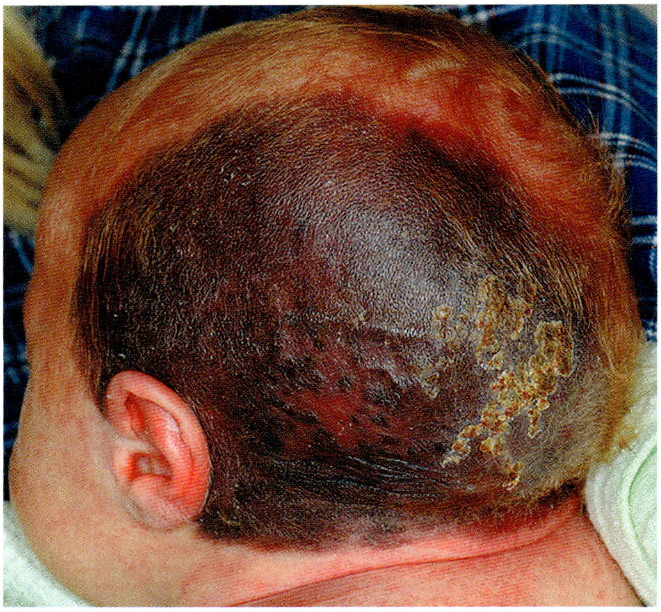

Fig. 9.15 Giant congenital melanocytic nevus with erosions. Surface erosion and crusting was present at birth and healed rapidly over a few weeks with topical care.

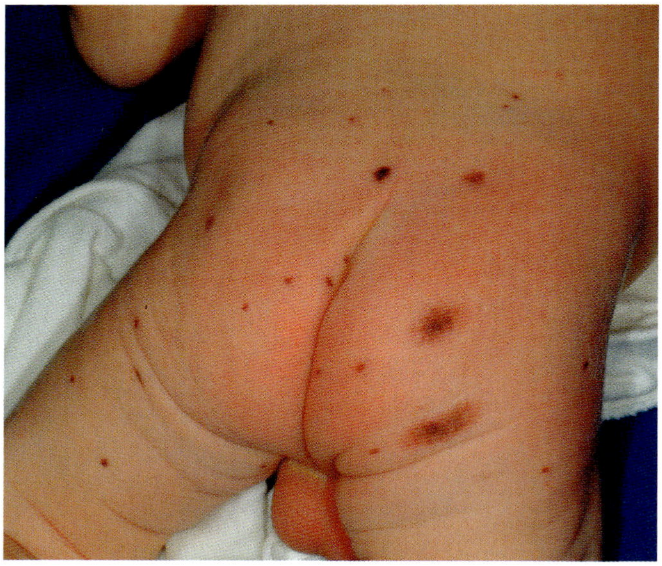

Fig. 9.16 Satellite melanocytic nevi. This patient had a giant nevus of the scalp.

associated with cosmetic disfigurement, an increased risk of MM, and underlying NCM (see later). These lesions often have associated "satellite" nevi that may be disseminated over the entire skin surface. Satellite nevi are usually tan to brown macules or papules, with varying degrees of hypertrichosis (Fig. 9.16). They may be present at birth or continue to develop during infancy.[36] Another feature seen in some large and giant CMN are proliferative nodules, which are benign dermal nodules that may raise clinical concern for MM. These nodules appear to be much more common than MM in CMN, are often multiple, and rarely ulcerate; histologic evaluation reveals distinct features and lower mitotic counts compared with MM.[49] Immunohistochemistry and fluorescence *in situ* hybridization were studied in an effort to identify features that further distinguish between proliferative nodules and childhood-onset MM but were not helpful in this regard.[50]

The congenital nature of nevi is one of several known risk factors for MM, but the exact magnitude of risk remains controversial, especially for small and medium-sized lesions. All congenital nevi should be considered potential precursors to melanoma. The lifetime risk in small and medium-sized lesions seems low, typically estimated at less than 1%, and if melanoma occurs, it tends to occur during adulthood.[12,51,52] This risk compares with a current overall lifetime risk for MM in the United States of 2.3%.[53] Factors that might increase the level of concern include atypical clinical features (e.g., deeply or irregularly pigmented or rapidly growing), an abnormal nevus phenotype, or a strong family history of MM. The risk of malignant transformation of congenital nevi in Black patients is extremely small.[54]

The risk of MM in large and giant CMN appears to be significantly greater than that for small and medium-sized lesions, with melanoma often (but not always) occurring before the age of 5 years.[55,56] It is unclear whether axial lesions pose a greater risk than those occurring on the extremities, as traditionally suggested.[57] When melanoma occurs in patients with large or giant CMN, it may occur within the skin or in extracutaneous sites such as the central nervous system.[58,59] When developing in the skin, these melanomas may occur in the dermis or deeper subcutaneous tissues, making detection more challenging. Development of melanoma in satellite lesions is exceedingly unlikely.[58] The overall lifetime risk of development of MM in patients with large CMN has been reported to range from 0% to 31% but is best estimated at between 2% and 10%.[55,56,60–62] In two large systematic reviews of the published data on melanoma risk in CMN, the rate of melanoma was 2% to 2.5% in large CMN and 3.1% in giant CMN.[61,62] However, others suggest that in giant CMN with satellite lesions, the lifetime risk may be as high as 10% to 15%.[63] In addition to melanoma, other malignancies may occur with increased rates in these patients, including rhabdomyosarcoma, liposarcoma, malignant peripheral nerve sheath tumor, and other sarcomas.[34,58]

Large and giant CMN, particularly those on the head, neck and back, may be associated with a condition termed *neurocutaneous melanosis* (NCM). NCM, as well as melanoma risk, appears to be more common in patients with greater numbers of satellite nevi (and not as correlated with posterior axial location as once believed).[64–66] Patients with NCM have a proliferation of nevus cells in the central nervous system (leptomeningeal melanocytosis) and are predisposed to seizures, MM of the central nervous system (CNS), and neurologic symptoms related to increased intracranial pressure or spinal cord compression. Treatment is often sought for symptoms during the first 3 years of life, including lethargy, irritability, headache, recurrent vomiting, seizures, increased head circumference, bulging anterior fontanel, photophobia, papilledema, neck stiffness, and occasionally nerve palsies, particularly of cranial nerves VI and VII. Magnetic resonance imaging (MRI) of NCM reveals focal areas of high signal on T1-weighted images in one or multiple areas of the brain, including the temporal lobes, cerebellum, pons, and medulla.[67,68] T2 shortening may also occur.[68] In one study, 45% of neurologically asymptomatic children with giant congenital nevi had these radiologic findings.[67] However, a questionnaire-based study of 186 patients with large congenital nevi who were imaged revealed that only 4.8% of those with positive MRI findings for NCM were asymptomatic.[69] Hence the exact prevalence of asymptomatic NCM remains unclear. Other findings in children with NCM may include dorsal spinal arachnoid cysts and amygdalar neuromelanosis (which may be associated with intractable seizures).[70–74] Overall, the prognosis for *symptomatic* NCM is poor, with more than 90% of patients dying of the disease and around 70% of those dying before 10 years of age.[59,75]

The management of CMN must be individualized for each patient. There are many factors that must be considered in the decision-making process regarding surgical excision of such lesions. These include location of the nevus, size, cosmetic issues (and potential psychosocial ramifications), and the risks of anesthesia, MM, and neurocutaneous melanosis.[76] There appears to be less consensus regarding the role of surgical excision of small and medium-sized CMN than that of large lesions. Small congenital nevi with uniform pigmentation, smooth texture, and lack of nodules can be clinically monitored, whereas lesions with atypical or deep pigmentation or uneven textures may warrant surgical excision given the heightened difficulty of melanoma detection in this setting.[34] Other risk factors, such as a strong family history of MM or the presence of numerous atypical-appearing nevi, may influence the decision regarding surgical removal of small and medium-sized CMN. Lesions located in areas that may be difficult to follow clinically, such as the scalp or groin, may be better served by excision, although in the case of benign-appearing lesions, this decision may be delayed until the child is older and the procedure can be performed under local anesthesia.

Large CMN are often treated with full-thickness surgical excision. The primary reason for this recommendation is the potentially decreased risk of malignant transformation, although controlled studies supporting this hypothesis are lacking.[76,77] Unfortunately, excision of large lesions does not usually result in complete removal of all nevus cells, and melanoma may still develop from this residual tissue. In addition, melanoma may develop with increased incidence at extracutaneous sites in these patients, and the significance of NCM (if present) must also be factored into this decision. Many still advocate for surgical excision in an effort to reduce the risk of malignancy,[78,79] whereas others highlight that treatment must be tailored to achieve the optimal cosmetic result, with nonsurgical management and partial excisions representing viable options in some settings.[80] Removal of these lesions has been refined with the use of tissue expanders and skin grafting, but multiple procedures are usually required. Partial thickness removal techniques (e.g., dermabrasion, dermatome excision, curettage, chemical peels, and laser therapy) have been advocated by some, but the impact of these procedures on malignant transformation or clinical surveillance of the lesion must be further defined. They may, however, be reasonable considerations when more aggressive procedures are impractical. There is no consensus on the timing of surgical procedures for large and giant CMN. Although many experts advocate for early referral and initiation of excisional therapy, other considerations may come into play, including anesthesia concerns surrounding neurocognitive effects on the developing brain. Ongoing prospective studies in this arena will hopefully clarify the optimal use and timing of sedation and anesthesia in young children as it pertains to procedures deemed to be elective or nonurgent.[77,81–84]

Close periodic clinical surveillance is important for all patients with CMN and may be aided by serial photography and dermatoscopic evaluation. Parent education in the importance of sun protection, sunscreen use, and danger signs of atypical nevi or melanoma (see later) is vital. Risks of malignant transformation should be discussed, and parents and patients should be allowed to reach an informed decision regarding therapy. Educational materials regarding moles, melanoma, and sun protection are useful and may be obtained from the American Academy of Dermatology (www.aad.org). A multidisciplinary approach must be employed for families of children with large congenital nevi. This includes the primary care physician, dermatologist, plastic surgeon, and diagnostic radiologist. Emotional support should be provided, and the family should be given information on support groups. One such organization is Nevus Outreach (www.nevus.org), which was founded by parents of children with large CMN and offers an annual family conference, newsletters, and a social support network.

ATYPICAL NEVI/FAMILIAL ATYPICAL MULTIPLE MOLE–MELANOMA SYNDROME

Atypical nevi, also known as *dysplastic nevi*, are defined based on their clinical and/or histologic appearance. These acquired nevi, which often do not present until at or after puberty, are regarded as markers and potential precursors for MM. The incidence of histologically confirmed atypical nevi in patients younger than 18 years of age is very low,[85] although in children who come from melanoma-prone families, their incidence seems much higher.[86] Clinically these lesions share some or all of the features of MM (Box 9.1). These include larger size and irregularities of color, texture, or borders (Fig. 9.17). Atypical nevi are often larger than common acquired nevi, usually measuring 6 to 15 mm in diameter, and display marked lesion-to-lesion variability, often with a cobblestone appearance or a dark, central papular component surrounded by a lighter tan and flatter periphery (the "fried egg" appearance, Fig. 9.18). Other patterns of clinically atypical

Box 9.1 Risk Factors for Malignant Melanoma in Children

- Familial atypical multiple mole–melanoma (FAMMM) syndrome
- Xeroderma pigmentosum
- Congenital melanocytic nevi
- Atypical (dysplastic) nevi
- Personal history of melanoma
- Family history of melanoma
- High numbers of melanocytic nevi
- Fair complexion
- Excessive sun exposures
- History of blistering sunburns
- History of immunosuppression

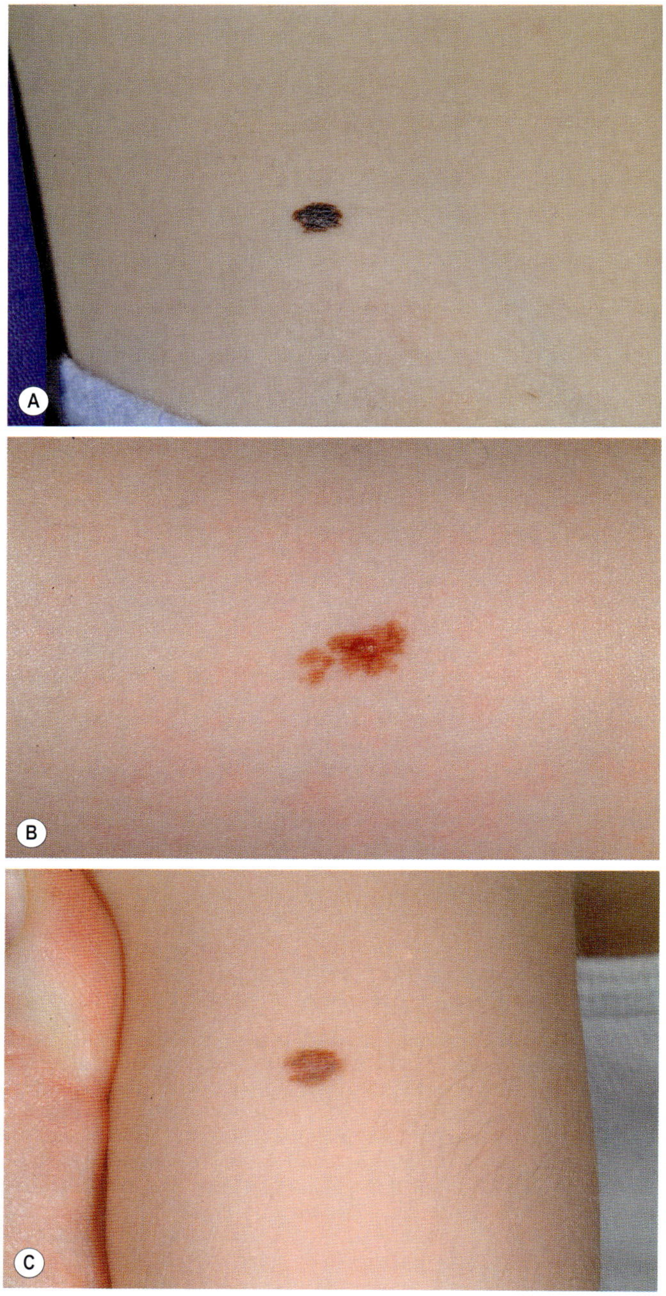

Fig. 9.17 (A–C) Atypical melanocytic nevi. These lesions revealed clinically atypical features, including asymmetry and border and color irregularity. All of them were histologically benign.

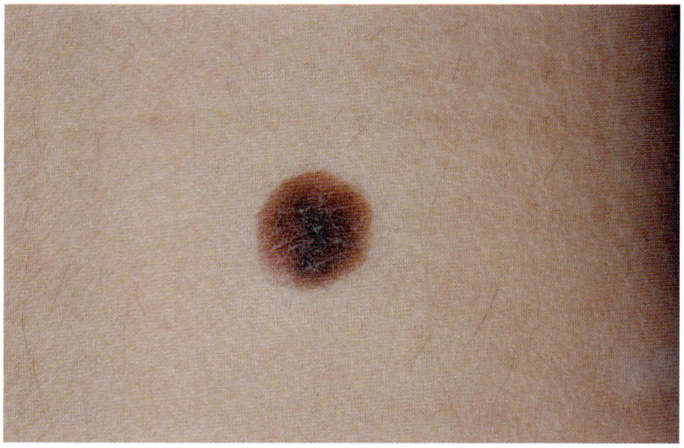

Fig. 9.18 "Fried egg" melanocytic nevus. Note the elevated, dark brown papule centrally and surrounding tan macular area.

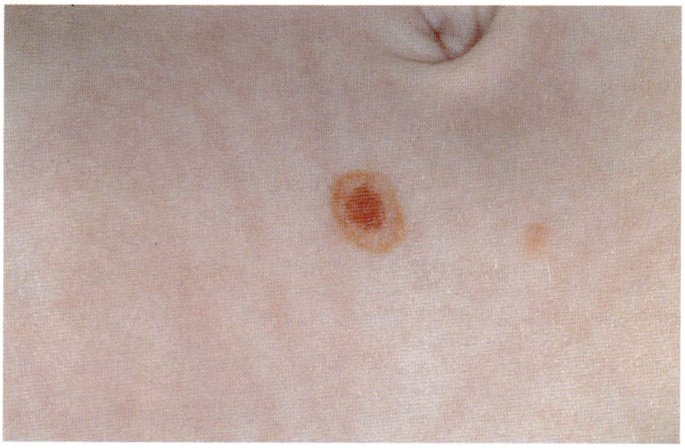

Fig. 9.19 Cockade nevus. This pattern refers to a central darkly pigmented portion surrounded by an intervening rim of minimal to no pigmentation and an outer rim of darker pigment, giving a target-like appearance. These nevi are usually benign.

nevi include the eclipse nevus (tan to hypopigmented center with a darker brown peripheral rim and irregular outer border) and the cockade nevus (target-like morphology with a central pigmented region, an intervening hypopigmented area, and an outer rim of pigmentation; Fig. 9.19).[87] These patterns may occur more with greater incidence on the scalp of children (see later).

Atypical nevi may occur anywhere, especially on sun-exposed sites, but also commonly occur on covered areas such as the back and in unusual locations such as the buttocks, breasts, and scalp.[88] In fact, a fairly high proportion of nevi removed from the scalp may demonstrate histologic features of atypical nevi.[24,89] Individuals with atypical nevi have been demonstrated to have an increased risk of melanoma despite the presence or absence of a family history of melanoma.[90,91] A distinct clinical phenotype characterized by numerous (>100) small, darkly pigmented atypical nevi has been described and termed the *cheetah* phenotype.[92] Longitudinal follow-up study of such patients is very challenging given the similar clinical appearance of several histologic patterns ranging from benign to cytologically atypical.[92]

Scalp nevi in children deserve special mention because they may be a source of anxiety for parents and clinicians alike. These lesions, which are more common in boys, tend to be somewhat larger in size and may often reveal irregular borders and some color variations (Fig. 9.20). The observed patterns may include the fried-egg, cockade, and eclipse phenotypes discussed previously, as well as clinically benign nevi patterns. Although scalp melanoma does occur in children, it seems that the majority of these lesions are benign; however, they may reveal mild to moderate atypia microscopically. Dermatoscopic (magnified light) examination may be helpful in demonstrating benign patterns (e.g., globular or reticular–globular pigmentation and perifollicular hypopigmentation).[93] It should be remembered that although the majority of scalp nevi in children are benign, their presence may suggest an increased risk for the development of numerous melanocytic nevi, which itself is a risk factor for MM.[94]

The familial atypical multiple mole–melanoma (FAMMM) syndrome is a disorder of autosomal dominant inheritance in which atypical nevi develop during the late second to third decade of life.[95] It was originally described in 1978 by Clark et al.[96] when they noted individuals with increased numbers of melanocytic nevi that

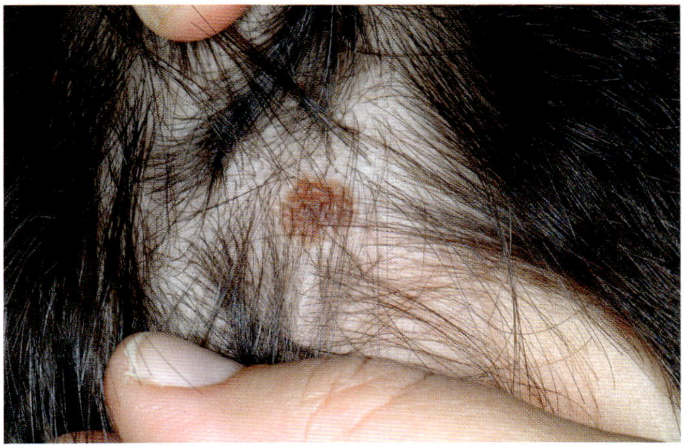

Fig. 9.20 Scalp nevus. These nevi may be larger and often reveal irregular borders and color variation, although the majority of them are histologically benign.

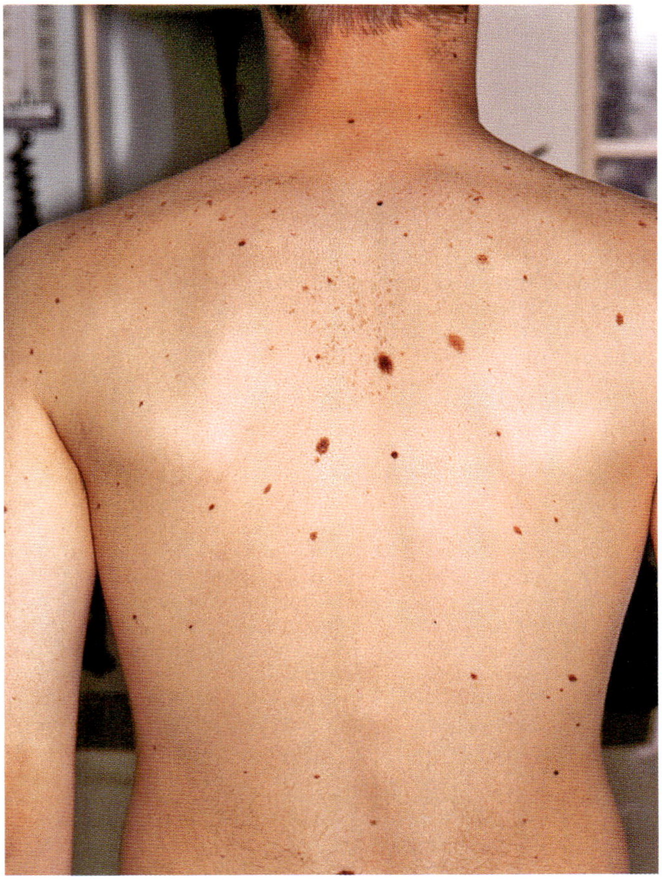

Fig. 9.21 Multiple atypical melanocytic nevi (familial atypical multiple mole–melanoma type). This adolescent boy had a family history of atypical nevi and malignant melanoma.

displayed atypical clinical and histologic features. Since the original description, FAMMM syndrome has been better characterized as a hereditary cancer predisposition syndrome, entailing not only an increased risk of MM but also other cancers in some kindreds, especially pancreatic cancer.[97–99] FAMMM syndrome is characterized by the familial occurrence of melanoma in combination with multiple dysplastic nevi (>50) in first-degree relatives, although around 10% of the melanoma patients may have very few to no dysplastic nevi.[100,101] It has been estimated that individuals with a family history of FAMMM syndrome and atypical nevi have nearly a 100% lifetime risk of acquiring MM. Importantly, patients with FAMMM syndrome may develop melanoma on normal skin despite the high numbers of atypical nevi.[102] In addition to melanoma of the skin, these individuals may develop intraocular melanoma. Observations of families displaying the association of pancreatic cancer and melanoma have led to the alternative terminology of *FAMMM–pancreatic cancer (FAMMM–PC) syndrome*. The phenotype of these families is variable, however, with several reported members lacking the dysplastic nevus phenotype. Some have therefore suggested the possibility of two distinct hereditary cancer syndromes, FAMMM–PC and the pancreatic cancer/melanoma syndrome (PCMS).[103]

The classic features of FAMMM syndrome are high numbers of melanocytic nevi, often more than 50, some of which are atypical and often have large variability in size (Fig. 9.21), that occur in the setting of a family history of MM in one or more first- or second-degree relatives.[88] Identification of at-risk children is vital because melanoma may occur before 20 years of age in up to 10% of individuals.[12] Although most of the atypical nevi develop during or after adolescence, prepubertal children may occasionally show the atypical nevus phenotype, particularly in scalp nevi. In fact, the development of scalp nevi during childhood, as well as large nevus counts early in life, may represent early indicators of increased risk for the atypical mole phenotype later in life.[86,104]

There are several known melanoma susceptibility loci, most notably the p16 *CDKN2A* gene on chromosome 9, which is a tumor suppressor gene responsible for melanoma susceptibility in some kindreds with FAMMM syndrome.[95] Up to 45% of familial melanomas are associated with germline mutations in *CDKN2A* or *CDK4*.[104] Deletion of p16 may play a role in the development of atypical nevi as an early event, as well as in the development of MM (see later).

Management of the patient with atypical nevi should include a thorough family history, total body inspection, and a regular clinical follow-up examination every 6 to 12 months, depending on the individual patient. Patients with FAMMM syndrome should undergo total body skin examinations every 3 to 6 months, and for children in these families, screening should begin in late adolescence.[104] Patients (and parents) should be educated regarding sun protection, regular skin self-examination, and atypical features of nevi, and surgical excision should be performed for lesions with concerning features. A helpful guideline in monitoring children with many nevi is the "ugly duckling" principle, which dictates that a lesion that stands out from the rest (i.e., markedly darker pigmentation, more irregularity of texture or borders) should be more closely scrutinized and considered for removal. Epiluminescence microscopy (dermatoscopy, dermoscopy) is a useful noninvasive instrument that provides magnification of nevi and may be useful in differentiating benign from atypical lesions. It is most often used by dermatologists, and its use requires training and experience to provide acceptable sensitivity and reliability. Serial photography of nevi may also be a useful adjunct in the longitudinal follow-up study of patients with multiple or atypical nevi.

MALIGNANT MELANOMA

The incidence of MM, the most deadly form of skin cancer, continues to rise, and although childhood MM continues to be rare, the incidence in this population may also be rising.[105,106] The overall lifetime risk of melanoma is estimated at around 1 in 45 individuals,[107] which is an alarming increase from the incidence of 1 in 1500 estimated in 1935.[108] The challenges of diagnosing MM in children are multiple and include lack of recognition, hesitancy to perform skin biopsies in children, and poor reliability in making the histopathologic diagnosis in this population.[109] Melanoma in individuals younger than 20 years of age accounts for only 1% to 3% of all MM, and prepubertal cases are even rarer, accounting for 0.3% to 0.4% of all cases.[110–112] Despite this rarity, the course of melanoma, when it does occur in a child, has similar prognostic implications to MM in adults.[111,113,114] Importantly, in recent decades, the incidence of pediatric melanoma was estimated to be increasing at an estimated 1% to 4% per year.[115] However, a review of SEER cancer registry data from 2000 to 2010 for age-adjusted incidence rates of MM in children and adolescents (younger than 20 years) revealed a decreasing incidence, possibly attributable to effective public health measures and improved sun protection behavior.[116] Interestingly, many lesions previously thought to be melanomas of childhood are now recognized to be benign Spitz nevi (see later). Congenital MM represents a small subset of all pediatric MM and is extremely rare, with only 23 cases reported in the English literature between 1925 and 2002.[111] It most commonly arises in a congenital melanocytic nevus and less commonly is *de novo* or related to transplacental transmission of MM from the mother.

MM most commonly affects individuals with fair skin, blue eyes, and red or blond hair, particularly those of Celtic origin whose pigment cells have a limited capacity to synthesize melanin. Approximately 50% to 65% of MM arises in a preexisting nevus. Although melanomas may occur in Black individuals, the incidence is extremely low compared with that of Whites. In Blacks, tumors usually arise in areas that are lightly pigmented, especially the mucous membranes, nailbeds, or the sides of the palms and soles. Exposure to high levels of sunlight in childhood seems to be a strong determinant of risk for MM, although adult sun exposure also plays a role.[117] Some studies have not supported this "critical risk period" hypothesis of ultraviolet radiation exposure, suggesting that sun protection education should be directed at the entire population with equal effort rather than concentrating solely on younger age groups.[118] However, maintaining a stringent focus on childhood sun protection still seems reasonable because a large proportion of overall lifetime sun exposure is likely to occur during these years.[119] Other risk factors for pediatric melanoma include xeroderma pigmentosum (see Chapter 19), immunosuppression, and history of treatment for other childhood cancers.

The genetics of MM continue to be elucidated, and it is now established that molecular defects in both tumor suppressor genes and oncogenes may be pathogenetically linked to melanoma.[120] Mutations in the *CDKN2A* (p16) gene predispose a patient to the FAMMM syndrome (see earlier) and have also been noted in families in which only one or two individuals are affected by MM.[121] A subset of melanoma-prone families with *CDKN2A* mutations also manifests an increased risk of pancreatic cancers (as discussed earlier).[99,120] Activating mutations in one of two Ras/mitogen-activated protein kinase pathway genes, *BRAF* (including *BRAF V600*) or *NRAS*, are present in up to 80% to 90% of melanomas.[122,123] Some of the other genes potentially mutated in melanoma include *PTEN*, *CDK4*, *CCND1*, *c-KIT*, *p53*, *EphA2*, *ERBB4*, *GRIN2A*, *GRM3*, *MEK1*, *MEK2*, *MITF*, β-catenin, *TERT-p*, and various apoptosis genes.[122–125]

Melanoma is classically categorized according to its clinical and histologic features. The most common forms are superficial spreading, nodular, lentigo maligna (usually confined to adults), and acral lentiginous melanoma. However, pediatric cases of MM often cannot be neatly classified into one of these categories. Pediatric melanoma seems to follow the same distribution patterns as adult melanoma, with head and trunk lesions predominating in boys and arm and leg lesions predominating in girls. Risk factors for pediatric MM are listed in Box 9.1. Some experts have suggested that pediatric melanoma be classified (based on clinical, dermoscopic, and histopathologic features) as spitzoid or nonspitzoid types (see also Spitz Nevus later in this chapter).[126]

The classic signs of MM are summarized in Table 9.1. Melanoma typically presents with a rapidly enlarging papule or nodule, most often brown to brown-black (Fig. 9.22), although blue, red, or white discoloration may also be noted. Importantly, a significant proportion of pediatric melanomas may present in an amelanotic (i.e., pink, white, red, or a combination of these colors) fashion; in one series of MM in children and adolescents, 45% of the lesions were amelanotic.[127,128] A halo of hypopigmentation or depigmentation may be present around a primary lesion of MM, although most often these halos occur in the setting of benign nevi (see Halo Nevus section). Melanomas often reveal asymmetry and irregularity of the borders, especially scalloping or notching, and tend to be larger than benign nevi, often (but not always) larger than 10 mm in diameter. Bleeding, itching, ulceration, crusting, and pain may be present. In a single-center

Table 9.1 Clinical Features (ABCDE Signs) of Malignant Melanoma

Clinical Feature*		Comment
A	Asymmetry	The two halves of the lesion are not alike
B	Border irregularity	Borders notched, scalloped, irregular
C	Color changes	Especially blue, red, black, white
D	Diameter >6 mm	Size of a pencil eraser; not applicable to congenital nevi, which are often >6 mm early in their evolution
E	Enlargement	Evolutionary change in the lesion

*See text for important discussion of features that may be more specific to pediatric melanoma.

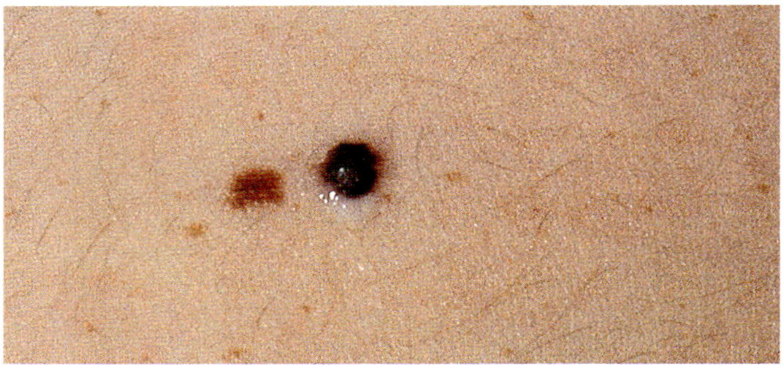

Fig. 9.22 Malignant melanoma. This small, black papule was noted on a 10-year-old boy with fair skin and red hair; excision confirmed a nodular malignant melanoma.

retrospective review of 70 children (younger than 20 years of age) with melanoma or other atypical melanocytic tumors, several clinical features were highlighted that may contradict the traditional ABCD portion of the ABCDE criteria (as shown in Table 9.1). These include the amelanotic (flesh-colored, pink, or red) nature of the lesions, bleeding, uniformity of color, small diameter (often <6 mm) and *de novo* development (as opposed to arising in an existing nevus).[129] These characteristics should be kept in mind when evaluating children with atypical "bumps" and may facilitate earlier recognition of (and hence therapy for) pediatric MM.

Lymph nodes may be palpable and if present are an ominous prognostic sign, suggesting metastatic spread. When MM goes undetected and undiagnosed, the lesion proliferates locally and may spread by satellite lesions or extend through the lymphatics or bloodstream, from which it may eventually invade any organ of the body. Once metastatic disease occurs, the prognosis of MM significantly declines.

Early detection of melanoma is germane to long-term survival. The survival rate for children and adults have traditionally been believed to be similar (see more later), and the primary determinants of prognosis have traditionally been tumor thickness and depth of invasion[108,113]; the presence or absence of ulceration are included in the American Joint Committee on Cancer staging system for MM as another important prognostic criterion (the presence of ulceration correlating with poorer prognosis).[130] Pediatricians (or other primary care providers of children) are in a good position to observe pigmented skin lesions over time in their patients. Early referral should be considered for any melanocytic lesion that displays substantial growth changes, especially if asymmetry, ulceration, or other atypical features are present. Melanoma is diagnosed by histopathologic examination of skin tissue from biopsy. When MM is suspected, full-thickness excision of the lesion should be performed because the depth of the lesion must be fully visualized to assess this prognostic indicator. Shave biopsies or excisions should be avoided in the removal of concerning pigmented lesions.

Although there is a lack of consensus on the management of pediatric melanoma, clinical approaches used in adults have also been useful for children. Surgical excision is the initial step in melanoma management, and one study demonstrated improved overall survival and disease-free survival when initial surgical treatment is performed at a comprehensive cancer center.[131] Once the diagnosis of MM is confirmed, the site is reexcised with appropriate margins (0.5 to 2 cm), depending on tumor depth in the initial specimen, and the disease must be adequately staged. Clinically suspected lymph nodes are surgically removed and histologically evaluated. Developments in tracer techniques have enabled sampling of the first lymph node draining the affected skin site (the "sentinel" lymph node), which assists in determining whether to proceed with regional lymph node dissection for further staging and therapy. This technique, which is called *sentinel lymph node biopsy* (SLNB) and usually performed concurrently with reexcision of the primary lesion, allows for accurate staging of the regional lymph nodes with minimal morbidity.[113] The most recent primary cutaneous MM management guidelines of the American Academy of Dermatology recommend consideration for SLNB in patients with cutaneous melanoma greater than 0.8 mm thickness (or <0.8 mm if ulceration is present), as well as those less than 0.8 mm without ulceration if other high-risk microscopic features are present.[132]

The usefulness of SLNB in children continues to be debated. In a series of 126 patients younger than 21 years of age who were diagnosed with MM, sentinel lymph node metastases were present in 29%, yet the survival was equal to or better than that reported for adults, suggesting that the biology of pediatric melanoma may be different from that in adult melanoma.[115] It appears that lymph node metastases and thicker tumors may be more common in younger children (younger than 10 years of age) with MM.[133] In addition to histopathologic analysis and lymph node examination, staging for pediatric MM may also include computed tomography (CT), positron emission tomography (PET), and PET-CT scanning in patients with thicker lesions to evaluate for distant metastases.[134]

Treatment of more advanced stages of MM includes chemotherapy, radiotherapy, and immunotherapy, although the results have been somewhat discouraging.[135] Adjuvant interferon α-2b therapy has received much attention in the treatment of high-risk melanoma in adults, with reports of improved disease-free survival and overall survival rates with use of the Kirkwood regimen (high-dose therapy for 4 weeks followed by a lowered dose for 48 weeks). Recommendations for use of this agent in children have primarily been extrapolated from the adult data, and although its use is potentially effective, it may be associated with some toxicities at higher doses, which may be limiting when treating the pediatric melanoma patient.[136,137] The benefit of adjuvant interferon in pediatric melanoma remains unknown, with large randomized trials lacking.[138] Immunotherapeutic approaches to MM include melanoma vaccines, cytokine therapy, and immunotherapy with monoclonal antibodies, and these and other approaches continue to be the topics of active investigation.[139] Traditional chemotherapy regimens have shown minimal activity against melanoma.[106] Biologic agents such as high-dose interleukin-2 (IL-2) have resulted in durable responses in some adult patients, but experience in children is limited.[134] More recently, treatments that target growth factor pathways or molecular targets have received increasing attention, including *BRAF* inhibitors such as dabrafenib and vemurafenib and MEK inhibitors such as trametinib.[140] The combination of *BRAF* and MEK inhibition appears to provide greater benefit than *BRAF* inhibitor monotherapy in adults.[141] Immune checkpoint inhibitors such as ipilimumab, pembrolizumab, and nivolumab have also been approved in adults with advanced melanoma. None of these treatments have been well studied in pediatric melanoma.

The prognosis for pediatric melanoma is strongly correlated with initial stage, along with important factors such as tumor thickness, ulceration, and lymph node status. In a review of data from the National Cancer Database of 3158 patients aged 1 to 19 years with melanoma, average 5-year survival rates were 98.7% (*in situ* disease), 93.6% (localized invasive disease), 68% (regionally metastatic disease), and 11.8% (distant disease).[142] Some studies have found decreased survival in prepubescent patients with MM, whereas others have found no difference or a better prognosis in this group.[134,143] In a retrospective cohort study of pediatric and adolescent melanoma diagnosed between 1998 and 2011 using the National Cancer Database, multivariate analyses revealed that pediatric (defined as 1 to 10 years) MM patients have longer overall survival than adolescent (defined as 11 to 20 years) and adult (21 years or older) patients. The findings in this study and others suggest that further study is required to assess age-based differences in melanoma outcomes.[144]

SPITZ NEVUS

Spitz nevus is a distinct subtype of melanocytic nevus that occurs primarily in children. The importance of the Spitz nevus, which was formerly known as *benign juvenile melanoma*, lies in its histologic differentiation from MM. This lesion was originally recognized in 1948 when Dr. Sophie Spitz realized that a subset of juvenile melanomas did not behave in the same fashion as adult melanomas.[145] Spitz nevi have subsequently been identified as a distinct nevus variant, occurring most commonly on the face of children and adolescents.

Spitz nevi present usually as a smooth-surfaced, hairless, dome-shaped papule or nodule with a distinctive red-brown color (Fig. 9.23). They are most often solitary, although multiple clustered (agminated, Fig. 9.24) or disseminated lesions have been described.[146,147] They may vary in size from a few millimeters to several centimeters, although most range from 0.6 to 1 cm in diameter. The lesion may be so red that the differential diagnosis for some includes pyogenic granuloma or early juvenile xanthogranuloma. The presence of brown pigmentation (Fig. 9.25), either with regular clinical examination or when examined through a glass slide compressing the surface (diascopy), may be useful in confirming the melanocytic nature of the lesion. Surface telangiectasia may also be a prominent feature. In some lesions, particularly those on the extremities, the red color is replaced by a mottled brown to tan or black appearance, often with verrucous surface changes and irregular borders. Clinically it is this type of lesion that is most easily confused with MM (Fig. 9.26). Dermoscopy of Spitz nevi may reveal several patterns, including the starburst pattern, which reveals radial pseudopods at the periphery and is seen in more than half of cases, and the vascular pattern with dotted or comma vessels.[148]

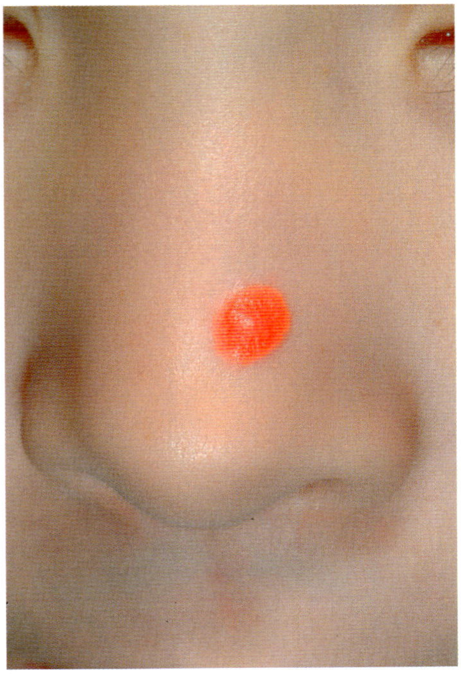

Fig. 9.23 Spitz nevus. This patient had the erythematous type of Spitz nevus on her nose.

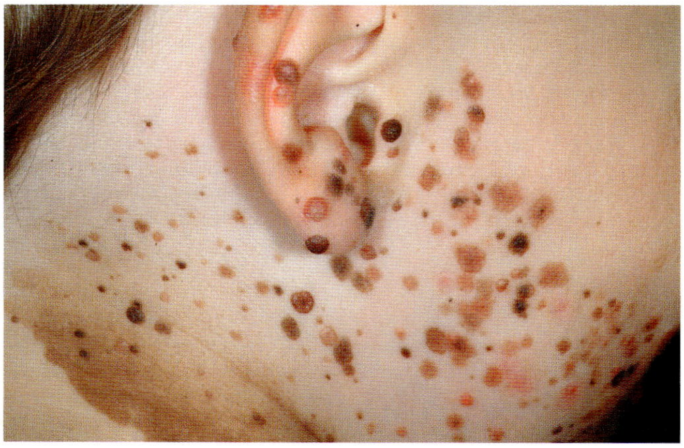

Fig. 9.24 Agminated Spitz nevi. This child had multiple lesions of the lateral cheek, ear, and neck, several of which were excised, revealing characteristic histologic features of Spitz nevus.

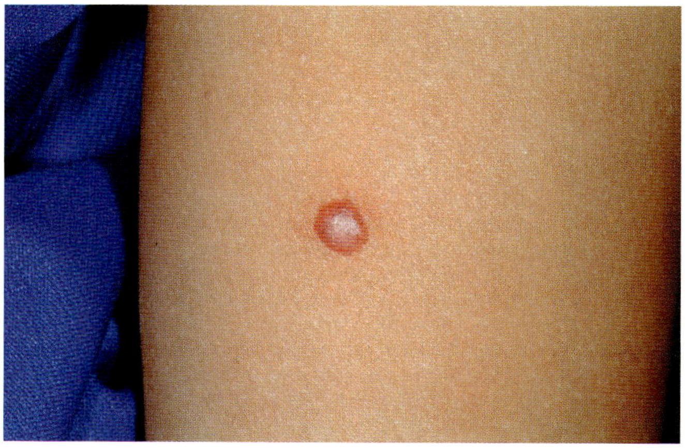

Fig. 9.25 Spitz nevus. This pink papule reveals brown speckling, which was easier to see when pressure was applied with a glass slide (diascopy).

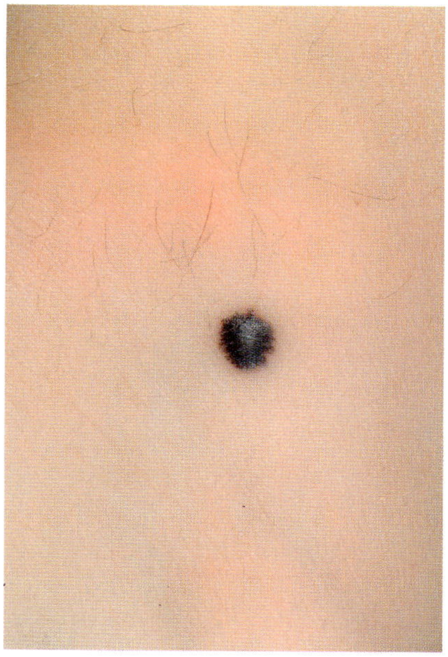

Fig. 9.26 Spitz nevus. The dark brown or black type is most often confused clinically with malignant melanoma.

Although most Spitz nevi behave in a benign fashion, local recurrence after excision may occur in as many as 5%.[149] It has been suggested by some that occasional Spitz nevi are malignant in origin and have the potential for more aggressive biologic behavior. Whether these represent a subtype of Spitz nevus or a "spitzoid" MM is unclear. It is obvious that some Spitz nevus–like lesions may pose substantial diagnostic difficulties especially when atypical features are present, even among dermatopathology experts.[150] These lesions have been variably called *spitzoid tumor of uncertain malignant potential* or *atypical spitzoid tumor.* A grading system has been proposed for Spitz nevi with atypical features, and application of such a system may be useful in guiding management for patients with atypical Spitz tumors.[151] *BRAF* mutations have occasionally been observed in a subset of Spitz nevi, suggesting that this finding should not be relied upon for distinguishing Spitz nevus from melanoma[152]; however, Spitz tumors typically have no mutations in *BRAF, NRAS,* or *KIT,* three commonly activated oncogenes in MM.[153] The expression of cell cycle and apoptosis regulators in Spitz nevi appears to more closely parallel the findings in benign nevi rather than melanoma.[154] Activating mutations in *HRAS* have been found in Spitz nevi (around 20%), as have kinase fusions, which may be found throughout the spectrum of these lesions from benign Spitz nevi to spitzoid melanomas.[153,155] Fluorescent *in situ* hybridization (FISH) using probes for chromosomal loci has been used in an attempt to predict biologic behavior in atypical spitzoid tumors: gains in 6p25 or 11q13 and deletions in 9q21 have been shown to correlate with more aggressive clinical behavior.[156] Deletions in 9q21 appear to correlate most with lymph node spread and distant metastasis.[157] A distinct type of atypical spitzoid tumor is characterized by inactivation of *BAP1,* often in conjunction with a mutation in *BRAFV600E.*[158,159] Mutations in *BAP1 (BRCA1-associated protein-1)* were initially found in aggressive uveal melanomas and subsequently found to also be associated with mesothelioma, atypical melanocytic tumors (described as atypical Spitz tumors, BAP-omas, or melanocytic *BAP1*-mutated atypical intradermal tumors), melanoma, and renal cell carcinoma. This increased malignancy risk related to germline *BAP1* mutations has been referred to as *BAP1 cancer syndrome* or *BAP1 tumor predisposition syndrome.*[160,161]

The management of Spitz nevi is controversial. Many experts recommend excision of these lesions on the basis of uncertainty in their biologic behavior, occasional reports of aggressive potential, and the increasing observation of the amelanotic nature of many melanomas in children. Others advocate for watchful waiting, reserving excision for lesions that demonstrate atypical features or those of psychosocial significance. When these lesions are excised, however, complete removal is advisable. More importantly, surgical specimens should be examined by a dermatopathologist or pathologist experienced in the diagnosis of melanocytic lesions and familiar with Spitz nevi. If an excised lesion is diagnosed unequivocally as a Spitz nevus without atypical features, no further therapy is necessary. However, because incompletely removed lesions may recur and result in a histopathologic appearance that may be more likely to be misinterpreted as MM, conservative reexcision is recommended for lesions with positive margins noted on the initial biopsy, especially if any atypical features are present.

HALO NEVUS

A halo nevus is a unique skin lesion in which a centrally placed, usually pigmented nevus becomes surrounded by a 1- to 5-mm halo of hypopigmentation or depigmentation (Fig. 9.27). These lesions are common in children and young adults. The cause of the spontaneous loss of pigmentation is unknown but appears to be related to an immunologic destruction of melanocytes and nevus cells that shares the immunophenotypic pattern of vitiligo.[162,163] Adding support to this hypothesis is the fact that several patients with halo nevi have a tendency toward the development of vitiligo (see Chapter 11; Fig. 9.28). In one series, 26% of 208 children with vitiligo had concomitant halo nevi, and the vitiligo was more likely to be of the generalized type.[164] Histologic examination of halo nevi reveals reduction or absence of melanin and a dense inflammatory infiltrate around the central nevus. Although compound or intradermal nevi are the tumors most commonly associated with the halo phenomenon,

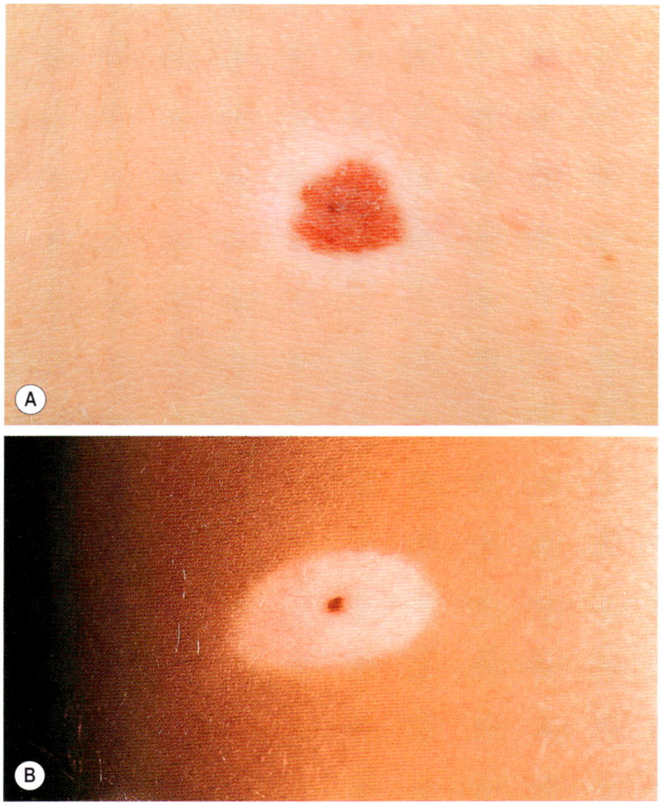

Fig. 9.27 Halo nevi. **(A)** Small halo surrounding a small congenital nevus. **(B)** Larger halo surrounding an acquired compound nevus.

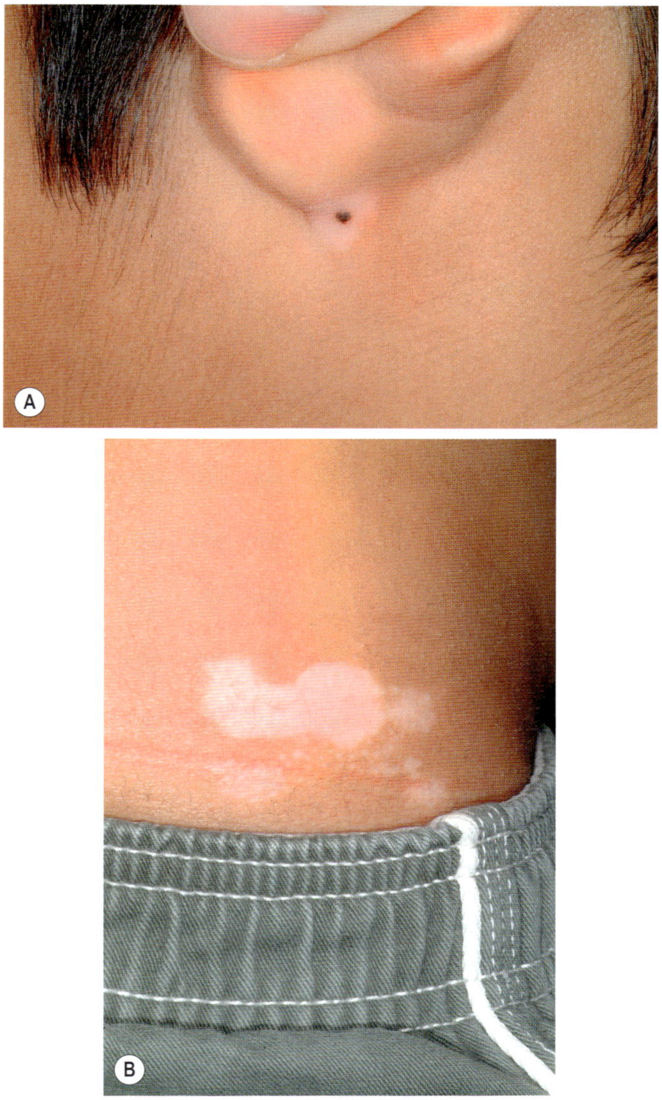

Fig. 9.28 Halo nevus with vitiligo. **(A)** Small halo nevus in the inferior ear crease. **(B)** The same patient had generalized depigmented macules and patches consistent with vitiligo, as seen here on the flank.

it may also occur around blue nevi, Spitz nevi, neurofibromas, melanomas, and metastatic lesions of melanoma. Giant CMN may also reveal the halo phenomenon with pigment regression and, at times, self-destruction.[165,166]

Typical halo nevi are notable for loss of pigmentation in the nevus, with a pink appearance and, commonly, eventual disappearance of the original melanocytic lesion. Occasionally, darkening of the central nevus may occur.[167] Halo nevi may appear on almost any cutaneous surface, but the site of predilection for most lesions is the trunk, particularly the back. In most patients, eventual repigmentation of the halo occurs over a period of months to years.

Halo nevi tend to be benign, although the halo phenomenon may occur around lesions revealing varying degrees of histologic atypia.[168] Potential concern has been raised over reports of MM exhibiting the halo phenomenon and the increased incidence of halo nevi in adults with melanoma.[169] In a survey of pediatric dermatologists, no diagnoses of MM in pediatric patients with halo nevi were noted.[169] In a series of 124 halo nevi from children and adults that were excised and had undergone histopathologic examination, most occurred in adolescents and young adults, and, importantly, the majority were nondysplastic.[170] Clinical features that may suggest an increased probability of an atypical melanocytic lesion within a halo include the ABCDE diagnostic criteria of melanoma (see Table 9.1) and asymmetry or irregularity of the surrounding depigmentation. Any patient with a halo nevus, especially if multiple halo lesions are present, should receive a complete skin and mucous membrane examination to assess for melanocytic lesions revealing atypical features. Patients with the halo nevus phenomenon, concomitant vitiligo, and ocular melanoma have been described,[171] but in general ophthalmologic evaluation is not routinely indicated. If the melanocytic lesion in the central portion of a halo reveals concerning or atypical features, complete excision should be performed. If, on the other hand, the central lesion has benign characteristics, excision is unnecessary and the lesion may be observed at intervals until it has resolved.

NEVUS SPILUS

Nevus spilus is a solitary, flat, brown patch of melanization dotted by smaller dark brown to black macules (Fig. 9.29). This relatively common lesion, although usually present at birth, may first become noticed during infancy, childhood, or even later. However, clinical and histologic data suggest that these lesions are most likely a subtype of CMN.[38] The earliest findings are usually similar to a café-au-lait patch, with eventual development of the secondary superimposed darker melanocytic lesions. Nevi spili may vary in size from 1 to 20 cm in diameter and may appear on any area of the face, trunk, or extremities without relation to sun exposure. Subtle hypertrichosis may occasionally be present (Fig. 9.30). Although the darker melanocytic components of these lesions have the potential to develop MM, the incidence of this transformation appears to be low.[172,173] Histologic evaluation of a nevus spilus usually reveals components of junctional and congenital nevi.[38,172] Patients with nevus spilus should be

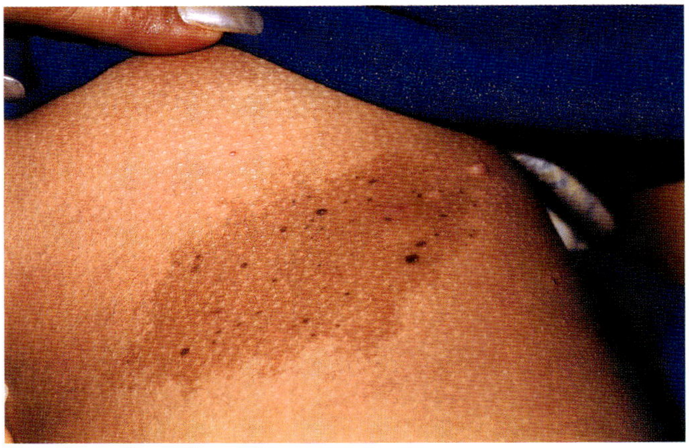

Fig. 9.29 Nevus spilus. A tan patch is studded with numerous darker brown macules and papules.

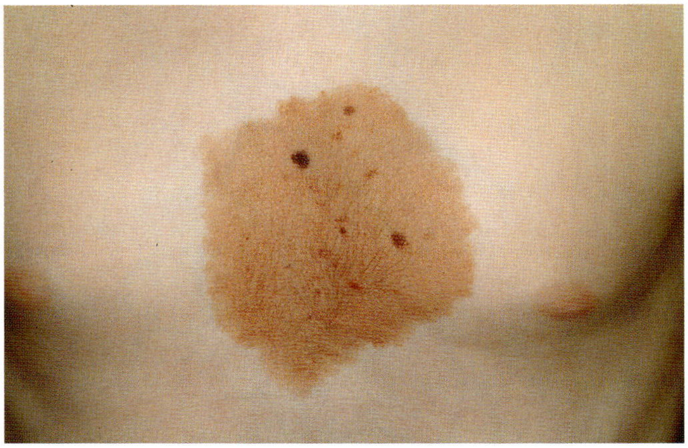

Fig. 9.30 Nevus spilus. This larger patch on the chest of a young boy reveals numerous superimposed nevi along with mild hypertrichosis.

monitored longitudinally with serial clinical examinations and, if possible, photographic surveillance. Any areas revealing atypical clinical features should be selectively excised and subjected to histologic evaluation, but widespread prophylactic excision seems unwarranted.[36] These lesions (especially when larger) have also been called *speckled lentiginous nevi* (SLN). Although they usually occur in isolation, they may sometimes be associated with other organ abnormalities as part of a syndrome such as phakomatosis pigmentovascularis (see Chapter 12), phakomatosis pigmentokeratotica (PPK), or SLN syndrome (see later).

BECKER MELANOSIS

Becker melanosis, also known as *Becker nevus*, is an acquired, unilateral hyperpigmentation usually involving the upper trunk of adolescent boys. Occasionally it may present very early in life (as early as birth) and may be distributed in other locations, including the extremities.[174] This pigmentation, which is caused by increased melanization of the epidermis and not by nevocellular proliferation, may be associated with hypertrichosis (Fig. 9.31) and occasionally proliferation of smooth muscle derived from erector pili muscles. Becker melanosis is discussed in more detail in Chapter 11.

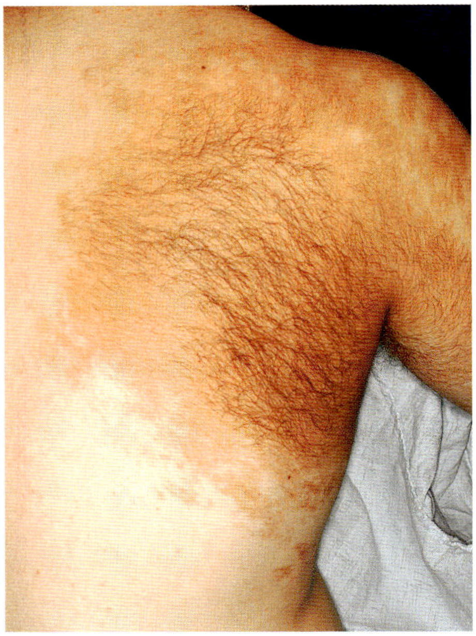

Fig. 9.31 Becker melanosis. This adolescent boy has hyperpigmentation of the upper back and shoulder with extension onto the right upper chest in association with surface hypertrichosis.

Tumors of the Epidermis

Tumors of the epidermis range in spectrum from benign lesions to those that are malignant. Benign tumors appear much more often than malignant lesions in children, and the latter, when they do occur, may be overlooked or the diagnosis delayed.

EPIDERMAL NEVI

Epidermal nevi (EN) are benign congenital lesions characterized by hyperplasia of epidermal structures. They are usually apparent at birth or become noticeable during early childhood, affect both sexes equally, and are known by several descriptive names, including *nevus verrucosus*, *nevus unius lateris*, and *ichthyosis hystrix*. In addition, EN can be divided into nonorganoid (keratinocytic) nevi and organoid EN, such as nevus sebaceus or follicular nevi. Although the exact cause of EN is unknown, activating fibroblast growth factor receptor 3 (*FGFR3*) mutations have been demonstrated in some,[175–177] as have mutations in the p110 α-subunit of *PI3K (PIK3CA)*, *HRAS*, *KRAS*, and *NRAS*.[178–180]

Keratinocytic EN (often referred to simply as *EN*) may be slightly or darkly pigmented and unilateral or bilateral in distribution. They often favor the extremities, although they may occur anywhere on the cutaneous surface. EN are usually distributed in a mosaic pattern of alternating stripes of involved and uninvolved skin. This pattern is termed *Blaschko lines* and occurs as a result of migration of skin cells during embryogenesis. Disorders that occur along the Blaschko lines usually reveal a linear pattern on the extremities and a wavy or arcuate pattern on the trunk. Although a single EN is most common, multiple lesions may be present, sometimes in association with the epidermal nevus syndrome (ENS; see later). The localized form is often present at birth and presents as a tan to brown, velvety or verrucous (warty) papule or plaque. There may be a single lesion (Fig. 9.32) or multiple lesions, and a linear configuration is common (Fig. 9.33). Over time, EN may become quite elevated, verrucous, or papillomatous (Fig. 9.34). One subtype of epidermal nevus has been termed the *acanthosis nigricans form of EN* and is characterized by a clinical (Fig. 9.35) and histologic resemblance to acanthosis nigricans.[181]

The term *nevus unius lateris* has been used traditionally to describe extensive unilateral lesions. Nevus unius lateris may present as a single or spiral linear, verrucous lesion or at times as an elaborate, continuous, or interrupted pattern affecting multiple sites (Fig. 9.36) and occasionally involves more than half of the body. *Systematized epidermal nevus* has been used to describe extensive lesions that are bilateral and in which truncal involvement predominates.

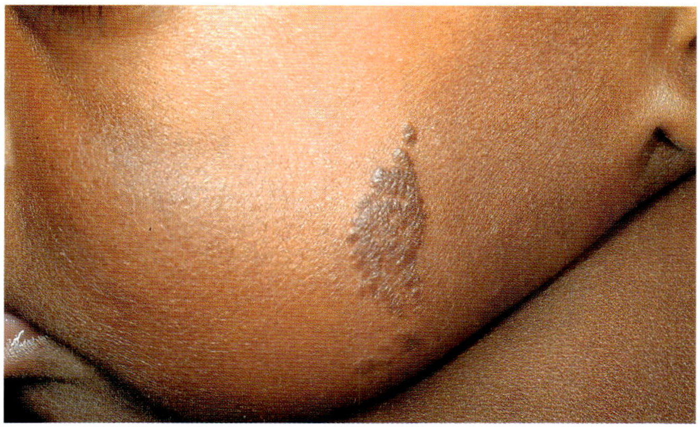

Fig. 9.32 Epidermal nevus. This multifocal, verrucous plaque was present since birth.

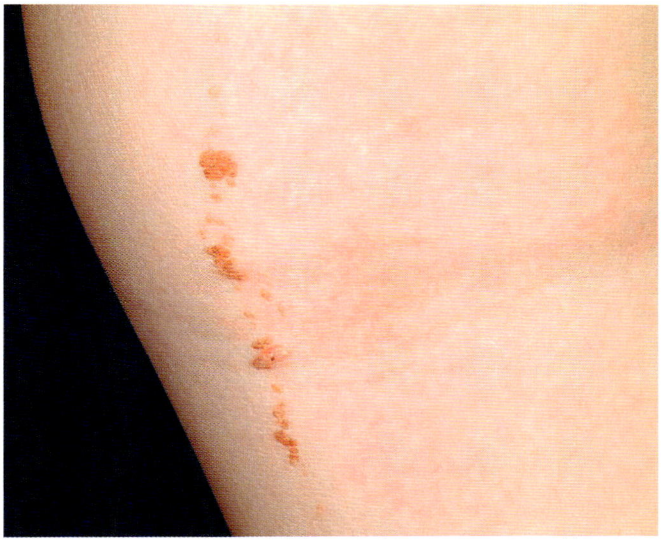

Fig. 9.33 Epidermal nevus. Note the warty nature and linear configuration.

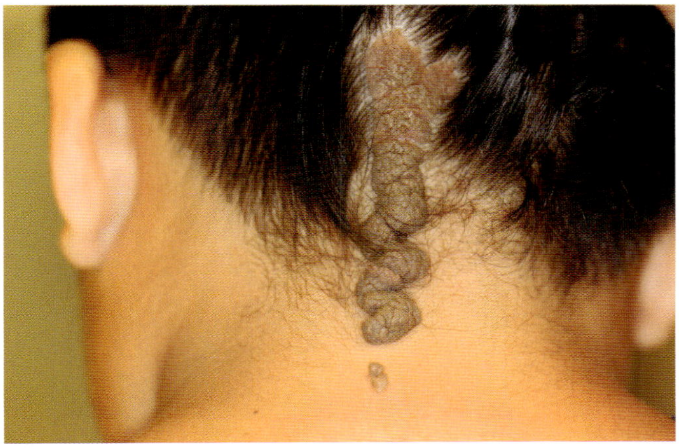

Fig. 9.34 Epidermal nevus. Note the thickened, papillomatous nature of this lesion in a 7-year-old boy.

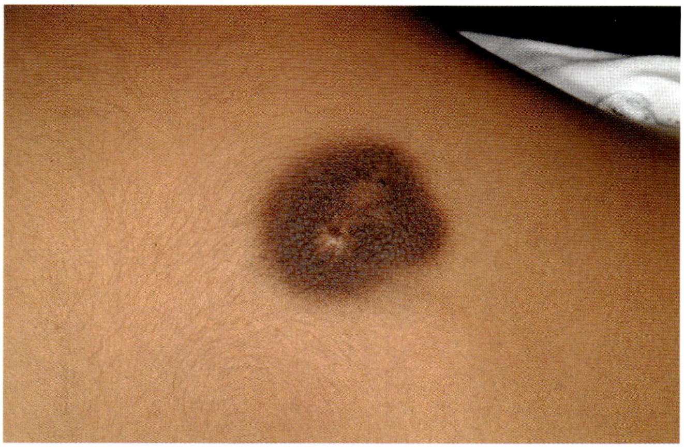

Fig. 9.35 Acanthosis nigricans form of epidermal nevus. This form of epidermal nevus reveals a well-demarcated area of velvety thickening, as classically seen with more widespread acanthosis nigricans.

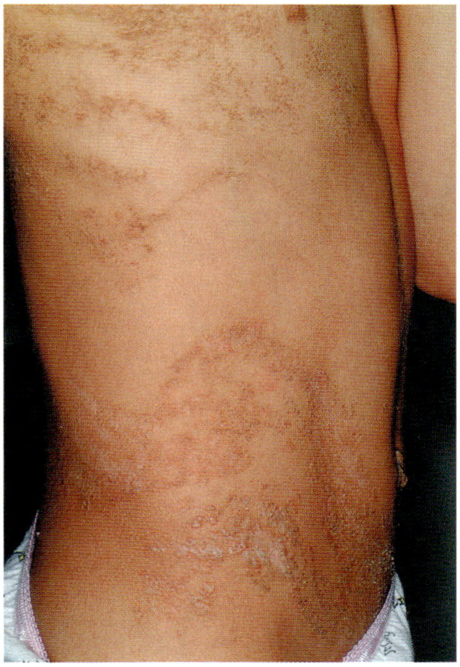

Fig. 9.36 Nevus unius lateris. Numerous linear and whorled lesions were present on the right side of this 10-year-old girl.

EN may reveal a variety of histologic features. Importantly, those that reveal epidermolytic hyperkeratosis, a distinct pattern of clumping of keratin filaments in the suprabasal cells of the epidermis, imply a mosaic disorder of keratin genes (typically keratins 1 and 10). Patients with this condition, especially when skin involvement is extensive, may transmit these mutations to offspring, resulting in a more widespread ichthyosiform condition termed *epidermolytic ichthyosis* and *epidermolytic hyperkeratosis* (also known as *bullous congenital ichthyosiform erythroderma*; see Chapter 5).[182] These EN may be clinically indistinguishable from other EN or may be lighter in color and thinner (Fig. 9.37).

EN are challenging to treat, given the observation that most superficial destructive therapies are followed by recurrence of the lesions. These superficial therapies have included cryotherapy with liquid nitrogen, dermabrasion, electrodesiccation, and laser ablation. In a

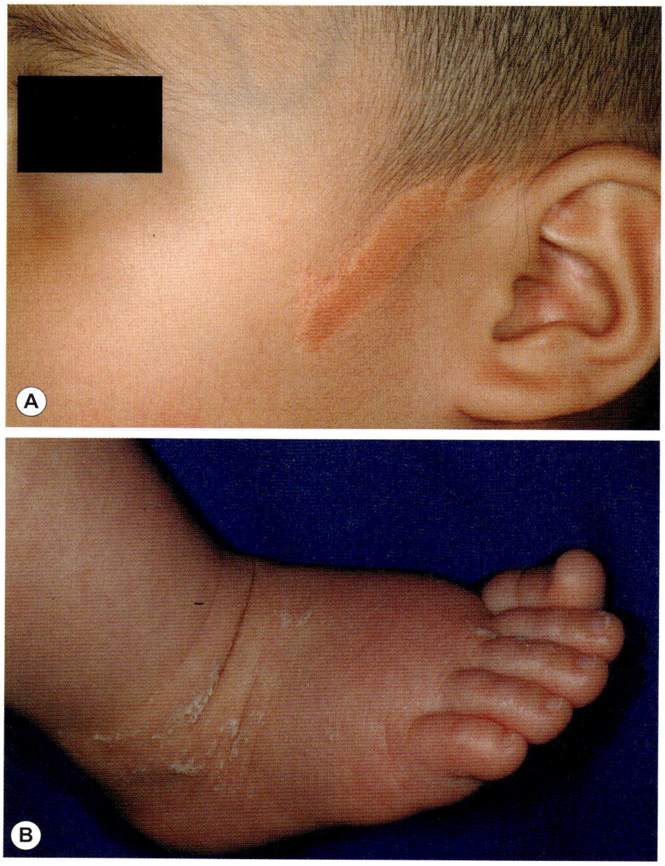

Fig. 9.37 Epidermal nevi, epidermolytic hyperkeratosis type. **(A)** This lesion presented as a linear yellow-tan plaque, similar to a keratinocytic epidermal nevus or nevus sebaceus. **(B)** This lesion presented as a thin, pink to tan, slightly hyperkeratotic plaque; note the extension to the distal dorsal foot and third toe. Both lesions demonstrated epidermolytic hyperkeratosis on histologic evaluation (see text).

series of 71 treated lesions, cryotherapy of small EN resulted in an excellent response in 90%.[183] Carbon dioxide (CO_2) laser therapy may offer excellent results, but response to therapy is unpredictable.[184] Staged CO_2 laser ablation has been used successfully, both with and without preceding surgical debulking.[185] Topical therapies used with variable success include retinoids, 5-fluorouracil, steroids, and podophyllin, among others. Photodynamic therapy with methyl-aminolevulinate was reportedly successful in a young girl, although hypertrophic scarring occurred.[186] Full-thickness surgical excision or deeper destructive procedures (such as deep dermabrasion) appear effective at removing these hamartomas but are generally limited to smaller, more localized lesions. Because these lesions may continue to extend during childhood, surgical intervention should be delayed until the full extent of the process is determined, if feasible.

EPIDERMAL NEVUS SYNDROME

ENS is a sporadic association of EN with abnormalities in other organ systems. Some believe that this syndrome is actually a group of several syndromes, each with distinguishing cutaneous and extracutaneous features. Happle suggests that the five well-defined ENSs are Schimmelpenning syndrome, nevus comedonicus syndrome, pigmented hairy ENS, Proteus syndrome (see Chapter 12), and congenital hemidysplasia with ichthyosiform nevus and limb defects (CHILD) syndrome (see Chapter 5).[187] Keratinocytic ENS also merits inclusion on this list.[188] Regardless, patients who fall into the spectrum of having an ENS generally have organoid or nonorganoid EN in conjunction with defects in the CNS, eyes, musculoskeletal system, connective tissue, and occasionally other organ systems. The manifestations of ENS are believed to represent genomic mosaicism with the effects of the genetic defect(s) and timing of the mutation during development determining the spectrum of clinical involvement.[152,188]

Phakomatosis pigmentokeratotica (PPK) has been used to describe the association of speckled lentiginous nevus with an epidermal nevus that has sebaceous differentiation and is accompanied by skeletal and neurologic abnormalities.[189] Neurologic findings may include mental retardation, seizures, deafness, dysesthesia, and ocular findings such as ptosis and strabismus; skeletal features include bony hypoplasia, kyphoscoliosis, and hemiatrophy.[190] It has been suggested that patients with PPK may have systemic features suggestive of either Schimmelpenning syndrome (extensive sebaceous nevi, mental retardation, seizures, coloboma, lipodermoids of the conjunctiva, skeletal defects, and vascular abnormalities) or what has been termed *SLN syndrome* (presenting with SLN, hyperhidrosis, sensory and motor neuropathy, nerve palsy, and spinal muscular atrophy).[191,192]

Examples of extracutaneous abnormalities seen in patients with ENS include seizures, mental retardation, hemiparesis, hypotonia, cranial nerve palsies, developmental delay, deafness, kyphosis, scoliosis, limb hypertrophy, hemihypertrophy, facial bone deformity, macrocephaly, ocular lipodermoids, coloboma, corneal changes, cortical blindness, cataracts, and retinal changes.[187,188,193,194] CNS imaging may reveal hemimegalencephaly, agenesis of the corpus callosum, cerebral heterotopia, cortical agyria or microgyria, or Dandy–Walker malformation; brainstem and cerebellar malformations and neonatal medulloblastoma have also been reported.[195,196] In addition, hypophosphatemic vitamin D–resistant rickets has been observed in patients with ENS, and in some reports the hypophosphatemia improved after surgical revision of the EN.[197–200] It has been suggested that some EN may produce a phosphaturic substance that contributes to this association.[197,198] *Cutaneous skeletal hypophosphatemia syndrome* (CSHS) is the contemporary nomenclature for the association of epidermal (or melanocytic) nevi with hypophosphatemic rickets, elevated levels of fibroblast growth factor-23 (a regulator of both phosphate and vitamin D homeostasis), and *RAS* mutation; recent reports have suggested that excision or ablation of the nevi in these patients is not necessarily correlated with recovery from hypophosphatemia.[199] Hyponatremia has also been observed as an early manifestation in a patient with ENS.[201] Cardiac and genitourinary defects may also be associated.

The features of the cutaneous lesions in ENS range from large unilateral nevus unius lateris–like lesions to diffusely distributed, whorled lesions (Figs. 9.38 and 9.39) involving variable degrees of the skin surface or linear, orange-yellow plaques as seen in nevus sebaceus of Jadassohn (see Nevus Sebaceus section). Plaques of dilated follicular

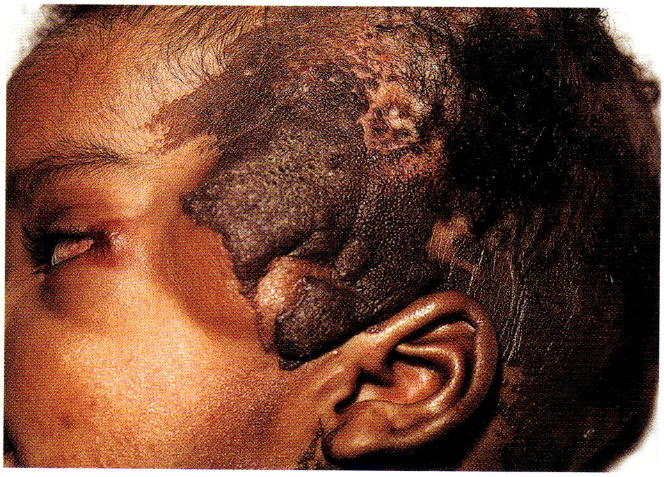

Fig. 9.38 Epidermal nevus syndrome. This infant had numerous widespread epidermal nevi in conjunction with multiple congenital anomalies.

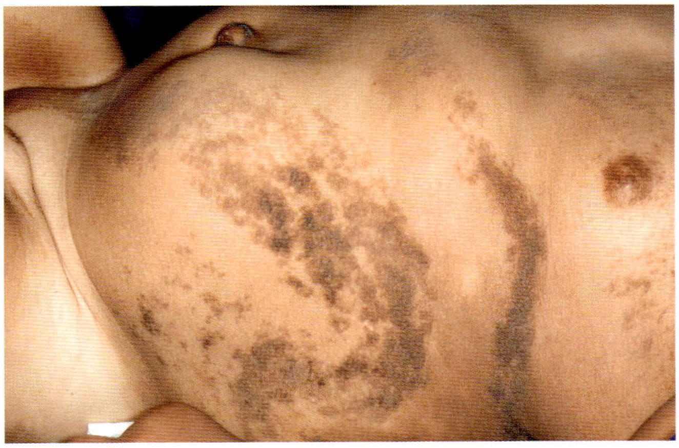

Fig. 9.39 Epidermal nevus syndrome. Multiple, whorled verrucous plaques are present in this child with multiple musculoskeletal, central nervous system, and ophthalmologic defects as well as profound developmental delay.

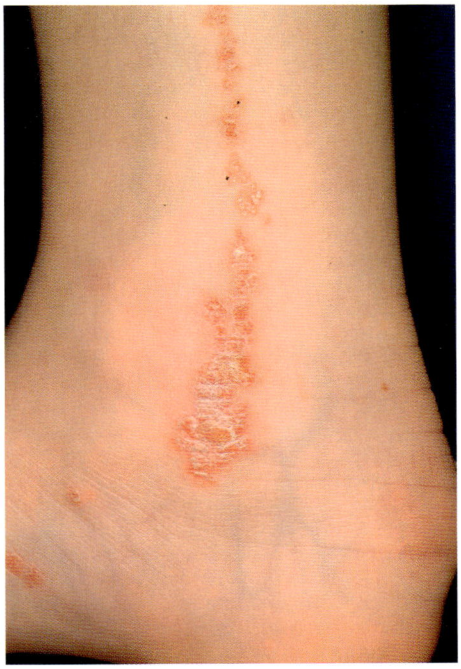

Fig. 9.40 Inflammatory linear verrucous epidermal nevus. Multiple red, scaly papules coalescing into a linear plaque on the medial leg, malleolus, and foot of a 7-year-old girl.

pits filled with keratin may be seen in the nevus comedonicus type of ENS, and extensive Becker nevus is seen in the pigmented hairy type of ENS. In the CHILD syndrome, a unilateral inflammatory epidermal nevus with a sharp midline demarcation and an affinity for body folds is seen in conjunction with the characteristic ipsilateral hypoplasia of limbs and other organ defects. Patients with Proteus syndrome have verrucous EN in association with partial gigantism, macrocephaly, and vascular malformations.

Patients with large or extensive EN require careful medical, family, and developmental histories and thorough physical evaluation, with particular emphasis on the musculoskeletal, neurologic, ocular, and cardiovascular examinations. Management of ENS should be multidisciplinary, including a dermatologist, pediatrician, neurologist, ophthalmologist, and plastic surgeon, with use of other subspecialists as necessary. EN can be treated as noted earlier, although treatment is even more challenging given their extensiveness in this setting. Malignant transformation of EN is rare but may occur, both in syndromic and nonsyndromic lesions, and includes basal cell carcinoma or squamous cell carcinoma, depending on the type of epidermal nevus.

INFLAMMATORY LINEAR VERRUCOUS EPIDERMAL NEVI

Inflammatory linear verrucous epidermal nevi (ILVEN) appear to be a unique variant of epidermal nevus that presents as a chronic pruritic process with erythematous, scaly, and verrucous papules that coalesce into linear plaques (Fig. 9.40). These lesions are often present at birth or may appear during early childhood and most often occur on an extremity. They are notable for their chronic and intermittent course and resistance to therapy.[202] Occasionally lesions may spontaneously improve or resolve only to eventually reappear. The differential diagnosis of ILVEN includes linear psoriasis, lichen striatus, linear lichen planus, verrucous epidermal nevus, and porokeratosis. ILVEN can usually be confirmed by the clinical course, morphologic appearance of lesions, intense pruritus, and resistance to therapy.

Treatment of ILVEN is difficult, as discussed previously for EN. Topical or intralesional corticosteroids may reduce inflammation and pruritus and produce a temporary remission, but the lesions generally recur. Topical retinoids, 5-fluorouracil, calcineurin inhibitors (e.g., tacrolimus or pimecrolimus), CO_2 laser therapy, and vitamin D derivatives (e.g., calcitriol) have been used with varying results.[203–205] Oral retinoid therapy may be an option, as may photodynamic therapy with methylaminolevulinate, both of which have been described in adults with ILVEN.[206,207] Patients with extensive and symptomatic ILVEN have been treated surgically, with tissue expansion, serial full-thickness excisions, and split-thickness skin grafting with excellent outcomes.[208]

BASAL CELL CARCINOMA

Basal cell carcinoma (BCC) is a slow-growing, usually nonmetastasizing but invasive malignant skin tumor with varying clinical patterns that may be triggered by ultraviolet radiation exposure. This disorder arises from the basal cells of the epidermis or its appendages and is most commonly seen in persons of middle age. BCC is the most common form of skin cancer, and although rarely seen in children, it can occur in childhood and must be considered even in the very young.[209,210] However, misdiagnosis must also be considered in a child because several benign hamartomas of follicular differentiation (trichoepithelioma, trichoblastoma, trichofolliculoma) may histologically appear similar to BCC to the inexperienced pathologist.

When the diagnosis of BCC is confirmed in a child, one must consider an associated predisposing condition such as basal cell nevus syndrome (BCNS, or Gorlin syndrome, see later), xeroderma pigmentosum (see Chapter 19), Bazex syndrome, Rombo syndrome (see Chapter 7), albinism (see Chapter 11), or an underlying nevus sebaceus of Jadassohn (see Nevus Sebaceus section). Other genetic skin disorders that may entail an increased risk for BCC include Bloom syndrome, Werner syndrome, Rothmund–Thomson syndrome, Muir–Torre syndrome, Brooke–Spiegler syndrome, Cowden syndrome, and some immunodeficiency disorders.[211] Children treated with irradiation for malignancy or with solid organ transplantation may develop BCC years to decades after the treatment.[209,212] In a review of childhood cancer survivors who were subsequently diagnosed with BCC, the majority of tumors developed between 20 and 39 years of age, and the risk was noted to be increased when patients received radiation doses to the skin of more than 1 Gy.[213] BCC lesions have occasionally been reported as sporadic cases in children without any underlying predisposition and appear to be most often located on the head, back, and chest.[209,214–216] The diagnosis of BCC in childhood is often delayed because of a low index of suspicion.

The majority of BCCs have a predilection for the upper central part of the face. Although they may arise without apparent cause, prolonged exposure to the sun is a predisposing factor, particularly in individuals with a fair skin phenotype. BCC may occur in several clinical forms. Noduloulcerative BCC, the most common type, begins as a small, elevated, translucent papule or nodule with telangiectatic vessels on its surface. It may enlarge, develop central necrosis, and result in an ulceration surrounded by a pearly rolled border. Although this form usually occurs as a single lesion, patients who develop this form of basal cell tumor often are likely to develop other such lesions. Superficial BCC presents as an erythematous, scaly, minimally elevated papule or plaque that may have superficial crusting. Often multiple, these lesions tend to occur on the trunk or extremities, expand slowly, and are easily mistaken for lesions of psoriasis, dermatitis, or tinea. Pigmented BCCs are similar to noduloulcerative lesions but also contain irregular brown pigmentation that may simulate the appearance of a nevus or MM. Sclerosing or morpheaform BCC presents as a firm, yellow-white waxy papule or plaque with an ill-defined border and absence of the translucent rolled edge. Tumors of this type have been known to arise in early childhood and may grow for years before attracting medical attention.

In the pediatric patient who is diagnosed with a BCC, a thorough history and physical examination should be performed with attention to the regional lymph node examination. An evaluation for an associated predisposing condition should be performed when indicated. No single method of therapy is applicable to all BCC lesions. The goal, as with any skin tumor, is for permanent cure with the best functional and cosmetic result. Curettage and electrodesiccation is a simple office therapy most commonly used by dermatologists for low-risk, small BCC in areas without a dense hair pattern. Excision (with or without Mohs micrographic surgery) is the treatment of choice for childhood-onset BCC.[209] Radiation therapy can be an effective treatment but is not desirable in children (and contraindicated in the setting of BCNS, discussed later in this chapter, because it may increase the risk for invasive BCC).[210] Other treatment modalities include cryotherapy, CO_2 laser therapy, photodynamic therapy, systemic retinoids, topical chemotherapy (e.g., topical 5-fluorouracil), and biologic response modifiers. The latter include imiquimod, a topical immune response modifier demonstrated to be effective against superficial BCCs and small nodular BCCs.[217] This agent promotes innate immune responses and exhibits antitumor as well as antiviral effects, having been initially approved for the treatment of anogenital condylomata. Experience with these therapeutic methods in childhood BCC is primarily anecdotal. Vismodegib, an oral inhibitor of the Sonic hedgehog signaling pathway (see later) has been reported for BCC in childhood,[218] although most of the experience with this agent is in treatment of adults with this tumor. Sun protection and skin self-examination education are vital.

BASAL CELL NEVUS SYNDROME

BCNS (also known as *Gorlin syndrome* or *nevoid BCC syndrome*) is an autosomal dominant disorder with complete penetrance and variable expressivity characterized by childhood onset of multiple BCCs and associated with other abnormalities, including odontogenic jaw cysts, bifid ribs, and intracranial calcification.[219–222] The most obvious cutaneous feature in patients with BCNS is the appearance of multiple BCCs early in life. These basal cell epitheliomas are indistinguishable on histopathologic examination from ordinary BCCs. The diagnostic criteria for BCNS are shown in Box 9.2. In a consensus statement from an international colloquium on BCNS, a modification of the diagnostic criteria was suggested such that medulloblastoma, typically desmoplastic, be included as a major (rather than a minor) criterion.[223]

The skin lesions of BCNS may appear as early as the first year of life but have a mean age of onset of around 20 to 23 years.[121,222] They may occasionally present in a congenital fashion or during infancy.[224] They involve, in decreasing order of incidence, the face, neck, back, trunk, and upper extremities. The distribution of BCCs may differ by gender, with male patients having more in the facial M-zone (forehead, temples, periorbital areas, and nose), upper back, neck, and upper extremities and female patients having more lesions located in the scalp, upper and lower back, and lower extremities.[225] The BCCs in BCNS may range in number from one to well over a thousand. In addition, patients with BCNS may develop skin lesions that appear similar to nevi or seborrheic keratoses and tend to follow a more benign course, although after puberty the cutaneous lesions of BCNS tend to be more aggressive. The BCC lesions appear as flesh-colored to pink or tan dome-shaped papules that measure 1 to 10 mm (Fig. 9.41, *A*).

Box 9.2 Diagnostic Criteria for Basal Cell Nevus Syndrome*,†

Major Criteria

- Multiple basal cell carcinomas (>5 in a lifetime or a BCC before 30 years)
- Lamellar calcification of the falx (or clear evidence of calcification in an individual younger than 20 years)
- Jaw keratocyst (odontogenic keratocyst, confirmed histologically)
- Palmar or plantar pits (>2; may be most easily seen after soaking of the hands and feet in warm water)
- First-degree relative with BCNS

Minor Criteria

- Macrocephaly
- Childhood medulloblastoma
- Cleft lip/palate
- Rib/vertebral anomalies: bifid, splayed, missing or extra ribs; bifid, wedged, or fused vertebrae
- Preaxial or postaxial polydactyly
- Cardiac or ovarian fibroma
- Lymphomesenteric or pleural cysts
- Ocular anomalies (cataract, coloboma, microphthalmia)

Modified from High A, Zedan W. Basal cell nevus syndrome. Curr Opin Oncol 2005;17:160–6; and Evans DG, Farndon PA. Nevoid basal cell carcinoma syndrome. GeneReviews® [Internet]. Seattle (WA): University of Washington, Seattle; 2002 (updated 2013).

BCC, Basal cell carcinoma; *BCNS*, basal cell nevus syndrome.

*Diagnosed when an individual has two major criteria and one minor criterion *or* one major criterion and three minor criteria.

†See text for further discussion.

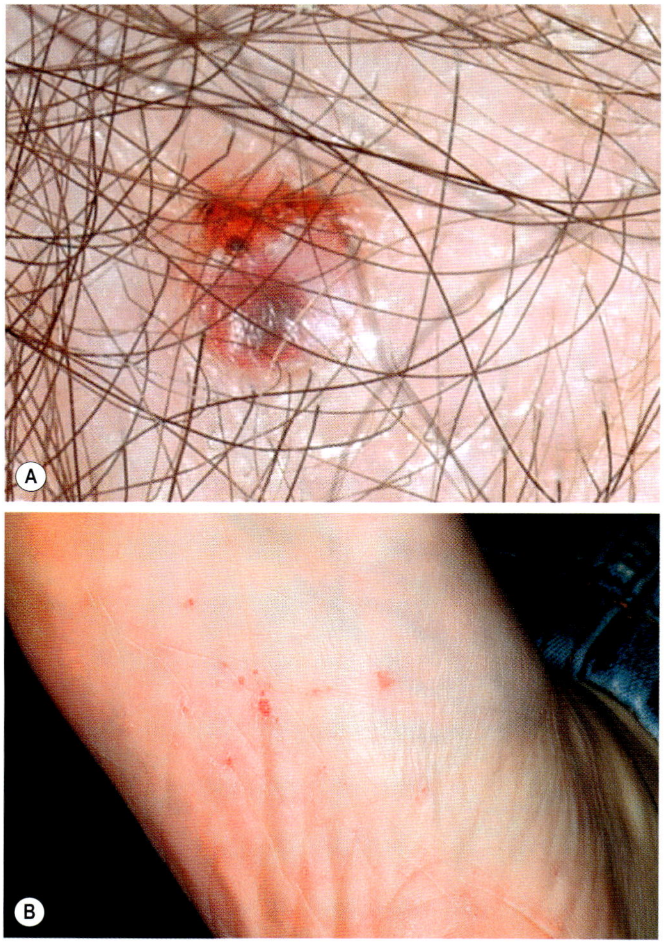

Fig. 9.41 Basal cell nevus syndrome (BCNS). **(A)** Pigmented basal cell carcinoma on the scalp of a 12-year-old girl. **(B)** Shallow erythematous depressions (pits) on the plantar surface of an adult female with BCNS.

Secondary changes such as ulceration, crusting, and bleeding rarely occur before puberty, but if left untreated these lesions can become extremely destructive. Unlike ordinary BCCs, BCNS-associated lesions are not typically believed to be induced by prolonged exposure to sunlight. However, in a prospective clinical registry of patients with BCNS, both age and number of sunburns were significantly associated with the severity of lifetime BCC.[226]

In addition to nevoid BCCs, affected individuals have a characteristic facies with coarse features, broad nasal root, hypertelorism, cleft palate, and cutaneous stigmata beyond the BCCs. These include multiple small facial milia, comedones, large epidermal cysts, lipomas, fibromas, and café-au-lait macules. Shallow 2- to 3-mm palmar and plantar pits (Fig. 9.41, *B*), a characteristic feature of the syndrome, are seen in 70% to 90% of affected individuals. They may become more prominent after immersion of the hands or feet in water. These defective areas of keratinization usually first appear during the second decade of life or later. Palmar and plantar pits tend to have associated erythema, which on casual observation appears as multiple small red spots on the palms and soles.

Odontogenic jaw cysts occur in around 75% of patients and may present with painless swelling, jaw pain, abnormal taste, or a discharge in the mouth. The first jaw cyst often occurs before the age of 20 years, and symptoms referable to these lesions are often the presenting complaint. Jaw cysts occurring in patients with BCNS present earlier in life than those occurring in patients without BCNS.[227] The cysts may be multiple and may result in loosening and loss of teeth. Patients with BCNS may become edentulous at an early age.

Musculoskeletal anomalies present in 60% to 80% of patients and include macrocephaly, frontoparietal bossing, high-arched palate, and broad nasal bridge.[221] Other abnormalities include splayed or bifid ribs, mandibular and maxillary bone cysts, prognathism, kyphoscoliosis, Sprengel deformity, cervical or thoracic vertebral anomalies, spina bifida, pectus excavatum and carinatum, and shortened fourth metacarpals.

The most common neurologic abnormality is calcification of the falx cerebri, which is seen in up to 90% of patients with BCNS. In addition, mental retardation, electroencephalographic abnormalities, agenesis of the corpus callosum, seizures, hydrocephalus, and deafness may occur. Other associations include anosmia, renal malformations, endocrinopathy, and blindness. Patients with BCNS appear to have a predisposition to malignancy, especially medulloblastoma, which may present early in life.[228] The desmoplastic subtype of medulloblastoma in children younger than 2 years of age is considered by some a major diagnostic criterion for the diagnosis of BCNS.[228,229] This desmoplastic variant has a favorable prognosis.[230] Ovarian and cardiac fibromas and meningiomas also occur at an increased rate in these patients. The latter occur in 14% to 24% of females with BCNS, and are often bilateral and calcified (compared with sporadic ovarian fibromas, which tend to be unilateral and noncalcified).[231]

The molecular cause of BCNS has been elucidated. Mutations in the human patched genes (*PTCH1* or rarely *PTCH2*) and the *SUFU* gene have been identified in patients with BCNS, with *PTCH1* being responsible for approximately 85% of cases.[232–236] *PTCH1* is located on chromosome 9q and encodes a transmembrane receptor that represses growth factor gene transcription. The gene product of *PTCH1* functions as a tumor suppressor, and *PTCH1* mutations results in dysregulation of several genes known to play a role in both organogenesis and carcinogenesis via the Sonic hedgehog (Shh) signaling pathway.[237] Mutations in *SUFU*, a gene that encodes a component of the same pathway, have been identified in BCNS patients lacking a mutation in *PTCH1* and appear to be associated with a higher risk of medulloblastoma, meningioma, and ovarian fibroma than seen in BCNS patients because of *PTCH1* mutation.[235,238] Mutations in these Shh pathway genes and other genes closely related to Shh signaling may act in an additive or multiplicative manner to give rise to the phenotypic variability characteristic of BCNS.[239]

The management of patients with BCNS must be multidisciplinary and individualized. Genetic counseling is important given the autosomal dominant mode of inheritance. Family members judged to be at risk may be screened with skeletal surveys, dental radiographs, and neurologic evaluation (both clinical and radiographic). Molecular diagnosis is also possible (GeneDx, Gaithersburg, MD, USA), with a sensitivity around 60% to 75%. Removal of cutaneous BCC may be accomplished with the same techniques as discussed earlier, and general anesthesia may be required for treatment of multiple lesions. Systemic retinoids (e.g., isotretinoin) may be useful in preventing BCCs, but its use must be balanced by potential side effects and in female patients the known teratogenicity. In addition, if the retinoid is discontinued, the patient may show rapid disease progression. Vismodegib, an inhibitor of the Shh signaling pathway approved for treatment of locally advanced or metastatic BCC, has been shown to reduce the BCC tumor burden and block growth of new lesions in patients with BCNS, though its potential benefit has been limited by adverse events that led to discontinuation by more than 50% of patients in one study, and the increased risk for squamous cell carcinoma after therapy highlights the need for continued vigorous skin surveillance if it is used.[240,241]

It is recommended that all pediatric patients with BCNS be monitored by a medical geneticist who ensures all appropriate referrals and follow-up evaluations. Patients require regular follow-up examinations with a dermatologist, pediatric dentist or oral surgeon, and ophthalmologist, as well as referral to a neurologist and psychologist as indicated. Annual vision, hearing, and speech screenings; routine developmental screening at well-child visits; and baseline brain MRI, digital panoramic radiograph of the jaw, and spinal films are also recommended.[223] Annual brain MRI is recommended until 8 years of age, beyond which the risk of medulloblastoma greatly decreases.[223]

SQUAMOUS CELL CARCINOMA

Squamous cell carcinoma (SCC) is a malignant tumor of the epidermis rarely seen in children. Occasionally it may arise in normal skin, but generally it is seen in skin that has been injured by sunlight, trauma, thermal burn, or chronic inflammation. The highest incidence rates occur in individuals with a fair skin phenotype, with skin that is at risk for sunburn.[242] Children who develop SCC often have an underlying predisposing condition, including xeroderma pigmentosum (see Chapter 19), human papillomavirus infection (especially in the immunocompromised host), or a history of organ transplantation, chemotherapy with immunosuppression, tanning bed use, or radiation therapy. In addition, scars related to recessive dystrophic epidermolysis bullosa (RDEB, see Chapter 13) may be predisposed to the development of SCC. Although these RDEB-associated tumors generally do not present until the third or fourth decade, they may occasionally occur during childhood.[243] SCC has also been reported to occur within the lesions of pansclerotic morphea of childhood.[244] Rarely, pediatric SCC may present as a mucosal tumor, in areas such as the tongue, palate, gingiva, larynx, or floor of the mouth.[245]

The most common sites for SCC are the face (in particular the lower lip and pinna of the ear) and the dorsal aspect of the hands and forearms. Lesions usually present as red, scaly papules or plaques, often with induration. Telangiectasias may be present, as may ulceration or necrosis. Lesions that arise *de novo* usually appear as solitary, slowly enlarging, firm nodules with central crusting, underlying ulceration, and an indurated base. The histologic evaluation of SCC offers prognostic information based on the depth of the lesion and the cytologic features and degree of differentiation of the cells.

The prognosis for SCC of the skin is quite variable. Easily cured small lesions arising in sun-damaged skin have a low propensity to metastasize. Lesions arising in burn scars, prior radiation fields, and chronic wounds (e.g., ulcers or epidermolysis bullosa scars; see Chapter 13) tend to be more aggressive with higher rates of metastases. Complete excision is the treatment of choice for SCC. Other treatment options that may be considered include electrodesiccation and curettage, cryotherapy, photodynamic therapy, and Mohs micrographic surgery. Sun protection and skin self-examination education are vital for SCC prevention.

KERATOACANTHOMA

Keratoacanthoma (KA) is an epithelial tumor that may be clinically and histologically indistinguishable from SCC. These lesions are considered by many to be benign, and they often involute spontaneously without therapy. However, given rare reports of extensive local destruction and metastases, some consider KAs to be a variant of SCC. KAs are usually seen in older adults with rare reports of neonatal or childhood involvement.[246,247] Multiple KAs characteristically have their onset in adolescence or early adult life and may occur in several clinical settings such as Ferguson Smith, Muir–Torre, or Witten–Zak syndromes. Generalized eruptive KA with the sudden onset of multiple lesions may also occur (termed the *Grzybowski type*).[248] KA may also occur in the setting of xeroderma pigmentosum.[249]

KA presents as a firm, dome-shaped nodule that generally measures 1 to 3 cm or more. The center contains a horny plug or is covered by a crust that conceals a central keratin-filled crater. The nodule generally grows rapidly and reaches its full size within 2 to 8 weeks. After a period of quiescence that may last for 2 to 8 weeks, most lesions heal spontaneously over several months with only a slightly depressed, somewhat cribriform scar in the previously affected area.

The main problem in the diagnosis of KA is its differentiation from SCC. In most cases the rapid evolution and typical clinical appearance help to establish the correct diagnosis. Because the architecture of the lesion is as important as the cellular characteristics, full excisional biopsy is recommended to enable appropriate histopathologic evaluation. The treatment of KA is usually approached with a view toward its spontaneous resolution. Its close resemblance to SCC, however, often results in excisional biopsy. Other reported treatment options include intralesional corticosteroids, topical imiquimod, intralesional methotrexate, topical 5-fluorouracil, cryotherapy, electrodesiccation and curettage, and radiation therapy.[250–254]

Tumors of the Oral Mucosa

WHITE SPONGE NEVUS

White sponge nevus is a rare, autosomal dominant condition that most often affects the oral mucosa and less commonly the mucosae of other regions. It presents as exuberant, asymptomatic white plaques on the buccal mucosae (Fig. 9.42), palate, gingivae, or sides of the tongue. Other regions that may be involved include the nasal, vaginal, labial, and anal mucosae. In some instances, the plaques may be quite thickened with fissures and folds, and occasionally a raw, denuded surface may be evident. White sponge nevus may be present at birth or may have its onset any time from infancy through adolescence. The lesions are most commonly misdiagnosed as candidiasis in young children.[255] It reaches its maximum severity during adolescence or early adulthood, and the lesions are entirely asymptomatic and often noted incidentally during examination. Both genders are equally affected. The differential diagnosis of white sponge nevus may include oral leukoplakia, pachyonychia congenita, dyskeratosis congenita, cheek biting, chemical burn, syphilis, betel nut or tobacco use, and lichen planus.

Defects in the genes for keratins 4 and 13 have been demonstrated to be responsible for white sponge nevus.[256,257] This disorder is generally benign and asymptomatic and requires no specific therapy. White sponge nevus should not be confused with focal epithelial hyperplasia (Heck disease), a rare disorder of the oral mucosa of children believed to be caused by infection with human papillomavirus, especially types 13 and 32. In patients with Heck disease, the mucosa of the lower lip is most commonly involved and reveals soft papules and plaques that tend to regress spontaneously over several months.

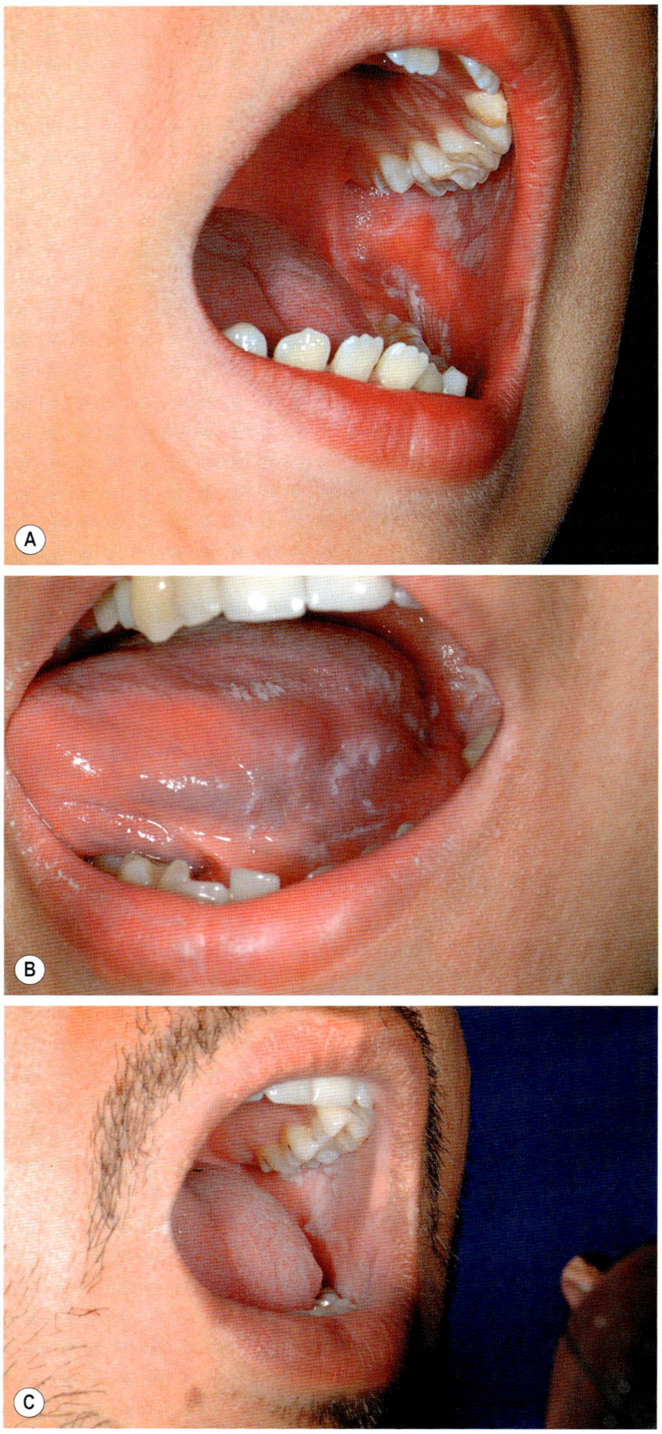

Fig. 9.42 Oral white sponge nevus. This 4-year-old boy **(A)**, his two brothers, one of whom is pictured in **(B)**, father **(C)**, and uncle all had similar white plaques of the oral mucosa.

LEUKOPLAKIA

Leukoplakia is a term generally used to describe a white plaque involving the oral mucosa that cannot be easily removed by scraping or rubbing with a cotton swab or tongue blade. It is a nonspecific term inconsistently applied to a variety of lesions of different etiology, including white sponge nevus, pachyonychia congenita, dyskeratosis congenita, hereditary benign intraepithelial dyskeratosis, hereditary mucoepithelial dysplasia, and many others. It is also used to describe white changes on the vulva of females, where its use is equally nonspecific.

Oral leukoplakia is the terminology usually used to describe a condition seen most often in adults and is related to a variety of factors, including trauma, poor oral hygiene, chronic irritation, and use of tobacco products. It may occasionally be seen in children and has been reported in pediatric patients with HIV infection.[258,259] The clinical presentation is notable for either focal or more diffuse involvement with white plaques of the buccal mucosae, hard or soft palate, lateral surfaces of the tongue, and the floor of the mouth. Mucosal biopsy with histopathologic evaluation is usually necessary to confirm the exact diagnosis, and treatment depends on the cause. Meticulous attention to oral hygiene is useful regardless of the cause. Because oral leukoplakia may have malignant potential (eventuating into SCC), long-term follow-up observation is indicated, with repeat tissue biopsy when necessary.

Tumors of the Epidermal Appendages

NEVUS SEBACEUS

Nevus sebaceus of Jadassohn is a common congenital lesion that occurs mainly on the face and scalp. These lesions are usually solitary and present as a well-circumscribed, hairless plaque. They are generally present at birth but may first be noted during early childhood and rarely in adult life. Although rare familial forms have been reported, these hamartomas tend to be sporadic. Multiple nevi sebaceus may occur in association with cerebral, ocular, and skeletal abnormalities as part of an ENS. This association has been termed *Schimmelpenning syndrome*.[187] Somatic mutations in *HRAS* and *KRAS* have been demonstrated in lesions of nevus sebaceus.[180,260]

Classic nevus sebaceus presents as a hairless, yellow to tan plaque on the scalp or face (Figs. 9.43 and 9.44). The surface may be verrucous or velvety, and the lesions are often oval or linear. In some patients, hyperpigmentation may be a prominent feature, making the distinction from a verrucous epidermal nevus difficult. Nevus sebaceus may vary in size from a few millimeters to several centimeters in length. Their yellow color is related to sebaceous gland secretion, and often this color becomes less prominent after infancy. The lesions tend to enlarge proportionate with growth of the child, until puberty when they may become significantly thicker, more verrucous, and more greasy in appearance (Fig. 9.45) as a result of hormonal stimulation of the sebaceous glands within them. Papillomatous projections may occur, sometimes simulating the appearance of verruca vulgaris.

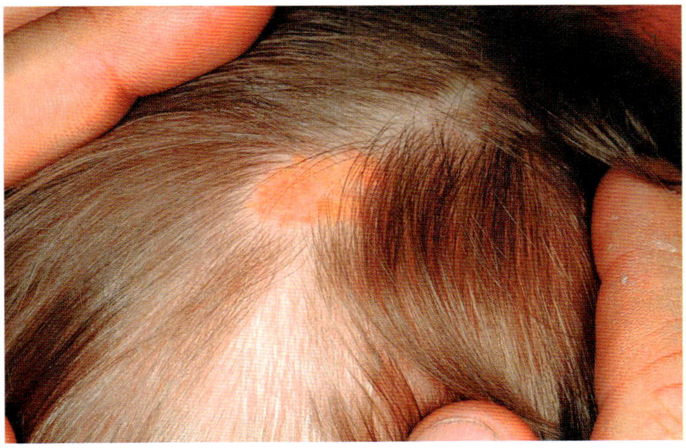

Fig. 9.43 Nevus sebaceus. Yellow-orange, hairless plaque on the scalp.

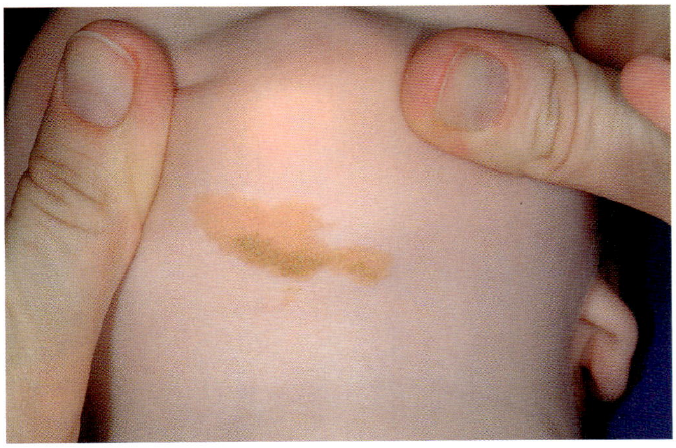

Fig. 9.44 Nevus sebaceus. Linear yellow verrucous plaque on the inferior chin of an infant.

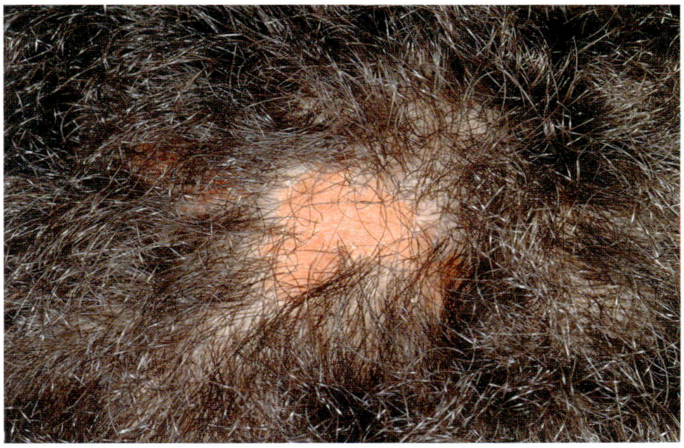

Fig. 9.45 Nevus sebaceus. The lesion in this adolescent boy demonstrates verrucous (warty) changes that are common with older age.

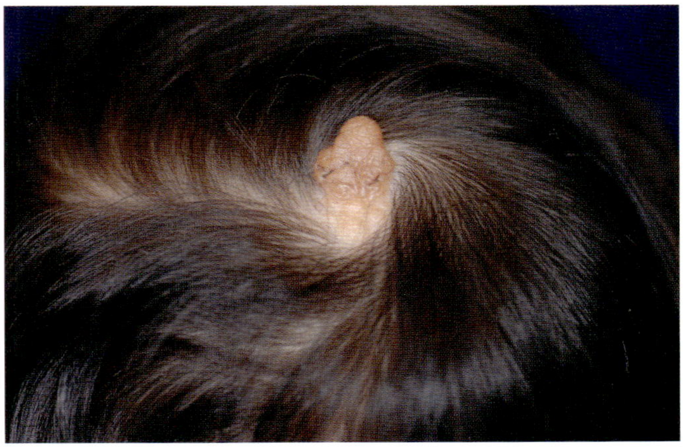

Fig. 9.46 Nevus sebaceus with syringocystadenoma papilliferum. This verrucous, exophytic papule developed on the surface of a previously flat nevus sebaceus.

Surgical excision, the treatment of choice for nevus sebaceus, has traditionally been recommended out of concern for the development of secondary malignant neoplasms within these lesions. Multiple secondary appendageal neoplasms may occur within nevus sebaceus, including syringocystadenoma papilliferum (the most common secondary benign neoplasm; Fig. 9.46), apocrine cystadenoma, spiradenoma, and trichoblastoma.[261–263] The secondary tumor that raises the most concern, however, is BCC, which in the past was estimated to occur in anywhere from 6.5% to 50% of lesions depending on the source.[264] More recent investigations have documented that the incidence of BCC is actually quite low, and in fact trichoblastoma (a benign proliferation that appears to be quite common) may be easily mistaken for BCC.[262,265–267] Other tumors that have been reported within lesions of nevus sebaceus include KA, leiomyoma, piloleiomyoma, SCC, apocrine hidrocystoma, apocrine carcinoma, malignant melanoma, eccrine poroma, and malignant eccrine poroma.[268–270] Malignant degeneration is usually heralded by the appearance of a discrete nodule with or without ulceration.

The timing of surgery in those patients for whom it is chosen is controversial. Many factors need to be considered, including size and location of the nevus, its cosmetic significance, and the risk-to-benefit ratio of general anesthesia (needed early in life) versus local anesthesia (a possibility when surgery for smaller lesions is delayed until later childhood or adolescence). These decisions must be made by the parents (and patient, where appropriate) with input from the involved physicians. The practitioner should provide parents with the objective data and allow them to make this personal decision, offering support and guidance as necessary.

NEVUS COMEDONICUS

Nevus comedonicus is a rare type of organoid nevus with a hair follicle origin. These lesions are often present at birth, or they may become evident over the first decade of life. There is no racial or sexual predisposition. Nevus comedonicus presents as a plaque primarily composed of hyperkeratotic papules and horny plugs (resembling the comedones of acne vulgaris) with varying degrees of erythema (Fig. 9.47). Lesions are most common on the face, neck, trunk, and upper extremities and are often linear or band-like in distribution (Fig. 9.48). They tend to grow as the child matures, and large lesions extending above the surrounding cutaneous surface may give a grater-like feeling to the skin. There is a spectrum of involvement with nevus comedonicus, from simple comedonal lesions to those with significant inflammation, cysts, and even scarring.[271] Secondary infection and abscess formation rarely occur.[272]

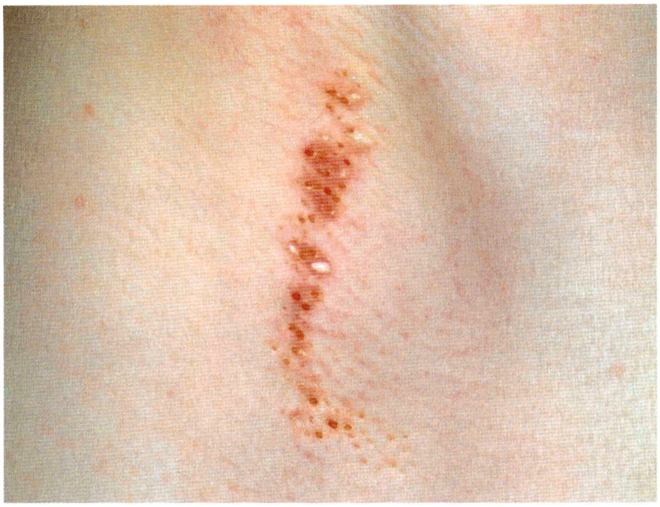

Fig. 9.47 Nevus comedonicus. Multiple open (blackheads) and closed (whiteheads) comedones in a linear distribution in the axilla of a 2-year-old boy.

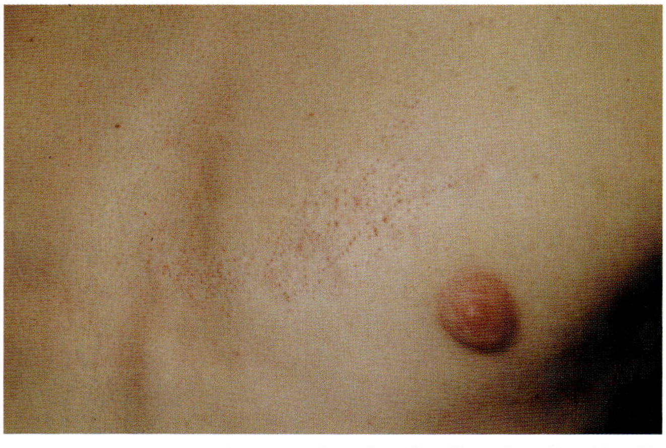

Fig. 9.48 Nevus comedonicus. Multiple open comedones (blackheads) in a wavy streak on the chest of an 18-year-old boy.

The differential diagnosis of nevus comedonicus includes nevus sebaceus, acne neonatorum, and in older patients, comedonal acne. Although the lesions usually occur as a sporadic finding, multiple or extensive lesions may be associated with abnormalities in other organ systems as part of the nevus comedonicus type of ENS.[187,273,274]

Management of nevus comedonicus is challenging. Topical retinoids, ammonium lactate lotion, or topical antibiotics may each be useful for some patients. Pore strips have been reported useful for removal of the keratin plugs.[275] However, most medical therapies are ineffective, and the definitive therapy for cosmetically significant lesions is surgical excision.

TRICHOEPITHELIOMA

Trichoepitheliomas may occur as a benign, autosomal dominantly inherited disorder characterized by the presence of multiple small lesions occurring primarily on the face or as a solitary nonhereditary tumor seen in early adult life or occasionally during childhood. *Brooke-Spiegler syndrome* (BSS) has traditionally been used to describe an autosomal dominant disorder characterized by numerous trichoepitheliomas, cylindromas (see also Cylindroma section), and spiradenomas, all benign skin appendageal tumors. *Multiple familial trichoepithelioma* (MFT) refers to an autosomal dominant disorder characterized by numerous trichoepitheliomas involving the central face and often starting during childhood. The term *trichoblastoma* has been used to denote benign neoplasms of follicular differentiation. Some consider these two conditions to be interchangeable, with others considering trichoepithelioma to be one type of trichoblastoma.

Multiple trichoepitheliomas generally begin during early childhood or around puberty as small, firm, flesh-colored papules and nodules on the face (Fig. 9.49), particularly in the nasolabial folds and over the nose, forehead, upper lip, and eyelids and occasionally the scalp, neck, trunk, scrotum, and perianal area. The lesions measure 2 to 5 mm in diameter, are firm, and have a translucent sheen. Occasionally, telangiectatic vessels are present over the rounded translucent surface of larger lesions. Trichoepitheliomas may enlarge slowly, reaching up to 5 mm on the face and ears and up to 2 to 3 cm in other sites; they often coalesce to form nodular aggregates. Mutations in the *CYLD* gene, a tumor suppressor gene, appear to be the genetic basis for MFT, BSS, and familial cylindromatosus (FC; also known as *turban tumor syndrome*), a disorder characterized by multiple cylindromas as the only tumor type (see also Cylindroma section).[276–280]

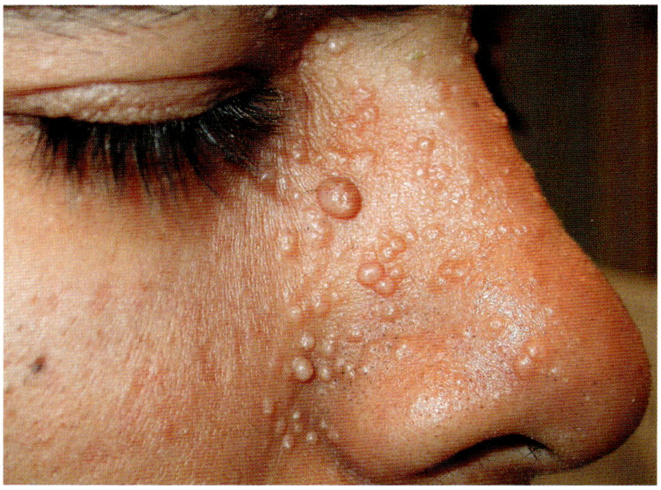

Fig. 9.49 Multiple trichoepitheliomas. Multiple flesh-colored papules of the medial cheek and nose. (Courtesy Keren Horn, MD.)

Solitary, nonhereditary trichoepitheliomas usually develop during the second or third decade of life and generally appear on the face. They may also be distributed on the scalp, neck, trunk, upper arms, or thighs. Solitary lesions appear as firm, flesh-colored papules and papulonodules and generally reach 5 mm or slightly larger in diameter.

Desmoplastic trichoepithelioma is a variant that presents as an indurated, flesh-colored to red papule or plaque with an elevated annular border and central depression. It occurs most commonly on the face, especially the cheek. Although most commonly seen in early adulthood, desmoplastic trichoepitheliomas may appear during the second decade, are much more common in females, and may occur in a familial fashion.[281] In one report, desmoplastic trichoepithelioma was initially mistakenly diagnosed as SCC.[282]

Although trichoepitheliomas are benign lesions, treatment may be cosmetically desirable, and at times biopsy is indicated to differentiate the lesion from other cutaneous neoplasms. Surgical excision is the treatment of choice, although electrodesiccation, cryotherapy, radiotherapy, dermabrasion, and laser therapy have also been used.[278]

TRICHILEMMOMA

Trichilemmoma is another benign appendageal neoplasm derived from the hair follicle. These lesions may be solitary or multiple and present as flesh-colored papules or nodules, occasionally with a verrucous (wart-like) surface. The most common location for trichilemmomas is the face, although genitals are another common site and they can occur anywhere on the cutaneous surface. A desmoplastic form (desmoplastic trichilemmoma) may occur, and at times the deeper component of these lesions may histologically simulate invasive carcinoma.[283] Treatment of these benign lesions may be accomplished with surgical excision or ablative procedures when desired.

Multiple trichilemmomas have clinical significance because they may be seen in the setting of the multiple hamartoma syndrome known as *Cowden syndrome* (CS). This autosomal dominant disorder is characterized by hamartomas in multiple organ systems including skin, breast, thyroid, gastrointestinal (GI) tract, endometrium, and brain.[284] Mucocutaneous lesions, which are present in nearly all patients, include multiple trichilemmomas, palmoplantar keratoses, oral papillomatosis, and sclerotic fibromas.[284,285] Pigmented macules of the genitalia, café-au-lait macules, acanthosis nigricans, skin tags, lipomas, and vascular malformations may also occur in CS.[285,286] Other benign extracutaneous manifestations include fibrocystic breast disease, breast fibroadenomas, thyroid adenomas, goiter, neuromas, meningiomas, and intestinal polyposis. Lhermitte–Duclos disease, considered to be a component of CS, results in hamartomatous growths arising in the cerebellum and presents with headache, ataxia, and visual disturbance. Patients with CS also have an increased risk of certain malignancies, especially those of the breast (up to 30% to 50% of female patients) and thyroid gland (nonmedullary thyroid carcinoma, 3% to 10%).[284,287] Skeletal abnormalities may include macrocephaly, scoliosis, and pectus excavatum. Patients may also have mental retardation.

Management of patients with CS consists of early recognition, specialist referral, treatment for cutaneous lesions (as needed/available), genetic counseling, and appropriate cancer surveillance, which should include breast self-examination, regular physician examinations, mammography, breast MRI, and thyroid ultrasound.[288]

Mutations in the tumor suppressor gene *PTEN*, which encodes a tumor suppressor phosphatase involved in cellular regulation, have been detected in patients with CS as well as in patients with Bannayan–Riley–Ruvalcaba syndrome (BRRS; see later and Chapters 11 and 12), *PTEN*-related Proteus-like syndrome (see Chapter 12), adult Lhermitte–Duclos disease, and autism-like disorders associated with macrocephaly.[287] CS and BRRS share many similarities, including the mucocutaneous findings of facial trichilemmomas, acanthosis nigricans, lipomas, palmoplantar keratoses, pigmented macules of the genitalia, and oral papillomatosis.[286] Mucocutaneous neuromas have been highlighted as another overlap finding that may be seen in both CS and BRRS, and gastrointestinal polyposis is also seen.[289,290] Macrocephaly and developmental delay are also seen in BRRS. The identification of kindreds with both diseases in the family, as well as identical *PTEN* mutations and overlapping clinical features, suggested that CS and BRRS may represent different phenotypic expressions of the same disease.[284,286,291] The disorders thus far attributable to *PTEN* mutations have been collectively referred to as *PTEN hamartoma tumor syndrome*.[292] In a series of 47 pediatric patients with *PTEN* mutations, the most common presenting features included macrocephaly, developmental delay, intellectual disability, and autism spectrum disorder.[293] In a prospective study of 368 individuals meeting criteria for CS and with confirmed germline *PTEN* mutation, incidence ratios were elevated not only for breast and thyroid cancer but also for colorectal cancer, kidney cancer, and melanoma, suggesting the need for surveillance for these malignancies in this patient cohort as well.[294] Tumor development in PTEN hamartoma tumor syndrome may be early, as noted in a series of 34 children (younger than 21 years) studied retrospectively. In this group, thyroid carcinoma was diagnosed as early as 7 years of age and renal cell carcinoma at 11 years of age.[295]

TRICHOFOLLICULOMA

Trichofolliculoma is an uncommon benign appendageal neoplasm, again of hair follicle derivation, that usually occurs as a solitary lesion. Trichofolliculomas most often involve the head and neck regions of adults but may occur during childhood. Trichofolliculomas present as a 2- to 10-mm, slow-growing, flesh-colored or pearly papule or nodule with a smooth surface. There is often a central pore with a protruding woolly or cotton-like tuft of hair (a highly diagnostic clinical feature). On occasion the protruding hairs may be so fine that a magnifying lens may be required to detect their presence. Treatment of trichofolliculoma by local surgical excision generally produces a good cosmetic outcome.

PILOMATRICOMA

Pilomatricoma (also known as *calcifying epithelioma of Malherbe* or *pilomatrixoma*) is a benign tumor derived from the hair matrix that usually develops within the first 2 decades of life. Pilomatricomas usually present as solitary lesions of the face, neck, upper trunk, or upper extremities. The two most common locations in studies appear to be the head and neck and the upper extremities.[296,297] Clinically, pilomatricomas appear as flesh-colored to white, firm papules or papulonodules that may have an overlying pink to blue hue (Fig. 9.50). They are generally very hard as a result of calcification and may demonstrate a positive "teeter-totter sign," whereby downward pressure directed at one end of the lesion causes the other end to spring upward in the skin. Another useful sign is the "tent sign," whereby multiple facets and angles (resembling a tent) are visualized when the skin overlying the lesion is stretched (Fig. 9.51).

Pilomatricomas range in size from 5 mm to more than 5 cm in diameter, with an average size of 1 to 1.5 cm.[298] Although pilomatricomas are usually not hereditary, familial cases have been recognized,

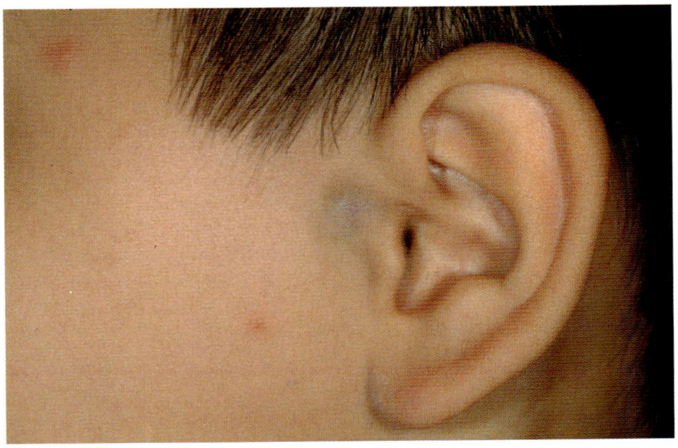

Fig. 9.50 Pilomatricoma. This preauricular blue papulonodule was very firm to palpation.

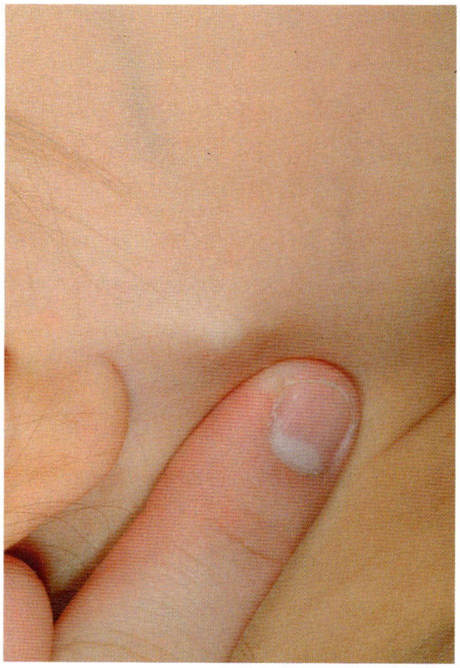

Fig. 9.51 Pilomatricoma. This lesion exhibits the "tent sign" as the adjacent skin is stretched.

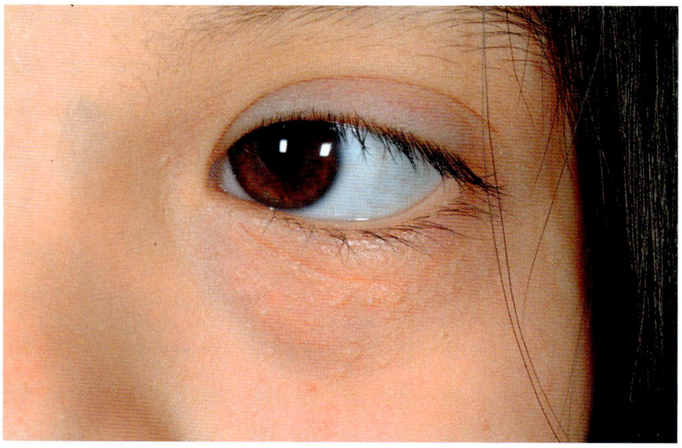

Fig. 9.52 Syringomas. These multiple, flesh-colored small papules were present bilaterally in the inferior periorbital regions of this young girl with Down syndrome.

and some familial forms have been associated with myotonic dystrophy, an uncommon autosomal dominant disorder characterized by hypotonia, muscle wasting, cataracts, hypogonadism, progressive mental retardation, and frontal baldness.[299–301] Multiple pilomatricomas have also been noted in patients with Gardner syndrome, Rubinstein–Taybi syndrome, and trisomy 9.[302–305] *Constitutional mismatch repair deficiency* (CMMR-D), a syndrome caused by mutations in the DNA mismatch repair genes *PMS2, MSH6, MSH2,* or *MLH1,* is a childhood cancer predisposition syndrome in which individuals are at increased risk of developing hematologic malignancies, brain tumors, and gastrointestinal cancer. Importantly, cutaneous findings in these patients may include multiple pilomatricomas, in addition to café-au-lait macules (which may mimic neurofibromatosis) and hypopigmented macules.[306,307] Other potential associations with multiple pilomatricomas include Turner syndrome and Kabuki syndrome.[308] Other variants of pilomatricomas include cystic-appearing lesions, in which hemorrhage may result in blue-red translucent nodules with rapid enlargement; perforating pilomatricomas; pilomatrix carcinoma (extremely rare); and extruding pilomatricomas (draining lesions that spontaneously discharge a chalky material containing calcium). Activating mutations in the β-catenin gene, *CTNNB1,* a participant in the Wnt signaling pathway, have been identified in pilomatricomas.[309] In patients with multiple pilomatricomas, mutations in the adenomatous polyposis coli *(APC)* gene have been identified.[310] Several cohorts with multiple familial pilomatricomas and no demonstrable underlying syndrome or association have been reported.[311]

Pilomatricomas may occasionally develop inflammation or swelling and may be painful when subjected to pressure on the affected region of skin. Definitive therapy is accomplished by surgical excision. Patients with multiple lesions or familial disease should be examined and monitored closely for potentially associated disorders, especially myotonic dystrophy, CMMR-D, and Gardner syndrome. Importantly, the onset of myotonic dystrophy may not occur until adulthood, and molecular diagnosis is possible.[300]

SYRINGOMA

Syringomas represent benign tumors of eccrine (sweat gland) structures and are predominantly seen in females. The lesions may occur at any age but commonly present initially during puberty or adolescence as small, firm, flesh-colored to yellow, translucent 1- to 3-mm papules (Fig. 9.52). They are usually multiple but may occasionally be solitary. In more than half of patients the lesions are located on the lower eyelids. Other common locations include the lateral neck, chest, abdomen, back, upper arms, thighs, and genitalia. Syringomas occur with increased incidence in patients with Down syndrome. They may occasionally occur in an eruptive fashion and tend to be influenced by hormones, as evidenced by increased size during pregnancy or the premenstrual period and enlargement in women receiving hormone therapy.

Syringomas gradually enlarge until they attain their full size and then persist, with little tendency for spontaneous resolution. Although they are benign, they may be of significant cosmetic concern. Treatment, however, is difficult. Therapeutic options include electrodesiccation, cryosurgery with liquid nitrogen, or local surgical excision. CO_2 laser ablation and trichloroacetic acid have also been found useful.[312]

ECCRINE POROMA

Eccrine poromas are benign cutaneous tumors that generally arise from the intraepidermal eccrine sweat duct unit. They occur most often during middle age or later but have been noted to develop as early as 12 years of age. Eccrine poromas present as firm papules, plaques, or nodules, and may be flesh colored to red. They are usually solitary, and range in size between 2 and 12 mm in diameter. They most commonly occur on the plantar surface of the foot and occasionally on the palms, fingers, neck, or trunk. In some lesions, the appearance is quite vascular and may simulate pyogenic granuloma. A striking clinical feature is the presence of a cup-shaped shallow depression from which the tumor grows and protrudes. Malignant eccrine poroma, also known as *eccrine porocarcinoma*, is a very rare tumor usually occurring in adults, although pediatric cases have been reported.[313] The treatment of choice for eccrine poroma is surgical excision.

CYLINDROMA

Cylindromas (also known as *turban tumors*) are benign neoplasms of either eccrine or apocrine origin and characterized by firm, rubbery, pink to bluish plaques and nodules. They may range in size from a few millimeters to several centimeters and are located primarily on the scalp and occasionally the face, trunk, or extremities. Cylindromas may occur singly or in multiples, and occasionally they coalesce to result in large mosaic tumors. Multiple lesions may occur as part of the autosomal dominant BSS (with multiple trichoepitheliomas and occasionally other appendageal tumors; see Trichoepithelioma section). This disease has been mapped to 16ql2–13, and mutations in the *CYLD* gene have been identified in families with this disorder.[314,315] Treatment consists of surgical excision, although CO_2 laser surgery has also been demonstrated useful.[316] Cylindromas are almost invariably benign, although malignant transformation has been rarely reported.

Dermal Tumors

ANGIOFIBROMA

Angiofibromas are benign dermal neoplasms that may occur as isolated or multiple lesions. The term *angiofibroma* actually describes the histologic appearance of these lesions (which reveals dermal fibroplasia and dilated blood vessels), but they may present in a variety of clinical fashions. Clinical subtypes include fibrous papules, pearly penile papules, and periungual fibromas. Another presentation pattern is that of multiple facial angiofibromas, which are commonly seen in patients with tuberous sclerosis (see Chapter 11), in which setting they have been erroneously referred to as *adenoma sebaceum*; multiple endocrine neoplasia type 1 (see Chapter 23); and Birt–Hogg–Dube syndrome (characterized classically by fibrofolliculomas, trichodiscomas, and acrochordons).[317]

A fibrous papule presents as a solitary, flesh-colored shiny papule, most often on the nose of adults. The differential diagnosis may include intradermal nevus, BCC, or another appendageal tumor. These lesions are treated with shave excision or electrocautery. Pearly penile papules present as tiny, flesh-colored to white papules on the glans penis of postpubertal men. They are most commonly distributed along the corona, and their importance lies in distinguishing them from genital condylomata (often a source of anxiety for the affected individual). This distinction is usually quite simple given their appearance, multiplicity, and localization. Treatment of pearly penile papules is unnecessary. Periungual fibromas present as flesh-colored to pink filiform growths arising from the proximal nailfold region (Fig. 9.53). Although they occasionally occur sporadically, multiple lesions are pathognomonic for tuberous sclerosis.

CONNECTIVE TISSUE NEVUS

Connective tissue nevus (also known as *connective tissue hamartoma*) is a localized hamartoma of either dermal collagen or elastic fibers or both. These benign skin lesions may be sporadic or hereditary and can be seen as a component of several syndromes. For instance, the shagreen patch and fibrous forehead plaque seen in tuberous sclerosis (see Chapter 11) are both forms of connective tissue nevi. In addition, the palmoplantar cerebriform hyperplasia that occurs in patients with Proteus syndrome (see Chapter 12) represents excess collagen and thus could also be classified under this umbrella term. This section discusses primarily the sporadic, nonsyndromic form of connective tissue nevus.

These lesions usually present as asymptomatic, flesh-colored dermal plaques composed of multiple papules. They may be quite subtle (Fig. 9.54), or they may be associated with significant thickening, cobblestoning, or cerebriform changes (Fig. 9.55). Solitary plaques may occur anywhere on the cutaneous surface, and multiple lesions are often distributed symmetrically on the back, buttocks, and extremities. The differential diagnosis may include smooth muscle hamartoma (see Congenital Smooth Muscle Hamartoma section).

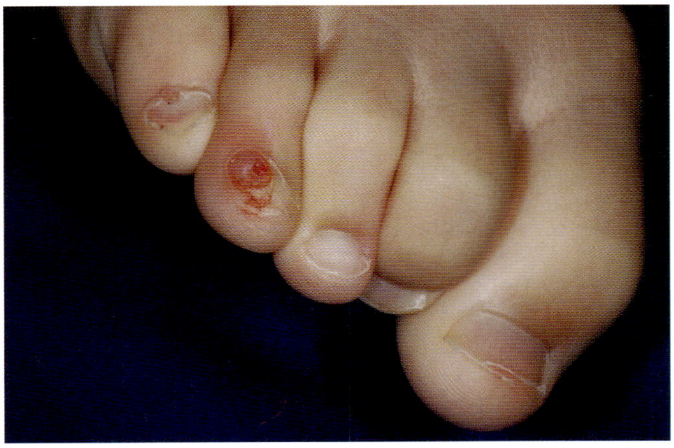

Fig. 9.53 Periungal fibroma. This pink papule arising from the proximal nailfold of the fourth toe occurred in a young boy with tuberous sclerosis. It was associated with nail dystrophy and intermittent bleeding. Note the smaller fibroma on the fifth toe as well.

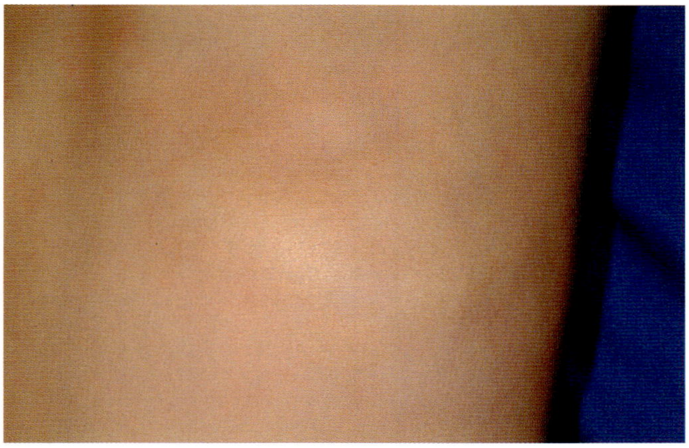

Fig. 9.54 Connective tissue nevus. This flesh-colored dermal plaque on the back of a school-aged boy had been present for several years.

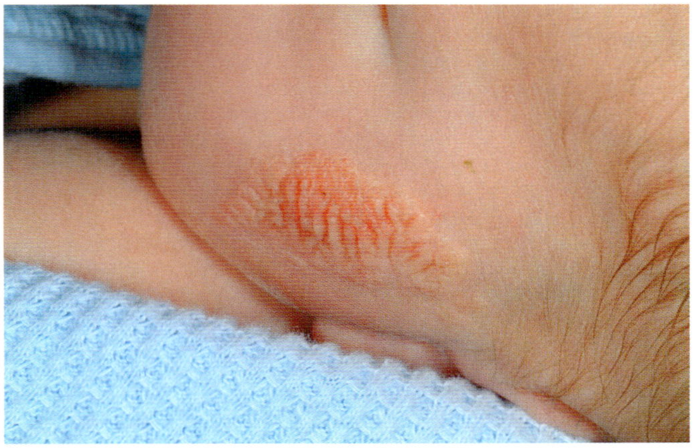

Fig. 9.55 Connective tissue nevus. A cerebriform, fleshy plaque on the cheek of a newborn boy.

Another form of connective tissue nevus, dermatofibrosis lenticularis disseminata, has been reported in association with a specific bone dysplasia termed *osteopoikilosis*. This association is also known as Buschke–Ollendorff syndrome (see Chapter 6). The cutaneous lesions in this setting usually appear in adult life, but their onset has also been reported during the first year or early childhood. They appear as flesh-colored to yellow papules, usually a few millimeters in size, distributed on the trunk, buttocks, and extremities. They often represent hamartomas of elastic tissue (elastomas) histologically. The bony lesions are usually asymptomatic and are often noted incidentally as focal sclerotic areas on bone radiographs. They may occasionally be mistaken for foci of metastatic malignancy, highlighting the importance of familiarity with this disorder and its associated skin lesions.

Connective tissue nevi are generally asymptomatic and not usually of cosmetic significance. If the diagnosis is unclear, incisional biopsy is useful. Surgical excision is otherwise unnecessary.

MASTOCYTOSIS

The term *mastocytosis* refers to a group of clinical disorders characterized by the accumulation of mast cells in the skin and at times other organs of the body. It may appear at any time from birth to middle age. Overall, in approximately 55% of patients, the onset occurs before the age of 2 years, and for 10% the onset is between 2 and 15 years of age.[318] In 75% to 90% of pediatric mastocytosis patients, disease onset occurs before 2 years of age, with congenital onset in up to 25%.[319,320] The growth and regulation of mast cells is dependent on stem cell factor, which is the ligand for the protein product of the *c-KIT* gene. Studies have documented *c-KIT* mutations in adult patients with mastocytosis, most often in codon 816 (exon 17), and activating *c-KIT* mutations have also been demonstrated in pediatric mastocytosis, occasionally in the same region but also in exons 8, 9, or 11.[321,322] Although mastocytosis is generally a sporadic disorder, familial cases have been reported.[323–325]

The clinical spectrum of cutaneous mastocytosis includes mastocytomas (single or multiple), urticaria pigmentosa (also called *maculopapular cutaneous mastocytosis*), bullous mastocytosis, diffuse cutaneous mastocytosis, and telangiectasia macularis eruptiva perstans (TMEP). An international task force on mastocytosis recently suggested eliminating TMEP as a variant and dividing urticaria pigmentosa into two groups: a monomorphic variant with small maculopapular lesions (more common in adults than in children) and a polymorphic variant with larger and asymmetric lesions (typical of pediatric disease).[322] The traditional classification of adult disease includes indolent mastocytosis, mastocytosis with an associated hematologic disorder, mast cell leukemia, and lymphadenopathic mastocytosis with eosinophilia.[318] Alternatively, for either pediatric or adults patients, mastocytosis may be divided into cutaneous and systemic forms with the potential for overlap between these two. Although the disease may be classified by several different schemas, there appear to be some fairly consistent differences between adult and pediatric mastocytosis. These include the following for pediatric disease: earlier onset, usually within the first 2 years of life; rare occurrence of TMEP; tendency toward spontaneous improvement; rare association with hematologic disorders; and rare infiltration of other organs aside from the skin.[320,323,326]

Although the classification of mastocytosis is often confusing, it can be somewhat simplified when considering the typical childhood presentations. Children most commonly present with mastocytomas (either solitary or multiple), urticaria pigmentosa, or, occasionally, diffuse cutaneous mastocytosis. All three of these childhood forms may display vesicular or bullous variants. Vesiculation is presumably related to histamine- or other chemical mediator-induced transuding leakage in a group susceptible to blister formation by less secure attachments of the epidermis to the underlying dermis.[327]

The diagnosis of all forms of cutaneous mastocytosis is aided by the phenomenon known as the *Darier sign*. This finding, a hallmark of the disorder, is seen in 90% of patients with skin disease and consists of localized erythema and urticarial wheals (Fig. 9.56) that develop after gentle mechanical irritation, such as might be induced by rubbing with a tongue blade or the blunt end of a pen or pencil. This urtication develops within a few minutes after the stimulus and may persist as long as 30 minutes to several hours. Occasionally, blister formation may result. It should be noted, though, that the Darier sign may be negative in mastocytosis, especially in patients with entirely flat lesions at baseline. Occasional systemic reactions, including hypotension, have been observed after elicitation of the Darier sign.

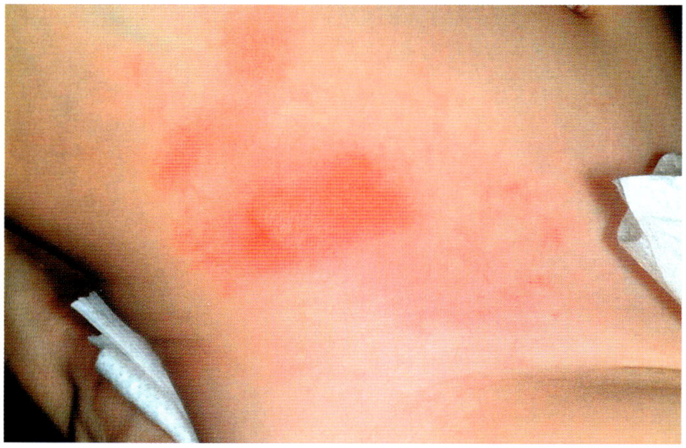

Fig. 9.56 Darier sign in mastocytosis. Edema and surrounding erythema developed within minutes after firmly stroking this lesion.

Box 9.3 Potential Triggers of Mast Cell Degranulation

- Physical
  Exercise, heat, hot baths, hot beverages, cold exposure, sunlight, stress
- Medications (systemic)
  Aspirin, alcohol, morphine, codeine, dextromethorphan, NSAIDs, opiates, amphotericin B, thiamine
- Medications (topical)
  Polymyxin B
- Medications sometimes used with general anesthesia
  D-tubocurarine, scopolamine, decamethonium, gallamine, pancuronium
- Local anesthetics
  Tetracaine, procaine, methylparaben
- Radiographic contrast
  Iodine-containing contrast media
- Venoms
  Snakebites, bee stings, jellyfish stings
- Foods
  Egg white, crawfish, lobster, chocolate, strawberries, tomatoes, citrus, ethanol

NSAIDs, Nonsteroidal antiinflammatory drugs.

Mast cell mediators include histamine, prostaglandin D_2, heparin, tryptase, chymase, leukotrienes, and others. Cutaneous symptoms related to release of these mediators in the setting of mastocytosis may include flushing, blistering, and itching. Systemic symptoms may include nausea, abdominal pain, diarrhea, bone pain, hypotension, and less often, pulmonary signs. Whereas the extent and density of cutaneous lesions may correlate with systemic symptoms in adults, such a correlation is lacking in children with mastocytosis.[328] There are many potential triggers of mast cell degranulation, including physical stimuli, drugs, and foods, and these are listed in Box 9.3. Most of these triggers are clinically insignificant in children with more mild forms of the disease, but exposures should be minimized in those at the more severe end of the spectrum or with a history of related systemic symptoms. A disease severity index, referred to as the *Scoring Mastocytosis (SCORMA) index*, has been developed and was demonstrated to correlate with the serum tryptase level in pediatric and adult cutaneous mastocytosis.[329] This index incorporates extent of surface area involvement, lesion intensity, and subjective symptoms (e.g., flushing, diarrhea, pruritus).

Mastocytomas are a common type of childhood mastocytosis. They may be either solitary or multiple and present as flesh-colored to yellow-orange-tan papules (Fig. 9.57) or plaques. Some lesions may have a bruise-like appearance, and others may present in similar fashion to café-au-lait macules.[326] They may range in size from a few millimeters to several centimeters and are present at birth in around 40% of patients.[330] In the remainder they generally appear by 1 year of age. The surface of the lesion often reveals a *peau d'orange* (orange peel–like) appearance (Fig. 9.58), and the Darier sign is notoriously positive. Occasionally, stroking or rubbing of even a solitary lesion may provoke symptoms of flushing or colic. Mastocytomas may occur on any part of the body but are noted most often on the arms, neck, and trunk. A history of intermittent blistering of the affected area may be obtained, and in this setting misdiagnosis of bullous impetigo or herpes simplex infection is common. The tendency toward vesiculation tends to disappear within 1 to 3 years. Although the course of mastocytomas is generally benign and the lesions usually involute over several years, there have been reports of solitary mastocytosis eventuating in generalized urticaria pigmentosa.[331]

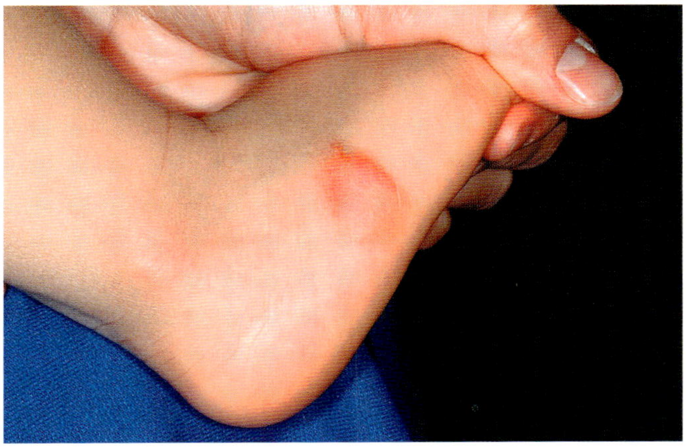

Fig. 9.57 Solitary mastocytoma. An edematous plaque with mild surrounding pigmentation.

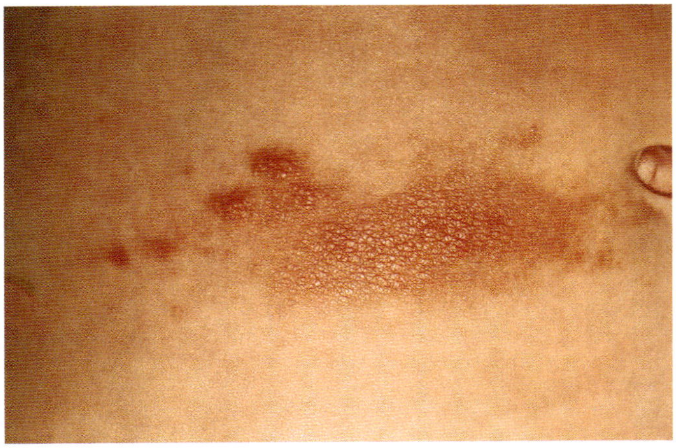

Fig. 9.58 *Peau d'orange* appearance of a mastocytoma. This plaque-like mastocytoma shows the characteristic surface changes.

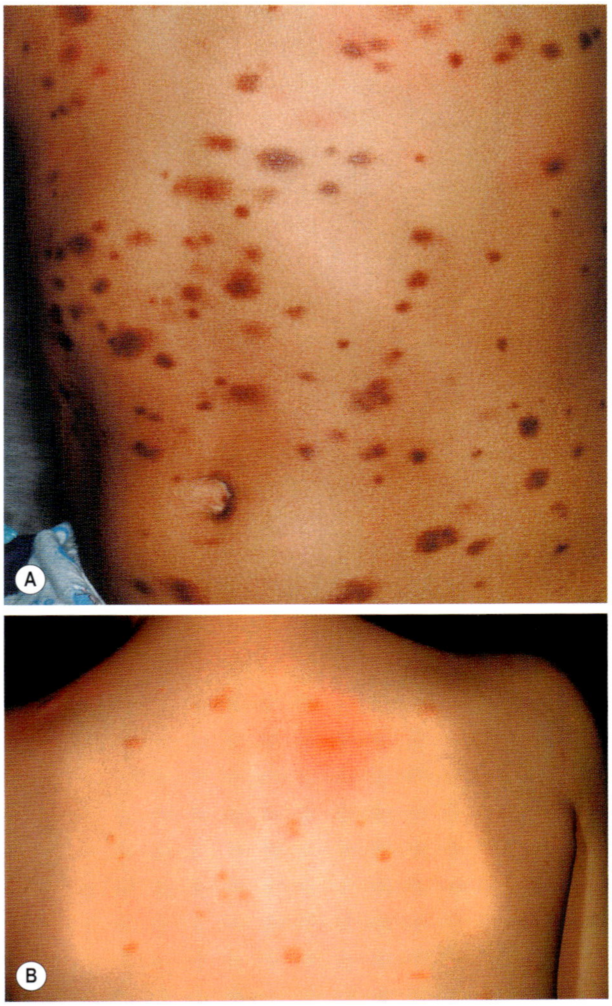

Fig. 9.59 Urticaria pigmentosa. **(A)** Multiple hyperpigmented macules and papules in this 2-year-old girl. **(B)** Light tan macules and papules in a school-aged boy. Note the Darier sign, which occurred after rubbing the lesion.

Urticaria pigmentosa is the most common presentation of mastocytosis. It presents with multiple, well-demarcated, tan to red-brown macules and papules (Fig. 9.59) that may occur anywhere on the cutaneous surface. Mucous membranes may be involved, and palms and soles are usually spared. Some lesions may have a purpuric quality, and occasionally a yellow coloration is noted. There may be tens to hundreds of lesions ranging in size from a few millimeters to several centimeters. The Darier sign is positive, and dermatographism may be present in 30% to 50% of patients. The lesions of urticaria pigmentosa may become vesicular or bullous (Fig. 9.60), a presentation termed *bullous mastocytosis*. These blisters may result in pain and secondary infection but generally heal without scarring. Beyond the age of 2 years, bullous changes are unusual.[318]

Diffuse cutaneous mastocytosis is a less common variant of mastocytosis, especially in children. This presentation is characterized by diffuse infiltration of the skin by mast cells with skin that may appear grossly normal, thickened, doughy, reddish-brown, or *peau d'orange* in texture (Fig. 9.61). There may be a yellow, carotenoderma-like color present, and occasionally these patients present with extensive bullous eruptions. Patients with the diffuse cutaneous form appear to have the highest rate of systemic disease and may experience intense generalized pruritus, flushing, temperature elevation, vomiting, diarrhea, abdominal pain, GI ulceration, or respiratory distress. Overt shock may occur in this form of mastocytosis.

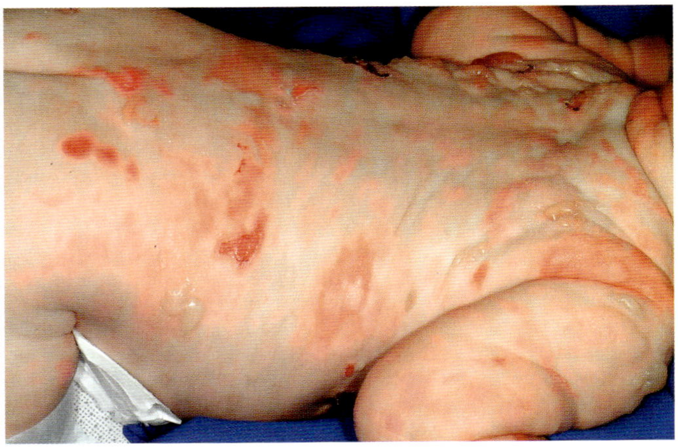

Fig. 9.60 Bullous mastocytosis. This 8-month-old girl had widespread mastocytosis with blister formation. Note the diffuse distribution of infiltrative plaques, *peau d'orange* changes, superficial erosions, and intact bullae of the shoulders, upper back, and flank.

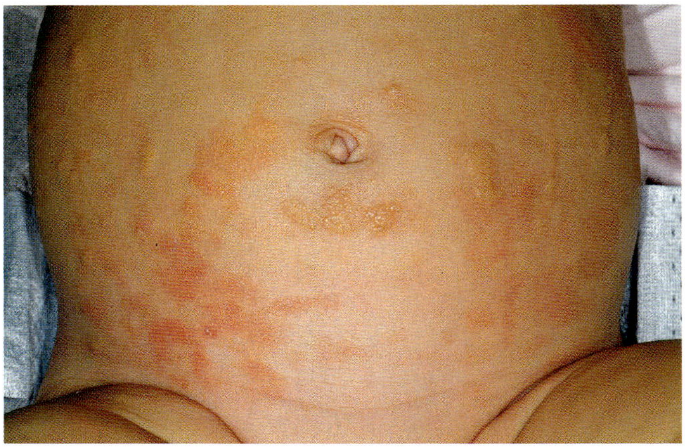

Fig. 9.61 Diffuse cutaneous mastocytosis. This child had diffuse erythematous yellow plaques and *peau d'orange* surface changes.

Box 9.4 Anesthesia Considerations in Pediatric Mastocytosis Patients

Ensure adequate familiarity of anesthesiologist with pediatric mastocytosis and preparedness to treat possible adverse events during anesthesia
Review detailed history of clinical drug reactions before anesthesia
Consider obtaining baseline serum tryptase, which may be useful to do the following:
- Suggest systemic mastocytosis (and concomitant higher risk of anesthetic reaction), if extreme elevation
- Diagnose possible anesthesia-related adverse events, if significantly elevated from baseline

Avoid preoperative drug skin testing
Continue scheduled maintenance mastocytosis medications
Consider administration of incremental (vs. single boluses) of necessary agents known to be mast cell degranulators
Administer NSAIDs with caution and only in the absence of a history of sensitivity
Consider patient positioning to minimize mechanical pressure on skin during anesthesia

Modified from from Carter MC, Uzzaman A, Scott LM, et al. Pediatric mastocytosis: routine anesthetic management for a complex disease. Anesth Analg 2008;107:422–7; and Ahmad N, Evans P, Lloyd-Thomas AR. Anesthesia in children with mastocytosis: a case based review. Paediatr Anaesth 2009;19(2):97–107.
NSAIDs, Nonsteroidal antiinflammatory drugs.

Systemic mastocytosis is markedly more common in adults than in children with mastocytosis. The most commonly involved systems are GI and skeletal, although the lungs, kidneys, lymph nodes, myocardium, pericardium, liver, spleen, and bone marrow may also be affected. Skeletal lesions may consist of radiopacities, radiolucencies, or a mixture of both. These changes are quite rare in children with the disorder.[332] Hepatomegaly, splenomegaly, and lymph node enlargement may also occur. GI symptoms include abdominal pain, diarrhea, nausea, and vomiting. GI hemorrhage may occasionally occur and is often secondary to gastritis or peptic ulcer disease. Children with the diffuse cutaneous form of mastocytosis may be at particular risk for this complication.[318] The "mastocytosis syndrome" results from massive histamine release with symptoms including bronchospasm, headache, flushing, diarrhea, pruritus, and hypotension. It occurs most often in infants or young children with the diffuse cutaneous form of the disease, and death may occasionally result.

The increased risk of development of a hematologic malignancy is a major concern in adults with mastocytosis, but significant hematologic consequences in children are fairly rare.[333] In a series of 15 patients with pediatric mastocytosis who were observed for approximately 20 years, some bone marrow specimens revealed increased mast cells, but this finding was not predictive for disease severity or persistence of symptoms. Furthermore, none of the patients in this series developed hematologic malignancy. The authors recommended bone marrow studies only in children with evidence of systemic disease including organomegaly, elevated tryptase, or unexplained peripheral blood abnormalities.[334] In a systematic review of more than 1700 pediatric mastocytosis patients, however, 0.7% of patients progressed to mast cell sarcoma or mast cell leukemia, and a fatal outcome (related to these malignancies or other systemic involvement) was noted in 3% of patients, highlighting the importance of close clinical follow up.[320]

Anesthetic management of pediatric patients with mastocytosis has traditionally been viewed as complex and risky given the nature of the disease, the degranulation effects of some anesthetic agents, and the reported adult literature. Published reports, however, suggest that pediatric patients with cutaneous (versus, systemic) mastocytosis are at fairly low risk for major anesthesia-related complications.[335,336] Anesthesia considerations for patients with pediatric mastocytosis are listed in Box 9.4.

The diagnosis of pediatric mastocytosis is often based on the characteristic cutaneous findings and a positive Darier sign. Although it is usually a straightforward diagnosis, atypical or unusual presentations or those lacking skin involvement may pose a diagnostic challenge. When skin lesions are present, the diagnosis can be confirmed with skin biopsy, which reveals an accumulation of mast cells in the dermis. Special immunohistochemical stains such as Giemsa, toluidine blue, anti-CD117, or tryptase antibodies may be useful in confirming the mast cell nature of the infiltrate. Biopsy of the bone marrow or GI tract may be necessary if such organ involvement is suspected and the patient lacks cutaneous lesions.

Indirect methods for diagnosing mastocytosis are also available. Measurement of serum tryptase, a protease produced by mast cells, is helpful in supporting the diagnosis.[337] Two forms (α and β) have been identified and measuring both of these mediators can be useful for correlation with the extent of mast cell disease. However, even persistently elevated levels of serum tryptase in children with mastocytosis is likely not indicative of systemic disease, and there appears to be no correlation with prognosis.[320,332,338] Urinary histamine and its metabolites may also be helpful. High levels of urinary N-methylhistamine may be suggestive of more extensive involvement.[339] Urinary N-methylimidazoleacetic acid is another histamine metabolite that is useful as a chemical marker for the disease.[340]

Extensive laboratory or radiographic studies or invasive diagnostic procedures in pediatric patients with mastocytosis are generally not indicated. However, in patients with extensive disease (e.g., extensive urticaria pigmentosa or diffuse cutaneous mastocytosis), complete blood cell count with peripheral smear and blood chemistry studies should be performed with occasional follow-up tests. Other diagnostic studies such as abdominal ultrasound, endoscopy, bone scan, or bone marrow biopsy should be reserved for patients in whom specific symptoms suggest systemic disease.[318,333,334]

The course and prognosis of mastocytosis depends on the clinical subtype, severity of disease, and age of onset. In general, the prognosis for childhood mastocytosis is favorable in most patients. Symptoms are estimated to improve by adolescence in up to 50% of patients,[341] but complete resolution may occur less often than previously believed. In one study, 5 of 33 children had complete resolution, and 21 of the 33 had improvement by adolescence.[342] In the previously mentioned series of 15 pediatric patients with mastocytosis studied longitudinally over 20 years, complete regression of disease occurred in 67%, and another 20% experienced major regression of symptoms.[334] Another longitudinal study noted that early regression (by 12 years) was associated with fewer mastocytosis lesions, with greater number of lesions correlating with late resolution (past 12 years).[343]

The treatment of mastocytosis is primarily symptomatic because no specific therapy or cure currently exists for this disorder. Patients (and/or their parents) should be counseled about the disease, its natural history, differences between pediatric and adult mastocytosis, and possible triggers of mast cell degranulation (see Box 9.3). Nonsedating histamine type 1 (H1) receptor antagonists are a good initial treatment of choice and include cetirizine, levocetirizine, loratadine, and fexofenadine. The long half-life and nonsedating nature of these medications offer advantages over traditional antihistamines. In patients with severe involvement or symptoms, a classic H1 antagonist (e.g., hydroxyzine, diphenhydramine, and cyproheptadine) may be useful. The addition of an H2 antagonist (i.e., cimetidine, ranitidine, famotidine) may be considered, especially in patients with flushing or marked GI symptoms.

Oral cromolyn sodium has been found useful in treating GI symptoms of mastocytosis, although controlled studies in children are lacking. Ketotifen, a mast cell stabilizer unavailable in the oral form in the United States, has shown promise in alleviating symptoms. Psoralen plus ultraviolet A light (PUVA) therapy has been demonstrated useful in urticaria pigmentosa, diffuse cutaneous mastocytosis, and systemic mastocytosis.[344,345] This therapy is more challenging though, and has a higher risk-to-benefit ratio in children. Aspirin and nonsteroidal antiinflammatory drugs (NSAIDs), although they may induce mast cell degranulation, may paradoxically be used to reduce prostaglandin-dependent flushing in some patients. Although topical agents are not typically effective, some mastocytomas have been noted to improve or disappear after therapy with a potent topical corticosteroid under occlusion. Additionally, two patients were reported whose mastocytomas responded to topical pimecrolimus cream in conjunction with a daily oral antihistamine.[346] A brief course of oral corticosteroids (e.g., 1 mg/kg per day of prednisone or prednisolone for 4 to 6 weeks) may be quite effective for symptomatic patients but obviously is not an appropriate long-term therapy. Cyclosporine and interferon α-2b have been used in some adults with more aggressive forms of mastocytosis, and imatinib (a tyrosine kinase inhibitor used in the treatment of some malignancies) was reportedly effective in a young adult with pediatric-onset, indolent systemic mastocytosis.[347] Midostaurin, an oral multiple tyrosine kinase inhibitor, was recently approved for treatment of adults with aggressive systemic mastocytosis and mastocytosis associated with hematologic malignancy or mast cell leukemia.[348,349] Lastly, patients (and parents of children) at risk for recurrent hypotensive episodes or mastocytosis syndrome should have a premeasured epinephrine pen kit (EpiPen or EpiPen Jr) with them at all times for emergency use. Information regarding patient support groups and education for pediatric mastocytosis (www.mastokids.org) should be given.

GRANULOMA ANNULARE

Granuloma annulare (GA) is a fairly common skin disorder characterized by papules or nodules grouped in a ring-like or circinate configuration. Although GA may occur on any part of the body, it often involves the lateral or dorsal surfaces of the hands, feet, wrists, and ankles. Patients may have solitary lesions or multiple sites of involvement. GA may occur at any age and is especially common in school-aged children.

The cause of GA is unknown. Various studies have suggested a possible association between GA and diabetes mellitus, but this hypothesis remains controversial and some studies refute it.[350–352] There appears to be a greater risk of dyslipidemia in adult patients with GA, notably the generalized form; in one case-control study, adults with GA had four times the odds of developing dyslipidemia (including significant differences in total cholesterol, triglycerides, and low-density lipoprotein cholesterol levels) compared with age- and sex-matched controls.[353] This association has not been confirmed in children. Other purported associations have included tetanus or bacille Calmette–Guérin (BCG) vaccination, hepatitis B infection, *Borrelia* infection, Hodgkin disease, leukemia, or a hypersensitivity reaction to an unidentified antigen.[354–357] In some individuals, GA has been noted after trauma, sun exposure, and insect bites.

GA most classically presents with an annular, smooth, nonscaly plaque with a border composed of numerous small papules (Figs. 9.62 and 9.63). Patients are often misdiagnosed with tinea corporis and have previously failed topical antifungal therapy. Early lesions begin as smooth, flesh-colored to pink papules that slowly enlarge peripherally and undergo central involution to form the classic rings with clear centers and elevated borders. Lesions may range in size from 5 mm to several centimeters.

There are several clinical variants of GA. A generalized form may occur, in which patients have multiple, disseminated, small papular lesions. Perforating GA presents as grouped papules, some of which have a central umbilication or crusting and scaling. This form is seen mainly on the extremities. Subcutaneous GA (Figs. 9.64 and 9.65) is

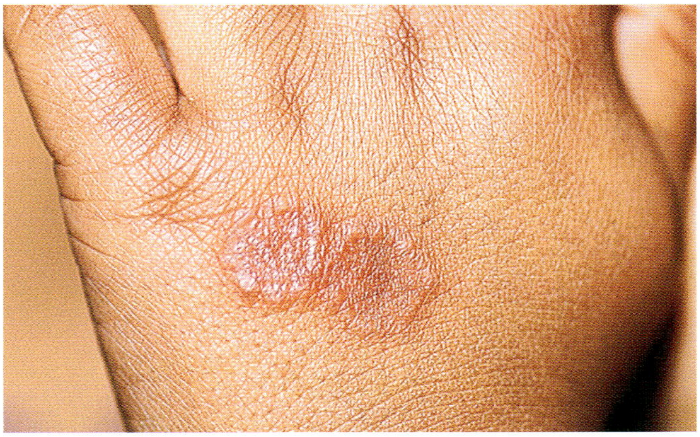

Fig. 9.62 Granuloma annulare. Annular, flesh-colored, nonscaly plaques.

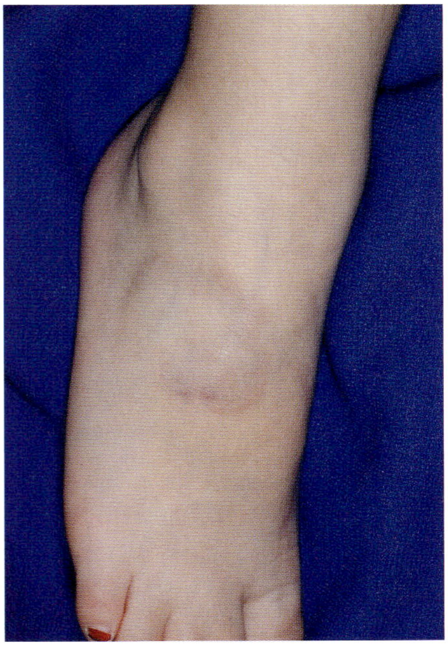

Fig. 9.63 Granuloma annulare. This patient has a semiannular, flesh-colored to pink plaque on the dorsal foot.

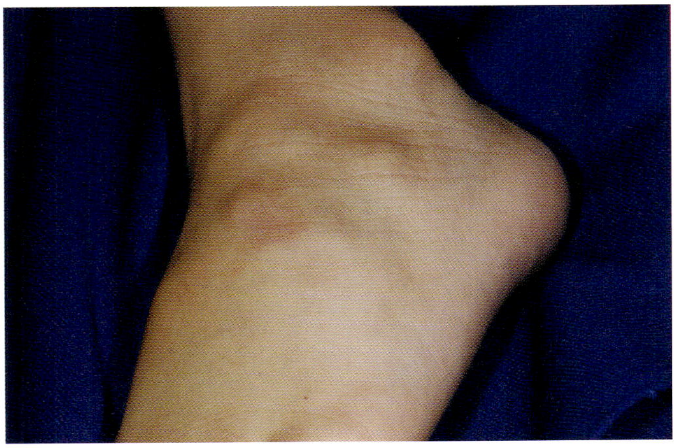

Fig. 9.64 Subcutaneous granuloma annulare. Subcutaneous nodules on the dorsolateral foot.

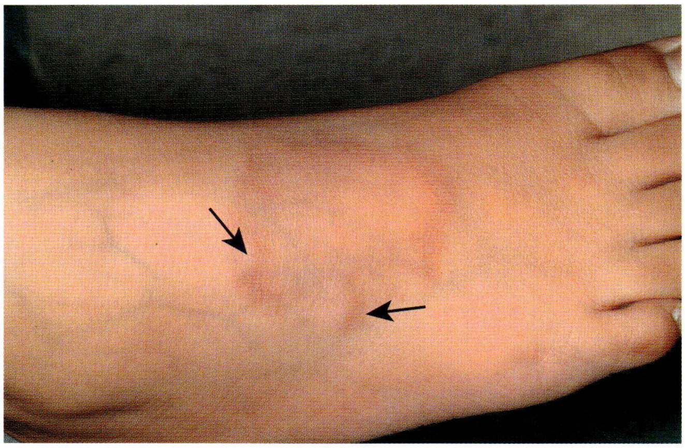

Fig. 9.65 Granuloma annulare. This patient's plaque reveals both cutaneous and subcutaneous *(arrows)* involvement.

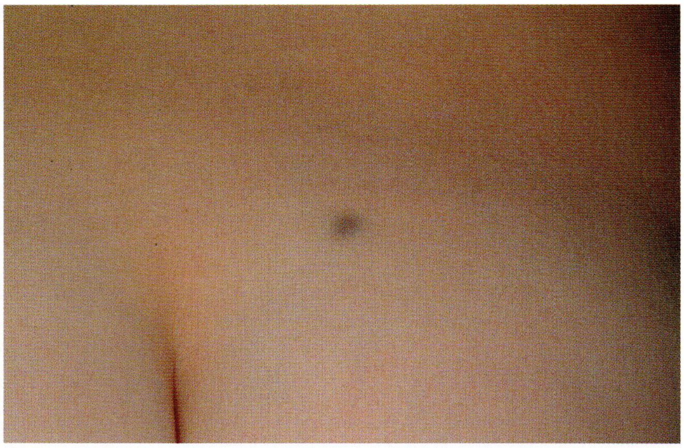

Fig. 9.66 Dermatofibroma. This gray-brown papule on the right superior buttock was very firm to palpation and showed a "dimple sign" with lateral pinching (see text for discussion).

an important subtype in children, in whom it is most common. This form presents as subcutaneous nodules, distributed mainly on the feet, anterior tibial surfaces, fingers, hands, and scalp.[358,359] Penile lesions have also been rarely reported.[360] These lesions are usually painless and only occasionally slightly tender. The differential diagnosis of these lesions may include rheumatoid nodules, trauma, foreign body reaction, infection, and malignancy. Incisional biopsy is often necessary to confirm the diagnosis, unless there are classic cutaneous GA lesions present elsewhere on the skin surface. Ultrasound with color Doppler may be useful and reveals a hypoechoic nonvascularized subcutaneous mass that may adhere to fascia or periosteum but does not invade underlying planes.[361]

Lesions of GA usually disappear spontaneously without sequelae and within several months to years. There is no satisfactory therapy for GA, but because the lesions are nearly always asymptomatic, watchful waiting is often acceptable. Topical corticosteroids, either ointments, creams, or impregnated into tape, may be effective but are limited by their potential in causing skin atrophy. Intralesional corticosteroid injection has also been used in some patients. Cryotherapy has been used, as have a variety of systemic agents (including isotretinoin, prednisone, dapsone, doxycycline, and cyclosporine), but the risk-to-benefit ratio is generally not justified for these drugs. Occasionally the lesions spontaneously regress after skin biopsy. Until the association with diabetes mellitus is clearly established or refuted, patients with GA should be monitored by their primary physician for signs or symptoms, and if there is any concern or a strong family history, testing should be considered. Serum lipid testing should be considered in patients with more generalized involvement.

NEUROFIBROMA

Neurofibromas may appear as isolated, usually single lesions in a healthy individual or as a cutaneous marker of dominantly inherited type 1 neurofibromatosis (NF1, von Recklinghausen disease; see Chapter 11). Lesions not associated with NF1 are discussed here.

Neurofibromas are benign tumors composed of neuromesenchymal tissue, including Schwann cells, endoneurial and perineurial cells, and other cellular components. They often present during young adulthood and occasionally early in life. Clinically, a neurofibroma presents as a soft, flesh-colored, solitary papule or papulonodule. They may occasionally be red, blue, or brown. They range in size from 2 mm to 2 cm, and with further growth they become globular, pear-shaped, pedunculated, or pendulous. Neurofibromas exhibit a positive "buttonhole" sign that is felt to be pathognomonic, whereby direct pressure on top of the lesion results in easy invagination into the

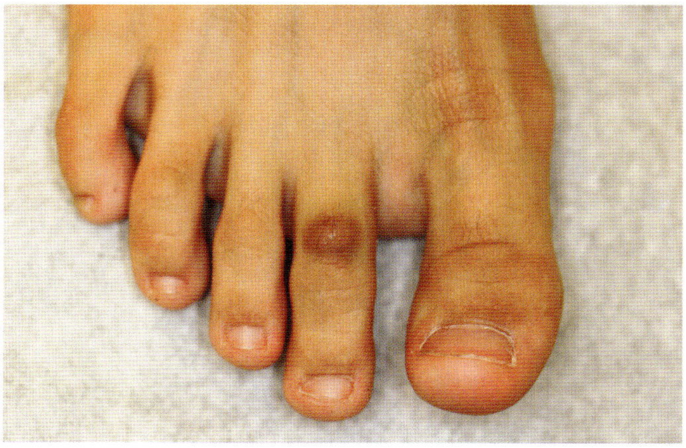

Fig. 9.67 Dermatofibroma. This firm tan-brown papule on the second toe of a 7-year-old girl presented at 1 year of age, was asymptomatic, and grew only proportionate to her growth.

dermis. This sign may be useful in differentiating neurofibromas from intradermal nevi or dermatofibromas.

When multiple neurofibromas are present, the diagnosis of NF1 must be considered. The presence of café-au-lait macules, axillary or inguinal freckling, or a plexiform neurofibroma lends further support to this diagnosis. Plexiform neurofibroma presents as a large, lobulated nodular plaque that may have a "bag of worms" consistency on palpation. These lesions are considered pathognomonic for NF1 (see Chapter 11). Sporadic neurofibromas are best treated with surgical excision.

DERMATOFIBROMA

Dermatofibroma (fibrous histiocytoma) is a benign neoplasm of connective tissue generally seen in adults; occasionally it occurs in children. It presents as a small, well-defined dermal nodule that is firmly fixed to the skin but freely movable over the subcutaneous fat. There is often a tan to brown color of the surface (Fig. 9.66). Dermatofibromas may be found on any part of the body and are common on the extremities (Fig. 9.67), particularly the anterior surface of the leg. They range in size from 1 mm to 2 cm. A useful diagnostic feature is the "dimple sign," whereby pinching the lesion results in downward displacement.

The differential diagnosis may include melanocytic nevus or cyst. Although treatment of dermatofibromas is unnecessary, surgical excision may be performed for cosmetic purposes or diagnostic confirmation.

DERMATOFIBROSARCOMA PROTUBERANS

Dermatofibrosarcoma protuberans (DFSP) is a slowly growing fibrohistiocytic tumor with intermediate malignant potential seen primarily in adults between the second and fifth decades of life. These lesions tend to be locally invasive, have a high recurrence rate after excision, and occasionally result in metastatic disease. Pediatric and even congenital cases are occasionally observed, although most lesions present during the second to fifth decades of life.

DFSP usually begins as erythematous to blue papules and nodules that increase in size and may ultimately become multinodular and protuberant. Some lesions present as atrophic plaques. Ulceration may be present. The majority of lesions occur on the trunk or proximal extremities (Fig. 9.68), and the scalp, neck, and face are occasionally involved. During infancy or early childhood, DFSP may be misdiagnosed as a vascular malformation or tumor given the vascular appearance of many lesions. (Fig. 9.69)[362,363] Other initial impressions may include keloid, dermatofibroma, morphea, scar, or epidermal cyst.[364] Significant variability in presentation appears to be common with congenital lesions, which are rare but well documented.[363] The median time from onset to diagnosis in a series of pediatric DFSP was 36 months.[365] Multicentric DFSP may occur in patients with adenosine deaminase–deficient severe combined immunodeficiency.[366]

DFSP has been linked to a chromosomal translocation, t(17;22)(q22;q13), which fuses the collagen type 1, alpha 1 *(COL1A1)* and *PDGFβ* genes.[367] This translocation can be found in tumor tissue via cytogenetic analysis, FISH, or polymerase chain reaction testing.[365] The treatment of choice for DFSP is complete surgical excision with adequate margins. In recent years, Mohs micrographic surgery (MMS) has evolved as the therapeutic standard of care, and it has been demonstrated to offer superior cure rates, smaller surgical margins, and fewer surgical sessions compared with wide local excision in treating congenital DFSP.[290,368] MMS in conjunction with a vacuum-assisted closure system has been reported as useful for treatment of pediatric DFSP, with associated decreased rates of infection and complications.[369]

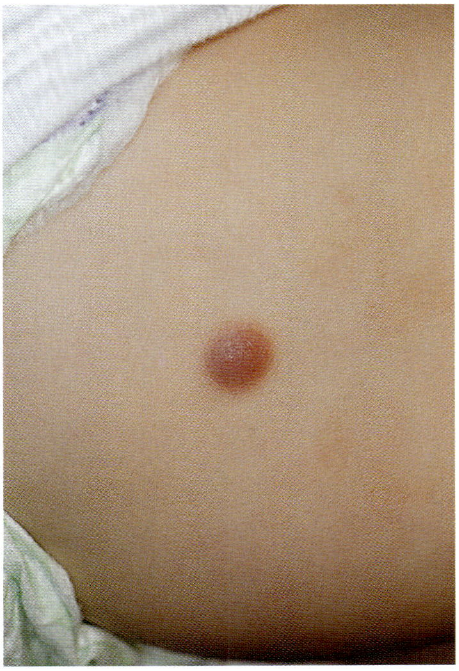

Fig. 9.68 Dermatofibrosarcoma protuberans (DFSP). This red nodule was present at birth on the proximal thigh of this young boy. Punch biopsy revealed changes of DFSP, and it was ultimately treated with complete surgical excision.

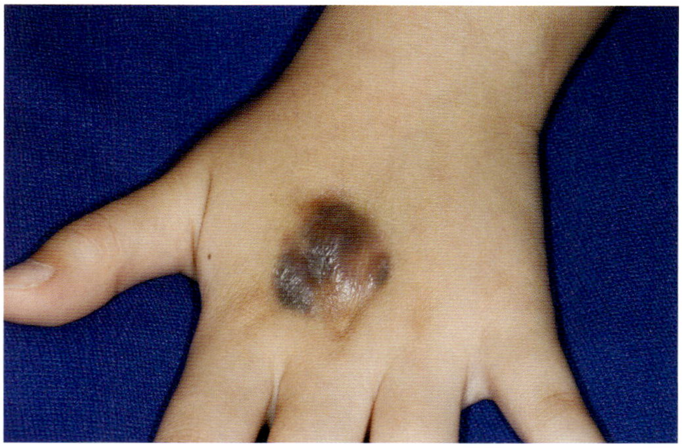

Fig. 9.69 Dermatofibrosarcoma protuberans (DFSP). This purple-pink nodule on the hand of a 9-year-old girl had been slowly growing since 3 years of age. Excision revealed changes of DFSP, with positive deep margins, necessitating repeat surgery with wide margins.

However, it appears that MMS is rarely used in children,[370] likely related to the complexities of different sites of care between adults and children in many centers and the need for concomitant pediatric anesthesia when this procedure is performed in those at the younger end of the age spectrum. Radiation therapy and imatinib have been recommended when clear surgical margins are unobtainable, the tumor recurs, or there is concern about metastases.[371,372] In patients with DFSP, lifelong clinical follow-up care is recommended given the risk of recurrence; however, metastatic spread is fortunately quite rare.[373] Several larger series have revealed an overall favorable prognosis for pediatric DFSP.[365,374,375]

Fibromatoses

The fibromatoses are a group of disorders marked by fibrous and fibrohistiocytic proliferations in the skin. These disorders may represent neoplastic or reactive processes and tend to be benign, although several have the potential for recurrence after excision. In this section, three pediatric fibromatoses are discussed.

RECURRING DIGITAL FIBROMA OF CHILDHOOD

Recurring digital fibroma of childhood (RDFC; also known as *recurring infantile digital fibromatosis*) is a rare, benign childhood fibromatosis. It usually occurs on the dorsal and lateral aspects of the fingers and toes and presents at birth or less commonly during infancy or later childhood. The majority of lesions are present by 12 months of age.[376] Interestingly, the thumbs and great toes are usually spared.

RDFC presents as flesh-colored to slightly erythematous papules and nodules (Fig. 9.70). Lesions are usually multiple and tend to affect multiple digits. They may become as large as 2 cm in size. Joint deformities and lateral deviation or flexion deformities may occasionally be associated.[376,377]

The cause of RDFC is unknown, and although a viral etiology was once postulated based on eosinophilic inclusion bodies seen on histologic examination, there appears to be little evidence in support of this hypothesis.[378] Management of RDFC is controversial. Arguments in favor of a conservative watchful waiting approach include the observation that many lesions spontaneously regress over a few years, that excision of the lesions does not alter the natural history of the joint disease (when present), and that excision is often followed by recurrence.[379] However, some assert that surgical excision is indicated to prevent continuous growth and involvement of deeper tissues and because some lesions do not spontaneously resolve. Medical approaches including topical imiquimod, intralesional fluorouracil, and topical or intralesional corticosteroids have yielded inconsistent

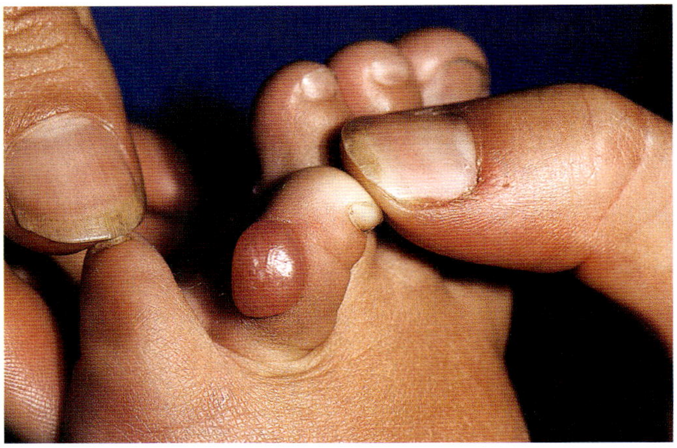

Fig. 9.70 Recurring digital fibroma of childhood. A firm, erythematous tumor on the lateral surface of the fourth toe.

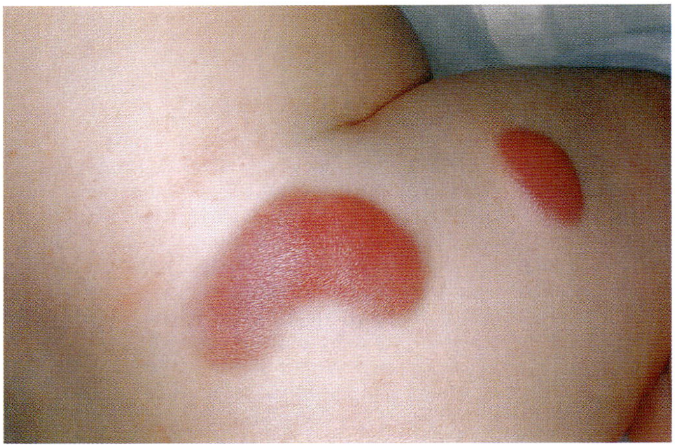

Fig. 9.72 Multiple myofibromas. Firm, rubbery nodules and plaques on the thigh of an infant.

results.[380] For smaller lesions without functional impairment, it seems that conservative management of RDFC is most appropriate.

INFANTILE MYOFIBROMATOSIS

Infantile myofibromatosis (IM) is a term used to describe several fibrous disorders (including solitary, multicentric, and generalized IM) that represent variants of the same process. Patients with these conditions have neoplasms composed of myofibroblasts, a distinct cell type that appears to also be involved in RDFC (see the previous section). The solitary form accounts for roughly half of all cases of infantile myofibromatosis.[381] Some cases of IM may mimic congenital infantile fibrosarcoma, and in these patients, molecular analysis for the *ETV6–NTRK3* gene fusion transcript (present in some infantile fibrosarcomas) may be useful.[299,382] Both autosomal recessive and autosomal dominant forms of multicentric and generalized IM have been reported. Missense mutations in *PDGFRB*, which encodes the platelet-derived growth factor receptor-β, as well as mutations in *NOTCH3* have been identified in several families with autosomal dominant IM, and mutations in *NDRG4* has been found in a family with autosomal recessive inheritance.[383–385]

In IM, fibrous nodules may occur in skin, subcutaneous tissue, skeletal muscle, and bone. Most patients have solitary lesions *(solitary IM)*, and the most common sites of involvement are the head and neck regions.[386] The myofibromas, which are often congenital,[387] appear as flesh-colored to purple, firm or rubbery papules (Fig. 9.71), nodules, or plaques. The differential diagnosis of a solitary myofibroma may include infantile hemangioma, histiocytoma, mastocytoma, and infantile digital fibroma. Visceral involvement is rare when the cutaneous lesion is solitary.

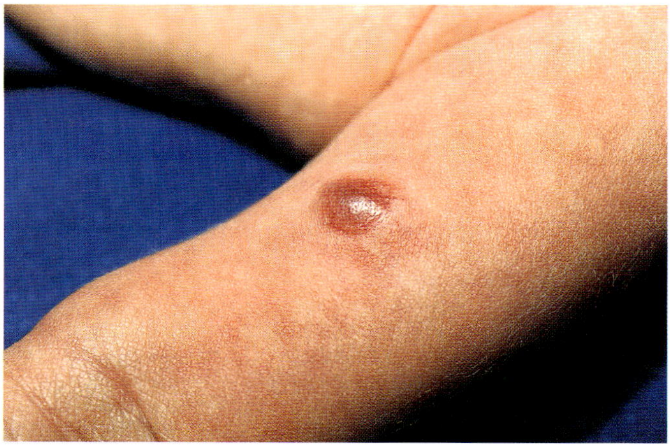

Fig. 9.71 Solitary myofibroma. This lesion was congenital and spontaneously resolved by 1 year of age.

Patients with multiple myofibromas may have *multicentric IM* or *generalized IM*, which often present with scattered cutaneous and subcutaneous tumors (Fig. 9.72) in addition to lytic bony lesions. The multicentric form usually involves lesions limited to skin, subcutaneous tissues, bone, and muscle, whereas the generalized form includes visceral involvement and has a very poor prognosis as a result of visceral dysfunction.[381]

Radiography of IM involving bones classically reveals multiple radiolucent areas in the metaphyseal regions but may also reveal osteopenia, lytic lesions, and fractures.[388,389] Visceral involvement in the generalized form may include lesions in the GI tract, lungs, kidneys, spleen, lymph nodes, meninges, nerves, thyroid, adrenal gland, and heart. Spinal canal involvement has also been reported.[390] Although the lesions do not tend to be locally aggressive or metastasize, their space-occupying nature in some anatomic regions may interfere with vital functions. The differential diagnosis of multiple myofibromas includes hemangiomatosis, juvenile xanthogranulomas, cutaneous metastases (e.g., from neuroblastoma or leukemia), mastocytosis, and sarcomas.

Because the cutaneous and subcutaneous nodules of IM tend to regress spontaneously, surgical excision is typically indicated only for diagnostic confirmation, to alleviate obstruction or potential trauma, or to treat lesions in which the clinical course is prolonged and progressive. Patients with lesions limited to skin and bone have a good prognosis. Those with disseminated multiorgan involvement, especially when including viscera (generalized IM), have a higher incidence of morbidity and mortality. Chemotherapy has been used for patients with severe involvement (and a regimen of low-dose vinblastine and methotrexate has been reported as useful while minimizing chemotherapy-related toxicity); imatinib has been reported for patients with *PDGFRB* mutations.[391,392] Later recurrence of disease in adulthood has been occasionally observed.[384]

FIBROUS HAMARTOMA OF INFANCY

Fibrous hamartoma of infancy is a rare, benign, soft tissue tumor that usually presents during the first 2 years of life. One in four cases is congenital, and around 90% occur within the first year of life.[393] It appears to be more common in boys and has a predilection for the upper trunk, axillae, upper extremities, groin, or genitalia.[394]

Fibrous hamartoma presents as a painless, flesh-colored subcutaneous nodule or nodular plaque (Fig. 9.73). Most cases are solitary, although multiple lesions may occur. They may be mobile or appear to be fixed to underlying tissues. The size of fibrous hamartoma is usually less than 4 to 5 cm, although significantly larger lesions have been reported.[395] The clinical differential diagnosis may include infantile

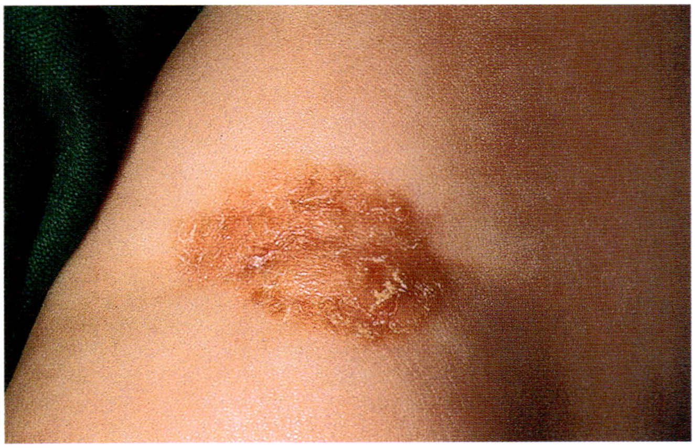

Fig. 9.73 Fibrous hamartoma of infancy.

myofibromatosis (see previous section), calcifying aponeurotic fibroma, fibrolipoma, juvenile hyaline fibromatosis, and malignant soft tissue sarcomas such as fibrosarcoma or rhabdomyosarcoma.[396] The natural history of fibrous hamartoma is characterized by slow growth, although rapid growth of lesions has been reported.[393] Histologic examination of biopsy tissue reveals the characteristic triad of tissues: adipose, fibrous, and myxoid mesenchymal tissue. Up to one-fourth of lesions may histologically mimic an entity called *giant cell fibroblastoma*, and rarely some regions may appear sarcomatous.[397]

The treatment of choice for fibrous hamartoma of infancy is full surgical excision, although for excessively large lesions this may not be a feasible option. Local recurrence may occur in up to 15% of cases and is often noted within a few months after the primary surgery.[398] In lesions left untreated, growth continues until around 5 years of age, at which time it plateaus.[399]

Tumors of Fat, Muscles, and Bone

LIPOMAS

Lipoma, one of the most common benign tumors, is composed of mature fat (adipose) cells. It can be seen at any age but usually occurs at or after puberty. Lesions may be present on any part of the body but predominantly involve the subcutaneous tissues of the neck, shoulders, back, and abdomen. They may be single or multiple, and their size is variable with a characteristic soft, rubbery or putty-like consistency. Microscopic examination reveals encapsulated tumors of adipose tissue with essentially the same appearance as that of normal subcutaneous fat.

A rare nevoid variety, *nevus lipomatosus superficialis* (Fig. 9.74), is characterized by clusters of soft, flesh-colored to yellow-orange papules, nodules, or plaques often located on the buttocks, lumbosacral region, or thighs. These lesions are often present at birth (Fig. 9.75) or develop over the first decade of life. Another lipoma variant, angiolipoma, is clinically indistinguishable except that the lesions are often tender or painful and have a greater tendency to be multiple. Angiolipomas occur primarily in teenagers and young adults and commonly present on the upper extremities or trunk.

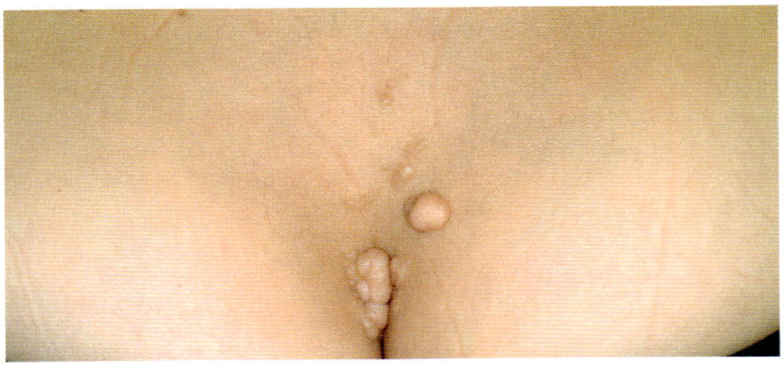

Fig. 9.74 Nevus lipomatosus superficialis. This soft, multilobulated plaque was present at birth in the superior gluteal cleft region.

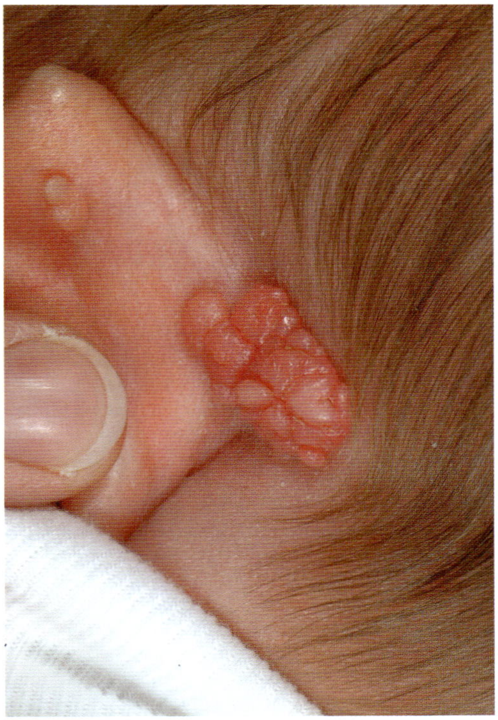

Fig. 9.75 Nevus lipomatosus superficialis. A congenital soft, fleshy, pink to orange plaque in the posterior auricular crease of an infant boy.

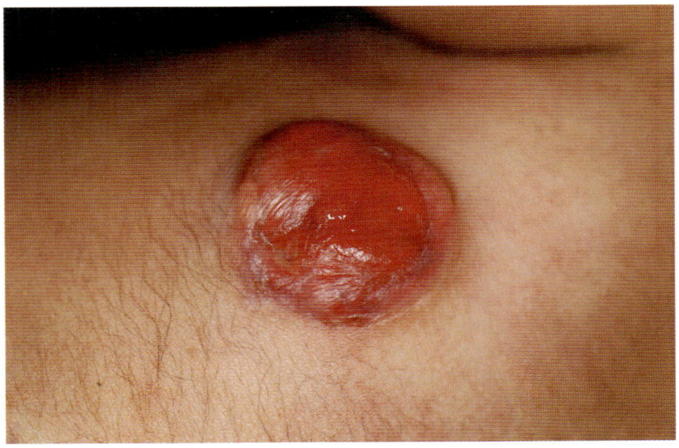

Fig. 9.76 Lipoblastoma. This congenital red tumor on the back developed ulceration and had originally been erroneously diagnosed as an infantile hemangioma. Biopsy results were characteristic of lipoblastoma, and the lesion was completely resected surgically.

Lipoblastoma deserves mention here because it may occasionally mimic the presentation of lipoma or other soft tissue tumors. Lipoblastoma is a benign soft tissue neoplasm seen primarily in infants and young children that is derived from embryonic adipose tissue. The median age at presentation in a review of the literature was 22.6 months.[400] Lipoblastoma presents as a rapidly growing subcutaneous or cutaneous tumor, primarily on the extremities.[401] It may also present as a vascular-appearing mass, which may mimic infantile hemangioma (Fig. 9.76), and the clinical differential diagnosis may also include myofibroma, fibrous hamartoma of infancy, and dermatofibrosarcoma protuberans.[400] Complete surgical excision is the treatment of choice, but recurrence is common. Fortunately, lipoblastomas typically behave in a benign fashion without metastatic spread.

Lipomas and the discussed variants are benign lesions. Surgical excision is generally curative and is indicated for lesions that are painful or of cosmetic significance or for those lesions for which the diagnosis is uncertain (although incisional biopsy is another option in this setting). Three syndromes that have lipomas as a component will be briefly discussed: BRRS, encephalocraniocutaneous lipomatosis, and the Michelin tire baby syndrome.

Bannayan–Riley–Ruvalcaba Syndrome

BRRS, or Bannayan–Zonana syndrome, is an autosomal dominant, multiple hamartoma syndrome caused by mutations in the *PTEN* gene. The hallmark of BRRS is macrocephaly. Patients also have multiple subcutaneous or visceral lipomas and vascular malformations. Pigmented macules of the penis are common. Facial trichilemmomas as described in Cowden syndrome may also be seen, and the same *PTEN* mutations have similarly been described in this syndrome (see earlier this chapter). *PTEN hamartoma tumor syndrome* is the terminology currently used to describe a collection of rare syndromes (including BRRS, Cowden syndrome, and some cases of Proteus syndrome) characterized by germline mutations in this tumor-suppressor gene.[402,403] Other clinical findings in BRRS include oral papillomas, acral (palmoplantar) keratoses, acanthosis nigricans, joint hyperextensibility, scoliosis, pectus excavatum, and downslanting palpebral fissures. Hypotonia, developmental delay, and hamartomatous intestinal polyps may also occur.[284] The latter may result in chronic anemia, diarrhea, failure to thrive, or small bowel intussusception.[404] Careful phenotyping has suggested that BRRS and Cowden syndrome represent one condition with variable expression and age-related penetrance.[405]

Encephalocraniocutaneous Lipomatosis

Encephalocraniocutaneous lipomatosis (ECCL, also known as *Haberland syndrome*) is a rare neurocutaneous syndrome characterized by mental retardation and unilateral skin and ocular lesions with ipsilateral cerebral malformations. The cutaneous lipomas in ECCL are most often limited to the scalp and may be accompanied by alopecia. A smooth, hairless fatty tissue nevus of the scalp is considered a hallmark finding and has been termed *nevus psiloliparus*.[406] Other cutaneous lesions may include skin tags, especially on the eyelids or along a line from the outer canthus to the tragus. Various ocular abnormalities, including eyelid defects, epibulbar or limbal dermoids (also called *choristomas*), scleral desmoid tumors, and corneal clouding, may occur.[407,408] CNS malformations are variable and include intracranial or spinal lipomas (most common), hemisphere asymmetry, cortical dysplasia, cysts, ventricular dilation, calcifications, and corpus callosum abnormalities.[409] Seizures are common and tend to start during infancy, and the developmental status of affected patients is varied, ranging from normal to profoundly delayed.[406,410] MRI of the brain and spine in patients with ECCL may reveal intracranial lipomas (often at the cerebellopontine angle), spinal lipomas, enlarged ventricles, widening of arachnoid spaces, arachnoid cysts, cortical dysplasia, and asymmetric cerebral atrophy.[411] The differential diagnosis includes Proteus syndrome, epidermal nevus (nevus sebaceus) syndrome, oculoectodermal syndrome, and oculocerebrocutaneous syndrome. Mutations in *FGFR1* cause ECCL, and *KRAS* mutation has been reported in one patient (as well as in patients with oculoectodermal syndrome, who have ocular and skin features that overlap with ECCL).[412,413]

Michelin Tire Baby Syndrome

Michelin tire baby syndrome (or *Michelin tire syndrome*) is a term used to describe a very rare disorder of newborns characterized by numerous, conspicuous cutaneous folds (Fig. 9.77), presumably caused by excessive fat. Elastic fiber abnormalities have also been noted on ultrastructural examination of lesional skin (see Chapter 6).[414] The terminology is derived from the resemblance of affected patients to the mascot for the tire manufacturer Michelin. This disorder has also been referred to as *congenital symmetric circumferential skin creases*, and it has been reported in both autosomal dominant and recessive forms.[415] Other histologic abnormalities that have been noted in these patients include nevus lipomatosis and smooth muscle hamartoma. A variety of extracutaneous defects including developmental delay or mental retardation, facial dysmorphism, microcephaly, musculoskeletal anomalies (including rocker-bottom feet, metatarsus abductus, and lax joints), hirsutism, hemiplegia, hemihypertrophy, chromosomal abnormalities, abnormal ears, cardiac and genital anomalies, and neurologic abnormalities may be associated, although there is significant phenotypic variability. Michelin tire baby syndrome may represent a nonspecific clinical presentation related to a variety of different causes.[416] A phenotype consisting of circumferential skin creases in association with cleft palate, dysmorphic facial features, growth delay, and intellectual disability has been termed *circumferential skin creases Kunze type* and has been associated with mutations in the *TUBB* or *MAPRE2* genes.[417] Spontaneous improvement in the numerous folds typically occurs with increasing age.[418]

CONGENITAL SMOOTH MUSCLE HAMARTOMA

Congenital smooth muscle hamartoma is a benign skin disorder characterized by a proliferation of smooth muscle within the reticular dermis. It may be seen within or without an associated Becker nevus (see Pigmented Lesions section). Smooth muscle hamartoma, when presenting independent of Becker nevus, appears as a localized, slightly elevated, flesh-colored to faintly hyperpigmented plaque. The lesions may be extremely subtle on examination, but a useful feature is mild overlying hypertrichosis (Fig. 9.78) that may best be visualized with side lighting using a penlight or otoscope head. Rubbing of the plaque may cause a "pseudo-Darier" sign, with transient piloerection and the appearance of gooseflesh-like surface changes (Fig. 9.79).

Although most lesions are congenital, they may not be noted until childhood or even early adulthood. Smooth muscle hamartoma is nearly always asymptomatic and rarely of cosmetic significance. Surgical excision is curative but rarely necessary.

LEIOMYOMAS

Leiomyomas represent benign tumors principally derived from cutaneous smooth muscle. The majority of these lesions arise from arrector pili muscles, the media of blood vessels, or smooth muscle of the scrotum, labia majora, or nipples. Although found among all age groups, leiomyomas generally occur during the third decade of life and are relatively uncommon in childhood.

Cutaneous leiomyomas may be solitary or multiple and generally present as pink, red, or dusky brown, firm dermal nodules of varying size. They are subject to episodes of paroxysmal spontaneous pain. When multiple, leiomyomas are usually red-brown to blue, firm intradermal nodules (Fig. 9.80) with a translucent or waxy appearance. They tend to occur on the back, face, or extensor surfaces of the extremities and are usually arranged in groups. Enlarging lesions may coalesce to form plaques with an arcuate or linear configuration. Multiple leiomyomas may be associated with common uterine fibroids, an autosomal dominant association termed *multiple cutaneous and uterine leiomyomatosis syndrome* (MCUL, formerly known as *Reed syndrome*). This disorder, as well as another autosomal dominant hereditary leiomyoma syndrome, *hereditary leiomyomatosis and renal cell cancer* (HLRCC), are both caused by heterozygous mutations in the fumarate hydratase *(FH)* gene.[419,420] Earlier-onset (compared with sporadic) uterine leiomyomas, in addition to cutaneous leiomyomas, are seen in patients with HLRCC.[421,422]

Leiomyomas may be classified as hereditary or nonhereditary types and are characterized by unencapsulated tumors of smooth muscle bundles and masses with an irregular arrangement. Cutaneous leiomyomas have been divided into three types:

1. Piloleiomyomas, the most common type, and typically the most painful
2. Solitary genital or mammary leiomyomas, derived from the smooth muscle of the nipple and genital regions (referred to as the *dartoic type*)
3. Angioleiomyomas, arising from the tunica media of the blood vessels and embryonic muscle rests and most often found on the lower leg.

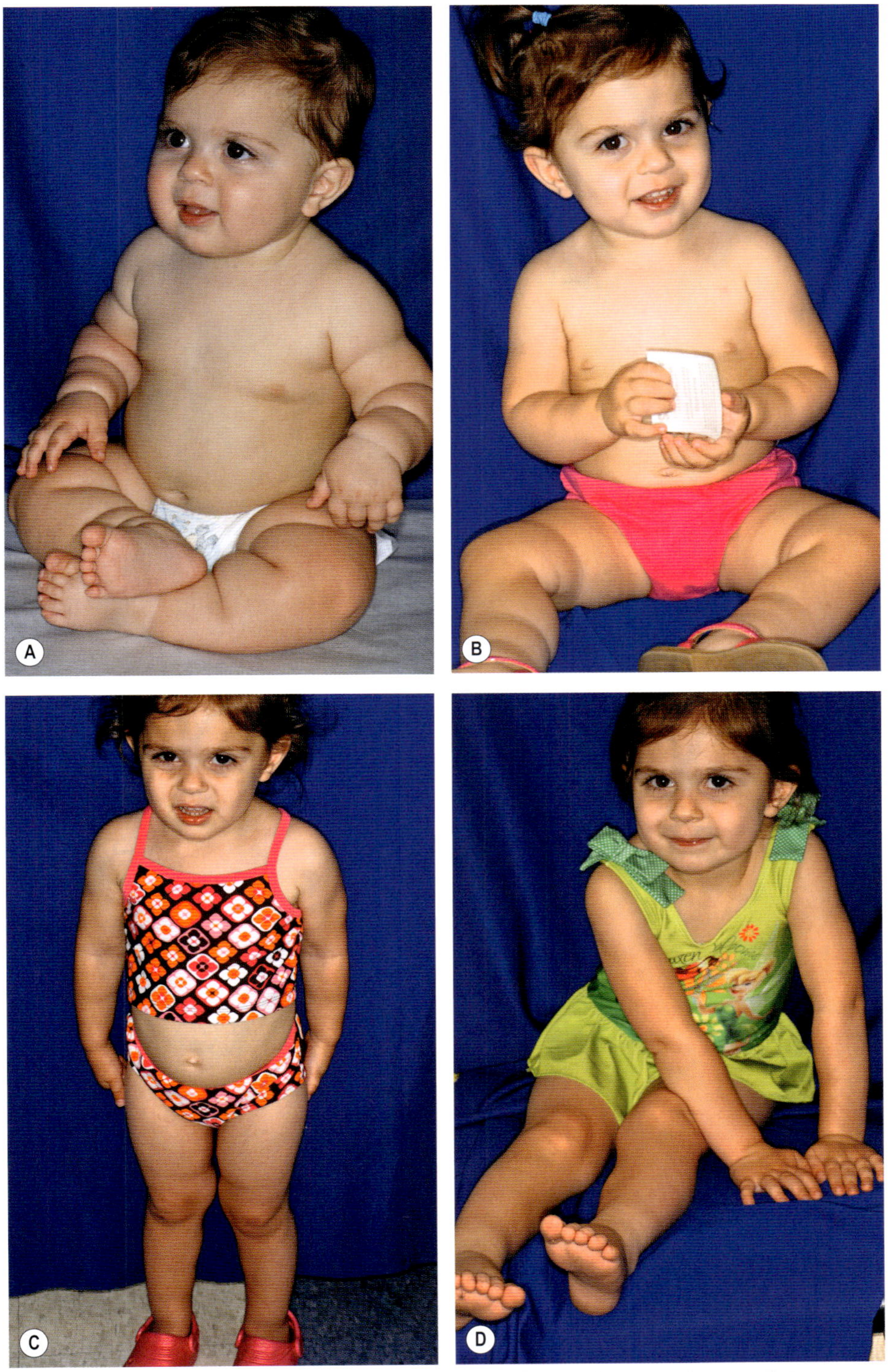

Fig. 9.77 Michelin tire syndrome. This young girl had excess skin folds since early infancy **(A)**, with gradual normalization as she aged **(B–D)**. Her history was otherwise notable only for mild linear growth delay, which also improved.

Leiomyosarcoma, a rare soft tissue sarcoma, occurs primarily in older individuals and may have histologic overlap with leiomyoma. Clinically, these sarcomas are larger than leiomyomas and present as nondescript subcutaneous masses that may enlarge rapidly and ulcerate. Metastases, when they occur, generally spread through the bloodstream and lymphatics, and lung involvement is common. The histologic features most useful in distinguishing these tumors from benign leiomyomas are high cellularity, cytologic atypia, and obvious mitotic figures.

Leiomyomas are benign but have a high incidence of recurrence after removal. Surgical excision is the treatment of choice and is curative for smaller, localized tumors. When multiple leiomyomas are present, therapy is challenging and has included CO_2 laser ablation.

GRANULAR CELL TUMOR

Granular cell tumor (GCT, also known as *myoblastoma*) is an uncommon tumor that occurs most often as a solitary nodule in the head and

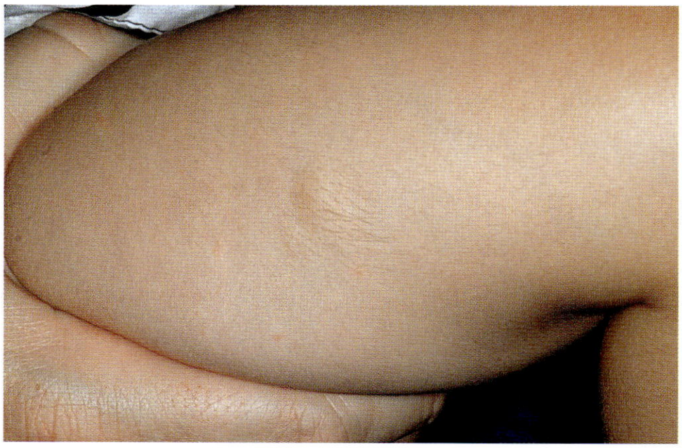

Fig. 9.78 Smooth muscle hamartoma. Note the mild hypertrichosis overlying this flesh-colored, dermal plaque.

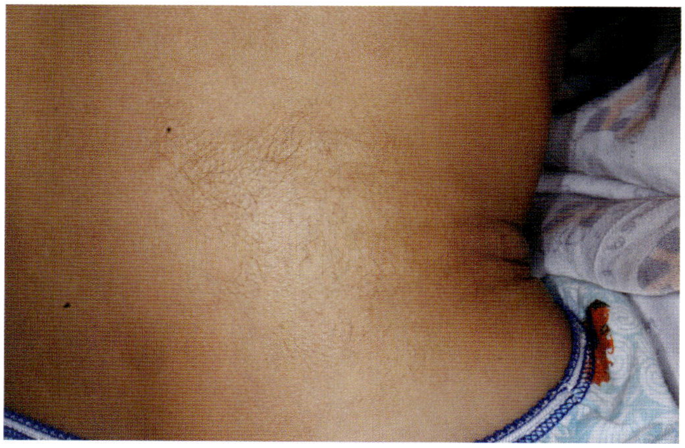

Fig. 9.79 Smooth muscle hamartoma. This plaque on the right flank of this 5-year-old girl was congenital in nature. Note the associated "gooseflesh" appearance and mild surface hypertrichosis.

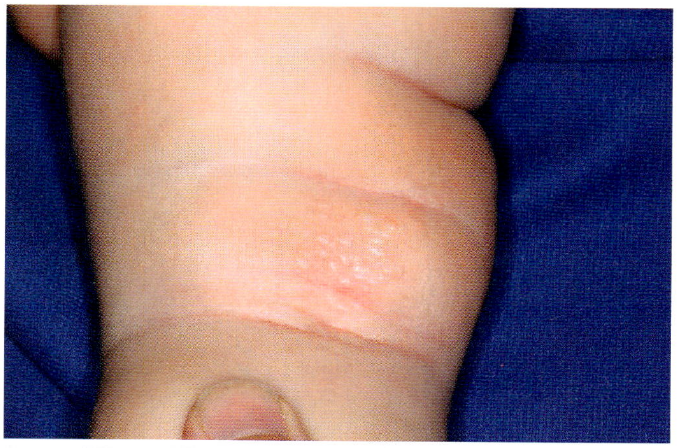

Fig. 9.80 Leiomyomas. This 5-month-old boy had clusters of flesh-colored to pink dermal papules in the popliteal region and the inguinal crease, confirmed on histologic testing to represent piloleiomyomas.

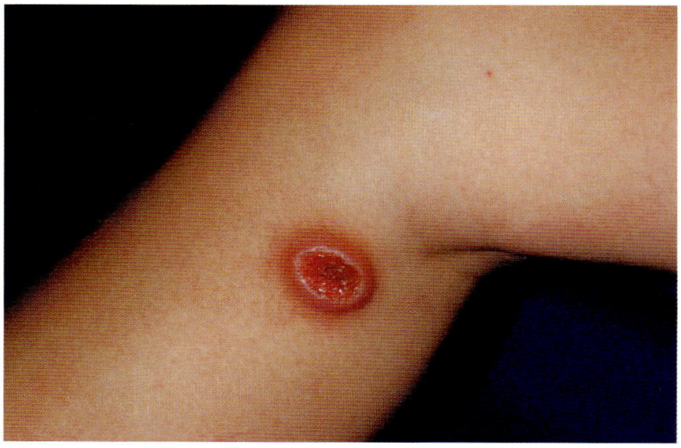

Fig. 9.81 Granular cell tumor. This ulcerated nodule presented on the leg of a 2-year-old girl. Skin biopsy revealed changes consistent with granular cell tumor, and complete resection was performed, without recurrence.

neck regions and especially on the tongue. It is rare overall in children. GCT with ulceration has been reported, including in children, and occurs primarily on the extremities (Fig. 9.81) and in the genital region.[423,424] Laryngeal involvement may occur in the posterior or anterior larynx, vocal folds, and arytenoids.[425] Patients with multiple tumors have been reported, occasionally in association with NF1.[426] Immunohistochemical findings that help to confirm the diagnosis include positive reactions for S100, NSE, CD68, and vimentin. Congenital epulis represents a granular cell tumor of the gingivae in a newborn that is usually marked by spontaneous involution. The origin of granular cell tumors is believed to be neural, with a Schwann cell derivation hypothesized but not proven. Complete surgical excision is the treatment of choice.

CALCINOSIS CUTIS

Calcinosis cutis is a general term for calcium deposition in the skin. It may be related to abnormal calcium or phosphorus metabolism or damage to the dermal collagen, or it may be idiopathic in origin.[427] It may be focal or widespread. Calcinosis cutis has traditionally been divided into the following subtypes: dystrophic, idiopathic, metastatic, and iatrogenic. Tumoral calcinosis is another distinct subtype. Calcinosis occurring in association with some inherited disorders (such as pseudoxanthoma elasticum, Ehlers–Danlos syndrome, and Werner syndrome) is discussed elsewhere.

Dystrophic calcinosis cutis occurs after trauma or inflammation in the skin. This form may also be noted in the setting of diseases that predispose to deposition of calcium in the skin, such as juvenile dermatomyositis (Fig. 9.82; see Chapter 22, Figs. 22.35 and 22.36), scleroderma, and systemic lupus erythematosus. Calcium deposition in the skin may occur years before other stigmata of dermatomyositis become noticeable,[428] although more typically the calcifications occur years after the disease onset. In dystrophic calcinosis cutis, calcium and phosphorus metabolism are normal. Clinically, patients exhibit firm to rock-hard papules or larger subcutaneous plaques. Elbows, knees, and shoulders are common locations. Secondary ulceration and transepidermal elimination of calcium may occur (presenting as white, chalky material protruding from the affected area). In calcinosis universalis, as may be seen in juvenile dermatomyositis, extensive subcutaneous deposits of calcium occur, and patients may appear to have an exoskeleton. This form has a particularly poor prognosis. Patients with the calcinosis cutis, Raynaud phenomenon, esophageal dysfunction, sclerodactyly, and telangiectasia (CREST) variant of scleroderma present with painful, calcified papules and nodules over bony prominences and distal digits (Fig. 9.83). Dystrophic calcinosis cutis can also be seen in the setting of some porphyrias, notably porphyria cutanea tarda, which is rarely encountered in children.[429]

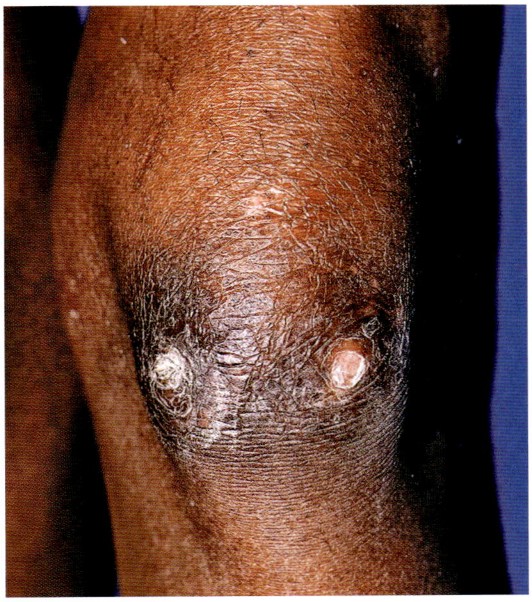

Fig. 9.82 Calcinosis cutis in juvenile dermatomyositis. This patient had painful, firm nodules of both knees and both elbows.

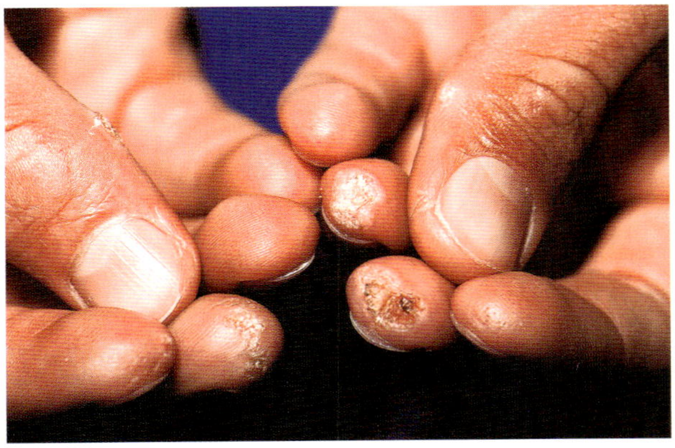

Fig. 9.83 Calcinosis cutis in CREST (calcinosis cutis, Raynaud phenomenon, esophageal dysfunction, sclerodactyly, and telangiectasia) syndrome. Painful, firm deposits with overlying skin breakdown are seen on the distal digits of this teenaged girl with CREST syndrome.

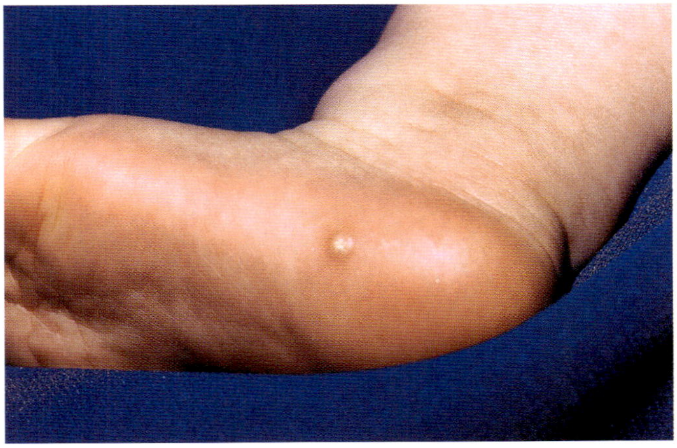

Fig. 9.84 Heel-stick calcinosis cutis. Firm, white papulonodule at the site of prior heel-stick procedures.

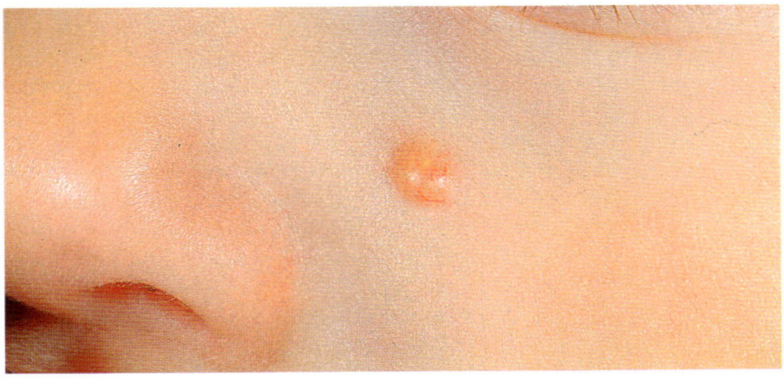

Fig. 9.85 Subepidermal calcified nodule. Solitary, firm, white to flesh-colored papulonodule on the cheek.

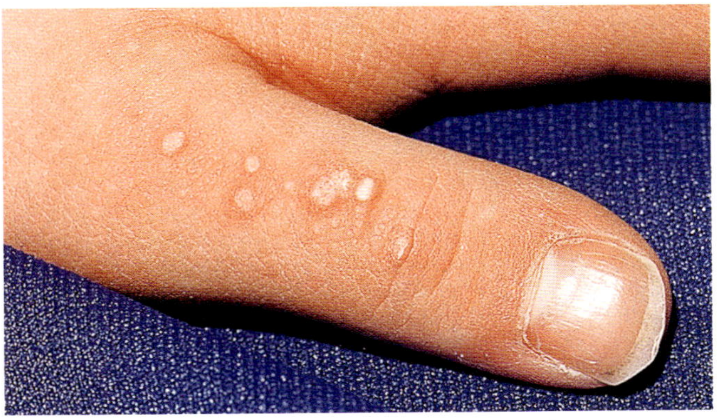

Fig. 9.86 Milia-like idiopathic calcinosis cutis in Down syndrome. These firm, white papules were asymptomatic.

A common setting for dystrophic calcinosis cutis is in infants after heel-stick procedures (*heel-stick calcinosis*; see also Chapter 2). These calcifications appear as firm, white to yellow papules on the heels (Fig. 9.84) and are most often seen in high-risk neonates after multiple needle sticks to these locations.[430] They can also occur in healthy neonates after only a single heel stick.[431]

Idiopathic calcinosis cutis occurs in individuals who have normal calcium and phosphorus metabolism and have no history of trauma or underlying inflammatory diseases. It may occur in various areas of the body, most commonly the scrotum (scrotal calcinosis), face, and female genitalia. Labial calcinosis cutis presents as white papules or nodules on the labia majora and is important to recognize because it may be misdiagnosed as a condition associated with potential sexual abuse (e.g., condylomata or molluscum).[427] A subepidermal calcified nodule is a solitary, white to flesh-colored, firm papule or papulonodule (Fig. 9.85), most commonly occurring in children. These lesions are often seen on the face. Milia-like idiopathic calcinosis cutis presents with small, white papules that may discharge a chalk-like substance. These lesions occur most commonly on the hands (Fig. 9.86) and feet and are usually seen in patients with Down syndrome.[432,433]

Metastatic calcinosis cutis occurs when calcium deposits form in the skin and soft tissue of patients who have altered metabolism of calcium or phosphorus. One association is chronic renal failure, which results in hypocalcemia with resultant secondary hyperparathyroidism with increased mobilization of both calcium and phosphate. Hypervitaminosis D and milk-alkali syndrome are other potential causes of metastatic calcinosis cutis. Calciphylaxis, or calcifying panniculitis, is a severe disorder characterized by vascular calcification with resultant ischemic necrosis of skin and soft tissue. It may result in gangrene and sepsis, and the mortality rate is high.

Tumoral calcinosis presents with calcifications in juxtaarticular sites, predominantly on extensor surfaces. These grow over months to years and often recur after surgical removal.[434] These lesions may attain a fairly large size (up to 20 cm) and may result in disfigurement or impaired function. This disorder may occur sporadically or in an autosomal dominant fashion and usually affects otherwise healthy adolescents.

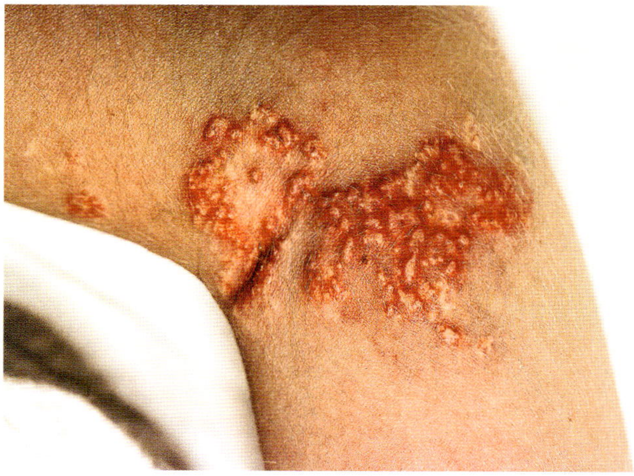

Fig. 9.87 Calcinosis cutis after extravasation injury.

Iatrogenic calcinosis cutis occurs when there is a precipitation of calcium salts in the skin. It most commonly occurs after extravasation of calcium gluconate or calcium chloride. It presents as yellow-white plaques (Fig. 9.87) that often reveal secondary inflammation. Lesions are most commonly (but not always) located around sites of prior intravenous line insertions.[435] Central ulceration may occur. These lesions tend to resolve over 4 to 6 months. Calcinosis cutis has also been reported after application of calcium chloride–containing electrode paste for electroencephalography, electromyography, and brainstem auditory evoked potential recordings.[436]

Treatment of calcinosis cutis is challenging and may include surgical excision, curettage, low calcium and phosphate diet, and administration of aluminum hydroxide, diltiazem, colchicine, or etidronate (a bisphosphonate). Systemic warfarin therapy has been shown to be helpful for small calcified deposits but not with larger or long-standing lesions. Other reported treatments in various settings have included minocycline, ceftriaxone, intravenous immunoglobulin, probenecid, intralesional steroid injection, and CO_2 laser.[437] The underlying disorder, if present, should be treated.

OSTEOMA CUTIS

Cutaneous ossification (bone formation) is a rare phenomenon, especially in children, that may occur in a variety of settings. It may be primary or secondary. The term *osteoma cutis* is nonspecific but has traditionally been used to refer to a primary form of spontaneous bone formation in the skin associated with Albright hereditary osteodystrophy (AHO) or as an isolated idiopathic occurrence. Secondary cutaneous ossification occurs in areas of inflammation or neoplastic tissue and may also be seen in any disorder where calcification is present and in benign skin tumors or cysts.

AHO (see Chapter 23) is a genetic condition that may present with diffuse cutaneous ossification in conjunction with pseudohypoparathyroidism (when hormonal resistance and obesity are present) or pseudo-pseudohypoparathyroidism (when these features are lacking). Classic AHO patients tend to be short and obese with a variety of dysmorphic features, including a classic foreshortening of the fourth and fifth metacarpals and metatarsals.

Progressive osseous heteroplasia (POH) is a rare disorder characterized by progressive ossification of skin, muscle, and connective tissue that may result in significant functional and cosmetic deformity. It usually begins in infancy, tends to be progressive, and may lead to joint ankyloses and growth retardation.[438,439] It can be distinguished from another ossification disorder, *fibrodysplasia ossificans progressiva* (FOP), by the presence of cutaneous ossification, the absence of congenital malformations of the skeleton (especially bilateral great toes, which are characteristic of FOP), the absence of intermittent tumor-like swellings (which begin in the first decade of life in children with FOP), the asymmetric distribution of lesions, and the predominance of intramembranous (seen in POH) rather than endochondral (seen in FOP) ossification.[440,441] Patients with FOP progress to develop an armament-like bony encasement, resulting in marked immobility. In both these disorders, calcium and phosphorus metabolism are normal, in distinction to patients with AHO. The prognosis of FOP is poor, whereas the prognosis of POH is variable. *Plate-like osteoma cutis* (POC) presents in infancy with one or a few areas of cutaneous ossification. These lesions tend to remain fairly localized, and these patients do not have abnormalities in calcium or phosphorus metabolism or other associated defects. The prognosis in POC tends to be good.

As can be seen, disorders of ossification may have a variety of presentations and severities. Several of these disorders may be linked to inactivation in the *GNAS* gene (also known as *GNAS1*), including isolated osteoma cutis, AHO, pseudohypoparathyroidism types 1a, 1b, and 1c, pseudo-pseudohypoparathyroidism, and POH.[442–445] Miliary osteomas of the face present as small, firm, flesh-colored to white or blue papules on the face. They have been observed in patients both with and without a history of acne vulgaris.

SUBUNGUAL EXOSTOSIS

Subungual exostosis is a solitary hard nodule that occurs on the terminal border of the distal phalanx of a finger or toe. Although the great toe tends to be the most commonly afflicted, this disorder may involve other toes or occasionally a finger. However, fifth-toe involvement is unusual.[446] Subungual exostosis is a benign osteochondroma that occurs primarily in the second or third decade of life. Patients may report a history of preceding trauma, although for many this history is lacking.

Subungual exostosis presents as a pink or flesh-colored, 5- to 15-mm exophytic papulonodule that projects from the distal portion of the affected digit (Fig. 9.88, *A*). The surface of the lesion may become hyperkeratotic. Pain is common, and the portion of the nail overlying the lesion may be lifted and in some instances become detached. The differential diagnosis includes wart, pyogenic granuloma, glomus tumor, epidermoid carcinoma, and amelanotic melanoma. The bony consistency on palpation will usually suggest the correct diagnosis, and plain radiography (Fig. 9.88, *B*) can usually confirm it, revealing an exostotic tumor arising from the dorsal aspect of the tip of the distal phalanx.[446]

Surgical excision, with curettage of the base, is the treatment of choice for subungual exostosis. Recurrences happen occasionally.

Miscellaneous

EPIDERMAL CYST

Epidermal cyst (epidermoid cyst, epidermal inclusion cyst) is a discrete, slow-growing nodule that may appear any time after puberty and most commonly occurs on the face, scalp, neck, trunk, or scrotum. This is a true cyst with an epithelial lining. The term *sebaceous cyst* is an antiquated misnomer for this common tumor.

Epidermal cysts present as well-demarcated, firm to slightly compressible nodules, measuring from a few millimeters to several centimeters. An overlying central punctum, through which keratinous, foul-smelling debris may be extruded, is characteristic. Occasionally the lesions become inflamed, but true secondary infection is quite rare. Such inflammation occurs when rupture of the cyst wall occurs, and this is a common scenario prompting a visit to the physician.

Tiny epidermal cysts are termed *milia* (see Chapter 2). These lesions tend to be multiple, 1 to 2 mm in size, and white in color. In addition to occurring sporadically in healthy newborns, they may occur after abrasion trauma to the skin or in the course of bullous disorders such as epidermolysis bullosa and porphyria. Multiple cysts on the scrotum may occur and occasionally result in calcinosis cutis (see Calcinosis Cutis section). Pilar cysts (trichilemmal cysts, wens) are epidermal cysts that occur on the scalp, and chalazions represent analogous cystic tumors of the eyelids that develop from meibomian glands.

An important association with multiple epidermal cysts is Gardner syndrome. This autosomal dominant condition is characterized by cutaneous cysts and intestinal polyposis. Gardner syndrome is a form

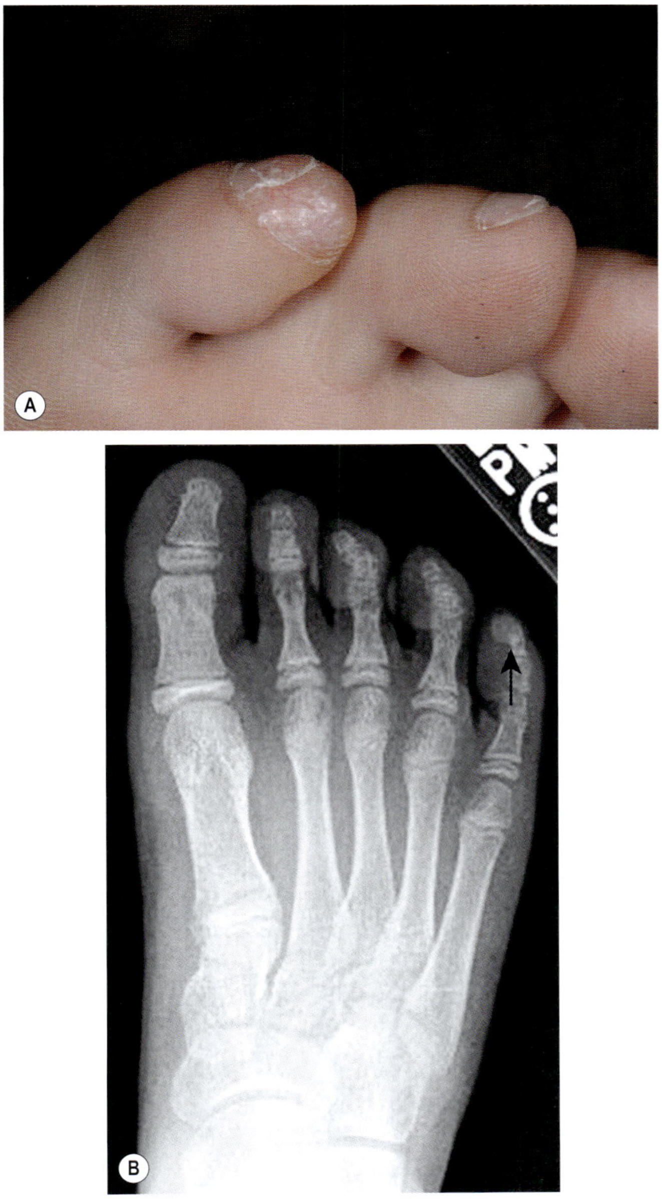

Fig. 9.88 Subungual exostosis. **(A)** This rock-hard nodule of the distal fifth digit was painful. **(B)** Radiographic evaluation revealed a well-demarcated bony projection projecting off the tip of the affected phalanx *(arrow)*. Surgical excision was curative, with histologic testing revealing trabecular bone with a cartilage cap, consistent with osteochondroma.

of *familial adenomatous polyposis* (FAP), an inherited colorectal cancer syndrome characterized by hundreds of adenomas involving the large bowel with progression (if untreated) to colorectal cancer by the fourth decade.[447,448] The term *Gardner syndrome* is used to describe the colonic manifestations of FAP in association with several extracolonic manifestations, but genotype-phenotype correlation studies have led some to suggest that the term is obsolete.[448,449] The epidermal cysts in Gardner syndrome, which are the most common cutaneous manifestation, are usually multiple, often present during early childhood, and can occur in any location, although they tend to occur most often on the face, scalp, and extremities. Multiple pilomatricomas may also be seen in patients with Gardner syndrome.[438] Other findings include

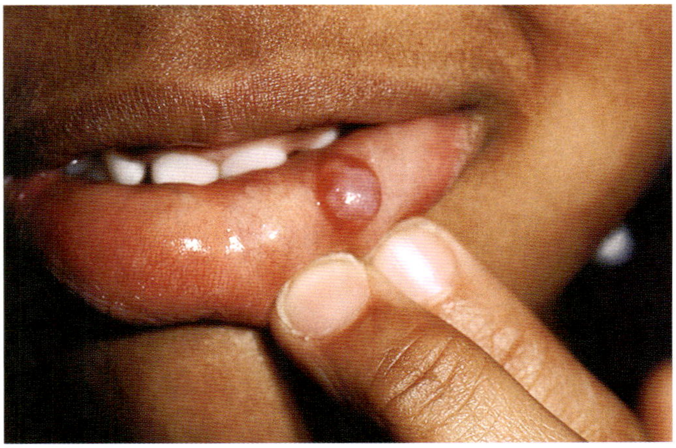

Fig. 9.89 Oral mucocele. This lesion was ultimately excised because of continued enlargement.

desmoid tumors (the second leading cause of mortality, following metastatic colorectal cancer), osteomas, fibromas, lipomas, abnormal dentition, thyroid tumors (especially papillary thyroid carcinoma), and congenital hypertrophy of the retinal pigment epithelium (CHRPE).[450,451] The latter finding is often present at birth or during early infancy, is seen in up to 90% of FAP patients, and as such usually precedes the development of intestinal polyposis.[447] Hepatoblastoma, a rare pediatric liver tumor, also occurs with increased frequency in these patients.[452] Both FAP and Gardner syndrome have been mapped to *APC*, a tumor suppressor gene.[447,448,453]

Malignant degeneration (squamous cell or BCC) of epidermal and pilar cysts is rarely reported. Treatment consists of surgical excision with an attempt to remove the entire epithelial lining of the cyst to minimize the chance of recurrence.

MUCOCELE (MUCOUS CYST)

Mucoceles (mucous cysts of the oral mucosa) present as soft, white to blue, solitary asymptomatic lesions, usually on the mucous surface of the lower lip and occasionally on the gingivae, tongue, or buccal mucosa. They are usually less than 1 cm in diameter and translucent (Fig. 9.89), containing a clear viscous fluid. In a review of 56 pediatric patients with mucoceles, the most common intraoral sites of involvement were the lower lip, tongue, and floor of mouth.[454] Mucoceles are the result of minor trauma, causing rupture of a mucous duct and extravasation of sialomucin into the tissues. Treatment options include surgical excision, incision, and drainage followed by coagulation of the sac, CO_2 laser ablation, or cryosurgery. Occasionally lesions may rupture spontaneously, although this is usually followed by eventual recurrence.

CONGENITAL LINGUAL MELANOTIC MACULE

Melanotic macules of the oral mucosae include oral and labial melanotic macules, which are most often seen in young and middle-aged adults. The congenital lingual melanotic macule presents as a well-circumscribed, hyperpigmented macule (or macules) on the dorsal tongue (Fig. 9.90). Histopathologic evaluation reveals increased basal layer melanin with some pigment-laden macrophages but normal melanocyte number and no nests of melanocytes, as would be expected in a congenital melanocytic nevus.[455] However, given the location and challenge in performing a tongue biopsy, most suggest close clinical follow-up, with consideration for biopsy only if significant changes occur.[456,457] These lesions tend to grow proportionately with the child, and in some cases lightening may be noted with aging.[458]

DIGITAL MUCOUS CYST

Digital mucous cyst (myxoid cyst) is a focal accumulation of mucin that presents as a soft, translucent, pink to blue, dome-shaped nodule

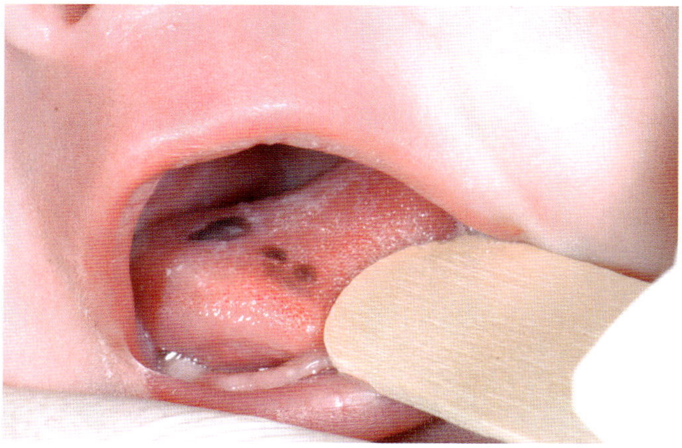

Fig. 9.90 Congenital lingual melanotic macule. These dark brown macules on the dorsal tongue were congenital in onset for this 7-week-old healthy boy.

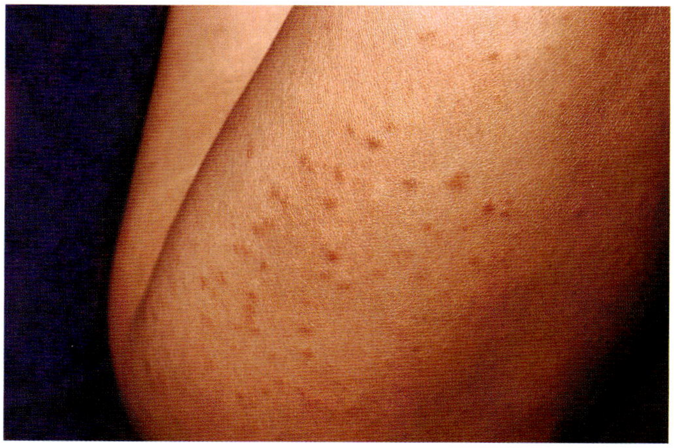

Fig. 9.91 Steatocystoma multiplex. Yellow-tan, small papules of the forearm in this patient who also had lesions on the chest.

on the dorsal aspect of the distal interphalangeal joint or proximal nailfold. Occasionally the overlying nail plate reveals a longitudinal depression distal to the cyst. There is controversy over whether these lesions arise from degenerative changes or as a direct extension from the underlying joint space. Regardless, there appears to be a metabolic derangement of fibroblasts with increased production of hyaluronic acid in sites exposed to friction or minor trauma. In some patients there may be a communication between the cyst and the underlying joint space.

Surgical excision is usually effective, but recurrences are common. Other therapeutic options include corticosteroid injection, cryosurgery, repeated incision and drainage, sclerosing therapy, and CO_2 laser ablation.[459–462]

STEATOCYSTOMA MULTIPLEX

Steatocystoma multiplex (SM) is a disorder characterized by numerous, 2- to 4-mm moderately firm, yellow to flesh-colored cutaneous cysts located primarily on the chest and occasionally the face, genitals, arms (Fig. 9.91), and thighs. The disorder has a high familial tendency and is often inherited in an autosomal dominant fashion. Lesions often appear or become larger around the time of puberty. In some patients there may be overlap with eruptive vellus hair cysts (see Chapter 7), and both conditions seem to originate from the pilosebaceous duct.[463] SM may also occur in association with pachyonychia congenita (see Chapter 7), and both conditions may be caused by mutations in keratin 17.[464,465] In addition, persistent infantile milia at times may be associated with both SM and eruptive vellus hair cysts and may represent a disorder with predisposition to multiple pilosebaceous cystic lesions.[466]

The lesions of SM are rarely symptomatic but occasionally may be of cosmetic concern to the patient. Treatment can be accomplished with surgical excision or cyst puncture with evacuation of the contents. Other reported approaches include CO_2 laser therapy, oral isotretinoin, and cryotherapy.[467]

CLEAR CELL PAPULOSIS

Clear cell papulosis (CCP) is a rare entity that occurs primarily in children (typically younger than 5 years of age) and presents with asymptomatic hypopigmented macules and flat papules, which may range in number from a few to more than 100. The lesions are most commonly distributed over the lower abdomen and along the embryologic milk line. A patient with exclusive involvement of the lower extremities has been reported.[468] CCP was originally reported in 1987 by Kuo et al.[469] in two young brothers. The differential diagnosis may include anetoderma, scars, postinflammatory hypopigmentation, vitiligo, hypopigmented macules of tuberous sclerosis, pigmentary mosaicism, flat warts, pityriasis lichenoides chronica, idiopathic guttate hypomelanosis, hypopigmented cutaneous T-cell lymphoma, and progressive macular hypomelanosis.[470,471] Histologically benign–appearing clear cells are found in the epidermis, especially along the basal layer, and stain positive for GCDFP-15, a glycoprotein found in breast cystic disease fluid.[472] They may also stain positive for cytokeratin, carcinoembryonic antigen, mucin, and epithelial membrane antigen.[473,474] The cells are felt to be analogous to Toker clear cells of the nipple, which may be seen in up to 83% of normal nipples at autopsy.[475] Because Paget cells are also typically positive for several of the same immunohistochemical stains, several recommend surveillance to ensure that CCP is not a precursor of primary intraepidermal or extramammary Paget disease.[473] Treatment is not typically recommended for CCP, given its asymptomatic nature and the spontaneous resolution that occurs in the majority of patients (seen in 85% of patients in one large series with a median follow-up duration of 11.5 years).[471]

KELOID

Keloids, which are benign dermal tumors characterized by invasive growth of fibroblasts and increased synthesis of collagen, represent an exaggerated connective tissue response to skin injury. They are rare in infancy, and their incidence increases throughout childhood, reaching a maximum between puberty and 30 years of age. Black individuals and other darkly pigmented persons are more susceptible to keloids than individuals with fair skin, and the tendency toward keloid formation often runs in families.

Early lesions are pink, smooth, and rubbery (Fig. 9.92) and may be tender. With increasing age, keloids become less erythematous, more pigmented (Fig. 9.93), and firmer to palpation. Although they may occur anywhere on the skin surface, keloids are most common on the earlobes, upper chest, and back and in wounds located in areas under tension. In a series of 40 pediatric keloids, the head (especially the earlobe) and neck regions were most commonly affected.[476] As opposed to hypertrophic scars, keloids often persist at the site of injury, often recur after excision, and always overgrow the original boundaries of the wound.[477]

Treatment of keloids is notoriously difficult and often ineffective. In fact, lesions not uncommonly become larger after attempts at therapy. Regardless, these lesions are a source of much psychosocial anxiety and suffering for patients, and hence therapy is often attempted. Intralesional injection of corticosteroid (usually triamcinolone acetonide) is the most commonly used treatment and often requires multiple injections. This therapy is most effective for smaller lesions. Surgery is generally not recommended, given the propensity for lesions to recur or even worsen, but it is often used given the lack of other consistently effective therapies. It is often combined with adjunctive therapies such as steroid injections, silicone sheeting, and compression. Keloid core

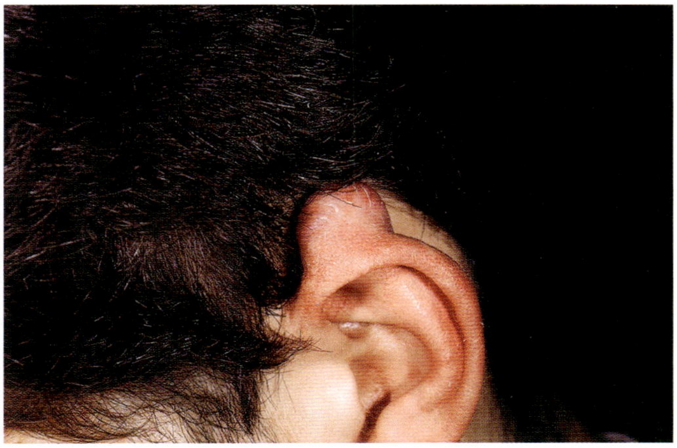

Fig. 9.92 Keloid. This early lesion is erythematous and only slightly firm to palpation.

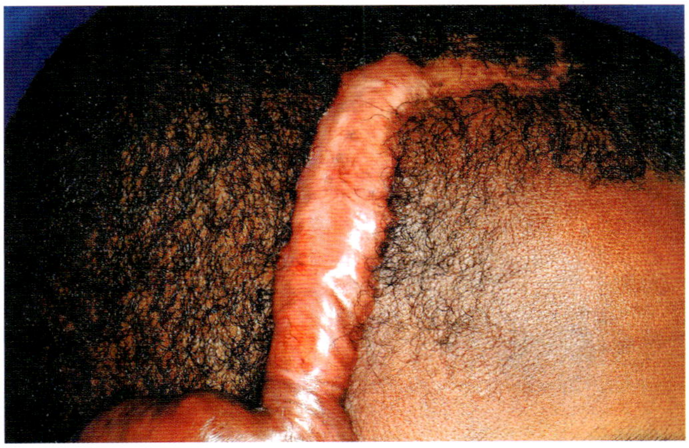

Fig. 9.93 Keloid. This older keloid is very firm and hyperpigmented; it had recurred after an initial attempt at surgical removal.

extirpation, a surgical approach involving excision of the inner core followed by a keloid rind flap, may be a more effective approach.[477] Other therapeutic options, each used with varying levels of success, include radiotherapy; pulsed dye, argon, or CO_2 laser therapy; and intralesional injections of bleomycin, interferon, mitomycin C (usually topically applied), or fluorouracil. Silicone gel and silicone sheeting have been used with variable success to treat both keloids and hypertrophic scars, but their mechanism of action remains unclear. It appears that the increased wound hydration that occurs with occlusive therapies may prompt keratinocytes to alter growth factor secretion and thereby may affect fibroblast regulation.[478] Several authorities, including a multidisciplinary expert group, recommend silicone products as the gold standard, first-line therapy.[479] Intralesional verapamil injections and topical imiquimod cream have also been used in combination with surgical excision.[478,480] Compression therapy via the use of compression garments may be helpful but can be difficult in terms of patient adherence and tolerability.[481] Targeted therapies directed at components of the fibrosis cascade are being studied and offer hope of newer treatment options once translated for clinical practice.[482]

The complete list of 482 references for this chapter is available online at http://expertconsult.inkling.com.

Key References

Scope A, Marchette MA, Marghoob AA, et al. The study of nevi in children: principles learned and implications for melanoma diagnosis. J Am Acad Dermatol 2016;75:813–23.

Souta E, Eliades PJ, Shannon K, et al. Hereditary melanoma: update on syndromes and management. J Am Acad Dermatol 2016;74:395–407.

Lorimer PD, White RL, Walsh K, et al. Pediatric and adolescent melanoma: a National Cancer Data Base update. Ann Surg Oncol 2016;23:4058–66.

Asch S, Sugarman JL. Epidermal nevus syndromes: new insights into whorls and swirls. Pediatr Dermatol 2018;35:21–9.

Hansen-Kiss E, Beinkampen S, Adler B, et al. A retrospective chart review of the features of PTEN hamartoma tumour syndrome in children. J Med Genet 2017;54(7):471–8.

Schena D, Galvan A, Tessari G, et al. Clinical features and course of cutaneous mastocytosis in 133 children. Br J Dermatol 2016;174(2):411–13.

Krengel S, Scope A, Dusza SW, et al. New recommendations for the categorization of cutaneous features of congenital melanocytic nevi. J Am Acad Dermatol 2013;68:441–51.

Alikhan A, Ibrahimi OA, Eisen DB. Congenital melanocytic nevi: where are we now? Part I. Clinical presentation, epidemiology, pathogenesis, histology, malignant transformation, and neurocutaneous melanosis. J Am Acad Dermatol 2012;67:495.e1–17.

Ibrahimi OA, Alikhan A, Eisen DB. Congenital melanocytic nevi: where are we now? Part II. Treatment options and approach to treatment. J Am Acad Dermatol 2012;67(4):515.e1–13.

Marghoob AA, Agero ALC, Benvenuto-Andrade C, et al. Large congenital melanocytic nevi, risk of cutaneous melanoma, and prophylactic surgery. J Am Acad Dermatol 2006;54(5):868–70.

Neier M, Pappo A, Navid F. Management of melanomas in children and young adults. J Pediatr Hematol Oncol 2012;34(2):S51–4.

Sugarman JL. Epidermal nevus syndromes. Semin Cutan Med Surg 2007;26:221–30.

Efron PA, Chen MK, Glavin FL, et al. Pediatric basal cell carcinoma: case reports and literature review. J Pediatr Surg 2008;43:2277–80.

Briley LD, Phillips CM. Cutaneous mastocytosis: a review focusing on the pediatric population. Clin Pediatr 2008;47(8):757–61.

10 Histiocytoses and Malignant Skin Diseases

CHAPTER OUTLINE

The histiocytoses are a broad group of disorders characterized by an abnormal proliferation of the histiocyte, a type of progenitor cell in the bone marrow (Box 10.1).[1] Some clinically relevant types of histiocytes include the Langerhans cell, the dermal dendrocyte, and cells of mononuclear cell/macrophage lineage. Several histiocytoses are discussed in this chapter. Malignant disorders to be discussed include hematologic malignancies (including leukemia, lymphoma, and Hodgkin disease), neuroblastoma, and some sarcomas.

Langerhans Cell Histiocytosis

Langerhans cell histiocytosis (LCH) is the term used to describe a disorder characterized by infiltration of Langerhans cells into various organs of the body. Older synonymous terms, which are now largely obsolete or unnecessary, include histiocytosis X, eosinophilic granuloma, Letterer–Siwe disease, Hand–Schüller–Christian disease, and Hashimoto–Pritzker disease.[2] The term *histiocytosis X* was coined by Lichtenstein in 1953 to identify three related clinical entities of unknown etiology and characterized by histiocyte proliferation.[3] This classification included the triad of Letterer–Siwe disease, Hand–Schüller–Christian disease, and eosinophilic granuloma. The *X* in this original nomenclature was used to denote the unknown derivation of the histiocyte involved in this disorder. Ultrastructural studies eventually confirmed the relationship of these three different presentations by showing the Langerhans cell to be the proliferative cell in each of them. LCH may occur at any age, from newborn to elderly, although the peak incidence appears to be between the ages of 1 and 4 years.[4]

Normal Langerhans cells are derived from the bone marrow and are a type of dendritic cell found primarily in the epidermis (as well as mucosal epithelia, thymus, esophagus, and lung). They are involved in antigen presentation for the skin- and mucosa-associated immune systems and are identified by strong staining with S100 (a neuronal protein) and cluster designation (CD) la (a cell surface marker). Langerhans cells also have a characteristic organelle, the Birbeck granule, which is visible on electron microscopy. The function of this organelle remains unknown. Immunohistochemical demonstration of Langerin (CD207), a mannose-specific lectin found in association with Birbeck granules, has also been demonstrated useful for diagnostic confirmation of LCH.[5] The pathologic cells in LCH share phenotypic and immunohistochemical features with normal Langerhans cells, but are derived from immature myeloid precursors.[6]

Although numerous etiologies have been proposed for LCH, the pathogenesis remains obscure. Hypothetic causes include somatic mutations, infection (especially viral), immune or cytokine dysregulation, and programmed cell death (apoptosis).[4–8] Whether LCH is a neoplastic versus a reactive disorder also remains debated. The cells in LCH have been demonstrated to be clonal, and such monoclonality has been demonstrated both in multisystem disease and with solitary organ involvement. Although this clonality suggests that LCH may be a neoplastic process with variable biologic behavior, the exact significance and implications remain controversial.[4,5] There are arguments both in favor of and against LCH being a neoplastic process.[9] Mutations in *BRAF-V600E* have been identified in around 40% to 70% of neoplastic cells from biopsy tissues in various series[10,11] and have been associated with higher-risk features and poorer response to first-line therapy.[12] Other reported mutations have included *MAP2K1*, *MAP3K1*, and *ARAF*.[6,13]

LCH may involve multiple organ systems, the most common being the skin and the bones. Table 10.1 lists the spectrum of organ involvement. The older classification system was based on the involved organ systems such that *eosinophilic granuloma* referred to localized bone disease; *Hand–Schüller–Christian disease* the multifocal triad of bone (usually skull) lesions, exophthalmos, and diabetes insipidus (DI); and *Letterer–Siwe disease*, the acute or subacute disseminated form of the disease. Under the more modern classification, LCH is the umbrella term for the disease, with notation made of the various organ systems involved. Patients may have unifocal, multifocal, or disseminated disease. In general, patients with widespread, multiorgan involvement have the poorest prognosis and those with isolated bone LCH have the best prognosis.[14] Although skin-isolated disease does occur, it is relatively uncommon, and more often skin involvement is suggestive of concomitant or future multisystem disease. Organ involvement considered to portend higher risk includes the liver, spleen, and bone marrow.

Cutaneous involvement is quite common in LCH (second only to bone) and is often the presenting complaint. The spectrum of skin findings is listed in Table 10.2. The most classic presentation is that of a seborrheic dermatitis–like eruption with prominent involvement of the scalp, posterior auricular regions (Fig. 10.1), perineum, and axillae. The rash tends to be resistant to standard therapy, which is an important clue that should prompt consideration of the diagnosis. Erythematous, red-brown papules are often seen, especially on the scalp and in flexural areas, and may have secondary erosion, hemorrhage, or crusting (Figs. 10.2 and 10.3). Crusted papules on the palms and/or soles (Fig. 10.4) are another important feature, especially in infants in whom the diagnosis of scabies has been excluded. Although this finding has traditionally been felt to portend a poor prognosis, this observation has not been validated.

In neonates with LCH, vesiculopustular lesions (Figs. 10.5 and 10.6) tend to predominate and may be misdiagnosed as congenital varicella or herpes.[15] These lesions may become hemorrhagic or crusted. Petechiae and hemorrhage may also be present in association with the dermatitis or the papular lesions of LCH, and they may be seen both with and without associated thrombocytopenia. Other less commonly seen cutaneous presentations include nodules (especially

Box 10.1 Contemporary Classification of Histiocytoses

Langerhans (L group)

Langerhans cell histiocytosis (LCH)
Indeterminate cell histiocytosis (ICH)
Erdheim–Chester disease (ECD)
Mixed LCH/ECD

Cutaneous and mucocutaneous (C group)

Cutaneous:
- Juvenile/adult xanthogranuloma (JXG/AXG)
- Solitary reticulohistiocytoma (SRH)
- Benign cephalic histiocytosis (BCH)
- Generalized eruptive histiocytosis (GEH)
- Progressive nodular histiocytosis (PNH)
- Cutaneous Rosai–Dorfman disease (RDD)
- Necrobiotic xanthogranuloma (NXG)
- Cutaneous histiocytoses not otherwise specified

Cutaneous with major systemic component:
- Xanthoma disseminatum (XD)
- Multicentric reticulohistiocytosis (MRH)

Rosai–Dorfman disease and miscellaneous non-LCH histiocytoses (R group)

Rosai–Dorfman disease (RDD)
Other non-classified histiocytoses

Malignant group (M group)

Primary malignant histiocytoses (MH)
Secondary malignant histiocytoses (MH)
- Secondary to:
- Follicular lymphoma
- Lymphocytic leukemia/lymphoma
- Hairy cell leukemia
- Acute lymphoblastic leukemia
- Histiocytosis or other hematologic neoplasia

Hemophagocytic lymphohistiocytosis and macrophage activation syndrome (H group)

Primary hemophagocytic lymphohistiocytosis (HLH)
Secondary HLH
- Secondary to:
- Infection
- Malignancy
- Rheumatologic conditions (includes macrophage activation syndrome, MAS)
- Other causes

Adapted from Emile JF, Abla O, Fraitag S, et al. Revised classification of histiocytoses and neoplasms of the macrophage-dendritic cell lineages. *Blood* 2016;127(22): 2672–81.

the congenital "skin-limited" presentation seen in some neonates) (Fig. 10.7) and granulomatous, ulcerative lesions.[16] Box 10.2 lists some cutaneous clues to the diagnosis of LCH.

Mucosal involvement may occur in patients with LCH, especially those with more disseminated involvement. Gingival erythema, erosions, and hemorrhage may be seen. In some infants, gingival and oral mucosal erosions with premature eruption of teeth (Fig. 10.8) may be the initial manifestations of LCH.[17] Loosening of the teeth may occur as a result of severe gingivitis, especially when there is concomitant bony involvement of the alveolar ridge and jaw. Involvement of the external auditory canals may result in chronic otitis externa.

Bone lesions are very common in patients with LCH, and when occurring in the setting of multisystem disease with high-risk organ involvement, may portend a better prognosis.[18] When they occur, pain (with or without swelling) is the most common presenting complaint, and patients may complain of discomfort both during activity and when at rest.[14] Bony involvement occurs most commonly in the skull, followed by the long bones of the extremities and the flat bones (pelvis, vertebrae, ribs). Radiographic studies usually reveal single or multiple lytic lesions of bone (Fig. 10.9) that often have a "punched-out" appearance.[17] Proptosis may result from orbital wall involvement, and the radiographic appearance may simulate mastoiditis when there is involvement of the mastoid process.[4] Middle-ear extension may cause destructive changes with resultant deafness, and chronic otitis media may also occur as a result of mastoid and temporal bone disease. Vertebral body involvement may result in compression with the radiographic finding of vertebra plana (Fig. 10.10). Plain radiographs are usually sufficient for diagnosing bony LCH, but computed tomography (CT), magnetic resonance imaging (MRI), and technetium (Tc)-99

Table 10.1 Organ Involvement in Langerhans Cell Histiocytosis

Organ	Comment
Skin	Often the initial presenting sign; often suggestive of multisystem disease
Bone	Painful swelling common; most commonly unifocal; incidence: skull > long bones > flat bones (ribs, pelvis, vertebrae); may mimic multiple myeloma on imaging
Lymph nodes	Cervical most common
Liver	Considered "risk organ"
Spleen	Considered "risk organ"
Lungs	Diffuse micronodular pattern on radiography
Gastrointestinal tract	
Thymus	
Bone marrow	Considered "risk organ"; pancytopenia portends a poor prognosis
Gingivae, buccal mucosa	Swelling, erythema, erosions, petechiae
Kidney	
Endocrine glands	Diabetes insipidus (pituitary involvement) most common
Central nervous system, excluding pituitary gland	

Table 10.2 Cutaneous Manifestations of Langerhans Cell Histiocytosis

Presentation	Comment
Scaly red-brown papules	Especially in scalp, flexural areas; may have associated crusting; may be umbilicated or lichenoid; palm and sole involvement common
Erythematous, scaly dermatitis	May simulate seborrheic dermatitis
Erosion or ulceration	Common secondary finding, especially in fold areas and in mucosal sites (oral, genital mucosae)
Petechiae, hemorrhage	With or without associated thrombocytopenia
Vesiculopustular lesions	Most common in neonates; may simulate congenital varicella or herpes; often have hemorrhagic crusts
Red nodules or plaques	Less common
Granulomatous plaques	Rare
Nail involvement	Rare; may include pustules, hemorrhage, nail plate grooves, paronychia, pitting

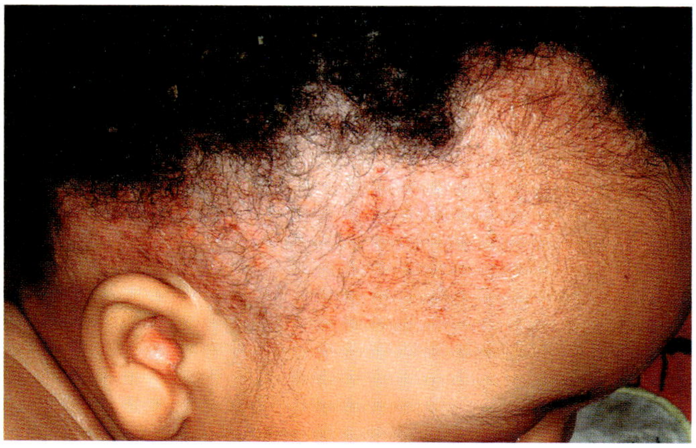

Fig. 10.1 Langerhans cell histiocytosis. Erythematous, crusted papules and plaques, with accentuation in the posterior auricular scalp.

bone scans may also be useful, especially in the setting of multifocal osseous disease.[19]

The classic triad (historically Hand–Schüller–Christian disease) of skull lesions, DI, and exophthalmos is the prototype for multifocal LCH, but many other organs may be involved in this setting. Disseminated LCH (historically Letterer–Siwe disease) is the most serious form of the disorder, differing only in extent and severity from multifocal involvement.[17] Lymph node involvement may be seen with localized or widespread LCH, and most often the cervical nodes are involved. Hepatosplenomegaly, biliary cirrhosis, and liver dysfunction may occur. Pulmonary LCH may present with cough, hemoptysis, dyspnea, or pain and is most common in the third decade of life.[4] Pulmonary involvement may also be asymptomatic, especially in younger children. Chest radiography reveals a diffuse micronodular or reticular pattern, and pneumothoraces may result. Gastrointestinal tract involvement may present as anorexia, malabsorption, vomiting, diarrhea, and failure to thrive. However, gastrointestinal involvement may be asymptomatic and thus is at times overlooked. Thymus abnormalities have been reported and may present with enlargement of the gland on chest radiography. Bone marrow involvement may result in pancytopenia, and concomitant hypersplenism may contribute to

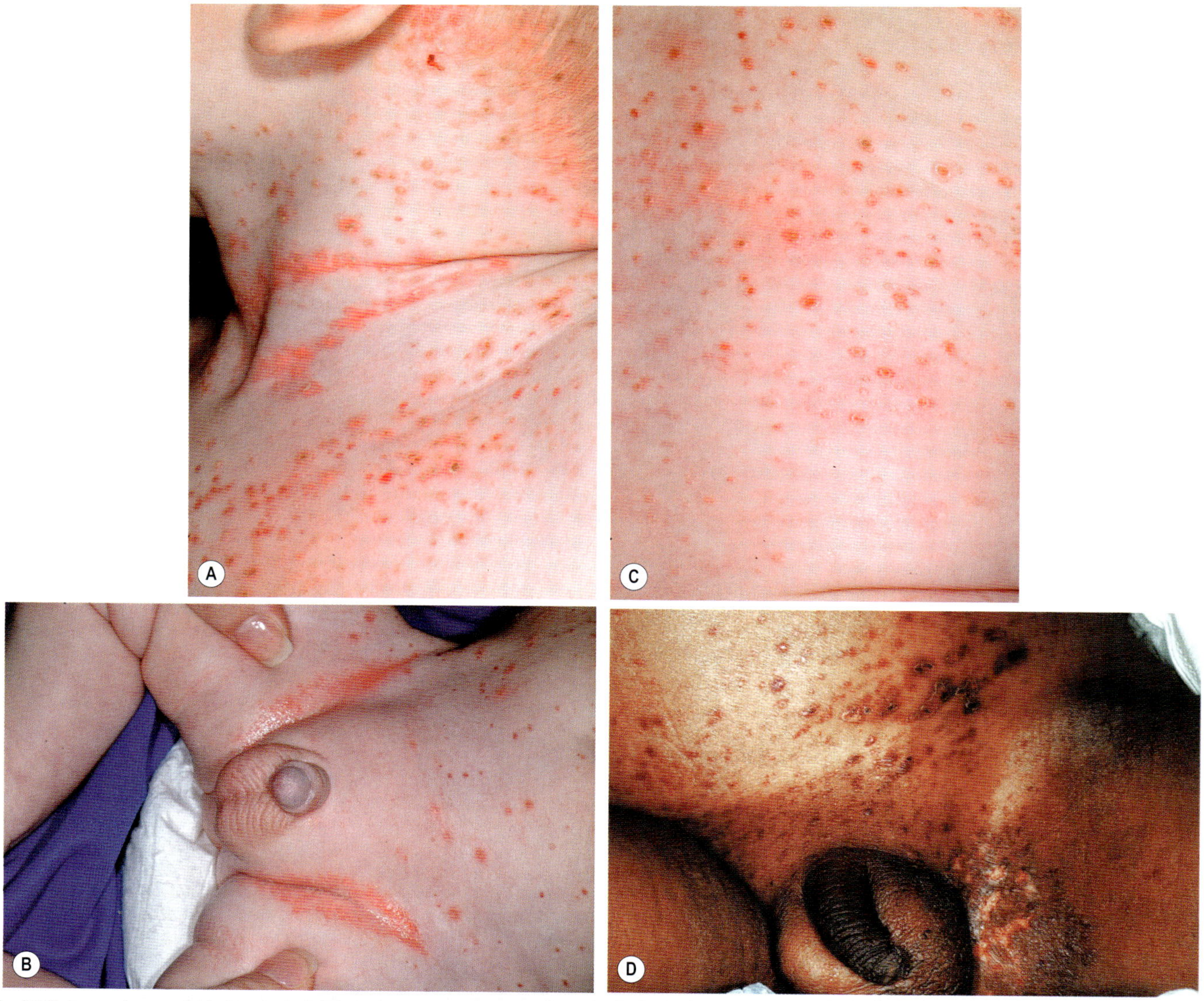

Fig. 10.2 Langerhans cell histiocytosis (LCH). **(A–C)** Erythematous and eroded papules in the neck fold, inguinal creases, and over the trunk. Note the associated crusting, purpura, and umbilicated nature of some of the papules. **(D)** Eroded, erythematous, and hemorrhagic papules in the groin of this infant with disseminated LCH. Note the associated jaundiced appearance, a result of massive liver involvement.

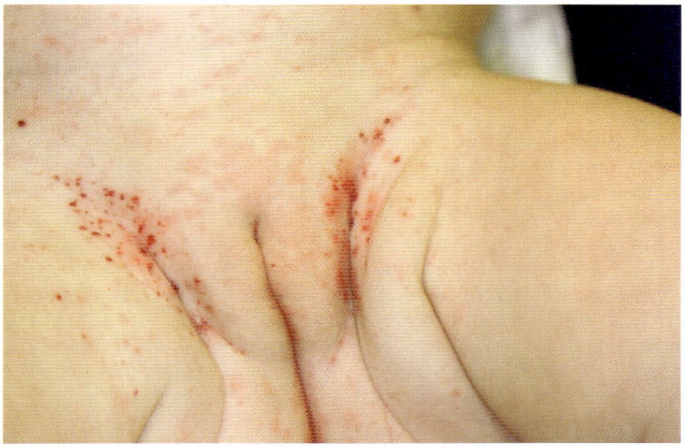

Fig. 10.3 Langerhans cell histiocytosis (LCH). Markedly hemorrhagic papules in the inguinal creases of a 10-month-old female.

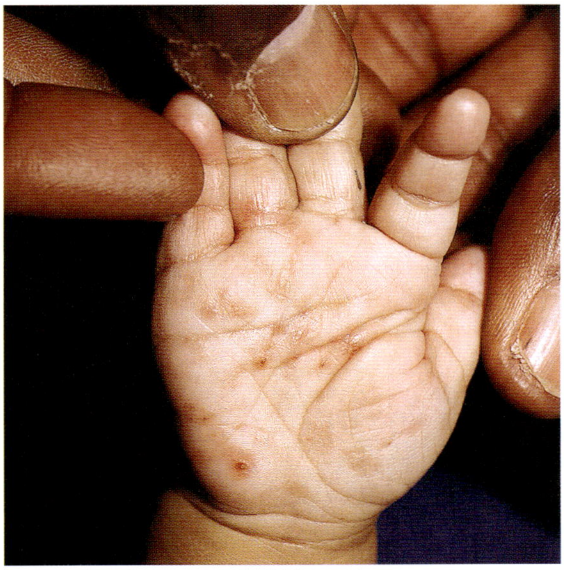

Fig. 10.4 Langerhans cell histiocytosis (LCH). Erythematous, crusted papules on the palm in this newborn with congenital multisystem LCH.

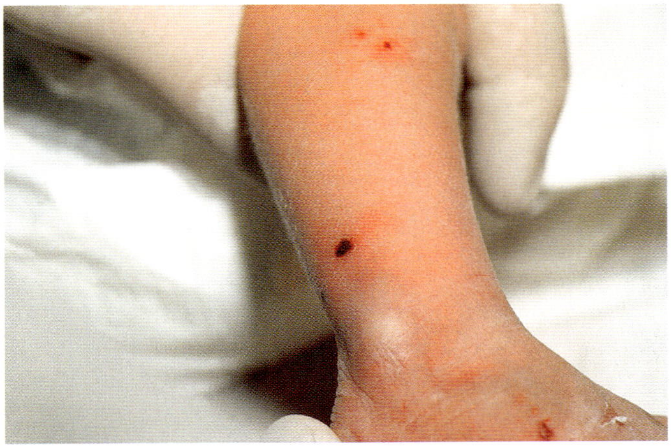

Fig. 10.5 Neonatal Langerhans cell histiocytosis (LCH). Hemorrhagic papules and papulovesicles in a neonate with congenital cutaneous LCH.

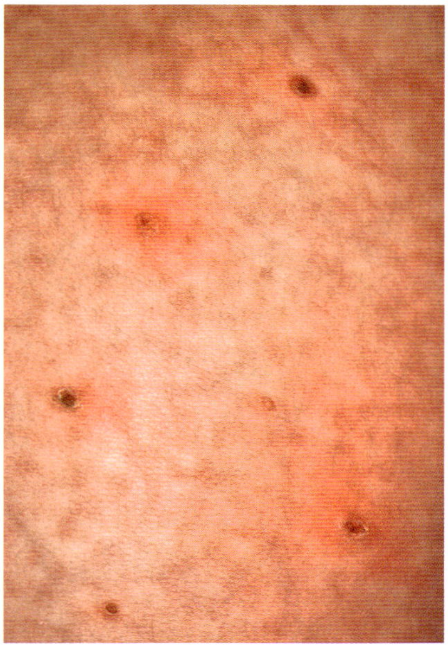

Fig. 10.6 Neonatal Langerhans cell histiocytosis (LCH). These crusted, vesicular lesions were initially felt to be suggestive of neonatal varicella in this 10-day-old female. Biopsy confirmed LCH.

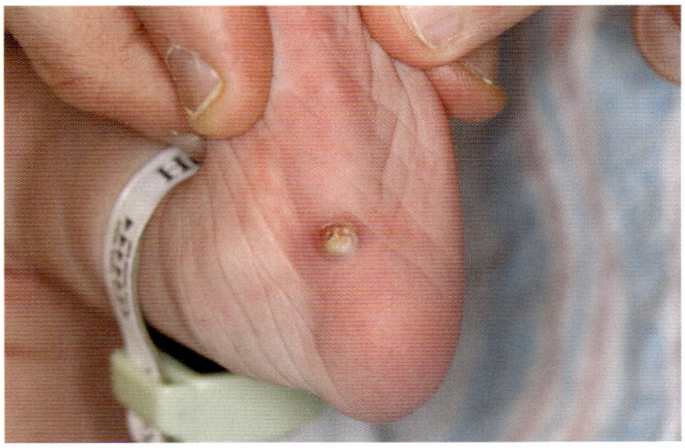

Fig. 10.7 Congenital Langerhans cell histiocytosis (LCH). This papulonodule on the plantar surface was one of just two lesions in a newborn girl. Skin biopsy confirmed the diagnosis of LCH, systemic evaluation was negative for other organ involvement, and the lesions resolved spontaneously over several months, without recurrence.

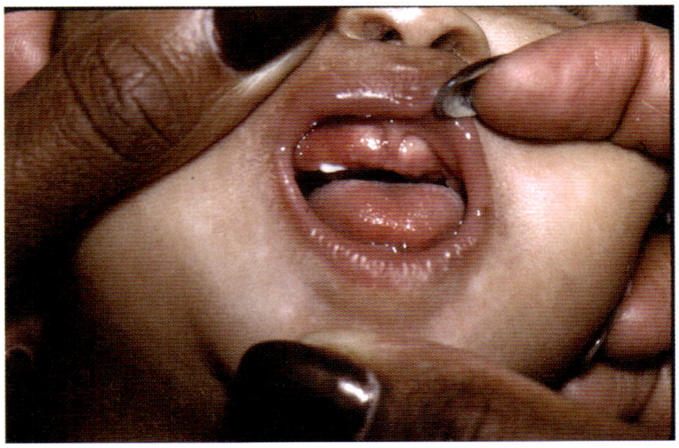

Fig. 10.8 Natal teeth in neonatal LCH. Dental eruption was noted on the upper (shown here) and lower gingivae of this newborn (same infant as shown in Fig. 10.4) with multisystem LCH.

Box 10.2 Cutaneous Clues to Langerhans Cell Histiocytosis

Recalcitrant seborrheic dermatitis–like eruption
Localization of rash to scalp, posterior auricular regions, perineum, axillae
Eroded papules in flexural areas
Petechial or purpuric papules
Crusted papules on palms and/or soles (scabies preparation negative)
Hemorrhagic vesiculopustular lesions (especially in neonates)
Any of these lesions in combination with lymphadenopathy

life-threatening sepsis and hemorrhage.[4,17] Nonspecific constitutional symptoms, including fever, weight loss, and malaise, are common in patients with multiorgan involvement.

Central nervous system (CNS) involvement in LCH may include infiltration of the hypothalamic–pituitary region, which can result in DI even years after the initial diagnosis. DI seems to develop more often in patients with bony involvement of the skull and multisystem disease.[4] Posterior pituitary infiltration may be evident on MRI as absence of a normally bright signal in the posterior pituitary gland or thickening of the pituitary stalk.[20] Growth retardation may result from anterior pituitary involvement, and growth hormone deficiency, which is relatively uncommon, may occur and was noted in 6% of patients in one large series.[21,22] Other manifestations of CNS involvement include hyperreflexia, dysarthria, cranial nerve defects, and, rarely, seizures. Progressive or rarely, acute ataxia has been observed as a complication.[23] Basilar invagination, which is associated with hydrocephalus and usually occurs as part of the Arnold–Chiari malformation or in patients with diseases that result in bone softening (i.e., osteogenesis imperfecta), has been reported in long-term survivors with LCH.[24] MRI is useful in diagnosing CNS disease. Positron emission tomography (PET) scan has been demonstrated useful in identifying areas with altered metabolism related to CNS LCH and may provide a tool for longitudinal involvement in some patients.[25] Neuropsychologic deficits that may occur in children with LCH include cognitive deficiencies and deficits in memory, attention and concentration, and perceptual-organizational capabilities.[26] Cognitive defects are noted especially in patients with multisystem LCH with CNS involvement.[27] Psychiatric deterioration and cognitive defects may both be more common in patients who develop cerebellar involvement.[28]

Congenital self-healing reticulohistiocytosis deserves special mention. This entity, also known as *Hashimoto–Pritzker disease* or *congenital self-healing LCH (CSHLCH)*, is marked by the congenital presence of LCH lesions, usually papules and nodules,[29] which may break down in the center and form crater-shaped ulcers. Systemic signs are often absent, and the lesions involute over a few months and are usually gone by 12 months.[29] There may be some distinct histologic features, but not always. It is generally accepted that CSHLCH is a variant of LCH and that most patients have a favorable prognosis. However, patients do not always have disease limited to the skin and thus require an evaluation for systemic involvement. In addition, reports of cutaneous and systemic relapse (including DI) months to years after resolution of the skin lesions highlight the importance of vigilant long-term follow-up observation, as one would do for patients with classic LCH.[5,30,31]

Erdheim–Chester disease is a rare, systemic histiocytosis characterized by xanthomatous or xanthogranulomatous infiltration of tissues and a cellular phenotype that is CD68 positive but CD1a and S100 negative.[32] It may present in a fashion similar to LCH, including bony involvement, although it most commonly causes osteosclerosis affecting the metaphyseal regions of the long bones (and presenting with bilateral knee and ankle pain). The cutaneous lesions are best characterized as a variant of juvenile xanthogranulomas (JXGs) (see later), and the clinical findings in the skin usually consist of xanthelasma-like lesions on the eyelids.[33] Annular plaques with central atrophy have also been observed.[34] Erdheim–Chester disease occurs predominantly in adults. In the recently revised histiocytoses classification, Erdheim–Chester disease is grouped together with LCH, given similarities in clinical findings and similar activating mutations of genes in the mitogen-activated protein kinase (MAPK) pathway.[35]

LCH is diagnosed by examination of tissue specimens from affected organs. Skin is a readily accessible organ for biopsy in patients who have cutaneous involvement. Routine histologic sections reveal an infiltrate of typical Langerhans cells, which can be confirmed by positive S100, CDla, or Langerin immunostaining. Electron microscopy, although rarely performed now because of the availability of special stains, reveals the characteristic Birbeck granules within the cytoplasm of the cells. The prognosis for patients with LCH is quite variable and dependent on many factors, including the extent of risk of organ

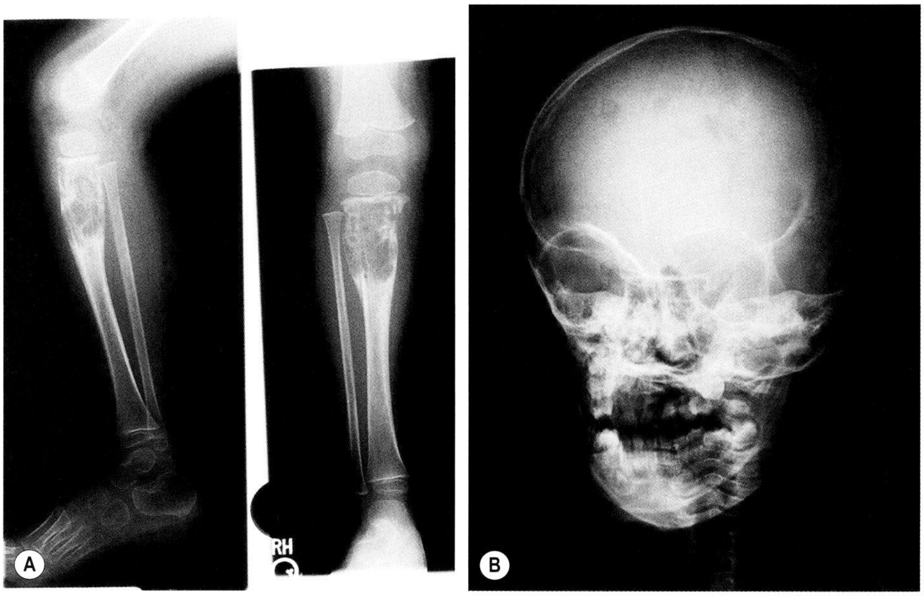

Fig. 10.9 Langerhans cell histiocytosis. Plain radiography reveals multiple lytic lesions in the tibia **(A)** and the skull **(B)** of a 4-year-old child with disseminated disease.

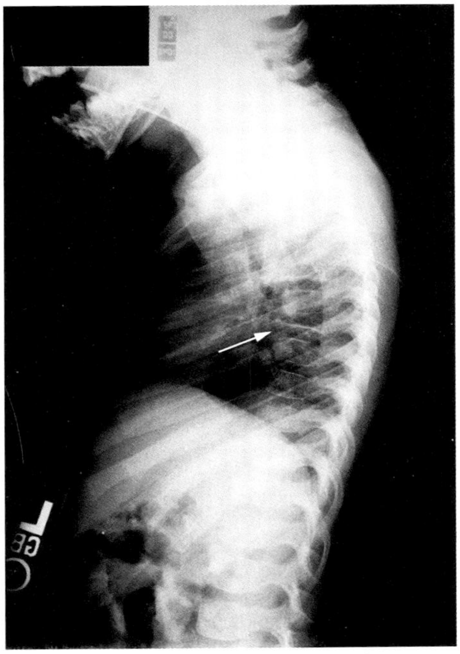

Fig. 10.10 Langerhans cell histiocytosis. Plain radiography demonstrates vertebral body compression (vertebra plana, *arrow*) in the same patient as that shown in Fig. 10.9.

Box 10.3 Recommended Evaluation of the Patient with Suspected Langerhans Cell Histiocytosis

Physical examination, including growth parameters
Laboratory evaluation:
- Complete blood cell count
- Coagulation studies
- Electrolytes
- Erythrocyte sedimentation rate
- Hepatic function testing
- Urine osmolality

Complete skeletal radiographic survey
Chest radiography
More specific studies as guided by initial results (i.e., bone marrow examination, pulmonary function testing, lung biopsy, liver biopsy, panoramic dental films, CT or MRI of the CNS, endocrine evaluation); some recommend abdominal ultrasound in young children (assessing size/structure of liver/spleen and abdominal lymph nodes)

Modified from Satter EK, High WA. Langerhans cell histiocytosis: A review of the current recommendations of the Histiocyte Society. *Pediatr Dermatol*. 2008;25(3):291–295. Also adapted from Haupt R, Minkov M, Astigarraga I, et al. Langerhans cell histiocytosis (LCH): Guidelines for diagnosis, clinical work-up, and treatment for patients till the age of 18 years. *Pediatr Blood Cancer*. 2013;60:175–184.
CNS, Central nervous system; *CT*, computed tomography; *MRI*, magnetic resonance imaging.

involvement and initial response to therapy. In general, the younger the age at diagnosis, the shorter the event-free survival and overall survival rates, although this association does not appear to be as strong as once believed.[36] Interestingly, neonates with isolated cutaneous lesions tend to do very well. Other prognostic factors include the type and number of disease sites, organ dysfunction, and response to therapy.[37] Single-system disease has an excellent prognosis overall.[38–40] Morbidity and mortality in LCH may be related to progressive disease or late sequelae, which include skeletal defects, dental problems, DI, growth failure or other endocrinopathies, hearing loss, and CNS dysfunction.[31] DI, which presents with polyuria and polydipsia, occurs in around 15% to 25% of patients and may even occur as a late complication in patients who present with "skin-limited" disease or CSHLCH.[36–41]

The recommended evaluation for the patient suspected of having LCH is shown in Box 10.3. Clinical stratification based on extent of disease has been recommended as follows: single-organ-system disease (unifocal or multifocal), multiorgan disease (without organ dysfunction), and multiorgan disease (with organ dysfunction). The latter category, multiorgan disease with organ dysfunction, is further stratified as low risk (skin, bone, lymph node, pituitary) or high risk (lung, liver, spleen, hematopoietic cells). Patients with single-organ-system disease seem to have the best outcome and a low reactivation rate.[22]

Therapy for LCH depends on the extent of disease. In patients with disease limited to the skin, observation alone is often appropriate, because the lesions may resolve spontaneously. Topical corticosteroids are only occasionally effective. Topical treatment with nitrogen mustard may be used, and in patients with severe skin disease, systemic therapy as is given for multiorgan LCH may be considered. Treatment for disease limited to bone is dictated by the extent of bone involvement and symptomatology. Single-bone lesions may resolve spontaneously, and simple observation is appropriate in this setting in patients who are not experiencing pain.[4,17] Painful lesions may be treated with curettage, surgical excision, or intralesional steroid injection. Localized radiation therapy is another treatment option.

In patients with more extensive LCH, there is a variety of therapeutic options. Most patients are treated with systemic chemotherapy, most commonly vinblastine or etoposide. These two agents have been found equally effective in the treatment of multisystem LCH.[42] Prednisone or methylprednisolone is commonly used during the induction phase of therapy for patients with multisystem LCH. Other reported therapies include cyclosporine A, 2-chlorodeoxyadenosine, interferon-α, cladribine, cytarabine, clofarabine, and allogeneic bone marrow or cord-blood transplantation.[43–49] Targeted therapy for LCH is an area of research focus, including *BRAF* inhibitors (vemurafenib, dabrafenib) and *MEK* inhibitors (trametinib, cobimetinib).[6,49,50]

LCH is a potentially fatal disorder that can be recognized and diagnosed early based on the characteristic cutaneous manifestations. The skin signs may appear alone or in combination with systemic disease, and all patients require a thorough evaluation for extracutaneous involvement before they can be diagnosed as having skin-limited disease. Although there is often a delay in the diagnosis of patients with LCH, becoming familiar with the cutaneous clues (see Box 10.2) will optimally position the pediatrician or other pediatric healthcare provider to recognize the disorder. Patients with LCH are usually treated by a pediatric oncologist, and all patients require long-term surveillance for late sequelae or relapse.

Juvenile Xanthogranuloma

JXG is a fairly common form of non-LCH histiocytosis. It is generally a benign, self-limited disease of infants, children, and occasionally adults. Lesions occur most often in skin, although extracutaneous disease may occasionally be present. Most JXGs occur early in life, and the true incidence may be underestimated because many of them may go undiagnosed or misdiagnosed as other common skin tumors such as nevi. JXG seems to be derived from dermal dendrocytes, and although the term *xantho-* appears in the name, there is no association of this condition with hyperlipidemia or other metabolic abnormalities.[51]

JXG presents as a firm, round papule or nodule, varying in size from 5 mm to 2 cm, with giant lesions (i.e., up to 5 or 10 cm) occasionally seen. Some authors have divided JXG into a "micronodular" form (lesions <10 mm) and a "macronodular" form (lesions >10 mm). Early JXGs are erythematous (Fig. 10.11) to orange or tan (Fig. 10.12), but with time they become more yellow in color (Figs. 10.13 and 10.14). Lesions may be solitary (up to 90% of all patients with JXG[52]) or, less commonly, multiple (Fig. 10.15), and they are usually asymptomatic. Ulceration and crusting may occasionally occur. The head, neck, and trunk are the most common areas to be involved. Lesions may also occur on mucous membranes or at mucocutaneous junctions (mouth, vaginal orifice, and perineal area). Oral lesions occur on the lateral aspects of the tongue, gingival, buccal mucosa, and midline hard palate and may ulcerate and bleed. Oral lesions may appear verrucous,

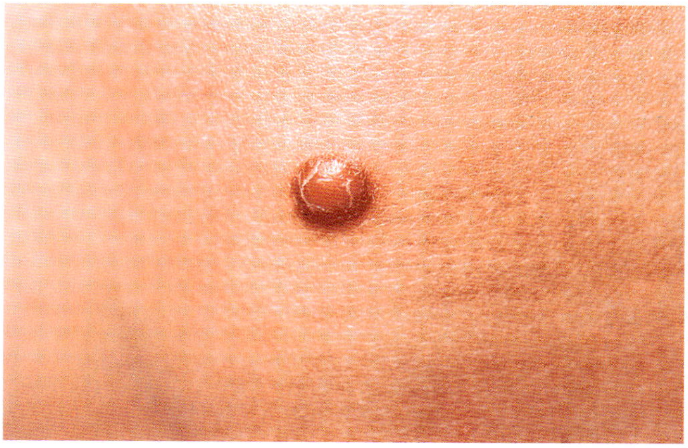

Fig. 10.11 Juvenile xanthogranuloma. An early lesion demonstrates erythema and mild surface scaling.

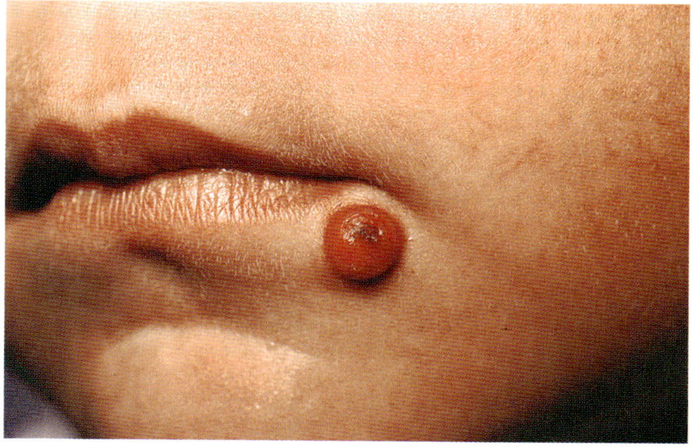

Fig. 10.12 Juvenile xanthogranuloma. This early lesion reveals a red to orange color.

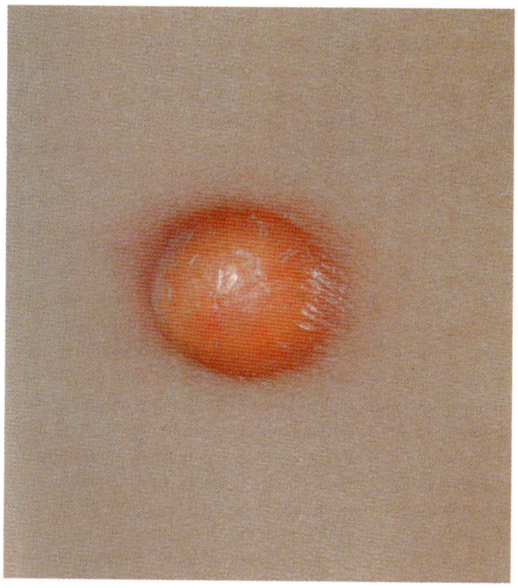

Fig. 10.13 Juvenile xanthogranuloma. An established lesion revealing the characteristic yellow to orange-brown appearance.

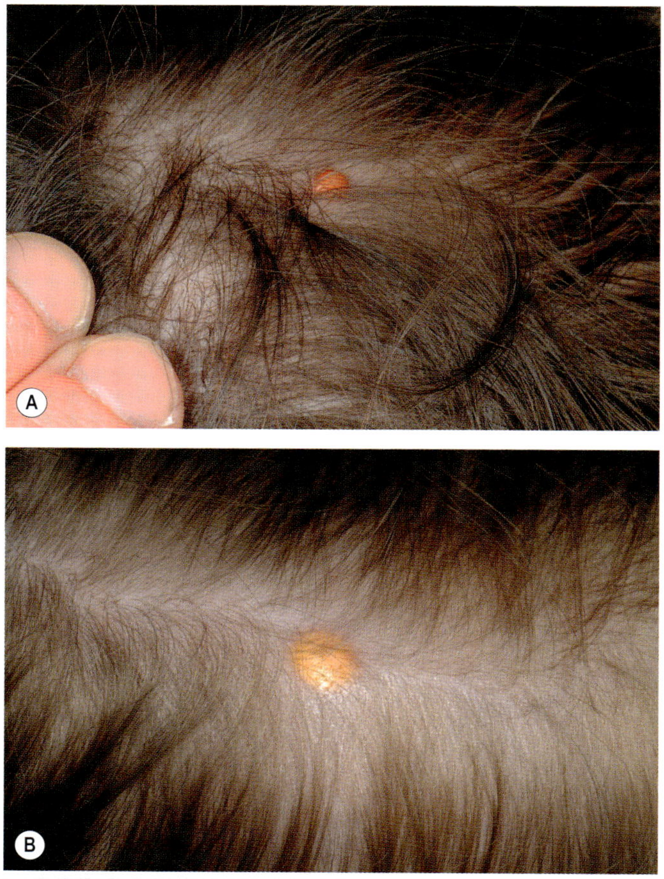

Fig. 10.14 Juvenile xanthogranuloma. Solitary yellow, dome-shaped nodular papule **(A)** and plaque **(B)**, both distributed on the scalp.

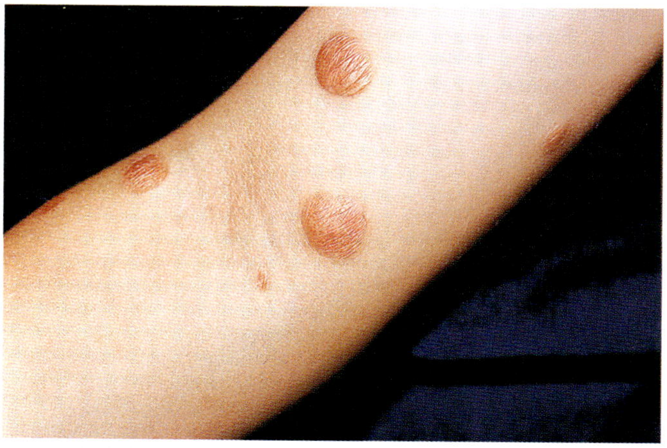

Fig. 10.15 Juvenile xanthogranuloma. Multiple lesions, with spontaneous involution evident, were present in this 11-year-old boy. Note the fibrofatty tissue residua.

pedunculated, umbilicated, or fibroma-like.[53] Typically, the lesions of JXG present at birth (20%) or during the first 6 months of life, and they may persist or continue to erupt for years.[54]

Histologic evaluation of JXG tissue reveals a dense dermal infiltrate of foamy histiocytes, foreign body cells, and the characteristic Touton giant cells, which are virtually pathognomonic for the condition. The Touton giant cell is a giant cell with a central wreath of nuclei and a peripheral rim of eosinophilic cytoplasm.[55]

Lymphocytes and eosinophils are often seen, and the histiocytes in JXG are S100 and CDla negative on special staining.

Extracutaneous involvement occasionally occurs with JXG. The eye is the most common organ of involvement second to the skin. The iris is the site most often involved, and potential complications of ocular JXG include hyphema, glaucoma, or blindness.[56] Patients may complain of eye redness, irritation, or photophobia. Children believed to be at greatest risk for ocular JXG include those 2 years of age or younger and those with multiple skin lesions.[56] However, the risk of eye involvement in children with cutaneous JXG overall appears quite low.[57] Intramuscular JXG presents as a deep, soft tissue lesion that may have imaging features similar to those of malignant tumors of infancy.[58] This form tends to affect exclusively infants and toddlers and occurs as a solitary lesion in skeletal muscles of the trunk.[59] Other sites of extracutaneous involvement include lung, liver, testis, pericardium, spleen, CNS, bone, kidney, adrenal glands, and larynx.[51,55] Solitary as well as multiple cranial, intracranial, and intracerebral lesions have rarely been reported, including one patient who experienced leptomeningeal spread and several who required therapy with chemotherapy and steroids.[60–64] Intracranial and cranial JXG have been reported in conjunction with *BRAF-V600E* mutations, suggesting that these lesions may be better classified as part of the LCH/Erdheim–Chester disease spectrum.[65] Intraspinal JXG with spinal cord compression has been reported.[66] Systemic JXG generally exhibits a benign clinical course but may occasionally be fatal, especially when the liver is involved.[52] There are rare reports of JXG in association with LCH, suggesting a possible common progenitor cell and overlap within the histiocytic spectrum of disorders.[67–69]

An important association is that of JXG and childhood leukemia. The most common association has been with juvenile chronic myelogenous leukemia (JCML), which may be seen with increased incidence in patients with multiple JXG lesions. It has been noted that several such reported patients also had café-au-lait macules and a family history of type 1 neurofibromatosis (NF).[70] A systematic review of the literature revealed that the frequency of the triple association of JXG, JCML, and NF is 30- to 40-fold higher than expected, and it was estimated that children with NF and JXG have a 20- to 32-fold higher risk for JCML than do patients with NF who do not have JXG.[71] However, in a retrospective case-control study comparing children with NF and malignancy to those with NF without malignancy, the presence of JXG was not associated with increased malignancy risk,[72] and the vast majority of patients with multiple JXG, even those with associated NF, do not develop JCML. The role of surveillance complete blood cell counts is controversial in this setting, and most practitioners monitor these patients primarily with regular, thorough physical examinations.

JXG usually runs a fairly benign course, with spontaneous regression occurring over 3 to 6 years. Pigmentary alteration, atrophy, or "anetoderma-like" changes may persist in areas of prior skin involvement. Although rare cases lasting until adulthood have been reported, generally those that have their onset early in life manifest complete spontaneous healing. The risk of complications is fairly high when ocular involvement is present. For this reason, once the disease has been confirmed in the eye, therapy should be initiated. Intraocular JXG is treated with intralesional or systemic steroids, radiation therapy, or excision.[73,74] Lesions limited to skin require no therapy, although surgical excision is occasionally performed for diagnostic or cosmetic purposes. Systemic involvement is treated if it interferes with vital functions and has shown response to chemotherapy regimens similar to those used in LCH.[51,52,75]

Xanthoma Disseminatum

Xanthoma disseminatum (XD), a rare disorder of mucocutaneous xanthomatous lesions, is another non-LCH histiocytosis. This disorder usually occurs in adults, although it may have its onset during childhood.[76,77] Patients have numerous (sometimes hundreds) round to oval, yellow-orange or brown papules, nodules, and plaques. They occur primarily on the face and the flexural and intertriginous surfaces, including the neck, antecubital fossae, periumbilical area, perineum, and genitalia. The lips, eyelids, and conjunctivae may be involved, and xanthomatous deposits have also been observed in the mouth and upper respiratory tract (epiglottis, larynx, and trachea), occasionally leading to respiratory difficulty.[78,79] Facial lesions may become exuberant and may cause disfiguration.[80] Osseous lesions, presenting radiographically as well-demarcated areas of osteolysis, may be present,[80] and synovitis and arthritis have been reported.[81] Ocular mucosal lesions may result in blindness. Liver involvement is occasionally present.[82] When XD involves the CNS, it is characterized by infiltration of the pituitary gland and is termed *xanthomatous hypophysitis*, and may result in DI, hyperprolactinemia, or hypopituitarism.[83] On histology, XD reveals a dermal infiltrate of foamy histiocytes and multinucleated giant cells, and stains are positive for CD68 and negative for S100 and CD1a.

As with JXG, there is no perturbation in lipid metabolism in patients with XD, although it has been rarely reported in affected children.[83,84] DI occurs in many patients with the disorder, although more often adults than children,[85] and severe laryngeal involvement may necessitate tracheostomy. The lesions of XD often persist indefinitely but have been known to involute spontaneously.[86] Treatment of the cutaneous lesions has been performed with cryotherapy, excision, and carbon dioxide laser ablation.[87] Despite the normolipemic nature of XD, lipid-lowering agents have been utilized in some patients with reported improvement.[88,89] Respiratory tract involvement, when severe, may justify a more aggressive approach with localized radiation therapy or chemotherapy. More recently, cladribine and imatinib have been reported as effective therapeutic options.[90,91]

Benign Cephalic Histiocytosis

Benign cephalic histiocytosis (BCH) is a self-healing, cutaneous, non-LCH histiocytosis that classically involves the face and head. The average age of onset is 15 months, and 45% of cases occur in infants under 6 months of age.[92] Clinically, BCH is characterized by small, 2- to 6-mm, yellow-brown macules and minimally elevated papules (Fig. 10.16). The lesions may occasionally coalesce to give a reticulate pattern.[93] BCH most commonly occurs on the face and head (more than 80% of 45 patients in one review) and less commonly on the neck and trunk, although in one series over 80% of patients had lesions on the proximal extremities or trunk.[94,95] The extremities, buttocks, and pubic area may be involved later in the course.[92] The differential diagnosis may include flat warts, micronodular JXG, LCH, multiple melanocytic nevi, and urticaria pigmentosa.

The diagnosis of BCH can be confirmed by skin biopsy, which reveals a histiocytic infiltrate with negative stains for S100 and CDla. Electron microscopy is useful in confirming the diagnosis, because the cells classically reveal intracytoplasmic comma-shaped or worm-like bodies and the absence of Birbeck granules,[93,96] clearly differentiating it from LCH.

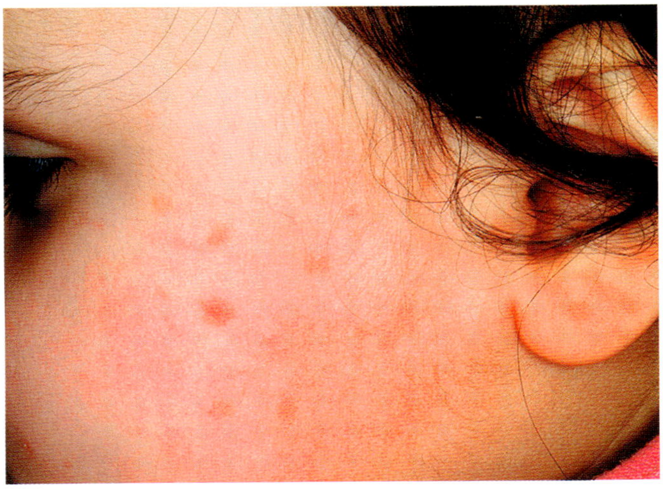

Fig. 10.16 Benign cephalic histiocytosis. Faintly tan to erythematous macules and papules on the cheek.

There is significant clinical overlap between some of the non-LCH histiocytoses. Some authors have considered BCH to be a variant of generalized eruptive histiocytoma (GEH) (see later). In addition, there are reports of BCH progressing into JXG,[97,98] and although BCH tends to be limited to the skin, there are some reports of associated internal involvement. One patient with BCH developed DI 1 year later with infiltration of the pituitary stalk on imaging.[99] In another patient with classic lesions of BCH on the face, lytic lesions in the skull, spine, and tibia were demonstrated to be LCH on tissue examination.[100] These clinical observations again highlight the potential overlap among the histiocytic syndromes.

BCH generally runs a benign course with spontaneous healing, often leaving behind flat or atrophic pigmented scars. Treatment is unnecessary, but given the clinical variation in presentation and overlap with other histiocytic syndromes, clinical follow-up observation for progression or internal involvement is advisable.

Necrobiotic Xanthogranuloma

Necrobiotic xanthogranuloma, a rare disorder usually reported in adults, is characterized by sharply demarcated, indurated plaques and nodules that are usually yellow to red-brown or violaceous and have a predilection for periorbital areas, the trunk, and proximal extremities.[101] Lesions vary in size, may at times be as large as 10 cm or more in diameter, and often ulcerate and heal with areas of atrophy and telangiectasia. Ocular involvement is fairly common and includes ectropion, ptosis, keratitis, uveitis, proptosis, and orbital masses. Visceral lesions of necrobiotic xanthogranuloma may involve the heart, skeletal muscles, larynx, spleen, and ovary. A hallmark of this disease is an associated paraproteinemia, immunoglobulin (Ig) G monoclonal gammopathy. The course of necrobiotic xanthogranuloma is chronic and progressive and may be associated with proliferation of plasma cells in the bone marrow or multiple myeloma. Reported treatment options include systemic or intralesional corticosteroids, cytotoxic drugs, radiation therapy, thalidomide, rituximab, infliximab, interferon alpha, hydroxychloroquine, azathioprine, plasmapheresis, and extracorporeal photopheresis.[102] Intravenous immunoglobulin has been reportedly useful in some patients.[103] Surgical removal of lesions is associated with a high recurrence rate.[104]

Generalized Eruptive Histiocytoma

GEH is a rare, self-healing histiocytosis characterized by recurrent crops of small, yellow to red-brown papules on the face, trunk, extensor extremities, and, rarely, mucous membranes. The lesions number in the hundreds and tend to occur in a symmetric distribution. They resolve over months with hyperpigmented macules left in their place. As a result of the continuous development of new lesions, however, the disorder may persist indefinitely. Although generally regarded as a disorder of adults, GEH has been seen in childhood and even in infants as young as 1 month of age.[105]

The differential diagnosis includes JXG (which may be very difficult to differentiate histologically from early lesions of GEH), LCH, BCH, and urticaria pigmentosa. XD has developed in a child with the prior diagnosis of GEH.[76] No treatment is generally necessary for this disorder. However, because there is considerable overlap within non-LCH histiocytoses, patients should be monitored carefully for the development of signs or symptoms of other organ involvement. Isotretinoin treatment has been reported in a patient with GEH, with transient improvement but eventual recurrence.[106]

Progressive Nodular Histiocytoma

Progressive nodular histiocytoma is characterized by a widespread eruption of hundreds of yellow-brown, 2- to 10-mm papules and deeper, larger subcutaneous nodules. Conjunctival, oral, and laryngeal lesions may occur. The face typically is heavily involved with numerous coalescent lesions, which may result in a leonine appearance. New lesions progressively occur, and ulceration is common. Occasionally, bleeding may occur within the subcutaneous nodules, resulting in marked pain.[107] Lesions of progressive nodular histiocytoma histologically show features typical of xanthogranuloma, and some authors suggest that this entity and JXG may represent a variation of the same process.[108] Treatment for this condition is difficult and includes excision of large or symptomatic lesions, chemotherapy with vinblastine, and electron beam therapy.

Multicentric Reticulohistiocytosis

Multicentric reticulohistiocytosis is a rare systemic disorder of unknown cause. It is characterized by cutaneous lesions and a destructive arthritis and is seen almost exclusively in adults (mean age at diagnosis of 40 to 50 years) with rare reports of pediatric disease.[109–112] The skin lesions present as firm red-brown papules and nodules, most often distributed on the hands, fingers, lips, ears, and nose; proximal and distal interphalangeal joint involvement is common with the cutaneous nodules.[113] Facial disfigurement may occur, with cartilaginous destruction and the appearance of a leonine facies. The coral bead sign refers to the presence of a chain of papules along the cuticle.[107] Nodular lesions on the arms, elbows, and knees may occur and at times resemble rheumatoid nodules.[114] Mucous membrane involvement may occur in up to one-half of patients. They most often present on the lips, buccal mucosa, nasal septum, tongue, palate, and gingivae.

Joint involvement is the presenting sign in more than half of the patients and is highly destructive. It may involve any joint, especially the interphalangeal joints, and coexisting synovitis is common. Shortening of the digits may occur with a "telescopic" or "opera-glass" deformity. Rheumatoid arthritis may be mistakenly diagnosed in some patients. Microscopic examination of skin, bone, or synovial tissue reveals a characteristic histiocytic process with multinucleated giant cells and a "ground-glass" appearance. Visceral involvement may include pleural effusion, pulmonary fibrosis, pericardial effusion, congestive heart failure, salivary gland enlargement, muscle weakness, lymphadenopathy, and gastric ulcer.[115] Multicentric reticulohistiocytosis may regress spontaneously over 6 to 8 years, but for many patients the articular destruction results in permanent joint deformities. The response of this disorder to therapy is often disappointing, with treatments including nonsteroidal antiinflammatory agents, corticosteroids, cyclophosphamide, chlorambucil, methotrexate, hydroxychloroquine, infliximab, tocilizumab, bisphosphonates, and interferon.[107,115–120]

Hemophagocytic Lymphohistiocytosis

Hemophagocytic lymphohistiocytosis (HLH; also known as *hemophagocytic syndrome)* refers to a condition characterized by fever, wasting, jaundice, and hepatosplenomegaly resulting from diffuse infiltration of phagocytizing histiocytes in various tissues.[121] This disorder is heterogeneous in its etiologies, which include a familial form (familial HLH) and a secondary/reactive form that may be associated with a variety of infectious agents (most notably viral, bacterial, or parasitic), malignancy, and collagen vascular disorders.[122,123] These have also been referred to as *genetic* and *acquired* forms of HLH. The infection-associated form is seen primarily in immunocompromised patients with evidence of preceding viral (usually Epstein–Barr virus [EBV]) infection, in which case it is also known as *virus-associated hemophagocytic syndrome.* The other viral agents reported in association with HLH include cytomegalovirus, enterovirus, and parainfluenza virus.[122,123] The term *malignant histiocytosis* refers to tumors with anaplastic histology for which other tumor types have been excluded by immunophenotyping. There are *primary* and *secondary* forms, with the latter seen in association with another hematologic neoplasm.[1]

HLH has been observed as a complication of allogeneic hematopoietic stem cell transplantation and in association with hematologic malignancies.[121,124] There also seems to be a relationship between EBV-associated HLH and EBV-associated T-cell lymphoma, with HLH representing the major cause of death in these patients.[121] Lymphoma-associated hemophagocytic syndrome (LAHS) is a rarely reported variant of HLH that has been described in the setting of systemic and cutaneous lymphomas, including subcutaneous panniculitic T-cell lymphoma (SPTCL) and epidermotropic cutaneous T-cell lymphoma, in which case it often occurs several years after the lymphoma diagnosis.[125] The pathway most commonly implicated in familial HLH is that of perforin-dependent cytotoxicity, an essential function of natural killer and cytotoxic T lymphocytes. The genetic forms of HLH have been shown to be related to mutations in any of several genes involved in this pathway, including *PRF1, UNC13D, Munc18-2, Rab27a, STX11, SH2D1A, STXBP2*, and *BIRC4*.[126–128] HLH may also be related to a primary immunodeficiency syndrome.[129] Macrophage activation syndrome (MAS; see Chapter 22) is a severe condition with features very similar to HLH that is seen in association with the systemic form of juvenile idiopathic arthritis and, less often, other autoimmune inflammatory diseases.[130] Box 10.4 summarizes the various subtypes of HLH.[129,131] Recently, a diagnostic tool was developed and validated to assist in discriminating primary HLH from MAS related to systemic juvenile idiopathic arthritis, helping practitioners identify patients who may benefit most from functional and genetic testing.[132]

Diagnostic criteria for HLH are shown in Table 10.3. The cutaneous manifestations seen in patients with HLH are variable. Most common is a transient, generalized maculopapular eruption. Petechial and purpuric macules, generalized erythroderma, and morbilliform erythema may also occur.[133] Although the skin findings are not specific, their presence in the patient with a supportive history and/or the concomitant findings of fever, lymphadenopathy, hepatosplenomegaly, and cytopenias should prompt consideration for this diagnosis. The most common hematologic findings are leukopenia and thrombocytopenia, and coagulopathy is fairly common.[122] Other findings may include liver dysfunction and elevated triglyceride, lactate dehydrogenase (LDH), and ferritin levels. Fibrinogen levels are often decreased. The clinical differential diagnosis may include extramedullary hematopoiesis (as may be seen with a variety of infectious or malignant disorders) and metastatic lesions from an underlying malignancy. LCH and myofibromatosis may also be in the differential.[133] Skin biopsy may be useful in eliminating some diagnoses, but the histologic findings are often nonspecific, and the changes of erythrophagocytosis are often absent in skin specimens. Examination of bone marrow or other solid organ (lymph node, spleen, liver) biopsy tissue may be necessary to confirm the diagnosis. In one series of children with HLH, bone marrow aspiration revealed hemophagocytosis in 85%.[134] HLH has a high mortality rate, although chemotherapy, steroids, intravenous immunoglobulin, and hematopoietic stem cell transplantation may offer hope for some patients. Etoposide and dexamethasone often induce clinical remission of the inflammatory symptoms, and improved survival has been noted with newer reduced-intensity transplant conditioning protocols. Cyclosporine A has been utilized to inhibit T-cell activation.[127,129]

Box 10.4 Subtypes of Hemophagocytic Lymphohistiocytosis

Genetic Forms

- Familial hemophagocytic lymphohistiocytosis (FHL)
  - FHL1–FHL5
- Immunodeficiency disorders
  - Griscelli syndrome type 2
  - Chediak–Higashi syndrome
  - Hermansky–Pudlak syndrome type 2
  - X-linked proliferative syndrome (XLP), types 1 and 2
  - IL-2 inducible T-cell kinase (ITK) deficiency

Acquired Forms

- Viral (especially EBV and other herpes viruses)
- Other infections (bacterial, fungal, parasitic)
- Malignancy (peripheral lymphomas, cutaneous lymphomas, leukemia, myeloma, some solid tumors)
- Immunosuppression (post–organ transplantation or post-HSCT)
- Autoimmune disease (systemic-onset JIA, SLE, spondyloarthropathies, Kawasaki disease; termed *macrophage activation syndrome*)

Modified from Rosado FGN, Kim AS. Hemophagocytic lymphohistiocytosis: An update on diagnosis and pathogenesis. *Am J Clin Pathol*. 2013;139:713–727; and Bode SFN, Lehmberg K, Maul-Pavicic A, et al. Recent advances in the diagnosis and treatment of hemophagocytic lymphohistiocytosis. *Arthritis Res Ther*. 2012;14:213.

EBV, Epstein–Barr virus; *HSCT*, hematopoietic stem cell transplantation; *JIA*, juvenile idiopathic arthritis; *SLE*, systemic lupus erythematosus.

Table 10.3 Diagnostic Criteria for Hemophagocytic Lymphohistiocytosis (HLH)

A patient meets criteria for HLH if either A or B are fulfilled:

A. Molecular diagnosis is consistent with HLH

B. Five of the following eight criteria:

Criterion	Comment
1. Fever	
2. Splenomegaly	
3. Cytopenias affecting two of three lineages	Hemoglobin <9 g/dL (or <10 g/dL in infant) Platelets $<100 \times 10^9$/L Neutrophils $<1 \times 10^9$/L
4. Elevated triglycerides and/or decreased fibrinogen	Fasting triglycerides ≥265 mg/dL Fibrinogen <1.5 g/L
5. Hemophagocytosis	In bone marrow, spleen, or lymph nodes
6. Low or absent NK-cell activity	Per local laboratory reference range
7. Elevated ferritin	Varies; from ≥500 μg/L to ≥10,000 μg/L, depending on reference
8. Elevation in soluble CD25 (IL-2 receptor)	≥2400 U/mL

Adapted from Erker C, Harker-Murray P, Talano JA. Usual and unusual manifestations of familial hemophagocytic lymphohistiocytosis and Langerhans cell histiocytosis. *Pediatr Clin N Am* 2017;64:91–109; Mehta RS, Smith RE. Hemophagocytic lymphohistiocytosis (HLH): a review of literature. *Med Oncol* 2013;30:740; Otrock ZK, Hock KG, Riley SB, de Witte T, Eby CS, Scott MG. Elevated serum ferritin is not specific for hemophagocytic lymphohistiocytosis. *Ann Hematol* 2017;96(10):1667–72.

Sinus Histiocytosis with Massive Lymphadenopathy (Rosai–Dorfman Disease)

Sinus histiocytosis with massive lymphadenopathy (SHML, or Rosai–Dorfman disease) is a rare disorder of reactive proliferation of histiocytes in the sinuses of lymph nodes. It occurs primarily in children, who show massive painless bilateral lymphadenopathy, especially cervical. Extranodal involvement may occur, and when it does, the head and neck region is the most common site, with a predilection for the nasal cavity and paranasal sinuses.[135] Papules and nodules are the most common skin lesions, and purely cutaneous SHML may occasionally occur.[136,137] The lesions of SHML often involute spontaneously, although surgical or medical therapy (which may include radiation, corticosteroids, or chemotherapy) may be indicated for lesions that are symptomatic, extensive, compromising vital organ function, or cosmetically deforming.[135] There are isolated reports of patients with both SHML and lymphoma.[138,139] Mutations in *NRAS, KRAS, MAP2K1*, and *ARAF* have been identified in lesional tissues from SHML patients,[140] and germline mutations in *SLC29A3* have been noted in familial SHML.[141]

Cutaneous Pseudolymphoma

Cutaneous pseudolymphoma (CPL; lymphocytoma cutis, lymphadenosis benigna cutis, Spiegler–Fendt pseudolymphoma, cutaneous lymphoid hyperplasia) refers to a benign process that may clinically and/or histologically mimic lymphoma. CPL may occur at any age, but most characteristically develop during early adult life. The diagnosis is nonspecific and does not imply the etiology. Some of the various causes of this process are listed in Box 10.5.

One of the most common etiologic categories of CPL is drugs. Many classes have been implicated, including anticonvulsants, antipsychotics, anxiolytics, antihypertensives, angiotensin-converting enzyme inhibitors, β-blockers, calcium channel blockers, antibiotics, cytotoxic agents, antihistamines, lipid-lowering agents, and some biologic agents.[142,143] The anticonvulsant hypersensitivity syndrome, or drug rash with eosinophilia and systemic symptoms (DRESS) (see Chapter 20), is a prototype for such a reaction, presenting with fever, lymphadenopathy, edema, hepatosplenomegaly with hepatitis, and a diffuse cutaneous eruption that may reveal histologic changes of pseudolymphoma.

Typically, CPL presents as a more localized process with papules, nodules, and tumors in the skin. The lesions are flesh-colored to red or violaceous (Fig. 10.17) and may be single or multiple. They are usually not associated with a drug ingestion, and they may reach up to 4 or 5 cm in size with continued enlargement. The most common locations are the face, ears, and scalp, with occasional involvement of other body regions. Borrelial lymphocytoma, which follows infection with the Lyme disease agent *Borrelia burgdorferi*, occurs primarily in Europe and usually presents with red nodules involving the ear lobe and areola.[144] CPL resulting from past scabies infestation (scabies nodules) presents as erythematous to red-brown papules and nodules, usually in an infant previously treated for scabies (Fig. 10.18). These lesions may persist for several months after adequate therapy for the infestation. CPL may occasionally be noted in association with molluscum contagiosum (see Chapter 15, Fig. 15.46), a common childhood viral infection.[145]

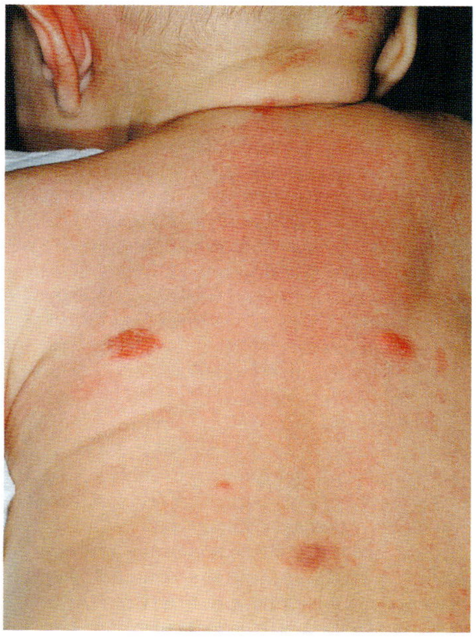

Fig. 10.18 Nodular scabies. Erythematous papulonodules with mild scaling in a 10-month-old infant who was treated for scabies 3 months before.

Box 10.5 Some Causes of Cutaneous Pseudolymphoma

Idiopathic
Arthropod bite reaction
Drug reaction
Contact dermatitis
Infestation (i.e., scabies nodules)
Lymphomatoid papulosis
Borrelia burgdorferi
Treponema pallidum
Tattoo pigment
Vaccinations
Actinic reticuloid/photosensitivity
VZV infection
HIV infection
Molluscum contagiosum

HIV, Human immunodeficiency virus; *VZV*, varicella zoster virus.

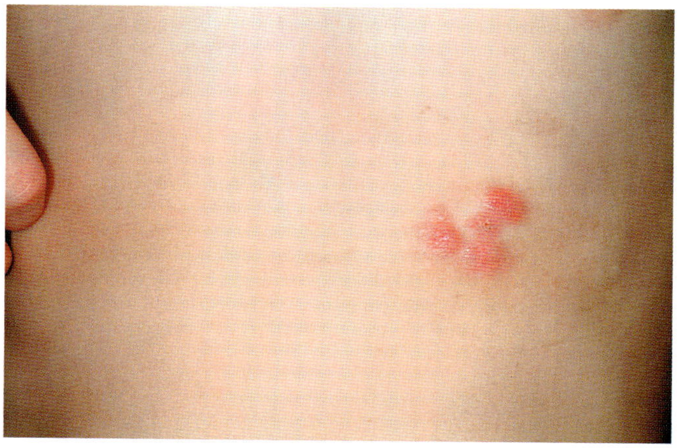

Fig. 10.17 Cutaneous pseudolymphoma. Infiltrative, erythematous papules and nodular plaques on the chest of a 7-year-old boy.

A more disseminated form of CPL may occur; it usually appears in adults and presents with firm, red to violaceous papules and nodules with a more diffuse distribution. These lesions may grow rapidly, are prone to recurrence, and tend to persist throughout life. Actinic reticuloid is a severe, chronic photosensitive dermatosis that occurs primarily in older men and presents with erythematous to violaceous, lichenified papules and plaques on sun-exposed skin. It is categorized as a form of CPL by several authors.

The diagnosis of CPL is based upon the combination of clinical features, histologic evaluation, and often immunohistochemical and/or gene rearrangement studies.[142] At times, the microscopic findings of CPL may be very difficult to differentiate from cutaneous lymphoma and consist of a mixture of B, T, or mixed lymphocytes with macrophages and dendritic cells.[146] Treatment of CPL depends on the underlying etiology. Removal of any offending drug or physical stimulus that is identified may be sufficient. In idiopathic cases, lesions may involute spontaneously over months to years. For persistent lesions, treatment options include topical agents (corticosteroids, tacrolimus, imiquimod), intralesional corticosteroids, interferon-alpha, cryosurgery, surgical excision, local radiation therapy, photodynamic therapy, photochemotherapy, and antimalarial (i.e., hydroxychloroquine) and cytotoxic agents.[142,143,147] Antibiotics appropriate for Lyme disease are indicated for treatment of borrelial lymphocytoma.

Leukemia Cutis

Leukemia is the most common malignancy of childhood. Cutaneous findings in leukemia may be primary (i.e., leukemic infiltrates in the skin) and secondary (i.e., Sweet syndrome, see Chapter 20; pyoderma gangrenosum, see Chapter 25; opportunistic infections). Cutaneous leukemic infiltrates may be known by a variety of names, including leukemia cutis, granulocytic sarcoma, and chloroma. *Myelosarcoma* is the more contemporary term for any extramedullary infiltrate with myeloid blasts.[148] Hence, leukemia cutis is a form of myelosarcoma that results from infiltration of the epidermis, dermis, or subcutaneous tissues by neoplastic leukocytes or their precursors. Although biopsies of lesions of leukemia cutis may suggest the diagnosis, the findings may mimic a variety of inflammatory or neoplastic diseases. Therefore immunophenotyping and examination of peripheral blood smears and bone marrow aspirates are often required in an effort to confirm the diagnosis.

Cutaneous involvement may be associated with various types of childhood leukemias, including acute lymphoblastic leukemia (ALL), acute myeloid leukemia (AML, also called *acute nonlymphocytic leukemia [ANLL]*), and chronic leukemias (i.e., chronic myeloid leukemia [CML] and chronic lymphoblastic leukemia [CLL]). In general, leukemia cutis is associated with a grave prognosis, the exception being in patients with congenital leukemia (see later). Cutaneous leukemic infiltrates are most common with the myeloid leukemias (between 3% and 30% of patients, depending on the subtype), especially acute myelomonocytic and monocytic leukemia.[148–150] Gingival hypertrophy is a notable feature seen with these subtypes of leukemia, less so with other acute leukemias, and rarely with chronic leukemias.[149] Leukemia cutis is less common in patients with ALL (around 1% to 3%); in these cases, it seems to be most common on the head and may be an early manifestation in children in both standard-risk and high-risk categories.[149,151] It has been reported in conjunction with facial nerve palsy as the presenting symptom of T-cell ALL.[152] Leukemia cutis may also occur in patients with myelodysplastic syndrome, usually before or simultaneously with identifiable leukemic transformation in the peripheral blood or bone marrow.[153,154] Rarely leukemia cutis may present as a manifestation of secondary leukemia after prior chemotherapy.[155]

The clinical appearance of leukemia cutis is variable. Lesion types include macules, papules, plaques, nodules, ecchymoses, erythroderma, palpable purpura, ulcers, bullous lesions, and urticaria-like lesions.[149] A "seborrheic dermatitis–like" presentation with scaling and papules of the scalp was observed in a 7-month-old with AML in remission.[156] Brown macules and nodules exhibiting a positive Darier sign and mimicking mastocytosis have been noted.[153] The most characteristic lesions of leukemia cutis are flesh-colored to erythematous (Fig. 10.19) to violaceous (Fig. 10.20) papules, nodules, and plaques that may become purpuric (especially with coexisting thrombocytopenia). Leukemia cutis lesions may localize to sites of skin trauma, burns, surgical sites, or sites of cutaneous infections. When presenting in the neonate, widespread lesions of leukemia cutis are part of the "blueberry-muffin baby" differential (see Congenital Leukemia Cutis later).

The clinical features of the skin lesions are not distinct for the different types of leukemias. However, certain subtypes may be more likely to result in cutaneous infiltrates with certain characteristics. For example, granulocytic sarcoma (or chloroma) presents as a rapidly growing, firm nodule that at times has a green hue. This tumor is usually associated with AML, and the greenish color is related to myeloperoxidase in the granulocytes. Granulocytic sarcoma may occur in patients with known AML, in those with a myeloproliferative disorder with an impending blast crisis, or in patients without any

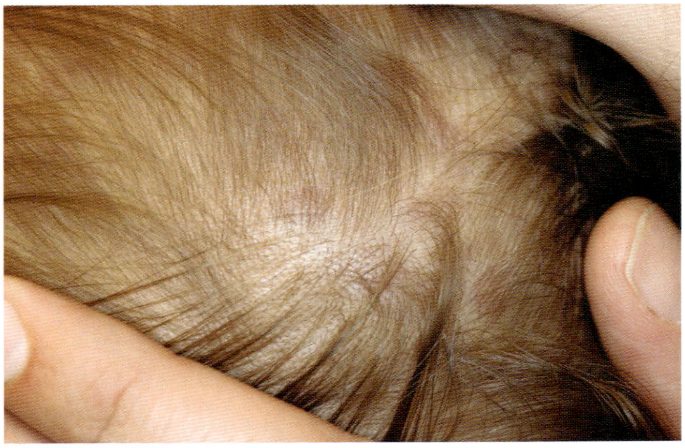

Fig. 10.20 Leukemia cutis. This 10-month-old, previously healthy boy presented with a 6-day history of fever, irritability, and new nodules on the scalp. Complete blood cell count revealed marked neutropenia with 21% circulating blasts, and bone marrow subsequently confirmed the diagnosis of acute myelocytic leukemia. Note the numerous subtle violaceous nodules.

known hematologic disease.[150] At times leukemia cutis may precede (or occur in the absence of) systemic leukemia. This phenomenon, in which there is cutaneous infiltration of leukemic cells in the absence of blood or bone marrow findings, is termed *aleukemic leukemia cutis (ALC)*, and the cutaneous lesions can sometimes precede the systemic malignancy (most commonly AML) by years.[157] Evaluation of the patient with ALC should include bone marrow aspiration, fluorescence *in situ* hybridization (FISH), and cytogenetic studies, and although some patients undergo spontaneous resolution, many oncologists treat with similar induction and consolidation chemotherapy regimens as used in acute leukemia.[158]

CONGENITAL LEUKEMIA CUTIS

Congenital leukemia is defined as leukemia presenting at birth or within the first month to 6 weeks of life. Congenital leukemia cutis, as compared with later-onset leukemia cutis, is believed to be quite common in the setting of this malignancy, with incidence estimates in the literature ranging between 25% and 30% of patients with congenital AML.[159] The cutaneous lesions range in size from a few millimeters to several centimeters and are usually red to brown to violaceous papules and nodules (Figs. 10.21 and 10.22). This latter

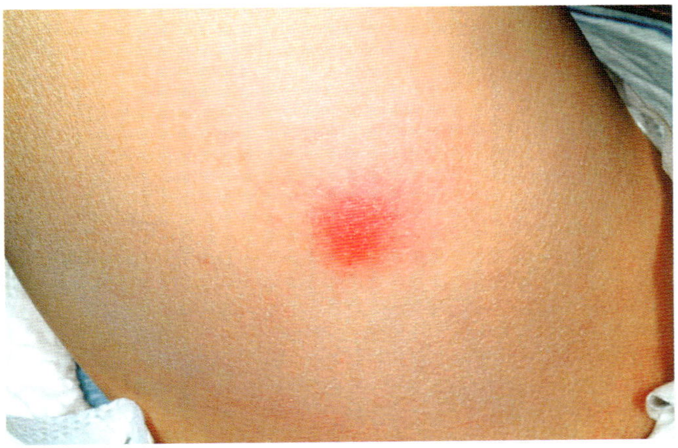

Fig. 10.19 Leukemia cutis. Erythematous nodule in a 3-year-old with diagnosed acute lymphocytic leukemia.

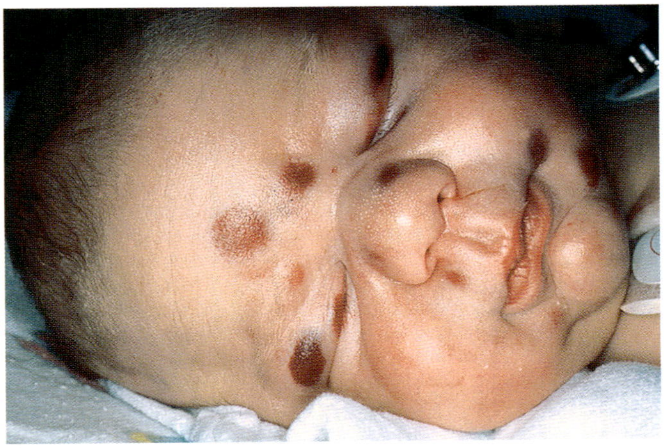

Fig. 10.21 Congenital leukemia cutis. Congenital acute lymphocytic leukemia with cutaneous facial lesions. (Courtesy Anne Lucky, MD.)

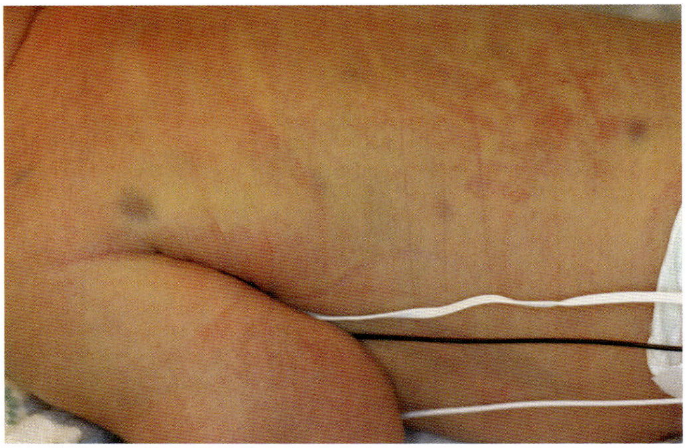

Fig. 10.22 Congenital leukemia cutis. This 2-day-old male had numerous congenital violaceous papules and nodules. Skin biopsy revealed histology and immunophenotyping consistent with metastatic lesions of monocytic leukemia.

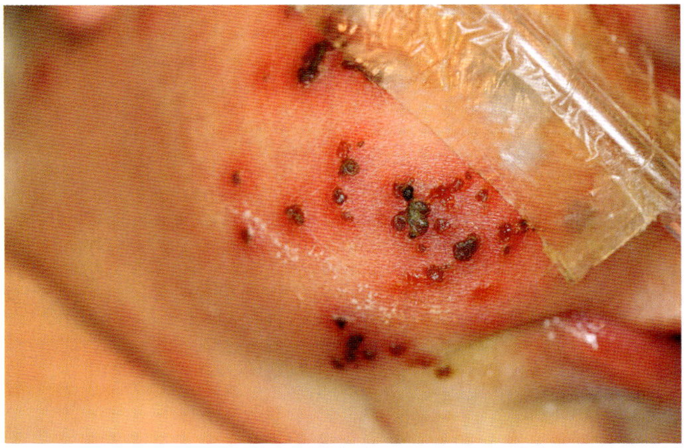

Fig. 10.23 Vesiculopustular eruption in a patient with Down syndrome and a transient myeloproliferative disorder. This 7-day-old had numerous vesicles and crusted vesiculopustules on his bilateral cheeks in conjunction with high numbers of circulating blasts. Both the skin and hematologic findings normalized spontaneously without the development of leukemia.

Box 10.6 Causes of Blueberry-Muffin Cutaneous Lesions in a Newborn

- Neoplastic infiltrates
  - Leukemia
  - Neuroblastoma
  - Histiocytosis
- Extramedullary hematopoiesis
  - Congenital infection
    - Rubella
    - Toxoplasmosis
    - Cytomegalovirus
    - Parvovirus B19
  - Anemia
    - Hemolytic disease of the newborn
    - Hereditary spherocytosis
    - ABO incompatibility
    - Twin–twin transfusion syndrome[GC90]
- Transient myeloproliferative disorders:
  - With Down syndrome
  - Without Down syndrome

clinical presentation in the neonate (with multiple violaceous papules and nodules) has been termed *blueberry-muffin baby*, and such skin findings may represent malignant cutaneous infiltrates or any of several possible causes of extramedullary hematopoiesis. Box 10.6 lists the various causes of blueberry-muffin skin lesions. As with noncongenital leukemia cutis, cutaneous infiltrates are more common with the myelogenous type of congenital leukemia.[159] Congenital leukemia cutis is felt to portend a poor prognosis, although some reports describe occasional spontaneous remission.[160,161] However, because late relapses have been noted in some of these patients, they deserve close long-term follow-up observation. Occasionally infants with congenital leukemia cutis may have a solitary nodule.[162,163]

Patients with Down syndrome have an increased risk of hematologic aberrations, including leukemia, leukemoid reaction, and transient myeloproliferative disorder. A leukemoid reaction is a temporary overproduction of leukocytes in response to infection, hemolysis, or other stress. Transient myeloproliferative disorder, which is also self-limited, is similar except that there is no identifiable trigger.[164] Patients with Down syndrome who have a leukemoid reaction or transient myeloproliferative disorder have been described with pustular or vesiculopustular skin eruptions, and smears or biopsies of these lesions have revealed immature myeloid forms.[164,165] This vesiculopustular presentation (Fig. 10.23) is quite distinct from the typical papules and nodules that occur with leukemia cutis. The significance of this eruption is unclear, and the findings resolve without therapy as the hematologic disorder subsides. However, true leukemia may develop months to years later, and therefore long-term follow-up monitoring is again indicated.

Lymphomatoid Papulosis

Lymphomatoid papulosis (LyP) is a benign, recurrent, self-healing dermatosis with histologic features suggesting lymphoma.[166–168] It is considered to be within the spectrum of lymphoproliferative disorders that ranges from pityriasis lichenoides to cutaneous T-cell lymphoma and has been included as a separate group in classifications of lymphomas.[169]

The disorder is manifested by numerous reddish-brown papules or, less commonly, vesiculopustules that are most often noted on the trunk and proximal extremities but occasionally on the hands and feet, scalp, and genitalia (Fig. 10.24).[170] Regional distribution has been described in children, although more generalized spread may occur after several years.[171] Lesions characteristically develop hemorrhagic necrotic centers and crusting and gradually involute with residual hyperpigmentation or hypopigmentation. Occasionally, varioliform scars or large ulcerating nodules (Fig. 10.25), plaques, or nonulcerating papules occur. Although individual lesions evolve over a period of several weeks to 1 month or more, tend to appear in crops, and sometimes disappear spontaneously within a few weeks to months, the entire course of the disorder may be prolonged and last for years. The disorder is generally asymptomatic.

LyP must be distinguished clinically and histopathologically from arthropod bites, pityriasis lichenoides et varioliformis acuta (PLEVA), pseudolymphoma, and lymphoma.[172]

The classic histopathologic picture of LyP in children is characterized by a heavy infiltrate of scattered large CD30+ CD15− cells that resembles Hodgkin disease in a background of inflammatory cells (type A), although variants resembling mycosis fungoides (type B), anaplastic large T-cell lymphoma (type C), and mixtures of these lymphomas have been described.

In 10% to 20% of adult patients, malignant lymphoma develops, and adults with LyP are also at increased risk for developing nonlymphoid malignancies.[173,174] In a report of 35 pediatric patients with LyP, 9% of them developed non-Hodgkin lymphoma during a mean follow-up period of 9 years.[168] In another series of 251 children and adolescents with LyP, 14 developed lymphoma, either before, with, or after the LyP, again emphasizing the need for long-term surveillance.[175]

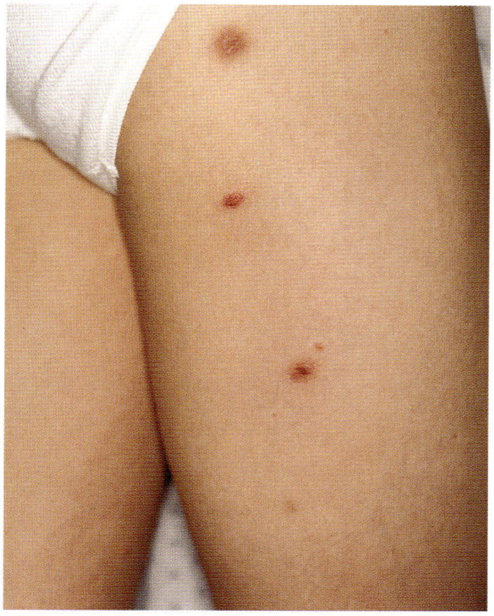

Fig. 10.24 Lymphomatoid papulosis. Reddish-brown papules, most commonly noted on the proximal extremities and trunk. This picture shows lesions in different stages of evolution from development of necrotic centers and crusting to resolution.

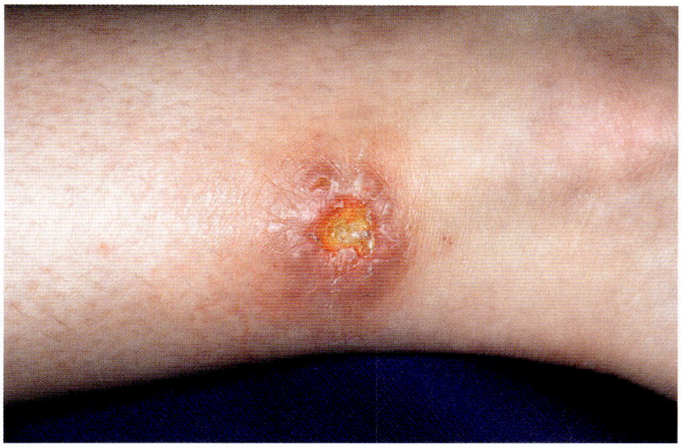

Fig. 10.25 Lymphomatoid papulosis. Ulcerating nodule.

Treatment is generally unnecessary except for cosmetic reasons because of the asymptomatic nature and tendency toward spontaneous clearance. The sometimes aggressive nature of lymphomatoid papulosis may lead to the misdiagnosis of lymphoma and chemotherapeutic treatment.[169] Application of ultrapotent topical corticosteroids twice daily for 2 to 3 weeks followed by weekly pulses has resulted in near clearance.[176] Other described therapies have included systemic steroids, methotrexate, systemic antibiotics, and phototherapy (psoralen and ultraviolet A [PUVA] and ultraviolet B [UVB]), although they usually do not lead to sustained complete remission. In one retrospective series of first-line treatments in adult and pediatric patients, however, those treated with phototherapy achieved a longer disease-free survival.[177]

Lymphoma Cutis

Lymphoma involving the skin is quite rare in children. The most common form of cutaneous lymphoma is cutaneous T-cell lymphoma

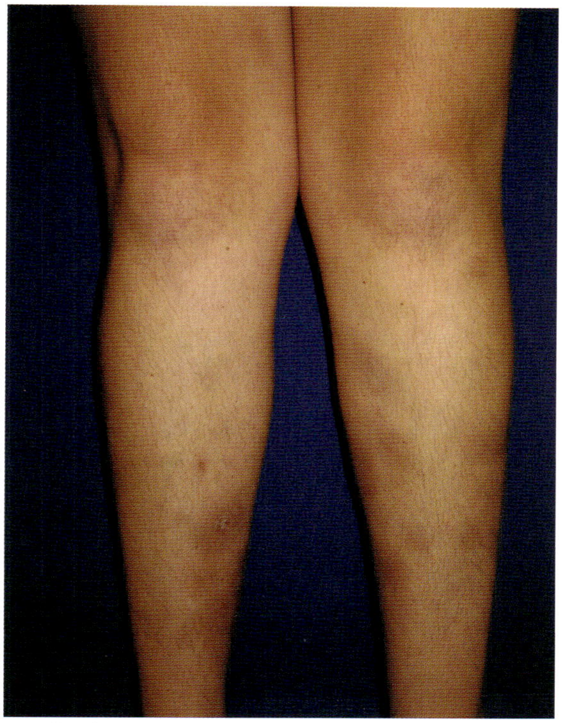

Fig. 10.26 Subcutaneous panniculitic T-cell lymphoma. Multiple tender nodules occurred on the lower extremities of this otherwise-healthy 12-year-old female. (Courtesy Joan Guitart, MD.)

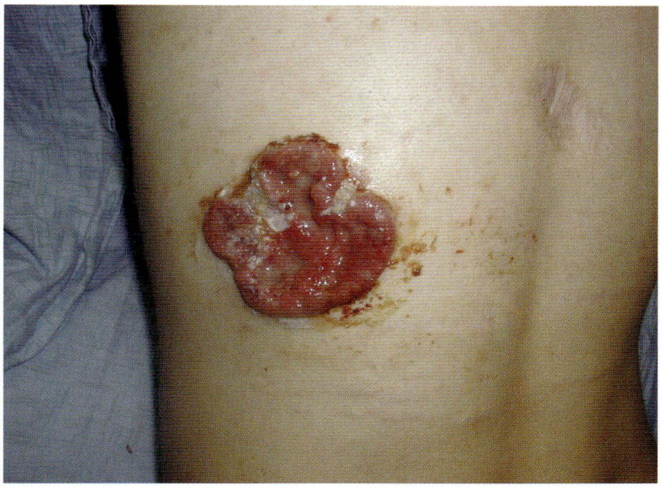

Fig. 10.27 Anaplastic large cell lymphoma. A large ulcerated tumor on the back of a 17-year-old male. Note the atrophic scar at a site of previous involvement (Courtesy Joan Guitart, MD.)

(CTCL; mycosis fungoides; see later). Other forms of lymphoma cutis include subcutaneous panniculitic T-cell lymphoma (SPTCL), anaplastic large cell lymphoma (ALCL), cutaneous B-cell lymphoma, natural killer–cell lymphoma, angiocentric CTCL, and Hodgkin lymphoma. Some types of lymphoma that can also have skin involvement but are not be discussed here include lymphoblastic lymphoma, marginal zone lymphoma, Burkitt lymphoma, and human T–lymphotropic virus (HTLV)-1–associated lymphoma. Lymphoma cutis may be a primary cutaneous process, or skin involvement may be associated with a systemic lymphoma. In patients with non-Hodgkin lymphoma overall, cutaneous involvement occurs in 1% to 5% of cases, and skin as the primary site (primary cutaneous lymphoma) is quite rare.[178–180]

Head and neck involvement is the most common pattern of cutaneous lymphoma in children.[178–180] The second most common site of involvement appears to be the abdomen.[178] Most patients present with solitary nodules in the skin, and less often multiple nodules are present. Papules or plaques are occasionally seen. The lesions are usually 5 to 10 cm in diameter, erythematous, and firm. SPTCL is a T-cell lymphoma that presents with subcutaneous nodules or nodular plaques and is most commonly seen in young adults (rarely in children). It may rarely present as diffuse cutaneous edema without nodules.[181] This tumor involves the subcutaneous fat in a manner similar to panniculitis and presents with multiple subcutaneous, inflammatory, poorly demarcated plaques and tender nodules, ranging in size from 0.5 to 10 cm. The lesions are most commonly localized to the lower extremities (Fig. 10.26) and occur less often on the trunk and upper extremities.[182,183] Ulceration may occasionally occur. Systemic symptoms include fever (most common), malaise, chills, and weight loss, and most patients have cytopenias, especially anemia.[184,185] The clinical presentation of SPTCL may mimic several processes, including lupus panniculitis and erythema nodosum, and hence this disorder may elude diagnosis.[186] SPTCL has been associated in some patients with hemophagocytic syndrome, and concomitant histiocytic cytophagic panniculitis has been observed.[187,188] Hence in any child with panniculitis and laboratory values suggestive of possible hemophagocytic syndrome, investigations for T-cell lymphoma should be performed. Treatments for SPTCL include watchful waiting, corticosteroids or other immunosuppressive agents, and multiagent chemotherapy (most often the CHOP regimen [cyclophosphamide, hydroxydoxorubicin, Oncovin, prednisone]); in patients without associated hemophagocytic syndrome, there is a favorable prognosis.

Ki-1/CD30-positive ALCL is a form of lymphoma that may simulate a metastatic carcinoma or malignant histiocytosis.[189,190] A significant proportion of patients with ALCL are children or young adults. Patients show signs of fever, wasting, lymphadenopathy, and often cutaneous lesions. Skin involvement may consist of fleeting eruptions or more specific lesions, usually painful nodules, that occasionally undergo spontaneous involution.[189,191] In 36% of children in one series with peripheral lymph node involvement, lymphomatous infiltration of contiguous skin occurred and presented as erythematous, thickened, desquamating, and ulcerative plaques.[192] Primary cutaneous ALCL (C-ALCL) presents as a rapidly evolving cutaneous tumor, often with ulceration (Fig. 10.27). It is most often solitary but may occur in regional or generalized forms.[193] ALCL is a high-grade non-Hodgkin lymphoma that has a relatively good prognosis with early multiagent chemotherapy.[190,192] The primary cutaneous form is often treated with excision or radiation without chemotherapy, because some studies have shown that chemotherapy does not affect the rates of recurrence or survival.[194,195] Biopsies of affected skin reveal large, atypical lymphoid infiltrates that stain positive with the activation antigen Ki-1, also known as *CD30*.

The systemic form of ALCL (S-ALCL) has been further divided into anaplastic lymphoma kinase (ALK)-positive and ALK-negative types, based on staining for this fusion protein. ALK-positive S-ALCL tends to have a better prognosis than the ALK-negative subtype and is the primary type of this systemic lymphoma to occur in children. C-ALCL is typically ALK-negative, but primary cutaneous ALK-positive ALCL has been reported in children and may follow a relatively benign course.[196] ALCL with a leukemic presentation has also been reported in children, and is associated with significant mortality and considered a high-risk lymphoma.[197]

Cutaneous B-cell lymphoma is fairly rare, even though B-cell lymphomas represent the majority of non-Hodgkin lymphomas occurring in lymph nodes. As with T-cell lymphomas, B-cell lymphomas may involve the skin in a primary fashion or be secondary in relation to dissemination of nodal disease. Hence complete staging and evaluation are indicated for any patient diagnosed with a cutaneous B-cell lymphoma. This form of lymphoma cutis is notoriously rare in the pediatric population. The clinical presentation of B-cell lymphoma cutis includes papules, plaques, and tumors, occasionally with associated ulceration. The head, neck, upper trunk, and extremities seem to be sites of predilection in most patients, although some subtypes favor the lower extremities. Primary cutaneous marginal zone B-cell lymphoma is an indolent lymphoma that, when occurring in pediatric patients, usually presents in teenagers; lesions are most often located on the extremities.[198,199]

Natural killer–cell (CD56+ NK/T-cell) lymphoma is classically an aggressive nasal lymphoma, although patients can also have cutaneous plaques and subcutaneous nodules. This neoplasm may occur in a primary cutaneous or secondary form, and these two variants show considerable clinicopathologic differences, with a more favorable prognosis associated with primary skin disease.[200] This neoplasm occurs primarily in older adults, seems to have an association with EBV infection, and usually is associated with a high mortality rate. Angiocentric CTCL is an unusual T-cell lymphoma of childhood that presents with a vesiculopapular eruption that may mimic hydroa vacciniforme (see Chapter 19).[201] It occurs mainly in children from Asia and Latin America and may be related to EBV infection.

Hodgkin lymphoma is a fairly common childhood lymphoma that often occurs before adolescence. It rarely occurs before the age of 5 years, and there is another peak of involvement later in adulthood. In the majority of cases, Hodgkin lymphoma, which is now classified as a B-cell lymphoma, is initially limited to the lymph nodes, with superficial lymph nodes more commonly initially involved than visceral lymph nodes. It presents as painless lymph node enlargement, usually in the neck. Hodgkin lymphoma is histologically characterized as one of several subtypes, and staging depends on the extent of lymph node involvement and the presence or absence of constitutional symptoms. Skin involvement resulting from infiltration of the malignant cells is quite rare (<1%), but nonspecific secondary findings may occur and include pruritus, purpura, ichthyosis, and pigmentary changes. When specific cutaneous lesions are present, they are usually pink to red-brown or violaceous papules or nodules that may coalesce to form larger plaques or tumors.

The treatment of cutaneous lymphomas can be planned only after thorough evaluation and staging for the extent of extracutaneous disease. Occasionally patients with low-grade neoplasms with limited involvement may be appropriately managed by watchful waiting. Therapeutic options otherwise include radiotherapy, chemotherapy, surgical excision (i.e., for localized primary cutaneous tumors), and newer cytokine and biologic therapies.

Cutaneous T-Cell Lymphoma

CTCL (mycosis fungoides [MF]) is a primary cutaneous lymphoma that occurs primarily in adults. Although approximately 75% of patients are diagnosed after the age of 50,[202] onset of the disease during childhood may occur in 0.5% to 5% of cases.[202,203] It has been diagnosed in patients as young as 22 months of age[202] and is suspected to have started in patients as young as 10 months of age.[204] Many factors may contribute to the seemingly lower incidence of CTCL in children, including lack of recognition of its occurrence and hesitancy to perform skin biopsies in younger patients. Delay in diagnosis is most common in the youngest age group (0 to 3 years old), and the average time to diagnosis is 5 years.[204,205] The possibility of CTCL should be considered in the setting of chronic dermatoses recalcitrant to therapy, and serial skin biopsies may be necessary.[206] In general, patients who have CTCL during childhood are more likely to have limited disease and as a result seem to have a better disease-specific survival rate than older patients with CTCL.[202,207] In a series of 74 patients under the age of 30 years with CTCL, overall survival was very high (97.2%), and progressive disease was noted in 26%. Favorable prognostic features included the hypopigmented variant (see later) and younger age, and progressive disease was associated with older age, Black race, the poikilodermatous variant, and advanced-stage disease.[208] Some studies, however, have found no statistically significant differences in the course between early childhood– and adult-onset disease.[209] Table 10.4 lists the updated staging and classification for CTCL.

The clinical presentation of CTCL is quite variable. Most pediatric patients have erythematous, scaly patches, papules, and plaques (Fig. 10.28) with variable degrees of pruritus. Thin, erythematous,

Table 10.4 Updated TNMB Staging/Classification of Cutaneous T-Cell Lymphoma

Stage	Skin (T)*	Nodes (N)†	Visceral (M)‡	Blood (B)§
IA	1	0	0	0, 1
IB	2	0	0	0, 1
IIA	1–2	1, 2	0	0, 1
IIB	3	0–2	0	0, 1
III	4	0–2	0	0, 1
IIIA	4	0–2	0	0
IIIB	4	0–2	0	1
IVA1	1–4	0–2	0	2
IVA2	1–4	3	0	0–2
IVB	1–4	0–3	1	0–2

Adapted from Olsen E, Vonderheid E, Pimpinelli N, et al. Revisions to the staging and classification of mycosis fungoides and Sezary syndrome: a proposal of the International Society for Cutaneous Lymphomas (ISCL) and the cutaneous lymphoma task force of the European Organization of Research and Treatment of Cancer (EORTC). *Blood* 2007;110(6):1713–22; Wilcox RA. Cutaneous T-cell lymphoma: 2016 update on diagnosis, risk-stratification and management. *Am J Hematol* 2016;91(1):151–65.

BSA, Body surface area; *TNMB,* tumor, nodes, metastasis, blood.

*Skin: T0, clinically suspicious lesions; T1, limited papules or plaques (<10% BSA); T2, generalized papules or plaques (>10% BSA); T3, one or more tumors; T4, generalized erythroderma (confluence of erythema covering ≥80% BSA).

†Nodes: N0, no clinically abnormal peripheral lymph nodes; N1, clinically abnormal peripheral lymph nodes, histopathology Dutch grade 1; N2, clinically abnormal peripheral lymph nodes, histopathology Dutch grade 2; N3, clinically abnormal peripheral lymph nodes, histopathology Dutch grade 3–4.

‡Visceral: M0, no visceral organ involvement; M1, visceral involvement confirmed by pathology.

§Blood: B0, atypical circulating cells (Sézary cells) not present (<5%); B1, low blood tumor burden (>5% are Sézary cells); B2, high blood tumor burden (≥1000/μL Sézary cells).

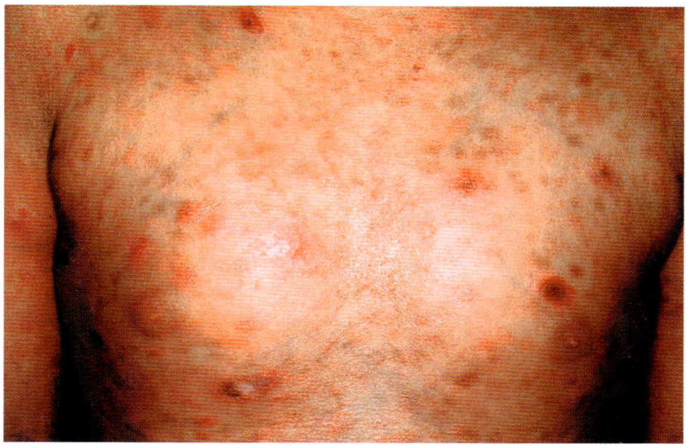

Fig. 10.28 Cutaneous T-cell lymphoma. Erythematous macules, papules, plaques, and nodules in this 6-year-old male. Skin biopsy revealed an atypical T-cell infiltrate with similar circulating cells noted in the blood.

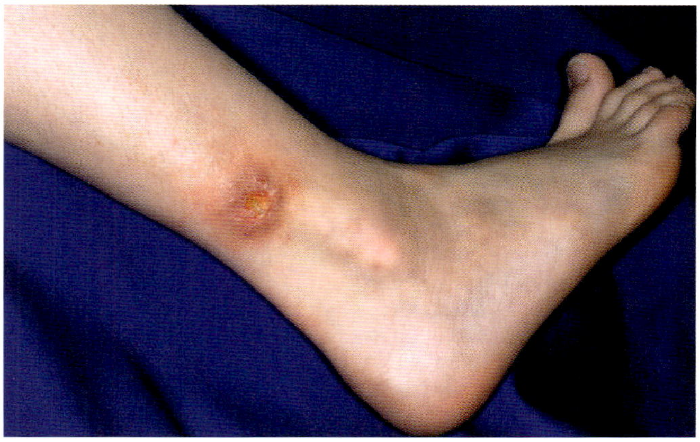

Fig. 10.29 Lymphomatoid papulosis in a patient with cutaneous T-cell lymphoma (CTCL). This 10-year-old male with a long history of patch- and plaque-stage CTCL developed intermittent self-healing ulcerative nodules that were noted to be CD30+ on histologic evaluation.

atrophic patches on the trunk and buttocks are a classic presentation. At times, central clearing develops and the lesions assume serpiginous, arciform, horseshoe, or other bizarre shapes. The lesions of CTCL may simulate many other skin disorders, including atopic dermatitis, psoriasis, parapsoriasis, hypopigmenting or depigmenting disorders (i.e., vitiligo or pityriasis alba; see later), and pityriasis lichenoides.[210,211] Some patients show changes of poikiloderma characterized by the combination of hyperpigmentation and hypopigmentation, atrophy, and telangiectasia. Although the lesions themselves may not be pathognomonic for CTCL, their chronic nature and history of recalcitrance to therapy often prompt further diagnostic investigations. Skin nodules and tumors, which may grow aggressively and occasionally ulcerate, are an uncommon presentation of pediatric CTCL and are more often seen in adult and elderly patients. Occasionally, focal skin nodules may intermittently occur superimposed on a background of patch- or plaque-type CTCL, with CD30+ cells and a self-limited clinical course consistent with lymphomatoid papulosis[212] (Fig. 10.29). Occasionally, patients exhibit skin findings suggestive of pigmented purpuric dermatosis.[213,214] In some patients, the entire cutaneous surface may become infiltrated, producing thickened red skin with or without scaling and with islands of normal skin often remaining for a time before the universal erythroderma becomes complete.

Hypopigmented CTCL is a variant of the disease that occurs most commonly in children and appears to be the most common pediatric presentation, especially in Blacks and Asians.[208,215] It tends to present most often in patients with black or darkly pigmented skin, although more fair-skinned individuals may also manifest these findings.[216–218] Patients with this form of CTCL show hypopigmented macules and patches (Fig. 10.30) that are usually asymptomatic. The clinical appearance most often simulates disseminated pityriasis alba, tinea versicolor, or postinflammatory hypopigmentation. Lesions may be round, arcuate, or gyrate, and often there is some subtle overlying scale.[203] Histologically, biopsies of hypopigmented lesions show the same features as the inflammatory lesions of CTCL, although on immunophenotyping, the infiltrate may be shown to be composed predominantly of CD8+ T cells rather than CD4+ T cells,[219] and there may be lack of fibroplasia and lichenoid infiltrate.[220]

Granulomatous slack skin (GSS) is an extremely rare form of CTCL characterized by the insidious onset of papules and violet-colored plaques with progression to pendulous skin masses.[221] The lesions appear erythematous, wrinkled, and cutis laxa–like, and are most commonly distributed in the axillary and inguinal regions. There is a male predominance in the literature.[203] Histologically, a granulomatous T-cell infiltrate is seen along with fragmentation of elastic fibers.[222] GSS occurring in pediatric patients may progress to CD30+ large cell lymphoma and may be more aggressive than the same disorder when it presents in adults.[198]

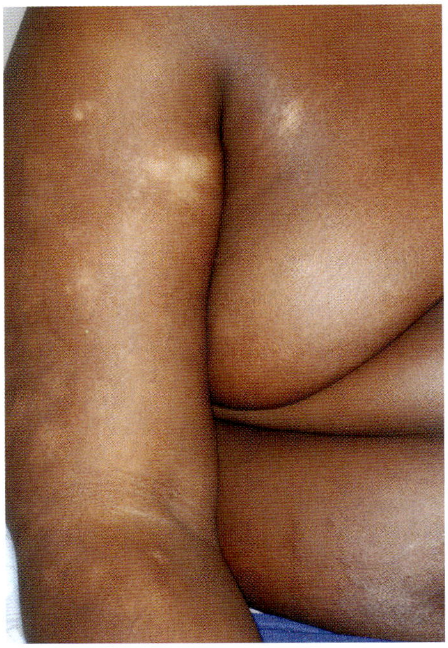

Fig. 10.30 Hypopigmented cutaneous T-cell lymphoma. Scattered hypopigmented macules and patches were present diffusely in this 13-year-old male with biopsy-confirmed cutaneous T-cell lymphoma.

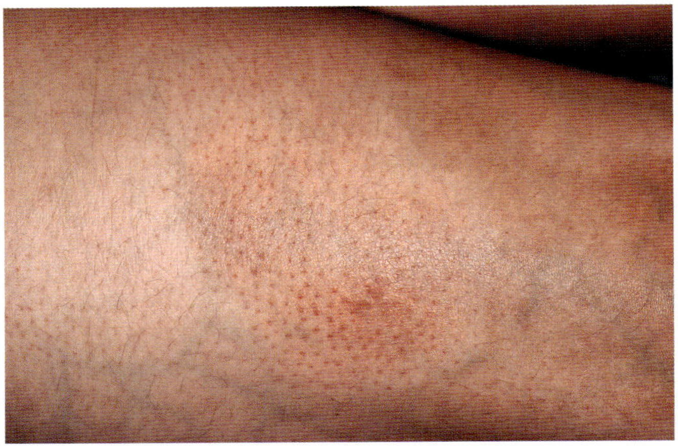

Fig. 10.31 Follicular mucinosis. This hypopigmented patch with superimposed follicular erythematous papules was present on the leg of a young boy with a known history of cutaneous T-cell lymphoma.

Follicular mucinosis (alopecia mucinosa) (see Chapter 7) has also been seen as a feature of CTCL, primarily in adults. Although it occasionally occurs as a manifestation of the disorder in children, in the majority of patients (children and adults <40 years), it is generally regarded as a benign condition not associated with CTCL. In a series of 31 children with follicular mucinosis, 12 fulfilled criteria for CTCL, and the vast majority responded to treatment with mild- to moderate-potency topical corticosteroids.[223] In another series of 11 patients with the condition, 3 were found to have CTCL based on immunophenotyping and/or T-cell–receptor gene cell rearrangement.[224] Follicular mucinosis presents as well-demarcated, flesh-colored to hypopigmented patches with prominent superimposed follicular papules (Fig. 10.31), often with associated hair loss. It occurs most commonly on the lower extremities, although it may also involve the trunk or face, and there are usually multiple lesions. Although most cases in childhood represent a benign self-limiting process, when lesions are persistent or other suggestive features are present, evaluation for possible CTCL should be considered. Folliculotropic-type CTCL (also known as follicular MF, or FMF) is defined as CTCL with folliculotropism on histologic examination, with or without follicular mucinosis; it was the second most common type (following the hypopigmented type) in a large series of pediatric patients with CTCL.[225] Pityriasis lichenoides–like CTCL presents with erythematous papules with scaling and crusting that simulate pityriasis lichenoides chronica or pityriasis lichenoides et varioliformis acuta (see Chapter 4).[226,227]

Sézary syndrome, which is characterized by erythroderma, lymphadenopathy, and circulating atypical lymphocytes (Sézary cells), is felt to be a systemic variant of CTCL. It is rare in children. The cutaneous eruption is scaly, pruritic, and resistant to multiple therapies. As with many forms of CTCL, repeat skin biopsies may be necessary to confirm the diagnosis.

The diagnosis of CTCL is established based on the histologic findings of skin biopsy tissue in conjunction with immunohistochemical studies. Although there are characteristic histologic features in well-developed disease, biopsy findings in patients with early involvement may be difficult to distinguish from other, more benign processes such as inflammatory dermatoses.[203] Immunohistochemical studies usually reveal an infiltrate of CD4+ T cells with loss of CD7+ (leu-9) cells. Southern blot analysis and polymerase chain reaction (PCR) may be used to evaluate for T-cell receptor γ gene rearrangement, which is seen in many, but not all, CTCL specimens.[228] A more specific technique, combining PCR and denaturing gradient gel electrophoresis (DGGE), demonstrates more sensitivity for detecting clonality but poorer specificity, because it may detect rearrangements in a subset of patients with chronic dermatitis.[229]

There is a variety of treatment options for children with CTCL, but no standard protocols exist, pediatric experience with several of the treatments is limited, and the ideal therapy remains unclear. Potent topical corticosteroids are often sufficient for limited patch- or plaque-stage CTCL, but patients must be monitored for adrenal suppression and cutaneous atrophy.[230] Narrowband UVB therapy may offer similar results as those seen in adults and has the potential advantages of being well tolerated in children, having fewer unpredictable phototoxic reactions and requiring shorter treatment sessions.[231] It is often recommended as a first-line therapy for children with CTCL, and in a series of 28 pediatric patients (the majority of whom had the hypopigmented variant of CTCL and all of whom had stage I disease), narrowband UVB therapy offered complete or partial response in 86%, with a subsequent course of treatment needed in 58% and no disease progression noted over a median follow-up period of 43 months.[232] Topical nitrogen mustard has demonstrated efficacy in adults with patch- or plaque-stage disease, and long-term follow-up studies have confirmed its safety.[233] PUVA photochemotherapy is effective but may be difficult and have limiting side effects in children. Topical PUVA has been demonstrated useful in children with patch- and plaque-stage disease.[234] Other therapies used for CTCL include carmustine, imiquimod, tazarotene, electron-beam therapy, systemic chemotherapy, denileukin diftitox (a fusion toxin), interferon, photopheresis, and bexarotene (a systemic rexinoid, a cousin of the retinoids). Young patients with CTCL may have an increased risk of Hodgkin lymphoma and hence should be monitored on a long-term basis.

Neuroblastoma

Neuroblastoma, a tumor derived from primitive cells of the sympathetic nervous system, is the most common malignant tumor affecting infants in the first month of life and accounts for 30% to 50% of all tumors occurring in the newborn period.[235] It is a tumor with large variability in its clinical presentation and natural history. Neuroblastoma may regress spontaneously (particularly in infants), mature into a benign ganglioneuroma, or result in extensive metastatic disease with a poor prognosis.[236] These tumors typically present as an abdominal mass because of liver infiltration with malignant cells and may originate in the adrenal medulla, visceral ganglia, or paravertebral

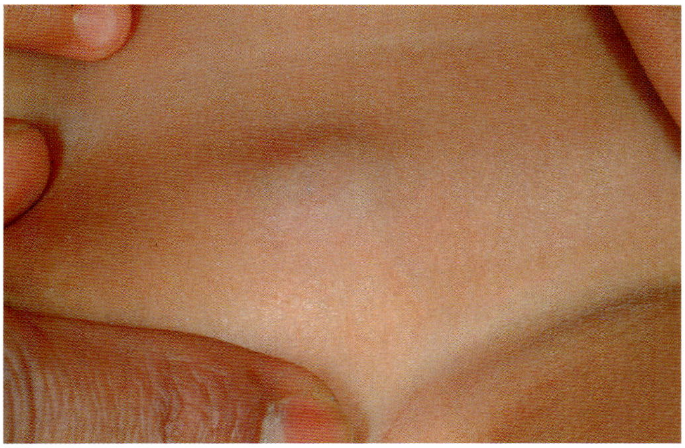

Fig. 10.32 Neuroblastoma with cutaneous metastases. This male infant had numerous firm, blue subcutaneous nodules that revealed neuroblastoma on histologic examination. He was found to have a large retroperitoneal primary tumor with disseminated metastatic disease.

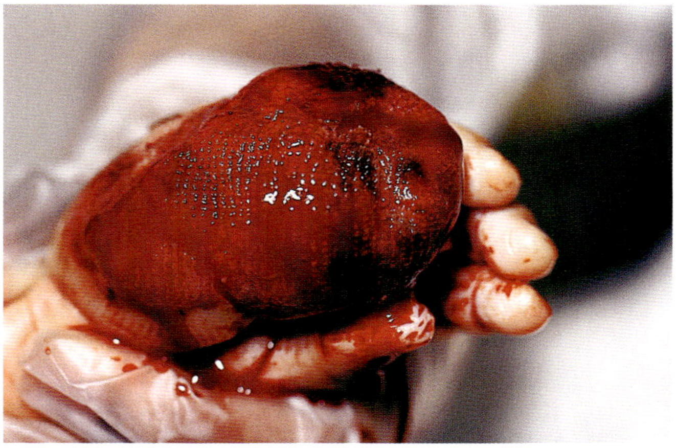

Fig. 10.33 Fibrosarcoma. This congenital, vascular, friable mass was initially thought to be an infantile hemangioma; it grew rapidly and ultimately required full excision with amputation.

sympathetic ganglia. Mutations that have been associated with neuroblastoma include *Phox2b* (mainly familial cases) and *ALK*, with germline genetic variants (which may predispose to sporadic disease) identified in *LINC00340*, *BARD1*, *LMO1*, *DUSP12*, *DDX4*, *LIN28B*, *HACE1*, and *TP53*.[237]

Cutaneous metastases of neuroblastoma are seen in around 2% of all patients and 32% of those with a neonatal presentation. These skin lesions, which may be the presenting sign of the disease, appear as firm, blue-purple papules and nodules (Fig. 10.32). When occurring in a neonate, they fall into the spectrum of blueberry-muffin lesions (see Box 10.6). The catecholamines produced by the tumor cells may result in the classic blanching and peripheral halo of erythema noted after firm stroking. Subcutaneous nodules mimicking deep infantile hemangiomas have also been observed.[238] When cutaneous metastases of neuroblastoma are encountered in the infantile period, it confers a more favorable prognosis than other patients with metastatic neuroblastoma, although tumor biology is the most critical prognostic consideration.[235,239] This favorable effect on prognosis is most apparent for children 17 months of age and younger with cutaneous metastases.[240] Very hard subcutaneous nodules arising from the skull and orbital ridges are caused by skeletal metastases. Orbital metastases may result in the classic presentation of periorbital ecchymoses, so-called "raccoon eyes." Another ocular finding is that of heterochromia irides, which is related to involvement of the ophthalmic sympathetic nerve.

Staging of neuroblastoma is based on clinical and radiographic extent of disease and surgical resectability. Tumor tissue is usually necessary to confirm the diagnosis, and when cutaneous lesions are present, skin biopsy with histologic evaluation, immunophenotyping, and genetic analysis may be indicated. Measurement of urine and serum catecholamines or metabolites, CT and/or MRI, bone marrow aspirate and biopsies, and iodine-123 metaiodobenzylguanidine (MIBG) scintigraphy are recommended as part of the staging evaluation.[241] Treatment recommendations range from observation only to intensive multimodal therapy, including chemotherapeutic, immunotherapeutic, and biologic therapies, as well as surgery and radiotherapy; targeted therapies (i.e., oral tyrosine kinase inhibitors for patients with documented *ALK* mutations) are also being studied.[242]

Rhabdomyosarcoma

Rhabdomyosarcoma is the most common soft tissue sarcoma in children and adolescents, accounting for 50% of all soft tissue sarcomas in those under 15 years of age and 4.5% of all cases of childhood cancer.[243–245] It is a malignant soft tissue neoplasm of skeletal muscle origin and is seen primarily in the first and second decades of life. Although rhabdomyosarcoma is not typically a primary skin tumor, it is included in this section, because it may simulate other cutaneous tumors, may extend or metastasize to the cutaneous surface, and may initially present to the pediatrician or other pediatric healthcare provider. Mutations associated with rhabdomyosarcoma may include *TP53*, *NRAS*, *KRAS*, *HRAS*, *PIK3CA*, *CTNNB1*, and *FGFR4*.[246]

Rhabdomyosarcoma usually presents as an asymptomatic mass that is occasionally painful.[247] The head and neck, especially the nasal cavity and paranasal sinuses, are the most common sites of involvement in children. The genitourinary tract and extremities are other common sites of predilection.[245] Patients may present with small to large nodules or rapidly expanding swellings. The surface may be flesh-colored to erythematous and at times may appear vascular with prominent vessel markings. The differential diagnosis may include infantile hemangioma, vascular malformation, fibrosarcoma (Fig. 10.33), cyst, infection, or other inflammatory or neoplastic process. Perianal rhabdomyosarcoma may mimic perirectal abscess.[248] *Primary cutaneous rhabdomyosarcoma* refers to a tumor that arises in the dermis or subcutis with no other identifiable primary tumor elsewhere and that tends to display aggressive behavior in both adults and children.[249] Congenital alveolar rhabdomyosarcoma is a rare subtype, with more than 50% of patients presenting with multiple cutaneous metastases[250] (Fig. 10.34). Tumor-specific translocations such as *PAX3-FOXO1* and *PAX7-FOXO1* are detected in the majority (70% to 80%) of cases, and the disorder is invariably fatal.

Treatment of rhabdomyosarcoma consists primarily of surgery, radiation therapy (including both traditional and newer options such as intensity-modulated, proton beam, and brachytherapy), and chemotherapy; it is hoped that targeted molecular agents will offer more promise in the future.[251–253] Although challenging, the overall 5-year survival rate of children and adolescents with both nonmetastatic and metastatic rhabdomyosarcoma approaches 80%.[254]

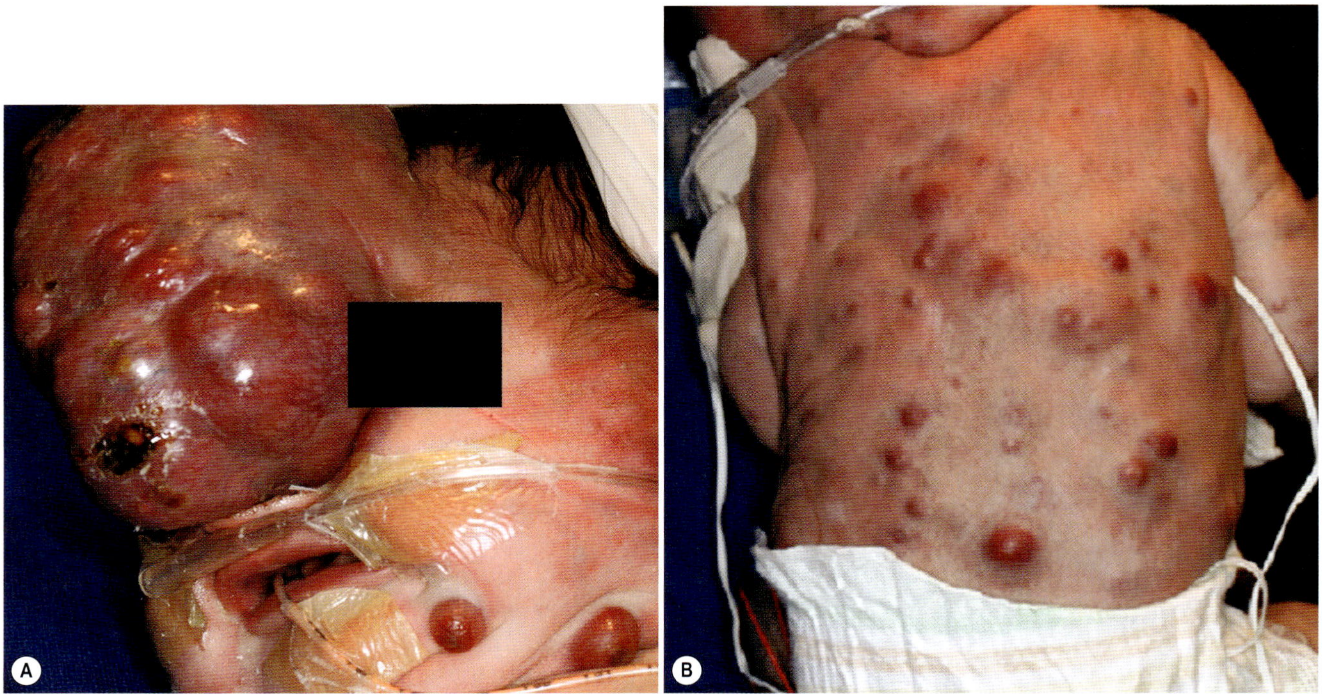

Fig. 10.34 Congenital alveolar rhabdomyosarcoma. This newborn female presented with a large congenital facial mass **(A)** with numerous cutaneous **(B)** and internal metastases; histopathologic evaluation of tissue biopsy confirmed the diagnosis of rhabdomyosarcoma, alveolar subtype. She expired on day 17 of life.

The complete list of 259 references for this chapter is available online at http://expertconsult.inkling.com.

Key References

Krooks J, Minkov M, Weatherall AG. Langerhans cell histiocytosis in children. History, classification, pathobiology, clinical manifestations, and prognosis. J Am Acad Dermatol 2018;78:1035–44.

Rigaud C, Barkaoui MA, Thomas C, et al. Langerhans cell histiocytosis: therapeutic strategy and outcome in a 30-year nationwide cohort of 1478 patients under 18 years of age. Br J Haematol 2016;174:887–98.

Emile JF, Abla O, Fraitag S, et al. Revised classification of histiocytoses and neoplasms of the macrophage-dendritic cell lineages. Blood 2016;127(22):2672–81.

Kempf W, Kazakov DV, Belousova IE, et al. Paediatric cutaneous lymphomas: a review and comparison with adult counterparts. J Eur Acad Dermatol Venereol 2015; 29(9):1696–1709.

Virmani P, Levin L, Myskowski PL,et al. Clinical outcome and prognosis of young patients with mycosis fungoides. Pediatr Dermatol 2017;34(5):547–53.

Iehara T, Hiyama E, Tajiri T, et al. Is the prognosis of stage 4s neuroblastoma in patients 12 months of age and older really excellent? Eur J Cancer 2012;48(11):1707–12.

Weitzman S, Egeler RM. Langerhans cell histiocytosis: update for the pediatrician. Curr Opin Pediatr 2008;20:23–9.

Postini AM, Brach del Prever A, Pagano M, et al. Langerhans cell histiocytosis: 40 years' experience. J Pediatr Hematol Oncol 2012;34(5):353–8.

Bode SFN, Lehmberg K, Maul-Pavicic A, et al. Recent advances in the diagnosis and treatment of hemophagocytic lymphohistiocytosis. Arthritis Res Ther 2012; 14:213.

Nijhawan A, Baselga E, Gonzalez-Ensenat A, et al. Vesiculopustular eruptions in Down syndrome neonates with myeloproliferative disorders. Arch Dermatol 2001;137:760–3.

Taggart DR, London WB, Schmidt ML, et al. Prognostic value of the stage 4s metastatic pattern and tumor biology in patients with metastatic neuroblastoma diagnosed between birth and 18 months of age. J Clin Oncol 2011;29(33): 4358–64.

Monclair T, Brodeur GM, Ambros PF, et al. The International Neuroblastoma Risk Group (INRG) staging system: an INRG task force report. J Clin Oncol 2009; 27(2):298–303.

Loeb DM, Thornton K, Shokek O. Pediatric soft-tissue sarcomas. Surg Clin N Am 2008;88:615–27.

11 Disorders of Pigmentation

CHAPTER OUTLINE Disorders of Abnormal Pigmentation | Disorders of Hyperpigmentation

Although chiefly of cosmetic significance, disorders of pigmentation are among the most conspicuous and thus can have profound psychosocial implications for pediatric patients. The most important pigments in skin are melanin, reduced and oxygenated hemoglobin, and carotene. Melanin is a pigment produced by melanocytes, specialized dendritic cells derived from the neural crest that migrate to the basal layer of the epidermis during embryogenesis. Melanocytes synthesize and package melanin within discrete membrane-bound organelles called *melanosomes*, which are then transferred via melanocytic dendrites to surrounding keratinocytes of epidermis and hair follicles; on average, there is one melanocyte to every 36 surrounding keratinocytes.[1–4,5] Variations in skin color among different individuals reflect the number and size of mature melanosomes, not the number of melanocytes.

Four stages of melanosome maturation have been described and can be distinguished by ultrastructural examination:

1. Membrane vesicles that contain no visible pigment (stage I or premelanosomes)
2. More elongated vesicles with an ordered internal membrane but no pigment (stage II melanosome)
3. The presence of melanin on ordered internal fibers (stage III melanosome)
4. Structures so full of melanin that the luminal structures cannot be seen (mature or stage IV melanosomes).

Darkly pigmented individuals have more numerous, larger, singly dispersed melanosomes, whereas individuals with light pigmentation have fewer, smaller melanosomes that are aggregated into complexes and are more rapidly degraded.[6] The presence of melanin, which caps cell nuclei in the epidermis, protects against ultraviolet (UV) radiation and associated cutaneous damage, including pigmented nevi,[7] actinic damage, and cutaneous neoplasia.

Melanin exists in two forms in human skin: brown-black eumelanin and yellow-red pheomelanin. Melanin biosynthesis is primarily regulated by tyrosinase, a copper-dependent enzyme that allows the initial conversion of tyrosine to dihydroxyphenylalanine (DOPA). Eumelanin synthesis involves increased levels of tyrosinase activity, higher pH,[8] and additional melanogenic enzymes such as tyrosinase-related protein (TRYP)-1 and dopachrome tautomerase (DCT; formerly called *TRYP-2*), both regulators of distal steps in the pathway to melanin and/or stabilizers of tyrosinase. Pheomelanin synthesis, however, requires addition of a cysteinyl group that accounts for the yellow-red color and is associated with reduced tyrosinase activity, low pH, and absence of TRYP-1, DCT/TRYP-2, and P protein (pink-eyed dilution protein).

The ratio of eumelanin to pheomelanin, as well as the total content of melanin, is higher in skin types V to VI (the darkest skin colors) than in skin types I and II (the lightest skin colors, most at risk for burning with UV light exposure). Pheomelanin levels tend to be greatest in individuals with bright red hair, whereas eumelanin is the predominant pigment in individuals with brown or black hair.[9]

Genetic polymorphisms affect overall pigmentation, as well as the risk of developing ephelides (freckles), nevi, and melanoma (Box 11.1). The main determinant to the type of pigment formed by melanocytes is the genotype of *MC1R*, encoding the G-protein–coupled α−melanocyte-stimulating hormone (α-MSH) receptor. Among the allelic variants in *MC1R* are R-alleles (approximately 18% of Whites) and r-alleles (approximately 27% of Whites). In Whites, R-alleles are strongly associated with the red hair color (RHC) phenotype, which includes red hair, fair skin, freckling, and an increased risk of both nonmelanoma and melanoma skin cancers.[5,10] RHC is a recessive trait that requires having two R-allele variants.

Having the SLC45A2/MATP 374L variant is typical of those from African and Asian populations, as well as Europeans with olive skin and dark hair. In contrast, the 374F variant is found in more than 95% of light-skinned Europeans. The *SLC24A5*/NCKX5 A111T change is found in virtually all persons of European descent, whereas the 111A allele is universally found in dark-skinned individuals of African descent. MATP and NCKX5 are melanocyte membrane-bound ion transport proteins, highlighting the role of active pumping of ions in melanin production. Reduction in MATP activity (as occurs in oculocutaneous albinism type 4) lowers melanosome pH and reduces tyrosinase activity. Reduction in NCKX5 activity (as occurs in oculocutaneous albinism type 6) impairs melanosome maturation and melanin biosynthesis. Skin color is also altered by nonpathogenic variants in *KITLG*, which encodes the ligand for the c-KIT receptor, known to regulate the number of melanocytes in development and cutaneous melanin distribution.[11] Single nucleotide polymorphisms (SNPs) in *KITLG* have been associated with darker skin color in Blacks (rs642742*T/C) and blonde hair in northern Europeans (rs12821256). The rs12203592*T SNP in *IRF4* (interferon regulatory factor 4) is linked strongly to dark hair color but light eyes, reduced ability to tan, more pigmented nevi during adolescence (in homozygotes), and an increased risk of melanoma and solar elastosis in adults. The *IRF4* rs12203592*C SNP, in contrast, is common in Asian and African populations. *IRF4* (in collaboration with the master regulator of melanogenesis, *MITF* [microphthalmia transcription factor]) is a driver of tyrosinase expression. Increased numbers of nevi have also been linked to variants in *IRF4* and *MITF*, as well as with other genes are involved in melanogenesis (*MTAP*, *PLA2G6*, *CDKN2A*, and *CDK4*).[12]

In all races the dorsal and extensor surfaces are relatively hyperpigmented, and the ventral surfaces are less pigmented. This is most evident in races with darker skin (Blacks, Hispanics, and Asians). The separation of the dorsal and ventral pigmentation is most conspicuous on the extremities (Voigt–Futcher lines) (Fig. 11.1).[13] This differentiation of dorsal and ventral pigmentation is present from infancy and persists throughout adulthood. Approximately 75% of Blacks and 10% of Whites have at least one line of pigmentary demarcation.

Disorders of Abnormal Pigmentation

Disorders of decreased pigmentation may be classified as follows:

1. Genetic or developmentally controlled disorders, in which pigmentation tends to be abnormal from birth or early infancy

Box 11.1 Determinants of Pigmentation Based on Genetic Polymorphism

Hair, Skin, and Eyes

MC1R (melanocortin receptor 1) R allele on both genes: red hair color (RHC) phenotype
 Red hair, fair skin, freckling, higher risk of skin cancer
TYR (tyrosinase)
TYRP1 (tyrosinase-related protein-1)
DCT (dopachrome tautomerase)
HERC2/OCA2 (P protein)
IRF4 (interferon regulatory factor 4)
MITF (microphthalmia transcription factor)

Skin Color

SLC45A2/MATP (membrane-associated transporter protein)
SLC2A5/NCKX5 (Na/Ca/K exchange protein)
KITLG (ligand for c-KIT receptor)

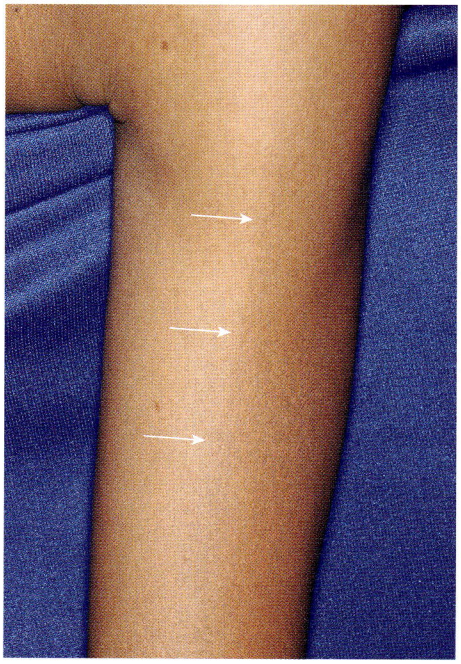

Fig. 11.1 Voigt–Futcher line. This persistent line of demarcation separates dorsal and ventral pigmentation.

2. Disorders associated with depigmentation or loss of previously existing melanin

Genetic disorders of decreased pigmentation include tuberous sclerosis, piebaldism, Waardenburg syndrome (WS), and albinism. Acquired disorders of decreased pigmentation include vitiligo, postinflammatory hypopigmentation, pityriasis alba, and tinea versicolor. Hypopigmentary disorders may be further divided into patterned and unpatterned groups. Patterned forms of decreased pigmentation include pityriasis alba, hypopigmented mycosis fungoides/cutaneous T-cell lymphoma, tinea versicolor, postinflammatory hypopigmentation, leprosy, pinta, tuberous sclerosis, pigmentary mosaicism, vitiligo, piebaldism, and the Waardenburg and Vogt–Koyanagi syndromes. Unpatterned decreases in pigmentation may be seen in albinism, phenylketonuria, and the silvery hair syndromes.

VITILIGO

Vitiligo, an acquired form of patterned loss of pigmentation,[14,15] affects approximately 1% of the population.[16] Although rarely congenital, its onset in about half of affected patients is before the age of 20 years and in one-quarter before 8 years of age.[17–19] The disorder has a prevalence of 7% to 12% among first-degree relatives, 6% among siblings, and 23% among monozygotic twins,[20] but a 2012 study suggested a family history of vitiligo in approximately 30% of patients.[21] Relative to postpubertal onset (after 12 years of age), prepubertal onset is associated with a greater likelihood of a family history of vitiligo and a personal history of atopic dermatitis.[21] Autoimmune disorders are seen with significantly increased incidence in immediate family members of affected individuals, most commonly vitiligo itself,[17] but other autoimmune disorders (particularly hypothyroidism and alopecia areata) occasionally occur in pediatric patients with vitiligo.[22–24] Thyroid autoimmune antibodies have been described in 11% of patients.[22,25,26] Although theoretically individuals with vitiligo should have a higher risk of skin cancer, studies have shown either no increase or a protective effect of vitiligo on the development of melanoma and nonmelanoma skin cancer.[27]

Vitiligo is a polygenic, multifactorial disorder that involves at least 16 susceptibility genes[28–30] encoding a variety of proteins involved in regulation of the adaptive and innate immune systems, as well as tyrosinase, the principal vitiligo autoimmune antigen. $CD4^+$ T-regulatory (Treg) cells play a role in preventing and regulating autoimmune disease, and patients have reduced number and/or function of Tregs[31] in vitiliginous skin. The role of insufficient Treg cells is further emphasized by the increased risk of developing vitiligo in patients with IPEX syndrome (immune polyendocrinopathy and X-linked syndrome; see Chapter 3), who lack Treg cells, and the reversal of vitiligo with Treg cell transfer in animal models.[32] The other population of cells that seems to play a role are tissue-resident memory T cells (T_{RM}), which may explain disease reactivation at the same site.[33] T_{RM} cells persist in the skin and do not circulate, enabling a fast memory immune response. Patients with vitiligo have circulating T cells that are skewed toward T helper 1 (Th1) cell polarization,[34] and circulating CXCL10 is increased.[35] Autoantibodies that can destroy melanocytes have also been detected in serum samples of patients with vitiligo, further emphasizing that alterations are not limited to lesional skin.

Vitiligo has been divided into several subtypes based on the distribution of lesions. In descending order of incidence in pediatric patients, these include generalized, focal, segmental, acrofacial, mucosal, and universal. Although usually considered to be a bilateral disorder, vitiligo may be asymmetric, especially with segmental vitiligo. Segmental vitiligo, which accounts for 5% to 16% of cases overall, occurs more often in children than in adults. It tends to develop and progress within 0.5 to 2 years but then stabilizes without further intervention. In segmental vitiligo, the depigmentation is confined to a localized, usually unilateral area, commonly on the face (Figs. 11.2 and 11.3). Occasionally, children have segmental involvement preceding the more typical generalized form.

In the generalized form, the location, size, and shape of individual lesions vary considerably, yet the overall picture is characteristic. Lesions usually appear as partially or completely depigmented ivory-white macules or patches, usually with well-defined, sometimes hyperpigmented, convex borders[40] (Figs. 11.4 through 11.7). They tend to have an oval or linear contour and range in size from several millimeters to large patches. Rarely, extensive or near-total depigmentation of the body (universal or total vitiligo) occurs (see Fig. 11.5). In 75% of affected individuals, the first lesions occur as depigmented spots on exposed areas such as the dorsal surfaces of the hands, face, and neck. Other sites of predilection include the body folds (the axillae and groin), body orifices (the eyes, nostrils, mouth, navel, areolae, genitalia, and perianal regions (see Figs. 11.6 and 11.7), and areas over bony prominences such as the elbows, knees, knuckles, and shins (see Fig. 11.4). Approximately 12% of patients show white hairs (leukotrichia or poliosis) (Fig. 11.8; see Fig. 11.2) within areas of vitiligo or as the predominant manifestation (follicular vitiligo),[41] especially notable when there is scalp involvement.

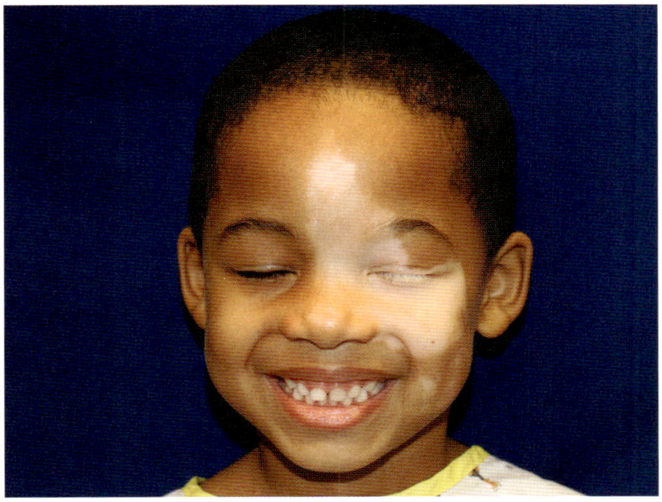

Fig. 11.2 Segmental vitiligo. Unilateral depigmented patch that also involves the left periorbital area and eyelashes.

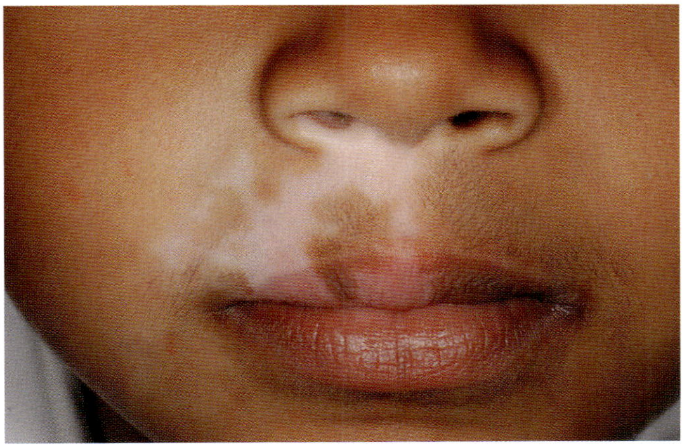

Fig. 11.3 Segmental vitiligo. Segmental distribution of depigmentation on the right side of the philtrum and upper lip. Note the sharp midline demarcation.

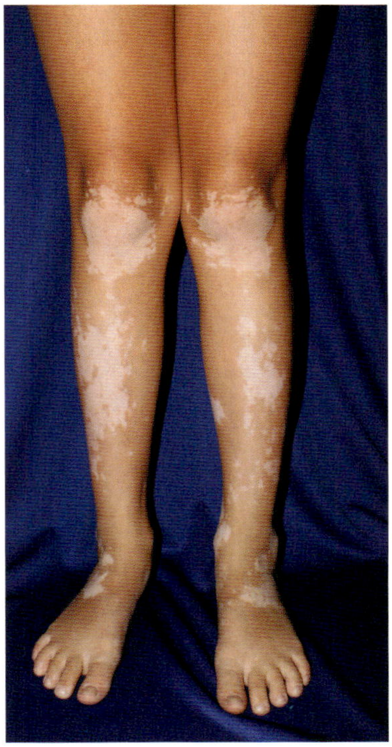

Fig. 11.4 Vitiligo. Symmetric depigmentation of the knees and lower extremities. The dorsal aspect of the feet and hands are particularly hard to repigment.

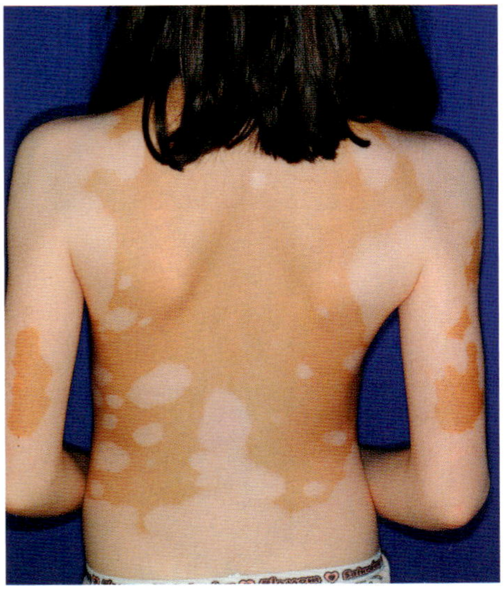

Fig. 11.5 Vitiligo. Extensive depigmentation in this 13-year-old girl. Virtually all of her skin was depigmented, except for the pigmented areas on the back. After years of unsuccessfully trying to stimulate repigmentation, at 16 years of age this girl and her parents elected to initiate 20% monobenzyl ether of hydroquinone.

Patients with vitiligo, especially those with prepubertal onset,[21] commonly show halo nevi,[42] pigmented nevi surrounded by a zone of depigmentation (Fig. 11.9) (see Chapter 9, Fig. 9.27 and 9.28). The discovery of a halo nevus and particularly multiple halo nevi[43] should prompt the search for vitiligo elsewhere.[44] The molecular mechanism for development of halo nevi parallels that of the development of vitiligo.[38]

The Koebner phenomenon (development of a lesion after trauma) has been described in approximately 15% of affected children with vitiligo, particularly related to sunburn. A 2003 study showed that skin friction induces melanocyte detachment in persons with vitiligo but not in individuals with normal skin, further emphasizing the role of trauma in triggering new lesions.[45] Other individuals associate the onset of vitiligo with periods of severe physical or emotional trauma.

Ordinarily the diagnosis of vitiligo is not difficult, especially when there is symmetric depigmentation about the eyes, nostrils, mouth, nipples, umbilicus, or genitalia. In fair-skinned individuals, it may be difficult to differentiate areas of vitiligo from the adjacent normal skin. In such cases, examination under Wood light in a darkened room may help delineate a contrast between normal and depigmented skin. When the diagnosis is in doubt, the distribution of lesions, the age at onset, the presence of a convex hyperpigmented border, and the characteristic sites of predilection may help establish the correct diagnosis.[46]

Lesions of postinflammatory hypopigmentation are typically hypopigmented, not depigmented, and patients usually provide a

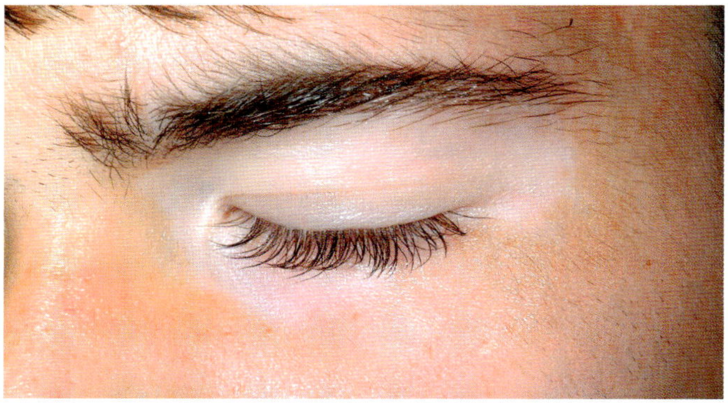

Fig. 11.6 Vitiligo. Periorbital depigmentation. Although eyebrows and eyelashes are occasionally affected as well (poliosis), in this boy the hair has retained its pigmentation. The perioral and perinasal areas are also commonly affected on the face.

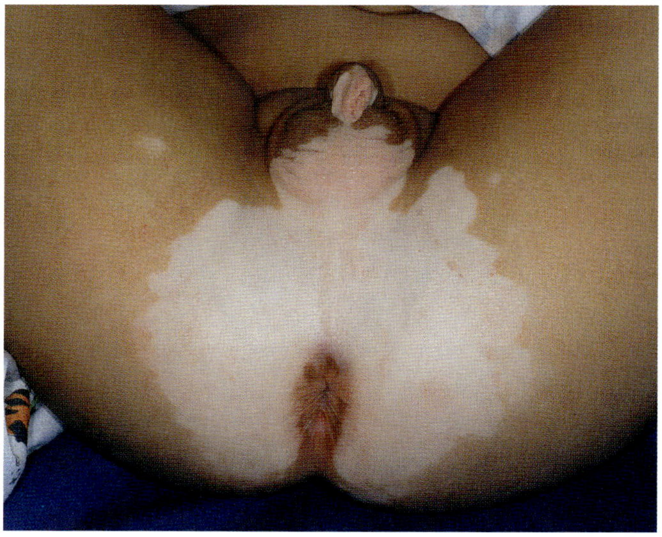

Fig. 11.7 Vitiligo. The vitiligo was limited to the genital and perianal areas in this Black boy.

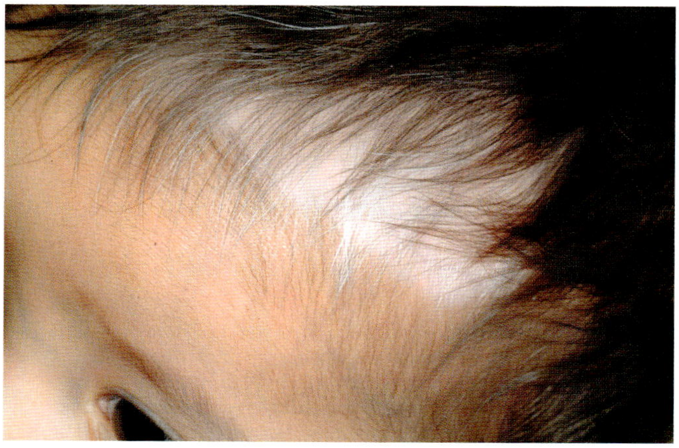

Fig. 11.8 Vitiligo with poliosis. When the hair in the affected area is white, there is a decreased likelihood of repigmentation.

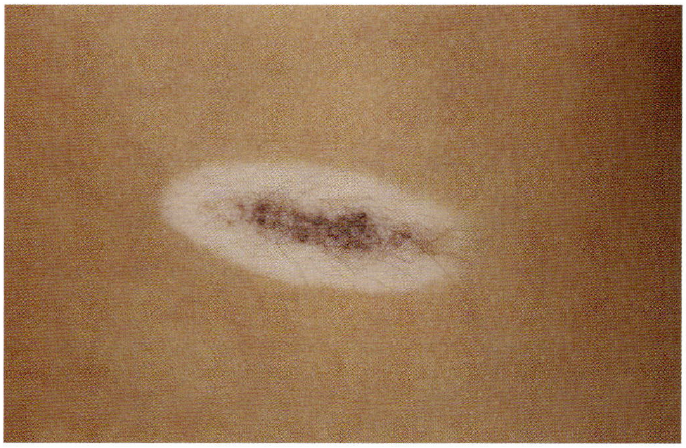

Fig. 11.9 Vitiligo. Halo nevi are commonly seen in children with vitiligo and can partially or fully clear the nevus. Any patient with a halo nevus should be completely examined for the possibility of vitiligo elsewhere. The mechanism of clearance of pigmentation in vitiligo and halo nevi is thought to be the same.

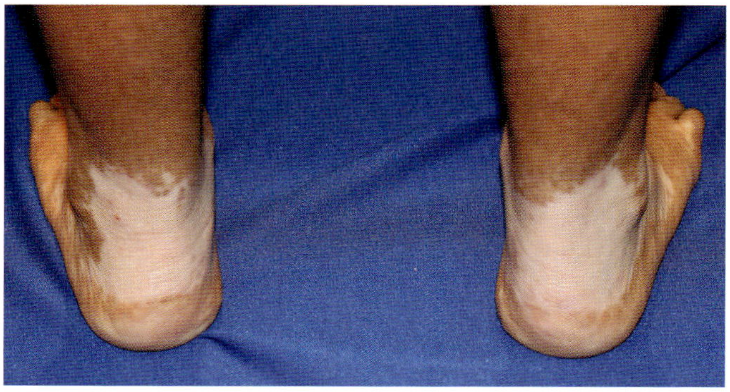

Fig. 11.10 Vitiligo characteristically localizes to joint areas and sites of frictional trauma.

history of previous localized inflammation. However, it is not uncommon to see residual depigmentation in severe atopic dermatitis, especially in darker-skinned patients and involving the wrists, hands, ankles, and feet (Fig. 11.10). Nevus depigmentosus tends to be a well-defined, usually hypopigmented patch that may be present at birth or appear during infancy as normal pigmentation increases but is subsequently stable (see Fig. 11.24). Pityriasis alba is a hypopigmentary disorder and may be further differentiated by its common distribution on the face, upper arms, neck, and shoulders and its occasional fine adherent scale (see Chapter 3, Fig. 3.38). Lesions of tinea versicolor may be differentiated by their discrete or confluent small, round hypopigmented macules; their fine scales; and their typical distribution on the trunk, neck, upper arms, or particularly in pediatric patients, the face (see Chapter 17, Figs. 17.38 and 17.39). The demonstration of hyphae on microscopic examination of epidermal scrapings is confirmatory (see Fig. 17.41). The diagnosis of cutaneous T-cell lymphoma of the hypopigmented type should be considered in adolescents with more extensive hypopigmented macules resembling pityriasis alba (see Chapter 10, Fig. 10.30).[47]

The presence of a white forelock and the pattern of depigmentation suggest a diagnosis of piebaldism or WS (see Figs. 11.18 and 11.21). Most individuals with WS show characteristic facial features. The diagnosis of albinism (see Oculocutaneous Albinism section) may be established by its presence at birth and by the fact that normal eye color is retained in vitiligo (but not in albinism); in addition, hair on glabrous skin in the patient with vitiligo, in contrast to that in the patient with albinism, often retains most of its pigment (see Fig. 11.12). Adolescents with GM3 synthase deficiency progressively develop depigmented patches as well as acral lentigines.[48] The hypopigmented macules of tuberous sclerosis (see Fig. 11.23, *A*) usually lack the characteristic milk-white appearance of lesions of vitiligo, are present at birth or during the first years of life, do not change with age, and have a normal number of melanocytes (with reduction in size of melanosomes and melanin granules within them) in contrast to the absence or decrease in number of melanocytes in patients with vitiligo.

The course of vitiligo is variable. Long periods of quiescence may be interrupted by periods of extension or partial improvement. Complete spontaneous repigmentation is very rare, and in one study, more than 50% repigmentation occurred in only 2.4% of patients over 6 months.[49] At least partial repigmentation is more likely in children with lesions of recent onset and during the summer months because of increased exposure to UV light. Loss of pigmentation in lesions that have at least partially repigmented is common in temperate climates during the winter months. The repigmentation process proceeds slowly, although children tend to respond with more permanent and complete repigmentation than adults. Repigmentation most commonly appears as small, freckle-like spots of repigmentation, reflecting the migration of melanocytes from the hair follicle (Fig. 11.11). As such, the chance of repigmentation in a site is greater if pigmentation of regional hairs is retained. Diffuse repigmentation of lesions or repigmentation from the margins has also been described. The preferential tendency to repigment the face and neck versus other body sites has been attributed to the high density of hair follicles at these sites, as well as exposure to UV light. In contrast, sites lacking or poor in hair follicles, such as the dorsal surfaces of the fingers, hands, feet, and the volar aspect of the wrists, do not respond as well as other areas.

Quality-of-life studies have shown that children with vitiligo have impaired social development as young adults, stressing the importance of intervention.[50–53] Risk factors associated with the highest risk for quality-of-life impairment are age (15 to 17 years), location (face and legs), and greater extent of involvement.[54] The impact of vitiligo can be particularly devastating in darker-skinned individuals, and in some societies individuals with vitiligo face tremendous discrimination. In one study, anxiety was observed in 42% of caregivers of children with vitiligo, even higher than that in caregivers of children with atopic dermatitis or psoriasis, and was correlated with poor quality-of-life scores in the children.[55] Patients with vitiligo and their families can find support through the National Vitiligo Foundation (www.vitiligofoundation.org or www. nvfi.org).

Full repigmentation is challenging, especially in children with more extensive involvement and when vitiligo involves more recalcitrant areas.[56,57] At least partial repigmentation can often be accomplished by first-line therapy, the twice-daily application of mid- to high-potency topical corticosteroids or topical calcineurin inhibitors (tacrolimus ointment, pimecrolimus cream).[58–60] The skin of the head and neck responds best to both of these treatment modalities. Overall, 40% to 90% of pediatric patients show a response to these treatments within a 6-month trial period. Moderate- to high-potency steroids can theoretically be associated with systemic absorption, especially if applied over large body surface areas or on the head and neck continuously,[24,61,62] so some suggest a discontinuous regimen (e.g., only 15 days a month) to reduce the risk; that said, evidence of local adverse events with topical treatment of vitiligo is rare. Application of a topical calcineurin inhibitor, especially for facial vitiligo, eliminates the risk of cutaneous atrophy and ocular toxicity carried by application of topical corticosteroids. However, hyperpigmentation in sun-exposed areas has been described after use of tacrolimus ointment.[63] Topical application of vitamin D_3 analogues (calcipotriene, calcipotriol) has also been used but has the potential to be more irritating. Although topical antiinflammatory therapy has been standard, one study described good to excellent repigmentation in 65% of 400 children treated with minipulses of oral methylprednisolone on 2 consecutive days weekly and fluticasone ointment twice daily.[64] A study in adults has shown that low-dose oral methotrexate gives equivalent results to oral corticosteroid minipulses.[65]

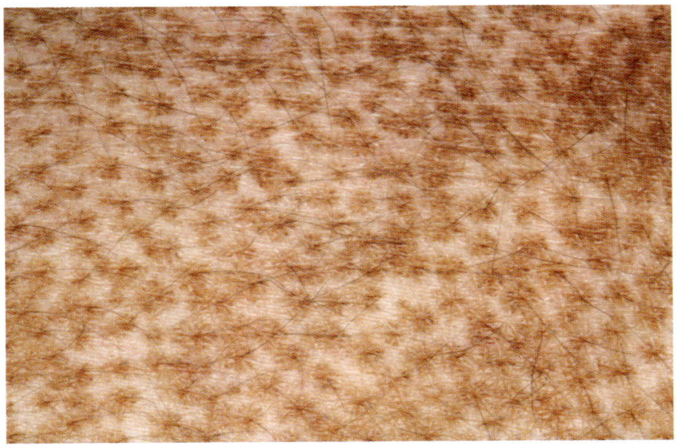

Fig. 11.11 Vitiligo. Note the perifollicular pattern of repigmentation.

Targeted immunotherapy, based on the recognized activation of the IFN-γ–CXCL10 chemokine axis, is under investigation for vitiligo.[66–70] Given that this axis signals through the JAK-STAT pathway, commercially available oral JAK inhibitors (tofacitinib and ruxolitinib) have been found to improve vitiligo in anecdotal reports. However, discontinuation leads to loss of the repigmentation, suggesting that chronic use would be necessary. Trials to evaluate efficacy and safety of oral and topical JAK inhibitors are in progress, but early evidence suggests that the combination of narrowband UVB (nbUVB) with JAK inhibition may be more effective than JAK inhibition alone.[71]

The repigmentation of lesional skin can be stimulated most effectively by exposure to UV light,[72] generally in combination with topically applied antiinflammatory medications (including topical calcineurin inhibitors[73] or vitamin D_3 analogues). Phototherapy is usually the treatment of choice if topicals are ineffective or for extensive involvement. Avoidance of burning with phototherapy is important because cutaneous burning can lead to further depigmentation via the Koebner phenomenon. Most commonly, nbUVB is used because it has been shown to be as effective as psoralen and UVA (PUVA)[72] therapy,[74–77] which is now rarely used in children because of its toxicity. nbUVB phototherapy is largely reserved for older pediatric patients who are highly motivated and completely informed about their chances for improvement with these therapies.[78] Treatment is traditionally two to three times weekly, beginning at a relatively low dose and increasing by about 20% each treatment until slight erythema is reached. Overall, 45% to 60% achieve at least 75% repigmentation.[77] The face and neck are most responsive,[79] whereas bony prominences and acral and mucosal sites usually have a poorer response. Should there not be a good response within 6 months, nbUVB can be stopped.[80] In 2017 the Vitiligo Working Group published recommendations for phototherapy use.[72] The group noted that 7 to 10 year olds are generally able to comply with phototherapy, including standing in the booth and keeping the goggles in place and eyes closed; however, in some situations, younger children are able to undergo phototherapy with an accompanying parent. The optimal frequency was thought to be three times weekly, although twice was acceptable. Given how cumbersome determining minimal erythema dose (MED) is, recommended initial dosing is 200 mJ/cm^2, regardless of skin type, increasing by 10% to 20% per treatment to a maximal acceptable dose of 1500 mJ/cm^2 for the face and 3000 mJ/cm^2 for the body. Response should be assessed after 18 to 36 exposures, with 48 the minimal number of exposures before calling lack of response. Dosing should be adjusted based on erythema and its severity. Once complete repigmentation is achieved, the frequency of nbUVB can be tapered.

Given the busy schedule of adolescents and difficulty in managing frequent office visits, home nbUVB[72,81] is an option for consideration. Numerous choices are available, ranging from handheld to full-length, cabinet-style machines. Patients must be good candidates for in-office phototherapy (motivated and able to comply), be willing to return to clinic for reevaluations, and ideally start the phototherapy in an office setting. Efficacy of in-office and at-home use has been found to be similar for vitiligo in adults.[82,83] Nevertheless, parents must be carefully instructed on home use, including about safety issues, which are low with good patient education. The major barrier for home phototherapy is insurance coverage, even though the costs overall are no greater than in-office therapy.

Targeted high-intensity[84] medium-band (304 to 312 nm) UVB light is a newer phototherapy option that has been shown to induce rapid repigmentation without full-body exposure. In a study in 27 Chinese children with 95 patches, 86% of patches showed some repigmentation and 37% at least 50% pigmentation after 10 treatments (given twice weekly) and the percentage with at least 50% pigmentation increased to 54% after 20 treatments. As with standard nbUVB, best results were seen on the face and trunk and in active (versus stable) vitiligo lesions. Similarly, the 308-nm monochromatic excimer laser (in the UVB range) is for more localized lesions.[85] The best responses to excimer laser are at sites that also respond best to nbUVB, with the dorsal aspect of the hands and feet, genital area, and suprapubic area the most difficult sites to repigment.[86] In one study of chronic stable vitiligo, more than 50% of patients showed more than 75% repigmentation.[87] Responses to the excimer laser may be improved by concurrently using antiinflammatory therapy.[88–90] Treatment with the combination of topical tacalcitol (vitamin D derivative) and excimer laser for 12 sessions (over 12 weeks) was significantly more effective than the excimer laser treatments alone.[91] The combination of excimer laser, topical tacrolimus, and short-term systemic steroid led to 75% or greater repigmentation in more than 50% of 159 patients with segmental vitiligo.[92]

Afamelanotide is a potent synthetic analogue of α-MSH that has been studied as an adjunctive agent with nbUVB. In a small study of adult vitiligo, patients achieved 49% repigmentation at 5 to 6 months of nbUVB treatment when a tiny pellet of dissolving afamelanotide was implanted subcutaneously monthly versus 33% with phototherapy alone (greater trend toward improvement with the implant); hyperpigmentation, itch, and nausea were adverse events.[93] Oral antioxidant treatments (e.g., *Polypodium leucotomos* extract, α-lipoic acid, and Gingko biloba) have also been used as adjuncts to improve the results of phototherapy. The use of pseudocatalase was based on the demonstration of decreased enzymatic and nonenzymatic oxidants in the skin of patients with vitiligo.[94] Although in one retrospective uncontrolled study twice-daily full-body application of pseudocatalase cream coupled with daily low-dose nbUVB stopped vitiligo progression and led to more than 75% repigmentation in 93% of treated children,[95] most experience with pseudocatalase cream has been disappointing.

Surgical modalities are based on the autologous grafting of nonlesional epidermis or cultured melanocytes from healthy skin sites to depigmented areas that have been deepithelialized by full surface ablative procedures.[96–101] Chinese cupping has been studied as a technique to induce blisters for capturing donor melanocytes.[102] Grafting has been demonstrated to lead to at least 75% repigmentation in 30% to 90% of patients and is most successful for more localized lesions.[103,104] Although minigrafting with or without UV light exposure has shown success, especially in patients with facial grafts and with segmental and limited stable disease subtypes,[105,106] these approaches are time consuming, costly, and can result in recurrence of vitiligo (including at the donor site), scarring, infection, and keloids in at-risk patients; grafting should only be considered for stable vitiligo in selected adolescents at sites that are resistant to medical treatment. In a 2018 trial, the direct application after dermabrasion of combined epidermal and follicular cell suspensions proved to be more efficacious than epidermal cell suspensions alone[107] based on extent and rapidity of repigmentation, color match, patient satisfaction, number of melanocyte stem cells, and expression of factors that promote repigmentation.

When treatment is unsatisfactory, lesions can be hidden by the use of camouflage therapy,[108] which has been shown to improve the quality of life in children with vitiligo.[52,109] Camouflage can be achieved most effectively with cosmetics (e.g., Cover FX, Dermablend, or Covermark), but aniline dye stains, such as Vitadye (Elder) and quick-tan preparations[110] have also been used.

In those recalcitrant cases in which vitiligo has progressed to such an extent that more than 50% of the body is involved (particularly in those persons in whom only a few islands of normal skin remain), an attempt at depigmentation with 20% monobenzyl ether of hydroquinone (Benoquin) may be considered.[111] Such patients should be reminded that the depigmentation is permanent, requiring lifelong vigilant use of sun protection. Because of the permanence of depigmentation therapy, this treatment is not generally offered to preadolescent patients.

VOGT–KOYANAGI–HARADA SYNDROME

Vogt–Koyanagi–Harada syndrome is a rare autoimmune disorder characterized by bilateral granulomatous uveitis, alopecia, vitiligo, poliosis, dysacousia (in which certain sounds produce discomfort), deafness, and sometimes meningeal irritation or encephalitic symptoms.[112,113] Usually seen in adults in the third and fourth decades of life,[114] the disorder also occurs in children and adolescents.[115,116] Drug-induced Vogt–Koyanagi–Harada–like syndrome has resulted[117–119] from treatment with nivolumab (targets PD-1 signaling), vemurafenib (BRAF), and dabrafenib (BRAF)/trametinib (mitogen-activated protein kinase [MEK]).

The bilateral uveitis occurs in all patients and generally takes a year or more to clear. The uveitis is often accompanied by choroiditis and optic neuritis. As the uveitis begins to subside, poliosis (in 80% to 90%), usually bilateral vitiligo (in 50% to 60%), alopecia (in 50%), and temporary auditory impairment develop. A prodromal febrile episode with lymphocytosis, encephalitic or meningeal symptoms, and increased pressure of the cerebrospinal fluid may precede the bilateral uveitis. Poliosis may be limited to the eyebrows and eyelashes or may also involve the scalp and body hair. The pigmentary changes, which generally appear 3 weeks to 3 months after the onset of the uveitis, tend to be permanent. Although most patients show some recovery of visual acuity, the majority of children and adolescents have a residual visual defect related to the development of cataracts, glaucoma, choroidal neovascularization, and subretinal fibrosis.[120]

Early and aggressive systemic corticosteroids are the primary intervention, but refractory cases may respond to cyclosporine, methotrexate, or tumor necrosis factor (TNF) inhibitors.[121–123] Lack of response to an initial TNF inhibitor does not preclude response to a different TNF inhibitor.[124] In one child, the facial depigmentation improved with topical steroids and tacrolimus.[125]

ALEZZANDRINI SYNDROME

Alezzandrini syndrome is a rare disorder of unknown origin that primarily seen in adolescents and young adults. Possibly related to Vogt–Koyanagi–Harada syndrome, it is characterized by unilateral degenerative retinitis with visual impairment followed after an interval of months or years by bilateral deafness and unilateral vitiligo and poliosis, which appear on the side of the retinitis.[126,127]

OCULOCUTANEOUS ALBINISM

Albinism is a group of inherited disorders of melanin synthesis manifested by a congenital decrease of pigmentation of the skin, hair, and eyes.[128,129] Although some classifications include nonsyndromic and syndromic (e.g., silvery hair and Hermansky–Pudlak syndromes) forms, the pigmentary changes are very different among these disorders. Most albinism is oculocutaneous, but affected individuals may have ocular albinism, usually an X-linked recessive form caused by mutation in *OA1/GPR143*, with the abnormal pigmentation limited to the eye. An oculocerebral syndrome with hypopigmentation (Cross–McKusick–Breen syndrome) is characterized by oculocutaneous albinism (OCA), microphthalmos, spasticity, and mental retardation.[130] A newly described lysosomal storage disorder, characterized by cutaneous (but not ocular) albinism, developmental delay, organomegaly, and enteropathy has been linked to a dominant gain-of-function missense mutation in *CLCN7*, encoding a transporter that regulates lysosomal pH; lysosomal structures, including melanosomes, are hyperacidic in the disorder.[131] Although albinism associated with immunodeficiency is primarily seen in the silvery hair syndromes (especially Chédiak–Higashi and Griscelli type 2), immunodeficiency is a feature of OCA associated with short stature (as a result of mutations in *LAMTOR2*)[132] and in Hermansky–Pudlak syndrome (HPS) type 2 (and occasionally HPS-9 and -10), all related to the requirement for secretion of lysosomes and cytosolic granules for cytotoxic T-cell and natural killer cell function, antigen presentation to T cells, and neutrophil antimicrobial activity.[133]

Nonsyndromic Oculocutaneous Albinism

Nonsyndromic oculocutaneous albinism (OCA) encompasses seven subtypes (Table 11.1) with decreased or absent melanin biosynthesis in the melanocytes of the skin, hair follicles, and eyes.[134–136]

OCA affects 1 in 17,000 persons in the United States. The highest prevalence (as high as 1% of the population) occurs in the indigenous Cuna tribe on the San Blas Islands off the coast of Panama. Affected Cuna children have been called *moon children* because they have marked photosensitivity and photophobia and prefer to go outdoors only at night. In some African tribes, the frequency is 1:1500. OCA is characterized by varying degrees of unpatterned reduction of pigment in the skin and hair, translucent irides, hypopigmented ocular fundi, and an associated nystagmus. Melanocytes and melanosomes are present in the affected skin and hair in normal numbers but fail to produce normal amounts of melanin. Regardless of subtype, affected individuals require vigorous sun protection of the skin and eyes and are at risk of adverse psychosocial effects because of the cosmetic aspects of albinism, especially in children from darker-skinned backgrounds. In addition to the stigma and potential social isolation, affected individuals in Africa (primarily OCA2) have been maimed or killed because of the myths associated with albinism (contagion, body parts with magical and medicinal powers, intercourse with an affected woman will cure human immunodeficiency virus [HIV] infection).[137,138]

In the past, albinism was divided into tyrosinase-negative and tyrosinase-positive forms based on the ability (tyrosinase-positive) or inability (tyrosinase-negative) of plucked hair to become pigmented in the presence of tyrosine or DOPA. Tyrosinase-negative albinism, now called *type I albinism (OCA1)*, results from absence (OCA1A) or partial reduction of the activity (OCA1B) of tyrosinase, the critical enzyme in melanin formation (see Table 11.1).[139] The underlying genetic bases for most forms of tyrosinase-positive albinism are also known. Type II albinism (OCA2) results from the absence of P protein.[140] OCA3 from absence of TRYP1,[141,142] and OCA4 from mutations in membrane-associated transporter protein (MATP).[143,144] OCA types 5 through 7 have been only been described in one to a few families (see Table 11.1).[145–148] The mutated gene underlying OCA5 has been mapped to 4q24. OCA6 results from mutations in *SLC24A5*/NCKX5 (Na^+/Ca^++/K^+ exchange protein) and OCA7 from mutations in ***LRMDA*** (also called *C10ORF11*), encoding the leucine-rich melanocyte differentiation-associated protein.

Table 11.1 Forms of Oculocutaneous Albinism

Type	Percentage of Patients Worldwide	Mutation	Function of Affected Gene	Comments
OCA1A	50%	TYR (absence) = tyrosinase negative	Rate-limiting steps in melanin formation; hydroxylates L-tyrosine to L-DOPA and L-DOPA to DOPA-quinone	1:40,000; most severe cutaneous and ocular defects; highest risk of skin cancer; most common type in Whites
OCA1B		TYR (decreased)	Critical enzyme in melanin formation	Subtypes: yellow mutant (yellow hair); platinum (metallic tinge); minimal pigment (only eyes darken)
OCA1-TS		TYR (mutation site functions at higher temperatures)	Temperature sensitive	Melanin at cooler sites (arms, legs) Occurs in Siamese cats
OCA2	30%	P protein	Transmembrane protein that is key for melanosome biogenesis and normal processing and transport of TYR and *TRYP1*	1:36,000 (Whites); TYR-positive; includes Brown albinism (1:3900–1:10,000; most common form in patients of African origin; more pigment with advancing age); also includes red OCA2 with concomitant *MC1R* gene mutation and red hair
OCA3 (Rufous)	3%	*TRYP1*	Catalyzes oxidation of 5,6-dihydroxyindole-2-carboxylic acid monomers into melanin and stabilizes TYR so it can leave endoplasmic reticulum for incorporation into melanosomes	1:8500 Africans; reddish-bronze color to skin and hair
OCA4	17%	*MATP/SLC45A2*	Membrane transporter in melanosomes and regulates pH	Rare (Whites); 1:, 000 Japanese (27% of OCA in Japan); resembles OCA2
OCA5		Unknown (4q24)	—	One Pakistani family
OCA6		*SLC24A5*	Na^+/K^+/Ca^++ solute carrier protein involved in melanosome maturation and melanin biosynthesis	Heterogeneous extent of pigmentation
OCA7		*LRMDA*	Melanocyte differentiation	Rare; skin color lighter only when compared with relatives

LRMDA, Leucine-rich melanocyte differentiation associated protein; *MATP,* membrane-associated transporter protein; *OCA,* oculocutaneous albinism; *P protein,* pink-eyed dilution protein; *TS,* temperature sensitive; *TYR,* tyrosinase; *TRYP1,* tyrosinase-related protein 1.

Individuals with OCA1A are unable to produce melanin at all and show white skin, white hair, and blue irides regardless of familial skin coloration.[149] Hair may show a slight yellow tint with advancing age because of denaturation of hair keratins. Similarly, ocular abnormalities are most severe with OCA1A. Eye findings include photophobia (with squinting), nystagmus (which typically develops at 6 to 8 weeks of age), strabismus, and decreased visual acuity[150]; patients with OCA1A are often legally blind. The optic fibers are misrouted, resulting in monocular vision, which is usually not altered by surgical correction of the nystagmus or strabismus.[151] Although neurologic development is otherwise generally normal, an increased risk of attention-deficit/hyperactivity disorder (ADHD) has also been described.[152] Actinic damage (cutaneous atrophy, telangiectasia and wrinkling, actinic cheilitis, actinic keratoses) and malignant skin tumors (especially squamous cell carcinoma and nodular basal cell carcinoma but also melanomas) typically are first seen in affected young adults[153] but may present during childhood if the skin and eyes are not protected.

Patients with OCA1B have been divided into different phenotypic subgroups (see Table 11.1) that occur because of differences in degree of tyrosinase activity and the localization of the mutation within the *TYR* gene. In the yellow mutant form, the hair turns yellow in the first few years and a golden blond to light brown by the end of the second decade. Patients with platinum OCA develop small amounts of pigment with a metallic tinge in late childhood. Those with minimal-pigment OCA show darkening of the eyes with time, but the skin remains without pigmentation. Individuals with temperature-sensitive OCA1B are born with white skin and hair and blue eyes. Usually during the second decade of life, however, areas with lower temperature (especially hair at acral sites on the upper and lower extremities) are able to produce melanin, because the tyrosinase activity is only inactivated above 35° C. This interesting phenotype is shared with that of the Siamese cat, a breed that also results from temperature-sensitive tyrosinase activity.

The OCA2 type of albinism, which includes tyrosinase-positive albinism and brown OCA, is the most common form and is usually the type that occurs in Black individuals (Fig. 11.12). The phenotype may vary from a slight to moderate decrease in pigmentation of the skin, hair, and eyes. With time, however, pigmented nevi may develop at sun-exposed sites (Fig. 11.13) and vision may improve.[154] These individuals can also have problems with their eyes and an increased risk of cutaneous malignancy, but significantly less than that seen in individuals with tyrosinase-negative albinism. Although the degree of pigment dilution in affected individuals is variable, the diagnosis is usually easily established in those who have striking pigment loss or relative pigment dilution when compared with unaffected siblings or parents. Some patients with OCA2 have red hair, which has been shown to result from concomitant mutations in the melanocortin 1 receptor.[155] OCA2 has also been described in approximately 1% of patients with Angelman syndrome or Prader–Willi syndrome, disorders that result from deletion of the long arm of chromosome 15, the site of the *P* gene. Prader–Willi syndrome results from deletion of the paternal chromosome at 15q and is characterized by hyperphagia with obesity, hypogonadism, and mental retardation. In contrast, Angelman syndrome results from deletion of the maternal chromosome at 15q and is characterized by microcephaly, severe mental retardation, ataxia, and inappropriate laughter. Pigment dilution occurs when both copies of the *P* gene are mutated or deleted. Interestingly, duplication of the 15q chromosomal region has been associated with generalized skin hyperpigmentation.[156]

Rufous OCA or OCA3 presents as "ginger" red hair, a reddish-bronze color of skin, and blue or sometimes brown irides. This form may be underreported because the decrease in pigmentation is slight and may be undetectable in lighter-skinned patients. OCA4 is now considered one of the most common forms in Japan,[157] and affected individuals resemble patients with OCA2.[143]

Patients with albinism should be monitored by an ophthalmologist in addition to the dermatologist. Glasses may help the poor vision, and contact lenses and tinted glasses may ameliorate the photophobia. Nystagmus may be helped by surgery of the eye muscles or contact lenses; eye patching may be needed for the strabismus. High-contrast written material, large-type textbooks, and computers that can enlarge text are all helpful for patients with poor visual acuity. Early actinic changes, keratoses, basal cell carcinomas,[158] and particularly squamous cell carcinomas are common; the risk of melanoma (often amelanotic)[159] is also increased, and it can even occur in infants.[160] Dermoscopic and reflectance confocal microscopy can help to distinguish benign nevi from melanoma.[161–163] Thus individuals with cutaneous albinism must learn to avoid sunlight exposure, wear sunglasses, and use protective clothing and sunscreen preparations on exposed surfaces. The National Organization for Albinism and Hypopigmentation (NOAH) is a national support group for patients and their families (www.albinism.org).

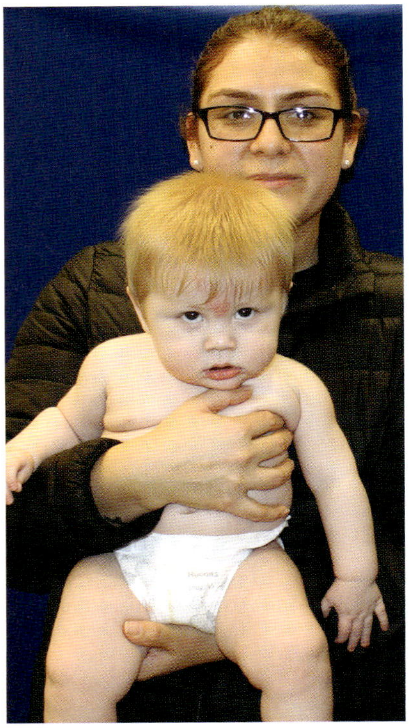

Fig. 11.12 Albinism. This Hispanic boy has type II albinism (OCA2; mutations in *P* gene) with light skin and yellow hair. Note his dark-haired mother.

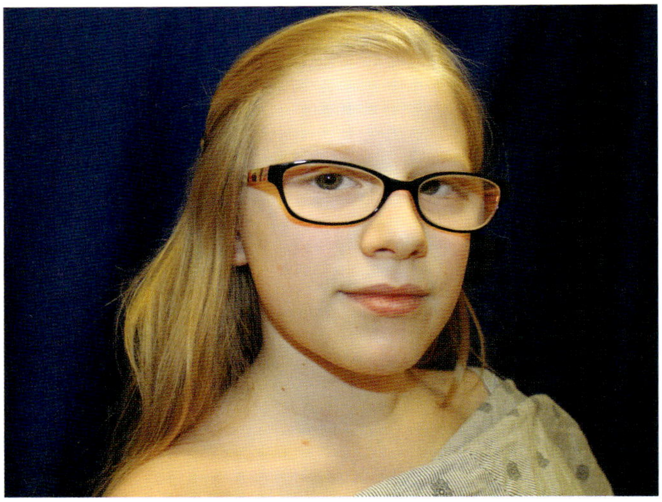

Fig. 11.13 In type II albinism, pigmentation can develop with time, including in pigmented nevi.

Table 11.2 Clinical Features of Hermansky–Pudlak Syndrome

Type	Mutation	Underlying Cause	Findings Associated with the Cutaneous Pigment Dilution
HPS-1 HPS-4	*HPS1* (82% of HPS in Puerto Ricans; 37% in non–Puerto Ricans) *HPS4*	BLOC-3 deficiency: HPS1 and HPS4 associate in a complex (BLOC-3) that regulates biogenesis of melanosomes, platelet dense bodies, and the lung lamellar body	Nystagmus, decreased visual acuity; prolonged bleeding; pulmonary fibrosis (typical onset in young adults); granulomatous colitis (up to one-third of patients)
HPS-2 HPS-10	*AP3B1* (~10% of non–Puerto Ricans) and *AP3D1* (rare)	AP-3 deficiency: *AP3B1* and APSD1 encode subunits of AP-3, which mediates protein trafficking into transport vesicles of the lysosome (and is thus also involved in immune function)	Nystagmus, decreased visual acuity; prolonged bleeding; congenital neutropenia and impaired NK cell cytotoxicity; recurrent bacterial and viral infections; conductive hearing loss; fibrosing lung disease (30%–50%) beginning during childhood; seizures in HPS-10
HPS-3 HPS-5 HPS-6	*HPS3* (~20% in Puerto Ricans and ~12% in non–Puerto Ricans) *HPS5* (~9% in non–Puerto Ricans) *HPS6* (~16% in non–Puerto Ricans)	BLOC-2 deficiency: HPS3, HPS5, and HPS6 are associated in a complex (BLOC-2) that localizes tyrosinase and *TRYP1*, allowing them to function normally	Nystagmus, decreased visual acuity; mild extraocular manifestations (bleeding, skin pigmentation)
HPS-7 HPS-8 HPS-9	*DTNBP1* *BLOC1S3* *BLOC1S6/PLDN*	BLOC-1 deficiency*: Dysbindin, BLOC1S3, and BLOC1S6 are subunits of BLOC-1 and also involved in skin melanosome biogenesis and platelet function	Nystagmus, decreased visual acuity; prolonged bleeding (may not be a feature with *BLOC1S6* mutation)

BLOC, Biogenesis of lysosome-related organelles complex; *DTNBP1*, dystrobrevin binding protein 1; *HPS*, Hermansky–Pudlak syndrome.
*Deficiency of subunits of BLOC-1 (BLOC1S5/*MUTED*, *BLOC1S4/CNO*, *KXD1*, *SNAPIN*) have not yet been reported in humans.

HERMANSKY–PUDLAK SYNDROME

Hermansky–Pudlak syndrome (HPS) is a group of at least nine autosomal recessive disorders (HPS1–9) characterized by pigment dilution, a hemorrhagic diathesis secondary to a platelet storage pool defect, and ceroid-lipofuscin depositions within the reticuloendothelial system, oral and intestinal mucosae, lung, and urine.[164–165] HPS is a disorder of biogenesis of melanosomes and other lysosome-related organelles[166–168] including platelet dense granules (Table 11.2), and all of the mutations found are in genes encoding components of protein complexes (e.g., *BLOC-1, BLOC-2, BLOC-3*, and *AP-3*) that regulate vesicle trafficking in these organelle systems.[169] HPS is most commonly seen in Hispanics from Puerto Rico (1:1800 to 1:400 persons; HPS-1 and sometimes HPS-3), in persons of Dutch origin, and in East Indians from Madras. The platelet defect in patients with HPS does not produce a severe problem in children. Its expression, however, can be aggravated by ingestion of aspirin and other prostaglandins. Special precautions and sometimes platelet transfusions must be given to avoid excessive bleeding after minor trauma or dental surgery.

The diffuse pigmentary features of the skin and eyes of individuals with HPS include pigmentary dilution of the skin and often the irides with hair that has a peculiar sheen, although not as silvery as in Chédiak–Higashi syndrome (CHS), another syndrome of dysfunction of lysosome-related organelles. Hair shafts show homogeneous distribution of melanin without clumping.[170] The degree of generalized pigment loss is quite variable in intensity, ranging from white skin to brown and light to brown eyes. Ocular pigmentation generally correlates with cutaneous pigmentation. Ocular findings include nystagmus, photophobia, and decreased visual acuity (usually 20/50 to 20/400). Extensive ecchymoses are a common clinical manifestation (Fig. 11.14). The bleeding diathesis also commonly manifests as epistaxis and menometrorrhagia. Patients with both HPS and systemic lupus erythematosus have been described.[171] Life-threatening complications of HPS, other than the bleeding diathesis, have been described in certain subtypes and are unusual in most affected children. These include granulomatous colitis (which may resemble metastatic Crohn's disease),[172,173] progressive pulmonary fibrosis,[174] and, less commonly, cardiomyopathy and renal failure. Pulmonary fibrosis is primarily a feature of HPS-1 but has been described in children in HPS-2.[175] Immunodeficiency is a primary feature of HPS-2 but has also been described in *AP3D1* mutations (in association with seizures)[176,177] and *HPS9* (which has not been associated with a bleeding diathesis).[178,179] Patients with deficiency of BLOC-2 (HSP-3, -5, -6) tend to have milder disease, including less of a bleeding diathesis, and may be hard to distinguish from oculocutaneous albinism.[180,181] However, a severe bleeding tendency has been described in a patient with *HSP6* mutation.[182]

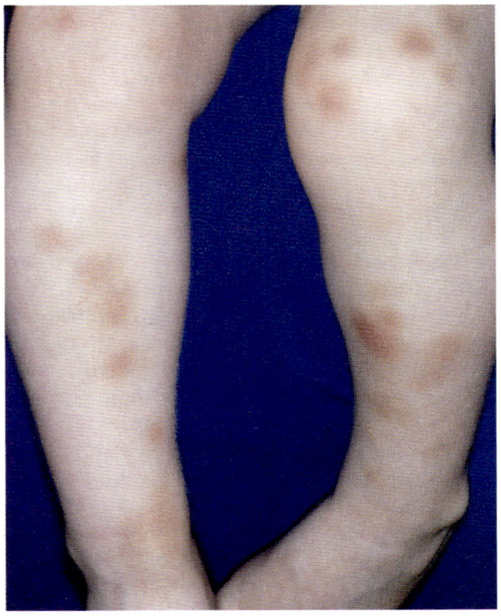

Fig. 11.14 Hermansky–Pudlak syndrome. The legs of this baby show both the pigmentary abnormality and extensive ecchymoses as a sign of the bleeding diathesis.

The life expectancy is 30 to 50 years of age. Sun protection and annual skin examinations should be recommended. Glasses or contact lenses can help to correct the refractive errors. Bleeding from skin wounds may be stopped with thrombin-soaked Gelfoam, and desmopressin (DDAVP) has been administered for tooth extraction and other invasive procedures. Transfusions of platelets or erythrocytes are occasionally required. Lung transplantation may be required because of the pulmonary fibrosis,[183] and the enterocolitis is severe in 15%, often requiring infliximab. [184] The neutropenia may respond to granulocyte colony-stimulating factor (G-CSF).

Phenylketonuria

Phenylketonuria results from deficiency in phenylalanine hydroxylase, the enzyme that converts phenylalanine to tyrosine (see Chapter 24). Although rarely an issue because of widespread perinatal Guthrie testing, untreated patients with phenylketonuria may develop generalized hypopigmentation of the hair, skin, and/or eyes compared with family members, related to the deficiency of tyrosine, the substrate for melanin. Neurologic features predominate (mental retardation, seizures, hyperreflexia), but patients may also show dermatitis and, rarely, focal morphea-like skin lesions. Treatment is by avoidance of dietary phenylalanine.

SILVERY HAIR SYNDROMES

Three syndromes, CHS, Griscelli syndrome (GS), and Elejalde syndrome (probably a subset of GS), are autosomal recessive disorders characterized by an early silvery sheen to the hair, relative pigmentary dilution of skin with a grayish coloration, and in some patients ocular hypopigmentation.[165]

Chédiak–Higashi Syndrome

Patients with CHS usually have a characteristic silvery sheen to the hair and skin, with a skin color that may appear lighter than that of other family members.[185,186] In affected individuals of family backgrounds of darker skin, however, the skin of acral, sun-exposed areas (ears, nose) may become intensely hyperpigmented (Fig. 11.15) or show only speckled hypopigmentation.[187,188] Decreased iris pigmentation results in an increased red reflex and photophobia. Strabismus and nystagmus are common, but visual acuity is usually normal. Inflammation and ulceration of the oral mucosa, especially of the gingivae, have been described.

The immunodeficiency of patients with CHS leads to infectious episodes. These episodes are associated with fever and predominantly involve the skin, lungs, and upper respiratory tract. The most common organisms found are *Staphylococcus aureus, Streptococcus pyogenes*, and pneumococcus. The skin infections are primarily pyodermas, but infections with these organisms that result in deeper ulcerations resembling pyoderma gangrenosum have been reported.

Approximately 50% to 85% of patients with CHS undergo an "accelerated" lymphohistiocytic phase during the first decade of life, characterized by widespread visceral tissue infiltration with lymphoid and histiocytic cells that are sometimes atypical in appearance.[189,190] Hepatosplenomegaly, lymphadenopathy, pancytopenia, jaundice, a leukemia-like gingivitis, and pseudomembranous sloughing of the buccal mucosa are associated features. The thrombocytopenia, platelet dysfunction, and depletion of coagulation factors may lead to petechiae, bruising, and gingival bleeding. Granulocytopenia and anemia are found in 90% of patients during the accelerated phase. Neurologic manifestations may range from seizures to cranial nerve palsy to loss of consciousness. Viral infection, particularly from Epstein–Barr virus (EBV) infection, has been implicated in causing the accelerated lymphohistiocytic phase. The pigmentary changes that help to distinguish the CHS-related accelerated phase must be distinguished from autoimmune hemophagic syndromes and familial hemophagocytic lymphohistiocytosis (genetic defects in the cytolytic granule-dependent exocytosis pathway such as perforin). Neutropenia is common, and neutrophils are deficient in chemotactic and bactericidal capability. Selective deficiency of natural killer (NK) cells is characteristic. These immune abnormalities have been thought to cause the increased susceptibility to infections and the lymphohistiocytic phase.

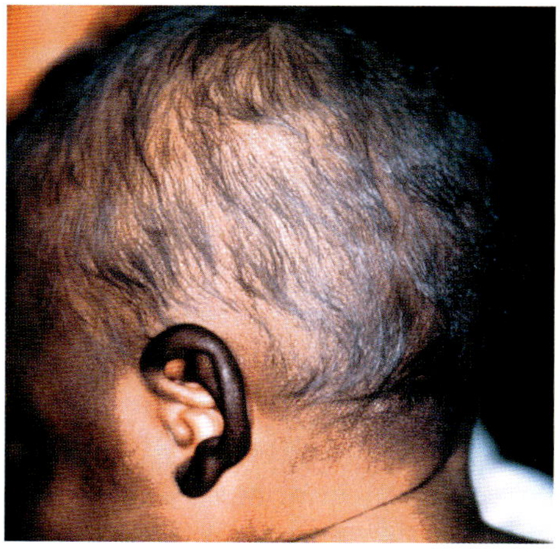

Fig. 11.15 Chédiak–Higashi syndrome. Note the silvery sheen to the hair and the intense pigmentation of the ear in this affected 8-month-old boy.

Patients who survive into early adulthood may develop progressive neurologic deterioration, particularly with clumsiness, abnormal gait, paresthesias, and dysesthesias. Peripheral and cranial neuropathies and occasionally a form of spinocerebellar degeneration may occur.

CHS results from biallelic mutations in *LYST*, a lysosomal transport protein that regulates the fusion of primary lysosome-like structures. The skin pigmentary disorder has been attributed to the inability of melanosomal fusion and transfer to keratinocytes, leading to giant melanosomes within melanocytes. Giant granules are found in circulating leukocytes, melanocytes of skin and hair, renal tubular epithelial cells, central nervous system (CNS) neurons, and other tissues. In the hair shaft, these giant melanosomes are smaller than those of GS and regularly spaced (Fig. 11.16, *A*). Skin biopsy specimens, however, show small granules of melanin uniformly distributed throughout the epidermis.[191] The giant granules within phagocytic cells of affected children cannot discharge their lysosomal and peroxidative enzymes into phagocytic vacuoles. Of note, patients with leukemia may show granules that resemble those of CHS in leukocytes.

The mean age of death for patients with CHS without immune reconstitution is 6 years of age. Fatality usually results from overwhelming infection or hemorrhage during the accelerated phase. Approximately 10% to 15% of affected patients have a milder clinical phenotype and survive into adulthood but tend to develop the progressive neurologic dysfunction.[192] Early bone marrow or stem cell transplantation is the treatment of choice for patients with a human leukocyte antigen (HLA) match. Bone marrow transplantation reverses the immunodeficiency and prevents the often-fatal accelerated phase but has no effect on pigmentation or on neurologic deterioration. Otherwise, management of the disorder is largely supportive. Antibiotics help to control the recurrent infections, and immunoglobulin or immunosuppressive agents have been administered in an attempt to control the lymphohistiocytic or hemophagocytic phases. Splenectomy has been advocated in patients with the accelerated phase unresponsive to other forms of therapy.

Griscelli Syndrome

Children with Griscelli syndrome are often diagnosed as well by their silvery hair. Three subsets of patients with GS have been described based on clinical manifestations and underlying gene defects. Two of these subsets are caused by mutations in genes close to each other on chromosome 15q21, *myosin Va* (type 1) and *RAB27A* (type 2).

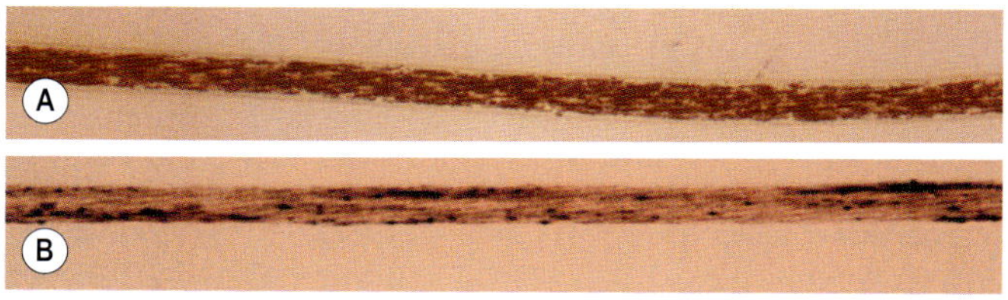

Fig. 11.16 Silvery hair syndromes. The giant melanosomes are easily seen in the hair shaft of individuals with Chédiak–Higashi syndrome (CHS) **(A)** and Griscelli syndrome **(B)**. Note the more regular spacing of the melanosomes in the hair from a patient with CHS.

Myosin Va encodes a protein that binds organelles such as melanosomes to actin. *RAB27A* is a guanosine triphosphate (GTP)–binding protein involved in the movement of melanosomes. Melanocytes are unable to transfer melanosomes to epidermal cells, and ultrastructural examination of skin biopsy specimens reveals accumulation of melanosomes in melanocytes but few in surrounding keratinocytes.

Patients who have uncontrolled activation of T lymphocytes and macrophages (hemophagocytic syndrome) and immune deficits (especially reduction in T-cell cytotoxicity and cytolytic granule exocytosis) have mutations in *RAB27A*,[193] whereas those patients with neurologic problems and without immune abnormalities or hemophagocytosis tend to have *myosin Va* mutations.[194] Cutaneous necrotizing granulomas have been described in children with *RAB27A* mutations and likely reflect the associated immunodeficiency but require comprehensive search for infection.[195] Elejalde syndrome (neuroectodermal melanolysosomal disease), characterized by similar abnormal pigmentation in the skin and hair and severe neurologic dysfunction (seizures, severe hypotonia, ocular abnormalities, and mental retardation) but no immunodeficiency or hemophagocytosis,[196,197] is now considered a subset of GS type 1.[198,199] Rare patients with neurologic abnormalities with or without hemophagocytosis have shown a *RAB27A* mutation.[196,200] Type 3 GS shows a phenotype restricted to the pigmentary defects and results either from mutation in the gene that encodes melanophilin *(MLPH)* or from a deletion in the F-exon of *myosin Va*.[201–204]

Patients with GS, especially GS type 2, may be difficult to distinguish clinically from patients with CHS, because the silver-gray hair and skin color (Fig. 11.17), recurrent episodes of fever with or without infection, increasing hepatosplenomegaly as a result of lymphohistiocytic infiltration, and progressive neurologic deterioration may be part of the clinical spectrum of both disorders.[205] In contrast to CHS, the lymphohistiocytic infiltration tends to occur in the first year of life. Blood smears show pancytopenia but, in contrast to the patients with CHS, no leukocyte inclusions. Microscopic examination of hair shows clumping of pigment in the hair shaft similar to that of CHS but with larger, more irregularly spaced macromelanosomes (see Fig. 11.16, *B*). Skin biopsy specimens show irregular pigment distribution in the basal layer, with areas devoid of pigmentation alternating with areas of large, dense granules.[191]

Intervention is similar to that of CHS, primarily through hematopoietic stem cell transplantation. Given the lack of success of transplantation in patients with mutations in *myosin Va*,[206] restriction of transplantation to patients with *RAB27A* mutations has been suggested. Early transplantation can prevent complications including the neurologic sequelae.[207,208]

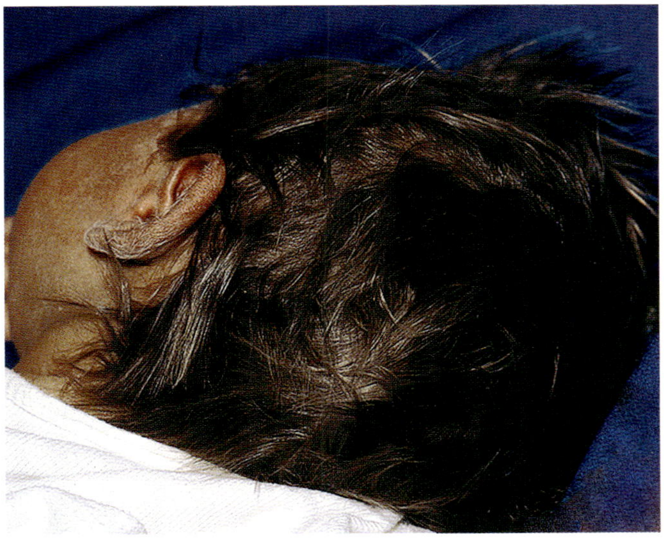

Fig. 11.17 Griscelli syndrome. The silvery hair suggests the reason for this child's hepatosplenomegaly and pancytopenia. The child died before bone marrow transplantation could be performed.

PIEBALDISM

Piebaldism is an autosomal dominant disorder characterized by congenital patterned areas of depigmentation, including a white lock of hair above the forehead (the white forelock) in most affected individuals.[209–211] The disorder usually results from mutations in the *KIT* protooncogene, which encodes a cell-surface receptor for the stem cell/mast cell growth factor[212]; deletions in *SNAI2/SLUG* (encoding snail homolog of 2), a transcription factor, have also been described.[213] The clinical manifestations of piebaldism may be explained by the resultant defective migration of melanoblasts from the neural crest to the ventral midline and a defect in the differentiation of melanoblasts to melanocytes. The distinctive patterns of hypopigmentation or depigmentation usually persist unchanged throughout life, but affected individuals with progressive depigmentation,[214] response to UV light and partial repigmentation,[215,216] or repigmentation during infancy[217,218] have occasionally been described.

The white forelock, with a depigmented triangular patch of the scalp and forehead (widest at the forehead with the apex pointing backward), occurs in 80% to 90% of individuals with piebaldism (Fig. 11.18). Depigmented areas on the forehead often include the whole or inner portions of the eyebrows and eyelashes and extend to the root of the nose. Hypopigmented or depigmented areas have also been noted commonly on the chin, anterior neck, anterior portion of the trunk (Fig. 11.19) and abdomen, and on the anterior and posterior aspects of the mid-arm to the wrist and the mid-thigh to mid-calf. Typical of the lesions of piebaldism are islands of normal and increased pigmentation within the hypomelanotic areas and sometimes hyperpigmented borders (Fig. 11.20). Intertriginous freckling and multiple café-au-lait (CAL) macules may occasionally be noted in patients and do not reflect the concurrence of piebaldism and neurofibromatosis (NF) type 1 or Legius syndrome but rather the tendency for concurrent hyperpigmented macules.[219,220]

The depigmentation of piebaldism can be differentiated from that of vitiligo by the usual presence at birth, lack of convex borders, and predilection for ventral surfaces in contrast to the predilection on

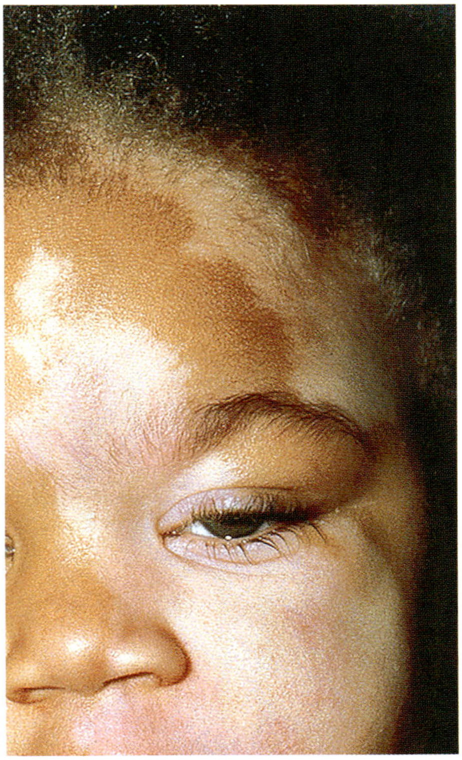

Fig. 11.18 Piebaldism. This young girl shows the white forelock with depigmentation on the forehead as two triangular patches. The left cheek is also depigmented.

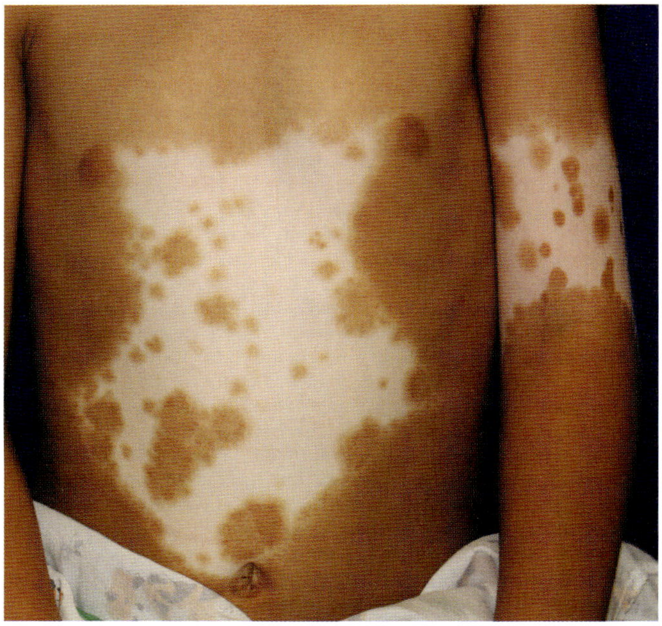

Fig. 11.19 Piebaldism. Sharply demarcated congenital depigmentation with islands of pigmentation. The left volar arm, but not the right, was involved.

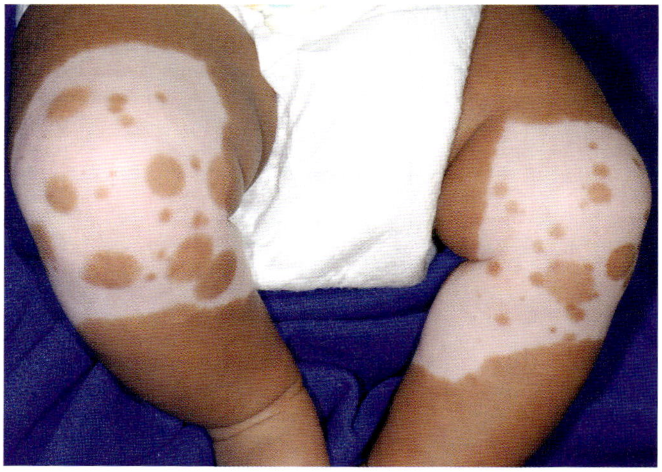

Fig. 11.20 Piebaldism. Note the sharply demarcated areas of depigmentation with the islands of normal pigmentation within the depigmented areas.

exposed areas, body orifices, areas of trauma, and intertriginous regions in vitiligo. The typical facial characteristics of type I WS are not seen in patients with piebaldism, although sensorineural deafness has rarely been described in piebaldism.[221] Biallelic homozygous mutations in *c-KIT* have been described from affected consanguineous parents; affected neonates show generalized depigmentation of the skin and hair, blue irides, and profound sensorineural deafness.[222] Incomplete penetrance has been described (e.g., a parent without evidence of piebaldism who has children with piebaldism and shares the *c-KIT* mutations).[223]

Treatment consists of cosmetic masking of areas of leukoderma[110] and vigorous sun protection. In the rare patients who show increased pigmentation after UV exposure, phototherapy may be considered. Reepithelialization by grafting from suction blisters and autologous cultured or noncultured epidermis, with or without laser, has provided permanent repigmentation. [100,224–226]

WAARDENBURG SYNDROME

Waardenburg syndrome (WS) is a heterogenous group of autosomal dominant disorders characterized by heterochromia irides, a white forelock, cutaneous depigmentation, and, in many patients, congenital sensorineural deafness.[227–230] WS reportedly accounts for 2% to 5% of cases of congenital deafness.[231] Four major subtypes of WS have been described (Tables 11.3 and 11.4).

Individuals with type I WS, the most common form, have characteristic facial features including a broad nasal root and lateral displacement of the medial canthi and lacrimal puncta of the lower eyelids (dystopia canthorum) (Fig. 11.21). [232,233] For clinical diagnosis, an individual must have two major criteria or one major plus two minor criteria to be considered affected (see Table 11.3). Dystopia canthorum can be confirmed by a W index of greater than 1.95 (see Table 11.3).[227] Congenital, usually nonprogressive, sensorineural hearing loss occurs in 47% to 58% of affected individuals, whereas the white forelock and cutaneous depigmentation occur in approximately 45% and 30%, respectively. The white forelock may be present at birth, may appear later (typically during teenage years), or may become pigmented with time. The heterochromic irides and/or hypoplastic (often brilliant) blue eyes (Fig. 11.22) are less common than the hair or skin depigmentation. Type I WS results from loss-of-function mutations in *PAX3*, a gene

Table 11.3 Diagnostic Criteria for Type I Waardenburg Syndrome

Two major criteria or one major plus two minor criteria allows for the diagnosis of WS type I

Major Criteria	Minor Criteria
White forelock, hair depigmentation	Skin depigmentation
Pigmentary abnormality of the iris	Synophrys/medial eyebrow flare
Dystopia canthorum, W index* > 1.95	High/broad nasal root
Congenital sensorineural hearing loss	Hypoplastic alae nasi
Affected first-degree relative	Gray hair before 30 years old

WS, Waardenburg syndrome.
*W index: The measurements necessary to calculate the W index (in mm) are as follows: the inner canthal distance (a), the interpupillary distance (b), and the outer canthal distance (c).
Calculate $X = (2a - 0.2119c + 3.909) / c$.
Calculate $Y = (2a - 0.2479b + 3.909) / b$.
Calculate $W = X + Y + a / b$.

Table 11.4 Subtypes of Waardenburg Syndrome

Disorder	Inheritance	Gene(s)	Other Comments
WS1	AD	*PAX3*	Most common form; dystopia canthorum
WS2	AD	*MITF, SOX10, SLUG, KITLG, KIT*	No facial dysmorphism; high risk of hearing loss; iris heterochromia
WS3	AD/AR	*PAX3*	Associated limb abnormalities
WS4A	AD/AR	*EDNRB*	Aganglionic megacolon
WS4B	AD/AR	*EDN3*	Aganglionic megacolon
WS4C	AD	*SOX10*	Aganglionic megacolon
PCWH	AD	*SOX10*	Severe hypotonicity with central nervous system and peripheral nerve abnormalities

AD, Autosomal dominant; *AR*, autosomal recessive; *EDN*, endothelin; *EDNRB*, endothelin receptor beta; *PCWH*, peripheral demyelinating neuropathy, central dysmyelination, Waardenburg syndrome, and Hirschsprung disease.

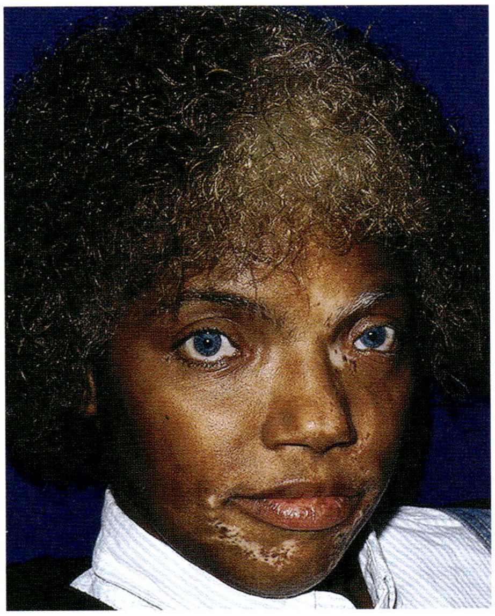

Fig. 11.21 Waardenburg syndrome, type I. Note the white forelock, dappled skin, broad nasal root, and dystopia canthorum. This young woman also had an affected son.

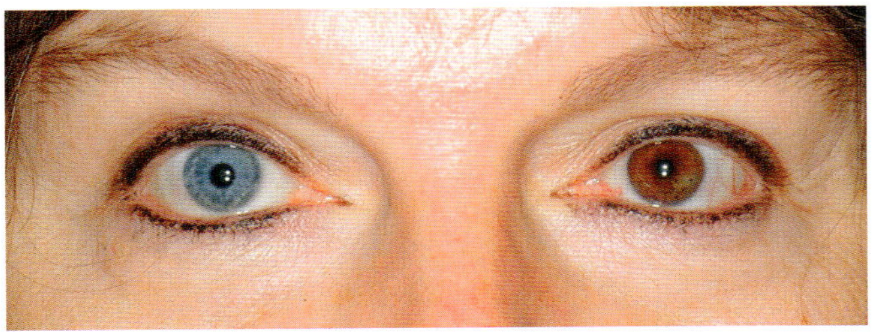

Fig. 11.22 Waardenburg syndrome, type II. This affected individual shows iris heterochromia with the brilliant blue iris. She had sensorineural deafness but none of the facial features seen in type I Waardenburg syndrome.

critical for both melanocyte migration and facial embryogenesis.[233,234] Neural tube defects ranging from sacral dimples to myelomeningocele have been described, although in the minority of patients.[235] Although the role of folic acid deficiency is unclear, folic acid supplementation before and during pregnancy is recommended for carriers. Several families have reported cleft lip and palate or vestibular symptoms.

Type II WS is a heterogeneous group of disorders that commonly shows the iris pigmentary changes (almost all patients, particularly the blue irides) and deafness (80%) of WS type I but not the facial characteristics.[236] Mutations in the microphthalmia-associated transcription factor *(MITF)* gene have been described in 15% to 21% of patients with type II WS, and the underlying mechanism may be haploinsufficiency of MITF.[237] Tietze syndrome, also linked to uniallelic *MITF* mutations, was originally characterized by generalized, albino-like pigmentary deficiency and hearing loss but no iris heterochromia; subsequent studies have shown clinical variability within families with heterozygous *MITF* mutations, ranging from a generalized decrease in pigmentation to patchy loss to no cutaneous manifestations in association with profound hearing loss and blue irides.[236] Patients with WS2 may have strabismus. Freckling in sun-exposed areas without depigmentation is common, especially among patients of Asian descent.[236–238] Other patients with type II WS have mutations in *SOX10* (15%, encoding sex-determining region Y [*SRY*]–box 10) or *SNAI2/SLUG* (as in piebaldism), transcription factors critical for the migration and development of neural crest cells, or even less often in *KITLG* or *KIT*.[238,239] Type III WS is an extreme presentation of type I WS with musculoskeletal abnormalities and a greater risk of associated neural tube defects.[240] Some but not all patients with type III WS have homozygous mutations in *PAX3*. Type IV WS includes the pigmentary defects and sensorineural deafness in association with absence of enteric ganglia in the distal part of the intestine (Hirschsprung disease); presentation with chronic constipation beginning in the neonatal period is not unusual.[241,242] Facies are normal. Mutations have been described in three genes: *EDN3*, *EDNRB*, and *SOX10*, encoding endothelin 3,[243] endothelin B receptor,[244] and Sox 10, respectively.[245] Patients with *SOX10* mutations may also have severe hypotonicity with seizures[246] and other CNS and peripheral nerve abnormalities because of the important role of *SOX10* in glial cell development.[247] All of the forms of WS show marked variability of clinical characteristics, even within families and in monozygotic twins,[248] and subtle features may be seen, especially in WS1. The white forelock may be a feature of several other genetic and acquired disorders, but most commonly piebaldism.[249] Iris heterochromia has also been described in HPS.[250]

TUBEROUS SCLEROSIS COMPLEX

Tuberous sclerosis complex (TSC) is an autosomal dominant disorder with variable expressivity that occurs in as many as 1 in 6000 to 1 in 10,000 persons.[251–254] Up to 70% of patients are thought to have new mutations. The disorder results from mutation in one of two different genes, *TSC1* (encoding hamartin; approximately 20% of patients) and *TSC2* (encoding tuberin; approximately 60% of patients); gene mutations have not been discovered in 10% to 25% of affected individuals. Tuberin and hamartin form a complex that suppresses cell growth through regulation of several signaling pathways, most importantly the mammalian target of rapamycin (mTOR) pathway signaling through switching Rheb from an active (GTP-bound) to inactive (guanosine diphosphate [GDP]–bound) state.[253] In general, patients with mutations in *TSC1* have milder disease.[255] The disorder is characterized by the development of hamartomas of the skin, brain, eye, heart, kidneys, lungs, and bone (Box 11.2).[253] A variety of cutaneous features, including hypopigmented macules, angiofibromas, fibrous tumors, and periungual and gingival fibromas, may be seen.

The earliest sign in most patients is the presence of hypopigmented macules (white spots), which show normal numbers of melanocytes, but reduced pigmentation because of constitutive activation of the mTORC1 pathway and reduced MITF expression, which is not seen in nonlesional skin.[256,257] It is most likely that loss of *TSC1* or *TSC2* heterozygosity occurs in a melanoblast lineage cell that leads to the clonal patches of hypopigmentation. Three or more hypopigmented macules are seen in 97% of

Box 11.2 Features of Tuberous Sclerosis

Pathogenic mutation in *TSC1* or *TSC2* *or* two major features *or* one major feature + two minor features = definite tuberous sclerosis
One major feature + one minor feature = probable tuberous sclerosis
One major feature *or* two or more minor features = possible tuberous sclerosis

Major Features

- Hypopigmented macules ≥5 mm across (≥3)
- Angiofibromas (>3) or fibrous cephalic plaque
- Shagreen patch (connective tissue nevus)
- Ungual fibromas (≥2)
- Cortical dysplasias
- Subependymal nodules
- Subependymal giant-cell astrocytoma
- Cardiac rhabdomyoma
- Multiple retinal hamartomas
- Angiomyolipomas (≥2)
- Lymphangioleiomyomatosis

Minor Features

- "Confetti" skin lesions
- Intraoral fibromas (>2)
- Dental enamel pits (>3)
- Multiple renal cysts
- Nonrenal hamartomas
- Retinal achromic patch

patients at birth or shortly thereafter, although the appearance of additional lesions as late as 6 years of age has been described.[258] Once present, the hypopigmented macules tend to be persistent and stable in shape and relative size but may become less apparent during adulthood. Wood lamp examination in a completely darkened room may be useful in accentuating the macules in fair-skinned children. The white spots most commonly occur on the trunk, but hypopigmented tufts of scalp or eyelash hair meet the criterion for a hypopigmented macule. They range in size from a millimeter to several centimeters and number from a few to more than 75; 18% to 20% of individuals with TSC have 1 or 2 hypopigmented macules. The hypopigmented macules (Fig. 11.23) are often round ("thumbprint"), confetti-like hypopigmented macules (particularly over the pretibial areas), oval, linear, or lance-ovate shape ("ash leaf spots").

Lesions of vitiligo tend to be depigmented and show a bright white coloration with Wood lamp examination. The hypopigmented white spots of TSC are most difficult to distinguish from nevus depigmentosus (also called *nevus achromicus;* Fig. 11.24), which occurs in 1.6% to 4.7% of children,[259,260] suggesting that the majority of young children with a white spot do not have TSC. Nevus depigmentosus may be present at birth or appear during early infancy as normal pigmentation increases and then persists. Despite its name, most nevus depigmentosus lesions are hypopigmented, not depigmented. Most individuals will have a solitary lesion of nevus depigmentosus, but multiple lesions and segmental forms of nevus depigmentosus have been described. Nevus depigmentosus and the hypomelanotic macules of TSC must also be distinguished from nevus anemicus, a developmental anomaly characterized by a circumscribed round or oval patch of pale or mottled skin[261] (see Chapter 12, Fig. 12.60).

Cutaneous angiofibromas (adenoma sebaceum), which are hamartomas composed of fibrous and vascular tissue, appear in 75% of cases. They typically develop between 2 and 6 years of age and continue to increase in number. However, they have been described at birth or as late as the mid-20s. These lesions characteristically are 1- to 4-mm, pink to red, dome-shaped papules with a smooth surface. They occur on the nasolabial folds, cheeks, and chin and sometimes more extensively on the face (Fig. 11.25). The upper lip is relatively spared, except immediately below the nose. The angiofibromas in affected adolescents may be masked by or misdiagnosed as acne. Their distribution is usually symmetric but may be asymmetric, especially in patients with a mosaic form of TSC.[262,263]

Fibrous cephalic plaques overall occur in 36% of patients, with most a solitary plaque less than 5 cm in diameter.[264] The forehead is the most common site (39%; Fig. 11.26), but plaques may be found on the scalp (31%), rest of the face (27%), or neck (3%). In 71% of those in whom the age of onset is known, the plaque was congenital. In 14% to 20% of patients, connective tissue nevi/collagenomas also develop on the trunk, especially in the lumbosacral area, and most commonly during later childhood or adolescence (shagreen patches or *peau de chagrin* lesions) (Fig. 11.27). In one study, more than half of adults with TSC had at least one connective tissue nevus on the trunk or thighs and more than half of these individuals had two or more.[265] They vary from smaller than 1 cm to palm sized. Collagenomas are usually slightly raised, with focal depression at follicular openings, leading to comparison with pigskin,

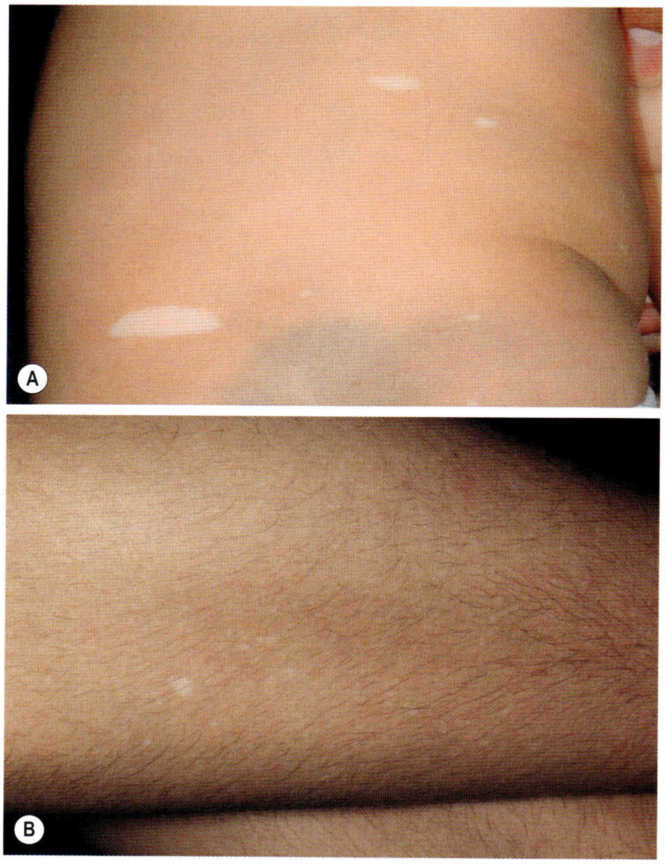

Fig. 11.23 Tuberous sclerosis. **(A)** Several lance-ovate ("ash-leaf") and "thumbprint" white macules are noted on this infant's back. **(B)** Confetti-like macules on the lower extremities in a 13-year-old boy.

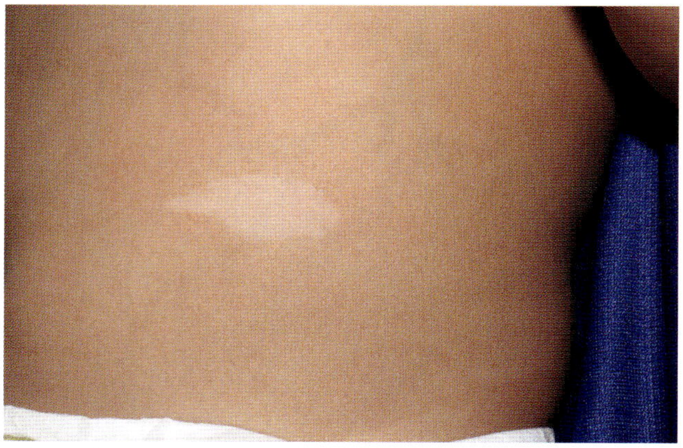

Fig. 11.24 Nevus depigmentosus. Well-demarcated patch of hypopigmentation that tends to be round or oval in configuration. Nevus depigmentosus, also known as *nevus achromicus,* may be noted at birth or may become apparent during infancy.

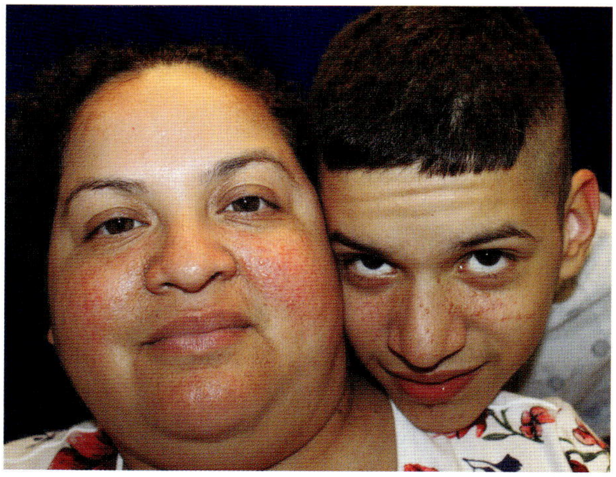

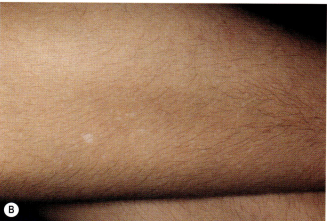

Fig. 11.25 Tuberous sclerosis. Both mom and son are affected with this autosomal dominant disorder. Facial angiofibromas (formerly called *adenoma sebaceum*) are typically 1- to 4-mm, skin-colored to red, dome-shaped papules with a smooth surface. The facial angiofibromas largely involve the cheeks and nose with relative sparing of the upper lip.

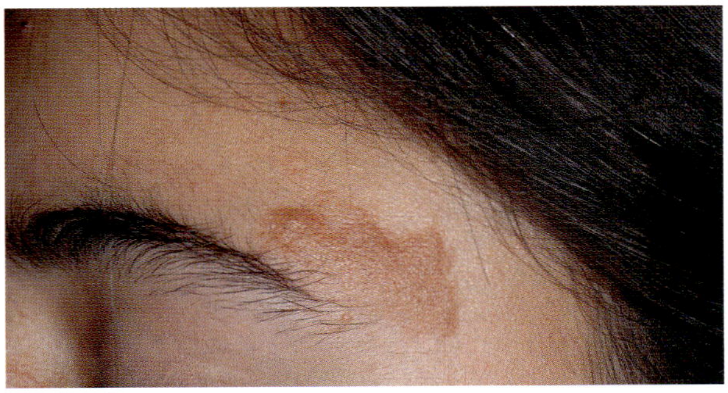

Fig. 11.26 Tuberous sclerosis. The fibrous cephalic plaque may be present at birth and, together with the hypopigmented macules, may allow a definitive diagnosis of tuberous sclerosis.

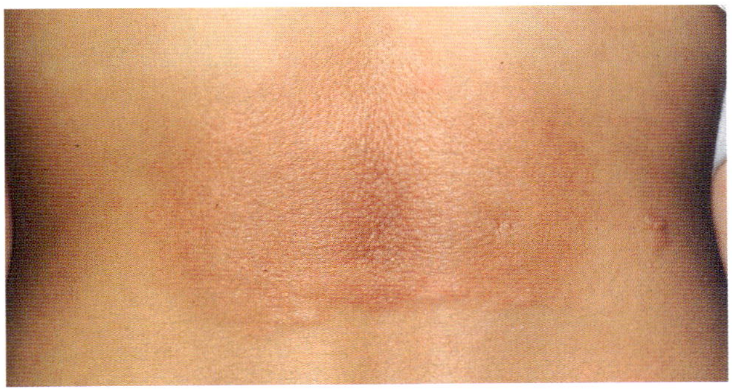

Fig. 11.27 Tuberous sclerosis. The shagreen patch is characteristically found at the lumbosacral area and has a *peau d'orange* texture.

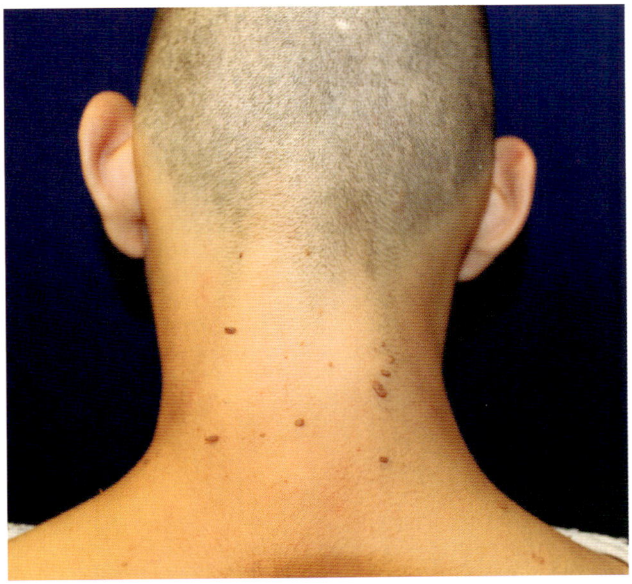

Fig. 11.28 Tuberous sclerosis. Acrochordons can be large and numerous, including in younger children.

elephant skin, orange peel, or gooseflesh. Acrochordons are reported to be more common (Fig. 11.28), including in affected children.[266] Fibromas under (Fig. 11.29, *A*) or around (Fig. 11.29, *B*) the nails of the fingers and especially the toes (subungual and periungual fibromas, respectively, sometimes called *Koenen tumor*) and on the gums and other intraoral sites (intraoral fibromas; Fig. 11.30) are also considered pathognomonic. Seen in up to 80% of patients,[267] these fibromas do not tend to appear until after puberty but may be the only sign of TSC.[268]

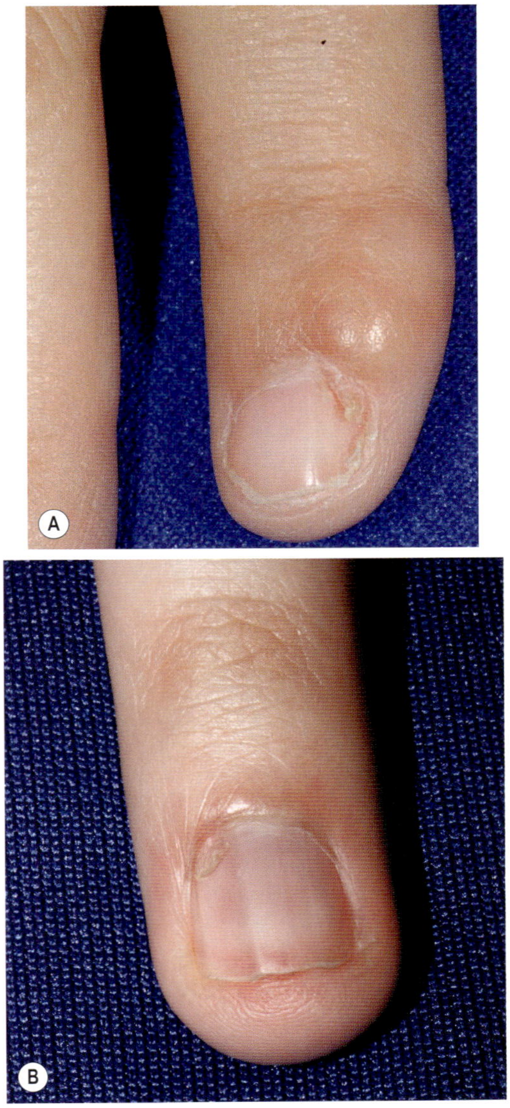

Fig. 11.29 Tuberous sclerosis. **(A)** Subungual fibroma on the fourth finger of this adolescent boy. **(B)** Periungual fibroma in an adolescent; note the deformity of the nail.

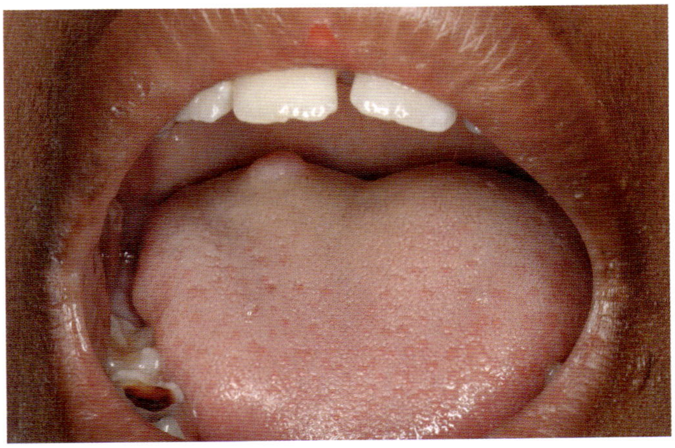

Fig. 11.30 Tuberous sclerosis. Intraoral fibroma.

Confetti-like hypopigmented macules have been noted in 6% of patients with multiple endocrine neoplasia (MEN) type 1[269] and multiple angiofibromas in 43% to 88% of adolescents and adults with MEN1 (see Chapter 23).[269,270] Facial angiofibromas in patients with MEN1 tend to be fewer in number than in patients with TSC, may involve the upper lip or vermilion border, and fail to cluster in the nasolabial folds. Collagenomas have been observed in 72% of patients with MEN1.[269] Patients with MEN1 are at high risk for the development of parathyroid, pituitary, pancreatic, and duodenal tumors.[271] Multiple facial angiofibromas with onset during adulthood have also been noted in patients with Birt–Hogg–Dubé syndrome,[272] but facial fibrofolliculomas or trichodiscomas are more typical.[273] Multiple biopsy-proven angiofibromas without other signs and with negative molecular testing have been described.[274] Having one to a few facial fibrous papules is common in normal adults and may begin during adolescence; they resemble angiofibromas and have been shown to have activated mTOR signaling as well.[275]

The systemic lesions of TSC may produce severe symptoms and possibly death. Seizures, seen in 80% to 90% of patients with TSC, may begin as infantile spasms in which sudden repetitive myoclonic contractions of most of the body musculature are combined with flexion, extension, opisthotonos, and tremors. By 2 or 3 years of age, focal or generalized seizures and mental retardation may become evident. Extensive CNS involvement leads to hypsarrhythmia (salaam seizures) with electroencephalographic findings of multifocal high-voltage spikes and slow chaotic waves. Later in life the seizure pattern may change to a *petit mal* variety, and in less severe cases generalized or focal motor seizures may develop.

Retardation may be mild or severe and appears in 62% of affected individuals. The severity of mental retardation correlates well with the age of seizure onset. In approximately 90% of patients with TSC, the brain shows areas of cortical dysplasia (including cortical "tubers" and white matter migrational abnormalities). These areas of cortical dysplasia can calcify and be visible on skull radiographs as curvilinear opacities. Periventricular or subependymal nodules may be seen by computed tomography (CT) or magnetic resonance imaging (MRI) scanning before calcification occurs.[276,277] Subependymal nodules are not malignant but may enlarge to cause obstructive hydrocephalus.

By the end of the first decade of life, 80% of patients show renal involvement. Renal hamartomas (angiomyolipomas) occur in about 70% of patients, and larger ones may lead to hemorrhage; of note, angiomyolipomas may be found in other organs as well, and having at least two angiomyolipoma without organ specificity is a major diagnostic feature. With advancing age, 20% to 30% of patients develop multiple bilateral renal cysts resembling those of polycystic kidney disease. These cysts can occur in individuals with *TSC1* or *TSC2* mutations, but a subset of individuals with aggressive renal cysts have deletions involving both *TSC2* and the contiguous polycystic kidney disease *(PKD1)* genes.[278] Abdominal ultrasound or scans are able to detect renal hamartomas or cysts in asymptomatic patients. Cardiac rhabdomyomas are most commonly present in the ventricles prenatally or in infancy and tend to regress spontaneously.[279] Although usually asymptomatic, rhabdomyomas may be associated with congestive heart failure, murmurs, cyanosis, arrhythmias, and sudden death, particularly during the first year of life. Two-dimensional echocardiography is a noninvasive technique that allows detection of asymptomatic cardiac rhabdomyomas.

The eyes may have characteristic retinal lesions (gliomas) referred to as *phakomas*. These retinal hamartomas have been described in 30% to 50% of patients. Funduscopy may show one of two types of lesions: multiple, raised, mulberry-like lesions on or adjacent to the optic nerve head, or flat, disk-like lesions in the periphery of the retina. Pulmonary lymphangioleiomyomatosis occurs overall in 2.3% of individuals with TSC, particularly in women between the ages of 20 and 40 years.[280] Affected individuals experience shortness of breath, hemoptysis, or pneumothorax and show diffuse interstitial infiltrates with cystic changes by CT examination. About 85% of patients with TSC have osseous manifestations with the bones, particularly those of the hands and feet, demonstrating cysts and periosteal thickenings. At least three dental pits (seen as punctate, round or oval, 1- to 2-mm randomly arranged enamel defects), particularly in the permanent teeth, are another marker of TSC and may be visualized better with use of dental disclosing solution.

The diagnosis of TSC may be difficult, because many affected individuals have subtle manifestations. However, the appearance of characteristic skin lesions in children, especially with seizures, retardation, or both, should lead to genetic testing to establish a diagnosis of TSC (see Box 11.2).[254,281] Patients with cutaneous features and mosaicism may not have a detectable mutation by blood analysis.[282] Family history should be assessed (with careful clinical and sometimes imaging examination of family members), and other components of the evaluation include MRI of the brain, renal ultrasound, cardiac echocardiography in infants and young children, and, in some cases, ophthalmologic examination and chest radiography for honeycombing of the lungs.

The prognosis of TSC depends on the severity of the disorder and the presence of neurologic involvement.[283] The leading causes of premature death, status epilepticus and bronchopneumonia, are related to the associated neurologic issues. Seizures can be controlled by anticonvulsant therapy in many patients, and prevention of seizures early in life has been shown to lower the risk of developmental delay and retardation. With routine MRI evaluations and the availability of microscopic surgery for neoplastic brain lesions, patients are surviving longer and have a better quality of life. Neurosurgical intervention may be required in patients with signs of increased intracranial pressure such as visual disturbances, papilledema, vomiting, or headaches. Sun protection is important for patients, not just at the sites of the hypopigmented macules but also to prevent facial angiofibromas, which show second-hit mutations in TSC genes with a UV-signature mutation that is not seen in *TSC* germline mutations, in 50% of patients.[284]

The facial angiofibromas may be a cosmetic problem that responds to cryosurgical, surgical, or laser therapy.[285] Mammalian TOR inhibitors such as rapamycin and everolimus cause regression of astrocytomas, renal angiomyolipomas, and pulmonary lymphangioleiomyomas, as well as facial angiofibromas[286,287] and fibrous cephalic plaques. A meta-analysis of 16 reports also noted improvement in 94% of 84 patients with use of a variety of topical formulations of compounded topical rapamycin 0.003% to 1% (ointment, gel, solution, cream; none commercially available).[288–292] In the largest double-blind, randomized trial of 179 patients (mean age 20 years), improvement was greatest with nightly application of 1% versus 0.1% rapamycin versus vehicle[293] and during the first month of the 6-month trial. There was no measurable absorption, and adverse events occurred in 10% (primarily mild application site erythema/irritation and itch/pain). In another trial, reduction to three times per week maintenance was insufficient to maintain improvement.[294] Topical rapamycin has been used for maintenance after laser or surgical therapy of facial angiofibromas and produced improvement in early ungual fibromas[295] and fibrous cephalic plaques (after 3 to 9 months of therapy).[294,296] The Tuberous Sclerosis Alliance (at www.tsalliance.org) and the Tuberous Sclerosis Association (of the United Kingdom, at www.tuberous-sclerosis.org) are among the groups that offer support for patients with TSC.

CHEMICALLY INDUCED DEPIGMENTATION

A number of chemical agents are known to cause depigmentation after topical exposure.[297] Among these compounds are the rubber antioxidant monobenzyl ether of hydroquinone, hydroquinone photographic developer, azo dyes, para-phenylenediamine/PPD,[298] diphenylcyclopropenone, phenolic germicidal agents (paratertiary butylphenol and amylphenol), hydroxyanisole, and 4-tertiary butyl catechol (an additive to polyethylene film). These compounds tend to share a benzene ring with a hydroxyl side chain that is also shared by tyrosine, the amino acid building block of melanin, suggesting competitive inhibition of tyrosinase. However, these chemicals can induce melanocyte toxicity directly by activating the cellular stress response (with secretion of HSP70) and unfolded protein response, inducing reactive oxygen species, and activating $CD8^+$ T cells in genetically predisposed individuals, as occurs in vitiligo.

Hypo- and Depigmentation from Medications

Depigmentation has also occurred after injections of triamcinolone or application of high-potency corticosteroids[299] and in the periorbital area after injection of botulinum A toxin.[300] The methylphenidate patch for attention-deficit/hyperactivity disorder has led to persistent skin depigmentation or hypopigmentation at or near the application site from 2 to 4 years after medication initiation, in most cases without previous inflammation.[301] Lanaprost, a prostaglandin analogue that is more typically associated with increased pigmentation, may paradoxically depigment periocular skin when used intraocularly for glaucoma.[302] The most common cause for drug-induced hypo- and depigmentation are targeted anticancer agents. A systematic review and meta-analysis of 36 clinical trials demonstrated pigmentary changes in the skin in 18% and hair in 21%.[303] Hypopigmentation and depigmentation of hair have been reported for inhibitors of epidermal growth factor receptor (EGFR), Bcr-Abl (especially dasatinib),[304] vascular endothelial growth factor receptor (VEGFR), and PD-1 (pembrolizumab, nivolizumab). Hypopigmentation and depigmentation of skin have been described from use of the same groups (especially Bcr-Abl inhibitor imatinib)[305] and also the BRAF inhibitor vemurafenib and interleukin-2.[303] Oral ingestion of chloroquine[306] and arsenic have also led to depigmentation. A progressive generalized decrease in pigmentation has been reported after drug reaction to sulfonamide.[307]

IDIOPATHIC GUTTATE HYPOMELANOSIS

Idiopathic guttate hypomelanosis is a common disorder of adults, and its incidence increases with increasing age.[308] It occasionally occurs in children and is more common in female individuals, although the latter may represent reporting bias. More striking in individuals with darker pigmentation, the lesions of idiopathic guttate hypomelanosis are characteristically 0.5- to 6-mm sharply defined, porcelain white macules. They are asymptomatic and once present do not tend to change. The macules most commonly occur on the extensor forearms and on the shins. The diagnosis is usually made clinically, and no treatment is effective. The underlying cause is unknown, although sun exposure is thought to be a trigger. Several therapies have been suggested with variable success, among them chemical peels, topical retinoids, cryotherapy, dermabrasion, laser abrasion, minigrafts, and intralesional triamcinolone. CO_2 and Er:YAG fractional lasers proved superior to tretinoin in one trial.[309] Excimer laser has also been used with promising results in a left-right comparison trial,[310] and 5-fluorouracil tattooing has even been suggested.[311]

Because idiopathic guttate hypomelanosis is unusual in children, other disorders must be considered. *Eruptive hypomelanosis* features uniform, symmetric, well-demarcated hypopigmented macules, most often on the extensor surface. They erupt days to weeks after signs of an upper respiratory infection, sometimes with lymphadenitis and pharyngitis.[312,313] The hypopigmented lesions are typically larger than those of guttate hypomelanosis. The disorder resolves spontaneously within 2 to 8 weeks and requires no intervention. *Leukoderma punctata* is a rare complication of phototherapy, which resolves spontaneously when phototherapy is discontinued.[314] Bier spots (also called *physiologic anemic macules*; see Chapter 12) are light-colored, typically irregularly shaped macules on the extensor surfaces that reflect excessive vasoconstriction and improve with limb elevation[315]; no therapy is needed.

POSTINFLAMMATORY HYPOPIGMENTATION

Postinflammatory hypopigmentation (or leukoderma) may be associated with a wide variety of inflammatory dermatoses or infections.[316,317] This relative pigmentary deficiency may be noted after involution of certain inflammatory skin disorders, particularly burns, bullous disorders, infections, eczematous or psoriatic lesions, and pityriasis rosea (see Fig. 3.17). In the inflammatory dermatoses, the intensity of the inflammatory reaction may bear little relationship to the development of postinflammatory leukoderma. Postinflammatory depigmentation can follow intense inflammatory lesions, as seen in severe atopic dermatitis with intense scratching (particularly on the dorsal aspect of the hands and feet), discoid lupus erythematosus, or burns.

Postinflammatory hypopigmentation is generally self-limiting, clearing after months to years. It often becomes cosmetically obvious in individuals with darker skin, particularly during summer months, because the preferential darkening with UV light exposure of surrounding skin accentuates the hypopigmentation.

Although the pathophysiology of postinflammatory hypopigmentation is unclear, it is postulated that the hypopigmentation is caused when keratinocytes injured by the inflammatory process are temporarily unable to accept melanosomes from the melanocyte dendrites. No therapy is effective, but the condition tends to improve with time.

Pityriasis alba (see Chapter 3) is a common cutaneous disorder characterized by asymptomatic, sometimes scaly hypopigmented patches on the face, neck, upper trunk, arms, shoulders, and at times the lower aspect of the trunk and extremities of children and young adults (see Fig. 3.38). Seen predominantly in children 3 to 16 years of age, individual lesions vary from 1 to several centimeters in diameter and have sharply delineated margins and a fine, branny scale. Although the cause is unknown, this disorder appears to represent a nonspecific dermatitis. Postinflammatory hypopigmentation is commonly seen in children with atopic dermatitis, psoriasis (see Chapter 4, Fig. 4.21), pityriasis lichenoides, and contact dermatitis; in the latter, the pattern of the hypopigmentation may provide the clue to the contactant.[318] Postinflammatory hypopigmentation must be distinguished from hypopigmented mycosis fungoides, which often presents during childhood or adolescence (see Chapter 10). Lesions characteristically are on the trunk and inner thighs and have associated scale. Multiple biopsies may be required to make the diagnosis.

Tinea versicolor (pityriasis versicolor; see Chapter 17) is a common condition often found on the upper part of the trunk and neck of young adults. Caused by overgrowth of a yeast that normally inhabits skin, *Pityrosporum orbiculare (Malassezia furfur)*, the condition is characterized by small, either hypopigmented or occasionally hyperpigmented macules, particularly on the trunk and upper arms. The round, individual lesions often coalesce. Facial involvement is more common in affected children than in older individuals. The hypopigmentation results from the production of azelaic acid, which inhibits tyrosinase; the hyperpigmentation is postinflammatory (see Figs. 17.33 and 17.34).

Sarcoidosis (see Chapter 25) is a granulomatous disorder of unknown origin with widespread manifestations involving the skin and many of the internal organs. In addition to the characteristic yellowish-brown, flesh-colored, pink, red, and reddish-brown to black or blue lesions, subcutaneous nodules, and infiltrated plaques, the spectrum of sarcoidal skin lesions includes hypomelanotic macules and papules. Measuring up to 1.5 cm in diameter, these hypopigmented lesions reveal sarcoid-type granulomas on cutaneous biopsy.

Leprosy (Hansen disease; see Chapter 14), a chronic infection in which the acid-fast bacillus *Mycobacterium leprae* has a special predilection for the skin and nervous system, can be divided into several types depending on the patient's cellular immune response to *M. leprae*. Tuberculoid leprosy shows characteristic well-defined anesthetic hypopigmented lesions and thickened and palpable peripheral nerves. Lepromatous leprosy, in contrast, more commonly shows nodules or diffuse infiltrates, especially on the eyebrows and ears, resulting in a leonine facies. A granulomatous infiltrate on microscopic examination of cutaneous lesions and, particularly in the lepromatous lesions, demonstration of *M. leprae* on cutaneous smear or biopsy specimen generally confirm the diagnosis.

Pinta (see Chapter 14) is a treponemal infection caused by *Treponema carateum*. Seen almost exclusively among the dark-skinned population of Cuba and Central and South America, the disorder is commonly found in children of parents afflicted with this disorder. The cutaneous manifestations may be divided into primary, secondary, and tertiary stages. The late dyschromic stage takes several more years to develop. These lesions have an insidious onset and usually appear during adolescence or young adulthood. They consist of slate-blue hyperpigmented lesions that after a period of years become widespread and are replaced by depigmented macules resembling those seen in patients with vitiligo. Lesions are located chiefly on the face, waist, and areas close to bony prominences (elbows, knees, ankles, wrists, and the dorsal aspect of the hands). These depigmented lesions of pinta can be differentiated from those of other depigmented disorders by the presence of pigmented lesions, histologic examination of lesional specimens, identification of antibodies directed against *T. carateum* by serologic testing, and darkfield examination.

GENETIC RETICULATE PIGMENTARY DISORDERS

Reticulate pigmentary disorders are a group of disorders with hyper- and/or hypopigmented macules that vary in size, many of which are hereditary and present during the pediatric years. They are divided by their often distinctive distribution of the mottled pigmentary pattern, features beyond pigmentation, and underlying gene mutations. However, classification within this group of reticulate pigmentary disorders can be challenging because of variability of features and overlap among subtypes.

DYSCHROMATOSES

Two major forms of dyschromatoses have been described: dyschromatosis symmetrica hereditaria (DSH; reticulate acropigmentation of Dohi) and dyschromatosis universalis hereditaria (DUH), both of which are seen most commonly in Japanese and Chinese individuals (in about 2 per 100,000 individuals).[319] These disorders show only pigmentary manifestations and affected individuals are almost always otherwise healthy. The reticulate hyperpigmentation of these disorders tends to appear spottier than the more net-like reticulated hyperpigmentation of disorders like dyskeratosis congenita (see Chapter 7), Rothmund–Thomson (see Chapter 19), and Kindler (see Chapter 13) syndromes. The differential diagnosis of these dyschromatoses includes other disorders with more of a macular pigmentation (such as xeroderma pigmentosum [see Chapter 19], Kitamura reticulate acropigmentation, and dyschromic amyloidosis [Table 11.5]). Keratin disorders with hyperpigmentation also tend to have a more net-like reticulated pigmentation (e.g., epidermolysis bullosa simplex with mottled pigmentation [see Chapter 13], Dowling–Degos disease, Naegeli–Franceschetti–Jadassohn syndrome and dermatopathia pigmentosa reticularis).

DSH is an autosomal dominant disorder characterized by symmetrically distributed, pinpoint to pea-sized hyperpigmented and hypopigmented macules on the dorsal aspects of the distal extremities and face.[320] Lesions first appear during infancy or early childhood, commonly spread until adolescence, and persist throughout the lifespan.

Table 11.5 Disorders with Reticulate Hyperpigmentation (and Sometimes Hypopigmentation)

Disorder	Inheritance	Gene	Onset	Features	Other Comments
Familial forms of amyloidosis		Unknown	Early childhood	Generalized hyperpigmentation with tiny generalized hypopigmented macules	AD form: focal subepidermal amyloid deposition in biopsies
Amyloidosis cutis dyschromica	AD			Carriers of X-linked form: along lines of Blaschko, resembling incontinentia pigmenti	
X-linked reticulate hyperpigmentation	XL	POLA1	Infancy	XL form: failure to thrive, developmental delay, seizures, hemiplegia, colitis, gastroesophageal reflux, inguinal hernia, urethral stricture, dental anomalies, hypohidrosis, photophobia, corneal clouding, skeletal changes	XL form: often no amyloid in biopsies of children
Dowling–Degos disease	AD	Keratin 5; *POFUT1*; *POGLUT1*	Early adolescence to adulthood	Reticulate pigmentation of flexures, neck, and sometimes generalized; sometimes pitted perioral scars and comedo-like follicular plugs	No acantholysis More generalized reticulated pigmentation in EBS with mottled pigmentation (KRT5 mutations; see Ch. 13)
Familial progressive hyperpigmentation and hypopigmentation	AD	*KITLG*	Birth or early infancy; increase in number with time	Face, neck, trunk, limbs with reticulate hyperpigmentation as well as diffuse background hyperpigmentation; café-au-lait macules and freckling; sometimes larger hypopigmented macules	Called *familial progressive hyperpigmentation* if no hypopigmentation; distinguish from NF1 and Legius syndrome
Dyschromatosis symmetrica hereditaria	AD	*ADAR1*	Infancy to early childhood	Hyperpigmented and hypopigmented small macules on dorsum of hands and feet	
Dyschromatosis universalis hereditaria	AD	*ABCB6*	First months of life (starts on trunk)	Generalized pigmented macules; may involve palms and soles, oral mucosa, and nails (dystrophy with pterygium)	
Galli–Galli disease	AD	Keratin 5	Early adolescence	Reticulate pigmentation of flexures	Moderate to severe suprabasal acantholysis in biopsies
Kitamura disease	AD	*ADAM10*	First to second decade	Acral reticular pigmentation with subtle atrophy, palmar pits, and rete ridge breaks	

Table 11.5 Disorders with Reticulate Hyperpigmentation (and Sometimes Hypopigmentation)—cont'd

Disorder	Inheritance	Gene	Onset	Features	Other Comments
Dyskeratosis congenita (see Ch. 7)	Esp. XL	Esp. *DKC1*	Late childhood	Net-like pigmentation, esp. in sun-exposed areas, often poikilodermatous; associated with mucosal leukokeratosis, nail dystrophy, risk of bone marrow failure, mucosal squamous cell carcinomas	Nine known genes can be mutated; can be AD or AR
Naegeli–Franceschetti–Jadassohn syndrome	AD	*KRT14*	First 2 years	Reticulate hyperpigmentation, primarily of abdomen, perioral, and periocular areas; palmoplantar keratoderma, absence of dermatoglyphics, onychodystrophy, hypohidrosis, dental anomalies Pigmentation fades during adolescence	
Dermatopathia pigmentosa reticularis	AD	*KRT14*		Pigmentation, primarily truncal distribution; nonscarring alopecia; palmoplantar keratoderma, absence of dermatoglyphics, onychodystrophy, hypohidrosis	

AD, Autosomal dominant; *ADAM10,* a disintegrin and metalloproteinase domain-containing protein 10; *ADAR1,* adenosine deaminase acting on RNA 1; *AR,* autosomal recessive; *DCK1,* dyskerin; *EBS,* epidermolysis bullosa simplex; *Esp.,* especially; *KITLG,* KIT ligand; *KRT,* keratin; *NF,* neurofibromatosis; *POFUT1,* protein O-fucosyltransferase 1; *POGLUT1,* protein O-glucosyltransferase 1; *XL,* X-linked.

Molecular studies have uncovered mutations in ribonucleic acid (RNA)–specific adenosine deaminase (*ADAR1*, also called *DSRAD*).[321–324] Mutations in *ADAR1* also cause type 6 Aicardi–Goutieres syndrome (AGS), usually an autosomal recessive disorder that has neurologic features (and sometimes chilblains, see Chapter 22), but not reticulate pigmentation. Nevertheless, a few cases of heterozygous or compound heterozygote mutations in *ADAR1* has been described with both pernio or typical AGS and the reticulate pigmentation of DSH,[325,326] and occasional patients with DSH and uniallelic mutations in *ADAR1* have had neurologic disease.[327,328] DSH has been treated with miniature punch grafting and excimer light therapy.[329]

Reticulate acropigmentation of Kitamura is another autosomal dominant disorder characterized by reticulated or lentiginous hyperpigmentation (not hypopigmentation) localized primarily to the dorsal areas of the hands and feet. It is caused by mutations in *ADAM10*.[330,331] Lesions have their onset is during childhood and tend to be more atrophic than those of DSH. Pits on the palms, soles, and dorsal surface of the fingers and toes are associated.[332] Histopathologic features may also help to distinguish RAK from DSH.[333]

DUH is an autosomal dominant disorder (rarely recessive) in which patients show hyperpigmented and hypopigmented macules of various shapes and sizes with a mottled appearance in a different distribution from DSH (Fig. 11.31). In DUH, skin lesions appear within the first months of life, predominantly on the trunk, and subsequently generalize, including the palms and soles in some cases. The oral mucosa may be involved, and nails may show dystrophy with pterygium formation. Some patients have been described with ocular abnormalities. The numbers of melanosomes is normal, and the disorder presumably reflects increased melanocyte activity. DUH is caused by mutations in *ABCB6*.[334] The hyperpigmented lesions of DUH have been treated with Q-switched alexandrite laser.[335]

Dyschromatoses resembling DUH may also be caused by heterozygous mutations in *KITLG*, encoding KIT ligand (familial progressive hyperpigmentation and hypopigmentation)[336–338] or *SASH1* (SAM and SH3 domain-containing protein 1), a tumor suppressor gene.[339,340] *SASH1* mutations on both alleles lead to the reticulate hypopigmentation and hyperpigmentation in association with alopecia, palmoplantar keratoderma, nail dystrophy, dental anomalies, skin ulcers, and recurrent squamous cell carcinoma.[341]

Reticulated hyperpigmentation is also seen in X-linked reticulate pigmentary disorder (also called *Partington syndrome* or *familial cutaneous amyloidosis*).[342] During the first months of life, affected boys tend to develop chronic diarrhea, failure to thrive, bronchiectasis, and recurrent pneumonias. By early childhood, the generalized reticulate to confluent hyperpigmentation with tiny intermingled hypopigmented macules appears.[343] Later xerosis, hypohidrosis, enterocolitis that resembles inflammatory bowel disease, corneal inflammation and scarring, recurrent urethral strictures, and dental anomalies may manifest. The disorder features a distinctive facies with arched eyebrows and an upswept frontal hairline. Skeletal changes may include delayed bone age and shortened metacarpals. Melanophages and amyloid material in the papillary dermis have been demonstrated in skin biopsies of some affected adults. Pigmentation distributed along the lines of Blaschko in female carriers resembles the pigmented streaks and whorls of incontinentia pigmenti. The disorder results

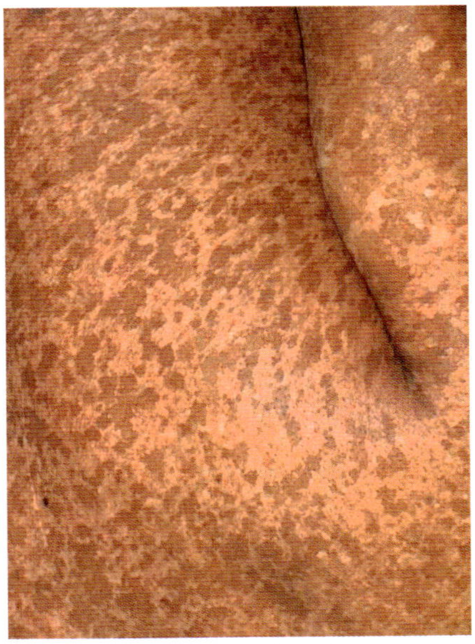

Fig. 11.31 Dyschromatosis universalis hereditaria. Reticulated hyperpigmented and hypopigmented macules of various shapes and sizes on the trunk. (Courtesy Drs. S. Worobec and S. Reddy.)

from a recurrent intronic mutation in *POLA1*, which encodes the catalytic subunit of DNA polymerase-α.[344] *POLA1* is responsible for synthesis of RNA:DNA primers during DNA replication and also directly regulates type I interferon synthesis and responses. Familial dyschromic amyloidosis with only the pigmentary abnormalities may also be inherited in an autosomal dominant manner with incomplete penetrance,[345,346] but the underlying genetic cause of this dominant form is unknown.

Dowling–Degos disease and its acantholytic variant Galli–Galli disease are autosomal dominant disorders with a spectrum of localization from the flexural/intertriginous areas (neck, axillae, submammary area, groin, antecubital fossae) to generalized involvement. These disorders typically first manifest during adulthood. Loss-of-function heterozygous mutations in the head region of *KRT5* (keratin 5),[347] *POFUT1* (protein-O-fucosyltransferase 1), or *POGLUT1* (protein O-glucosyltransferase 1)[348,349] are responsible. In the more localized form from *KRT5* mutations, reticulated pigmentation and sometimes erythematous erosive papules tend to be flexural and may be associated with comedonal lesions and pitted acneiform facial scars.[350] A phenotype resembling flexural Dowling–Degos disease with hidradenitis suppurativa has been described in association with a mutation in *PSENEN*, encoding the γ-secretase subunit of the protein presenilin enhancer.[351] In addition to trunk and flexural areas, patients with *POFUT1* mutations and more generalized manifestations tend to show involvement of the acral regions, sometimes with palmar pits and disrupted dermatoglyphics, whereas those with *POGLUT1* mutations show more widespread involvement of the extremities.

Naegeli–Franceschetti–Jadassohn syndrome and dermatopathia pigmentosa reticularis are autosomal dominant disorders with reticulate hyperpigmentation, palmoplantar keratoderma, absence of dermatoglyphics, onychodystrophy, and decreased sweating with lifelong heat intolerance. Both disorders result from heterozygous nonsense or frameshift mutations in *KRT14* that increase the susceptibility of keratinocytes to apoptosis.[352,353] In Naegeli–Franceschetti–Jadassohn syndrome, the reticulated hyperpigmentation is present during the first 2 years of life and primarily involves the abdomen, perioral, and periocular areas.[354] The pigmentation commonly fades during adolescence and may disappear altogether. A severe enamel defect with early loss of teeth is associated, and patients may have acral blistering. The pigmentation in dermatopathia pigmentosa reticularis is primarily in a truncal distribution and is associated with nonscarring alopecia.[355,356] Epidermolysis bullosa simplex with mottled pigmentation (see Chapter 13) also results primarily from heterozygous mutations of the head region of *KRT5*, further highlighting the role of this region of keratin 5 in melanosome transfer.

The hyperpigmentation in all of these disorders is nonpalpable in contrast to the hyperpigmented papules and plaques of confluent and reticulated papillomatosis of Gougerot and Carteaud, an asymptomatic disorder of hyperkeratotic hyperpigmented papules in a reticulated pattern.[357] Seen primarily in adolescents and young adults, this disorder usually occurs on the upper anterior trunk, often in individuals with acanthosis nigricans (see Chapter 23, Figs. 22.39 and 23.29).

POIKILODERMA

The term *poikiloderma (poikiloderma atrophicans vasculare)* is used to describe a triad of telangiectasia, atrophy, and reticulated dyschromia (hyperpigmentation and hypopigmentation). The disorder may be seen in patients with poikiloderma congenitale (Rothmund–Thomson syndrome), xeroderma pigmentosum, Bloom syndrome (see Chapter 19); poikiloderma with neutropenia (Clericuzio-type),[358] dyskeratosis congenita (see Chapter 7); Kindler syndrome (Chapter 13); juvenile dermatomyositis (see Chapter 22); and cutaneous T-cell lymphoma (see Chapter 10). Actinic, thermal (see Erythema Ab Igne section, Chapter 20), and radiation damage can also leave poikilodermatous changes. Histopathologic examination of areas of poikiloderma reveals varying degrees of epidermal hyperkeratosis and atrophy, hydropic degeneration of the basal layer, varying numbers of pigment-laden melanophages, and a lymphocytic band-like or perivascular infiltration in the dermis. Management consists of early recognition, avoidance of sun exposure, and the use of protective clothing and topical sunscreen preparations in an attempt to arrest progression of the dermatosis.

INCONTINENTIA PIGMENTI

Incontinentia pigmenti (Bloch–Sulzberger syndrome) is an X-linked disorder that predominantly affects the skin, teeth, CNS, and eyes.[359–361] The disorder results from mutations in nuclear factor-κB (NF-κB) essential modulator (*NEMO; IKBKG*), a gene localized to the X chromosome. In approximately 80% of patients the mutation is a rearrangement in the *NEMO* gene that eliminates its activity.[362,363] Less commonly, affected girls (often with milder disease) have a missense or splice mutation in the *NEMO* gene, particularly involving exon 10; these girls with hypomorphic mutations in NEMO (e.g., missense, splice site) are at risk of having a son with hypohidrotic ectodermal dysplasia with immunodeficiency (see Chapter 7). *De novo* mutations occur in 65% of patients.[364] The mutation in *NEMO* prevents the activation of NF-κB, which is a regulator of cell proliferation, inflammation, and TNF-α-induced apoptosis. Approximately 97% of patients are female, suggesting that the disorder is lethal to affected hemizygous male individuals.[365] Male patients with Klinefelter syndrome (XXY genotype) or with incontinentia pigmenti as a mosaic condition have been described.[366–370] Mosaicism[371] in males can result in father-to-daughter transmission of germline IP.[372,373] Affected girls show functional mosaicism because of the random inactivation early in embryologic development of one of the X chromosomes (lyonization). As such, the cutaneous lesions of incontinentia pigmenti tend to follow lines of Blaschko, representing the clonal outgrowth of cells that express the affected allele. The variable severity and expression of clinical involvement in the eyes and brain reflect the random activation of the affected X allele in these tissues.

The disorder generally appears at birth or shortly thereafter (90% of patients have cutaneous lesions within the first 2 weeks of life; 96% have their onset before the age of 6 weeks). Although the cutaneous lesions have four distinct phases, their sequence is irregular and overlapping of stages is common (Box 11.3).

The first phase of incontinentia pigmenti begins with inflammatory vesicles or pustules that develop in crops over the trunk and extremities, often persisting for months. These may range from largely papules with scattered vesicles to pustules (Fig. 11.32). Biopsy of a blister during this vesicular stage reveals epidermal vesicles filled with eosinophils, and 74% of affected neonates show eosinophilia (from 18% to 89%). The vesicles clear spontaneously through cellular apoptosis and repopulation by normal keratinocytes. However, the vesicular phase may be reactivated focally, especially in infants and after infection, immunization, or physical trauma; less commonly, erythematous whorls without vesiculation may occur in older individuals.[374–377] Treatment with topical corticosteroids[378] or tacrolimus[379] may halt the progression of the vesicular phase, although lesions ultimately clear spontaneously.

In 70% of patients, the vesicular stage is followed by a verrucous phase characterized by irregular, linearly arrayed warty

Box 11.3 Manifestations of Incontinentia Pigmenti

- X-linked dominant disorder; random X-chromosome inactivation dictates extent of disease
- Mutations in NF-κB essential modulator *(NEMO)*
- Approximately 97% of patients are females; probably lethal in males; living males usually represent somatic mosaicism
- Four cutaneous phases that may overlap
  - Inflammatory vesicles or bullae
  - Verrucous lesions
  - Streaks of hyperpigmentation
  - Streaks of atrophy/hypopigmentation
- May have cicatricial alopecia and nail dystrophy
- Eosinophilia in >70% of patients (often lasts for 4 to 5 months)
- Systemic manifestations
  - Dental
  - Ocular
  - Central nervous system

NF-κB, Nuclear factor kappa B.

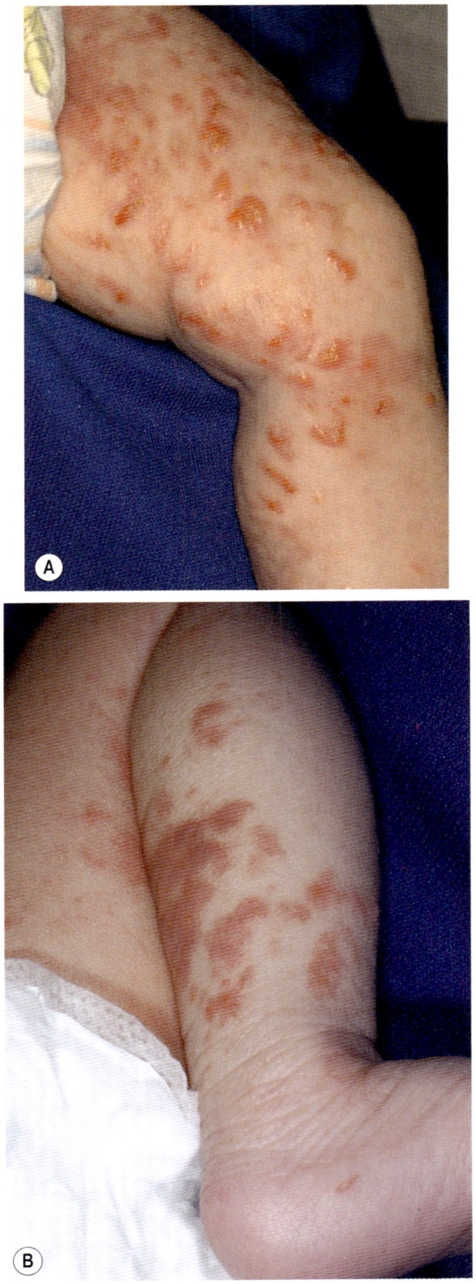

Fig. 11.32 Incontinentia pigmenti. **(A)** The lesions of incontinentia pigmenti tend to follow a curvilinear pattern along lines of Blaschko, lines of the embryologic development of ectoderm, as a manifestation of functional mosaicism (i.e., the X chromosome with the mutation in the *NEMO* gene is the activated X chromosome in the skin at these sites). The lesions of the vesicular phase may range from largely papular with a minor vesicular component to vesiculopustular as shown here and occasionally to bullous. **(B)** Sometimes the lesions of incontinentia pigmenti do not show a linear pattern.

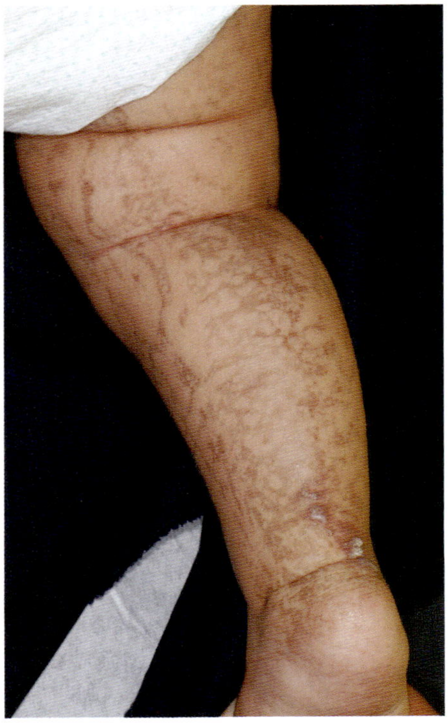

Fig. 11.33 Incontinentia pigmenti. Characteristic slate-brown lines on the legs may coalesce in areas and more closely resemble Chinese writing figures or a reticulated pattern than linear streaks. The hyperpigmentation usually fades by late in childhood. Note the warty papules of the verrucous phase, which are most commonly found on the hands and feet.

papules on one or more extremities and often on the hands and feet (Fig. 11.33). This stage resolves spontaneously, usually within a period of up to 2 years.

During or shortly after this verrucous stage, the highly characteristic pigmentary phase occurs in approximately 80% of patients. Lesions typically are thin bands of slate-brown to blue-gray coloration arranged in lines and swirls on the extremities and trunk (see Fig. 11.33). These pigmentary bands may coalesce in areas and more closely resemble Chinese writing figures than linear streaks or whorls. When more linear, they must be distinguished from X-linked macular amyloidosis in carrier females.[380,381] Occasionally these bands appear purpuric at onset (Fig. 11.34), and this appearance has raised the question of child abuse.[382] These pigmentary lesions progress until the patient's second year of life, then stabilize and persist for years. By adolescence, they gradually fade and disappear in two-thirds of affected individuals. Biopsy sections from lesional skin show incontinence of pigment during this phase, leading to the name *incontinentia pigmenti*. Although the pigmentary changes were originally considered to be a postinflammatory phenomenon secondary to the vesiculobullous or verrucous stages, the pigment fails to follow the pattern, shape, or location of the vesicular or verrucous lesions.

A fourth phase is characterized by persistent atrophic streaks that are often hypopigmented (Fig. 11.35). Most commonly noted on the arms, thighs, trunk, and particularly the calves of affected individuals, these affected areas show diminished hair, eccrine glands, and sweat pores. These streaks are often subtle and may be accentuated by viewing with side lighting or by Wood lamp examination. Skin biopsy shows characteristic changes with scattered apoptotic cells, thickened dermis, and absence of hair follicles and sweat glands, allowing diagnosis in older individuals.[383]

Cicatricial alopecia is seen in 38% to 66% of patients (Fig. 11.36). It occurs most often near the vertex, does not necessarily relate to the previous presence of lesions at the site, and may be the only marker in older children and adults.[384] Nail dystrophy is present in 7% to 51% of affected individuals. In addition, painful grayish-white verrucous or keratotic subungual tumors are seen in up to 10%, usually during the second or third decades of life.[385] Uncommonly, patients develop keratoacanthomas[386] and rarely squamous cell carcinomas.[387,388] In one affected teenager with keratoacanthoma-like growths on the leg, four monthly intralesional methotrexate treatments led to clearance[386] after unsuccessful curettage and cryotherapy. Lytic defects may be seen on radiographs of the distal phalanges as well.

Noncutaneous manifestations occur in a high percentage of patients with incontinentia pigmenti. Some 70% to 95% of patients

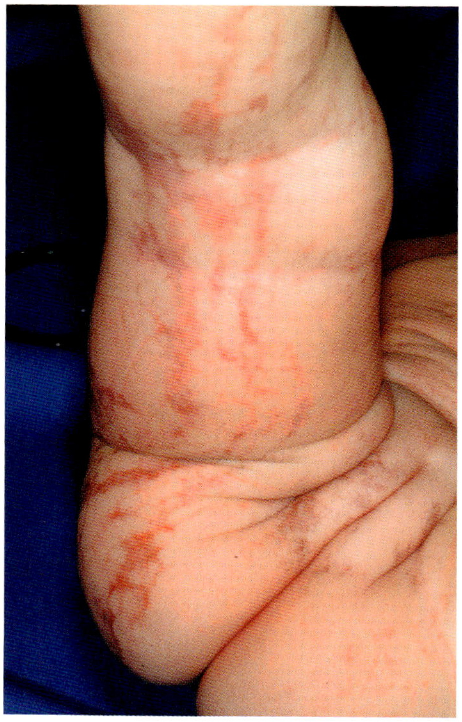

Fig. 11.34 Incontinentia pigmenti. The bands of brownish-gray pigmentation may initially appear purpuric, raising the question of child abuse.

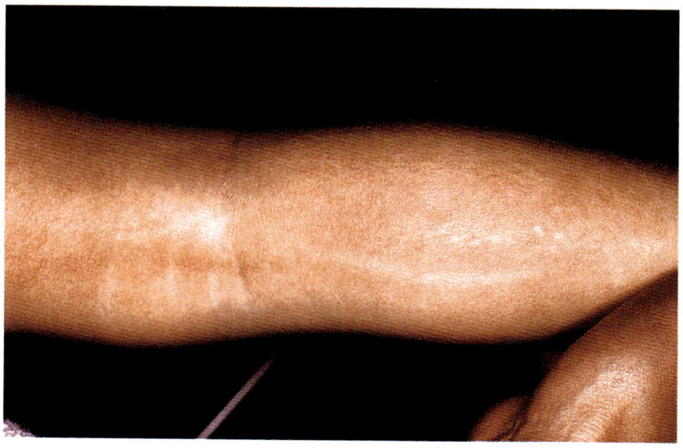

Fig. 11.35 Incontinentia pigmenti. Atrophic streaks that are often hypopigmented can be found in the minority of affected individuals. Most commonly noted on the arms and legs, these affected areas show diminished hair, eccrine glands, and sweat pores. The atrophic, hypopigmented streaks are often subtle and may be accentuated by viewing with side lighting or by Wood lamp examination.

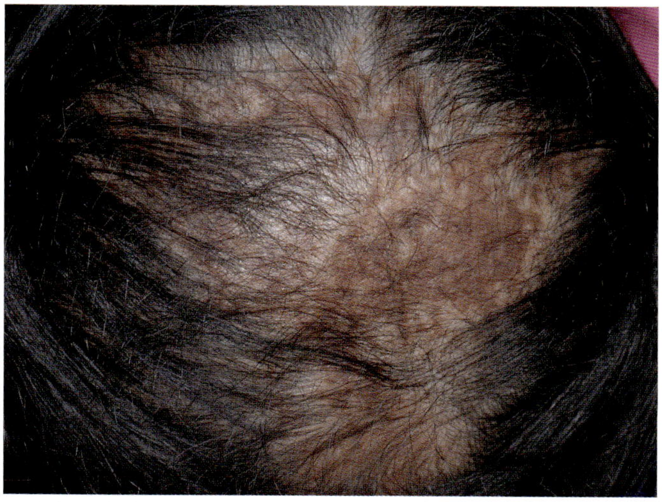

Fig. 11.36 Incontinentia pigmenti. Cicatricial alopecia most commonly appears near the vertex and does not necessarily relate to the previous presence of lesions at the site.

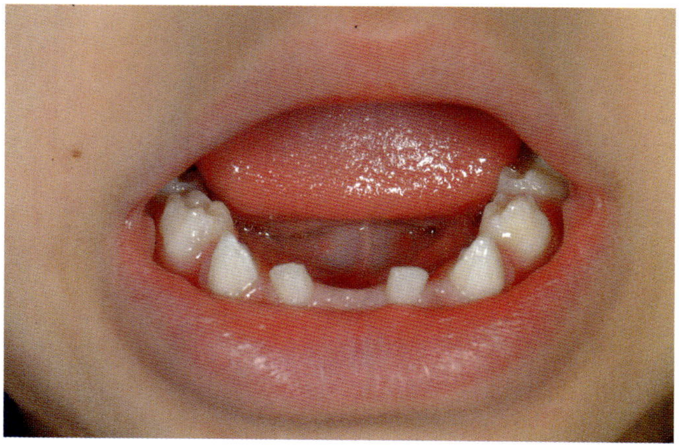

Fig. 11.37 Incontinentia pigmenti. Dental anomalies (delayed dentition, partial anodontia, pegged or conical teeth) occur in the majority of affected individuals. Interestingly, these dental changes mirror those of boys with hypohidrotic ectodermal dysplasia, a disorder that shares the NF-κB signaling pathway.

show dental anomalies (delayed dentition, partial anodontia, pegged or conical teeth)[389–391] (Fig. 11.37) reminiscent of those in boys with hypohidrotic ectodermal dysplasia (see Chapter 7). Ectodysplasin (which is usually mutated in boys with hypohidrotic ectodermal dysplasia), the ectodysplasin receptor, and *NEMO* all participate in NF-κB signaling, providing an explanation for these shared phenotypic features. In fact, boys with a form of ectodermal dysplasia with immunodeficiency (see Chapter 7) have mutations in *NEMO* that decrease its function but do not eliminate it.

Up to 30% of patients with incontinentia pigmenti demonstrate involvement of the CNS, most commonly seizures. [392,393] These seizures have been attributed to acute microvascular hemorrhagic infarcts,[394] although recurrent stroke has also been described.[395] Many such neonates are mistakenly thought to have neonatal herpes simplex infection because of the presence of vesiculopustular lesions and seizures. Overall, 7.5% have severe neurologic abnormalities, including continuing seizures, retardation, and spastic abnormalities.[361] Seizures during the first week of life have been associated with the worst prognosis for normal development. Learning disabilities are common.[396]

Ophthalmic changes are present in 37% of patients; 18% have strabismus, and an equal number demonstrate more serious eye involvement (cataracts, optic atrophy, or retinal neovascularization or detachment). The retinal neovascularization may regress with laser photocoagulation,[397] and preliminary studies of VEGF inhibitors appear promising.[398] Bilateral blindness has been described in 4% to 8% of individuals with incontinentia pigmenti. Occasionally, cardiopulmonary anomalies[397] and skeletal malformations (such as microcephaly, syndactyly, supernumerary ribs, hemiatrophy, or shortening of the arms or legs) occur.

The characteristic cutaneous lesions of incontinentia pigmenti allow early diagnosis and investigation for associated ocular and neurologic abnormalities. No special therapy is required for the skin lesions of incontinentia pigmenti, because they tend to clear spontaneously, but regular ophthalmologic evaluations are important.[398] If retinal involvement is discovered, early intervention with laser, cryotherapy, laser photocoagulation,[399] or intravitreal bevacizumab[400] should be initiated. If seizures or evidence of developmental delay appear, neurologic consultation is appropriate. High-dose glucocorticoids in the neonatal period have helped to control seizures recalcitrant to antiepileptics.[401] Dental evaluation by 2 years of age will allow investigation of missing or misshapen secondary teeth; prostheses can be made in patients with significant dental abnormalities.

Obtaining a history of cutaneous disorders during the neonatal and infantile periods and careful physical examination of mothers who may be carriers is important for genetic counseling. A mother of an affected individual who shows subtle manifestations is at increased risk for having another affected daughter (50% probability in daughters) and aborting a male fetus (50% probability in sons). Affected mothers may show subtle signs, most commonly hypopigmented, atrophic, hairless streaks along Blaschko lines (sometimes seen best by side lighting)[402] and sometimes a patch of cicatricial alopecia,[403] conical incisor, or nail dystrophy.[404] Sometimes carrier mothers show no signs, despite a history of a previous blistering disorder in the neonatal period. Prenatal diagnosis is possible, and preimplantation genetic diagnosis has been performed.[405] The Incontinentia Pigmenti International Foundation provides education and support (http://www.ipif.org/).

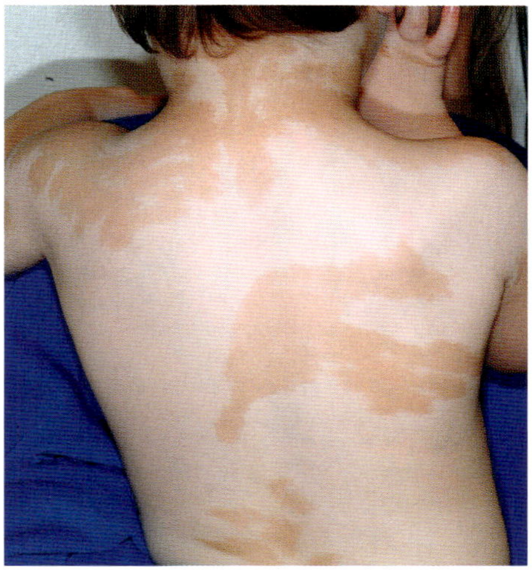

Fig. 11.39 Pigmentary mosaicism. Patterned hyperpigmented patches on the neck and trunk in a phylloid pattern. This child was otherwise normal.

PIGMENTARY MOSAICISM

The term *pigmentary mosaicism* is preferred for this heterogeneous group of disorders, characterized by patterned streaks of hypopigmentation and/or hyperpigmentation (Figs. 11.38 through 11.40). Old terms include hypomelanosis of Ito[406] (incontinentia pigmenti achromians), linear and whorled nevoid hypermelanosis,[407] and the segmental form of nevus depigmentosus.[408] The linear streaks and whorls tend to follow lines of mosaicism,[409] particularly the lines of Blaschko (lines of ectodermal embryologic development) in narrow or broad bands (92%), but less commonly along a phylloid pattern (3%) or patchy pattern (2%) of published cases in which the distribution was described.[410–412] Both hypopigmented and hyperpigmented streaks may be seen in the same individual. In a literature review of 651 patients, 43% had hyperpigmentation, 50% hypopigmentation, and 7% the combination.[412] The abnormal pigmentation was visible at birth in 46% and sometime during the first year of life in 75%. Among these reported patients, 56% had extracutaneous manifestations, most often developmental delay (54%), bone issues (38%), seizures or electroencephalogram abnormalities (37%), dysmorphic facial features (31%), and/or psychomotor retardation (16%). Having extracutaneous manifestations occurred more often with hypopigmentation (73%) or combined hyper- and hypopigmentation (83%) than with hyperpigmentation alone (32%) ($p < .001$). In another study, an unselected patient population with pigment mosaicism showed an incidence of associated abnormalities (particularly of the bones, eyes, and/or CNS) in only 30% of patients.[413] Given the propensity to report patients with more complex manifestations, it is likely that most patients do not have extracutaneous involvement by history and examination, especially

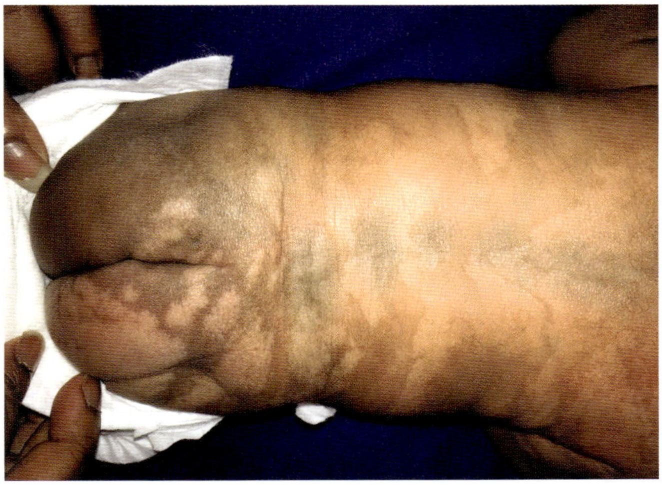

Fig. 11.40 Pigmentary mosaicism. Patterned hypopigmentation in an infant with multiorgan abnormalities due to Pallistoer–Killian syndrome with a small extra short arm of chromosome 12.

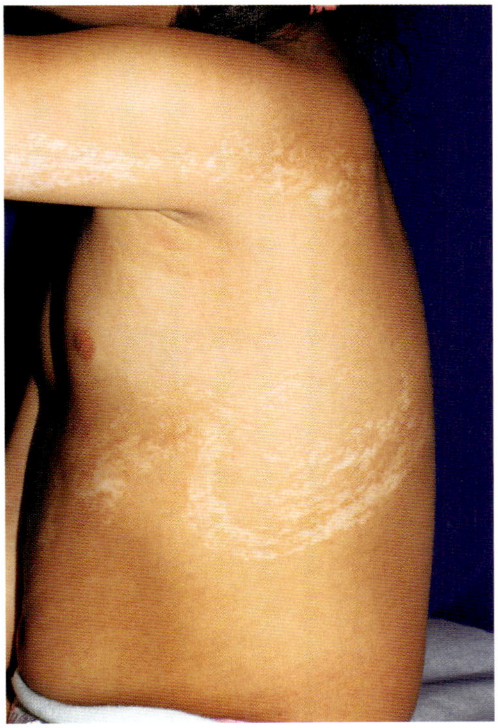

Fig. 11.38 Pigmentary mosaicism. Streaks of patterned hypopigmentation. The terms *incontinentia pigmenti achromians* and *hypomelanosis of Ito* are no longer used.

without widespread pigmentary mosaicism, and these children require no further investigation.

Mosaic conditions do not tend to be hereditary as mosaic disorders, although 7% of cases with a known family history claim to have an affected family member.[412] Structural and numerical chromosomal abnormalities[414–416] have been described in peripheral blood leukocytes and, occasionally, cultured fibroblasts or keratinocytes from 42% to 60% of affected pediatric patients, with 84% in a mosaic state. In general, more abnormalities are found with more extensive pigmentary mosaicism and associated noncutaneous abnormalities.[412,417–419] The greatest number of publications have cited abnormalities in chromosomes 7, 13, and 18, and the sex chromosomes. The molecular mechanism of pigmentary mosaicism, however, is currently unclear. Given the patterning primarily along Blaschko lines, the gene defect may lie within keratinocytes (e.g., pigment transfer) and possibly melanocytes, given that the patterns of melanocytic development are not as well delineated. As such, looking for mosaicism in blood or fibroblasts alone would be expected to yield less than evaluation of keratinocytes (or melanocytes) directly.

The streaks of hypopigmentation or hyperpigmentation along Blaschko lines of embryologic development must be distinguished from the hypopigmented or hyperpigmented streaks of incontinentia pigmenti. The term *incontinentia pigmenti achromians* for the streaks of hypopigmentation has been abandoned to avoid confusion because incontinentia pigmenti is unrelated. The lack of preceding vesicular or verrucous lesions of incontinentia pigmenti and the finding of increased melanin deposition at the basal cell layer in hyperpigmented streaks of pigment mosaicism (linear and whorled hypermelanosis) rather than the pigment incontinence of incontinentia pigmenti help to distinguish these disorders.[420] Epidermal nevi may present as flat brown streaks but more commonly are hyperkeratotic (see Chapter 9).

Disorders of Hyperpigmentation

Pigmented nevi are among the most common hyperpigmented lesions and are reviewed in Chapter 9, as are streaks of pigmentation involving the nails (longitudinal melanonychia; see Chapter 7). Treatment of hyperpigmented lesions with topical agents has generally been unsuccessful. Sun protection is a critical aspect of management in preventing darkening. Lasers have been used to treat a variety of hyperpigmented disorders in children,[421,422] in particular CAL macules, nevus of Ota, and other forms of dermal melanocytosis, Becker nevi, and tattoos. Several therapeutic sessions are required, and results are rarely permanent.

EPIDERMAL MELANOCYTE LESIONS

Freckles

Freckles (ephelides) are light brown, well-circumscribed macules, usually smaller than 3 mm in diameter, which appear in childhood, especially between 2 and 4 years of age, and tend to fade during the winter and adult life. Freckles are most common on the sun-exposed areas of the face (especially the nose and cheeks), shoulders, and upper back. Their presence correlates with fair skin, red hair, and an increased risk of developing melanoma.[423] In addition to the variants in *MC1R* as a major contributor toward freckle formation, variants in other genes (*ASIP, TYR, HERC2/OCA2, IRF4, BNC2*) have been implicated.

Freckles become darker and more confluent after UV light exposure in the sunburn spectrum (290 to 320 nm) as well as in the long-wave UV (UVA) range (320 to 400 nm). UVA light is not blocked by window glass and sunscreen agents that filter out only the sunburn spectrum. Freckles often become smaller, lighter, and fewer during the winter months. Histopathologic features of ephelides include increased melanin pigmentation of the basal layer without an increase in the number of melanocytes or elongation of the epidermal rete ridges.

Freckles bear cosmetic but no systemic significance. Treatment includes avoidance of sun exposure and appropriate covering makeup. Use of "full-spectrum" sunscreens that provide protection against both UVA and UVB light (e.g., with avobenzone or titanium dioxide) are more protective than sunscreens that only provide UVB protection. When desired, although seldom necessary, gentle chemical peels or laser may remove the superficial pigmentation and make many of the freckles less conspicuous.

Becker Nevus

Becker nevus (Becker melanosis), an irregular macular hyperpigmentation with hypertrichosis, is sometimes congenital, but more commonly appears later during childhood with accentuation during adolescence. Generally the first change is brown pigmentation that expands to 10 to 15 cm in diameter (about the size of a hand or larger) (Fig. 11.41). The outline is irregular and sometimes surrounded by islands of blotchy pigmentation. Although characteristically seen unilaterally on the upper half of the trunk, especially around the shoulder, it has also been reported in other areas on the trunk, forehead, cheeks, supraclavicular region, abdomen, forearm, wrist, buttocks, and shins and may be bilateral.[423,424] After a time (often 1 or 2 years), coarse terminal hairs appear in the region in affected males, usually at the site of the pigmentation (Fig. 11.42), suggesting androgenic stimulation. The intensity of pigmentation may fade somewhat as the patient becomes older, but the hyperpigmentation and hypertrichosis tend to persist for life. The disorder has been described much more commonly in males than females, likely because the hypertrichosis in males (but rarely in females) increases the likelihood of diagnosis.

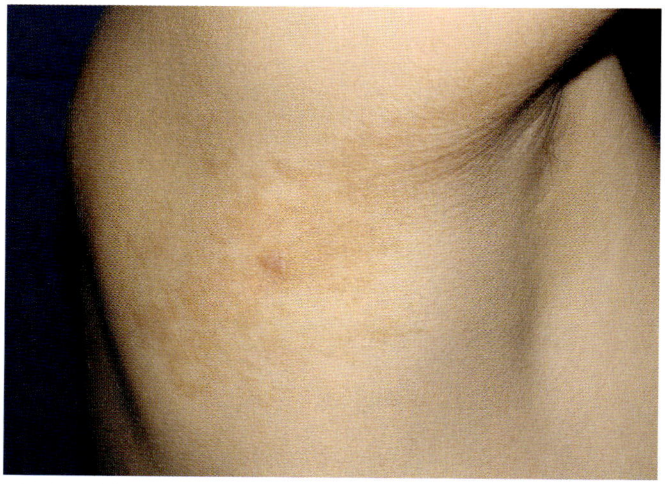

Fig. 11.41 Becker nevus. This light brown, irregularly bordered patch without hypertrichosis was noticed on the axillary area and shoulder of this 12-year-old boy.

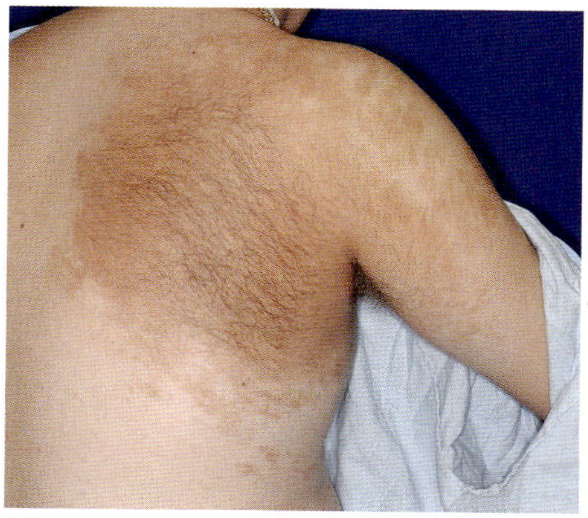

Fig. 11.42 Becker nevus. Large patch of grayish-brown pigmentation on the back with associated coarse terminal hairs. These lesions usually appear during late childhood or early adolescence on the upper trunk.

The underlying genetic basis for Becker nevus is somatic mosaicism of *ACTB*, encoding β-actin[426] Mutations tend to be hotspot mutations in R247, which can increase Hedgehog pathway signaling. Preliminary data using laser capture microdissection studies suggest that the arrector pili muscle is the altered tissue. The basis for the occurrence of familial cases[427,428] is unknown. Although most Becker nevi occur without other pathologic findings, association with a variety of other abnormalities (such as unilateral breast and areolar hypoplasia, focal acne, pectus carinatum, limb asymmetry, and spina bifida)[429,430] has been called *Becker nevus syndrome*.[427,431]

Histopathologic features reveal epidermal thickening, elongation of the rete ridges, and hyperpigmentation of the basal layer with increased melanocytes.[432] Malignant transformation does not occur. Treatment of this disorder is purely cosmetic and is generally discouraged. Laser therapy or excision usually does not improve the appearance. The hypertrichosis may be treated with laser depilation[433] (see Chapter 7).

Lentigines

Lentigines are small, tan, dark brown, or black flat, oval, or circular, sharply circumscribed lesions that usually appear in childhood and may increase in number until adult life. These may occur on sun-exposed areas (especially the face and dorsal aspect of the hands) as "lentigo simplex." Lentigines usually measure 3 to 15 mm in diameter and may occur on any mucocutaneous surface (Fig. 11.43) including the lips or conjunctivae. The pigmentation is uniform and darker than that seen in ephelides (freckles) and CAL macules, and the color is unaffected by exposure to sunlight. Lentigines are typically larger than freckles and smaller than a typical CAL macule and can be distinguished from freckles and CAL macules histologically.[434] Multiple facial lentigines can be an early sign of xeroderma pigmentosum, especially in association with a history of sunburning after limited sun exposure. Lentigines have rarely been described after use of topical tacrolimus.[435–437]

Lentigines that appear early in life may fade or disappear; those appearing later in life tend to be permanent. Treatment other than for cosmetic purposes is ordinarily not indicated. When desired, however, excision by a small punch biopsy, cryosurgery, or laser may be beneficial. Imatinib led to marked lightening of lentigines in a patient treated for familial gastrointestinal stromal tumor syndrome,[438] presumably because of its inhibitory effect on c-KIT activation.

Patients with speckled lentiginous nevus or segmental lentiginosis show patches of lentigines, usually overlying a slight increase in cutaneous pigmentation (Fig. 11.44). Eruptive, agminated Spitz nevi may be seen within a segmental lentiginosis.[439] Eruptive lentiginosis are characterized by a widespread eruption of several hundred lentigines, which may develop over a few months or years, usually in adolescents or young adults, without systemic manifestations. Some cases are postinflammatory and have been described after resolution of psoriatic plaques treated with methotrexate or ustekinumab[440–443] and nonsteroidal antiinflammatory drug–induced fixed drug eruption.[444] Azathioprine therapy has also been linked to eruptive lentiginosis. Inherited patterned lentiginosis is an autosomal dominant disorder of darker-skinned individuals with the onset of lentiginosis during infancy or early childhood. Lentigines occur on the face initially but can become widespread. Affected individuals are otherwise healthy.

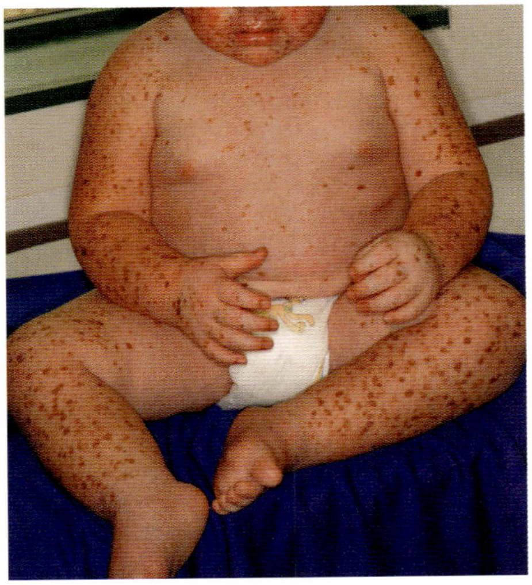

Fig. 11.43 Lentigines. This girl showed hundreds of lentigines, particularly on the face and extensor surfaces of the extremities. These sharply demarcated macules tend to be larger than a freckle but smaller than a café-au-lait spot and range in color from tan to black. Although one might consider LEOPARD syndrome or Carney complex in this girl, genetic testing showed no mutations in *PTPN11, RAF1, BRAF, MAP2K1*, or *PRKAR1A*.

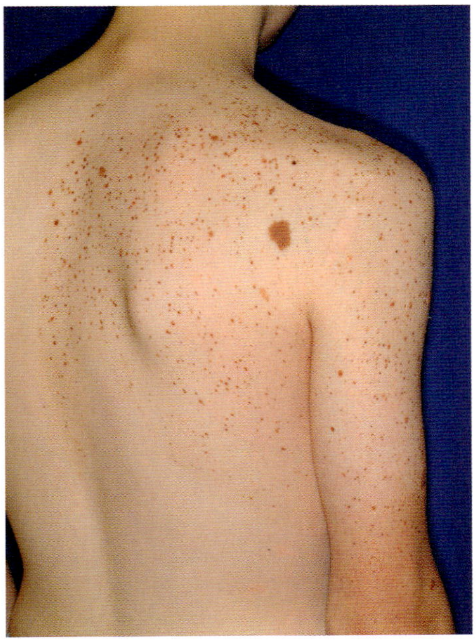

Fig. 11.44 Speckled lentiginous nevus. This large patch of lentigines of different sizes overlying an increase in cutaneous pigmentation may represent a mosaic form of multiple lentiginosis syndrome.

Localized or extensive lentiginosis may also be a component of a multisystem disorder. Although they may occur in children without medical problems, lentigines of the penis are characteristic of Bannayan–Zonana (Bannayan–Zonana–Ruvalcaba) syndrome, an autosomal dominant disorder that results from mutations in the *PTEN* gene and is allelic with Cowden syndrome (Fig. 11.45) (see Chapter 9). Other major features are macrocephaly and lipomas. Lentigines of the hands, feet, and buccal mucosa may also be a feature of Cronkhite–Canada syndrome, in which nail dystrophy, hair loss, and intestinal polyposis are other characteristics. Centrofacial lentiginosis (also called *centrofacial neurodysraphic lentiginosis* or *Touraine syndrome*) is an autosomal dominant process in which lentigines are first noted in the first year of life, particularly on the nose and cheeks. Patients with centrofacial lentiginosis may have associated mental retardation, congenital mitral valve stenosis, seizures, sacral hypertrichosis, coalescence of the eyebrows, high-arched palate, absent upper middle incisors, bony abnormalities, defective fusion of the neural tube (dysraphia), psychiatric disorders, dwarfism, and endocrine dysfunction.

The major lentiginous syndromes are Peutz–Jeghers syndrome, LEOPARD syndrome, and Carney complex.

Peutz–Jeghers Syndrome

The prevalence of this autosomal dominant disorder of mucocutaneous lentiginous macules and multiple hamartomatous intestinal polyps is approximately 1 in 100,000 individuals.[445] Mutations in the

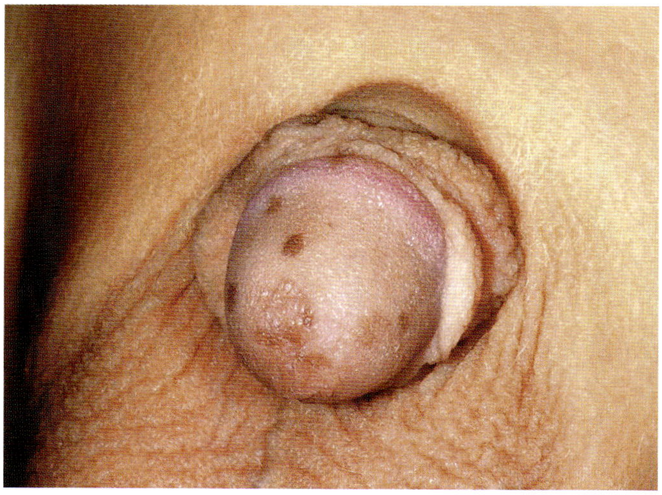

Fig. 11.45 Bannayan–Zonana–Ruvalcaba syndrome. Lentigines of the penis are characteristic of Bannayan–Zonana–Ruvalcaba syndrome, an autosomal dominant disorder that also commonly features macrocephaly and lipomas.

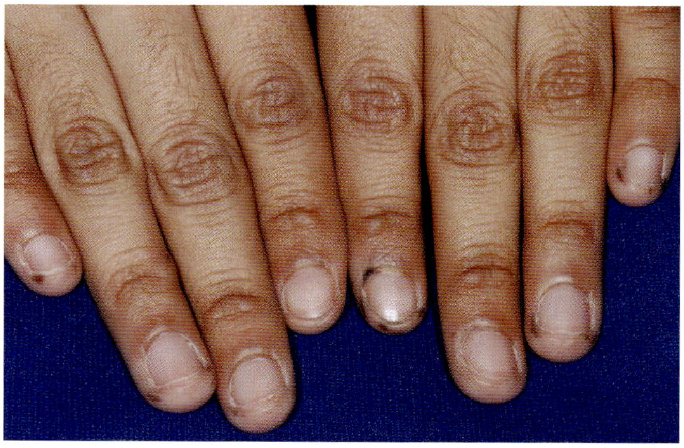

Fig. 11.47 Peutz–Jeghers syndrome. Lentigines on the fingers.

serine-threonine kinase *STK11/LKB1* gene have been found in 75% to 94% of cases.[445–447] Parental mosaicism (without mutations detected in blood samples) has been described.[448]

Characteristic bluish-brown to black spots, often apparent at birth or in early infancy, represent the cutaneous marker of this syndrome. These discrete, flat pigmented lesions are irregularly oval and usually measure less than 5 mm in diameter. They are most commonly seen on the lips (Fig. 11.46), buccal mucosa, nasal and periorbital regions, elbows, dorsal aspects of the fingers and toes (Fig. 11.47), palms, soles, and periumbilical, perianal, and labial regions; occasionally the gums and hard palate and on rare occasions even the tongue may be involved. An umbilical lentigo has been described at birth in an affected neonate.[449] The pigmented lesions on the skin and lips often fade after puberty; those on the buccal mucosa, palate, and tongue, however, persist.

The hamartomatous gastrointestinal polyps seen in this disorder may be found from the stomach to the anal canal, although the small bowel represents the most commonly involved portion of the intestinal tract. Polyps vary from minute pinhead lesions to those measuring several centimeters in diameter. They may occur in early childhood and even during the first year of life,[450] with one study showing a median age of presentation of 5 years; 50% of patients have symptoms in the first 2 decades of life, including abdominal pain, melena, or intussusception.[451,452] The most common symptom, recurrent attacks of colicky abdominal pain, is thought to result from recurring transient episodes of incomplete intussusception. A prospective multicenter study found a 15% risk of cumulative intussusception by age 10 years and 50% by age 20.[453] Hematemesis, although less common, may occur owing to involvement of the stomach, duodenum, or upper jejunum. Polyps of the nasal mucosae and gallbladder have occasionally been described, and rarely polyps involve the respiratory and urogenital tracts.[454]

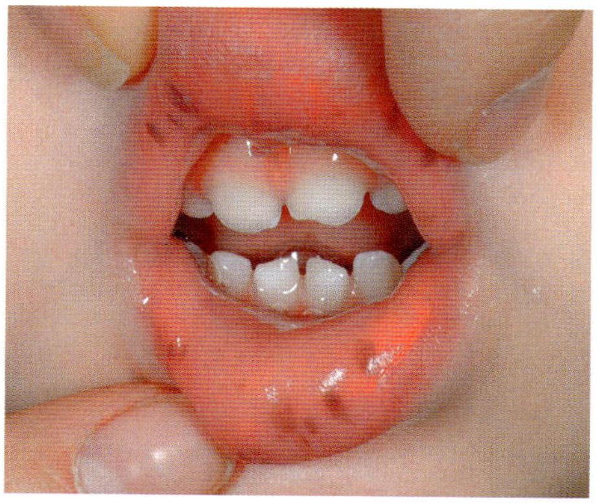

Fig. 11.46 Peutz–Jeghers syndrome. Characteristic bluish-brown to black spots were first noted in early childhood on the lips of this boy who later developed hamartomatous gastrointestinal polyps.

Although the polyps of Peutz–Jeghers syndrome are generally benign, adenocarcinomas of the gastrointestinal tract (stomach, small intestine, colorectum, pancreas, and biliary tract), breast and uterine cervical carcinomas, and gonadal sex tumors (Sertoli cell tumors of the testis and sex-cord tumors of the ovary) have been described.[446,455] Sertoli cell tumors can occur prepubertally and may present with gynecomastia.[456] Adenocarcinoma can be diagnosed during the first decade of life.[457] However, most cancers occur during adulthood[458] with a mean age of first cancer diagnosis of 41 years.[459] The lifetime cumulative risk for all cancers is 55% to 94% (up to 63-fold increased relative risk of that of the general population), although most commonly gastrointestinal cancer (2600-fold increased risk of small intestinal tumors).

In the past, therapeutic management focused on relief of symptoms and recurrent resections with the risk of malabsorption. The recommendation now is to remove polyps if technically feasible (especially if larger than 5 mm).[460–462] Initial screening is generally suggested by 8 years[463] with esophagogastroduodenoscopy, narrow-band imaging endoscopy,[464] or capsule endoscopy. If these are negative, colonoscopy can be put off until age 18 unless a concern arises. In a case series of 14 children, however, the median age of polyp detection was 5 years,[456] leading to the suggestion that initial screening occur at 4 to 5 years of age. Sertoli cell tumors should be sought prepubertally, but yearly evaluation of other organs at risk of malignancy (breast, thyroid gland, pancreas, uterus, and ovaries) should begin by the end of adolescence. The lentigines of Peutz–Jeghers syndrome have responded to laser[465] and intense pulsed light[466] therapies, although the lentigines not uncommonly recur.[467] The gynecomastia may respond to aromatase inhibition.[468]

Laugier–Hunziker syndrome is a benign pigmentary disorder that manifests as macular hyperpigmentation of the lips and buccal mucosa. Many patients also show long pigmented bands of the nails (melanonychia striata), but the visceral manifestations of Peutz–Jeghers syndrome are absent.[467,469,470]

Carney Complex

Carney complex comprises an autosomal dominant disorder that features the pigmentary abnormalities of lentigines, epithelioid blue nevi, and pigmented schwannomas.[471,472] Nevi, atrial myxoma, and neurofibroma ephelides (NAME)[473] and lentigines, atrial myxoma (which may present in childhood as an ischemic stroke),[474] and blue nevi (LAMB)[475] syndromes are included in Carney complex.[476–479] Most cases are sporadic. The group of disorders is considered a form of MEN, in that endocrine abnormalities and tumors are common features, especially pituitary adenomas, ovarian tumors,[480] testicular (Sertoli cell) tumors, and pigmented nodular adrenocortical disease, which may present as Cushing syndrome.[481,482]

Skin manifestations are seen in 80% of patients, most commonly lentigines that typically fade during adulthood in 70% to 75% of patients. The lentigines tend to appear peripubertally and most commonly involve the center of the face, especially the vermilion border of the lips (leading to the misdiagnosis of Peutz–Jeghers syndrome),[483] as well as the conjunctivae and occasionally the intraoral area. Peutz–Jeghers and Carney syndromes share several other features including the occurrence of gynecomastia and growth acceleration, as well as Sertoli cell tumors and tumors of the breast and thyroid. The blue nevi, including epithelioid blue nevi, occur in 40% of Carney complex patients. They tend to be multiple, most commonly on the face, trunk, and extremities, and characteristically are dome-shaped dark blue papules. Most epithelioid blue nevi in children are associated with Carney complex.[484] The lentigines and blue nevi are often accompanied by CAL spots. Multiple cutaneous myxomas occur in 30% to 55% of studied patients and are most commonly seen on the eyelids, ears, nipples, and external genitalia. They are usually diagnosed during the late teen years but can occur as early as infancy.[485,486] Patients often show myxomas of the oropharynx, heart, and breast and may develop other neoplasia of mesenchymal and neural crest origin. The typical psammomatous melanotic schwannomas occur in 10% of affected individuals and may involve the skin, posterior spinal nerve roots, gastrointestinal tract, and bone. Biopsy specimens of the blue nevi and schwannomas show characteristic histologic features.[487] Patients have been described both with predominantly cutaneous features[488] and without cutaneous lentigines. The most common endocrine tumors or overactivity include primary pigmented nodular adrenocortical disease (25% of patients),[489] growth hormone–producing pituitary adenoma (10% of patients), large-cell calcifying Sertoli cell tumor, and thyroid adenoma (up to 75% of patients). Development of carcinoma is rare. Recommended surveillance for affected individuals includes regular skin and physical examinations (including close monitoring of growth, pubertal staging, and palpation of thyroid and testes); at least annual echocardiograms beginning during infancy; serum levels of growth hormone, prolactin, and insulin-like growth factor-1 beginning in adolescence; and imaging studies.[472]

Mutations in the protein kinase A type I-α regulatory subunit (*PRKAR1A*)[490] occur in more than 70 % of patients. An additional 20% of families with Carney complex show linkage to 2p16 (gene not yet identified) and have a milder phenotype with later onset. Copy number gain in *PRKACB* has been described in one patient.[472]

Multiple Lentigines/LEOPARD Syndrome

Multiple lentiginoses/LEOPARD syndrome (also called *Noonan syndrome with multiple lentigines* [NSML]) is a RASopathy (Table 11.6) with a spectrum of manifestations ranging from generalized lentigines alone to the complete syndrome that characteristically shows lentigines, electrocardiographic abnormalities, ocular hypertelorism, pulmonic stenosis, abnormal genitalia, retardation of growth, and sensorineural deafness.[491–494] Mutations in *PTPN11* have been found in 90% patients; genotyping may be required to confirm the diagnosis. Rarely, affected individuals have mutations in *RAF1* (3%), *BRAF*, or *MAP2K1*.[495–498] Variable expressivity is seen within families, so some

Table 11.6 Features of RASopathies

Syndrome	Pigment Changes	Other Features	Gene(s)
Neurofibromatosis 1	Café-au-lait macules, freckling, pigmentation overlying cutaneous and plexiform neurofibromas	Macrocephaly, learning disabilities, Lisch nodules, short stature, skeletal abnormalities (esp. scoliosis, sphenoid wing dysplasia, and tibial pseudoarthrosis), renal and cerebral artery stenosis, aortic coarctation, tumors (neurofibromas, optic gliomas, MPNST, juvenile chronic myelogenous leukemia, pheochromocytomas, astrocytomas, glioblastomas, rhabdomyosarcomas, GI stromal tumors, carcinoid tumors, leiomyosarcomas)	*NF1* (neurofibromin)
Legius syndrome	Café-au-lait macules, freckling	Macrocephaly, learning disabilities; can have Noonan-like facies, pectus abnormalities, lipomas	*SPRED1*
Noonan syndrome	Multiple nevi	Macrocephaly, short stature, distinct facies, ulerythema ophryogenes, keratosis pilaris, pectus excavatum, webbed neck, mild cognitive impairment, cryptorchidism, craniosynostosis	*PTPN11, KRAS, SOS1, RAF1, NRAS, BRAF, RIT1, SOS2, LZTR1*
LEOPARD syndrome	Lentigines	Electrocardiographic abnormalities, ocular hypertelorism, pulmonic stenosis, abnormal genitalia, retardation of growth, and sensorineural deafness	*PTPN11, RAF1, BRAF, MAP2K1*
Noonan-like syndrome	Hyperpigmented macules	Noonan-like facies, cardiac defects, may have microcephaly, risk of juvenile myelomonocytic leukemia–like disorders	*CBL*
Noonan-like syndrome with loose anagen hair	Hyperpigmented macules	Macrocephaly, short stature, cardiovascular anomalies, mild cognitive impairment, fine, sparse, loose hair	*SHOC2, PPP1CB*
Cardiofaciocutaneous syndrome	Multiple pigmented nevi, lentigines	Distinctive facies, cardiovascular anomalies, failure to thrive, curly hair, ulerythema ophryogenes, keratosis pilaris, palmoplantar keratoderma, seizures, intellectual impairment	*BRAF, MAP2K1, MAPK2K2, KRAS*
Costello syndrome	None	Coarse facial features, flexible joints, loose skin, warts, curly hair, palmoplantar keratoderma, failure to thrive, short stature, developmental and intellectual delay, cardiovascular abnormalities, risk of tumors (rhabdomyosarcoma, ganglioneuroblastomas, bladder carcinoma)	*HRAS*
Capillary malformation-arteriovenous malformation syndrome	None	Capillary malformations and arteriovenous malformations	*RASA1, EPHB4*
Hereditary gingival fibromatosis	None	Gingival fibromatosis, dysmorphic facies with lip protrusion	SOS1

GI, Gastrointestinal; *LEOPARD*, lentigines, electrocardiographic conduction abnormalities, ocular hypertelorism, pulmonic stenosis, abnormal genitalia, retardation of growth, deafness; *MPNST*, malignant peripheral nerve sheath tumor.

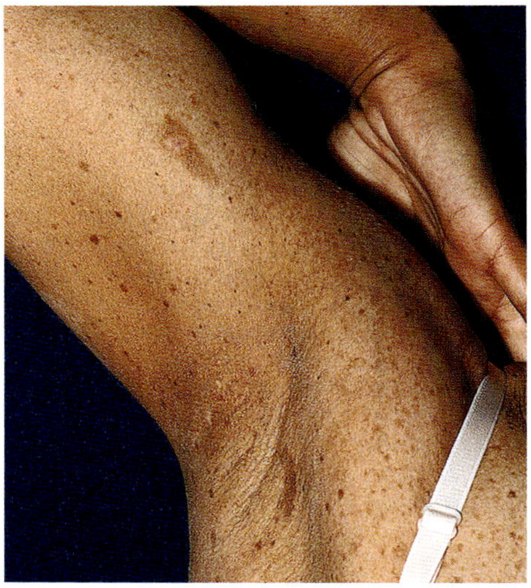

Fig. 11.48 Multiple lentiginosis/LEOPARD syndrome. Myriad lentigines with scattered café-au-lait macules overlying generalized hyperpigmentation in this adolescent with only cutaneous changes. In some individuals, the pigmentary changes are associated with a spectrum of visceral abnormalities, including lentigines, electrocardiographic abnormalities, ocular hypertelorism, pulmonic stenosis, abnormal genitalia, retardation of growth, and sensorineural deafness, leading to the term *LEOPARD syndrome.*

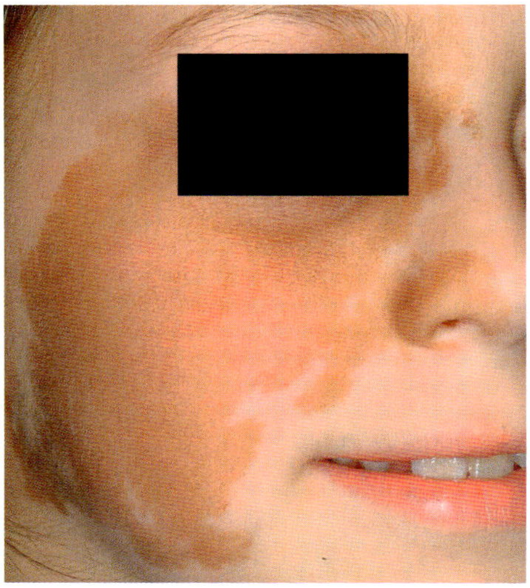

Fig. 11.49 Café-au-lait (CAL) spot. Round or oval patches of light brown pigmentation are common in children but usually are up to a few centimeters in diameter, in contrast to this larger CAL spot of the face. Although a rare disorder, the segmental distribution of the CAL spot should alert one to consider the possibility of McCune–Albright syndrome.

affected individuals show only the multiple lentigines or lentigines and cardiac disease,[499] whereas others show a variety of the visceral manifestations. Mutations in *SASH1* have been shown to be an alternative cause for familial multiple lentiginosis (allelic for *SASH1* mutations in dyschromatoses, see earlier).[500–502] Oral mucosae, palms, and soles can be involved, but there are no other manifestations.

Affected individuals typically are thin; show an elongated, marfanoid facies; and have CAL macules admixed within the myriad of lentigines (Fig. 11.48). The dark, 1- to 5-mm lentigines that define the syndrome often first appear at 4 to 5 years of age but then increase dramatically (to thousands of lentigines) by puberty. The cutaneous lesions tend to be concentrated on the neck and upper trunk, but they may also appear on the skin of the face and scalp, arms, palms, soles, and genitalia. The lentigines characteristically spare the mucosa. Occasionally formes frustes of this disorder occur, in which the characteristic lentigines are absent. In most patients, the CAL macules are present before the onset of the lentigines, leading to consideration of an alternative diagnosis of NF type 1 or its allelic variant with CAL spots and pulmonary valve stenosis, Watson syndrome.[503]

Cardiac abnormalities occur in about 85% of affected individuals—mostly hypertrophic cardiomyopathy (up to 75%), which usually appears during infancy and subsequently progresses. Pulmonary valve stenosis and conduction defects have been described in 10% and 7% of patients, respectively.[497] Skeletal aberrations may include retardation of growth (below the 25th percentile), hypertelorism, an elongated facies, pectus deformities (carinatum or excavatum), dorsal kyphosis, winged scapulae, and prognathism. Endocrine disorders include gonadal hypoplasia, hypospadias, undescended testes, hypoplastic ovaries, and delayed puberty. The hearing loss of LEOPARD syndrome is often congenital and is neurosensory, can be detected by early auditory evoked potentials, and is treated by cochlear implantation.[504]

Café-au-Lait Spots

CAL spots are large, round or oval, flat lesions of light brown pigmentation found in up to 33% of normal children; having a greater number of CAL spots is more common in children with darker skin color, but having more than five is rare other than in NF or Legius syndrome.[505–508] Commonly present at birth or developing soon thereafter, they vary from 1.5 cm or less in their smallest diameter to much larger lesions that may measure up to 15 to 20 cm or more in diameter (Fig. 11.49). CAL spots may rarely occur anywhere on the body. Neonatal blue-light phototherapy may increase the development of CAL spots in preschool children.[509]

The CAL spots of McCune–Albright syndrome are seen in approximately 50% of patients. They tend to be present during infancy or early childhood, with a predilection for areas with particularly bony prominences (the forehead, nuchal area, thorax, sacral areas, and buttocks). However, CAL spots may be seen elsewhere, including on the oral mucosae.[510] They are commonly unilateral, stopping abruptly at the midline and follow a dermatomal distribution. They tend to have irregularly jagged or serrated borders (described as resembling the coast of Maine, in contrast to the smooth-bordered CAL spots of NF, which have been compared to the coast of California). The McCune–Albright syndrome in its complete form is a triad characterized by CAL spots, polyostotic fibrous dysplasia, and endocrine dysfunction, often manifesting as precocious puberty (see Chapter 23, Fig. 23.26).[511] McCune–Albright syndrome is a mosaic disorder resulting from activating mutations in *GNAS*, but next-generation sequencing techniques enable detection of the low-abundance mutations in blood samples.[512]

CAL spots are increased in number in Russell–Silver syndrome,[513] a disorder that also features short stature, musculoskeletal abnormalities, craniofacial dysmorphism, and genitourinary malformations, as well as in multiple lentigines/LEOPARD syndrome (see Multiple Lentigines/LEOPARD Syndrome section and Fig. 11.48). Johnson–McMillin syndrome is an autosomal dominant disorder in which families show truncal CAL spots in association with facial nerve palsy and mild developmental delay.[514] Other disorders with increased numbers of CAL spots are ring chromosomes (chromosomes 7, 11, 12, 15, 17, 22), Cowden and Fanconi syndromes, TSC, and piebaldism.

Not uncommonly, infants may show what appears to be a CAL, but sometimes years later the CAL develops tiny more darkly hyperpigmented macules or papules. This lesion is called *nevus spilus* (see Chapter 9), and biopsy of the more darkly pigmented lesions will show typical features of pigmented nevi (see Figs. 9.29 and 9.30). Individuals with red hair or with parents of markedly different skin pigmentation may show hyperpigmented macules that resemble CAL spots. They can be differentiated by their often irregular shape, tendency to be less well defined than the CAL spots of NF, and the paler coloration of the hyperpigmentation. Observation of these CAL-like macules during the first 5 to 6 years of life should be performed. Ophthalmologic evaluations to seek the presence of concomitant Lisch nodules may help to distinguish NF. Lichen aureus, a form of pigmented purpuric eruption, can also be confused with a CAL but tends to show pinpoint petechiae and purpura on a hyperpigmented base[515] (see Chapter 12).

Neurofibromatosis

Neurofibromatosis is an autosomal dominant disorder characterized by an increased propensity toward the development of tumors, particularly of the nerve sheath.[516–518] NF encompasses three distinct disorders: NF type 1 (NF1; von Recklinghausen disease), NF type 2 (NF2; bilateral acoustic or central NF),[519] and schwannomatosis. The latter is characterized by painful peripheral (nonvestibular, nondermal) schwannomas and is largely diagnosed in adults.[520] More than 90% of cases of NF are NF1, which occurs in approximately 1 in 3000 births.[521–524] NF2 occurs in 1 in 25,000 to 40,000 individuals, and its diagnosis during childhood is unusual. Both disorders show variable expressivity; NF1 shows an approximately 50% rate of new mutations, whereas two-thirds of children with NF2 have an affected parent. Patients with NF1 have mutations in neurofibromin, a large GTPase-activating cytoplasmic protein that negatively regulates Ras activation.[518] The gene mutated in NF2, merlin or schwannomin, encodes a cytoskeletal protein that inhibits a serine/threonine kinase PAK1, which is essential for Ras transformation.[525]

The cutaneous manifestations of NF1 are of major importance,[526] and thus most discussion of NF in this chapter will focus on NF1. However, skin tumors are an important diagnostic clue for patients with NF2 and are often present months to years before other features. These tumors, predominantly schwannomas or neurofibromas, are the presenting sign in 27% of individuals with NF2 and eventually occur in 59% of patients.[527,528] A higher number of skin tumors has been correlated with a worse prognosis. CAL spots are found in 33% of individuals with NF2, but only 2% have six or more CAL spots. Although NF2 is commonly considered a disorder of adults, approximately 15% of patients with NF2 are diagnosed before 18 years of age,[529] and onset during childhood predicts a worse prognosis. The major criteria for NF2 are shown in Box 11.4. NF2 in children most commonly presents with hearing impairment (one-third of children) or cranial-nerve dysfunction (one-third of children). Tumor load is often extensive in pediatric patients (especially vestibular and cranial schwannomas, cranial meningiomas, and spinal cord tumors). Overall, 75% of affected children develop hearing loss. Removal of vestibular schwannomas does not preserve hearing, although early detection and smaller tumors are associated with a better prognosis. Visual impairment as a result of cataracts and amblyopia occurs in 83% of affected children. Treatment is primarily surgical. Auditory brainstem implants may partially restore hearing.[530]

Although NF1 is best known because of Joseph Merrick, the famed "Elephant Man" of the 1800s, he is now thought to have had Proteus syndrome, a disorder characterized by segmental overgrowth with asymmetry, macrocephaly, lipomas, linear verrucous epidermal nevi, and vascular malformations (see Chapter 12). The diagnostic criteria for NF1 (Box 11.5) have not been modified since 1988 and thus do not yet include having a pathogenic mutation in neurofibromin. These criteria are of limited value for young children who typically show only multiple CAL spots and in 50% of cases have no affected first-degree family member. As such, the diagnostic criterion of six or more CAL spots of greater than 5 mm in diameter prepubertally and more than 15 mm postpubertally probably indicates the presence of NF1 (Fig. 11.50)[531] but is not definitively diagnostic. About 95% of patients with NF1 meet these criteria by 8 years of age, and all meet it by age 20 years. Nevertheless, a 2017 analysis of children with multiple café-au-lait macules who were followed clinically or analyzed genetically showed an 80% risk of having NF1 if six or more CALs were present in children younger than age 29 months, whereas children older than 29 months with fewer than six CALs or at least one atypical CAL had only a 0.9% risk.[532] There is marked variability in the overall severity and progression of NF. It can cause serious problems and even death in the newborn, or it may produce only mild or insignificant problems during the lifetime of the affected individual.

Box 11.4 Diagnostic Criteria for Neurofibromatosis Type 2

Bilateral vestibular schwannomas seen by MRI scan
or
A first-degree relative with NF2
AND
Unilateral vestibular schwannoma
or
Two of the following criteria:
- Meningioma
- Glioma
- Schwannoma
- Juvenile posterior subcapsular cataract

Modified from Mulvihill JJ, Parry DM, Sherman JL, et al. NIH conference. Neurofibromatosis 1 (Recklinghausen disease) and neurofibromatosis 2 (bilateral acoustic neurofibromatosis): an update. Ann Intern Med 1990;113(1):39–52; and Nunes F, MacCollin M. Neurofibromatosis 2 in the pediatric population. J Child Neurol 2003;18(10):718–24.
MRI, Magnetic resonance imaging; *NF*, neurofibromatosis.

Box 11.5 Diagnostic Criteria for Neurofibromatosis Type 1

Must have two or more of the following:
Six café-au-lait macules that measure ≥0.5 cm before puberty and ≥1.5 cm in diameter in adults*
Freckling of the axillary and/or inguinal areas*
A plexiform neurofibroma *or* two or more dermal neurofibromas
Two or more Lisch nodules
Optic nerve glioma
Pathognomonic skeletal dysplasia (i.e., tibial or sphenoid wing dysplasia)
An affected first-degree relative

*Given the recognition that Legius syndrome is distinct from neurofibromatosis type 1 (NF1) clinically and genetically but shares two of the major features, having the cutaneous pigmentary lesions alone (café-au-lait spots and freckling) is insufficient for a definitive diagnosis of NF1.

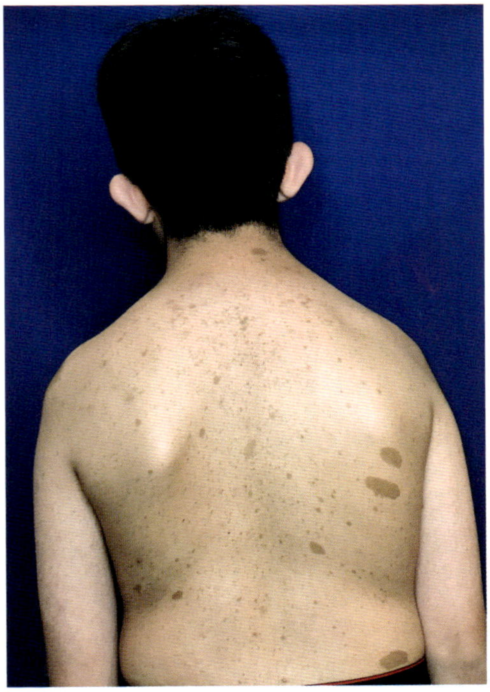

Fig. 11.50 Neurofibromatosis type 1 (NF1). The presence of six or more café-au-lait (CAL) spots larger than 0.5 cm in diameter in children and 1.5 cm in adolescents suggests the possibility of NF1, although having CAL spots alone does not allow for definitive diagnosis. This boy has features of Noonan syndrome as well (low-set, posteriorly rotated ears, low posterior hairline), a RASopathy with overlapping features.

Cutaneous Manifestations of Neurofibromatosis Type 1. CAL spots and dermal and plexiform neurofibromas are the characteristic cutaneous findings of pediatric NF1. The severity of cutaneous involvement is not indicative of the extent of disease in other organs. In fact, the number of CAL spots has been shown to be a function of germline sequence variants of other genes involved in pigment biology.[533]

CAL spots may occur anywhere on the body. They may be present at birth but often first appear during the first few months. They continue to increase in size and number during the first decade, especially the first 2 years of life. CAL spots in NF1 tend to have a greater melanocyte density and increased fibroblast secretion of stem cell factor than CAL spots without associated NF1.[534] Large CAL spots may be a sign of an underlying plexiform neurofibroma.

Another form of pigmentation, termed *axillary freckling* (Crowe sign), also serves as a valuable diagnostic aid in the early recognition of NF (Fig. 11.51).[535] Axillary freckling appears as multiple 1- to 4-mm CAL spots in the axillary vault. These most commonly appear between 3 and 5 years of age. Lack of sun exposure in this area prevents confusion with true freckles. These freckles are also commonly seen in the inguinal region and may be more generalized. Overall, almost 90% of affected children have intertriginous freckling by 7 years of age.

Multiple CAL spots and axillary and/or inguinal freckling are features of Legius syndrome (sometimes called *NF type 1–like syndrome*), which results from mutations in *SPRED1*. *SPRED1* interacts directly with Ras and is involved in its function. Although the clinical features during childhood generally do not allow Legius syndrome to be distinguished from NF1, distinction is important prognostically because Legius syndrome has been associated with macrocephaly, learning disabilities, and, uncommonly,[536] other clinical issues (e.g., the Noonan-like facies, pectus excavatum or carinatum, and lipomas), but not with the cutaneous or plexiform neurofibromas, NF1 osseous lesions, or symptomatic optic-pathway gliomas.[537] Almost 2% of individuals with a previous diagnosis of NF1 are now thought to have Legius syndrome. Although CAL spots and freckling have been distinct criteria that, if both present, allow the definitive diagnosis of NF1, the discovery that Legius syndrome presents with these two criteria has led to the suggestion that multiple CAL spots and freckling be combined into a single criterion for diagnosis.[538]

NF1 is also characterized by dermal (cutaneous) neurofibromas (cNFs), which represent tumors primarily composed of Schwann cells, mast cells, and fibroblasts. The cell of origin for these cNFs is dermal Schwann cell–like skin-derived precursor (SKP) cell. However, the milieu and other cells are important in encouraging growth. cNFs usually appear in late childhood or adolescence, although they are sometimes observed before 5 years of age. Their appearance is commonly associated with puberty and pregnancy, and they have been noted in 84% of affected adults.[539] They tend to grow rapidly and then are quiescent. They are soft in consistency, may range in size from a millimeter to several centimeters in diameter, and often have an overlying violaceous, pink, or blue hue (Fig. 11.52). They may be sessile or pedunculated. With pressure from a finger, dermal neurofibromas may be invaginated, a sign called *buttonholing*. "Pseudoatrophic macules" and "red-blue macules" are unusual variants of dermal neurofibromas that show replacement of dermal collagen with neural tissue and thick-walled blood vessels in the superficial dermis overlying the neurofibroma, respectively. By adulthood, dermal neurofibromas may number from a few to hundreds, with a progressive increase in size and number as the patient becomes older. Neurofibromas may occur anywhere on the body with no specific site of predilection. Not uncommonly, patients complain of itchiness at the site of a dermal neurofibroma, perhaps related to the presence of mast cells.

Plexiform neurofibromas (pNFs) also arise from SKP cells through loss of the normal neurofibromin allele, leading to loss of heterozygosity in the setting of NF1 and resultant uncontrolled growth.[540,541] pNFs may be superficial or deep and occur in 25% to 40% of children.[542,543] They often are oriented along the length of a nerve and involve several fascicles. They may be barely palpable, may be quite firm, or may become huge with a "bag of worms" consistency. Plexiform neurofibromas not uncommonly are present at birth and have a predilection to involve the extremities. Commonly, a large CAL spot, often with irregular borders, overlies the plexiform neurofibroma (Fig. 11.53); hypertrichosis maybe associated as well (Fig. 11.54). Underlying soft tissue and bone hypertrophy (Fig. 11.55) or bone erosion may be seen, especially with growth of the pNF. Biochemical factors and epigenetic change, rather than additional genetic mutations, are thought to underlie tumor growth. Plexiform neurofibromas may at times cause pain, muscle weakness, atrophy, or slight sensory loss. Given the hyperpigmentation and associated hypertrichosis, a plexiform neurofibroma may be confused with a congenital nevus, Becker nevus, or smooth muscle hamartoma. Orbital plexiform neurofibromas present with eyelid swelling and ptosis,[544] leading to amblyopia in 62% of affected children.[545] Isolated plexiform neurofibromas have been described in patients without NF1, although the possibility of mosaicism should be considered (Fig. 11.56).

Although a benign course for cutaneous neurofibromas is usual, plexiform neurofibromas can transform into malignant peripheral nerve sheath tumors (MPNSTs), which occur in 8% to 13% of affected individuals, peak in their occurrence during the second and third decades of life, and are the primary cause of early mortality. In contrast

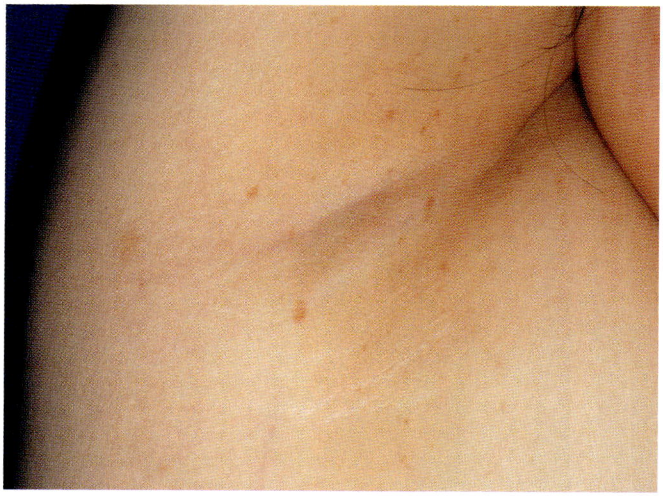

Fig. 11.51 Neurofibromatosis type 1 (NF1). Axillary freckling (Crowe sign) is present in 20% to 50% of individuals with NF1 and commonly appears between 3 and 5 years of age. Although the presence of both axillary freckling and multiple café-au-lait spots currently allows a definitive diagnosis of NF1, these features are also seen in Legius syndrome.

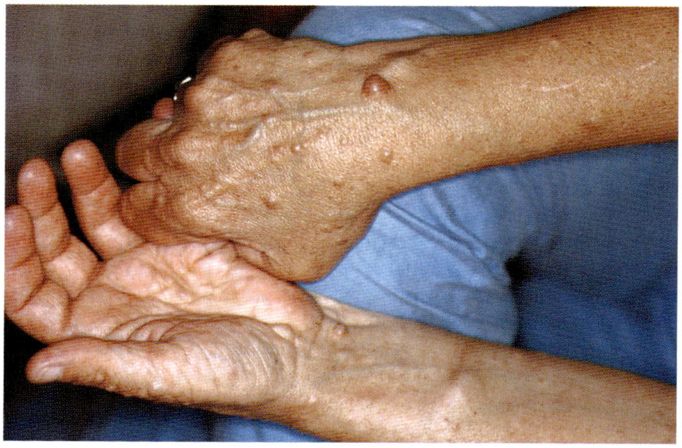

Fig. 11.52 Neurofibromatosis type 1. Dermal and subcutaneous neurofibromas are rarely found before adolescence. These tumors, which originate from Schwann cells, increase in number progressively thereafter.

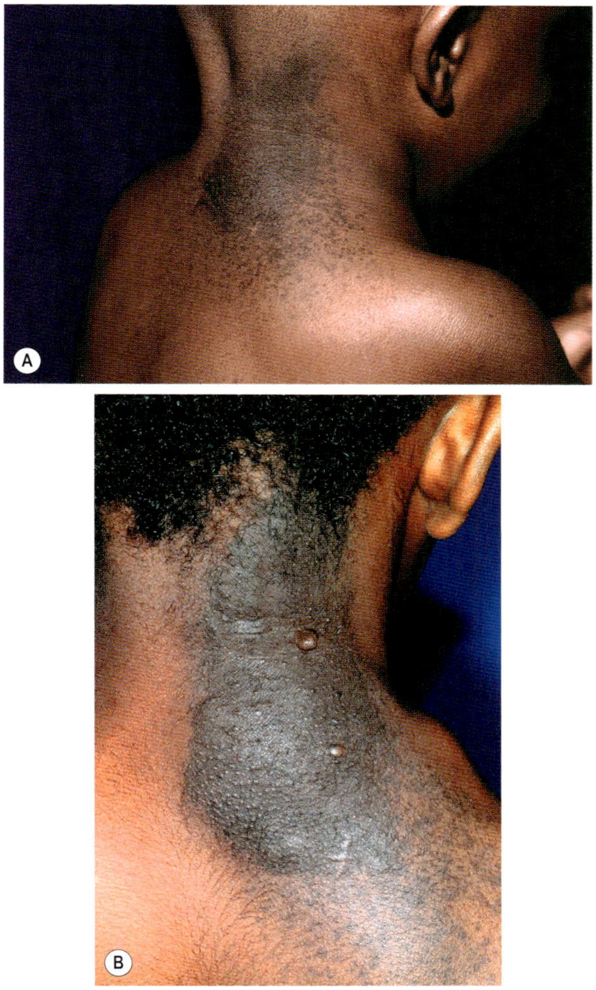

Fig. 11.53 Neurofibromatosis type 1. **(A)** Plexiform neurofibromas are commonly present at birth and can resemble giant café-au-lait spots, although borders are often more irregular. **(B)** With advancing age, plexiform neurofibromas may enlarge and become more elevated with a firm or "bag of worms" consistency. **(A)** A plexiform neurofibroma in a 3-year-old boy, and **(B)** the same plexiform neurofibroma when the child is 11 years of age. This boy passed away as a teenager from a malignant peripheral nerve sheath tumor at a different site.

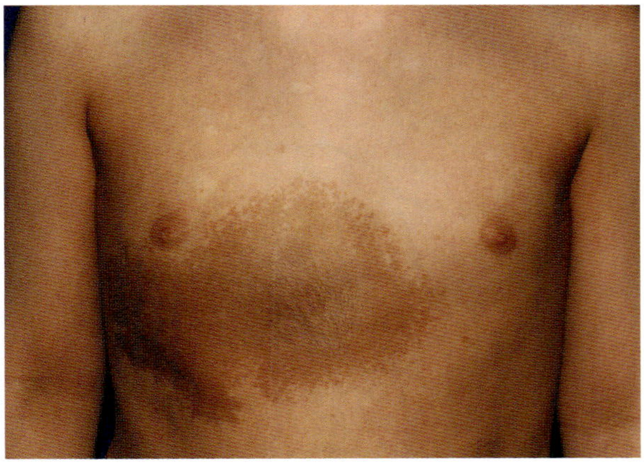

Fig. 11.54 Neurofibromatosis type 1. This plexiform neurofibroma is hypertrichotic and could be confused with a Becker nevus (except for the other features of NF1). Subtle nevus anemicus can also be seen on the upper chest.

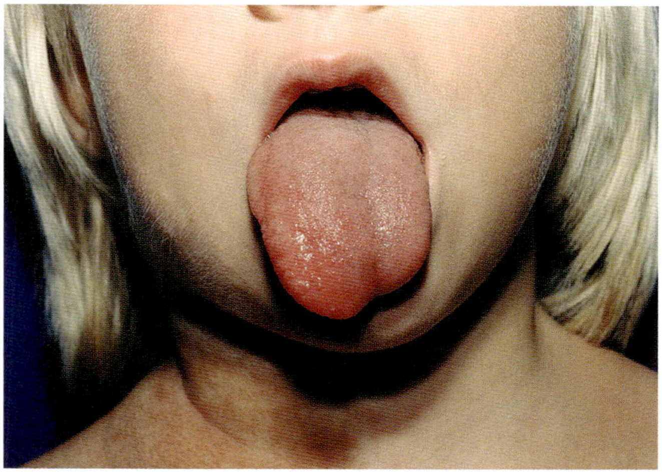

Fig. 11.55 Neurofibromatosis type 1. This plexiform neurofibroma of the tongue led to discomfort and difficulty with both speech and mastication. Note the cheek and neck involvement.

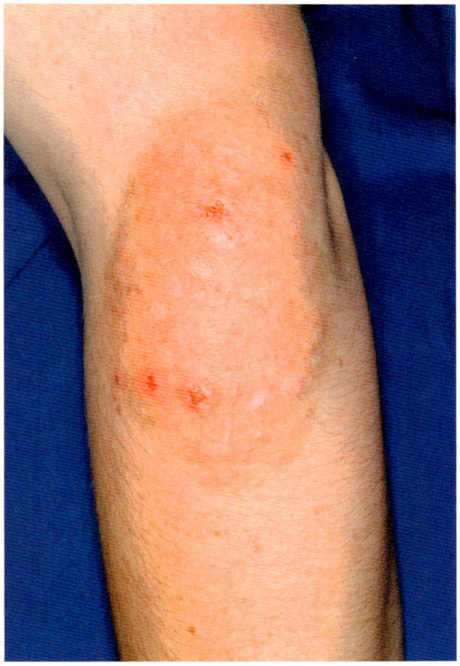

Fig. 11.56 Plexiform neurofibroma without neurofibromatosis type 1 (NF1). Occasionally, typical plexiform neurofibromas occur in individuals without evidence of NF1; mosaicism should be considered.

to cNFs and pNFs, atypical NFs and MPNSTs usually show deletions in *CDKN2A/CDKN2B*, which encode key cell cycle inhibitors.[546] MPNSTs often have a mutation in p53 as well.[547] Malignant degeneration may be heralded by rapid enlargement, pain, change in texture, and neurologic deficit. Positron emission tomography (PET)–CT imaging of MPNSTs can distinguish benign neurofibromas from MPNSTs. Prognosis is poor, with 5-year survival rates of 34% to 60%.

Two other skin changes in NF1 are juvenile xanthogranulomas (JXGs) and nevus anemicus.[548] JXGs (see Chapter 10) are yellow dome-shaped papules (Fig. 11.57) found overall in up to 37% of affected children with a mean age of onset of 24 months of age.[542,549,550] Most children have more than one JXG (mean 3), and 90% clear by a mean age of 47 months. Nevus anemicus (see Chapter 12) tends to be present at birth or infancy and has been described in 9% of children with

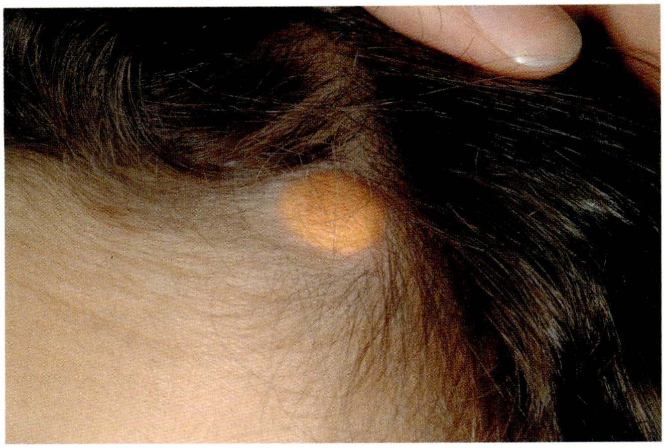

Fig. 11.57 Neurofibromatosis type 1. Juvenile xanthogranulomas (JXGs) are seen in up to 37% of affected children, are usually multiple (mean of three per patient), occur with a mean age of onset of 24 months of age, and tend to clear about 2 years later. Some have suggested that having both JXGs and café-au-lait spots should allow a definitive diagnosis of NF1.

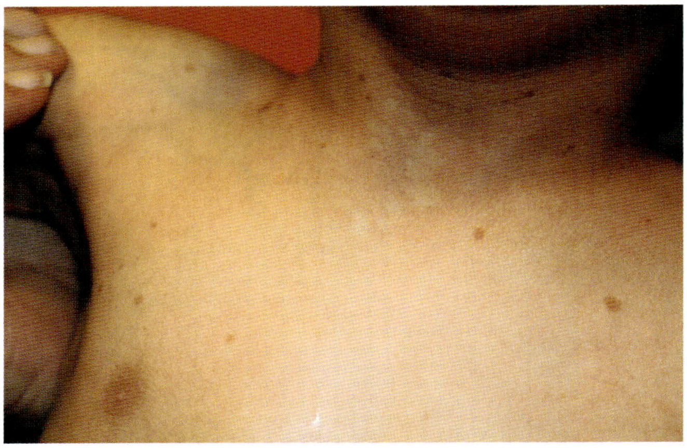

Fig. 11.58 Neurofibromatosis. Nevus anemicus is clearly seen on the neck. This is a more recently recognized association with neurofibromatosis.

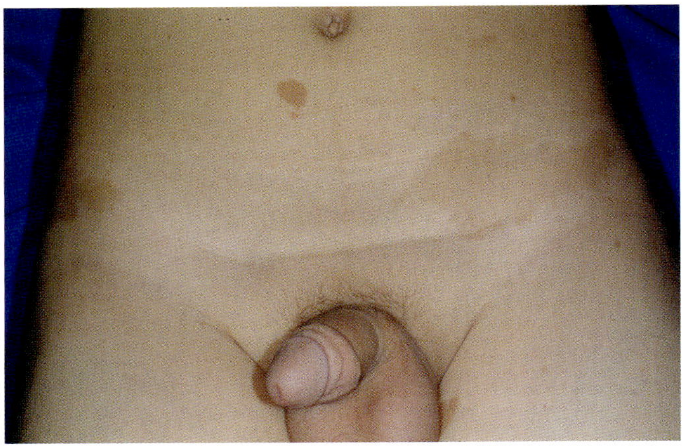

Fig. 11.59 Neurofibromatosis type 1. Precocious puberty in a 5-year-old boy with an optic chiasm/hypothalamic glioma.

NF[551] and 35% of those younger than 2 years of age (Fig. 11.58; see Fig. 11.54).[550] Nevus anemicus is a pale patch that becomes more easily visible when the skin is rubbed or warmed, which leads to vascular dilation in the surrounding skin. These skin signs may add to the suspicion of NF1 in an infant (nevus anemicus) or young child (JXG) with only CAL spots and may become new criteria for RASopathies.[552]

Systemic Manifestations of Neurofibromatosis. Other than the CAL spots, learning disability is the most common manifestation of NF1 in children.[553–555] Learning disability, which occurs in 30% to 70% of affected children, includes nonverbal and verbal disability as well as attention-deficit/hyperactivity disorder, which can lead to the poor development of social skills.[556] Diagnostic criteria for autism spectrum disorders have been found in 30% of children with NF1.[557] Another common sign is the occurrence of enhanced intensity of T2 signals in brain MRI examinations in the basal ganglia, brainstem, internal capsule, and cerebellum (unidentified bright objects; 43% to 93%).[558]

The ocular manifestations of NF1 include plexiform neurofibromas, Lisch nodules, optic gliomas, and choroidal nodules. Lisch nodules are asymptomatic yellowish-brown melanocytic hamartomas on the iris that cause no problem with vision. These Lisch nodules are found in more than 90% of affected adults but in only 43% of children younger than 12 years of age. They are best detected by slit-lamp examination, although dermoscopy may aid in diagnosis and larger ones may be seen without magnification as beige spots on a dark iris or darker spots on a light iris. Their presence virtually ensures the diagnosis of NF1, but their absence does not discount the diagnosis. Choroidal nodules are detectable in 71% to 100% of children with NF1 by near-infrared reflectance[559,560] and are not found in Legius syndrome,[561] suggesting that they may be a better criterion for diagnosis in young children.[562] Optic gliomas occur in approximately 15% of children with NF1 and are more indolent than optic gliomas in individuals without NF1. Precocious puberty has been described in up to 40% of patients with gliomas of the posterior chiasm and hypothalamic areas (Fig. 11.59).[563] Overall, only 33% of patients with optic gliomas develop symptoms or signs such as decreased visual acuity or visual-field defects, proptosis, strabismus, or optic-nerve pallor. A total of 35% of those with symptomatic optic gliomas eventually require treatment, specifically for their progressive loss of vision, gross disfigurement (e.g., from proptosis), or poor weight gain with diencephalic syndrome. Chemotherapy with carboplatin and vincristine is still the treatment of choice, despite modest outcome. Surgical resection is used for cosmetic palliation, and radiation therapy is avoided because of the risk of second malignancy treatment.[564–566] Bevacizumab, an anti-VEGF monoclonal antibody, has led to rapid improvement in some cases, and MEK inhibitors are considered salvage treatment.[566,567]

Progression in optic gliomas usually occurs by 6 to 7 years of age, suggesting that annual eye examinations can thereafter be spaced to every 2 years until adulthood. Although routine baseline MRIs are not necessary, imaging should be performed if abnormalities are found on ophthalmologic evaluation or in the face of signs of a problematic optic glioma.[565] Spontaneous regression of optic gliomas may occur.[568]

Brain tumors may lead to neurologic abnormalities.[569] Other than optic pathway gliomas, brainstem gliomas (pilocytic astrocytomas) are the most common intracranial neoplasms[570] but usually behave less aggressively than histologically identical tumors patients who do not have NF1. Because of the indolent nature of these tumors, conservative management with close follow-up monitoring is recommended. In one series of 13 children with meningiomas, 28% had NF1.[571] More severe developmental delay occurs in only 5% of patients and has been associated with total deletion of the neurofibromin gene[572]; these patients also have facial dysmorphism and large numbers of neurofibromas.

Skeletal manifestations are most commonly bone dysplasias, pectus deformity, and scoliosis. Even without osseous abnormalities, children and adolescents with NF1 have decreased bone mineral density.[573] Although not among the diagnostic criteria, spinal deformities, particularly scoliosis or kyphosis, may occur in at least 10% of patients, and pectus deformities occur in approximately 24% of patients.[574,575] The dystrophic form of scoliosis almost always develops before 10 years of age and then progresses, usually involving the lower cervical and upper thoracic spine, and is associated with dysplastic changes of the

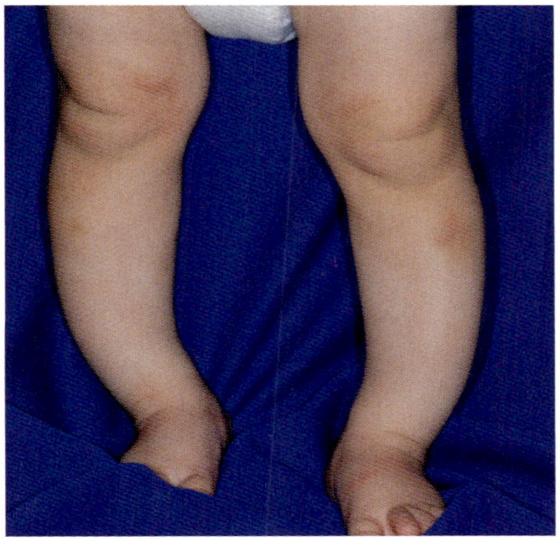

Fig. 11.60 Neurofibromatosis type 1. Bilateral tibial bowing without evidence of pseudoarthrosis in an affected infant.

vertebral bodies. Tibial dysplasia (congenital bowing), pathognomonic for NF1, presents as anteromedial bowing of the tibia (Fig. 11.60), usually during the first year of life, and has been described in about 1% to 4% of affected children. The cortex of the bone is thinned, and the medulla is sclerotic.[576] Fractures may occur at the site, leading to pseudoarthrosis. Sphenoid wing dysplasia occurs in 3% to 7% of children with NF1 and may manifest as pulsating exophthalmos. Nonossifying fibromas have also been described in association with multiple CAL spots (Jaffe–Campanacci syndrome); this group of patients has a high risk of recurrent fractures and significant resultant deformity and disability.[577]

Other features of NF1 that may be seen during childhood are short stature (10%; especially slowed growth acceleration during puberty),[578] frequent headaches (30% to 40%), macrocephaly (24%), and, rarely, hypertension (1%). Short stature most often occurs without evidence of neuroendocrine problems.[579,580] The macrocephaly is usually not associated with hydrocephalus, although aqueductal stenosis has rarely been reported. In children, hypertension usually relates to renal artery stenosis, a form of NF1 vasculopathy[581]; in adults with hypertension and NF1, pheochromocytoma should be suspected. Stenosis or occlusion of several other arteries may occur, leading to cerebral vascular accidents, aneurysms, and even sudden cardiac death.[582,583] Small telangiectatic vessels often form around the stenotic area of the cerebral arteries, leading to a "puff of smoke" (moyamoya) on cerebral angiography. Watson syndrome is an allelic variant of NF 1 with associated pulmonic stenosis, and NF1–Noonan syndrome combines the features of Noonan syndrome (ocular hypertelorism, low-set ears, downslanting palpebral fissures, webbed neck, and pulmonic stenosis) with NF1, usually with mutations in neurofibromin and not *PTPN11*, the gene usually associated with Noonan syndrome.

NF1 is associated with an 8% to 13% lifetime risk of developing malignancy. In addition to the development of MPNSTs, nonlymphocytic leukemias, rhabdomyosarcoma, and lymphoma are described with increased incidence in affected children. Although JXGs have been described in association with juvenile chronic myelogenous leukemia, few patients with NF1 and JXGs have leukemia.[584]

Therapy of Neurofibromatosis Type 1. Management for most children with NF1 is anticipatory guidance, genetic counseling, and surveillance for potential complications. If available, referral to a multidisciplinary clinic that specializes in seeing individuals with NF1 is optimal. Baseline screening tests, except for ophthalmologic examinations, are not recommended. Monitoring and early intervention for learning disabilities is important. Complete physical examinations should be performed at least twice yearly, including measurements of height, weight, head circumference, and blood pressure; careful palpation for tumors; and assessment for scoliosis or other bony deformities. Methylphenidate has been shown to be helpful for the attention-deficit issues in children with NF1.[585]

Dermal neurofibromas may be excised, but plexiform neurofibromas usually cannot be removed in their entirety.[586] Surgical debulking may be undertaken for tumors that are disfiguring, interfere with function, or are subject to irritation, trauma, or infection. MEK inhibition has been shown to decrease both neurofibroma and MPNST size and prolong survival in preclinical studies[587]; decreased tumor size was noted in all 11 children treated with selumetinib, an MEK1/2 inhibitor.[588] Larger clinical trials and anecdotal reports are showing promise.[589–591] Mast cells appear to play a critical role in the initiation and progression of plexiform neurofibromas, and imatinib has led to an at least 20% decrease in tumor size within 6 months in 26% of patients.[592,593] Treatment with oral sirolimus (mTOR inhibitor) improved pain associated with pediatric plexiform neurofibromas but caused no shrinkage in one study,[594] and everolimus only reduced the tumor volume in a small percentage of adults with disfiguring neurofibromas.[595]

Genetic counseling is another important aspect of treatment, because there is a 50% chance of transmitting NF with each pregnancy. Mutations can be found by multistep mutation detection in more than 95% of individuals with NF1.[518,596] Mosaicism with postzygotic mutation in neurofibromin, however, is not uncommon.[597,598] Affected patients may show mosaic-generalized NF1, which is indistinguishable clinically from germline mutations with generalized manifestations or mosaic-localized NF1. Even patients with more localized evidence of mosaic ("segmental") NF1 often have the requisite six or more CALs within the localized area of involvement[599] (Fig. 11.61). Mosaicism for *SPRED1* mutations has also been described and is difficult to distinguish clinically from mosaic NF1 when other features of NF1 are not present.[600] Although CAL spots are the most common manifestation of mosaic NF1 in children, other cutaneous manifestations (freckling, dermal and plexiform neurofibromas) or noncutaneous manifestations (pseudoarthrosis, sphenoid wing dysplasia, optic glioma, Lisch nodules) in the localized area may also occur.[601] Individuals with mosaic forms of NF1 who also have germline involvement (more common with mosaic-generalized NF1) may have offspring with full NF1, with an up to 50% probability with each pregnancy. A national support group, the National Neurofibromatosis Foundation (www.nfnetwork.org and www.ctf.org), offers patient information and support.

ERYTHEMA DYSCHROMICUM PERSTANS

Erythema dyschromicum perstans (ashy dermatosis) is an acquired chronic, progressive bluish to ash-gray hyperpigmentation that can affect individuals of both sexes from childhood through adulthood. Although more common in darker-skinned individuals, several light-skinned affected children have been described.[602,603] In one study of

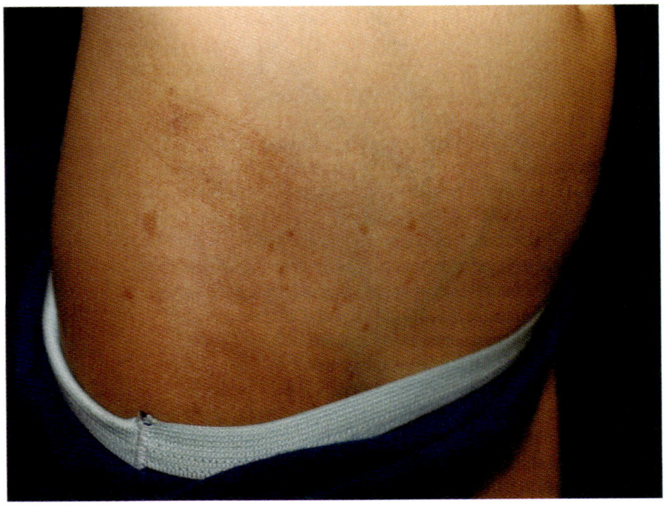

Fig. 11.61 Segmental neurofibromatosis. Note that there are more than six café-au-lait macules, even within the segmental area.

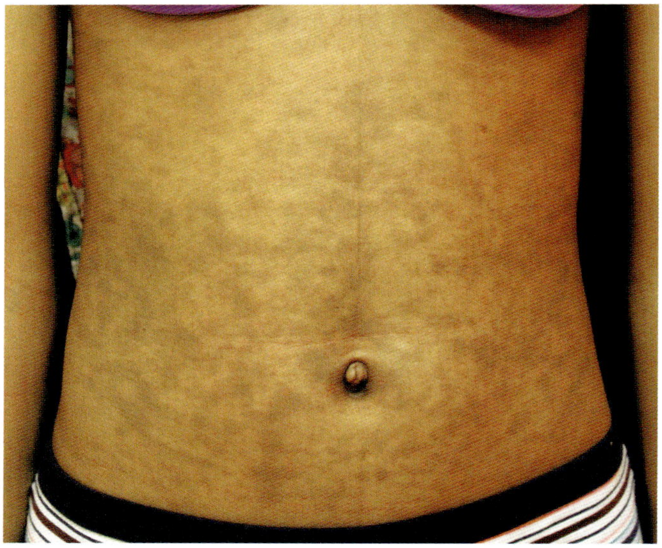

Fig. 11.62 Erythema dyschromicum perstans. Oval slate-gray macules, all oriented along the same axis, on the trunk of this otherwise healthy girl. In children with erythema dyschromicum perstans, the hyperpigmented macules often clear spontaneously after years.

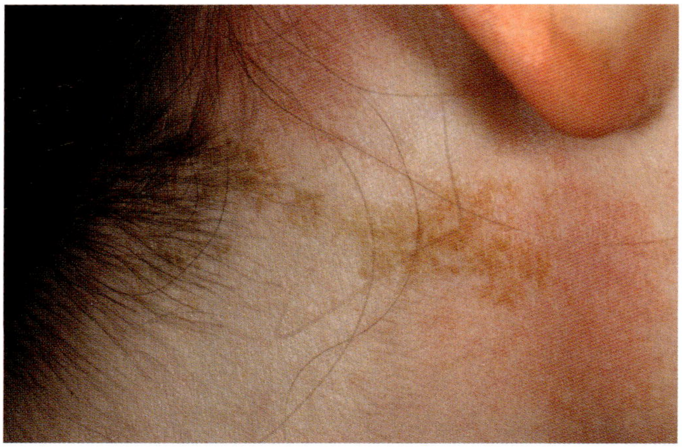

Fig. 11.63 Retention hyperkeratosis. Persistent focal patches of hyperpigmentation and mild skin thickening, especially on the neck and near joints, represent retained scale and can be removed easily by gently scrubbing with an alcohol pad. Parents often erroneously consider this a sign of inadequate cleansing.

68 cases, 7% were in the first decade and 15% in the second decade of life.[604] The cause of erythema dyschromicum perstans remains unknown. Lesions usually begin as slate-gray macules (Fig. 11.62) but occasionally show a transient, slightly raised erythematous border. Generally seen on the trunk (69% of cases), upper limbs (40%), neck (38%), and face (32%), lesions may also occur on other areas, rarely occur on the mucosae,[605] and are not described on the scalp, palms, or soles. Lesions vary from a few millimeters to many centimeters in diameter and often cover extensive areas. Lesions are usually distinct but can be confluent. Multiple linear lesions of erythema dyschromicum perstans have been described that follow the lines of Blaschko,[606] and lesions may be unilateral.[607]

This disorder must be differentiated from the postinflammatory hyperpigmented lesions of tinea versicolor, pityriasis rosea, and fixed-drug eruption, which usually show brown rather than grayish pigmentation. Idiopathic eruptive macular pigmentation is differentiated by the development of brown (rather than grayish) nonconfluent macules of the trunk, neck, and proximal extremities; the absence of preceding inflammation; the lack of exposure to a medication; and basal cell hyperpigmentation without damage to the keratinocytes and without dermal mast cells in biopsy sections. Lichen planus pigmentosus tends to occur primarily on the face and has a fluctuating course. Histologic features of erythema dyschromicum perstans depend on the stage of the lesion. Older lesions show pigment incontinence, but early lesions may show hydropic degeneration of epidermal cells and a lichenoid infiltrate of lymphocytes.

The dermatosis is asymptomatic but chronic. There are frequent exacerbations with extension into previously uninvolved areas. Therapy is generally unsuccessful, although there are reports of improvement with topical tacrolimus (with and without laser), isotretinoin, dapsone, clofazimine, nbUVB, laser, and isotretinoin. Most cases in children clear spontaneously within a few years.[602,608]

POSTINFLAMMATORY HYPERPIGMENTATION

Postinflammatory hyperpigmentation is one of the most common causes of hyperpigmentation and is characterized by an increase in melanin formation after cutaneous inflammation.[609–613] Ordinary postinflammatory hyperpigmentation is of relatively short duration and tends to persist for several months after the original cause has subsided. Examples include the pigmentation after physical trauma, friction, primary irritants, eczematous eruptions, lichen simplex chronicus, acne vulgaris, and dermatoses such as pityriasis rosea, psoriasis, fixed drug eruptions, photodermatitis, and pyoderma. Individuals with dark complexions and those who tan easily after UV light exposure show the greatest degree and longest persistence of this form of postinflammatory hyperpigmentation. Pigmentation can be epidermal or dermal, and the former fades more quickly. Epidermal pigmentation tends to be light to dark brown but dermal pigmentation gray to black. Residual pigmentation after improvement in lesions of lupus erythematosus, lichen planus, and lichenoid drug eruptions tends to be dermal because these disorders involve disruption of the basal layer and dermal–epidermal junction, with melanin incontinence, uptake into dermal melanophages, and more pronounced and persistent discoloration (see Chapter 4, Figs. 4.43 and 4.51).

Topical antiinflammatory medications are appropriate if inflammation is ongoing.[614,615] If areas of postinflammatory hyperpigmentation can be protected from further UV light exposure, fading gradually occurs over a period of months to years. Most patients do not respond to topical agents or resurfacing procedures as well as patients with melasma (see later).[616,617] However, those with epidermal pigmentation tend to respond better to topical retinoid, hydroquinone, azelaic acid, and/or peeling agents (e.g., glycolic acid or salicylic acid). In general, combination therapy is more effective than monotherapy. Although in general the treatment of postinflammatory hyperpigmentation (especially dermal) is difficult, the Q-switched neodymium:yttrium-aluminum-garnet (Nd:YAG) and erbium-doped lasers have shown the most promising results.

Retention Hyperkeratosis

Because melanin is transferred to epidermal cells, thickened epidermis often appears hyperpigmented. Focal patches of hyperpigmentation and mild skin thickening are not uncommon at fold areas (such as the ankle) and on the neck and represent retention hyperkeratosis (sometimes called *scurf*) (Fig. 11.63). These persistent patches can be removed easily by gently scrubbing with an alcohol pad.

MELASMA

Melasma is a term applied to a patchy dark-brown to black hyperpigmentation located primarily on the cheeks and forehead and occasionally the temples, upper lip, and neck.[610,618] Seen in up to 20% of women, including adolescents, this disorder has been termed the *mask of pregnancy*. However, typical melasma also can occur in males[619,620] (overall 10%) and in females who are neither pregnant nor taking oral contraceptives. Increasing evidence suggests a role for UV-induced photoaging in the disorder. Phenytoin (Dilantin) has also been implicated. Nevertheless, melasma associated with pregnancy often clears within a few months after delivery, only to recur with subsequent pregnancies. Oral contraceptive–induced melasma may persist for up to 5 years after discontinuation of the medication.

Because sun exposure tends to trigger and intensify this hyperpigmentation, the disorder characteristically becomes more prominent in the summer months.[621] Both UVA and visible light have been implicated, emphasizing the need for physical sunscreen use and use of sun-protective clothing. In addition, treatment of melasma consists of discontinuation of potentially responsible medications and the use of topical medications.[616,617] The gold standard of treatment is hydroquinones (inhibit tyrosinase), compounds with tretinoin (0.05% to 0.1%), and mild topical steroids. Concurrent sun protection is critical to prevent further hyperpigmentation in patients using hydroquinones. Because continuous use of hydroquinone bleaching creams or lotions can result in excessive pigmentary loss or ochronosis-like hyperpigmentation, once the desired degree of depigmentation is achieved, hydroquinone therapy should be discontinued. The combination of pulsed dye laser with this trio of topical agents may give a superior result. Twice-daily application of azelaic acid 15% to 20% is less efficacious but causes less irritation.[622] Other topical agents that have been used are tranexamic acid (also used orally),[623] kojic acid, plant extracts (such as licorice or orchid extracts, soy, arbutin, and silymarin), ascorbic acid, N-acetylglucosamine, and niacinamide.[617] Chemical peels (e.g., with tretinoin or trichloroacetic acid) and laser therapy, especially with Q-switched Nd:YAG, may also be helpful.[624,625] These preparations often require 3 to 4 months before a therapeutic effect is achieved.

METABOLIC CAUSES OF HYPERPIGMENTATION

Cutaneous changes often are helpful in the diagnosis of several endocrine disorders, including Addison disease (see Figs. 23.6 and 23.7), hyperthyroidism (see Fig. 23.2), hypothyroidism, acromegaly, and Cushing syndrome (see Chapter 23). More than two-thirds of patients with chronic hepatic disease (cirrhosis or prolonged bile-duct obstruction) also have some degree of cutaneous hyperpigmentation. Of these, diffuse darkening of the skin is perhaps the most common. Blotchy areas of brown hyperpigmentation occasionally may be seen, and accentuation of normal freckling and areolar hyperpigmentation may appear. Progressive, diffuse blotchy hyperpigmentation in addition to hair lightening has been described with cobalamin (vitamin B_{12}) deficiency from homozygous mutations in *ABCD4*, which encodes a transporter involved in processing cobalamin.[626] Polycystic kidney disease and other chronic renal disease may be accompanied by diffuse yellowish-brown skin discoloration, especially on the face and hands. Although urinary chromogens and carotenemia may be present, melanin pigmentation also has been implicated.

Hemochromatosis

Hemochromatosis is a familial iron storage disorder characterized by cutaneous hyperpigmentation that usually manifests between 40 and 60 years of age. Type 2 or the juvenile form of hemochromatosis typically presents during childhood, although some have a late onset beyond 30 years of age.[627] An autosomal recessive disorder, the juvenile form is usually caused by mutations in *HJV*, encoding hemojuvelin (HFE2A), and occasionally in *HAMP*, encoding hepcidin (HFE2B).[628,629] Hemojuvelin and hepcidin are involved in iron metabolism. The most common type overall results from mutations in *HFE*, which, although not symptomatic during childhood, leads to increases in the mean concentration of iron, ferritin levels, and transferrin saturation in children carrying mutant alleles (40% of children in one study).[630]

Hyperpigmentation is seen in almost every patient with hemochromatosis and, in conjunction with abdominal pain, is often the presenting sign. The increased pigmentation is produced by melanin and not by the deposition of iron in the skin. It appears initially in the exposed areas before it becomes diffuse and is most intense in the skin of the face, arms, body folds, and genitalia. Mucous membranes (the gums, palate, and buccal mucosa) and sometimes the conjunctivae are involved in 15% to 20% of affected persons. The skin is soft, dry, thin, shiny, and of fine texture. Spider angiomas are present in 60% to 80% of affected individuals, and palmar erythema is common. Facial, axillary, thoracic, and pubic hairs are scant or absent. Cardiomyopathy, evidence of hypogonadism, and reduced glucose tolerance are seen by young adulthood. The hepatic cirrhosis characteristic of adult-onset hemochromatosis, however, is less clinically relevant in type 2 hemochromatosis, and icterus is unusual.[631]

Secondary hemochromatosis (hemosiderosis) with associated hyperpigmentation may be seen in patients with anemia who receive numerous blood transfusions. In such instances, visceral fibrosis is unusual, diabetes mellitus is uncommon, and hypogonadism is not present.

The diagnosis of metabolic hemochromatosis is suggested by the presence of cutaneous hyperpigmentation in patients with a history of diabetes and sometimes hepatic cirrhosis. Elevated levels of serum ferritin and transferrin saturation confirm the diagnosis.[632] The demonstration of parenchymal iron distribution by skin, liver, and gastric biopsies and the presence of hemosiderin in urinary sediment are helpful. Skin biopsy specimens show increased melanin in the basal layer and deposition of iron in the upper cutis (especially in macrophages, endothelial cells of capillaries, and the propria of eccrine glands).

The clinical course of untreated hemochromatosis is characterized by tissue destruction, malfunction of involved organs, and eventual death. Symptomatic treatment of the diabetes, liver dysfunction, and cardiac symptoms and quarterly phlebotomies, when initiated early, commonly result in clinical and pathologic improvement. Dietary restriction of iron is impractical, and chelating agents to date have been of little value.

Ochronosis

Alkaptonuria (ochronosis) is an inborn error of tyrosine metabolism in which homogentisic acid, an intermediate product in the metabolism of phenylalanine and tyrosine, accumulates in the tissues, and is excreted in the urine because of a lack of homogentisic acid oxidase. This autosomal recessive disorder usually first becomes manifest in the third decade with scleral blue-black pigmentation (Osler sign). Affected children rarely show Osler sign, and the characteristic dark urine is usually not noted because the color change only occurs with sitting for 1 to 2 h, especially in an alkaline environment.[633,634] Dark urine in the discarded diaper may be the first sign in infants. Skin pigmentation first becomes visible around the fourth decade of life, especially on ear cartilage, eyelids and other facial areas, intertriginous areas, and over tendons. Nails may be stained brown. Around this time, the ochronotic arthropathy from pigment deposition also starts to develop and involves the weight-bearing joints (spine, knees) most commonly. The mean age of joint replacement is 55 years, of development of renal stones 64 years, of cardiac valve involvement 54 years, and of coronary artery calcification 59 years. The diagnosis can be confirmed by alkalinizing the urine (e.g., with sodium hydroxide), which leads to the typical black color; the homogentisic acid is detected by enzymatic spectrophotometry or gas liquid chromatography. Treatment with ascorbic acid twice daily may reduce the connective tissue damage, and affected children have also been placed on a low-protein diet. Nitisinone therapy may decrease homogentisic acid production.[635] Endogenous ochronosis has been improved by erbium-doped YAG laser resurfacing and deep focal point treatment to remove areas of residual deep pigment.[636]

Exogenous ochronosis resembles its endogenous counterpart clinically and histologically but is not hereditary and has no internal manifestations.[637] The condition usually occurs in Black patients from exposure to hydroquinones and is characterized by asymptomatic hyperpigmentation of the face, neck, back, and extensor surfaces of the extremities. Less commonly, exogenous ochronosis has been described after exposure to antimalarials or products containing resorcinol, phenol, mercury, or picric acid.[638]

HYPERPIGMENTATION CAUSED BY HEAVY METALS

The systemic absorption of chemicals can also cause discoloration of the skin. Although the incidence of hyperpigmentation owing to exogenous heavy metals has decreased in recent years, limited exposure to such preparations still occurs, and metallic hyperpigmentation may still be seen in children as well as adults.

Argyria occurs after long-term ingestion or excessive application of silver preparations and presents as localized or widespread bluish-gray or slate-colored discoloration of the skin produced by the deposition of silver within the dermis. The condition is more pronounced on exposed parts of the body—namely the face, forearms, and hands—but may also occur in the sclerae, oral mucous membranes, and lunulae of the nails. Argyria has been increasingly described because of the promotion of colloidal silver–based products for their immunostimulant, antimicrobial, and antiinflammatory properties. The antimicrobial properties are proportional to the bioactive silver ion released and its availability to interact with bacterial or fungal cell membranes.[639] These "health food" products deliver primarily inactive metallic silver, not the antimicrobial ionized form. Colloidal silver and silver sulfadiazine cream, for example, have high levels of silver release with relatively low levels of ionized silver,[640] and silver deposition has been seen at the sites of burns and epidermolysis bullosa wounds.[641,642]

Ionized silver dressings are used for wound care[639] and, although they often cause temporary superficial silver staining of the stratum corneum, are thought only to cause low local silver levels. A study in adults with chronic wounds, however, showed increased levels after just 1 month of treatment in half the subjects.[643] An adolescent girl with osteosarcoma who had limb salvage and placement of a silver-coated megaprosthesis developed intense blue-gray pigmentation along the surgical incision line 1 year after surgery from slow release of the silver.[644]

Cases with more extensive hyperpigmentation have been described after chronic ingestion of silver-containing water[645] or colloidal silver[646] or widespread topical application of silver sulfadiazine[641,647] or colloidal silver. Localized staining can be seen periorbitally and on the eyes from ophthalmic preparations containing silver. Small, localized blue macules that resemble blue nevi may be detectable at sites of acupuncture,[648–650] exposure to silver earrings,[651,652] or nasal piercing.[653]

The diagnosis of argyria is based on clinical examination and history of exposure and may be confirmed by cutaneous biopsy of affected areas, which shows fine, small round refractive silver granules throughout the dermis, especially around eccrine glands. *In vivo* reflectance confocal microscopy shows a hyperrefractile network with a periadnexal pattern.[654] Increased amounts of melanin may be seen in the basal layer of the epidermis, as well as within macrophages in the upper dermis. Treatment of argyria depends on recognition of the disorder, discontinuation of the use of the silver-containing preparation, and avoidance of sunlight exposure. The dermal hyperpigmentation is usually irreversible, although picosecond alexandrite laser may improve some cases of local deposition.[653,655]

Chrysiasis (gold-induced hyperpigmentation) is a rare cutaneous disorder induced by the administration of gold salts followed by exposure to UV light[656,657] or Q-switched laser.[658–660] The pigmentation is bluish gray or purplish and is similar to that seen in argyria except that the hyperpigmentation is more prominent around the eyes, is limited to areas of light exposure, and does not affect the sclerae and oral mucous membranes. Other cutaneous manifestations are seen in up to 20% of individuals on gold therapy, which is most commonly administered for rheumatoid arthritis. These include morbilliform, eczematous, urticarial, bullous, purpuric, lichen planus–like, and pityriasis rosea–like eruptions. The histopathologic features of gold-induced hyperpigmentation consist of small, black, round or oval, irregularly shaped gold particles located in a perivascular distribution and in dermal histiocytes.

Chronic exposure to mercury systemically may result in acrodynia (pink disease), a disorder of infants and young children characterized by leg cramps; headaches; hypertension; excessive perspiration; itching; swelling; redness and peeling of the hands, feet, and nose (and sometimes a papulovesicular eruption); weakness of the pectoral and pelvic girdles; and nerve dysfunction in the lower extremities.[661] However, exposure to topically applied mercury may lead to slate-gray pigmentation in areas of topical application. The discoloration is exaggerated in the areas of skin folds and is permanent.[662]

DRUG-INDUCED HYPERPIGMENTATION

Hyperpigmentation may be induced by chronic exposure to medication and tends to be worsened by sun exposure. The diagnosis of a drug eruption is based almost entirely on history and physical examination. The main drugs implicated in causing skin pigmentation are nonsteroidal antiinflammatory drugs, minocycline, antimalarials,[663] amiodarone, diltiazem,[664] cytotoxic drugs, imatinib,[665] heavy metals (see Hyperpigmentation Caused by Heavy Metals section), clofazimine, and psychotropic drugs (imipramine,[666,667] amitriptyline, and chlorpromazine). Clinical features are variable according to the triggering molecule and have a large range of patterns and shades. Bluish-gray discoloration is most common and especially prominent at sites of exposure to UV light. The condition is most commonly seen in the pediatric population in adolescents who have been taking minocycline for acne, with the blue discoloration usually notable at sites of acne scarring and on the oral mucosae and shins (Fig. 11.64).[668] Three subgroups have been described based on clinical appearance and histopathologic correlates: type I (blue-gray pigmentation in scars), type II (blue-gray pigmentation in previously normal skin, especially of the shins), and type III (brown discoloration at sun-exposed sites).[669] Biopsy specimens tend to show pigmentation within dermal macrophages, often localized to vessels and adnexal structures.

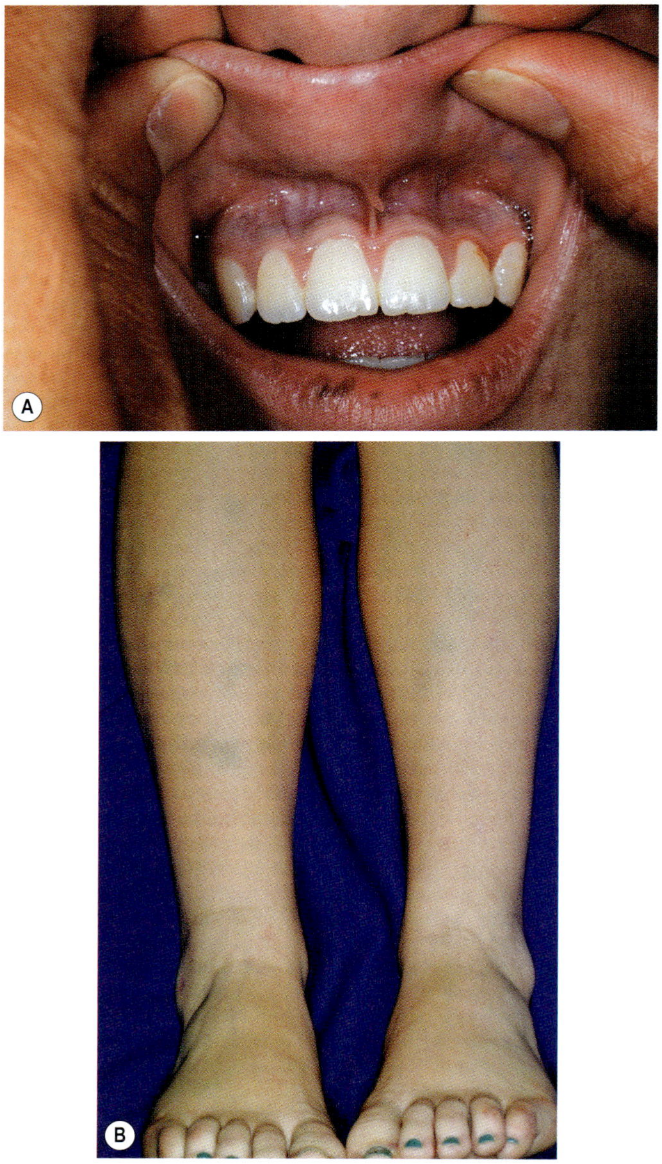

Fig. 11.64 Minocycline-induced hyperpigmentation. Bluish-gray discoloration on the oral mucosae **(A)** and shin **(B)** of adolescents administered minocycline for acne. This girl had blue discoloration of the gingivae, hard palate, and lips.

Treatment involves interruption of therapy and sun avoidance, although laser, particularly the alexandrite 755 nm laser, may be useful.[670,671] These measures are often followed by fading of lesions, but pigmentation may persist for a long time or even be permanent.[672]

The plaques of fixed drug eruptions are circumscribed, usually round or oval, often edematous and sometimes bullous, usually pruritic, and reddish-purple. Drug-induced hyperpigmentation tends to recur in the same location after the readministration of certain drugs, particularly sulfonamides, tetracyclines, acetaminophen, phenolphthalein, barbiturate derivatives, and antineoplastic agents such as cyclophosphamide. Histopathologic examination of lesions of the hyperpigmented phase of fixed drug eruptions reveals an increase in the amount of melanin in the basal layer of the epidermis and within macrophages of the upper dermis and is helpful in confirming the diagnosis.

Carotenemia

Carotenemia (sometimes called *carotenoderma*) is a yellowish-orange discoloration of skin caused by the ingestion of excessive quantities of carotene-containing foods, particularly carrots, squash, pumpkin, yellow turnips, sweet potatoes, peaches, apricots, papayas, mangos, egg yolk, and even green beans.[673–675] The condition is seen primarily in infants and occasionally in older children and adults.[676] The color is most prominent on the palms and soles; in the nasolabial grooves; on the forehead, chin, upper eyelids, postauricular areas, and anterior axillary folds; and over areas of pressure such as the elbows, knees, knuckles, and ankles (see Chapter 23, Fig. 23.4). Lack of involvement of the sclerae and mucous membranes coupled with the absence of pruritus and lack of color change in the urine or stool helps rule out the presence of hepatic or biliary jaundice. Lycopene, a red-colored carotenoid pigment found in fruits and vegetables, especially ripened tomatoes, beets, chili beans, and various fruits and berries, may cause a reddish-yellow discoloration of the skin (lycopenemia).

Carotenemia is a benign disorder in infants, and no intervention is required. Rarely carotenemia may be a sign of systemic disease, especially hypothyroidism, weight-loss diets or anorexia, or diabetes. The diagnosis of carotenemia is confirmed by the presence of high carotene levels in the presence of normal serum bilirubin. If the coloration is problematic, reduction of dietary intake of carotene-containing foods to normal levels or correction of the underlying disorder usually results in gradual improvement within 4 to 6 weeks. Rarely children will show a genetic defect in the metabolism of carotenoids that is more recalcitrant to dietary intervention.[677,678]

DERMAL MELANOCYTOSES

Congenital Dermal Melanocytosis (Formerly Called *Mongolian Spots*)

Congenital dermal melanocytosis is characterized by flat, deep brown to slate gray or blue-black, often poorly circumscribed, large macular lesions generally located over the lumbosacral areas, buttocks (Fig. 11.65), and occasionally the lower limbs, back, flanks, and shoulders of normal infants. These patches are seen in 75% to 90% of individuals of African descent and Native-American babies, 62% to 86% of Asians,[679–682] 70% of the Hispanic population, and 10% of White infants. The dermal melanocytosis is present at birth, tends to fade during the first 2 to 3 years of life, and only occasionally persists into adulthood. Extrasacral location, multiple patches, large size (>10 cm in diameter), and darker color are associated with persistence beyond 1 year.

The lesions of congenital dermal melanocytosis may be single (50% of babies) or multiple and vary from a few millimeters to 10 cm or more in diameter. They represent collections of spindle-shaped melanocytes located deep in the dermis, probably as the result of arrest during their embryonal migration from the neural crest to the epidermis. The slate-blue to blue-black color depends on the Tyndall effect (a phenomenon in which light passing through a turbid medium such as the skin is scattered as it strikes particles of melanin). Long-wavelength light rays (red, orange, and yellow) tend to be less scattered and therefore continue to pass downward into the lower levels of the skin; colors of shorter wavelengths (blue, indigo, and violet) are scattered to the side and backward to the skin surface, thus creating the blue-black

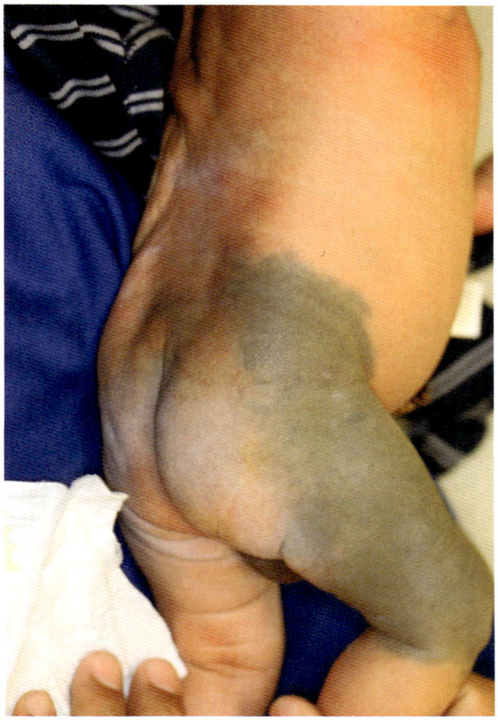

Fig. 11.65 Congenital dermal melanocytosis. Large blue-gray patches over the lumbosacral area, buttocks, and thigh of a Black baby. These spots often fade or clear within the first few years of life.

or slate-gray discoloration. A halo is typically seen around a café-au-lait macule superimposed on an area of dermal melanocytosis, as can be seen with NF1; the molecular mechanism for this phenomenon is unknown.[683]

In some children, new patches of dermal melanocytosis appear after birth and should not be confused with bruises. Their persistence, coloration, shapes, and lack of tenderness should be discriminating.[684] However, large and numerous spots may be seen in lysosomal storage disorders, among them GM1 gangliosidosis type 1, Hunter syndrome, and Hurler syndrome.[685–689] In these children, the spots often fade but not until at least the second decade of life.[686,] Because congenital dermal melanocytosis is benign and usually clears spontaneously, therapy is unnecessary.

Nevus of Ota and Nevus of Ito

The nevus of Ota (nevus fuscoceruleus ophthalmomaxillaris) represents a usually unilateral, irregularly patchy, blue to bluish-gray to brown discoloration of the skin of the face supplied by the first and second divisions of the trigeminal nerve.[690,691] It typically involves the periorbital region, temple, forehead, malar area, and nose (Fig. 11.66). About two-thirds of patients with this disorder have a patchy bluish discoloration of the sclera of the ipsilateral eye (see Fig. 11.66) and occasionally the conjunctiva, cornea, and retina. Palatal involvement has been described in up to 18% of affected individuals.[692] In about 5% of cases, the nevus of Ota is bilateral rather than unilateral, and in rare instances, the lips, pharynx, and nasal mucosa are similarly affected.

Although most commonly seen in Asians (0.02% to 0.8%),[693] nevus of Ota is not uncommonly seen in persons of African descent. Unlike congenital dermal melanocytosis, which tends to disappear with time, the cutaneous coloration of nevus of Ota generally persists and often shows a speckled rather than a uniform discoloration. In more than 50% of cases,[693] the lesions are congenital; the remainder usually appear during the second decade of life. Scleral melanocytosis alone is a much more common finding, which can progress and then recede with advancing age. In a study of Chinese children, only

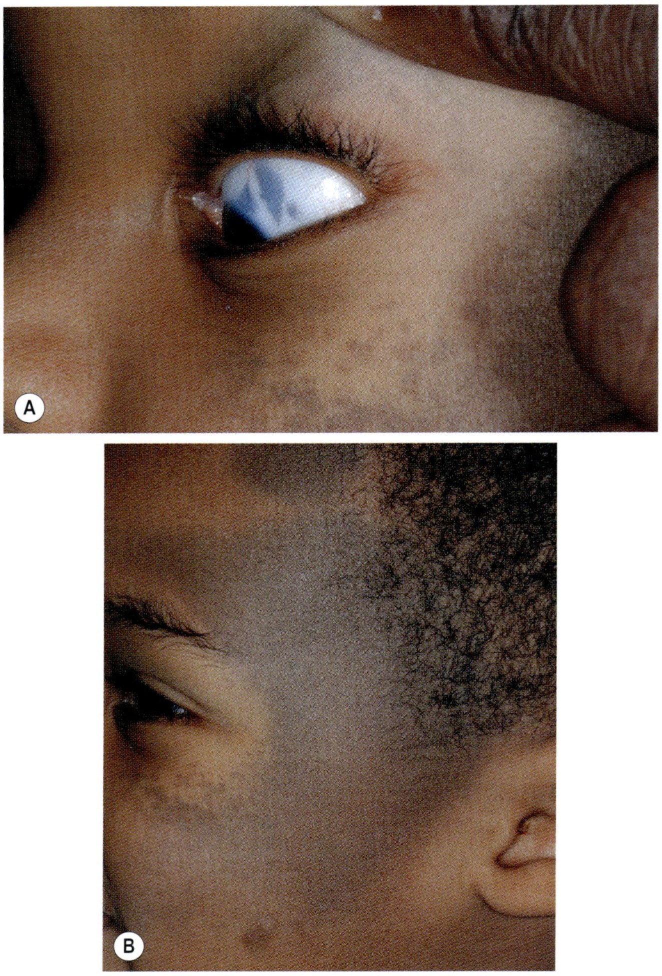

Fig. 11.66 Nevus of Ota. Unilateral, irregularly patchy, brownish-gray discoloration of the sclera (A) and periorbital region (B).

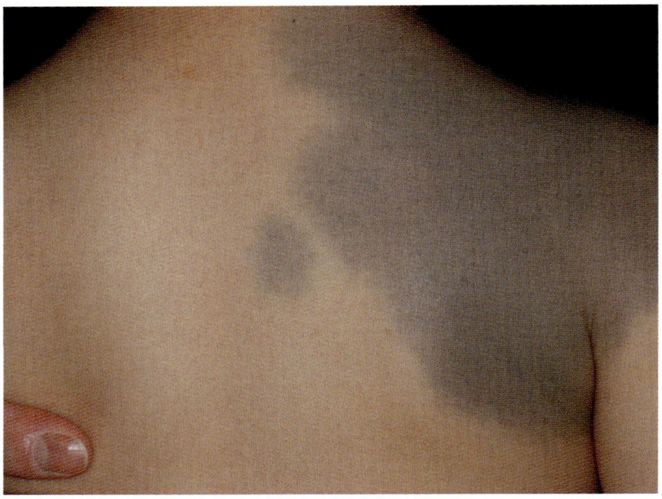

Fig. 11.67 Nevus of Ito. Blue patch on the shoulder.

4% to 5% were found to have scleral melanocytosis during the first year of life, but that number increased to 45% by 6 years of age with 78% of cases bilateral[694]; only 12% of the children continued to show evidence of scleral melanocytosis by 18 years of age.

The nevus of Ito (nevus fuscoceruleus acromiodeltoideus) has the same features as the nevus of Ota except that the pigmentary changes tend to involve the shoulder (Fig. 11.67), supraclavicular areas, sides of the neck, and upper arm, scapulae, and deltoid regions. It may occur alone or may be seen in conjunction with the nevus of Ota.

As in congenital dermal melanocytosis, biopsy sections of the nevus of Ota and nevus of Ito show elongated dendritic melanocytes scattered among the collagen bundles. The melanocytosis, however, often appears higher in the dermis than those seen in ordinary Mongolian spots.

Although these lesions do not disappear spontaneously, changes in color may occur. Darkening of lesions has been noted during and after puberty. These disorders are generally benign. However, glaucoma has been described in 10%,[695] and melanoma, most commonly of the eye (choroid, orbit, iris, ciliary body, and/or optic nerve) but also of the skin, brain, and meninges, has rarely been reported.[695–699] Long-term dermatologic and ophthalmologic follow-up monitoring is needed. In one patient, gene profiling revealed *GNAQ* mutations in both the nevus and the melanoma, with evidence of *BAP1* and *TP53* (p53) mutations developing in regions with melanoma.[700]

Laser therapy may improve the appearance of nevus of Ota, especially the Q-switched alexandrite laser and fractionated Nd:YAG.[701–703] Multiple sessions are required, but resultant scarring is rare and recurrences have only been reported after complete clearance in 0.6% to 1.2%. One complication in individuals with darker skin types is postinflammatory hypopigmentation; vigorous sun protection is imperative, and pretreatment with hydroquinone is sometimes used. Involvement on the zygomatic arch or frontal forehead regions responds better than periorbital pigmentation.[704–706] Cosmetic cover-up may also be used.

Dermal Melanocytosis with Vascular or Pigmented Lesions

Congenital dermal melanocytosis, nevus of Ota, and nevus of Ito can be seen with vascular malformations (most often nevus flammeus [including with Sturge–Weber] or cutis marmorata telangiectatica congenita as *phakomatosis pigmentovascularis* or *phakomatosis cesioflammea* and *phakomatosis cesiomarmorata*, respectively; see Chapter 12).[707–711] Mosaic activating mutations in GNA11 and GNAQ in both vascular and melanocytic cells are responsible for phakomatosis pigmentovascularis.[712]

BLUE NEVI

Blue nevi are a heterogeneous group of congenital and more often acquired melanocytic tumors.[713] Most often seen are common blue nevi and cellular blue nevi, although there may be histologic overlap between these types.[714] The nevi appear blue-gray clinically because of the deep (dermal) location of the melanin pigment and the Tyndall effect (selective absorption of longer wavelength components of light by melanin with reflection of the shorter blue components). Blue nevi are thought to result from the arrested embryonal migration of melanocytes bound for the dermal–epidermal junction. It is thus possible that the blue nevi, congenital dermal melanocytosis, and the nevi of Ota and Ito are closely related and possibly represent different stages of the same physiologic process.

The common blue nevus (also called the *classic* or *dendritic blue nevus*) presents as a small, round or oval, dark blue or bluish-black, smooth-surfaced, sharply circumscribed, slightly elevated dome-shaped papule, nodule, or plaque (Fig. 11.68). Most common blue nevi range from 2 or 3 mm to 10 mm (<1 cm) in diameter. Although usually single, they may be multiple at different sites or agminated. Lesions may be present at birth but may appear at any age. Although common blue nevi may occur on any part of the body, areas of predilection include the buttocks, dorsal aspect of the hands and feet, scalp, and the extensor surfaces of the forearms. They also may occur on the face, bulbar conjunctiva, mucous membranes, and the hard and soft palates. Agminated blue nevi has been described in association with underlying soft tissue hypertrophy and associated hypertrichosis.[715]

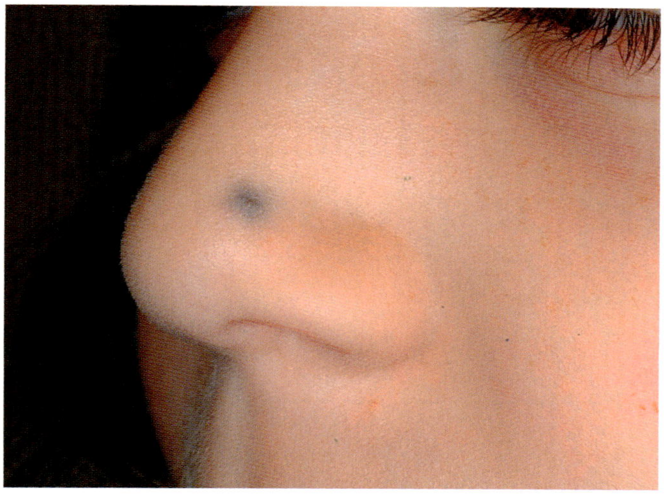

Fig. 11.68 Blue nevus. Acquired navy blue papule on a girl's nose.

Once a common blue nevus appears, it usually remains static and persists throughout life. Although fading of color and some degree of flattening may occur with time, malignant degeneration of this form of blue nevus is rare. When a diagnosis of malignant melanoma is considered, the common blue nevus can be differentiated from it by the presence of normal skin markings over the lesion, in contrast to the loss of such markings in lesions of malignant melanoma, the homogeneity of coloration and the smooth borders on routine examination, and the presence of a bluish-gray homogeneous lesion by dermoscopic evaluation.[716]

Cellular blue nevi tend to be larger and generally measure more than 1 cm in diameter. They are usually located on the scalp, buttocks, and sacrococcygeal areas and occasionally the dorsal aspect of the hands and feet. The plaque-type variant of blue nevus is a subset that is present at birth or develops during early childhood, occurs most commonly on the scalp, and may enlarge during puberty. The cellular blue nevus carries a higher risk of malignant transformation than the common blue nevus, but malignant transformation is still rare. Malignant blue nevi are locally aggressive but spread to regional lymph nodes in about 5% of individuals.

The classification of other forms of blue nevi is controversial.[717] Blue nevi may be hypochromic (sclerotic, hypomelanotic, and amelanotic forms), eruptive (particularly after sunburn on the upper central chest, shoulders, and V of the neck), or targetoid (preferentially on the back of the hands or feet, leading to a misdiagnosis of melanoma). Many show clinical and histologic features of more than one form, particularly combinations of variants of blue nevi with common or Spitz nevi (see Chapter 9). The deep penetrating nevus (usually has its onset after the first decade of life), epithelioid blue nevus (most commonly seen in individuals with Carney complex), and pigmented epithelioid melanocytoma show features of both blue nevi (intradermal location, pigmentation) and Spitz nevi (epithelioid morphology).[718] Molecular studies are likely to refine classification. *GNAQ* is mutated in 53% to 83% of blue nevi[719] and GNA11 in an additional 15%. However, deep penetrating nevi show *HRAS* mutations as seen in Spitz nevi rather than *GNAQ* or *GNA11* mutations,[720] suggesting reclassification of deep penetrating nevi with Spitz nevi.

Benign-appearing blue nevi do not require excision. If the diagnosis is in question, biopsy can be performed. Histopathologic examination of common blue nevi reveals greatly elongated spindle-shaped melanocytes, mainly in the middle and lower thirds of the dermis, which results in the blue coloration. In addition to spindle-shaped melanocytes, cellular blue nevi also have nodular islands of melanocytes.

The complete list of 720 references for this chapter is available online at http://expertconsult.inkling.com.

Key References

Ainger SA, Jagirdar K, Lee KJ, et al. Skin pigmentation genetics for the clinic. Dermatology 2017;233(1):1–15.

Rodrigues M, Ezzedine K, Hamzavi I, et al. New discoveries in the pathogenesis and classification of vitiligo. J Am Acad Dermatol 2017;77(1):1–13.

Ezzedine K, Eleftheriadou V, Whitton M, et al. Vitiligo. Lancet 2015;386(9988):74–84.

Kaplan J, De Domenico I, Ward DM. Chédiak-Higashi syndrome. Curr Opin Hematol 2008;15:22–9.

Oiso N, Fukai K, Kawada A, et al. Piebaldism. J Dermatol 2013;40(5):330–5.

Northrup H, Krueger DA. Tuberous sclerosis complex diagnostic criteria update: recommendations of the 2012 International Tuberous Sclerosis Complex Consensus Conference. Pediatr Neurol 2013;49(4):243–54.

Krueger DA, Northrup H, International Tuberous Sclerosis Complex Consensus Group. Tuberous sclerosis complex surveillance and management: recommendations of the 2012 International Tuberous Sclerosis Complex Consensus Conference. Pediatr Neurol 2013;49(4):255–65.

Zhang J, Li M, Yao Z. Updated review of genetic reticulate pigmentary disorders. Br J Dermatol 2017;177(4):945–59.

Scheuerle AE, Ursini MV. Incontinentia pigmenti. In: Adam MP, Ardinger HH, Pagon RA, et al., editors. Gene Reviews® [Internet]. Seattle (WA): University of Washington; 1993–2019. 1999 Jun 8 [updated 2017 Dec 21].

Kromann AB, Ousager LB, Ali IKM, et al. Pigmentary mosaicism: a review of original literature and recommendations for future handling. Orphanet J Rare Dis 2018;13(1):39.

Williams VC, Lucas J, Babcock MA, et al. Neurofibromatosis type 1 revisited. Pediatrics 2009;123:124–33.

Hernandez-Martin A, Duat-Rodriguez A. An update on neurofibromatosis type 1: not just cafe-au-lait spots, freckling, and neurofibromas. An update. Part I. Dermatological clinical criteria diagnostic of the disease. Actas Dermosifiliogr 2016; 107(6):454–64.

Barnhill RL, Cerroni L, Cook M, et al. State of the art, nomenclature, and points of consensus and controversy concerning benign melanocytic lesions: outcome of an international workshop. Adv Anat Pathol 2010;17:73–90.

12 Infantile Hemangiomas, Vascular Malformations, and Other Vascular Disorders of Infancy and Childhood

Classification of Vascular Lesions

Vascular birthmarks, or congenital vascular anomalies, are common lesions that may present in a variety of fashions. There has traditionally been a significant amount of confusion regarding the nomenclature of these lesions, and the term *hemangioma* was widely used in the medical literature in reference to a variety of different vascular anomalies.[1,2] In 1982, Mulliken and Glowacki proposed a classification system for vascular anomalies based on clinical and cellular features.[3] This classification was further refined 6 years later in a book,[4] and in 1996 it was adopted as the official classification system for vascular anomalies by the International Society for the Study of Vascular Anomalies (ISSVA). This nomenclature revolutionized the classification of vascular lesions and is the basis for continued study into the causes of these lesions and their therapy. The ISSVA classification was updated in 2014, reflecting the expanded spectrum of relevant disorders identified after publication of the initial classification.[5]

According to the updated ISSVA classification system (Box 12.1), vascular birthmarks are divided into the categories of tumors and malformations. Vascular tumors, which have been divided into *benign*, *locally aggressive/borderline*, and *malignant* forms, are neoplasms of the vasculature. The benign category includes infantile hemangioma (the most common vascular tumor), congenital hemangiomas, tufted angioma, and pyogenic granuloma (PG). Kaposiform hemangioendothelioma and Kaposi sarcoma are examples of locally aggressive/borderline types, and angiosarcoma is the predominant malignant form.

Vascular malformations represent anomalous blood vessels without any endothelial proliferation or cellular turnover. In distinction to infantile hemangioma (IH), these lesions tend to be present immediately at birth and persist for a lifetime. Vascular malformations are further classified as *simple*, and then according to their predominant components (e.g., capillary malformation [CM], also known as port wine stain [PWS]; salmon patch), venous malformation (VM), lymphatic malformation (LM), and arteriovenous malformation (AVM)/arteriovenous fistula; *combined* (CM + VM, CM + LM, CM + LM + VM, etc.); *of major named vessels*; and *associated with other anomalies*. Fig. 12.1 pictorially demonstrates the different natural histories of IHs and vascular malformations.

This chapter includes discussion of vascular tumors and tumor syndromes, vascular malformations and malformation syndromes, disorders associated with vascular dilation, and a few miscellaneous disorders of the cutaneous vasculature.

Vascular Tumors and Tumor Syndromes

INFANTILE HEMANGIOMA

IH, or hemangioma of infancy, is the most common benign soft-tissue tumor of childhood. Although estimates vary, it occurs in around 2% to 12% of infants.[6–10] Female infants are three times more likely to have IHs than male infants, and the incidence is increased in premature neonates. Although they occur in all races, IHs appear to be less common in those of Black or Asian descent.[11] Multiple gestation pregnancy, advanced maternal age, placenta previa, and preeclampsia also appear to be risk factors for IH.[12] Although they are traditionally considered to be sporadic lesions, autosomal dominant segregation (with incomplete penetrance) or maternal transmission has been suggested.[13,14] Comparison of twin pairs with regard to IH has revealed no significant difference in concordance (both infants having IH) between monozygotic and dizygotic twins.[15] These lesions vary considerably in their appearance and significance, related to their size, depth, location, growth pattern, and stage of evolution. Older descriptive terms for IH include *strawberry*, *cavernous*, and *capillary hemangiomas*. These terms are no longer useful and should not be used in the era of more specific vascular lesion nomenclature, as discussed earlier and shown in Box 12.1. Although IHs may occur on any part of the body, they most commonly involve the head and neck regions. Facial hemangiomas have been noted to have a nonrandom distribution, with the majority of lesions occurring on the central face at sites of development fusion.[16] Four primary segments of facial IH distribution have been identified, as shown in Table 12.1.[17]

The pathogenesis of IH is not yet completely understood. Positive endothelial cell staining with erythrocyte-type glucose transporter (GLUT)–1 protein has been noted in lesions during all of the growth phases.[18] It is absent in other vascular lesions such as vascular malformations and hemangioendotheliomas. This protein is normally expressed in the microvascular endothelia of blood–tissue barriers such as the brain, retina, placenta, and endoneurium.[11] As such it has been suggested that IH may originate from invading angioblasts that have differentiated toward a placental cell type or from embolized placental cells, although some data refute a placental trophoblastic origin for these lesions.[19] Further evidence of a potential relationship between human placenta and IH includes the high level of transcriptome similarity between these tissues[20] and the higher incidence of pathologic placental findings observed from pregnancies resulting in a child with IH compared with those resulting in healthy infants without IH.[21] Other endothelial cell markers shared between IH and placental tissue

Box 12.1 Contemporary Classification of Vascular Anomalies (ISSVA 2014 Classification)

Vascular Tumors

Benign

Infantile hemangioma/hemangioma of infancy
Congenital hemangiomas (RICH, NICH, PICH)
Tufted angioma
Spindle cell hemangioma
Epithelioid hemangioma
Pyogenic granuloma

Locally Aggressive or Borderline

Kaposiform hemangioendothelioma
Retiform hemangioendothelioma
Papillary intralymphatic angioendothelioma (Dabska tumor)
Composite hemangioendothelioma
Kaposi sarcoma

Malignant

Angiosarcoma
Epithelioid hemangioendothelioma

Vascular Malformations

Simple

Capillary (CM) (e.g., port wine stain, telangiectasia, CMTC, salmon patch/nevus simplex)
Venous (VM) (includes common, familial, glomuvenous, others)
Lymphatic (LM) (includes macrocystic, microcystic, primary lymphedema, others)
Arteriovenous (AVM) and arteriovenous fistula (sporadic or syndromal)

Combined

CM + VM, CM + LM, CM + AVM
LM + VM
CM + LM + VM
CM + LM + AVM, CM + VM + AVM
CM + LM + VM + AVM

Of Major Named Vessels

Affect veins, arteries or lymphatics; usually of large caliber

Associated with Other Anomalies

Associated with anomalies of bone, soft tissue (usually overgrowth, rarely undergrowth) or viscera

Modified from Wassef M, Blei F, Adams D, Alomari A, Baselga E, Berenstein A, et al. Pediatrics 2015;136(1):1–12.
CMTC, Cutis marmorata telangiectatica congenita; *NICH*, noninvoluting congenital hemangioma; *PICH*, partially involuting congenital hemangioma; *RICH*, rapidly involuting congenital hemangioma.

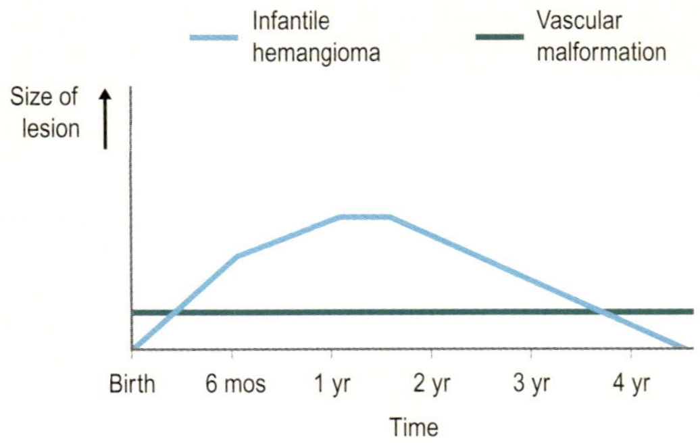

Fig. 12.1 Natural history of infantile hemangioma and vascular malformation.

include Lewis Y antigen, FcγRII, and merosin. The Wilms tumor 1 (*WT1*) gene was found to also stain proliferative vascular tumors, including IH.[22,23] Aside from the placental embolization theory of pathogenesis, other hypothesized causes for IH development include a somatic mutation in a gene mediating endothelial cell proliferation and hypoxia-induced stress that triggers overexpression of angiogenic factors such as vascular endothelial growth factor (*VEGF*).[24]

Hemangiomas may occur as superficial, deep, or mixed lesions representing their soft-tissue depth. The clinical appearance of the lesion depends on the type of hemangioma present. Superficial IHs, when well formed, present as bright red to scarlet, dome-shaped to plaque-like to lobulated papules, plaques, and nodules (Figs. 12.2 through 12.6). They may partially blanch with pressure and are rubbery or noncompressible on palpation. Deep IHs usually present as subcutaneous, partially compressible nodules and tumors, often with an overlying blue hue, prominent venous network, or telangiectasias (Figs. 12.7 through 12.9). These lesions may be warm to palpation.

Table 12.1 Distribution Patterns of Facial Infantile Hemangiomas

Segment Number/Name	Distribution	Comment
1 Frontotemporal segment	Lateral forehead Anterior temporal scalp Lateral frontal scalp Upper eyelid	Potentially greater risk of associated brain anomalies when PHACES syndrome present
2 Maxillary segment	Lateral cheek Upper lip Spares philtrum, preauricular area	
3 Mandibular segment	Preauricular area Mandible Chin Lower lip	Potentially greater risk of cardiac defects when PHACES syndrome present
4 Frontonasal segment	Medial frontal scalp/forehead Nasal bridge Nasal tip/ala Philtrum	

Modified from Haggstrom AN, Lammer EJ, Schneider RA, et al. Patterns of infantile hemangiomas: new clues to hemangioma pathogenesis and embryonic facial development. Pediatrics 2006;117(3):698–703.
PHACES, Posterior fossa malformations, hemangioma, arterial anomalies, cardiac defects, eye anomalies, and sternal defects.

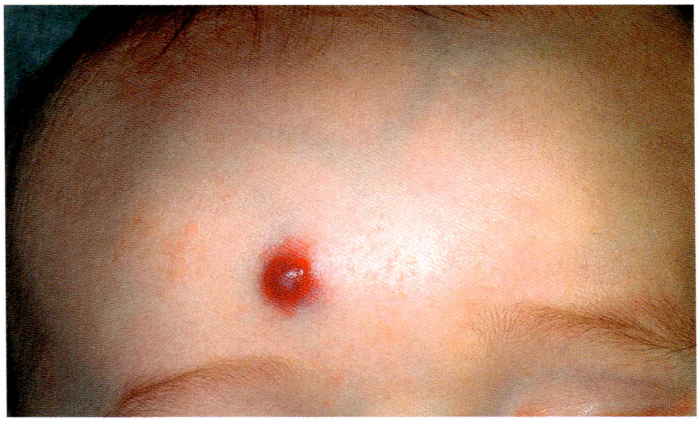

Fig. 12.2 Hemangioma, superficial: forehead.

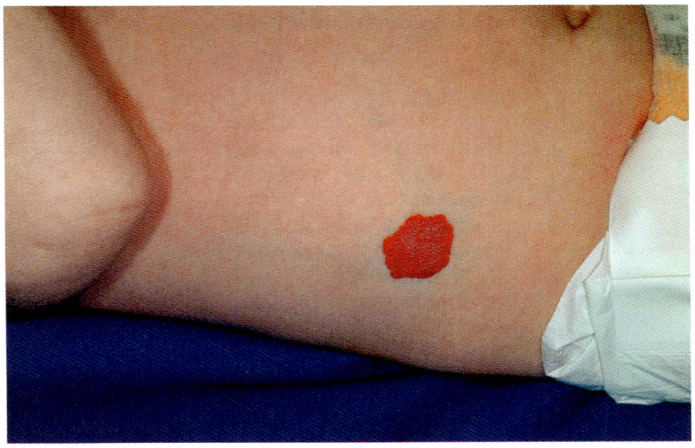

Fig. 12.3 Hemangioma, superficial: trunk.

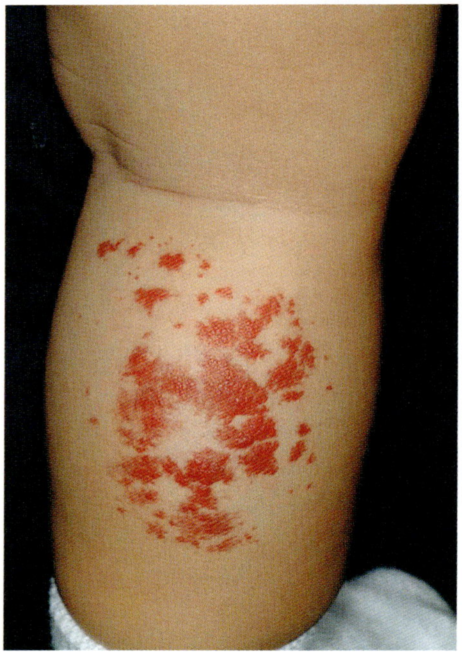

Fig. 12.4 Hemangioma, superficial. Note the patchy nature of this lesion, which eventually became confluent.

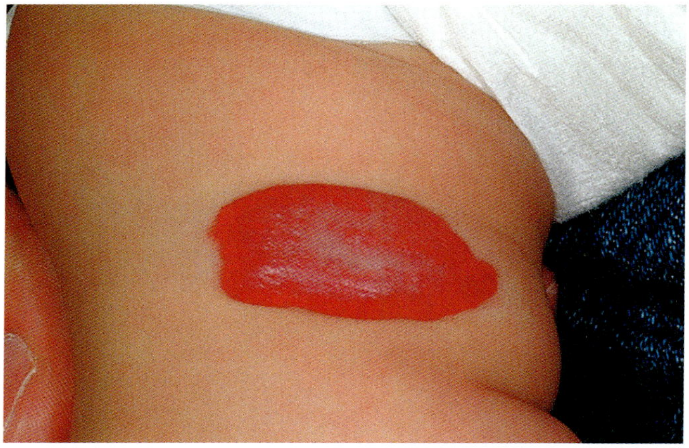

Fig. 12.5 Hemangioma, superficial: leg.

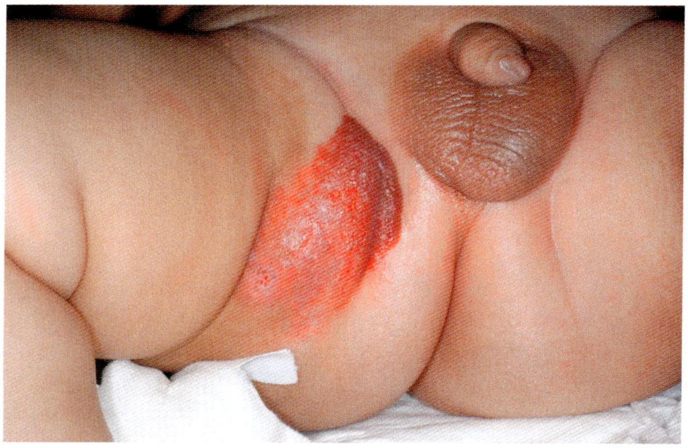

Fig. 12.6 Hemangioma, superficial. Note the early ulceration of the lateral inferior portion.

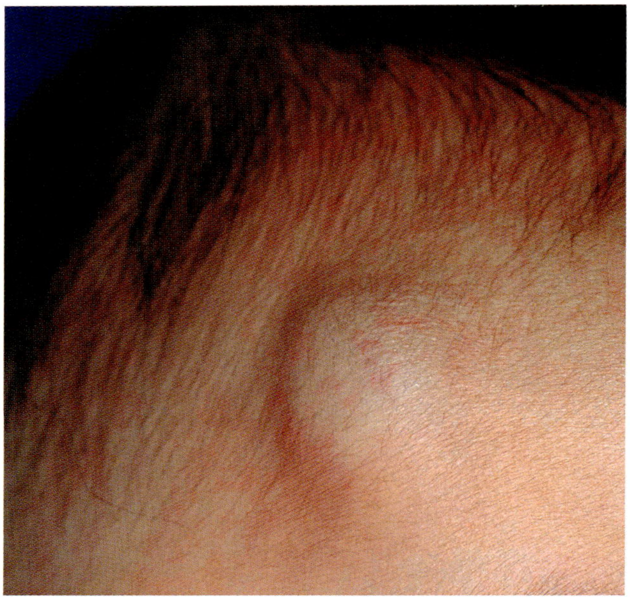

Fig. 12.7 Hemangioma, deep. Note the subtle blue hue and surface telangiectasias.

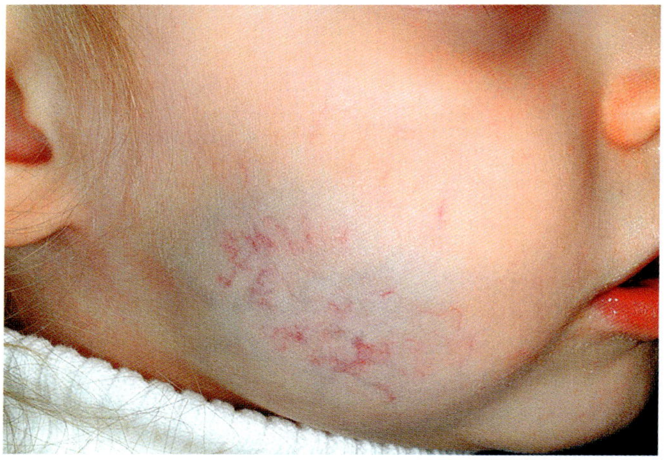

Fig. 12.8 Hemangioma, deep. This larger lesion shows the characteristic deep-blue hue and surface telangiectasia.

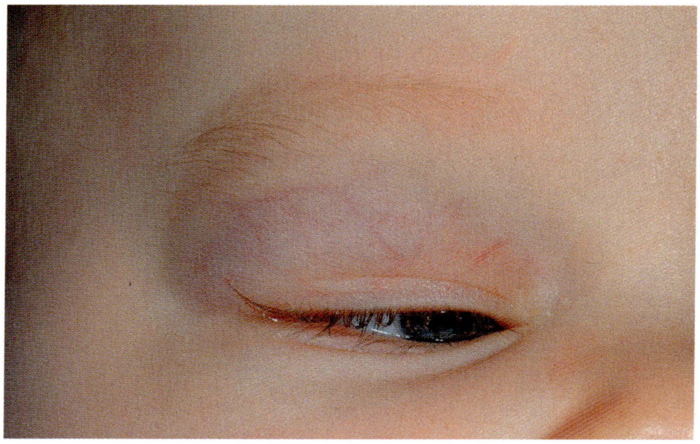

Fig. 12.9 Hemangioma, deep. This small, deep lesion resulted in mechanical ptosis, necessitating therapy out of concern for light-deprivation amblyopia. Note the overlying surface telangiectasias.

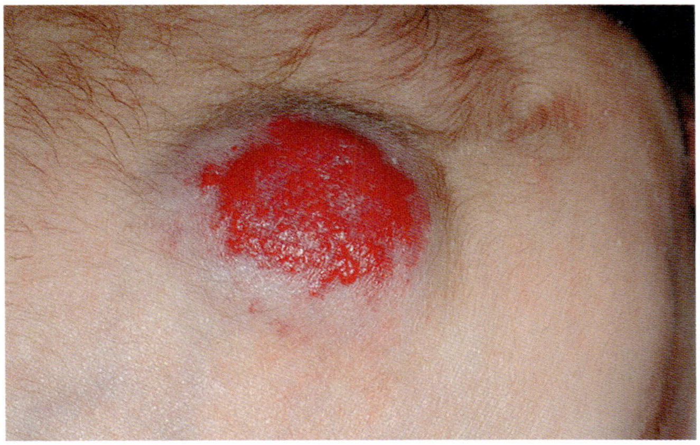

Fig. 12.10 Combined hemangioma. Note the larger, deep component and the bright red, superficial component of this combined lesion.

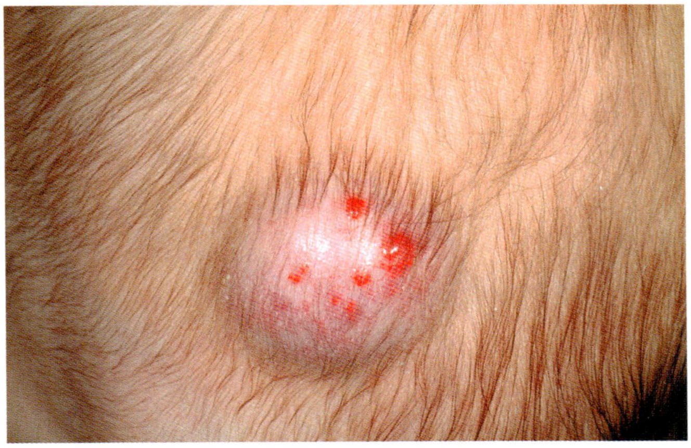

Fig. 12.11 Combined hemangioma. This lesion is predominantly deep, with studding of the surface with small, superficial components.

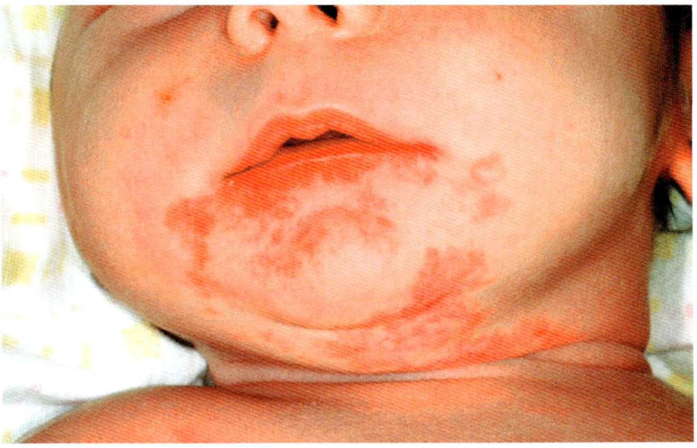

Fig. 12.12 Hemangioma precursor, telangiectasias. This lesion might initially be diagnosed as a port wine stain; within 4 weeks it was thickening, with eventual ulceration of the lip.

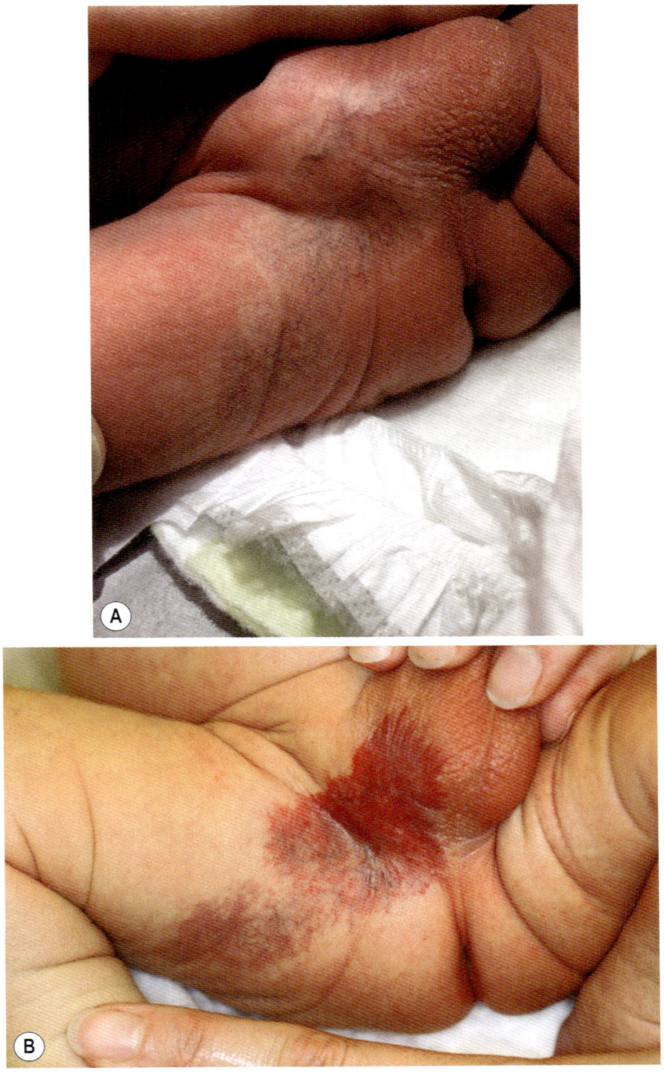

Fig. 12.13 Hemangioma precursor, pallor and telangiectasias. This 2-day-old boy presented with a vasoconstricted patch (pallor) with telangiectasias **(A)**. Follow-up evaluation at 2.5 weeks of age revealed changes consistent with proliferative infantile hemangioma **(B)**. (A courtesy Andrew Sagan, MD.)

Combined IHs have both a superficial component and a deep component and occur in up to 25% to 30% of patients.[25] They present with both the superficial, bright red component and a deeper, blue nodular component (Figs. 12.10 and 12.11). Hemangiomas may also be divided into subtypes based on their anatomic configuration. Focal lesions are discrete, usually round lesions that appear to arise from a single focal point. Segmental lesions (see later) involve a more broad anatomic unit that may be determined by embryonic placodes. Indeterminate lesions are difficult to classify into one of the preceding two subtypes.

Hemangiomas may present with a variety of precursor lesions, and in up to 50% of affected infants these premonitory marks may be evident at birth.[11] They include areas of telangiectasias (Fig. 12.12), pallor (Fig. 12.13), ecchymotic macules (Fig. 12.14), and even ulceration (Figs. 12.15 and 12.16).[26] Fully formed IHs may occasionally present at birth and are termed *congenital hemangiomas*. These lesions are discussed in more detail later.

The natural history of IH is characteristic. It is notable for a period of growth (the proliferative phase), a period of stability (the plateau phase), and a period of spontaneous regression (the involutional phase). The majority of IHs first become evident at 2 to 3 weeks of life, with potential continued growth until around 9 to 12 months of age. The majority of growth, however, occurs during the first 5 months of age (with 80% of growth completed by 3 months), and in those that continue to grow beyond this age, the growth rate is markedly slower.[27] Occasionally, lesions have a proliferative phase that lasts for longer than 1 year, sometimes as long as 18 to 24 months. Deep IHs tend to exhibit both a delayed onset of growth and a sustained, longer growth phase.[27] The onset of the involutional phase, which is difficult to predict in any given patient, is marked by a color change from bright red to dull red, purple, or gray (for superficial

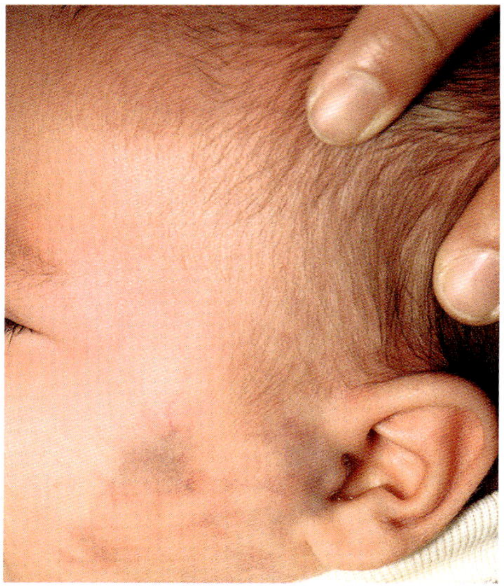

Fig. 12.14 Hemangioma precursor, ecchymosis. This bruise-like appearance may be seen before hemangioma proliferation occurs.

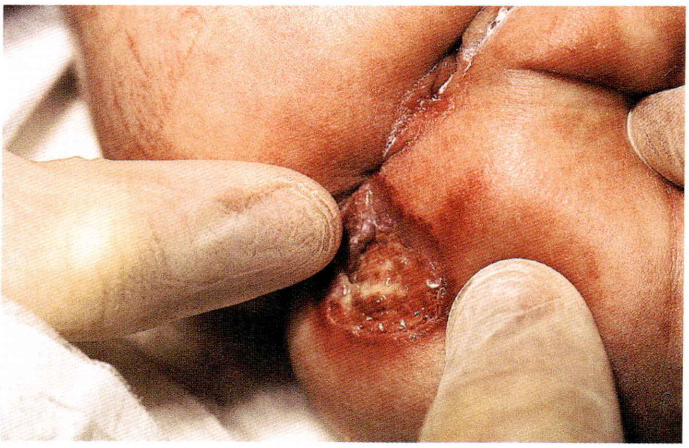

Fig. 12.15 Hemangioma precursor, ulceration. This 2-day-old newborn had this perianal ulceration; at 3 weeks of age, the ulceration was healing and the lesion had the classic appearance of a superficial hemangioma.

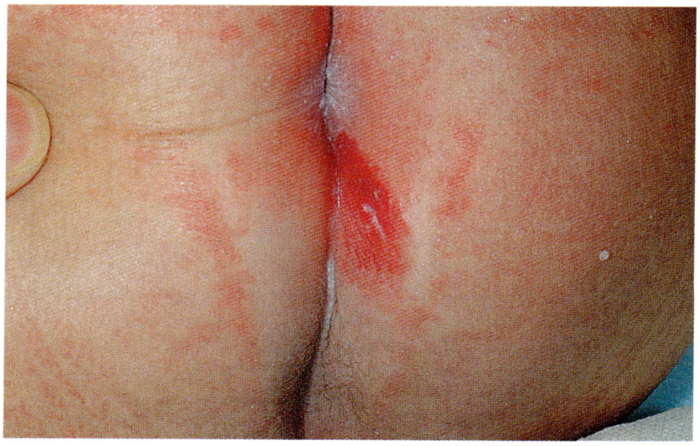

Fig. 12.16 Hemangioma precursor, ulceration. This perianal lesion presented at 1 week of age as a vascular plaque with ulceration.

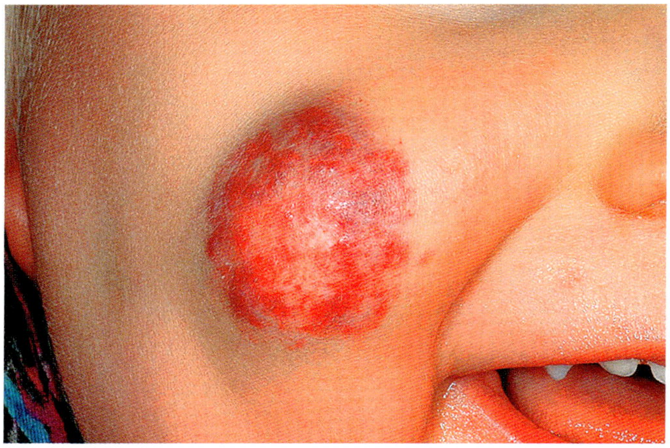

Fig. 12.17 Hemangioma, involution phase. Note the patchy vascular appearance in this involuting lesion in a 2-year-old boy.

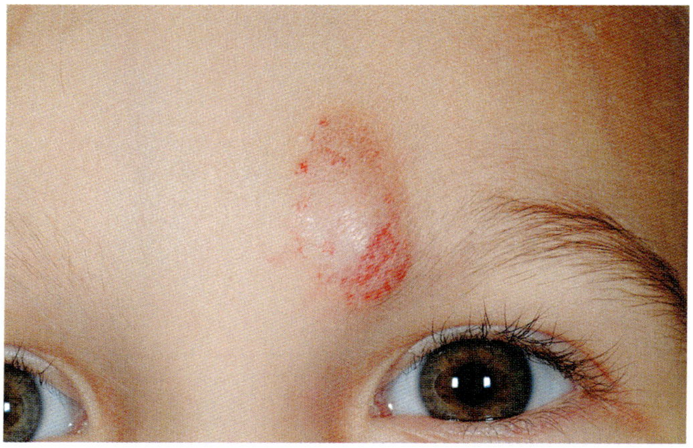

Fig. 12.18 Hemangioma, involution phase. The redness has largely resolved and the lesion flattened in this 3-year-old female.

lesions) (Figs. 12.17 and 12.18). It may be more difficult to appreciate early involution in deep IH, but with time these lesions become smaller/flatter, more compressible, and less warm. It was traditionally suggested that completed involution of IH occurs at a rate of 10% per year, such that 30% have involuted by 3 years of age; 50% by 5 years of age; 70% by 7 years of age, and more than 90% by 9 or 10 years of age.[11,25,28,29] It is now believed that the regression phase is completed in 90% of patients by 4 years (but maybe longer for deep IH).[24,30,31] However, it should be remembered that involution does not necessarily imply totally normal skin. Possible residual changes after IH involution include telangiectasias (Fig. 12.19), atrophy (Fig. 12.20), scarring (Fig. 12.21), and fibrofatty masses (Figs. 12.22 and 12.23). These possibilities must be explained thoroughly to the parents of patients with IH.

Treatment decisions regarding an IH must incorporate many factors. These include the size and location of the lesion or lesions (see later), the age of the patient and growth phase of the hemangioma, associated findings, and the perceived potential for psychosocial distress both for parents and for the patient later in life. The latter is quite difficult to predict but must be seriously considered in the patient with a conspicuous IH, especially if it is facial. These lesions may be associated with parental disbelief, fear, mourning, and social stigmatization.[32] Various instruments have been developed to help measure disease burden and quality of life (QoL) in patients and families with IH and have suggested that parents experience a high burden of disease and that certain clinical characteristics (such as location on the head and neck, being in the proliferative phase, and requiring treatment) correspond to a greater impact on QoL.[33,34]

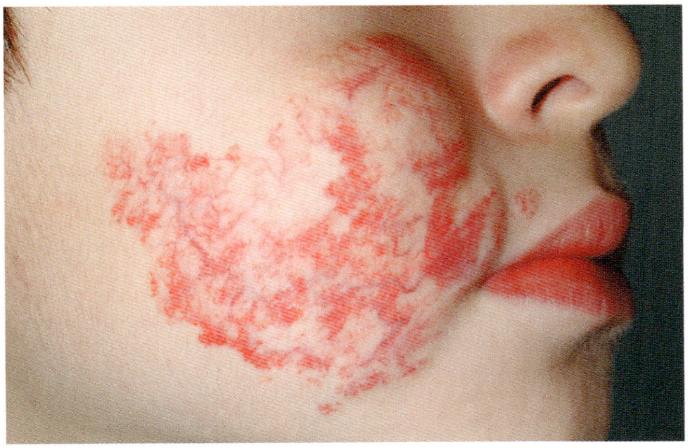

Fig. 12.19 Hemangioma, involuted. This lesion demonstrates the residual telangiectasias that may persist after involution of the hemangioma.

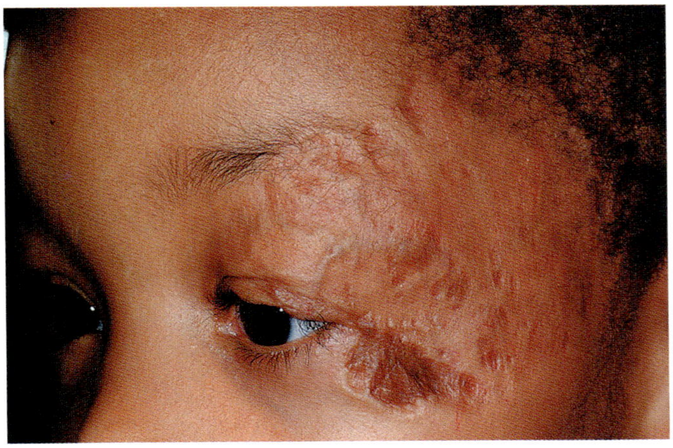

Fig. 12.20 Hemangioma, involuted. This hemangioma was very large with complete obstruction of the visual axis and secondary ulceration. After involution, atrophy and scarring are both evident.

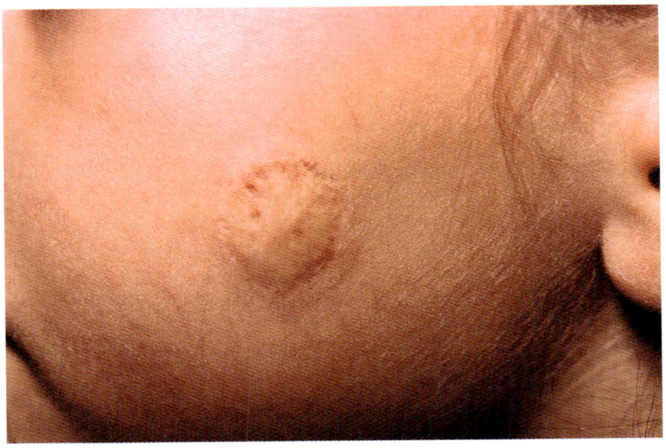

Fig. 12.21 Hemangioma, involuted. Residual scarring and atrophy are evident in this fully involuted lesion.

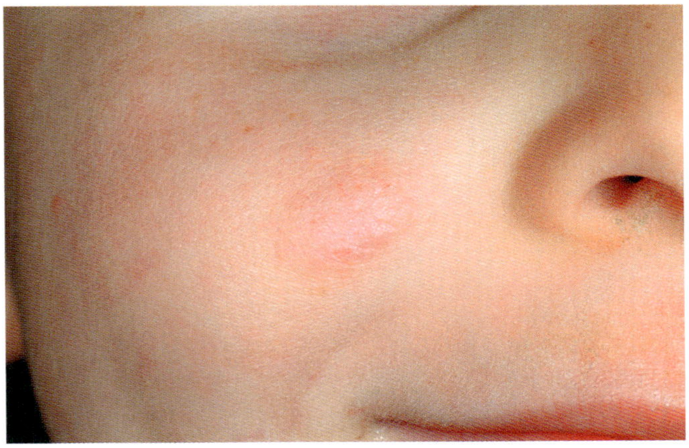

Fig. 12.22 Hemangioma, involuted. The cheek of this 4-year-old boy shows the residual fibrofatty tissue that may remain after involution.

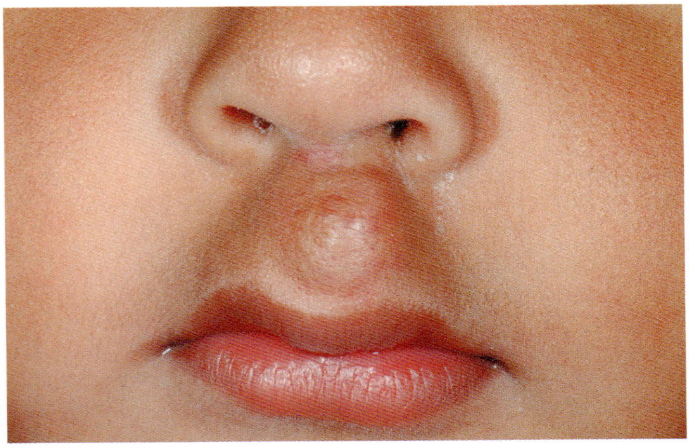

Fig. 12.23 Hemangioma, involuted. This philtrum lesion has involuted, but fibrofatty residua remain.

A hemangioma severity scale (HSS) has been developed and validated. HSS incorporates the factors described earlier, as well as risk for associated structural anomalies, complications, pain, and likelihood of disfigurement; testing of the HSS on large cohorts of infants with IH has suggested that a cutoff value of 10 to 11 or higher may be appropriate as a triage instrument for propranolol therapy and that a HSS score of 6 or greater merits referral to an IH specialist.[35–37] The major goals of management should be to prevent or reverse life- or function-threatening complications; prevent disfigurement; minimize psychosocial stress; avoid overly aggressive procedures; and adequately prevent or treat ulceration to minimize infection, pain, and scarring.[38] Treatment decisions can be challenging and must include parental input and a thorough risk-to-benefit analysis. Hemangiomas for which further evaluation, referral to a specialist, or therapy should be considered are listed in Box 12.2. (These are discussed in more detail under Clinical Variants and Associated Syndromes.)

Treatment options for IH are listed in Table 12.2, and clinical practice guidelines for the management of infantile hemangiomas have recently been published.[39] Probably the most useful principle in the treatment of these lesions is that of *active nonintervention*. This term implies that the physician inquires about the parents' knowledge of the condition, offers education regarding natural history and therapeutic indications, and offers anticipatory guidance and support. Active nonintervention is an appropriate "therapy" for the majority of IHs and can be offered by the pediatrician or primary care physician in most instances. Serial photography may be useful for parents of children with hemangiomas to document the gradual spontaneous involution, which may be subtle and underappreciated by them.[25] Referral to support groups and informational resources, such as the Hemangioma Investigator Group (www.hemangiomaeducation.org), Vascular Birthmarks Foundation (www.birthmark.org), or the National

Box 12.2 Hemangiomas: Considerations for Evaluation, Referral, and/or Therapy

- Life threatening
- Function threatening
  - Periocular
  - Nasal tip
  - Ear (extensive)
  - Lips
  - Genitalia, perineum
  - Airway
  - Hepatic
- Large facial
- Large anogenital/perineal
- "Beard" distribution*
- Ulcerating
- Lumbosacral
- Multiple

*See text for discussion.

Table 12.2 Treatments for Infantile Hemangioma*

Treatment	Comment
Active nonintervention	Emotional support and guidance; distribution of patient education materials and referral to informational and support networks
Local wound care	When ulcerated: topical antibiotic, nonstick wound dressings, compresses, becaplermin gel
Oral antibiotics	When secondary infection present
Pain control	When ulcerated: may require temporary use of narcotic analgesics
Oral β-blockers	Usually propranolol 2–3 mg/kg per day; risks include bradycardia, hypotension (both usually asymptomatic), hypoglycemia, bronchospasm, hypothermia, nightmares
Topical β-blockers	Most often timolol gel-forming ophthalmic solution, 0.1%–0.5%, applied two to three times daily; may be useful for smaller, localized and/or superficial IH
Topical corticosteroids	Potent formulations; may be useful for localized, superficial IH
Intralesional corticosteroids	Usually triamcinolone; localized bulky lesions; caution with periocular IH
Oral corticosteroids	Traditional gold standard for systemic therapy; prednisone or prednisolone, 2–4 mg/kg per day; far less used in era of β-blocker therapy
Laser therapy	Usually PDL; mainly useful for ulcerated IH or residual surface vascularity (e.g., telangiectasias) persisting after involution
Vincristine	Severe, treatment-resistant or life-threatening IH; requires venous access; risks include myelosuppression, peripheral neuropathy, extravasation necrosis
Interferon-α	Subcutaneous injection; severe, treatment-resistant, or life-threatening IH; risk of spastic diplegia
Surgical excision	Useful in select situations, (e.g., incomplete resolution, disfiguring facial lesions, smaller complicated IH refractory to medical therapy)

IH, Infantile hemangioma; *PDL*, pulsed-dye laser.
*See text for more discussion.

Organization of Vascular Anomalies (www.novanews.org), is useful for parents of these children.

The standard of care for IH requiring systemic therapy is oral propranolol. This nonselective β-blocker, which is traditionally used for cardiac indications such as hypertension or arrhythmia, was incidentally noted to result in marked shrinkage of IHs when administered in two children who had a cardiac indication and who also happened to have hemangiomas.[40] Subsequently these effects were confirmed in several more patients reported by the same authors as well as in several other open-label series, prospective studies, and retrospective reviews.[41–47] In the years after the initial report, propranolol evolved to become the therapy of choice for most clinicians with expertise in the treatment of IH. A multicenter, prospective, international, placebo-controlled study of oral propranolol for IH was subsequently completed and culminated in the approval of propranolol for treating IH by the US Food and Drug Administration (FDA) as well as the European Medicines Agency.[48] It is the first FDA-approved medication for this indication. The mechanism of action of propranolol in this setting is unclear, although most attribute the effects to some combination of vasoconstriction, inhibition of proangiogenic growth factors (including vascular endothelial growth factor, basic fibroblast growth factor, and matrix metalloproteinase-9), regulation of the renin-angiotensin system, and induction of apoptosis.[49,50] It is most often started at around 1 mg/kg per day, with the dosage gradually titrated up to 2 to 3 mg/kg per day divided into two to three doses daily. The FDA approval of propranolol hydrochloride suggests a target dose of 3.4 mg/kg per day divided into two daily doses; however, many experts use lower target doses if efficacy is noted. Potential side effects include hypotension, bradycardia, bronchospasm, hypoglycemia, hypothermia, and nightmares/night terrors, and this agent should be administered under close supervision with attention to these possible toxicities.[51] Propranolol has been used for IH in premature infants and has demonstrated both efficacy and safety.[52–53] Rebound growth or recurrence of IH after propranolol therapy has been increasingly recognized and may occur in 6% to 25% of patients; this risk seems greatest in those who discontinue therapy before 9 months of age and in those with IH on the head and neck and of the segmental, deep, or mixed types.[54–56] The time between discontinuation of therapy and appreciation of rebound is typically 3 to 6 months, and most lesions respond well to a second course of propranolol. Although propranolol therapy tends to be most effective during the early proliferative phase of IH (e.g., first 6 months), lesions in the postproliferative phase may also respond to treatment.[57]

Hypoglycemia has surfaced as one of the most relevant (and preventable) potential toxicities of oral propranolol therapy, and the highest risk period for this effect is in the morning after the overnight fast that occurs during sleep.[58] The mechanism for the development of hypoglycemia is likely related to β-blocker–mediated inhibition of gluconeogenesis and glycogenolysis, mandatory components of physiologic glucose homeostasis. Measures to decrease this risk include always giving propranolol with food, holding therapy during periods of illness or decreased oral intake, and the avoidance of fasting for longer than 8 hours (which may require nighttime awakenings for feeding).[59,60] Parents should be taught to recognize early warning signs of hypoglycemia, including shakiness, sweating, anxious appearance, and coldness. Table 12.3 list some guidelines for the use of propranolol in the treatment of IH. A systematic review of propranolol safety in the treatment of IH found the therapy to be well tolerated overall, with most adverse events considered nonserious, transient, and manageable.[61] Concerns about potential detrimental effects on learning, memory, and motor development related to propranolol therapy for IH in young infants have been suggested by some authors.[62,63] Although still controversial, several studies have been reassuring, finding no increased cognitive or other developmental risks, growth impairment or psychological problems in children as far out as 7 years from treatment with propranolol for IH.[64–67]

Other β-blockers have also been studied as treatment for IH and may have a lower adverse event risk profile given they do not cross the blood–brain barrier. These include nadolol, a nonselective β-blocker, and atenolol, a selective β1 antagonist. Nadolol was demonstrated to be efficacious in a comparative trial against propranolol and has the potential advantages of decreased central nervous system (CNS) side effects such as nightmares.[68,69] Atenolol, which also entails a lower risk of CNS-related concerns, has shown efficacy in the treatment of IH and, given its β-receptor selectivity, may be associated with less risk of bronchospasm; it was found to be at least as effective as oral propranolol in a retrospective noninferiority trial.[70–72]

After the discovery of propranolol's efficacy in treating IH, several investigators reported the use of a topical nonselective β-blocker timolol for small, uncomplicated superficial hemangiomas. Topical timolol maleate gel-forming ophthalmic solution is classically used for the treatment of glaucoma, but reports have described its efficacy

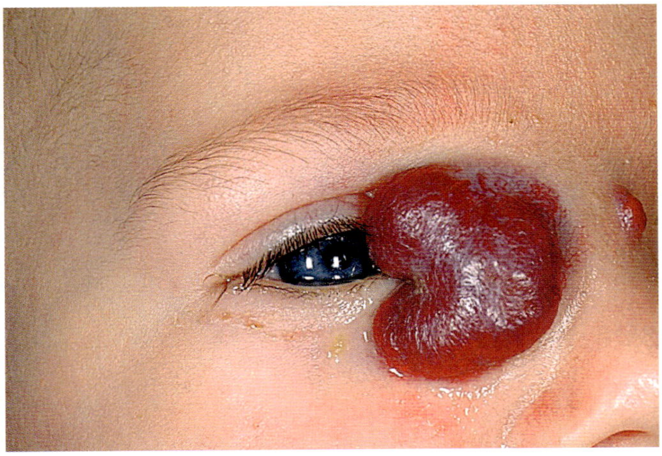

Fig. 12.28 Hemangioma, periocular. This large hemangioma was obstructing the visual axis secondary to its size and location.

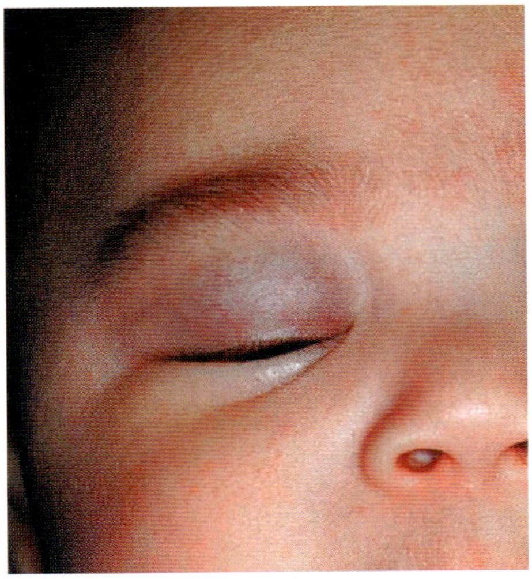

Fig. 12.29 Hemangioma, periocular. Superior eyelid hemangiomas may result in ptosis, with a risk for light-deprivation amblyopia.

be relatively insignificant when small, but larger lesions (Fig. 12.28) may result in a variety of ocular complications. In addition, any periorbital IH may be indicative of deeper, retrobulbar involvement, which may or may not present with unilateral proptosis. Light-deprivation amblyopia may result from visual axis obstruction, most commonly in the setting of significant upper eyelid lesions that result in mechanical ptosis (Fig. 12.29). Astigmatism may occur if the IH compresses the globe and may result in permanent amblyopia.[11] In a retrospective study of 96 patients with periocular IH, lesions larger than 1 cm, with a deep component, and with involvement of the upper eyelid were significantly associated with astigmatism and amblyopia.[104] Rarely, IH situated near a tear duct may block the drainage system and result in matting and conjunctivitis.[82] Because of these concerns, any child with a periorbital IH should undergo ophthalmologic examination. If there are functional or anatomic ophthalmologic concerns, systemic therapy is usually indicated.

Nasal tip/bridge IHs (Fig. 12.30) often require specialist consultation because of their propensity to distort the nasal anatomy (Fig. 12.31), resulting in permanent disfigurement. Slow involution of these lesions may pose significant psychosocial distress to the older child, and the splaying of nasal cartilage combined with redundant fibrofatty tissue after involution may result in the "Cyrano" nasal deformity (Fig. 12.32). The nasal crease sign is a linear, gray atrophic crease in the inferior columella that may occur with segmental facial IH involving the nose (Fig. 12.33) and that may portend imminent cartilage destruction and

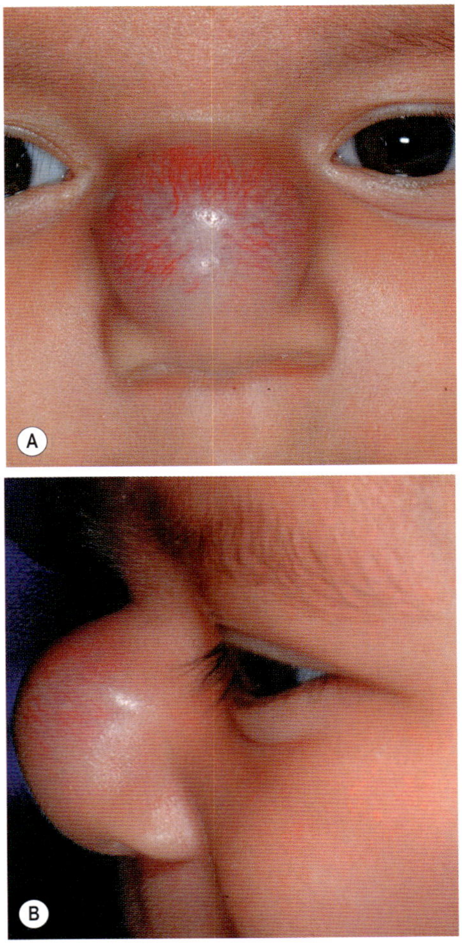

Fig. 12.30 Hemangioma, nasal bridge. This large lesion of the nasal bridge **(A)** results in significant bulbous distortion of the nose **(B)** and is likely to leave residual deformity.

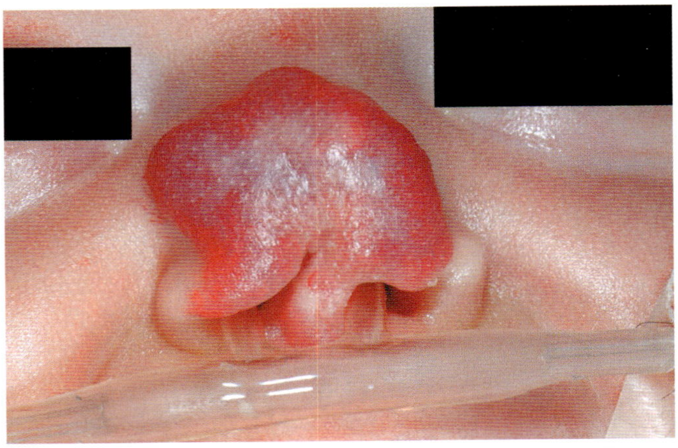

Fig. 12.31 Hemangioma, nose. This large nasal lesion resulted in destruction of nasal cartilage and erosion of the columella in this extremely premature infant girl.

nasal collapse.[105] It is for these reasons that therapy is often indicated for nasal IH.

Hemangiomas located on the lips tend to involute slowly and are more at risk for ulceration and bleeding. These changes may in turn contribute to increased pain, feeding difficulties, and permanent scarring. Ear IHs may also be cosmetically disfiguring (Fig. 12.34) and,

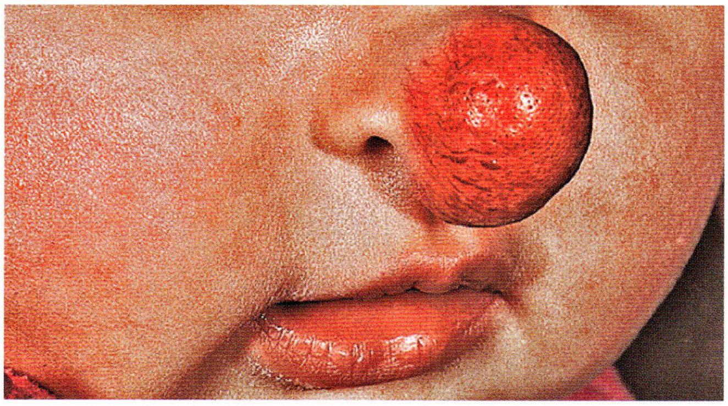

Fig. 12.32 Hemangioma, nasal tip. Large nasal tip lesions like this one may leave significant fibrofatty residua, resulting in a "Cyrano" deformity.

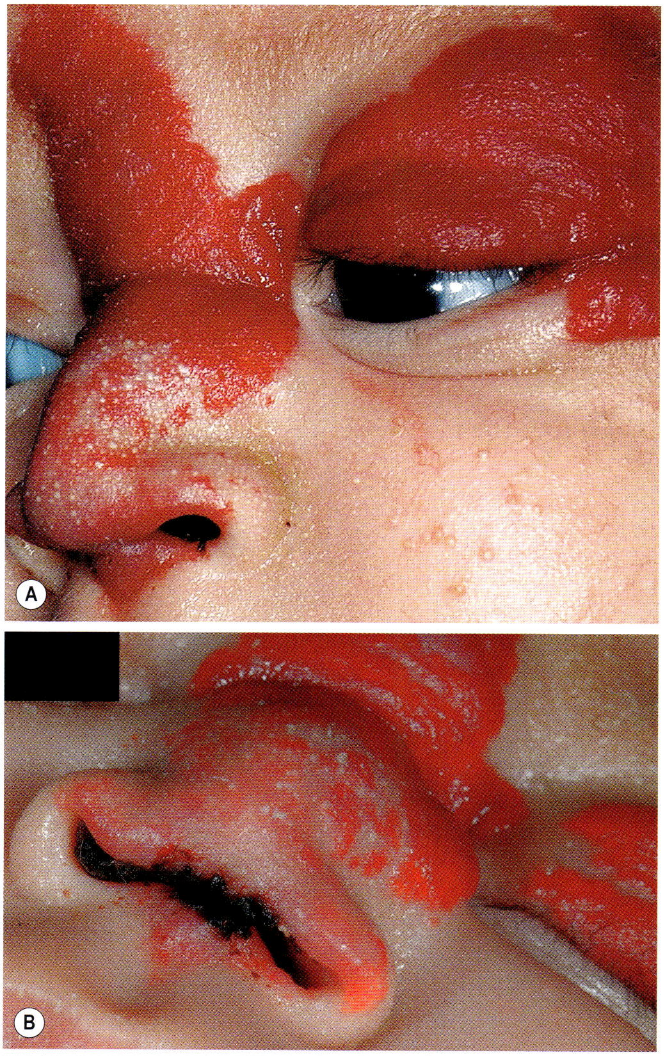

Fig. 12.33 Hemangioma, nasal crease sign. This infant girl had a segmental facial hemangioma involving the left forehead, periorbital region, glabella, nasal bridge, and nose. At 11 days after noting this linear gray atrophic crease **(A)** she returned to clinic with complete destruction of the nasal septum and columella and nasal collapse **(B)**.

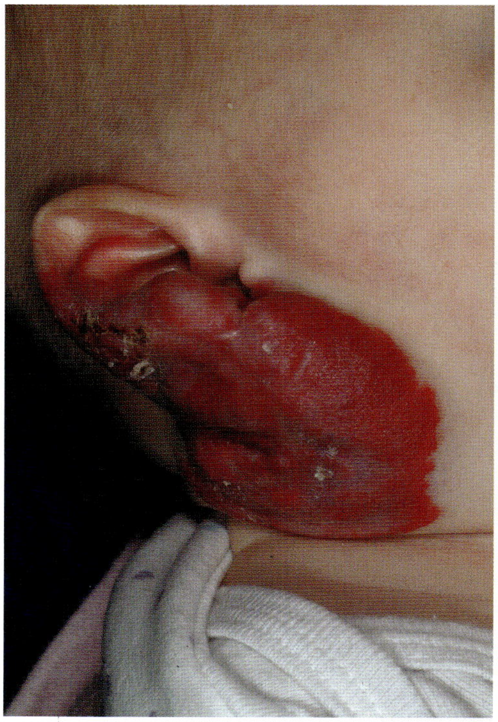

Fig. 12.34 Hemangioma, ear. This large hemangioma encompassed much of the ear as well as part of the adjacent neck. Ear hemangiomas this significant may result in permanent ear deformity and, occasionally, conductive hearing loss.

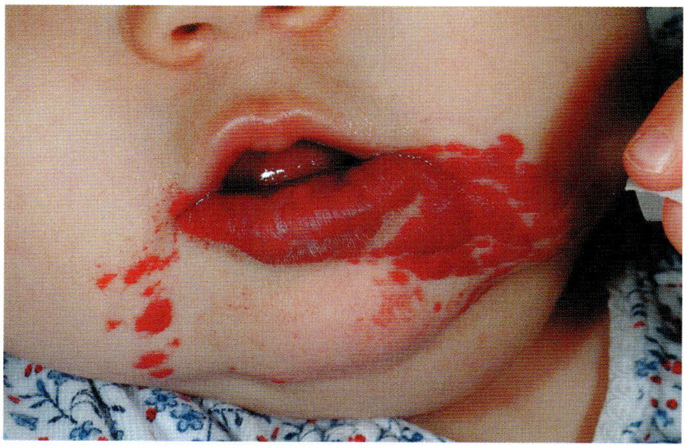

Fig. 12.35 Hemangioma, beard distribution. Lesions involving the lower lip, chin, neck, or mandibular regions have a greater risk of airway involvement, as was seen in this female infant.

when large, may obstruct the auditory canal and result in conductive hearing loss.

Hemangiomas that involve the neck, lower lip, chin, preauricular, and mandibular areas (beard lesions) (Fig. 12.35) are clinically important because of the increased risk of associated airway lesions in these patients. In one study, patients with more extensive IHs in this location had up to a 63% incidence of subglottic or upper-airway hemangiomatosis.[106] In another series, beard IH presenting as telangiectatic lesions and those involving more medial regions (lower lip, chin, anterior neck, and sternum) appeared more likely to be associated with subglottic IH.[107] Airway IH may also occur in the absence of cutaneous IH. Infants with symptoms are usually brought for treatment within the first few months of life with croup-like cough,

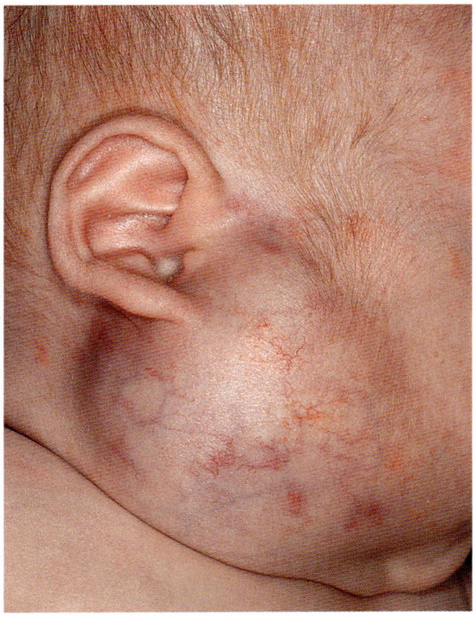

Fig. 12.36 Hemangioma, parotid. This large subcutaneous tumor with a blue hue and surface telangiectasias was characteristic for a parotid infantile hemangioma. These lesions tend to grow significantly and regress more slowly, and often require systemic therapy.

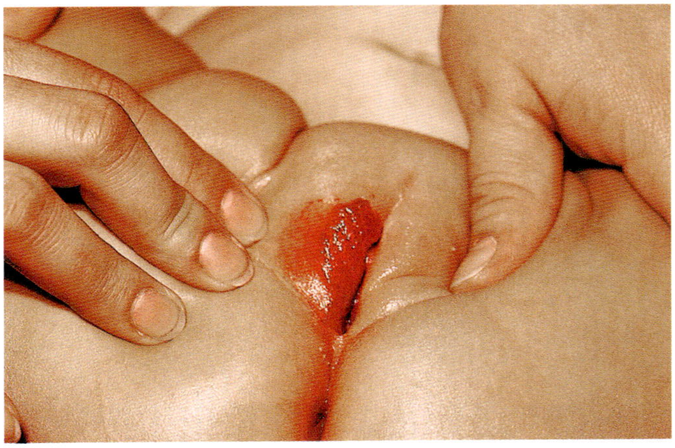

Fig. 12.37 Hemangioma, genital. This labial lesion is at increased risk for surface breakdown given its location.

hoarseness, and biphasic stridor. Any infant with extensive IH in this distribution or symptoms of upper-airway obstruction should be immediately referred for direct visualization of the airway with laryngoscopy. Treatment options in this setting may include propranolol, corticosteroids, laser therapy, surgical excision, and, occasionally, tracheotomy.

Parotid IHs often present as mixed superficial and deep lesions with a prominent deep component of swelling with an overlying blue hue (Fig. 12.36). These lesions tend to grow significantly and may involute more slowly than IHs in other locations. They may have a poorer response to pharmacologic therapy, although propranolol has been demonstrated to be effective in many patients.[108–111] Genital (Fig. 12.37) and perineal IHs are problematic because of ulceration, with the concomitant risks of bleeding, infection, permanent scarring, and pain. When these lesions are larger or segmental, the possibility of associated developmental anomalies of the external genitalia, anorectal region, genitourinary tract, spine, and spinal cord must be considered (see PELVIS syndrome). Hepatic IHs may be associated with significant morbidity and mortality and are discussed further in the Diffuse Neonatal Hemangiomatosis section.

Lumbosacral IHs (Fig. 12.38) are important because they may signal underlying occult spinal dysraphism or spinal cord defects. Tethering of the spinal cord is one of the more common associations,[112] and this anomaly may result in permanent neurologic sequelae without release. Other common findings include spinal lipoma, intraspinal hemangioma, and sinus tracts.[113] In a prospective study of 41 patients with lumbosacral IHs who underwent magnetic resonance imaging (MRI) examination, intraspinal abnormalities were detected in 21 patients, with a positive predictive value of IH for spinal dysraphism of 51.2%. An increased risk for spinal anomalies correlated with IH ulceration and the presence of additional cutaneous anomalies (including gluteal cleft asymmetry or deviation, sacral dimple, skin appendage, lipoma, dermal melanocytosis, dermal sinus, and aplasia cutis). Importantly, 35% of patients with an isolated lumbosacral IH had spinal dysraphism and 42% of children with normal ultrasound scans who then underwent MRI evaluation had spinal anomalies, highlighting the potential risk of relying on ultrasonography as a screening tool for high-risk infants.[114] In addition to spinal anomalies, sacral IH may also be associated with various congenital anorectal or urogenital anomalies, as discussed with genital and perineal lesions.[115] This association is discussed in more detail later (see PELVIS syndrome). Any infant with a lumbosacral IH, especially when it is large or of the segmental type or when other cutaneous stigmata are present, should be considered for MRI to assess for underlying abnormalities.

Segmental hemangiomas are lesions that involve a broad anatomic region (Fig. 12.39; see Fig. 12.38) or a recognized developmental unit.[116] They are often unilateral and sharply demarcated at the

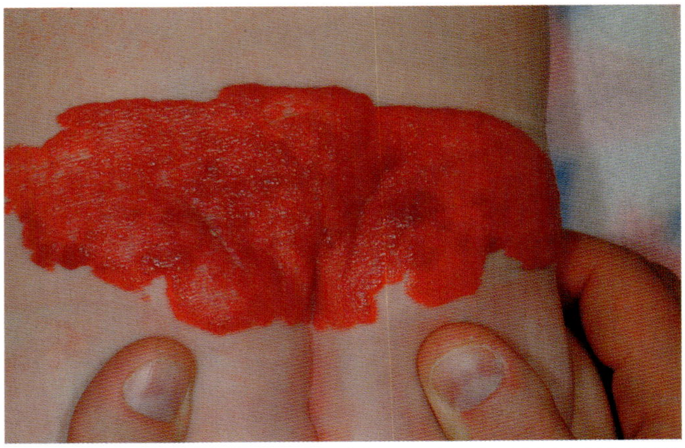

Fig. 12.38 Hemangioma, lumbosacral. This large segmental lesion would have an increased risk of association with underlying spinal dysraphism or spinal cord defects. Magnetic resonance imaging in this child was normal.

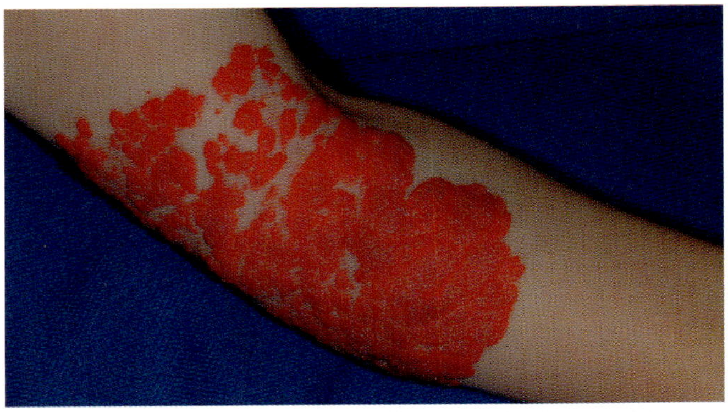

Fig. 12.39 Hemangioma, segmental. This superficial hemangioma occupied a large surface area of the distal arm and proximal forearm.

Table 12.4 PHACES Syndrome: Consensus-Derived Diagnostic Criteria

Manifestation (Organ/Location)	Major Criteria	Minor Criteria
Posterior fossa malformations (brain)	Dandy–Walker complex Other hypoplasia/dysplasia of mid/hind brain	Midline brain anomalies Malformation of cortical development
Hemangioma (skin)*	N/A	N/A
Arterial anomalies (cerebrovascular)	Anomaly of major cerebral or cervical arteries† Dysplasia of large cerebral arteries (kinking, looping, tortuosity or dolichoectasia) Arterial stenosis or occlusion‡ Absence/moderate to severe hypoplasia, or aberrant origin/course of large cerebral/cervical arteries Persistent carotid-vertebrobasilar anastomosis	Aneurysm of any cerebral arteries
Cardiac anomalies/**c**oarctation of the aorta (cardiovascular)	Aortic arch anomalies ▪ Aortic coarctation ▪ Dysplasia (kinking, looping, tortuosity, dolichoectasia) ▪ Aneurysm ▪ Aberrant origin of subclavian artery with or without vascular ring	Ventricular septal defect Right or double aortic arch Systemic venous anomalies
Eye abnormalities (ocular)	Posterior segment anomalies ▪ Persistent hyperplastic primary vitreous ▪ Persistent fetal vasculature ▪ Retinal vascular anomalies ▪ Morning glory disc anomaly ▪ Optic nerve hypoplasia ▪ Peripapillary staphyloma	Anterior segment anomalies ▪ Microphthalmia ▪ Sclerocornea ▪ Coloboma ▪ Cataract
Sternal clefting/**s**upraumbilical abdominal raphe (ventral/midline)	Anomaly of midline chest/abdomen ▪ Sternal defect ▪ Sternal pit ▪ Sternal cleft ▪ Supraumbilical raphe	Hypopituitarism Ectopic thyroid Midline sternal papule/hamartoma

Modified from Metry D, Heyer G, Hess C, et al. Consensus statement on diagnostic criteria for PHACE syndrome. Pediatrics 2009;124(5):1447–56; and Garzon MC, Epstein LG, Heyer GL, Frommelt PC, Orbach DB, Baylis AL, et al. PHACE syndrome: Consensus-derived diagnosis and care recommendations. J Pediatr 2016;173:24–33.

N/A, not applicable.

*Often extensive facial/plaque-like/segmental; occasional airway or other organ involvement.

†Internal carotid, middle cerebral, anterior cerebral, posterior cerebral aa. or vertebrobasilar aa.

‡With or without moyamoya collaterals.

DEFINITE PHACES syndrome:

Hemangioma >5 cm diameter of head/scalp PLUS 1 major criterion OR 2 minor criteria, OR

Hemangioma of neck, upper trunk or trunk & proximal upper extremity PLUS 2 major criteria.

POSSIBLE PHACES syndrome:

Hemangioma >5 cm diameter of head/scalp PLUS 1 minor criterion, OR

Hemangioma of the neck, upper trunk or trunk & proximal upper extremity PLUS 1 major OR 2 minor criteria, OR

No hemangioma PLUS 2 major criteria.

midline, although exceptions occur. Segmental IHs are most commonly located on the face. They seem to have a higher rate of complications and entail a greater risk for functional compromise and associated abnormalities such as urogenital anomalies or **p**osterior fossa malformations, **h**emangioma, **a**rterial anomalies, **c**ardiac defects, **e**ye anomalies, and **s**ternal defects (PHACES) syndrome (see the following paragraph).[116] In addition, they are more often complicated by ulceration.[16] The association of segmental IH with GI (typically lower GI) bleeding has been highlighted and appears to occur most often in the setting of PHACES syndrome with aortic dysplasia.[117]

PHACES syndrome or PHACES association (Online Mendelian Inheritance in Man, 606519) is a constellation of clinical findings associated with extensive facial IH. Table 12.4 outlines the consensus-derived diagnostic criteria and various features seen in this syndrome. The majority of patients with PHACES syndrome are female.[118,119] Although the pathogenesis of this syndrome is unclear, it appears to be a developmental "field defect" that arises around the seventh to tenth week of gestation.[120] In a large cohort of patients with the syndrome, greater reported rates of preeclampsia and placenta previa than expected in the general population were noted; these are also known risk factors for IH in general, and hence their significance as risk factors for PHACES syndrome is unclear.[121]

The facial IHs in patients with PHACES syndrome are usually large and segmental (Fig. 12.40) and may be unilateral or bilateral. They usually follow an aggressive growth pattern, and ulceration is common

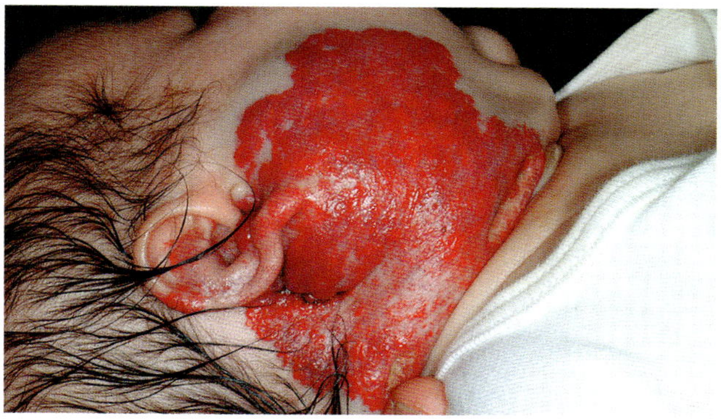

Fig. 12.40 Hemangioma, facial. Giant lesions like this one may be associated with the PHACES (posterior fossa malformations, hemangioma, arterial anomalies, cardiac defects, eye anomalies, and sternal defects) syndrome.

(Fig. 12.41).[118] There may be a dermatomal distribution, although these dynamic lesions should not be confused with the static vascular malformations (PWSs) associated with Sturge–Weber syndrome (see later). When there is "beard" area involvement, airway hemangiomatosis should be considered. Hemangiomas may also occur in other

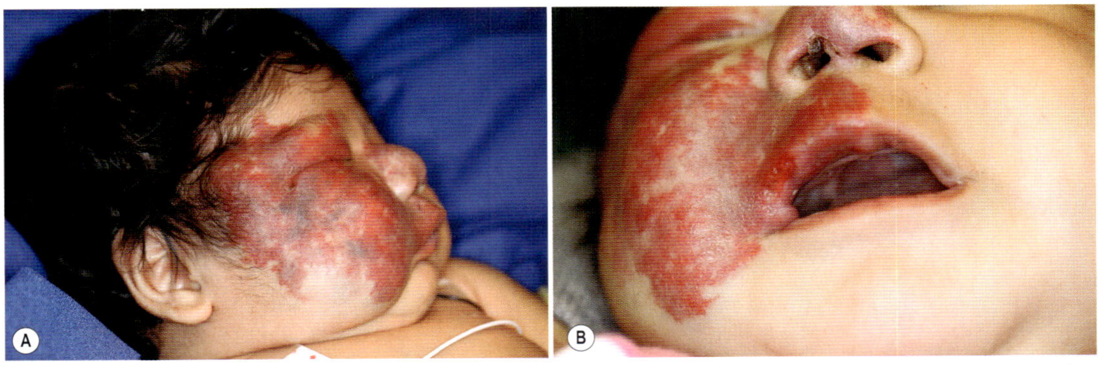

Fig. 12.41 Hemangioma with PHACES (posterior fossa malformations, hemangioma, arterial anomalies, cardiac defects, eye anomalies, and sternal defects) syndrome. This female infant presented with this large right-sided segmental facial hemangioma **(A)**, which developed ulceration of the right upper lip and nasal tip/columella **(B)**. She was found to also have intracranial arterial anomalies.

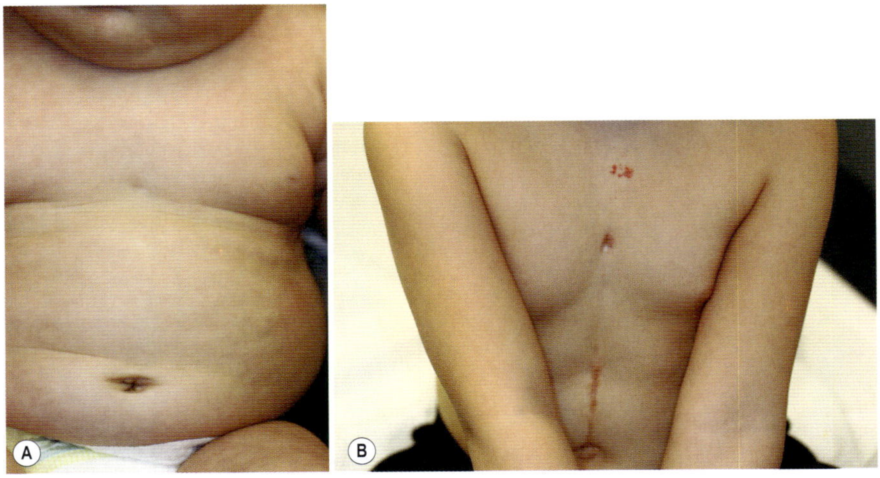

Fig. 12.42 PHACES syndrome with ventral developmental defects. **(A)** Sternal pit in a female infant with telangiectatic facial hemangiomas and multiple intracranial vascular anomalies. **(B)** Sternal pit/cleft and supraumbilical abdominal raphe in a 4-year-old female with partially involuted hemangiomas (note telangiectatic patch on upper midchest) and hypoplastic and tortuous cerebrovasculature. (B courtesy Brandi Kenner-Bell, MD.)

nonfacial locations in the setting of PHACES syndrome, most notably the upper torso and extremities.[122] Patients with large facial IHs (as well as those involving the scalp, neck, upper trunk, and proximal upper extremity), especially in the presence of ventral developmental defects such as sternal clefting or abdominal raphe (Fig. 12.42), should be screened for this syndrome with MRI or magnetic resonance angiography (MRA) of the brain and neck, echocardiography, ophthalmologic examination, and close neurologic and head circumference examinations. Direct airway visualization should be considered if the infant has extensive involvement in the beard area or symptoms of upper airway obstruction. In one prospective study, 31% of infants with a large facial IH measuring at least 22 cm^2 met diagnostic criteria for PHACES syndrome.[123]

Anomalies of the cervical and cerebral vasculature are commonly noted in PHACES syndrome, and these patients appear to have a progressive arterial vasculopathy with risk of arterial ischemic stroke (AIS).[124] Regressive changes in the vascular anomalies have also been noted in some patients.[125] Common CNS structural abnormalities include Dandy–Walker malformation, cerebellar hemisphere hypoplasia (ipsilateral to the hemangioma), and arachnoid cysts.[126,127] Aortic arch anomalies, especially aortic coarctation, are the most commonly noted cardiac abnormalities in PHACES syndrome and tend to be complex and anatomically atypical. These anomalies may remain asymptomatic in the first days of life until the ductus arteriosus closes, at which time they may result in severe hemodynamic consequences.[128] Box 12.3 lists the recommended evaluation for the infant deemed to be at risk for PHACES syndrome. Diagnostic criteria for PHACES syndrome have been published.[129] The greatest risk for morbidity in PHACES syndrome appears to be related to anomalies of the aorta and medium-sized arteries of the head, neck, and chest. Other findings in patients with this syndrome include headaches (may be severe), hearing loss, speech-language delay, dysphagia/feeding difficulties, dental enamel hypoplasia, and a variety of endocrinologic

Box 12.3 Recommended Evaluation of the Infant at Risk for PHACES Syndrome

Baseline

Thorough physical examination, including the following:
- Cutaneous (including assessment for ventral developmental defects)
- Cardiac (including pressure measurements in all four extremities)
- Respiratory (e.g., for stridor, hoarseness of cry, tachypnea)
- Neurologic (e.g., for hypotonia, developmental delay)
- Abdominal (e.g., for hepatomegaly, abdominal bruit)

MRI/MRA of the brain and neck
Echocardiography
Ophthalmologic evaluation
Thyroid function testing

If Indicated

MRI/MRA of the chest (if aortic arch abnormalities suspected)
Other endocrine evaluations (e.g., for growth hormone deficiency, hypopituitarism, diabetes insipidus)
Airway evaluation/direct laryngoscopy

MRA, Magnetic resonance angiography; *MRI*, magnetic resonance imaging; *PHACES*, posterior fossa malformations, hemangioma, arterial anomalies, cardiac defects, eye anomalies, and sternal defects.

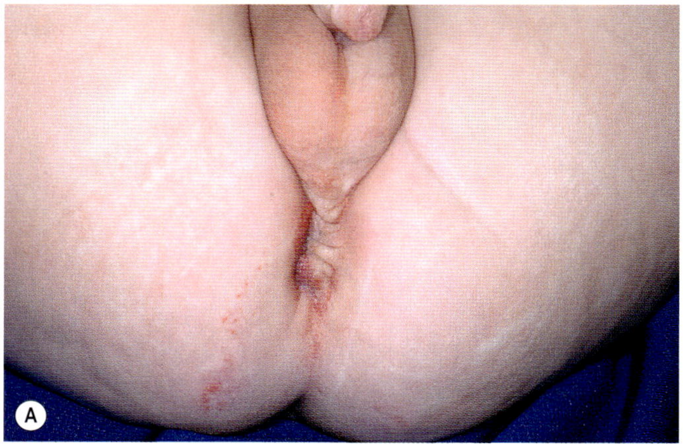

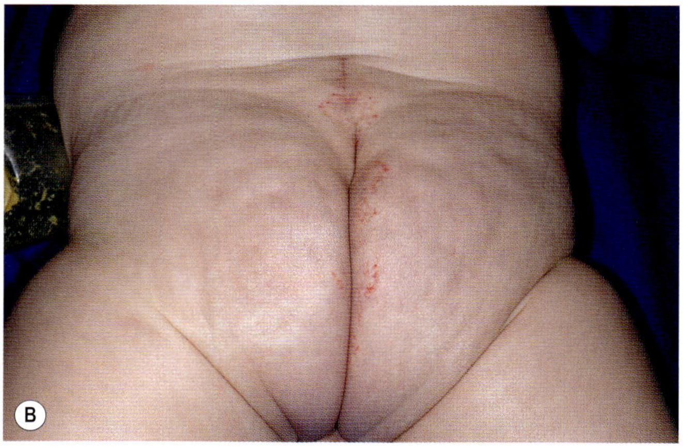

Fig. 12.43 PELVIS (perineal hemangioma, external genitalia malformations, lipomyelomeningocele, vesicorenal abnormalities, imperforate anus, and skin tag) syndrome. This infant has an infantile hemangioma with minimal growth involving the perineum **(A)**, buttocks, and lumbosacral back **(B)**. His history was also notable for imperforate anus, tethered spinal cord, and a filar lipoma. Note the midline lumbosacral scar related to his cord-untethering surgery.

defects, including thyroid dysfunction, hypopituitarism with growth hormone deficiency, hypogonadotropic hypogonadism, and adrenal insufficiency.[129–131]

PELVIS syndrome has been used to describe infants with perineal IH in association with a variety of other malformations involving the genitourinary and GI tracts, lumbosacral spine, and spinal cord.[132] The acronym *PELVIS* stands for **p**erineal hemangioma, **e**xternal genitalia malformations, **l**ipomyelomeningocele, **v**esicorenal abnormalities, **i**mperforate anus, and **s**kin tag. This association has also been known as *SACRAL syndrome*, which stands for **s**pinal dysraphism, **a**nogenital anomalies, **c**utaneous anomalies, and **r**enal and urologic anomalies associated with **a**ngioma of **l**umbosacral localization.[133] This phenotype has also been expanded to include IHs involving not only the perineum but also the lumbosacral region, genitalia, and/or lower extremity by a group that suggested the terminology *LUMBAR association*, for **l**ower body IH and other cutaneous defects, **u**rogenital anomalies/**u**lceration, **m**yelopathy, **b**ony deformities, **a**norectal malformations/**a**rterial anomalies, and **r**enal anomalies.[134] In this series, the IHs were noted to often be segmental as well as of the "minimal growth" phenotype (Fig. 12.43; also see later). Other cutaneous findings that may be present include lipoma, skin tag, caudal appendix, hair tuft, and sacral dimple. PELVIS/SACRAL/LUMBAR syndrome has been likened to PHACES syndrome, although it affects the lower half of the body and should be considered in any infant with a segmental IH (including those with minimal growth) affecting the anogenital, lumbosacral, or lower extremity regions.

Abortive hemangioma refers to IHs that exhibit very little (if any) proliferation during the period of expected growth. These lesions typically present as reticulated vascular patches, often with fine telangiectasias, occasionally as grouped telangiectases overlying normal-appearing skin, or as blue patches with a peripheral halo.[135] Small foci of typical bright red, superficial IH may be present around the periphery (Fig. 12.44). Other terms that have been used to describe these lesions include *plaque-telangiectatic hemangiomas, macular hemangioma with PWS-like appearance, reticular IH, minimal-growth hemangiomas*, and *IHs with minimal or arrested growth (IH-MAGs)*.[136,137] Several authors have confirmed these lesions to be IH in origin via positive GLUT-1 immunostaining of biopsy specimens. IH-MAGs tend to present more commonly on the lower half of the body than typical IHs and may be associated with ulceration, especially when occurring in the anogenital area.[137] They have also been reported in association with soft-tissue hypertrophy, particularly on the extremities.[138]

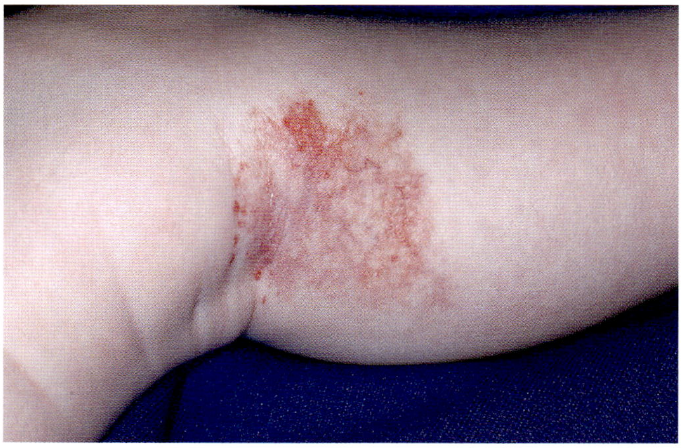

Fig. 12.44 Abortive hemangioma (infantile hemangioma with minimal or arrested growth). This telangiectatic vascular patch presented on the medial calf of this 5-month-old boy. Note the scattered brighter red vascular macules and papules around the periphery, a classic feature in some of these lesions.

Congenital IHs are lesions that are fully formed at birth. These lesions may follow the typical time course of IH, may have a more accelerated involution phase, or may persist unchanged. *Noninvoluting congenital hemangioma (NICH)* is a specific subtype of IH also known as a *congenital nonprogressive hemangioma*. These lesions may be diagnosed *in utero*, are fully formed at birth, and do not show the postnatal proliferation characteristic of IH.[139] Clinically, NICH lesions are round to ovoid, pink to purple tumors with overlying prominent telangiectasias and peripheral pallor (Fig. 12.45).[140] Importantly, these lesions also do not undergo the spontaneous involution typical of IH and hence appear to be a distinctive type of vascular lesion. Interestingly,

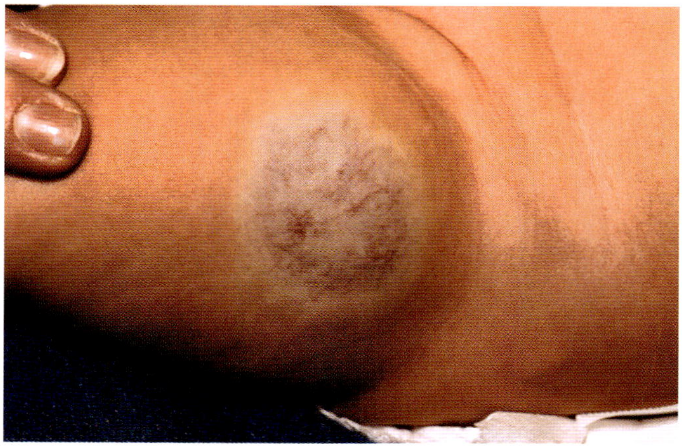

Fig. 12.45 Hemangioma, noninvoluting congenital. Characteristic features include prominent surface telangiectasias and a peripheral rim of pallor.

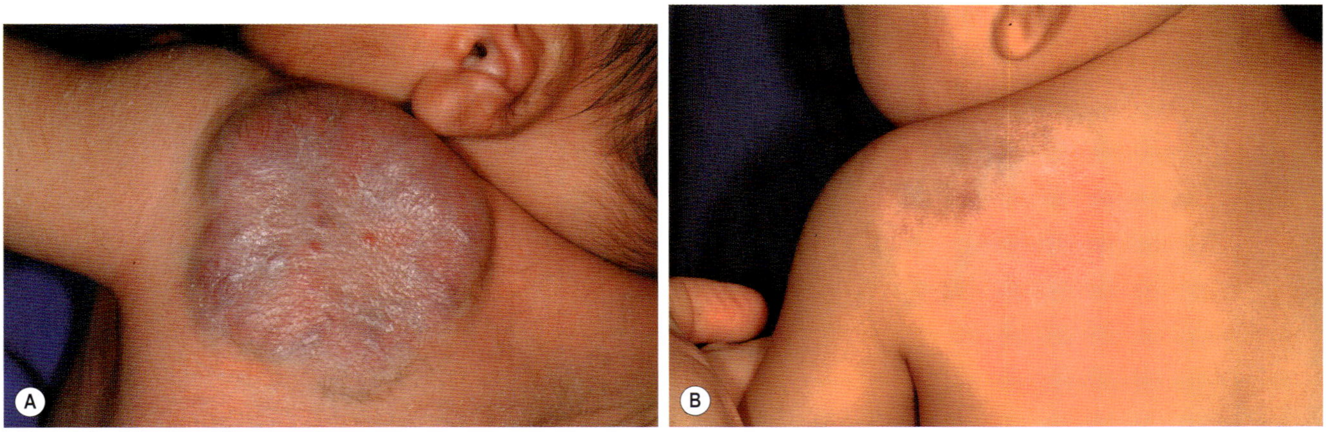

Fig. 12.46 Hemangioma, rapidly involuting congenital. This hemangioma was fully formed at birth **(A)** and involuted completely by 1 year of age **(B)**.

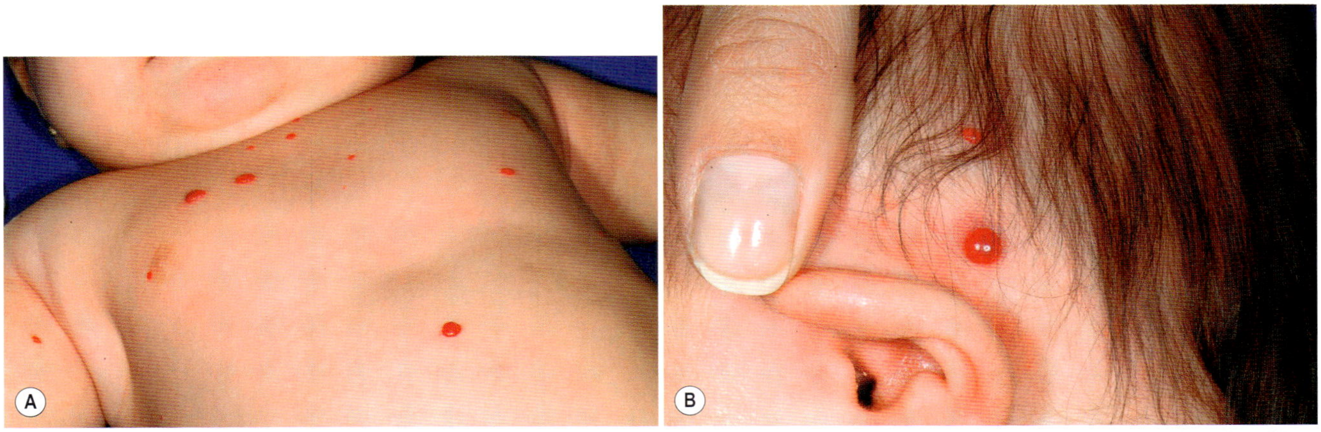

Fig. 12.47 Hemangiomatosis, benign. This infant had multiple small lesions as shown on the trunk **(A)** and scalp **(B)** and no internal involvement.

NICH lesions also have a different histologic appearance and are not immunoreactive for GLUT-1.[139]

Rapidly involuting congenital hemangioma (RICH) is the term used to describe a congenital IH that undergoes rapid involution early in life. These tumors may present similar to a NICH or may have the appearance of a typical IH. They may also present as small to large tumors with a red, violaceous, or gray appearance that may mimic other vascular (e.g., kaposiform hemangioendothelioma [KHE]; see Kaposiform Hemangioendothelioma section) or malignant (e.g., rhabdomyosarcoma, fibrosarcoma) neoplasms. They often involute completely by 12 to 15 months of age (Fig. 12.46) and may leave behind dermal and subcutaneous atrophy.[141] RICH lesions may present as atrophic violaceous plaques, suggesting *in utero* involution.[142] Lesions that begin and behave as a RICH but that involute only partially and then assume the appearance of a NICH have been termed *partially involuting congenital hemangiomas (PICHs)*.[143]

Diffuse Neonatal Hemangiomatosis

Diffuse neonatal hemangiomatosis (disseminated neonatal hemangiomatosis) describes multiple cutaneous lesions in conjunction with extracutaneous organ involvement. It must be differentiated from benign neonatal hemangiomatosis, in which the infant has multiple cutaneous lesions without any symptomatic visceral lesions or complications.[144,145] Patients with either type of hemangiomatosis may have only a few or up to hundreds of cutaneous IHs (Figs. 12.47 and 12.48). Some authors advocate for the terminology *multifocal IH with or without extracutaneous disease*, noting that many cases reported in the literature as diffuse neonatal hemangiomatosis may actually represent other entities such as multifocal lymphangioendotheliomatosis with thrombocytopenia (see later this chapter).[146]

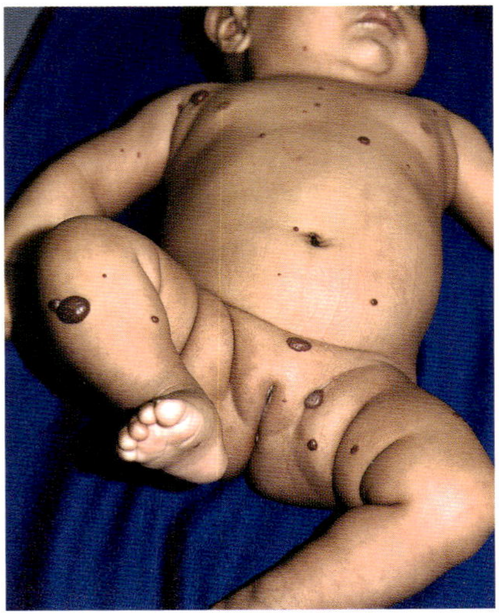

Fig. 12.48 Hemangiomatosis, diffuse. This infant had variably sized lesions and liver hemangiomatosis.

Although past data suggested that the risk of internal involvement could be predicted by the number of cutaneous IHs, the traditional recommendation for internal imaging in patients with five or more lesions was more anecdotal than evidence based. Subsequently, in a prospective study comparing 151 infants with five or more IHs to

50 infants with between one and four IHs, hepatic hemangiomas were identified on hepatic ultrasound in 16% (24) of the infants with five or more cutaneous IHs and in none of the control group with one to four cutaneous IHs. The study also revealed that preterm (<37 weeks' gestational age) delivery, multiple gestation, lower birthweight, *in vitro* fertilization, placental anomalies, and preeclampsia each occurred more often in infants with more than five cutaneous IHs, but on multivariate analysis only preterm delivery and lower birthweight were associated with having five or more cutaneous IHs. Of the 24 infants with hepatic hemangiomas, only two required therapy specifically for this finding.[147] This study confirmed that infants with five or more IHs are at greater risk for hepatic hemangiomas (and should be evaluated with liver ultrasound) and that the majority of those with hepatic involvement remain asymptomatic and do not require therapy.

Although the most common extracutaneous site for IH in patients with diffuse hemangiomatosis is the liver, multiple other organs can be involved, including the intestine, brain, eyes, spleen, oral mucosa, kidney, and lungs.[148,149] The diagnosis of hepatic hemangiomatosis is usually made clinically and radiographically, because liver biopsy is undesirable as a result of the risk of bleeding. Liver lesions may be asymptomatic or present with hepatomegaly and congestive heart failure, the latter of which is believed to be the result of arteriovenous (AV) shunting, which leads to increased venous return and increased cardiac output. Occasionally anemia or thrombocytopenia are present.

Three patterns of liver hemangiomatosis have been proposed: focal, multifocal, and diffuse.[150] Focal lesions are well defined and solitary on imaging and are most often clinically asymptomatic. They usually are not accompanied by cutaneous lesions and tend to involute rapidly. Multifocal liver hemangiomas present as multiple spherical tumors, which may be asymptomatic or can result in high-output cardiac failure secondary to AV shunting. These lesions involute after the same course as seen with cutaneous IH. Diffuse lesions are extensive, may result in near-total replacement of hepatic parenchyma, and may be associated with serious complications including vessel compression, respiratory decompensation, abdominal compartment syndrome, and multiorgan system failure.[150] These lesions may also be associated with severe hypothyroidism. The transient hypothyroidism associated with hepatic IH is caused by hemangioma production of the thyroid hormone inactivating enzyme, type 3 iodothyronine deiodinase. Evaluation reveals elevated thyroid-stimulating hormone (TSH), normal to decreased free thyroxine (fT4), decreased free triiodothyronine (fT3), and increased reverse T3 (rT3). Higher-than-normal replacement doses of levothyroxine may be required to achieve euthyroid status in these infants.[151,152]

Abdominal ultrasonography with Doppler studies is the diagnostic modality of choice, although MRI or computed tomography (CT) may occasionally be necessary. Treatment options may include optimization of cardiac function, corticosteroids, propranolol, interferon-α, vincristine, cyclophosphamide, embolization, hepatic artery ligation, hepatic resection, and liver transplantation.[11,150] Propranolol has been increasingly reported as an effective therapy for hepatic IH, and in most patients improvement in the liver lesions correlates with resolution of heart failure and improvement or resolution in the associated hypothyroidism, when present.[153,154] Infants with diffuse liver hemangiomas should undergo thyroid hormone monitoring and replacement as necessary. Most visceral hemangiomas, like the cutaneous lesions, grow during infancy and in surviving children regress during early childhood. Other evaluations that may be useful in the investigation for diffuse hemangiomatosis include complete blood cell counts, stool examinations for occult blood, liver function studies, urinalysis, echocardiography, electrocardiography, and CNS imaging when clinically indicated.

KASABACH-MERRITT PHENOMENON

Kasabach–Merritt phenomenon (KMP; also known as *Kasabach–Merritt syndrome*) is characterized by thrombocytopenia (owing to platelet trapping), coagulopathy, and microangiopathic hemolytic anemia in association with a rapidly enlarging vascular lesion. It was traditionally felt to be a complication of IH but is now well established to be associated with vascular tumors other than IH, namely KHE and tufted angioma.[155] These lesions have characteristics that clinically distinguish them from hemangiomas (see later). KMP occurs most often within the first few weeks of life and presents with sudden enlargement of the vascular lesion, ecchymosis, prolonged bleeding, epistaxis, hematuria, or hematochezia.[156] The cutaneous lesions show purpura, edema, induration, and an advancing ecchymotic margin (Fig. 12.49).[157] In addition to thrombocytopenia, other laboratory findings include anemia, hypofibrinogenemia, elevated D-dimers, fragmentation of erythrocytes on manual smear, and prolonged coagulation studies. The mortality rate is high, from 10% to 30%.

Kaposiform Hemangioendothelioma

KHE is a locally aggressive vascular tumor, so named because of the histologic resemblance to Kaposi sarcoma. It presents as a firm, subcutaneous nodule or plaque that expands rapidly and often has a violaceous discoloration (Fig. 12.50).[25,158] Although KHE usually presents in infancy, it may appear months to years later.[159] In addition to involvement of the skin, KHE may involve the deep soft tissues (Fig. 12.51) and the bone.[160] The consensus-derived treatment recommendation for KHEs that require therapy based on growth or symptoms, but without KMP, is oral prednisolone with or without adjunctive aspirin.[161]

Tufted Angioma

Tufted angioma (TA) is actually named after its histologic appearance, which reveals groups of dermal capillary tufts. These lesions present clinically as erythematous, annular nodules, or plaques, often with

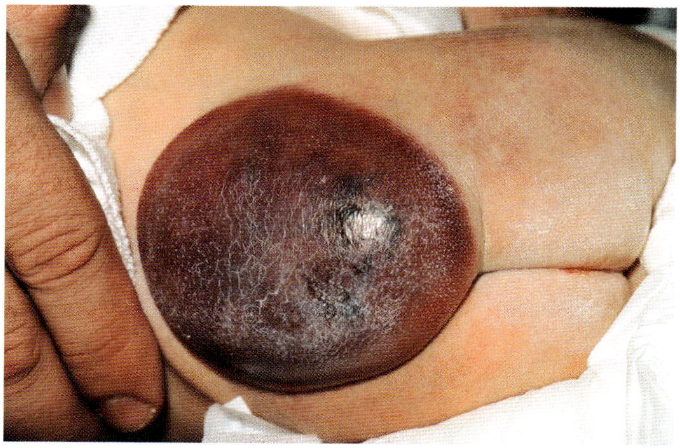

Fig. 12.49 Kasabach–Merritt phenomenon. Note the deep purple color of this vascular tumor, which suddenly enlarged and became firm, with accompanying thrombocytopenia.

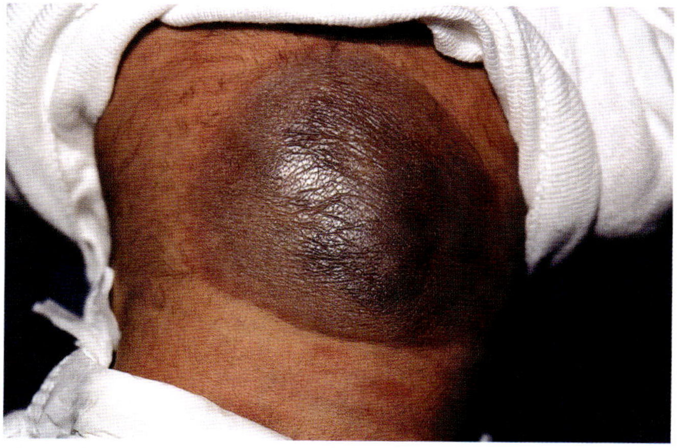

Fig. 12.50 Kaposiform hemangioendothelioma. These tumors are characteristically deep purple in color and may be associated with Kasabach–Merritt phenomenon.

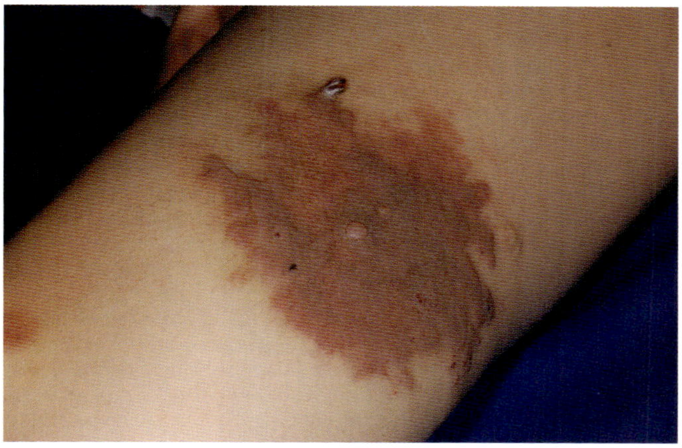

Fig. 12.51 Kaposiform hemangioendothelioma. This tumor on the medial thigh of a 10-year-old boy had been present since early infancy and extended to the deeper subcutaneous tissues. He never developed Kasabach–Merritt phenomenon. Note the secondary pyogenic granuloma–like papule that developed at the superior border.

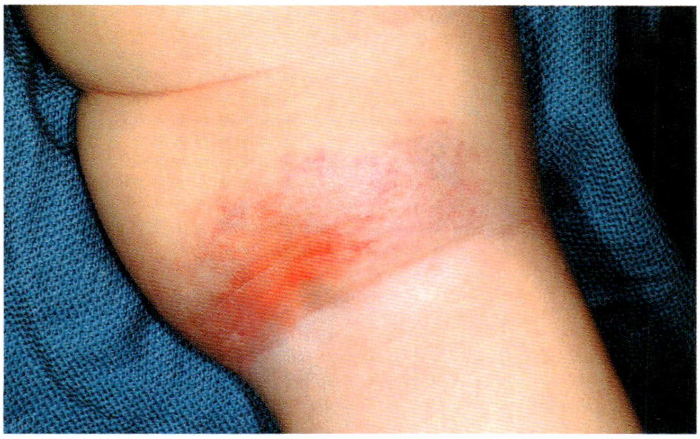

Fig. 12.52 Tufted angioma. This vascular plaque was mildly indurated to palpation. (Courtesy Annette Wagner, MD.)

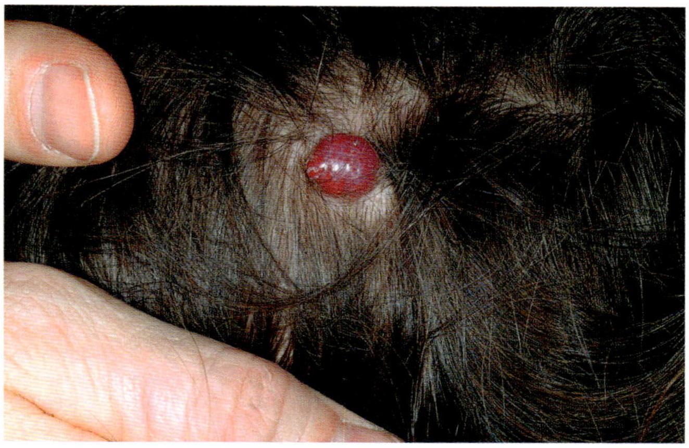

Fig. 12.53 Pyogenic granuloma. An acquired, vascular papule.

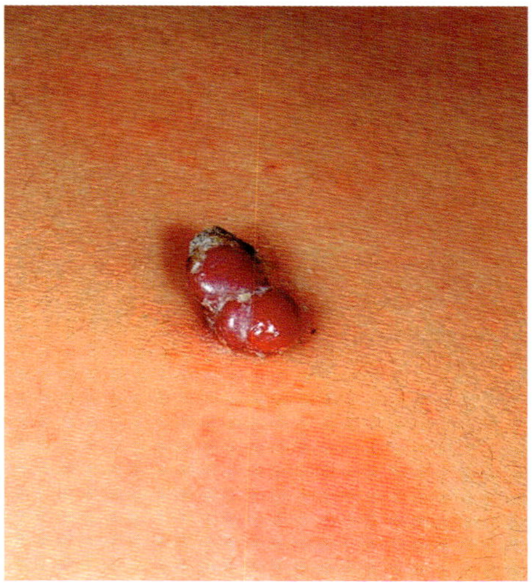

Fig. 12.54 Pyogenic granuloma. This lesion is multilobulated.

induration (Fig. 12.52).[162,163] Although these lesions may spontaneously involute over years, they tend to persist or gradually progress in most patients. Both KHE and TA are usually easily distinguished clinically from IH, although in some patients either of the former two may mimic the latter. Treatment with low-dose aspirin has been advocated as safe and effective for TA lesions that are large or symptomatic yet not associated with KMP.[164]

Treatment for KMP is challenging. Multiple different regimens have been reported without randomized studies to support or refute their efficacy. It seems clear that a multidisciplinary approach is optimal, including medical and surgical components of diagnosis and therapy.[157] Hematologic therapies include red blood cell transfusions, administration of fresh frozen plasma and cryoprecipitate, and antiplatelet therapy. Many experts recommend minimization of platelet transfusions given the risks of further platelet trapping and further expansion of the tumor. High-dose corticosteroids, antifibrinolytics, interferon-α, vincristine, sirolimus, cyclophosphamide, and antiplatelet therapy (particularly dual platelet blockade such as ticlopidine and aspirin) have been most often advocated.[165–169] Corticosteroid monotherapy appears to be effective in only a small subset of patients.[170,171] Vincristine was demonstrated useful in a retrospective study of 15 patients with KMP based on increased platelet count and fibrinogen level and decreased size of the tumor.[172] Four of these patients had a relapse and were again treated successfully with the agent.[172] Vincristine in combination with corticosteroids is considered first-line treatment for many experts, including the expert panel consensus-derived recommendation for KHE complicated by KMP.[161,165,167] Combination vincristine and ticlopidine, without or with aspirin (vincristine-aspirin-ticlopidine [VAT] therapy), has been reported useful in several patients with KMP.[173,174] The alternative mTOR inhibitor everolimus was reported very effective in two patients with KHE, one of whom had associated KMP and another with a treatment-resistant tumor involving the femur.[175,176] Early surgical intervention with full resection has been advocated for smaller lesions where this modality is feasible.[156] Other reported treatments include embolization, compression (usually in combination with other medical therapies), and radiation therapy.[171,177–181] Transcatheter arterial embolization plus vincristine was reported effective in a cohort of 17 infants with corticosteroid-resistant KMP.[182] Propranolol was associated with clinical response in only 25% of patients with KMP in one series, suggesting the need for further study of this agent; however, it was reportedly useful when dosed at higher levels than typically used for IH or when used in combination with corticosteroids.[183–185]

PYOGENIC GRANULOMA

Pyogenic granuloma (PG) is a common acquired vascular lesion of the skin and mucous membranes in infants and children. It presents as a bright red to red-brown, raised, slightly pedunculated or sessile papulonodule (Figs. 12.53 and 12.54). The base of sessile lesions may reveal a peripheral collarette of scale (Fig. 12.55). Although its appearance is usually solitary, PG may occasionally present as several lesions. In addition, secondary PG-like proliferations may occasionally

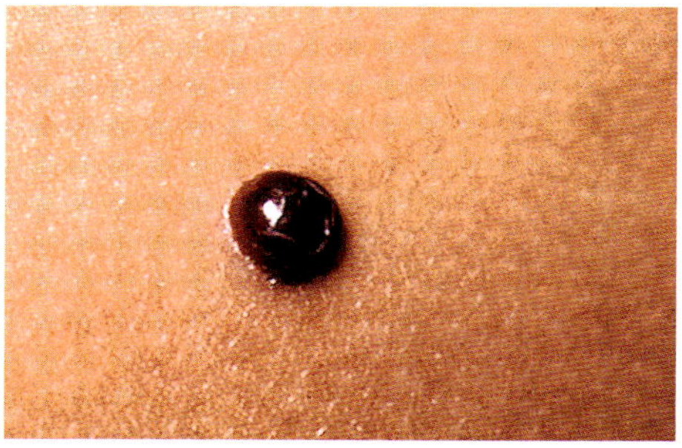

Fig. 12.55 Pyogenic granuloma. This lesion demonstrates the collarette of skin around the base of the lesion.

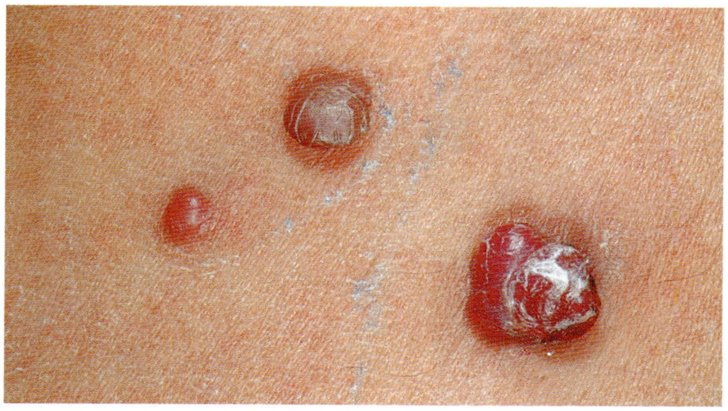

Fig. 12.56 This young girl with Klippel–Trénaunay syndrome has multiple, pyogenic granuloma–like papules overlying a port wine stain of her lower extremity.

occur on the surface of an existing PWS (Fig. 12.56), usually in the older child or young adult. Multiple, or "agminated," PG lesions have been reported in the setting of preexisting congenital vascular stains as well as in areas of preceding scalding burns.[186,187] PG is at risk for superficial ulceration and bleeding, which usually brings the patient to medical attention. The pathogenesis of PG is unknown. Despite the name, the lesions are not considered infectious. Although they may occur on any skin surface, they most commonly appear in areas subject to trauma, especially the hands, fingers, forearms, face, and occasionally the mucosal surfaces of the mouth. They have been described on the penile shaft after circumcision.[188] Although histologic evaluation is usually not necessary for diagnosis, pathologic examination reveals changes similar to those of a well-circumscribed IH.

The traditional therapy for PG is simple shave excision followed by treatment of the base with electrodesiccation, which achieves hemostasis and seems to help prevent recurrence. PDL therapy may be useful for the treatment of smaller lesions,[189] and the continuous wave/pulsed carbon dioxide (CO_2) laser has also been demonstrated effective.[190] Topical imiquimod cream, an immune response modifier, may be helpful in some patients.[191,192] Timolol solution, a topical β-blocker as discussed earlier in the section on IH, has also been reported effective in the treatment of PG.[193–195]

BACILLARY ANGIOMATOSIS

Bacillary angiomatosis (BA) is an exanthem characterized by cutaneous vascular lesions in association with *Bartonella* (previously *Rochalimaea*) infections. *Bartonella* species also cause cat-scratch disease, prolonged fever, hepatosplenic disease, ocular manifestations (including Parinaud oculoglandular syndrome), encephalopathy, hemolytic anemia, osteomyelitis, endocarditis, glomerulonephritis, and pulmonary disease.[196] BA occurs primarily in immunocompromised individuals and was originally described (and once seen quite commonly) in patients with acquired immunodeficiency syndrome (AIDS).[197] It has been rarely documented in immunocompetent children.[198,199] BA is caused by *B. henselae* and *B. quintana*, and transmission is via the body louse, a cat scratch, or cat fleas. The lesions may involve various tissues, including brain, bone, lymph nodes, GI tract, respiratory tract, and bone marrow. Osseous lesions are most commonly seen with *B. quintana* infection, and visceral involvement is caused almost solely by *B. henselae*.[200] However, skin lesions are the most common manifestation, may be caused by both species, and present as disseminated red to purple papules generally no larger than 1 to 2 cm in diameter. The clinical differential diagnosis may include PG and Kaposi sarcoma. Occasionally, BA may present with ulcerative lesions.[201] Liver peliosis is a similar condition affecting the liver and lymph nodes and usually caused by *B. quintana*.

The diagnosis of BA is confirmed by tissue biopsy with histologic examination, which reveals vascular proliferation and plump endothelial cells with the infecting bacilli identified on Warthin–Starry stain. Culture, polymerase chain reaction (PCR) studies, and serologic testing can also be useful in confirming the diagnosis. The possibility of human immunodeficiency virus (HIV) infection should be considered if BA is diagnosed. The disorder usually responds to antibiotic therapy with erythromycin, azithromycin, clarithromycin, levofloxacin, doxycycline, or rifampin.[202,203]

GLOMUS TUMOR

Glomus tumor (glomangioma, glomuvenous malformation) is a benign vascular lesion that usually presents as a blue papule or nodule. It represents a relatively uncommon hamartoma of the glomus body, which is a temperature-regulating AV shunt that bypasses the usual capillary bed of the dermis. The glomus cell, which proliferates in this disorder, is a modified smooth-muscle cell. Rarely seen in infants, these lesions may be solitary or multiple and occur in children as well as adults. Occasionally, nodular or plaque-like lesions may also occur.

Solitary glomus tumors, which represent 90% of all lesions,[204] do not appear to have a familial tendency. They are characterized by the clinical triad of paroxysmal pain, local tenderness, and cold sensitivity. Solitary lesions present as a blue-red nodule (Fig. 12.57) from 1 mm to several centimeters in size. They most often appear on the upper extremities, particularly the nailbeds, and occasionally on the lower extremities, head, neck, or penis. Although the cause is unknown, some lesions appear to be associated with previous trauma. The differential diagnosis of a solitary glomus tumor includes VM, blue nevus, melanoma, dermatofibroma, and leiomyoma. If occurring in an infant, IH may also be in the differential.

In contrast to the solitary type, multiple glomus tumors (often referred to as *glomuvenous malformations*) are often dominantly transmitted, may be painful or painless, and vary from a few lesions to several hundred. The familial nature may not be obvious because family members may have small lesions and never seek treatment.[205] They are relatively more common in children than adults, and although they can occur anywhere on the cutaneous surface, the majority involve the lower extremities. They may be regionally distributed or

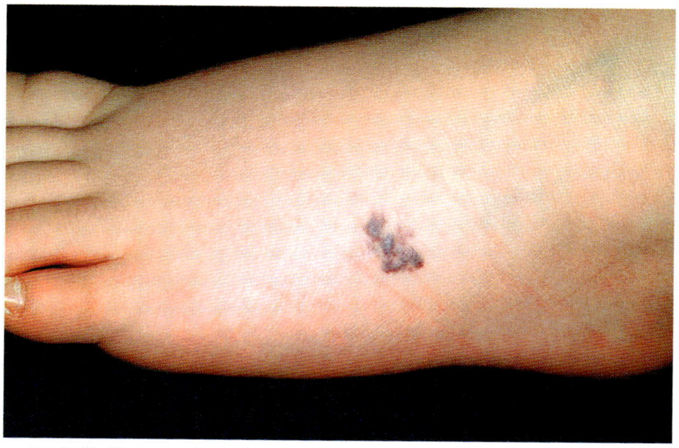

Fig. 12.57 Solitary glomus tumor. (Courtesy Sarah Chamlin, MD.)

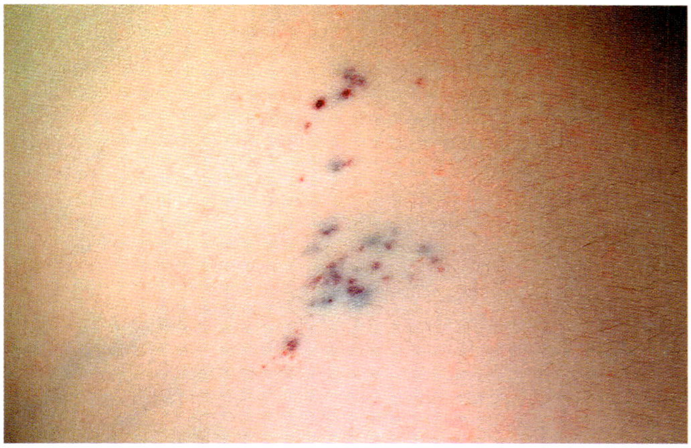

Fig. 12.58 Multiple glomus tumors. This patient had multiple blue papules and papulonodules.

generalized, and segmental patterns of presentation have been reported.[206,207] Affected individuals usually have truncating mutations in the glomulin *(GLMN)* gene.[208] Multiple glomus tumors appear as blue-purple, flat to dome-shaped papules, plaques, and nodules (Fig. 12.58) that vary from a few millimeters to several centimeters in size. The differential diagnosis of multiple glomus tumors includes leiomyomas, diffuse hemangiomatosis, and blue rubber–bleb nevi. Multiple glomus tumors, preferentially involving the fingers and toes, have been reported in individuals with neurofibromatosis type 1.[209,210]

A congenital variant of glomus tumor *(plaque-type glomus tumor* or *glomuvenous malformation)* has been described and is characterized by a blue-red, nodular plaque that may be painful, may show atrophy centrally, and tends to grow proportionate with the child's growth.[204,211] Congenital facial plaque-like glomus tumors may mimic VMs and can be quite disfiguring.[212]

Treatment of glomus tumors consists primarily of surgical excision, although this is not a feasible option for patients with multiple lesions and recurrence tends to be common. Sclerotherapy has been used with some success, as have CO_2 lasers.[213] Subungual glomus tumors are usually treated successfully with periungual or transungual surgical excision, although residual nail deformities may result.[214]

HEMANGIOPERICYTOMA

Hemangiopericytoma is a rare tumor that occurs in both an adult and a childhood form, although children account for fewer than 10% of all cases.[215] Congenital lesions are occasionally observed.[216,217] This tumor arises from pericytes, which are smooth-muscle cells that surround capillaries and postcapillary venules. Skin, subcutaneous, and muscular tissues may be involved, and any part of the body can be affected, the most common location being the lower extremities. Some experts suggest that a majority of lesions previously called *hemangiopericytomas* actually represent solitary fibrous tumors (originating from fibroblasts), and there is a likely relationship between these tumors and infantile myofibromatosis.[218,219]

Hemangiopericytoma may present in a variety of fashions without a distinctive or pathognomonic appearance. It often presents as a deep soft-tissue mass with slow growth. It may be flesh colored or have a blue-red hue. Multicentric lesions have been described in infants and tend to behave in a fashion similar to their solitary counterparts.[219,220] The diagnosis of hemangiopericytoma is based on the cellular and architectural features on tissue histologic examination.

The prognosis of this tumor in childhood is variable. It appears that children younger than 1 year of age (in which case, it is termed *infantile hemangiopericytoma* or the *congenital/infantile form of hemangiopericytoma)* have a better prognosis with a high response to chemotherapy. In children older than 1 year of age, the tumor behaves more similarly to those in adults and may be more aggressive.[215] Treatment consists of complete surgical resection when feasible, as well as radiotherapy and, when more extensive, chemotherapy.[218]

ANGIOLYMPHOID HYPERPLASIA WITH EOSINOPHILIA

Angiolymphoid hyperplasia with eosinophilia (ALHE) is an uncommon vascular proliferation disorder occurring most commonly in young adult women and only rarely in children. It presents as a subcutaneous mass of the head and neck region, especially around the ears or on the scalp. Regional lymph node enlargement and eosinophilia may be present, and treatment is usually by surgical excision, although observation, cryotherapy, laser ablation, steroids, radiation, and chemotherapy have been reported.[221]

Kimura disease is a closely related, yet distinct, chronic inflammatory disorder that occurs primarily in young Asian males. It is characterized by the triad of painless subcutaneous nodules in the head or neck region, blood and tissue eosinophilia, and elevated serum immunoglobulin (Ig) E levels.[222] Clinically, the lesions of Kimura disease present as solitary or multiple, purple-red papules, nodules, or deep swellings. The parotid and submandibular glands may be involved,[223] as may the oral mucosa, scalp, ears, or orbit. Unilateral cervical lymphadenopathy is commonly present. Laboratory evaluation consistently reveals eosinophilia and increased IgE.[224] Pediatric Kimura disease may be associated with nephritic syndrome, urticaria, and eczema.[225]

ALHE and Kimura disease may be confused with a variety of other entities, most commonly malignancies such as lymphoma, salivary gland tumors, or histiocytosis. These disorders histologically reveal vascular proliferation with eosinophils and mast cells, and their etiology remains unclear. Trauma may precede its onset, and it has been reported as a rare complication of ear piercing.[226] Treatment options for ALHE include surgical excision (although recurrence is common), steroids, chemotherapy, pulsed dye laser therapy, and radiation; propranolol was reported as effective in a young adult woman with the condition.[227,228]

Vascular Malformations and Malformation Syndromes

SALMON PATCH

The salmon patch (nevus simplex) is the most common vascular lesion of infancy. It occurs in 30% to 40% of all newborns and appears as a flat, dull pink, macular lesion on the posterior neck and scalp (Fig. 12.59), glabella (Fig. 12.60), forehead, upper eyelids, and occasionally the nose or nasolabial regions. When seen on the nape of the neck, it is commonly referred to as a *stork bite* and when on the forehead/glabella as the *angel kiss.* Although the salmon patch represents the most common form of CM, it is felt by many to be a form of persistent fetal circulation rather

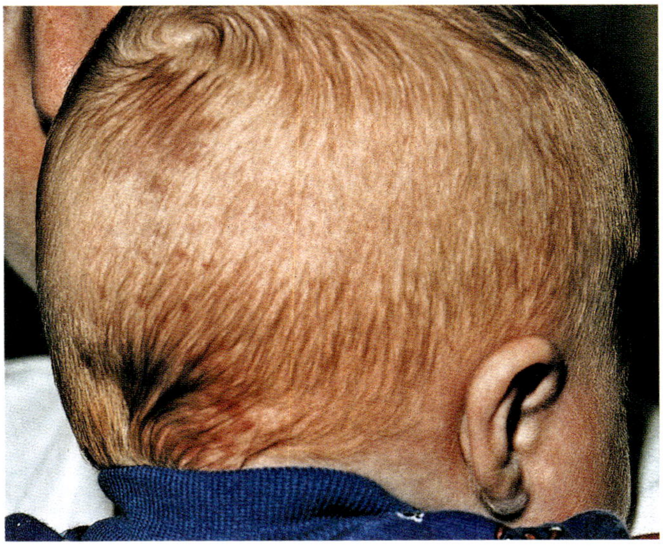

Fig. 12.59 Salmon patch. Faint, vascular macules of the occipital scalp.

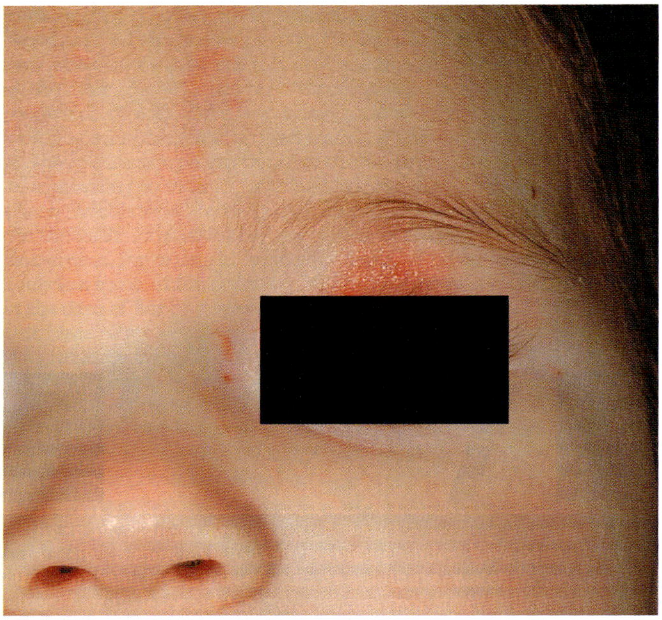

Fig. 12.60 Salmon patch. This blanchable vascular patch of the glabella and forehead becomes more prominent with crying or increased body temperature. Note the associated stain over the left superior eyelid.

than a true malformation. Although older nomenclature may include salmon patch under the category of PWS, this terminology should not be used because these lesions have distinct natural histories and differing significance in terms of potential syndrome associations. Salmon patches are usually isolated lesions without other associated findings. Nuchal or occipital stains may occasionally develop an associated overlying dermatitis (Fig. 12.61), which may respond to topical corticosteroids or PDL treatment, if necessary.[229]

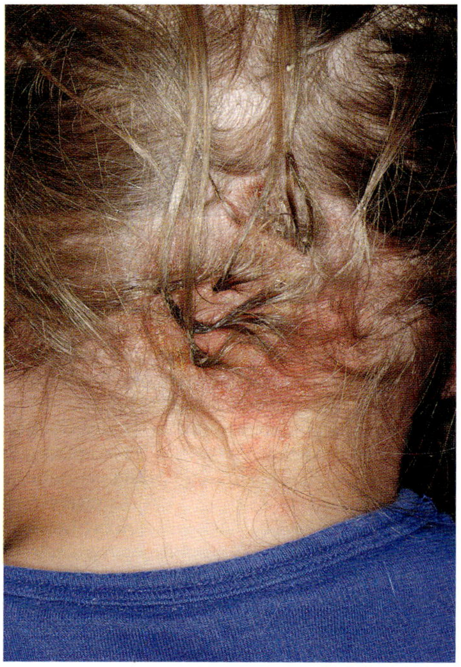

Fig. 12.61 Inflammatory nuchal salmon patch. This young girl developed dermatitis overlying her congenital salmon patch. Note the central purulence, which represented secondary bacterial superinfection. The dermatitis resolved after treatment with topical steroids and oral antibiotics.

No treatment is usually necessary for salmon patches, because 95% of facial lesions fade within the first 1 to 2 years of life. Lesions on the posterior neck or scalp (also known as *Unna nevus*) may fade, although some of these persist indefinitely. Because they are usually covered by hair, these lesions do not typically pose a cosmetic problem. Parents should be educated regarding the common finding of "reappearance" or accentuation of facial lesions during episodes of crying, breath-holding, straining with defecation, or physical exertion.

NEVUS FLAMMEUS/PORT WINE STAIN

Nevus flammeus, or PWS, is a congenital CM that may occur as an isolated lesion or in association with a variety of syndromes. These lesions present as macular (nonpalpable) stains with a pink (Fig. 12.62) to dark red (Fig. 12.63) color. Although an early PWS may be indistinguishable from an IH, these lesions are usually distinguished by their congenital presence and their static nature without the rapid proliferation and thickening that characterizes hemangiomas during the first months of life. PWS may darken progressively over many years, and occasionally lesions develop secondary proliferative (PG-like) vascular blebs on their surface (see Fig. 12.56). They may also become somewhat thickened and raised later in life. PWSs are often, but not always, unilateral, and the most common site of involvement is the face, although they may occur on any cutaneous surface.

The significance of PWS is twofold: the potential cosmetic impact of the lesion (especially facial PWS) on the developing child, and the

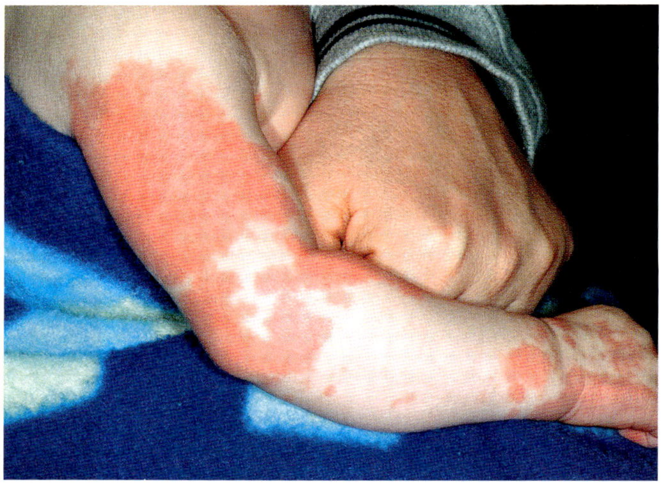

Fig. 12.62 Port wine stain: arm/hand.

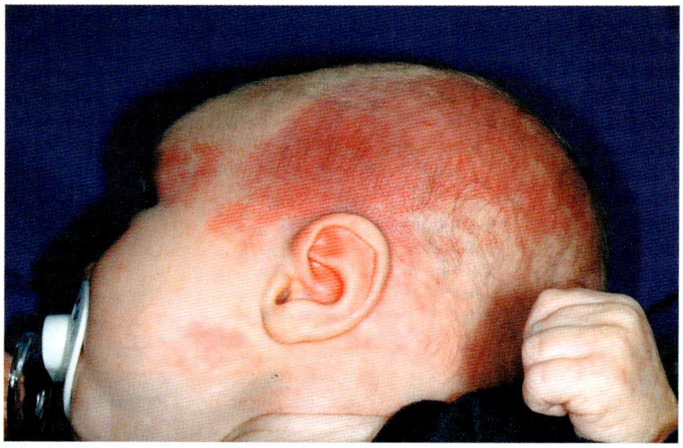

Fig. 12.63 Port wine stain: face/scalp.

Box 12.4 Port Wine Stain–Associated Syndromes

Sturge–Weber syndrome
Klippel–Trénaunay syndrome
Parkes Weber syndrome
Phakomatosis pigmentovascularis
Proteus syndrome
CLOVES syndrome
Macrocephaly–capillary malformation (M-CM) syndrome
Capillary malformation–arteriovenous malformation (CM-AVM) syndrome
Diffuse capillary malformation with overgrowth (DCMO)
Cobb syndrome
Bannayan–Riley–Ruvalcaba syndrome
Beckwith–Wiedemann syndrome
Von Hippel–Lindau disease
Rubinstein–Taybi syndrome
Wyburn-Mason syndrome
Roberts syndrome
Coat disease

CLOVES, Congenital lipomatous overgrowth, vascular malformations, epidermal nevi, and scoliosis/skeletal and spinal anomalies.

potential for syndrome associations. Box 12.4 lists some syndromes that may have PWS as a component. Several of these will be discussed later.

PWS lesions show little tendency toward spontaneous improvement or involution, and traditional therapy was limited to the use of tinted "cover-up" cosmetics (such as Covermark or Dermablend). Laser therapy has revolutionized the treatment of these lesions, and the flashlamp-pumped tunable PDL is the most accepted laser for PWS treatment.[230] PDL allows the targeting of short bursts of energy at intravascular hemoglobin (because of the specific wavelength of the emitted light) within the lesional vessels while sparing other tissue components and thus allowing for precise therapy. The absorbed light is converted into thermal energy, which leads to the coagulation of blood vessels. Treatment of PWS with PDL can be performed in the office or in conjunction with general anesthesia, depending on the size and location of the lesion and the age of the patient. Smaller, more localized lesions are often treated in the clinic setting without anesthesia. Concerns have been raised about repeated episodes of general anesthesia in young children and the potential effects on learning and behavioral outcomes.[231] In one retrospective review of patients who had received multiple rounds of anesthesia specifically for treatment of vascular anomalies before the age of 4 years, prevalence rates of attention-deficit/hyperactivity disorder (ADHD), anxiety, behavior problems, and motor or speech delay were similar to those reported in the US population.[232] However, other studies not specific to treatment of vascular lesions have suggested an increased risk of learning disability and ADHD, with decrease in cognitive ability and academic achievement, primarily in those who received multiple exposures before 3 years of age,[231] and animal studies support detrimental effects of general anesthetics on the growth and development of the very young brain.[233] This is an area of ongoing investigation, and in the interim it is prudent for clinicians to discuss potential risks with caretakers of young children, allowing for well-informed decisions regarding treatment under general anesthesia. Use of topical anesthetics for these lesions is often avoided given the associated blanching of vessels, which makes the stains more challenging to accurately treat.[230]

PDL therapy is usually performed over several sessions separated in time by 6 to 8 weeks and can be quite effective in lightening these lesions, thereby minimizing their cosmetic and psychosocial significance. Although there may be psychological benefits of PDL therapy of facial PWS early in life,[234] studies evaluating efficacy as a function of patient age have yielded mixed results. Some authors have reported optimal treatment response in patients younger than 1 year of age, whereas others have found no evidence that treatment during early childhood is more effective than treatment at a later age.[235,236] In general, lesions over bony areas of the face (e.g., the forehead), lateral cheeks, chest, and proximal arms seem to respond best to PDL therapy, whereas those over the midface and distal extremities respond less well.[230] PWS of the central face may not respond as well as those located in more lateral locations, possibly because of the deeper location and greater diameter of the vessels in the former distribution.[237,238] Hypertrophic PWS respond more poorly to PDL.[239] When PDL is being considered for PWS, it is important for the patient and parents to understand that complete clearance is rare and 20% to 30% of PWSs are resistant to the treatment.[240] Topical rapamycin in conjunction with PDL has been reported to increase the efficacy of the laser therapy.[241]

Sturge–Weber Syndrome

Sturge–Weber syndrome (SWS; encephalofacial or encephalotrigeminal angiomatosis) is a neuroectodermal syndrome characterized by a PWS in the distribution of the first (ophthalmic) branch of the trigeminal nerve (V1) in association with leptomeningeal angiomatosis (presenting usually with seizures) and glaucoma. There are rare reports of patients with classic brain and ophthalmic findings of SWS in the absence of a facial PWS.[242–245] A somatic activating mutation in *GNAQ* (specifically, a single-nucleotide variant c.548G>A, p.Arg183Gln) has been identified as the cause behind SWS and has also been found in a significant number of individuals with nonsyndromic PWS.[246–248]

Patients with SWS have a PWS that has classically been described as occurring in a V1 distribution (Fig. 12.64) but may also have "multidermatomal" or more extensive cutaneous involvement. Overall it appears that approximately 7% to 8% of patients with a trigeminal or "high-risk" (hemifacial, forehead) PWS have associated imaging findings, glaucoma, and/or seizures.[249,250] Involvement of the region of the V1 dermatome seems to be consistent in all patients.[245] Involvement of the other trigeminal dermatomes may be useful in predicting the risk of SWS. In one study, involvement of V1, V2, and V3 was associated with an increased incidence of SWS, as was bilateral trigeminal involvement.[245,249] Another study comparing unilateral to bilateral facial PWS found a higher incidence of glaucoma and leptomeningeal angiomatosis with bilateral involvement and greater risk of CNS involvement when there was complete (versus incomplete) involvement of V1.[251] Although the exact innervation of the lower eyelid is controversial (V1 versus V2), it seems that involvement of both upper and lower eyelids portends a significantly higher risk of SWS.[245,249] When PWS lesions are unilateral, there is usually a sharp demarcation at the midline. More recently it has been suggested that the PWS of SWS do not correspond to trigeminal dermatomes but rather to areas delineated by somatic mosaicism[252] or embryonic vasculature of the face.[253] According to these contemporary observations,

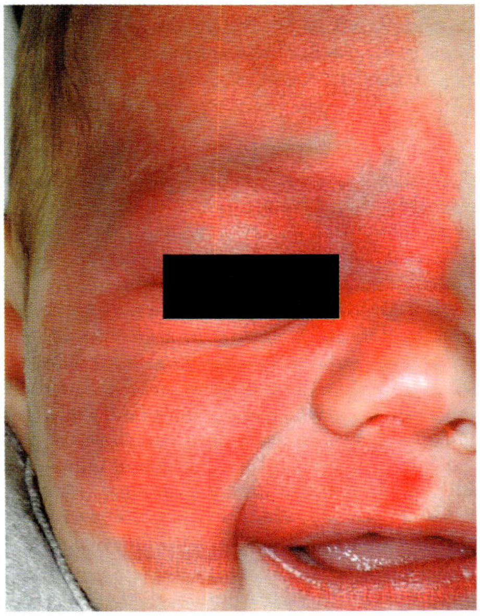

Fig. 12.64 Port wine stain. This lesion involves both the V1 and V2 trigeminal dermatomes in this infant with Sturge–Weber syndrome. (Courtesy Annette Wagner, MD.)

hemifacial and forehead (either medial or lateral) involvement portend the greatest risks for SWS.[252,253]

CNS disease is another component of SWS. Seizures are the most common CNS feature and often have their onset during the first year of life. The seizures of SWS may be difficult to control, and both early onset and increased seizure intensity are associated with future developmental and cognitive delay.[245,254,255] Headaches (including migraines), stroke-like episodes, focal neurologic impairments, cognitive deficits, and emotional and behavioral problems including depression, violent behavior, and self-inflicted injury are also more common in SWS.[245,256] Low self-esteem is common in relation to the facial PWS.

Leptomeningeal angiomatosis is a classic component of the syndrome, and lesions are commonly ipsilateral to the cutaneous vascular stain. Cerebral atrophy is a common radiologic finding, as is enlargement of the choroid plexus and venous abnormalities. Size of the PWS has been shown to correlate with the ipsilateral size and severity of brain involvement by angiomatosis and atrophy, as well as neurologic impairment.[257] MRI is the modality of choice for identifying these changes, although CT scans are better at detecting the classic cortical calcifications, which are also seen.[258] These calcifications follow the convolutions of the cerebral cortex and are characterized by double-contoured parallel streaks of calcification ("tram lines"). Intracerebral calcifications may be visible during early infancy and can often help confirm the diagnosis before other characteristic features are present. Diffusion MRI, postcontrast fluid-attenuated inversion recovery (FLAIR) imaging, and high-resolution blood oxygen level–dependent (BOLD) magnetic resonance venography may be useful in the imaging of suspected SWS.[256] Electroencephalography (EEG) is a good option for assessing abnormal brain activity in young children and may be useful in identifying patients at risk for future neurologic symptoms. However, a concerning EEG should always be followed by appropriate radiographic imaging.[259] Transcranial Doppler ultrasound measurement of cerebral blood flow, which may be decreased in SWS patients, may be useful in predicting neurologic progression.[260]

Ocular involvement occurs in around 60% of patients with SWS.[245] Glaucoma is the most common ocular finding, and it may present at any time between birth and the fourth decade. It may be unilateral or bilateral, with the latter being more common in patients with bilateral facial PWS. Vascular malformations of the eye in patients with SWS may involve the conjunctiva, episclera, choroid, and retina.[261] Other eye findings include nevus of Ota, buphthalmos, and blindness.[262]

Care of the child with SWS should be multidisciplinary. Dermatologic, neurologic, and ophthalmologic follow-up care is indicated, and the primary care provider must provide anticipatory guidance and support. Other specialty services may become necessary, including plastic surgery, neurosurgery, interventional radiology, and physical and occupational therapy. Referral to support organizations is useful. The Sturge–Weber Foundation (www.sturge-weber.org) provides education and support to individuals with this condition and other disorders associated with PWS.

The primary aim of treatment in SWS is the minimization or elimination of seizure activity because seizures may result in significant neurologic and developmental consequences. Referral to a pediatric neurologist is recommended, and although some advocate for early presymptomatic MR imaging in the setting of high-risk facial PWS, one large literature review suggests against this recommendation given the lack of data to confirm improved neurodevelopmental outcomes.[263] Although the primary management for seizures is with pharmacologic agents, surgical therapy may become necessary. Visually guided lobectomy with excision of the angiomatous cortex is considered the primary surgical approach in a patient with focal lesions.[264] Hemispherectomy is often advised for patients with intractable seizures and unihemispheric involvement. This radical therapy is often successful, with decreased seizure activity and, in some patients, cognitive and behavioral improvement.[265,266] Presymptomatic therapy with low-dose aspirin has been advocated by some for young children before the onset of seizures or strokes in an effort to decrease the incidence of these complications and optimize neurodevelopmental outcome.[259,267,268] The modified Atkins diet and ketogenic diet have been used in some patients to help control seizures.[259,269]

Phakomatosis Pigmentovascularis

Phakomatosis pigmentovascularis (PPV) is a term used to describe the association of a nevus flammeus (PWS) with a pigmented nevus or, in some cases, a nevus anemicus. PPV has traditionally been classified into four types. A fifth type of PPV was subsequently proposed as the concomitant findings of cutis marmorata telangiectatica congenita (CMTC) and dermal melanocytosis (formerly called Mongolian spots).[270] The traditional classification of PPV is shown in Table 12.5. In 2005 a simpler classification was proposed that includes only three types: *phakomatosis cesioflammea* (blue spots and nevus flammeus); *phakomatosis spilorosea* (nevus spilus and nevus flammeus); and *phakomatosis cesiomarmorata* (blue spots and cutis marmorata telangiectatica congenita).[271] Although the cause of PPV remained unknown for years, mosaic activating mutations in *GNA11* and *GNAQ* have been found in some patients with PPV and extensive dermal melanocytosis.[272] Nevus anemicus is a distinct vascular birthmark characterized by blanching of cutaneous blood vessels, hence presenting as a "white" (actually vasoconstricted) patch of skin (Fig. 12.65) that becomes unnoticeable when the surrounding skin is blanched with a glass slide (diascopy). These lesions may occur as part of PPV (types II, III, and IV) but may also be seen as sporadic lesions.

The most common form of PPV is type II (cesioflammea type), consisting of nevus flammeus and congenital dermal melanocytosis (including former Mongolian spots, nevus of Ota) (Fig. 12.66). Without extracutaneous involvement, the subtype designation *a* is used (e.g., PPV type IIa). When systemic involvement is present, the subtype designation *b* is used (e.g., PPV type IIb). Systemic involvement usually consists of similar changes to those seen in SWS or Klippel–

Table 12.5 Traditional Classification of Phakomatosis Pigmentovascularis*

Type†	Findings
I	Nevus flammeus + epidermal nevus
II	Nevus flammeus + dermal melanocytosis ± nevus anemicus
III	Nevus flammeus + nevus spilus ± nevus anemicus
IV	Nevus flammeus + dermal melanocytosis + nevus spilus ± nevus anemicus
V	Cutis marmorata telangiectatica congenita + dermal melanocytosis

*See text for further discussion.
†Further subdivided into *a*, skin abnormalities only; *b*, skin abnormalities and systemic abnormalities.

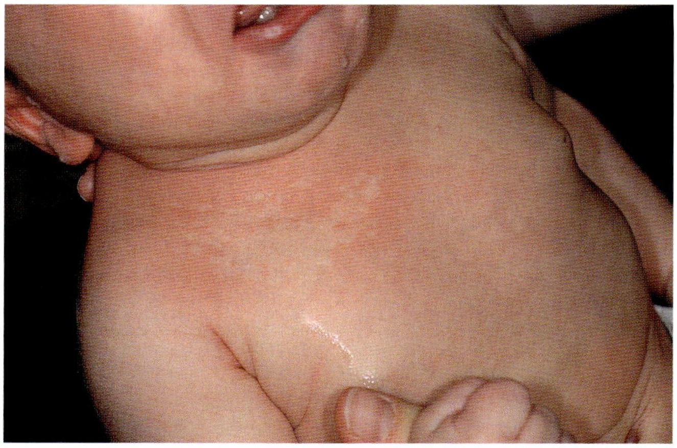

Fig. 12.65 Nevus anemicus. Note the well-demarcated patch of hypovascular blanching on this infant's upper chest. This area became more prominent with crying, as during this photograph.

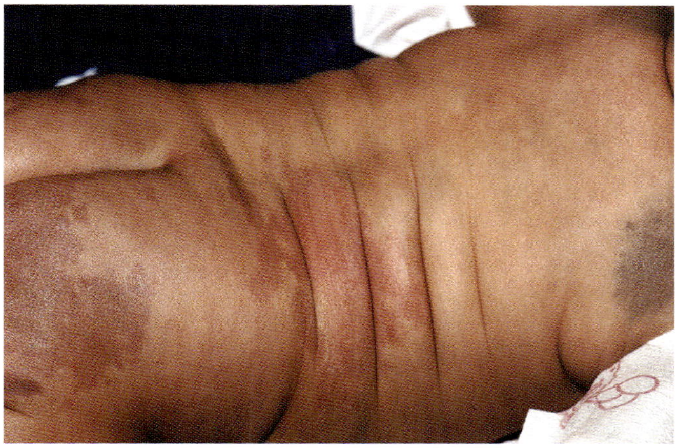

Fig. 12.66 Phakomatosis pigmentovascularis type II. This infant has port wine stains in combination with congenital dermal melanocytosis (lesions formerly known as Mongolian spots and nevus of Ito).

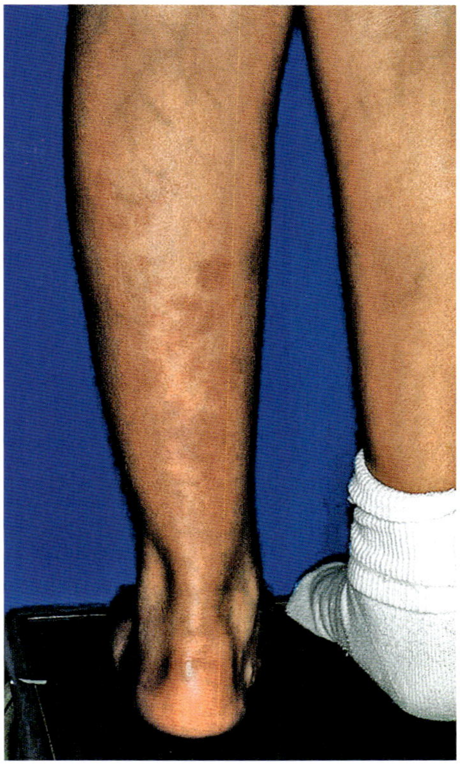

Fig. 12.67 Klippel–Trénaunay syndrome. Lower extremity port wine stain with mild hemihypertrophy.

Trénaunay syndrome.[273] This involvement is usually related to the body surface area affected by the vascular lesion.[274] In one series, nevus of Ota was a common associated finding.[275] Neurologic involvement in PPV may include psychomotor retardation, seizures, cerebral atrophy, and hydrocephalus, and ophthalmologic associations include conjunctival melanocytosis, episcleral vascular malformations, and glaucoma.[276,277] Other potential associations include asymmetric growth or overgrowth, scoliosis, spinal dysraphism, and kidney anomalies.

Therapy for the cutaneous lesions of PPV is generally not necessary, although PDL treatment may be useful for the nevus flammeus. Lesions of dermal melanocytosis may or may not fade spontaneously with time.

Klippel–Trénaunay and Parkes Weber Syndromes

Klippel–Trénaunay (KT) syndrome is a sporadic disorder characterized by the triad of vascular malformation, venous varicosity, and hyperplasia of soft tissue and bone. The vascular malformation is most often capillary in nature, although other vessel types may also be involved. The various lesions of KT syndrome are usually distributed on the same extremity, although other areas may be involved. The lower extremity is the most common location affected. When AVMs are also present, patients have been invariably referred to as having Klippel–Trénaunay–Weber (KTW) syndrome or Parkes Weber syndrome.[278] KT syndrome has been confirmed in some patients to be associated with mutations in *PIK3CA* (see more in next section).[279–281]

Patients with KT syndrome exhibit a CM that may vary from fairly localized, faint lesions to extensive, bright red or purple stains (Figs. 12.67 and 12.68). These lesions are usually present at birth or become evident during early infancy. Prominent superficial veins may be present, and venous varicosities often develop with aging, being present in nearly all patients older than 12 years of age.[278] These varicosities may become quite large and tortuous and may predispose patients to episodes of thrombophlebitis. Hypertrophy of the affected body part is another component of the syndrome and usually presents with increased limb girth and length (Fig. 12.69). The majority of this hypertrophy is related to soft tissue and fat overgrowth, although bony hypertrophy is also observed.[278] Although the cause of this overgrowth is unknown, local hyperemia and augmented arterial flow related to the vascular abnormalities are hypothesized causal factors. Digital anomalies may also be present in patients with KT syndrome and include macrodactyly, syndactyly, ectrodactyly, clinodactyly, and camptodactyly.[282]

Lymphatic disease seems to be more common than originally thought in patients with KT syndrome. This component may be manifested as lymphangiectasia, large LMs, lymphedema, vascular blebs (Fig. 12.70), and pseudoverrucous papules. Patients with sharply demarcated and "geographic" vascular stains may have an increased likelihood of lymphatic involvement.[283]

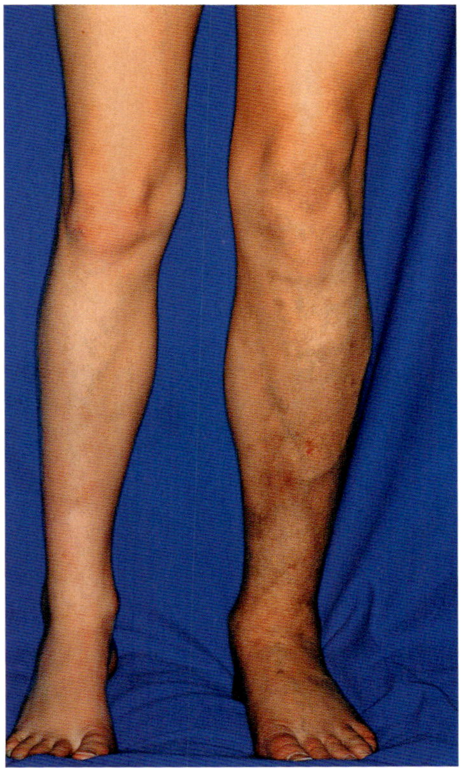

Fig. 12.68 Klippel–Trénaunay syndrome. This patient has the characteristic triad, including port wine stain, hemihypertrophy, and venous varicosities. (Courtesy Sarah Chamlin, MD.)

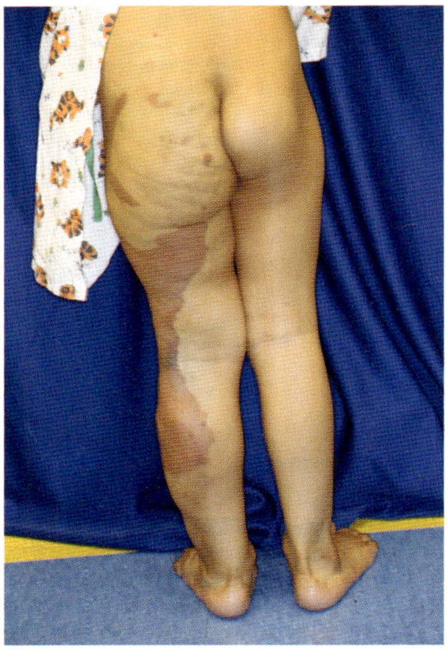

Fig. 12.69 Klippel–Trénaunay syndrome. This young girl has hemihypertrophy and vascular malformations, including capillary (well-demarcated red stains on the skin, as shown here), venous, and lymphatic types. Multiple vascular blebs were also present on the medial thigh.

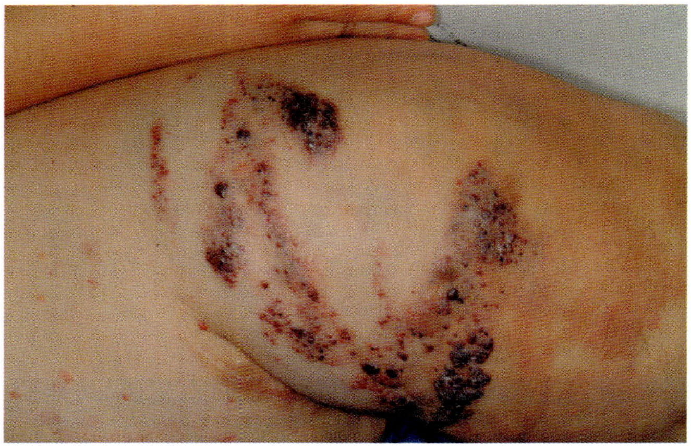

Fig. 12.70 Klippel–Trénaunay syndrome with vascular blebs. Note the purple, translucent papules overlying the vascular stain on the lower extremity of this young boy.

Complications of KT syndrome, in addition to occasional thrombophlebitis as mentioned previously, include coagulopathy, congestive heart failure (in the presence of hemodynamically significant AVM), pulmonary embolism, stasis dermatitis, cutaneous ulcerations, and bleeding. Vascular malformations may occasionally involve the GI tract, liver, spleen, genitourinary tract, and heart, and life-threatening GI bleeding has been reported.[284] Orthopedic difficulties related to the overgrowth include compensatory scoliosis and hip dislocation. Facial involvement may result in premature dental eruption, facial asymmetry, and malocclusion.[285] Pain is a potentially debilitating problem for patients with KT syndrome and may be related to multiple causes, including superficial or deep thrombosis, cellulitis, calcifications, arthritis, and neuropathic origins.[286] Treatments for KT syndrome are primarily supportive and may include compression garments, chronic pain therapy, laser therapy for the cutaneous stains, and vascular/orthopedic surgical procedures as needed. The clearest indication for surgical therapy is leg-length discrepancy projected to exceed 2 cm at skeletal maturity, which can be treated with epiphysiodesis in the growing child.[287] Physical and occupational therapy should be considered, and referral to the Klippel–Trénaunay Support Group (www.k-t.org) is strongly encouraged. In addition, there are a variety of resources available for individuals who require different shoe sizes (including www.oddshoe.org, www.oddshoefinder.com, and the National Shoe Retailers Association at www.nsra.org).

Proteus Syndrome

Proteus syndrome is a rare and sporadic disorder characterized by postnatal segmental overgrowth of multiple tissues. This overgrowth may involve the skin and subcutis, connective tissues, CNS, and viscera.[288] The involvement characteristically occurs in a patchy (mosaic or segmental) and asymmetric pattern. Proteus syndrome was named after the Greek god Proteus, who had the ability to assume various forms to avoid capture.[289] Joseph Merrick, whose life was characterized in the story *The Elephant Man*, is believed to have had Proteus syndrome, although he was originally thought to have had neurofibromatosis type 1. A mosaic activating mutation in *AKT1*, which encodes the AKT1 kinase, has been identified in several individuals with Proteus syndrome.[290] Previously a potential association with somatic mutations in the tumor suppressor gene *PTEN* (see Chapter 9) was suggested, although some now designate this cohort as having **s**egmental **o**vergrowth, **l**ipomatosis, **AVM**, and **e**pidermal **n**evus (SOLAMEN) syndrome.[291]

Cutaneous manifestations of Proteus syndrome include connective tissue hamartomas that primarily involve the palms and soles and result in cerebriform hyperplasia (Fig. 12.71). Lipomas and extensive fatty hyperplasia may be found in the subcutaneous tissues as well as more diffusely, at times involving body cavities, muscles, and limbs, and regional absence of fat may also occur. Epidermal nevi are common. A variety of cutaneous and subcutaneous vascular malformations may occur, including capillary, venous, and LMs. Patchy hypoplasia of the dermis may occur, resulting in prominent cutaneous venous structures.[292]

Other features of Proteus syndrome include disproportionate overgrowth that may involve the extremities, hands, feet, digits (macrodactyly; Fig. 12.72), skull (macrocephaly, exostoses), vertebrae, external auditory meatus, and viscera.[293] Dysmorphic facial features are occasionally present and include dolichocephaly, elongated facies, low nasal bridge, downslanting palpebral fissures, and wide or anteverted nares. Adenomas of the ovaries or parotid glands may occur with increased incidence in patients with Proteus syndrome. Hemimegalencephaly is the most common CNS finding, and ocular manifestations may include strabismus, nystagmus, high myopia, cataracts, and retinal pigmentary abnormalities.[294,295]

Diagnostic criteria for Proteus syndrome, which include general nonspecific criteria (mosaic distribution of lesions, sporadic occurrence, and progressive course) as well as multiple specific criteria, may be useful both clinically and in the research arena.[296] Evaluation and management of the patient with Proteus syndrome may include skeletal survey, MRI of clinically affected areas, and consultation with dermatology, genetics, and orthopedic specialists when necessary. Both the medical and emotional aspects of the disorder must be considered. Supportive counseling and referral to the Proteus Syndrome Foundation (www.proteus-syndrome.org) are useful.

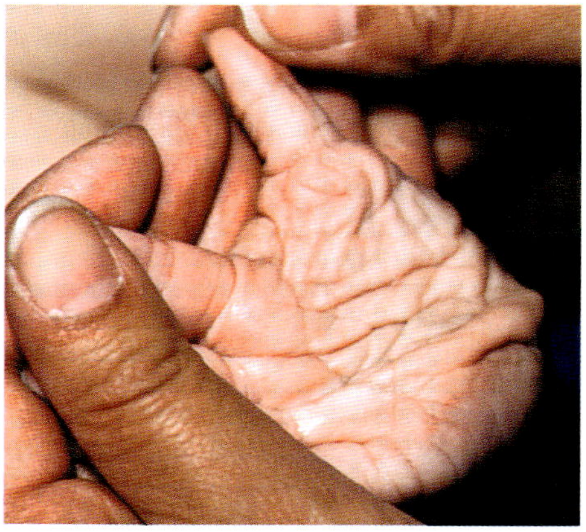

Fig. 12.71 Proteus syndrome, cerebriform palmar hyperplasia.

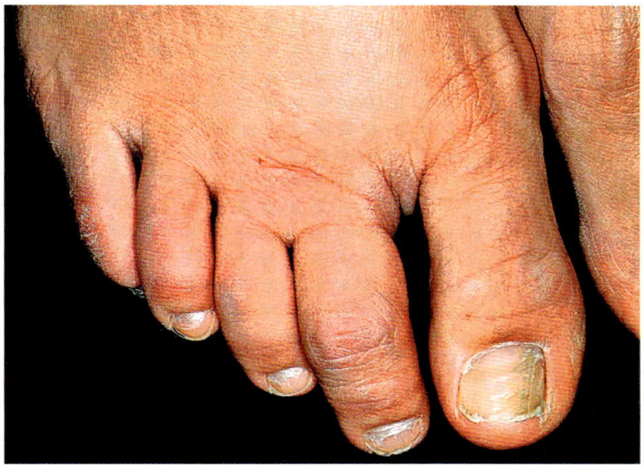

Fig. 12.72 Proteus syndrome, macrodactyly. Note overgrowth of the second toe.

CLOVES Syndrome and *PIK3CA*-Related Overgrowth Spectrum

CLOVES syndrome refers to an overgrowth syndrome characterized by congenital lipomatous overgrowth, vascular malformations, epidermal nevi, and scoliosis/skeletal and spinal anomalies. Originally termed *CLOVE syndrome* by Sapp et al., the suggestion for expanding the acronym to *CLOVES* was made by Alomari one year later based on observations of associated spinal and skeletal involvement.[297,298] Patients with this disorder are often born with lipomatous masses involving the thoracic and abdominal regions among other areas. They may have slow-flow vascular malformations such as capillary, lymphatic, and venous malformations but may also have spinal or paraspinal fast-flow lesions consistent with AVMs, and these lesions may result in spinal cord injury, including myelopathy.[299] Linear epidermal nevi are present and may be extensive. Musculoskeletal defects often involve the hands and feet (most commonly overgrowth, macrodactyly, or sandal gap toe deformity) but may also include scoliosis, spina bifida, vertebral anomalies, congenital hip dysplasia, pectus excavatum, facial skeletal anomalies, patellar chondromalacia, and rib defects. Neurologic manifestations may include tethering or AVM of the spinal cord, spasticity, paresis, agenesis of the corpus callosum, hemimegalencephaly, neuronal migration defects, and neural tube defects.[300,301] Although there is some significant overlap in the clinical features of CLOVES and Proteus syndromes, there are several distinguishing features in CLOVES syndrome, including the lack of cerebriform connective tissue hamartomas of the palms and soles, the progressive enlargement (and recurrence after resection) of the lipomatous masses, and the presence of paraspinal high-flow vascular lesions.[300] Given the potentially increased risk of Wilms tumor in patients with CLOVES syndrome, quarterly abdominal ultrasonography should be considered until age 7 years.[302]

CLOVES syndrome has been ascribed to postzygotic mutations in *PIK3CA*, a gene involved in the PI3K-AKT growth-signaling pathway. Various segmental overgrowth disorders have been described in association with mutations in this gene and have been termed *PIK3CA-related overgrowth spectrum (PROS)*.[303] Other disorders that fall under this mutation umbrella include KT syndrome, fibroadipose overgrowth, isolated lymphatic malformations, fibroadipose vascular anomaly, and some megalencephaly syndromes, including macrocephaly–capillary malformation syndrome (see later), hemimegalencephaly, and dysplastic megalencephaly.[279,280,301,303] Because *PIK3CA* is known to be a cancer predisposition gene, long-term cancer surveillance strategies should be considered in patients with these disorders.[280] Targeted therapy via *PIK3CA* inhibition is a promising potential treatment strategy and was demonstrated helpful in improving disease symptoms, including shrinkage in vascular tumors, improvement in hemodynamic parameters and scoliosis, and decreased pain and fatigue, in 19 patients with PROS.[304]

Macrocephaly–Capillary Malformation Syndrome

The combination of CMTC-type skin changes and macrocephaly, occurring along with other findings such as abnormal somatic growth (asymmetry or overgrowth), craniofacial and skeletal anomalies, developmental delay, neonatal hypotonia, neurologic abnormalities with abnormal findings on neuroimaging, mental retardation, syndactyly/polydactyly, joint hypermobility, and connective tissue abnormalities, was originally termed *macrocephaly-CMTC*.[305,306] Subsequently, however, it was suggested that the vascular lesions seen in this setting are more consistent with reticulate PWSs and that this constellation is more appropriately termed *macrocephaly–capillary malformation syndrome (M-CM)*.[307,308] Other names for this entity include *megalencephaly–capillary malformation syndrome* and *megalencephaly–capillary malformation–polymicrogyria syndrome (MCAP)*. Centrofacial capillary malformations seem to be common in patients with this syndrome and most notably involve the nose, glabella, lip, and philtrum.[307,308] The most common findings on neuroimaging include ventriculomegaly, cavum septum pellucidum, cerebellar tonsillar herniation, megalencephaly, and cerebral and/or cerebellar asymmetry.[309,310] It is unclear whether patients with M-CM are at increased risk for Wilms tumor.[311]

Diffuse Capillary Malformation with Overgrowth

The term *diffuse capillary malformation with overgrowth (DCMO)* has been proposed to describe patients with extensive capillary stains in association with proportionate overgrowth.[312] These infants have congenital stains that may be reticulate or more homogeneous. Soft tissue or bony overgrowth develops and does not appear to correlate to the location of the vascular stains. In a series of 73 patients, most overgrowth was limited to an extremity, with hemihypertrophy occurring less commonly. Digital anomalies included syndactyly, sandal gap toe deformity (widened first interdigital web space), and macrodactyly.[312] These patients tended to do well overall, without noted developmental delay. Although the risk of Wilms tumor in this patient group remains unclear, in one retrospective review of 67 patients with DCMO seen over an 18-year period, no cases were reported.[311]

Capillary Malformation–Arteriovenous Malformation Syndrome

Capillary malformations occurring in a familial fashion were demonstrated to be associated with the *CMC1* locus on chromosome 5q in 2002 and subsequently shown to be associated with inactivating mutations in the gene *RASA1*.[313,314] These individuals were also shown to have a predisposition toward the development of AVMs (see Arteriovenous Malformation section), AV fistulae, or Parkes Weber syndrome, and this autosomal dominant disorder was subsequently named *capillary malformation–arteriovenous malformation (CM-AVM) syndrome*. The hallmark skin lesions are CMs that are typically multiple (Fig. 12.73) and occur in a haphazard distribution; may reveal pink, red, brown, or gray coloration; and occasionally have an associated white halo.[315,316] These white halos may be an early finding reflective of AVM.[317] They are often present at birth but may continue to develop during childhood, a key feature that should suggest the need to consider this diagnosis. Mucosal CMs (e.g., of the tongue, lips, or conjunctivae) may also occur in CM-AVM syndrome.[318] It is generally believed that CM-AVM syndrome is underrecognized.

The AVMs in CM-AVM syndrome may be cutaneous, subcutaneous, intramuscular, intraosseous, or cerebral, and arteriovenous fistulae (AVFs) may also be present. Occasionally one patient may have two or more AVMs or AVFs. The most common locations for AVMs are the extremities, intracranial and intraspinal regions, face, and neck.[318] Aneurysmal malformation of the vein of Galen has been described.[316] Spinal AVMs or AVFs have also been recognized in association with CM-AVM syndrome and *RASA1* mutation,[319] highlighting the importance of both brain and spine imaging (as well as mutation analysis) for patients in whom the disorder is suspected.[320] More recently, a genome-wide linkage study on a CM-AVM family, with whole-exome sequencing on nine unrelated families, led to identification of mutations in *EPHB4*, a gene that encodes a transmembrane receptor expressed in endothelial cells during vascular development.[321] The authors proposed the name *CM-AVM2* to distinguish this presentation from *CM-AVM1*, which is associated with *RASA1* mutations. Clinically, CM-AVM2 differs in that Bier spots (see later in this chapter) are more common, the large CMs may have a pale central region, and telangiectasias (mainly lips, perioral, and upper trunk) are present.

Bannayan–Riley–Ruvalcaba Syndrome

Bannayan–Riley–Ruvalcaba syndrome (BRRS) is an autosomal dominant, multiple hamartoma syndrome caused by mutations in the

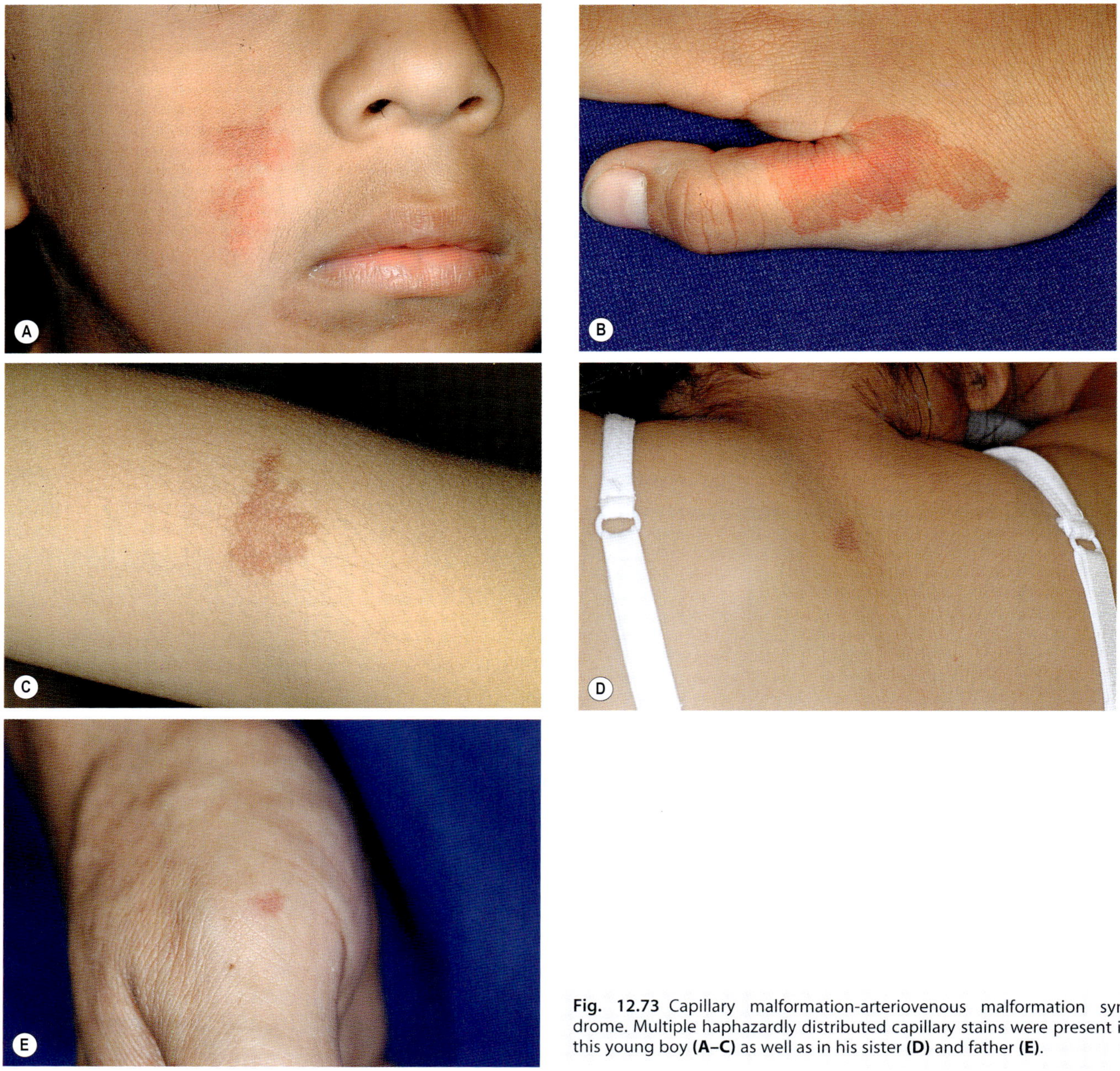

Fig. 12.73 Capillary malformation-arteriovenous malformation syndrome. Multiple haphazardly distributed capillary stains were present in this young boy **(A–C)** as well as in his sister **(D)** and father **(E)**.

PTEN gene. This syndrome is one of the so-called *PTEN hamartoma tumor syndromes*, which also include Cowden syndrome (see Chapter 9), Lhermitte–Duclos syndrome, and some cases of Proteus syndrome. The hallmarks of BRRS are macrocephaly, lipomas, penile lentigines (most notably involving the glans penis; Fig. 12.74), developmental delay, and vascular malformations. The latter have been inconsistently described in the literature as "hemangiomas" or "angiomas" but are actually vascular malformations usually of the capillary type. AVM has also been described in patients with BRRS.[322] Cowden syndrome and BRRS are considered allelic disorders and share several clinical features, possibly including the predisposition to malignant tumors known to exist in the former.[323,324] Some consider these two disorders to be one condition with variable expression and age-related penetrance.

Cobb Syndrome

Cobb syndrome (cutaneomeningospinal angiomatosis) consists of the association of a cutaneous vascular malformation with a vascular malformation (often an AVM) involving the same metamere of the spinal cord. The cutaneous and spinal cord lesions usually correspond within a segment or two of the involved dermatome.[325] The skin lesions present as a dermatomal CM with or without a deeper vascular component and occasionally with hyperkeratosis of the surface suggestive of an angiokeratoma. The importance of recognizing this cutaneous lesion lies in the resultant ability to image the spine and refer a patient for neurosurgical therapy before symptoms ensue. Neurologic symptoms related to the spinal cord vascular malformation may include root pain, motor dysfunction, paresthesias, and spastic paralysis.[325,326]

Evaluation of the patient with a dermatomal CM should include MRI of the corresponding region of the spinal cord with consideration for spinal angiography. Treatment options may include surgery (when feasible), endovascular embolization, radiation, and steroid therapy, and the goal of therapy is to minimize neurologic sequelae by reducing mass effect, venous hypertension, and vascular steal.[327]

Beckwith–Wiedemann Syndrome

Beckwith–Wiedemann syndrome (BWS) is a genetic overgrowth syndrome characterized most classically by visceromegaly, macroglossia, abdominal wall defects, various developmental malformations (including genitourinary tract and ear), hemihyperplasia, and neonatal

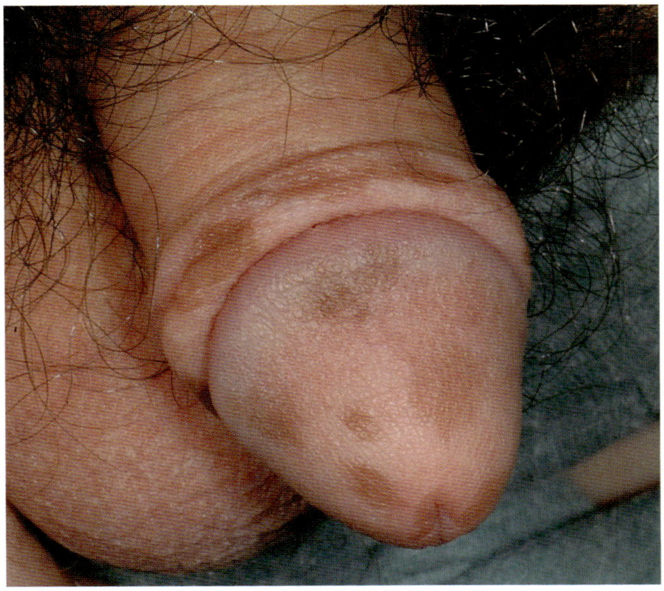

Fig. 12.74 Penile lentiginosis. Tan to brown macules and patches on the glans penis and prepuce, such as those noted in this teenaged boy, may be associated with Bannayan–Riley–Ruvalcaba syndrome.

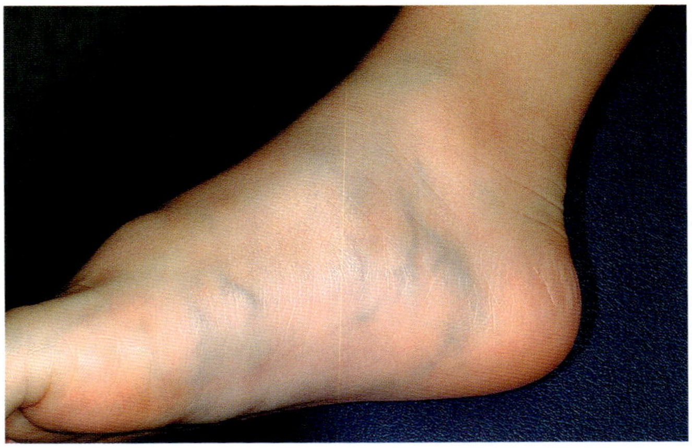

Fig. 12.75 Venous malformation. Note venous prominence of the medial and plantar surfaces and the swelling of the dorsal foot.

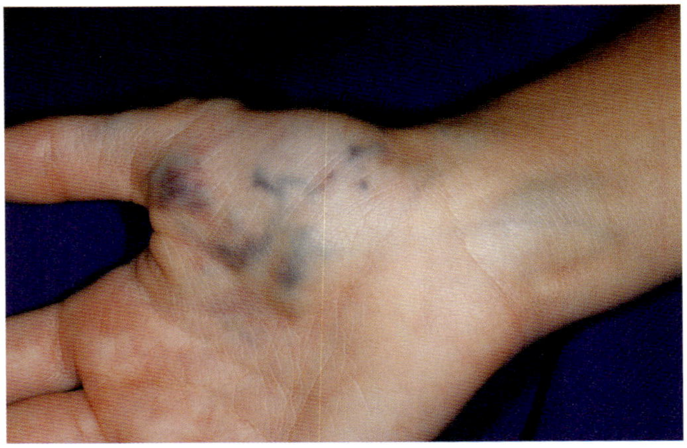

Fig. 12.76 Venous malformation. This palmar lesion in a 15-year-old boy gradually increased in size over years, with extension to the proximal thumb and volar wrist (note blue-colored swellings). He was ultimately referred for sclerosing therapy.

hypoglycemia. It is the most common of the overgrowth syndromes.[328] BWS is a multigenic disorder with dysregulation and unbalanced expression of imprinted genes residing in the 11p15.5 region.[329] The inclusion of BWS in this section relates to the common occurrence of a facial CM involving the midforehead, glabella, and upper eyelids. This malformation may extend to involve the nose and upper lip in some patients.

The most notable clinical features of BWS, which are variable, include omphalocele, macrosomia, and macroglossia. Overgrowth may be generalized or limited to specific body regions and may be associated with an advanced bone age. In addition to omphalocele, other abdominal wall defects include umbilical hernia, prune-belly sequence, and inguinal hernia. Visceromegaly may involve the kidneys, liver, spleen, and pancreas. Hypoglycemia is the most common laboratory finding and tends to regress during early infancy. Patients with BWS have an increased risk of malignant tumors including Wilms tumor, adrenocortical carcinoma, neuroblastoma, rhabdomyosarcoma, and hepatoblastoma.[330] The cumulative risk of such embryonal tumors during the first decade is estimated at 8% to 10%.[331] Perinatal features include prematurity, polyhydramnios, enlarged placenta, distended abdomen, and large fetal size.[328] Prenatal ultrasound may be useful in detecting the latter four features, enabling an early diagnosis of the syndrome.[328]

VENOUS MALFORMATION

Venous malformation (VM) is a fairly common slow-flow type of vascular malformation present at birth. Various inaccurate names have been used to describe these lesions in the literature, including *venous angioma, cavernous angioma,* and *cavernous hemangioma.* It should be remembered that VM, like all vascular malformations, is a nonproliferative collection of abnormal vessels distinct from IH and other proliferative vascular tumors. They usually grow with the child. Although these lesions are present at birth, they occasionally may not become obvious until later in life. In addition, VM may rapidly enlarge after trauma, and occasionally this may be the initial presentation.

VM tends to present as blue to purple nodules in the skin (Figs. 12.75 and 12.76). Surrounding veins may be prominent, and calcified phleboliths may be present within the lesion. These are the result of spontaneous local venous thrombosis within the malformation. Most VMs are asymptomatic, although they may occasionally become painful in association with their gradual enlargement and pressure on surrounding structures. Although most VMs are isolated, they may occur in association with other syndromic features such as in Maffucci syndrome and blue rubber bleb nevus syndrome (BRBNS) (see later).

VM can occur in any body location, although head and neck lesions tend to be the most extensive.[332]

The diagnosis of VM can be confirmed with CT, MRI (with or without venography), or Doppler ultrasonography. Plain radiographs may reveal the calcifications associated with phleboliths (which present as painful, firm nodules). Other complications of VM (in addition to thromboses) include disfigurement with psychosocial distress (Fig. 12.77), pain, limitation of motion, bleeding coagulopathy (usually localized intravascular coagulopathy [LIC]), and functional compromise related to location of the lesion. LIC typically presents with pain and elevation of the D-dimer and variable fibrinogen levels.[333] Treatment for VM is difficult and may include compression with elastic stockings (which helps limit swelling, decrease pain, and decrease the risk of coagulopathy in extremity lesions), surgery, physical therapy, and percutaneous sclerosing therapy. Low-dose aspirin therapy or low-molecular-weight heparin may be useful in patients at risk for thrombotic changes or LIC within the lesions. A multidisciplinary approach to therapy is desirable, with the goals of improving cosmesis, decreasing pain, limiting bony deformities, and maintaining function.

Maffucci Syndrome

Maffucci syndrome is a rare, congenital, nonhereditary disorder characterized by the combination of dyschondroplasia and vascular malformations. The cutaneous lesions in this disorder are compressible, red-blue papules and nodules most consistent with VMs. They may develop thrombi and phleboliths, with the associated calcifications

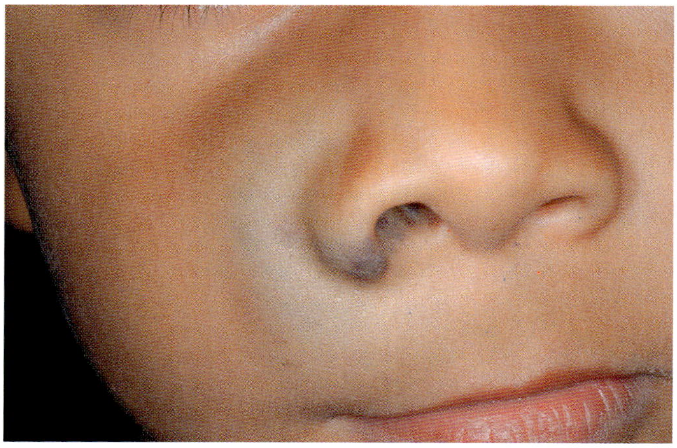

Fig. 12.77 Venous malformation. This blue nodular plaque involved the right medial cheek and lateral naris, and became more disfiguring as this young boy grew older, posing a psychosocial concern.

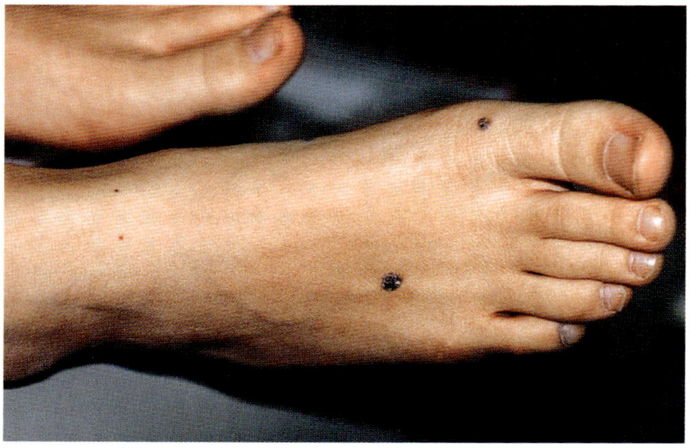

Fig. 12.78 Blue rubber bleb nevus syndrome. This patient has multiple blue-purple, compressible papules and papulonodules.

visible on plain radiography.[334] These vascular malformations may occur anywhere on the skin surface but are often more extensive on one side of the body and have a preference for the hands and feet.[335] In addition to these lesions, LM[336] and spindle-cell hemangioendothelioma[337] (a proliferative vascular tumor) are occasionally present. The vascular malformations of Maffucci syndrome may involve extracutaneous sites in some patients, including mucosal regions, bones, the respiratory tract, and the GI tract.

In addition to the vascular malformations, patients with Maffucci syndrome have enchondromas, which are the result of a developmental abnormality in cartilage formation (dyschondroplasia). These lesions start to develop during early infancy in conjunction with the vascular anomalies. They present as hard nodules over areas of long bones, hands, fingers, and feet. Occasionally they may enlarge and become so numerous as to result in grotesque deformity. Radiographically, enchondromas appear as irregular cystic lucencies. Other progressive skeletal abnormalities (marked bony deformities, pathologic fractures) may occur, as may neurologic deficits related to cerebral encroachment of skull enchondromas.

A significant risk in patients with Maffucci syndrome is that of malignancy, especially chondrosarcoma, which tends to arise from preexisting enchondroma lesions (up to 40% of which may transform into chondrosarcomas).[338] Other malignancies may also occur with increased incidence in these patients. Intracranial chondrosarcoma may rarely occur.[339] Maffucci syndrome has been shown to be caused by somatic mosaic mutations of *IDH1* and *IDH2*.[340] Ollier disease (enchondromatosis), which may be confused with Maffucci syndrome and is also caused by mutations in *IDH1* and *IDH2*, presents with enchondromas only (without the vascular malformations) and entails a significantly lower rate of malignant transformation.[340,341]

Blue Rubber Bleb Nevus Syndrome

Blue rubber bleb nevus syndrome (BRBNS; also called *Bean syndrome*) is a rare disorder characterized by the presence of cutaneous and GI VMs. Other visceral organs may occasionally be involved. Although usually a sporadic disorder, autosomal dominant inheritance has been reported.[342] Double *(cis)* somatic mutations (two mutations on the same allele) in *TEK*, the gene encoding TIE2, have been identified in individuals with BRBNS, in contrast to somatic point mutations in *TEK* in patients with sporadically occurring multifocal VM.[343] Some of the VMs in BRBNS may have a lymphatic component.

Patients with BRBNS have signs at birth or during early childhood of numerous blue to purple, soft, compressible nodules (Fig. 12.78). The lesions range in size from a few millimeters to 4 cm. Any area of the skin may be involved, as well as mucosal surfaces of the mouth and genitalia. With time, the lesions increase in both size and number. One of the diagnostic features is the ability to compress the nodules, leaving an empty wrinkled sac that then refills rapidly on withdrawal of the pressure. GI involvement is characterized by hematemesis or melena with chronic anemia. The small bowel is the most common site of GI tract involvement, but lesions can occur anywhere from the mouth to the anus.[342] Blood loss may at times be severe, necessitating transfusion, and intestinal intussusception may occur.[344] Various orthopedic complications caused by adjacent VMs may occur and include bowing and pathologic fractures. CNS involvement with vascular malformations may also be a component of the syndrome.[345,346]

BRBNS may be diagnosed based on the clinical presentation, although other diagnostic studies may be necessary and may include CT, MRI, barium studies, skin biopsy, and upper and lower GI tract endoscopy. Capsule endoscopy and intraoperative enteroscopy have been reported as useful for thorough investigation of the small bowel.[347] Treatment of the condition is primarily supportive and may include iron replacement, transfusions, endoscopic sclerotherapy, band ligation or laser photocoagulation, and resection of severely involved portions of the GI tract. The response to pharmacologic agents is variable. Subcutaneous octreotide, a somatostatin analog used to decrease splanchnic blood flow in patients with GI bleeding, may be useful in decreasing the need for blood transfusion.[348] Other reported agents include corticosteroids, interferon-α, and vincristine.[349] Favorable response to oral sirolimus has also been reported, with decreased pain and improvement in lesion size and quality of life.[350,351]

Fibroadipose Vascular Anomaly

Fibroadipose vascular anomaly (FAVA) describes a rare condition manifested by a painful intramuscular lesion of an extremity. It most commonly presents in the calf or forearm, and most patients complain of severe pain.[352] The most common misdiagnosis is that of a muscular VM; FAVA differs from intramuscular VM by the solid fibrofatty replacement of the affected muscle, with phlebectasia and significant morbidity. The pain of FAVA tends to be constant (as opposed to the intermittent pain reported in VMs) and may result in contractures. Treatment is challenging and may include physical therapy, casting/splinting, sclerosing therapy, intralesional steroid injections, oral sirolimus, and surgery.[352,353]

ARTERIOVENOUS MALFORMATION

AVMs are rare fast-flow vascular malformations consisting of both arterial and venous components with AV shunting. These lesions may vary in their clinical presentation, from macular erythema to thin vascular plaques to larger pulsating nodules or masses with an audible bruit. They typically range from stage I (pink patches or macules that may mimic a CM) to stage IV (larger lesions characterized by the presence of cardiac compromise). A bruit may be appreciated on auscultation or with bedside Doppler ultrasonography and supports the diagnosis. AVMs preferentially involve the head and neck, followed by the extremities, and they are typically congenital in nature.[354] AVMs may display aggressive growth patterns and result in functional or cosmetic deformity and, in some patients, cardiovascular compromise related to increased blood flow. They are the most endangering type of vascular anomaly. Potential associations with AVMs include CM-AVM syndrome, Parkes Weber syndrome, Cobb syndrome, and hereditary hemorrhagic telangiectasia (all are discussed elsewhere in this chapter). Diagnostic confirmation of an AVM may involve ultrasound with color Doppler study, CT or MRI evaluation, or arteriography. Treatment is notoriously challenging and includes percutaneous embolization (considered first-line therapy), surgical excision, and amputation. Embolic agents typically used include ethanol, n-butyl cyanoacrylate glue, and Onyx (an ethylene vinyl alcohol copolymer). Multidisciplinary management is advisable when available.

Disorders of Lymphatic Vessels

The lymphatic system is a complex network of thin-walled vessels responsible for carrying tissue fluid to the venous system.[355] Anomalies of the lymphatic system may include lymphedema and LMs. Lymphedema occurs as a result of aplasia or hypoplasia of lymphatic channels or obstruction of lymphatic pathways. LMs are slow-flow malformations that occur as a result of hyperplasia of the lymphatic network. Older terms for LMs are common in the literature, including *lymphangioma*, *cavernous lymphangioma*, *lymphangioma circumscriptum*, and *cystic hygroma*. These malformations are probably best described in accordance with the modern classification as *LMs* and further classified as macrocystic, microcystic, or combined.

LMs are composed of interconnected lymphatic channels and present differently depending on the size of these aberrant vessels. LMs may remain undiagnosed for years and may initially present after trauma with resultant enlargement, hemorrhage, or secondary infection.

Macrocystic LMs are composed of large interconnected lymphatic channels and cysts. They have been most commonly referred to as *cystic hygromas* or *cavernous lymphangiomas* in the literature. They may occur in any location, although the head, neck, axilla, and chest are the most common sites. Although macrocystic LM was once considered a diagnostic sign of Turner syndrome, it is now known that these lesions may be associated with other karyotypic abnormalities and malformation syndromes.[355] Other potential associations include Down syndrome, trisomy 18, trisomy 13, and Noonan syndrome. Teratogens may also be associated with macrocystic LM. These lesions are typically present at birth, and may be recognized antenatally on prenatal ultrasound.[356]

Macrocystic LM presents as a large, somewhat translucent mass lying under normal-appearing skin (Fig. 12.79). It enhances with transillumination. Acute hemorrhage within an LM may result in swelling, tenderness, and purple discoloration. Diagnostic confirmation can be made with ultrasound, CT, or MRI examination. Prenatal and neonatal complications include lymphedema, facial deformity, and effusions (pleural, pericardial, abdominal). Hydrops fetalis, heart failure, respiratory compromise, and intrauterine demise may occasionally occur. Treatment options for macrocystic LM typically include surgical excision; serial aspirations; and sclerosing therapy with bleomycin, OK-432 (Picibanil), ethanol, sodium tetradecyl sulfate (STS), or doxycycline.[356–360] Oral sildenafil, which selectively inhibits phosphodiesterase-5 and is normally used for pulmonary hypertension and erectile dysfunction, resulted in marked reduction in size in 3 young children with large LMs and subsequently in 6 of 7 children in one open-label study and in 14 of 21 children with head and neck LM in another study.[361–363] One report described improvement in LM in three patients treated with oral propranolol, with partial responses in two patients with KT syndrome with lymphatic components.[364]

Microcystic LMs are a more common form of LM, representing microscopic aggregations of small lymphatic channels. These lesions usually present as cutaneous plaques or nodules with superimposed changes in the overlying skin. These surface changes consist of erythematous to flesh-colored papules that may be somewhat translucent (Fig. 12.80), accounting for the traditional analogy with frog spawn. The differential diagnosis of the superficial component of microcystic LM may include warts, molluscum contagiosum, herpes simplex, herpes zoster, and epidermal nevus. Perianal lesions may be misdiagnosed as anogenital condylomata.[365] Hemorrhage may occur within the superficial component (Fig. 12.81), and intermittent swelling or bruising may be a feature. Other complications include intermittent leakage of lymph fluid, inflammation, and secondary infection.

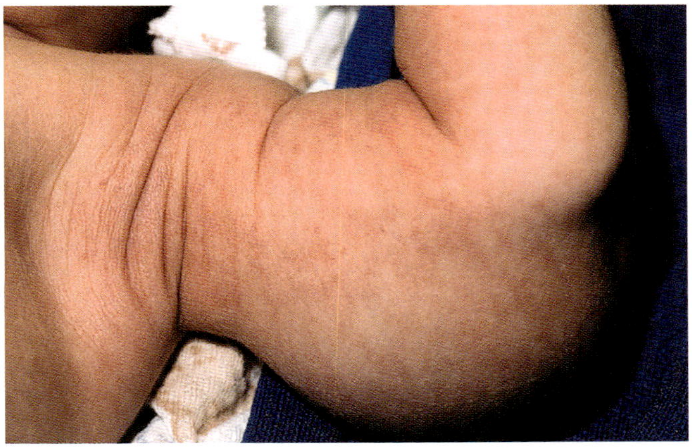

Fig. 12.79 Macrocystic lymphatic malformation.

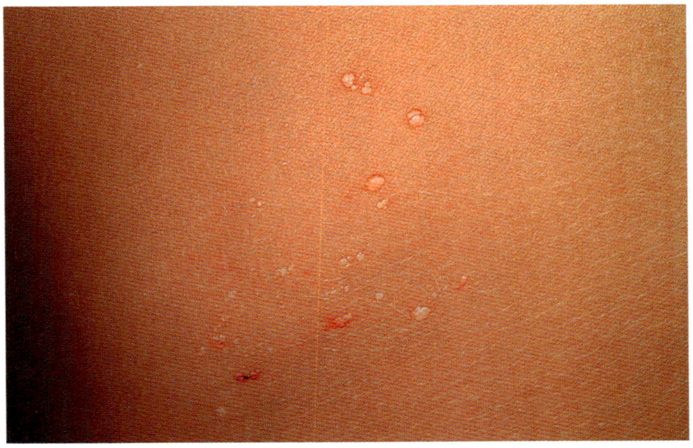

Fig. 12.80 Microcystic lymphatic malformation. Note the multiple flesh-colored, translucent papules with hemorrhagic changes in some of the lesions.

Microcystic LMs often present during infancy and may involve any area of the skin or mucosa. Oral lesions are quite common, most often involving the tongue (Fig. 12.82) or cheek. Microcystic LM is often (but not always) treatable by surgical excision, but consideration should be given to a possible larger deep component.

LYMPHEDEMA

Lymphedema refers to a set of conditions characterized by interstitial accumulation of lymphatic fluid and may be primary or secondary (Table 12.6). Primary lymphedema is related to anatomic abnormalities in the lymphatic system, which may include hypoplasia of vessels, absence of lymphatic valves, and/or impaired contractility of the structures. Secondary lymphedema, which results in disruption or obstruction of lymphatic pathways, arises as a consequence of disease, surgery, or radiotherapy.[366,367] Primary lymphedema most often involves the lower extremities, whereas upper extremity involvement is more common in secondary lymphedema.

Lymphedema presents as edema of the affected extremity. Early in the course the involved region is puffy (Fig. 12.83), whereas later in the course the area becomes more fibrotic and indurated. Secondary cutaneous changes may be present, including a *peau d'orange* appearance of the overlying skin, pigmentary changes, and recurrent episodes of cellulitis. When a lower extremity is involved, swelling of the dorsal aspect of the foot (Fig. 12.84) is common with a characteristic

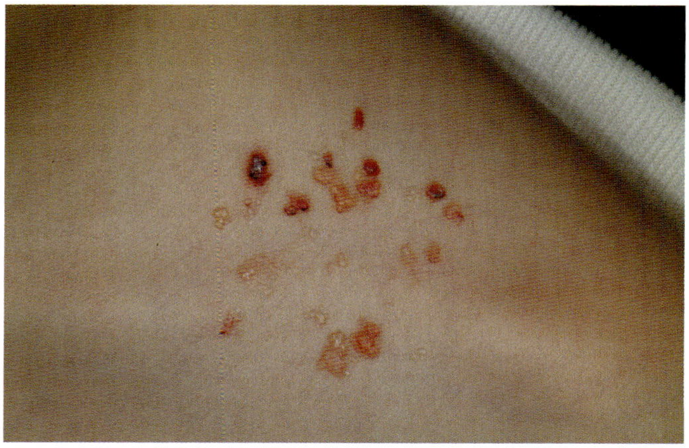

Fig. 12.81 Combined microcystic/macrocystic lymphatic malformation with hemorrhage. There are numerous surface blebs (microcystic component), many of which reveal hemorrhage.

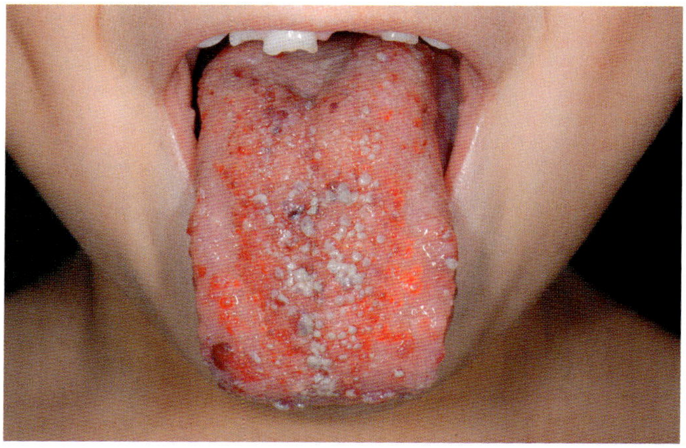

Fig. 12.82 Microcystic lymphatic malformation of the tongue. This boy has extensive involvement of his tongue with translucent papules, several of which reveal hemorrhage. The white color of some lesions relates to maceration from the moist environment of the mouth.

blunt, "squared off" appearance of the digits.[366] The staging system for lymphedema includes stages 0 or Ia (subclinical state without appreciable swelling) through III (lymphostatic elephantiasis with or without pitting and with trophic skin changes such as acanthosis, deposition of fat and fibrosis, and warty overgrowths).[368]

Congenital lymphedema may involve a single extremity (upper or lower) or multiple limbs, and the changes are present at birth. Lymphedema praecox, which usually occurs in girls around the time of puberty, presents as edema of the foot or ankle or rarely with upper extremity involvement.[369] Milroy disease is an inherited form of lymphedema, usually occurring with an autosomal dominant pattern of transmission, most commonly resulting from mutations in *FLT4/VEGFR3* (see Table 12.6). Limb swelling in all extremities is possible, although bilateral lower extremity lymphedema is most typical.[370]

The diagnosis of lymphedema is usually a clinical one. Useful findings include edema, fibrosis, *peau d'orange* appearance of the skin, and a positive Stemmer sign (inability of the examiner to tent the skin at the base of the digits in the involved extremity).[367] In cases where further diagnostic confirmation is necessary, available options include indirect radionuclide lymphoscintigraphy, lymphangiography, MRI or CT imaging, and Doppler ultrasonography. Therapy for lymphedema includes massage (manual lymphatic drainage), elevation, compression garments, physical therapy and exercise, and meticulous skin care in an effort to prevent skin breakdown and infection. Intermittent pneumatic compression may be useful. Surgical approaches are reserved for patients with severe disease who have failed conservative

Table 12.6 Classification of Lymphedema

Type	Comment
PRIMARY	
Congenital lymphedema	Single extremity or multiple limbs
Lymphedema praecox	Pubertal or postpubertal females
Lymphedema tarda	Usually after 35 years of age
Milroy disease	AD form of congenital familial lymphedema; linked most commonly to mutations in *FLT4* gene (VEGFR3)
Lymphedema-distichiasis	AD; lymphedema in association with distichiasis (supplementary row of eyelashes); linked to mutations in *FOXC2* gene
Hypotrichosis-lymphedema-telangiectasia	AD; linked to mutation in *SOX18* gene
Hennekam lymphangiectasia-lymphedema syndrome/mental retardation	AR; linked to mutation in *CCBE1*
Hereditary lymphedema II (Meige disease)	AD; linked to mutation in *GJC2* (CX47)
Primary lymphedema, myelodysplasia (Emberger syndrome)	AD; linked to mutation in *GATA2*
Fetal chylothorax	AR, de novo; linked to mutation in *ITGA9*
SECONDARY	
Lymphedema Occurring after Disruption of Lymphatic Pathways by:	
Disease	Filariasis
Surgery	Lymph node dissection
Radiation therapy	
Burns	
Pregnancy	
Large/circumferential wounds to the extremity	

Modified from Rockson SG. Lymphedema. Am J Med 2001;110(4):288–95; Rockson SG. Diagnosis and management of lymphatic vascular disease. J Am Coll Cardiol 2008;52:799–806; Murdaca G, Cagnati P, Gulli R, et al. Current views on diagnostic approach and treatment of lymphedema. Am J Med 2012;125:134–40; and Brouillard P, Boon L, Vikkula M. Genetics of lymphatic anomalies. J Clin Invest 2014;124(3):898–904.
AD, Autosomal dominant; *AR*, autosomal recessive.

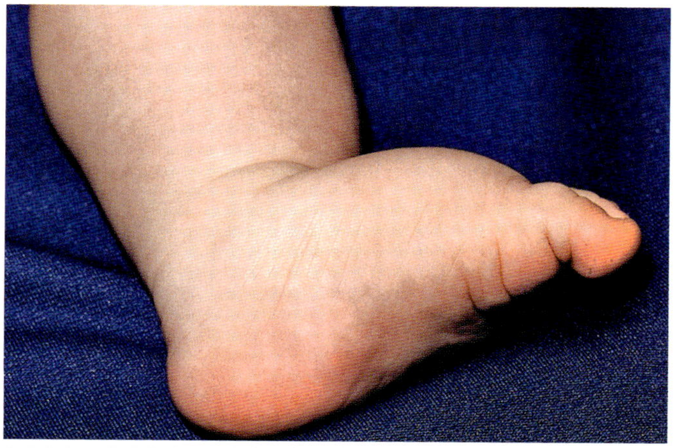

Fig. 12.83 Congenital lymphedema. Note the fullness of the dorsal aspect of the foot in this infant boy.

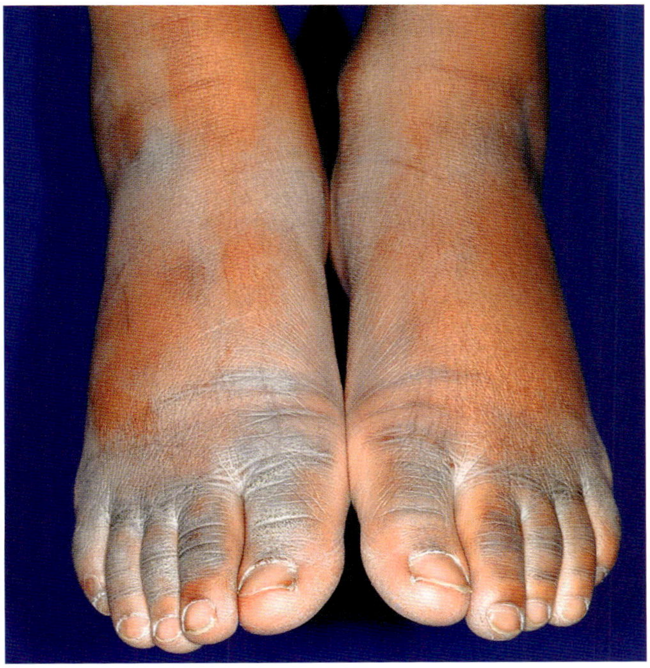

Fig. 12.84 Lymphedema. This 10-year-old girl had long-standing, non-pitting edema of her feet bilaterally.

measures and include excision of lymphedematous tissues, use of a lymphatic collector or interposition vein segment to restore lymphatic continuity, and microsurgical lymphaticovenous anastomoses. Suction-assisted lipectomy uses liposuction techniques to remove additional subcutaneous tissues from the suprafascial compartment and may decrease the risk of recurrent cellulitis.[371] Pharmacologic therapy is of limited use but may include diuretics, benzopyrones (including rutosides and bioflavonoids), and antimicrobial agents (as needed).

GORHAM SYNDROME

Gorham syndrome (Gorham–Stout disease, disappearing bones, vanishing bone disease, massive osteolysis) is a rare condition of unknown origin characterized by progressive bony destruction with intramedullary proliferation of thin-walled vascular structures. Many affected patients have cutaneous vascular lesions as well. Although there is no consensus on the nature of these vascular elements, several authors have proposed that they represent lymphatic vessels.

Patients with Gorham syndrome are usually children or young adults, and they have pathologic fractures and/or bone pain. Nearly any bone may be involved, but most common are the ribs, scapula, clavicle, humerus, pelvis, spine, femur, skull, and mandible.[372,373] It may occur in a focal fashion with spread to contiguous bony structures and occasionally with multicentric, widespread involvement. Nonskeletal manifestations include respiratory distress, pleural effusions, ascites, and chylothorax. Chylothorax is an uncommon but often fatal complication of Gorham syndrome and may be associated with malnutrition, lymphocytopenia, and infection.[372] The diagnosis of Gorham syndrome is confirmed by the finding of osteolytic changes on radiography without reparative bone formation and in the absence of soft-tissue mass and by histologic evaluation of biopsied material.[374]

The natural history of Gorham syndrome is variable, and therapy is difficult. Surgical resection, bone grafting, fractionated radiation therapy, and chemotherapy have all been used with variable results. Oral sirolimus has been demonstrated useful in these patients.[375–377]

MULTIFOCAL LYMPHANGIOENDOTHELIOMATOSIS WITH THROMBOCYTOPENIA

Multifocal lymphangioendotheliomatosis with thrombocytopenia (MLT; also known as *cutaneovisceral angiomatosis with thrombocytopenia*) is a condition characterized by multifocal, congenital, and progressive vascular papules and nodules involving the skin and GI tract in association with severe GI bleeding and thrombocytopenic coagulopathy.[378] Histologically these vascular lesions reveal collections of ectatic, thin-walled vessels lined by hobnailed endothelial cells and may express markers such as *CD31*, *D2-40*, and *LYVE-1*, which suggest they are consistent with lymphatic differentiation.

Clinically MLT presents with multiple vascular lesions that are red to brown to purple macules (Fig. 12.85), papules, and nodules varying in size from a few millimeters to several centimeters. They may number in the hundreds, may have a scaly surface, and may be indurated, suggesting deeper dermal or subcutaneous involvement. GI tract bleeding may be severe, and endoscopy reveals diffusely distributed mucosal vascular lesions in the stomach and the small and large intestines. Thrombocytopenia is usually present with normal to slightly elevated coagulation studies (prothrombin and partial thromboplastin times) and variable values for fibrinogen and D-dimer in patients reported to date. Other organs of potential involvement include the lungs, synovium, muscle, bone, eye, bone marrow, spleen, and brain.

Treatment for MLT is challenging, and therapies reported to date (with variable response) have included corticosteroids, interferon-α, blood product transfusions, octreotide, aminocaproic acid, thalidomide, propranolol, intravenous immunoglobulin, bevacizumab, suture ligation of GI tract lesions, sirolimus, colectomy, and, in one patient who developed portal hypertension and decompensating liver function, orthotopic liver transplantation.[378–384]

ANGIOKERATOMAS

Angiokeratomas are skin lesions characterized by ectasia (dilation) of the superficial vessels of the dermis and hyperkeratosis of the overlying epidermis. They present as hyperkeratotic, dark red (Fig. 12.86) to purple or black papules measuring between 1 and 10 mm in diameter, occasionally larger. Several types of angiokeratoma are recognized,

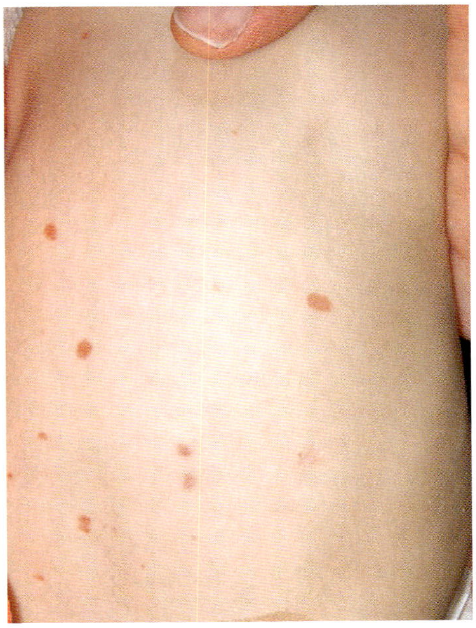

Fig. 12.85 Multifocal lymphangioendotheliomatosis with thrombocytopenia. This neonate had multiple cutaneous vascular macules as well as multiple gastrointestinal lesions with severe bleeding and thrombocytopenia. (Courtesy Beth A. Drolet, MD.)

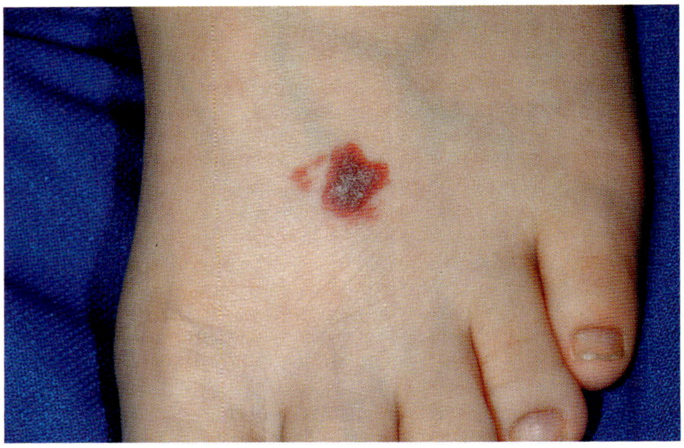

Fig. 12.86 Angiokeratoma. This was an isolated lesion in an otherwise healthy 14-year-old girl.

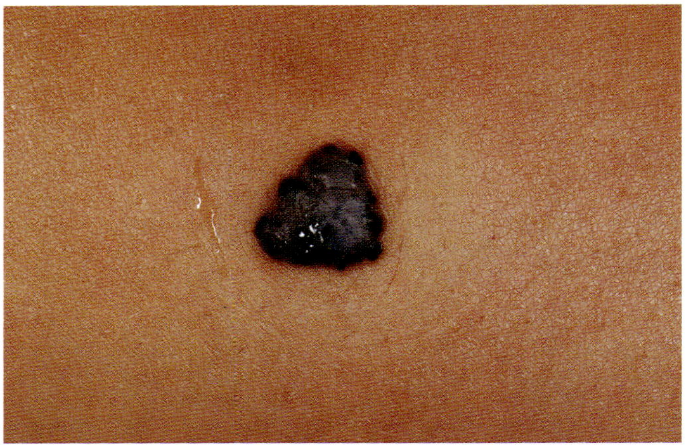

Fig. 12.87 Angiokeratoma. This purple to black firm plaque developed on the knee of a 12-year-old girl. Microscopic evaluation of the excised tissue revealed changes of angiokeratoma.

and although these lesions usually occur sporadically, they may occasionally be associated with potentially serious metabolic disease.

Solitary or Multiple Angiokeratomas

Solitary or multiple angiokeratomas usually occur on the lower extremities of young adults. They are blue to black (Fig. 12.87) and may sometimes be confused with malignant melanoma. These lesions may be related to preceding trauma or injury.

Angiokeratoma Circumscriptum

Angiokeratoma circumscriptum presents as a plaque composed of multiple, clustered red to purple papules. These lesions may be present at birth or develop during childhood.

Angiokeratoma of Mibelli

Angiokeratoma of Mibelli occurs on the dorsal fingers or toes or in interdigital spaces. These lesions appear during childhood or adolescence, are more common in females, and are inherited in an autosomal dominant fashion.

Angiokeratoma of Fordyce

Angiokeratoma of Fordyce is a condition that presents with numerous red to purple papules on the scrotum or vulva of adults. Scrotal lesions may be seen in association with varicocele or inguinal hernia.

Although these forms of angiokeratoma occur in the absence of associated serious abnormalities, the lesions may occasionally be seen in the setting of potentially serious metabolic disorders.

Angiokeratoma Corporis Diffusum

Angiokeratoma corporis diffusum (ACD) is the name used to describe lesions that present as numerous dark red to black papules distributed primarily on the abdomen (Fig. 12.88), genitals, buttocks, and thighs (Fig. 12.89; "bathing-trunk" distribution). The most common disorder associated with ACD is Fabry disease (FD; also known as *Anderson–Fabry disease*), a rare X-linked recessive disorder caused by deficient α-galactosidase A. The genetic cause is a mutation in the *GLA* gene (encoding α-galactosidase A), most often point mutations but occasionally small and large deletions or insertions.[385] Males with FD have an accumulation of glycosphingolipids, especially globotriaosylceramide, which results in dysfunction of the heart, kidneys, and nervous system.[386] Acral paresthesias and acral or abdominal pain occur, often within the first decade of life, and may respond to treatment with carbamazepine. Other findings in FD include corneal and lenticular opacities, hypohidrosis, progressive neuropathy, progressive renal and heart failure, and cerebral artery thrombosis.[387] The risk of stroke is estimated to be 5.5- to 12.2-fold higher than that expected in the general population, and transient ischemic attacks are common.[388] The angiokeratomas of FD may number in the thousands and tend to cluster in the iliosacral areas, on the scrotum, and around the umbilicus. The first lesions commonly appear on the scrotum and must be differentiated from angiokeratoma of Fordyce. A majority of patients have pinpoint macular purplish spots on the lips, particularly near the

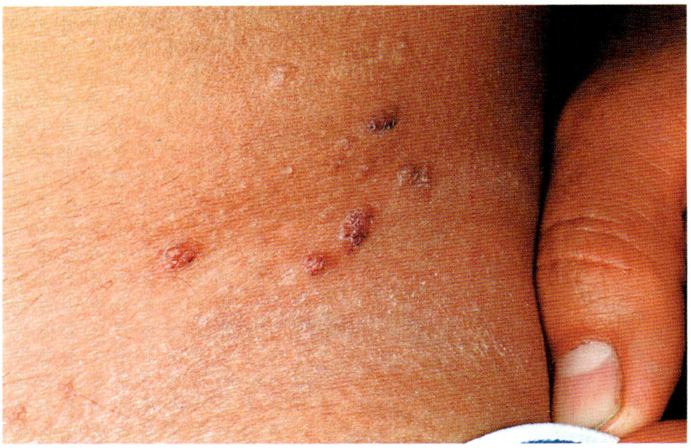

Fig. 12.88 Angiokeratoma corporis diffusum in Fabry disease. This 19-year-old man had multiple lesions involving the trunk, groin, and thighs.

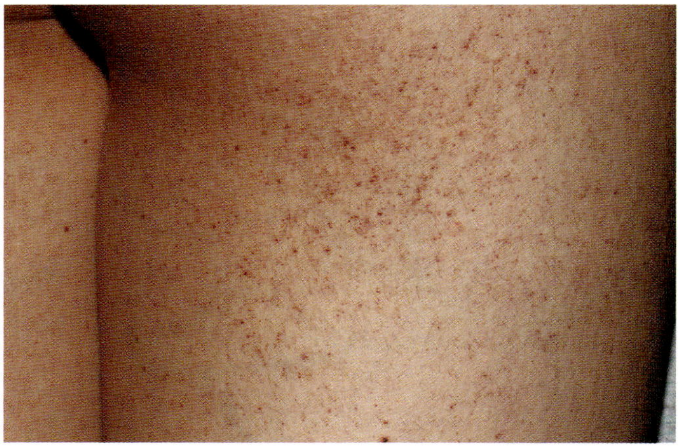

Fig. 12.89 Angiokeratoma corporis diffusum in Fabry disease. This 12-year-old boy presented with multiple dark red macules and papules on the thighs (shown here), buttocks, scrotum, and lower trunk and complained of lower extremity pain and paresthesias. His leukocyte α-galactosidase activity was markedly diminished, confirming the diagnosis of Fabry disease.

vermilion border of the lower lip. These lesions are smaller than those on the skin. The tongue is generally not affected, but hemoptysis and epistaxis have been reported with involvement of the buccal and nasal mucosae. In addition to the typical cutaneous lesions, fine telangiectasias have been described in the axillae and on the upper chest. Enzyme replacement therapy (ERT) with recombinant α-galactosidase A (available as agalsidase α and agalsidase β) is available for treatment of FD, although it may not lead to complete resolution of symptoms in all patients. When started early in life, however, ERT may halt and even reverse the progressive multiorgan deterioration seen in patients with FD and improve quality of life.[389,390]

There are other inherited lysosomal storage diseases that may have associated angiokeratomas of the skin. Fucosidosis is an autosomal recessive lysosomal storage disease in which deficiency of α-fucosidase results in multisystem accumulation of oligosaccharides and glycosphingolipids.[391] This disorder is characterized by progressive neuromotor deterioration, seizures, coarse facial features, dysostosis multiplex, visceromegaly, and growth retardation. Recurrent respiratory infections may also occur. The predominant cutaneous feature of fucosidosis is ACD, which may resemble that seen in FD. In distinction to the lesions of FD, however, the angiokeratomas associated with fucosidosis tend to occur earlier in life, usually around 5 years of age and display a more generalized distribution. Other dermatologic features reported in fucosidosis include hypohidrosis or hyperhidrosis, cutaneous vascular abnormalities, and transverse nail bands.[391] Fucosidosis is caused by a mutation in the *FUCA1* gene.

Other metabolic disorders that may be associated with ACD include GM1 gangliosidosis, galactosialidosis, β-mannosidosis, sialidosis, Schindler disease type II, and aspartylglycosaminuria. All these conditions are inherited in an autosomal recessive fashion, and the diagnosis is made by urine oligosaccharide analysis or enzyme assay.

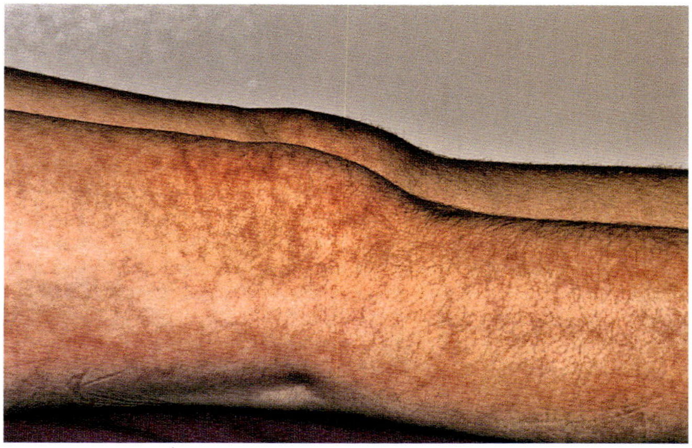

Fig. 12.90 Livedo reticularis.

Box 12.5 Associations with Livedo Reticularis

- Autoimmune diseases
- Coagulation disorders
- Hematologic aberration or malignancy
- Hormone-secreting tumors
- Arterial occlusive diseases
- Sneddon syndrome (cerebral ischemic arterial disease)
- Antiphospholipid antibody syndrome
- Systemic vasculitis
- Paraproteinemia
- Drugs

Disorders Associated with Vascular Dilation or Constriction

LIVEDO RETICULARIS

Livedo reticularis is a mottled or reticulated, blue-red discoloration of the skin that occurs predominantly on the lower extremities (Fig. 12.90) and less commonly on the trunk or upper extremities. Ulceration may occasionally occur. Although the pathogenesis of livedo reticularis is unclear, the changes seem to be related to slow blood flow and decreased oxygen tension. Exposure to cold environments usually intensifies this vascular pattern. The distinction between livedo reticularis and cutis marmorata may be clinically difficult, although cutis marmorata tends to disappear with rewarming and may be seen as a normal finding in up to 50% of infants.

The significance of livedo reticularis lies in its possible association with a variety of systemic disorders (Box 12.5; see Chapter 22). Associated disorders may include coagulopathies, autoimmune diseases (including systemic lupus erythematosus, dermatomyositis, rheumatoid arthritis, and scleroderma), systemic vasculitides (including polyarteritis nodosa, granulomatosis with polyangiitis [formerly Wegener granulomatosis], and Churg–Strauss syndrome), arterial occlusive disease, and antiphospholipid antibody syndrome. Sneddon syndrome is characterized by the association of livedo reticularis and cerebral ischemic arterial events such as stroke or transient ischemic attack.[392,393] These patients may have associated antiphospholipid antibodies. Moyamoya disease, a rare chronic cerebrovascular occlusive disease involving the circle of Willis, has also been reported in conjunction with cutaneous livedo reticularis in a child.[394] In rare instances, recurrent small ulcerations may develop on the lower legs and feet primarily in adults with idiopathic livedo reticularis and has been termed *livedo vasculitis* or *livedoid vasculopathy*. Mild hypertension and edema of the legs, ankles, and feet may occur in this setting. A variant of this disorder *(atrophie blanche)* is characterized by white atrophic areas, hyperpigmentation, and ulceration with telangiectatic vessels at their periphery. Atrophie blanche usually occurs on the ankles and dorsal feet in young to middle-aged women but may also occasionally occur in children (Fig. 12.91).

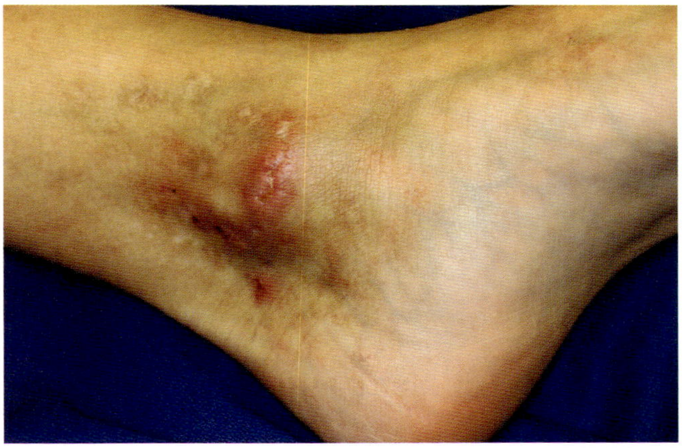

Fig. 12.91 Atrophie blanche (livedoid vasculopathy). This 10-year-old girl developed recurrent painful ulcerations that healed with atrophic ivory white scars, over the bilateral medial and lateral malleoli. Biopsy confirmed changes consistent with atrophie blanche, and extensive laboratory evaluations were unrevealing. She responded well to pentoxifylline but continued to develop intermittent mild flares.

Although there is no specific treatment for livedo reticularis, therapeutic options include avoidance of cold, anticoagulant therapy (especially for patients with ulceration), and treatment of the underlying associated condition. Reported treatment options for livedoid vasculopathy include antiplatelet, anticoagulant, antithrombotic, and fibrinolytic medications; anabolic steroids; hyperbaric oxygen therapy; psoralen plus ultraviolet A (PUVA); and intravenous immunoglobulin.[395,396]

FLUSHING AND THE AURICULOTEMPORAL NERVE SYNDROME

Flushing, a transient diffuse erythema of the blush areas (the face, neck, and/or adjacent trunk), is caused by dilation of superficial cutaneous blood vessels mediated by neural mechanisms or the direct action of a vasodilator substance on vascular smooth muscles. Flushing can be caused by emotion; the ingestion of alcoholic or hot beverages; food additives such as sulfites, nitrites, and monosodium glutamate (MSG) in what has been termed the "Chinese restaurant syndrome"; calcium channel blockers such as nifedipine; disulfiram (Antabuse); carcinoid syndrome (a disorder caused by a neoplasm that produces large amounts of serotonin and bradykinin); and other tumors that produce catecholamines such as neuroblastoma, renal cell carcinoma, or ganglioneuroma.

The auriculotemporal nerve (Frey) syndrome is a phenomenon characterized by unilateral (rarely bilateral) flushing, sweating, or both in the distribution of the auriculotemporal nerve. These changes usually occur in response to gustatory or olfactory stimuli. Frey syndrome is believed to be related to increased irritability of the cholinergic fibers and possibly to misdirected regeneration of fibers during the healing that comes after trauma. It may result after parotid surgery, CNS disease (cerebellopontine angle tumors), cervical sympathectomy, and radical neck dissection.[397] When it occurs in one of these settings, it is usually in an adult.

Frey syndrome in infants and children is less common and is most often noted after the introduction of solid food.[398] It may occasionally be misdiagnosed as a food allergy reaction,[398,399] although the unilaterality of the eruption in most cases should distinguish it from an allergic process. In one retrospective review, unnecessary dietary eliminations were initially recommended in 21% of patients.[400] Table 12.7 lists some features that help to distinguish food allergy from pediatric Frey syndrome. In children the presentation of Frey syndrome is often limited to facial flushing (without sweating), and these changes occur most often after ingestion of fruits (especially citrus fruits and apple), candy, or a favorite food. Perinatal birth trauma from forceps-assisted delivery with subsequent damage to the auriculotemporal nerve may be responsible in many pediatric cases, especially when unilateral in presentation.[400] In those with no history of trauma to the parotid area, congenital aberration of the auriculotemporal nerve pathway between parasympathetic and sympathetic fibers is suspected. The gustatory flushing of Frey syndrome has also been observed in patients with type 1 neurofibromatosis and facial plexiform neurofibromas.[401] The clinical presentation is that of bright erythema extending in a patch from the corner of the mouth toward the preauricular cheek and as far as the frontotemporal scalp (Fig. 12.92) that occurs within a few seconds after ingestion of the responsible food. The changes resolve spontaneously over 30 to 60 minutes, and therapy is unnecessary. Spontaneous resolution may occur after a period of time and often is the case in children with Frey syndrome. In adults with severe forms of the disorder, treatments have included topical antiperspirants or anticholinergic ointments and botulinum toxin injections.

ERYTHROMELALGIA

Erythromelalgia (also known as *erythermalgia*) is a rare condition characterized by paroxysmal intense burning pain, erythema, and warmth of the skin. It most often involves the distal limbs, especially the feet but also the hands. It may occur in primary or secondary forms and is quite uncommon in childhood. When it does occur in children, it is usually idiopathic.[402,403] Secondary erythromelalgia has been reported in association with various disorders including hematologic diseases (e.g., polycythemia, malignancy, spherocytosis, and thrombotic thrombocytopenic purpura), embolic disease, cardiovascular disease, connective tissue disorders (including lupus erythematosus, rheumatoid arthritis, and vasculitis), infectious diseases, neurologic disease, and musculoskeletal disease, and as a drug-induced condition.[404] In patients with an associated myeloproliferative disorder, the findings of erythromelalgia may precede the diagnosis by months to years.[405] Inherited erythromelalgia has been demonstrated to be caused by gain-of-function mutations in *SCN9A*, which encodes the voltage-gated sodium channel protein $Na_v1.7$.[406,407] These channels are preferentially expressed in primary sensory neurons of the

Table 12.7 Useful Features for Distinguishing Food Allergy from Pediatric Frey Syndrome

	Food Allergy	Frey Syndrome
Laterality	Often bilateral	Usually unilateral (occasionally bilateral)
Distribution	Patchy and irregular; often diffuse, not just facial	Segmental distribution within areas innervated by auriculotemporal nerve (usually a stripe from mouth angle toward frontotemporal scalp); limited to face
Skin lesions	Urticaria	Flushing (typically without sweating in children)
Pruritus	Present	Absent
Angioedema	May be present	Absent
Other findings	May have respiratory or GI symptoms, anaphylaxis	None
Implicated foods	Commonly cow's milk, egg, soy, wheat, peanuts, tree nuts, fish, shellfish	Commonly citrus fruits, green vegetables, candy (especially sour), child's favorite foods
History	May have associated personal or family history of atopy	May have history of forceps-assisted delivery

Modified from Sethuraman G, Mancini AJ. Familial auriculotemporal nerve (Frey) syndrome. Pediatr Dermatol 2009;26(3):302–5.
GI, Gastrointestinal.

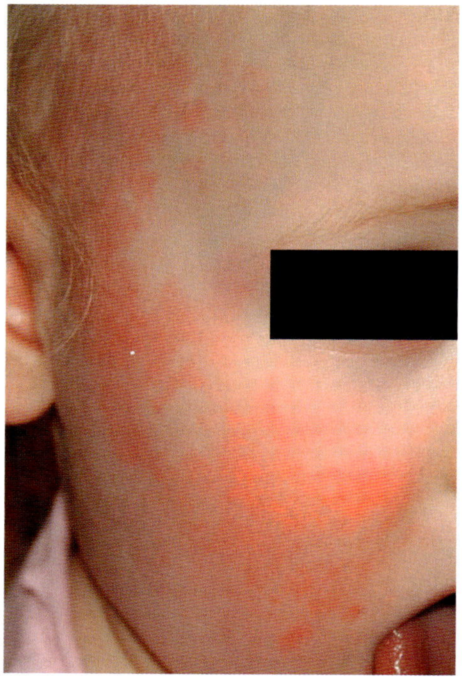

Fig. 12.92 Auriculotemporal nerve (Frey) syndrome. Facial flushing extended from the mouth angle to the frontotemporal scalp in this young girl just seconds after ingestion of solid foods (in this instance, fruit snacks).

dorsal root and trigeminal ganglion and sympathetic ganglion neurons.[408] Erythromelalgia is believed to be part of the same disease spectrum as small fiber neuropathy, the latter of which presents with sensory symptoms such as neuropathic pain and autonomic dysfunction, and is related to abnormalities in thin myelinated Aδ-fibers and unmyelinated C-fibers.[409]

Erythromelalgia presents with striking erythema and warmth of the affected distal extremity that is worsened by heat and relieved by cooling and elevation. The affected skin may have a purple hue. It is most often bilateral, although it may occasionally be unilateral. Occasionally proximal extension of the warmth and redness up the extremity are noted. Less often the face, ears, or nose may be affected.[410] When severe, erythromelalgia may have a profound effect on QoL and sleep quality and may disrupt work and social functioning.[404] In a review of 32 pediatric patients with erythromelalgia, physical activity was limited in 66%, with 13% of patients becoming wheelchair-bound as a result of the condition, and school attendance was adversely affected in 34% of the patients.[410] Multiple therapies have been used for erythromelalgia with variable (and usually minimal) success. These include cooling, topical anesthetic agents (including lidocaine patches), aspirin, serotonin reuptake inhibitors, tricyclic antidepressants, anticonvulsants, calcium channel blockers, sympathetic blocks, sympathectomies, intravenous lidocaine, mexiletine, and psychotherapy.[403,404,411,412] Patients should be cautioned against overuse of ice or ice packs, cold water, and fans given the risk of immersion foot, which presents with increased mottling, edema, maceration, bullae, and even erosions or ulcers.[413]

Red ear syndrome (erythromelalgia of the ears, auricular erythromelalgia) deserves mention here. This entity presents with a painful, burning, bright red ear (Fig. 12.93) that occurs paroxysmally and is usually unilateral. Both ears may occasionally be involved. Some have termed this presentation *otomelalgia* given its similarity in presentation to erythromelalgia. Red ear syndrome may represent a migraine variant and in fact may be associated with classic symptoms of migraine headache.[414] Other potential associations include irritation of the third cervical root, temporomandibular joint dysfunction, or thalamic syndrome.[415] Patients with this presentation may respond to therapies directed at migraine headache or a tricyclic antidepressant.[416] Cool compresses of the ears often relieve discomfort acutely during an episode.[417]

ANGIOSPASTIC MACULES (BIER SPOTS)

Angiospastic macules, also known as *Bier spots*, are asymptomatic, pale, irregularly shaped small anemic macules that were initially identified after brachial artery compression, when a surgeon (Augustus Bier) noted white spots on a cyanotic background, which appeared on the forearm and hand.[418] They are most often found on the extensor lower and upper extremities but may be generalized. They are most often found incidentally, and present as 1- to 10-mm pale macules

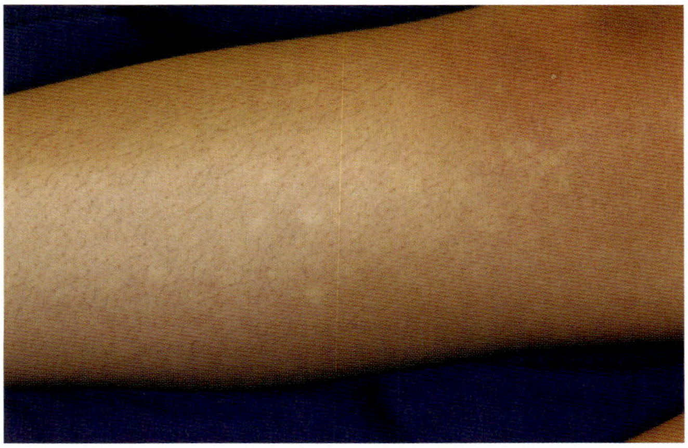

Fig. 12.94 Angiospastic macules (Bier spots). Note the multiple anemic, pale small macules on the lower extremity of a healthy teenaged girl.

overlying the normal pink background skin (Fig. 12.94). Lower extremity lesions become more prominent with standing, and upper extremity lesions become more prominent when the arms are hanging down; the spots disappear with blanching of the surrounding skin (e.g., with diascopy). Bier spots appear related to small vessel vasoconstriction. Although they have been reported during pregnancy and there have been some reports of disease associations, including scleroderma renal crisis, cryoglobulinemia, aortic hypoplasia, CM-AVM syndrome, and lymphoma, the vast majority occur in otherwise healthy individuals and are idiopathic.[418–422] An association of Bier spots with cyanosis and an urticarial-like eruption (BASCULE syndrome) has been identified and is notable for associated pruritus in some patients, presence of cyanosis, and edema of the affected extremities.[423,424] Skin biopsy is typically unnecessary for Bier spots, and there is no effective therapy.

CUTIS MARMORATA TELANGIECTATICA CONGENITA

CMTC (congenital generalized phlebectasia) is a condition characterized by either localized or generalized reticulate erythema. Although the clinical findings may resemble physiologic cutis marmorata, the changes of CMTC do not disappear with rewarming and may be associated with other abnormalities.

Patients with CMTC exhibit skin changes either at or shortly after birth. Clinical examination reveals red to violaceous, reticulate, marbled, or mottled patches (Figs. 12.95 and 12.96). The nature of the skin changes may include prominent veins, telangiectasias, and atrophy. The changes may be limited to a localized region of the body or an extremity or may show a diffuse pattern of involvement. When localized,

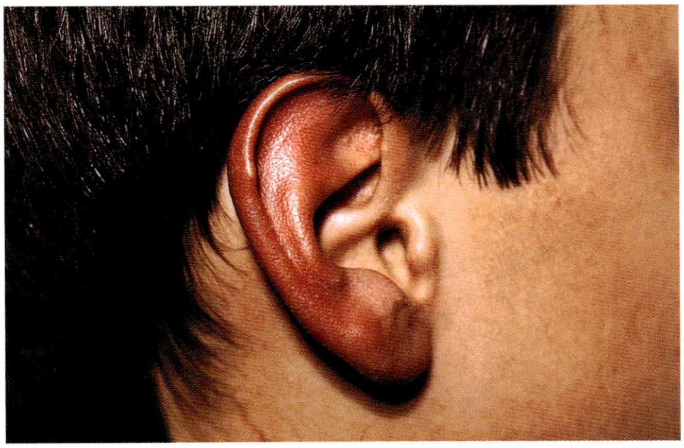

Fig. 12.93 Red ear syndrome. This young boy had recurrent episodes of painful burning and redness of the ear.

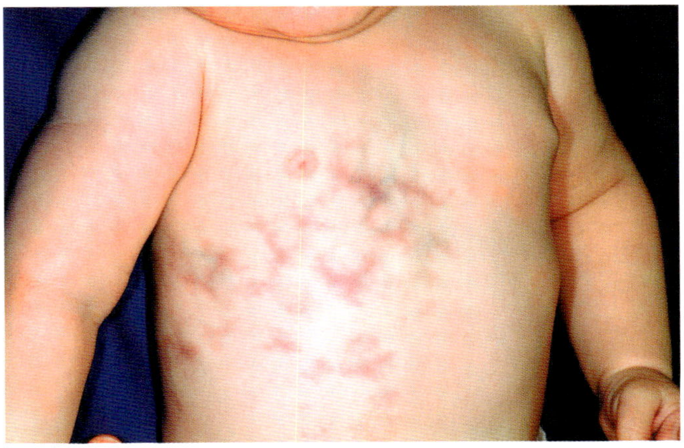

Fig. 12.95 Cutis marmorata telangiectatica congenita. The reticulate mottling was limited to the chest in this newborn male.

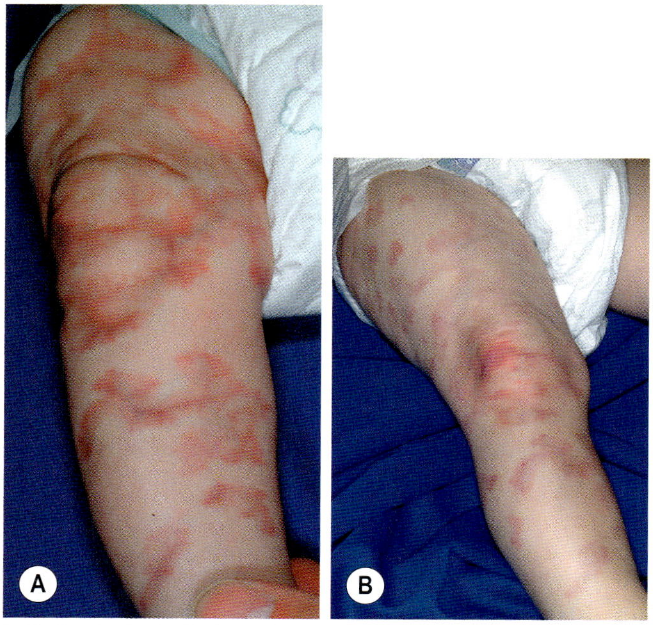

Fig. 12.96 Cutis marmorata telangiectatica congenita. **(A)** This blue-purple, reticulate mottling on the leg of this 2-month-old boy does not disappear with rewarming, which distinguishes it from typical cutis marmorata. **(B)** Marked fading was noted at 2 years of age.

the distribution tends to be segmental with a sharp demarcation at the midline.[425] The skin changes are accentuated by a decrease in the ambient temperature. CMTC lesions may resemble livedo reticularis or cutis marmorata, and occasionally ulceration may be present. The color of the skin lesions may vary from light pink to dark purple.

Additional anomalies may occasionally be present in patients with CMTC. A common finding is body asymmetry, especially limb hypoplasia on the affected side.[426,427] Limb hyperplasia may also occasionally occur. Limb length discrepancy may be present, and was noted in 51% of 69 patients with CMTC in one series.[428] Other vascular anomalies may be present in patients with CMTC, most commonly PWS and less often IH.[425,426,429] SWS has been reported in some patients. Ophthalmologic abnormalities include glaucoma, retinal pigmentation, and retinal detachment. Neurologic abnormalities may include macrocephaly, seizures, hydrocephalus, and psychomotor retardation.[305,426,427] Adams–Oliver syndrome is a genetically heterogeneous disorder characterized by CMTC in association with distal transverse limb defects and aplasia cutis congenita of the scalp. Despite the potential associations, most patients with CMTC have only minor associated anomalies or disease limited to the skin. The incidence of associated findings is unclear and varies in the literature from 18% to 89%.[426,430] In the authors' experience, the majority of patients do not have associated anomalies. The syndrome previously referred to as *macrocephaly-CMTC* was subsequently renamed *M-CM syndrome* once it was recognized that the vascular stains in this condition are actually reticulate PWSs (and not CMTC). This entity is discussed in more detail earlier in this chapter.

The pathogenesis of CMTC is unclear. Histologic examination, when skin biopsy has been performed, reveals dilated capillaries and veins in the dermis. Vascular proliferation analogous to that seen with IH has been reported.[431] The clinical diagnosis of CMTC is usually straightforward. The differential diagnosis may include reticulate PWS, KT syndrome, and disorders with pronounced cutis marmorata such as homocystinuria, Down syndrome, Divry–Van Bogaert syndrome, and Cornelia de Lange syndrome.[425,432] It is important to recognize that CMTC-like lesions may also occur in the setting of neonatal lupus erythematosus.[433] Diffuse genuine phlebectasia (Bockenheimer syndrome) is a rare disorder characterized by large venous ectasias usually limited to an extremity. This disorder is unlikely to be confused clinically with CMTC.

The natural history of CMTC is notable for gradual fading of the cutaneous lesions in most patients. When improvement occurs it tends to be within the first several years of life.[429] Treatment is unnecessary, and in fact PDL therapy seems less effective for these lesions than it is for CMs (e.g., PWSs). Ophthalmologic evaluation is probably unnecessary in most patients but should be considered when there is facial involvement with the vascular process. Referral to a neurologist should be made if neurologic symptoms or features of a complex, multiorgan syndrome are present.

TELANGIECTASES

Telangiectases are permanent dilations of capillaries, venules, or arterioles in the skin that may disappear on diascopy (gentle pressure with a microscope slide). Many processes affecting the blood vessel endothelium and its supporting structure can lead to the development of this common vascular lesion. Some of these are primary disorders of the blood vessels themselves for which the cause is unknown. Others are secondary and are related to a known disturbance, such as aging, sun exposure, radiation, or a systemic disorder in which they may serve as a useful diagnostic clue. Although telangiectases are usually a sporadic finding without associated underlying abnormalities, a benign hereditary form has also been described. Medical intervention is usually unnecessary, but PDL therapy may be considered for cosmetic purposes.

Spider Angioma

The spider angioma (nevus araneus) is the best-known type of telangiectasia. It is characterized by a central vascular papule with symmetrically radiating thin branches ("legs") (Fig. 12.97). Spider angiomas appear most commonly on exposed areas of the face, upper trunk, arms, hands, and fingers, and occasionally on the mucous membranes of the lip and nose. They usually blanch with diascopy only to refill and reappear once the glass slide is removed. The central body is an arteriole that at times may reveal pulsations with diascopy.

Although spider angiomas can be associated with liver disease, pregnancy, and estrogen therapy, they are commonly idiopathic and may occur in up to 15% of normal children and young adults. The etiology of spider angiomas in patients with liver disease is unclear, but they seem to be related to alcoholism and impaired liver function.[434]

Whereas some spider angiomas may regress spontaneously, in many individuals they tend to persist indefinitely. Treatment options, when desired, include electrocoagulation or PDL therapy.

Angioma Serpiginosum

Angioma serpiginosum is a rare condition that manifests as multiple punctate erythematous lesions. It seems to represent a vascular malformation, although vascular proliferation has been reported. The condition is reported most often in young females.

Angioma serpiginosum presents as pinpoint red to violaceous macules that often extend in a gyrate or serpiginous pattern (Fig. 12.98).[435]

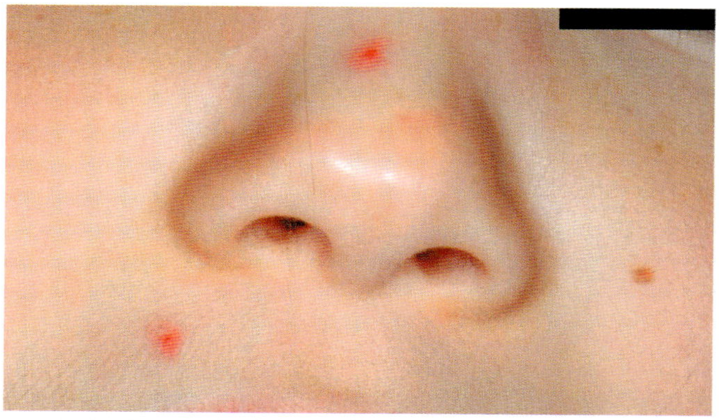

Fig. 12.97 Spider angioma. Note lesions on the nasal bridge and the right upper lip.

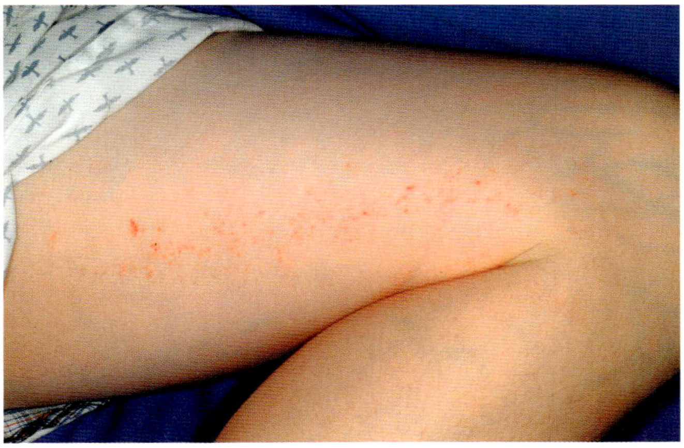

Fig. 12.98 Angioma serpiginosum.

There is often some background erythema. The lesions may occasionally appear purpuric and may be confused with various purpuric dermatoses.[436] The disorder is usually localized, and the most common distribution is on the lower extremities, although more extensive involvement may be seen.[437] Angioma serpiginosum tends to be asymptomatic.

Individual puncta of angioma serpiginosum may disappear, but complete spontaneous clearing of lesions is rare. Treatment with the PDL therapy often leads to improvement or resolution.[437,438] The 532 nm potassium-titanyl phosphate (KTP) laser has also been reported effective in treating the condition. [439]

Hereditary Hemorrhagic Telangiectasia

Hereditary hemorrhagic telangiectasia (HHT; also called *Osler–Weber–Rendu syndrome*) is an autosomal dominant vascular disorder characterized by mucocutaneous telangiectases and a bleeding diathesis, as well as arteriovenous malformations (AVMs) in the lungs, brain, and liver. It has been estimated to affect approximately 1 in 5000 to more than 10,000 individuals.[440–442] Two molecular subtypes of HHT are recognized: HHT1 and HHT2. HHT1 is known to be caused by mutations in the endoglin gene *ENG*, and HHT2 by mutations in the activin receptor-like kinase 1 *(ALK1/ACVRL1)* gene.[443,444] Mutations in *SMAD4* give rise to juvenile polyposis/HHT (JPHT). Although there is significant overlap between the clinical findings in HHT1 and HHT2, there appears to be a difference in the rates of underlying vascular anomalies.

Patients with HHT most commonly experience epistaxis and anemia, the latter usually being the result of GI blood loss. The epistaxis may begin in early childhood (an estimated 50% report having nosebleeds by 10 years of age) and is often mild during the pediatric years; the characteristic mucocutaneous telangiectases often do not appear until 5 to 30 years after the epistaxis, often during adolescence or even later.[441,445] These vascular lesions have a predisposition for certain anatomic sites, including the lips, ears, oral cavity (especially tongue and palate), palms, fingers, soles, and nasal mucous membranes. Lesions may be present under the nails. The telangiectases in HHT are often described as *punctate* or *macular* (versus the more classic spider variety with a central core and peripheral radiating vessels). Epistaxis occurs spontaneously on more than one occasion, and nighttime bleeds are particularly suspicious for HHT.[446] Other mucous membranes may also be involved, and hemorrhage may occur from any involved mucosal site. Although the distribution of lesions and associated bleeding diathesis are clinically suggestive of HHT, it may occasionally be difficult to distinguish the cutaneous lesions from those seen in benign disorders such as generalized essential telangiectasia. In addition, the classic distribution of HHT-associated telangiectases may not be observable until the third or fourth decade of life,[440] further compounding the challenge of rendering an early diagnosis.

AVMs may occur in patients with HHT and may be responsible for significant morbidity and even death. Pulmonary and cerebral AVMs are the most classically recognized lesions, although hepatic and spinal AVMs also occur. In a prospective cross-sectional survey of 44 children between 1 and 18 years of age and seen in a multidisciplinary HHT center, cerebrovascular malformations were found in 7, pulmonary AVMs in 20, and liver AVMs in 23. Importantly, size was the most important predictive factor of complication, with large lesions being associated with complications and small lesions being of low clinical significance.[448] Previously "silent" lesions in the lung or brain may hemorrhage, and pulmonary lesions are particularly worrisome because of the risks of hypoxemia or embolism of particulate matter through right-to-left shunts, with neurologic sequelae.[446] Pulmonary AVMs appear less common in HHT2 than in HHT1.[440] Catastrophic intracranial hemorrhage has been reported in infants and children with HHT who were not suspected of having the disease despite family histories of the syndrome.[448] Screening for pulmonary and cerebral AVMs, when clinically indicated, may include chest radiography, pulse oximetry, blood oxygen determination, and high-resolution CT, MRI, and MRA. Transthoracic contrast echocardiography with agitated saline contrast (echo bubble study) appears to be a sensitive test for pulmonary AVMs and is being increasingly used as an initial screen for HHT. Hepatic AVMs in patients with HHT do not appear to pose the same risk for catastrophic events as compared with pulmonary or cerebral lesions.[44] Patients may also be at risk for vascular lesions in the primarily upper GI tract, which may lead to GI bleeding.

The diagnosis of HHT generally relies on history, clinical examination, and review of family history. The Curacao criteria for diagnosis of HHT include epistaxis, mucocutaneous telangiectases, visceral AVMs, and positive first-degree family history; the diagnosis is *definite* if three criteria are present, *possible/suspected* if two criteria are present, and *unlikely* if fewer than two criteria are present.[446]

Deoxyribonucleic acid (DNA) diagnostic testing is technically difficult and costly, but mutation testing is available for diagnosis of an affected individual and for prenatal diagnosis. Newborn screening by endoglin protein expression and mutation analysis of umbilical vein endothelial cells may allow early identification of affected newborns.[449] Treatment of HHT is dictated by the extent of mucocutaneous and organ involvement. Therapies for epistaxis include embolization, laser ablation, and septal dermoplasty, as well as some pharmacologic alternatives such as estrogen receptor modulators, desmopressin (DDAVP), and antifibrinolytic agents. GI tract bleeding is treated with surgical or medical therapies, including hormones, danazol, iron replacement, and octreotide. Treatments for lung, cerebral, and hepatic AVMs depend on the extent of involvement and may include medical therapies, surgery, embolization, and transplantation. Antiangiogenic agents such as bevacizumab (a VEGF antagonist) have been used but may be associated with inconsistent efficacy, relapse, or undesirable side effects.[450]

Unilateral Nevoid Telangiectasia

Unilateral nevoid telangiectasia is a condition characterized by multiple telangiectases in a dermatomal distribution. The condition may be congenital or acquired and may be sporadic or associated with medical conditions (such as chronic liver disease), physiologic states (e.g., puberty, pregnancy), or medications (usually estrogen hormonal therapy).[451–452] Although the cause is controversial, it may be related to an increased level of estrogen receptors in involved skin.[452]

The condition presents with numerous skin telangiectases in a unilateral distribution, especially involving the upper body or extremities (Fig. 12.99). A dermatomal distribution may or may not be evident. Unilateral nevoid telangiectasia occurs most often in females during pregnancy or puberty. When it occurs in adult men, it is often in association with alcoholic cirrhosis. It has also been reported in association with hepatitis C virus.[452] Treatment is unnecessary, although PDL therapy has been demonstrated to be useful.[453]

Ataxia-Telangiectasia

Ataxia-telangiectasia (A-T; or Louis-Bar syndrome) is a multisystem autosomal recessive disorder characterized by oculocutaneous telangiectases, cerebellar ataxia, a profound humoral and cellular immunodeficiency, progressive respiratory failure, and a predisposition toward hematologic malignancy. A-T is caused by a mutation in the A-T mutated *(ATM)* gene, which maps to chromosome llq. The protein

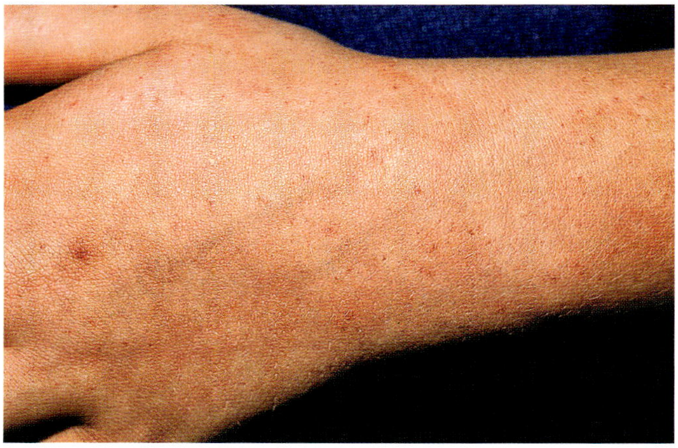

Fig. 12.99 Unilateral nevoid telangiectasia. These telangiectatic macules were limited to the hand, forearm, and upper arm.

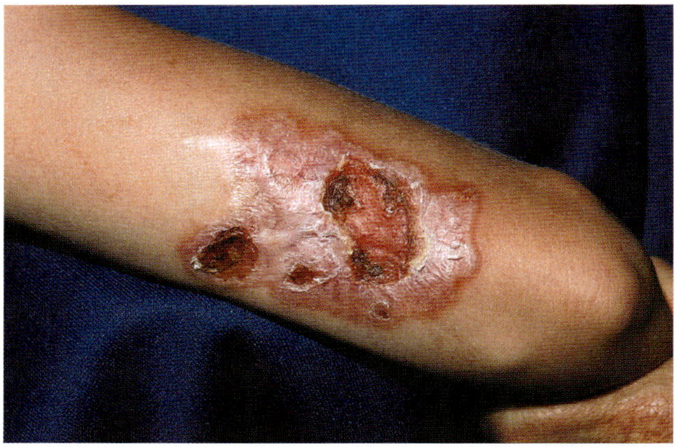

Fig. 12.101 Ataxia-telangiectasia, granulomas. These granulomatous skin lesions are very resistant to therapy.

product of this gene is a nuclear protein involved in the early recognition and response to double-stranded DNA breaks.[454]

There is considerable phenotypic variability in patients with A-T, and patients may differ significantly in their rate of progression or appearance of features.[455] The initial clinical manifestation is often truncal ataxia, which may present as early as infancy.[456] Other neurologic features include choreoathetosis, dysarthria, myoclonic jerks, and oculomotor abnormalities. Affected patients may display drooling; peculiar eye movements; a sad, mask-like facies; and a stooped posture with drooping shoulders and the head tilted forward and to the side. Progressive joint contractures and confinement to a wheelchair by the second decade is not unusual.

The mucocutaneous telangiectases are a variable feature of A-T but not uncommonly help lead to the correct clinical diagnosis. They usually appear around 3 to 5 years of age, most often on the medial and lateral bulbar conjunctivae. Skin telangiectases develop primarily on sun-exposed sites including the ears, cheeks, neck (Fig. 12.100), arms, and upper chest. Other body regions may be affected, and occasionally the cutaneous telangiectases are quite subtle. Other cutaneous findings may include subcutaneous fat loss, progeroid (premature aging) changes of skin and hair, and diffuse hair graying. Segmental, patchy hypopigmentation and hyperpigmentation have been observed,[457] and patients without the telangiectases have been reported.[458] Noninfectious cutaneous granulomas (Fig. 12.101), which present as erythematous plaques, nodules, and ulcers, are a fairly common cutaneous feature in patients with A-T.[459,460] They are usually located on the extremities, with the second most common site being the face. The granulomas less commonly involve the trunk.[461] These lesions tend to be persistent but may be improved by intralesional injections of triamcinolone or short courses of oral corticosteroids (which must be used cautiously given the underlying risk of infection). Some have suggested that these noninfectious lesions are caused by immune dysregulation and its effects on wound healing and tissue repair.[461]

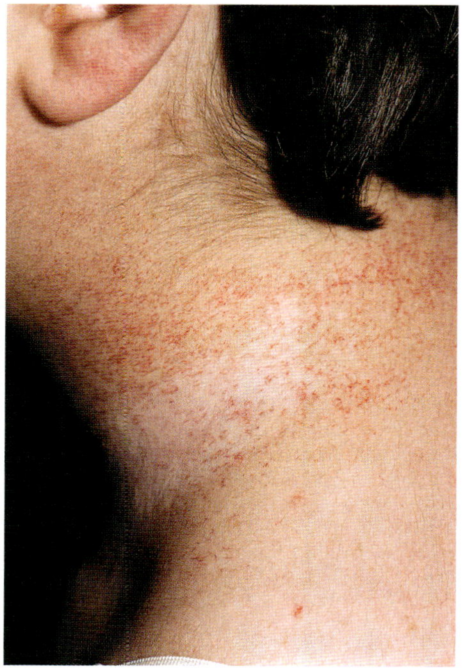

Fig. 12.100 Ataxia-telangiectasia, telangiectasias. (Reproduced with permission from Bolognia JL, Jorizzo JL, Rapini RR. Dermatology. Philadelphia: Mosby; 2003.)

Chronic sinopulmonary infections occur in the majority of patients with A-T. Bronchiectasis with respiratory failure may occur and is the most common cause of death. Growth failure and mental retardation may also occur. Several immunologic defects have been reported in patients with A-T, including decreased IgA, IgE, and IgG and multiple defects in cell-mediated immune responses. Decreased thymic output and skewed T- and B-cell receptor repertoires have been observed.[462]

Lymphoid malignancies occur with markedly increased incidence in patients with A-T. These include Hodgkin disease, non-Hodgkin lymphoma, and leukemia. There appears to be a four- to fivefold increased rate of T-cell tumors compared with B-cell tumors in patients who have A-T.[463] In those with Hodgkin disease there is a reduced survival compared with Hodgkin disease in the general population.[464] Of the non-Hodgkin lymphomas, diffuse large B-cell lymphomas account for the majority, and T-cell acute lymphoblastic leukemia is the most common form of leukemia.[463,465]

The diagnosis of A-T usually rests on the clinical findings. Elevated levels of α-fetoprotein (AFP) and carcinoembryonic antigen support the diagnosis. Early measurement of the AFP level in any child with unexplained ataxia, especially if there is also a history of frequent respiratory tract infection and/or oculocutaneous telangiectasias are present, has been advocated.[466] Molecular diagnosis and prenatal diagnosis are possible but the testing is complicated, and the familial mutation must be known. Treatment for A-T is largely supportive, including antimicrobial therapy for infection, early therapy for bronchiectasis, neurodevelopmental follow-up care and therapy, and aggressive surveillance for malignancy. Vigorous photoprotection is vital because A-T patients have a lowered threshold for the development of skin malignancies, and radiation use for treatment of hematopoietic malignancy should be minimized when feasible. Death is usually the result of chronic bronchiectasis with pulmonary insufficiency and/or pneumonia (55%) or malignancy (15%).

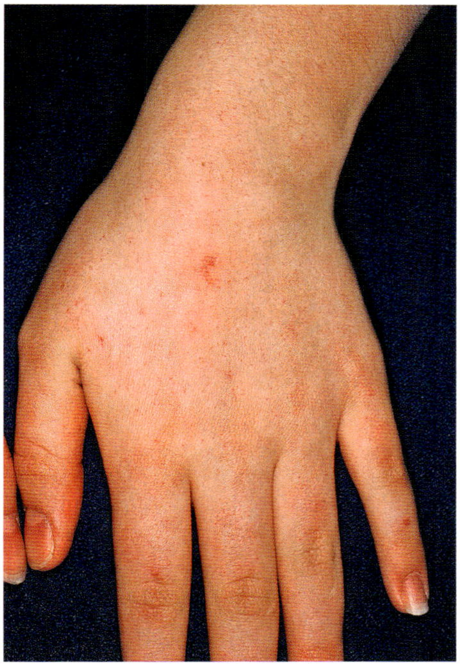

Fig. 12.102 Generalized essential telangiectasia. This patient had a widespread distribution of telangiectasias without any bleeding diathesis.

Generalized Essential Telangiectasia

Generalized essential telangiectasia is a disorder of multiple cutaneous telangiectases without a bleeding diathesis. The condition is notable for a widespread distribution of lesions (Fig. 12.102), progression and/or permanence of the telangiectases, accentuation by dependent positioning, and absence of other epidermal or dermal skin changes (e.g., atrophy, purpura, or dyspigmentation).[467] The most common site of involvement is the lower extremities, and the disorder is more common in females. Oral mucosal and conjunctival telangiectases have occasionally been reported. Although the cause of generalized essential telangiectasia is unknown, some have suggested a possible autoimmune diathesis.[468] Treatment for this condition is unnecessary. In patients who desire therapy for cosmesis, pulsed-dye or Nd:YAG laser treatment appears effective.

Pigmented Purpuric Eruptions

Pigmented purpuric eruptions (PPEs; pigmented purpura, pigmented purpuric dermatosis, progressive pigmented purpura) comprise a group of dermatoses characterized by cutaneous petechiae, purpura, and often a yellow-brown pigmentation. Histologically these disorders all reveal inflammation of the superficial dermal capillaries (capillaritis) without frank vasculitis. Table 12.8 lists the five different subtypes of PPE. The cause of PPE is unknown, and although they occur primarily in adults, they may also occur in children. Proposed associations with PPE include capillary fragility, cell-mediated immune responses, hepatitis B and C infection, and medication reactions.[469–471] The vast majority of children with PPE are healthy and have no associated medical condition.

Schamberg disease is the prototype for PPE, being the most common type and the most common to present in children. Although rare, it may even occur in infants.[472,473] The primary lesion is a red-brown punctuate macule, and multiple such lesions ("cayenne pepper spots") occur at the border of red-brown patches (Fig. 12.103).[470,474] The most common location is the lower extremities, although more widespread involvement may occur. Schamberg disease has been associated with the ingestion of several medications, including aspirin and acetaminophen. In addition there are rare reports of an association

Table 12.8 Subtypes of Pigmented Purpuric Eruptions

Type	Comment
Schamberg disease	Red-brown patches with petechiae ("cayenne pepper spots"); mainly lower extremities
Majocchi disease	Also called *purpura annularis telangiectodes*; punctate, perifollicular; telangiectases present; tend to become annular and hyperpigmented
Lichen aureus	Rust-yellow lichenoid papules and papules; often linear or along Blaschko lines; fairly common in children
Eczematid-like purpura of Doucas and Kapetanakis	Generalized; eczematous, with lichenification and pruritus present
Pigmented purpuric lichenoid dermatitis of Gougerot and Blum	Red-brown, lichenoid papules and plaques; very rare in children

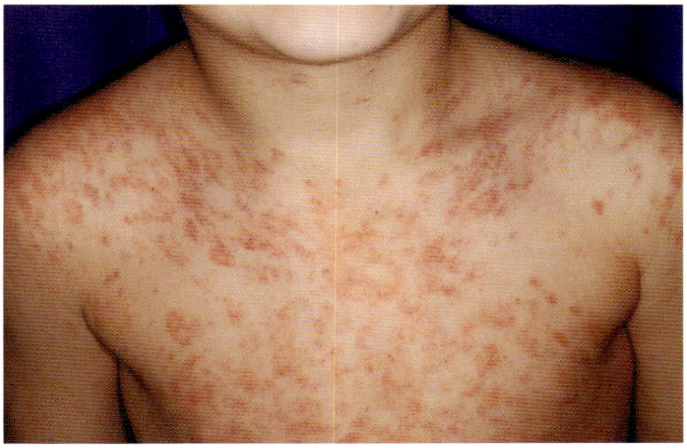

Fig. 12.103 Pigmented purpuric eruption, Schamberg disease. Multiple red-brown patches with numerous petechiae ("cayenne pepper spots"). This 6-year-old boy had generalized involvement and was largely asymptomatic.

between pigmented purpura-like eruptions and progression to cutaneous T-cell lymphoma (mycosis fungoides).[475,476] Although seemingly rare, these reports highlight the need to consider this diagnosis in patients (especially adults) with unusually persistent PPE.

Majocchi disease is an annular variant of PPE, presenting with punctuate, perifollicular petechiae, telangiectases, and hyperpigmented annular patches (Fig. 12.104). It occurs primarily in adolescents and younger adults and occurs on the lower extremities as well as the trunk and upper extremities.

Lichen aureus is a unique type of PPE in its presentation. Patients have lichenoid papules that coalesce to form plaques, often with a linear distribution or in some cases, distribution along the lines of Blaschko. The color of the lesions varies from pink to rust-yellow (Fig. 12.105) to purple, and again the lower extremities are the favored site of involvement.

Eczematid-like purpura of Doucas and Kapetanakis is usually a generalized form of PPE with eczematous changes and pruritus. Lichenification (skin thickening with accentuated skin markings) occurs as a result of frequent scratching. Pigmented purpuric lichenoid dermatosis of Gougerot and Blum presents with red-brown, polygonal lichenoid papules with telangiectases.

There are no satisfactory treatments for PPE. In cases where a drug reaction is possible, withdrawal of the offending agent may induce regression. Treatments used with variable success have included

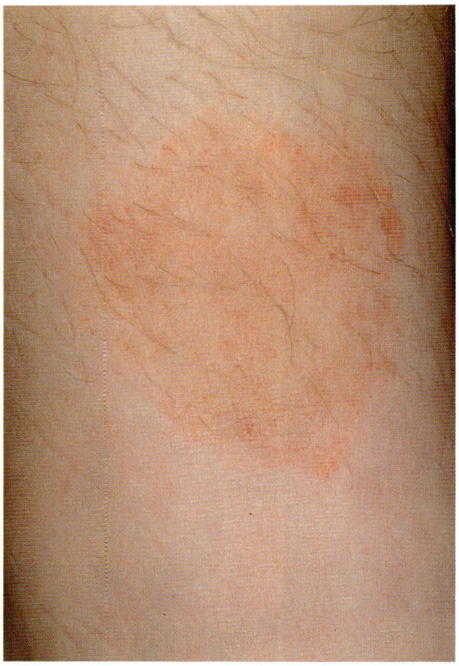

Fig. 12.104 Pigmented purpuric eruption, Majocchi disease. Pink-tan patches with petechiae and mild central clearing were present on the lower legs of this adolescent boy.

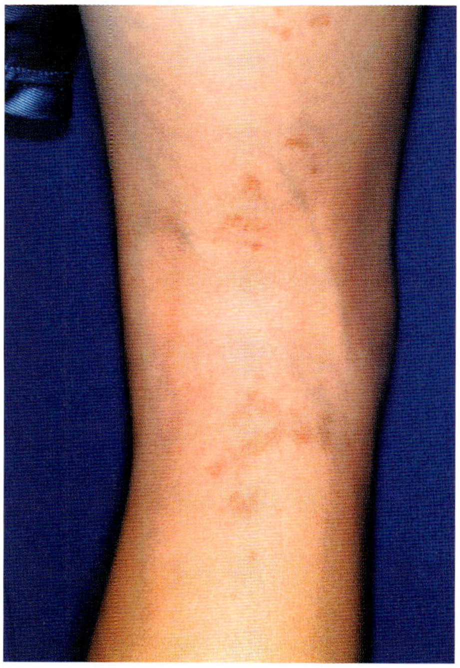

Fig. 12.105 Pigmented purpuric eruption, lichen aureus. These golden-tan macules and patches distributed in a linear fashion revealed pinpoint petechial macules with diascopy (viewing through a glass slide while applying pressure).

topical and systemic corticosteroids, antihistamines, and psoralens and PUVA light therapy. Therapy with ascorbic acid (vitamin C) and bioflavonoids (specifically rutoside or rutin) as well as narrowband ultraviolet B (UVB) phototherapy has also been reported as useful in open-label studies.[477–480] Two young adults with extensive PPE responded to pentoxifylline therapy.[481]

Purpura Fulminans

Purpura fulminans (PF) is a rare condition of microvascular thrombosis characterized by acute, rapidly progressive hemorrhagic necrosis of the skin and disseminated intravascular coagulation. The potential etiologic associations with PF are listed in Box 12.6. It occurs most often in association with severe bacterial (especially meningococcal and *Staphylococcus aureus* septicemia) or viral infection or as a postinfectious syndrome after infections such as varicella or scarlet fever.[482,483] In the latter instance it usually occurs 10 days to 1 month after the infection. PF has also been described in association with invasive pneumococcal and acute West Nile virus infections.[484,485] It may also be associated with congenital deficiencies of proteins C or S, which are vitamin K–dependent glycoproteins with antithrombotic properties. In fact, infection-associated PF may be partly the result of acquired deficiencies in these proteins.[486,487] Factor V Leiden, which is a mutated version of factor V, has been shown to be associated with activated protein C resistance, an increased risk of thrombotic events, and exacerbated PF in patients with meningococcal disease.[482,488] PF is associated with significant morbidity and is occasionally fatal, especially in the presence of concomitant meningococcal disease. Survivors often undergo amputation of the involved extremities and experience severe scarring.[489]

PF presents with erythematous macules that progress rapidly into purpura and ecchymoses, often with sharp irregular borders. The lesions are tender, enlarge rapidly, and coalesce with the development of central necrosis, hemorrhagic blebs (Fig. 12.106), and a

Box 12.6 Etiologic Associations with Purpura Fulminans

Severe Acute Infection
Neisseria meningitidis
Staphylococcus aureus
Streptococcal infections (including invasive pneumococcal)
Plasmodium falciparum
Others

Postinfectious
Varicella
Streptococcal infections
Others

Inherited Disorders of Coagulation
Homozygous protein C deficiency (neonatal PF)
Homozygous protein S deficiency (neonatal PF)
Factor V Leiden mutation

Medication Related
Coumarin-induced skin necrosis

Other
Sepsis
Disseminated intravascular coagulation
Trauma
Malignancy
Obstetric complications
Hepatic failure
Immunologic reactions

Modified from Chalmers E, Cooper P, Forman K, et al. Purpura fulminans: recognition, diagnosis and management. Arch Dis Child 2011;96:1066–71; Price VE, Ledingham DL, Krumpel A, Chan AK. Diagnosis and management of neonatal purpura fulminans. Semin Fetal Neonatal Med 2011;16:318–22; and Thornsberry LA, LoSicco KI, English JC. The skin and hypercoagulable states. J Am Acad Dermatol 2013;69:450–62.
PF, Purpura fulminans.

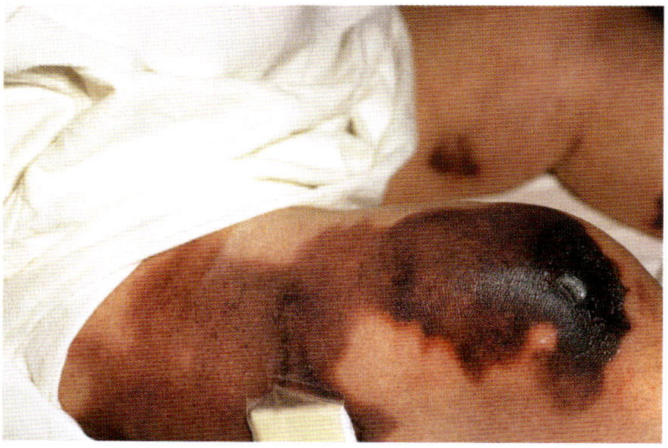

Fig. 12.106 Purpura fulminans. Ecchymotic patches and plaques with necrosis and a hemorrhagic bulla over the knee.

raised edge with surrounding erythema. The ecchymotic lesions are most commonly distributed on the lower extremities and buttocks, with occasional involvement of the trunk and upper extremities. Deep extension with muscle necrosis and bone involvement may occur. Mucous membranes are usually spared. Chills, fever, tachycardia, anemia, and prostration are common. Visceral involvement is less common but may include CNS and retinal vessel thrombosis, hematuria, and GI hemorrhage. Adrenal gland thrombosis may result in Waterhouse–Friderichsen syndrome. Skin and muscle necrosis may be severe enough to require grafting, and digital or limb ischemia may necessitate amputation. Epiphyseal growth plate necrosis in a growing child may result in limb foreshortening.[490] Newborn infants with protein C or S deficiency or factor V Leiden have clinical features of PF within 24 hours after birth and are at high risk for widespread thrombosis of capillaries and venules.[491] Children younger than 4 years of age and those with the factor V Leiden mutation appear to be at increased risk for severe disease and amputation.[483]

Laboratory evaluation in the patient with PF reveals decreased fibrinogen and thrombocytopenia. The prothrombin time and partial thromboplastin time are prolonged, and fibrin degradation products are increased. Protein C, protein S, and antithrombin III levels are decreased. Histologic evaluation of the skin lesions reveals dermal vascular thrombosis and hemorrhagic necrosis.[490]

The treatment for PF depends on the underlying disorder or associated infection. Initial management consists of fluid resuscitation, ventilatory and inotropic support, and antibiotic administration when indicated.[492] Administration of proteins C and S (e.g., in the form of fresh frozen plasma or protein C concentrate) may prevent progression of lesions that are not yet necrotic.[486,493] Repeated infusions may be necessary because of the short half-life of protein C.[486] Antithrombin III concentrate has been administered to some patients. Concomitant heparin has been advocated by some (but not by others), especially when there is evidence for large vessel venous thrombosis. Long-term administration of oral anticoagulants is often necessary in patients with congenital protein C or S deficiency. Packed red blood cell transfusion, platelet transfusion, and cryoprecipitate may each need to be considered in certain patients. Surgical modalities include debridement, autologous skin grafting, tissue and muscle flaps, amputation, skin allografts, and tissue-engineered skin.[494,495]

Gardner–Diamond Syndrome

Gardner–Diamond syndrome (autoerythrocyte sensitization syndrome, painful bruising syndrome, psychogenic purpura) is a rare disorder characterized by painful bruising and usually seen in patients with emotional or psychiatric disturbance. Historically the disorder was ascribed to a sensitization reaction to the patient's own erythrocytes, hence the alternative nomenclature *autoerythrocyte sensitization syndrome*.[496] The majority of patients with Gardner–Diamond syndrome are adolescent or adult females, with only occasional reports of involved males.

The disorder is characterized by recurrent episodes of spontaneous, painful ecchymoses that are often precipitated by emotional stress. The lesions may vary in size and may involve any part of the cutaneous surface. Most patients report a burning sensation initially. The lesions of Gardner–Diamond syndrome tend to resolve over weeks only to recur again with time. GI symptoms may also be present, including pain, nausea, vomiting, diarrhea, and bleeding.[497]

The cause of this condition remains unclear. In the original reports, patients were noted to have a positive reaction to intradermal injection of their own erythrocytes, which resulted in an ecchymosis.[498] The significance of this finding has been questioned in some subsequent reports, and the immune nature of the condition remains speculative. A number of psychiatric disorders have been observed in association with the cutaneous findings, including depression, anxiety, impulse-control issues, adjustment disorders, hypochondriasis, hysterical and borderline personality disorders, conversion disorder, and obsessive-compulsive behavior.[496,497] There is no universally effective treatment for Gardner–Diamond syndrome, which has a chronic unremitting course, and psychiatric evaluation is advisable.[499] Psychotropic medications, hypnotherapy, and psychotherapy have been successfully used in some patients.[500]

Scurvy

Scurvy, which is caused by vitamin C deficiency, is relatively rare in developed countries, although there are several cases described in the literature in children with an inadequate dietary intake of this vitamin.[501] Clinicians caring for children and adolescents must therefore be aware of this disease and its clinical presentation.

Vitamin C (ascorbic acid) is a vital component of the human diet because of the inability of humans to derive it from glucose via gluconolactone oxidase.[502] Ascorbic acid is found primarily in fresh fruits, vegetables, and vitamin supplements. When deficiency of this vitamin occurs in a developed country, it is usually in the elderly, indigent, drug- or alcohol-abusing, or food-faddism populations or those with GI disorders or poor dentition.[502,503] Children at risk include those in neglectful social situations, with neurodevelopmental disabilities or psychiatric illnesses, with severe food allergies or GI disease, with a history of iron overload from multiple transfusions, and with unusual dietary habits or with parents who are food faddists.[501–507] There are multiple reports of scurvy in children with autism and, in that setting, a long-standing history of extreme food selectivity with a diet low in fruits and vegetables.[508–512] Because ascorbic acid is a cofactor in the synthesis of collagen and collagen is a vital component of the pericapillary network in the skin, capillary fragility results from deficiency of this nutrient.

Clinical manifestations of scurvy include fatigue, petechiae, ecchymoses, purpura, and perifollicular hemorrhages. The latter finding is considered pathognomonic for the condition. In addition, follicular hyperkeratosis and "corkscrew hairs" may be noted. Purpura often occurs on the lower extremities but may also involve other body regions. Gingival findings include swelling, bleeding, and loosening of teeth. Bony fractures appear to be more common in pediatric patients when compared with adults, and arthralgias, joint swelling, and hemarthrosis may occur. Other findings include GI bleeding, conjunctival and intraocular hemorrhage, alopecia, and epistaxis. In some patients, musculoskeletal discomfort and weakness may be presenting features, and they may complain of lower extremity pain, a limp, or refusal to bear weight.[502,505,506,512] Cardiovascular manifestations of scurvy may include cardiac hypertrophy, postural hypotension, syncope, and possibly hypertension.[502] Pulmonary hypertension may be the presenting feature.

Scurvy is usually diagnosed clinically, with the differential diagnosis including hematologic malignancy, vasculitis, infection, coagulopathy, child abuse, and factitial disorder.[501] Extensive involvement of the legs may resemble stasis dermatitis. A serum ascorbic acid level is usually confirmatory (when less than 11 μmol/L), although this value may be normal if the patient has had recent intake of vitamin C. Concomitant vitamin deficiencies (especially calcium, vitamin B_{12}, or iron) may also be present.[503] Radiographic findings may include ill-defined sclerotic and lucent metaphyseal bands around the knee and osteopenia with a ground glass appearance on plain radiographs; magnetic resonance imaging may reveal increased T2 signal in marrow cavities of the metaphyses (especially adjacent to the knee joint), periosteal elevation and edema, and subperiosteal hematoma.[507,513,514] The clinical symptoms usually respond promptly to vitamin C replacement, with dosages for infants and children ranging from 100 to 300 mg/day.

The complete list of 518 references for this chapter is available online at http://expertconsult.inkling.com.

Key References

Wassef M, Blei F, Adams D, et al. Vascular anomalies classification: recommendations from the International Society for the Study of Vascular Anomalies. Pediatrics 2015;136(1):1–12.

Haggstrom AN, Drolet BA, Baselga E, et al. Prospective study of infantile hemangiomas: demographic, prenatal, and perinatal characteristics. J Pediatr 2007;150(3):291–4.

Haggstrom AN, Lammer EJ, Schneider RA, et al. Patterns of infantile hemangiomas: new clues to hemangioma pathogenesis and embryonic facial development. Pediatrics 2006;117(3):698–703.

Chang LC, Haggstrom AN, Drolet BA, et al. Growth characteristics of infantile hemangiomas: implications for management. Pediatrics 2008;122:360–7.

Krowchuk DP, Frieden IJ, Mancini AJ, et al. Clinical practice guideline for the management of infantile hemangiomas. Pediatrics 2019;143(1):e20183475.
Leaute-Labreze C, Roque ED, Hubiche T, et al. Propranolol for severe hemangiomas of infancy. N Engl J Med 2008;358(24):2649–51.
Leaute-Labreze C, Hoeger P, Mazereeuw-Hautier J, et al. A randomized, controlled trial of oral propranolol in infantile hemangioma. N Engl J Med 2015;372:735–46.
Darrow DH, Greene AK, Mancini AJ, et al. Diagnosis and management of infantile hemangioma. Pediatrics 2015;136(4):e1060–104.
Drolet BA, Frommelt PC, Chamlin SL, et al. Initiation and use of propranolol for infantile hemangioma: report of a consensus conference. Pediatrics 2013;131:128–40.
Haggstrom AN, Drolet BA, Baselga E, et al. Prospective study of infantile hemangiomas: clinical characteristics predicting complications and treatment. Pediatrics 2006;118(3):882–7.
Garzon MC, Epstein LG, Heyer GL, et al. PHACE syndrome: consensus-derived diagnosis and care recommendations. J Pediatr 2016;178:24–33.
Horii KA, Drolet BA, Frieden IJ, et al. Prospective study of the frequency of hepatic hemangiomas in infants with multiple cutaneous infantile hemangiomas. Pediatr Dermatol 2011;28(3):245–53.
Stier MF, Glick SA, Hirsch RJ. Laser treatment of pediatric vascular lesions: port wine stains and hemangiomas. J Am Acad Dermatol 2008;58:261–85.
Shirley MD, Tang H, Gallione CJ, et al. Sturge-Weber syndrome and port wine stains caused by somatic mutation in *GNAQ*. N Engl J Med 2013;368(21):1971–9.
Dutkiewicz AS, Ezzedine K, Mazereeuw-Hautier J, et al. A prospective study of risk for Sturge-Weber syndrome in children with upper facial port wine stain. J Am Acad Dermatol 2015;72:473–80.
Yeung KS, Ip JJK, Chow CP, et al. Somatic *PIK3CA* mutations in seven patients with *PIK3CA*-related overgrowth spectrum. Am J Med Genet 2017;Part A 173A:978–84.
Garzon MC, Huang JT, Enjolras O, et al. Vascular malformations. Part I. J Am Acad Dermatol 2007;56:353–70.
Garzon MC, Huang JT, Enjolras O, et al. Vascular malformations. Part II. Associated syndromes. J Am Acad Dermatol 2007;56:541–64.

13 *Bullous Disorders of Childhood*

CHAPTER OUTLINE **Hereditary Blistering Disorders**

Blisters or bullae are round or irregularly shaped lesions of the skin or mucous membranes that result from the accumulation of fluid between the cells of the epidermis and sometimes between the epidermis and dermis. The term *bullae* refers to blistering lesions 0.5 cm in diameter or larger; those smaller than 0.5 cm in diameter are called *vesicles*. The classification of bullous or vesiculobullous disorders is based on clinical morphology and examination of biopsied specimens of lesional or perilesional skin by light microscopy, immunofluorescence analysis, and electron microscopy. In general, the skin of infants and children is more susceptible to blister formation than that of adults, and bullous disorders may manifest differently based on age.[1]

Hereditary Blistering Disorders

EPIDERMOLYSIS BULLOSA

The term *epidermolysis bullosa (EB)* refers to a group of inherited disorders characterized by bullous lesions that develop spontaneously or as a result of varying degrees of friction or trauma.[2–4] The various subtypes of inherited disorders of skin fragility result from mutations in 38 different genes.[5] In the newest classification, established at a consensus meeting in 2019, heritable disorders with skin fragility were subdivided into "disorders with skin fragility" (peeling disorders, erosive disorders, hyperkeratotic disorders, and a connective tissue disorder with blistering) and "classical EB" (based on the level of skin cleavage and clinical features as simplex, junctional, dystrophic, and Kindler syndrome) (Fig. 13.1).[6] Disorders can be further considered as nonsyndromic (i.e., with any extracutaneous manifestations, such as failure to thrive, anemia, and cardiomyopathy, as secondary) or syndromic (i.e., with the extracutaneous manifestation as part of the disorders, such as cardiomyopathy, muscular dystrophy, or pyloric atresia). Subsequent classification is based on the genotype, mode of inheritance, and clinical phenotype, including distribution of lesions and presence of scarring, and the relative severity of cutaneous and extracutaneous involvement.

In EBS (epidermolytic EB) the blister cleavage occurs within the epidermis, and healing usually occurs without scarring. In junctional EB (JEB) the skin separates in the lamina lucida of the dermal–epidermal junction, and blistering leads to atrophic scarring. In dystrophic (dermolytic) EB (DEB) the blister forms in the papillary dermis below the basement membrane, and patients form scars and milia. EB with congenital absence of skin (formerly called *Bart syndrome*) can be seen at birth with any of the major forms of EB (Fig. 13.2), although it occurs most commonly with dystrophic forms of EB. Neonates most commonly show congenital localized absence of skin on the lower extremities. EB acquisita (EBA) is an acquired immune-mediated blistering disorder that can resemble DEB (see Epidermolysis Bullosa Acquisita section). It usually presents in adulthood, although cases in children and neonates have been described.

Immunofluorescence mapping on skin biopsy samples was traditionally used to confirm the diagnosis of EB and to determine the subtype based on the level of cleavage from localization of known antigens in the skin and the presence of structural proteins associated with EB. Biopsies, if performed for immunomapping, are ideally taken from the edge of a lesion freshly induced by rotating the skin with a moist Q-tip. Light microscopic evaluation of biopsy sections is generally not useful, except for rare types (such as for showing the intraepidermal erosions from desmosomal defects in the erosive disorders of skin fragility). Whole-exome sequencing has largely replaced mapping because it allows concurrent analysis of all genes known to be mutated in EB and now is quite cost-effective, especially compared with sequencing individual genes.[7] The disadvantage is that exome sequencing still takes at least a month for results, whereas immunomapping studies may be performed within days, providing the family and healthcare team with faster prognostic information. Of note, some genetic changes in EB are intronic and require other genetic analysis for detection.

The overall incidence of EB is 1 in every 50,000 births, although the simplex forms comprise the majority of cases. A national EB registry was established in the United States and has generated data beneficial to many families who have children with EB. The Dystrophic Epidermolysis Bullosa Research Association (DEBRA), a national (www.debra.org) and international (www.debra-international.org) group, is dedicated to research and support for patients with all forms of EB and their families. A validated scoring system is available for EB severity, the EB Disease Activity and Scarring Index (EBDASI).[8]

EPIDERMOLYSIS BULLOSA SIMPLEX

EBS is characterized by blisters that develop in areas of trauma and most commonly results from defective keratin filaments.[9,10] Because the blister cleavage is intraepidermal, lesions usually heal without scarring. The most common forms are localized EBS (formerly called *Weber–Cockayne disease*), intermediate EBS (formerly called *Koebner type*), and severe EBS (formerly called *Dowling–Meara EBS* or *EBS herpetiformis*) (Table 13.1).[4] These are predominantly inherited as autosomal dominant disorders, although autosomal recessive forms have been described.[11–13]

Classical Epidermolysis Bullosa Simplex

EBS most commonly results from mutations in the genes encoding keratin 5 and keratin 14 (the keratins expressed in basal cells). Keratins are the most abundant proteins of epidermal keratinocytes, and keratin pairs are critical for the filamentous network that provides integrity to epidermal cells. When a point mutation occurs in one of the keratin alleles, resulting in a change in one amino acid, the abnormal keratin protein is still able to form filaments, but these filaments are abnormal. The abnormal filaments do not provide adequate structural integrity to the cell, and as a result, the cell lyses. Cytolysis of epidermal basal cells is the essential histologic feature of all forms of EBS resulting from keratin gene mutations. Electron microscopic examination shows cleavage through the basal layer (above the periodic acid–Schiff-positive basement membrane of the epidermis). In the severe generalized form, clumping of tonofilaments and displacement of nuclei are seen ultrastructurally. The risk of cell lysis and the trauma required to elicit the blistering depend on the site of the mutation and how critical that gene region is for resultant keratin function. The sites of mutations in generalized severe EB simplex are those most critical for keratin function (end-terminal rod domains), whereas the sites mutated in the localized type are less critical.

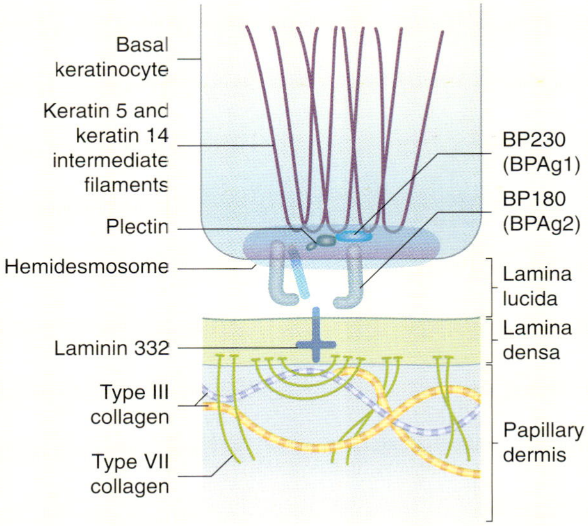

Fig. 13.1 Schematic of the structural elements of the basal keratinocytes, basement membrane zone, and upper dermis.

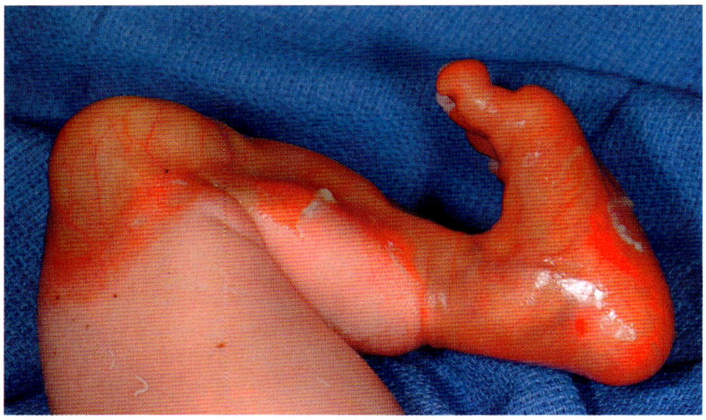

Fig. 13.2 Epidermolysis bullosa (EB). Congenital localized absence of skin, also known as *Bart syndrome,* is now known to be a pattern seen in any of the three major subsets of EB. This baby with Bart syndrome has a form of junctional EB, but denudement at birth is most often seen in babies with dystrophic EB and occasionally EB simplex.

Severe EBS (formerly Dowling–Meara) is the most severe form of EBS from keratin gene mutations (Table 13.2). During the newborn period, the generalized blisters tend to be large and may be difficult to distinguish from those of the severe dystrophic or junctional forms of EB despite the relatively good overall prognosis of babies with this form (Fig. 13.3).[14] Many young infants also show a significant inflammatory reaction in association with blistering and the formation of transient milia at sites of healed blisters, a finding usually characteristic of the dystrophic forms. The characteristic small, clustered (herpetiform) blisters may be seen in neonates, especially on the proximal extremities or trunk, but are more commonly noted during infancy and later childhood (Fig. 13.4). Blistering tends to decrease during later childhood and adulthood, and hyperkeratosis of the palms and soles may develop by 6 or 7 years of age, especially in those younger children with significant palmoplantar blistering (Fig. 13.5). During the neonatal period and early infancy, the extensive blistering may prove life-threatening. After this period, however, the blistering is rarely a threat to life. As with all types of EB, pigmented nevi may occur *(EB nevi)* (Fig. 13.6). EB nevi are dark, irregular hyperpigmented patches that

Table 13.1 Nomenclature of Epidermolysis Bullosa Simplex Subtypes

Subtype	Gene Defect/Abnormal Protein(s)
AUTOSOMAL DOMINANT	
EBS, localized (formerly Weber–Cockayne)	*KRT5, 14*/keratins 5 or 14
EBS, intermediate	*KRT5, 14* keratins 5 or 14 *PLEC*/plectin (formerly Ogna)
EBS, severe	*KRT5, 14* keratins 5 or 14
EBS, with mottled pigmentation	*KRT, 14*/keratin 5
EBS, migratory circinate erythema	*KRT, 14*/keratin 5
EBS, intermediate with cardiomyopathy	*KLHL24*/Kelch-like member 24
AUTOSOMAL RECESSIVE	
EBS, intermediate or severe	*KRT5, 14*/keratins 5 or 14
EBS, intermediate	*PLEC*/plectin
EBS, localized or intermediate – BP230 deficiency	*DST-e*/BP230, BPAg1e, dystonin-e
EBS, localized or intermediate – exophilin 5 deficiency	*EXPH5*/exophilin 5 (Slac2-b)
EBS, intermediate with muscular dystrophy	*PLEC*/plectin
EBS, severe with pyloric atresia	*PLEC*/plectin
EBS, localized with nephropathy	*CD151*/tetraspanin 24 (formerly tetraspanin 151)

EBS, Epidermolysis bullosa simplex.

Table 13.2 Characteristics of the Major Forms of Epidermolysis Bullosa Simplex*

Type	Clinical Manifestations
EBS, localized (formerly Weber–Cockayne)	Easy blistering on palms and soles May be focal keratoderma of palms and soles in adults ≈25% show oral mucosal erosions Rarely show reticulated pigmentation, especially on arms and trunk and punctate keratoderma (EBS with mottled pigmentation)
EBS, intermediate (formerly Koebner)	Generalized blistering Variable mucosal involvement Focal keratoderma of palms and soles Nail involvement in 20% Improves with advancing age
EBS, severe (formerly Dowling–Meara or EB herpetiformis)	Most severe in neonate, infant; improves beyond childhood Large, generalized blisters; later, smaller (herpetiform) blisters Mucosal blistering, including esophageal Nails thickened, shed but regrow May have natal teeth
EBS, with mottled pigmentation	Reticulated hyperpigmentation, especially on arms and trunk Punctate keratoses and keratoderma

EB, Epidermolysis bullosa; *EBS,* epidermolysis bullosa simplex.
*Resulting from *KRT5/14* variants.

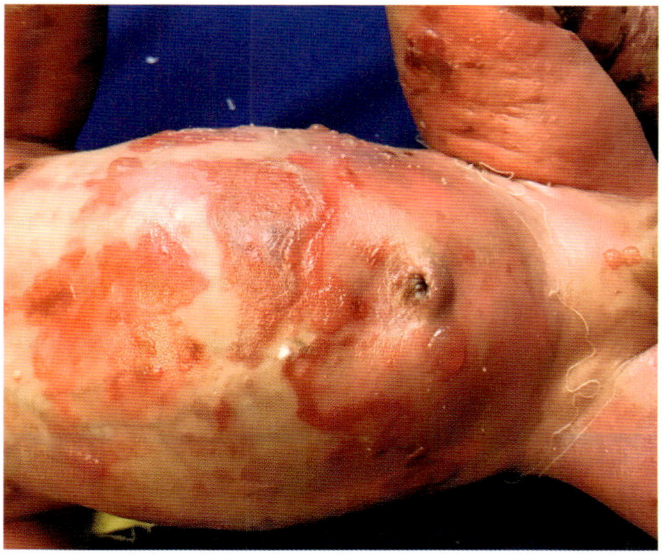

Fig. 13.3 Generalized severe epidermolysis bullosa (EB) simplex. During the infantile periods the blistering is often severe and generalized, making distinction clinically from other forms of EB difficult.

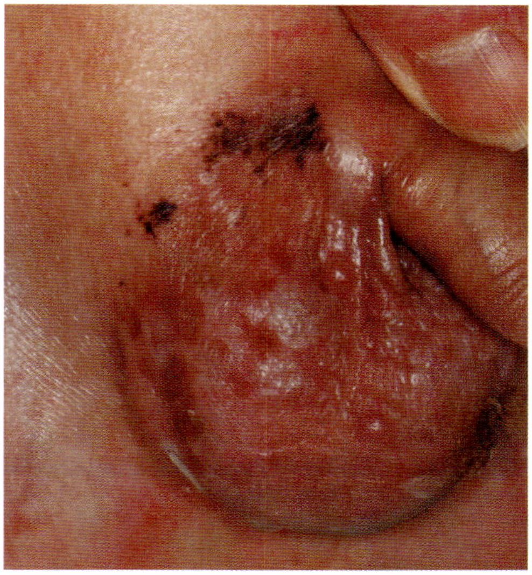

Fig. 13.6 Generalized severe epidermolysis bullosa simplex. EB nevi can occur in any type of EB and can appear atypical, particularly because of the irregular borders. EB nevi can change shape and sometimes clear spontaneously.

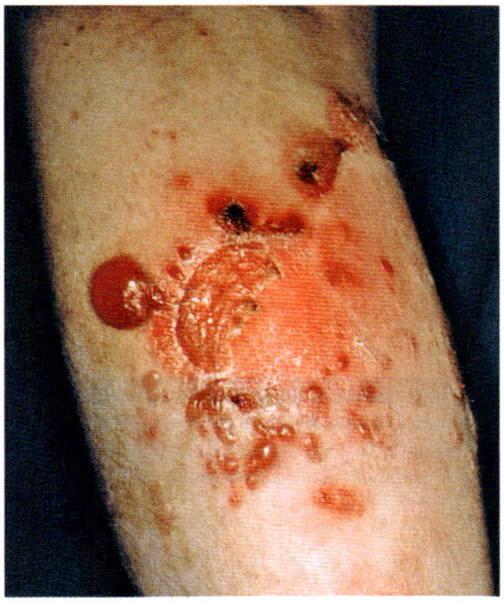

Fig. 13.4 Generalized severe epidermolysis bullosa (EB) simplex. With advancing age, the blisters often become smaller and more clustered (herpetiform) in this form of EB. Blisters may be hemorrhagic and quite inflamed.

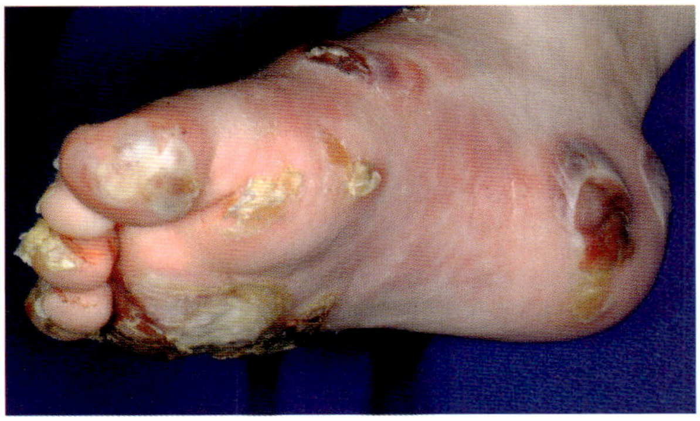

Fig. 13.5 Generalized severe epidermolysis bullosa simplex. Blistering on the palms and soles may be severe, but palms and soles show thickening with advancing age that is likely protective.

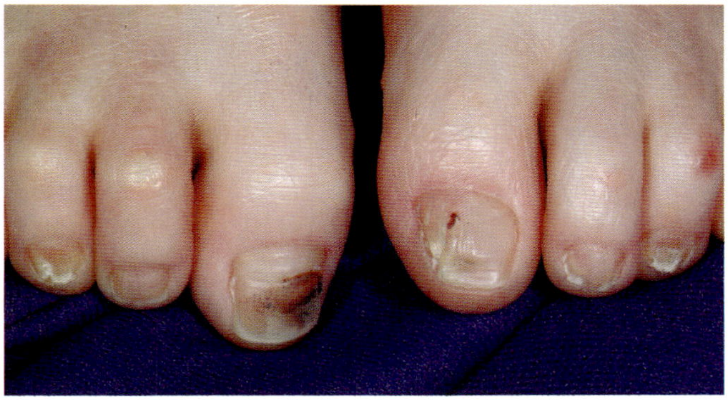

Fig. 13.7 Generalized severe epidermolysis bullosa simplex. Nails commonly show hemorrhagic blistering with residual, but transient dystrophy.

may be worrisome dermoscopically[15] but show benign nevi or increased basal pigment deposition histologically[16,17] and typically clear spontaneously during the subsequent months to years. Nail involvement with sloughing, hemorrhage, and transient dystrophy is common in the generalized severe form (Fig. 13.7). Oral and esophageal mucosal blistering may occur and cause problems with feeding and obtaining adequate nutrition, especially with the markedly increased caloric needs of more severely affected infants and younger children. Ocular mucosal blistering is less common, but natal teeth have been described.

Intermediate EBS (formerly Koebner EBS) is characterized by generalized blistering of skin, most notable at sites of friction (see Table 13.2). Extensive blistering in the neonatal period and early infancy increases the risk of sepsis and may be life-threatening. In general the tendency toward blistering tends to improve with advancing age, particularly by the teenage years. Hyperhidrosis is common, and mild to moderate hyperkeratosis of the soles is often present. Although erosions of the mucous membranes may be seen in the newborn as a result of vigorous sucking, mucosal involvement is generally mild and the nails are rarely affected, in contrast to the generalized severe form. Involvement of the conjunctiva and cornea has rarely been described.

Localized EBS (formerly Weber–Cockayne EBS) is the most common clinical variant (see Table 13.2). A relatively high threshold of frictional trauma is required to induce blister formation. Bullae are usually confined to the hands and feet (primarily the palms and soles; Fig. 13.8); they are often first seen in infants but may not appear until adolescence or early adulthood. The bullae are usually associated with trauma, occur more readily in hot weather with sweating of the feet, and do not tend to be seriously debilitating, although activities that involve trauma to the feet are often restricted. Associated hyperhidrosis is common and may exacerbate blistering. Keratoderma of the palms and soles occurs with advancing age, especially in children with more plantar-area trauma (Fig. 13.9), but tends to be milder than with other keratinopathies, such as epidermolytic ichthyosis from *KRT1* mutations or pachyonychia congenita. Lesions heal rapidly without scarring, nail involvement rarely occurs, and the mucous membranes do not tend to be involved. In young children, blisters may develop on the knees from the frictional trauma of crawling. In adolescents and young adults, blisters often occur on the feet after long hikes or dancing or on the hands after a game of tennis or golf.

EBS with mottled pigmentation is characterized by a mottled, reticulated pigmentation (Fig. 13.10), particularly of the trunk and neck, in association with mild acral blistering (see Table 13.2). Patients often show small verrucous papules of the hands and feet and palmoplantar keratoderma.[18] The mutations that lead to EBS with mottled pigmentation tend to be at the head region of *KRT5* or *KRT14* (most often a mutation that changes the 25th amino acid of keratin 5),[19,20] suggesting that this site on the keratin protein is vital for the transfer of pigment from melanocytes to keratinocytes. Migratory circinate EBS (see Table 13.1) is characterized by small blisters on the hands, feet, and legs with migratory circinate erythema and often postinflammatory hyperpigmentation.[21] Mucosal and nail involvement have not been described. The migratory circinate form has been linked to specific frameshift mutations in the V2 tail region of *KRT5*.

Autosomal recessive EBS from mutations in *KRT5/KRT14* can present with localized to generalized blistering. It can result from biallelic mutations in *KRT5* or *KRT14*, or can be digenic, with a combination of a mutation each in *KRT5* and *KRT14*; in the latter, parents may be mildly affected or have normal skin.[22]

Autosomal dominant EBS can also occur from mutations in *KLHL24*. Blistering tends to be mild but is often present at birth and results in skin atrophy and scarring (Fig. 13. 11). Distinguishing features include dyspigmentation, dystrophic nails, sparse hair (especially after the first decade), variable oral involvement, follicular atrophoderma, dilated cardiomyopathy,[23,24] and neurologic abnormalities, including seizures. Mutations in *KLHL24*, encoding Kelch-like protein 24, affect the initiation codon region and result in an increase in ubiquitination and thus accelerated degradation of keratin.[25,26] The increase in keratin 15, which can also form heterodimers with keratin 5, is thought to be compensatory.

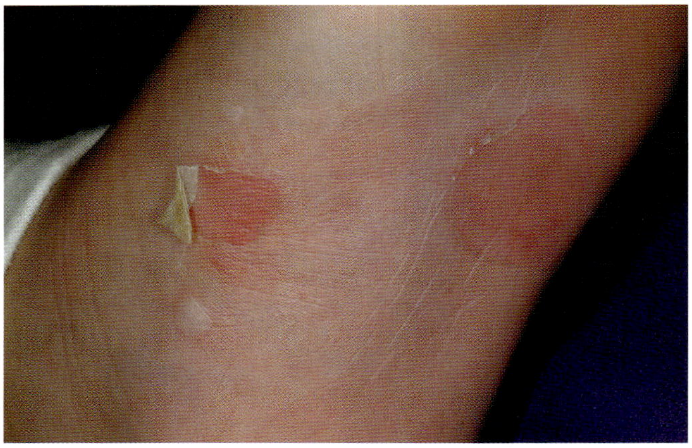

Fig. 13.8 Localized epidermolysis bullosa simplex. Note the superficial blistering with both intact bullae and denuded skin. This form tends to be limited to the palms and soles.

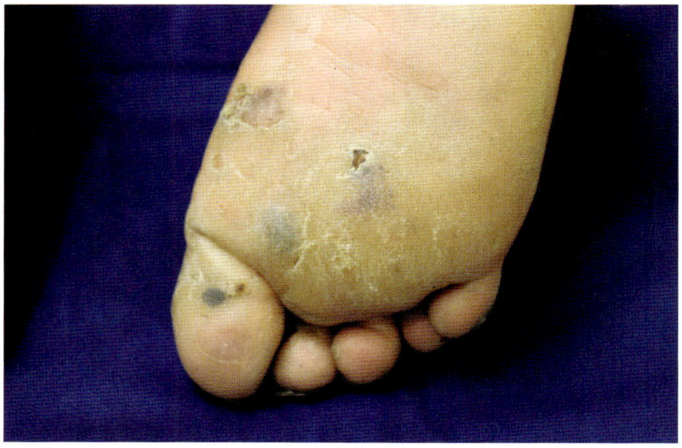

Fig. 13.9 Localized epidermolysis bullosa simplex. This adolescent participated actively in sports that traumatized his feet, despite the blistering and pain, and his keratoderma was more extensive than typical cases.

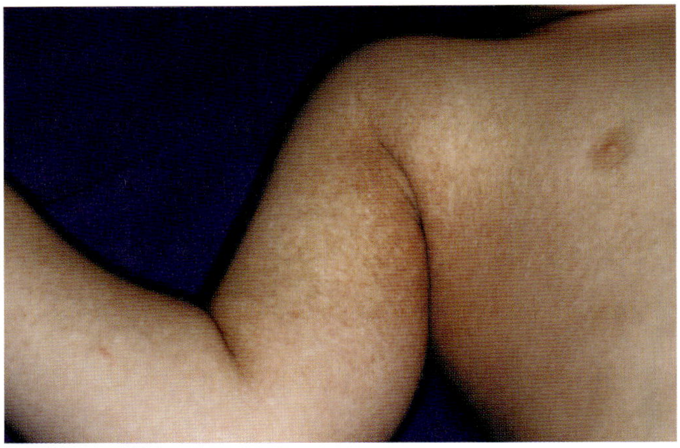

Fig. 13.10 Epidermolysis bullosa simplex with mottled pigmentation. The reticulated pigmentation may be bothersome to affected individuals, but the mild acral blistering is not problematic.

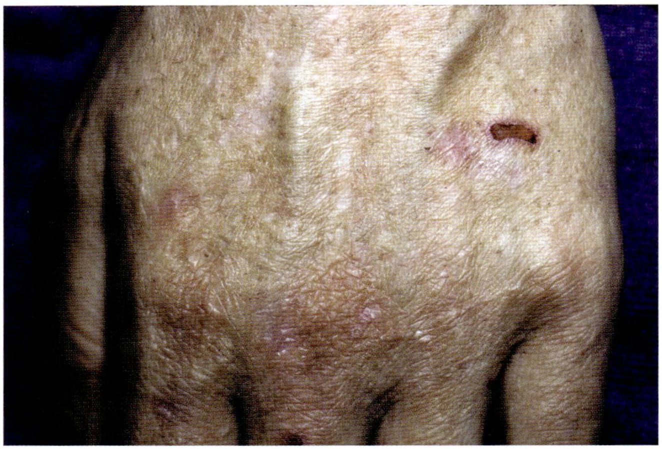

Fig. 13.11 Epidermolysis bullosa simplex, intermediate, with cardiomyopathy. This patient with a *KLHL24* variant experienced relatively mild blistering as a child, but had more dyspigmentation and atrophy (including follicular atrophy) of residual lesions than typical EB simplex. As an adult, she has been monitored for cardiomyopathy, but has none to date.

Mutations in the gene encoding plectin *(PLEC)* can lead to either autosomal dominant or recessive EBS.[27,28] The dominant form (called *EBS-Ogna* in the past) predominantly has acral blistering, although more generalized blistering has been described. Affected individuals characteristically bruise easily and may show onychogryphosis. Autosomal recessive forms are usually associated with muscular dystrophy or pyloric atresia. EBS with muscular dystrophy presents in the neonatal or infantile period with generalized blisters, but the onset of muscular dystrophy varies from infancy to adulthood. Patients may show ptosis, granulation tissue with stenosis of the respiratory tract, and focal keratoderma. The mutations of EBS with muscular dystrophy cluster in exon 31, which is spliced out in one of the two isoforms of plectin, explaining the much milder phenotype of EBS with muscular dystrophy.[29] EBS with pyloric atresia presents with the same widespread congenital absence of skin (especially on the extremities), generalized blistering, and pyloric atresia as in JEB with pyloric atresia (from variants in genes encoding integrin α6 or integrin β4, see later). Malformed pinnae and nasal alae, joint contractures, and cryptorchidism are other shared features. Plectin interacts with α6β4 integrin, providing a rationale for similar clinical manifestations.

Autosomal recessive EBS (EBS-AR BP230) may result from mutations in DST-e (dystonin-e), the epidermal isoform of bullous pemphigoid (BP) antigen (BPAG1e or BP230).[30,31] Affected individuals experience blistering and erosions beginning in infancy, usually localized to the ankles and feet; however, an intermediate-severity form of EBS associated with prurigo papules has been associated with *DST* mutations.[32]

Autosomal recessive EBS (EBS-AR exophilin 5) may also occur due to mutations in *EXPH5*, encoding exophilin-5 (or SLAC2b), which is a protein involved in vesicle transport.[33] Small, localized erosions and bleeding primary affect sites of trauma, primarily the lower back, knees, and ankles. Mottled pigmentation has been associated.[34] Exophilin-5 co-localizes with integrin β4 at the keratinocyte periphery and affects its adhesion to the laminin-332 matrix. Ultrastructural studies show typical perinuclear cytoplasmic vesicles in addition to keratin filament clumping and acantholysis (which is occasionally seen in EBS related to keratin gene mutations).[35,36]

EBS localized with nephropathy is associated with biallelic mutations in *CD151*, which encodes a tetraspanin expressed in keratinocytes at the dermal–epidermal junction. Cutaneous features are pretibial blistering (sometimes more widespread), poikiloderma,[37,38] and acrogeria. Tetraspanin 24 (formerly called *tetraspanin 151*) is a component of basement membranes that forms complexes with integrins, including α3β1 and α6β4 in skin. Patients also have oral erosions, nail dystrophy, early-onset alopecia and loss of teeth, nasolacrimal duct stenosis, esophageal webbing and strictures, and corneal vascularization. An important feature is protein-wasting nephropathy, given the important role of tetraspanin 24 in glomerular function and renal tubules.

Erosive, Peeling, and Hyperkeratotic Disorders with Skin Fragility

Biallelic mutations in *DSP, PKP1*, and *JUP*, all encoding desmosomal proteins, can lead to autosomal recessive **erosive disorders with skin fragility** associated with suprabasal cleavage and acantholysis in histologic sections (Table 13.3). Mutations in the C-terminal domain of *DSP* lead to generalized denudement at birth with absence of hair and nails (formerly called the *lethal acantholytic form of EB*, or *LAEB*).[39,40] Frank blisters are not seen, but the skin peels in sheets (Fig. 13.12). Mucosal sloughing is severe, and affected neonates may be born with teeth. All babies to date have died in the neonatal period. Cardiomyopathy is usually associated. Mutations have been described in the C-terminal domain of *DSP*. Less deleterious mutations in *DSP* also cause skin fragility and woolly hair syndrome (see Chapter 7), characterized by superficial erosions and crusting with woolly hair, palmoplantar keratoderma, and cardiomyopathy.

Mutations in *JUP*, encoding plakoglobin, manifest at birth as generalized erythroderma with superficial peeling and erosions. Patients have alopecia, dystrophic nails, and recurrent infections and generally die in the neonatal period, but without cardiac issues.[41,42] As with other mutations in desmosomal components, a milder form allows survival but the development of generalized erosions, sparse woolly hair, and focal keratoderma.

Plakophilin deficiency (skin fragility and ectodermal dysplasia syndrome) results from mutations in *PKP1*, the gene encoding plakophilin-1.[43–46] Affected patients show generalized erythroderma at birth with blistering. The soles are often most disabling, with palmoplantar keratoderma and painful fissures. Superficial erosions and crusting are prominent in the perioral area, and tongue fissures have been described. The hair tends to be short, sparse, and woolly, and the nails are thickened and dystrophic. Affected individuals show variable hypohidrosis, blepharitis, and growth retardation.[44] Plakophilin-1 is a structural component of the desmosomes that allows cell–cell adhesion; biopsies of affected skin show acanthosis, acantholysis, widening of the space between keratinocytes, and few poorly formed desmosomes.[47]

Table 13.3 Classification and Affected Genes in Other Disorders with Skin Fragility and Intraepidermal Cleavage

Type	Inheritance	Gene Defect/Abnormal Protein(s)
Peeling skin disorders (see Chapter 5)	Autosomal recessive	*CAST*/calpastatin *CDSN*/corneodesmosin *CSTA*/cystatin A *CTSB*/cathepsin B *DSG1*/desmoglein 1 *FLG2*/filaggin 2 *SERPIN8/serpin* protease inhibitor 8 *SPINK5*/LEKTI *TGM5*/transglutaminase 5
Erosive disorders	Autosomal recessive	*DSC3*/desmocollin 3 *DSG3*/desmoglein 3 *DSP*/desmoplakin *JUP*/plakoglobin PKP1/plakophilin 1
Hyperkeratotic disorders: keratinopathic ichthyoses (see Chapter 5)	Autosomal dominant	*KRT1, KR2, KRT10*/ keratins 1, 2, 10
Keratinopathic ichthyoses (see Chapter 5)	Autosomal recessive	*KRT10*/keratin 10
Pachyonychia congenita (see Chapters 5 and 7)	Autosomal dominant	*KRT6A, KRT6B, KRT6C, KRT16, KRT17*/keratins 6A, 6B, 6C, 16, 17

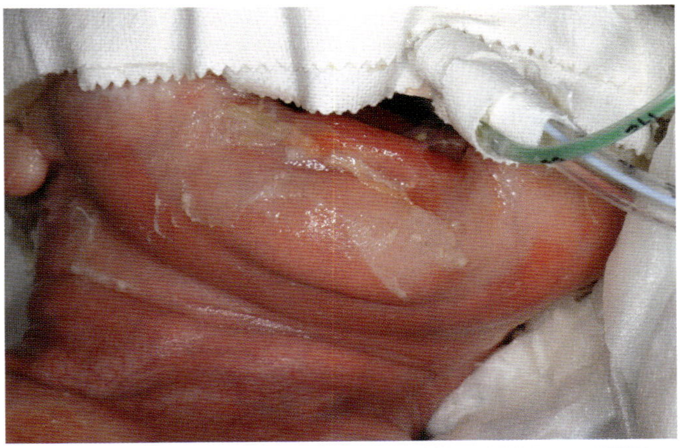

Fig. 13.12 Suprabasal acantholytic epidermolysis bullosa simplex. Note the sheet-like peeling of skin on the chin. This baby, who died as a neonate, had total body denudement, extensive mucosal sloughing, and complete alopecia from a mutation in *DSP*.

Several disorders result in peeling of skin without erosion (see Table 13.3). An acral peeling skin syndrome results from mutations in TGM5, the gene encoding transglutaminase 5. The subcorneal cleavage can be confused with localized EB on the hands and feet.[48] Several additional disorders present with peeling skin in an acral or generalized distribution; these result from biallelic pathogenic variants in genes encoding calpastatin, cathepsin B, cystatic A, corneodesmosin, desmoglein 1 (SAM syndrome), filaggrin 2, LEKTI (Netherton syndrome), and serine protease inhibitor 8 (serpin B8) (see Chapter 5). Inherited keratinopathies of suprabasal keratinocytes can also present with blisters, but in association with predominant hyperkeratosis. These include the epidermolytic ichthyoses (caused by mutations in KRT1, KRT2, and KRT10) (see Chapter 5) and pachyonychia congenita (caused by mutations in KRT6A, KRT 6B, KRT6C, KRT16, and KRT17) (see Chapter 7).

Junctional Epidermolysis Bullosa

Junctional EB (JEB) is a group of mechanobullous disorders in which the cleavage plane occurs in the lamina lucida at the junction of the epidermis and dermis (Table 13.4).[49,50] Encompassing a spectrum from severe, life-threatening disease to relatively mild involvement, various subtypes of this disorder have been described, each transmitted in an autosomal recessive manner (see Table 13.4). Certain missense mutations affecting only one allele (autosomal dominant) of *LAMB3* have resulted in only dental manifestations,[51] and of *COL17A1* have led to dental issues and blistering[52] or corneal erosions (termed *epithelial recurrent erosion dystrophy [ERED]*).[53]

Early diagnosis of the JEB subtype is critical for determining prognosis and is now based primarily on genotyping, although immunomapping is also helpful (detects the level of cleavage and absence of lamina lucida proteins). Immunomapping studies of sections from skin adjacent to a freshly induced blister show cleavage at the lamina lucida level. Electron microscopic evaluations reveal markedly reduced or absent hemidesmosomes, anchoring structures that span the lamina lucida of the basement membrane of skin and mucosae.

In the severe form of JEB (formerly called *JEB-Herlitz*), blistering begins at birth and death occurs in 45% by 1 year of age and 54% by 2 years of age.[54] Survival into adulthood is common for most other forms of JEB, but has only occasionally been described for individuals with the severe type of JEB.

Severe JEB is characterized by the generalized distribution of blisters and large erosions, mainly on the buttocks, perioral area, trunk, and scalp (Table 13.5). Blistering is almost always present at birth (see Fig. 13.2). Blistering of the fingertips with sloughing of the nails (Fig. 13.13) and perioral involvement (Fig. 13.14) with sparing of the lips are important, if not diagnostic, features of the junctional forms of EB. Granulation tissue, especially of the perioral and periungual regions, is characteristic of this severe form (and of laryngoonychocutaneous [LOC] syndrome), and is usually present by a few years of age. Sites of healing tend to be atrophic but show far fewer milia than the dystrophic forms. The mucous membranes are affected,

Table 13.4 Classification and Causes of Junctional Epidermolysis Bullosa*

Type	Gene Defect/Abnormal Protein(s)
JEB, severe (formerly Herlitz)	*LAMA3, LAMB3, LAMC2*/laminin 332
JEB, intermediate (formerly non-Herlitz)	Mild mutation: laminin 332 *COL17A1*/type XVII collagen
JEB, localized	*COL17A1*/type XVII collagen *ITGA6, ITGB4*/integrin α6β4 *LAMA3, LAMB3, LAMC2*/laminin 332 *ITG3*/integrin α3
JEB, localized, inversa	*COL17A1*/type XVII collagen
LOC syndrome	Laminin 332, α3 chain
JEB, with pyloric atresia (syndromic)	*ITGA6, ITGB4*/integrin α6 or β4
JEB, with respiratory and renal involvement (syndromic)	*ITGA3*/integrin α3
JEB with nephropathy (syndromic)	*CD151*/tetraspanin 24

JEB, Junctional epidermolysis bullosa; *LOC*, laryngoonychocutaneous syndrome.
*All forms of JEB are autosomal recessive.

Table 13.5 Characteristics of Major Forms of Junctional Epidermolysis Bullosa

Type	Clinical Manifestations
JEB, severe (formerly Herlitz)	50% of patients die by 2 years old Blisters heal with atrophic scarring but no milia Periungual and finger pad blistering, erythema Blistering of oral and esophageal mucosae Laryngeal and airway involvement with early hoarseness Later, perioral granulation tissue with sparing of lips Anonychia Dental enamel hypoplasia, excessive caries Growth retardation Anemia
JEB, intermediate (formerly non-Herlitz)	Less severe, but similar manifestations to Herlitz type, including dental, nail, and laryngeal involvement Granulation tissue is rare Perinasal cicatrization Less mucosal involvement Alopecia Anemia but not as severe as JEB, generalized severe
JEB, localized	Localized blisters without residual scarring or granulation tissue Minimal mucosal involvement Dental and nail abnormalities as in JEB, generalized severe
JEB, with pyloric atresia	Usually lethal in neonatal period Generalized blistering, leading to atrophic scarring May be born with large areas of cutis aplasia No granulation tissue Nail dystrophy or anonychia Pyloric atresia, genitourinary malformations Rudimentary ears Dental enamel hypoplasia (survivors) Variable anemia, growth retardation, mucosal blistering

JEB, Junctional epidermolysis bullosa.

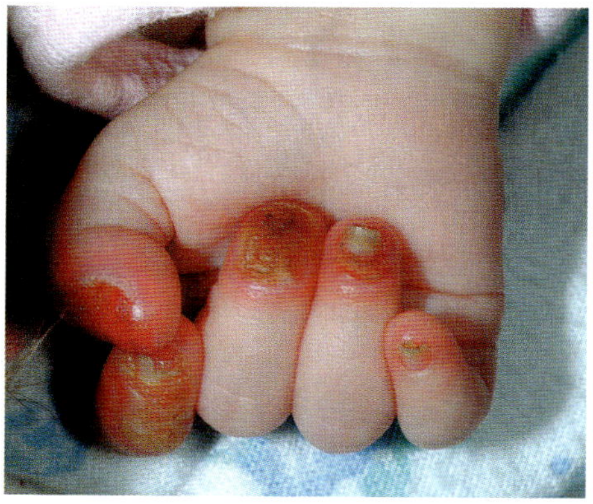

Fig. 13.13 Generalized severe junctional epidermolysis bullosa (JEB). Blistering of the fingertips with periungual erythema and sloughing of the nails is characteristic of JEB.

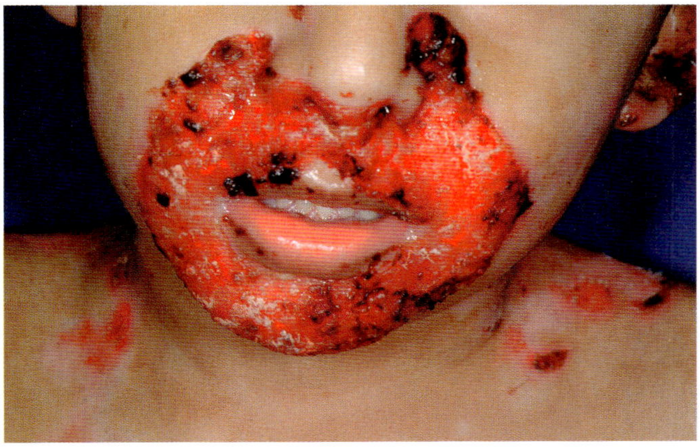

Fig. 13.14 Generalized severe junctional epidermolysis bullosa. Perioral blistering with formation of granulation tissue is characteristic. Note that the lips are relatively spared, but the teeth show enamel dysplasia.

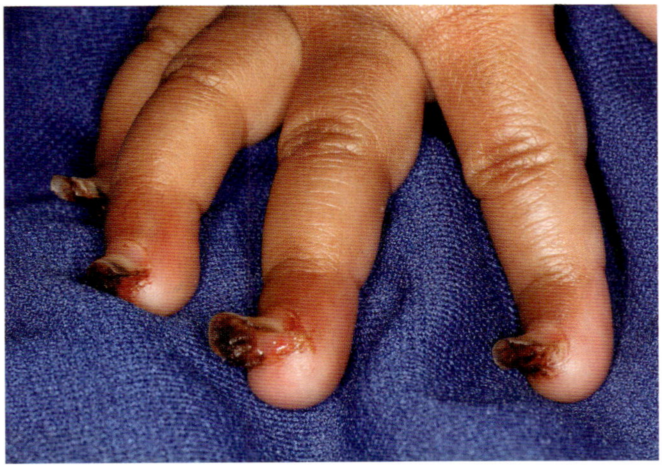

Fig. 13.15 Junctional epidermolysis bullosa, localized. This girl with biallelic variants in *LAMC2* has mild sparse blistering but severe acral involvement, including granulation tissue of all of her nailbeds.

especially the oral mucosae. Hoarseness and laryngeal involvement are common, and airway involvement may lead to death. The genitourinary and gastrointestinal tracts are often affected as well. The teeth are dysplastic, and a cobblestone appearance to the dental enamel is characteristic. Severe growth retardation and recalcitrant anemia are common. Biallelic mutations in JEB usually affect a gene encoding one of the three chains of laminin 332 (*LAMA3* [17% of patients], *LAMB3* [59%], and *LAMC2* [12%], encoding α3, β3, and γ2 chains, respectively).[55]

Generalized intermediate or localized JEB may also result from less deleterious mutations in one of the laminin 332 genes (Fig. 13.15). The localized form, LOC syndrome (Shabbir syndrome),[56,57] is usually due to mutations in the α3 chain of laminin 332, although *LAMB3* mutations may be causative.[58] LOC syndrome occurs most often in the Punjab region of India and Pakistan. It features excessive granulation tissue of the larynx (leading to hoarseness and potentially airway obstruction), conjunctival granulation tissue (leading to symblepharon, corneal scarring, and potentially blindness), and erosive blisters most commonly on the face and neck. Death is common because of respiratory tract involvement. JEB inversa presents with blisters predominantly in intertriginous areas (axillary areas and groin). Mucosal blistering tends to be variable in extent but less than in the generalized forms.

Generalized intermediate JEB (previously called *non-Herlitz JEB* or *generalized atrophic benign EB [GABEB]*) most commonly affects the gene encoding BP180 (collagen XVII; *COL17A1*) but occasionally reflects at least one missense mutation in a gene encoding laminin 332 (leading to a milder phenotype than with two highly deleterious gene changes). In general, features tend to be less severe than in the severe generalized form, but granulation tissue is rarely seen, and EB nevi are common. Diffuse alopecia (scarring or nonscarring) is a key feature of this form (Fig. 13.16), and narrowing of the nares is often seen. Squamous cell carcinoma (SCC) only occasionally occurs in the severe generalized form of EB, in contrast to recessive dystrophic epidermolysis bullosa (RDEB), contributing to the greater lifespan.

JEB with pyloric atresia results from mutations in either α6 integrin *(ITGA6)* or its hemidesmosome partner, β4 integrin *(ITGB4)*.[29] Blistering is generalized at birth, often with large areas of cutis aplasia. Other features in addition to pyloric atresia, such as rudimentary and malformed ears (Fig. 13.17) and genitourinary tract malformations,

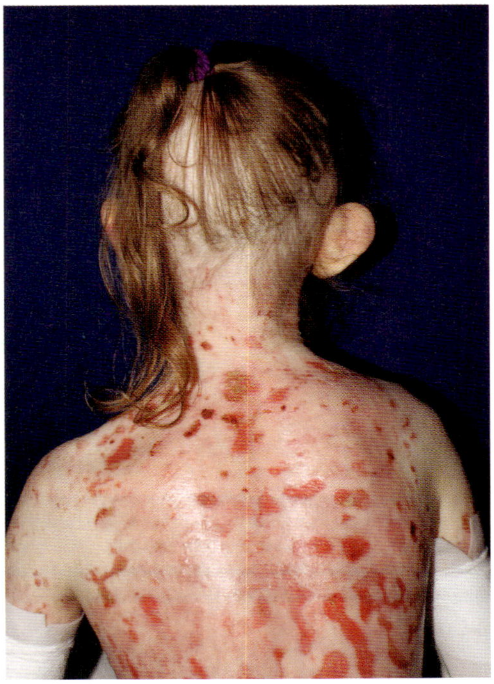

Fig. 13.16 Junctional epidermolysis bullosa, intermediate. Generalized blistering and progressive alopecia in this 12 -year-old girl with biallelic *COL17A1* variants.

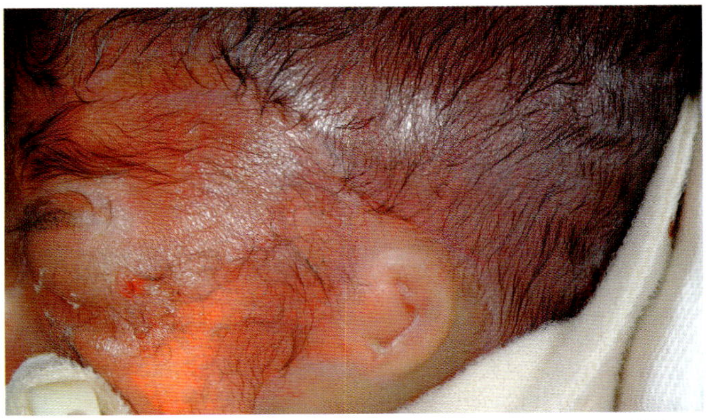

Fig. 13.17 Junctional epidermolysis bullosa, pyloric atresia type. The rudimentary ears and extensive denudement of the extremities is typical of this type of epidermolysis bullosa. This baby had a mutation in the gene encoding integrin β4.

attest to the important role of $\alpha6\beta4$ integrin in the development of the pylorus, ears, and genitourinary tract. Several cases of severe blistering at birth with milder involvement thereafter and a favorable outcome after pyloric atresia repair have been described, especially with mutations in *ITGB4*,[59,60] which should be considered in decision-making in the first weeks of life. EB with pyloric atresia can also result from plectin abnormalities[61] and can similarly be associated with urologic abnormalities (see EBS from *PLEC* mutations, earlier). Heterozygous missense mutations in *ITGB4* may cause an autosomal dominant disorder with nail dystrophy, late-onset mild skin fragility with acral blistering, and sometimes mucosal granulation tissue.[62]

Interstitial lung disease, nephrotic syndrome, and epidermolysis bullosa (ILNEB) is a form of syndromic JEB that results from homozygous mutations in *ITGA3*, encoding[63] integrin $\alpha3$. Integrin $\alpha3$ forms heterodimers with integrin $\beta1$ and plays important roles in basement membrane assembly and wound healing. Cutaneous blistering begins during the first months of life and is associated with dystrophic nails with distal onycholysis and fine, sparse hair, but not with mucosal blistering. Renal disease is variable and can include congenital nephrotic syndrome, glomerulosclerosis, cysts, and malformations. Most affected infants have renal disease and die within the first months of life.[64]

Dystrophic Epidermolysis Bullosa

The scarring (dystrophic) types of EB are predominantly divided into dominant dystrophic epidermolysis bullosa (DDEB) and RDEB forms, and their various subtypes are based on severity, distribution, and characteristics (Tables 13.6 and 13.7). All forms of DEB affect anchoring fibrils, critical elements for epidermal–dermal cohesion, and most result from mutations in type VII collagen.[65–67]

The one exception to collagen VII as the underlying mutated gene is a syndromic dystrophic blistering disease is *connective tissue disorder with skin fragility*, resulting from biallelic variants in *PLOD3*, encoding lysyl hydroxylase 3 (LH3), a key enzyme in the posttranslational modification of type VII collagen.[68,69] LH3 glycosylates the hydroxylysine group of collagen VII and is reduced in the skin of all RDEB patients.[70] Patients with *PLOD3* mutations present with trauma-induced blistering (extremities, ears) beginning during infancy, delayed wound healing, and dystrophic nails, as well as poor growth, developmental delay, several eye abnormalities, dysmorphic facies, connective tissue abnormalities (prominent knees, scoliosis, osteopenia, flexion contractures of the elbows and carpometacarpal joints, talipes equinovarus, and webbing at fold areas), and variable deafness and dilatation of blood vessels. The level of blistering is below the lamina densa, and the extent of reduced and abnormal-appearing anchoring fibrils is variable. The early blistering distinguishes this syndromic form of EB from connective tissue disorders, particularly the spondylocheirodysplastic form of Ehlers–Danlos syndrome, which results from mutations in *PLOD1* (see Chapter 6).

In general, the dominant forms are considerably less severe; affected individuals are generally healthy, are of normal stature, and show limited blistering of the skin. The severe generalized form of RDEB, conversely, is severe and incapacitating. Functional deformities of the hands and feet result from extensive scarring, growth and development are retarded, and profound anemia and hypoalbuminemia are standard.

Table 13.7 Characteristics of Major Forms of Dystrophic Epidermolysis Bullosa*

Type	Clinical Manifestations
Dominant dystrophic	Onset at birth to early infancy Blistering predominates on dorsum of hands, elbows, knees, and lower legs Milia associated with scarring Some patients develop scar-like lesions, especially on the trunk 80% have nail dystrophy
Recessive dystrophic, severe generalized	Present at birth Widespread blistering, scarring, milia Deformities: pseudosyndactyly, joint contractures Severe involvement of mucous membranes, nails; alopecia Growth retardation, poor nutrition Anemia Mottled, carious teeth Osteoporosis, delayed puberty, cardiomyopathy, glomerulonephritis, renal amyloidosis, IgA nephropathy Predisposition to squamous cell carcinoma in heavily scarred areas
Recessive dystrophic, generalized intermediate	Generalized blisters from birth with milia, scarring Less anemia, growth retardation, mucosal but more esophageal issues with advancing age

IgA, Immunoglobulin A.
*COL7A1 variants.

Table 13.6 Classification and Cause of Dystrophic Epidermolysis Bullosa

Type	Gene Defect/Abnormal Protein(s)
AUTOSOMAL DOMINANT	
DDEB, intermediate DDEB, localized DDEB, self-improving (bullous dermolysis of newborn) DDEB, pruriginosa (DDEB-pr)	*COL7A1*/collagen VII
AUTOSOMAL RECESSIVE	
RDEB, severe RDEB, intermediate RDEB, localized (RDEB-loc) RDEB, inversa (RDEB-I) RDEB, self-improving RDEB, pruriginosa (RDEB-pr)	*COL7A1*/collagen VII

DDEB, Dominant dystrophic epidermolysis bullosa; *LH3*, lysyl hydroxylase 3; *RDEB*, recessive dystrophic epidermolysis bullosa.

Dominant Dystrophic Epidermolysis Bullosa

Dominant dystrophic epidermolysis bullosa (DDEB) usually presents at birth or shortly thereafter. There is great phenotypic variability, even within families.[71] Some cases present as isolated milia, nail changes (DDEB, localized, nails only), blistering limited to the acral areas of the hands and feet, or prurigo papules. In some individuals with mild disease, the diagnosis is not recognized until manifestations appear in adulthood. Interestingly, a large deletion of approximately 40% of *COL7A1* has led to a mild form of DDEB, with the expression of a shorter collagen VII protein that could still assemble and function.[72]

Nevertheless, the typical features are blisters, with resultant scars and milia, primarily involving the extensor areas of the extremities and the dorsal surface of the hands (Figs. 13.18 and 13.19). Nail thickening, dystrophy, or complete nail destruction are seen in 80% of cases (Fig. 13.20).[73] Although mucous membrane lesions appear in 20% of cases, they tend to be mild and not problematic. The teeth and hair are generally not affected, and physical development is normal.

DEB pruriginosa (DEB-Pr) is a poorly understood form of DEB (usually dominant) with the onset of severe associated pruritus and

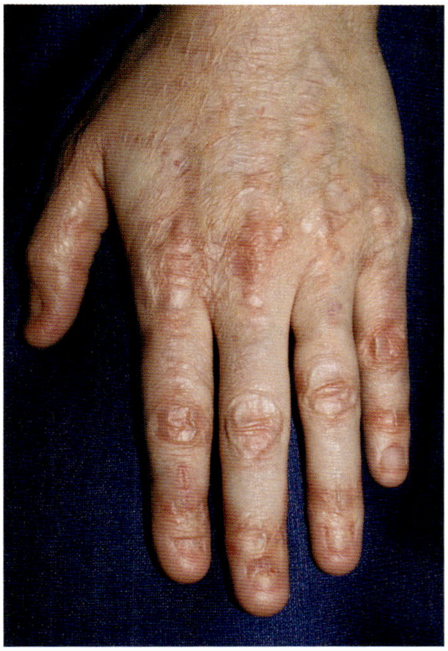

Fig. 13.18 Dominant dystrophic epidermolysis bullosa (DDEB). Blistering was limited to the dorsal aspect of the hands and feet, as well as elbows, knees, and anterior lower legs in this adolescent. Note the residual discoloration and scarring.

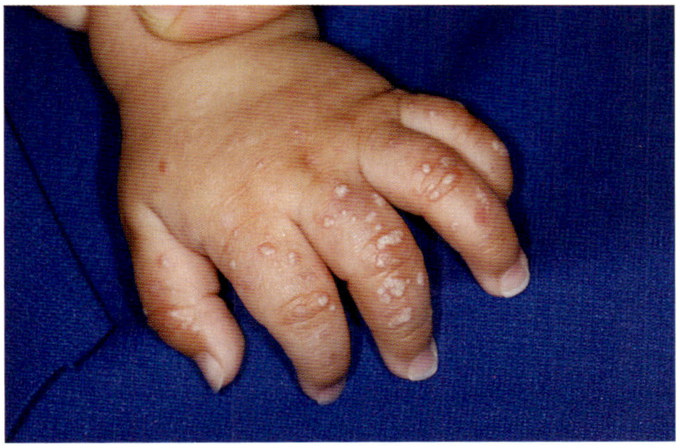

Fig. 13.19 Dominant dystrophic epidermolysis bullosa. Milia on dorsal aspect of the hand of this infant.

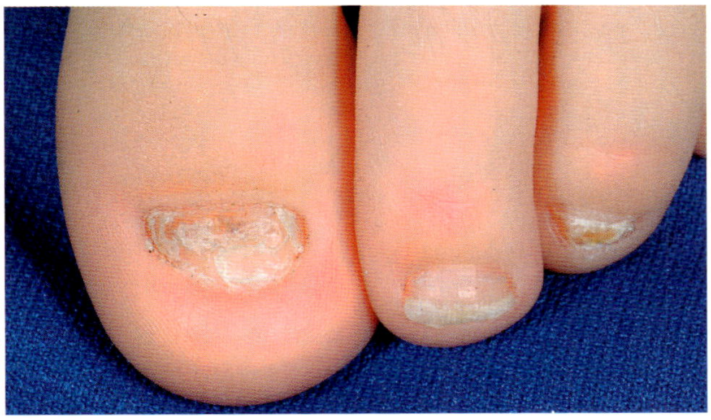

Fig. 13.20 Dominant dystrophic epidermolysis bullosa. Nail dystrophy, especially of the toenails, is commonly seen in individuals with dominant dystrophic epidermolysis bullosa (DDEB).

prurigo-like, scarred vesicles and papules primarily of the pretibial areas (Fig. 13.21). Onset is often delayed until adolescence or adulthood[74] in patients with typical features of DDEB during childhood.[75–78]

The self-improving form (formerly called *bullous dermolysis of the newborn*) shows skin blistering, often extensive, at birth or in early infancy (Fig. 13.22). However, blistering dramatically improves during the first months to 2 years of life, and affected individuals usually have only mild residual atrophy, scarring, and nail dystrophy thereafter. The disorder results from certain mutations in *COL7A1* that lead to the milder phenotype and can be inherited in a dominant or recessive manner. Characteristically, epidermal cells show intracytoplasmic retention (rather than secretion) of type VII collagen.[79]

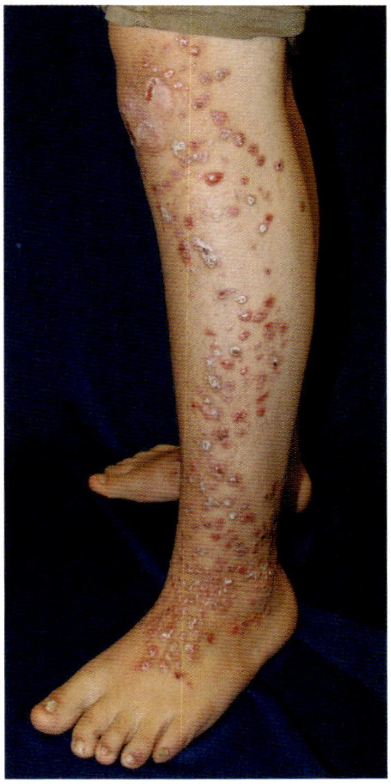

Fig. 13.21 Epidermolysis bullosa pruriginosa. A subset of individuals with dominant dystrophic epidermolysis bullosa (DDEB) develop EB pruriginosa during adolescence or adulthood, although the underlying cause is unknown. The pruriginous lesions are predominantly on the lower extremities and are extremely pruritic.

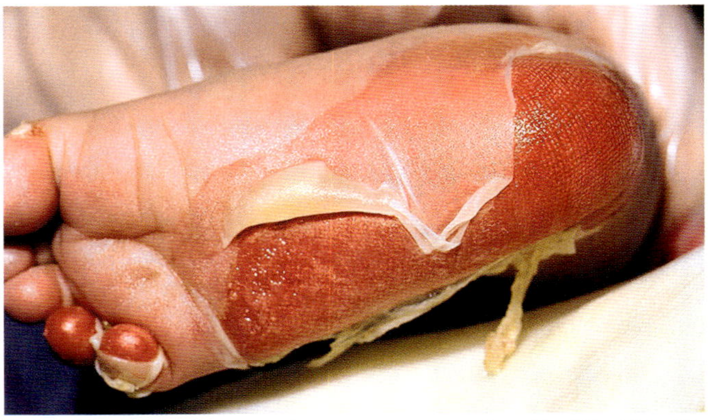

Fig. 13.22 Transient bullous dermolysis of the newborn. After extensive blistering of the lower extremity at birth, no further blisters developed. Immunomapping showed the split to be in the upper dermis, and staining for type VII collagen was reduced.

Recessive Dystrophic Epidermolysis Bullosa

Children with severe RDEB (formerly called the *Hallopeau–Siemens type*) have a severe, life-altering bullous disease characterized by widespread dystrophic scarring and deformity and by severe involvement of mucous membranes. RDEB may manifest as a less severe form (intermediate RDEB), with less severe blistering of the skin and mucosae that may be mistaken for DDEB (Fig. 13.23). Individuals with this milder form often begin to have increasing problems with mucosae, especially esophageal function, in adolescence. Blistering in RDEB inversa tends to be localized to the intertriginous axial, lumbosacral, and acral sites, in addition to extensive mucosal involvement, including esophageal strictures and external auditory canal stenosis.

Although any area of the skin may be involved in infants with generalized severe RDEB, the most commonly affected areas are the hands, feet, buttocks, scapulae, face, occiput, elbows, and knees. In older children the hands, feet, knees, elbows, and posterior neck and/or upper mid-back (Fig. 13.24) are most commonly involved. Bullae may be hemorrhagic, and large areas, especially on the lower extremities, may be completely devoid of skin. When a blister ruptures or its roof peels off, a raw, painful surface is evident. The Nikolsky sign (production or enlargement of a blister by slight pressure or the production of a moist abrasion by slight pressure on the skin) is often positive. Fluid contained in bullae, although at first sterile, may become secondarily infected (Fig. 13.25), which can lead to sepsis; *Staphylococcus aureus* and *Pseudomonas aeruginosa* are the most common organisms.

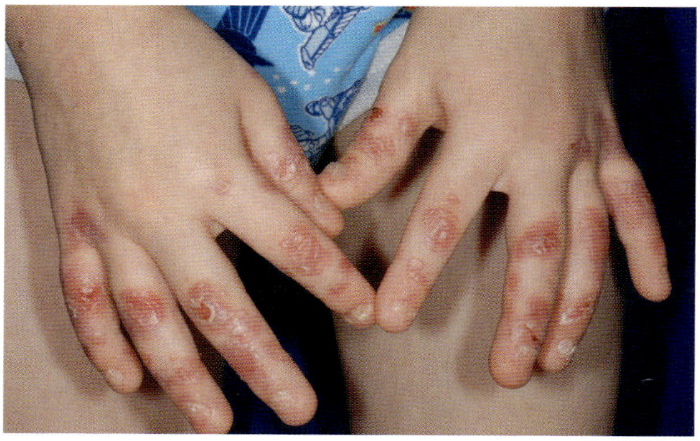

Fig. 13.23 Generalized intermediate recessive dystrophic epidermolysis bullosa. This boy and his brother had mild involvement of the hands, feet, and legs with nail dystrophy. The sites and appearance of lesions resembled dominant dystrophic epidermolysis bullosa, but the involvement in his brother and subsequent genotyping showed the biallelic mutation in *COL7A1*.

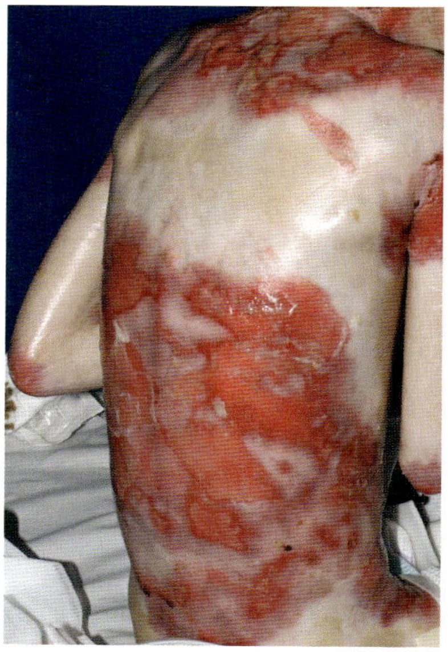

Fig. 13.24 Recessive dystrophic epidermolysis bullosa (RDEB). This young girl demonstrates the "shawl sign" of RDEB, as well as relative sparing of the mid-back.

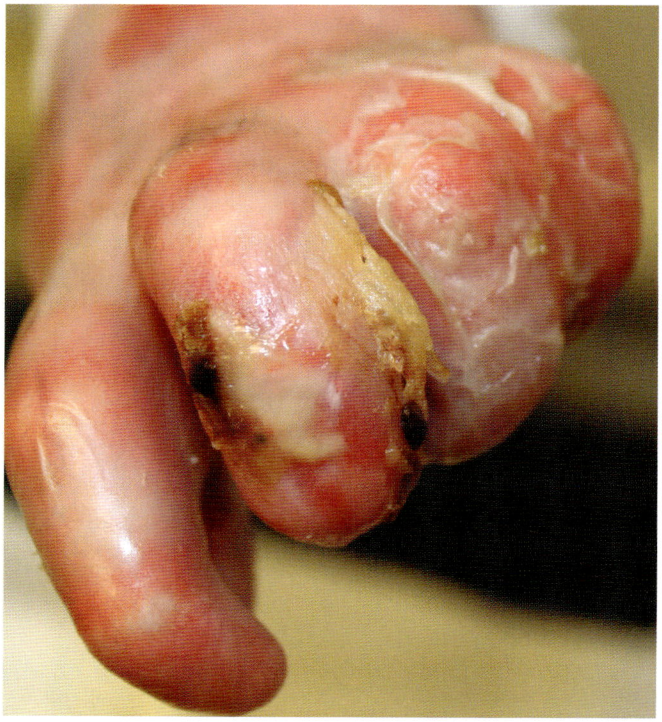

Fig. 13.25 Recessive dystrophic epidermolysis bullosa (RDEB). Infection in RDEB is common, initially *S. aureus* and, with advancing age, *P. aeruginosa* as well. This girl had recurrent infection of the fingers. Note the purulence from *S. aureus* infection.

Bullae are often followed by atrophic scars and varying degrees of hyperpigmentation or hypopigmentation. Milia overlying the scars are characteristic. EB nevi are common (see earlier). The hands and lower aspects of the legs are particularly susceptible to severe blistering and scarring. The fingers and toes may become fused, with resultant pseudosyndactyly in which the digits become bound together by a glove-like epidermal sac, with resulting claw-like clubbing or mitten-like deformities (Fig. 13.26). The fingers and toes become immobile (usually during the first years of life), and the wrists, elbows, knees, and ankles may become fixed in a flexed position from contractures, leading to immobility and often confinement to a wheelchair.

Oral mucosal involvement occurs soon after birth (Fig. 13.27), leading to dysphagia and limiting the ability to suck well. Erosions of the esophagus may at times result in segmental stenosis (most often in the upper third) with consequent difficulty in swallowing. Gastroesophageal reflux disease often occurs, especially presenting as effortless vomiting. Constipation is common and may be related to anal fissuring, inadequate dietary fiber, and administration of iron. Affected children are reluctant to eat and often fail to thrive, given their increased nutritional needs due to loss of protein and other nutrients through wounds. As the child grows older, there is a tendency for the disease to become less severe, but the affected individual also soon learns to avoid hot drinks, rough foods, and large particles that might produce blistering of the mouth, pharynx, or esophagus. Typically, patients show microstomia due to intraoral scarring and a frenulum that is bound down. The eyes may develop blisters with associated ocular inflammation and later corneal scarring, potentially leading to visual impairment.[80] Hoarseness, aphonia, and even laryngeal stenosis may result from laryngeal blistering and scarring. Bone mineralization is low in patients with EB, particularly those with RDEB,

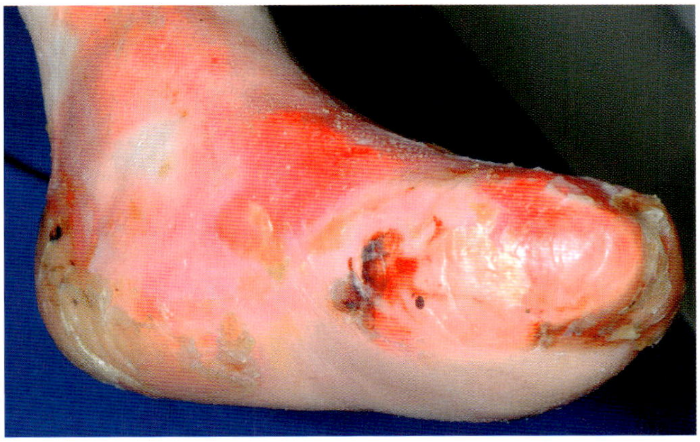

Fig. 13.26 Recessive dystrophic epidermolysis bullosa. Pseudosyndactyly or mitten deformity of the foot in this young boy with extensive atrophic scarring.

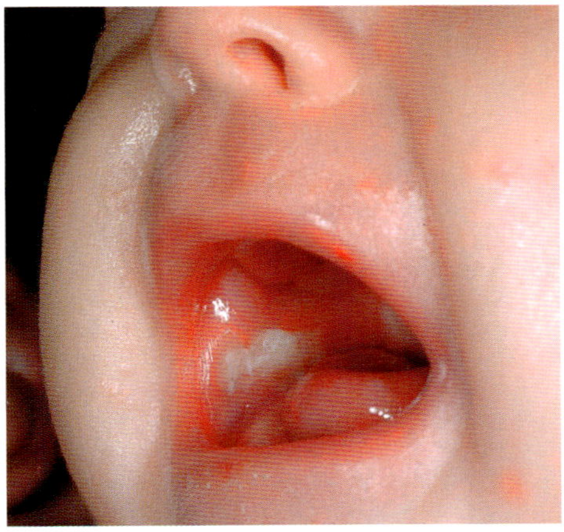

Fig. 13.27 Recessive dystrophic epidermolysis bullosa. Oral mucosal blistering in a neonate.

probably due to a combination of insufficient nutrition, reduced physical activity, and chronic inflammation.[2,81]

The teeth in RDEB are particularly susceptible to early and commonly severe caries. The progressive intraoral scarring leads to microstomia and decreased salivation.[2,82] Even routine dental care may cause the eruption of bullae and erosions on the lips, gingivae, and oral mucosa. The nails may show severe dystrophy or complete absence of nails. Scalp and body hair may be sparse, and there may be patches of cicatricial alopecia.[83]

In patients with the severe generalized form of RDEB, death may occur during infancy or childhood as a result of septicemia, pneumonia, or renal failure. Patients with RDEB (and rarely DDEB) have an increased risk of glomerulonephritis, renal amyloidosis, and immunoglobulin (Ig) A nephropathy.[2,84–86] The tremendous loss of fluid, blood, and protein through the skin coupled with malnutrition can lead to hypoalbuminemia and anemia. Dilated cardiomyopathy is an uncommon complication (4.5% by 20 years of age)[87] but may be fatal, especially in the presence of concurrent chronic renal failure. The cause of the cardiomyopathy may be multifactorial, including from transfusion-associated iron overload, viral myocarditis, and deficiency of selenium and carnitine. Other complications of RDEB include erosions and scarring of the anal area (often resulting in severe discomfort, chronic constipation, or soiling), urethral stenosis, urinary retention, hypertrophy of the bladder, and occasionally hydronephrosis.[3,84]

Patients with RDEB (and, to a much lesser extent, JEB and DDEB) show a progressively increasing risk of developing cutaneous SCCs with advancing age; in a recently described Australian cohort, the earliest age of development was 16 years with a cumulative risk of developing SCC of 76% by 35 years of age.[88,89] In another study the accumulative risk of SCC in RDEB was 13% by 20 years of age.[2] The SCCs tend to occur in heavily ulcerated and scarred areas of skin.[90] Lesions are predominantly over joints and on the distal extremities and present as nodular lesions or nonhealing ulcers.[91,92] Suspicious masses should be biopsied to distinguish SCCs from benign lesions such as verruciform xanthoma.[93,94] SCCs rarely appear on the tongue or esophagus. Cutaneous carcinomas tend to be locally aggressive, often requiring amputation, and almost 70% metastasize,[95] often leading to death within 4 to 5 years after SCC development. The genetic mutations found in RDEB SCCs are similar to those alterations found in ultraviolet light–related cutaneous SCCs.[95] Melanoma may arise in children with RDEB, whereas the risk of developing basal cell carcinomas seems to be increased in adults with generalized severe EBS.

Although death during childhood is most common with JEB (median age 4 to 6 months)[54] due to sepsis, failure to thrive, and respiratory failure, children with RDEB generally survive the neonatal and infantile periods but succumb to infection later during childhood or to aggressive cutaneous carcinomas during adulthood.

KINDLER SYNDROME

Kindler syndrome has been classified as mixed EB because the blistering arises at multiple levels within and/or beneath the basement membrane zone. Kindler syndrome is characterized by generalized progressive poikiloderma, congenital acral skin blistering, diffuse cutaneous atrophy (Fig. 13.28), skin fragility, webbing of the fingers and toes with digital tapering that can resemble scleroderma, nail dystrophy, oral mucosal lesions, and photosensitivity, sometimes within minutes after exposure.[96–98] Early atrophy on the dorsal surface of the hands (resembling finely wrinkled paper, not follicular atrophoderma) helps distinguish Kindler syndrome from other forms of EB.[99] Other features are hyperkeratosis of the palms and soles; leukokeratosis; ectropion; red, friable, hyperplastic gingivae; constipation and sometimes severe colitis; stenosis of the esophagus, larynx, anus, vagina, and urethral meatus; and phimosis.[100] Although the photosensitivity and blister formation seem to decrease with age, the atrophic scarring and poikiloderma increase after adolescence. The incidence of SCC of the acral skin or mouth is increased after the age of 30 years.

Treatment of this disorder requires the avoidance of trauma and the proper use of emollients, appropriate sun protection, and the judicious use of antibiotics to prevent secondary infection. Regular dental care and surveillance for early malignancies are important, as are iron replacement if the patient is anemic and management of the stenoses and colitis. The gene mutated in Kindler syndrome is *FERMT1* (formerly called *KIND-1*), which encodes fermitin family homolog 1 (FFH1) protein or kindlin-1, a focal adhesion protein that regulates keratinocyte cell adhesion, motility, and stem cell homeostasis.[101–104]

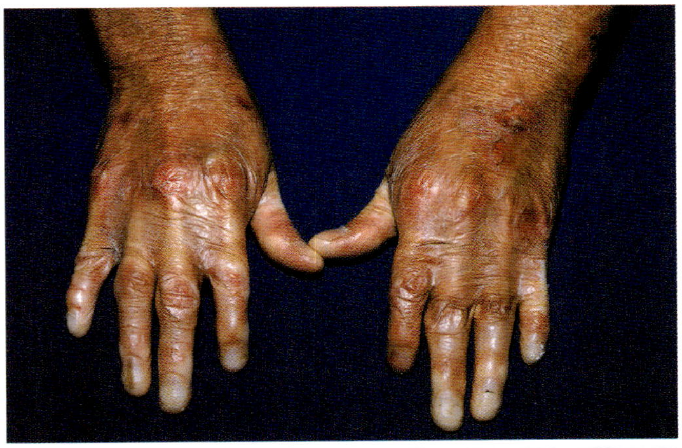

Fig. 13.28 Kindler syndrome. This boy shows poikiloderma, cutaneous atrophy, webbing of the fingers, and nail dystrophy.

Treatment of Epidermolysis Bullosa

EB is a group of disorders in which multidisciplinary care provides the best option for the patient, especially in patients with more severe disease.[105] Currently, treatment of EB is largely palliative, with protection from friction or overheating, avoidance of abrasion and constriction, control of secondary infection, nutritional supplementation, and pain control.[106–108]

As in any inherited disorder, it is the responsibility of the physician to inform parents of the risks of transmitting genetic abnormalities.[109] When the condition is determined by a dominant gene (as in DDEB)[110,111] and a parent is affected, the risk of the disorder in siblings is 50%. In a family in which a child manifests abnormalities because of a recessive gene (as in RDEB), parents risk a 25% possibility with each pregnancy of the disorder occurring in future offspring. Appropriate genetic counseling, however, depends on accurate diagnosis. For example, some recessive forms of EB may result from uniparental isodisomy (i.e., inheriting two copies of a mutated gene from a single parent), in which case the chances of having another affected child is <1%.[112,113] Similarly, a dominant disorder in which the genetic mutation occurs in the early postzygotic period has no greater chance of occurring in a sibling than in the general population; however, if one of the parents has germline mosaicism, the risk is higher.[114–116] Because the clinical course of many forms of EB is variable, especially during the neonatal and infantile periods, it is recommended that patients be carefully evaluated as early as possible with genotyping, if accessible, although immunofluorescent mapping can provide important information as well. Prenatal diagnosis of all forms of EB is now available using molecular techniques, but is easiest if the gene defect is known in that family.[117] Preimplantation diagnosis has been performed and is an option that utilizes *in vitro* fertilization to ensure a normal fetus without the risk of abortion.[118,119]

The psychosocial effects of EB, especially the more severe forms, on the affected individual and family are among the most dramatic of any skin disease.[109] Affected children are concerned about having itchy skin, being in pain, having difficulty with participation, failing to understand others, and feeling different.[120] Parents of affected children worry about the child being different, the child suffering pain, feeling uncertain about the future, restrictions on employment and leisure, problems with organizing care, being constantly on duty, family problems, the ignorance and lack of skills of alternative care providers, and resistance by the child to care.[121] These problems should be discussed and psychological support for patients and their families offered as part of optimal care. In addition, the economic impact on the family of a child with EB can be devastating, not merely from the cost of medication, dressings, and in-patient and outpatient medical care but also because of the tendency for one parent to stop working to care full-time for the child, leading to loss of income.[122]

Practical Measures to Reduce Blistering. Because blisters result from mechanical injury, measures should be taken to relieve pressure and prevent unnecessary trauma. During hospitalization and procedures, care must be taken to educate the healthcare team about EB and the required adjustments in care to minimize skin and mucosal trauma.[123] Clothing should be soft and worn inside out. Labels that may rub the skin should be removed. Velcro closures are less traumatizing than other traditional closures. Mittens can be worn to minimize self-induced trauma. A cool environment and lubrication of the skin to decrease surface friction are helpful in the reduction of blister formation. A water mattress and a soft fleece covering will also help limit friction and trauma. Applying nonstick dressings (such as Mepilex Lite) under electrocardiogram (ECG) leads and other adhesive surfaces prevents adhesive contact directly with the skin, and foam dressings can also be used as a cushion beneath blood pressure cuffs. Occupational therapy is important for maintaining function, particularly hand dexterity, and learning to prevent physical injury. Neoprene pads can be applied to protect areas of contact, and sheepskin liners can be made for seats and as modified grips. When blisters occur, extension may be prevented by aseptically puncturing the wound with a needle and releasing blister fluid. The roofs of blisters should be left intact whenever possible to protect the underlying skin.

Shoes should be soft and fit well; leather shoes with leather linings, ideally with external seams (e.g., moccasins), are usually recommended.[109] During the summer, canvas shoes and jelly sandals are the best choices. Shoes should be large enough to accommodate dressings and minimize friction. Insoles can be made from cooling gel, sheepskin, or protective dressings.

In patients with EBS, keeping palms and soles cool and dry helps minimize blistering, especially during hot weather. Hyperhidrosis is often a concomitant feature, and measures to minimize the increased blistering associated with hyperhidrosis can be helpful. These include applying 20% aluminum chloride hexahydrate at night and gently drying the area with a cool hair dryer, wearing socks that absorb moisture,[109] and sprinkling affected areas with absorbent powder such as Zeasorb. For extreme cases and in older patients with the localized form of EBS, injections of botulinum toxin A have been helpful.[124] Silver-impregnated socks can also decrease infections and increase foot comfort.

Daily to every-other-day baths can help reduce crusting and discomfort. In one study of 16 children with primarily RDEB, saltwater baths (0.9% sodium chloride/normal saline, made by adding 1.5 pounds pool salt per 35-gallon tub) led to a significant reduction in pain and pain medication use in 91% and 66%, respectively.[125] The bathtub can be lined with a thick towel, and affected babies can be lifted and moved on a soft pad. Topical application of protective petrolatum to eroded areas is helpful.

Protective dressings should be applied to eroded areas to promote healing and increase comfort. Use of dressings that do not adhere to wounds is critical to prevent further denudation when dressings are changed. In the neonatal period, petrolatum-impregnated gauze is commonly used with extra ointment applied to prevent adherence to the wound. The choice of dressings thereafter depends on access, wound exudation, and personal choice. Most use a nonadherent thin contact layer, topped with a padded secondary dressing. Tape and any significant pressure to skin must be avoided. Dressings can be held in place by a third layer of rolled gauze or loose self-adherent wraps with tape only applied to the dressing itself or by stockinette. DEBRA, the patient support organization, provides product names and recommendations for physicians and patients (http://www.debra.org/careproducts#contact). Among products often used in contact with the skin are nonadherent foams and hydrogels. Draining wounds need absorbent dressings, such as hydrofibers, calcium alginates, and foam products. Although nonadherent absorbent pads such as Telfa are inexpensive, they often stick to wounds with serous or purulent drainage, requiring vigorous soaking or greasing for removal without denudement.[126,127] A type I collagen dressing was shown to improve wound healing in RDEB in a small number of patients. Many advocate that dressings be carefully placed between the digits in children with RDEB to slow the development of pseudosyndactyly (Fig. 13.29), although the ameliorative effect of this practice has not been tested.

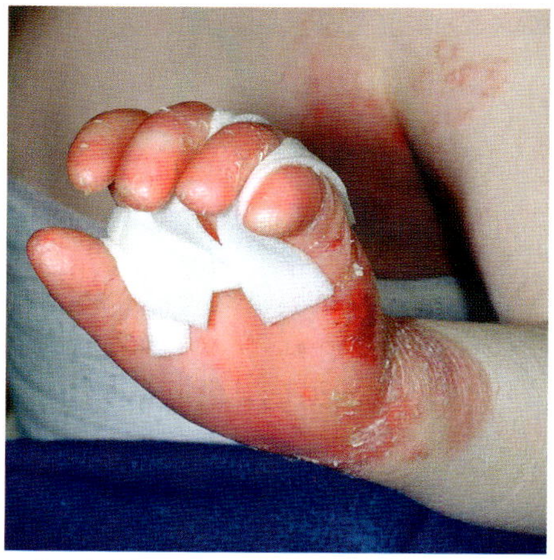

Fig. 13.29 Recessive dystrophic epidermolysis bullosa (RDEB). Nonadherent dressings should be placed between the fingers and toes of children with RDEB to reduce the risk of pseudosyndactyly. Note the scarred skin and anonychia.

Sterile precautions must be taken when changing dressings to reduce the risk of bacterial infection. Dressings with silver have helped patients with recurrent infections, but application of silver sulfadiazine has been associated with argyria.[128,129] Families need to weigh the antiinfective benefits with the risk of potentially high blood levels of silver.[130] Bacteriostatic dressings with methylene blue and crystal-violet dyes (such as Hydrofera blue) and medical-grade honey[131] are also available. It should be noted that children with EB have developed contact allergy to topically applied ointments or dressings, which may be difficult to diagnose given the challenge of doing patch testing.[132]

Crusted or purulent areas should be cultured and treated based on the sensitivity of organisms. Infection may require administration of systemic antibiotics, but antibiotics should only be used for clinical infection because of the high risk of development of resistance and given the baseline reduction in microbial diversity in EB wounds.[132] Choice of antibiotic (based on organism sensitivity), but not the decision to use an antibiotic, should be based on culture results, because most patients are colonized by *S. aureus* and/or *P. aeruginosa* in the absence of infection. Gentamicin soaks (480 mg/L saline) or acetic-acid soaks (diluted white vinegar) have been used to decrease the overgrowth of *Pseudomonas* and staphylococcal organisms. The risk of sepsis with cutaneous infection is high in neonates and infants, and patients should be monitored carefully.

Topical and systemic steroids are generally not useful for patients with EB and should be avoided in view of their increased risk of systemic absorption and promotion of side effects, including increased risk of infection. However, short courses of low- to moderate-strength topical steroids are sometimes useful for pruritus. The severely pruritic prurigo lesions of EB pruriginosa are traditionally managed by application of potent steroids, often under occlusion, but oral thalidomide[133,134] and cyclosporine[135–137] have also been used. In addition, a potent topical steroid is the treatment of choice for localized areas of exuberant granulation tissue in JEB (for example, periungual).[138] In two children who were unresponsive to potent topical steroids,[139] topical timolol 0.5% ophthalmic drops applied twice daily to wounds led to full or almost complete healing in the wounds.

Pain control is an important component of EB care, especially in affected infants. Changing of dressings at blistered sites is excruciatingly painful for patients, yet must be performed from a few times weekly to up to twice daily, depending on the extent of drainage and the presence of infection. Evidence-based guidelines from DEBRA International for pain care were published in 2014.[140] Among the stronger recommendations are that anxiolytics and analgesics (nonsteroidal antiinflammatory drugs [NSAIDs] and acetaminophen) be used for procedural pain and fear. Tramadol and other opioids are also used, but the common side effects of opioids—constipation and pruritus—are significant baseline problems in EB. Methadone should only be used under guidance from a pain specialist, given its risk of QT interval prolongation and dosing challenges. For older children, acetaminophen with codeine, oral midazolam, or morphine have been used before dressing changes and baths to improve tolerance. Because the pain has a burning quality that resembles neuropathic pain, gabapentin is often used. Topical anesthetics can be applied before venipuncture and other procedures to reduce local discomfort. Medications should be coupled with cognitive behavioral techniques, particularly distraction and breathing techniques,[141] relaxation training, and biofeedback. Many patients claim benefit in healing and discomfort from the use of cannabidiol (CBD), especially topical CBD oil, but to date no studies have been done, and over-the-counter CBD is not regulated to assure safety and verify the stated formulation.

Overall, 85% of patients with EB complain of pruritus, which can be more problematic on a 5-point Likert scale than pain.[142] The itch is less problematic with EBS than with the more severe JEB and DEB types and can interfere with sleep. Exacerbants are healing wounds, a hot environment, infection, high humidity, and stress. Antihistamines and topical creams and ointments are of limited value,[106,143] but short-term courses of mid-potency topical steroids and, as second-line agents, antidepressants (such as mirtazapine) and low-dose gabapentin or pregabalin can be considered.[106] Serlopitant, a neurokinin-1 inhibitor, is currently being tested in EB as an antipruritic.

Nutritional supplementation is critical for patients with the more severe forms of EB to prevent failure to thrive, which has been linked to mortality in 20.5% of patients with generalized severe JEB by 2 years of age. The loss of protein, iron, and blood through the open areas of skin leads to hypoalbuminemia and deficiency of iron and trace minerals. Furthermore, the chronic disruption of the epithelial lining of the small intestine leads to gross malabsorption of nutrients, and the pain with ingestion of food decreases intake. Consultation with a nutritionist is important to maximize caloric and protein intake and provide specific nutrients and vitamins such as iron, zinc, and vitamin D_3. High consumption of milk products can serve as a source of protein, calcium, and vitamin D, and is important because 64% of patients with generalized severe RDEB are osteoporotic.[144] The reduction in bone mineral density results from the combination of poor nutrition, decreased ultraviolet exposure, reduced mobility and weight-bearing, and delayed puberty. Noncontact sports are recommended to strengthen muscles and bones; more physically active children tend to have more autonomy and less dependency on a wheelchair. Food aversion, especially for children who predominantly use their gastrostomy as a source of nutrition, is a confounding factor; speech therapists can help teach children to eat (a complication of early gastrostomy use). Oral iron may be poorly tolerated by the gastrointestinal tract, and constipation is a potential issue; intravenous administration of iron or blood transfusions may be needed to maintain a hemoglobin (Hgb) level of at least 8 g/dL in severely affected children. Soft nipples such as the Haberman feeder should be used, with the opening enlarged to minimize the need for sucking. The lips should be protected with petrolatum before initiating feeding. In general, nasogastric tube feeding should be avoided, or if necessary, a tube suitable for long-term feeding should be used. Placement of a button gastrostomy tube should be considered in infants who start to drop off their growth curve as a means of supplemental feeding to increase caloric intake and as an alternative route to oral feeding, especially for severe generalized forms of JEB and RDEB.[145] Twice-yearly dental visits are recommended, and daily care is important to decrease the risk of caries; teeth can be cleaned with soft, moist gauze or a soft toothbrush and rinses of chlorhexidine[146]; some advocate for use of an enamel-promoting toothpaste (such as MI Paste). Endosseous implants have been placed successfully in patients with EB.[147]

Dysphagia is the major symptom of esophageal involvement in RDEB.[148] It may result from a reversible inflammatory reaction or from a permanent stricture. Barium studies demonstrate esophageal lesions; endoscopy, however, is not recommended. Softening of the diet for several weeks may result in modest to marked improvement of symptoms. If conservative management fails to result in proper nourishment, esophageal dilation, ideally through fluoroscopic guidance, should be performed and may be repeated if stenosis recurs.[149] Esophageal perforation is the most serious complication of dilation. Surgery is an alternative, through colonic interposition and resection of localized strictures with end-to-end anastomosis, but the procedures carry a high risk. Gastroesophageal reflux may be exacerbated by esophageal dilation but responds to medical management with thickening of the milk, histamine 2 receptor (H2)-blockers, proton pump inhibitors, or promotility agents. Constipation is usually managed by maintaining adequate fluid intake and dietary fiber and by administering laxatives such as polyethylene glycol 3350 (MiraLAX). Restoration of function in severe fusion and flexion deformities of the hands and feet can often be helped by physiotherapy and appropriate plastic surgery, especially to separate the thumb and straighten digits.[150] However, partial recurrence is the norm, especially on the nondominant hand. Healing in these "degloving" procedures may be facilitated by application of biologic dressings with the tissue-engineered skin substitutes and epidermal grafts to the wounds.[151–153]

Individuals with EB may have "revertant mosaicism," in which a second gene change in a localized area leads to functional and clinical normalization (see Fig. 13.30),[165,166] or nonrevertant mosaicism, in which a gene change in some, but not all, somatic cells either leads to a mosaic dominant disorder (one allele affected) or converts a carrier state into a recessive disorder (both alleles affected) at the involved sites, as has recently been described for RDEB.[167] Detection of normal-appearing skin sites, which are most common in generalized intermediate JEB because of mutations in *COL17A1*, allows an unlimited source of cultured keratinocytes, fibroblasts, or even iPSCs for stem cell transplantation or for grafting.[166,168]

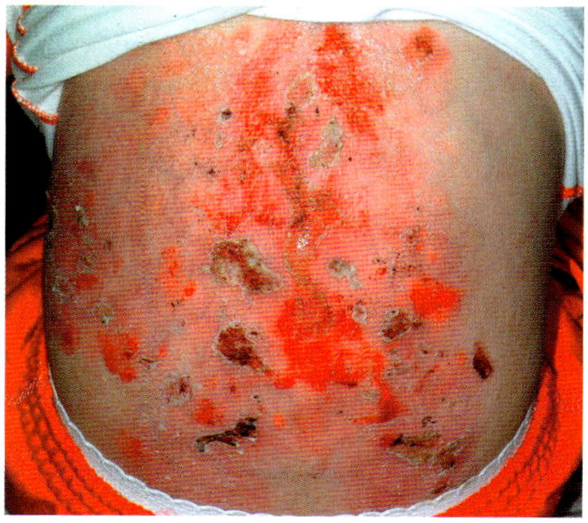

Fig. 13.30 Recessive dystrophic epidermolysis bullosa with revertant mosaicism. Note that the right side of the back shows no blistering, in contrast to the extensively blistered and scarred left side of the back. This clear area of revertant mosaicism only became visible for assessment after years of blistering and residual inflammation and scarring.

Ablative fractional laser resurfacing has shown promising results in managing pseudosyndactyly[154] and accelerating wound healing.[155] Anesthesia management for procedures is complicated,[156] especially given the microstomia of RDEB, but may include mask anesthesia, endotracheal tube, intravenous sedation, and local anesthetic blocks.[157,158]

Clinical surveillance through complete skin examination should be performed starting in later adolescence to search for SCCs. Self-monitoring should also be taught with photography, especially because full examination at the medical visit is sometimes challenging. Wounds that fail to heal or appear atypical, especially in affected adults, deserve biopsy to consider the possibility of SCC. Guidelines for best practices related to surveillance and diagnosis, tumor evaluation, surgical and nonsurgical treatment, use of prosthetics, and end-of-life care were published in 2016.[159] Of paramount importance is psychological support after a diagnosis of SCC is made. Early intervention using full-thickness excision with wide margins is usually first-line therapy.[106,160,161] Mohs surgery offers no long-term benefit in decreasing local recurrence, metastases, or death. Amputation is required in 42% of patients with RDEB and SCC, with approximately equal outcomes on the hands and legs. Surgical debulking and radiation therapy are palliative to reduce pain or bleeding, but radiation should be delivered in small fractions to reduce the risk of skin desquamation. The benefit of chemotherapy may be outweighed by the risks, and use should be considered carefully. Cetuximab (epidermal growth factor receptor [EGFR] antagonist) has controlled SCC metastasis and may be of benefit for palliation in advanced cancer.[162,163]

Management of EB represents a huge unmet need, and several experimental approaches are currently being investigated. These range from gene therapy with grafting, to protein replacement, to trying to accelerate wound healing or reduce fibrosis (Box 13.1; details in online version).

Box 13.1 Experimental Approaches for Treating EB (see Online Details)

- Gene therapy
  - Grafting after gene correction or replacement (viral, nonviral)
  - Grafting through expansion of revertant mosaic cells
  - Stem cell transplantation
  - Intradermal injection of gene-corrected fibroblasts
  - Topically applied gene therapy
- Cell therapy
  - Intradermal injection of allogenic fibroblasts
- Pharmacologic approaches
  - Readthrough for null mutations (topical, intravenous gentamycin)
  - Protein replacement therapy (recombinant type VII collagen)
  - Inhibition of inflammatory cytokines
  - Fibrosis reduction
  - Acceleration of wound healing

Experimental Approaches for Treating EB[164]

Gene Therapy. For patients without revertant mosaicism, gene correction or replacement will be required. Transplantation of retroviral gene-corrected cultured epidermal stem cells from a patient with non-Herlitz JEB was first described in 2006, resulting in long-term graft persistence without blistering.[169,170] Retrovirus-transduced gene-corrected keratinocyte grafts have also been applied to seven adults with RDEB, 50% of greater healing of wounds persistent by 2 years after transplantation but few of the controls without the transduced epidermal sheets.[171] Cells from a patient with RDEB have been made into induced pluripotent stem cells (iPSCs), corrected by adenovirus-associated genome editing and after removal of any cells with mutations predisposing to cancer, allowed to differentiate into keratinocytes.[172] By selecting for stem cells and lack of cancer predisposition of transplanted cells, risks are minimized. A concern about keratinocyte gene therapy is the likelihood that only limited areas of skin could be transplanted. However, stem cell–derived keratinocyte gene therapy was recently used to replace more than 80% of the skin of a boy with generalized intermediate JEB resulting from mutations in *LAMB3*.[173] Designer nucleases, such as CRISPR/Cas9, allow gene modification through excision and replacement of a precise gene sequence and have been used to introduce the normal *COL7A1* gene to produce type VII collagen in RDEB-cultured 3D skin equivalents,[174] as well as to correct *LAMB3* mutations *in vitro* in JEB[175] cells. As efficiency of introduction of CRISPR/Cas9 into keratinocyte stem cells increases, these experimental data will likely translate to human trials.

Topical application of multiple copies of COL7A1 integrated into an inactivated herpes simplex virus has shown promise in early phase trials. Antisense oligonucleotides have been used *in vitro* to skip specific exons in mutant *COL7A1* RNA to restore synthesis of normal, but slightly shorter, collagen VII in human cells and DEB mice.[176–178]

Cell Therapy. Intradermal injection of allogeneic fibroblasts temporarily stimulates increased expression of type VII collagen from patient (not donor) fibroblasts, especially in patients who have RDEB with less severe disease.[179–181]

Bone Marrow Transplantation. Stem cell transplantation has shown promise in some (but not all) patients with RDEB,[164,182] but does not appear promising for JEB. Through the introduction of mesenchymal stem cells and reduced-intensity conditioning regimens, toxicity has been greatly reduced. Stem cell transplantation of autologous cells after gene correction holds promise for more global replacement of abnormal genes.

Pharmacologic Approaches

READTHROUGH. In patients with null mutations (46% of patients with RDEB), the aminoglycoside gentamicin may enhance "readthrough," essentially skipping the stop codon and allowing full-length gene expression. The efficacy of this approach has now been demonstrated *in vitro*[183] and in small numbers of RDEB patients with nonsense mutations[184] after intravenous, topical, and intradermal administration of gentamicin. Most recently, this approach has been shown to be valuable as well in JEB keratinocytes in restoring laminin 332.[185] The potential for renal and ototoxicity from systemic levels of gentamicin continues to be a potential concern, but intravenous administration for 2 weeks has led to improvement that is sustained for months, suggesting that intermittent courses can be administered to minimize potential toxicity. Amlexanox, an antiinflammatory medication that has been used topically to treat aphthous ulcers and now is in trials for oral administration for type 2 diabetes, was recently shown to increase readthrough by a different mechanism (as an inhibitor of nonsense-mediated mRNA decay) to the same or greater extent than gentamicin, leading to expression of full-length type VII collagen.

PROTEIN REPLACEMENT THERAPY. Recombinant type VII collagen, whether intralesional, intravenous, or topical, has been shown to home to the dermal–epidermal junction of wounded skin in mouse models and decrease blistering.[186–189] Intradermally injected recombinant type VII collagen is currently approved for early human trials; studies with intravenous and topical administration are planned. One potential concern is that overexpression of type VII collagen in RDEB SCC cell keratinocytes increased cell invasion,[190] raising the caution that giving high concentrations of type VII collagen may increase cancer-associated risks.

INHIBITORS OF INFLAMMATION. Diacerein cream, an inhibitor of interleukin-1β, a cytokine shown to be increased in EBS, was shown in a small randomized, placebo-controlled, crossover trial to reduce significantly the number of blisters in EBS, but did not reach its primary endpoint in a phase 3, double-blind, randomized, placebo-controlled trial.[191]

REDUCTION OF FIBROSIS. Transforming growth factor beta (TGF-β) activity is elevated in injured RDEB skin and is thought to contribute to the progressive scarring with fibrosis and joint contractures. Losartan, a drug commonly used for hypertension, inhibits excessive TGF-β signaling and TGF-β-induced inflammation, and has been shown to halt fibrosis and subsequent fusion of the digits in RDEB mouse models[192]; clinical trials in humans are ongoing.

EXPERIMENTAL APPROACHES TO PROMOTE WOUND HEALING THYMOSIN β4 PEPTIDE. This facilitates actin polymerization and may be helpful for wound healing; it is currently in double-blind trials for JEB and DEB.[193] Application of sunflower oil with a betulin-rich triterpene extract from birch bark (Oleogel-S10)[194] met its primary endpoint for efficacy in a double-blind, randomized, placebo-controlled phase 3 study. Although allantoin 6% looked promising in smaller trials, the pivotal phase 3 controlled clinical trial with 169 patients did not show evidence of benefit vs. those treated with placebo.[164]

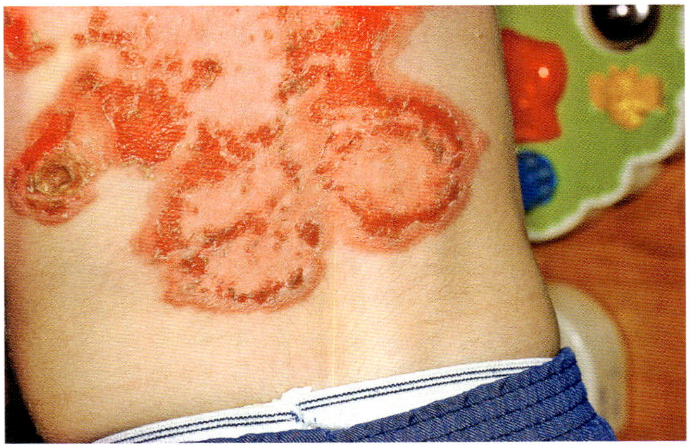

Fig. 13.31 Pemphigus vulgaris. The cutaneous bullae and erosions are uncommon in children. The most common manifestation of pemphigus vulgaris is oral mucosal blistering. (Courtesy Moise Levy, MD.)

Immune-Mediated Blistering Disorders

The chronic nonhereditary bullous diseases of childhood are a group of rare, largely autoimmune disorders with autoantibodies directed against structural components of the skin.[1] The most common autoimmune blistering disorder in children is linear IgA dermatosis,[195,196] but the most common diagnosis requiring hospitalization for an autoimmune blistering disorder in children is pemphigus.[197] Immune-mediated blistering disorders can occur at any age, including in the neonatal period, because of transplacental passage of maternal antibodies (especially pemphigus vulgaris, pemphigus foliaceus, and bullous pemphigoid).[198] Diagnosis is based on clinical characteristics and histologic and immunofluorescent features of skin biopsy specimens.[199] Treatment of autoimmune blistering disorders usually requires systemic immunosuppressive agents. In general, pemphigus, mucous membrane pemphigoid, and EBA are more challenging to manage.

PEMPHIGUS

Pemphigus is a term applied to a group of severe, chronic, sometimes fatal blistering disorders characterized by flaccid bullae that develop on normal-appearing skin and mucous membranes. Pemphigus can be classified into pemphigus vulgaris, pemphigus foliaceus, pemphigus herpetiformis, IgA pemphigus, drug-induced pemphigus, and paraneoplastic pemphigus. The blister formation in pemphigus results from acantholysis, which is loss of cohesion between epidermal cells due to intercellular edema and the loss of intercellular bridges in the lower epidermis. The structural components against which autoantibodies are generated in pemphigus are all components of desmosomes.

Pemphigus Vulgaris

Pemphigus vulgaris is a potentially life-threatening chronic vesiculobullous disease characterized by flaccid bullae and persistent erosions, with a predilection for middle-aged individuals. Approximately 5% of cases of pemphigus are pediatric.[200] The prognosis is better in children than in adults.[201] The cutaneous lesions of pemphigus vulgaris favor the seborrheic areas (the face, scalp, neck, sternum, axillae, groin, and periumbilical regions) and pressure areas of the feet and back (Fig. 13.31). The oral mucosae are affected in 95% of patients and are the initial site in the majority of patients, often months before the appearance of skin lesions. Intact blisters are rarely seen on the oral mucosa, because they rupture soon after formation, leaving raw, denuded, painful erosions that heal slowly. Other mucosal surfaces, the anogenital areas, conjunctivae,[202] vermilion borders of the lips, pharynx, larynx, and esophagus may be similarly involved. Pemphigus in children can involve the ileum, leading to protein-losing enteropathy, which has been reported in several children from Japan.[203,204] Because a majority of patients with proven pemphigus vulgaris have painful oral erosions for weeks to months before they develop the characteristic bullous eruption (and the disease may be limited to mucosae), children with severe recurrent mucocutaneous lesions or chronic erosive mucous membrane disease should be examined carefully.[205] Mucosal biopsy should be performed if skin lesions are not present.

The primary cutaneous lesions of pemphigus vulgaris appear as vesicles or bullae that arise on erythematous plaques or normal-appearing skin. The initial lesions may remain localized to one area of the skin or mucous membrane for weeks or months before other areas of the skin are involved. With the onset of new lesions, the patient may experience some pruritus, burning, or local discomfort. Blisters generally measure 1 cm or less at onset but may increase by peripheral extension to several centimeters in diameter. Lateral pressure applied to the normal-appearing skin at the periphery of a lesion results in lesional extension and shearing of skin (the Nikolsky sign). This phenomenon, a manifestation of defective epidermal cohesion, is not pathognomonic of pemphigus, because the Nikolsky sign may also be seen in patients with superficial forms of EB, Stevens–Johnson syndrome, and toxic epidermal necrolysis. Vertical pressure may also produce peripheral extension of lesions. The blisters rupture easily, and the resultant erosions are painful, bleed easily, and heal slowly. Scaling and crusting are common, and patients commonly are misdiagnosed as having impetigo or infected seborrheic dermatitis.

A variant of pemphigus vulgaris, pemphigus vegetans, is differentiated by the hypertrophic granulomatous tissue (vegetations) after healing and the predilection for the face, flexural, and intertriginous areas.[206] Patients commonly show small pustules at the periphery of ruptured bullae.[207]

Diagnosis of pemphigus is based on clinical presentation and histopathology consistent with pemphigus and either a positive direct immunofluorescent (DIF) or serologic detection of autoantibodies against epithelial surface antigens (by indirect immunofluorescent [IIF] assays or enzyme-linked immunosorbent assay [ELISA]). Biopsy should be taken of a recent (<24 hours old) small vesicle or edge of a bulla (with two-thirds perilesional skin) for routine histologic analysis; perilesional skin (within 1 cm of a recent lesion) is best for DIF analysis. The earliest histologic change is intercellular edema with loss of cohesion between epidermal cells, resulting in the formation of clefts and bullae in a suprabasal location. The basal cells, although separated from one another, remain attached to the dermis with a resultant "row of tombstones" appearance. A rapid Tzanck smear will show acantholytic cells, but is generally not useful.[208] DIF tests on biopsied samples show IgG and complement bound to intercellular areas of the epidermis. IIF studies of the serum of patients with pemphigus vulgaris show IgG antibodies binding to the intercellular spaces. The targeted structural antigen in patients with only mucosal pemphigus is desmoglein 3, a desmosomal component expressed in the mucosa and lower region of the epidermis, and the presence of antibody can be tested by ELISA. ELISA tends to be positive in more than 90% of patients and generally correlates with disease activity.[209] Desmoglein 1 can compensate for desmoglein 3, and antibodies against both desmogleins must be present for both mucosal and skin blistering to occur in pemphigus. ELISA assays with antidesmoglein 1, and to a lesser extent antidesmoglein 3, antibodies have correlated with disease activity better than IIF assays in some studies.[210–213] Increases in antidesmoglein antibody titers may precede clinical flares, and decreases in titer correlate with clinical responses.

A transient form of pemphigus vulgaris, neonatal pemphigus vulgaris, may be seen in neonates of pregnant women with circulating antidesmoglein 3 antibodies, even without active mucocutaneous disease. Blistering subsides in affected neonates within a few weeks, concomitant with the catabolism of maternal antibodies.[214–217]

Pemphigus Foliaceus

Pemphigus foliaceus (superficial pemphigus) is a more superficial form of pemphigus.[218] The disease most commonly affects middle-aged persons and, although rare in children, is more common than pemphigus vulgaris in prepubertal children. The disorder in children is more benign than in adults and the course is milder than that of pemphigus vulgaris.

Bullae are usually small and flaccid. They rupture easily and, because of their superficial location, leave shallow erosions. Slowly spreading crusted plaques thought to be impetigo but resistant to oral antibiotics are the most common presenting manifestation (Fig. 13.32). Patients often show an arcuate configuration to lesions. Common areas of erosive involvement include the scalp,[219] face, upper chest, abdomen, and back. Bullae are more likely to be intact if located on the lower extremities. Patients generally are not severely ill, but may rarely complain of pruritus, pain, and burning. At times, however, the clinical picture may progress to resemble that of a severe, generalized exfoliative dermatitis. Oral lesions are rarely seen in pemphigus foliaceus and, when present, usually consist of small, superficial, often inconspicuous erosions.

Histologic findings in pemphigus foliaceus are similar to those of pemphigus vulgaris and demonstrate epidermal bullae and intercellular acantholysis. The acantholysis seen in pemphigus foliaceus is more superficial and occurs in the upper epidermis, usually in the granular layer or just beneath it, with resultant formation of clefts in a superficial, often subcorneal, location. DIF shows intracellular deposition of IgG and C_3 that is indistinguishable from that of pemphigus vulgaris. The targeted antigen is desmoglein 1, a desmosomal component localized to the suprabasal keratinocytes, which is also the target of bacterial exfoliative toxins in patients with bullous impetigo and staphylococcal scalded skin syndrome (see Chapter 14).[220] Although desmoglein 1 is also found in the mucosa, desmoglein 3 at this location provides stabilization, and patients with pemphigus foliaceus, as a result, do not tend to have oral mucosal lesions (a phenomenon referred to as *desmoglein compensation*).[221] Exclusively, IgG antibodies to desmocollins have also been linked to childhood pemphigus foliaceus.[222] Neonatal pemphigus has been described in babies of mothers with sporadic pemphigus foliaceus and high titers of antidesmoglein 1 antibodies.[223–225]

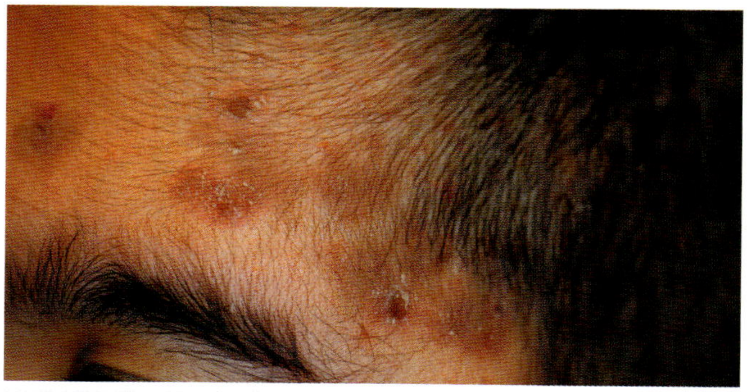

Fig. 13.32 Pemphigus foliaceus. Children with pemphigus foliaceus are often thought to have impetigo and treated unsuccessfully with courses of antibiotics as a result; the target of this immunobullous disorder, desmoglein 1, is the same target as the exfoliatin produced by *S. aureus* infection.

Pemphigus herpetiformis is a form of pemphigus that may resemble dermatitis herpetiformis, with polymorphic clinical lesions that range from urticarial to bullous and no mucosal lesions. In the six pediatric patients reported to date, two had antibodies tested and both were targeting desmoglein 1.[226] Drug-induced pemphigus herpetiformis has been described.[227]

Pemphigus erythematosus (Senear–Usher syndrome) is a variant of pemphigus foliaceus in which lesions often localize to the butterfly area of the face, the scalp, upper chest, and back. Patients may show detectable antinuclear antibodies.[228,229] Fogo selvagem (endemic pemphigus; Brazilian pemphigus) is a variant of pemphigus foliaceus found in tropical regions but is clinically and immunologically indistinguishable from sporadic pemphigus foliaceus.[230] Certain human leukocyte antigen (HLA) alleles and exposure to certain blood-sucking insects are risk factors. Patients with fogo selvagem show pathogenic antidesmoglein 1, IgG4, and IgM autoantibodies,[231,232] which may develop as a result of antigenic mimicry initiated by an environmental stimulus in predisposed persons.[233] Endemic in Brazil, and to a lesser extent in other South American countries, 15% of patients are children. The striking distribution of lesions on sun-exposed skin, its burned appearance, and the painful burning sensation in lesions (more so than in sporadic pemphigus foliaceus) are responsible for the name *fogo selvagem* (Portuguese, meaning *wildfire*). In chronic cases, hyperpigmentation, hyperkeratosis, and loss of hair over the scalp and body are prominent features of this disorder. Neonatal pemphigus has not been observed in infants born to mothers with active fogo selvagem because IgM and IgG4 do not cross the placenta.[234]

Drug-Induced Pemphigus

Drug-induced pemphigus is particularly rare in children. The most commonly implicated oral agents are penicillamine and captopril (both thiol drugs), but other drugs have also been associated (Box 13.2). Sulfhydryl groups are thought to interact with the sulfhydryl groups in desmogleins 1 and 3, thus modifying the antigenicity of the desmoglein. In contrast to other types of drug reactions, drug-induced pemphigus often requires several months of exposure to the medication before onset. Initially a nonspecific morbilliform, annular, or urticarial eruption may be seen, eventually evolving after a variable latency period into the blistering process. The disorder typically resembles pemphigus foliaceus more often than pemphigus vulgaris. Oral lesions are rare. Topical imiquimod has been described to trigger pemphigus foliaceus in several adults and, more recently, a 5-year-old girl.

Immunoglobulin A Pemphigus

Immunoglobulin A (IgA) pemphigus, characterized by the intercellular deposition of IgA rather than IgG autoantibodies, has been divided into the subcorneal pustular dermatosis form and intraepidermal neutrophilic IgA dermatosis based on the subcorneal or intraepidermal localization of the blister histologically. Both conditions clinically show vesicles, small bullae, and pustules overlying well-circumscribed erythema. IgA pemphigus resembling pemphigus vegetans has also been described.[235] The youngest reported patient was 1 month of age.[236] The autoantigen for the subcorneal pustular dermatosis form has been shown to be the desmosomal protein desmocollin 1.[237] Although circulating antibodies against either desmoglein 1 or desmoglein 3 have been identified in patients with intraepidermal

Box 13.2 Causes of Drug-Induced Pemphigus

- β-blockers
- Captopril
- Ceftazidime
- Imiquimod (topical)
- Penicillamine
- Penicillin
- Progesterone
- Rifampin
- Sulfasalazine

neutrophilic IgA dermatosis, other patients have shown no identifiable autoantigen.[238–240]

The pustular form may be the same disorder as subcorneal pustular dermatosis (Sneddon–Wilkinson disease), a condition that rarely occurs in children, although it has been described in individuals as young as 7 weeks of age.[241] The disease generally begins with small pustules or vesicles on an erythematous base. Occasionally only vesicles may be present, but these soon change into sterile pustules. The pustules tend to appear in crops and spread to large parts of the body, forming large circinate or gyrate patterns that coalesce to form serpiginous patterns, especially on the abdomen, axillae, and groin. Individual lesions tend to last for periods of 5 days, with new lesions appearing as others disappear. As the pustules resolve, they are replaced by a superficial leafy scale or crust. After the eruption resolves, a faint, blotchy, brown hyperpigmentation without atrophy or scarring remains. The condition is benign and is characterized by remissions and exacerbations that may last for 5 to 8 years. Histopathologic examination of an intact lesion of subcorneal pustular dermatosis reveals a subcorneal blister filled almost entirely with neutrophilic polymorphonuclear leukocytes, but immunofluorescence analysis shows no immunodeposits.

Paraneoplastic Pemphigus

Paraneoplastic pemphigus, a rare autoimmune disorder associated with malignancy, has been described occasionally in children.[242,243] In one study of 92 patients with known age, only one was a child (11 years old).[244] The majority of pediatric patients have underlying Castleman disease, a lymphoproliferative disorder characterized by massive growth of lymphoid tissue usually located in the retroperitoneum or mediastinum.[245,246] Sarcoma, T-cell lymphoblastic lymphoma, and myofibroblastic tumor may also underlie paraneoplastic pemphigus; occasionally no underlying tumor is detected.

All patients tend to show intractable stomatitis, particularly involving the labial mucosa and resembling the labial manifestations of Stevens–Johnson syndrome. Two-thirds of patients show conjunctival involvement, sometimes leading to symblepharon and visual impairment. Skin changes can be bullous and/or may resemble lichen planus or erythema multiforme. The trunk and extremities are most commonly involved. Palmoplantar involvement and paronychial inflammation, which may result in nail shedding, are commonly seen. Mucosae of the tracheobronchial system are also involved, and respiratory involvement with the development of bronchiolitis obliterans may be fatal.[247]

Biopsies show intraepithelial acantholysis, keratinocyte dyskeratosis, and basal cell vacuolar changes, combining the histologic features of pemphigus and Stevens–Johnson syndrome. DIF is often negative, but immunoblots show several circulating autoantibodies directed against a variety of epidermal proteins, particularly of the desmogleins and plakin family (BP antigen 1, DSP, envoplakin, and periplakin), but also to the protease inhibitor α2-macroglobulin-like protein 1 (A2ML1).[244,248]

Paraneoplastic pemphigus must be distinguished from Stevens–Johnson syndrome, toxic epidermal necrolysis, pemphigus vulgaris, bullous and cicatricial forms of pemphigoid, lichen planus pemphigoides, and mucosal infections from herpes or *Candida*. Once the diagnosis is suspected in a child or adolescent, evaluation for malignancy should be initiated. Complete physical examination, particularly of the liver, spleen, and lymph nodes, complete blood count, serum protein electrophoresis, and computerized tomographic scans of the chest, abdomen, and pelvis should be performed to seek evidence of malignancy.

Treatment of Pemphigus

A support group for patients with pemphigus can be accessed at www.pemphigus.org. The latest guidelines for treatment suggest that corticosteroids and anti-CD20 monoclonal antibodies/rituximab are first-line treatment.[249] Systemic corticosteroids are given either as high doses orally (1 to 1.5 mg/kg per day) or, in more refractory cases, as intravenous pulses.[250,251] In one study, intervention led to complete recovery in only 18% of children, although partial improvement with minor relapses was seen in 79%.[252] The majority of children with pemphigus developed serious side effects from their immunosuppression, including cushingoid features in 65% and growth retardation in 50%, stressing the need for steroid-sparing agents.[253–255]

Rituximab (with short-term, low-dose prednisone) has been shown in a double-blind, randomized, comparator trial to be superior in its outcome of proportion of patients in remission at 24 months than high-dose corticosteroid therapy alone in adults with newly diagnosed pemphigus.[256] Rituximab has now been used for children as young as 18 months of age[257] with dramatic clinical results and long-term remission.[258,259] In one study with 10 children, complete remission was achieved with single-agent rituximab by a mean of 21 weeks; relapses occurred in about half of the children, but a repeat cycle led to good response when used.[258] The most common dosing regimen is 375 mg/m^2 weekly for 4 weeks, but a two-dose regimen of 375 mg/m^2 given 15 days apart has also been used. Infusion reactions are the most common side effect. Hypogammaglobulinemia, low antimicrobial antibody titers, and angioedema have also been reported in children. There is a risk of infection and sepsis.

Other steroid-sparing agents for pemphigus vulgaris are dapsone (which may be sufficient for milder cases),[260] mycophenolate mofetil (600 to 1200 mg/m^2 per day),[261,262] cyclosporine (3 to 5 mg/kg per day), methotrexate,[263] azathioprine (2 to 4 mg/kg per day),[264] or high-dose intravenous immunoglobulin[265,266] and can be added to allow the corticosteroid to be tapered. However, each of these agents has significant potential side effects. For oral lesions of the gingivae, a technique involving 1 hour of exposure to topical steroid ointment–soaked cotton balls has been described.[267]

Pemphigus foliaceus is a milder disorder. Suprapotent topical corticosteroids may be effective in some patients, but often treatment with dapsone with or without systemic corticosteroids (initially 1 mg/kg per day) may be required for clearance. In all forms of pemphigus, therapy should be tapered gradually as tolerated when improvement is noted, which may require several months in severe cases.[268] Although patients with Brazilian pemphigus (fogo selvagem) may respond to antimalarial therapy (quinine or quinacrine), systemic corticosteroids continue to be the treatment of choice. Once the disease has cleared, pemphigus foliaceus has a lesser tendency to recur than pemphigus vulgaris. Rituximab has been used as a third-line agent for adults with pemphigus foliaceus, but the response rate is lower than in pemphigus vulgaris.[269] It has been used for refractory pediatric cases as well and is generally well tolerated.[270]

Drug-induced pemphigus usually clears with treatment of the pemphigus and withdrawal of the offending medication. IgA pemphigus in children usually responds to treatment with dapsone or sulfapyridine within 24 to 48 hours, but tends to be more difficult to control with steroids and other systemic antiinflammatory agents. Oral retinoids have been used in patients with IgA pemphigus who do not respond to systemic administration of corticosteroids and dapsone.[271]

Patients with paraneoplastic pemphigus often have their condition clear or improve significantly with surgical removal of the Castleman disease, but not until 6 to 18 months after tumor removal. The prognosis is much worse with malignant neoplasms. The majority of patients succumb within months of the diagnosis, usually to respiratory failure or secondary infection. Aggressive treatment of the malignancy coupled with immunosuppressive therapy, such as the combination of systemic corticosteroids and cyclosporine, should be initiated but may not affect the prognosis. Plasmapheresis has been used in conjunction with corticosteroids and tumor resection.[272]

BULLOUS PEMPHIGOID

BP is a blistering disorder characterized by large, tense, subepidermal bullae that appear on normal-appearing or erythematous skin.[273] Although usually seen in elderly persons, BP may also occur occasionally in infants[274] and children,[275–278] the youngest reported being a 1-month-old infant.[277,279] Several infantile cases have been described after vaccination[280–284] or primary varicella infection.[285] Childhood BP has been described as a manifestation of chronic renal allograft rejection.[286] BP is more common in girls than in boys. It may be more localized, especially to the hands and feet and feet of infants or to the genital region, but it also may be generalized, especially after infancy.

The disorder often starts as mild to moderate pruritus with urticarial or erythematous plaques that evolve over weeks to months into large, tense, sometimes hemorrhagic bullae. Lesions may appear on normal skin or on an erythematous base. The blisters commonly occur at the periphery of annular or polycyclic erythematous plaques. Bullae typically measure 0.25 to 2 cm in diameter. The lower abdomen, anogenital region (including the vulva), and flexural areas of the arms and legs are most often involved, although bullae not uncommonly occur on the face in children. The Nikolsky sign is characteristically absent, and blisters do not extend or increase in size as they do in patients with pemphigus vulgaris. Blistering of the palms and soles is seen in virtually all affected infants,[279] whereas penile involvement is more common in older children.[274,277,287,288] Bullous and vesicular lesions may be on the dorsal aspect of the hands.[289,290] The bullae tend to be tenser and more inflamed than those of pemphigus vulgaris (Fig. 13.33), and the course of BP is more indolent than that of pemphigus vulgaris, including spontaneous remission.[291] Blisters resolve without scarring. Pemphigoid vegetans has been described during childhood, resembling pemphigus vegetans.[292] Oral lesions are seen in approximately 25% of patients with BP, especially in older children.

Variants include cicatricial pemphigoid, which affects mucosal surfaces, and a localized form (chronic pemphigoid of Brunsting–Perry), which is generally limited to the head and neck. The predominant localization of blisters in cicatricial pemphigoid is mucosal[293] (Fig. 13.34), with only 25% of patients showing skin involvement, particularly on the face, neck, and upper chest. Recurrent bullae are seen in the oral mucosa, conjunctivae, and other mucous membranes such as those of the nasopharynx, esophagus, larynx, genitalia,[294] and anus.[295] Oral involvement often takes the form of a desquamative gingivitis,[296] and ocular involvement may not occur until many years after the onset of the condition. Eye involvement often presents as dryness of the eyes with a feeling of chronic, intractable conjunctival irritation. Conjunctival involvement can lead to entropion, trichiasis (in-growing eyelashes), symblepharon, dryness of the cornea, corneal ulceration, and in 25% of patients, blindness. Esophageal lesions may result in stricture formation. Laryngeal lesions, when present, can be life-threatening. Adhesions of the genitourinary region may lead to phimosis in boys and narrowing of the vaginal opening in affected girls. Lichen planus pemphigoides is an overlapping disease in which the lichen planus develops first[297]; most cases respond to dapsone (see Chapter 4).

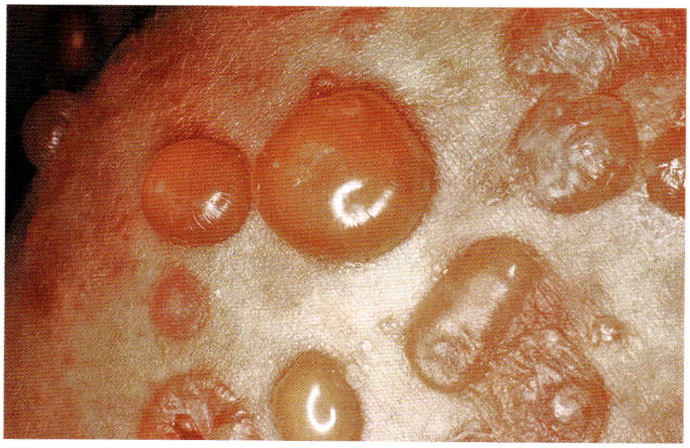

Fig. 13.33 Bullous pemphigoid. Large, tense bullae are seen on the lower region of the abdomen in this 13-year-old boy.

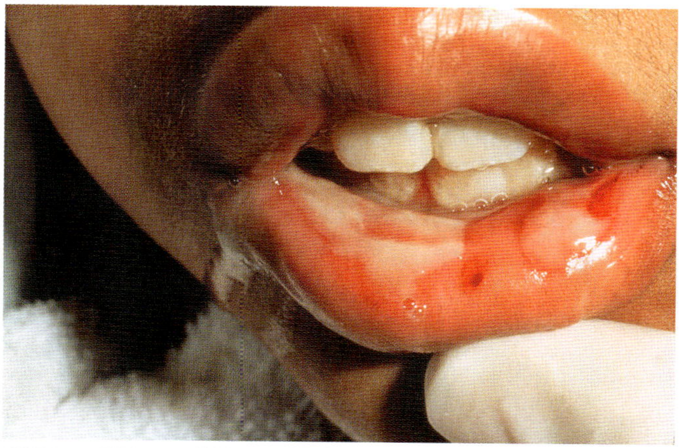

Fig. 13.34 Cicatricial pemphigoid. This 3-year-old boy showed blistering of the oral and ocular mucosae. Early diagnosis is critical to prevent the scarring and permanent blindness. The minority of patients with this condition show cutaneous involvement.

Biopsy specimens of cutaneous lesions show subepidermal blister formation generally without papillary microabscesses (an important diagnostic feature of dermatitis herpetiformis [DH]). Eosinophils are often seen in sections, and peripheral eosinophilia is common. DIF reveals deposition of C_3 and IgG at the lamina lucida of the basement membrane zone. Although indirect testing of serum for circulating IgG anti-basement membrane zone antibodies (IIF) is positive in 72% of children, antibody titers do not correlate with clinical disease activity. These circulating immune deposits bind to the roof of salt-split skin, in which the cleavage runs through the lamina lucida of the basement membrane. Antibodies are most commonly directed against the *NC16A* domain of BP180 antigen (collagen XVII) but may be directed against BP230.[287] ELISA assays have been shown to be more sensitive and just as specific as IIF.[298]

Potent topical corticosteroids may be effective for localized areas of involvement and in patients who are mildly affected.[299] In general, systemic corticosteroids are the mainstay of treatment (1 to 2 mg/kg per day) with dapsone (1 to 2 mg/kg per day) used as a steroid-sparing agent. Sulfapyridine (60 to 150 mg/kg per day), azathioprine, mycophenolate mofetil,[300] intravenous immunoglobulin,[280,301] and rituximab[257] have also been used as steroid-sparing agents and in steroid-resistant cases.[302] Erythromycin (50 mg/kg per day) or clarithromycin (10 mg/kg per day)[303] with or without nicotinamide (25 to 40 mg/kg per day) has been beneficial in some children, presumably due to its antiinflammatory effects. Omalizumab, which targets IgE, has been effective as a steroid-sparing agent.[304,305] Rarely plasma exchange and extracorporeal photochemotherapy have been used for childhood BP.[306] The disorder typically remits in most children within a year and has an excellent prognosis, in contrast to the more chronic disease in adults that is associated with greater morbidity and mortality.

Pemphigoid Gestationis

Pemphigoid gestationis (formerly called *herpes gestationis*) usually presents during the second or third trimester of pregnancy or in the immediate postpartum period.[307] It occurs in 1:50,000 pregnancies. Maternal skin lesions often start at the umbilical area and spread to the abdomen and thighs. Before the development of bullae, initial lesions may be pruritic, eczematous, or erythema multiforme–like erythematous papules and plaques. The face and mucosae are usually spared.[308] The disorder can start for the first time with any pregnancy but tends to recur in subsequent pregnancies. Although the eruption tends to clear in the majority of patients within a few days of delivery, it can persist for many months after delivery. Mild recurrences occasionally have been noted to appear at the time of menstruation, in women who take oral contraceptives, and in women with choriocarcinomas and hydatidiform moles. Cutaneous involvement of the newborn has been noted in about 10% of infants born to mothers with this disorder (Fig. 13.35); on the basis of immunofluorescent findings, a high percentage of newborns have been noted to have subclinical forms of pemphigoid gestationis as well.

The immunopathologic hallmark of pemphigoid gestationis is deposition of C_3, with or without IgG, distributed in a linear band along the basement membrane. The targeted antigens in skin are BP180 and, less commonly, BP230.[309]

The course of pemphigoid gestationis is characterized by alternating exacerbations and remissions. Systemic corticosteroids are the most reliable mode of therapy and with certain precautions are generally

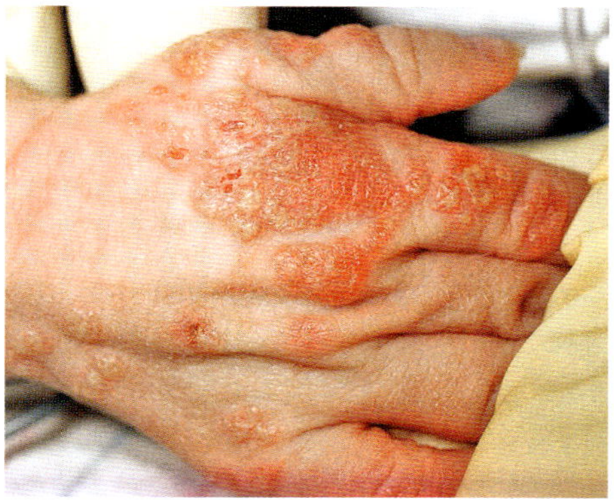

Fig. 13.35 Pemphigoid gestationis. Cutaneous involvement of the newborn has been noted in about 10% of infants born to mothers with this disorder. In the neonate the condition subsides within several weeks as maternal antibodies wane. (Courtesy Moise Levy, MD.)

considered safe for both mother and fetus, especially after the first trimester of pregnancy. Alternate-day dosage, if possible, is preferable to daily treatment. To avoid fetal adrenal suppression, dosages should be reduced to a minimum during the final weeks of pregnancy. Intravenous immunoglobulin is an alternative intervention.[310] The cutaneous lesions in infants with this disorder generally remit within several weeks and do not require therapy. Although there may be an increased risk of prematurity or intrauterine growth restriction, pemphigoid gestationis does not result in an increased mortality risk for the mother or the fetus.

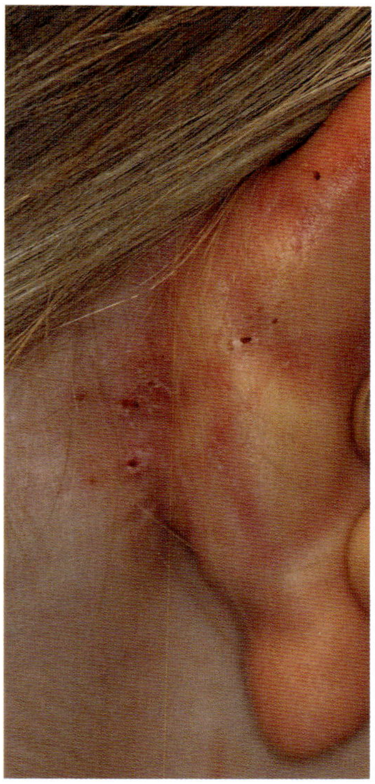

Fig. 13.36 Dermatitis herpetiformis. Note the tiny excoriated papules behind the ear. This patient had involvement of the elbows and buttocks as well. Often primary lesions are not seen because of their rapid excoriation.

DERMATITIS HERPETIFORMIS

Dermatitis herpetiformis (DH; Duhring disease) is characterized by an intensely pruritic papulovesicular and sometimes bullous eruption that responds dramatically to orally administered doses of sulfones or sulfapyridine.[311] Although the disorder may affect infants and children, DH generally occurs during the second to fifth decades of life. It is most common in individuals of Northern European descent and is rare in Blacks. DH is considered the cutaneous form of celiac disease and affects about 5% to 17% of patients with celiac disease.[312,313]

Diagnosis of this disorder cannot be based solely on the morphologic aspects and distribution of lesions, but on the constellation of clinical appearance, histopathologic characteristics, immunofluorescent findings, serologic testing, and response to therapy. The major environmental trigger is ingested gluten and particularly its gliadin component. IgA antibodies develop against gliadin but also two structurally homologous autoantigens: tissue transglutaminase (tTG; widely distributed; most important for celiac disease) and epidermal transglutaminase (eTG or transglutaminase 3; epidermis-specific and most important for DH).[314–317] Virtually all patients with DH have intestinal sensitivity to gluten, but the minority show gastrointestinal symptoms. Of children with DH, 16% have chronic diarrhea, 10% have iron-deficiency anemia, and growth retardation is rare.[318,319]

DH tends to affect the extensor surfaces: the elbows, knees, sacrum, buttocks, and shoulders, and occasionally affects the face, eyelids, facial hairline and retroauricular areas (Fig. 13.36), posterior nuchal area, and scalp. Lesions are usually grouped and symmetric in distribution with centrifugal extension and vesicles predominantly at the periphery. In association with the onset of intense pruritus or burning, erythematous and, at times, urticarial lesions may develop. Characteristic of this disorder are minute, clear, relatively tense vesicles that measure from 0.3 to 4 mm in diameter. These vesicles rupture easily, either spontaneously or when scratched. Not uncommonly, the grouped ("herpetiform") vesicles and papules are seen amid excoriated papules and postinflammatory hypopigmentation and hyperpigmentation. The palms, flexor fingers, and soles may show hemorrhagic, purpuric, or petechial lesions with active DH,[320–322] found in 64% in one pediatric study.[323] Palmoplantar hyperkeratosis, chronic urticaria, and prurigo have been described in atypical cases. The general course of this disorder is chronic (often lasting 5 to 10 years or more) with frequent exacerbations and remissions.

Childhood DH can be confused with arthropod bites, dermatitis, urticaria, scabies, and pityriasis lichenoides et varioliformis acuta. Serum IgA anti-transglutaminase 3 levels have been proposed as a screening test for DH, although confirmation of the diagnosis requires lesional biopsy for routine histologic evaluation and, most importantly, perilesional biopsy (within 1 cm away) for immunofluorescent analysis. Subepidermal microabscesses with accumulations of neutrophils and eosinophils are found at the tips of the dermal papillae by routine histology. IgA is seen at the tips of the dermal papillae in a granular pattern by immunofluorescent microscopy of perilesional skin.[324] Patients should be eating a gluten-containing diet for biopsy or any serologic testing, or false-negative results may occur. If the DIF testing on biopsy sections is negative but the clinical presentation is typical, serologic testing showing antibodies against tTG and endomysial antibodies (or, even better, the more sensitive anti-eTG or deamidated antigliadin, if available) can allow a provisional diagnosis and lead to a trial of medical and dietary intervention.

Sulfones (dapsone) and sulfapyridine are effective in relieving the symptoms and suppressing the eruption of DH in children as well as adults. Dramatic relief from the use of these agents, often as early as 24 to 48 hours after initiation, is often helpful in making the diagnosis. The recommended initial dosage for dapsone is 0.5 mg/kg per day. If no response is seen in a week, the dosage can be increased by 0.5 mg/kg per day to a maximum of 2 mg/kg per day, assuming blood counts are normal before each dosage increase. Once existing lesions have been suppressed, the dosage may be tapered to a minimal level (usually 12.5 to 50 mg/day). Baseline blood counts and glucose-6-phosphate dehydrogenase (G6PD) levels are important before initiating therapy. Blood counts should be repeated at least monthly for the first 6 months. Side effects are uncommon but can include hemolytic anemia (especially seen in patients with G6PD deficiency, a contraindication to use), agranulocytosis, methemoglobinemia (manifested most commonly by headache and fatigue but sometimes by bluish discoloration of the face, mucous membranes, and nails), nausea, vomiting, headache, giddiness, tachycardia, psychoses, anemia, leukopenia, fever, exfoliative dermatitis, liver necrosis, lymphadenitis, and peripheral neuropathy. Topical dapsone 5% may be helpful for limited disease.[325] Iodide can worsen DH and should be avoided (e.g., potassium iodides in expectorants).[326]

If at all possible, a gluten-free diet should be instituted. With a gluten-free diet alone, children experience remission in approximately 11 months, although clearance of IgA deposits can take years. Reintroduction of gluten leads to rapid clinical deterioration. Adherence to a gluten-free diet for at least 5 years is also thought to lower the increased risk of developing lymphoma (most commonly involving the gastrointestinal system and non-Hodgkin lymphoma). Adherence is particularly difficult, however, in affected adolescents. Support and information about DH and gluten-free diets can be found online (http://www.celiac.org/celiac-disease/dermatitis-herpetiformis/; http://www.dermatitisherpetiformis.org.uk).

LINEAR IMMUNOGLOBULIN A BULLOUS DERMATOSIS

Linear IgA bullous dermatosis of childhood (chronic bullous disease of childhood; LABD) usually has its[327] onset during the first decade of life, particularly during preschool years.[328–330] The prevalence in Germany in 2014 was approximately 24 per million children, and much more common than other autoimmune blistering disorders.[200] Spontaneous remission usually occurs after several months to 3 years and almost always before the onset of puberty. IgA nephropathy is a rare complication.[331] It can follow an infection or represent a manifestation of drug hypersensitivity, especially to antibiotics such as vancomycin, amoxicillin-clavulanate, and trimethoprim-sulfamethoxazole or nonsteroidal antiinflammatory agents, generally 1 to 13 days after the first dose.[332–334]

LABD is characterized by large, tense, clear or hemorrhagic bullae measuring 1 to 2 cm in diameter on a normal or erythematous base. The eruption is widespread, and areas of predilection include the face, scalp, lower part of the trunk (including the genitalia and pubis), buttocks, inner thighs, legs, and dorsal aspect of the feet (Fig. 13.37). The bullae may form characteristic annular or rosette-like lesions composed of sausage-shaped blisters resembling a cluster of jewels surrounding a central crust: the string-of-pearls sign (Fig. 13.38). Pruritus is a variable feature and may be mild to moderate, intense and distressing, or completely absent. Mucous membrane lesions occasionally occur, especially in neonatal LABD, with both oral and ocular lesions described.[335]

Histologically, LABD is characterized by subepidermal bullae with edema of adjacent dermal papillae and a dermal infiltrate of polymorphonuclear leukocytes, eosinophils, and mononuclear cells. A subepidermal blistering disease, it may be indistinguishable both clinically and histologically from BP[336] or DH, but the immunofluorescent finding of linear IgA deposits, typically in the lamina lucida zone of the dermal–epidermal junction of perilesional skin, confirms the diagnosis.[337,338] Circulating IgA basement membrane–zone antibodies are found in up to 80% of patients and usually bind the epidermal side of salt-split skin. Antibodies are most commonly directed against a 120-kDa fragment of BP180/collagen XVII (also called *linear IgA disease antigen-1 [LAD-1]*) and, less commonly, a 97-kDa fragment that is generated from the 120-kDa fragment.[339] Type VII collagen is the major antigen for the sublamina densa type. Some children with clinically typical LABD show "mixed immunobullous disease of childhood," in which both IgG and IgA autoantibodies are detected.

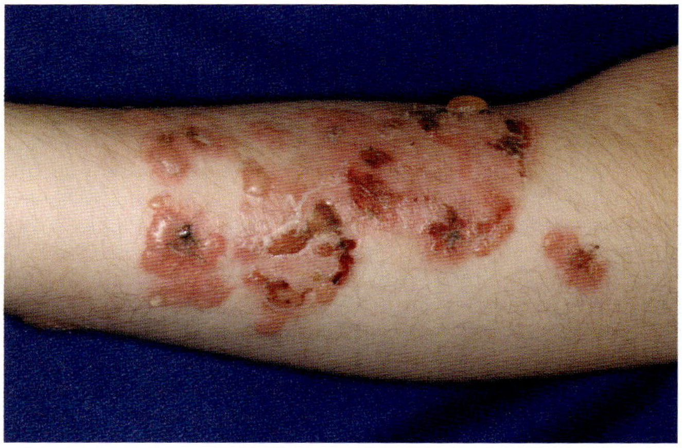

Fig. 13.37 Chronic bullous disease of childhood. Clear or hemorrhagic bullae are commonly found on the legs, as well as the face, lower part of the trunk, and genitalia.

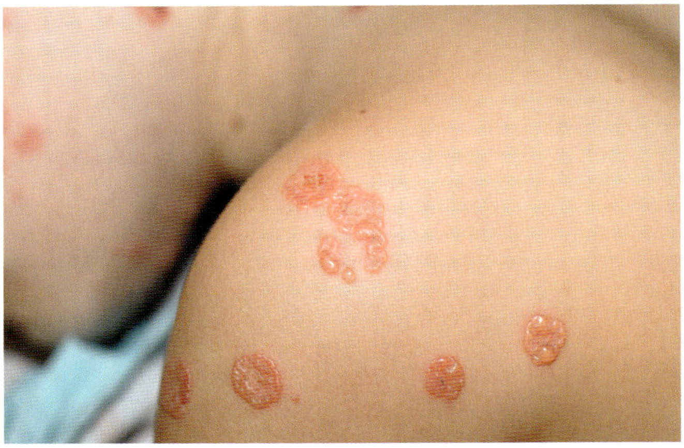

Fig. 13.38 Chronic bullous disease of childhood. The bullae may form characteristic annular or rosette-like lesions resembling a cluster of jewels surrounding a central crust: the string-of-pearls sign. (Courtesy Dr. Brandon Newell).

Response to therapy is generally favorable.[340] Dapsone, as in DH, is the drug of choice, although patients have responded to administration of erythromycin, dicloxacillin, or sulfonamides.[341–344] Children have also responded to administration of nicotinamide, with or without antibiotics.[345] Responses to antibiotics, however, are often transient, and their use has been advocated initially while awaiting results of diagnostic tests or in patients unable to take dapsone and sulfapyridine.[346] If response to dapsone or antibiotics is inadequate, sulfapyridine, systemic corticosteroids, and mycophenolate mofetil are alternative therapies.

EPIDERMOLYSIS BULLOSA ACQUISITA

Epidermolysis bullosa acquisita (EBA; acquired EB) is a subepidermal blistering disorder that largely affects adults. EBA has recently been classified into five subtypes: (1) classical/mechanobullous (with scarring and milia formation (Fig. 13.39) reminiscent of DDEB); (2) nonclassical/nonmechanical (BP-like); (3) MM-EBA (predominantly mucous membranes; (4) Brunstein–Perry (head and neck); and (5) IgA-EBA.[347] Approximately 40 cases in children have been described.[348] A neonate with EBA from transplacental transfer of antibody has been described (Fig. 13.40).[349] Blisters may be hemorrhagic or serous and tend to be localized to sites of trauma or pressure, especially on the extensor areas of the extremities. Oropharyngeal mucous membrane erosions are commonly seen; the conjunctival, esophageal, and anogenital mucous membranes are less commonly involved, although blindness may result. The nails may be dystrophic, and scarring alopecia may be seen.

The condition results from the deposition of IgG and, less commonly, IgA[350,351] autoantibodies directed against type VII collagen (see Fig. 13.1).[352] Type VII collagen is a structural component of anchoring fibrils that is missing or abnormal in children with RDEB or DDEB, respectively. Immunofluorescence examination shows the linear deposition of IgG and sometimes C_3 at the lower lamina densa or sublamina densa zones of the basement membrane. IIF shows IgG binding to the dermal side of salt-split skin (e.g., beneath the lamina lucida). Immunoblotting analysis shows binding to a 290-kDa protein

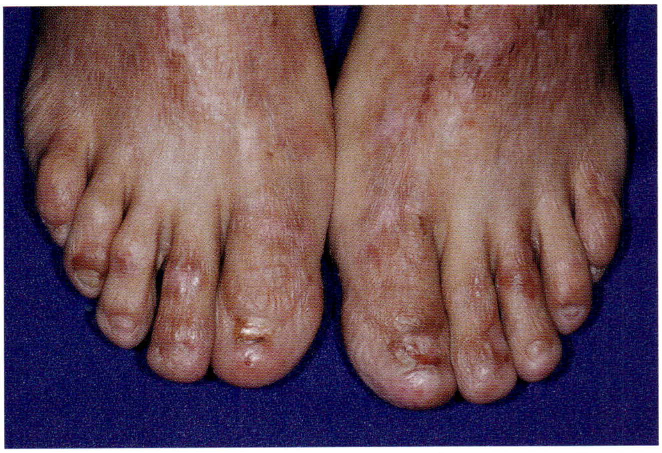

Fig. 13.39 Epidermolysis bullosa acquisita (EBA). This disorder may resemble dystrophic epidermolysis bullosa (DEB). Note the scarring, milia, and nail dystrophy. The immunodeposits in patients with EBA are directed against collagen VII, the same protein missing or dysfunctional in patients with DEB.

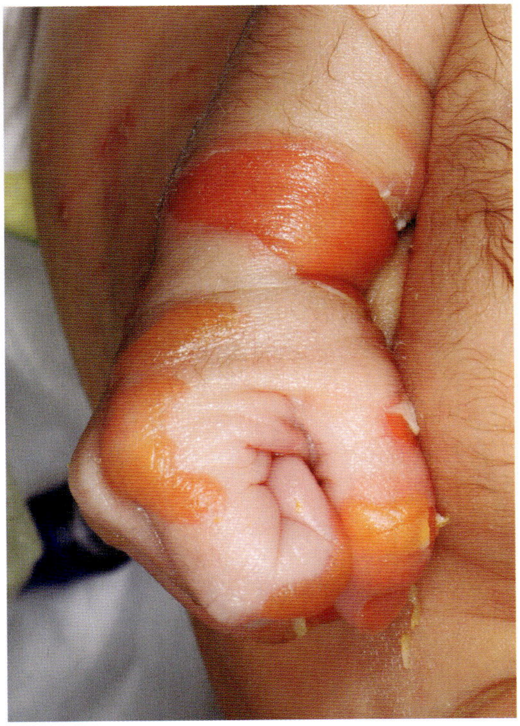

Fig. 13.40 Epidermolysis bullosa acquisita (EBA). This baby developed EBA by transplacental passage of maternal antibodies against type VII collagen. The tense blisters shown resulted in neonatal denudement and subsequent milia formation, as in dystrophic epidermolysis bullosa.

that corresponds to type VII collagen and recognition primarily of the NC1 noncollagenous domain of type VII collagen; however, children may show antibodies directed against additional domains, particularly children with EBA younger than 10 years of age with the inflammatory phenotype.[353] However, ELISA detection of anti-Col7 IgG autoantibodies (especially full-length C7) is more sensitive than western blotting and IIF on salt-split skin.[354,355] Biochip technology to screen for EBA shows good correlation with ELISA.[356]

EBA has been reported in patients with mild recessive[357] and dominant[358] DEB. A patient with RDEB and only nail dystrophy during childhood developed EBA at 24 years of age, whereas a patient with DDEB had relative quiescence after childhood and developed florid EBA at 63 years old. Both had high levels of circulating anti–type VII collagen antibodies and deposition in skin. Although circulating anti–type VII collagen antibodies are detected in more than half of patients with dystrophic EB, positive DIF and clinical signs of EBA in association with inherited EB are rare.

EBA has also been described in association with celiac disease[359] and during squaric acid dibutyl ester immunotherapy for scalp alopecia areata.[360] In the latter situation, it regressed with treatment discontinuation and initiation of corticosteroids and dapsone and did not recur after medication withdrawal, suggesting a relationship to treatment.[360]

EBA has a chronic course with flares but seems to have a better prognosis in children than in adults. Dapsone and corticosteroids are first-line therapy and often lead to remission within about 2 years[361,362]; mycophenolate mofetil may be steroid-sparing. Rituximab is now also used for treatment-resistant EBA.[363,364] Childhood IgA-mediated EBA has responded to mycophenolate mofetil.[351] Colchicine, infliximab, photophoresis,[365] rituximab,[366] and intravenous immunoglobulin have been helpful for some patients.[368] The recent demonstration that T cells are critical in initiation of EBA[352] and that a mouse model responded to TNF inhibition[369] suggests that T-cell–directed immunomodulatory strategies may be effective in the future.[369]

BULLOUS SYSTEMIC LUPUS ERYTHEMATOSUS

Similar to patients with EBA, patients with systemic lupus erythematosus (SLE) who manifest immune-mediated bullae show antibodies directed against type VII collagen.[370–373] However, the clinical manifestations more closely resemble those of BP or DH. Black adolescents and young women are most often affected, with a mean age of onset of 22 years.[374] Occasionally bullous SLE is the presenting sign of lupus,[375–378] but more typically it develops in a patient with known SLE (see Chapter 22). Typical lesions are pruritic vesicles and tense bullae with occasional erythematous macules and papules (Fig. 13.41).[379] Cases have been described resembling Stevens–Johnson syndrome/toxic epidermal necrolysis[380] or may present as annular collections of vesicles and bullae.[381] Lesions tend to leave postinflammatory hypopigmentation or hyperpigmentation. Sun-exposed areas are most commonly involved, but flexor and extensor skin surfaces, as well as oral mucosae, may be affected. Bullous

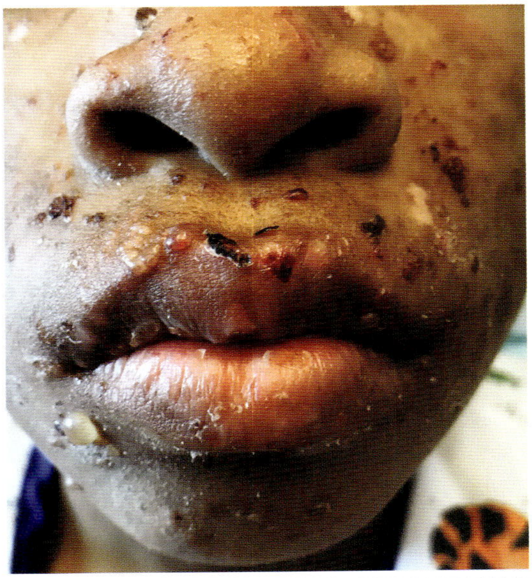

Fig. 13.41 Bullous systemic lupus erythematosus. Pruritic vesicles and tense bullae develop and may leave intense postinflammatory hypopigmentation or hyperpigmentation. The bullous component of systemic lupus erythematosus is most often treated with dapsone. (Courtesy Dr. Lacey Kruse.)

SLE in a linear pattern following Blaschko lines has been described in a child.[382]

Immunofluorescence examination shows deposition of IgG and sometimes IgM, IgA, or C_3 at the basement membrane and upper dermis. Granular, linear, and mixed patterns have all been described. Prognosis is usually favorable and is largely determined by the course of the associated SLE. Most patients generally respond quickly to dapsone therapy (in contrast to EBA), but rituximab[383] and intravenous immunoglobulin[384] have also been used in refractory cases. Administration of systemic corticosteroids with or without additional immunosuppressive agents (e.g., methotrexate, mycophenolate mofetil, azathioprine, cyclophosphamide, or cyclosporine) has led to variable response.

The complete list of 384 references for this chapter is available online at http://expertconsult.inkling.com.

Key References

Fine JD, Mellerio JE. Extracutaneous manifestations and complications of inherited epidermolysis bullosa. Part I. Epithelial associated tissues. J Am Acad Dermatol 2009;61:367–84, quiz 385–366.

Fine JD, Mellerio JE. Extracutaneous manifestations and complications of inherited epidermolysis bullosa. Part II. Other organs. J Am Acad Dermatol 2009;61:387–402, quiz 403–384.

Fine JD, Bruckner-Tuderman L, Eady RA, et al. Inherited epidermolysis bullosa: updated recommendations on diagnosis and classification. J Am Acad Dermatol 2014;70(6):1103–26.

Fine JD, Johnson LB, Weiner M, et al. Cause-specific risks of childhood death in inherited epidermolysis bullosa. J Pediatr 2008;152:276–80.

El Hachem M, Zambruno G, Bourdon-Lanoy E, et al. Multicentre consensus recommendations for skin care in inherited epidermolysis bullosa. Orphanet J Rare Dis 2014;9:76.

Cohn HI, Teng JM. Advancement in management of epidermolysis bullosa. Curr Opin Pediatr 2016 Aug;28(4):507–16. doi:10.1097/MOP.0000000000000380.

Uitto J, Bruckner-Tuderman L, McGrath JA, et al.. EB2017—progress in epidermolysis bullosa research toward treatment and cure. J Invest Dermatol 2018;138(5):1010–16. doi:10.1016/j.jid.2017.12.016.

Marathe K, Lu J, Morel KD. Bullous diseases: kids are not just little people. Clin Dermatol 2015 Nov-Dec;33(6):644–56. doi:10.1016/j.clindermatol.2015.09.007.

Sansaricq F, Stein SL, Petronic-Rosic V. Autoimmune bullous diseases in childhood. Clin Dermatol 2012;30(1):114–27.

Kasperkiewicz M, Schmidt E. Current treatment of autoimmune blistering diseases. Curr Drug Discov Technol 2009;6:270–80.

Hull CM, Liddle M, Hansen N, et al. Elevation of IgA anti-epidermal transglutaminase antibodies in dermatitis herpetiformis. Br J Dermatol 2008;159:120–4.

14 Bacterial, Mycobacterial, and Protozoal Infections of the Skin

The normal skin of healthy infants and children is resistant to invasion by most bacteria because the cutaneous surface provides a dry mechanical barrier from which contaminating organisms are constantly removed by desquamation. Under normal conditions the skin is sterile at delivery and for a short period thereafter. During the process of vaginal birth it acquires organisms from the birth canal, which gradually increase in number during the first 10 days of life. If the newborn is delivered by cesarean section, however, the cutaneous surface remains sterile until after delivery but soon becomes exposed to bacteria from human contactants and fomites.

Almost any organism may live on the cutaneous surface under appropriate conditions. A complete list of transient organisms accordingly would include virtually all microorganisms found in the human environment. The number of species composing the resident flora, however, is relatively small and consists predominantly of Gram-positive organisms and a few Gram-negative species, including *Cutibacterium acnes* (formerly *Propionibacterium acnes*, normally found in high concentrations around the pilosebaceous follicles of the face and less commonly the axillae and forearms), aerobic diphtheroids (*Corynebacterium minutissimum* and *Corynebacterium tenuis*), *Staphylococcus epidermidis*, micrococci, and anaerobic Gram-positive cocci. Others include Gram-negative bacilli (*Escherichia coli*, *Proteus*, *Enterobacter*, and *Pseudomonas*, among others), found uncommonly on normal skin except in the moist intertriginous areas of the groin, axillae, and toe webs, and *Staphylococcus aureus*, a common pathogen that appears to usually be seeded from the carrier state in the anterior nares.

Because the cutaneous surface is continuously exposed to microorganisms, it is most helpful to distinguish among transient, resident, and pathogenic flora. The transient flora consists of multiple organisms that are deposited on the skin from the environment, presumably do not proliferate, and are removed easily by washing or scrubbing of the affected area. The resident flora consists of a smaller number of organisms that are found more or less regularly in appreciable numbers on the skin of normal individuals, multiply on the skin, form stable communities on the cutaneous surface, and are not easily dislodged. Pathogenic bacteria, not ordinarily a regular part of this flora, persist on the skin if there is continuous replacement from some internal or external source or if the integrity of the skin is disrupted by injury or disease. It should be noted that the mere presence of potentially pathogenic bacteria in a cutaneous lesion does not necessarily prove the demonstrable organism to be a cause of bacterial infection.

Children have a more varied cutaneous flora than adults and often harbor soil bacteria on their skin. Prepubertal children lack sebum and accordingly have fewer diphtheroid organisms than adults. It is estimated that 10% to 30% of individuals are nasal carriers of *S. aureus* and that 70% to 90% are transient carriers.[1,2] Such coagulase-positive staphylococci are not considered part of the normal cutaneous flora of glabrous skin in adults, but are common transients acquired from carrier sites such as the anterior nares and perineum. In a 1-year study of 333 healthy preschool children ages 3 to 6 years, 34% of nasal swab samples yielded *S. aureus* from 185 (55%) carriers, and based on consecutive genotype analysis, 15% of the children were classified as persistent carriers (the remaining were considered to be intermittent carriers).[3] In newborns, the primary predictor of *S. aureus* (as well as group B streptococcus) carriage is maternal carriage of these organisms.[4,5]

The introduction of a vast array of antibiotics and chemotherapeutic agents has affected striking changes in the management of bacterial infections. With increased use of these agents, the focus of attention has shifted to identifying the specific bacterial cause and its antimicrobial sensitivity pattern, when feasible, permitting the appropriate choice of antibacterial agent(s). In purulent skin infections, it is relatively easy to obtain adequate specimens for examination and culture. With dry or crusted lesions, the yield will be greatest if the crust is gently lifted off and cultures are obtained from the moist underlying surface. In nonpurulent infections like erysipelas or cellulitis, past recommendations were for aspiration of the most active zone (not the surrounding area of erythema) with a 25-gauge needle attached to a syringe containing sterile saline without added preservatives. This procedure, unfortunately, has a very high false-negative rate, and often the clinician in this setting is forced to rely on clinical features or other diagnostic findings.

Bacterial Infections

IMPETIGO

Impetigo is a common, contagious superficial skin infection caused by streptococci, staphylococci, or both. Although seen in all age groups, the disease is most common in infants and children. Lesions may involve any body surface but occur most often on the exposed parts of the body, especially the face, hands, neck, and extremities.

There are two classic forms of impetigo: bullous and nonbullous (or crusted). Nonbullous impetigo accounts for more than 70% of cases.[6] It begins with a 1- to 2-mm erythematous papule or pustule that soon develops into a thin-roofed vesicle or bulla surrounded by a narrow rim of erythema. The vesicle ruptures easily with release of a thin, cloudy, yellow fluid that subsequently dries, forming a honey-colored crust, the hallmark of nonbullous impetigo (Fig. 14.1). The infection is easily spread by autoinoculation (Fig. 14.2) through fingers, towels,

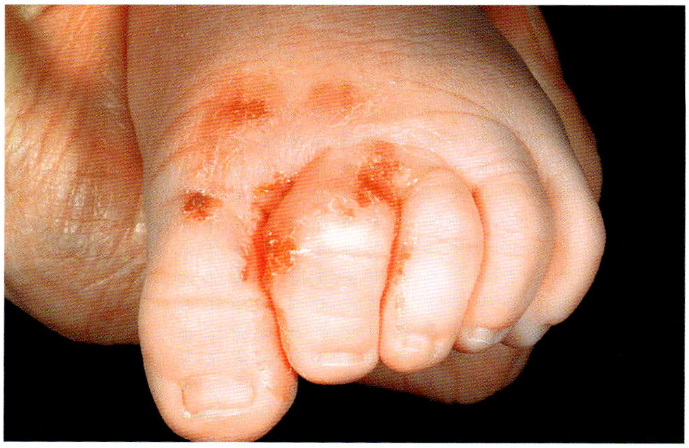

Fig. 14.1 Nonbullous (crusted) impetigo. Erythematous papules with honey yellow-colored crusting.

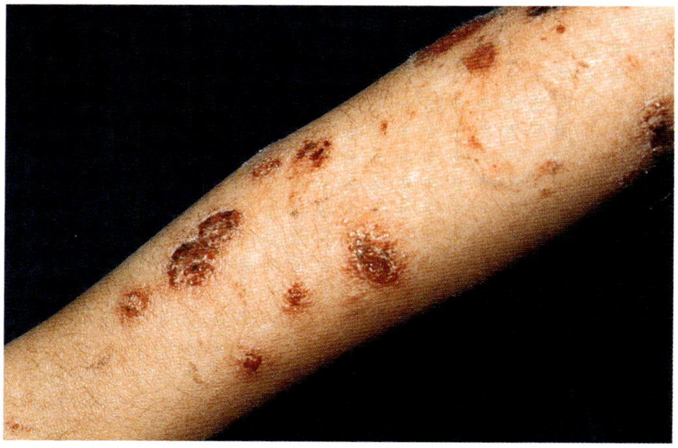

Fig. 14.2 Nonbullous (crusted) impetigo. These multiple lesions have spread as a result of autoinoculation.

or clothing, with resultant satellite lesions in either adjacent areas or other parts of the body. Individual lesions may extend peripherally with central clearing, resulting in annular or gyrate morphologies. Nonbullous impetigo historically was caused primarily by group A β-hemolytic streptococci (GABHS) but now is also most commonly caused by *S. aureus*, except for endemic tropical regions, where GABHS may still predominate.[6–8] Anaerobic organisms may also be recovered from lesions of nonbullous impetigo.[7]

Bullous impetigo, which is nearly always caused by *S. aureus*, presents as flaccid, thin-walled bullae or, more commonly, tender, shallow erosions surrounded by a remnant of the blister roof (Figs. 14.3 and 14.4). Common locations include the diaper region (Fig. 14.5), face, and extremities. Lesions of bullous impetigo can be thought of as a localized form of staphylococcal scalded skin syndrome (SSSS) (see Staphylococcal Scalded Skin Syndrome section), the characteristic lesions being the result of the same exfoliative toxin as implicated in that condition. Neonatal pustulosis (see Chapter 2), another condition favoring the diaper region and other fold areas in infants, is usually caused by *S. aureus* and presents with small pustules on an erythematous base that rupture easily upon swabbing.

Fever and regional lymphadenopathy may occur later in the course of impetigo but appear to be more common with the nonbullous type caused by GABHS. Potential complications of both bullous and nonbullous impetigo include sepsis, osteomyelitis, septic arthritis, lymphadenitis, and pneumonia.[6] Cutaneous streptococcal disease may be associated with guttate psoriasis, scarlet fever, and poststreptococcal glomerulonephritis when a nephritogenic strain of GABHS is implicated.

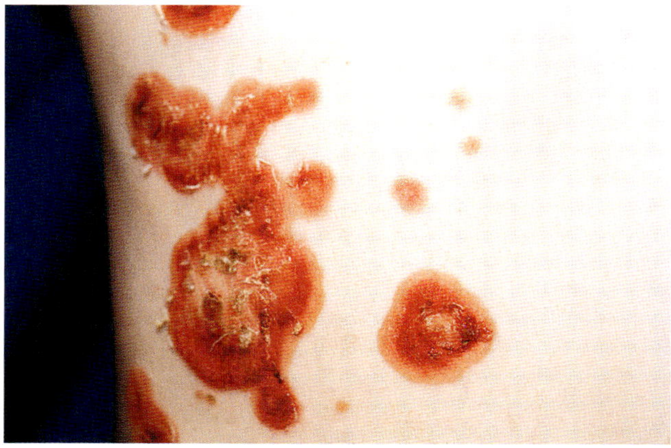

Fig. 14.3 Bullous impetigo. Multiple tender, erythematous patches with a peripheral collarette, representing remnants of the blister roof.

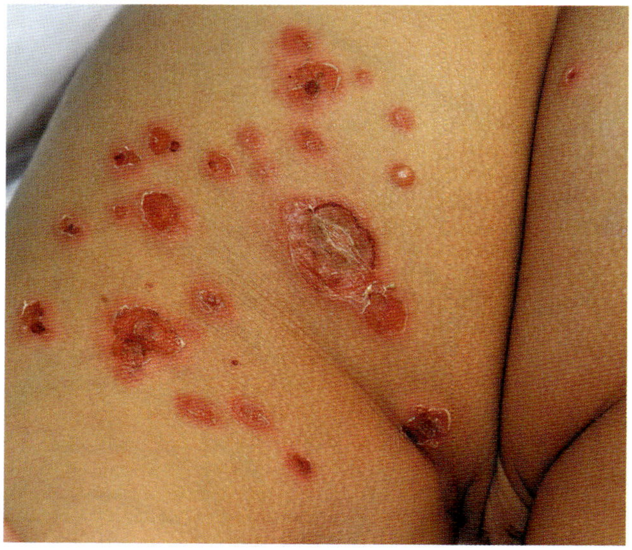

Fig. 14.4 Bullous impetigo. Thin-walled vesicles and shallow erosions with peripheral collarettes and mild crusting on the buttock and posterior thigh.

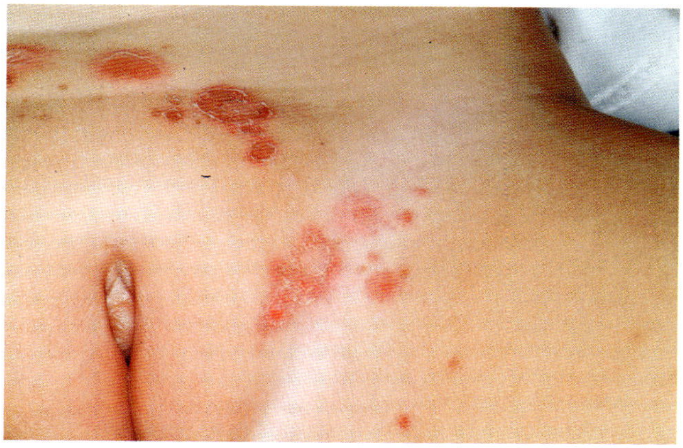

Fig. 14.5 Bullous impetigo. Inguinal and suprapubic involvement in an infant female. Lesions of bullous impetigo prefer this location in diapered infants.

An important reservoir for staphylococci is the upper respiratory tract of asymptomatic persons. Asymptomatic nasal carriage occurs in 20% to 40% of normal adults and up to 80% of patients with atopic dermatitis. The perineum is another common site of carriage, albeit not as common as the nares. These carriers spread the agent to the skin of infants and young children, probably with their hands. The reservoir for streptococci involved in skin infections appears to be skin lesions of other individuals, not the respiratory tract of affected or asymptomatic persons. Factors such as trauma and insect bites probably contribute to the pathogenesis of this infection.

Treatment for impetigo depends on the clinical presentation. Untreated, the disorder may last for 2 to 3 weeks with continuous spread and development of new lesions. In severe cases there may be large, crusted vegetations with deep extension and ulceration. Gentle cleansing, removal of crusts, and drainage of blisters and pustules may help prevent local spread of disease. If crusts are firmly adherent, warm soaks or compresses are useful.

Topical antibiotics may be useful in the treatment of mild, localized disease caused by *S. aureus*. With streptococcal or more severe staphylococcal infections, however, systemic antibiotics produce a swifter response and fewer failures. Bacitracin, polymyxin, gentamicin, and erythromycin are all effective topical agents and are relatively nonallergenic. Bacitracin, however, is a potential contact allergen, and this should be remembered in patients treated with this agent who develop worsening erythema and evidence of contact dermatitis.[9,10] In addition, treatment failures are common when bacitracin is used for impetigo.[11] Neomycin is another effective topical agent, although reports of contact allergy have traditionally appeared to be more common with this agent than with other topical antimicrobials (see Chapter 3). Mupirocin exerts a high level of bactericidal activity against a broad spectrum of Gram-positive organisms, including *S. aureus* and GABHS, and has little or no potential for irritation, side effects, or cross-reaction with other antibiotics. It is effective against methicillin-resistant *S. aureus* (MRSA), although some resistance to mupirocin has emerged in recent years, especially after prolonged use.[12–15] In a study of 249 children with documented *S. aureus* isolates on culture, 31% of all isolates were resistant to mupirocin; some factors that correlated with resistance included prior mupirocin use, MRSA, and atopic dermatitis.[16] Some studies have demonstrated equal or greater effectiveness of topical mupirocin over oral erythromycin in the treatment of impetigo in children.[17,18] Mupirocin is typically applied three times daily for 7 to 10 days.[19] Nasal carriage of *S. aureus* may be reduced with the use of intranasal mupirocin, which should be considered in known carriers with recurrent impetigo or in the setting of epidemic outbreaks. Retapamulin, a pleuromutilin-class topical antibiotic for the treatment of skin and skin-structure infections, has been demonstrated effective against both *S. aureus* and GABHS and is another treatment option for localized impetigo.[20,21] Retapamulin is also active against MRSA and many anaerobes, including *Propionibacterium* species, *Bacteroides* species, and *Clostridium* species.[19] The benefits of retapamulin include its lower propensity toward the development of resistance and twice-daily dosing.[22] Ozenoxacin is a novel topical quinolone cream for impetigo and has shown efficacy in both bullous and nonbullous types and against both *S. aureus* (including MRSA) and GABHS.[23,24]

Oral therapy for impetigo should be with an agent that covers both *S. aureus* and GABHS because distinguishing between these etiologies clinically is often not possible. In areas with a low prevalence of erythromycin-resistant *S. aureus*, erythromycin ethylsuccinate or erythromycin estolate are reasonable options. If known erythromycin resistance is present in the community, alternative oral agents with a good track record include a penicillinase-resistant penicillin (i.e., cloxacillin or dicloxacillin), amoxicillin plus clavulanic acid, a first-generation (i.e., cephalexin) or second-generation (i.e., cefprozil) cephalosporin, clindamycin, or in some cases, other macrolide antibiotics (i.e., clarithromycin or azithromycin). Oral therapy is used by most clinicians when the involvement is more widespread and/or severe.

In severe or recalcitrant cases, a skin swab for bacterial culture and sensitivity testing should be performed. The epidemiology of community-associated MRSA (CA-MRSA) (see later) infection must be considered in this setting, as highlighted by multiple observations of the increased prevalence of this pathogen. These patients often lack traditional risk factors for MRSA, and the isolates may be more susceptible to clindamycin and trimethoprim-sulfamethoxazole.[25,26]

A review of the National Ambulatory Medical Care Survey data on office visits for impetigo from 1997 to 2007 revealed that a majority of the 4 million patients were treated by nondermatologists (pediatricians, internists, emergency room and family physicians) and systemic antibiotics were the most commonly prescribed therapy, followed by topical antibiotics.[27] A Cochrane review found that topical mupirocin and topical fusidic acid (not available in the United States) were equally or more effective than oral treatment in the studies that met their inclusion criteria.[28] This highlights a potential opportunity for physician education, because increased utilization of topical therapy for patients with more limited impetigo could decrease the morbidity associated with oral antibiotic treatment, in line with the principles of antibiotic stewardship.

Lesions of impetigo caused by GABHS are shallow and usually heal well, and rheumatic fever does not occur after streptococcal skin infection. In contrast, acute glomerulonephritis and scarlet fever can occur after cutaneous streptococcal infection. As in the case of nephritis after streptococcal pharyngitis, only certain serologic types, different from those producing nephritis as a sequalae of streptococcal pharyngitis, appear to result in this complication of cutaneous infection.[20] This complication is uncommon except for certain epidemics resulting from nephritogenic strains of streptococci. Although systemic antibiotics help eliminate cutaneous streptococci, they do not appear to prevent glomerulonephritis caused by streptococcal impetigo. In general, however, with the changing bacteriology and the fact that staphylococci are a more common cause of both types of impetigo, concerns about postimpetigo glomerulonephritis have been greatly reduced.

METHICILLIN-RESISTANT *STAPHYLOCOCCUS AUREUS* INFECTIONS

The epidemiology of *S. aureus* skin and soft-tissue infections (SSTIs) has changed over recent decades, with an increasing prevalence of CA-MRSA infections observed in both the United States and elsewhere. Since the initial descriptions of children lacking predisposing risk factors with CA-MRSA infection in the late 1990s, marked increases in *S. aureus* isolates with this characteristic were observed, both in endemic and epidemic forms. By the middle of the first decade of the twenty-first century, up to 50% of community-associated *S. aureus* infections in many US centers were being identified as MRSA.[29] Increases in the number of children hospitalized with MRSA infections were also observed, but fortunately, the mortality rate for these children remained relatively low.[30] In recent years, the trend in *S. aureus* in adults has been a decline in the proportion caused by MRSA. One study reviewing *S. aureus* susceptibility data in pediatric patients over 2005–2014 suggested that a similar trend exists, with a decreasing proportion of MRSA infections (primarily SSTIs), although increased clindamycin resistance was documented.[31] Another study of *S. aureus* isolates in Chicago over 2006–2014 also suggested a decrease in the incidence of MRSA SSTI in both adults and children.[32] However, another review of invasive MRSA infections (defined as isolation of MRSA from a normally sterile body site) in children between 2005 and 2010 showed that these infections, which appear to predominate in young infants and black children, experienced an increase in incidence.[33] These data highlight the importance of considering regional trends and susceptibility patterns when deciding on empiric therapies (or awaiting testing results).

MRSA originated after the introduction of a mobile genetic element, staphylococcal chromosomal cassette (SCC) carrying the *mecA* gene, into strains of methicillin-sensitive *S. aureus* (MSSA). This gene encodes an altered penicillin-binding protein.[34] In distinction to hospital-associated MRSA, CA-MRSA is generally classified as such when there is no history of prior MRSA infection or colonization, when the positive culture was obtained in the outpatient setting or isolated within 48 hours of hospitalization, and when the patient lacks an exposure history (i.e., to a healthcare facility, chronic care facility, or indwelling catheter).[29,34] Molecular characteristics of the isolate are also useful in distinguishing the strains. Many CA-MRSA strains

Box 14.1 Clinical Associations with Community-Associated MRSA Infection

Skin/soft-tissue infections (SSTIs)	Pneumonia/empyema
Folliculitis	Lymphadenitis
Furuncles	Otitis media/externa
Carbuncles	Osteomyelitis
Impetigo	Thrombophlebitis
Pustulosis (neonates)	Septic arthritis
Cellulitis	Bacteremia
Abscesses	Pyelonephritis
Paronychia	Toxic shock syndrome
Staphylococcal scalded skin syndrome	Endocarditis
Necrotizing fasciitis/myositis	Epidural abscess

Modified from Miller LG, Kaplan SL. Staphylococcus aureus: A community pathogen. Infect Dis Clin N Am. 2009;23:35–52; Paintsil E. Pediatric community-acquired methicillin-resistant Staphylococcus aureus infection and colonization: Trends and management. Curr Opin Pediatr. 2007;19:75–82; Kirkland EB, Adams BB. Methicillin-resistant Staphylococcus aureus and athletes. J Am Acad Dermatol. 2008;59:494–502.
MRSA, Methicillin-resistant *S. aureus*.

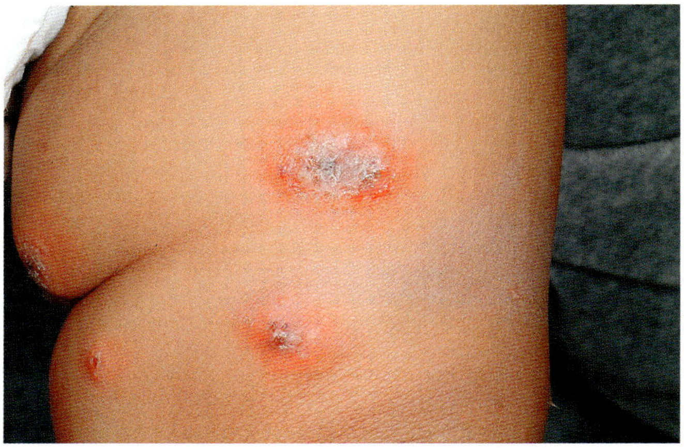

Fig. 14.6 Community-associated methicillin-resistant *Staphylococcus aureus* infection (CA-MRSA). This 1-year-old girl exhibited an acute onset of multiple tender, fluctuant nodules. Incision and drainage revealed exudate that grew MRSA.

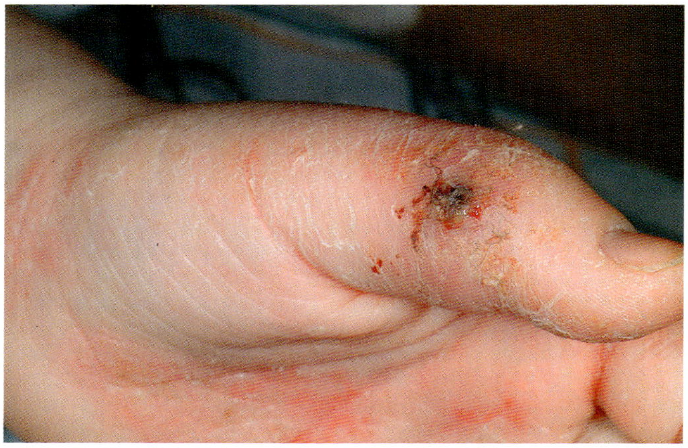

Fig. 14.7 Community-associated methicillin-resistant *Staphylococcus aureus* (CA-MRSA). This 6-year-old girl with a history of atopic dermatitis had an acute onset of a painful, fluctuant nodule over the thumb. Culture of the drainage revealed MRSA, and the infection cleared with an appropriate systemic antibiotic.

produce Panton–Valentine leukocidin (PVL), a toxin that kills neutrophils, although this toxin is also produced by some of the other more-sensitive strains of *S. aureus*.[35,36] The exact role of PVL in CA-MRSA infections remains controversial, although it appears to be increasingly associated with follicular infections (see Furuncles and Carbuncles section).

CA-MRSA infections seem to disproportionately affect children, young adults, and individuals from ethnic minority and low socioeconomic groups.[37] Spread is facilitated by crowding, skin-to-skin contact, skin compromise, and shared personal hygiene items. Cutaneous CA-MRSA infections are common in athletes, most notably collegiate football players.[38] The potential clinical manifestations associated with CA-MRSA infection are listed in Box 14.1. The constellation of disorders caused by infection with CA-MRSA have been grouped under the designation of SSTIs. Empiric outpatient therapy decisions for CA-MRSA infections should incorporate the type and site of infection, prevalence of the organism in the community, and local antibiotic susceptibility patterns.[37] Abscesses (including furuncles and carbuncles), which are collections of pus within the dermis and deeper skin layers, are a common manifestation of CA-MRSA infection (Figs. 14.6 and 14.7) and are most commonly located on the buttocks.[39] Incision and drainage of abscesses is often useful and sometimes sufficient as monotherapy for purulent uncomplicated infections. However, better studies are required to determine the role of antibiotics in treating abscesses that have been adequately drained.[40]

The most commonly utilized oral antibiotics in the United States are trimethoprim-sulfamethoxazole, clindamycin, doxycycline, linezolid, rifampin, and the fluoroquinolones. Fusidic acid is also utilized in the United Kingdom, Australia, and other countries.[41] Inducible clindamycin resistance has increased in recent years and should be considered when testing reveals clindamycin susceptibility and erythromycin resistance. In these instances, a "D test" should be performed and used to guide the choice of therapy. In a prospective randomized study of oral clindamycin versus oral trimethoprim-sulfamethoxazole for uncomplicated staphylococcal skin infections (77% of which were MRSA), the cure rate was similar in both groups.[42] Management of colonization has been attempted with intranasal mupirocin and skin disinfection (i.e., with chlorhexidine washes), with variable success.[43] Persistent colonization with MRSA in outpatients is associated with increased household colonization pressure (colonization of household contacts).[44] There is a high rate of recurrent colonization after clearance of MRSA SSTIs.[45] In addition, MRSA colonization and infection have been increasingly observed in companion animals, especially cats and dogs, and may serve as reservoirs for human infection.[46–48]

ECTHYMA

Ecthyma is a deep or ulcerative type of pyoderma commonly seen on the lower extremities and buttocks of children and is caused most often by GABHS. It may occur as small punched-out ulcers or a deep spreading ulcerative process. The disorder begins in the same manner as impetigo, often occurring after infected insect bites or minor trauma, but penetrates through the epidermis to produce a shallow ulcer. The initial lesion is a vesiculopustule with an erythematous base and firmly adherent crust. Removal of the crust reveals a lesion deeper than that seen in impetigo with an underlying saucer-shaped ulcer and raised margin (Fig. 14.8). The lesions are painful and heal slowly over a few weeks, often with scar formation. When multiple, lesions of ecthyma may be confused with child abuse related to cigarette burns. *S. aureus* (including MRSA) may occasionally be cultured from the lesions, and epidemic outbreaks have been reported, occasionally in association with poststreptococcal glomerulonephritis or other systemic sequelae.[49,50] Treatment consists of warm compresses and the appropriate systemic antibiotic.

Ecthyma gangrenosum is a cutaneous finding that may be seen in patients with *Pseudomonas aeruginosa* bacteremia. Most of the affected individuals have an underlying immunodeficiency (either congenital or acquired) or a history of cancer chemotherapy. There are reports of ecthyma gangrenosum in apparently healthy, immunocompetent children (often with diaper-area involvement), but the diagnosis should prompt a thorough investigation for occult immunodeficiency.[51,52] Neutropenia may be a risk factor for ecthyma gangrenosum. The characteristic lesions are hemorrhagic papules with a pink

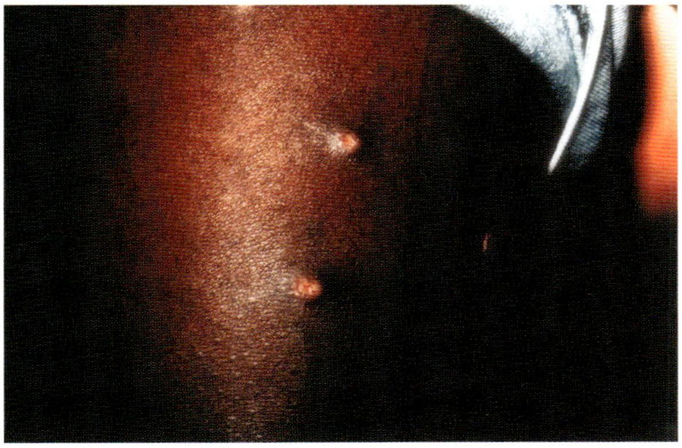

Fig. 14.8 Ecthyma. Well-demarcated, punched-out ulcers on the thigh of this 10-year-old boy.

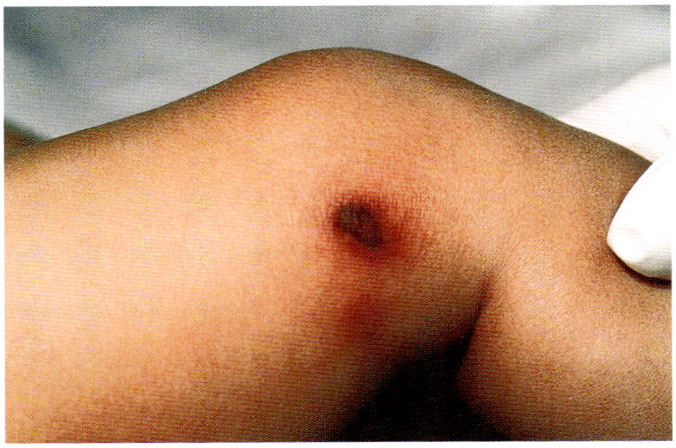

Fig. 14.9 Ecthyma gangrenosum. These hemorrhagic, necrotic skin lesions were accompanied by *Pseudomonas aeruginosa* bacteremia in this immunosuppressed child being treated with chemotherapy.

or violaceous rim (Fig. 14.9) that progress to bullae, ulcers, and necrotic plaques. Eschar formation eventually occurs (Fig. 14.10), and old lesions heal with scarring. The diagnosis can be confirmed by Gram stain and bacterial culture of lesions or blood cultures, which are positive for *P. aeruginosa*. Treatment with appropriate antipseudomonal therapy (i.e., aminoglycoside and an antipseudomonal penicillin) should be instituted early.

FOLLICULITIS

The term *folliculitis* refers to an infection of hair follicles. The clinical appearance varies according to the location and depth of follicular involvement. Deeper follicular infections (furuncles and carbuncles) are discussed later. Superficial folliculitis (Bockhart impetigo), an infection of the follicular ostium, begins with superficial small, yellow-white pustules, often with a narrow red areola (Fig. 14.11) and a hair shaft protruding from the center of the lesion. It occurs most commonly in children and usually is seen on the buttocks (Fig. 14.12) and extremities, especially the thighs. Most lesions are painless, occur in crops, and heal over 7 to 10 days with postinflammatory hyperpigmentation. *S. aureus* is by far the most common pathogen; other possible etiologies include streptococci, Gram-negative organisms, and even dermatophytes. In immunocompromised children, commensal organisms may cause folliculitis, including *Pityrosporum* and *Demodex* (see Chapter 18). Superficial folliculitis is not always infectious in origin. "Sterile folliculitis" may be seen after skin contact with oil or other occlusive products and results in follicular plugging and inflammation. A classic example of sterile folliculitis is the scalp pustulosis occasionally associated with application of hair oils.

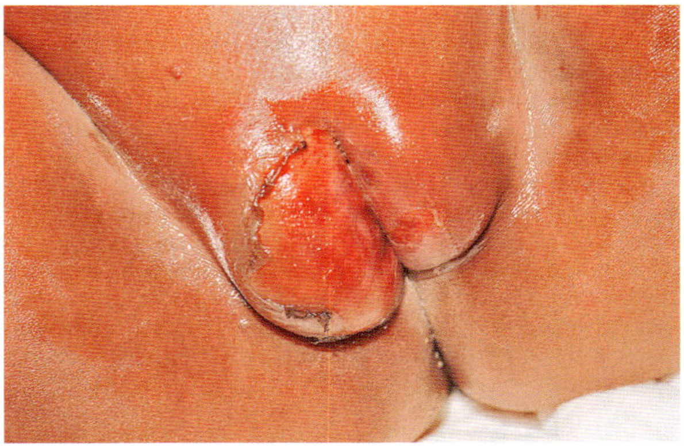

Fig. 14.10 Ecthyma gangrenosum. This child with congenital immunodeficiency developed thick eschars, which required a diverting colostomy and eventual skin grafting.

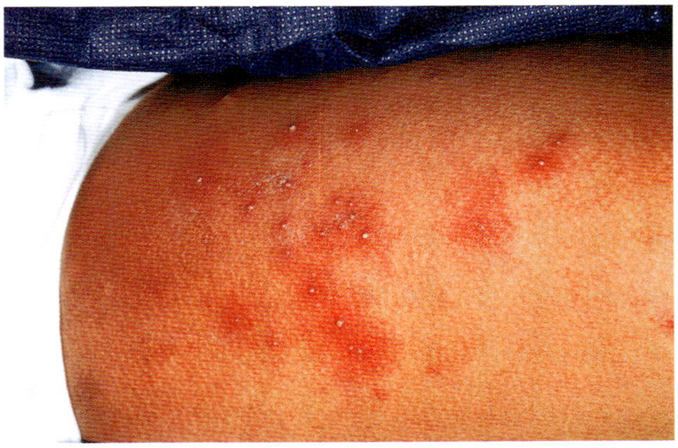

Fig. 14.11 Bacterial folliculitis. Erythematous, follicular papulopustules.

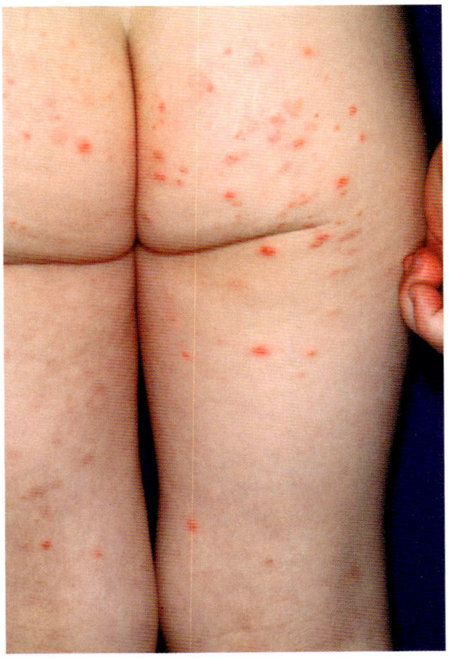

Fig. 14.12 Bacterial folliculitis. Erythematous follicular papules and papulopustules on the buttocks and posterior thighs of a young boy. This is the most common location for bacterial folliculitis in children.

Superficial folliculitis usually responds to gentle cleansing with antibacterial soaps and the application of topical antibiotics such as clindamycin, erythromycin, or mupirocin. More extensive or resistant cases should be treated with a systemic antibiotic (a penicillinase-resistant penicillin or cephalosporin, depending on local resistance patterns). In such instances, bacterial culture should be obtained before the initiation of systemic therapy. Sodium hypochlorite (bleach) baths or washes on a twice- to three-times weekly basis may be useful for individuals or families with recurrent folliculitis or furunculosis (see later), although some newer data suggest that this nonirritating concentration may not truly be antibacterial. The typical recommended concentration for bleach baths is ¼ to ½ cup of bleach (around 5% to 6% sodium hypochlorite) dissolved in a full bathtub (around 40 gallons) of water.

Folliculitis Barbae

Folliculitis barbae (sycosis barbae) is a term used to describe a deep-seated folliculitis of the beard area involving the entire depth of the follicle and perifollicular region (Fig. 14.13). A pruritic papule is usually the initial lesion, with the process spreading from one follicle to another by trauma from scratching and/or shaving. The disorder is characterized by follicular papules and pustules and with progression, erythema, crusting, and boggy infiltration of the skin. Although occasionally other bacteria may be isolated, the etiology is usually *S. aureus*. The use of an electric rather than traditional razor or complete avoidance of shaving can sometimes be helpful in prevention and treatment of this condition. Warm compresses and topical antibiotics are often sufficient to control minor forms of sycosis barbae. If the condition is severe or recurrent, several weeks of systemic antibiotics may be necessary.

Pseudofolliculitis Barbae

Pseudofolliculitis barbae (PFB) (see Chapter 7) is a common, noninfectious inflammatory disorder of the pilosebaceous follicles of the beard that may be confused with sycosis barbae. PFB (commonly referred to as *razor bumps*) is caused by shaved hairs that curve inward with resultant penetration of the skin, followed by an inflammatory foreign body reaction. This form of folliculitis is seen particularly in Blacks and other populations (i.e., Hispanic, Middle Eastern) with tight curly hair. The incidence in Black men is estimated to be as high as 40% to 80%.[53] PFB presents with follicular, erythematous to hyperpigmented papules in regions where recurrent shaving occurs, most commonly the neck and cheeks. Mild cases may be managed by careful shaving hygiene and occasionally by changing from a traditional to an electric razor. The traditional recommendation for discontinuation or minimizing the frequency of shaving, which was touted to be effective but which is not always acceptable to the patient, has more recently been questioned. Some now recommend daily shaving with "light strokes," use of a preshave skin preparation regimen with a gentle cleanser, liberal use of shaving foam/gel, use of an advanced multiblade razor, and use of an after-shave product containing moisturizing ingredients.[54] Other treatment options include chemical depilatory or eflornithine cream (in an effort to decrease shaving necessity), topical retinoids or glycolic acid, topical steroids, benzoyl peroxide, and topical (and less commonly oral) antibiotics.[55] Epilation laser therapy (see Chapter 7) has been demonstrated to be effective for the condition,[56,57] and other procedural options include surgical depilation, chemical peels, laser therapy, photodynamic therapy, and punch excision.[53,58]

Pseudomonal Folliculitis (Hot Tub Folliculitis)

Pseudomonal folliculitis is a form of folliculitis caused by *P. aeruginosa* that occurs after exposure to poorly chlorinated hot tubs, whirlpools, or swimming pools. It has also been reported in association with a contaminated water slide,[59] a contaminated loofah sponge,[60] swimming in a children's pool filled with well water,[61] after exposure to household rubber gloves used for cleaning,[62] and after shower or bath exposure.[63,64] It is characterized by erythematous, follicular pustules and vesiculopustules that occur most often on the trunk, buttocks, and legs (Fig. 14.14), especially in sites occluded by swimming garments. Lesions usually develop within 1 to 2 days after exposure. Mild constitutional symptoms may be present, including fever, malaise, headache, and arthralgias. More serious associations, including urinary tract infection and pneumonia, have also been reported.[65,66] Lesions of hot tub folliculitis generally subside spontaneously over 7 to 10 days. Antipseudomonal antibiotic therapy (i.e., with ciprofloxacin) may be necessary in severe cases. Preventive measures include maintenance of appropriate chlorination, frequent water changes, and thorough scrubbing of whirlpool baths and hot tubs with each water change. Importantly, 21% of 108 water and swab samples of hot tubs and indoor swimming pools were positive for *P. aeruginosa* in one study, and 96% of these isolates were multidrug resistant.[67] The Centers for Disease Control and Prevention recommend maintaining the concentration of free chlorine in swimming pools to between 1 and 3 parts per million (ppm) and the pH at 7.2 to 7.8.[68]

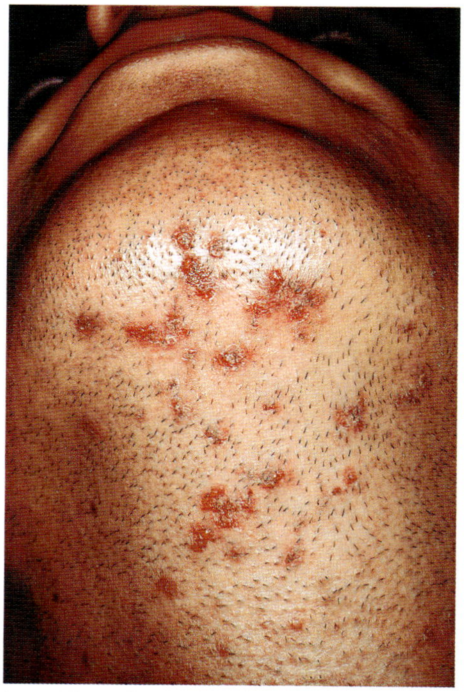

Fig. 14.13 Folliculitis barbae. Follicular papules, pustules, and crusting with autoinoculation caused by shaving.

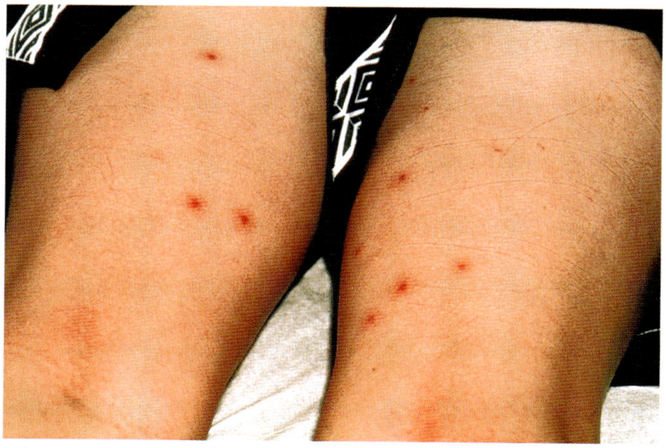

Fig. 14.14 Pseudomonal (hot tub) folliculitis. Erythematous, follicular papules and papulopustules of the thighs, correlating with areas covered by the swim garment.

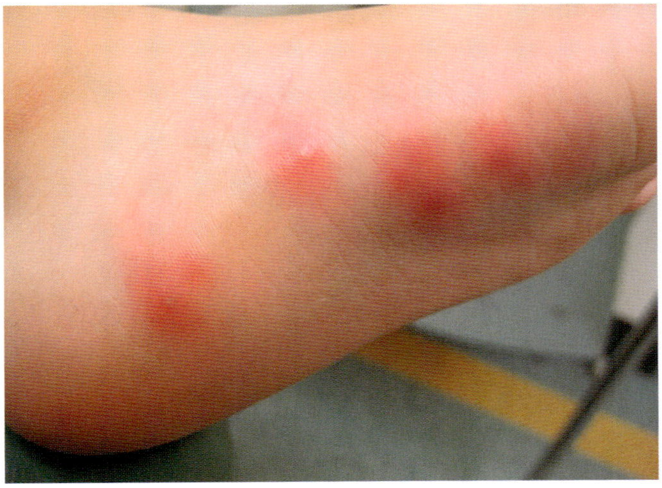

Fig. 14.15 *Pseudomonas* hot foot syndrome. Tender papules and papulopustules on the plantar foot. Culture of a swab from one of the pustules grew out *P. aeruginosa*. (Courtesy John J. Van Aalst, MD.)

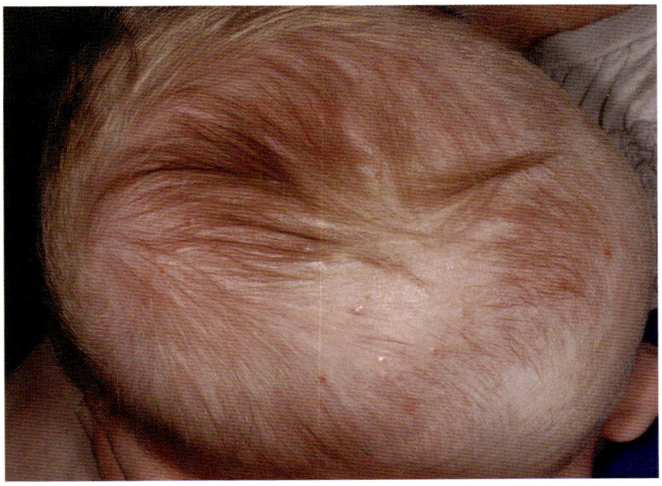

Fig. 14.16 Eosinophilic folliculitis of infancy. This 8-week-old girl had recurrent, pruritic, follicular papules and papulopustules on the scalp in conjunction with a peripheral eosinophilia. She was ultimately diagnosed with hyper-IgE syndrome.

Hot hand–foot syndrome (also known as *Pseudomonas hot foot syndrome*) presents with painful, erythematous palmoplantar nodules (Fig. 14.15) after exposure to water containing a high concentration of *P. aeruginosa* and may be seen in conjunction with hot tub folliculitis.[69,70] When pustules are present, the organism can be easily cultured from skin swab material. An epidemic occurred in children exposed to the same community wading pool with a floor that was coated with abrasive grit and which, along with the inlets and a drain, yielded *P. aeruginosa* on culture.[71] This disorder may be related to (or the same condition as) idiopathic palmoplantar hidradenitis of childhood (see Chapter 20). Similar palmoplantar inflammatory lesions have been reported in otherwise healthy children infected with *Mycobacterium abscessus*, also in association with exposure to public swimming pools (see Nontuberculous ["Atypical"] Mycobacterial Infections section).

Eosinophilic Pustular Folliculitis/Eosinophilic Folliculitis of Infancy

Eosinophilic pustular folliculitis (EPF; Ofuji disease) is a dermatosis of unknown cause characterized by erythematous patches with follicular papules and pustules, often in an annular or serpiginous arrangement, with occasional peripheral eosinophilia and leukocytosis. It was classically reported in Japanese individuals, although it may be seen in people of diverse ethnic backgrounds, and men appear to be affected more than women.[72] Although this disorder is not bacterial in origin, it is included here because it is in the differential diagnosis of folliculitis. EPF may involve any surface area, including the face, trunk, and extremities. A form of EPF is recognized as an extremely pruritic dermatosis in adult patients with human immunodeficiency virus (HIV) infection, usually presenting late in the course of infection.[73]

A distinct form of EPF occurs in otherwise healthy infants and toddlers and has been called *eosinophilic folliculitis of infancy*. It presents with recurrent crops of itchy follicular pustules of the scalp (most commonly; Fig. 14.16), trunk, and extremities with eventual spontaneous involution (see Chapter 2). The outbreaks occur in a cyclical fashion and may last from 3 months to 5 years, occasionally longer. Peripheral eosinophilia may be present.[74] Whereas adults tend to have annular, serpiginous, or polycyclic lesions, the prominent scalp involvement and failure to form annular rings appear to distinguish the infantile form. Occasionally, eosinophilic folliculitis of infancy may be a presenting feature of the hyperimmunoglobulin-E (hyper-IgE) syndrome (see Chapter 3).[75]

Treatment options for EPF include topical corticosteroids, antihistamines, oral erythromycin, dapsone, indomethacin, colchicine, topical tacrolimus, and ultraviolet B (UVB) phototherapy, which have each been used with variable success. The majority of patients respond to treatment with the former two agents; in one study of 51 patients treated with low- to medium-potency topical steroids, 46 (90%) responded well.[76] The other treatments have been demonstrated successful but carry a greater risk of adverse effects.

FURUNCLES AND CARBUNCLES

Furuncles (or "boils") are painful, deep infections of the hair follicle in which purulent material extends into the dermis and subcutaneous tissues, forming perifollicular abscesses (see earlier). These lesions have a tendency toward central necrosis and suppuration. They are caused by *S. aureus* and are seen most often in older children and adults. They usually develop from a preceding folliculitis with deeper extension into the dermis and subcutaneous tissue. Chronic carriers of *S. aureus* are particularly predisposed,[77] and familial spread of PVL-producing MSSA isolates has been observed and may be associated with greater numbers and more intensely erythematous lesions.[78] Furuncles caused by CA-MRSA infection have increased in incidence in the United States and are strongly related to production of the PVL virulence factor.[79] Furuncles are most common in areas of skin that are hairy and subject to friction and maceration, particularly the back, axillae, thighs, buttocks, and perineum. They present as tender, red nodules (Fig. 14.17) that gradually become fluctuant and, if untreated, may have a purulent blood-tinged discharge. There is a high rate of contagion in patients with furunculosis.

Carbuncles are larger, deep-seated staphylococcal abscesses composed of aggregates of interconnected furuncles that drain at multiple points on the cutaneous surface (Fig. 14.18). They are usually seen in males on the posterior neck, back, thighs, and buttocks and extend into the deeper dermis and subcutaneous tissues, reaching a larger size than furuncles (up to 10 cm in diameter). They undergo necrosis and suppuration more slowly than furuncles and may present with severe pain and constitutional symptoms. Several factors predispose to the development of furuncles and carbuncles (Box 14.2).

The treatment of furuncles and carbuncles depends on the extent and location of lesions. The mainstay of therapy is systemic antistaphylococcal antibiotics with incision and drainage of fluctuant lesions. Cultures with sensitivity testing should be considered, especially in geographic areas with an increasing prevalence of staphylococcal resistance. Lesions caused by MRSA may respond (as discussed) to incision and drainage alone. Topical antibiotics (as discussed for impetigo and folliculitis) are not sufficient for the treatment of furuncles and carbuncles, given the depth of the process. The triple regimen of chlorhexidine skin disinfection (21 days), mupirocin applied to the nares (5 days), and oral clindamycin (21 days) was found to be very

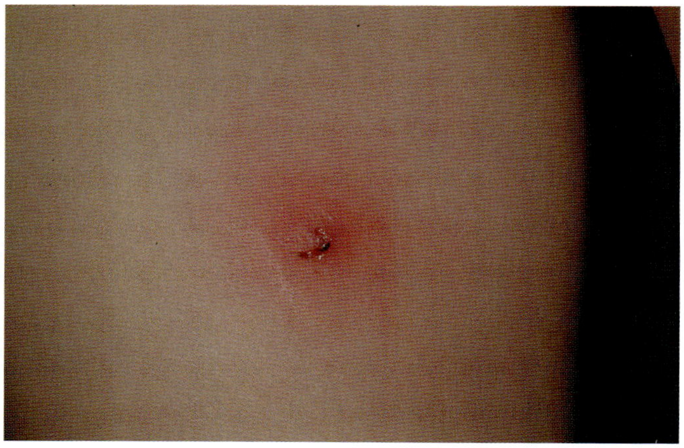

Fig. 14.17 Furuncle. This tender, fluctuant papulonodule was located on the thigh in a patient who also had folliculitis on the buttocks.

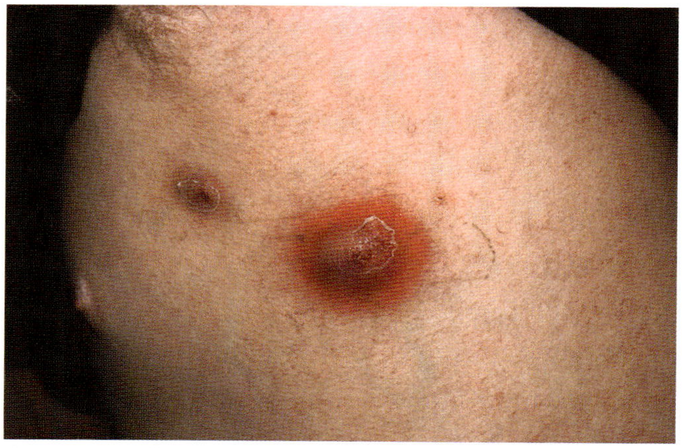

Fig. 14.18 Carbuncle. Large, tender, erythematous nodule on the lateral trunk of this 14-year-old overweight male patient. Note the adjacent, smaller furuncle.

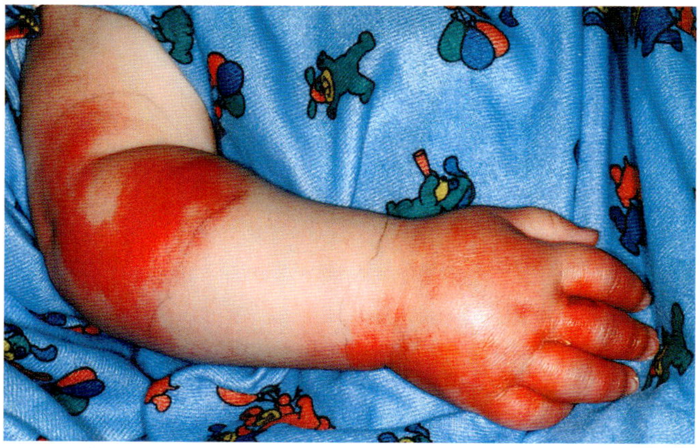

Fig. 14.19 Cellulitis. Erythematous patches and plaques with edema involving the arm of this 18-month-old male patient. Note the multifocal nature and partial clearing as a result of parenteral antibiotic therapy.

Box 14.2 Predisposing Factors for Furuncles and Carbuncles

- Physical contact with other infected individuals
- Family history of furuncles/carbuncles
- Diabetes mellitus
- Obesity
- Alcoholism
- Scabies
- Hematologic disorders, including anemia
- Immunodeficiencies, including hyper-IgE syndrome
- Malnutrition
- Chemotherapy
- Corticosteroid therapy
- Local skin trauma (abrasions, cuts, excoriations)
- Atopic dermatitis
- Debilitated state

effective with a prolonged remission in nearly 90% of patients in an open-label study that included patients with both MSSA and MRSA furunculosis.[80] Many practitioners recommend dilute sodium hypochlorite baths or washes for patients with recurrent disease (see Folliculitis section).[81] Lastly, attention to predisposing factors with appropriate treatment or modification (as feasible) is indicated.

CELLULITIS

Cellulitis is an acute infection of the skin, particularly the subcutaneous tissues, characterized by poorly demarcated erythema, warmth, swelling, and tenderness. The borders of cellulitis are not elevated or sharply defined, which helps contrast it from the more superficial form called *erysipelas* (see Erysipelas section). Cellulitis is a common public health burden, with hospitalization frequently undertaken.[82]

Cellulitis is a dermal and subcutaneous infection that usually occurs after some form of skin trauma, including puncture wounds, lacerations, dermatitis, burns, varicella, or dermatophyte infections. It presents with markedly red, tender, warm swelling of the skin with an infiltrated appearance (Fig. 14.19), and the most common location is the lower extremities. Constitutional symptoms, including malaise and fever, are often present. The most common causes of cellulitis are *S. aureus* and GABHS, although occasionally other bacterial agents may be implicated. MRSA appears to be a rare cause of nonsuppurative cellulitis when extrapolated from staphylococcal patient-colonization data, although colonization may not be a primary risk factor in the pathogenesis of this infection.[83] In young children, particularly those under 2 years of age, *Haemophilus influenzae* type b (Hib) was traditionally implicated in a facial cellulitis termed *buccal cellulitis*, although this form is now less common since licensure of the conjugated Hib vaccine.[84] Buccal cellulitis characteristically reveals a dusky red to blue discoloration of the involved skin. Children with *H. influenzae* cellulitis may be quite toxic, with accompanying upper respiratory tract symptoms and bacteremia or septicemia. *Streptococcus pneumoniae* is another potential etiology of facial cellulitis in children, occurring especially in those under 36 months of age who are at risk for pneumococcal bacteremia. Because 96% of the serotypes (in one large series of *S. pneumoniae* facial cellulitis) are included in the 13-valent pneumococcal conjugate vaccine (PCV13) recommended for routine vaccination in infants 2 months of age and older (as well as the prior heptavalent conjugated vaccine), this cause of cellulitis is becoming less relevant.[85,86] Lastly, in children younger than 3 months of age, cellulitis is most commonly caused by group B streptococci (GBS) and is more likely to be associated with invasive disease, including bacteremia and meningitis.[87] These children require blood, urine, and cerebrospinal fluid (CSF) sampling and cultures as part of their initial evaluation.

Periorbital cellulitis is a unique form of cellulitis that deserves special mention here, given the potential confusion with orbital cellulitis and the associated complications. Periorbital (preseptal) cellulitis is a form of the disease that presents with erythema and swelling of the periorbital tissues. It may appear after skin trauma, in which case it is usually caused by *S. aureus* or GABHS infection, or may result from cutaneous spread of pathogens from the paranasal sinuses or bloodstream, where it may result from Hib or *S. pneumoniae* infection. If the infection traverses the orbital septum (a continuation of the periosteum of the bony orbit to the margins of the upper and lower eyelids), it may result in *orbital cellulitis*, a more serious condition that may be complicated by abscess formation or cavernous sinus thrombosis.[88]

Patients with orbital cellulitis may experience proptosis, ophthalmoplegia, and decreased visual acuity in addition to the cutaneous findings. Computed tomography (CT) and ophthalmologic examinations are indicated if orbital cellulitis is suspected. The microbiology of periorbital and orbital cellulitis has also changed with the advent of Hib immunization, and Hib is now an uncommon cause of these disorders, being supplanted by streptococcal species (including *S. pneumoniae* and GABHS) and *S. aureus*.[89–91] In a retrospective study of 85 children with periorbital or orbital cellulitis, the majority of isolates were MRSA, 85% of which were PVL positive.[92] However, a retrospective review of 101 children in Canada diagnosed with orbital cellulitis revealed that of the 30 patients who required surgical drainage, 4 (13.3%) grew *H. influenza* from abscess fluid, highlighting that this pathogen still remains an occasional cause of this infection.[93]

Treatment of cellulitis depends on the clinical presentation and knowledge (and identification, when possible) of the affecting organisms. The diagnosis of cellulitis is generally a clinical one, although fine-needle aspiration with Gram stain and bacterial culture may be helpful when unusual organisms are suspected (i.e., the immunocompromised host).[77] Knowing the epidemiology of various etiologic agents in specific presentations and age groups is important in initiating appropriate therapy, as skin surface swab cultures may be misleading and blood cultures are usually negative (less than 8% in one large systematic review).[82,94] Antibiotic therapy that covers GABHS and *S. aureus* will be appropriate in most cases of routine, nonfacial cellulitis. Typical options for nonpurulent cellulitis (more likely to be caused by GABHS) include cephalexin, dicloxacillin, penicillin VK, amoxicillin/clavulanate, and clindamycin.[82,95] For patients with purulent cellulitis (more likely to be caused by *S. aureus*), empiric treatment options include cephalexin, dicloxacillin, amoxicillin/clavulanate, trimethoprim-sulfamethoxazole, doxycycline, and clindamycin.[82,96] In geographic areas with high rates of CA-MRSA, antibiotic selection should include coverage against this organism. There is no consensus on the choice between oral and intravenous antibiotics, although blood cultures, intravenous antibiotics, and hospitalization have traditionally been recommended for children at high risk for cellulitis complications (i.e., immunocompromised), and it is recommended that patients with systemic signs of infection (temperature $>38°$ C, tachycardia, tachypnea, or abnormal white blood cell count with $>12{,}000$ or $<4{,}000$ cells/μL) be treated parenterally.[82,95] Short-course intravenous antibiotic therapy has been used in emergency department (ED) settings but may be associated with a higher failure rate and longer ED stay.[97]

In children with facial or periorbital cellulitis, the possibility of *S. pneumoniae* and Hib infection should be considered in conjunction with the patient's age and immunization status, and antibiotics should be chosen accordingly. Imaging (most often contrast-enhanced CT or diffusion-weighted magnetic resonance imaging [MRI]) is recommended in these patients to define the extent of involvement and help guide appropriate therapy.[98] In infants younger than 3 months of age with cellulitis, GBS should be presumed as a potential etiologic agent, and in these infants, as well as the patient with periorbital or orbital cellulitis who is young, toxic, or shows signs of meningeal irritation, laboratory evaluation for sepsis and meningitis should be performed. Hospitalization with parenteral antibiotic therapy (and ophthalmologic consultation in those with orbital cellulitis) is indicated in these latter settings.

ERYSIPELAS

Erysipelas is a superficial cellulitis of the skin with marked lymphatic involvement, resulting in most cases from GABHS. The organism usually gains access by direct inoculation through a break in the skin, but occasionally hematogenous infection may occur. The initial lesion begins as a small area of erythema that gradually enlarges to reveal a characteristic warm, painful, shiny, bright red infiltrated plaque with a distinct and well-marginated border. The face, scalp, and hands are the most common sites of involvement, although erysipelas may involve any skin surface. Penicillin, or a macrolide antibiotic in patients with penicillin allergy, is the drug of choice for therapy. In occasional patients, *S. aureus* may be a co-pathogen, in which case antimicrobial therapy directed against this organism is necessary. Erysipelas-like erythema may occasionally be the presenting sign of familial Mediterranean fever (see Chapter 25).[99]

PERIANAL STREPTOCOCCAL DERMATITIS

Perianal streptococcal dermatitis (PSD, also known as *perianal dermatitis, perianal cellulitis, perianal streptococcal cellulitis,* and *streptococcal perianal disease*) is a well-defined entity that may be often overlooked. It presents as sharply circumscribed perianal erythema with occasional fissures, purulent discharge, and/or functional disturbances.[100] GABHS is the etiology in most cases of PSD, although *S. aureus* and coliform bacteria have also been recovered.[101,102] An epidemic outbreak in a daycare center has been reported.[103] In one series of 26 patients with perianal dermatitis, *S. aureus* was the most common isolate and clinically was notable for concurrent papules and pustules on the buttocks and extension of the erythema to the adjacent buttock skin.[104]

The skin findings in PSD are variable, from a dry pink appearance to bright red erythema (Fig. 14.20) with a wet surface and occasionally the presence of a white pseudomembrane.[105] The surface is often tender to touch, and associated symptoms include rectal itching or discomfort, painful defecation, blood-streaked stools, and constipation. In males, balanoposthitis (Fig. 14.21) or in females, vulvovaginitis may be present.[106] Fever is notoriously rare in patients with PSD. Streptococcal pharyngitis may concomitantly be present in patients

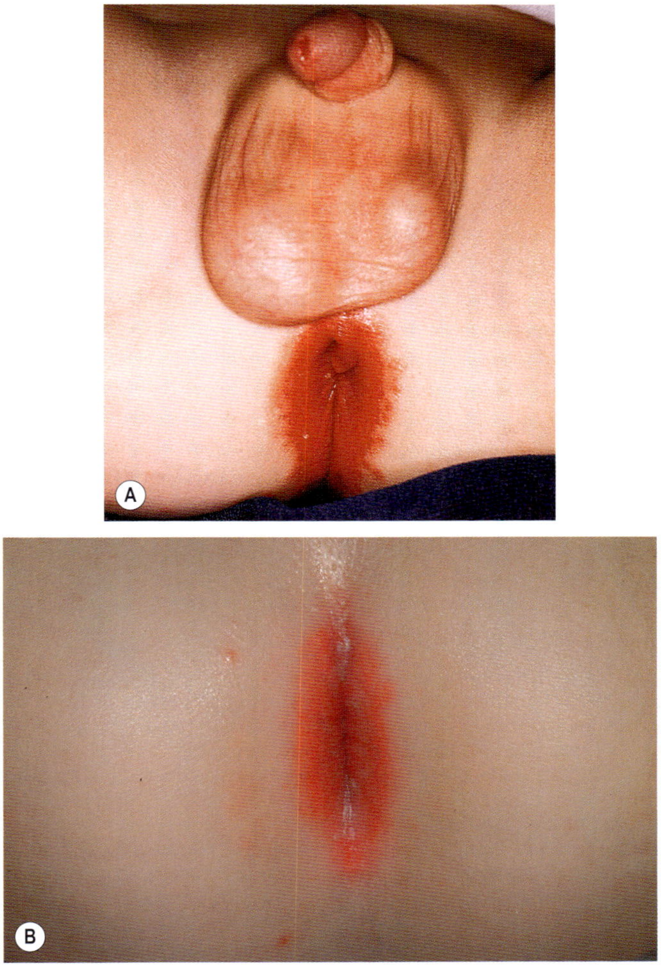

Fig. 14.20 Perianal streptococcal dermatitis. Bright red erythema with a moist, tender surface **(A)** and pink maceration with mild exudate or pseudomembrane **(B)**. Both patients were tender to palpation and had painful defecation.

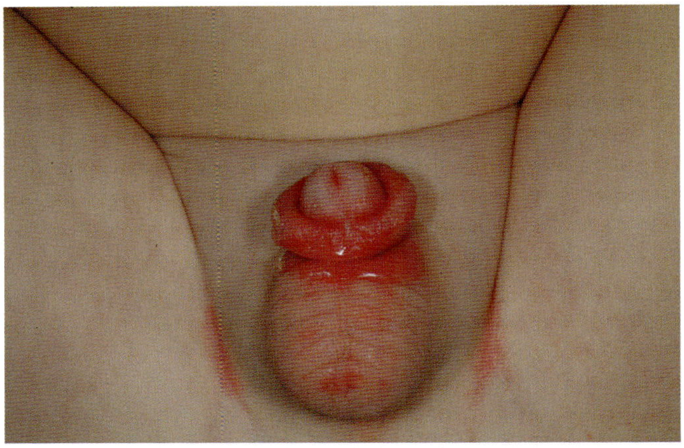

Fig. 14.21 Balanoposthitis. Inflammation and edema of the foreskin and glans penis (balanoposthitis) along with erosive intertrigo of the scrotum/penile shaft occurred in this infant male, who also had classic perianal streptococcal dermatitis.

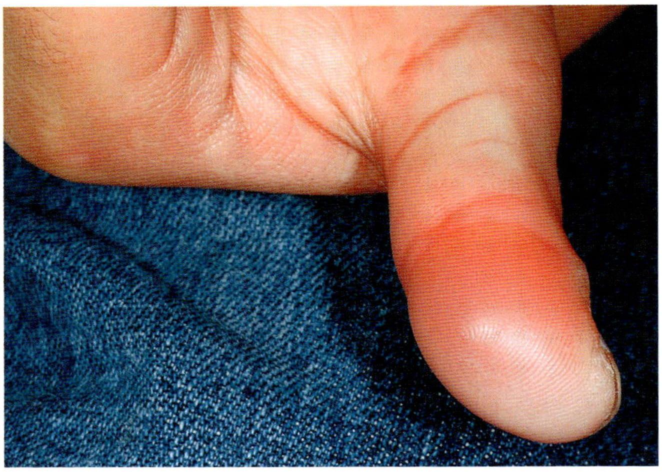

Fig. 14.22 Blistering dactylitis. Edema and a tense bulla on the thumb of this 7-year-old girl. Culture of the blister fluid yielded *Staphylococcus aureus* rather than the more commonly seen group A β-hemolytic streptococci.

with PSD, but the exact associations between pharyngitis, PSD, and streptococcal colonization is unclear.[105] There is some suggestion that specific GABHS isolates may have a tropism for perineal tissues, but the mechanism of infection is not yet clear.[106] Guttate psoriasis (see Chapter 4), which is classically associated with streptococcal pharyngitis, may also be associated with PSD, and in any patient with new-onset guttate psoriasis, a thorough anogenital examination should be performed. Pediatric autoimmune neuropsychiatric disorder associated with streptococcal infection (PANDAS)–like presentation has been suggested as potentially linked to PSD in some children.[107]

The differential diagnosis of PSD is broad and includes psoriasis, candidiasis, seborrheic dermatitis, cutaneous Crohn's disease, pinworm infestation, and sexual abuse. The diagnosis can be confirmed by bacterial culture of a perianal swab, but when performing cultures to confirm the diagnosis of PSD, it is important to notify the laboratory of the microbe (GABHS) in question, because several labs utilize media selective for enteric pathogens with rectal swabs. Treatment with oral penicillin V, amoxicillin, a first-generation cephalosporin, or a macrolide or azalide (i.e., erythromycin, clarithromycin, or azithromycin) for patients allergic to penicillin is usually effective, with or without concomitant topical mupirocin. Some have suggested, however, that the risk of clinical recurrence is greater in patients treated initially with penicillin or amoxicillin.[108] Oral cefuroxime was demonstrated to be more effective than penicillin in one study and is another reasonable option.[109] If staphylococcal infection seems more probable clinically or is isolated in culture, the antibiotic regimen should be adjusted accordingly.

BLISTERING DACTYLITIS

Blistering dactylitis (also known as *blistering distal dactylitis*) is a unique bullous manifestation of GABHS infection or, occasionally, other bacteria, including *S. aureus* and GBS.[110–112] It is rarely reported in association with MRSA infection.[113] In its classic form, blistering dactylitis presents as a painful, tense, superficial blister on an erythematous base (Fig. 14.22), most often located over the volar fat pad of the distal phalanx of a finger or several fingers. It is most common in children between the ages of 2 and 16 years, although it is also reported in adults, most notably immunocompromised ones. The blisters may occasionally extend to involve the dorsal surfaces of the fingers. Systemic manifestations, including fever, are rare. The differential diagnosis of blistering dactylitis includes bullous impetigo, herpetic whitlow, traumatic blistering, burns, and epidermolysis bullosa. Coexistent whitlow and blistering dactylitis have been reported.[114] The diagnosis is confirmed by Gram stain and culture of blister fluid. If herpes infection is suspected, direct fluorescent antibody testing, polymerase chain reaction (PCR), or viral culture should be performed. Streptococcal blistering dactylitis is successfully treated with penicillin or erythromycin, but given recognition of the increasing role that staphylococci may play in the etiology, empiric antimicrobial therapy to cover for both organisms is recommended.

NECROTIZING FASCIITIS

Necrotizing fasciitis (NF) is a rapidly progressive, potentially fatal, necrotizing infection of the skin and subcutaneous tissues commonly associated with severe systemic toxicity. Over the years it has been known by several different names, including *hospital gangrene*, *acute infective gangrene*, *streptococcal gangrene*, *gangrenous erysipelas*, *synergistic necrotizing cellulitis*, and *Meleney ulcer*. A popular term in the lay media is *flesh-eating bacteria disease*. Although usually caused by GABHS, NF may be polymicrobial in nature and has been reported in association with other streptococci, *S. aureus*, *P. aeruginosa*, *Klebsiella* species, *E. coli*, *Enterobacter cloacae*, *Serratia* species, *Proteus* species, *Enterococcus*, a variety of anaerobic agents including *Clostridium* species and *Bacteroides* species, and even *Vibrio* species.[115–119] CA-MRSA has been described as a potential monomicrobial cause of NF.[120] The disorder is most common in individuals with decreased local resistance (skin trauma, surgery, varicella), malnutrition, or chronic disease. NF is far less common in children, but the timely diagnosis in this population remains a challenge, partially attributed to the lack of a "toxic" appearance and nonspecific features early on in the disease process.[121,122] In neonates, NF has been observed in association with omphalitis, balanitis, mammitis, fetal scalp monitoring, and postoperative complications, with omphalitis being the most common.[123,124]

NF most commonly presents on an extremity and is characterized by pain, edema, and erythema with exquisite tenderness to palpation. These changes quickly progress through several sequential stages, including ecchymosis, bullae, necrosis (Fig. 14.23), gangrene, and with deep and extensive infection, overlying skin anesthesia.[116] The inflammation extends deeply along fascial planes, highlighting the importance of rapid diagnosis and surgical exploration. Laboratory findings include leukocytosis, elevated serum creatine kinase level, hyponatremia, coagulopathy, and bacteremia. Fever, shock, and altered mental status typically develop within 48 hours. The most serious complication of NF is streptococcal toxic shock syndrome (TSS) (see later), which is characterized by hypotension, renal impairment, coagulopathy, liver abnormalities, respiratory distress, and a diffuse erythematous cutaneous eruption. Clinical clues that suggest NF over cellulitis include intense pain (often out of proportion to the clinical examination), rapid progression, bullae, necrosis, and lack of a rapid response to antibiotic therapy. Additionally, higher fever, heart rate, respiratory rate, and C-reactive protein (a value >7 mg/dL was highly

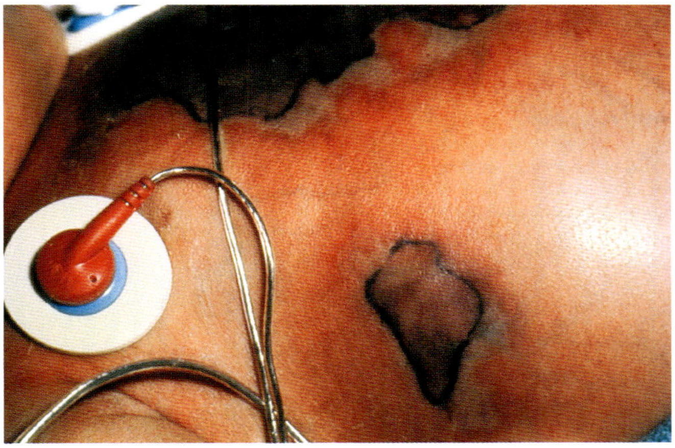

Fig. 14.23 Necrotizing fasciitis. Erythema and necrosis of the abdominal wall are seen in this severely ill toddler.

sensitive and specific for NF in one retrospective study) may help to distinguish this disorder from cellulitis.[125] Imaging studies may be useful in confirming the diagnosis, especially if soft-tissue gas is present, although this is not a consistent finding. MRI may be useful in distinguishing NF from uncomplicated infective fasciitis.[126] Confirmation of infection can be accomplished with Gram stain and culture of blister fluid, lesion discharge or tissue, blood culture, and PCR analysis for pyrogenic exotoxin B on tissue biopsy specimens.[117]

Prompt thorough surgical debridement of necrotic tissue is of prime importance in the management of patients with this disorder, because without exploration and debridement, the mortality rate approaches 100%.[127] Additionally, greater delays in time to initial surgical debridement are associated with increased mortality in children, as in adults with similar infections.[128] Antimicrobial therapy should be initiated immediately, and the chosen agents should have activity against Gram-positive (including MRSA), Gram-negative, *Clostridium*, and anaerobic organisms.[116,119] Clindamycin in particular seems to be quite effective as part of the antimicrobial regimen, given its ability to suppress both toxin and M protein synthesis.[118] Antimicrobial therapy should be adjusted based on the results of Gram stain and bacterial cultures of the surgical specimen. In addition to these specific therapies, fluid resuscitation and blood pressure/blood product support are often indicated. The roles of hyperbaric oxygen therapy and intravenous immunoglobulin (IVIG) remain controversial, with the latter being used primarily in the setting of GABHS infection with TSS.

NOMA

Noma (cancrum oris, necrotizing ulcerative stomatitis) is a rare, progressive, destructive infection usually involving the soft and hard tissues of the oral and paraoral structures. Most reported cases of noma are in children who are severely malnourished or chronically debilitated, and the disease tends to be most common in sub-Saharan Africa, South America, and Asia. The peak ages of incidence are between 1 and 4 years.[129] The triad of malnutrition, poor oral hygiene, and periodontal disease contributes to the increased incidence in these locations.[130] It is usually caused by anaerobic organisms, including *Fusobacterium* species, *Prevotella intermedia*, *Actinomyces* species, *Peptostreptococcus micros*, and *Borrelia* species and is characterized by a gangrenous, ulcerative infection of the gingivae, buccal mucosa, and eventually the cheeks and jaw.

The initial stage of noma is characterized by a painful, small, purple-red lesion that becomes indurated and progresses to edema, necrosis, and ulceration. With expansion, underlying bone involvement occurs with resultant loss of dentition as well as soft facial tissues. It may progress rapidly over days. Bony sequestrations of the mandible or maxilla may occur. Patients may also have fever, tachycardia, tachypnea, and anorexia, and their medical history may reveal recurrent fevers, diarrhea, and history of parasitic and/or viral infections.[131] Treatment of noma includes antibiotics, wound care, and debridement with eventual surgical reconstruction. Without treatment, the mortality rate is 70% to 90%, and survivors suffer the long-term sequelae of orofacial mutilation and functional impairment.[132] Rehydration, attention to electrolyte balance, and nutritional rehabilitation to correct protein and micronutrient deficiencies are other important aspects of therapy.[131] *Necrotizing ulcerative gingivitis (acute necrotizing gingivitis)* is a related gingival infection that presents with rapid onset of gingival interdental necrosis, pain, bleeding, and halitosis and may precede the onset of noma.[133,134]

Noma neonatorum is a gangrenous process of the mucocutaneous junctions of the nose, eyelids, oral cavity, and anogenital region in low-birthweight infants usually caused by *P. aeruginosa*. Most patients also have *Pseudomonas* sepsis, and the mortality rate without antimicrobial therapy is extremely high. Noma neonatorum, which is also more common in developing countries, was so named because of the clinical and histologic similarity to noma. However, there is significant overlap with the clinical presentation of ecthyma gangrenosum. Although some of the reported infants had immunodeficiency, it was either absent or not tested for in the majority of published cases. Noma neonatorum may represent a neonatal form of ecthyma gangrenosum.[135] It has been reported in association with multidrug-resistant *P. aeruginosa* strains.[136]

MENINGOCOCCEMIA

Meningococcal infection, caused by the Gram-negative diplococcus *Neisseria meningitidis*, is a major world health problem in children under 5 years of age and is the leading cause of bacterial meningitis in children. Four serogroups of *N. meningitidis*—B, C, Y, and W—account for more than 90% of cases of meningococcal disease in the United States, and in infants and children under 60 months of age, approximately two-thirds of cases are caused by serogroup B.[137] Person-to-person spread of *N. meningitidis* usually occurs through inhalation of droplets of infected nasopharyngeal secretions by direct or indirect oral contact.[138] Meningococcal disease typically presents between 1 and 14 days after nasopharyngeal acquisition of *N. meningitidis*, but the incubation can be under 4 days. [137,139]

Acute meningococcemia may present in a variety of ways, from transient fever to fulminant disease. After an upper respiratory prodrome, patients develop high fever and severe headache. If meningitis develops, stiff neck, nausea, vomiting, and coma may be present. Up to two-thirds of patients develop a skin eruption, most classically a petechial rash of the skin and mucous membranes. Other cutaneous morphologies include macular, morbilliform, and urticarial eruptions, as well as a gray-colored acrocyanosis. The petechiae are usually small, stellate, and gray-purple (Fig. 14.24) with a raised border and slightly depressed, vesicular, or pustular center.[140] The trunk and lower extremities (especially ankles and wrists) are common sites of predilection, whereas the palms, soles, and head tend to be spared. Mucosal surfaces, including the palpebral and bulbar conjunctivae, may be involved. More extensive hemorrhagic lesions are seen in fulminant meningococcal infections, and a progressive increase on all areas of the body may be followed by coalescence of lesions to form large purpuric patches with sharply marginated borders. These may progress to bullae, necrosis with sloughing, and eventual eschar formation. Autoamputation related to digital ischemic necrosis is a potential complication. Consumptive coagulopathy may be present and when occurring in the setting of progressive cutaneous hemorrhage and necrosis is termed *purpura fulminans*.[141] This finding portends a poor prognosis for the patient with meningococcemia. Three important clinical features that are suggestive of early acute meningococcal disease are leg pain, cold hands and feet, and abnormal skin color.[142]

Chronic meningococcemia is a rare form of meningococcal infection that is unusual in children. It is characterized by intermittent episodes of skin lesions in conjunction with fever, migratory joint pain, myalgia, and episcleritis. The cutaneous lesions seen in the majority of patients appear in crops coincident with or after the fever. Individual lesions are usually macular and occasionally purpuric or pustular and histologically reveal leukocytoclastic vasculitis. Because of potential confusion with other infectious or collagen vascular illnesses, a high index of suspicion is necessary.[143] Patients with

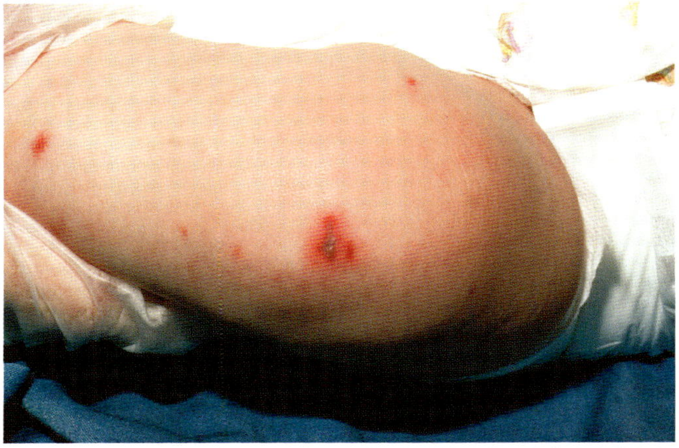

Fig. 14.24 Meningococcemia. Erythematous macules and papules with petechiae, purpura, and early skin necrosis.

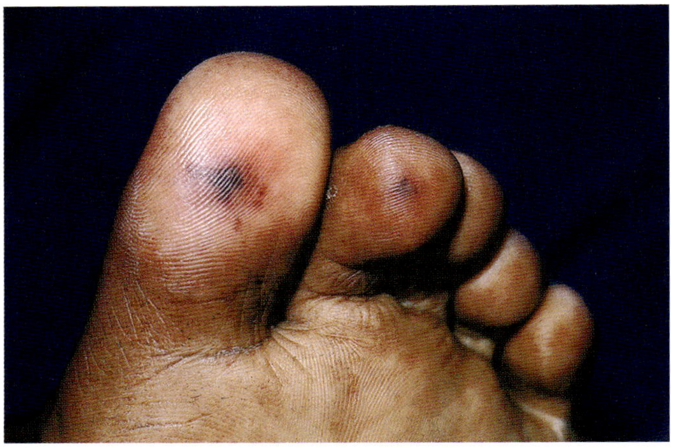

Fig. 14.25 Gonococcemia. Hemorrhagic, erythematous papules and nodules involve the distal digits in this 17-year-old female patient with disseminated gonococcal infection and underlying systemic lupus erythematosus.

complement deficiencies, especially of the terminal complement system (C5-9), have an increased risk of both acute and chronic meningococcal infections.[144]

The differential diagnosis of meningococcemia includes gonococcemia, Henoch–Schönlein purpura, rickettsial diseases, enteroviral infections, erythema multiforme, atypical measles, hypersensitivity vasculitis, and other bacterial septicemias or meningitides. The diagnosis is confirmed by culture of the blood and CSF. Isolation of meningococci from the nasopharynx is presumptive, but not diagnostic, because asymptomatic carriage is not uncommon. Petechial lesions can be smeared and examined for the presence of Gram-negative diplococci and may be cultured for organisms. Serologic assays that can detect *N. meningitidis* capsular polysaccharide antigen in CSF, urine, serum, and other bodily fluids are also available. A serogroup-specific PCR test to detect *N. meningitidis* is used routinely in the United Kingdom and some other European countries, and may be useful in patients who receive antimicrobial therapy before cultures have been obtained.[137] The diagnosis of chronic meningococcemia is best confirmed by blood culture taken during a febrile episode, although several cultures may be necessary.[145]

Meningococcal disease is treated with penicillin G, but at the time of presentation, the initial choice of antimicrobials should be based on the clinical differential diagnosis and local antibiotic susceptibility patterns. Antibiotics with more expanded coverage such as cefotaxime or ceftriaxone are often used empirically in patients with sepsis or meningitis until the diagnosis is confirmed. In patients with a history of anaphylaxis to penicillin, meropenem or ceftriaxone is recommended.[137] Supportive therapy with fluid, pressor, and blood product support as indicated is vital. Chemoprophylaxis of close contacts of patients with invasive meningococcal disease is recommended within 24 hours of diagnosis of the index case; in children, the agents of choice are rifampin, ciprofloxacin, or ceftriaxone. Selective immunization is recommended for children 2 years of age and older in high-risk groups (asplenia, terminal complement deficiencies, or travel to endemic or epidemic areas). Routine immunization with one of two licensed quadrivalent vaccines is recommended for adolescents at the 11- to 12-year visit, with a booster given at 16 years of age, as well as students entering college who plan to live in dormitories and military recruits. Routine early childhood immunization is not recommended because of the low incidence of disease, the poor response in young children, the short-lived immunity, and the potential impaired response to subsequent vaccine doses in some serogroups.[137,146] However, children between 2 and 23 months of age with high-risk conditions (same ones as noted earlier for children over 2 years of age) should receive immunization.[137] Tissue injury from poor perfusion, vascular infarction, and gangrene may require surgical debridement, vacuum-assisted dressings, amputation, or disarticulation.[147]

GONOCOCCEMIA

Gonococcemia is associated with cutaneous lesions similar to those of meningococcemia and presents with fever, chills, arthralgia, and myalgia in patients with gonococcal septicemia. Symptoms of sexually transmitted gonococcal infection may or may not be present, including vaginitis, pelvic inflammatory disease, urethritis, proctitis, or pharyngitis. Hematogenous spread of *Neisseria gonorrhoeae* occurs in up to 3% of untreated persons with mucosal gonorrhea.[148] Skin lesions develop within 3 to 21 days of contact; are located primarily over joints of the distal extremities; and usually appear as petechiae, small erythematous or hemorrhagic papules (Fig. 14.25), or vesiculopustules. They usually heal spontaneously in 4 to 6 days. Patients with lupus erythematosus may be predisposed to infection with *N. gonorrhoeae*, and this may be attributable to the common co-occurrence of complement deficiencies in that population.[149] In the neonate, gonorrhea usually presents as conjunctivitis.

The causative agent, *N. gonorrhoeae*, is a Gram-negative diplococcus and may be demonstrated by smear, culture, or immunofluorescence studies of skin lesions or by culture of the blood, anogenital tract, pharynx, or joint fluid on Thayer–Martin medium (chocolate agar with the addition of antibiotics to inhibit normal flora and nonpathogenic neisserial organisms). Nucleic acid amplification studies (i.e., PCR) are also available and have a high sensitivity and specificity when performed on urethral or cervicovaginal swabs.[148]

The treatment of choice for uncomplicated infection is parenteral ceftriaxone and oral azithromycin. Oral cefixime is an option if parenteral ceftriaxone is unavailable. The alternative for individuals with cephalosporin allergy is intramuscular gentamicin and oral azithromycin. Importantly, if *N. gonorrhoeae* infection is confirmed in prepubertal children (outside of the newborn period) or adolescents who deny sexual activity, the possibility of sexual abuse must be considered.[148]

STAPHYLOCOCCAL SCALDED SKIN SYNDROME

SSSS is a term used to describe a blistering skin disease caused by the epidermolytic (or exfoliative) toxin (ET)–producing *S. aureus*. It was previously known as *Ritter disease* or *pemphigus neonatorum* and tends to occur most often in neonates and young children (most commonly in the 2- to 5-years age group).[150] Its severity may range from mild, localized blistering to widespread exfoliation. Mild cases are probably more common yet less often reported.[151]

The pathogenesis of SSSS relates to the production of ETs, of which there are two serotypes affecting humans: ETA and ETB. These toxins have high sequence homology and are both capable of cleaving the epidermis at the superficial level of the stratum granulosum. The pathogenic mechanisms of ETA and ETB have been clearly elucidated, and they have been shown to target desmoglein 1, a cell–cell adhesion molecule found in desmosomes of the superficial epidermis.[152–154] Desmoglein 1 is the same molecule targeted in the autoimmune blistering disease, pemphigus foliaceus (PF) (see Chapter 13).[152] Once it was determined that antibodies against desmoglein 1 cause PF, astute researchers hypothesized and eventually proved that the target of the staphylococcal ET was also desmoglein 1.[155] There are two main theories for the observation that SSSS preferentially affects neonates and children: lack of protection from antitoxin antibodies (which may be particularly predisposing in preterm infants) and decreased renal excretion of the toxin.[156,157] In adults, SSSS is quite rare and often occurs in the setting of immunosuppression, sepsis, renal failure, malignancy, heart disease, or diabetes.[158,159]

Outbreaks of SSSS have been reported in neonatal intensive care units and well-baby nurseries. In these settings, asymptomatic or clinically infected healthcare workers often act as carriers of the epidemic strain of *S. aureus*, and given the potential severity of infection in the premature infant, prompt recognition with institution of strict infection-control strategies is vital to prevent further nosocomial spread.[160,161] In a series of 39 neonates with SSSS, pneumonia was the most common complication, followed by myocarditis.[162]

SSSS generally begins with localized infection of the conjunctivae, nares, perioral region, perineum, or umbilicus. Separation of perioral crusts often leaves behind radial fissures around the mouth, resulting in the characteristic facial appearance of SSSS (Figs. 14.26 and 14.27). Other infections that may serve as the initial nidus for SSSS include pneumonia, septic arthritis, endocarditis, or pyomyositis. Fever, malaise, lethargy, irritability, and poor feeding subsequently develop, and the generalized eruption begins. The rash is characterized by erythema that progresses to large, superficial fragile blisters that rupture easily, leaving behind denuded, desquamating, erythematous, and tender skin (Figs. 14.27 and 14.28). The eruption is most marked in flexural creases but may involve the entire surface area of skin. Extensive involvement of the hand/fingers in a "degloving" pattern, concerning for epidermolysis bullosa, has been reported.[163] The Nikolsky sign (progression of the blister cleavage plane induced by gentle pressure on the edge of the bulla) is positive. With extensive denudation of skin, patients may have decreased thermoregulatory ability, extensive fluid losses, and electrolyte imbalance and are at serious risk for secondary infection and sepsis. With appropriate management, the skin heals without scarring, given the superficial cleavage plane of the blisters.

SSSS is usually diagnosed based on the clinical presentation. The main differential diagnosis is toxic epidermal necrolysis (TEN), a severe exfoliative condition that is usually drug-induced and has a high mortality rate. The most helpful distinguishing feature of TEN is mucosal involvement, including of the mouth, conjunctivae, trachea, and genital mucosa, which is lacking in SSSS.[156] Other less common differential diagnoses include scalding burns, epidermolysis bullosa, graft-versus-host disease, nutritional-deficiency dermatosis, and bullous ichthyosis (in the neonate). The diagnosis of SSSS is confirmed by isolation of *S. aureus*. It must be remembered that the majority of blisters in SSSS are sterile, because they are caused by the hematogenous dissemination of the bacterial toxin and not the bacteria itself. The organism is most easily recovered from pyogenic (not exfoliative) foci on the skin, conjunctivae, nares, or nasopharynx. When the

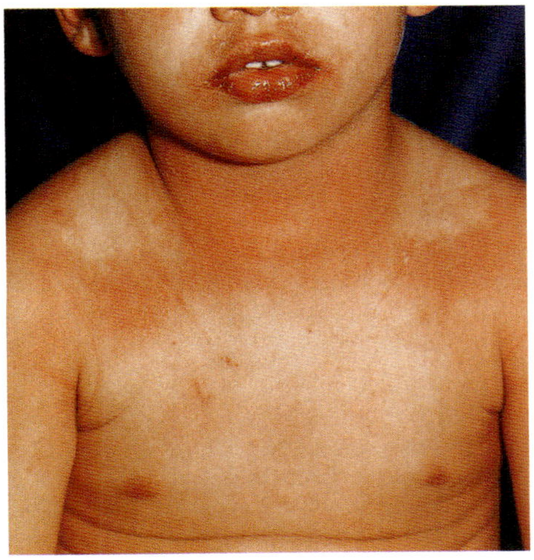

Fig. 14.26 Staphylococcal scalded skin syndrome. Periorbital (not shown) and perioral erythema and erythema of the neck folds and upper trunk in this 4-year-old boy with early infection.

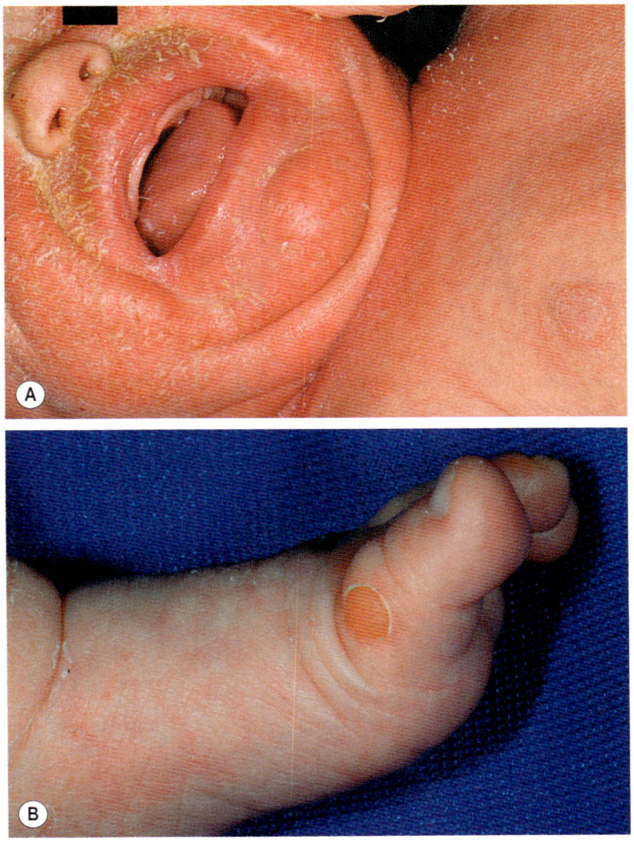

Fig. 14.27 Staphylococcal scalded skin syndrome. Facial and neck-fold erythema with desquamation, crusting, and perioral radial fissures **(A)** and a distant ruptured bulla on the toe **(B)** of an infant girl with the disorder.

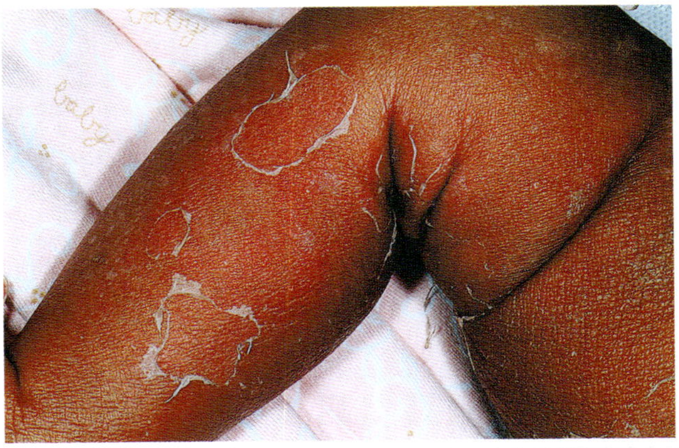

Fig. 14.28 Staphylococcal scalded skin syndrome. Diffuse peeling and erythema in a 4-week-old Black infant girl who also had *Staphylococcus aureus* isolated from her blood.

diagnosis remains in question, differentiation from TEN can be made by microscopic examination of a skin snip of the blister roof or a skin biopsy. In SSSS, cleavage occurs in the superficial epidermis at the level of the granular layer, whereas in TEN the split occurs below the dermal–epidermal junction.

Treatment of SSSS is directed at the eradication of toxin-producing staphylococci, thus terminating toxin production. A penicillinase-resistant penicillin, first- or second-generation cephalosporin, and clindamycin are all appropriate initial choices, with modification based on sensitivity testing. In patients with MRSA infection, parenteral vancomycin or other agents (as dictated by local resistance patterns) would be indicated. Because SSSS is usually a milder disease in older children, ambulatory therapy may be an option in this population. In neonates or in infants or children with severe infection, hospitalization is mandatory, with attention to fluid and electrolyte management, infection control measures, pain management, and meticulous wound care with contact isolation. In particularly severe disease, care in an intensive care or burn unit is required. Neutralizing antibodies that inhibit the binding of ETs to desmoglein 1 have been investigated, given concerns about the development of antibiotic-resistant, ET-producing staphylococci.[164] Administration of fresh frozen plasma or IVIG has also been reported,[165] but is not routinely advocated.

TOXIC SHOCK SYNDROME

TSS is an acute febrile illness characterized by fever, rash, hypotension, and multisystem organ involvement. Although classically described in menstruating women in relation to the use of superabsorbent tampons, TSS is now recognized in both menstrual and nonmenstrual forms, with the latter now being more common.[166] Nonmenstrual TSS may occur in association with surgical procedures, nasal packing, the postpartum state, and a variety of *S. aureus* infections.

TSS is caused by toxin-producing strains of *S. aureus*. Manifestations of the disease are mediated primarily by the TSS toxin (TSST-1) and staphylococcal enterotoxins (SEA, SEB, SEC). These toxins are capable of widespread polyclonal activation of T cells, which results in massive cytokine release and in the clinical picture of TSS. Both TSST-1 and the SEs are considered "superantigens," given their ability to activate T cells without intracellular processing and via specific binding to major histocompatibility complex (MHC) class II molecules.[167,168] MRSA (which can also produce TSST-1) appears to account for a small percentage of TSS cases.[169,170]

A prodrome of mild constitutional symptoms, including malaise, myalgias, and chills, often precedes the symptoms of TSS. Eventually, fever develops along with lethargy, diarrhea, chills, nausea, and altered mental status. Symptoms of hypovolemia, including hyperventilation, palpitations, and orthostatic dizziness, may be present.[171] Physical findings include high fever, hypotension, a diffuse rash, and pharyngitis with hyperemia of mucous membranes. The cutaneous eruption is a diffuse, macular erythroderma that is occasionally reminiscent of the rash of scarlet fever. Accentuation of the eruption in skin folds is a common finding, and in rare cases the inguinal or perineal regions may be the only skin surfaces involved.[172] Edema of the hands, feet, and face may be present, and desquamation of the affected skin surfaces (Fig. 14.29) eventually ensues. The nails may be shed, and telogen effluvium may occur up to several months later. Oral examination often reveals a strawberry tongue (Fig. 14.30), and palatal petechiae may be present. Diffuse myalgia is almost always present, and many patients complain of exquisite skin or muscle tenderness when they are touched or moved.

In addition to the fever, desquamating rash, and hypotension, evidence of multiorgan involvement is present. To meet the case definition of TSS, three or more of seven other organ systems must be involved (Box 14.3).[173] The diagnosis of TSS generally rests on clinical criteria, although isolation of *S. aureus* from a normally sterile site, especially if toxin production can be demonstrated, is supportive. Histopathologic findings on skin biopsy are not pathognomonic. The differential diagnosis of TSS includes streptococcal TSS (see later), Kawasaki disease (KD), scarlet fever, drug reaction, atypical measles, Rocky Mountain spotted fever, and other exanthematous illnesses. The presence of shock and multiorgan involvement is unusual in the other entities, except for streptococcal TSS, which usually has some distinguishing features. *Kawasaki disease shock syndrome (KDSS)* refers to the clinical presentation of hypotension and shock in patients with KD. Although KDSS and TSS may be difficult to differentiate during the acute phase of the disorders, distinguishing features of KDSS include lower hemoglobin concentration, higher platelet count, and more common presence of valvulitis (mitral or tricuspid regurgitation) and coronary artery lesions.[174]

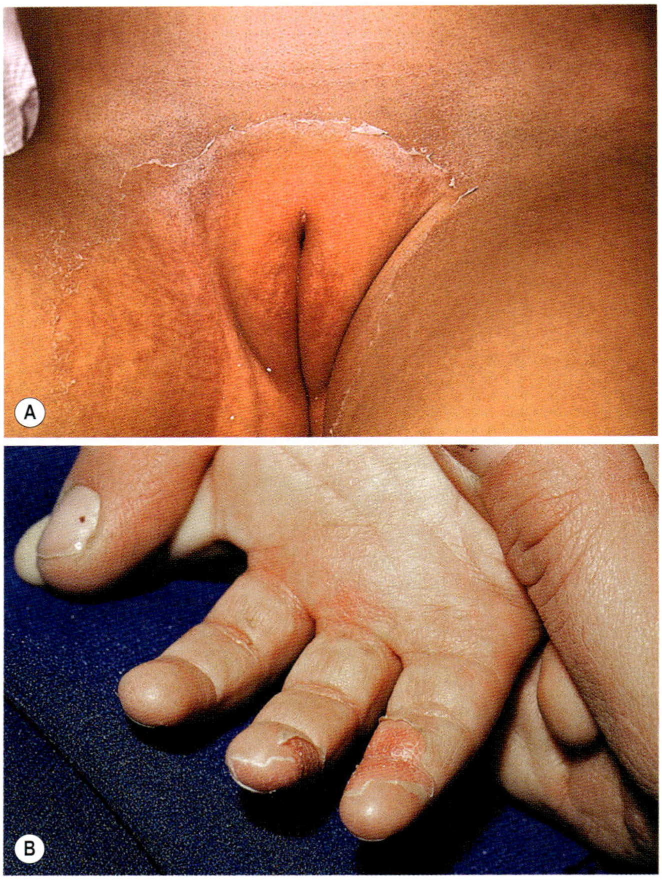

Fig. 14.29 Desquamation in toxic shock syndrome. Mild perineal **(A)** and digital **(B)** desquamation in a 3-year-old girl with toxic shock syndrome.

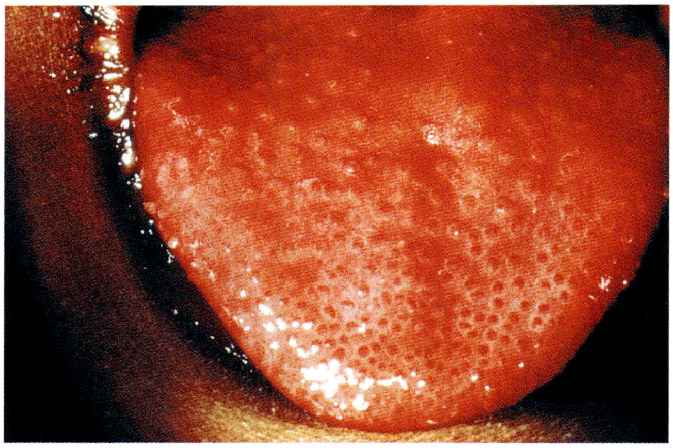

Fig. 14.30 Strawberry tongue in toxic shock syndrome. Hyperemia with prominent lingual papillae.

Box 14.3 Case Definition of Toxic Shock Syndrome

- Temperature >38.9° C (102° F)
- Diffuse macular erythroderma
- Desquamation, 1 to 2 weeks after onset, particularly of the palms, soles, fingers, and toes
- Hypotension (<5th percentile for age in children <16 years)
- Multisystem involvement (three or more of the following):
  - Gastrointestinal (vomiting, diarrhea)
  - Muscular (severe myalgia, increased creatine phosphokinase level)
  - Mucous membrane (vaginal, oropharyngeal, or conjunctival) hyperemia
  - Renal (elevated serum urea nitrogen or serum creatinine level more than twice the upper limit of normal, or urinary sediment with >5 WBC per field in absence of UTI)
  - Hepatic (total bilirubin, AST or ALT greater than twice the upper limit of normal)
  - Hematologic (platelet count ≤100,000/mm^3)
  - Central nervous system (disorientation, altered consciousness without focal neurologic signs when fever and hypotension are absent)
- Laboratory criteria: negative results on the following tests (if obtained):
  - Blood, throat, or CSF cultures (except blood culture may be positive for *S. aureus*)
  - Serologic tests for Rocky Mountain spotted fever, leptospirosis, or measles

Probable disease: meets laboratory criteria and four of the five bulleted (dark green) findings are present

Confirmed disease: meets laboratory criteria and all five of the bulleted (dark green) findings, including desquamation (unless patient expires before desquamation occurs)

ALT, Alanine aminotransferase; *AST*, aspartate aminotransferase; *CSF*, cerebrospinal fluid; *UTI*, urinary tract infection; *WBC*, white blood cell.

Modified From American Academy of Pediatrics. Group A streptococcal infections. In Kimberlin DW, Brady MT, Jackson MA, et al., et al. Red Book: 2018 Report of the Committee on Infectious Diseases. Elk Grove Village, IL: American Academy of Pediatrics; 2018:749–62 and Wharton M, Vogt RL, Buehler JW. Case definitions for public health surveillance. MMWR. 1990;39(RR-13):1–43.

A neonatal TSS-like disease has been reported, and in some of these patients MRSA was recovered.[175] When studied, several of these MRSA isolates were positive for TSST-1 production. Most of the reported neonates had a mild course with a fairly rapid recovery.[175]

Since the late 1980s a disease similar to TSS yet with some distinguishing features has been recognized. This disorder is associated with toxin-producing GABHS and is referred to as *streptococcal TSS*. Although the pathogenic mechanisms are not entirely clear, streptococcal pyrogenic exotoxins (SPEA, SPEB, SPEC), mitogenic factor, and streptococcal superantigen appear to be associated with the clinical findings.

Streptococcal TSS is similarly characterized by the acute onset of shock and multisystem organ failure, but unlike staphylococcal TSS, patients usually have a focal, invasive tissue or blood infection with GABHS (Box 14.4).[176] Most patients with streptococcal TSS have pain localized to an extremity in association with NF or myonecrosis. This pain is usually out of proportion to the clinical findings on physical examination. Varicella is a particularly important risk factor for invasive GABHS infections in children, and in the child with varicella who becomes febrile after having been afebrile or who has any fever beyond the fourth day of illness, GABHS infection should be considered.[177]

A prodromal illness with influenza-like symptoms is present in up to 20% of patients with streptococcal TSS. Subsequently shock develops rapidly, and often the patients develop renal impairment, disseminated intravascular coagulopathy, and an adult respiratory distress syndrome–like illness. Physical examination reveals a diffuse macular erythroderma and mucous membrane findings similar to those seen in staphylococcal TSS. Examination of the site of primary infection (usually an extremity) reveals localized swelling and erythema with eventual development of vesicles and hemorrhagic bullae.[178] Laboratory aberrations include leukocytosis, anemia, thrombocytopenia, elevation of serum creatinine and creatine phosphokinase, hypocalcemia, abnormal liver function studies, and evidence of disseminated coagulopathy. Streptococcal TSS presenting with purpura fulminans has been reported.[179] In one series of pediatric streptococcal TSS, one-quarter of the patients succumbed to the disease as a result of refractory shock and multiorgan failure; in half of these, death occurred within 24 hours of hospital admission.[180]

Box 14.4 Case Definition of Streptococcal Toxic Shock Syndrome[177]

Isolation of GABHS:

- From a normally sterile site (i.e., blood, CSF, joint fluid, pleural fluid, peritoneal fluid)*

OR

- From a nonsterile site (i.e., throat, sputum, vagina, open wound, skin lesion)†

AND

Hypotension (<5th percentile for age in children <16 years)

AND

- At least two of the following:
  - Renal impairment (creatinine >2 mg/dL or more than twice the upper limit for age)
  - Coagulopathy (platelet count ≤100,000/mm^3 and/or DIC)
  - Hepatic involvement (AST, ALT, or total bilirubin more than twice the upper limit for age)
  - Adult respiratory distress syndrome
  - Generalized erythematous rash with or without desquamation
  - Soft-tissue necrosis (i.e., necrotizing fasciitis or myositis or gangrene)

ALT, Alanine aminotransferase; *AST*, aspartate aminotransferase; *CSF*, cerebrospinal fluid; *DIC*, disseminated intravascular coagulopathy; *GABHS*, group A β-hemolytic streptococcus.

* Definite case: from a normally sterile site and both bulleted (dark green) findings.

From American Academy of Pediatrics. *Staphyloccus aureaus*. In Kimberlin DW, Brady MT, Jackson MA, et al., et al. Red Book: 2018 Report of the Committee on Infectious Diseases. Elk Grove Village, IL: American Academy of Pediatrics; 2018:733–45.

Management of TSS is similar for both staphylococcal and streptococcal disease. Supportive therapy (including aggressive fluid management), vasopressors, and antibiotics are the mainstays of therapy. Identification of sites of infection is vital, with appropriate drainage or in the case of streptococcal TSS, aggressive and early surgical exploration and debridement as indicated.[176] Many experts recommend combination antibiotic therapy that includes clindamycin, given its effects on protein (i.e., toxin) synthesis inhibition, although clindamycin should not be used alone.[177] IVIG may be beneficial when used in combination with antibiotics for TSS because IVIG blocks superantigen-induced T-cell activation. Use of IVIG should be considered in patients in whom there has been no clinical response within the first several hours of aggressive supportive therapy.[173,181]

CORYNEBACTERIAL INFECTIONS

Erythrasma is a superficial bacterial infection of the skin caused by *C. minutissimum*. It is characterized by asymptomatic, well-demarcated, reddish-brown, slightly scaly patches in the groin, axillae, gluteal crease, or inframammary regions and less often the interdigital spaces of the feet. Involvement of the vulvar mucosae has been observed.[182] Some 15% of erythrasma cases occur in children between 5 and 14 years of age. Erythrasma is often confused with a dermatophyte infection (i.e., tinea corporis), with which it may occasionally coexist. However, it can be differentiated from tinea infection by the characteristic coral-red fluorescence seen when viewed under Wood lamp illumination (because of the production of porphyrins by the corynebacteria). Erythrasma tends to be more common in patients who are overweight, the elderly, and patients with diabetes.[183] Culturing the organism is difficult and requires a special medium. Erythrasma may be treated with topical antibiotics, including erythromycin or clindamycin, although there is some evidence of increasing antibiotic resistance to the former.[184] Antibacterial soaps may help prevent recurrence. Oral antibiotic therapy is very effective and classically includes erythromycin, tetracycline, or newer-generation macrolide agents.[185] Single-dose clarithromycin therapy has been reported.[186] In one recent series of patients with erythrasma who had cultures and susceptibility testing performed, amoxicillin clavulanate was the systemic agent with the least demonstrated resistance and hence should also be considered as potential systemic therapy when indicated.[184] *C. minutissimum* has rarely been associated with more severe disease, including cellulitis and bacteremia.[187]

Trichomycosis axillaris (trichobacteriosis) is a superficial infection of the axillary and, less commonly, pubic hairs that results in adherent white or yellow concretions distributed irregularly along the hair shafts. *C. tenuis* is the causative agent for this condition and hence the traditional name *trichomycosis axillaris,* which implies a fungal infection, is a misnomer. The disorder usually occurs after puberty due to its association with axillary and pubic hair but then occurs with equal incidence in all postpubertal age groups. The most common sign of trichomycosis axillaris is the presence of red-stained perspiration on the clothing, and individuals with hyperhidrosis often complain of a particularly offensive axillary odor. The nodules of trichomycosis axillaris consist of bacterial elements embedded in an amorphous matrix, and Gram stain reveals thread-like Gram-positive bacteria. Affected areas only rarely fluoresce (as a pale yellow color) under Wood light examination. Treatment consists of shaving the hairs of the affected areas, using antiperspirants (to help decrease hyperhidrosis and growth of Gram-positive flora), and the application of topical antibiotics such as clindamycin or erythromycin. Benzoyl peroxide has also been demonstrated to be useful.

Pitted keratolysis is another superficial corynebacterial infection, in this case involving the plantar feet, lateral aspects of the toes, and occasionally the palms and finger web spaces.[188] It is characterized by erythema with shallow round pits (Fig. 14.31), crateriform depressions (Fig. 14.32) or shallow erosions most commonly involving weight-bearing portions of the feet. Malodor is common, and although the condition is usually asymptomatic, painful, plaque-like lesions have been reported in children.[189] Pitted keratolysis is caused by *Corynebacterium (Kytococcus) sedentarius* (formerly *Micrococcus* spp.), which produces extracellular enzymes capable of degrading human keratins.[190] The disorder has worldwide distribution and occurs most commonly in hot, tropical climates and in populations (i.e., homeless individuals, elite athletes) who experience repeated skin exposure to moisture and environmental hazards.[191,192] The diagnosis is fairly straightforward and based on clinical findings, although Gram stain of stratum corneum shavings can be used if necessary. Culture is generally not helpful, and Wood lamp examination may or may not reveal coral-red fluorescence. Pitted keratolysis is treated with topical erythromycin, clindamycin, or mupirocin. Clindamycin–benzoyl peroxide combination topical gel was very effective in an open-label study of four patients.[193] Treatment of the hyperhidrosis component with prescription-strength aluminum chloride products, 40% formaldehyde in petrolatum ointment, or other treatments directed towards hyperhidrosis may also be useful.

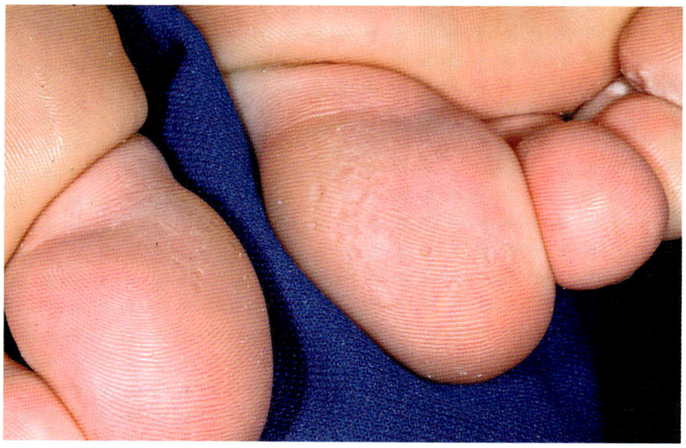

Fig. 14.31 Pitted keratolysis. Shallow pits of the plantar great toes in this adolescent boy. Malodor was also present.

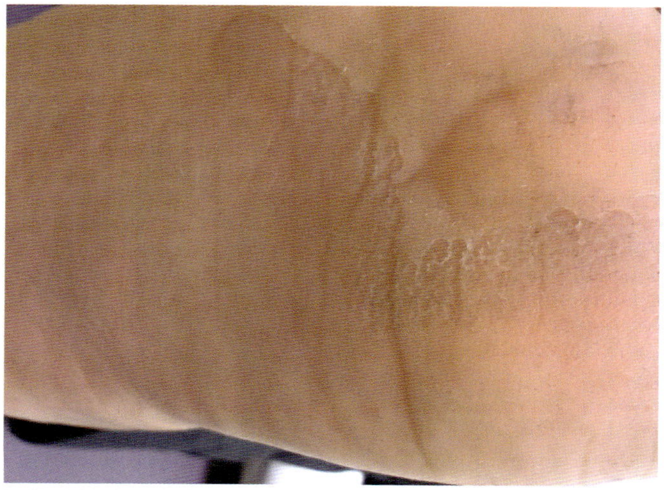

Fig. 14.32 Pitted keratolysis. Coalescing pits and crater-like depressions were present in this adolescent boy with extreme malodor and plantar discomfort.

ERYSIPELOID

Erysipeloid is an infection of traumatized skin, particularly the fingers, hands, or arms of individuals who handle meat, raw saltwater fish, shellfish, or poultry and in those who come into contact with certain animals, especially pigs, sheep, rabbits, chickens, turkeys, ducks, emus, pigeons, cows, guinea pigs, cats, dogs, fish, and shellfish.[194] As such, it is most commonly associated with occupations such as animal breeders, veterinarians, slaughterhouse workers, butchers, fishermen, fishmongers, cooks, and grocers.[195] It is caused by *Erysipelothrix rhusiopathiae (insidiosa)*, a Gram-positive bacillus that can survive for months in soil or decomposed organic material. Human infection with this organism can take one of three forms: the mild cutaneous infection erysipeloid, which may be confused clinically with erysipelas; a diffuse cutaneous form; and a serious systemic infection, usually septicemia or endocarditis.[196] Erysipeloid presents 1 to 7 days after inoculation as a painful, violaceous-red, sharply demarcated patch, usually on the hand or a finger. Burning, pain, or pruritus may be reported by the patient, and constitutional symptoms may occasionally be present. A diffuse, generalized eruption in regions remote from the site of infection, hemorrhagic vesicles, and regional lymphadenopathy may occasionally occur. Systemic complications are rare and include septicemia, endocarditis, septic arthritis, cerebral infarct, osseous necrosis, and pulmonary effusion. When endocarditis occurs, it tends to involve structurally damaged but native left-sided valves.[197]

The diagnosis of localized cutaneous erysipeloid can be difficult, because the organism does not grow well in culture and tissue biopsy findings are nonspecific. The yield in culture may be increased by using enriched blood culture and incubating with 5% to 10% carbon dioxide. Blood culture may be useful when systemic infection is present. PCR assays are also available to assist in the diagnosis. Although the vast majority of patients with untreated localized erysipeloid tend to recover spontaneously within 3 weeks, antibiotics such as penicillin, cephalosporins, erythromycin, and tetracyclines (among others) have been demonstrated to be effective.

Nontuberculous ("Atypical") Mycobacterial Infections

The nontuberculous mycobacteria (NTM), which have traditionally been referred to as *atypical mycobacteria,* include those species different from *Mycobacterium tuberculosis*. These slender, nonmotile, acid-fast organisms have a worldwide distribution and usually are nonpathogenic for humans. They are considered hardy, environmental saprophytes and can be isolated from soil, water, vegetation, animals, and hospital environments; tap water, though, serves as the main reservoir for humans.[198] Infection tends to occur in immunocompromised individuals (especially disseminated infections) or, when in the immunocompetent host, after an episode of skin trauma.[199] Six major clinical syndromes have been identified, including lung infection; lymphadenitis;

SSTI; disseminated infection; catheter-related infection; and chronic granulomatous infection of bones, joints, and tendon sheaths. Skin infection with NTM usually manifests as skin nodules, abscesses, papulopustules, or ulcers.[200] Systemic spread most often occurs in immunocompromised hosts. The diagnosis of NTM infection is usually confirmed by histology and tissue culture, with PCR and DNA gene sequencing being increasingly utilized.[201]

The NTM include *Mycobacterium marinum, Mycobacterium ulcerans, Mycobacterium fortuitum, Mycobacterium chelonae, Mycobacterium abscessus, Mycobacterium kansasii, Mycobacterium avium-intracellulare* (Mycobacterium avium complex), *Mycobacterium haemophilum*, and a variety of others that less commonly result in clinical infection. Those that will be discussed in this section are *M. marinum* (swimming pool granuloma), *M. ulcerans* (Buruli ulcer), and *M. fortuitum/M. chelonae/M. abscessus* (the "rapid growers"). Cervical lymphadenitis caused by NTM will also be briefly discussed.

M. marinum may result in a skin infection termed *swimming pool granuloma* or *fish tank granuloma*. The organism resides in stagnant water and seawater, as well as in natural pools and some heated pools in temperate climates. Exposure to fish tank water is another described source for inoculation and seems to be a fairly common mode of infection.[202,203] Abrasions from swimming pools or fish tanks and at times cuts sustained from cleaning fish may become infected with this NTM. *M. marinum* infections, sometimes unusually aggressive ones, have been increasingly reported in patients receiving anti–tumor necrosis factor therapy, including etanercept and infliximab.[204,205] Most lesions begin on an extremity, hand, or foot after an incubation period of 2 to 3 weeks. In some studies the incubation period may be longer, up to 9 months after inoculation.[206] Infection begins with a nodule or pustule that eventually forms an ulcer or abscess. Multiple secondary lesions develop, often in a linear, lymphatic (sporotrichoid) distribution (Fig. 14.33). Without therapy, the skin lesions resolve over 1 to 3 years with scarring. Potential associated complications include tenosynovitis, arthritis, and osteomyelitis, and in immunocompromised individuals severe disseminated infection may occur. The differential diagnosis includes cellulitis, sporotrichosis, syphilis, cutaneous leishmaniasis, tularemia, foreign body reaction, cat-scratch disease (CSD), neoplasia, and deep fungal infection. Skin biopsy reveals inflammation with tuberculoid granulomas, and culture of *M. marinum* from tissue (which may require 10 days to 6 weeks of incubation) confirms the diagnosis. Although purified protein derivative (PPD) skin testing may be positive, it is not diagnostic of *M. marinum* infection.

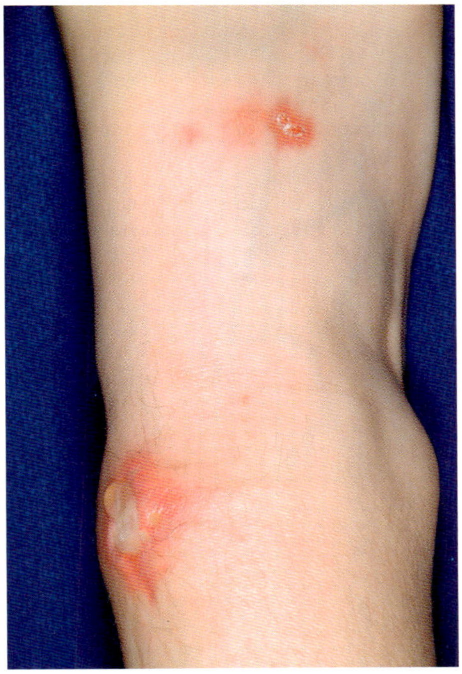

Fig. 14.33 *Mycobacterium marinum* infection. This boy developed nodules that subsequently ulcerated on the dorsal foot *(superior lesion in photograph)* and the medial ankle *(inferior lesion in photograph)*. The family had a large fish tank that they routinely cleaned in the bathtub used by the patient.

When a patient has cutaneous lesions suggestive of *M. marinum* infection, a thorough exposure history should be pursued and tissue biopsy performed. Although there is no completely satisfactory treatment for this infection, options used with variable success include tetracycline, minocycline, doxycycline, clarithromycin, trimethoprim-sulfamethoxazole, linezolid, and rifampin, alone or in combination with ethambutol.[199,202,207–209] Excision, curettage, and warm compresses are traditional treatment modalities that may be helpful for early or small lesions, but recurrences are common.

M. ulcerans may result in an ulcerating skin condition called *Buruli ulcer*, which is most common in Africa (heaviest burden in West and sub-Saharan Africa), Central and South America, and Asia. Buruli ulcer usually begins after a scrape by grass or a thorn and presents initially as a painless nodule that progresses to abscess formation and, eventually, a shallow ulcer. The favored site of distribution is a lower extremity. The ulcer persists for months to years and eventually heals spontaneously with scarring and lymphedema.[199] Contractures and limb deformities may occur, occasionally requiring amputations.[209] Surgery, hyperthermic therapy, and systemic antimicrobials have all been used with variable success. The World Health Organization (WHO)–recommended antibiotic therapy is rifampin and streptomycin for an 8-week course.[210]

M. fortuitum, M. chelonae, and *M. abscessus* are all referred to as *rapid growers*, given their distinctive ability to produce colonies in culture as soon as 5 to 7 days. They may result in clinical disease after trauma, the most notable association being abscess formation after surgery, especially within postsurgical scars. Skin findings reported with these organisms are diverse and, in addition to abscesses, include nodules, cellulitis, ulcers, sinus tracts, pustules and folliculitis.[210] Disseminated infection may occur in immunocompromised individuals. Children are more likely to experience infection with *M. fortuitum* than the other two rapidly growing NTMs, which are more commonly isolated from older individuals.[211] Treatment options for infection with a rapidly growing mycobacterial organism may include clarithromycin, amikacin, cefoxitin, linezolid, imipenem, sulfonamides, ciprofloxacin, and doxycycline.[212,213] There are increasing reports of *M. chelonae* infection after tattooing, with culture of the organism originating from premixed tattoo inks.[214–216] Inflammatory skin lesions (papules, pustules, and nodules) involving primarily the palms and soles have been observed in children in association with *M. abscessus* infection acquired from public swimming pools. This presentation has been designated by some as "*M. abscessus* hand-and-foot disease," and may have a prolonged latency (45 to 60 days) between exposure and onset, which is significantly longer than that typically seen with *Pseudomonas* hot foot syndrome (see earlier this chapter).[217,218] Lesions may occasionally occur in other sites, including elbows, knees, and trunk, and although this condition is self-limited, recurrences may appear. This observation has led some to recommend therapy with an appropriate agent such as clarithromycin when this diagnosis is suspected or confirmed.[218]

Cervical lymphadenitis resulting from NTM should be mentioned because it is the most common manifestation of infection with these agents in healthy, immunocompetent children. These patients usually experience nontender, unilateral cervical lymphadenopathy, although other sites may be involved, including the inguinal region, axilla, and lower limb.[219,220] There may or may not be a history of preceding local trauma, and the area may reveal overlying erythema (Fig. 14.34), violaceous discoloration, fluctuance, or drainage. The most common of the NTMs to cause cervical lymphadenitis is *M. avium-intracellulare*,[219,221] although *Mycobacterium haemophilum* appears to be increasing in incidence as another etiology in some areas.[222,223] Treatment options include surgery (with complete excision traditionally considered the gold standard), incision and drainage, and antimicrobial therapy including ethambutol, rifampicin, and clarithromycin. Observation alone is another option, given the complete resolution seen in most patients within 9 to 12 months.[224] Although surgical excision has long been considered the standard of care for NTM lymphadenitis, it carries up to a 10% risk of facial nerve

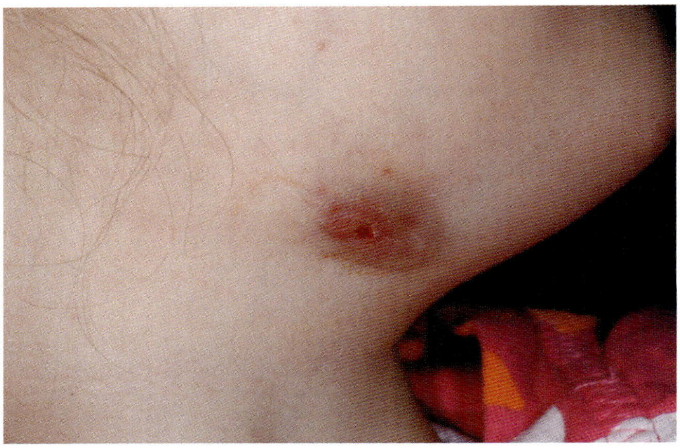

Fig. 14.34 Nontuberculous mycobacterial cervical lymphadenitis. This fluctuant, violaceous nodule developed in the inferior mandibular region of this otherwise-healthy 3-year-old girl. Occasional drainage had been noted by her parents, and the lesion improved gradually with clarithromycin therapy.

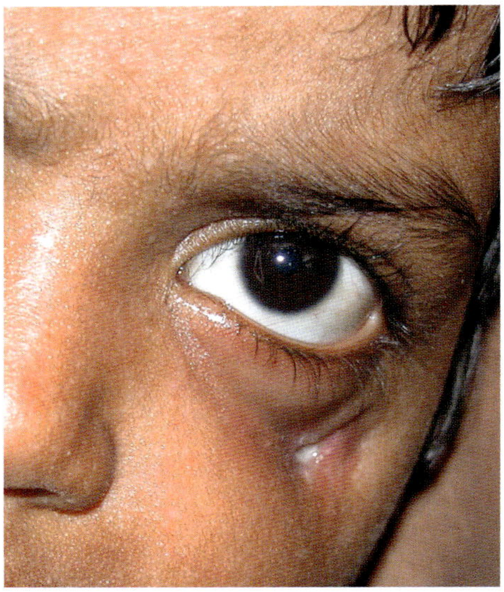

Fig. 14.35 Scrofuloderma. A discharging sinus is noted from the tuberculous focus in the underlying bone in this 4-year-old boy. (Courtesy Venkatesh Ramesh, MD.)

palsy, and more diversified treatment strategies, including the increased use of antimicrobial agents, are being observed.[225,226]

Tuberculosis of the Skin

The incidence of cutaneous tuberculosis (TB) was at one time declining due to the availability of effective antimycobacterial therapy, improvement in living standards, and vigorous preventive and therapeutic programs. However, it has reemerged in areas with a high incidence of HIV infection and multidrug-resistant pulmonary TB.[227,228] Children appear to be especially vulnerable to acquisition of both susceptible and resistant types of TB, and diagnosis of childhood TB is challenging.[229] Most published reports of childhood cutaneous TB are from developing countries, and the prevalence is high in India and Southeast Asia, with the highest prevalence reported in Pakistan.[230] Cutaneous TB can be acquired exogenously (inoculation tuberculosis), endogenously (i.e., skin breakdown over a subcutaneous focus such as a lymph node or bone infection), or via hematogenous spread of *M. tuberculosis* and may show a wide range of clinical presentations. The majority of cases of cutaneous TB are related to systemic involvement. In this section, several types of tuberculous skin lesions are reviewed. Of the lesions discussed, scrofuloderma and lupus vulgaris tend to be the most common types of cutaneous TB to occur in children.[231,232]

Primary tuberculous complex (tuberculous chancre, primary inoculation TB) develops as a result of inoculation of *M. tuberculosis* into the skin (and occasionally the mucosa) of an individual who has not previously been infected or who has not acquired immunity to the organism. This disorder occurs on exposed surfaces at sites of trauma (e.g., abrasion, insect bite, puncture wound, ritual circumcision, piercings, tattooing). The cutaneous lesion develops 2 to 4 weeks after inoculation. The earliest lesion is a brown-red papule that develops into an indurated plaque that may ulcerate. The edges of the ulcer are ragged and undermined, and thick adherent crusts may be present. When viewed through a glass slide producing pressure on the lesion (diascopy), these areas may have an "apple jelly" yellow-brown color. Marked regional lymphadenopathy may be associated with the skin lesion[233] and usually develops several weeks after the cutaneous lesion. Healing of the ulcer generally occurs over several weeks, but the regional lymphadenopathy may persist significantly longer and after weeks to months may soften and form sinuses that communicate with the skin surface (scrofuloderma, see later).

Tuberculosis verrucosa cutis (warty TB) is an externally acquired, relatively uncommon inoculation type of TB in individuals who have had previous contact with *M. tuberculosis* and thus have some degree of immunity. The inoculation usually occurs at sites of minor wounds or abrasions, and it occurs most often in adults with occupations that require the handling of patients with TB infections or tuberculous tissues, including pathologists ("prosecutor's wart") and butchers ("butcher's wart"). Lesions usually occur on the dorsal hands, fingers, or lower extremities. They begin as small violaceous papules that become hyperkeratotic and warty. Multiple lesions may occur, but the majority of lesions of tuberculosis verrucosa cutis are solitary.

Scrofuloderma refers to direct extension to the skin from underlying foci of tuberculous infection, and in addition to lymph nodes may occur overlying infection of the bone or joint. It is the most common form of cutaneous TB in children less than 10 years of age.[234] Scrofuloderma is manifested most commonly as painless swelling in the parotid, submandibular, supraclavicular, or lateral regions of the neck.[235] As the lesions grow, they may develop ulcers and sinuses (Fig. 14.35). *M. tuberculosis* can be easily identified by Gram stain and culture of the draining exudate. Untreated lesions of scrofuloderma may persist with little change for years and eventually heal with cicatricial bands. *Lupus vulgaris* is the most common form of cutaneous TB. It is a chronic, smoldering form of the infection and usually occurs in individuals with a high degree of sensitivity. Although lupus vulgaris can arise at the site of a primary inoculation, in the scar of scrofuloderma, or at the site of a bacillus Calmette–Guérin (BCG) vaccination, it generally appears in previously normal areas of skin. The most common location of involvement is the head and neck, and regional lymphadenopathy may be present in over half of the patients.[232] In children in India, this form of cutaneous TB most often occurs on the lower extremities and gluteal region.[230] Lupus vulgaris presents as small, soft, brown-red papules that enlarge and coalesce to form larger plaques with elevation and intensification of their brownish color. As in tuberculous chancre, the lesion shows a characteristic apple-jelly color on diascopy. The natural history of lupus vulgaris is marked by slow and limited growth over years or occasionally decades. Ulceration and atrophy may occur.[231,235] When ulceration occurs, it may be complicated by scarring and disfigurement, especially with nose and nasal cartilage involvement (Fig. 14.36). A mutilating form is marked by destructive skin lesions with invasion of underlying tissues. The differential diagnosis of lupus vulgaris includes sarcoidosis, cutaneous lymphoid hyperplasia, lupus erythematosus, halogenoderma, leishmaniasis, leprosy, deep fungal infections, and cutaneous malignancy.

Orificial TB is a rare manifestation of cutaneous TB occurring usually in individuals who are debilitated or immunocompromised. It affects the mucocutaneous junctions of the orifices (nose, mouth, anus, urinary meatus, and genitals) and is caused by autoinoculation of tubercle bacilli from secretions. Lesions present as shallow, painful ulcers with a granulating base and undermined edges, with swelling, edema, and inflammation of the surrounding mucosa. Painful ulcers

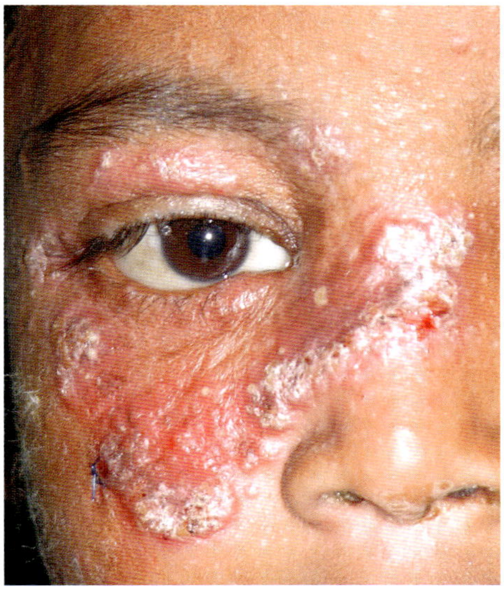

Fig. 14.36 Lupus vulgaris. This 7-year-old boy had an enlarging erythematous, infiltrative, scaly plaque of the nasal bridge, cheek, and periorbital region. Note the characteristic central scarring and peripheral activity. (Courtesy Venkatesh Ramesh, MD.)

of the mouth or other mucosal membranes in patients with visceral TB should arouse suspicion of this disorder. These patients are prone to progressive pulmonary, genitourinary, or gastrointestinal TB.

Miliary TB of the skin (tuberculosis cutis miliaris disseminata) is an extremely rare manifestation of fulminating pulmonary or meningeal TB. It is quite uncommon in children and in recent times is seen most often in the setting of adult HIV infection.[236,237] When present, the eruption is caused by hematogenous dissemination of *M. tuberculosis* to the skin in addition to multiple internal organs. Cutaneous lesions present as minute, symmetrically distributed, erythematous, red-brown macules, papules, or vesiculopustules. Purpuric lesions may occasionally be present. The course of miliary TB is usually fulminating and the mortality rate high.

Diagnostic options for cutaneous TB include smears, stains, and cultures of skin swabs, aspirates, and biopsy tissue. The Mantoux intradermal tuberculin test is commonly positive, but the reactivity does not correlate with disease activity.[232] Another screening test is the interferon gamma release assay (IGRA), which can be performed via the QuantiFERON TB Gold test or the T-SPOT.TB test. These tests, which quantify the release of interferon-γ in whole blood upon stimulation with *M. tuberculosis* antigens, have been demonstrated useful even in young children with latent or active TB and have the advantage of little to no effect of previous BCG vaccination on the results.[238,239] PCR amplification of *M. tuberculosis* DNA is a rapid, sensitive, and accurate technique for diagnosis and may be applied to paraffin-embedded skin biopsy tissue.[240,241] Any patient suspected of having cutaneous TB should be evaluated for active pulmonary disease with chest radiography, and HIV testing is also indicated.[242]

The treatment of all forms of cutaneous TB is similar to that used for active pulmonary TB. Current recommendations of the American Academy of Pediatrics include a 6-month regimen consisting of isoniazid, rifampin, ethambutol, and pyrazinamide for 2 months followed by 4 months of isoniazid and rifampin (with ethambutol or streptomycin added if drug resistance is a concern) or a 6-month regimen (for hilar adenopathy only) of isoniazid and rifampin.[243] Tuberculous meningitis is treated with a four-drug regimen for 2 months followed by isoniazid and rifampin for 7 to 10 more months.[243]

The Tuberculid Disorders

The tuberculid disorders are hypersensitivity reactions to *M. tuberculosis* and classically include erythema induratum, papulonecrotic tuberculid, and lichen scrofulosorum. Originally felt to be related to toxins or an allergic response to tubercle bacilli, they are now believed to be the result of hematogenous dissemination of organisms from an internal focus to the skin, where they incite a cutaneous inflammatory response. *Lupus miliaris disseminatus faciei* (formally described as a tuberculid) is probably more aptly described as a granulomatous disorder of the pilosebaceous units (see Chapter 8). A deep nodular form presenting on the lower extremities has been termed *nodular tuberculid* and seems to represent a hybrid between papulonecrotic tuberculid and erythema induratum.[244] The tuberculid disorders are notable for the usual absence of *M. tuberculosis* bacilli in skin biopsy (although PCR may occasionally be positive), positive tuberculin skin test, evidence of current or past TB, and response to anti-TB treatment regimens.[245] Once a tuberculid disorder has been diagnosed, a thorough evaluation for subclinical active TB should be initiated.[246]

Erythema induratum of Bazin is a chronic, recurring panniculitis (inflammation of the fat) that typically occurs on the calves of girls and young women. Although the association with TB has historically been controversial, the clinical and histopathologic features, ability to identify *M. tuberculosis* on PCR studies, and response to antituberculosis therapy seem to support a tuberculous etiology.[247–251] Lesions present as symmetric, tender, deep-seated nodules that develop into red-purple masses that tend to ulcerate (Fig. 14.37). The ulcers are irregular and shallow and heal with an atrophic scar. Erythema induratum tends to be chronic and recurrent; many patients have a personal or family history of TB. The tuberculin skin test is positive, but mycobacteria are seldom recovered from lesions by standard culture

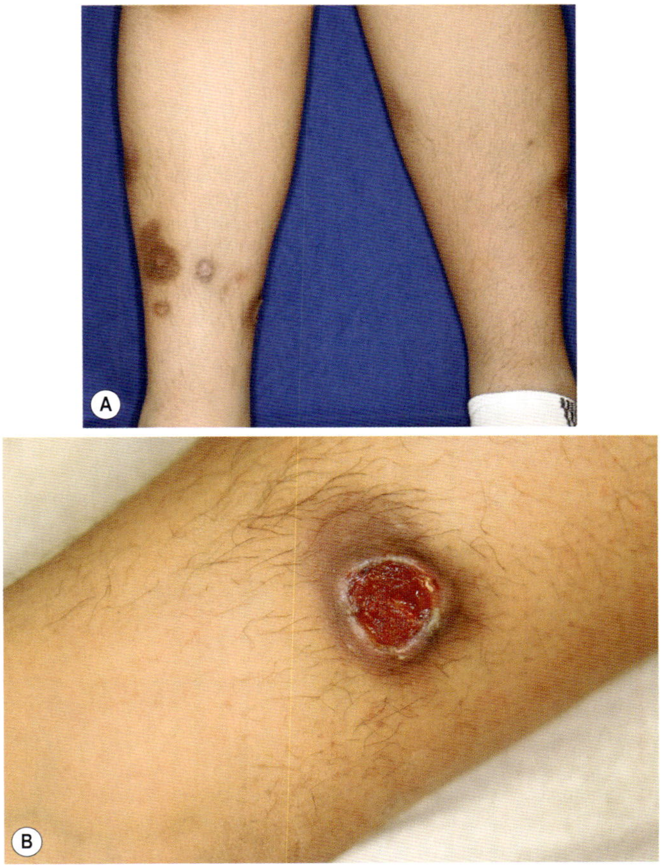

Fig. 14.37 Erythema induratum. This 14-year-old male patient had a 3-year history of recurrent indurated, violaceous, and hyperpigmented plaques **(A)** and nodules, some of which ulcerated **(B)**, located on the lower extremities. QuantiFERON gold was positive, histology revealed changes consistent with erythema induratum (and tissue cultures were negative), and he improved on quadruple antituberculous therapy. (Courtesy Duri Yun, MD, MPH.)

techniques. PCR analysis of skin biopsy specimens has been found to be rapid and sensitive in the diagnosis of this disorder.[249–251] Treatment of erythema induratum with combination antituberculous therapy is usually successful, although in untreated patients the lesions usually involute spontaneously over a period of years.

Papulonecrotic tuberculid is the most common tuberculid seen in children, although it is rarely seen in the United States. It is characterized by symmetric crops of dusky red, small papules and nodules with central necrosis or ulceration that crust and heal with superficial varioliform (smallpox-like) scarring.[252] Sites of predilection for papulonecrotic tuberculid include the extensor extremities (particularly the knees and elbows), the buttocks, and the lower trunk. Ear involvement may also be common, and pulmonary TB is usually present.[253] The lesions may clinically resemble those of varicella. As with erythema induratum, recovery of the organism from standard tissue culture is of low yield. Patients usually have a positive intradermal tuberculin skin-test reaction, and gene-amplification PCR performed on skin biopsy tissue is useful in confirming the diagnosis.[254] Papulonecrotic tuberculid usually responds promptly to antituberculous therapy. Simultaneous occurrence of papulonecrotic tuberculid and erythema induratum has been reported.[255]

Lichen scrofulosorum is characterized by clusters of lichenoid perifollicular papules on the trunk of children or young adults, usually in association with TB of lymph nodes, bones, and/or other organs or history of BCG vaccination.[256] Lesions are firm, 1- to 5-mm, flesh-colored to reddish-brown, flat-topped papules. Given its similarity to several other conditions, delay in diagnosis of lichen scrofulosorum is common.[257] The lesions tend to be asymptomatic and slowly resolve with antitubercular therapy.

Leprosy

Leprosy (Hansen disease) is a chronic infectious disorder of worldwide distribution in which the acid-fast bacillus *Mycobacterium leprae* has a special predilection for the skin and nervous system. Although the worldwide incidence of leprosy decreased significantly after the WHO recommendations for multidrug therapy (MDT), along with widespread BCG vaccination and public health initiatives, it is still somewhat prevalent in certain endemic areas, including India, Brazil, and Indonesia,[258] and the prevalence and incidence have plateaued since 2005.[259] Leprosy is rare in the United States, with around 85% of diagnosed cases occurring in immigrants, and the disease may mimic many common dermatologic and neurologic disorders.[260] It is considered one of the most important causes of peripheral neuropathy, with up to one-third of patients developing permanent nerve damage.[261]

Although there is no universal agreement on the classification of leprosy, the disorder is usually divided into several clinical subtypes depending on the patient's degree of cell-mediated immune response to *M. leprae* (Table 14.1). At one end of the spectrum is the lepromatous (LL) form of the disorder, the disfiguring disease most familiar to the public. In this variant patients are anergic to *M. leprae* and develop widespread disease involving the skin (Fig. 14.38), upper respiratory tract, sensory and motor nerves, eyes (superficial keratitis), testes, lymph nodes, and bone. Many bacilli are present in the tissues. Nodules or diffuse infiltrates, especially on the face and earlobes, produce the characteristic "leonine facies." Loss of eyebrows and eyelashes may also occur. At the opposite pole is tuberculoid leprosy (TT), a form that occurs in patients with a very high degree of immunity against *M. leprae*. In this variant, patients have only a single (or occasionally a few) large well-defined macule(s) or infiltrative plaques that show hypopigmentation and loss of sensation. The peripheral nerves, most commonly the ulnar, external popliteal, and great auricular nerves, are thickened and palpable, and patients may develop trophic disturbances and paralyses. Between these ends of the spectrum, borderline forms of the disorder are seen. Patients with borderline lepromatous leprosy tend to have the most extensive involvement of nerves. Due to the decreased sensation in affected areas, these patients are at risk for secondary infections and digital ulceration. Blindness occurs in around 5% of patients with leprosy.[262]

The incubation period of leprosy is typically very long and ranges from 3 months to 40 years (average, 2 to 4 years).[260] Early childhood disease often presents with solitary lesions that may occur on any exposed area of the skin, and childhood disease is most commonly indeterminate or at the tuberculoid end of the spectrum. The mode of transmission of leprosy remains unclear, although an upper respiratory route is suggested. Household contacts are the primary source of infection.[263]

Leprosy should be suspected in any patient from a leprosy-endemic area (or immigrants from such regions) who has chronic hypopigmented or infiltrative skin lesions, skin anesthesia, thickened nerves, or eye complaints. The diagnosis is confirmed by the identification of acid-fast bacilli in skin smears or biopsy material, and the histologic picture reveals a granulomatous infiltrate containing large foamy histiocytes (lepra cells) in the epidermis. Treatment should be directed by a clinician experienced in the care of patients with leprosy and preferably in a Hansen-disease center where feasible. Although therapeutic recommendations of the past called for monotherapy with dapsone, given increasing resistance to this approach, MDT is now recommended and includes other agents such as rifampin and clofazimine. In treated patients, 95% of all nerve function impairment develops within 2 years, supporting a decreased frequency for neurologic follow-up examination in patients without neurologic findings by that time.[264]

Leprosy reactions are fairly commonplace during treatment for the disease and are related to immune-mediated inflammation. They occur in 30% to 50% of patients.[265] These reactional states, which include reversal reactions (type 1 reactions) and erythema nodosum leprosum (ENL, type 2 reactions), may result in worsening of neural

Table 14.1 Classification of Leprosy (in Order of Decreasing Host Resistance)

Group	Clinical Features
Tuberculoid (TT) (mildest; high resistance)	A single or few localized anesthetic macules or plaques; hair loss within lesions; few, if any, organisms; peripheral nerve involvement common
Borderline tuberculoid* (BT)	Lesions similar to TT but more numerous; satellite papules around larger lesions (at times); hair and sensation diminished (but not absent) within lesions; peripheral nerve involvement common
Borderline borderline (BB)	Features of both TT and LL; more lesions than BT; borders vaguer; nerve involvement and satellite lesions common; many bacilli usually present
Borderline lepromatous (BL)	Multiple nonanesthetic, asymmetrically distributed annular plaques; may be surrounding papules; late neural lesions; leonine facies
Lepromatous (LL) (most severe; low or no resistance)	Generalized involvement (skin, mucous membranes, upper respiratory tract, reticuloendothelial system, adrenal glands, and testes); no neural lesions until late; no sensory or hair growth impairment; many bacilli in tissue
Indeterminate	Small number of hypopigmented macules; no thickened nerves or sensory impairment

*The three intermediate forms (BT, BB, and BL) are clinically unstable and may pass from milder to more severe states and vice versa.

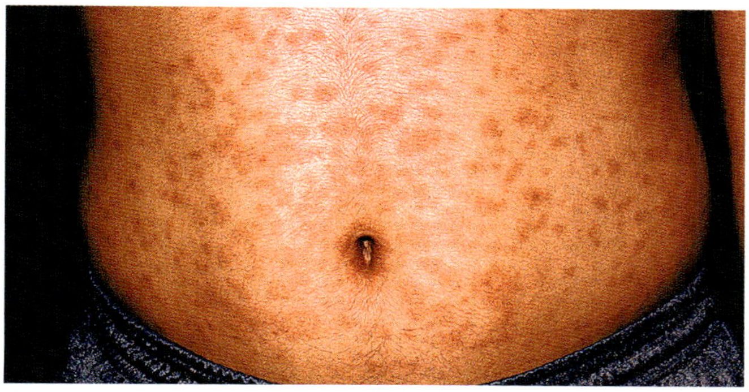

Fig. 14.38 Lepromatous leprosy. Erythematous, infiltrative patches and plaques that revealed many acid-fast bacilli in the skin biopsy specimen.

and skin lesions and significant tissue damage. These reactions are often treated with systemic corticosteroids, and in the case of ENL, thalidomide is a very effective agent.[266] Although there is no effective vaccination for leprosy, BCG vaccination has been demonstrated to be effective at protecting some populations from infection.[260,267]

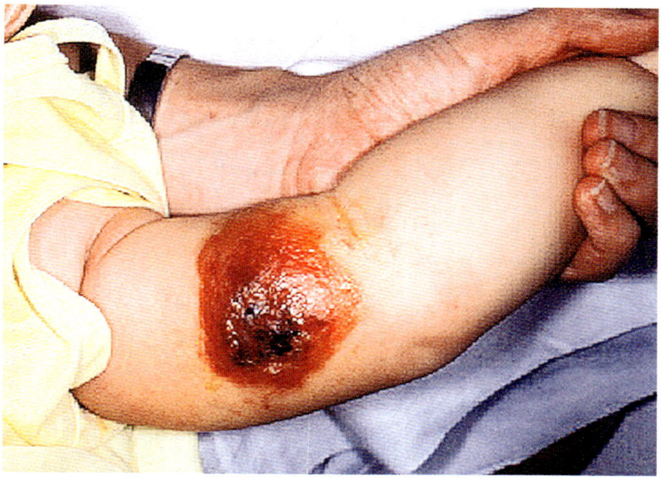

Fig. 14.39 Cutaneous anthrax in a child. Erythematous plaque with necrosis and eschar formation in a 7-month-old male. Anthrax bacilli were detected in biopsy tissue. (Reprinted with permission from Roche KJ, Chang MW, Lazarus H. Images in clinical medicine: Cutaneous anthrax infection. N Engl J Med. 2001;345(22):1611. © 2001, Massachusetts Medical Society. All rights reserved.)

Anthrax

Anthrax, an infection caused by the Gram-positive *Bacillus anthracis*, is occasionally transmitted to humans through contact with infected animals or animal products such as hides or wool. Whereas this mode of infection usually results in cutaneous anthrax, inhalation disease ("woolsorters' disease") has occurred in settings such as factories where processing of these products takes place.[268] Anthrax has long been considered a potential agent of biologic warfare, the significance of which was magnified by the events of September 11, 2001, and the following apparent bioterrorism involving the spread of *B. anthracis* via bioengineered spore-containing letters within the US postal system. These events highlight the importance of adequate education in and recognition of this infection and other potential biologic weapons of mass destruction. Some of the other potential "category A" biologic agents (those which pose the greatest risk due to easy dissemination and high mortality and which require special public health preparedness) include *Yersinia pestis* (plague), smallpox, *Francisella tularensis* (tularemia), botulinum toxin from *Clostridium botulinum* (botulism), and several viral hemorrhagic fevers.[269]

Clinical infection with *B. anthracis* usually takes one of three forms: inhalational, cutaneous, or gastrointestinal. The cutaneous form (malignant pustule) is responsible for 95% of the cases in the United States and is usually an occupational disease of farmers, butchers, veterinarians, and individuals who process animal products.[270] The spore is introduced via an abrasion or cut in the skin and develops into the primary lesion, which is a painless, pruritic papule. This papule progresses to develop small surrounding vesicles surrounded by a brawny, nonpitting edema. The vesicles rupture with the development of necrosis, and eventually a black eschar forms (Fig. 14.39) and overlies an ulcer. Nonnecrotic ulcerations may also be the presenting feature, as was observed in a patient affected by the 2001 terrorism attacks, and lesions may be solitary or multiple.[271] Low-grade fever, malaise, and headache are often present, and regional lymphadenopathy early in the course is common. Without therapy, this form is fatal in 20% of cases.[272] Cutaneous anthrax is rare in children and may be accompanied by anthrax meningitis or systemic spread of disease. Microangiopathic hemolytic anemia, hyponatremia, and coagulopathy were reported in a 7-month-old infant with cutaneous infection.[273]

Gastrointestinal anthrax forms after ingestion of undercooked meat from infected animals. In this case, the characteristic eschar forms in the gastrointestinal tract, usually the terminal ileum or cecum, and patients experience fever, nausea, vomiting, and anorexia. Severe abdominal pain (presenting as an acute abdomen), bloody diarrhea, sepsis, and death may ensue, with a mortality rate greater than 50%.

Inhalational anthrax is the most severe form of infection and is traditionally associated with a very high (>95%) mortality rate. Patients initially experience flu-like symptoms and progress to dyspnea, stridor, fever, and cyanosis. Meningitis, coma, and death may ensue.

The diagnosis of anthrax can be confirmed by Gram stain and culture of a skin lesion, CSF, or blood. Confirmatory studies are usually performed in a reference laboratory. Nasal swabs are used epidemiologically but are not a reliable method of diagnosis.[268,272] Serologic testing is useful for surveillance and confirmation of infection and requires acute and convalescent samples. A variety of real-time PCR assays exist for detection of *B. anthracis*, and an ultra-sensitive nanoparticle immunoassay has been developed.[274,275] Histopathologic examination of a skin biopsy specimen may also be useful, especially with the concomitant use of a tissue Gram stain.

Penicillin has been the drug of choice for anthrax for many decades, with penicillin resistance found only rarely in naturally occurring strains. Other antimicrobials with good activity against *B. anthracis* include ciprofloxacin, tetracyclines, macrolides, clindamycin, and cephalosporins. Some of these other agents may be more concentrated in the phagocyte and therefore may be more desirable.[276] The treatment of choice for bioterrorism-associated anthrax, however, is ciprofloxacin or doxycycline, even in children.[277] Postexposure prophylaxis is recommended in situations where there is a credible threat of exposure and includes 10 days of antimicrobial prophylaxis to local populations, as guided by the Centers for Disease Control and Prevention (CDC), followed by an additional 50 days of antibiotics and initiation of a three-dose anthrax vaccine series for those found to have had clear and significant exposure.[277]

Cat-Scratch Disease

Cat-scratch disease (CSD) is an acute, self-limited infection of children and young adults caused by the pleomorphic Gram-negative bacillus *Bartonella henselae*. *Bartonella* species, which are Gram-negative bacilli, result in a variety of diseases in humans, including Carrión disease, prolonged fever of unknown origin, encephalopathy, ocular disease, trench fever, and endocarditis. CSD is a benign cause of lymphadenitis in children and is usually transmitted from infected kittens to humans by means of a scratch or bite that is often recalled only in retrospect.[278] The domesticated house cat is the most important natural reservoir for *B. henselae*, and stray cats and kittens are more likely to be infected than are pet or adult cats, respectively.[279] It is estimated that up to half of domestic cats have antibodies to *B. henselae*, testing seropositive for the bacteria.[280] This organism has also been linked to bacillary angiomatosis (see Chapter 12), a vascular proliferative disease seen most commonly in individuals infected with HIV. CSD is most common in areas with warm climates and occurs most often in the fall and winter.[281] CSD is transmitted to humans via scratches and possibly bites from reservoir cats, and it is most common in children between 5 and 9 years of age.[282]

The most common clinical presentation of CSD is lymphadenopathy proximal to the site of a cat scratch or bite. However, the infection actually typically begins with a small papule or nodule within the original cat scratch line 3 to 10 days after the trauma. Over the following 1 to 2 weeks, the regional lymph nodes draining the region begin to enlarge (Fig. 14.40), reaching the point of maximal enlargement around 1 month after the initial injury.[283] Often the initial wound at the site of contact with the animal has resolved by the time the patient pursues medical care. The enlarged lymph nodes gradually decrease in size over a period of a few months in the absence of therapy. In up to 10% of patients, lymph nodes become erythematous and fluctuant, occasionally requiring needle aspiration.[281] In 85% of patients, only a single lymph node is involved.[280] Common locations for the lymphadenopathy of CSD include the neck, axillary, and inguinal regions.[284] In one large series, the most common sites of lymphadenopathy (in order of decreasing incidence) were the axilla, epitrochlear region, cervical region, submandibular region, and groin.[285] Biopsy of lymph nodes, when performed, reveals granulomas with multiple microabscesses.

Other features that may be present in patients with CSD include fever, headache, and malaise. *Parinaud oculoglandular syndrome* consists of unilateral granulomatous conjunctivitis with concomitant ipsilateral preauricular lymphadenopathy at the site of inoculation and represents the most common form of atypical CSD. This presentation appears to occur as a result of indirect inoculation of the organism into the eye rather than by direct contact through a cat scratch, as is typical of CSD. Other less common associations include neuroretinitis (presenting as acute-onset unilateral vision loss), encephalopathy/encephalitis, endocarditis, seizures, generalized lymphadenopathy, or prolonged fever. Bony involvement may present with osteomyelitis and may include lytic lesions of the cortex and/or inflammation of the marrow.[286] Immunocompromised individuals with *B. henselae* infection may develop a disseminated, invasive form of infection that involves multiple organs. *Bacillary peliosis* is the term used to describe reticuloendothelial organ involvement including the liver (peliosis hepatis), spleen, abdominal lymph nodes, and bone marrow.[281]

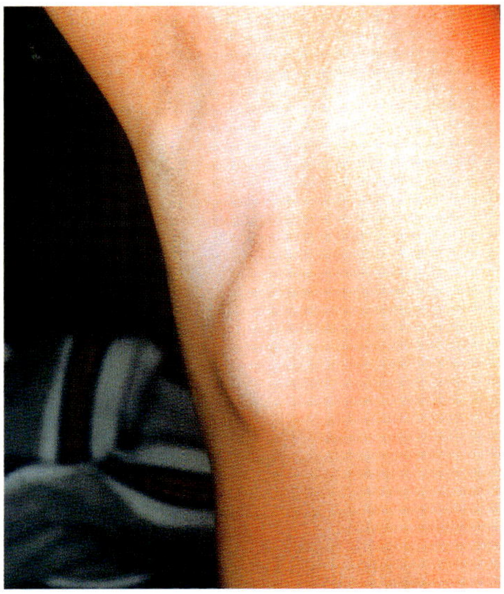

Fig. 14.40 Cat-scratch disease. Axillary lymphadenopathy in a 2-year-old boy with a crusted red papule at the primary inoculation site on the chest.

CSD is usually diagnosed based on the characteristic clinical presentation in combination with a history of recent contact with a cat. Diagnostic confirmation is provided by positive serologic studies for antibodies to *B. henselae* (an IgG antibody titer between 1:64 and 1:256 may suggest past or acute infection, and a titer >1:256 is consistent with acute infection).[287] Serology remains the most practical diagnostic tool for the laboratory detection of *B. henselae* infection.[280] Blood and tissue can be cultured, but the organism is slow growing and may be difficult to isolate. Identification of the organism in tissue samples stained with the Warthin–Starry silver stain lends further support to the diagnosis and may be useful in some settings. The most sensitive test available is *B. henselae* DNA sequence detection via PCR (applied to tissue or body fluids), but this modality is not readily available.[283]

Treatment of CSD in the immunocompetent host with uncomplicated disease is not always necessary, as it is a self-limited disease and studies demonstrating a significant advantage of therapy are lacking. However, treatment may shorten the period of symptomatic illness and may promote more rapid resolution of the clinical abnormalities.[283] *B. henselae* has been demonstrated to be susceptible to a variety of antimicrobial agents, including azithromycin (the recommendation of many clinician-researchers), clarithromycin, rifampin, doxycycline, ciprofloxacin, gentamicin, and trimethoprim-sulfamethoxazole. Disease in immunocompromised patients may be more serious, and thus antimicrobial therapy is usually recommended for at least 6 weeks, up to several months.[278,287] Surgical removal of lymph nodes is generally not indicated except in rare patients in whom the diagnosis is in doubt, in whom repeated aspirations fail to relieve pain, or in whom the inflammatory process persists without involution.

Disorders Resulting from Fungus-Like Bacteria

Actinomycosis and nocardiosis are disorders caused by actinomycetes, which are Gram-positive organisms that may resemble fungi both microscopically and macroscopically. Although these infections can occur at any age, they most often occur in adults. Although primary skin infection is rare, involvement of the cutaneous and subcutaneous tissues may result from contiguous spread from other sites or secondary infection of traumatized or injured skin, particularly in debilitated or immunodeficient individuals.

ACTINOMYCOSIS

Actinomycosis is a chronic suppurative infection caused by *Actinomyces israelii*, an anaerobic Gram-positive saprophyte of the tonsillar crypts, carious teeth, and female genital tract, and rarely by other *Actinomyces* species. Given their presence as normal flora, these organisms only become virulent when there is compromise of the mucous membranes or local ischemia.[288] Infection is often associated with dental procedures, trauma, or surgery.[289] This disorder is clinically characterized by the production of "sulfur granules" (1- to 2-mm aggregates of organisms surrounded by polymorphonuclear leukocytes with organisms in a radial arrangement around the periphery) from multiple draining sinuses.[290] It tends to occur in one of three areas: the cervicofacial region (most common), lungs, or intestinal tract. Some patients have mixed-organ involvement that may include the skin, brain, pericardium, and extremities.[291] Cervicofacial actinomycosis, seen most often in individuals with poor oral hygiene and carious teeth, begins when the infecting organism invades a traumatized oral mucous membrane. This form presents as soft-tissue swelling, usually over the mandibular region. It increases to form a brawny, erythematous nodule that discharges serosanguineous or purulent material through multiple sinus tracts, from which the characteristic sulfur-yellow granules consisting of masses of organisms can be demonstrated. Destruction of bone with periostitis and osteomyelitis may occur, and absence of regional lymph node involvement is characteristic.

Aspiration of the organism causes pulmonary infection that progresses through the pleura, causing draining sinus tracts of the chest wall. It may occur after esophageal disruption during surgery or nonpenetrating trauma, or may occur as a manifestation of extension of cervicofacial infection.[292] The abdominal form develops from the ileum, cecum, or appendix (in association with appendicitis) and is seen as draining sinuses, tracts, or subcutaneous abscesses extending to either the abdominal wall or the perineum. Primary infection of other body sites may affect the urinary tract, central nervous system (CNS), bones, and joints. A localized form, known as *mycetoma*, occurs most commonly on the feet or ankles of individuals who walk around barefoot (see Chapter 17).

Actinomycosis is diagnosed by isolation and identification of the causative organism in anaerobic culture. It may also be confirmed by observation of the highly characteristic sulfur granules (groups of delicate filaments, often with club-shaped ends) in purulent or biopsied materials. The course of actinomycosis is prolonged and characterized by closure of one sinus tract and the opening of another. Treatment is with intravenous penicillin G or ampicillin for 4 to 6 weeks followed by oral penicillin in high doses for 6 to 12 months.[292] Cervicofacial disease can sometimes be managed with oral therapy from the beginning of treatment. Surgical incision and drainage of abscesses and excision of fibrotic, avascular tissue are occasionally necessary. Alternative antibiotics for patients allergic to penicillin include tetracyclines, erythromycin, or clindamycin.

NOCARDIOSIS

Nocardiosis is a severe, primarily pulmonary infection caused by an aerobic Gram-positive, partially acid-fast, fungus-like filamentous bacteria, *Nocardia asteroides*. It is less often caused by *Nocardia braziliensis* or other species. Nocardiosis primarily affects men in the 30- to 50-year-old age group, although it has been increasingly recognized in infants and children. Disseminated disease has a significant morbidity and mortality and is more likely in immunosuppressed hosts. The organism is found worldwide in various environments, including water, dust, soil and decaying vegetation.

Nocardiosis may occur with several different presentations, including pulmonary, systemic, CNS, and skin/soft-tissue forms. It generally occurs through inhalation of contaminated dust, and the clinical picture is usually that of a primary pulmonary disease that resembles TB in its clinical and radiographic findings. These primary pulmonary infections may result in blood vessel erosion with subsequent hematogenous dissemination to other organs, including the skin. In those instances in which the skin is involved ($<15\%$ of cases), the most common lesions are abscesses of the chest wall with granulomatous lesions surrounding draining sinuses.[293] Primary cutaneous or subcutaneous nocardiosis is usually the result of traumatic implantation of foreign objects into the skin and often presents in immunocompetent hosts.[289,294] Once inoculated into the skin, it may present in a lymphocutaneous syndrome mimicking sporotrichosis, as a cellulitis-like picture, or as a mycetoma (large, draining mass).[295] Disorders that may predispose an individual to invasive disease include chronic granulomatous disease, organ transplantation, HIV infection, or diseases requiring long-term systemic steroid therapy; individuals who have received tumor necrosis factor inhibitors (particularly infliximab) are also at increased risk.[296] It is estimated that around one-third of total cases of nocardiosis in resource-rich settings occurs in transplant recipients, most notably after allogeneic hematopoietic stem cell transplantation.[297]

Nocardiosis should be considered in obscure pulmonary and meningeal syndromes and chronic suppurative disorders of the bones or skin. The diagnosis is established by the presence of organisms in smears or cultures of sputum, aspirated material collected from lesions, or biopsy material. Unfortunately, the diagnosis is seldom established until the disease is far advanced, given the slow growth rate of the organism. Molecular methods, such as 16S rRNA gene sequence analysis, can identify the organism to the species level.[296] The cornerstone of therapy for nocardiosis is sulfonamides (alone or as trimethoprim-sulfamethoxazole). Imipenem, meropenem, third-generation cephalosporins, amoxicillin clavulanate, amikacin, minocycline, and fluoroquinolones may be other options.[295,296] The overall mortality rate of nocardiosis is around 25% and is highest in those patients who have pulmonary involvement and those with immunocompromise.[298]

Treponemal Infections

SYPHILIS

Syphilis is an infectious disease caused by the spirochetal organism *Treponema pallidum*. It is transmitted primarily by sexual contact, with the next most common mode being vertical transmission across the placenta, which may result in congenital syphilis (see Chapter 2). Transmission via oral sex is possible if the infected partner has lesions on the oral mucosa.[299] After a steady decline in the number of cases of syphilis in the early 1970s, the incidence has fluctuated, with peaks and troughs occurring in approximately 10-year cycles, with the overall trend being toward increasing rates, especially in men who have sex with men (MSM).[300,301] Syphilis continues to be an important health problem throughout the world and, left untreated, may result in long-term neurologic, cardiovascular, and other systemic sequelae, as well as congenital syphilis in offspring of infected mothers. Some 15% to 40% of untreated patients develop recognizable late complications.[302] Currently more than 60% of new cases of syphilis occur in MSM (and in 2013, 75% of all primary and secondary syphilis occurred in MSM), and the HIV coinfection rate is high (up to 60% in some geographic locations) among patients with syphilis in the United States.[301–304] Importantly, syphilis infection increases the likelihood of acquiring and transmitting HIV.

Untreated acquired syphilis is characterized by a series of clinical stages that are summarized in Table 14.2. There may be considerable overlap of symptoms in the various stages, and the early stages may pass by undiagnosed. The incubation period for syphilis ranges from 5 to 90 days. Patients with early syphilis (primary, secondary, and the first year of latent syphilis) are considered infectious. The late latent (after the first year) and late (tertiary) stages, conversely, are considered noninfectious, rarely relapse, and tend to be destructive and scarring.

Primary syphilis usually manifests as a single, painless genital papule or, more commonly, ulcer (chancre), occurring on the labia or vaginal wall in females and the glans penis (see Fig. 14.41) in males. In homosexual men, anorectal ulcers are most common. Chancres

Table 14.2 Clinical Stages of Syphilis

Stage	Clinical Manifestations
PRIMARY	
	Painless papule or ulcer at site of inoculation Regional lymphadenopathy
SECONDARY	
	Generalized macular/papular rash, involves palms/soles Condylomata lata in intertriginous areas Mucous patches (oral cavity and/or genital tract) Patchy hair loss Constitutional symptoms (malaise, headache, low-grade fever) Occasional aseptic meningitis
LATENT	
	No symptoms, but specific antibody tests positive
TERTIARY (LATE)	
Cardiovascular	Aortic aneurysm (especially ascending aorta), AI, CAD
Neurosyphilis	CVA, paresis, psychiatric symptoms, ataxia, autonomic dysfunction, numbness, cranial nerve palsies, optic neuritis, dementia Tabes dorsalis: abrupt, severe radicular pain; ataxia; areflexia
Gumma	Inflammatory infiltrates in multiple organs, especially skin and bones

AI, Aortic valve insufficiency; *CAD*, coronary artery disease; *CVA*, cerebrovascular accident.

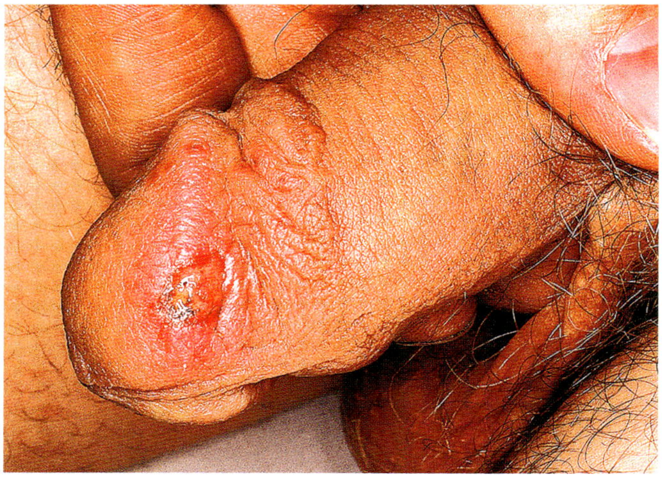

Fig. 14.41 Primary syphilis. Eroded chancre of the glans penis in a male with primary infection.

may occasionally be multiple, painful, purulent, or destructive.[305] Painless regional lymphadenopathy is often present, although there may occasionally be tenderness to palpation. The differential diagnosis of the primary syphilitic chancre includes other sexually transmitted diseases, including herpes simplex virus infection and chancroid (caused by *Haemophilus ducreyi*), which both tend to be differentiated by painful ulcers, as well as trauma, fixed drug eruptions, and Behcet disease.[306] Extragenital ulcers occur rarely in primary syphilis and when present occur most commonly on the fingers, tongue borders, or anus. If left untreated, the ulcer of primary syphilis heals spontaneously over 4 to 6 weeks.

Secondary syphilis develops 2 to 8 weeks after exposure in untreated individuals and is more common in females given the increased number of asymptomatic or undiagnosed primary lesions compared with men.[307] The primary chancre may still be present at the time of diagnosis of secondary syphilis. The classic cutaneous findings of this stage are characterized by a widespread macular and papular skin eruption that may occasionally be follicular or pustular. Examination reveals pink to erythematous, slightly scaly macules and papules that often involve the palms and soles, as well as flanks and arms. In dark-skinned individuals, the lesions tend to be hyperpigmented. The palm and sole lesions may appear as macular or hyperkeratotic red-brown papules or plaques (Fig. 14.42) and are often helpful in the differentiation between secondary syphilis and the primary differential diagnosis, pityriasis rosea. Other entities in the differential diagnosis include drug eruption, lichen planus, acute

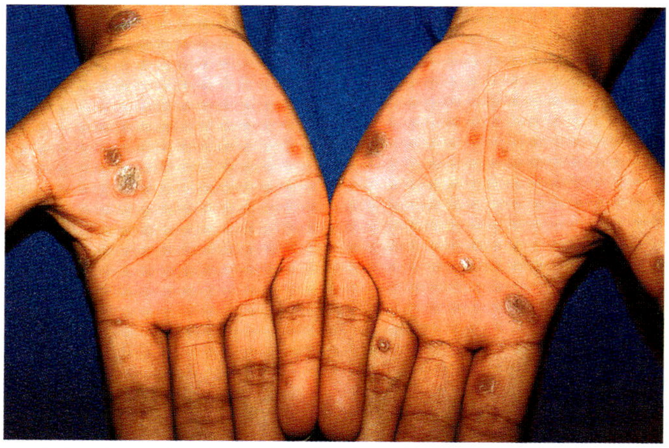

Fig. 14.42 Secondary syphilis. Crusted, hyperkeratotic, erythematous papules and plaques of the palms.

exanthems, tinea versicolor, sarcoidosis, Mucha–Habermann disease (pityriasis lichenoides), nummular eczema, and psoriasis.

Other mucocutaneous lesions seen in secondary syphilis include alopecia, mucous patches, and condyloma lata. Patchy alopecia may be present in up to 7% of patients and classically has a "moth-eaten" appearance. Mucous patches occur on the tongue, buccal mucosa, and lips and present as erythematous patches, often with associated erosion and a silvery-gray membrane. Condylomata lata are smooth, gray plaques found in warm and moist intertriginous zones in up to 20% of patients. These lesions are highly infectious and must be differentiated from genital warts (condylomata acuminata).

Systemic symptoms may also be present and include fever, headache, malaise, pharyngitis, and arthralgias. Ocular inflammatory conditions (including episcleritis, keratitis, and uveitis) may occur, as may aseptic meningitis, painless lymphadenopathy (especially epitrochlear), and hepatitis. A particularly aggressive form, termed *lues-maligna*, has been observed most often in the population infected with HIV.[308]

Cutaneous lesions of secondary syphilis usually heal without scarring, even in the absence of therapy, within 2 to 10 weeks. Residual hyperpigmentation or hypopigmentation may be present. Residual hypopigmentation on the skin of the neck has been termed the *necklace of Venus* (leukoderma colli).

Latent syphilis is a stage of the disease during which there are no clinical signs or symptoms or during which there are mild but generally unrecognized nonspecific symptoms such as malaise, anorexia, headache, sore throat, arthralgia, and low-grade fever. A diagnosis of latent syphilis is usually established on the basis of a positive serologic test after other stages of syphilis have been ruled out by physical and CSF examination. This stage is arbitrarily divided into early latent syphilis (occurring within 1 year of infection) and late latent syphilis (occurring after 1 year). Patients with early latent syphilis are considered to be infectious.

Tertiary (late) syphilis is divided into late benign syphilis (gumma), neurosyphilis, and cardiovascular syphilis (see Table 14.2). It appears in around 10% to 40% of untreated patients and after a latent period of 3 to 30 years or longer. Tertiary syphilis is extremely rare in children.

The hallmark lesions of late benign syphilis are the "gummas," and the skin is one of the most common organs of involvement, other common sites being the bone and liver. The cutaneous lesions present as superficial nodules or noduloulcerative plaques that may result in punched-out ulcers. Common sites of involvement include the extremities, face, scalp, sternum, and the sternoclavicular joints. Upon healing, hyperpigmentation and atrophic scarring may persist. When the palate or nasal mucosa is affected, destruction is often pronounced and may lead to perforation of the affected areas. Large gummas may have several perforations, and as the intervening bridges of skin break down and necrose, lesions tend to produce arched or scalloped margins with arciform and geographic patterns. Bone lesions occurring in this stage are marked by periostitis involving the cranial bones, tibia, and clavicle and present with nocturnal pain and local swelling.[300]

The diagnosis of syphilis depends on the combined findings from history, clinical examination, tissue examination, and serologic studies. *T. pallidum* cannot be cultured. Dark-field microscopy (on lesion exudate, nasal discharge, or tissue) is the gold-standard diagnostic method for primary syphilis, although it is not always readily available. Direct fluorescent antibody testing for *T. pallidum* has also been described for the diagnosis of primary syphilis. Both of these approaches, however, have been supplanted by serologic diagnostic methods, which are also the mainstay of laboratory diagnosis for secondary, latent, and tertiary syphilis. PCR-based testing is available but not yet in widespread use in the United States.

Serologic tests, which provide only indirect evidence of infection, are divided into nontreponemal and treponemal categories. The nontreponemal tests detect an antibody against cardiolipin that is present in the sera of many patients with syphilis. These examinations include the Venereal Disease Reference Laboratory (VDRL) slide test and the Rapid Plasma Reagin (RPR) card test. These examinations are inexpensive, rapid, and convenient but may result in false-positive reactions (i.e., with advanced age, malignancies, Lyme disease, chronic liver disease, pregnancy, systemic lupus erythematosus, and some viral or bacterial infections) and are limited in their sensitivity. The treponemal tests include fluorescent treponemal antibody absorption

(FTA-ABS), the *T. pallidum* chemiluminescent assay (TP-CIA), the *T. pallidum* enzyme immunoassay (TP-EIA), and *T. pallidum* particle agglutination (TP-PA) tests.[309] Treponemal tests measure specific antibodies formed by the host in response to infection with *T. pallidum*. They have a higher sensitivity and specificity than nontreponemal tests and are used as confirmation of diagnosis. Treponemal tests establish the high likelihood of a treponemal infection either at the present time or at some time in the past.[310]

Parenteral penicillin G benzathine is the mainstay of treatment for all forms of syphilis, with dosing regimens and duration of therapy varying based on stage of disease and the clinical manifestations that are present.[309] In patients with penicillin allergy, doxycycline, tetracycline, ceftriaxone, or azithromycin are potential alternatives.[311,312] The treatment of choice for congenital syphilis or neurosyphilis is aqueous crystalline penicillin G.[309] Patients under therapy for syphilis are generally assessed for response to therapy by serial quantitative nontreponemal tests. Patients with neurosyphilis require very close follow-up clinical and intermittent CSF examinations for at least the first 2 years after diagnosis.

PINTA

The endemic treponematoses are nonvenereal infections closely related to syphilis and include pinta, yaws, and bejel (endemic syphilis). The former two are briefly discussed here.

Pinta, a nonvenereal treponemal infection caused by *T. pallidum* subspecies *carateum*, occurs almost exclusively among the dark-skinned population of Central and South America (especially Mexico and Colombia) and Cuba.[313] Given the influx of migrants and refugees from Latin America in recent years, pinta should be considered in the differential diagnosis when clinically relevant.[314] It is transmitted by direct contact and is often seen in children of affected parents. Although transmission by insects is possible, this mode of exposure is considered to be exceedingly rare. Pinta is the only spirochetal disease that results in purely cutaneous manifestations.

There are three basic forms of pinta, termed *primary*, *secondary*, and *late*. The primary stage, seen on uncovered areas such as the face, arms, and legs, begins 1 to 8 weeks after inoculation as red papules that enlarge into oval or round erythematous scaly plaques measuring up to 10 cm in diameter. Small papules often become surrounded by satellite macules or papules that coalesce to form configurative patterns. Regional lymphadenopathy is common. After several months to years, secondary lesions (referred to as *pintids*) appear as small, scaly papules that coalesce into large, scaly plaques. Their color is initially red to violaceous, with progression to a slate-blue, brown, gray, or black hue.[315] In this stage, widespread involvement is present with coalescence of lesions. The differential diagnosis may include psoriasis, eczema, tinea corporis, syphilis, or leprosy. Lesions of primary and secondary pinta are highly infectious.

The late phase develops in 3 to 10 years and is characterized by irregular pigmentation with a range of different shades (correlating with the site of deposition of melanin in the dermis), resulting in a spotted and highly characteristic appearance. These lesions have an insidious onset, usually during adolescence or young adulthood, and are eventually replaced by depigmented patches closely resembling vitiligo. The most common sites of involvement are the bony prominences, including the wrists, elbows, and ankles. Periarticular skin atrophy and extensor surface hyperkeratosis is also common during this phase.[316]

The diagnosis of pinta is made by identification of *T. carateum* on dark-field examination or, more commonly, serologic testing. The serologic studies utilized for the diagnosis of pinta are the same as those utilized for venereal syphilis, and these diseases are immunologically and serologically indistinguishable.[317] Penicillin is the treatment of choice, with options similar to those of syphilis for patients with penicillin allergy.

YAWS

Yaws, caused by *T. pallidum* subspecies *pertenue*, is a nonvenereal treponemal disease endemic in many tropical regions that typically begins in childhood (usually before puberty). It is also transmitted by direct skin contact (nonsexual) and has been divided into primary, secondary, and tertiary stages. The primary stage is characterized by an erythematous papule that occurs within 2 to 4 weeks at the site of inoculation (the "mother yaw"), usually the legs, feet, or buttocks. It enlarges and becomes confluent with surrounding satellite nodules, with eventual ulceration. This stage is occasionally accompanied by constitutional symptoms, arthralgias, and lymphadenopathy. Spontaneous healing of the skin lesion eventually occurs with scarring, although it may take up to 6 months.[318]

Weeks to months after the primary lesion, secondary yaws occurs, presenting as smaller, widespread cutaneous papules ("daughter" yaws or framboesias) that tend to occur adjacent to body orifices. These lesions ulcerate and secrete infectious treponemes. This stage is characterized also by palmoplantar lesions, bone involvement, lymphadenopathy, and occasional neurologic and ophthalmologic abnormalities. Hyperkeratotic involvement of the palms and soles with painful fissuring is common. The latter may cause patients to walk on the sides of their feet, producing a characteristic gait known as *crab yaws*. If not treated in its early stages, yaws may become a chronic infection with frequent relapses and severe disfigurement with permanent bony deformities.[319]

Although the disorder generally terminates with the secondary stage, 10% of patients develop a late tertiary stage in which gummatous lesions occur. These lesions, which present 5 to 10 years after inoculation, may be locally destructive and lead to skin ulceration as well as deforming bone and joint sequelae. Late neurologic or ophthalmologic manifestations may occasionally present during the tertiary stage, but are not typical.

Yaws is usually diagnosed based on the characteristic clinical findings in an endemic region combined with dark-field microscopy or serologic studies. Again, the same serologic examinations used to diagnose venereal syphilis and pinta are utilized. Newer PCR-based diagnostic assays have been developed.[320] Treatment options include long-acting penicillin (benzathine penicillin), azithromycin, and tetracycline. Mass treatment of at-risk populations with a single dose of azithromycin has been part of the WHO strategy at yaws eradication and has been demonstrated effective.[321,322]

LYME DISEASE

Lyme disease is the most common vector-borne disease in the United States. It was first recognized in southeastern Connecticut in 1975 and is an immune-mediated multisystem disorder caused by the spirochete *Borrelia burgdorferi* sensu stricto. Lyme disease is transmitted by *Ixodes* species ticks, primarily *Ixodes scapularis* (the deer tick), in the United States. It occurs most commonly in areas where deer ticks are abundant and *B. burgdorferi* carriage is common, especially the coastal northeastern, mid-Atlantic, and northern central regions of the United States (in particular Wisconsin and Minnesota), as well as much of Europe and Northern Asia.[323] Lyme disease is rare in the Pacific states because of the low infection rate of *Ixodes pacificus* (the Western black-legged tick) with *B. burgdorferi*.[324] When cases occur in the western states, they are most common in northern California and Oregon. The geographic distribution of Lyme disease is expanding, and it is now considered endemic in Virginia.[325] In Europe, the vector is most often *Ixodes ricinus*, and the pathogenic *Borrelia* species are *Borrelia afzelii* and *Borrelia garinii*.[326] There is a bimodal age distribution of Lyme disease, with the initial peak occurring in children between the ages of 5 and 14 years.

Several factors are associated with the risk of transmission of *B. burgdorferi* from ticks to humans. Because organisms often remain dormant in the tick until multiplication and migration occur during feeding, the risk of transmission is low if the tick is removed within 24 hours of attachment. In addition, the proportion of infected ticks varies according to geographic location, and hence the risk of disease is low outside of endemic regions. The highest probability of transmission of infection occurs 48 to 72 hours after the onset of attachment.[327]

The clinical findings of Lyme disease were originally described as occurring in three stages, although now they are generally divided into two stages: early (divided into early localized or early disseminated) and late (Table 14.3). These correspond to the traditional stages I, II, and III. The onset of clinical manifestations usually occurs from 3 days to 4 weeks after the tick bite. However, because of the

Table 14.3 Clinical Manifestations of Lyme Disease

Stage of Disease	Clinical Findings
Early localized (stage I)	Erythema migrans (single) Constitutional symptoms (headache, myalgias, arthralgias, fatigue, fever) Lymphadenopathy
Early disseminated (stage II)	Erythema migrans (multiple) Lymphadenopathy Constitutional symptoms (headache, myalgias, arthralgias, fatigue, fever) Neurologic: facial (occasionally sixth) nerve palsy, meningitis, other neuropathies Cardiac: atrioventricular conduction defects, congestive heart failure, myocarditis, pericarditis Rheumatologic: arthritis
Late (stage III)	Neurologic: encephalopathy, encephalomyelitis, peripheral neuropathy Rheumatologic: arthritis Cutaneous: Borrelial lymphocytoma (aka lymphocytoma cutis, lymphadenosis benigna cutis), acrodermatitis chronica atrophicans

small pencil-point size of the *Ixodes* tick, only about 30% of patients recall having had a tick bite.

Early Localized Lyme Disease (Stage I)

The earliest manifestation of Lyme disease is usually a single skin lesion termed *erythema migrans (EM)*. It is felt that at this stage the spirochetal infection is restricted to the skin in most patients. EM begins with a red papule at the site of the bite and progresses to become a flat, erythematous patch. With peripheral expansion, there may be central clearing (although this appears to be much less commonly seen in the United States compared with Europe),[328] resulting in an annular patch (Fig. 14.43). This lesion usually is nonpalpable, and it is most commonly asymptomatic. Occasional variations include vesicular, urticarial, scaly, and purpuric presentations.[329] Systemic symptoms may be present and include fatigue, fever, chills, headache, myalgias, and arthralgias. Lymphadenopathy may also occur. Although EM may occur anywhere on the cutaneous surface, the thighs, groin, and axillae are particularly common sites of involvement. The lesions can be differentiated from those of tinea corporis and nummular eczema by rapid peripheral expansion, lack of scaling, and lack of pruritus. Other entities in the differential diagnosis may include cellulitis, contact dermatitis, arthropod bite hypersensitivity, or erythema multiforme.[328] The eruption of EM resolves spontaneously over several weeks even without therapy. Multiple EM lesions may be seen and usually correlate with spirochetemia and disseminated disease (see the following section).

Early Disseminated Lyme Disease (Stage II)

As the organism disseminates, patients may show additional signs or symptoms, including multiple lesions of EM (Fig. 14.44). The individual lesions are similar to the original EM lesion, although they tend to be less inflamed and do not extend as aggressively.[330] Multiple EM lesions occur in around 25% of infected children in the United States.[324] Constitutional symptoms are common during this stage of infection. Neurologic manifestations of early disseminated Lyme disease include peripheral neuropathy (especially cranial nerve VII palsy) and lymphocytic meningitis. Facial palsy is the most characteristic neuropathy and is reported in 40% to 50% of patients with neurologic involvement. Bilateral facial palsy, a quite rare presentation, should be highly suspicious for Lyme disease, especially when occurring in an endemic area. The facial palsy of Lyme disease usually resolves in 2 to 8 weeks with or without treatment. Other cranial and peripheral mononeuropathies are possible, albeit more common in adults than children,[329] and a Guillain–Barré-like syndrome has been reported. Because Lyme meningitis is fairly common in endemic regions between April and December, clinicians should include this on the differential diagnosis for children presenting with undifferentiated aseptic meningitis and CSF pleocytosis in this scenario.[331] Migratory arthralgia or frank arthritis may also occur, as may cardiac involvement. The latter is marked by first-, second-, or third-degree atrioventricular conduction defects or bundle branch blocks and, less commonly, carditis or congestive heart failure.[329] In children with early disseminated Lyme disease, predictive variables for carditis include older age, presence of arthralgias, and cardiopulmonary symptoms.[332] Given that conduction abnormalities may be clinically silent, electrocardiography should be performed in children presenting with early disseminated Lyme disease.[333]

Late Lyme Disease (Stage III)

The primary features of late Lyme disease, which occurs in 60% of untreated cases, are arthritis and neurologic disease. Fortunately, with better and earlier recognition of this disorder, manifestations of late disease have become much less common.[323] Cutaneous manifestations during late disease include lymphocytoma cutis and acrodermatitis chronica atrophicans (ACA) (see later). The arthritis is usually monoarticular or oligoarticular and tends to involve the knees most commonly, although migratory and small-joint involvement may be seen. The presentation may simulate that of juvenile

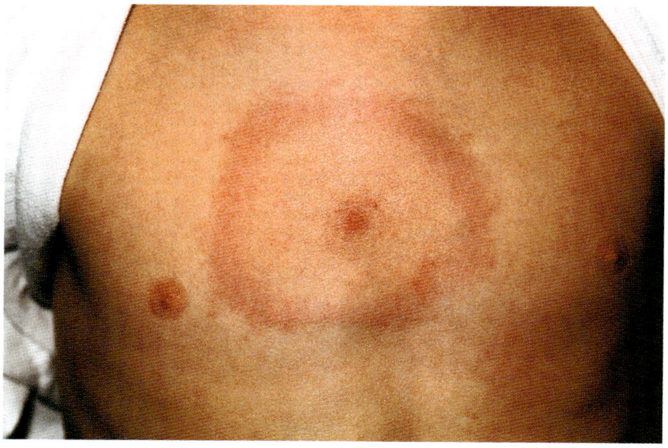

Fig. 14.43 Erythema migrans of Lyme disease. Expanding, erythematous, annular patch of early localized Lyme disease. A small red papule is seen centrally at the site of the tick bite.

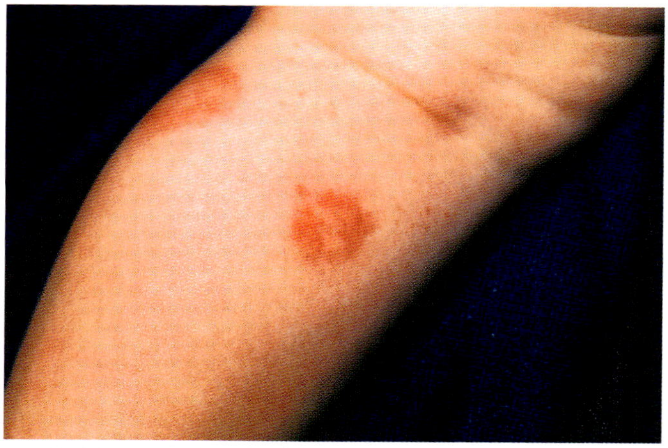

Fig. 14.44 Erythema migrans, multiple lesions. Multiple erythematous macules and patches were present in this child with early disseminated Lyme disease.

rheumatoid arthritis or an acute septic arthritis, and confusion with the latter may be compounded by the finding of markedly elevated joint-fluid leukocyte counts.[334] The most common neurologic sequelae of late disease are encephalopathy, encephalomyelitis, and sensorineural peripheral neuropathy, although late neurologic disease tends to be rare in children.

Other cutaneous manifestations that have been potentially linked to *B. burgdorferi* infection include linear morphea, lichen sclerosis et atrophicus, and lymphocytoma cutis (Borrelial lymphocytoma, lymphadenosis benigna cutis, cutaneous lymphoid hyperplasia). In Europe, *B. burgdorferi* infection has also been associated with Bannwarth syndrome (localized radicular pains accompanied by motor or sensory changes and occasionally lymphocytic meningitis), atrophoderma of Pasini and Pierini, eosinophilic fasciitis, and progressive facial hemiatrophy. ACA is reported primarily in Europe as a late manifestation of disease. It is characterized early by violaceous plaques followed by induration, hyperpigmentation, and atrophy of the skin on the distal extensor extremities and may be associated with concurrent arthritis and neuropathy.[330] This Lyme disease complication is associated primarily with infection by *B. afzelii*.[335] Borrelial lymphocytoma presents with plaques or nodules, classically on the earlobes or areolae but occasionally in other regions.[333]

Chronic Lyme disease (also known as *posttreatment chronic Lyme disease*) is a challenging and controversial entity from both a diagnostic and therapeutic standpoint. Two syndromes to occur in this context have been reported. The first consists of patients who continue to have symptoms similar to the pretreatment period despite appropriate therapy, especially joint complaints. The second syndrome to occur in this setting is similar to chronic fatigue syndrome or fibromyalgia, and patients present with complaints of extreme fatigue, myalgias, headache, polyarthralgias, and mood disturbances. Some patients are more symptomatic than others, possibly reflecting some sort of genetic influence, and although the disease does not tend to be destructive or progressive, its effects can be quite debilitating.[336] Chronic Lyme disease may be overdiagnosed as a result of equivocal test results, unreliable tests, or the misdiagnosis of associated psychiatric comorbidities.[337,338]

The diagnosis of Lyme disease relies upon clinical findings suggestive of the disease in combination with confirmatory laboratory testing. Antibody determinations are the most commonly utilized diagnostic examinations and include indirect immunofluorescence assays and enzyme-linked immunosorbent assays (ELISAs). Both can assess for IgM and IgG antibodies to *B. burgdorferi*. It must be remembered that patients with early localized Lyme disease are commonly seronegative for antibodies (with positive findings only in 25% to 40% of patients with localized EM lesions), and hence this testing is of minimal use in these patients and the diagnosis requires astute clinical judgment.[339] Serologic studies may also be limited by cross-reactivities with other organisms and high rates of seropositivity among asymptomatic persons in endemic areas.[340] Immunoblotting allows for more specific detection of antibodies and may be used in conjunction with the previously mentioned assays. The Study Group for Lyme Borreliosis (ESGBOR) of the European Society of Clinical Microbiology and Infectious Diseases (ESCMID) recommends clinical diagnosis of Lyme disease in patients presenting with EM, without laboratory testing.[341] Culture of *B. burgdorferi* is possible from tissue or fluid, but it is slow and difficult and requires special media that are not readily available. PCR studies for Lyme disease have been applied to a variety of tissues and fluids, but in general are neither approved nor widely available for this purpose and may result in false-positive results. Lyme urinary antigen capture tests are unreliable and should not be used.

The treatment of Lyme disease depends on the type of presentation and the age of the patient. In patients in whom the diagnosis of early Lyme disease is strongly suspected, treatment is initiated based on clinical findings, given the potential delays in laboratory confirmation. Doxycycline for 14 to 21 days is the treatment of choice for early localized disease in children older than 8 years of age. For those younger than 8 years of age, amoxicillin or cefuroxime for the same period is indicated.[342] Alternatives include azithromycin, erythromycin, or clarithromycin.[329,333] Early disseminated disease and late disease are treated with the same oral regimen but for 21 days. Persistent arthritis, carditis, or atrioventricular heart block are treated with the same oral agents as for early localized disease or parenteral ceftriaxone; meningitis is treated with oral doxycycline or parenteral ceftriaxone.[342] Occasionally, patients may develop intensification of symptoms during the first 24 hours of antibiotic therapy (a Jarisch–Herxheimer-like reaction), presumably caused by the host immune response to dying organisms. This reaction usually disappears in 1 to 2 days and is not an indication for discontinuation of therapy.

The hallmark of prevention for Lyme disease is tick avoidance. Simple measures to this end include avoidance of tick-infested areas, tucking pant legs into socks, and inspection for ticks after high-risk activities or exposures in endemic areas. The judicious use of chemical repellents such as N,N-diethyl-3-methylbenzamide (DEET), picaridin, or permethrin (see Chapter 18) on skin or clothing is also helpful. Because the *Ixodes* tick must be attached to the skin for at least 24 hours before infection is transmitted, daily inspection should be performed on individuals after exposure to potentially infested areas, and prompt tick removal by grasping the tick with a forceps, tweezers, or gloved fingers will help prevent transmission of the disease.[343] Removal should be performed without crushing the tick, and an effort should be made to leave no body parts behind. The bite site should be washed with soap and water to prevent secondary infection. Maintaining household pets as tick-free will also decrease the chance of transmission of tick-borne diseases.

Most experts recommend against serologic testing or prophylactic antibiotic therapy after a tick bite, especially for patients who have had ticks attached for less than 36 hours.[323] Most deer ticks, even in highly endemic areas for Lyme disease, are not infected with *B. burgdorferi*, and the overall risk of infection after a recognized deer-tick bite in such an area is less than 3%.[342] A vaccine for Lyme disease was available and approved by the US Food and Drug Administration for individuals between 15 and 70 years of age but was withdrawn in 2002 and is no longer available.

Protozoal Disorders

LEISHMANIASIS

The term *leishmaniasis* refers to three different diseases caused by the protozoan parasite of the genus *Leishmania*: cutaneous leishmaniasis (oriental sore, Delhi boil, Baghdad boil, Balkh sore), mucocutaneous leishmaniasis, and visceral leishmaniasis (kala-azar). These infections are characterized by diversity and complexity, and the majority of cases occur in Afghanistan, Algeria, Iran, Iraq, Saudi Arabia, and Syria (in the "Old World") and Brazil and Peru (in the "New World").[344] Leishmania is present in most tropical and subtropical countries due to characteristics of the sandfly vector (see later). In the United States, leishmaniasis is primarily seen in foreign travelers, immigrants, and military personnel returning from countries where it is endemic.[345] Travelers can become infected even after short stays in *Leishmania*-endemic areas,[346] and the increase in travel to endemic regions of South and Central America has led to an increase in the number of cases diagnosed in the United States.[347] Although there may be overlap in clinical presentations caused by specific species, in general Old World cutaneous leishmaniasis is caused by *Leishmania tropica* or *Leishmania major*; New World cutaneous disease by *Leishmania braziliensis*, *Leishmania mexicana*, or *Leishmania guyanensis*; mucocutaneous disease by *Leishmania braziliensis*, *Leishmania panamensis*, and *Leishmania guyanensis*; and visceral disease by *Leishmania donovani*.[348] There are, however, multiple other less common species of *Leishmania* as well.

Leishmaniasis is transmitted by the sandfly (*Phlebotomus* or *Lutzomyia* species), which lives in dark and damp places. Sandflies fly silently and are most active in the evening and at night. They are one-third the size of a mosquito. The infection is transmitted to humans (an accidental host) by the bite of the sandfly, which itself becomes infected after a blood meal from infected mammals (primarily rodents and dogs).[344,349] *Leishmania* species are obligate intracellular parasites of macrophages, by which they are phagocytosed after inoculation into the skin. They subsequently replicate within macrophages and spread throughout the reticuloendothelial system of the host.

Cutaneous leishmaniasis has a variety of clinical presentations, although the most common is an indolent skin ulcer. There are an estimated 1.2 to 1.5 million new cases of cutaneous disease each year, and the incidence may be increasing.[350,351] The incubation period after the bite of the sandfly is usually 2 to 4 weeks (but may be up to several years), and occasionally the infection may remain subclinical. The initial lesion is a papule that enlarges to form a painless ulcer with a raised margin and necrotic base (Figs. 14.45 and 14.46). Most often there are one to two lesions, although multiple lesions have been observed, and some patients may show a lymphangitic distribution similar to that of sporotrichosis.[346] Regional lymphadenopathy and secondary bacterial infection may occur, the latter of which is often associated with pain.[344] Most lesions of cutaneous leishmaniasis heal over months to years, leaving an atrophic scar.

Other presentations of cutaneous leishmaniasis include a dry ulcerative form that appears as a brown nodule that ulcerates more slowly and reveals an adherent crust; leishmaniasis recidivans, which is manifested by red to yellow-brown papules that appear in or close to a scar of an old lesion of cutaneous leishmaniasis; and a nonulcerating generalized form that may resemble lepromatous leprosy. Patients with this form of leishmaniasis present a public health hazard, because the skin is heavily infested and may act as a reservoir for transmission by the *Phlebotomus* fly.

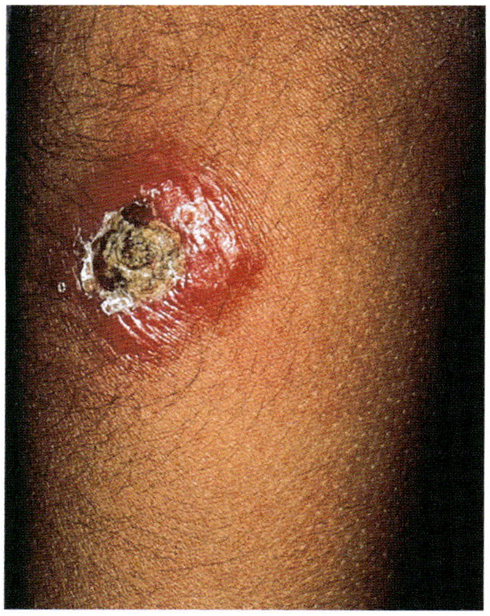

Fig. 14.45 Cutaneous leishmaniasis. An erythematous crusted plaque in a 4-year-old child. (Courtesy William Burrows, MD.)

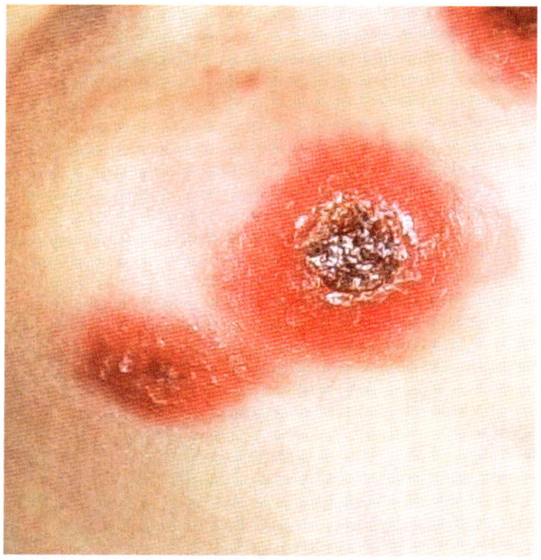

Fig. 14.46 Cutaneous leishmaniasis. Multiple erythematous papules and plaques with necrosis and crusting were present in this 2-year-old girl. *Leishmania tropica* was confirmed by PCR analysis. (Courtesy Ayelet Shani-Adir, MD.)

The differential diagnosis of cutaneous leishmaniasis includes foreign body reactions; tropical or traumatic ulcers; superinfected insect bites; myiasis; impetigo, ecthyma or furunculosis; fungal, viral, spirochetal, and mycobacterial infections; leprosy; sarcoidosis; and neoplasms such as basal cell carcinoma, squamous cell carcinoma, or lymphoma.[344,346,352] The diagnosis of leishmaniasis is usually made on the basis of the typical lesion(s) combined with a history of exposure or travel to an endemic region. Confirming the diagnosis can be challenging. Tissue biopsy for culture, smear, and histologic evaluation is useful. An impression smear is made by gently pressing the fresh biopsy tissue against a glass microscope slide, staining with Giemsa or hematoxylin and eosin (H&E) stain, and examining for amastigotes (intracellular organisms). Tissue specimens for culture must be plated on special culture, and the organisms can be typed by isoenzyme analysis in a reference laboratory, although the procedure is quite time consuming.[350] Alternative methods for diagnosis include needle aspirates, slit-skin smears, monoclonal-antibody tissue stains, and molecular techniques based on kinetoplast (a small portion of extranuclear material) DNA analysis. Serologic studies, which may be helpful in visceral or disseminated cutaneous disease, are usually of no value for localized cutaneous leishmaniasis. PCR-based diagnosis is available and is particularly useful in cases with a low parasite load (i.e., mucosal leishmaniasis). The CDC offers diagnostic services for leishmaniasis and will accept biopsy specimens (or prepared histopathology slides), aspirates, tissue impression smears (touch preparations), and dermal scrapings for evaluation.[354]

Mucocutaneous leishmaniasis results from hematogenous or lymphatic dissemination of organisms from skin to the nasopharyngeal mucosa. It often manifests years after resolution of cutaneous lesions of leishmaniasis.[346] Mucocutaneous leishmaniasis presents with chronic nasal symptoms and is followed by progressive nasopharyngeal destruction. Secondary bacterial infections with regional adenitis and lymphangitis are common, and occasionally the mucocutaneous lesions may be nodular and vegetative. Destruction of the nasal septum and nasopharynx may result in soft-tissue and cartilage erosion, with resultant deformities of the nose, lips, cheeks, pharynx, larynx, and palate that are often cosmetically debilitating.[353]

Visceral leishmaniasis may present with varied clinical findings and severity of illness. It infects an estimated 500,000 new individuals in less developed countries each year and may occur in large-scale epidemics, especially in east Africa and India.[354,355] The classic kala-azar syndrome, caused by *L. donovani*, results in fever, cachexia, hepatosplenomegaly, pancytopenia, and progressive deterioration. If left untreated, visceral leishmaniasis is often fatal. A common complication after therapy for kala-azar is "post-kala-azar dermal leishmaniasis." This disorder is characterized by macular, papular, and nodular skin lesions that usually begin around the mouth and subsequently generalize.[356]

Treatment of leishmaniasis depends upon the clinical presentation, and in fact there is no single optimal therapy for all forms. When considering treatment for cutaneous disease, it is important to remember that this form of leishmaniasis tends to heal spontaneously but that *L. braziliensis* has the potential to progress to mucocutaneous disease.[350] Therefore any patient with *L. braziliensis* confirmed as the etiologic agent or with a history of contracting the infection in an area endemic for this organism should receive adequate systemic therapy. The goals of therapy are to reduce scarring and prevent parasite dissemination.

Pentavalent antimonial drugs such as sodium stibogluconate (Pentostam) and meglumine antimoniate (Glucantime) remain the mainstay of systemic therapy. These agents are generally administered in the hospital, although controlled outpatient management is an acceptable alternative in some situations. Pentostam is available in the United States from the Drug Service of the CDC. Potential toxicities related to the antimonial agents include electrocardiographic abnormalities, hepatic toxicity, pancreatitis, and pneumonitis. Amphotericin B and its lipid formulations have shown efficacy in the treatment of leishmaniasis, especially in India, where antimonial resistance has been an increasing concern.[349,354] Other treatments utilized with varying degrees of success have included cryosurgery, surgical excision, topical paromomycin ointment, intralesional sodium stibogluconate, intralesional amphotericin B, photodynamic therapy, and pentamidine. High-dose oral fluconazole was demonstrated useful in the treatment of cutaneous leishmaniasis caused by *L. braziliensis*.[357] Other potentially promising treatments for visceral leishmaniasis that have been studied include the anticancer alkylphosphocholines miltefosine, edelfosine, and ilmofosine.[358,359] Miltefosine has been approved by the Food and Drug Administration for treatment of cutaneous disease caused by *L. braziliensis*, *L. guyanensis*, and *L. panamensis*.[360]

The complete list of 360 references for this chapter is available online at http://expertconsult.inkling.com.

Key References

Sutter DE, Milburn E, Chukwuma U, et al. Changing susceptibility of *staphylococcus aureus* in a US pediatric population. Pediatrics 2016;137(3):e20153099.
Fry S, Barnabas S, Cotton MF. Update on trends in childhood tuberculosis. Curr Opin Pediatr 2018;30:152–60.
Lipsett SC, Nigrovic LE. Diagnosis of lyme disease in the pediatric acute care setting. Curr Opin Pediatr 2016;28:287–93.
Shapiro ED. Lyme disease. N Engl J Med 2014;370(18):1724–31.
Atkins BL, Gottlieb T. Skin and soft tissue infections caused by nontuberculous mycobacteria. Curr Opin Infect Dis 2014;27:137–45.
Miller LG, Kaplan SL. Staphylococcus aureus: a community pathogen. Infect Dis Clin N Am 2009;23:35–52.
Odell CA. Community-associated methicillin-resistant *staphylococcus aureus* (CA-MRSA) skin infections. Curr Opin Pediatr 2010;22:273–7.
Endorf FW, Garrison MM, Klein MB, et al. Characteristics, therapies, and outcome of children with necrotizing soft tissue infections. Pediatr Infect Dis J 2012;31(3):221–3.
Amagai M, Yamaguchi T, Hanakawa Y, et al. Staphylococcal exfoliative toxin B specifically cleaves desmoglein 1. J Invest Dermatol 2002;118:845–50.
Lappin E, Ferguson AJ. Gram-positive toxic shock syndromes. Lancet 2009;9:281–90.
Centers for Disease Control and Prevention (CDC). Tattoo-associated nontuberculous mycobacterial skin infections: multiple states 2011–2012. MMWR Morb Mortal Wkly Rep 2012;61(33):653–7.
Florin TA, Zaoutis TE, Zaoutis LB. Beyond cat scratch disease: widening spectrum of *bartonella henselae* infection. Pediatrics 2008;121(5):e1413–25.

15 Viral Diseases of the Skin

CHAPTER OUTLINE		
	Herpes Simplex Virus Infection	**Cowpox and Pseudocowpox**
	Herpes Zoster	**Orf**
	Viral-Like Disorders of the Oral Mucosa	**Smallpox**
	Warts	**Acquired Immunodeficiency Syndrome in Children**
	Molluscum Contagiosum	

Viruses are ultramicroscopic organisms that grow only within living cells. The antigenic material responsible for viral immunologic reactions is present in the outer protein membrane (capsid) of the virus. The nucleoprotein core is composed of either deoxyribonucleic acid (DNA) or ribonucleic acid (RNA). Lacking ribosomes, viruses depend on the use of the host cells' enzyme systems, blending with metabolic material of the host cell and often remaining undetected until some stimulus incites the production of new viral particles.

Viral infections of the skin may present with varied morphologies, including papules, vesiculobullous lesions, ulcers, and tumors. This chapter will include a discussion of herpes simplex virus (HSV) infections, herpes zoster (HZ), viral-like disorders of the oral mucosa, and warts. Some poxvirus infections will be discussed, including molluscum contagiosum (MC), cowpox, pseudocowpox ("milker's nodules"), orf, and smallpox. Although human immunodeficiency virus (HIV) infection does not result in primary skin disease, a brief discussion of acquired immunodeficiency syndrome (AIDS) in children and its skin disease associations is included. Neonatal herpes infection is discussed in Chapter 2.

Herpes Simplex Virus Infection

The herpesvirus family includes HSV, Epstein–Barr virus (EBV), cytomegalovirus (CMV), varicella zoster virus (VZV), and human herpesviruses (HHV) 6 through 8. Aside from HSV, the other herpesviruses are implicated primarily in exanthematous illnesses. HSV infections are quite prevalent in both children and adults. HSV-1 and HSV-2 are double-stranded DNA viruses that primarily infect the epidermis or mucosal surfaces. After acute infection, the virus rapidly replicates and establishes latent infection in regional nerve ganglia, from which it occasionally reactivates.[1,2] These viruses rely on the host-cell nucleus for DNA replication, and hence when microscopic evaluations are performed on samples with infection, the characteristic cytologic inclusions are located within the nucleus.[3]

HSV-1 is primarily associated with oral and labial lesions, and HSV-2 with anogenital lesions, although the predilection of a specific viral serotype to a particular anatomic site has become more variable.[4] Primary HSV-1 infection is largely a childhood disease that affects the oral mucosa, pharynx, lips, and occasionally the eyes.[2] HSV-2 is primarily implicated in genital tract disease, with spread occurring via sexual contact or, most commonly in neonates, by passage through an infected birth canal (see Chapter 2). Although the mucocutaneous lesions caused by HSV-1 and HSV-2 are clinically indistinguishable, differentiation between the two serotypes can be made by viral culture, Western blot serologic testing, HSV-antigen detection with monoclonal anti-HSV antibodies, or polymerase chain reaction (PCR) studies. The Tzanck smear is a rapid and cost-effective diagnostic test, but is dependent on the experience of the examiner and cannot distinguish between HSV and VZV infections. Transmission of HSV is accomplished via exposure to infected mucous membranes or skin with active lesions or to mucosal secretions from an individual with active infection, but can also be transmitted via exposure to secretions from an asymptomatic person who is shedding the virus.[5]

Infection with HSV is classified as primary or recurrent. Primary infections occur in individuals without circulating antibodies and result from direct contact with infected secretions or actual mucocutaneous lesions. After an incubation of days to weeks, they may present as subclinical infection, characterized only by the development of antibodies, as a localized or generalized cutaneous eruption, or as a serious systemic infection with central nervous system or disseminated involvement. Most primary HSV infections are asymptomatic. Recurrent HSV infection occurs in individuals who were previously infected either clinically or subclinically. It is characterized by repeated episodes of mucocutaneous lesions at the same site or sites.

Topical and systemic antiviral agents commonly used to treat HSV infections are summarized in Table 15.1.

HERPETIC GINGIVOSTOMATITIS

Herpetic gingivostomatitis most commonly occurs in children between the ages of 10 months and 5 years, although it may occur at any age. It presents with small vesicles on an erythematous base that evolve into painful, shallow gray erosions and ulcerations (Fig. 15.1). The lesions most often involve the palate, tongue, and gingivae. Gingival swelling and easy bleeding may occur. Perioral lesions involving the lips, cheeks, and chin (Fig. 15.2) occur in up to three-quarters of patients.[6] Other common features include fever, drooling, eating and drinking difficulties, foul breath odor, and irritability. Cervical and submandibular lymphadenopathy is also quite common. Secondary bacteremia with group A β-hemolytic streptococci, *Staphylococcus aureus*, or other organisms may occasionally be a complication.[7] Associated hepatitis has been observed, most often in neonates and immunosuppressed patients with acute primary HSV-1 infection, but also rarely in immunocompetent children.[8]

The differential diagnosis of herpetic gingivostomatitis in a child includes herpangina, hand-foot-and-mouth disease, aphthous stomatitis, Behçet syndrome, pemphigus vulgaris, and Stevens–Johnson syndrome. The diagnosis can be confirmed by viral culture, direct fluorescent antibody studies, or PCR-based testing, when necessary. Although gingivostomatitis is usually caused by HSV-1, HSV-2 may cause a similar syndrome that usually occurs in adolescents and young adults who engage in oral–genital contact.[1] Such primary HSV-2 infection results in similar symptoms of gingivostomatitis and pharyngitis, which in some patients may be difficult to differentiate

Table 15.1 Topical and Oral Antiviral Medications Used for Herpes Simplex Virus Infections*

Drug	Formulation	Regimen	Indication/Comment
TOPICAL			
Acyclovir	5% cream (2 g, 5 g)	Apply 5 times/day	Recurrent HL; A: ≥12 years; 4 days; Rx
	5% ointment (15 g, 30 g)	Apply 6 times/day	Initial GH, localized HSV; A: adults; 7 days; Rx
Penciclovir	1% cream (1.5 g, 5 g)	Apply every 2 h (while awake)	Recurrent HL; A: ≥12 years; 4 days; Rx
Docosanol	10% cream (2 g)	Apply 5 times/day	HL; A: ≥12 years; treat until healed; OTC
ORAL (ALL RX)			
Acyclovir	200 mg capsule 400 mg, 800 mg tablet 200 mg/5 mL susp		A: ≥2 years
		400 mg TID (alternate: 200 mg 5 times/day)	Initial GH; 7–10 days
		400 mg TID (alternates: 800 mg BID, 200 mg 5 times/day)	Recurrent GH; 5 days
		400 mg BID	Suppression, recurrent GH; up to 12 months, then reevaluate
		75 mg/kg per day divided 5 times daily (max 1000 mg/day)	Initial GH or mucocutaneous HSV, 2–11 years old; 5–7 days
		1000 mg/day divided 5 times daily	Initial GH or mucocutaneous HSV (mild to moderate), 12 years and older; 7–10 days
		1000 mg/day divided 5 times daily	Recurrent GH or mucocutaneous HSV, 12 years and older; 5 days
		30 mg/kg per day divided every 8 hours	Suppression, GH or mucocutaneous HSV, 2–11 years old; up to 12 months
		800 mg/day divided every 12 hours	Suppression, GH or mucocutaneous HSV, 12 years and older; up to 12 months
Famciclovir	125, 250, 500 mg tablet		A: ≥18 years
		250 mg TID	Initial GH; 7–10 days
		1000 mg BID	Recurrent GH; 1 day
		250 mg BID	Suppression, recurrent GH; up to 12 months
		1500 mg single dose	Recurrent HL
Valacyclovir	500 mg, 1 g caplet		A: adults, and ≥12 years for HL
		1 g every 12 hours	Initial GH; 7–10 days
		500 mg every 12 hours	Recurrent GH; 3 days
		1 g once daily	Suppression, GH; up to 12 months
		2 g every 12 hours	HL; 1 day; both adults and children ≥12 years
		500 mg once daily	Suppression, HL; up to 4 months

A, Approved; *BID*, two times daily; *GH*, genital herpes; *HL*, herpes labialis; *HSV*, herpes simplex virus; *OTC*, over-the-counter; *Rx*, by prescription; *TID*, three times daily.
*Approved indications and regimens listed; often used off-label.

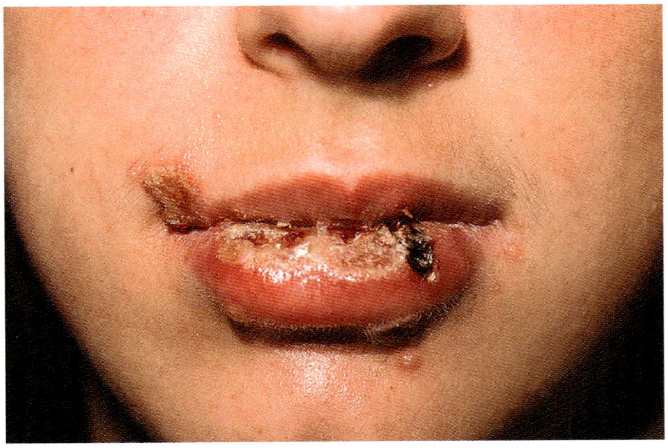

Fig. 15.1 Herpetic gingivostomatitis. Multiple erosions with crusting. Note the associated lesions involving the chin.

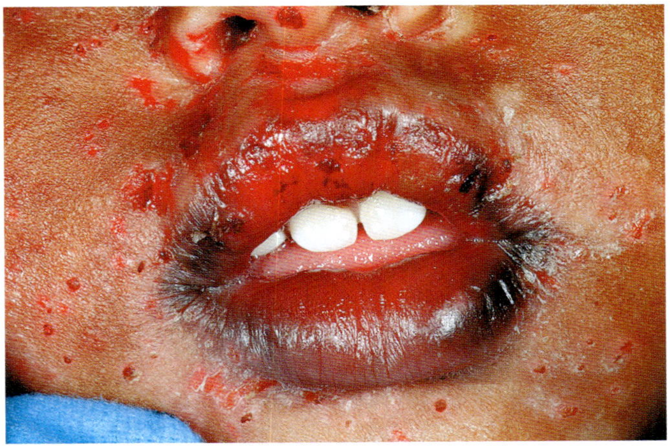

Fig. 15.2 Herpetic gingivostomatitis. Lip erosions with multiple perioral herpetic lesions.

from bacterial pharyngitis. Adolescents and young adults may also have primary HSV-1 gingivostomatitis.[9,10]

Although herpetic gingivostomatitis tends to be self-limited over 10 days to 2 weeks, dehydration may result from poor oral intake and excessive fluid losses, especially in younger children. In some patients, hospitalization may be required for intravenous hydration and pain control. Ambulatory treatment measures include supportive therapy with fluids and use of topical analgesics, anesthetics, or coating agents, including viscous lidocaine, diphenhydramine, milk of magnesia ("magic mouthwash"), Maalox, or Kaopectate.[11] Specific antiviral therapy with acyclovir is advocated by some; seems most effective when started within 3 days of disease onset; and may reduce the number of oral lesions, prevent the development of new lesions, diminish difficulties with eating and drinking, and reduce the rates of hospitalization in young children.[12–14]

OCULAR HERPES INFECTION

Primary HSV infection of the eye can result in a severe purulent conjunctivitis with edema, erythema, and vesiculation, with superficial erosion or ulceration of the cornea (epithelial keratitis). Ocular HSV infection is a leading cause of recurrent keratoconjunctivitis with associated corneal opacification and is one of the chief causes of corneal blindness in the United States.[1,11] This infection results from recurrent viral shedding from the trigeminal nerve reactivation and is more often caused by HSV-1. Patients with keratoconjunctivitis present with pain, photophobia, lacrimation, and eye discharge. Fluorescein testing may reveal dendritic lesions.[15] There may also be involvement of the eyelid (blepharitis). Deeper involvement of the cornea (stromal keratitis) or anterior uvea (iritis) may occur, and both are more serious and associated with a greater risk of visual loss. Children with HSV keratitis may have poorer visual outcomes than adults, are more often misdiagnosed, and are susceptible to amblyopia.[16] Ocular HSV infections may be unilateral or bilateral; patients with bilateral involvement tend to have a more protracted clinical course, and recurrences are more common.[17] Bacterial superinfection of herpetic keratoconjunctivitis is common. Acute retinal necrosis has rarely been reported in children.[18]

The diagnosis of herpetic keratoconjunctivitis can be confirmed with viral culture. Nested PCR studies, where available, seem to be superior to culture and can be performed on tear film or corneal scrapings.[19] The immunochromatographic assay (ICGA) kit utilizes a monoclonal antibody against HSV glycoprotein D and has high specificity (but lower sensitivity) when applied to corneal scrapings.[20] Ophthalmology referral is indicated, and treatment includes topical antiviral ophthalmic ointments or solutions and oral antiviral agents. Topical antiviral agents include trifluridine, vidarabine, and idoxuridine. In a series of 53 pediatric patients with HSV eye infections, 79% of those with keratitis had corneal scarring and 26% experienced vision impairment, highlighting the importance of prompt referral and therapy.[21] Recurrence of anterior-segment HSV is common in children, occurring in nearly 40% of 103 children in one series.[22] Penetrating keratoplasty (full-thickness cornea transplant) has been reported for pediatric HSV keratitis and was shown to improve the best-corrected visual acuity when not complicated by amblyopia.[23]

HERPES LABIALIS

Herpes labialis refers to herpetic infections occurring on the lips, most often the vermilion border. This is the most common type of recurrent herpes infection and represents the classic "cold sore." As with other types of recurrent infection, it occurs after reactivation of latent HSV in the cells of the trigeminal ganglia. Herpes labialis often presents initially with prodromal symptoms such as tingling, burning, or itching. After 1 to 2 days the cutaneous eruption appears as a localized cluster of small vesicles or erosions on an erythematous base (Figs. 15.3 and 15.4). Occasionally other areas of the face may be involved, and in immunocompromised individuals oral mucosal and/or severe involvement (Fig. 15.5) may be noted (see later). Topical and oral antiviral agents are useful in treating herpes labialis, especially when initiated within 1 to 2 days of the disease onset. Prophylaxis with oral

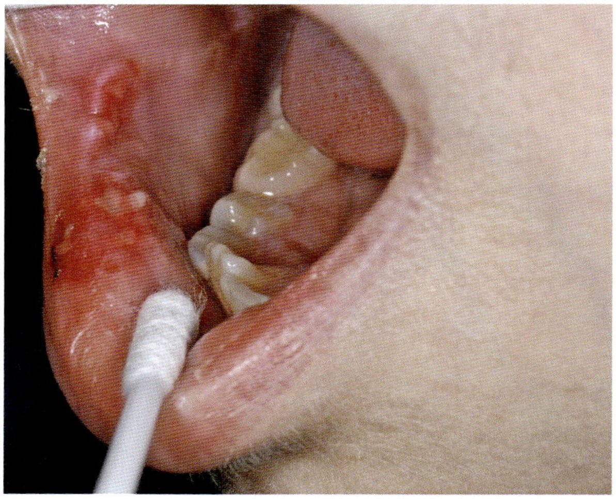

Fig. 15.3 Herpes labialis. Erythematous erosions clustered on the right lower lip in a patient with labial herpes. This young girl also had herpes-associated erythema multiforme (see Chapter 20).

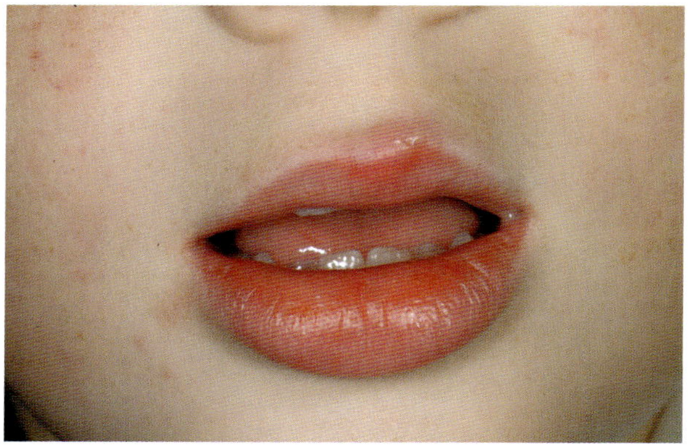

Fig. 15.4 Herpes labialis. This 7-year-old boy experienced burning and tingling of the upper vermilion border, which was followed a day later by these clustered vesicles on a red base.

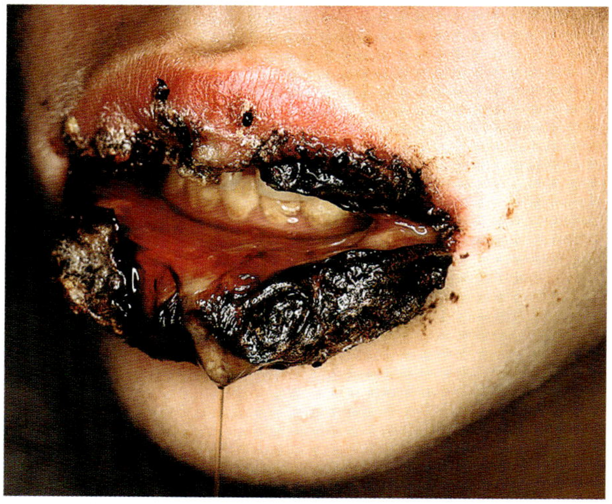

Fig. 15.5 Herpes labialis. Severe crusting and lip edema in a patient receiving cancer chemotherapy.

agents is advocated by many for patients with a history of multiple recurrences of herpes labialis.

GENITAL HERPES

Genital herpes (herpetic vulvovaginitis, herpes progenitalis) is one of the most widespread sexually transmitted diseases (STDs) in the developed world.[24,25] HSV-2 is primarily responsible for genital tract herpetic infections, and seroprevalence studies reveal rates as high as 60% to 90% in developing countries and 20% to 22% of the general population in developed countries.[2,26] The proportion of HSV-1 isolates in genital herpes is also increasing, especially in young adults and college students.[27] A large prospective study in young women demonstrated a primary HSV-1 infection rate of over twice that of HSV-2 and that it presented more often as genital rather than oral disease.[28] Given that the overall seroprevalence of HSV-1 in teenagers has decreased over the last few decades, an increasing number of adolescents lack protective HSV-1 antibodies when they become sexually active, which may be one factor leading to an increase in the frequency of HSV-1 genital herpes from oral–genital sex practices.[29] Risk factors that directly correlate with HSV-2 infection include race (higher risk in Blacks and Hispanics), age, years of sexual experience, lower family income, lower education level, number of sexual partners, and other STDs.[2] The diagnosis of genital HSV in a child should raise the suspicion of sexual abuse.[30] Maternal–fetal transmission of HSV may result in neonatal herpes, which is discussed in Chapter 2.

The majority of genital HSV infections are subclinical and go unrecognized by the host.[11] Symptomatic primary genital herpes presents with lesions 2 to 8 days after contact with an infected individual. In contrast, first-episode, nonprimary genital herpes (the initial episode of genital herpes in a host with a past history of nongenital herpes) may not present with signs or symptoms for several months.[25] The lesions of primary genital HSV are painful vesicles clustered on an erythematous base (Fig. 15.6) and distributed on the vulva, labia, vagina, perineum, penile shaft, glans penis, urethra, and, less often, the scrotum. In females, cervical involvement, intense soft-tissue swelling, and severe pain may be present. The vesicles rupture rapidly, leaving behind painful erosions or ulcers that may be associated with pruritus, dysuria, vaginal and urethral discharge, and tender inguinal lymphadenopathy. Pustules may occasionally be present. Systemic signs and symptoms may include fever, malaise, headache, and myalgias. Herpetic sacral radiculomyelitis with urinary or fecal retention and neuralgias may occur, as may aseptic meningitis.[1,11] Less common features of HSV infection include endometritis and salpingitis in women and prostatitis in men. The symptoms of genital HSV usually improve over 5 to 7 days, and the cutaneous lesions crust over and gradually heal over 2 to 4 weeks without therapy. HSV replicates locally and spreads to adjacent cells and is then transported to the neuronal cell bodies of

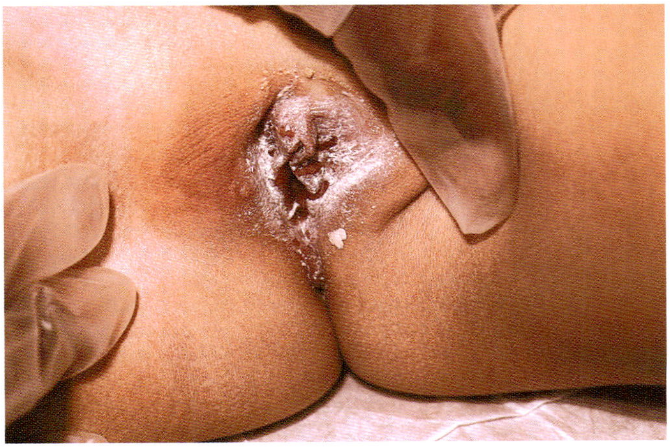

Fig. 15.6 Genital herpes. Vesicles on an erythematous base involving the right labia minora in a childhood victim of sexual abuse.

the dorsal root ganglion, where it establishes latent infection or is transported back to mucocutaneous sites, where it again replicates and leads to clinical findings.[31]

Genital herpes may show a heterogeneous clinical spectrum. Extragenital involvement may be seen, with lesions most commonly involving the buttocks, anal region, thighs, mouth, and fingers (see later).[2,24] Atypical morphologies may also be present, including deep and tender ulcers, single erosions, erosive urethritis, vulvar fissure, and penile edema.[24] A high index of suspicion must be maintained, especially in the immunocompromised host or in patients with features of other STDs. The differential diagnosis for genital herpes includes syphilis, chancroid, lymphogranuloma venereum, condylomata acuminate, Behçet syndrome, HZ, erosive candidiasis, and lichen sclerosis. Acute infection with EBV may also present with acute genital ulceration (see Chapter 16).

Recurrent genital HSV infection is characterized by less severe cutaneous lesions that are usually preceded by a prodrome of pain, tenderness, itching, tingling, or paresthesia. The vesicles are fewer in number, the duration of clinical findings is less than with primary disease, and recurrent disease may be less common with HSV-1 versus HSV-2 infection. Triggering factors for recurrent disease may include physical or emotional stress, febrile illness, and menstruation. Recurrence rates tend to be highest for the first years after the initial infection.[32] Asymptomatic (subclinical) HSV shedding is another feature of genital herpes and among individuals with genital HSV-2 infection, occurs on 10% to 20% of days.[29,31] The risk of subclinical shedding increases with the rate of symptomatic recurrences.

The diagnosis of genital herpes can be confirmed by viral culture, Tzanck preparation (cannot distinguish between HSV-1 and HSV-2), direct fluorescent antibody testing, Western blot serologic testing, or PCR. PCR assays for HSV are rapid and type-specific, highly sensitive, and competitive from a cost perspective.[29] Serologic screening for genital HSV infection in asymptomatic adolescents and adults is not recommended and is associated with a high rate of false-positive results and potential psychosocial harms.[33,34] Treatments for genital herpes include supportive care and antiviral therapy (see Table 15.1). Supportive measures include warm sitz baths, topical anesthetics, topical antibacterial ointments to prevent secondary infection, and oral analgesics. Education regarding the nature and risks of HSV infection and safe sex practices should be offered, and evaluation for other STDs should be considered when appropriate. An effective vaccine against HSV is highly desirable, and research toward this end is ongoing. Experimental vaccines contain recombinant glycoprotein subunits, attenuated or replication-defective virus vaccines, and those composed of plasmids expressing glycoprotein subunits. Vaccine development has been challenging, given the poor understanding of the mechanisms by which host immune responses fail to control HSV.[35–37]

The choice of antiviral therapy depends on the host immune status and the nature of the infection (primary or recurrent). Oral acyclovir, famciclovir, and valacyclovir may all help to speed healing, decrease symptoms, and decrease viral shedding. Long-term suppressive therapy in patients with frequent recurrences is useful in reducing both the rate and duration of flares. Although topical acyclovir ointment may offer some benefit for initial genital herpes infections, it offers little in the way of recurrent infections. Tenofovir, a nucleoside reverse transcriptase inhibitor used orally for the treatment of HIV in adults and children >2 years of age, was shown with topical pericoital application to reduce HSV-2 acquisition in women in one study, and in another study of vaginal application, decreased the quantity of vaginal HSV shed by 60%.[38,39]

CUTANEOUS HERPES AND ECZEMA HERPETICUM

Cutaneous HSV infection can occur on any body surface area. Involvement of the finger (herpetic whitlow) is discussed in the next section. Nonorolabial, nongenital involvement presents in a similar fashion, with clustered vesicles or erosions on an erythematous base (Figs. 15.7 and 15.8). The lesions may be misdiagnosed as impetigo or HZ. Occasionally, recurrent cutaneous HSV may present only with prodromal symptoms followed by skin erythema and edema but without the characteristic vesiculation. In some instances, patients with

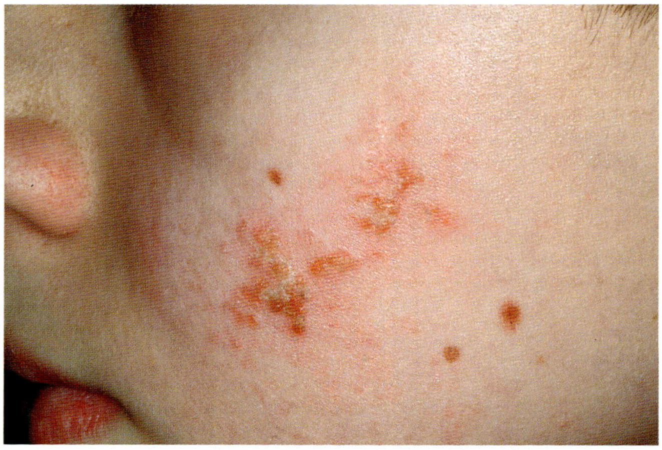

Fig. 15.7 Cutaneous herpes. Resolving vesicles and crusted papules overlying an erythematous base on the left cheek.

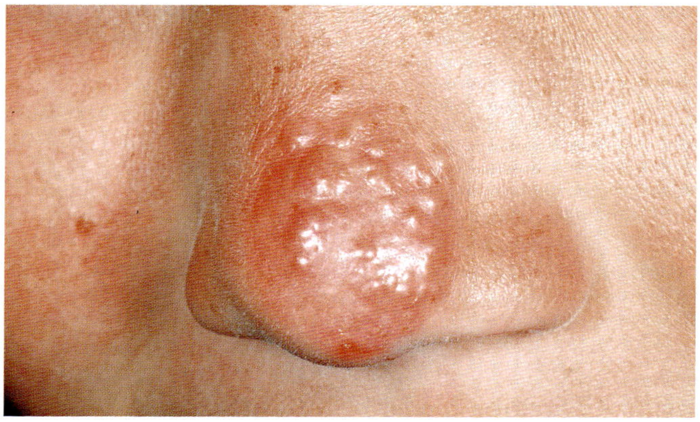

Fig. 15.8 Cutaneous herpes. Coalescing vesicles on a red base over the distal nose.

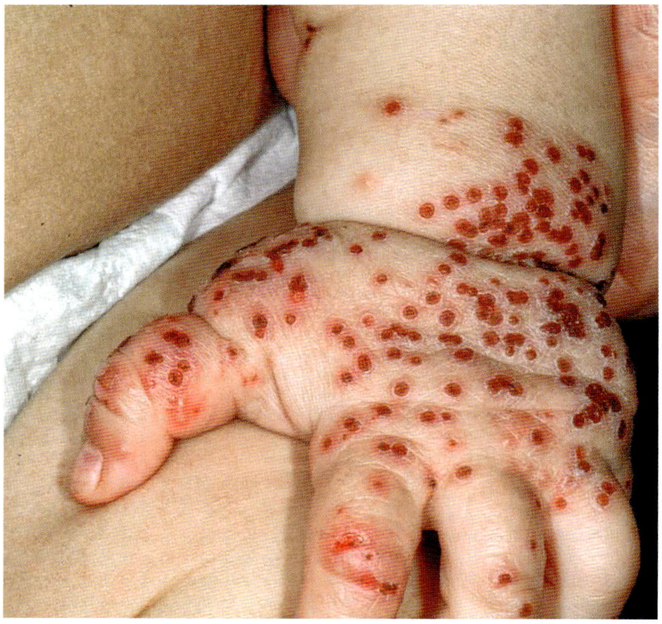

Fig. 15.9 Eczema herpeticum. This toddler with chronic atopic dermatitis had an explosive onset of fever and widespread vesicles with crusting in eczematous areas. Note the monomorphous nature and clustering of these crusted papules with a few intact small vesicles on the dorsal hand.

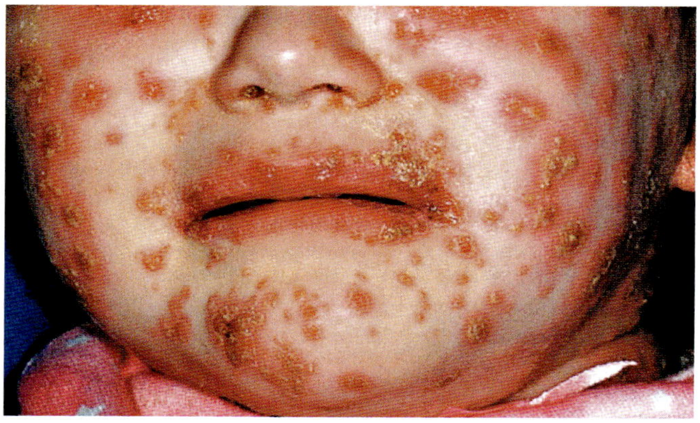

Fig. 15.10 Eczema herpeticum. These coalescing vesicles progressed rapidly in this young girl with atopic dermatitis.

recurrent cutaneous HSV may develop associated secondary bacterial infection or lymphangitis.

Eczema herpeticum (EH, or Kaposi varicelliform eruption; see Chapter 3) is a severe, disseminated HSV infection that occurs in individuals with atopic dermatitis or other chronic skin disease, including pemphigus, Darier disease, burns, and others.[40] Although the etiology of EH has not been clearly established, the impaired skin barrier associated with these diseases is believed to create a more permissive environment for viral invasion and binding to cellular receptors,[40] leading to a higher prevalence of EH with greater dermatitis severity.[41] Despite the high prevalence of atopic dermatitis (AD) in the general population and frequent exposure to HSV, EH is quite rare, possibly relating to a requirement for multiple additional host and environmental factors.[42] Single-nucleotide polymorphisms in the interferon regulatory factor 2 *(IRF2)* gene have been demonstrated to confer a greater risk of EH, possibly reflecting an abnormal immune response to HSV.[43] A type 2 immune response by virus-specific T cells has been suggested by analysis of cellular immune responses (specifically, measurement of interleukin 4 [IL-4] and interferon gamma [IFN-γ] expression and characterization of T-cell markers) in AD patients both with and without a history of EH.[44]

Patients with EH usually experience an abrupt onset of fever, malaise, and a widespread eruption of monomorphous vesicles and erosions (Figs. 15.9 and 15.10; see Chapter 3, Figs. 3.30, 3.31 and 3.32). The lesions are most prominent in areas of active dermatitis but especially tend to involve the head, neck, and trunk. Complications of EH include keratoconjunctivitis, secondary bacterial superinfection, fluid loss, and viremia. The mainstay of treatment for EH is systemic antiviral therapy, which for the majority of patients is most appropriately administered via intravenous delivery in the hospital. Early initiation of therapy is preferable, and delays in starting acyclovir therapy appear to be associated with increased length of hospital stay.[45] Other treatment considerations include hydration with attention to electrolyte balance, antibiotic therapy for secondary bacterial infection, and pain control. Meticulous skin care should be performed, with bland emollients applied during the early phase of barrier recovery, as well as the application of antiinflammatory agents for the underlying dermatitis. The timing of the latter remains controversial; although some have suggested that use of topical corticosteroids during active EH may adversely affect prognosis, a review of more than 1300 children admitted for treatment revealed no increase in length of stay when these agents were started at the time of admission.[46] Ophthalmologic evaluation is indicated when facial involvement is present. More extensive EH at presentation may be an indicator of an increased rate of repeated episodes.[47]

Erythema multiforme (see Chapter 20), an acute, self-limited reactive skin disease, has been associated with HSV infection in both children and adults. In prepubertal children with erythema multiforme, especially the recurrent type, HSV DNA was detected by PCR studies on skin biopsy specimens taken from the target lesions.[48,49] This finding was noted both in patients with a known history of HSV and in those without any such history. Prophylactic acyclovir may thus be useful in abrogating recurrences of erythema multiforme in children.

HERPETIC WHITLOW

Herpetic whitlow is a unique form of HSV infection involving the pulp of the distal phalanx (or multiple phalanges). It is seen most often in physicians, dentists, dental hygienists, and nurses who have contact with the mouth or genital regions of patients with herpetic lesions. It may also occur as a result of autoinoculation in patients with herpes labialis, herpes stomatitis, or genital herpes.[50] The virus is inoculated onto the skin of one or more fingers, resulting in a deep-seated, painful vesicular or bullous eruption with erythema (Fig. 15.11). Spontaneous resolution usually occurs over 3 weeks if the condition is left untreated. The differential diagnosis of herpetic whitlow may include blistering dactylitis, burns, and impetigo. The diagnosis is confirmed by viral culture or direct fluorescent antibody testing, and treatment with oral acyclovir or other antiviral agents may result in alleviation of pain and more rapid healing.

HERPES GLADIATORUM

Herpes gladiatorum is a term used to describe a widespread primary inoculation HSV infection occurring in contact sports enthusiasts such as wrestlers or rugby players. It may occur at some time in up to one-third of wrestlers and is characterized by grouped vesicles on an erythematous base. It has also been observed after shared use of boxing gloves believed to be contaminated by HSV-1, with lesions occurring over the knuckles.[51] The most common locations for herpes gladiatorum are the head (Fig. 15.12), neck, and upper extremities.[52,53] In addition to widespread cutaneous lesions, affected individuals may have fever, malaise, sore throat, anorexia, headache, weight loss, and regional lymphadenopathy. The cutaneous lesions of herpes gladiatorum may occasionally lack classic vesicles, in which case the differential diagnosis may include tinea corporis gladiatorum, impetigo, and atopic dermatitis.[53] EH may also occur with increased frequency in wrestlers.[54]

Herpes gladiatorum can be effectively treated with oral acyclovir, famciclovir, or valacyclovir. The duration of therapy necessary before allowing the athlete to return to competition is controversial, and evidence-based recommendations do not exist. Sharing of equipment and towels should be discouraged and appropriate cleaning of wrestling mats encouraged. Expert organizations recommend that wrestlers with visible, uncovered lesions be excluded from competition and that wrestling mats be disinfected between each match with an Environmental Protection Agency (EPA)–approved disinfectant active against both *S. aureus* and HSV-1.[55] Seasonal antiviral prophylaxis has been advocated by some in an effort to suppress recurrent outbreaks and reduce the risk of spread to susceptible teammates or opponents.[56,57] In one 10-year observational study of a 28-day high school wrestling camp, valacyclovir 1 gram taken once daily for the duration of the camp resulted in an 84% decrease in the probability of an HSV outbreak.[58]

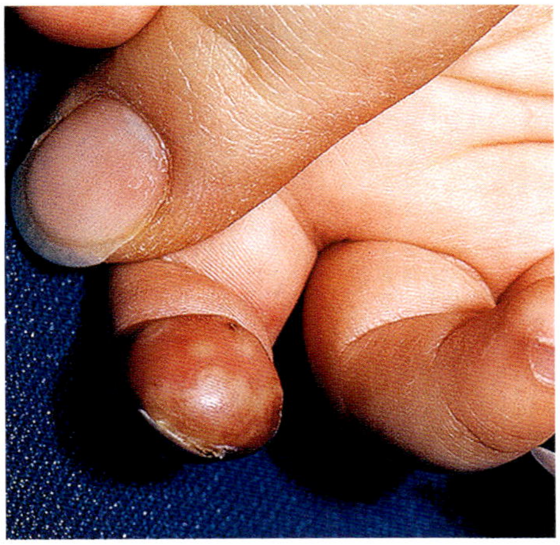

Fig. 15.11 Herpetic whitlow. Clustered, tender, deep-seated vesicles of the distal phalanx.

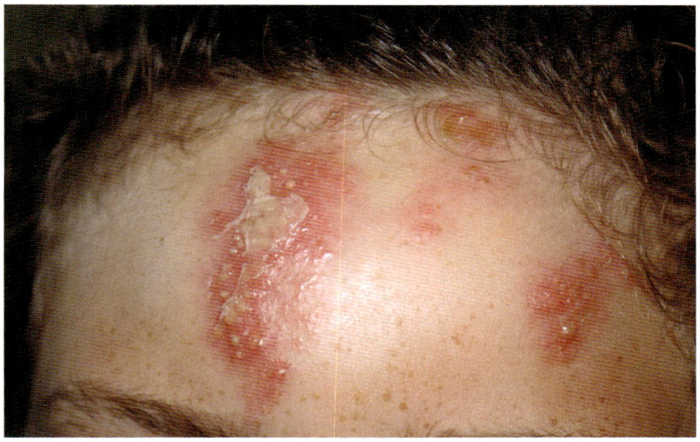

Fig. 15.12 Herpes gladiatorum. Widespread and often multifocal clusters of vesicles overlying an erythematous base, as shown here, occur in patients with cutaneous herpes simplex virus (HSV) infection related to contact sports. Common locations include the head, neck, and upper extremities.

HERPES IN THE IMMUNOCOMPROMISED HOST

Severe, chronic, and recalcitrant HSV infections may be seen in the setting of immunodeficiency. These settings include individuals with hematologic malignancy, those with a history of bone marrow or solid-organ transplantation, and those with HIV infection. Although these patients may develop common forms of HSV infection, their lesions may be more widespread and extensive. Persistent or recurrent ulcers are a common manifestation of HSV infection in patients with AIDS.[1] Large, persistent ulcers in patients infected with HIV should arouse suspicion for HSV, although the differential diagnosis may include syphilis and chancroid. Less common locations such as the buttocks and back are also more likely to be involved in these patients.[24] HSV lesions in immunocompromised hosts may also be verrucous, pustular, markedly crusted (Fig. 15.13), necrotic (Fig. 15.14), or exophytic.

In addition to cutaneous lesions, disseminated HSV may be noted in this patient population. Oropharyngeal involvement, esophagitis, tracheobronchitis, pneumonitis, hepatitis, pancreatitis, adrenal necrosis, and gastrointestinal tract and bone marrow involvement may occur.[1] These severe and/or disseminated infections may be caused by either HSV-1 or HSV-2.

Herpes Zoster

HZ (also called *zoster* or *shingles*) is an acute vesicular eruption caused by reactivation of a latent infection with VZV in the sensory ganglia. Although it is most often seen in elderly or immunosuppressed individuals, it may also occur in children. Although pediatric zoster is most common in immunocompromised children or those who had a primary intrauterine infection or acute varicella within the first year of life,[59] it may occasionally occur in children without any of these risk factors. Children with systemic lupus erythematosus and asthma may be more susceptible to developing HZ.[60,61] Neonatal HZ has rarely

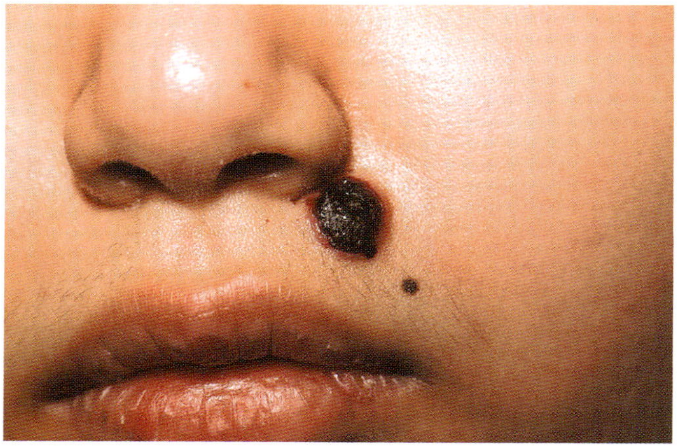

Fig. 15.13 Herpes in the immunocompromised host. This large, crusted plaque was culture positive for *Herpes simplex* in this 6-year-old girl receiving chemotherapy for leukemia.

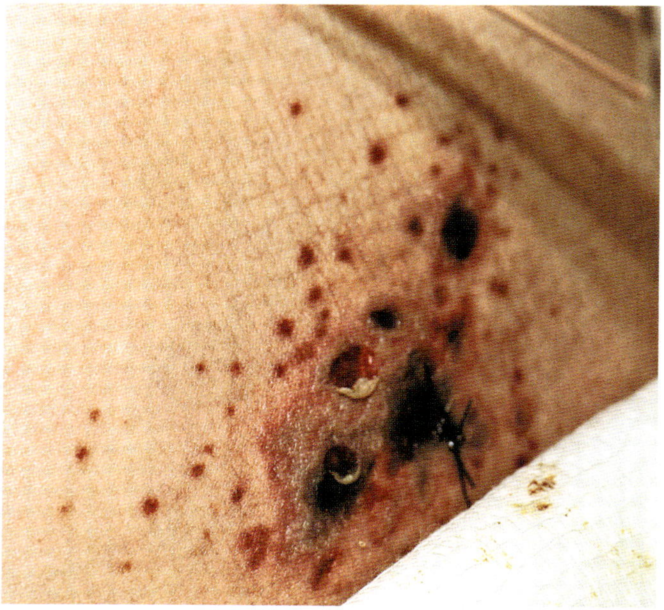

Fig. 15.14 Herpes in the immunocompromised host. Vesicles rapidly progressed to necrotic plaques in this young girl status post–bone marrow transplantation.

been reported, presumably in association with exposure to varicella zoster *in utero*. Due to licensure of the live attenuated Oka strain varicella vaccine, it has become clear that HZ may be caused by reactivation of the latent vaccine virus, even in children.[62,63] Studies of HZ incidence since implementation of the vaccination program in 1995 have yielded conflicting results, showing both increased incidence and no increase, and suggesting that there may be other unidentified risk factors for HZ that are changing over time.[64] In a review of 322 children with HZ, the incidence in vaccinated children (either wild type or vaccine strain) was 79% lower than in unvaccinated children (wild type only).[65] In one series of seven vaccinated children who developed HZ, the location correlated with the vaccination site, suggesting possible vaccine strain–related HZ with retrograde spread from the sensory nerves to the dorsal ganglion.[66]

HZ is characterized by vesicles and erythema clustered in a dermatomal distribution of one or more sensory nerves (Figs. 15.15 and 15.16). The most commonly affected dermatomes are the second cervical to second lumbar nerves (C2 to L2) and the fifth (Fig. 15.17) and

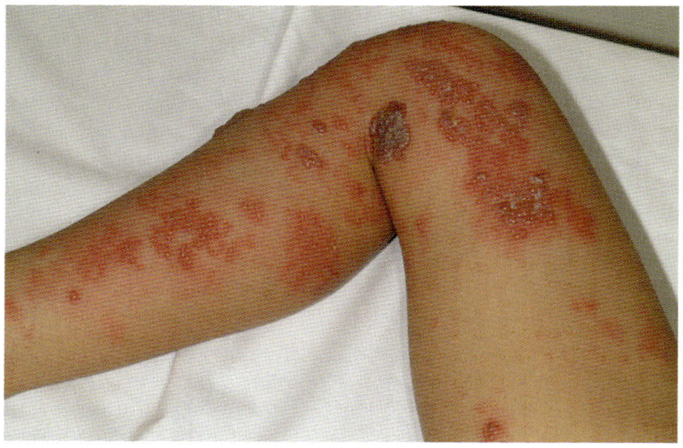

Fig. 15.15 Herpes zoster. Numerous clustered vesicles and bullae in a dermatomal distribution on the lower extremity of a 4-year-old girl who had been diagnosed with natural varicella at 2 months of age.

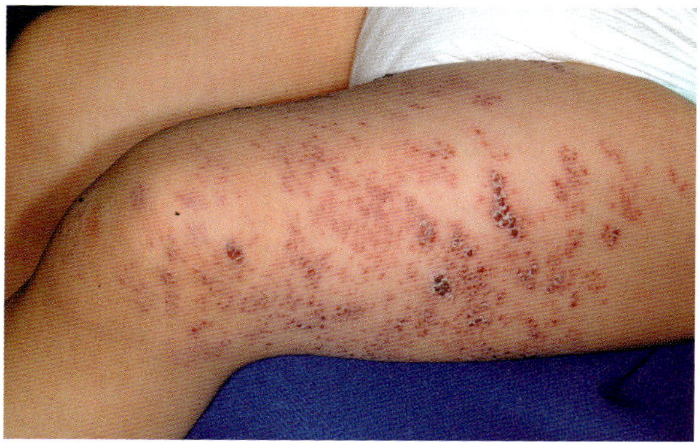

Fig. 15.16 Herpes zoster. Confluent vesicles and crusted vesicles with erythema in a dermatomal distribution on the left thigh. This immunized boy was otherwise healthy with no identifiable underlying predisposition.

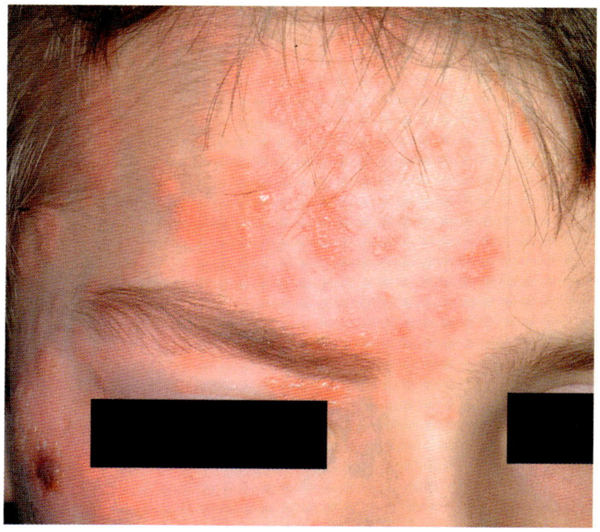

Fig. 15.17 Herpes zoster. Edema with erythema and vesiculation, distributed in a V1 and partial V2 distribution, in an 8-year-old boy. Corneal involvement may occur with this presentation.

seventh cranial nerves. Patients often complain of hyperesthesia, pain, and tenderness to light touch in the affected area(s), usually before any cutaneous findings are present. Although the eruption is usually unilateral with a sharp demarcation at the midline, occasional contralateral involvement is seen. It is not unusual to see a few randomly scattered vesicular lesions beyond the primary dermatomal involvement, and such scattered lesions do not necessarily constitute disseminated zoster.

Successive crops of new lesions with extension of the process may occur for up to 1 week, followed by crusting of the vesicles and healing over 1 to 2 weeks. In children the disorder tends to be milder, and healing often occurs rapidly, within a few days to 1 week.[67] In addition, in otherwise healthy children, postherpetic neuralgia (PHN, a delayed phenomenon of chronic pain and paresthesias in an area previously affected by HZ) is rare. PHN is more common in elderly patients and in those with a history of ophthalmic HZ (see later).[68]

Immunocompromised children with HZ may have more extensive involvement with a higher risk of viremia and visceral dissemination.[67] This may include pneumonia, encephalitis, hepatitis, and disseminated intravascular coagulopathy.[67,69] These patients may also have disseminated cutaneous involvement that presents in a fashion more typical of acute varicella and with no obvious dermatomal component.[69] The intensity of chemotherapy may affect the risk of HZ; in one series, more than half of the children with acute lymphoblastic leukemia receiving chemotherapy on high-risk protocols developed HZ during their course of treatment.[70] *Abdominal zoster* refers to the presentation of HZ as severe abdominal pain that precedes the development of cutaneous lesions. These patients are often explored surgically, and the condition is associated with a high incidence of abdominal visceral involvement. Children infected with HIV may have chronic or relapsing HZ or HZ with unusual cutaneous lesions (e.g., hyperkeratotic papules, ulcers, or necrotic plaques).

Infection associated with the ophthalmic branch of the fifth (trigeminal) nerve may involve the cornea with keratitis and uveitis and may lead to permanent damage. This presentation (termed *HZ ophthalmicus*) occurs when the nasociliary branch is involved and accordingly presents with cutaneous involvement of the nasal tip (Hutchinson sign).[71] This important sign should not be overlooked and should prompt rapid diagnosis, referral, and institution of therapy.

HZ of the maxillary division of the trigeminal nerve produces vesiculation of the palate, uvula, and tonsillar area. Involvement of the mandibular division produces vesicular involvement of the anterior aspects of the tongue, floor of the mouth, lips, and buccal mucous membranes. Involvement of the geniculate ganglion produces lesions on the tongue, ear, and skin of the auditory canal. When accompanied by Bell palsy and disturbances of hearing and equilibrium, it is part of the Ramsay Hunt syndrome.

The diagnosis of HZ is often a clinical one, and in typical cases further evaluations are generally unnecessary. In patients in whom diagnostic confirmation is indicated, direct detection with fluorescent antibody stains of vesicle-base scrapings is useful. Viral culture can be used, but VZV may take up to 1 week to induce cytopathic changes. The most sensitive method for confirming the diagnosis of VZV infection is use of PCR, especially on swabs taken from vesicular lesions. This testing is convenient and very accurate, with high sensitivity (approaching 100% with multiplex real-time PCR).[72,73] Real-time PCR analysis of salivary DNA may also be sensitive for diagnosing VZV in patients with HZ.[74] Serologic studies are considered less useful in the diagnosis of HZ.

Treatment for HZ consists of symptomatic measures and specific antiviral therapy (Table 15.2). Symptomatic care includes wet compresses, drying lotions (e.g., calamine), antihistamines, and analgesics. High-dose acyclovir decreases vesicle formation, time to crusting, and days of pain when instituted within 72 hours of onset of the exanthem. Acyclovir should be administered via the intravenous route in immunocompromised patients, given their greater severity of disease, or in any patient with disseminated or severe infection. Other antiviral options in immunocompetent patients or those with uncomplicated HZ include valacyclovir and famciclovir. An HZ vaccine is licensed for adults 50 years of age and older (although the Advisory Committee on Immunization Practices [ACIP] recommends it only for immunocompetent adults 60 years of age and older), with widespread vaccination desirable to help in the prevention of HZ and PHN in this population and in reducing the health and financial costs of HZ.[75-77] This vaccine is nearly identical to the varicella vaccine, except that the HZ vaccine contains 14 times as many virus particles.[78] Given that vaccine protection wanes completely after 10 years, future recommendations may include booster dosing after that time.[79]

Table 15.2 Systemic Antiviral Medications Used for Herpes Zoster*

Drug	Formulation	Regimen	Indication/ Comment
Acyclovir	200 mg capsule 400 mg, 800 mg tablet 200 mg/ 5 mL susp		A: ≥2 years
		800 mg 5 times/day	Adults and children ≥12 years; 7–10 days Pediatric HZ dosing: NE
	50 mg/ 1 mL IV	60 mg/ kg per day	IC <12 years; divide every 8 hours; 7–10 days
		30 mg/kg per day	IC ≥12 years; divide every 8 hours; 7–10 days
Famciclovir	125, 250, 500 mg tablet	500 mg 3 times/ day	A: ≥18 years; 7 days
Valacyclovir	500 mg, 1 g caplet	1 g 3 times/day	A: adults; 7 days

A, Approved; *HZ,* herpes zoster; *IC,* immunocompromised; *IV,* intravenous preparation; *NE,* not established.
*Approved indications and regimens listed; often used off-label.

Viral-Like Disorders of the Oral Mucosa

APHTHOUS STOMATITIS

Recurrent aphthous stomatitis (RAS; aphthous ulcers, canker sores) is one of the most common painful diseases affecting the oral mucosa of children. It has been reported in 5% to 25% of the general population, and there may be a genetic predisposition.[80,81] The etiology is not well understood, and treatment has traditionally been symptomatic. Aphthous stomatitis presents with single or multiple shallow erosions or ulcerations (Fig. 15.18) on the labial and buccal mucosae, gingivae, tongue, floor of the mouth, palate, or pharynx. Before the onset of the lesions, a tingling sensation may be present. After 24 to 48 hours, a focal erythema develops, followed soon thereafter by tiny, superficial gray-white erosions. Usually there are one to three lesions (minor RAS; 80% to 85% of cases), and the area of erosion increases and evolves into one or more sharply defined shallow ulcers covered by gray membranes and surrounded by sharp borders and slightly elevated, bright red areolae. Lesions usually measure 3 to 6 mm in diameter, and if left untreated, persist for 8 to 12 days (sometimes longer) and heal without scarring. Occasionally patients develop larger ulcerations, up to several centimeters in size with prolonged pain, fever, and healing with scarring. This variant has been termed *major RAS* (10% of cases; formally known as *Sutton disease*) and may be associated with dysphagia, malaise, and HIV infection.[82] Another form of aphthae, herpetiform RAS, occurs in 5% to 10% of patients with aphthous lesions and presents as clusters of pinpoint ulcers that simulate, but are not caused by, infection with HSV.[83]

Aphthous stomatitis is believed to be multifactorial in origin and may occur in response to a variety of triggering factors, including

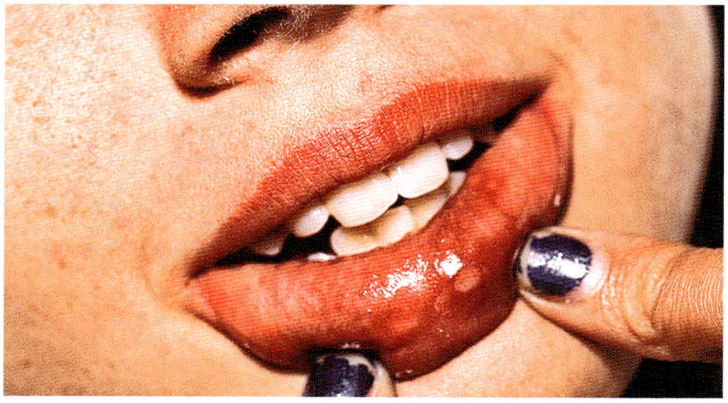

Fig. 15.18 Aphthous stomatitis. Multiple shallow erosions of the labial mucosa.

stress, trauma, hormonal changes, and infection. Cytokines are felt to play an important role, and polymorphisms in the genes for ILs lb and 6 may increase a patient's individual risk of RAS.[84] Human leukocyte antigen (HLA)–B52 and HLA-B44 antigens were found to be strongly associated with RAS in Israeli Arab youths.[85] Drug-induced RAS has also been suggested, especially in association with nonsteroidal anti-inflammatory drugs and β-blockers.[86] Both EBV and CMV have been hypothesized as potential infectious causes of RAS.[87,88] In the vast majority of cases, the etiology remains unknown.

The differential diagnosis (and/or potential associations) of RAS includes Behçet syndrome (see Chapter 25); inflammatory bowel disease (see Chapter 25); cyclic neutropenia; gluten-sensitive enteropathy; herpes simplex infection; candidiasis; vitamin/nutritional deficiencies (iron, folic acid, zinc, and vitamins B_1, B_2, B_6, and B_{12}); and the syndrome of periodic fever, aphthous stomatitis, pharyngitis, and cervical adenitis (PFAPA, Marshall syndrome) (see Chapter 25). PFAPA syndrome is characterized by high fevers (up to 41° C), aphthous ulcers, pharyngitis (which is usually culture negative), and cervical adenitis, and there is a familial predisposition.[89] A variant in the *CARD8* gene *(CARD8-FS)* is associated with classical PFAPA.[90] Associated symptoms include headache, nausea, vomiting, and abdominal pain.[83,91] The syndrome usually occurs in patients younger than 5 years of age, and flares recur at 21- to 42-day intervals. The fevers resolve over 24 to 48 hours spontaneously and often drop dramatically after even a single dose of oral corticosteroids. Other reportedly effective therapies have included cimetidine, colchicine, and tonsillectomy; the latter is particularly effective in patients with late-onset (>5 years) or incomplete PFAPA.[91–93] Overall, patients with PFAPA syndrome do well, with spontaneous resolution of the episodes within 3 to 5 years and without any long-term sequelae.

Treatments for RAS include primarily topical corticosteroids and topical and/or oral analgesics. Topical clobetasol, a potent corticosteroid, in a denture paste or oral analgesic base and applied two to three times daily, often results in remission and symptomatic relief.[94] Mixtures of diphenhydramine elixir and Kaopectate or Maalox have been used successfully, as have a variety of medical mouthwashes (e.g., chlorhexidine [Peridex] antibacterial oral rinse). Patients with severe manifestations of RAS may respond to the oral corticosteroids (usually short course), colchicine, thalidomide, or dapsone. Multivitamin administration has not been demonstrated useful in reducing the frequency or duration of RAS episodes.[95,96]

ACUTE NECROTIZING GINGIVITIS

Acute necrotizing gingivitis (acute necrotizing ulcerative gingivitis, trench mouth, Vincent stomatitis, Vincent angina) is a painful ulcerative disorder that chiefly affects adolescents and young adults. A related disorder termed *noma* (see Chapter 14) occurs when the infection spreads beyond the gingiva to involve other oral mucosal surfaces. Although acute necrotizing gingivitis was formerly common in schools and military establishments, it is quite rare in the United States and Western Hemisphere, perhaps due to improved oral and dental care. The cause of acute necrotizing gingivitis is often a mix of bacterial pathogens, including *Fusobacterium, Prevotella, Actinomyces*, and *Bacteroides* species and spirochetes. The condition occurs most commonly in patients with predisposing conditions such as malnutrition, poor oral hygiene, ethanol or tobacco use, or immunosuppression.

Clinical findings consist of painful gingivae that bleed easily and an inflamed, eroded, hemorrhagic oropharynx. Ulcerations are most common at the gingival margins and interdental papillae. The ulcers are covered by a grayish-white slough or pseudomembrane that can be removed, leaving behind a raw bleeding surface. Single or multiple papillae may be involved, and the ulceration can be very extensive. Associated features include lymphadenopathy, pain, bleeding of the gums, fever, and a foul breath odor.[97] Treatment of acute necrotizing gingivitis consists of debridement by a dentist or periodontist and broad-spectrum antibiotic therapy, usually penicillin, clindamycin, or erythromycin. Chlorhexidine or saltwater oral rinses may help alleviate discomfort. Attention to good oral hygiene and nutritional rehabilitation (where indicated) are important steps in prevention.

Warts

Warts (verrucae) are a common viral infection of the skin and mucosae caused by the human papillomavirus (HPV). These benign intraepidermal tumors most commonly occur in children and young adults, and their incidence has been estimated at 10%.[98,99] However, frequency estimates vary widely by study. In a cross-sectional study of 1465 primary schoolchildren, 33% had warts, whereas a population-based study using the US National Health Interview Survey found a childhood prevalence of 3.3%.[100,101] Although harmless and often self-involuting over years, warts are occasionally painful and may carry a negative social stigma. In addition, HPV may be associated with cutaneous and genital oncogenesis, particularly in immunosuppressed individuals.

There are four basic types of warts: verruca vulgaris, verruca plana, verruca plantaris, and condyloma acuminatum. Each of these will be discussed individually in the following sections. Most warts occur on the hands, fingers, elbows, and plantar surfaces of the feet. Patients with warts commonly autoinoculate themselves inadvertently with the subsequent appearance of multiple secondary lesions. A classic feature of cutaneous warts is that of koebnerization, whereby a linear constellation of lesions develops along the path of excoriation (Fig. 15.19).

HPV is transmitted via skin-to-skin contact or from fomites, where recently shed viruses may survive if the environment is warm and moist (e.g., locker room floors, pool decking, showers). The entry site is often an area of recent trauma or a skin region with subclinical

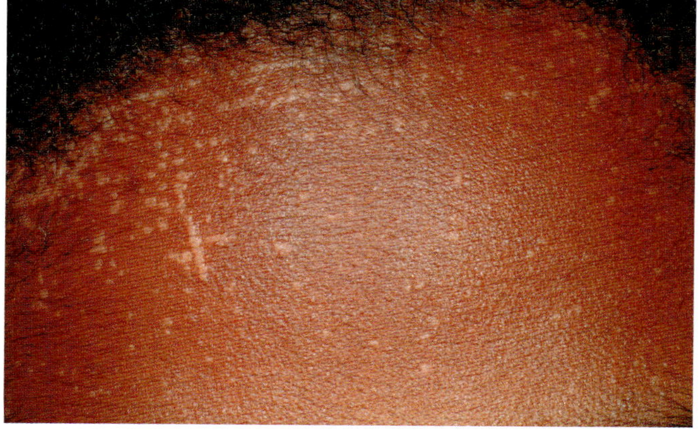

Fig. 15.19 Warts with koebnerization. Multiple small, verrucous papules with a linear clustering (Koebner phenomenon) were present on this child's forehead.

abrasion or fissuring. It has been shown that important environmental risk factors include having family members with warts and wart prevalence in classrooms, suggesting that preventive recommendations should perhaps focus on these sources more than public places.[100,102] The incubation period from inoculation to development of the wart may range from 1 to 6 months or more. Although the duration of warts is variable, one study documented that two-thirds of lesions resolve spontaneously within 2 years.[103] In another retrospective study of warts in children, 65% resolved by 2 years and 80% within 4 years, regardless of treatment.[104] The most important mechanism in wart regression appears to be cell-mediated immunity, with cytokines released by keratinocytes or immune system cells inducing an immune response against HPV.[105]

Over 200 HPV genotypes comprise this family of small double-stranded DNA viruses, and the various HPV types have been divided into two groups: cutaneous and mucosal. HPV can also be categorized into groups of "high risk" and "low risk" relating to their oncogenicity.[106,107] Mucosal types are recovered mainly in the genital tract, although other mucosae may be infected, including the respiratory tract, nose, conjunctiva, and mouth. Although the same HPV virus can cause various types of warts, there is often a correlation between the virus type and the clinical/morphologic characteristics of the lesions it causes. For instance, HPV types 1, 2, 4, and 7 are often associated with common warts (verrucae vulgaris); type 1 with deep palmar and plantar warts; types 3, 10, 28, and 41 with flat warts; types 5, 8, 17, and 20 (among others) with the autosomal recessive disorder epidermodysplasia verruciformis (EV) (see later); and types 6 and 11 with respiratory, conjunctival, and genital infection.[106] In addition, HPV types associated with a high risk for cervical cancer include 16, 18, 31, 33, 35, 39, 45, 51, 52, 56, 58, 59, 66, and 68, among others.[80] HPV types 16 and 18 are the most common high-risk types found in the female anogenital system and are seen in up to 70% of women with cervical cancer. In a study of HPV types and their relationships to patient characteristics, the most distinct clinical profile was noted with HPV-1, which was associated with infection in children younger than 12 years of age, plantar location, a duration of less than 6 months, and patients with fewer warts.[108] Laboratory diagnosis of routine HPV skin infection is usually unnecessary, and the diagnosis is usually straightforward. In instances where identification of the HPV genotype is necessary, Food and Drug Administration (FDA)–approved options include DNA-based assays (nuclear acid hybridization, real-time PCR, and signal amplification invader assay) and messenger RNA (mRNA)–based assays (transcription-mediated amplification). HPV genotyping on swabs of the skin overlying warts using a novel PCR assay has been shown to be a simple and highly sensitive approach to typing.[109]

VERRUCAE VULGARIS

Verrucae vulgaris (common warts) occur predominantly on the dorsal surface of the hands or periungual regions but may be seen anywhere on the cutaneous surface. Occasionally they may also occur on the oral mucosa. Common warts may occur as single or multiple lesions. They clinically present as flesh-colored, verrucous (rough surfaced) papules that may be dome-shaped (Fig. 15.20), exophytic (Fig. 15.21), or filiform (having a stalk; Fig. 15.22). Individual lesions may coalesce into larger plaques (Fig. 15.23). "Ring warts" may occur after overly aggressive therapies and are another example of koebnerization (Fig. 15.24). Oral lesions present as small, pink-white, soft papules and plaques of the labial, lingual (Fig. 15.25), buccal, or gingival mucosa. In Heck disease, multiple verrucous papules occur in a similar mucosal distribution (Fig. 15.26).

Periungual and subungual verrucae (Figs. 15.27 and 15.28) occur around and beneath nailbeds, particularly on the fingers of cuticle pickers and nail biters. These lesions, because of their location and susceptibility to trauma, often become irritated, infected, or tender and are often more resistant to therapy. Satellite lesions may appear, particularly near warts that have been irritated, manipulated, or incompletely treated. When the diagnosis of verruca is in doubt, gentle paring with a number 15 scalpel blade will reveal characteristic punctate black dots that represent thrombosed capillaries (Fig. 15.29).

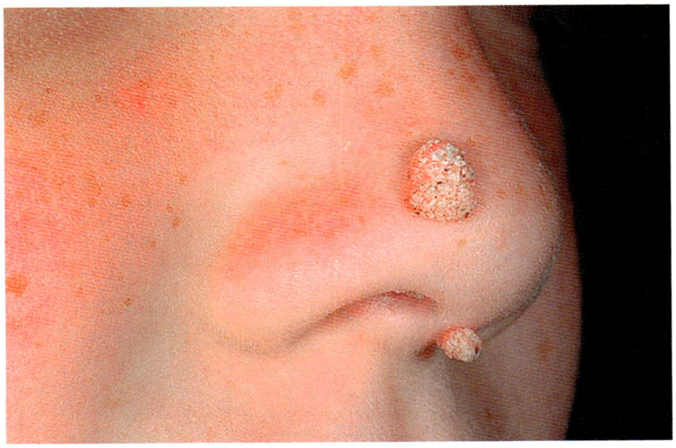

Fig. 15.20 Common warts. A dome-shaped lesion of the lateral nose and a filiform lesion of the columella.

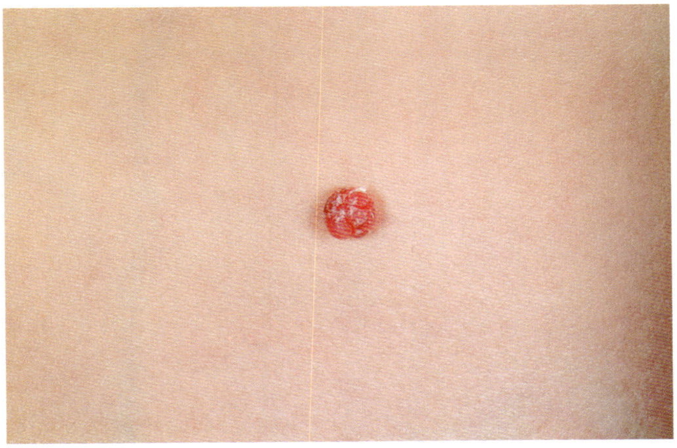

Fig. 15.21 Common wart. This lesion demonstrates the exophytic type of verruca vulgaris.

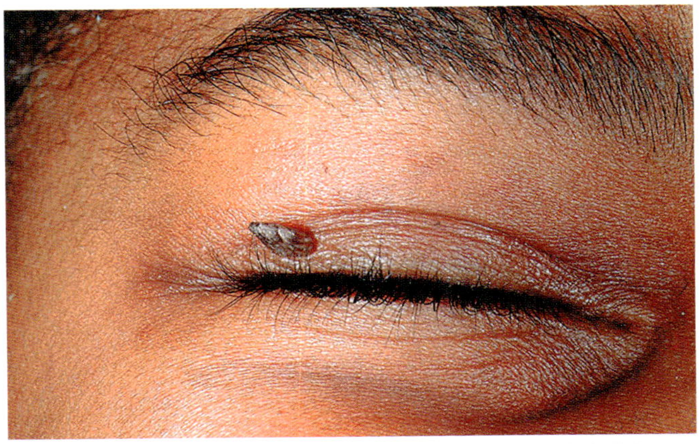

Fig. 15.22 Common wart. This lesion has a stalk and is termed a *filiform wart.*

VERRUCAE PLANA

Verrucae plana (flat warts) occur primarily on the face, neck, arms, and legs. They are usually seen as smooth, flesh-colored to slightly pink or brown, flat-topped papules measuring 2 to 5 mm in diameter (Figs. 15.30 and 15.31; see also Fig. 15.19). They vary from a few lesions to several hundred in any given individual. They may appear

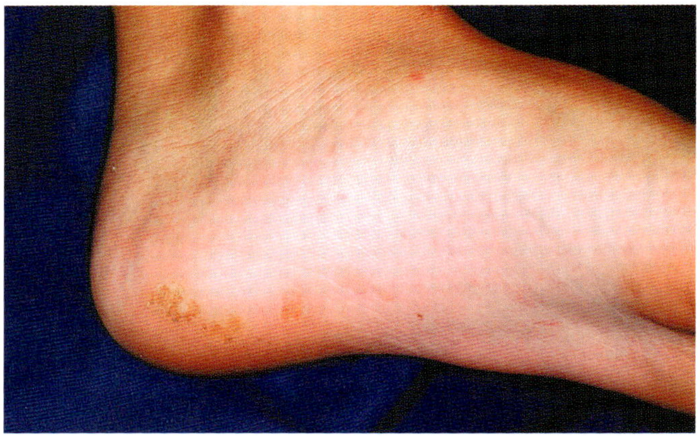

Fig. 15.23 Common warts. Multiple lesions coalesce into a mosaic plaque on the plantar surface.

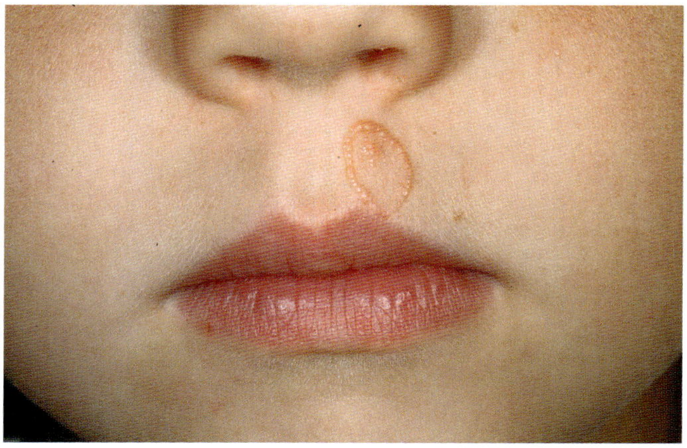

Fig. 15.24 Ring warts. This annular plaque composed of small verrucous papules developed after a marked blister response to therapy of a single wart above the upper lip.

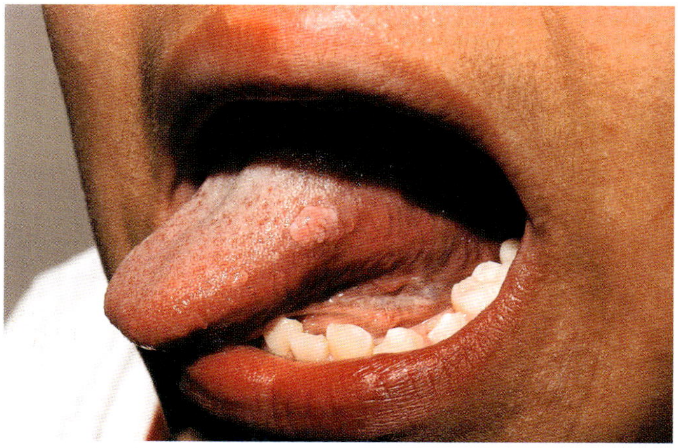

Fig. 15.25 Common warts affecting mucosa. This tongue lesion presented as a soft, verrucous papule.

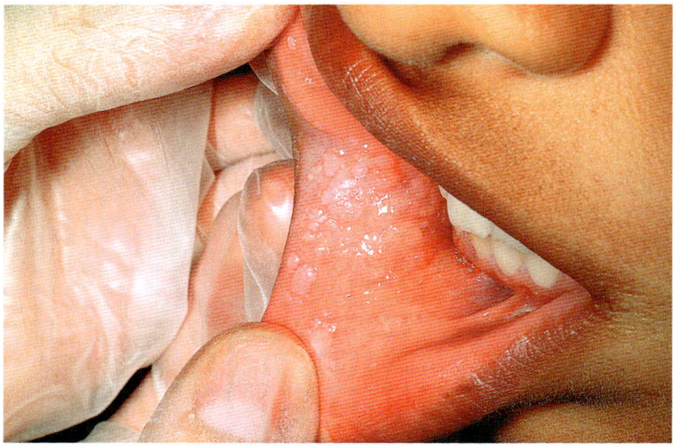

Fig. 15.26 Heck disease. Multiple soft, pink verrucous papules of the inner lip mucosa.

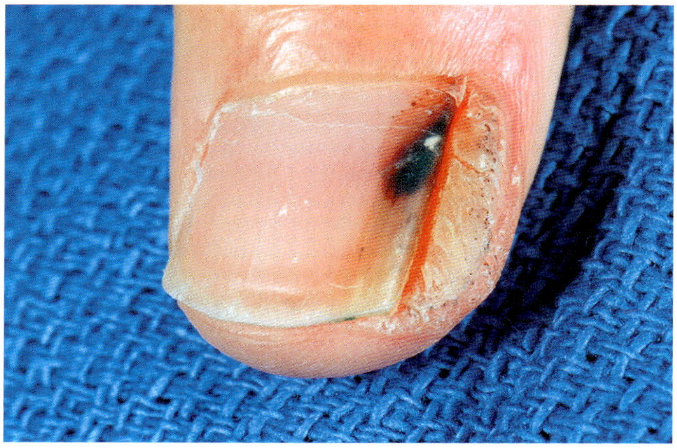

Fig. 15.27 Periungual warts. Verrucous papules of the lateral nailfold. Note adjacent subungual hemorrhage.

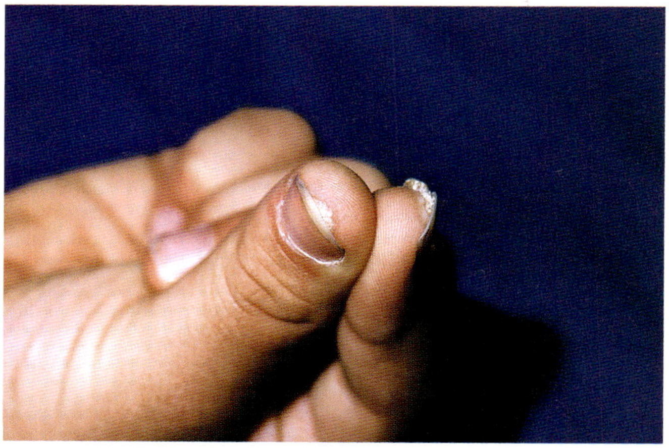

Fig. 15.28 Subungual warts. Verrucous papules of the distal thumb and index finger with extension under the nail plate.

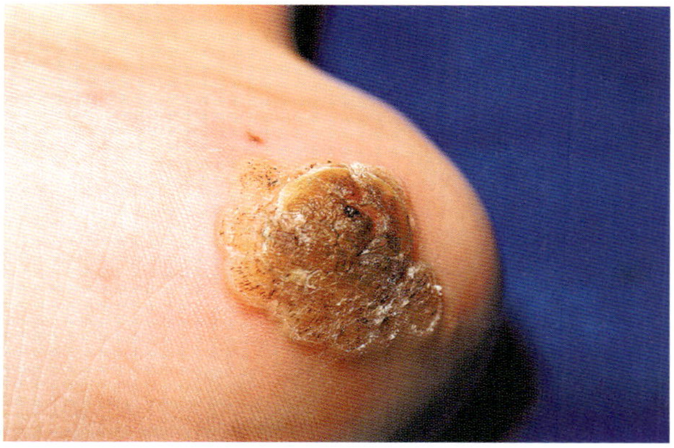

Fig. 15.29 Wart with thrombosed capillaries. Note the multiple black dots within this large mosaic plantar wart.

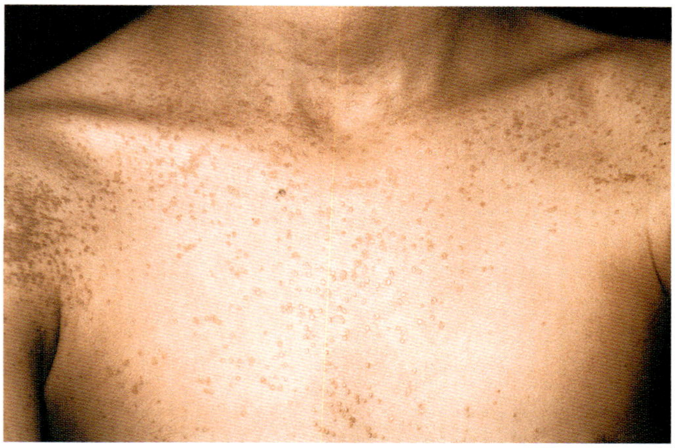

Fig. 15.31 Flat warts. Multiple disseminated flat papules in a patient infected with human immunodeficiency virus (HIV).

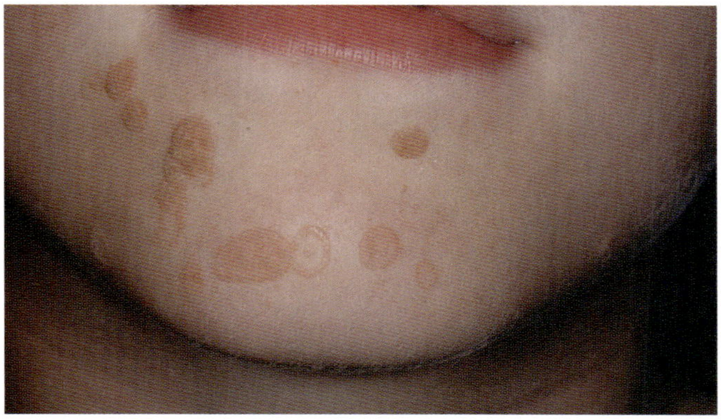

Fig. 15.30 Flat warts. Flat, verrucous papules on the chin of a 6-year-old boy. Note the scattered "ring warts," related to prior therapy with cantharidin.

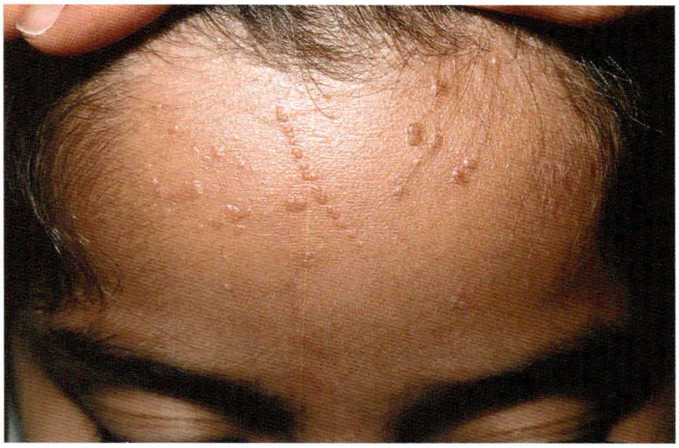

Fig. 15.32 Flat warts with koebnerization. Flat papules on the forehead, with a linear configuration (Koebner phenomenon) at sites of autoinoculation.

in the bearded areas of men and on the legs of women, because irritation from shaving tends to cause their spread. Contiguous warts may coalesce to form larger, plaque-like lesions. Again, linear arrangements of the papules in areas of scratching (koebnerization) are characteristic (Fig. 15.32; see also Fig. 15.19).

VERRUCAE PLANTARIS

Verrucae plantaris (plantar warts) occur on the plantar surfaces of the feet and tend to be the most symptomatic type of warts, as well as a therapeutic challenge. They usually occur on the weight-bearing areas of the heels, toes, and midmetatarsal areas (Fig. 15.33). Because of the pressure of walking, the lesions often develop an endophytic component and are very painful and tender. Coalescence of multiple lesions may result in mosaic warts (Fig. 15.34), and individual lesions may attain a large size (Fig. 15.35). It may occasionally be difficult to differentiate plantar warts from corns or calluses. Corns are localized hyperkeratoses that form over interphalangeal joints as the result of intermittent pressure and friction. Penetrating corns often appear at the base of the second or third metatarsal–phalangeal joint. They can be distinguished from plantar warts by the lack of thrombosed capillaries after paring and by their characteristic hard core. Soft corns are macerated hyperkeratotic lesions that persist at points of friction and pressure in intertriginous areas. They are usually seen on the lateral aspect of the toes or in the web spaces between the fourth and fifth toes.

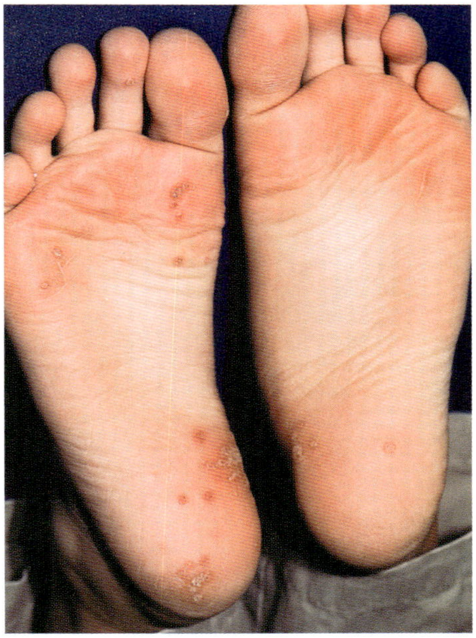

Fig. 15.33 Plantar warts. Verrucous papules on the plantar surfaces.

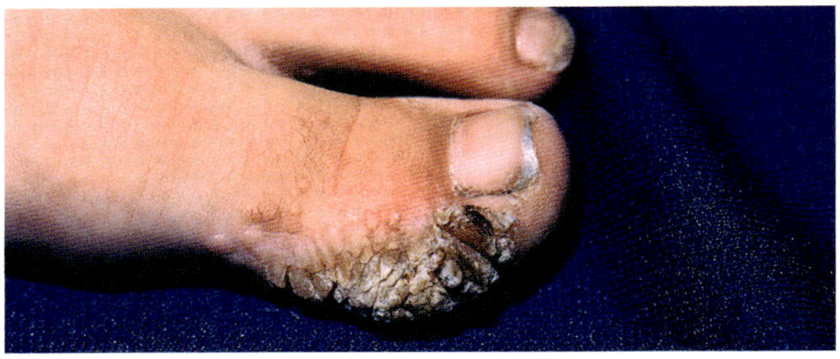

Fig. 15.34 Plantar warts, mosaic. Multiple verrucous papules coalesced into this giant, painful verrucous plaque.

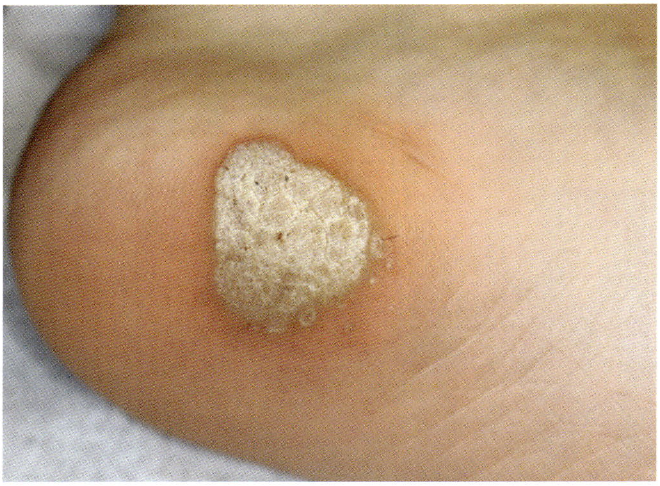

Fig. 15.35 Plantar wart. This lesion in a teenaged girl attained a large size and was quite painful with ambulation.

Black heel (talon noir, calcaneal petechiae) is a common condition that is often confused with plantar warts. In this disorder, superficial dermal capillaries are ruptured by the shearing action associated with sudden stops in athletic individuals, usually tennis, racquetball, or basketball players. Clinically it is characterized by clusters of brown or blue-black pinpoint petechial macules in the horny layer along the backs or sides of the heels or lateral edges of the feet. Gentle paring of the surface with a number 15 scalpel blade can help differentiate this condition from malignant melanoma, calluses, corns, and plantar warts.

CONDYLOMATA ACUMINATA

Condylomata acuminata (anogenital warts, anogenital HPV) are HPV-induced lesions of the anogenital tract and one of the most common STDs. The diagnosis of condylomata acuminata in a child is fraught with anxiety for parents and practitioners alike, and the implications regarding sexual abuse versus benign transmission are controversial and often unclear. Although condylomata often occur after sexual contact, other modes of acquiring the infection include vertical (perinatal) transmission, benign (nonsexual) heteroinoculation, and autoinoculation. In addition, fomite spread is another potential mode of transmission.[110]

Condylomata acuminata present most commonly in the perianal area as flesh-colored, soft, verrucous papules (Fig. 15.36) measuring 1 to 5 mm in diameter. The lesions are usually multiple, and "mirror image" lesions may be noted on each side of the anus. Other areas of involvement include the glans penis, penile shaft, scrotum, and vulva. Vaginal and cervical involvement are appreciable only with internal examination. Occasionally, lesions may enlarge rapidly and present as large, exophytic, cauliflower-like masses (Fig. 15.37). Childhood condylomata are usually incidentally noted during diaper changes, toileting, bathing, or physical examinations.[111] The lesions are usually asymptomatic, but irritation, bleeding, and pain may occur. The differential diagnosis of condylomata acuminata includes molluscum contagiosum, epidermal nevus, skin tag, and pseudoverrucous papules and nodules. Infantile perianal pyramidal protrusion is a pyramid-shaped, flesh-colored to pink soft-tissue swelling (Fig. 15.38) that appears in the medial raphe of girls and may represent a peculiar form of lichen sclerosus et atrophicus.[112,113] The distribution, appearance, and solitary nature of this lesion should distinguish it from condylomata.

The diagnosis of condylomata acuminata in a child should prompt consideration for the possibility of sexual abuse. In one large study of children with evidence of child sexual abuse, genital HPV infection was present in 13.7%.[114] However, it should be remembered that anogenital warts occur in large numbers of children as a result of innocent (nonsexual) or vertical transmission or from autoinoculation. Although HPV DNA typing is occasionally considered, it does not help in the differentiation between the various modes of transmission.[110,111] Although innocent autoinoculation or heteroinoculation from hand warts is common and the finding of such hand lesions in an adult contact or caretaker might be reassuring, fondling is a form of sexual abuse commonly seen in younger children, and thus the possibility of sexual abuse must still be considered.[115]

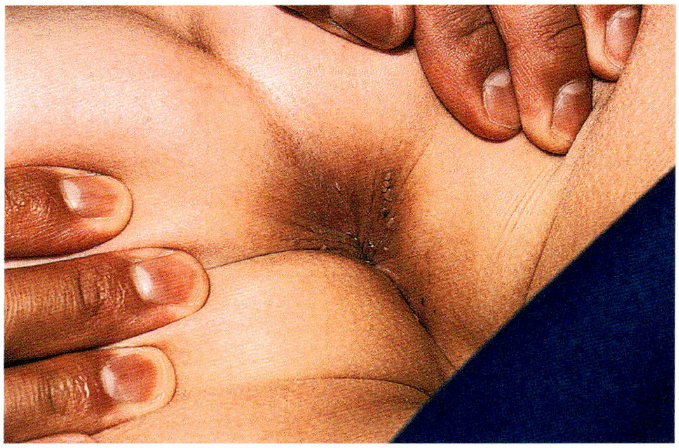

Fig. 15.36 Condylomata acuminata. Verrucous, brown papules in a perianal distribution.

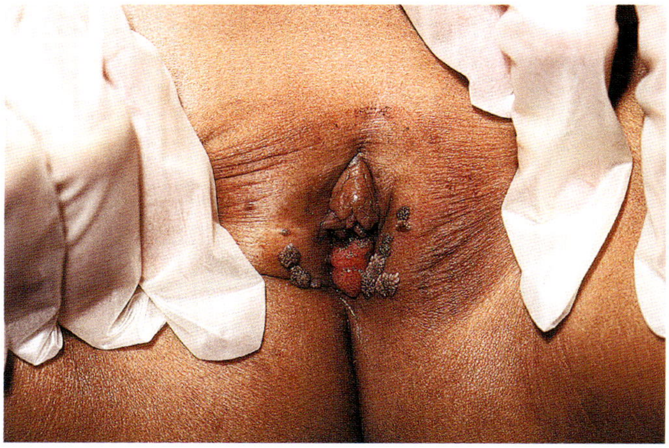

Fig. 15.37 Condylomata acuminata. Verrucous papules of the labial surfaces, with a large, vegetative lesion protruding from the vagina. This toddler had been sexually abused.

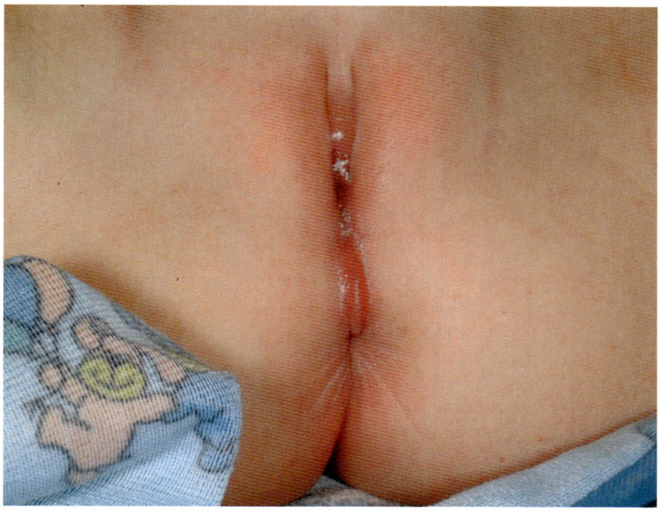

Fig. 15.38 Infantile perianal pyramidal protrusion. Pyramidal-shaped, fleshy papule of the midline raphe.

When a child is diagnosed with anogenital condylomata, a directed history should include the age of onset, history of maternal infection (genital warts or abnormal Papanicolaou [Pap] smear), and personal or family history of warts, as well as inquiries about the child's social environment and all caregivers.[115] Physical examination should be focused on findings suggestive of sexual abuse, and laboratory evaluation for other STDs should be performed if noninnocent HPV transmission is suggested. A behavioral and social assessment by a skilled professional should be considered. A summary of findings that should prompt referral to child protective services is shown in Table 15.3. The literature contains significant disagreement with regard to the prevalence of sexual abuse in children with condylomata, with estimates ranging variably from 4% to 91%.[111] Although sexual transmission of HPV may occur at any age, the risk seems greater in children over 3 to 4 years of age, and some experts recommend definitive reporting if this age criterion is met.[116–118] The Committee on Child Abuse and Neglect of the American Academy of Pediatrics (AAP) considers the presence of anogenital warts in children "suspicious" and recommends reporting to a child protective agency.[30]

The authors' personal approach is to consider nonsexual transmission of HPV if the child is under 3 years of age; if lesions developed within the first year of life; if the patient has other nongenital warts; if warts are present in close contacts, especially genital warts (or history of abnormal Pap smear) in the mother; and when there are no findings to suggest sexual abuse. If there is any suspicion of sexual abuse, referral to child protective services is initiated. In patients in whom there is uncertainty or where the situation is ambiguous, a social worker from the protective-services team should be enlisted early on in the evaluation for a formal structured interview. Although the diagnosis of sexual abuse must never be missed, "reflexive reporting" to child welfare authorities should be avoided, given the emotional devastation and destruction that may result. Practitioners need to balance the risk of missing a case of sexual abuse (if they do not report) against the decision to report the family, with the parents or caregivers potentially suffering false accusation and its ramifications, which in some cases may include losing parental custody.[119] If the practitioner evaluating the patient is uncomfortable in performing such an evaluation, referral should be made to a clinician with expertise for further evaluation.[111]

Table 15.3 Findings in a Child with Condylomata that Should Prompt Referral to Child Protective Services

Finding	Comment
Abuse suspected by parent(s)	Includes history of access to the child by a known sexual offender
Abuse disclosed by child	If child appropriately aged for interview (usually 3–4 years)
Child's behaviors suggestive	Includes nightmares, advanced sexual knowledge for age, acting out sexually with peers
Suggestive physical examination	Acute or chronic trauma (petechiae, bruising to the hymen, anal tears, absent hymen, anogenital scarring)
Findings of other sexually transmitted infection	May include gonorrhea, *Chlamydia, Trichomonas,* human immunodeficiency virus, hepatitis B and C, syphilis
Child older than 4 years	Some experts recommend routine referral

Modified from Sinclair KA, Woods CR, Sinal SH. Venereal warts in children. Pediatr Rev. 2011;32(3):115–121; Kingston M, Smurthwaite D, Dixon S, White C. Sex Transm Infect. 2017;93:267–269.

Treatment of condylomata acuminata in children (see the following section) is challenging for many reasons. In an interesting study of the natural history of these lesions in children, spontaneous resolution occurred in 54% of patients within 5 years of the diagnosis, suggesting that nonintervention is a reasonable initial approach to managing this condition, especially in asymptomatic patients.[120] Precise identification of the rate of spontaneous involution is challenging, however, because the majority of infected children receive some form of therapy.[121]

Treatment of Common Warts and Condylomata Acuminata

No specific antiviral therapy exists for HPV infections, and most wart treatments rely on destruction of the affected area of epidermal proliferation. Some newer methods of therapy are immunomodulatory in nature. Because spontaneous involution of warts may occur, watchful waiting is an appropriate consideration, especially in younger patients in whom destructive therapies are traumatic and poorly tolerated. When considering therapy for warts, every effort should be made to avoid overly aggressive or scarring therapies. Table 15.4 lists some of the treatment options for common, plantar, and planar warts and for condylomata acuminata. Several are discussed here in more detail.

Patients and parents must be reminded that even with apparent "cures" of warts or condylomata, latent HPV infection in grossly normal-appearing squamous epithelium beyond the areas of treatment may persist and results in a fairly high risk of recurrence. Whether warts should be treated depends on the patient's and parents' desires and the nature of the lesions. Those patients with warts that are painful, extensive, enlarging, subject to trauma, or cosmetically objectionable are most likely to be interested in therapy. If treatment is to be given, it should be harmless to the child, and if a painful therapy is being utilized, the child should be old enough to consent to the therapy. Parents occasionally request painful therapies (e.g., cryotherapy) for young children; this decision should be made only after a thorough discussion of the therapy, the pain involved, and its risk-to-benefit ratio. It should be emphasized that some modalities used for the treatment of warts in adults are neither feasible nor desirable for the treatment of warts in children. The choice of therapy will depend on the age, personality, and developmental status of the patient and the number, size, and location of the lesions.

Salicylic acid is available commercially under a variety of brand names and generics. It comes as liquids, gels, plasters, and pads. Salicylic acid preparations are applied directly to the wart surface and may be left on continuously or overnight. An effective form of combination therapy is to apply a salicylic acid liquid to the wart(s) and after drying occurs (5 minutes) to occlude the surface with duct tape. This treatment is placed on at bedtime, and the duct tape is removed the next morning. With removal of the tape, gradual debridement of the wart is performed, and the application is repeated nightly until the warts have resolved. Salicylic acid therapy may take from 2 to 12 weeks for complete wart resolution. A potential side effect of this therapy is maceration and irritation of the skin surrounding the wart. If this occurs, therapy should be held for 2 to 3 days to allow for resolution and then it is resumed. A compounded product of 17% salicylic acid and 2% 5-fluorouracil (Wart PEEL, NuCara Pharmacy, Coralville,

Table 15.4 Treatments for Warts and Condylomata Acuminata in Children

Treatment	Comment
WARTS	
Watchful waiting	Especially appropriate in young children
Topical salicylic acid	Available OTC; may be more effective when combined with duct tape occlusion
Cryotherapy	Both in-office and OTC available; in-office treatment typically more effective
Manual paring or filing	May minimize pain from plantar warts
Immunotherapy:	
Oral	Cimetidine; OL use (see text)
Topical	Imiquimod (home use; OL); SADBE, DCP
Laser therapy	Pulsed-dye laser potentially useful; CO_2 laser useful but scarring may result
Photodynamic therapy	Rarely utilized in children
Injection therapy	*Candida*/mumps antigens, MMR, bleomycin, interferon; rarely utilized in young children
Curettage, electrocautery	Rarely utilized in children
Topical retinoids	May be useful for flat warts; OL; often limited by irritation
Topical chemotherapy:	
5% 5-fluorouracil	OL use; may be useful for facial flat warts
2% 5-fluorouracil + 17% salicylic acid	Available from compounding pharmacy; useful for common and plantar warts; applied nightly with tape occlusion
Antiviral therapy:	
Cidofovir	OL use; typically used IV to treat CMV retinitis in immunocompromised patients; has been compounded as 1% topical cream for refractory warts
CONDYLOMATA	
Watchful waiting	Especially appropriate in young asymptomatic children
Chemovesicants	Podophyllin, TCA, podofilox
Immunotherapy:	
Oral	Cimetidine; OL use (see text)
Topical	Imiquimod; OL if <12 years
Cryotherapy	
Sinecatechins	Green tea extracts; 15% ointment approved for anogenital warts ≥18 years
Laser therapy	Rarely used for this indication in children
Surgery	Rarely used for this indication in children

CMV, Cytomegalovirus; *CO_2*, carbon dioxide; *DCP*, diphenylcyclopropenone; *IV*, intravenous; *MMR*, measles, mumps, and rubella vaccine; *OL*, off-label; *OTC*, over-the-counter; *SADBE*, squaric acid dibutylester; *TCA*, trichloroacetic acid.

IA) is available and quite effective when applied to common or plantar warts nightly under tape occlusion. Salicylic acid–based therapies are not typically recommended for facial or genital lesions.

Cryotherapy is a highly effective therapy for warts, albeit one that is painful and that may be unacceptably traumatic for younger patients. The most effective cryogen is liquid nitrogen, which has a vaporization temperature of −196° C.[115] Other agents such as dimethyl ether and propane (Histofreezer) and chlorodifluoromethane (Verruca-Freeze) achieve temperatures in the range of −40° to −80° C and appear to be less effective.[122] Liquid nitrogen is applied to the wart with a cotton-tipped applicator or via a spray gun for 10 to 20 seconds. The number of applications per treatment session depends on multiple factors, including the size of the wart, its location, past responses, and the style of the physician. The goal is to induce blister formation above the dermal–epidermal junction without causing a deep ulcer or significant necrosis to surrounding tissue. Therapy is often repeated at 3- to 4-week intervals and may be more effective when preceded by gentle debridement of warty tissue with a number 15 scalpel blade. Cryotherapy may be extremely uncomfortable, and some children will not accept this mode of therapy. Although a child can be held down for the procedure, this is an undesirable approach in most instances, and alternative treatments should be considered. Several over-the-counter cryotherapy wart removal products (e.g., Wartner, Compound W Freeze Off, Dr Scholl's Freeze Away) are available and use the combination of dimethyl ether and propane to freeze to −57° C. The cryogen is delivered by a foam pad attached to an applicator and held on the wart for 10 to 20 seconds.

Immunologic forms of wart therapy rely on the host immune system to mount a response against the HPV-induced lesions. Although these forms of therapy are not uniformly efficacious, they offer another option in the treatment of patients with warts. The most common form of oral immunotherapy is treatment with cimetidine, which is believed to possess immunomodulatory activity, including the ability to inhibit suppressor T-cell function, activate T helper (Th) l cells, and stimulate production of IL-2 and IFN-γ.[123,124] In one study, 32 children with warts were treated with cimetidine, 25 to 40 mg/kg per day divided into three or four doses, with an 81% clearance rate after 2 months of treatment.[123] Other studies of cimetidine and warts have shown conflicting results.[125–128] When utilized, most experts recommend 30 to 40 mg/kg per day divided into twice-daily doses. In general, the treatment is usually well tolerated with few, if any, side effects, and when effective, recurrences are rare.

Imiquimod is a topical immune-response modifier approved for the treatment of genital and perianal warts in patients 12 years of age or older. It is marketed in 5% and 3.75% creams (Aldara and Zyclara, respectively) and is applied to those lesions thrice weekly (on nonconsecutive days) to daily. Imiquimod has its therapeutic effect via induction of IFN-α and other cytokines in the skin.[129,130] Studies have suggested that the off-label use of this agent with more frequent application schedules (once daily for 5 weeks to twice-daily applications) may be useful in the treatment of common warts.[131,132]

Topical immunotherapy with squaric acid dibutylester (SADBE) is another option in the treatment of recalcitrant warts. Topical immunotherapy was initially described with dinitrochlorobenzene (DNCB) and subsequently with diphenylcyclopropenone (DCP). These agents are less desirable because of mutagenicity associated with the former and local side effects associated with the latter.[133] With SADBE immunotherapy, sensitization of (unaffected) skin is followed by the application of the solution to nonfacial warts. The therapy is painless and often effective, with complete clearance rates ranging from 58% to 84% in open-label studies.[133–136] Although in-office application has been traditionally utilized for topical immunotherapy, experience with at-home application of SADBE has demonstrated safety and high patient acceptance.[133]

Side effects of this treatment include allergic contact dermatitis (at either sensitization or treatment sites) and rarely urticaria. The hypothesized mechanism of action of this form of immunotherapy is generation of a delayed-type hypersensitivity reaction at the site of the wart and possibly a systemic antiviral effect, because even untreated lesions at distal sites may occasionally resolve.[133]

Intralesional immunotherapy is another reported treatment for warts. For this treatment, the warts are injected with skin test antigens (e.g., *Candida* or mumps antigen) or vaccines (e.g., measles, mumps, rubella [MMR]), typically at several visits, and when effective, warts at distant (untreated) sites may also improve.[137,138] This treatment, however, may be limited by pain and anxiety, especially in younger children.

Pulsed-dye laser therapy is another option for the treatment of recalcitrant warts. This laser, which is most often utilized in the treatment of vascular birthmarks, works by selectively destroying the blood vessels found within warts.[139] This therapy has a large advantage over carbon dioxide laser therapy in that it is nonscarring and the period of postoperative recovery is significantly shorter. Pulsed-dye laser therapy has been demonstrated to be quite effective in the treatment of warts, including common, plantar, and periungual types.[98,139,140] Its use, however, is best limited to lesions that are recalcitrant and have failed other therapeutic modalities.

Flat warts may be treated with a variety of modalities, although their small size, common location on the face, and occurrence in groups make aggressive therapies impractical. Treatment options for these lesions include light cryotherapy, imiquimod, topical retinoids (e.g., tretinoin or adapalene cream), oral cimetidine, topical chemotherapy (e.g., 5-fluorouracil cream), or topical immunotherapy.

Therapies for condylomata acuminata have been poorly studied in children. As mentioned, a significant portion of anogenital warts in the pediatric population may spontaneously involute over several years, and thus watchful waiting is an appropriate consideration. When therapy is desired, a commonly used regimen is that of either podophyllin or trichloroacetic acid (or the two in combination), which are applied in the office. These agents cause cytotoxic effects with resultant necrosis of the affected cells, and their use may be limited by local irritation. Podofilox solution or gel (Condylox) is a closely related compound marketed for application in the home setting. Podofilox, which is approved for use in adult patients, is applied twice daily for 3 consecutive days, although more limited regimens (e.g., once daily) are often recommended for children to try and avoid local irritation. Self-treatment with podofilox has shown greater efficacy and cost-effectiveness than office therapy with podophyllin.[141] Imiquimod, applied three times weekly on nonconsecutive days, is another option that has been demonstrated effective in the treatment of external genital and perianal warts.[142] This treatment is also occasionally limited by local irritation. Other treatments used occasionally for condylomata acuminata include cryotherapy, laser therapy,[143,144] oral cimetidine, topical immunotherapy,[145] 5-fluorouracil cream, and surgical ablation. The pain of cryotherapy often precludes its use for warts in this location for children. Sinecatechins ointment, derived from the extract of green tea leaves *(Camellia sinensis)*, is approved for adults with anogenital warts (applied three times daily) and has been used off-label successfully in children with the condition.[146,147]

Prevention of anogenital HPV infection is the goal of HPV vaccination. Three vaccines have been licensed in the United States, including a quadrivalent (types 6, 11, 16, and 18; Gardasil, Merck & Co.) vaccine initially approved for use in females 9 to 26 years of age and then in males 9 to 26 years of age; a bivalent (types 16 and 18; Cervarix, GlaxoSmithKline) vaccine initially approved for use in females 10 to 25 years of age; and a nine-valent (types 6, 11, 16, 18, 31, 33, 45, 52, 58; Gardasil 9, Merck & Co.) vaccine licensed for use in females and males 9 to 26 years of age.[148] The latter vaccine is the only one still being sold in the United States. These vaccines have subsequently been demonstrated useful in preventing related cervical precancerous lesions in females, anal precancerous lesions in males, and genital warts in both males and females.[149,150] The current recommendation of the AAP and the ACIP is for routine immunization of females and males, starting the series between 9 and 12 years of age (11 or 12 years of age per ACIP), and females through age 26 years and males through 21 years who were not previously immunized.[148,151] Vaccination is also recommended for men who have sex with men, transgender individuals, and those who are immunocompromised through 26 years of age.[148] It is important to emphasize that these vaccines do not provide benefit for established HPV infections, and they are most effective when administered before the first sexual contact.[152]

EPIDERMODYSPLASIA VERRUCIFORMIS

EV is a rare autosomal recessive disorder characterized by a genetically determined susceptibility to widespread and persistent infection of the skin with specific HPV types.[153] The most commonly implicated HPV serotypes are HPV-5 and HPV-8, although many other HPV types have been isolated from EV lesions, and in one review, HPV-3, -14, and -20 were also identified frequently.[154,155] Infections begin in early childhood, and malignant transformation (nonmelanoma skin cancer) occurs in approximately half of patients during adulthood. The predisposition to HPV infection is believed to be the result of an immunogenetic defect associated with generation of cytokines, which downregulate cell-mediated immunity, and possibly with low levels of IL-10.[156] The role of environmental factors (most notably ultraviolet [UV] irradiation) also appears to be important in the pathogenesis of the HPV-associated malignancies.[157] EV has been found to be caused by inactivating mutations in two adjacent, related genes, *EVER1/TMC6* and *EVER2/TMC8*, in approximately 75% of individuals with the disorder; other genetic mutations that have been associated with HPV susceptibility include *RHOH, MST-1, CORO1A,* and *IL-7*.[154] These genes encode transmembrane proteins located in the endoplasmic reticulum.[158,159] EV may represent a primary deficiency of intrinsic immunity to the EV-specific HPVs (β-papillomaviruses), in innate immunity, or in both.[159] There is also an acquired form of EV, which has been rarely reported, usually in the setting of HIV infection or other forms of immunosuppression.[160–162]

Patients with EV seek treatment during childhood with widespread, tinea versicolor–like, hypopigmented macules and/or flat verruca plana–like papules. These papules are red to red-brown and may coalesce into larger plaques. The most common locations for the warty lesions are the hands, extremities, and face, whereas the tinea versicolor–like lesions occur predominantly on the trunk.[157] When skin malignancy (usually squamous cell carcinoma) develops during adulthood, it is most often at sun-exposed sites, and these tumors are most often associated with HPV types 5 and 8. There is no specific therapy for EV. Protection from UV radiation with protective clothing and sunscreens and sun avoidance are vital. Close clinical surveillance for squamous cell carcinoma is recommended, with early surgical excision as needed. Experimental therapies have included interferon, imiquimod, cimetidine, photodynamic therapy, and systemic retinoids.[157,163]

RECURRENT RESPIRATORY PAPILLOMATOSIS

Recurrent respiratory papillomatosis (RRP; laryngeal papillomatosis) is a disorder of HPV-associated benign tumors of the larynx and at times other portions of the aerodigestive tract. It has a bimodal distribution, occurring in children ("juvenile-onset RRP") and young adults, with the childhood form being characterized by a more aggressive course and a high recurrence rate.[164] RRP is the most common benign neoplasm of the larynx in children and is usually caused by HPV types 6 and 11, which are both common genital tract HPV types.[165] Although the exact method of HPV acquisition in patients with RRP is not well established, it is most likely caused by maternal–fetal transmission (ascending *in utero* infection or direct contact in the birth canal) and, less likely, via postnatal acquisition.[166,167] However, even given the potential links among cervical HPV, vaginal delivery, and RRP, the utility of elective cesarean sections in mothers with genital tract HPV infection as a preventive measure remains controversial.[167–169] A maternal history of condylomas during pregnancy appears to be a risk factor for more severe RRP.[170] Fortunately, very few children overall who are exposed to genital HPV at birth develop symptoms of RRP.

Although the tumors of RRP are benign, significant morbidity may result from obstruction of the airway and potential malignant degeneration. RRP is usually diagnosed before the age of 5 years, and the clinical presentation often includes the triad of stridor, progressive hoarseness, and respiratory distress.[165] Other symptoms may include dyspnea, chronic cough, wheezing, recurrent upper respiratory infections, pneumonia, dysphagia, and failure to thrive.[171] Patients may be initially diagnosed with asthma, croup, or bronchitis. In some, the condition may go undiagnosed until frank respiratory distress develops with the resultant need for emergent tracheotomy. The condition is diagnosed with direct airway endoscopy or helical computed tomography, and the mainstay of therapy for RRP is surgery or laser therapy. Adjuvant treatments include IFN, photodynamic therapy, and antiviral therapy. Tracheostomy may be required in patients with more extensive disease. Intralesional cidofovir in combination with surgery has been advocated as an effective therapeutic combination, although efficacy has been questioned by some, and weight-based dosing limits are recommended.[172–175] It also appears that aggressive control of gastroesophageal reflux disease, when present, is vital, because it may contribute to the severity of RRP.[165,176] Immunization with the HPV vaccine may be associated with a decline in the incidence of juvenile-onset RRP, an effect that may increase with greater vaccine coverage in women of childbearing age; in one study of active immunization after the diagnosis of RRP, however, the clinical course in the year after vaccination was similar to the course in the year before vaccination, suggesting that the vaccine is not useful as treatment for established disease.[177–179]

Molluscum Contagiosum

Molluscum contagiosum (MC) is a common cutaneous viral infection in children caused by a member of the poxvirus family (*Molluscum contagiosum* virus, or MCV). Although MC is often an STD or associated with immunodeficiency (especially HIV infection) in adults, childhood disease tends to lack these associations. There has been a dramatic increase in MC over recent decades in the United States, with an 11-fold increase in patient visits for the disorder reported for one 18-year period.[180] In children, the infection is also quite prevalent, because the spread of virus through skin-to-skin contact and fomites is rapid and easy. MC occurs most often in school-aged children and especially those under 8 years of age. Although controversy exists, epidemiologic data suggest that MC may be transmitted via swimming pools as well as via fomites such as sponges and towels and in beauty parlors.[181–184]

Autoinoculation of the virus is a common mode of spread in affected patients. MC lesions tend to spread more rapidly in children with AD, possibly related to suppressed Th-cell responses. Congenital MC has been reported and likely represents vertical transmission of MCV.[185]

MC presents as pearly, flesh-colored to pink papules that often appear translucent (Figs. 15.39 through 15.41). The range in size is from 2 to 8 mm. A small central dell or depression may or may not be evident, and occasionally excrescences protrude from this central region (Fig. 15.42). Although single lesions may occur, MC most often presents with numerous clustered papules, and linear configurations (from koebnerization) may be present (Fig. 15.43). Although MC lesions may occur on any area of the skin surface, they are most common in areas of skin rubbing or moist regions, including the axillae, popliteal fossae, and groin. Genital and perianal lesions are also common, even in children, in whom the disorder is nearly always transmitted in a benign (nonsexual) fashion. Lesions may develop significant erythema (Fig. 15.44), which usually represents a host immune response against MCV and often heralds spontaneous involution. Occasionally, childhood MC may be marked by very high numbers of lesions (Fig. 15.45) or a giant size (Fig. 15.46). The latter may occasionally be confused with cutaneous pseudolymphoma (see Chapter 10), although MC is also considered to be one potential cause of pseudolymphomatous skin infiltration (and may be associated with CD30-positive lymphoid infiltrates).[186]

Surrounding dermatitis around MC lesions ("molluscum dermatitis") is common (Fig. 15.47), is considered one form of an id reaction, and may be misdiagnosed as eczema.[187] Importantly, the presence of molluscum dermatitis, if untreated, may propagate the cycle of infection when the patient scratches and subsequently autoinoculates the virus onto other regions. Complications of MC are rare but include secondary bacterial infection (Fig. 15.48), which is often secondary to scratching-induced impetiginization. In some patients with eyelid lesions, chronic conjunctivitis or superficial punctate keratitis may develop. Gianotti–Crosti syndrome–like reactions have been observed in some patients with MC and present with an eruption of monomorphous papules on the extensor extremities primarily and occasionally on the face, buttocks, or trunk. When this pattern presents, the papules are distinct from the underlying molluscum lesions (Fig. 15.49).[188]

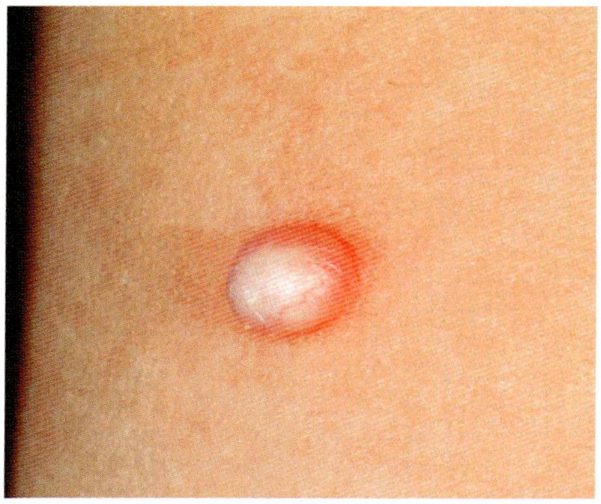

Fig. 15.39 Molluscum contagiosum. Solitary, dome-shaped pearly papule. Note the capped white plug.

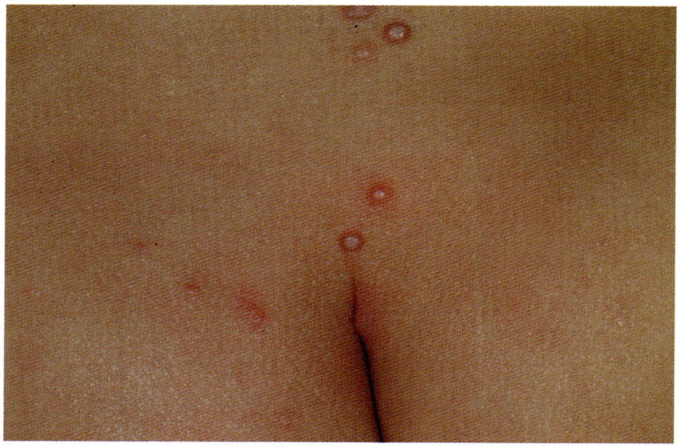

Fig. 15.40 Molluscum contagiosum. Multiple pearly, translucent papules on the lower back and superior buttocks. Note some flattened and resolved lesions.

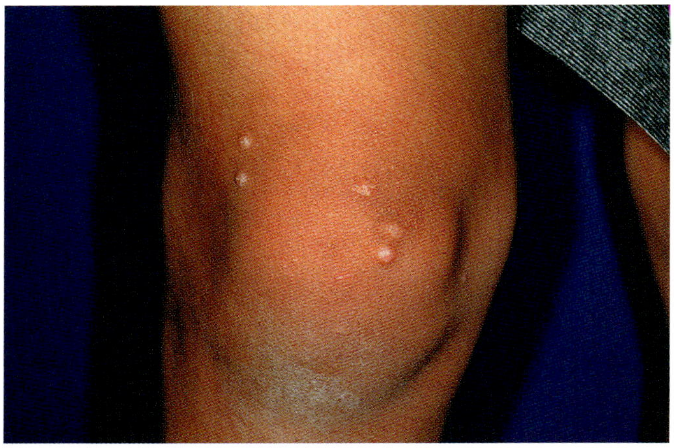

Fig. 15.41 Molluscum contagiosum. Pearly, umbilicated papules around the knee.

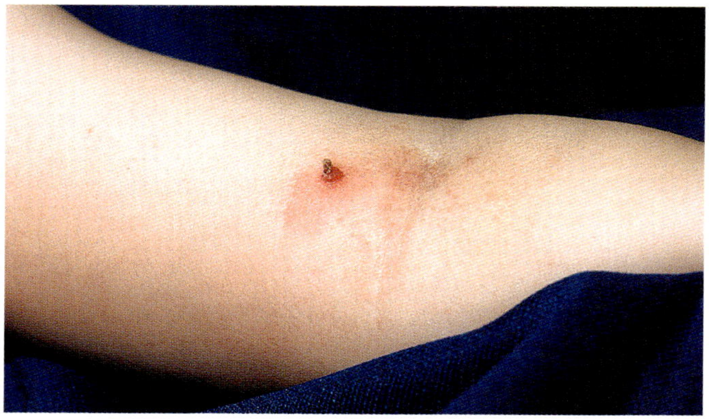

Fig. 15.42 Molluscum contagiosum. This solitary lesion with surrounding dermatitis demonstrates the central excrescence that may be present in some mollusca.

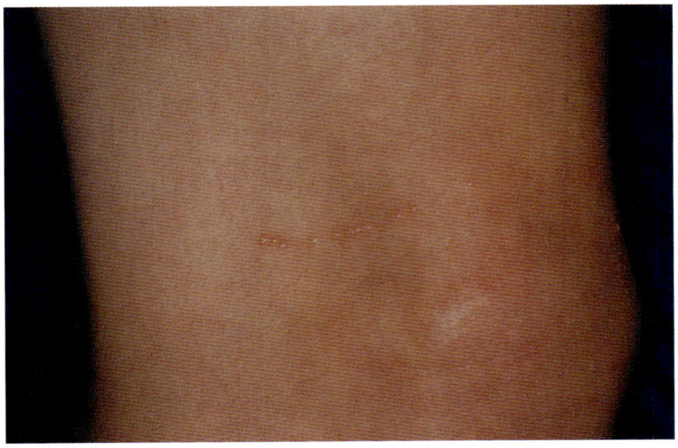

Fig. 15.43 Molluscum contagiosum with koebnerization. Linear configuration of lesions along a line of autoinoculation on the medial knee of a young boy.

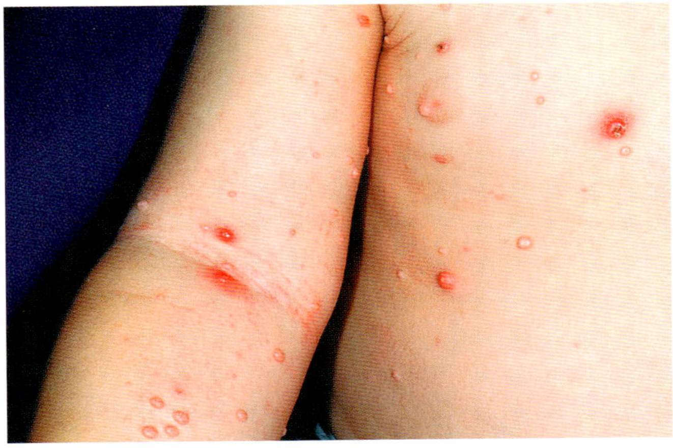

Fig. 15.44 Molluscum contagiosum with host immune response. The bright red appearance of several of the lesions is typical once an immune response is being mounted by the host. The inflamed lesions usually resolve over 2 to 3 weeks.

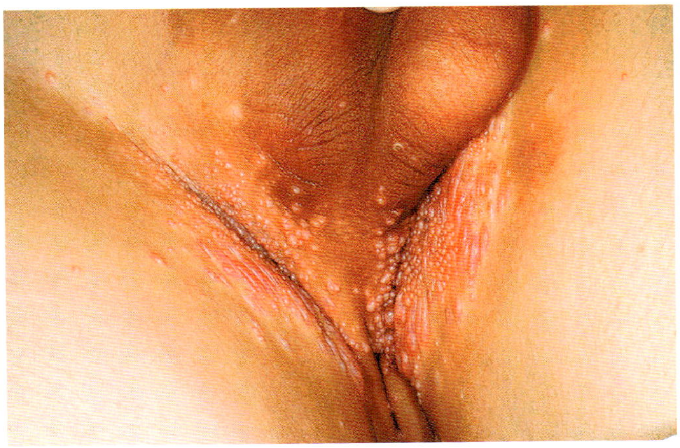

Fig. 15.45 Molluscum contagiosum in an immunocompromised host. This young boy receiving cancer chemotherapy had disseminated mollusca contagiosa, including multiple recalcitrant lesions in the groin.

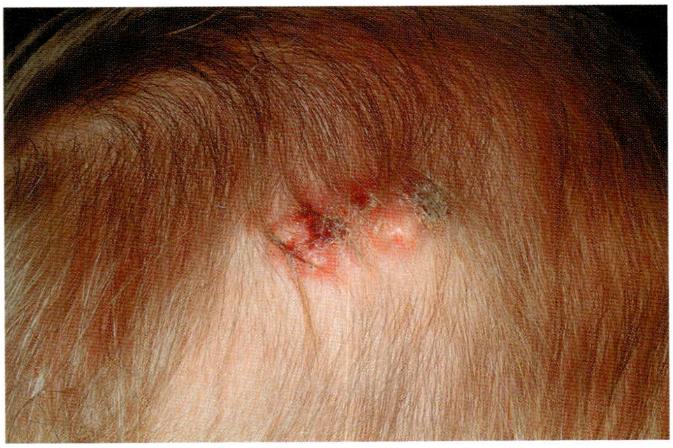

Fig. 15.46 Giant molluscum contagiosum. These two nodular plaques of the scalp turned out to be giant molluscum lesions. This pattern of presentation may be confused with other causes of cutaneous pseudolymphoma (see Chapter 10).

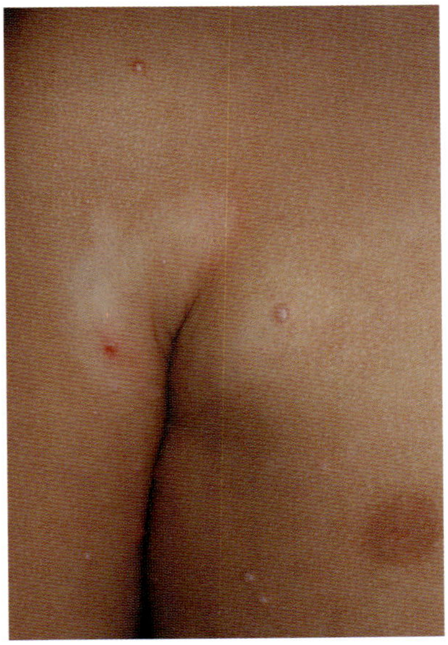

Fig. 15.47 Molluscum contagiosum with molluscum dermatitis. Note the surrounding mild dermatitis and postinflammatory hypopigmentation in this patient with skin of color.

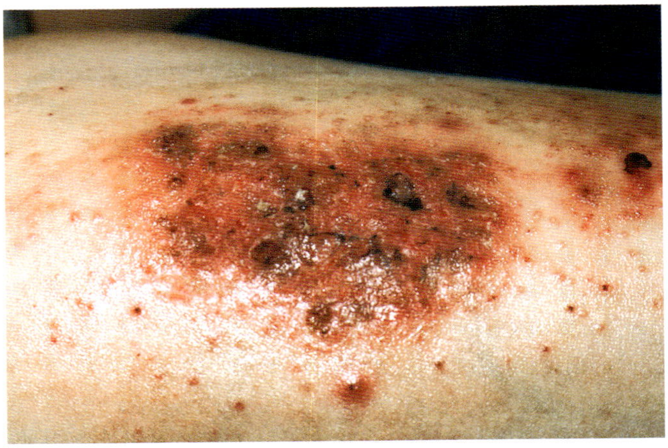

Fig. 15.48 Molluscum contagiosum with secondary bacterial infection. This patient with mollusca developed an associated dermatitis and eventual secondary infection with *Staphylococcus aureus*.

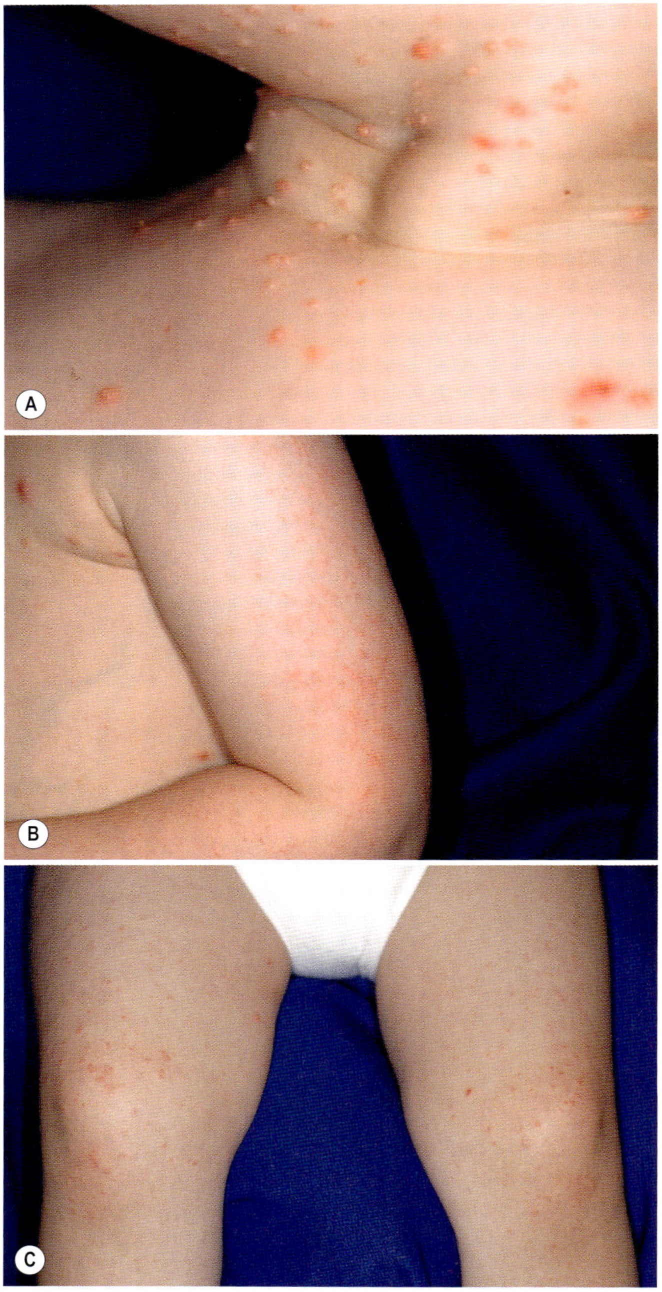

Fig. 15.49 Molluscum contagiosum and Gianotti–Crosti syndrome-like reaction. This 2-year-old boy had numerous lesions of molluscum, several of which were becoming inflamed **(A)** in conjunction with monomorphous papules on the extensor surfaces of the upper **(B)** and lower **(C)** extremities, suggestive of Gianotti–Crosti syndrome.

Spontaneous clearing of MC often occurs over years (with average time to resolution ranging between 6 and 16 months in published observational studies),[189] but parents and patients may request therapy for several reasons. These include the cosmetic significance of the lesions, pruritus, and epidemiologic concerns of other parents, teachers, or school nurses. In addition, in patients with an underlying atopic diathesis, the lesions may be more extensive and autoinoculation more significant, given the extensive pruritus. Traditional therapies (and those utilized in adults), such as curettage or cryotherapy, rely on destructive measures and may be traumatic for pediatric patients. Although curettage is not a preferred method of the authors, the pain of the procedure may be reduced by pretreatment of the lesional areas with topical anesthetic (lidocaine or lidocaine/prilocaine) cream. Care must be exercised, however, given reports of the latter (2.5% lidocaine/2.5% prilocaine, eutectic mixture of local anesthetics [EMLA] cream) associated with adverse events, including methemoglobinemia, hypoxemia, and seizures.[190,191] In these reports, however, the topical anesthetic had been applied in excess of the recommended use. The maximum dose and application area recommendations suggested by the manufacturer of EMLA cream are listed in Table 15.5. Lidocaine/prilocaine hydrogel has been reported as a safe and effective alternative for children undergoing therapy of MC, with onset of analgesia within 10 minutes of application, but is not available at this time in the United States.[192]

Table 15.5 Maximum Recommended EMLA Dose and Application Areas

Age and Body Weight*	Maximum Total Dose of EMLA (g)	Maximum Application Area (cm²)	Maximum Application Time (h)
0–3 months or <5 kg	1	10	1
3–12 months and >5 kg	2	20	4
1–6 years and >10 kg	10	100	4
7–12 years and >20 kg	20	200	4

EMLA, Eutectic mixture of local anesthetics, lidocaine/prilocaine.
*If patient is older than 3 months of age and does not meet minimum weight requirement, the maximum total dose of EMLA should be based on the patient's weight.

A highly effective and well-tolerated therapy for MC is the in-office application of cantharidin. Cantharidin is an extract from the blister beetle, *Cantharis vesicatoria*, and is known to induce vesiculation of the epidermis upon application to human skin.[193] Although concerns regarding the safety of cantharidin therapy have tempered its use for some, with appropriate application and patient education, it is usually very well tolerated and effective.[193–196] Among pediatric dermatologists surveyed, 92% reported satisfaction with cantharidin's efficacy in treating MC.[197] Although a prospective, blinded, placebo-controlled study of cantharidin did not demonstrate superiority of cantharidin over placebo during a 2-month observation period,[198] favorable results are often noted clinically, and this therapy continues to be a top choice for practitioners who treat these lesions.

A concentration of 0.7% or 0.9% cantharidin is usually used, and guidelines for the safe and effective use of this agent for the treatment of MC are listed in Box 15.1. Treatment results in blister formation within 24 to 48 hours, with healing over several days to 1 week. The extent of blistering is minimized by having the patient (or parent) rinse treated areas after a specified time after application, usually 2 to 6 hours.[195] Treatment of perioral or periocular facial lesions, mucosal sites, or occluded areas (e.g., diaper region) with this agent is not generally recommended. Cantharidin should be applied in the office only and by a physician or other qualified and well-trained health professional and should never be dispensed for home application.[199] If molluscum dermatitis is present, it should be cleared by use of a topical corticosteroid ointment before commencing with cantharidin therapy. Access to cantharidin has remained challenging in some regions of the United States, given intense scrutiny of pharmacy-compounding practices by the FDA. When available, however, cantharidin is considered by many practitioners to be a first-line treatment for this common condition in children.

Other methods of therapy that have been reported for MC include imiquimod cream, tretinoin cream, salicylic acid, α-hydroxy acids, tape stripping, pulsed-dye laser therapy, 5% potassium hydroxide, hydrogen peroxide, topical cidofovir, oral cimetidine, silver nitrate paste, and topical evening primrose oil.[131,181,193,200–211]

Imiquimod cream, approved for the treatment of genital warts, has been used off-label with different treatment regimens for MC, from three times weekly to application on a daily basis, with variable

Box 15.1 Guidelines for Treatment of Molluscum Contagiosum with Cantharidin

Patient and parent education (handouts useful)
Avoid treating lesions in the following sites:*
- Facial
- Mucosal
- Occluded

Treat 20 to 30 lesions maximum per treatment session
Application of cantharidin (0.7% or 0.9%):
- Vigorously shake bottle several times before opening to ensure even dispersal of cantharidin crystals within collodion base
- Use applicator stick or blunt (wooden) end of cotton-tipped applicator
- Apply single small droplet (sufficient to cover lesion) to each molluscum
- Avoid "painting"
- Let area dry for 3 to 5 minutes before patient gets dressed
- Do not occlude treated sites
- Treat initial lesion in a location that can be easily visualized by patient (to calm anxiety about the therapy)

Have patient bathe/rinse off all treated sites in 2 to 6 hours (may vary based on past response; 4 hours good starting point with first treatment; may rinse sooner if significant discomfort or if vesiculation is noted)
Acetaminophen or ibuprofen may be administered by parent, if needed, for pain
Bacitracin ointment applied to blisters twice daily until areas heal
Therapy repeated at 3- to 6-week intervals as needed

*Treatment of facial (but not periorbital) lesions can be considered on a case-by-case basis once the patient's initial response to cantharidin application has been assessed.

results. Several unpublished randomized controlled trials failed to show superiority of imiquimod over vehicle, although some smaller trials and observational studies have suggested potential efficacy.[212,213] The FDA, in the imiquimod prescribing information, states that the agent "did not show a statistically significant difference in complete clearance of baseline MC lesions from vehicle cream."[214] Topical tretinoin cream is a commonly used method (also off-label) for treating facial MC, although its use may be limited by its irritation potential.

Cowpox and Pseudocowpox

Cowpox is a rare zoonotic infection caused by the cowpox virus (CPXV), a DNA orthopoxvirus that is similar to the vaccinia and smallpox viruses. CPXV infections are limited largely to the United Kingdom and northern Europe, and their incidence has been increasing in both humans and animals.[215,216] Cowpox is transmitted by contact with infected animals, which may include cattle (from whom it may be transmitted as an occupational infection) and wild rodents, which serve as its natural reservoir.[217] After an incubation period of 1 to 3 weeks, a localized crusted nodule with ulceration or vesiculation forms and evolves through several stages to ultimately heal with a scar over several weeks. Flu-like symptoms may occasionally be present, and lymphadenopathy is common. Immunocompromised hosts may develop severe generalized infection, which may be fatal.[216] Although there is no accepted standard for therapy, cidofovir and some novel antiviral agents have been studied for patients with severe involvement, and measures to prevent secondary bacterial infection (e.g., wound care, topical and oral antibiotics) are recommended.[217]

Pseudocowpox (milker's nodule, paravaccinia) is a parapox virus infection seen worldwide usually occurring in dairy farmers and new milkers. It is caused by the paravaccinia virus. The infection is acquired from contact with the teats (the exit nipple of the udder) or nose of cattle infected with the virus, and children may occasionally acquire it. It may also occur in those who handle raw beef. Clinically, pseudocowpox is characterized by a single or several papules on the hands or fingers that develop after an incubation period of 5 to 15 days and progress through several stages: a macular or papular lesion becomes a vesicular lesion; then subsequently it progresses to a nodular stage with weeping; then it moves to a papillomatous or verrucous (warty) stage; and finally a dry crust develops, and healing occurs over 4 to 8 weeks. Typically, no scarring results. Secondary bacterial infection may occur in some patients. Occasionally, an erythema multiforme–like secondary eruption may occur, primarily in immunocompromised patients.[218,219] Treatment is similar to that discussed for cowpox.

The diagnosis of cowpox or pseudocowpox is usually made by the combination of the history of exposure and clinical examination. The differential diagnosis may include herpetic whitlow or other poxvirus infections (e.g., orf). If confirmation of the diagnosis is necessary, virus isolation and serologic studies may be useful. In addition, light or electron microscopic examination of skin biopsy tissue is useful, with the latter showing characteristic brick-shaped viral particles.[217,220]

Orf

Orf (ecthyma contagiosum, contagious ecthyma) is another parapox virus infection that normally infects sheep and goats (scabby mouth, sore mouth, contagious pustular dermatosis) and occasionally humans. Transmission is via contact with infected lesions in animals or fomites, including barn doors, fences, troughs, and shears.[220] Human orf has also been associated with household meat processing and animal slaughter, often in the setting of ethnic religious celebrations.[221] Clinically, orf usually presents with a solitary lesion (Fig. 15.50), although several lesions may be present. The onset usually follows a 3- to 7-day incubation period after exposure. The clinical stages of the skin lesions are identical to those described previously for cowpox and pseudocowpox. Associations include secondary bacterial infection, lymphadenopathy, lymphangitis, erythema multiforme–like eruptions, and recurrences in immunocompromised hosts.[222,223] Giant lesions of orf are occasionally reported.[224] Diagnostic modalities are the same as those discussed earlier, and in addition, a PCR method for diagnosis has been described[225] (see Cowpox and Pseudocowpox section) and is available through the Centers for Disease Control and Prevention (CDC) or state health departments. Treatment is supportive, and the lesions involute spontaneously over 4 to 8 weeks without scarring. Antibiotics should be given if secondary bacterial infection is present.

Smallpox

Smallpox (variola major) is an exanthematous disease but is included here with other poxvirus infections. The last case of endemic smallpox occurred in Somalia in 1977, and the disease was declared eradicated by the World Health Organization in 1980.[226] Variola virus, the etiologic agent of smallpox, has been maintained since that time in two

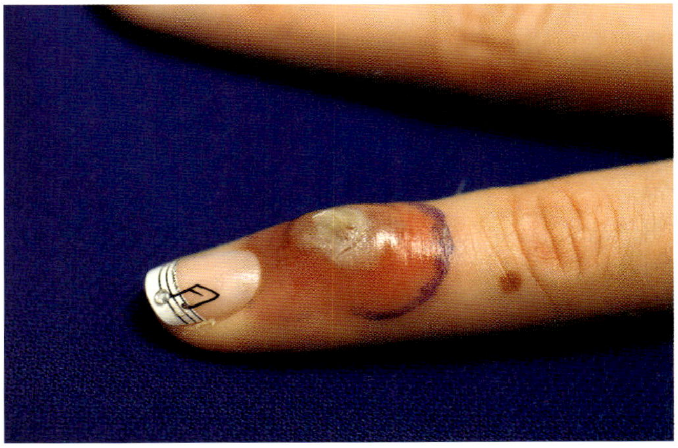

Fig. 15.50 Orf. An inflammatory nodule with superficial vesiculation and oozing on the distal index finger of a 16-year-old female patient. She had been bitten by a goat 3 weeks before while visiting a petting zoo.

high-security laboratories, the CDC in Atlanta and the Vektor Institute in Novosibirsk, Russia. However, concerns that some virus may exist outside of these laboratories and that it could potentially be used for a widespread bioterrorism attack remain. Routine vaccination for smallpox ended after the eradication declaration in 1980, and as such, a large population of susceptible persons now exists. The remaining protection of individuals who have received vaccination is unclear.

Smallpox begins with entry of the virus from respiratory droplets via the respiratory tract. It then travels to regional lymph nodes, where replication occurs. Viremia develops, and after an incubation period of 7 to 17 days, symptoms develop. These include high fever, malaise, severe headache, and backache. The temperature may be as high as 40° C. An enanthem precedes the exanthem and presents as erythematous macules on the oral mucosae, including the palate, tongue, and pharynx. The characteristic exanthem begins 1 to 2 days later with erythematous macules that progress to papules, then vesicles, and eventually pustules (Fig. 15.51) over 4 to 7 days. All lesions tend to be in the same stage of development, which is a useful feature in distinguishing smallpox from varicella (see Chapter 16) (Table 15.6). Skin lesions begin on the face and

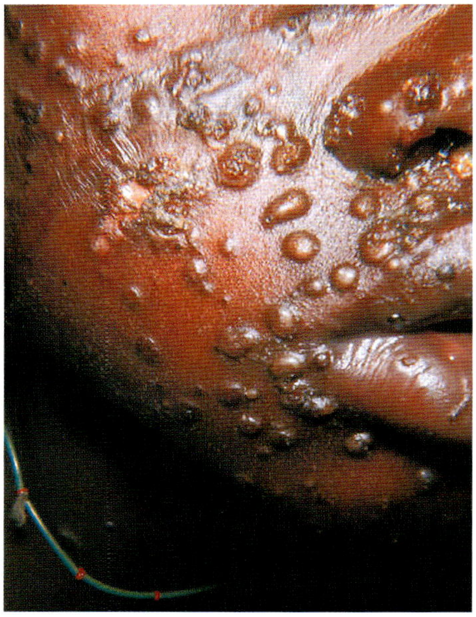

Fig. 15.51 Smallpox. Multiple tense pustules of the face in a patient from Ghana with smallpox. (Courtesy of the CDC, Dr. J. Noble Jr.)

Table 15.6 Distinguishing Features of Smallpox and Varicella

	Smallpox	Varicella
Prodrome	High fever, headache, backache, malaise	Mild fever, constitutional symptoms
Skin examination	Centrifugal distribution; pustules all in same stage of development; deep involvement	Central distribution; vesicles and crusted papules in different stages at one time; superficial
Scarring	Common; often severe	Occasional; usually mild (unless secondary bacterial infection)
Complications	Bacterial infection, pneumonia, arthritis, encephalitis, blindness, death	Bacterial infection; rarely pneumonia, encephalitis, arthritis

extremities with subsequent spread to the rest of the body and eventual widespread involvement. Crusting then begins around day 8 or 9 and is followed by healing with scarring. Complications of smallpox include secondary bacterial infection (usually associated with a second fever spike during the exanthem phase), pneumonia, arthritis, encephalitis, and death. Mortality in the past was as high as 30%, although it would probably be lower in developed countries with the availability of modern-day medical intervention. In survivors, blindness may occur because of viral keratitis or bacterial eye infection.

Variants of smallpox include hemorrhagic and malignant forms. In the hemorrhagic form, which is uniformly fatal (usually within the first 24 hours of the onset of symptoms), patients have high fever, abdominal pain, and then petechiae and hemorrhage of skin and mucous membranes.[227,228] The malignant form is similar but without progression of the rash from vesicles to pustules. Variola minor (alastrim) is a less severe variant of smallpox with fewer lesions and a milder course occurring in individuals with partial immunity.[227] These patients have a longer incubation period, milder prodrome, and lower mortality rate.[229]

Rapid diagnosis of smallpox is vital, because a single confirmed case could result in an international epidemic. State health officials should be contacted, and the tissue should be submitted to a Biological Safety Level 4 laboratory for processing.[226] The CDC should also be notified. Airborne and contact precautions should be strictly followed. Vesicular or pustular fluid, crusts (scabs), blood samples, and throat swabs should be collected as directed by regional or national health authorities. Methods for confirming the diagnosis of smallpox include cell culture, PCR, electron microscopy, serologies, and immunohistochemical stains. Collection of epidemiologic data is vital, and contacts must be identified so that a vaccine can be administered. The administration of a vaccine within 4 days of exposure may diminish the severity of the illness.

Therapy for smallpox consists first and foremost of isolation of the patient, who will remain infectious until approximately 10 days from the onset of the rash. Vaccination should be given, and meticulous skin and eye care, as well as hydration and nutrition support, is vital. No specific antiviral therapy exists for smallpox, although cidofovir has shown some benefit in the postexposure prevention of other poxvirus infections; other antiviral agents being investigated include brincidofovir and tecovirimat.[230–232]

The issue of smallpox vaccination has received much attention with the resurgence of interest in this disease. A vaccinia virus *(Orthopoxvirus vaccinia)* vaccine has been used to prevent infection with the smallpox virus. Concern about the variola virus potentially being used as a biologic weapon has resulted in the United States and some other countries deciding to stockpile live vaccinia virus vaccines (ACAM2000, Imvamune, and Aventis Pasteur Smallpox Vaccine [APSV]) to be provided to persons at high risk for infection in the event of a smallpox release.[233] Imvamune is an attenuated live virus vaccine that has been investigated for individuals who cannot safely receive ACAM2000.[234] In light of world events in the twenty-first century, several groups of individuals have received smallpox vaccination, including physicians from the CDC and eligible first responders and healthcare workers. New production of a smallpox vaccine has again been initiated, this time in tissue cell culture. The current recommended vaccination strategy is known as *ring vaccination* and also is referred to as *surveillance and containment.* In this strategy, if a single case of smallpox occurs, infected patients would be immediately isolated, and contacts would be identified and immunized by specially trained (and vaccinated) healthcare teams.

Complications of smallpox vaccination include local vaccination site reactions and more widespread reactions such as fever, generalized vaccinia, urticaria, erythema multiforme, encephalitis, and rarely death. Local reactions are common and include pustules at the vaccination site, bacterial superinfection, and lymphadenitis. In addition, pustular reactions at sites distant from the vaccination site occasionally occur from autoinoculation.

Eczema vaccinatum is a serious, potentially life-threatening side effect of smallpox vaccination occurring in individuals with AD or, less commonly, other skin disorders. It is caused by widespread dissemination of vaccinia and can occur in patients with either active or quiescent dermatitis.[235] The barrier disruption in these patients permits viral implantation, with subsequent spreading from cell to cell and occasionally

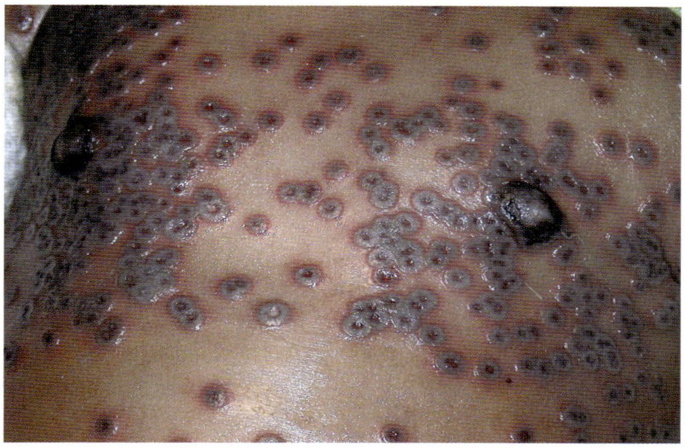

Fig. 15.52 Eczema vaccinatum. Extensive umbilicated papulopustules involving the chest and nipples of a 2-year-old hospitalized male patient. He had a history of atopic dermatitis and was exposed to vaccinia virus via household contact with a relative who had recently received the smallpox vaccination. (Courtesy Sarah Stein, MD.)

a viremic phase.[236] The lesions are similar in appearance to those associated with primary vaccination, but with extensive involvement they may become confluent (Fig. 15.52). Bacterial superinfection, shock, and death may occur, especially without the prompt administration of vaccinia immunoglobulin (VIG). Scarring is common. Because of the risks of eczema vaccinatum, individuals with AD should not receive elective vaccination if there is no risk of exposure to smallpox, and individuals who have regular contact with persons with AD should not receive vaccination unless they can avoid person-to-person contact until the scab separates from the vaccination site.[236] In addition to administration of VIG, patients with eczema vaccinatum may require treatment with cidofovir, ST-246, or other potent antivirals. Importantly, patients with eczema vaccinatum may shed large amounts of virus, and viable vaccinia virus may be present on inanimate objects in their environment, potentially causing inadvertent infection in other susceptible individuals exposed to those items.[237]

Childhood smallpox vaccination is a topic that has received considerable attention as part of the "pre-event" vaccination program. Of concern is the fact that children under the age of 5 years have historically had the highest rates of complications, especially for the most severe reactions.[226] In response to this and other data, the ACIP does not recommend routine smallpox vaccination for children and adolescents younger than 18 years of age, and the Committee on Infectious Diseases of the AAP has strongly endorsed further vaccine development and testing in children as well as adults.[229,238] A postevent vaccination strategy has been outlined and supports administration of single-dose, replication-competent smallpox vaccine (ACAM2000 or APSV) to persons with known exposure to smallpox virus, unless severely immunodeficient (e.g., bone marrow transplant recipients within 4 months of transplant, persons infected with HIV with CD4 cell count of <50 cells/mm^3, people with severe combined immunodeficiency, complete DiGeorge syndrome, or other severe immunocompromised states).[233] This recommendation includes persons with AD exposed to smallpox virus, given the risk for severe smallpox in this scenario likely outweighs the risk for experiencing a severe adverse event related to ACAM2000 vaccination.

Acquired Immunodeficiency Syndrome in Children

Infection with HIV type 1 occurs worldwide in adults and children, with the majority of new pediatric cases occurring in children living in sub-Saharan Africa (up to 2000 new cases per day). The number of children with AIDS is decreasing in the United States, due to better prevention of perinatal transmission, counseling, and the availability of effective therapies.[239,240] HIV-1 is an RNA retrovirus that infects $CD4^+$ T lymphocytes as well as other cells of the immune system. With the subsequent depletion of $CD4^+$ T cells, progressive immunocompromise occurs, leaving the patient at risk for a wide variety of infections, inflammatory conditions, and malignancies. AIDS is diagnosed when an infected patient has an opportunistic or other unusual or persistent infection as well as a $CD4^+$ T-cell count lower than 200 cells/mcL. There are two primary populations of childhood HIV infection, including those who acquire the virus through perinatal transmission and require care from the time of birth onward, and those who acquire HIV through risk behaviors, typically during adolescence.[240]

More than 90% of infant and childhood HIV-1 infections in the United States are the result of perinatal (mother-to-child) transmission (MTCT). The remaining children acquire the infection from blood-product exposure or risk behaviors such as unprotected sexual encounters or injection drug use. It is estimated that in the absence of antiretroviral therapy, approximately 30% of women infected with HIV-1 transmit the virus to their infants.[241] This can occur *in utero*, during delivery, or via breastfeeding after delivery. Maternal plasma viral load is one of the strongest predictors of perinatal transmission.[242] Infection with HSV type 2 or other STDs resulting in cervical or vaginal ulcers also increases the risk of transmission.[243] When infants acquire the infection via breastfeeding, it tends to occur within the first several months of life.[244] Formula feeding therefore is a desirable choice in this setting. The availability of treatments and the global commitment to prevent MTCT have positively affected the epidemiology of childhood HIV infection. In the United States, the number of infected infants per year has decreased from over 1800 to around 69 in 2013.[245] Combination antiretroviral drugs administered during pregnancy and labor have drastically reduced transmission rates to under 2%.[246]

Adolescents, on the other hand, are a population with a traditionally increasing rate of HIV-1 infection, although during 2010–2014, the rates of diagnosis decreased among persons aged 15 to 19 years in the United States.[247] Some of these patients acquired the infection perinatally and because of improved medical care are living longer than in the past. As a result, the number of vertically infected adolescents would be expected to increase over the years to come.[248] In others, high-risk behaviors such as intravenous drug abuse and unprotected sexual encounters place them at increased risk. Those at highest risk are homeless youth and those living in poverty, as well as young minority men who have sex with men. Victims of sexual abuse are another population of adolescent youth at high risk for HIV-1 infection. A high index of suspicion of HIV-1 infection should be maintained when an at-risk adolescent presents with a mononucleosis-like illness or persistent adenopathy.[239]

HIV-1 infection may present differently depending on the child's age. Although a detailed discussion of the clinical features is beyond the scope of this section, a brief review is included. Importantly, cutaneous and/or mucosal findings are often significant in the patient with HIV-1 infection or AIDS. These are listed in Table 15.7.

Acute HIV-1 infection may present with several nonspecific features, known as *acute HIV infection syndrome*. Symptoms may include fever, myalgias, fatigue, pharyngitis, weight loss, and headache, and because of the nonspecific nature of many of these, the infection often goes unrecognized.[249] Dermatologic features that may be seen during acute HIV infection syndrome include a mononucleosis-like, erythematous eruption; desquamation of palms and soles; urticaria; and alopecia. In addition, gastrointestinal symptoms are common during this acute illness and include abdominal pain, vomiting, and diarrhea.

In infants with HIV-1 infection, the most common features include *Pneumocystis jirovecii* (formerly *Pneumocystis carinii*) pneumonia (PJP), lymphoid interstitial pneumonitis (LIP), failure to thrive, recurrent infections (especially bacterial and candidal), and encephalopathy.[239] LIP occurs in the setting of EBV infection with chronic lymphoid pulmonary infiltrates and a "honeycomb" pattern on chest radiography. It may represent a unique immune response to coinfection with EBV and HIV,[250,251] and it usually responds to therapy with oxygen and steroids. Patients with LIP have a better prognosis than those with PJP, the latter of which is the most common AIDS-defining illness in children. The acute HIV infection syndrome may be absent in infants with HIV-1 infection.[248] Infants infected with HIV-1 are prone to gastrointestinal

Table 15.7 Mucocutaneous Manifestations of HIV-1/AIDS

Class	Type	Comment
Infections	Bacterial	Syphilis *Staphylococcus aureus*: impetigo, folliculitis, ecthyma, abscess *Pseudomonas aeruginosa*: folliculitis, ecthyma gangrenosum, abscess *Bartonella*: bacillary angiomatosis
	Mycobacterial	MAC: nodules, ulcers, pustules, folliculitis TB: scrofuloderma, papules, vesicles, ulcers, nodules, pustules, abscess Atypical mycobacteria: various skin findings
	Viral	HSV: typical or atypical (deep ulcers, thick crusts) VZV: primary varicella, herpes zoster CMV: perianal ulceration, vesicles, purpura, nodules EBV: oral hairy leukoplakia HPV: common warts, condylomata acuminate, epidermodysplasia verruciformis Molluscum contagiosum: often genitals/face or widespread; recalcitrant
	Fungal	*Candida albicans*: cutaneous, oral, esophageal, vulvovaginal *Pityrosporum ovale*: tinea versicolor Dermatophytes: tinea infections, onychomycosis Deep fungal infections: histoplasmosis, cryptococcosis, sporotrichosis, coccidioidomycosis *Penicillium marneffei*: various skin findings
	Protozoal	*Pneumocystis carinii*: occasional skin lesions
Infestations	Scabies	Classic findings or severe, crusted (Norwegian) form
	Amoeba	*Acanthamoeba, Naegleria* species: papules, nodules, ulcers
	Demodicidosis	*Demodex folliculorum*: folliculitis (often facial)
Inflammatory	Psoriasis	May be severe, widespread
	Reactive arthritis	NG urethritis, arthritis and skin changes: keratoderma blennorrhagicum, balanitis, oral ulceration
	Seborrheic dermatitis	More severe, more widespread
	Eosinophilic folliculitis	Sterile, pruritic follicular papules and pustules
	Drug eruption	May be severe; most often secondary to trimethoprim/sulfamethoxazole, penicillins, antituberculous medications; include morbilliform eruption, erythema multiforme, SJS; may also develop in response to cART
	Aphthous ulcers	
Idiopathic	Pruritus	Absence of primary cutaneous findings; may be severe
	Papular eruption	Pruritic, nonfollicular papules
	Ichthyosis	An acquired form of the disorder
	Xerosis	Severe skin dryness
	Nail changes	Clubbing, melanonychia, nail plate dystrophy
Malignant	Kaposi sarcoma	Skin and mucosal nodules, plaques; may metastasize; mainly homosexual/bisexual men; association with HHV-8
	Cutaneous lymphoma	Usually T-cell, less commonly B-cell, non-Hodgkin lymphoma
	Other skin cancers	Basal cell, squamous cell carcinoma; malignant melanoma

Data from Moylett EH, Shearer WT. HIV: clinical manifestations. J Allergy Clin Immunol 2002;110:3–16; Brodie SJ, de la Rosa C, Howe JG, et al. Pediatric AIDS-associated lymphocytic interstitial pneumonia and pulmonary arterio-occlusive disease: role of VCAM-1A/LA-4 adhesion pathway and human herpesviruses. Am J Pathol 1999;154(5):1453–64; McClain KL. Epstein-Barr virus and HIV-AIDS-associated diseases. Biomed Pharmacother 2001;55(7):348–52; Majaliwa ES, Mohn A, Chiarelli F. Growth and puberty in children with HIV infection. J Endocrinol Invest 2009;32(1):85–90; Shingadia D, Novelli V. Diagnosis and treatment of tuberculosis in children. Lancet 2003;3:624–32; Forsyth BW. Psychological aspects of HIV infection in children. Child Adolesc Psychiatr Clin N Am 2003;12(3):423–37; Phillips N, Amos T, Kuo C, et al. HIV-associated cognitive impairment in perinatally infected children: a meta-analysis. Pediatrics 2016;138(5):pii:e20160893.Epub 2016 Oct 11; Lazarus JR, Rutstein RM, Lowenthal ED. Treatment initiation factors and cognitive outcome in youth with perinatally acquired HIV infection. HIV Med 2015;16:355–61; Oleske JM. Review of recent guidelines for antiretroviral treatment of HIV-infected children. Int AIDS Soc USA 2003;11(6):180–4; Panel on antiretroviral therapy and medical management of HIV-infected children. Guidelines for the use of antiretroviral agents in pediatric HIV infection, <http://aidsinfo.nih.gov/contentfiles/lvguidelines/pediatricguidelines.pdf>; [accessed 11.19.18]; Van der Linden D, Callens S, Brichard B, et al. Pediatric HIV: new opportunities to treat children. Expert Opin Pharmacother 2009;10(11):1783–91; Safrit JT. HIV vaccines in infants and children: past trials, present plans and future perspectives. Curr Mol Med 2003;3(3):303–12; Leonard EG, McComsey GA. Metabolic complications of antiretroviral therapy in children. Pediatr Infect Dis J 2003;22(1):77–84; Davies MA, Gibb D, Turkova A. Survival of HIV-1 vertically infected children. Curr Opin HIV AIDS 2016;11:455–64; Rico MJ, Myers SA, Sanchez MR. Guidelines of care for dermatologic conditions in patients infected with HIV. J Am Acad Dermatol 1997;37:450–72; Mankahla A, Mosam A. Common skin conditions in children with HIV/AIDS. Am J Clin Dermatol 2012;13(3):153–66; Mittal S, Mendiratta V, Kumar P, et al. Mucocutaneous manifestations in Indian children with human immunodeficiency virus infection. Pediatr Dermatol 2013;30(6):e274–5; Katibi OS, Ogunbiyi AO, Oladokun RE, et al. Mucocutaneous disorders of pediatric HIV in South West Nigeria: surrogates for immunologic and virologic indices. J Int Assoc Prov AIDS Care 2016;15(5):423–31.

AIDS, Acquired immunodeficiency syndrome; *cART,* combination antiretroviral therapy; *CMV,* cytomegalovirus; *EBV,* Epstein–Barr virus; *HIV-1,* human immunodeficiency virus type 1; *HHV,* human herpesvirus; *HPV,* human papillomavirus; *HSV,* herpes simplex virus; *MAC, Mycobacterium avium* complex; *NG,* nongonococcal; *SJS,* Stevens–Johnson syndrome; *TB, Mycobacterium tuberculosis*; *VZV,* varicella zoster virus.

infections, enteropathy, and malabsorption. They may also have hepatosplenomegaly and lymphadenopathy. Primary infection with CMV may result in hepatitis, bone marrow failure, pneumonitis, or encephalitis. Perinatal HIV infection may also result in endocrine dysfunction with growth failure and pubertal delay.[252]

In children (those between 2 and 6 years of age), the most common features of HIV-1 infection are recurrent episodes of otitis media and sinusitis, recurrent bacterial infections, LIP, and encephalopathy. Other serious infections, including meningitis and osteomyelitis, may occur. Invasive disease caused by *Streptococcus pneumoniae* may occur, although this may become less common with the advent of routine pneumococcal immunization. Again, hepatomegaly and lymphadenopathy are common, and problems with weight gain and linear growth may be seen.

In older children and adolescents with HIV-1 infection, the most common signs and symptoms include *Candida* infections (e.g., oral thrush, vulvovaginitis, esophagitis), HZ, recurrent herpes simplex infection, parotitis, cryptosporidiosis, and infections with CMV and atypical mycobacteria. Nonspecific signs after acute HIV infection are common and may simulate those of EBV infection. Poor growth, pubertal delay, and HIV-associated wasting may all occur.

There are multiple other associations with HIV-1 infection. Metabolic disturbances may result in hyperlipidemia, body fat redistribution (with resultant lipodystrophy or lipoatrophy), insulin resistance, and hyperglycemia. Lipodystrophy appears to be propagated by the use of combination antiretroviral therapy (cART) (see later), which contributes to altered lipid metabolism.[249] Ocular manifestations include retinopathy, keratoconjunctivitis, keratitis, iridocyclitis, and retinal microvasculopathy. Infectious retinitis may be caused by CMV, VZV, *Toxoplasma*, or other agents. Cardiac manifestations of HIV-1 infection include effusion, myocarditis, endocarditis, dilated cardiomyopathy, and pulmonary hypertension. In addition to HIV-associated encephalitis, or AIDS encephalopathy, other neurologic complications include aseptic meningitis, peripheral neuropathy, Guillain–Barré-like syndrome, and myelopathy. Patients may also have genitourinary, rheumatologic, gastrointestinal, and hematologic manifestations and have an increased risk of malignancy, especially non-Hodgkin lymphoma. Tuberculosis occurs with increased incidence in patients infected with HIV-1 and has important epidemiologic significance both within the community and for the world at large. In fact, the incidence of tuberculosis worldwide has been increasing, due primarily to the incidence of HIV infection.[253] Psychological effects of HIV infection can be profound and may relate to the degree of illness, the threat of death, the association with substance abuse, and the social stigma associated with the disease.[254] A meta-analysis of cognitive impairment in perinatally infected children revealed an association between this form of HIV infection and deficits in working memory, executive function and processing speed, and possibly visual memory and visual-spatial ability.[255] In another retrospective study, initiating cART (formerly known as *highly active antiretroviral therapy* [HAART]) before the diagnosis of AIDS was associated with a significantly higher full-scale IQ.[256]

The diagnosis of HIV infection is based on clinical, immunologic, and serologic findings and the exclusion of other causes of immunodeficiency. Antibody-based tests include enzyme-linked immunosorbent assays (ELISAs), second-generation ELISAs, and confirmatory Western blotting. Direct detection assays include p24 antigen capture ELISA and DNA/RNA assays via PCR, *in situ* hybridization, or other hybridization assays. In infants under 18 months of age, anti-HIV antibody may be transplacental and therefore is not diagnostic of HIV infection (although a negative result suggests that the infant is uninfected). The diagnostic method of choice in infants therefore is HIV DNA PCR on peripheral blood lymphocytes.[248] Other laboratory tests that may be useful in the evaluation for HIV infection include complete blood cell counts with platelets, $CD4^+$ lymphocyte counts, serum chemistries, and urinalysis. Plasma HIV RNA (viral load) studies are useful in monitoring response to therapy and are the best indicator of risk for disease progression in children.[257]

The treatment of choice for children with HIV infection is a regimen of at least three agents from at least two classes of antiretroviral drugs.[258] These categories and some preferred agents/combinations for use in children include dual-nucleoside analog reverse transcriptase inhibitors (NRTIs), including abacavir with lamivudine or emtricitabine; tenofovir alafenamide with emtricitabine; tenofovir disoproxil fumarate with lamivudine or emtricitabine; zidovudine (formerly azidothymidine [AZT]) with lamivudine or emtricitabine; zidovudine with abacavir or didanosine; didanosine with lamivudine or emtricitabine; nonnucleoside analog reverse transcriptase inhibitors (NNRTIs), including nevirapine, efavirenz, and rilpivirine; and HIV protease inhibitors (PIs), including atazanavir/ritonavir, darunavir/ritonavir, and lopinavir/ritonavir.[239,258,259] Fusion inhibitors (enfuvirtide, maraviroc) interfere with the penetration of HIV into the target cells (maraviroc via binding to the chemokine receptor [CCR] type 5 receptor on CD4 Th cells), and integrase strand transfer inhibitors (dolutegravir, elvitegravir, raltegravir) block the viral integrase and insertion of the DNA copy of the viral genome into the host cell chromosome.[258,259] HIV vaccines intended to boost immunity toward the virus have been studied,[260] and adjunctive therapies such as intravenous immune globulin and cytokine therapy are occasionally utilized. The challenge of developing an HIV vaccine has been compounded by the poor host immune response to HIV infection, and to date, only one trial (RV144) has shown modest vaccine efficacy.[261,262]

Special considerations in treating young children infected with HIV include differences in body size; composition; and drug metabolism, distribution, and elimination (updated treatment guidelines for pediatric HIV infection can be found at www.aidsinfo.nih.gov/guidelines). In infants the best outcome is seen when antiretroviral therapy is immediately initiated after diagnosis. In older children or adolescents, the decision to start therapy is based on the viral load, $CD4^+$ lymphocyte count, and clinical status. Survival in children infected with HIV has improved notably with the introduction of cART, with a decrease in disease progression and mortality.[263,264] However, children seem to be more likely than adults to develop metabolic side effects of therapy, including lipodystrophy, dyslipidemia, insulin resistance, mitochondrial toxicity with lactic acidemia, and decreased bone mineral density. Interestingly, HIV-associated growth retardation, manifested by muscle wasting and decreased linear growth, appears to be minimized with the use of cART in children, although the long-term significance of these findings is unclear.[265]

The complete list of 268 references for this chapter is available online at http://expertconsult.inkling.com.

Key References

Fatahzadeh M, Schwartz RA. Human herpes simplex virus infections: epidemiology, pathogenesis, symptomatology, diagnosis and management. J Am Acad Dermatol 2007;57:737–63.

Gnann JW, Whitley RJ. Genital herpes. N Engl J Med 2016;375(7):666–74.

Reynolds MA, Chaves SS, Harpaz R, et al. The impact of the varicella vaccination program on herpes zoster epidemiology in the United States: a review. J Infect Dis 2008;197(Suppl. 2):S224–7.

Weinmann S, Chun C, Schmid DS, et al. Incidence and clinical characteristics of herpes zoster among children in the varicella vaccine era, 2005–2009. J Infect Dis 2013;208(11):1859–68.

Javed S, Javed SA, Tyring SK. Varicella vaccines. Curr Opin Infect Dis 2012;25:135–40.

Giuliano AR, Palefsky JM, Goldstone S, et al. Efficacy of quadrivalent HPV vaccine against HPV infection and disease in males. N Engl J Med 2011;364(5):401–11.

Moye VA, Cathcart S, Morrell DS. Safety of cantharidin: a retrospective review of cantharidin treatment in 405 children with molluscum contagiosum. Pediatr Dermatol 2014;31(4):450–4.

Narayanan N, Lacy CR, Cruz JE, et al. Disaster preparedness: biological threats and treatment options. Pharmacotherapy 2018;38(2):217–34.

Gray ME, Nieburg P, Dillingham R. Pediatric human immunodeficiency virus continuum of care. A concise review of evidence-based practice. Pediatr Clin N Am 2017;64:879–91.

Paintsil E, Andiman WA. Update on successes and challenges regarding mother-to-child transmission of HIV. Curr Opin Pediatr 2009;21(1):94–101.

16 *Exanthematous Diseases of Childhood*

CHAPTER OUTLINE

Several viral and bacterial illnesses may be accompanied by localized or generalized skin eruptions called *exanthems*. These eruptions may be the first manifestation of a disorder and often are the reason for parents and patients to pursue medical evaluation. Prompt recognition and diagnosis of exanthems is desirable and may dictate that other examinations be performed to assess for systemic associations. Although identification of the exact infectious agent is not always practical or possible, knowledge of the most common causes of the various exanthems is important from an epidemiologic perspective. For instance, when diagnosing a child with a parvovirus B19–related exanthematous disease, consideration of at-risk contacts (e.g., gravid females, individuals with hemolysis or conditions resulting in decreased red blood cell production) is vital.

The majority of childhood exanthems are caused by viruses and, less often, by bacterial or rickettsial agents. Most childhood exanthems are diagnosed and managed by primary care providers, and thus a thorough familiarity with both classic and atypical exanthems is desirable for the pediatric primary care practitioner. When evaluating the patient with an exanthem, several features should be considered, including the morphology of individual lesions, the distribution pattern, prodromal and concurrent symptoms, known exposures, associated enanthem (eruption of the mucous membranes), local epidemiology, and the findings of a thorough review of systems and physical examination. Whereas some exanthematous processes present with a characteristic patterning of lesion morphology and distribution, others may reveal no pathognomonic features, and the cutaneous findings must be taken into context with the overall presentation of the patient. Exanthems may be divided into erythematous, vesicular, and papular forms and have also been invariably described as *morbilliform* ("measles-like"), *rubelliform* ("rubella-like"), *scarlatiniform* ("scarlet fever–like"), or urticarial.[1] Pustular and petechial changes may occasionally be noted.

The classic childhood exanthems are listed in Table 16.1. These disorders were originally classified with a numeric designation in the early 1900s. Since then, much has been learned about the etiologic agents of the classic exanthems, and several newer exanthematous disorders have been described. This chapter includes a discussion of the classic exanthems; varicella; infectious mononucleosis (IM); and exanthems caused by enteroviruses, *Mycoplasma*, and rickettsial agents. In addition, nonspecific viral exanthems are discussed, as are some atypical exanthems, including papular acrodermatitis of childhood, unilateral laterothoracic exanthem (ULE), and papular-purpuric gloves-and-socks syndrome (PPGSS). Kawasaki disease, which may have clinical overlap with multiple exanthematous disorders, is discussed in Chapter 21. Acute generalized exanthematous pustulosis (AGEP), another exanthematous disorder, is discussed in Chapter 20.

Varicella (Chickenpox)

Varicella zoster virus (VZV) is a member of the herpesvirus family and the causative agent of both varicella (chickenpox) and herpes zoster (shingles, see Chapter 15). Varicella results from primary infection with VZV and is a highly communicable human disease. Once acquired, VZV becomes permanently established in the sensory ganglia in a latent form with intermittent reactivation in a dermatomal distribution, resulting in herpes zoster.[2] Although acute varicella is usually a self-limited infection, before extensive use of the varicella vaccine, most children had upward of 250 to 500 skin lesions, approximately 9000 to 11,000 children were hospitalized annually, and up to 100 individuals per year died of the disease or its complications.[3,4]

VZV is found worldwide, and annual epidemics occur most often during late winter and spring.[5] Varicella is highly contagious and is usually spread between the prodrome and the first 3 days of the skin eruption.[6] VZV is transmitted via respiratory droplets, then enters regional lymph nodes, and eventually a viremia ensues with more widespread dissemination. Primary infection elicits a humoral immune response with production of immunoglobulin (Ig) A, IgM, and IgG anti-VZV antibodies, the latter of which help protect against reinfection.[5] Patients are considered contagious until at least 5 days after onset of the rash or until all existing lesions are dry and crusted.

A live attenuated varicella vaccine (Oka strain) was introduced in 1995, and in 1996 the Advisory Committee on Immunization Practices (ACIP) recommended universal one-dose vaccination of all children at age 12 to 18 months, with catch-up vaccination of all susceptible children before age 13 years.[4] The ACIP and the American Academy of Pediatrics (AAP) expanded their recommendations to include use of the vaccine for postexposure prophylaxis and for some immunocompromised children.[3] The vaccine is also indicated in adults who are susceptible to varicella.

The varicella vaccine has been quite effective in decreasing the overall incidence of varicella, and in vaccinees who develop breakthrough disease ("breakthrough varicella"), the disease tends to be milder with fewer lesions that may remain papular rather than becoming vesicular.[3] In a 6-year case-control study of the effectiveness of the varicella vaccine over time, the effectiveness in the year after vaccination (97%) was greater than in years 2 through 8 after vaccination (84%), although most cases of breakthrough disease in vaccinees were mild.[7] Another study of the effectiveness of a one- versus two-vaccination regimen revealed high vaccine efficacy over 10 years for both groups (94.4% and 98.3%, respectively), and again, breakthrough disease was mild.[8] Despite these reports, severe breakthrough varicella has rarely been described and may occasionally be associated with other organ (pulmonary, central nervous system, hematologic, renal, hepatic, and ocular) involvement.[9]

Table 16.1 Classic Childhood Exanthems

Numerical Designation	Name(s)	Agent(s)	Comment
1	Measles, rubeola	Measles virus (paramyxovirus)	Markedly decreased incidence with vaccination; recent resurgence of epidemics of imported cases and disease occurring in unimmunized individuals in United States (see text)
2	Scarlet fever, scarlatina	GABHS	Toxin-mediated; complications may include glomerulonephritis, RF
3	German measles, rubella	Rubella virus (togavirus)	Rare in era of vaccination
4	Filatow–Dukes disease	?SA	No longer considered a distinct entity
5	Erythema infectiosum, fifth disease, slapped cheek disease	Parvovirus B19	Patients not contagious once rash is present
6	Exanthem subitum, roseola infantum, sixth disease	HHV-6 and HHV-7	Diffuse rash appears after abrupt defervescence

GABHS, Group A β-hemolytic streptococcus; *HHV*, human herpesvirus; *RF*, rheumatic fever; *SA*, *Staphylococcus aureus*.

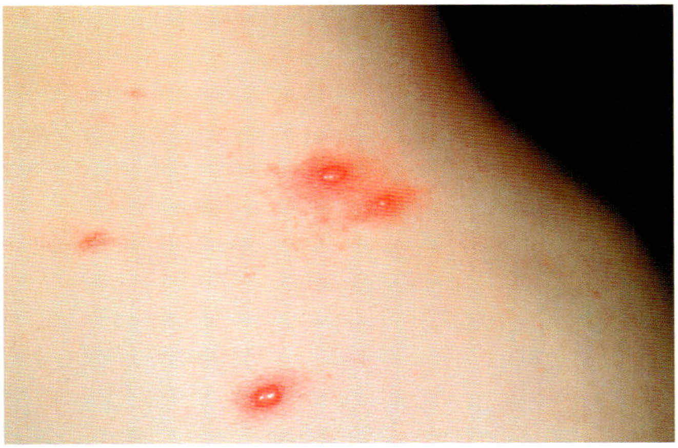

Fig. 16.1 Varicella. Note the early lesions consisting of erythematous macules and papules and the well-developed vesicular lesion.

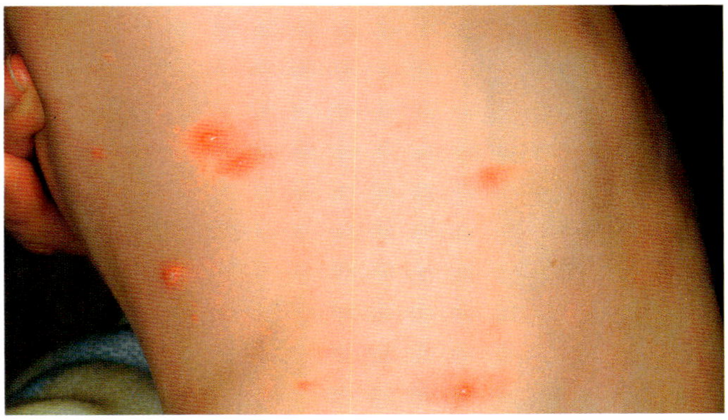

Fig. 16.2 Varicella. These well-developed lesions demonstrate why they have been likened to "dewdrops on a rose petal."

A decline in varicella-related hospitalizations for invasive group A β-hemolytic streptococcus (GABHS) infections was documented between the period of the prevaccine era and that of widespread vaccine use.[10] Although some studies have demonstrated lower effectiveness of the varicella vaccine than expected, overall, the data support its universal use.[11] In 2006, because of insufficient population immunity to prevent community transmission, the ACIP and AAP changed the varicella vaccine policy, recommending a universal two-dose vaccination program.[12] This two-dose vaccination regimen has been demonstrated highly effective against varicella outbreaks in public school students.[13]

The varicella vaccine is available as a monovalent vaccine (Varivax, Merck & Co, Kenilworth, NJ) and as part of a quadrivalent measles, mumps, rubella, varicella vaccine (MMRV; ProQuad, Merck & Co). Postlicensure studies have suggested a slightly increased risk of febrile seizures among children aged 12 to 23 months who received MMRV for their initial dose (versus separate MMR and varicella vaccines). A personal or family history of seizures is considered a precaution for use of MMRV, and unless a parent expresses strong preference for this vaccine, it is recommended that the first dose be administered as separate MMR and varicella vaccines.[14] For the second dose at any age or the first dose at ages 48 months and older, the combination MMRV vaccine is recommended.[15]

Primary varicella begins with a prodrome of fever, chills, malaise, headache, arthralgia, and myalgia. After 24 to 48 hours, the earliest skin lesions become evident, initially as red macules or papules (Fig. 16.1) that progress rapidly to a vesicular phase. The fully developed lesion has been likened to a "dewdrop on a rose petal" (Fig. 16.2). Varicella lesions present initially on the scalp, face, or trunk and then spread to the extremities. Older lesions crust over, and new lesions continue to develop, resulting in the pathognomonic finding of lesions in various stages being present at the same time (Fig. 16.3). New lesions continue to develop for 3 to 4 days, and by day 6, most lesions have crusted over. Patients with sunburn or dermatitis may develop a more severe exanthem. An associated enanthem may be present and consists of painful erosions in the oropharynx, conjunctivae, or vaginal mucosae. The lesions of varicella heal with hypopigmentation (Fig. 16.4) and scarring (Fig. 16.5), especially at sites of the initial lesions.

Varicella tends to be a mild, self-limited disease in most immunocompetent hosts. Complications, however, may occur. The most common complication is secondary bacterial superinfection, usually the result of *Staphylococcus aureus* or GABHS.[16] Invasive GABHS infections, including streptococcal toxic shock syndrome and necrotizing fasciitis, may rarely occur. Secondary bacterial infection usually presents as isolated secondary fever or localized symptoms, such as bulla (large blister) formation or cellulitis. Varicella gangrenosa is diagnosed when an area reveals rapidly progressing erythema, induration, and pain.[5] Peripheral gangrene may occur in the distal extremities.[17] Other skin-related complications include deep ulcerative lesions (Fig. 16.6), subcutaneous abscesses, and regional lymphadenitis. Patients under the age of 5 years who live in a household with older children seem to be at greatest risk for bacterial complications.[16] In patients who develop secondary bacterial infection, bacteremia may occur, as may pneumonia, arthritis, or osteomyelitis.

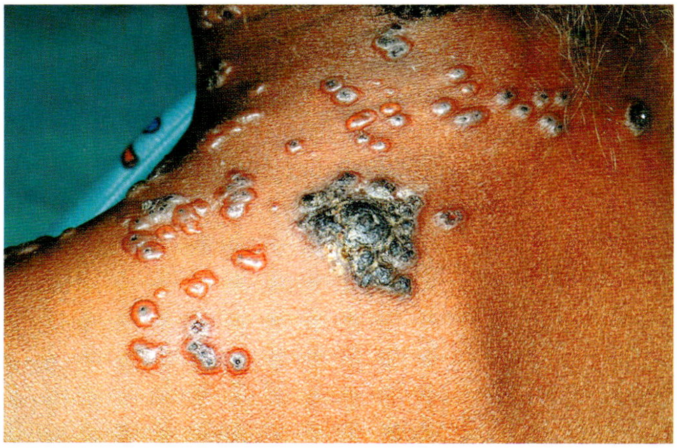

Fig. 16.3 Varicella. Various stages are present in this patient with human immunodeficiency virus (HIV) infection and varicella, including vesicles and crusted papules.

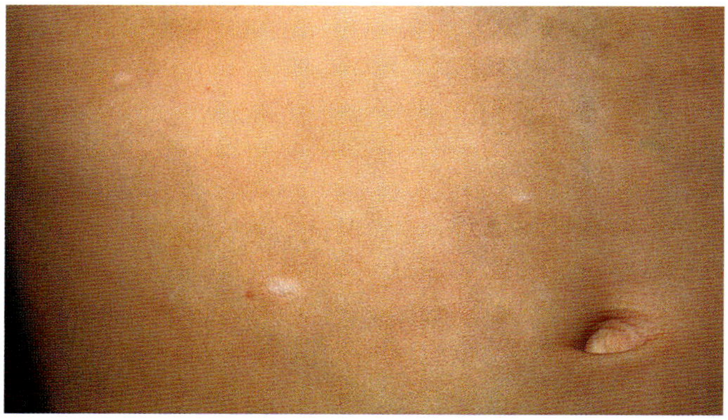

Fig. 16.4 Varicella scarring. Hypopigmented macules and scars are present in this patient with a history of varicella.

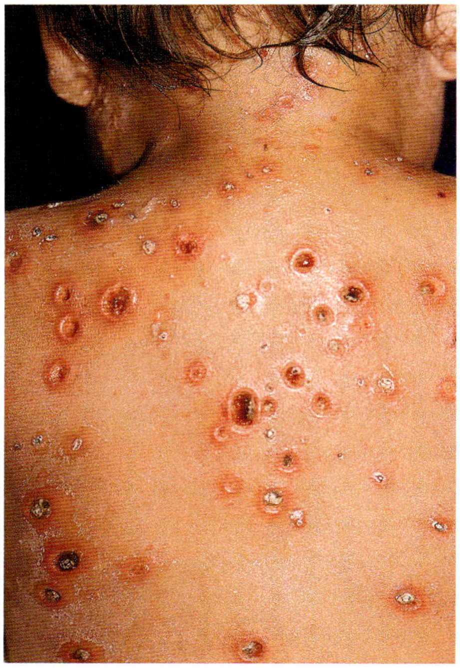

Fig. 16.5 Varicella scarring. Large, deep scars are present in this patient who had secondary bacterial infection of her primary varicella lesions.

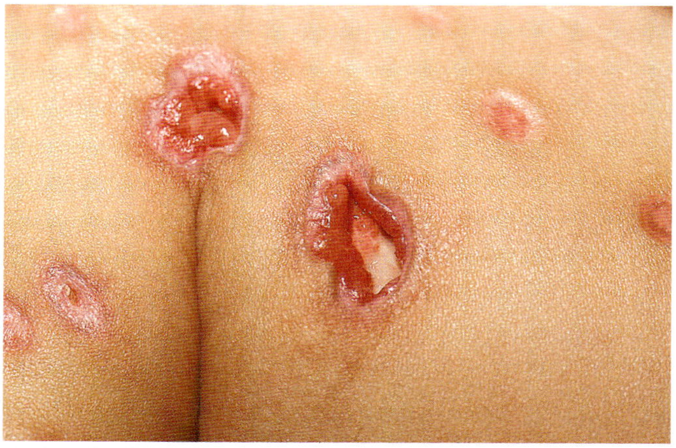

Fig. 16.6 Varicella, complicated. Deep, ulcerative lesions occurred in this young girl with underlying immunodeficiency and secondary infection of the skin with *Streptococcus pyogenes*.

Second to bacterial superinfection, the most common complication in patients with primary varicella is neurologic involvement. This may present as encephalitis, meningoencephalitis, cerebellar ataxia, transverse myelitis, or Guillain–Barré syndrome. Reye syndrome was a fairly common complication of varicella before the association with salicylates was identified. Reye syndrome (acute encephalopathy and fatty degeneration of the viscera) presents with decreased level of consciousness, vomiting, and abnormalities in liver function. The incidence of this complication has fallen dramatically following implementation of universal vaccination. Varicella pneumonia is the most common serious complication in adults but is rare in healthy children.[2,5] When it occurs during the course of childhood varicella, it is usually bacterial in origin. Severe pulmonary deterioration may occur, and it may occasionally be fatal.[18] Thrombocytopenia, arthritis, uveitis, nephritis, myocarditis, pancreatitis, and hepatitis may also occasionally occur. When arthritis occurs in this setting, it may be bacterial *(Streptococcus pyogenes* or *S. aureus)* or aseptic ("varicella arthritis") in origin. The latter is typically confined to a single joint, most commonly the knee, ankle, shoulder, or foot.[19] Purpura fulminans is a rare and life-threatening complication of varicella, and disseminated intravascular coagulopathy may occasionally occur.[20]

Immunocompromised hosts with varicella, including those with leukemia, lymphoma, or human immunodeficiency virus (HIV) infection; those receiving corticosteroids (>2 mg/kg per day of prednisone or equivalent); and those with a history of organ or bone marrow transplantation may have more serious disease and a higher incidence of complications. These individuals have an increased risk of disseminated varicella, with high fever, pneumonia, hepatitis, and encephalitis. Bacterial superinfection may also occur with increased incidence, and hemorrhagic complications of the disease are more common. Varicella during pregnancy poses an increased risk of serious disease to both the mother and the fetus (see Chapter 2). Pregnant females have a higher incidence of varicella pneumonia, and mortality from the disease is increased.

The diagnosis of primary varicella is usually based on the history and clinical findings. Laboratory confirmation, when desired, can be performed by either virologic or serologic methods. The diagnostic method of choice is polymerase chain reaction (PCR) testing of vesicular fluid or crusts, although early in the illness, PCR testing can also be performed on buccal swab material or saliva.[21] Direct fluorescent antibody testing, performed on cells scraped from the base of a fresh vesicle, is also useful, and although not as highly sensitive as PCR, is rapid and fairly sensitive.[22,23] Tzanck smears on skin scrapings identify multinucleated giant cells and confirm the diagnosis of herpesvirus infection but are not specific for VZV. Cell culture is unequivocally confirmatory but not ideal for VZV, given the prolonged time necessary for cytopathic effects to appear. Serologic studies looking for a fourfold or greater increase in IgG antibody between acute and convalescent samples can help in the diagnosis, but may not be reliable in immunocompromised individuals.

The treatment of varicella in otherwise-healthy children is usually symptomatic, with the goals being control of pain and pruritus and prevention of secondary superinfection. Supportive therapies include oral antihistamines for pruritus, acetaminophen for fever or pain, and topical care. Useful topical regimens may include cool compresses, oatmeal baths, and application of topical products such as bacitracin ointment, calamine lotion, pramoxine-containing preparations, or menthol-camphor (Sarna) lotion. Antibiotics should be given if secondary bacterial infection is present.

The decision regarding the use of antiviral therapy for primary varicella depends on several factors, including host immune status, the extent of the infection, and timing of the diagnosis. In general, routine use of antiviral agents for varicella in otherwise-healthy children is not recommended. Acyclovir, famciclovir, and valacyclovir are antiviral agents licensed for treatment of VZV infections, although famciclovir is not approved for primary varicella. Oral acyclovir has been suggested in some studies to decrease the severity of primary VZV infection, including a decrease in the days of fever, number of days of new lesion formation, total number of lesions, and pruritus. In a review of published studies on acyclovir treatment of varicella in otherwise-healthy children and adolescents, a reduction in the number of days with fever was noted, but the results were inconsistent with respect to the number of days to no new lesions, maximum number of lesions, and number of days to relief of itching.[23] In addition, no differences in the incidence of varicella complications between acyclovir and placebo groups were consistently noted.[24] Oral antiviral therapy should be considered, however, for healthy individuals who are at risk for moderate or severe disease, such as those over 12 years of age (especially unvaccinated), those with chronic skin or lung disorders, and those receiving therapy with salicylates (long-term courses) or corticosteroids (short, intermittent, or aerosolized courses).[21] When used in the treatment of varicella in otherwise-healthy patients, antiviral therapy should be started within 24 hours of the appearance of the rash. The use of oral antivirals for pregnant females with uncomplicated varicella remains controversial, although some experts recommend its use for those who develop it during the second or third trimester. Intravenous acyclovir is recommended for pregnant females with serious complications of varicella.[21]

In immunocompromised children, intravenous antiviral therapy with acyclovir should be administered and is most effective when initiated early in the course of the disease (preferably within 24 hours of the onset of the rash). Some experts endorse high-dose oral acyclovir in selected immunocompromised individuals who are perceived to be at a lower risk for severe disseminated varicella. Valacyclovir is also approved for treatment of primary varicella in children 2 to under 18 years of age; some experts have used this agent for treating selected immunocompromised patients.[21] In susceptible individuals with a known exposure to VZV, options include administration of varicella zoster immune globulin (VariZIG) or varicella vaccine. VariZIG is a high-titer preparation of VZV IgG that is given via the intramuscular route. It is recommended for susceptible individuals at high risk for infection and pregnant females who have been exposed to VZV (Box 16.1). VariZIG is best given within 48 hours of the exposure, but the US Food and Drug Administration (FDA) extended the approved period for which it can be given to up to 10 days.[5,21,25]

Box 16.1 Indications for Varicella Zoster Immune Globulin (VariZIG)

Types of exposure to varicella zoster:
- Residing in same household as infected patient
- Playmate: face-to-face indoor play
- Hospital: varicella in roommate; face-to-face contact with infected staff member or patient; visit by a person deemed contagious with varicella; intimate contact with person deemed contagious with zoster
- Newborn: onset of varicella (not herpes zoster) in mother from 5 days or less before delivery or within 48 hours after delivery

Candidates for VariZIG:
- Immunocompromised child without history of varicella or varicella immunization
- Susceptible pregnant female (no evidence of immunity)
- Newborn infant whose mother develops varicella (see earlier)
- Hospitalized premature infant:
  - ≥28 weeks' gestation, if mother lacks reliable history of varicella or serologic evidence of antibodies
  - <28 weeks' gestation or birthweight 1000 g or less, regardless of maternal history of varicella or serologic status

Modified from American Academy of Pediatrics. Varicella-zoster virus infections. In: Kimberlin DW, Brady MT, Jackson MA, Long SS, editors. Red Book: 2018 Report of the Committee on Infectious Diseases. Elk Grove Village, IL: American Academy of Pediatrics; 2018:869–83.

Rubeola (Measles)

In the prevaccine era, more than 500,000 cases of measles, or rubeola, were reported annually in the United States. After introduction of a live-virus vaccine in 1963, a significant reduction in the incidence of infection was noted. The MMR vaccine has been distributed in excess of 575 million doses and is one of the most widely used combination viral vaccines in the world.[26] However, a dramatic resurgence occurred from 1989 to 1990, and during this period the highest mortality since 1977 was noted.[27,28] Those affected most during these measles resurgences were preschool-aged children from the inner-city areas, especially those who were unvaccinated and from low-income families. A majority of the deaths occurring from measles infection during this period occurred in children aged 5 years or younger.[28] Other target populations during the measles resurgence included vaccinated school-aged children and college students, probably due to the insufficiency of a single vaccine dose and waning immunity.

In response to the measles resurgence of the 1980s, the Committee on Infectious Diseases of the AAP and the ACIP recommended an amendment to the previous vaccination schedule and suggested two doses of measles vaccination rather than one.[28,29] The current recommendation for measles vaccination calls for a two-dose schedule, with the first given at 12 to 15 months and the second at 4 to 6 years of age, and catch-up vaccination of children and adolescents as long as the two vaccinations are given at least 4 weeks apart.[30] Changes in the measles vaccination strategy resulted in a markedly diminished incidence of the disease in the United States, with 100 cases reported in 1999.[31] Although the incidence in the United States declined to extremely low levels compared with the prevaccine era, measles continues to be a major health problem worldwide, with an estimated 89,780 measles deaths in 2016.[32] Of the 100 cases reported in the United States in 1999, 33% were imported from other countries.[31] In developing countries, infants under 9 months of age who are too young to have received vaccination have a high incidence of measles, with more multisystem involvement and a greater risk of death.[33] Importantly, epidemics of measles continue to occur in the United States, Europe, Africa, and other regions. During January through July 2008, 131 measles cases were reported to the Centers for Disease Control and Prevention (CDC), and these occurred primarily in unvaccinated school-aged children.[34] The majority of these children were eligible for vaccination but had parents who chose not to have them vaccinated. In 2011, 222 measles cases were reported to the CDC, the majority of which were associated with importations from other countries, and more than 85% of cases occurring in individuals who were unvaccinated or had unknown vaccination status. In 2014, measles cases in the United States had risen to 644.[35] In early 2015 the United States experienced a large, multistate outbreak of measles infection linked to an amusement park in California. Among 110 of the earliest patients in this outbreak, 45% were unvaccinated, 5% had received only one dose of the vaccine, and 43% had unknown or undocumented vaccination status. Of the unvaccinated patients, 67% were intentionally unvaccinated because of personal beliefs (65% of these were children under the age of 18 years).[36] In 2017, 79 confirmed measles cases were reported to the Minnesota Department of Health, most of them Somali-American children, a community with declining vaccination coverage relating to concerns about an association with autism.[37,38] And as of April 2019, there were 704 reported cases of measles in the United States in 2019, representing the largest number reported in a single year since 1994.[39] Of the 13 outbreaks between January 1 and April 26, six of them were associated with underimmunized close-knit communities (accounting for 88% of all cases), including the 2018–2019 outbreak that occurred in Rockland County, New York, and nearby counties, affecting primarily individuals in orthodox Jewish neighborhoods with low school immunization rates.[40] Given these and other observations, maintaining high vaccination coverage and index of suspicion for measles and ensuring a rapid public health response at times of outbreaks are critical in the attempt to maintain measles elimination in the United States.[41,42] In response to the previously mentioned New York outbreak, the affected counties excluded unvaccinated students from school for 21 days after measles exposure and extended school exclusions to include all nonimmune students at schools with immunity rates <95%, as documented by two valid doses of MMR vaccine or serologic evidence of immunity.[40]

Measles is caused by a single-stranded ribonucleic acid (RNA) virus in the family Paramyxoviridae. Infection begins in the nasopharyngeal epithelium and, less commonly, through the conjunctivae. Transmission of measles is primarily via respiratory droplets and, less commonly, by small-particle aerosols.[43] The incubation period is around 10 to 14 days. From the initial site of infection, the virus enters the lymph nodes and lymphatics and multiplies within the reticuloendothelial system with a subsequent viremia.[33] The virus is then disseminated to multiple lymphoid tissues and other organs, including the skin, liver, and gastrointestinal tract.[44] Measles immunity includes cell-mediated, humoral, and mucosal responses. Measles antibodies are responsible for protection from future infection or reinfection.[33]

Measles classically presents with fever and the three Cs: cough, coryza, and conjunctivitis. The pathognomonic enanthem, Koplik spots, usually occurs during this prodromal period and presents with punctuate, gray-white to erythematous papules distributed on the buccal mucosa (Fig. 16.7). These lesions have been found to be highly predictive of confirmed measles,[45] although they are not always present. The skin eruption of measles usually begins 2 to 4 days after the prodrome, which may intensify several days before the onset of rash. It begins on the face (Fig. 16.8), especially the forehead, hairline, and behind the ears, and spreads downward onto the trunk (Fig. 16.9) and extremities. The lesions are erythematous to purple-red macules and papules that may become confluent and fade in the same order as their appearance, leaving behind coppery macules and desquamation. The diagnosis of measles should be considered in any child presenting with fever and an erythematous rash, especially with the earlier concomitant findings.[46]

Complications of measles include pneumonia, laryngotracheobronchitis, otitis media, stomatitis, gastroenteritis, myocarditis, and encephalitis. Pneumonia may be caused by the measles virus itself or be related to secondary bacterial or viral infection. Keratoconjunctivitis is common, especially in children with vitamin A deficiency, in which case it may result in blindness.[43] Measles complications occur in up to 40% of patients and tend to be more severe in patients at the extremes of age and in malnourished patients.[46]

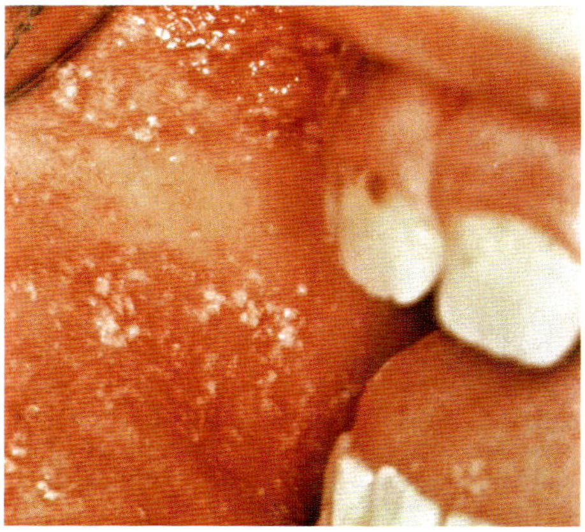

Fig. 16.7 Koplik spots. Gray-white papules of the buccal mucosa in a patient with measles.

Modified measles is measles occurring in a previously vaccinated individual. In this situation the prodrome is milder and of shorter duration, the exanthem is less prominent, and Koplik spots may be absent.[47] This presentation of measles may pose a diagnostic challenge, given the nonpathognomonic presentation. Atypical measles occurs rarely in contemporary times and is seen in individuals exposed to natural measles after vaccination with the killed measles vaccines. These vaccines were utilized for a short period in the 1960s in the United States and for more variable periods of time in other countries, including Canada and Sweden.[47] It has occasionally been reported in children who received the live attenuated vaccine.[48] Atypical measles presents with high fever, headaches, and myalgias and eventually the measles rash and often pneumonia. Hemorrhagic features may be present, and the exanthem may be confused with Rocky Mountain spotted fever (RMSF).

Subacute sclerosing panencephalitis (SSPE) is a delayed neurodegenerative disease characterized by seizures, personality changes, cognitive decline, motor dysfunction, coma, and death within 5 to 15 years of the

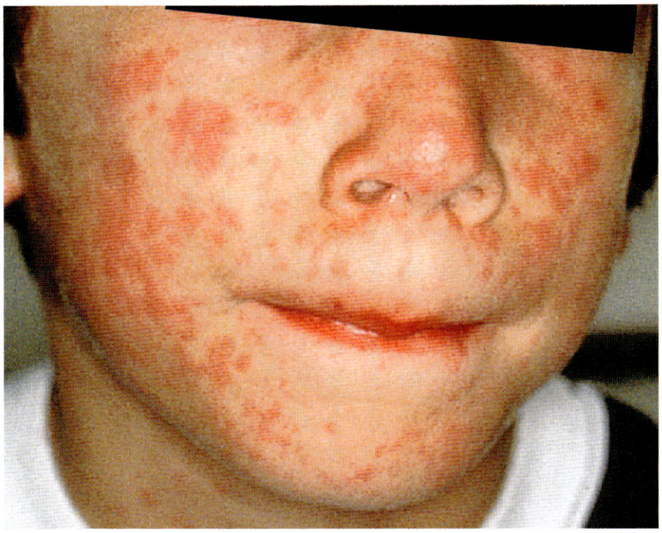

Fig. 16.8 Rubeola (measles). Erythematous macules and patches on the face early in the course of the disease.

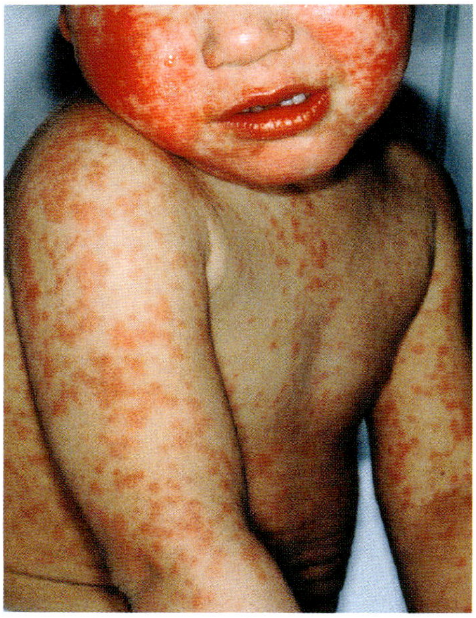

Fig. 16.9 Rubeola (measles). Intensely erythematous patches of the face with cephalocaudad spread onto the trunk and extremities.

measles diagnosis. It classically occurs many years later in 1 in 100,000 patients with measles, but fortunately has been dramatically decreased in incidence with widespread vaccination strategies.[43,49]

The diagnosis of measles is traditionally based upon the clinical presentation with laboratory confirmation. Acute and convalescent serologic studies documenting a fourfold increase in titer confirm the diagnosis of measles.[50] Culture can be performed on nasopharyngeal or conjunctival swabs, respiratory secretions, urine, or blood. PCR and semiquantitative real-time PCR assays have been developed, the latter being quite sensitive and specific and potentially useful in situations where early and rapid diagnosis is vital.[51] Measles is a notifiable disease and should be reported to the local health department in a timely fashion.

The treatment of uncomplicated measles is largely supportive, because specific antiviral therapies do not exist. Ribavirin, a synthetic nucleoside analog useful in the treatment of other paramyxovirus (respiratory syncytial virus) infections, has been utilized in severely ill or immunocompromised patients.[49,52] Antibiotics are useful in patients with secondary bacterial infections such as otitis media or bacterial pneumonia. Vitamin A supplementation is currently recommended by the World Health Organization (WHO) for all children diagnosed with measles, despite their country of residence, administered once daily for 2 days.[53] This recommendation is based on the observations that children in resource-limited countries appear to have decreased morbidity and mortality when treated with vitamin A and that some children diagnosed with measles in the United States have decreased levels; vitamin A appears to ameliorate the severity of diarrhea, possibly through a protective action on the epithelial lining of the gastrointestinal tract, increased mucous secretion, and enhanced local barriers to infection.[53,54] Hospitalized patients with measles should be kept in respiratory isolation for 4 days from the onset of the rash (and for the duration of the illness in immunocompromised hosts). Most patients will recover completely without sequelae and have lifelong immune protection against reinfection.

Scarlet Fever

Scarlet fever (scarlatina) is a bacterial exanthem that may at times be confused with a variety of viral exanthematous diseases. It is caused by GABHS and is primarily a disease of children between the ages of 1 and 10 years. It is very rarely diagnosed in infants. Transmission of GABHS is usually via respiratory secretions. The organism produces a variety of toxins referred to as *streptococcal pyrogenic exotoxins (SPEs)* (including serotypes A, C, and G to M) and can produce up to 11 serologically distinct superantigens, which include the SPEs, streptococcal superantigen, streptococcal M protein, and streptococcal mitogenic exotoxin Z_n. SPE B is another toxin that appears to have some superantigen properties, but also appears to be a cysteine protease.[55] The majority of the SPEs are encoded by bacteriophages. Epidemiologic changes over time in the types of SPEs produced appeared to correlate with changes in the severity of this disease. The shift from SPE-A– to SPE-B– and SPE-C–producing strains, which was seen early in the twentieth century, paralleled the decrease in morbidity and mortality from scarlet fever, as well as the decline in incidence and severity of acute rheumatic fever (ARF) in the United States.[56] However, ARF (a systemic inflammatory autoimmune reaction appearing 2 to 4 weeks after GABHS pharyngitis) and rheumatic heart disease (RHD; progressive valve damage) continue to burden many low- and middle-income countries, as well as some populations in higher-income countries. Immigration from countries where ARF and RHD are endemic to higher-income areas have resulted in an increased prevalence in some regions where they were once believed to be eliminated.[57] In the United States, the incidence of ARF is generally lower than in developing countries, but there have been some regional outbreaks, including an outbreak in Utah in the 1980s in which the incidence in children aged 3 to 17 years approached 12 per 100,000.[58] The incidence of ARF peaks between 5 and 15 years, and the risk of subsequent RHD is greater in women; the global health burden of these disorders continues to be significant, with a high prevalence in Africa, the Pacific region, Latin America, the Middle East, and Asia.[59] The revised Jones criteria for ARF are listed in Table 16.2.

Table 16.2 Revised Jones Criteria (2015) for Diagnosis of Acute Rheumatic Fever (ARF)*

	Major Criteria	Minor Criteria	Comment
Low-risk population†	Carditis (clinical and/or subclinical)	Polyarthralgia	
	Arthritis (polyarthritis only)	Fever (≥38.5° C)	
	Chorea	ESR ≥60 mm/hour and/or CRP ≥3 mg/dL	
	Erythema marginatum	Prolonged PR interval (age appropriate; in absence of carditis)	*Erythema marginatum:* evanescent pink patches/plaques with pale centers and serpiginous margins
	Subcutaneous nodules		*Subcutaneous nodules:* firm, painless nodules on extensor surfaces of joints, especially knees, elbows, wrists; also occiput, spinous processes
Moderate- and high-risk population‡	Carditis (clinical and/or subclinical)	Monoarthralgia	
	Arthritis (monoarthritis or polyarthritis; polyarthralgia)	Fever ≥38° C	
	Chorea	ESR ≥30 mm/hour and/or CRP ≥3 mg/dL	
	Erythema marginatum	Prolonged PR interval (age appropriate, in absence of carditis)	*Erythema marginatum:* see earlier
	Subcutaneous nodules		*Subcutaneous nodules:* see earlier

Adapted from American Academy of Pediatrics. Group A streptococcal infections. In: Kimberlin DW, Brady MT, Jackson MA, et al., editors. Red Book: 2018 Report of the Committee on Infectious Diseases. Elk Grove Village, IL: American Academy of Pediatrics; 2018:748–62; Gewitz MH, Baltimore RS, Tani LY, et al. Revision of the Jones criteria for the diagnosis of acute rheumatic fever in the era of Doppler echocardiography. A scientific statement the American Heart Association. Circulation 2015;131:1806–18.

CRP, C-reactive protein; *ESR*, erythrocyte sedimentation rate; *GABHS*, group A β-hemolytic streptococcus; *RHD*, rheumatic heart disease.

*All patients must have evidence of preceding GABHS infection

†Low-risk population: those with ARF incidence ≤2 per 100,000 school-aged children or all-ages RHD prevalence ≤1 per 1000 population/year (e.g., United States, Canada, Europe)

‡Moderate- and high-risk population: those with ongoing endemic ARF (e.g., Africa, Asia-Pacific, indigenous populations in Australasia)

For diagnosis of ARF:

- Initial ARF: 2 major OR 1 major + 2 minor criteria
- Recurrent ARF: 2 major OR 1 major + 2 minor OR 3 minor criteria

Scarlet fever presents with fever, throat pain, headache, and chills along with cutaneous findings. It is less commonly associated with streptococcal skin infection rather than pharyngitis. The primary distinction between GABHS pharyngitis and scarlet fever is the accompanying exanthem present in the latter. Oropharyngeal inspection reveals tonsillopharyngeal erythema, exudates, and petechial macules of the palate. During the first few days of illness, the tongue may reveal a white coating with red and edematous papillae projecting through (white strawberry tongue). By the fourth or fifth day, the coating peels off, leaving behind a red, glistening tongue studded with prominent papillae (red strawberry tongue).

The differential diagnosis of GABHS pharyngitis includes infection with viral agents (especially Epstein–Barr virus [EBV], mononucleosis), *Mycoplasma*, *Chlamydia*, and *Arcanobacterium haemolyticum*. In adolescents the differential diagnosis should include groups C and G *Streptococcus* species and *Neisseria gonorrhoeae*,[60] and in developing countries *Corynebacterium diphtheriae* may be implicated. *A. haemolyticum*, formerly known as *Corynebacterium haemolyticum*, is a Gram-positive bacillus that most often infects adolescents and young adults and may result in a syndrome of pharyngitis and a scarlatiniform exanthem.[61] The pharyngitis in these patients is usually severe (occasionally mistaken for diphtheria), and the exanthem may also occasionally mimic toxic shock syndrome, measles, urticaria, or erythema multiforme.[62,63] Infection with *A. haemolyticum* can occasionally be associated with bacteremia, severe sepsis, and soft-tissue infections (especially in patients with concomitant diabetes mellitus).[64,65] Lemierre syndrome, a condition characterized by pharyngitis, bacteremia (usually with anaerobic organisms including *Bacillus* and *Fusobacterium*), and thrombophlebitis of the internal jugular vein, has also been reported in association with this organism.[66]

Tender anterior cervical adenopathy is commonly present in patients with scarlet fever, and rhinorrhea and cough are usually absent. Some experts argue that presence of the latter two findings is a negative factor for the diagnosis of GABHS infection.[60] The exanthem of scarlet fever presents as a fine, erythematous, macular and papular eruption (Fig. 16.10) that has been described as "sandpapery." It involves the trunk and extremities and may be accentuated in flexural areas with a petechial component (Pastia lines). In darker-skinned individuals, the exanthem of scarlet fever may be more difficult to recognize and may consist only of punctate papules resembling cutis anserina ("goose flesh") (Fig. 16.11). Circumoral pallor may be a useful clinical sign and is visualized as a rim of pallor encircling the perioral area. The exanthem generally resolves over 4 to 5 days and often heals with desquamation (Fig. 16.12), which can occasionally occur in thick sheets, especially over the hands, feet, toes, and fingers (Fig. 16.13). An interesting observation is that the SPEs produced by GABHS contribute to the exanthem by their ability to stimulate a delayed-type hypersensitivity response that requires prior exposure of the host to the organism.[67]

Scarlet fever is diagnosed based on the clinical presentation in conjunction with results of laboratory testing. The gold-standard laboratory examination is throat culture with growth of GABHS.

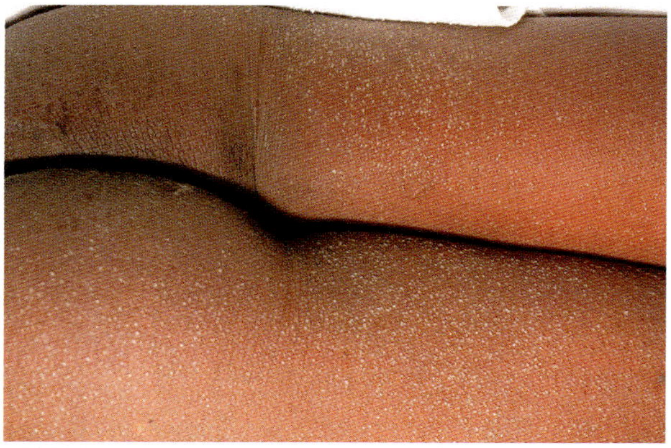

Fig. 16.10 Scarlet fever. Diffuse erythema with small, punctuate papules. This eruption has a sandpapery texture to palpation.

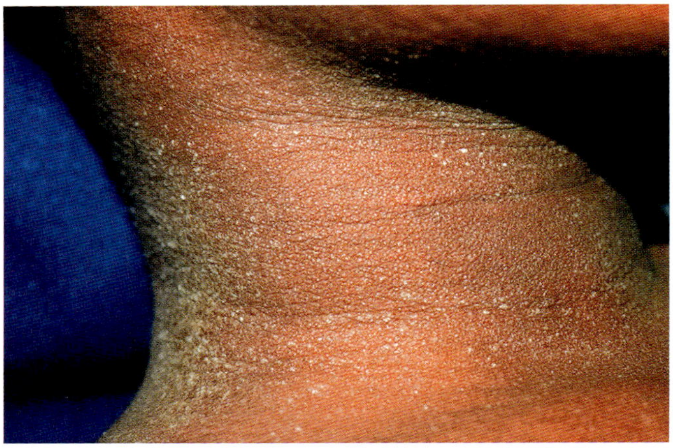

Fig. 16.11 Scarlet fever in a dark-skinned patient. The rash in this patient resembles "goose flesh." Note the early desquamation at some sites.

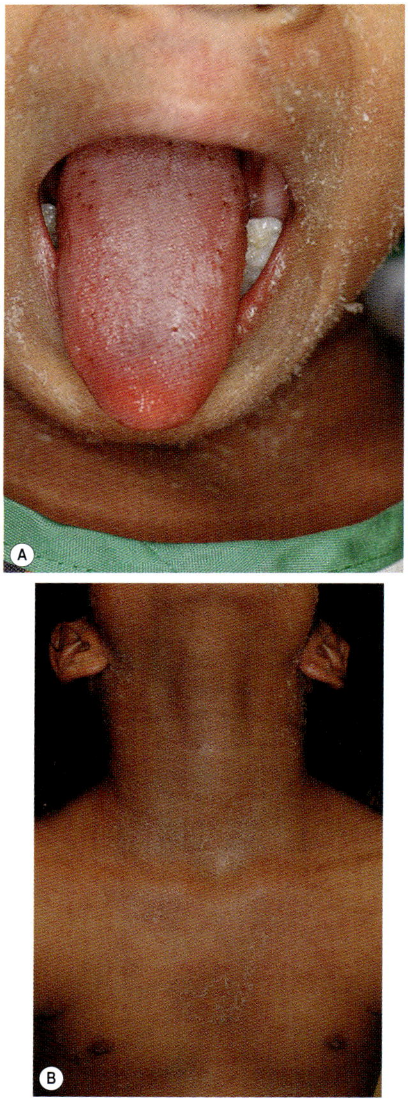

Fig. 16.12 Scarlet fever, subacute. This 4-year-old girl presented with a several-day history of sore throat and fever, and examination was notable for cervical lymphadenopathy, red strawberry tongue **(A)**, and faint diffuse erythema with marked desquamation **(B)**.

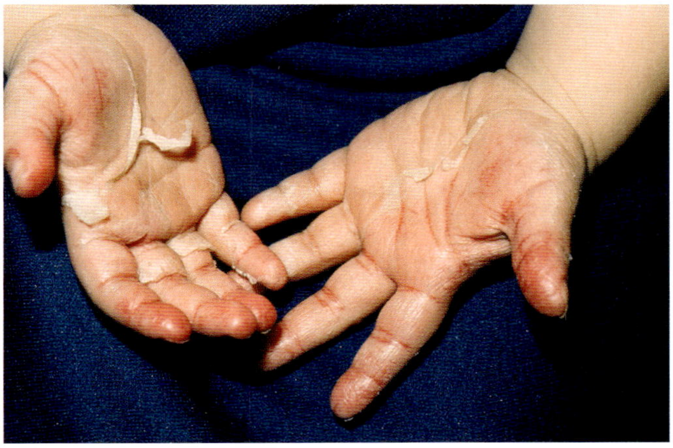

Fig. 16.13 Post–scarlet fever desquamation. Extensive peeling of the hands and digits occurred in this patient after treatment for scarlet fever.

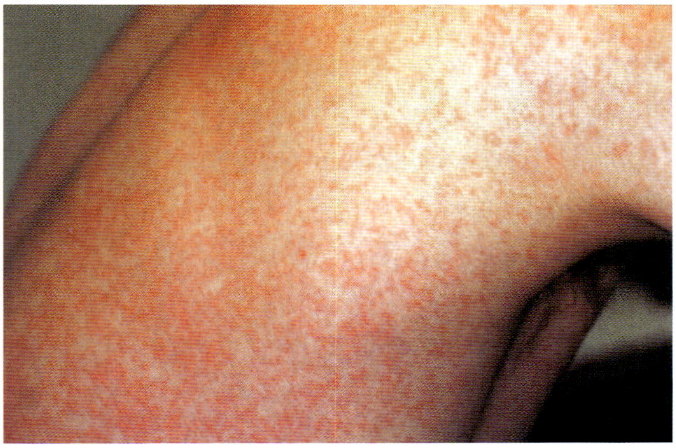

Fig. 16.14 Rubella. Nonspecific rose-pink macules and papules on the trunk of an adolescent male with German measles.

Rapid antigen detection (rapid strep testing), when properly performed, has a high sensitivity and specificity.[60] In addition, antistreptococcal serologies may occasionally be useful. Complications of scarlet fever include pneumonia, pericarditis, meningitis, hepatitis, glomerulonephritis, and ARF. In endemic regions, around 60% of patients with ARF go on to develop RHD.[68] Although the symptoms of GABHS pharyngitis and scarlet fever will often improve spontaneously, treatment more rapidly alleviates symptoms and, more importantly, is the primary mode of prevention for the subsequent occurrence of ARF. The prevailing theory regarding ARF prevention is that antimicrobial therapy should be started within 9 days from the onset of symptoms of GABHS pharyngitis.[60,69] In a review of an ARF prevention program in New Zealand entailing a vigorous school-clinic sore throat management approach with free care, antibiotics, and monitoring, a marked decline in the diagnosis of ARF in 5- to 12-year-old children was demonstrated.[70]

The drug of choice for the treatment of scarlet fever and GABHS pharyngitis is penicillin V, given for 10 days. Amoxicillin administered as a single daily dose has been demonstrated to be as effective as penicillin V or multiple daily doses of amoxicillin.[69] In patients allergic to penicillin, erythromycin or another macrolide (e.g., clarithromycin or azithromycin) or clindamycin may be utilized. Other options include a first-generation cephalosporin (as long as the history of penicillin allergy is nonanaphylactic in origin) or intramuscular penicillin G benzathine, which has the advantage of not being adherence-dependent but the disadvantage of being painful during administration.[69]

Rubella (German Measles)

Rubella, or German measles, is a viral exanthematous disease with a worldwide distribution. The incidence of rubella has greatly decreased since widespread rubella vaccination began in the United States in 1969. Before that time, epidemics occurred every 6 to 9 years, and major epidemics or pandemics occurred every 10 to 20 years.[71] The primary goal of the rubella vaccination program was to prevent fetal infection, which may have various effects, including miscarriage, stillbirth, and congenital rubella syndrome (CRS) (see Chapter 2). As of 2013, goals for rubella elimination had been established in two WHO regions, the Americas (by 2010) and the European region (by 2015), and accelerated control of rubella and prevention of CRS had been established for the Western Pacific region.[72,73] The African, Eastern Mediterranean, and Southeast Asia regions have not yet established goals for control or elimination of rubella.[74] In Japan, rubella outbreaks significantly increased in 2012 and 2013 with a corresponding increase in CRS. The effects of such outbreaks can be far-reaching, given the possibility of disease importation into other countries, and serve as a reminder of the need to maintain high levels of vaccination coverage and infectious disease surveillance.[72] In April 2015, the Pan American Health Organization announced the elimination of rubella and CRS from the WHO Americas region, making them the third and fourth diseases to be officially eliminated from the region, following smallpox in 1971 and polio in 1994.[75,76]

Rubella is caused by an RNA virus in the Togaviridae family. Humans are the only source of infection, and postnatal disease is spread through direct or droplet contact from nasopharyngeal secretions. Up to 50% of cases of rubella are asymptomatic, and mild, self-limited disease is common. The incubation period ranges from 14 to 23 days, and the mean age of rubella infection is 5 to 9 years.

Prodromal symptoms may occur, especially in adolescents and adults, and include low-grade fever, headache, malaise, eye pain, myalgias, sore throat, rhinorrhea, and cough. The prodrome usually presents 2 to 5 days before the exanthem appears. The skin eruption consists of erythematous to rose-pink macules and papules (Fig. 16.14) that tend to become confluent and most commonly involve the face and trunk. The eruption spreads in a cephalocaudad manner and begins to involute after 1 to 3 days, fading in the same order in which it appeared. After severe rubella eruptions, a fine flaky desquamation may be observed in areas of maximum involvement.

Generalized lymphadenopathy often occurs, especially in the suboccipital, postauricular, and cervical regions. Although this pattern of lymph node enlargement is highly characteristic of rubella, it is not pathognomonic and may occur in other disorders, including measles, varicella, adenovirus infection, and mononucleosis. Arthralgias and arthritis are common, especially in females, in whom they occur up to 52% of the time.[77] The most common joints affected are those of the fingers, wrists, and knees. Complete resolution of the joint symptoms may take up to several weeks, and chronic arthritis occasionally develops. A characteristic enanthem, Forschheimer spots, may be present in patients with rubella and presents with erythematous and petechial macules on the soft palate.[78] Other complications of rubella include encephalitis (which occurs in 1 in 6000 patients), myocarditis, pericarditis, and hepatitis.[50] Anemia, neutropenia, and thrombocytopenia may also occur, as may hemolytic uremic syndrome.

A clinical diagnosis of rubella is difficult to make, given the potential overlap with multiple other exanthematous diseases. Serologic tests are most useful in confirming the diagnosis of rubella. The presence of rubella-specific IgM antibody indicates recent infection, as does a fourfold or greater increase in titer between acute and convalescent serum taken 1 to 2 weeks apart.[50,79] The virus can be isolated from nasal specimens plated onto appropriate cell-culture media, and amplification of rubella virus RNA with PCR from throat or nasal swabs or urine can be useful for diagnosis, and although not currently FDA approved, is available in several laboratories.[79] The treatment of postnatal rubella is generally supportive. Hospitalized patients require contact isolation for 7 days after onset of the rash, and nonhospitalized children should be excused from school or day care.

The live-virus rubella vaccine, typically given as a component of the combination MMR vaccine, is typically recommended in the United States at 12 to 15 months of age, with a second dose at 4 to 6 years of age. The ongoing efforts of global rubella eradication campaigns will hopefully result in eventual worldwide elimination of the disease. Continued efforts to ensure the immunity of women of childbearing age will help to decrease the incidence of vertical transmission and CRS.

Filatow–Dukes Disease

In 1900, Dukes described what was believed to be a unique exanthem and contrasted it with rubella and scarlet fever.[80] This disorder was termed *fourth disease* and subsequently became known as Filatow–Dukes disease, given a similar description by Filatow 15 years earlier. The exanthem was described as bright red papules with a diffuse distribution, skin tenderness, and fever, and there was significant overlap with other exanthematous diseases, including staphylococcal scalded skin syndrome, scarlet fever, and rubella. Significant controversy followed the initial descriptions of fourth disease, and some authors propose that a distinct disorder never existed.[81] The possibility that epidermolytic toxin-producing staphylococci were the etiologic agent for the disorder described in the original reports has been suggested.[82] In general, researchers and practitioners alike have abandoned the idea of Filatow–Dukes disease representing a distinct entity.

Erythema Infectiosum

Erythema infectiosum (EI; fifth disease) is a common childhood exanthematous illness caused by parvovirus B19 (referred to as *B19*). Although parvoviruses are ubiquitous in nature and may cause significant disease in a wide range of animals, B19 is the only one resulting in human disease.[83] Several disorders have been linked to B19 infection in humans (Box 16.2), including EI, arthritis, aplastic crises, and fetal hydrops. B19 infection is common in most countries, and in the United States 60% of adults are seropositive for the virus.[84] Infection is most common in school-aged children, with approximately 20% of susceptible contacts in the school setting becoming infected during an outbreak.[85] The incubation period ranges from 4 to 21 days. In immunocompromised hosts, persistent bone marrow suppression may occur, resulting in severe cytopenias that may be misinterpreted as being related to malignancy relapse or drug reactions.[86]

In patients with classic EI, B19 infection is transmitted via the respiratory tract and is followed by a viremia that ends after 5 to 7 days with the production of IgM anti-B19 antibody. Prodromal symptoms such as headaches, fever, and chills are common during the viremic phase.[87] Respiratory symptoms may also be present. IgG antibody appears during the third week of illness and coincides with the appearance of the rash and arthralgias, and hence patients with the cutaneous findings of EI are not considered infectious. Outbreaks of EI occur primarily during the winter and spring.

Box 16.2 Clinical Associations with Parvovirus B19 Infection

- Asymptomatic infection
- Exanthematous disorders
    - Erythema infectiosum (fifth disease)
    - Papular-purpuric gloves-and-socks syndrome
    - Asymmetric periflexural exanthem
    - "Bathing trunk" exanthem
    - Petechial exanthems
- Other disorders
    - Arthritis
    - Transient aplastic crises
    - Chronic anemia
    - Refractory anemia after solid organ or stem cell transplantation
    - Hemophagocytic lymphohistiocytosis
    - Myelodysplastic syndrome
    - Fetal hydrops
    - Vasculitis
    - Neurologic disease, including arterial ischemic stroke, encephalopathy, encephalitis
    - Rheumatologic disease
- Liver failure
- Myocarditis

EI is the most recognizable B19-associated manifestation. It is also known as *"slapped cheek" disease*, given the characteristic fiery-red facial erythema (Fig. 16.15) that occurs 2 to 3 days after the prodromal symptoms. The cheeks are most prominently affected, with the nasal bridge and perioral areas usually being spared. This phase of the illness has been termed the *first stage*, and is subsequently followed by stages two and three. The differential diagnosis of the initial eruption of EI includes phototoxic reaction and systemic lupus erythematosus.

During stage two, the patient develops a lacy, reticulated eruption on the extremities and trunk 1 to 4 days after the facial rash. This eruption may be pruritic and is often evanescent. It often begins with a confluent pattern followed by central clearing, which results in the lacy and reticulated appearance (Figs. 16.16 and 16.17). The palms and soles are usually spared. The rash of the second stage of EI tends to fade over 2 to 3 weeks but may intermittently recur in response to environmental stimuli, including sunlight, warm temperatures (e.g., a hot bath), or physical activity. This intermittent waxing and waning represents the third stage of EI, and the duration is variable, usually 1 to 3 weeks.

Joint symptoms occur in 8% to 10% of children with EI but in up to 60% of adults with primary B19 infection, especially females.[83,88,89] The most commonly involved joints include the metacarpophalangeal joints, proximal interphalangeal joints, knees, wrists, and ankles. For most patients, the joint symptoms are transient and self-limited. Occasionally, affected children develop a chronic arthritis.[90] Some experts have suggested a potential association between B19 infection and rheumatic arthritis or other connective tissue diseases, although the strength of this association remains unclear.

B19 has a remarkable affinity for erythroid precursors, binding to a receptor known as *P antigen (globoside)*.[91] Direct infection of the red blood cell precursors results in a transient arrest in red blood cell production and resultant transient anemia. Transient aplastic crises may occur in patients

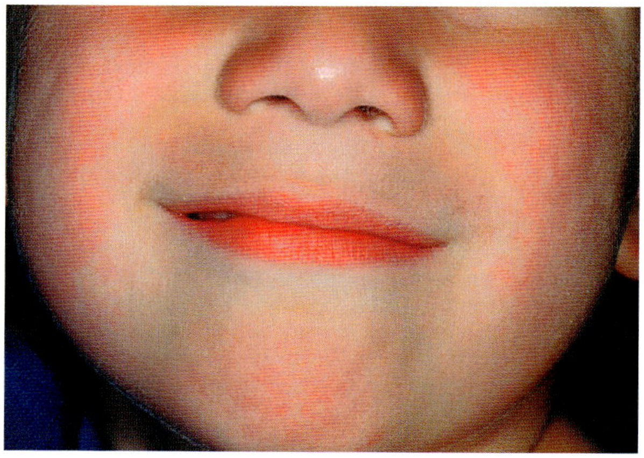

Fig. 16.15 Erythema infectiosum. Erythema of the bilateral cheeks, which has been likened to a "slapped cheeks" appearance.

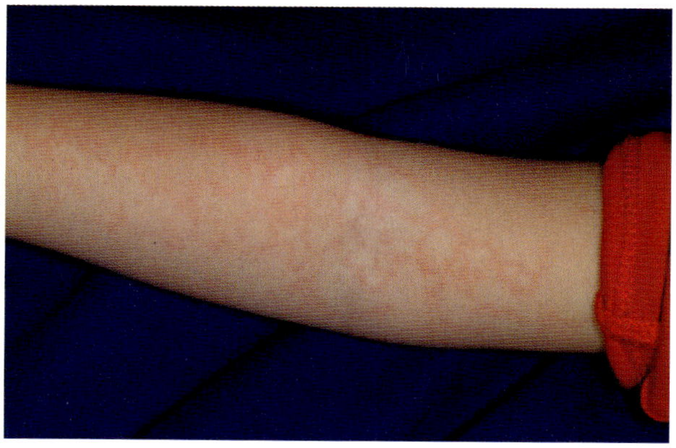

Fig. 16.16 Erythema infectiosum. Reticulate erythema on the upper extremity of a 4-year-old girl who also had bright erythema of both cheeks.

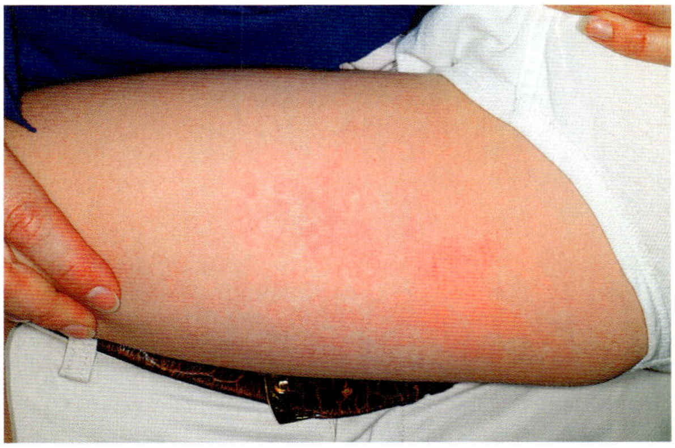

Fig. 16.17 Erythema infectiosum. Patchy erythema with reticulate changes of the inner thigh in a patient with erythema infectiosum.

suffering from disorders of decreased red blood cell production or increased red blood cell destruction or loss. Predisposing disorders include iron-deficiency anemia, spherocytosis, sickle cell disease, thalassemia, glucose-6-phosphate dehydrogenase deficiency, and pyruvate kinase deficiency. Although these episodes may be asymptomatic with spontaneous recovery, severe involvement may result in chills, pallor, weakness, fatigue, vasoocclusive crises, or congestive heart failure. Treatment with red blood cell transfusions may be indicated and for some patients is lifesaving.

Because B19 can cross the placenta, fetal infection is possible in nonimmune females with acute infection. Fetal infection with B19 may result in a variety of effects, occasionally even *in utero* fetal death. This epidemiologic consideration is important in caring for pediatric patients with B19-associated disorders. Fetal effects of B19 infection may include anemia (ranging from mild and self-limited to severe), high-output congestive heart failure, hydrops fetalis (generalized edema with ascites, pleural effusions, and polyhydramnios), and intrauterine fetal demise. Neonatal encephalopathy, encephalitis, cerebral migratory abnormalities, and meningitis have rarely been reported. The majority of pregnant women with B19 infection are asymptomatic, which makes the true incidence of fetal involvement difficult to determine.[87,92] When infected gravid females are symptomatic, they typically experience a biphasic illness with fever, headache, and myalgia followed 1 to 3 weeks later by arthritis or an exanthem.[93] It is estimated that 30% to 66% of adult females are immune to B19 infection,[92,94–96] and therefore their fetuses are not at risk. In the majority of fetuses who acquire acute infection *in utero*, the infection is self-limited and the infants are delivered asymptomatic and at term.[97] The greatest risk appears to be when infection is acquired before 20 weeks' gestation, and the majority of fetal losses occur between 9 and 28 weeks' gestation, mostly between 20 and 24 weeks.[92,98,99] The overall risk of B19-related fetal loss in pregnancies complicated by B19 infection is estimated around 1% to 9%.[92,96,100] Surviving infants tend to be healthy with normal development and neurologic outcome.[100,101] In one retrospective series of fetuses with confirmed B19 infection with anemia and/or hydrops, survival was 70% overall and 76% in those fetuses that received one or more transfusions.[102] B19-related teratogenicity has only rarely been reported.[101,103] The diagnosis of B19 infection during pregnancy can be confirmed by maternal B19 IgM and IgG antibodies or PCR assay (see later). These studies are usually corroborated with findings on prenatal ultrasonography, most often evidence of fetal anemia and hydrops.[104] PCR assays on fetal cord blood or amniotic fluid samples have also been utilized for diagnosis.[105] Management of severely afflicted fetuses with B19 infection includes fetal digitalization and *in utero* blood transfusions.

B19 may be associated with a variety of purpuric or petechial exanthems, including PPGSS (see later) and more generalized presentations. In one outbreak of petechial rashes, B19 was confirmed in 76% of 17 children, and the petechiae were widely distributed, often with accentuation in the axillary and inguinal regions as well as the distal extremities.[106] A similar purpuric or petechial presentation, with periflexural accentuation and arthralgias, has been observed in adults.[107] Some authors have suggested the terminology *parvovirus B19–associated purpuric-petechial eruption* for these polymorphous presentations that appear to correspond to the viremic phase of primary infection.[108] A B19-associated bathing-trunk exanthem has been described in children and adults, and presents with erythema and petechiae, with a predilection for the groin and, in some, the axillae.[109–111] A generalized exanthem with microvesicles has also been reported in a child.[112]

PAPULAR-PURPURIC GLOVES-AND-SOCKS SYNDROME

PPGSS is another viral exanthematous illness that in many (but not all) cases has been documented to be caused by B19. This rare disorder presents most often in young adults and less often in children and is usually diagnosed during the spring and summer months.[113,114] Patients with PPGSS present with the acute onset of rapidly progressive, symmetric swelling and erythema of the hands and feet, often with a petechial or purpuric component (Figs. 16.18 and 16.19). Bullous lesions are rarely present.[115] The eruption has a sharp demarcation at the wrists and ankles and is usually quite pruritic. A more diffuse, papular exanthem may occur elsewhere on the body. An associated enanthem consisting of hyperemia, petechiae, and erosions is often present and affects the soft and hard palate, pharynx, tongue, and inner lips.[113,116] The symptoms of PPGSS tend to be milder in children and adolescents compared with adults.[117]

Associated symptoms include fever, arthralgias, malaise, and respiratory or gastrointestinal complaints. Hematologic complications, including leukopenia and thrombocytopenia, are rarely observed.[113,116,118,119] Mononeuritis multiplex has been described in association with perineuritis noted on skin biopsy.[120] PPGSS resolves spontaneously over 1 to 2 weeks, and recurrences are rare. Importantly, the antibody response to B19 seen in PPGSS may differ from that observed in patients with EI, such that patients with the exanthem of PPGSS may still be viremic and therefore infectious.[113,116] The B19 VP2 structural protein has been demonstrated in the endothelial lining of dermal blood vessels in skin biopsies from patients with PPGSS.[121]

The diagnosis of B19 infections is often made clinically in patients presenting with classic EI. In immunocompetent children who are otherwise well, laboratory confirmation of B19 infection is usually unnecessary. Instances in which such confirmation may be indicated, however, include atypical presentations, immunocompromised hosts, individuals with hematologic diseases, and those who have been exposed to gravid females. Serologic studies, including enzyme immunoassays and radioimmunoassay, are useful in detecting anti-B19 IgM and IgG antibodies, and other useful tests include direct hybridization with deoxyribonucleic acid (DNA) probes, *in situ* hybridization, and PCR studies.[83,91,122] In immunocompetent children for whom diagnostic testing is preferred, detection of B19-specific IgM antibodies is the testing of choice; however, as serologic studies are not always reliable in those who are immunocompromised, PCR-based assays are recommended.[85] In a pregnant female who has been exposed to B19, serologic testing for IgM and IgG antibodies should be performed, and if acute infection is documented, serial fetal ultrasonography is usually indicated. As mentioned, maternal and fetal serum PCR techniques may be useful, especially when serologic study results are unclear,[123] and B19 antigen detection in amniotic fluid samples has also been described.[124]

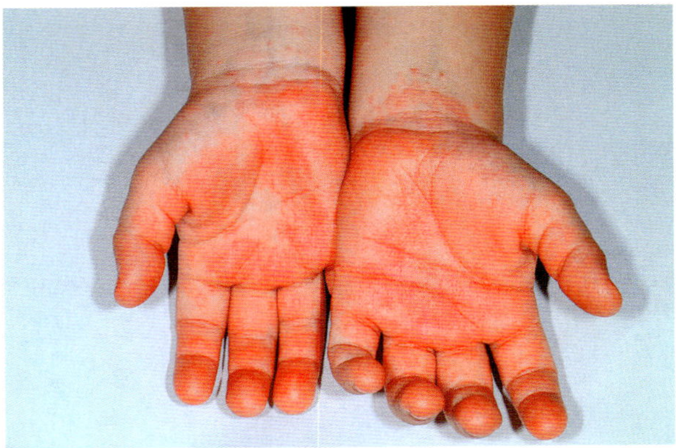

Fig. 16.18 Papular-purpuric gloves-and-socks syndrome. Petechial purpura of the palms in a patient with parvovirus B19 infection.

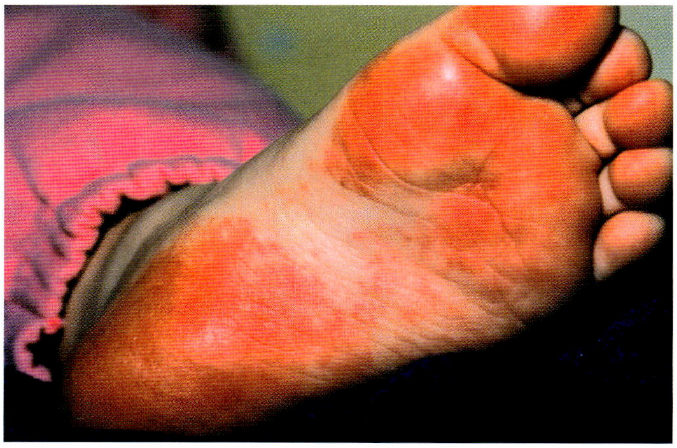

Fig. 16.19 Papular-purpuric gloves-and-socks syndrome. Erythema and petechiae of the plantar feet were accompanied by pruritus and sore throat in this young girl with parvovirus B19 infection.

Roseola Infantum

Roseola infantum (exanthem subitum, sixth disease) is a common childhood disease caused by human herpesvirus (HHV) type 6 or 7 (also called the *roseoloviruses*). HHV-6 and HHV-7 are ubiquitous members of the Herpesviridae family. These DNA viruses preferentially infect activated T cells, resulting in enhancement of natural killer cell activity and induction of numerous cytokines.[125] As with other herpesviruses, they become latent after primary infection and may reactivate during times of altered immunity.[126] Serologic studies have demonstrated that most children have been infected with HHV-6 before 3 years of age and with HHV-7 by 6 to 10 years of age.[125–127]

Transmission of HHV-6 and HHV-7 is believed to be primarily via saliva, and horizontal transmission between mother and child is well documented.[126] Persistent or intermittent excretion of HHV-6 in saliva and stool has been documented in parents of children who had documented primary infection, and in children who had exanthem subitum, one prospective study found maximum viral shedding at 3 to 7 months after the illness.[128,129] Although most newborns have transplacentally acquired antibodies, by 6 months nearly all have become seronegative and are therefore susceptible to infection.[125] HHV-6 has been divided into two variants, HHV-6A and HHV-6B. Most childhood infections are ascribed to the HHV-6B variant, and HHV-6A may be more commonly implicated in immunocompromised hosts.[130] The diagnosis of these infections can be made via virus isolation in peripheral blood mononuclear cell (PBMC) cultures, serologic studies, qualitative PCR, reverse transcriptase-PCR (RT-PCR), and real-time quantitative PCR. PCR-based diagnosis has been applied to a variety of body fluids and tissues, including plasma, whole blood, saliva, urine, cervical swabs, placenta, and PBMCs. RT-PCR can detect messenger RNA (mRNA), which is present only during active replication and hence may be useful in distinguishing between primary infection and past or latent infection.[131–133]

A broad range of conditions has been potentially linked to infection with HHV-6 and HHV-7 (Table 16.3).[125,127,130,134–138] By far, however, the best-recognized association for both agents is that of roseola infantum. Roseola is a mild exanthematous illness that most often occurs in children under 3 years of age. The classic presentation is that of high fever (38° to 41°C [101° to 106°F]) that lasts for

Table 16.3 Some Clinical Associations with HHV-6 and HHV-7 Infection

Condition	HHV-6, HHV-7, or Both	Comment
Roseola infantum	Both	HHV-6 more common
Fever	Both	Infants mainly
Febrile seizures	Both	In young infants; occasional status epilepticus
Otitis media	6	
Meningitis	6	
Encephalitis	Both	
Encephalopathy	6	Basal ganglia/white matter abnormalities on brain MRI; brainstem infarction rarely reported
Guillain-Barre syndrome	6	
Hepatitis	Both	
Lymphadenopathy	Both	
Lymphoproliferative disease	6	Proposed but unproven
Infections in patients who have had transplants	6	Viral reactivation seen in up to 50% after HSCT; may mimic acute GVHD or correlate with its onset; associated with more severe GVHD
Hemophagocytic syndrome (macrophage activation syndrome)	6	Especially in patients who have had transplants
Drug hypersensitivity syndrome	Both, but mainly 6	Proposed as complex interplay between drug reaction and HHV infection
HIV-1 cofactor	Both	Proposed but unproven
Pityriasis rosea	7	Controversial
Mononucleosis	Both	In adults
Myocarditis	6	
Rhabdomyolysis	6	
Multiple sclerosis	6	In adults; controversial

Data from Leach CT. Human herpesvirus-6 and -7 infections in children: agents of roseola and other syndromes. Curr Opin Pediatr 2000;12(3):269–74; Kimberlin DW. Human herpesviruses 6 and 7: identification of newly recognized viral pathogens and their association with human disease. Pediatr Infect Dis J 1998;17:59–68; Braun DK, Dominguez G, Pellett PE. Human herpesvirus 6. Clin Microbiol Rev 1997;10(3):521–67; Levy JA. Three new human herpesviruses (HHV6, 7 and 8). Lancet 1997;349:558–62; Tohyama M, Hashimoto K, Yasukawa M, et al. Association of human herpesvirus 6 reactivation with the flaring and severity of drug-induced hypersensitivity syndrome. Br J Dermatol 2007;157(5):934–40; Dharancy S, Crombe V, Copin MC, et al. Fatal hemophagocytic syndrome related to human herpesvirus-6 reinfection following liver transplantation: a case report. Transplant Proc 2008;40(10):3791–3; Mitani N, Aihara M, Yamakawa Y, et al. Drug-induced hypersensitivity syndrome due to cyanamide associated with multiple reactivation of human herpesviruses. J Med Virol 2005;75(3):430–4; Matsumoto H, Hatanaka D, Ogura Y, et al. Severe human herpesvirus 6-associated encephalopathy in three children: analysis of cytokine profiles and the carnitine palmitoyltransferase 2 gene. Pediatr Infect Dis J 2011;30(11):999–1001; Verhoeven DHJ, Claas ECJ, Jol-van der Zijde CM, et al. Reactivation of human herpesvirus-6 after pediatric stem cell transplantation. Pediatr Infect Dis J 2015;34(10):1118–27; Winestone LE, Punn R, Tamaresis JS, et al. High human herpesvirus 6 viral load in pediatric allogeneic hematopoietic stem cell transplant patients is associated with detection in end organs and high mortality. Pediatr Transplant 2018;22(2):doi:10.1111/petr.13084; Drago F, Ciccarese G, Parodi A. Atypical exanthems related to human herpesvirus-6 reactivations in transplant recipients. Transpl Infect Dis 2016;18:639–40; Tesini BL, Epstein LG, Caserta MT. Clinical impact of primary infection with roseoloviruses. Curr Opin Virol 2014;9:91–6; Wada A, Muramatsu K, Sunaga Y, et al. Brainstem infarction associated with HHV-6 infection in an infant. Brain Dev 2018; 40(3):242–6.

GVHD, Graft-versus-host disease; *HHV,* human herpesvirus; *HIV,* human immunodeficiency virus; *HSCT,* hematopoietic stem cell transplantation; *MRI,* magnetic resonance imaging.

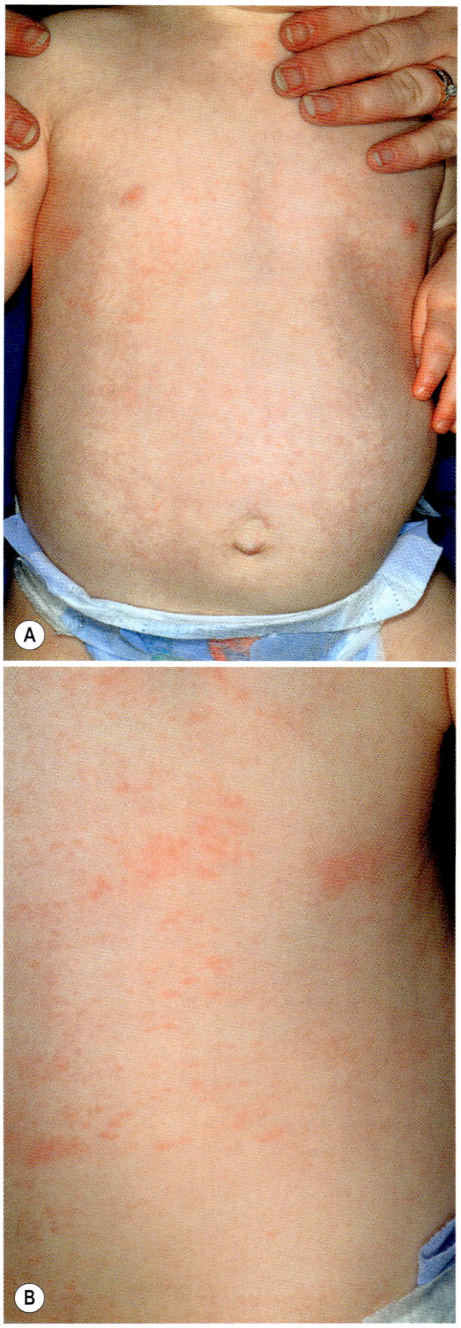

Fig. 16.20 Roseola infantum. **(A)** Erythematous, blanchable macules and papules in an infant who had a high fever for 3 days preceding the skin eruption. **(B)** On closer inspection, some lesions reveal a subtle peripheral halo of vasoconstriction.

3 to 5 days in an otherwise-well infant. With normalization of the temperature, the classic exanthem appears, initially on the trunk and eventually spreading to involve the extremities, neck, and face. The skin eruption is composed of fairly nondescript, erythematous, blanchable macules and papules (Fig. 16.20) that occasionally display a peripheral halo of vasoconstriction. The exanthem usually resolves over 1 to 3 days.

Associated signs and symptoms may include irritability, diarrhea, bulging fontanel, cough, cervical lymphadenopathy, and edematous eyelids.[139] Periorbital edema is quite common and when present in a febrile but otherwise well-appearing child may be a useful clue to the diagnosis during the preexanthematous stage. Nagayama spots are erythematous papules involving the mucosae of the soft palate and uvula and represent the enanthem that occurs in up to two-thirds of patients.[130,139] The differential diagnosis of the skin eruption in roseola infantum may include measles, scarlet fever, and rubella, although the temporal characteristics (rash after abrupt defervescence) are usually suggestive of roseola. Other entities on the differential diagnosis may include infection with enterovirus or adenovirus and a drug eruption.

Primary HHV-6 infection may also be asymptomatic or may present in a manner distinct from classic roseola infantum. Nonspecific fever in infants with or without otitis media may often be the result of HHV-6 infection.[140,141] First febrile seizures in young children may also commonly be associated with primary HHV-6 infection.[140,142] Other potential central nervous system complications include encephalopathy and encephalitis, which tend to occur during the preexanthematous stage and may be associated with long-term neurologic morbidity.[138,143] HHV-6–associated encephalitis has occurred in both immunocompetent and immunocompromised individuals. The prognosis is variable in these patients and ranges from complete recovery to severe neurologic sequelae or death.[144,145]

Solid organ and bone marrow transplant recipients are at increased risk of reactivation of the disease, which may be asymptomatic or present with rash, fever, encephalitis, pneumonitis, hepatitis, or bone marrow suppression.[146,147] HHV-6 reactivation is estimated to occur in approximately half of patients after allogeneic hematopoietic stem cell transplantation, correlates with the presence of acute graft-versus-host disease (GVHD), and is associated with greater severity of GVHD.[148,149] In some patients, the clinical presentation of HHV-6 reactivation may also mimic that of acute GVHD.[150] HHV-6 and HHV-7 reactivation has also been associated with drug reaction with eosinophilia and systemic symptoms (DRESS; see Chapter 20).[151–154]

Treatment for roseola infantum is unnecessary, and the illness usually spontaneously resolves without long-term sequelae. Although *in vitro* studies or clinical observations have suggested anti-HHV activity of ganciclovir, foscarnet, brincidofovir, cyclopropavir, cidofovir, and some others, these agents are rarely used clinically for patients with HHV-6 or HHV-7 infection, although intravenous ganciclovir and foscarnet have been proposed as first-line agents for treatment of HHV-6 encephalitis in transplant recipients.[155,156] Further research to identify effective treatment options is desirable, given the wide array of complications that may be associated with severe infection and, especially, infection in the immunocompromised host.

Other Viral Exanthems

NONSPECIFIC VIRAL EXANTHEMS

Although several exanthematous eruptions may present with characteristic features such as lesion morphology or distribution, the majority are somewhat nonspecific and may be difficult to distinctly categorize. These eruptions may be hard to distinguish from drug reactions or, in some younger patients, miliaria rubra (prickly heat). Unique defining characteristics such as an associated enanthem or symptom complex may be absent. Most nonspecific exanthems fall into the erythematous and/or papular categories, presenting with blanchable red macules and papules with a diffuse distribution (Fig. 16.21). Associated symptoms, which are generally nonspecific as well, may include fever, headache, myalgias, fatigue, and respiratory or gastrointestinal complaints.[157] Most nonspecific exanthems resolve without treatment over 1 week without long-term sequelae.

Common causes of nonspecific exanthems include nonpolio enteroviruses (see later) and respiratory viruses (e.g., adenovirus, rhinovirus, parainfluenza virus, respiratory syncytial virus, influenza virus). Other potential agents include EBV, HHV-6 and HHV-7, and parvovirus B19, although these agents more often result in distinct exanthematous illnesses, as discussed elsewhere in this chapter. In general, the majority of nonspecific exanthems occurring in the winter months are caused by the respiratory viruses, and those occurring during the summer months are most often caused by the enteroviruses.

Petechial exanthems, in particular, may pose a diagnostic dilemma to clinicians (given their potential association with life-threatening infections) and are associated with increased rates of hospitalization and diagnostic testing. Multiple viral organisms may be associated with a petechial exanthem, including parvovirus, respiratory syncytial virus, influenza and parainfluenza viruses, rhinovirus, EBV, cytomegalovirus (CMV), adenovirus, and enteroviruses. In a prospective study of children 0 to 18 years of age who had petechiae and signs or

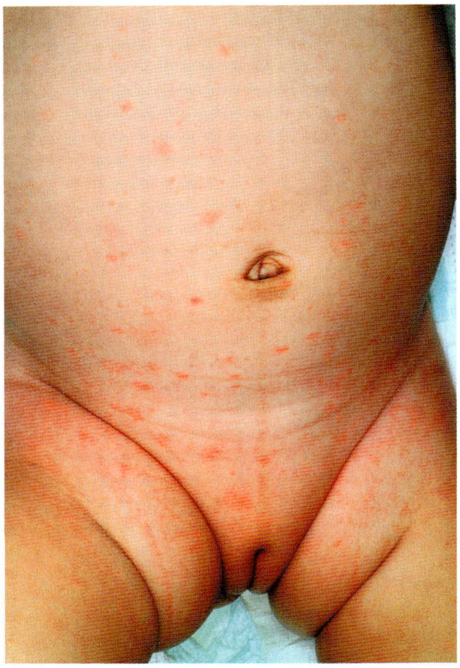

Fig. 16.21 Nonspecific viral exanthem. Nondescript erythematous macules and papules in an infant with a nonspecific symptom complex.

symptoms of infection, real-time PCR was utilized to identify a variety of viruses in nasopharyngeal aspirates. Of 58 patients with a petechial rash, 67% were positive for a viral pathogen, and 41% were notable for viral coinfections (two or more pathogens).[158] The most common pathogens in this study were CMV and EBV (18% each of the patients), followed by enteroviruses and rhinovirus (14% each of the patients). Influenza A H1N1 and human bocavirus were also noted fairly often (9% each of the patients). Distinguishing clinically between viral and bacterial processes may be challenging. The ability to rapidly diagnose viral infection via quantitative PCR, however, may help minimize unnecessary antibiotic therapy, invasive diagnostics, and hospitalizations.[158]

GIANOTTI–CROSTI SYNDROME

Gianotti–Crosti syndrome (GCS; papular acrodermatitis of childhood) was initially described in 1955 by Gianotti as an erythematous papular eruption symmetrically distributed on the face, buttocks, and extremities of children. A subsequent description by Crosti and Gianotti was made in 1956, and since then the disorder has been commonly known as *Gianotti–Crosti syndrome.* A viral etiology was suspected early on after the description of the disorder, and subsequently the notion of hepatitis B virus as a cause was hypothesized. It is currently well accepted that GCS is a distinct viral exanthem that may occur after infection with any of several viral agents, with hepatitis B being one possible (but uncommon) cause in certain parts of the world, especially Italy and Japan.[159]

GCS occurs predominantly in children between the ages of 1 and 6 years. Before the appearance of the exanthem, upper respiratory symptoms, fever, and lymphadenopathy may be present. The eruption is characterized by edematous, erythematous, monomorphous papules and occasionally papulovesicles distributed symmetrically over the face, buttocks (Fig. 16.22), and extensor surfaces of the upper (Fig. 16.23) and lower (Fig. 16.24) extremities. Occasionally the papules coalesce into larger, erythematous plaques (Fig. 16.25). Hemorrhagic changes or localized purpura (Fig. 16.26) may occasionally be present. The trunk is usually (but not always) spared in patients with GCS.[160] In most patients the skin eruption is asymptomatic, although mild pruritus may be present.

A viral etiology has long been suspected as the cause of GCS. In 1970 two independent groups confirmed the association with hepatitis B infection.[161,162] In these patients, the exanthem was

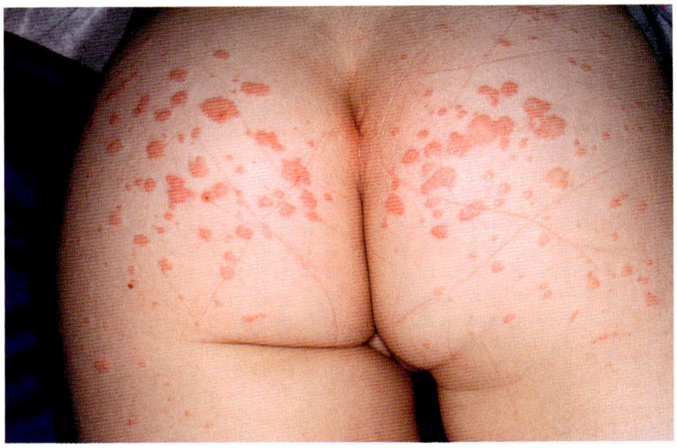

Fig. 16.22 Papular acrodermatitis of childhood. Erythematous, edematous papules symmetrically distributed on the bilateral buttocks.

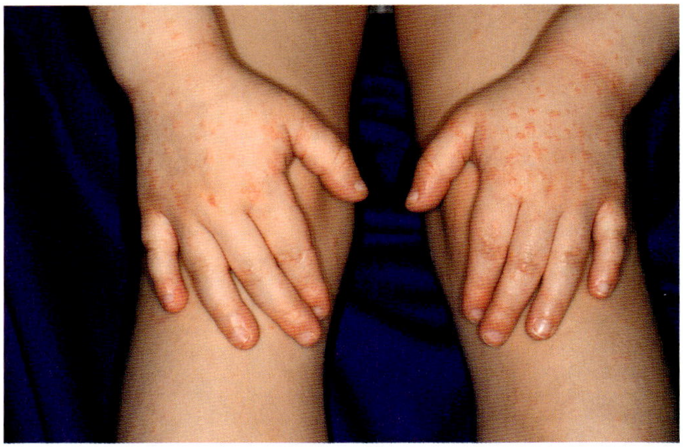

Fig. 16.23 Papular acrodermatitis of childhood. Monomorphous, erythematous papules of the dorsal hands in a young girl who had similar lesions on the face and the extensor surfaces of her arms and legs.

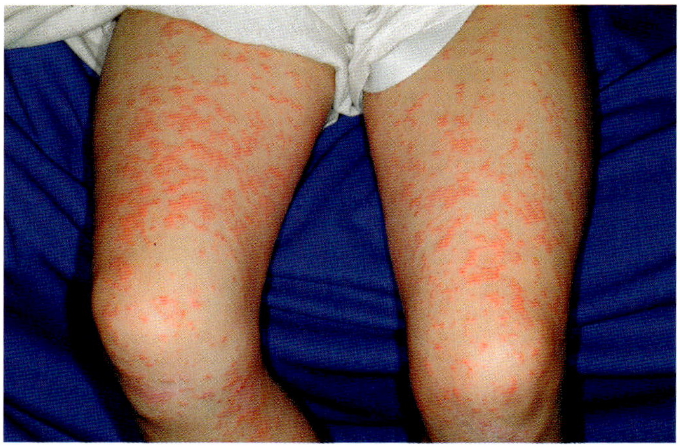

Fig. 16.24 Papular acrodermatitis of childhood. Erythematous, edematous papules of the thighs and knees in a patient with Gianotti–Crosti syndrome.

accompanied by acute anicteric hepatitis. In patients with hepatitis-associated GCS, hepatitis B surface antigen subtype ayw has been most classically implicated. Another term, *papulovesicular acrolocated syndrome (PVAS)*, was traditionally used to describe a similar presentation with a more vesicular component. It was once believed that this presentation was distinct based on the presence of pruritus and the lack of both hepatitis and a hepatitis B association. In a review of 308

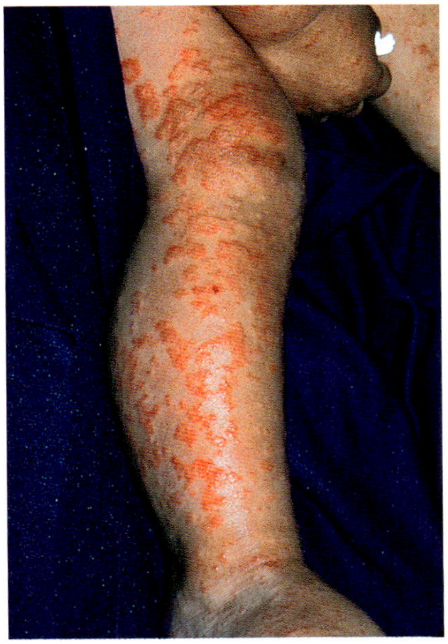

Fig. 16.25 Papular acrodermatitis of childhood. Erythematous papules coalesced into larger, edematous plaques in this patient.

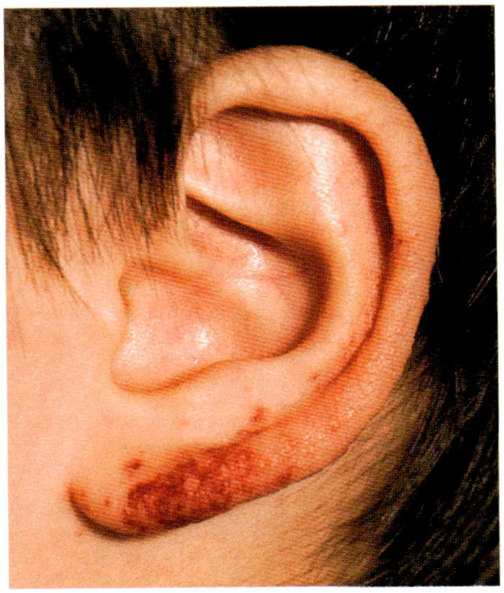

Fig. 16.26 Papular acrodermatitis of childhood. Localized purpura of the earlobe occurred in this patient with Gianotti–Crosti syndrome.

cases of GCS in Italy, however, distinction between GCS and PVAS was not clinically possible, nor was there a significant difference in the presentation or course as related to the etiologic agent (e.g., hepatitis B versus other viruses).[163]

Subsequently multiple viral agents have been implicated in causing GCS. These include EBV, which is believed to be the most common etiology in the United States, as well as CMV, Coxsackie viruses, respiratory viruses (adenovirus, respiratory syncytial virus, parainfluenza virus), parvovirus B19, rotavirus, and HHV-6.[159,163–171] A possible association with immunizations has also been suggested. Vaccination reports have included MMR, *Haemophilus*, oral polio, diphtheria-pertussis-tetanus, Japanese B encephalitis, varicella, and hepatitis B vaccines.[172–178] Recurrence of the eruption and accentuation of lesions at the site of vaccination have been observed.[179] There is also a report of GCS occurring in association with primary HSV-1 gingivostomatitis in a 3-year-old boy.[180] Children with atopic dermatitis and other atopic conditions (including allergic rhinitis/conjunctivitis, asthma, and urticaria) appear to have a greater risk ratio for developing GCS.[181] GCS-like reactions have been observed in some patients with molluscum contagiosum (see Chapter 15, Fig. 15.49)[182]; GCS seems

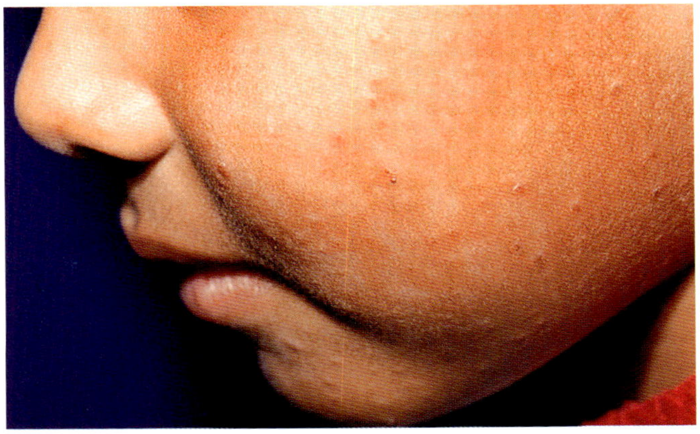

Fig. 16.27 Papular acrodermatitis of childhood, postinflammatory hypopigmentation. These postinflammatory changes are most common in patients with darker native complexions.

to be a distinct exanthem occurring in response to a variety of viral agents and possibly vaccinations, with hepatitis B being an extremely rare cause in the United States.

Treatment for GCS is supportive. Although the eruption is self-limited, it may take 8 to 12 weeks to resolve completely. Postinflammatory hypopigmentation (Fig. 16.27) may occasionally persist for several months after resolution of the exanthem. Routine laboratory studies for hepatitis are generally not warranted. However, a thorough history (including potential risk factors for hepatitis) and physical examination (with attention to the presence or absence of hepatosplenomegaly and lymphadenopathy) should be performed. Hepatitis serologies and liver function studies should be performed only in patients in whom there is a clinical suspicion.

UNILATERAL LATEROTHORACIC EXANTHEM

Unilateral laterothoracic exanthem (ULE; also known as *asymmetric periflexural exanthem of childhood* and *superimposed lateralized exanthem*) was initially described by Bodemer and de Prost in 1992 as a distinct exanthem presenting initially in a unilateral, localized fashion.[183] It was probably described years earlier when Brunner et al. described a "new papular exanthem of childhood" in 1962,[184] and in 1986 when Taieb et al. reported five children with a "localized erythema" similar to that described in ULE.[185]

ULE is most common in patients between 1 and 5 years of age, although it has been observed in older children and even adults. It usually occurs during the winter or spring, although it has been described year round.[184,186,187] In most patients, onset of the skin eruption is unilateral and on the trunk (Fig. 16.28), often with extension toward the axilla (Fig. 16.29) and, less often, around the inguinal region or on an extremity (Fig. 16.30). The lesions spread in a centrifugal fashion and often become bilateral, although they maintain a predominance on the initial side of involvement. The skin lesions in ULE may show various morphologies, including macules; papules; eczematous changes; and morbilliform, scarlatiniform, annular, or reticulate patterns. Some have described early lesions as consisting of a red papule surrounded by a pale halo.[186] Pruritus occurs in around 50% of patients. Vesicles and purpuric changes are rare. Desquamation is common during the healing stage, and postinflammatory pigment changes may also be present. Although skin biopsy is usually unnecessary, when performed, it has revealed a lymphocytic infiltrate with notable clustering around the dermal eccrine ducts.[186,188] The most common initial misdiagnosis is that of contact dermatitis. The clinical differential diagnosis of ULE may also include nonspecific exanthem, pityriasis rosea, scarlet fever, miliaria, EI, tinea, and GCS.

Associated features may include a prodrome consisting of low-grade fevers and respiratory or gastrointestinal symptoms. Fatigue and conjunctivitis may also be present. Enlarged axillary and/or inguinal lymph nodes are occasionally noted, and hepatosplenomegaly is generally absent. An associated enanthem has not been described with ULE.

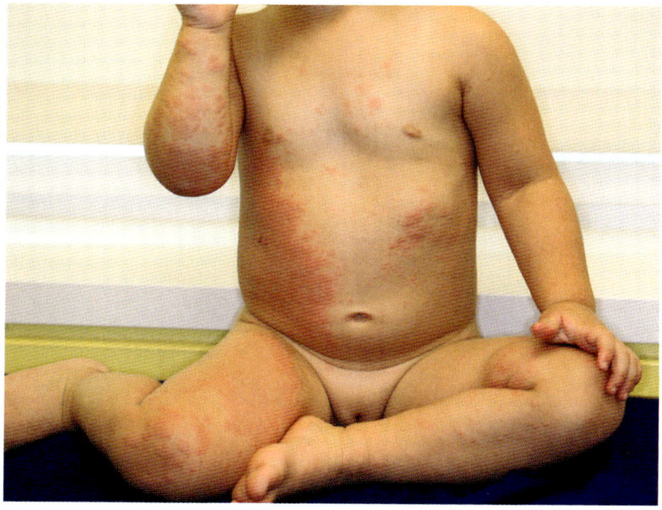

Fig. 16.28 Unilateral laterothoracic exanthem. Erythematous papules coalescing into plaques began on the right trunk in this 21-month-old female, with eventual spread to the right-sided extremities and, subsequently, lesser generalized involvement.

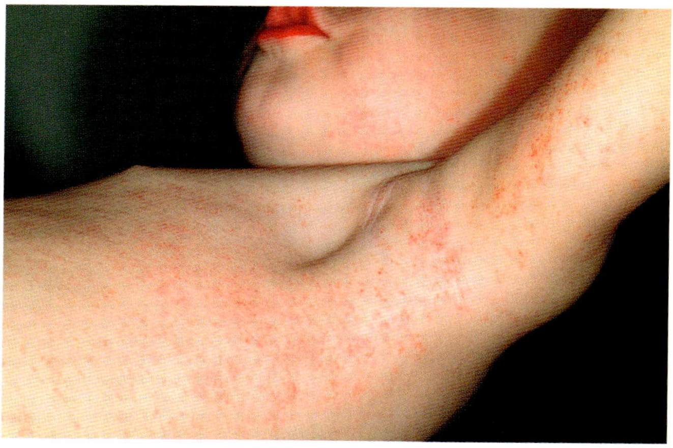

Fig. 16.29 Unilateral laterothoracic exanthem. Early involvement shows localization to the lateral trunk, axilla, and proximal inner arm in this patient.

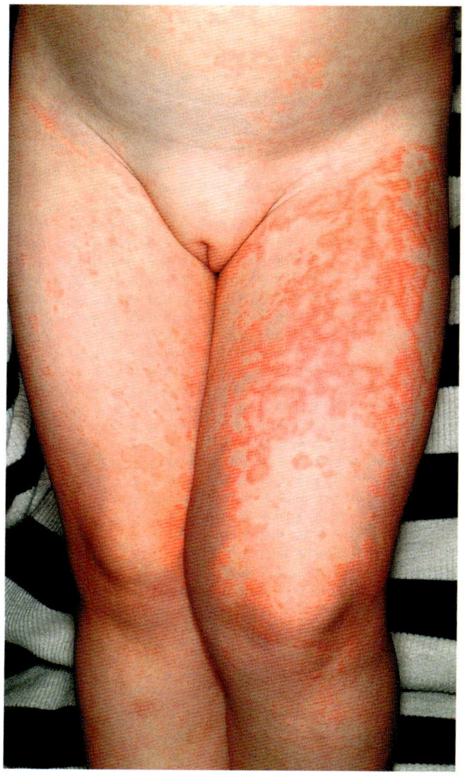

Fig. 16.30 Unilateral laterothoracic exanthem. The thigh was the initial site of involvement in this patient whose lesions demonstrate an erythema infectiosum–like morphology. (Courtesy Dr. Sarah Chamlin.)

The etiology of ULE remains unclear, although most favor a viral etiology. Early reports suggested *Spiroplasma* infection,[185] although this has not been confirmed in subsequent studies. In a prospective case-controlled study using throat, stool, blood, and skin samples, several microbiologic investigations were performed for viral and bacterial infection. No differences between cases and controls were noted, and no consistent etiologic agent was identified.[189] Although parainfluenza virus and adenovirus infection were diagnosed in six patients in one series, confirmation of a causal role is lacking.[187] ULE was observed in a 1-year-old girl who also had positive EBV PCR in peripheral blood, suggesting a possible association.[190] The appearance of ULE after the onset of molluscum contagiosum has also been reported, similar to GCS (see earlier).[191] ULE appears also to be a distinct presentation pattern in response to a variety of potential infectious agents.

The lesions of ULE resolve spontaneously, but similar to those of GCS, they may be delayed. Most often ULE resolves over 3 to 4 weeks, although in some patients it may take up to 8 weeks. Treatment is supportive.

ENTEROVIRAL EXANTHEMS

Enteroviruses (EV), a subgroup of the picornaviruses, may cause a variety of clinical syndromes with associated exanthems. Human EV are small, single-stranded RNA viruses that include echovirus (serotypes 1–7, 9, 11–21, 24–27, 29–33), Coxsackievirus A (serotypes A1–8, 9–13, 14, 16, 17, 19–22, 24), Coxsackievirus B (serotypes B1–6), EV (types 68–71, 73–88, 89–91, 93–99, 100–102, 104–107, 109, 111, 114, 116–118, and 119–121), and polioviruses (serotypes 1–3).[192] Human parechovirus (HPeV) was identified as a new group of picornaviruses in the 1990s and had been previously classified as echovirus 22 and 23.[193] These agents may cause gastroenteritis, respiratory infections, sepsis, meningitis, and encephalitis, particularly in neonates and young infants, and are not discussed further here.

The majority of EV infections seen in practice are benign and manifested by fever alone or distinct syndromes, including hand-foot-and-mouth disease (HFMD), herpangina, hemorrhagic conjunctivitis, and pleurodynia.[194] However, severe or life-threatening infections may also result from enteroviral infection, including meningitis, encephalitis, myocarditis, neonatal sepsis, and polio. Infections in neonates are often disseminated and may be difficult to differentiate from bacterial processes. Nonpolio enteroviruses are the leading cause of viral meningitis.[194,195] *Acute flaccid paralysis (AFP)*, characterized by the acute onset of limb weakness and classically associated with paralytic poliomyelitis, has emerged in recent years in association with nonpolio enterovirus infection, including EV68, EV71, and echovirus 11.[196,197] Spread of EV occurs person-to-person via the fecal–oral route and occasionally common source exposure (e.g., swimming pool water).[198] Enteroviral infections tend to predominate during the summer and fall, although sporadic cases may be seen throughout the year.

Nonspecific exanthems resulting from nonpolio EV are common and may present as macular and papular nonpruritic eruptions, with or without petechiae. When a petechial component is present, the clinical presentation may be confused with that of more serious infections such as meningococcemia. This diagnostic confusion may be exacerbated by the concomitant presence of aseptic meningitis, which may accompany enterovirus, Coxsackie virus, or echovirus infections.[47] Other exanthem patterns may include urticarial, scarlatiniform, zosteriform, and vesicular forms. Table 16.4 lists some exanthem/enanthem associations with the nonpolio enteroviruses.[199–209] Several are discussed in more detail in the following paragraphs.

Table 16.4 Some Reported Exanthem/Enanthem Associations with Enteroviruses

Exanthem	Comment
Hand-foot-and-mouth disease	Most common; Coxsackie virus A or B, enterovirus 71; atypical form with high numbers of vesicles on extremities, palms, soles, face, and buttocks may occur, especially in association with epidemics of Coxsackie virus A6 infection
Herpangina	Oral lesions and fever; Coxsackie virus A or B
Eczema coxsackium	Accentuation of erosions and vesicles in areas of skin previously or currently affected with AD
Hemorrhagic conjunctivitis	Eyelid edema, lacrimation, pain; Coxsackie virus A24 and enterovirus 70
Nonspecific exanthem	Any enterovirus
Gianotti–Crosti syndrome	Coxsackie virus A or B
Henoch–Schönlein purpura	Coxsackie virus B1
Still-like disease	Coxsackie virus B4
Zoster-like eruption	Echovirus 6
EI-like eruption	Echovirus 12
Congenital skin lesions	Coxsackie virus B3
Eruptive pseudoangiomatosis	Echovirus
AGEP	Coxsackie virus B4
Nail matrix arrest	Patients with preceding hand-foot-and-mouth disease

Data from Meade RH III, Chang T. Zoster-like eruption due to echovirus 6. Am J Dis Child 1979;133:283–4; Cherry JD, Bobinski JE, Horvath FL, et al. Acute hemangioma-like lesions associated with echo viral infections. Pediatrics 1969;44(4):498–502; Prose NS, Tope W, Miller SE, et al. Eruptive pseudoangiomatosis: a unique childhood exanthem? J Am Acad Dermatol 1993;29:857–9; Mancini AJ, Bodemer C. Viral infections. In: Schachner LA, Hansen RC, editors. Pediatric Dermatology. 3rd ed. London: Mosby; 2003:1059–92; Costa MM, Lisboa M, Romeu JC, et al. Henoch-Schönlein purpura associated with Coxsackie-virus B1 infection. Clin Rheumatol 1995;14(4):488--90; Sauerbrei A, Bluck B, Jung K, et al. Congenital skin lesions caused by intrauterine infection with Coxsackievirus B3. Infection 2000;28(5):326–8; Roberts-Thomson PJ, Southwood TR, Moore BW, et al. Adult onset Still's disease or Coxsackie polyarthritis? Aust NZJ Med 1986;16(4):509–11; Feio AB, Apetato M, Costa MM, et al. Acute generalized exanthematous pustulosis due to Coxsackie B4 virus. Acta Med Port 1997;10(6-7):487--91; Clementz GC, Mancini AJ. Nail matrix arrest following hand-foot-mouth disease: a report of five children. Pediatr Dermatol 2000;17(1):7–11; Bernier V, Labreze C, Bury F, et al. Nail matrix arrest in the course of hand, foot and mouth disease. Eur J Pediatr 2001;160(11):649–51; Balfour HH, May DB, Rottee TC, et al. A study of erythema infectiosum: recovery of rubella virus and echovirus 12. Pediatrics 1972;50(2):285–90.
AD, Atopic dermatitis; *AGEP,* acute generalized exanthematous pustulosis; *EI,* erythema infectiosum.

HFMD is the best-recognized enteroviral exanthem. It is a disorder of young children, most commonly affecting those between 1 and 4 years of age. HFMD has been linked to several nonpolio EV, including Coxsackie viruses A5, A6, A7, A9, A10, A16 (most common), B1, B2, B3, and B5; echovirus 4[210]; and enterovirus 71.[157] Patients have fever, malaise, and the characteristic exanthem, which consists of gray-white, vesicular lesions on the palms (Fig. 16.31) and soles (Fig. 16.32) and less often involving the dorsal or lateral surfaces of the hands and feet. A less specific macular and papular erythematous eruption may be present on the buttocks, thighs, and external genitalia. Occasionally a more diffuse vesicular eruption with lesions in areas other than the palms and soles may be present (Fig. 16.33). The enanthem of HFMD consists of vesicles and erosions of the buccal surfaces, palate, tongue (Fig. 16.34), uvula, gingivae, and anterior tonsillar pillars. These lesions are painful and lead to anorexia and occasionally dehydration. Cervical and submandibular lymphadenopathy may occasionally be present in patients with HFMD.

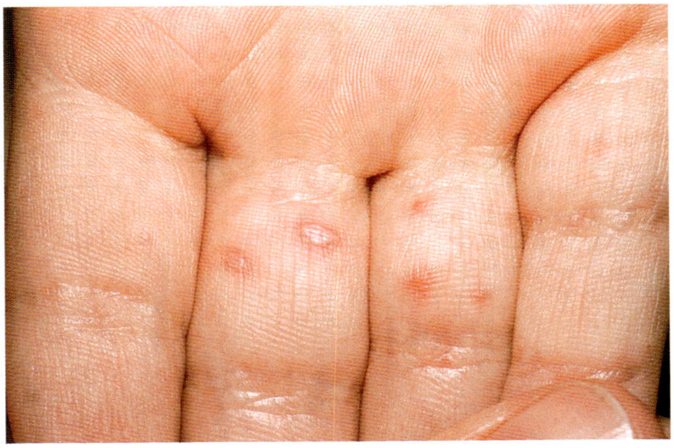

Fig. 16.31 Hand-foot-and-mouth disease. Deep-seated vesicles with erythema involving the palmar surface of the fingers.

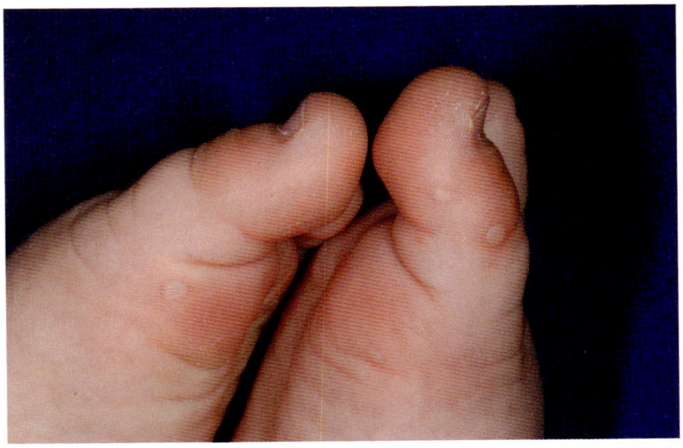

Fig. 16.32 Hand-foot-and-mouth disease. Erythematous deep-seated and superficial vesicles involved the plantar surface in this infant with erosions of the palate and uvula.

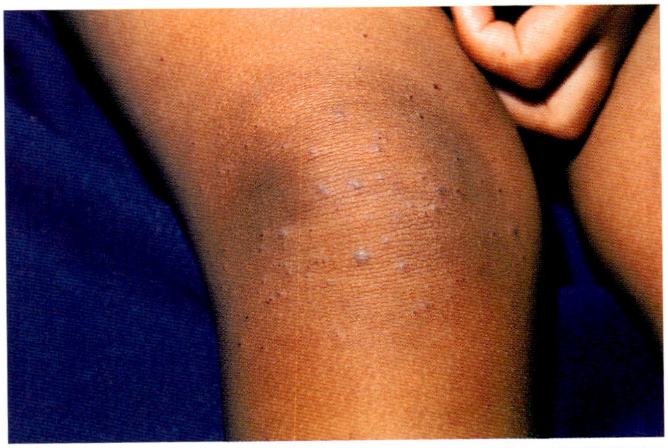

Fig. 16.33 Hand-foot-and-mouth disease. Red to purple vesicles involved the knees and elbows in this patient with classic lesions involving the mouth, palms, and soles.

Although the course of HFMD is most often benign and treatment is supportive, epidemics of enterovirus 71 infection in Asia highlight the potential seriousness of the disease. In these epidemics, severe disease was seen most often in children under 5 years of age, with the majority of deaths occurring secondary to pulmonary edema or

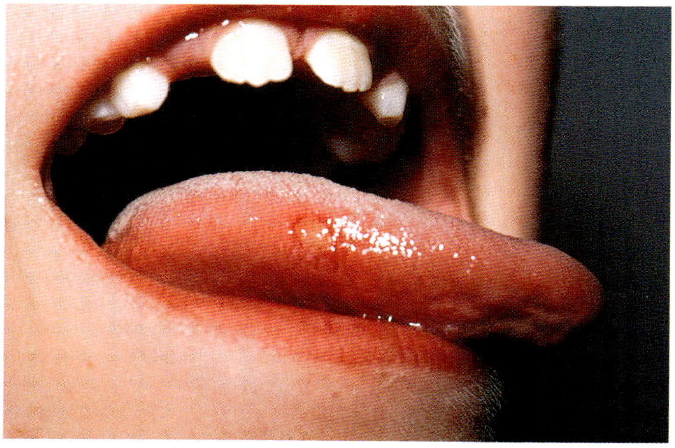

Fig. 16.34 Hand-foot-and-mouth disease. A painful erosion of the lateral aspect of the tongue.

pulmonary hemorrhage.[211] Other complications included encephalitis, aseptic meningitis, acute flaccid paralysis, myocarditis, and cardiorespiratory collapse.[211–213] The neurotropism of EV is demonstrated by the common finding of brain (especially brainstem) involvement on autopsy specimens from children who died of severe HFMD.[214]

Atypical forms of HFMD may occur, highlighted over recent years in the setting of epidemics of Coxsackie virus A6 infection, primarily in children but with some reported outbreaks in adults.[215–220] In these patients, extensive numbers of vesicles and erosions may occur on the extremities (Fig. 16.35), perioral face, groin, and buttocks, in addition to the more classic locations. Perioral involvement appears to be a distinguishing feature of atypical HFMD caused by Coxsackie virus A6 compared with extensive exanthems caused by other EVs, such as Coxsackie virus A16.[221] In patients with atopic dermatitis, accentuation of the blistering process may be noted in areas previously or concurrently affected with eczematous lesions. This observation has been termed *eczema coxsackium*,[215] and these patients may be mistakenly diagnosed as having eczema herpeticum (see Chapter 3). A similar accentuation of the viral exanthem may be seen in other areas of skin inflammation or injury, including sunburn, irritant dermatitis, tinea infection, or lacerations.

Post-HFMD nail matrix arrest with onychomadesis (nail shedding), initially reported in five children in 2000,[207] is now a well-recognized postinfectious association. It may present as Beau lines (transverse depressions in the nail plate) or complete separation of the nail plate from the nail matrix (Fig. 16.36). Although this observation has been seen after infection with a variety of EV, Coxsackie viruses A6, A10, B1, and B2 have been the most commonly confirmed.[222–226] The changes tend to occur around 30 to 40 days after the onset of HFMD and are followed by spontaneous regrowth of normal nail plates; cases often present with temporal clustering, reflecting local epidemics of enteroviral infection.[227]

Herpangina is a characteristic enanthem that may be caused by a variety of nonpolio EV, especially Coxsackie viruses A and B. It presents with fever, sore throat, and malaise, usually in children between 3 and 10 years of age. Inspection of the oral mucosa reveals gray-white vesicles and erythematous erosions involving the palate, uvula, and tonsillar pillars. Although it may occasionally be confused with acute herpetic gingivostomatitis, labial and skin involvement is much more common with HSV infection. Treatment for HFMD or herpangina consists of pain control and ensurance of adequate fluid intake to prevent dehydration. The lesions spontaneously resolve over 1 week. Handwashing by preschool-aged children and their caregivers was demonstrated to have a significant protective effect against community-acquired HFMD and herpangina during an enterovirus 71 outbreak in China.[228]

Echovirus exanthems have been variably described with a number of presentations and morphologies. Some of these include macular, vesicular, urticarial, and petechial eruptions; erythema multiforme; HFMD; and roseola-like exanthems.[47] Echovirus 6 has been associated with a dermatomal, vesicular eruption mimicking herpes zoster.[199] Echovirus type 9 infection may result in an illness with aseptic meningitis and a petechial eruption that may mimic meningococcemia.[229]

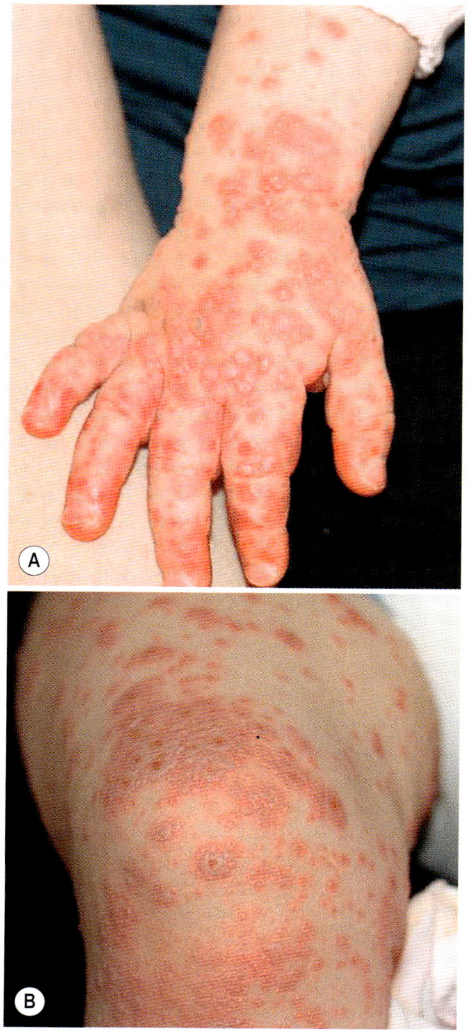

Fig. 16.35 Atypical enterovirus exanthem. This 3-year-old girl had fever and the acute onset of a vesicular eruption on her upper **(A)** and lower **(B)** extremities and her face with a perioral accentuation. Her skin manifestations coincided with a local Coxsackie virus A6 epidemic.

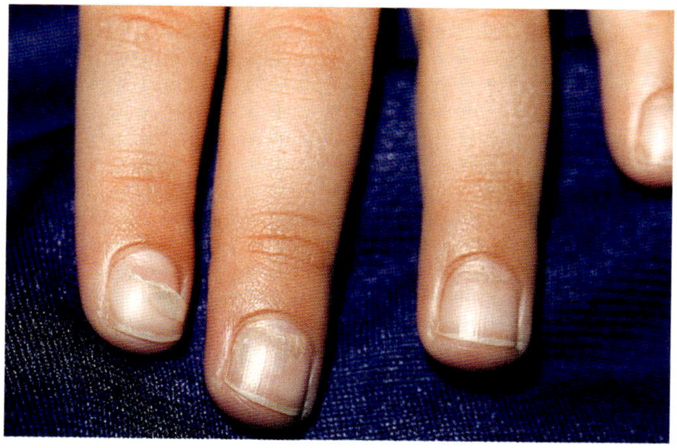

Fig. 16.36 Nail matrix arrest after hand-foot-and-mouth disease. Transverse ridging and eventual nail shedding occurred in this 5-year-old boy 2 months after having the enteroviral infection. The nails spontaneously grew back normally within several months.

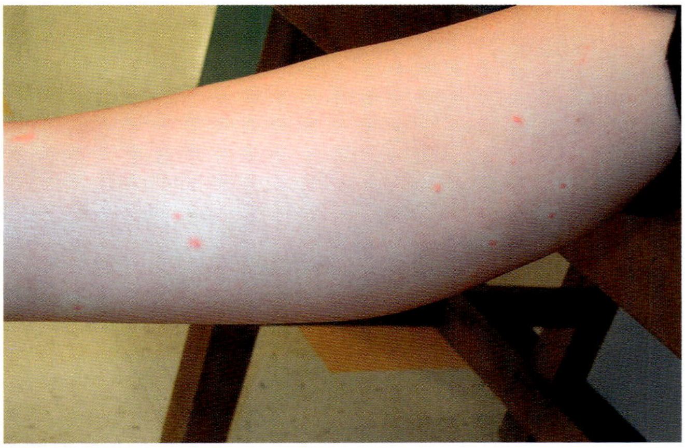

Fig. 16.37 Eruptive pseudoangiomatosis. This teenaged girl sought treatment in the summer with the acute onset of small, hemangioma-like papules. Note the surrounding halo of vasoconstriction surrounding each lesion. (Courtesy Dr. Andrew Sagan.)

Echovirus 16 was classically associated with a roseola-like exanthem referred to as *Boston exanthem*, which was one of the initial exanthems to be described and virologically confirmed. Approximately one-third of individuals with echovirus infection may develop a rubelliform eruption consisting of discrete pink-red macules that spread from the face and neck to the upper trunk and extremities. Some patients also have yellow or gray-white lesions on the oral mucous membranes that may resemble Koplik spots. Other symptoms that may be associated with echovirus infection include fever, gastrointestinal complaints, upper respiratory symptoms, and conjunctivitis.

Eruptive pseudoangiomatosis is an exanthem consisting of the acute onset of hemangioma-like lesions and possibly related to echovirus infection.[230] Cherry et al., in 1969, originally described four children with acute echovirus infection (two with echovirus 25 and two with echovirus 32) who developed such lesions with resolution occurring over 2 to 6 days.[200] Other affected children were subsequently described, all of whom presented with the acute onset and spontaneous resolution of angioma-like papules during the course of a viral illness.[201,231] The disorder has also been observed in adults.[232,233] The angiomatous papules in eruptive pseudoangiomatosis are often surrounded by a rim of blanching (Fig. 16.37), and histopathologic evaluation, when performed, has revealed dilated dermal blood vessels and plump endothelial cells without any increase in the number of blood vessels.[201,234] Associated symptoms have included fever, malaise, headache, diarrhea, and respiratory complaints. Although EV have not been confirmed as the etiology by other investigators, a viral cause continues to seem most likely. Familial outbreaks have been reported.[235] A similar presentation to eruptive pseudoangiomatosis, but with the angiomatous lesions arranged in annular configurations, has been described in association with adenovirus infection.[236] Recurrence of eruptive pseudoangiomatosis has occasionally been observed.[237]

INFECTIOUS MONONUCLEOSIS

IM is a common infection occurring during adolescence and is usually associated with EBV infection. Although most cases of IM are related to EBV infection, not all primary EBV infections manifest as IM.[238] The spectrum of disorders linked to EBV infection is shown in Box 16.3. Other etiologic agents of IM-like illness include CMV, hepatitis A, adenovirus, GABHS, *A. haemolyticum*, HHV-6, rubella virus, HIV, and *Toxoplasma gondii*.[239,240] Malignancy and drug reactions may also result in IM-like illnesses.[238]

Confirmation of EBV as the major cause of IM occurred in the late 1960s.[238,240] EBV is a member of the Herpesviridae family and as such is a large, DNA-containing virus with the ability to become latent after primary infection and with the potential for subsequent reactivation. The virus has tropism for both lymphocytes (especially B cells) and epithelial cells, with infection beginning in the oropharyngeal epithelial cells, which may shed the virus for up to 18 months after primary acquisition.[240,241] The primary transmission route is via saliva. Natural EBV infection occurs only in humans and results in lifelong infection.[242] It is estimated that more than 95% of adults are infected with EBV worldwide.

Primary EBV infection in infancy is mostly asymptomatic or presents with very mild, nonspecific symptoms such as upper respiratory tract symptoms, pharyngitis, lymphadenopathy, and fever. Epidemiologic studies suggest that most children have acquired EBV by 5 years of age in underdeveloped countries or lower socioeconomic classes, whereas primary infection occurs later in life (e.g., between 10 and 30 years) in developed countries and higher socioeconomic classes.[238,243] Older children and adolescents are more likely to develop clinical symptoms of IM after an incubation period of 4 to 7 weeks.

IM is generally a benign, self-limited illness characterized by fever, exudative tonsillopharyngitis, and lymphadenopathy. Malaise, fatigue, and headache are also common. The temperature may reach 40° C (104° F) and is often prolonged, lasting for 1 to 2 weeks. Physical examination may reveal splenomegaly, hepatomegaly, periorbital edema, palatal petechiae, jaundice, and a skin eruption. The lymphadenopathy is typically nontender and involves both the anterior and posterior cervical chains. Diffuse adenopathy is occasionally present. Historically, IM was divided into three syndromes: anginose, characterized by the classic triad of fever, pharyngitis, and lymphadenopathy; typhoidal, characterized by prolonged high fever; and glandular, characterized by mild pharyngitis, low-grade fever, and marked lymphadenopathy.

The skin eruption of IM is nonspecific; occurs in around 5% of patients; and may present as a macular, petechial, scarlatiniform, urticarial, or erythema multiforme–like rash.[240,243] After the administration of ampicillin or amoxicillin, however, 90% to 95% of patients develop an erythematous macular and papular eruption (Fig. 16.38) that may be related to ampicillin-antibody immune complexes resulting from B-cell activation.[244] This reaction occurs about 5 to 9 days after starting the antibiotic and does not appear to represent a true drug allergy.

Box 16.3 **Some Disease Associations with Epstein–Barr Virus (EBV)**

- Asymptomatic infection
- Infectious mononucleosis
- Diffuse exanthem, especially in patients receiving penicillin-class antibiotics
- Hematologic disorders:
  - Thrombocytopenia
  - Agranulocytosis
  - Hemolytic anemia
- X-linked lymphoproliferative syndrome
- EBV-associated hemophagocytic lymphohistiocytosis
- Lymphoproliferative disorders in immunocompromised patients
- Central nervous system infections:
  - Aseptic meningitis
  - Encephalitis
  - Myelitis
  - Optic neuritis
  - Cranial nerve palsies
  - Guillain–Barré syndrome
  - Seizures
- Gianotti–Crosti syndrome
- Chronic EBV infection
- Acute genital ulceration
- Hydroa vacciniforme
- Oral hairy leukoplakia
- Pneumonia
- Orchitis
- Myocarditis/ECG abnormalities
- Rhabdomyolysis
- Chronic liver disease
- Neoplastic disorders:
  - Burkitt lymphoma
  - Nasopharyngeal carcinoma
  - B- or T-cell lymphoma (including AIDS-associated B-cell lymphomas)
  - Extranodal NK/T-cell lymphoma, nasal type
  - Hodgkin disease
  - Hepatocellular carcinoma

AIDS, Acquired immunodeficiency syndrome; *ECG*, electrocardiography; *NK*, natural killer.

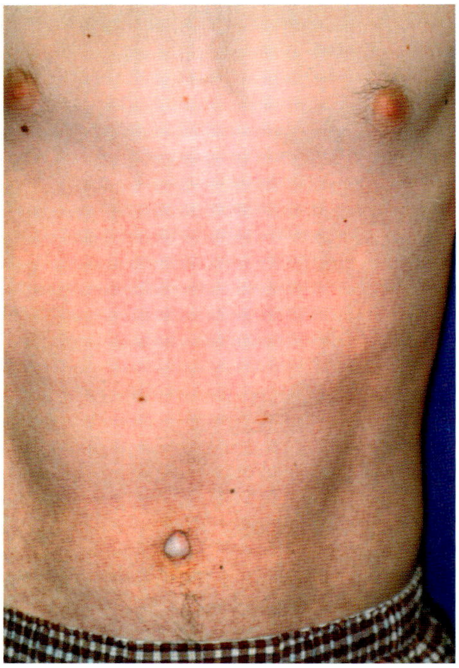

Fig. 16.38 Infectious mononucleosis. A diffuse, erythematous macular and papular eruption occurred in this adolescent male after receiving amoxicillin therapy.

Table 16.5 Epstein–Barr Virus–Specific Serology Interpretation

	VIRAL CAPSID ANTIGEN (VCA)			
Status	**IgG**	**IgM**	**Early Antigen**	**EBNA**
No past infection	−	−	−	−
Acute IM	+	+	±	−
Convalescent IM	+	±	±	±
Past infection	+	−	Low + or −	+
Reactivated/ chronic	++	±	++	±

Adapted from Peter J, Ray CG. Infectious mononucleosis. Pediatr Rev 1998; 19(8):276–9; Godshall SE, Kirchner JT. Infectious mononucleosis: complexities of a common syndrome. Postgrad Med 2000;107(7):175–86; Jenson HB. Acute complications of Epstein-Barr virus infectious mononucleosis. Curr Opin Pediatr 2000;12:263–8; American Academy of Pediatrics. Epstein-Barr virus infections (infectious mononucleosis). In: Kimberlin DW, Brady MT, Jackson MA, Long SS, editors. Red Book: 2018 Report of the Committee on Infectious Diseases. Elk Grove Village, IL: American Academy of Pediatrics; 2018:334–38.

EBNA, Epstein–Barr virus nuclear antigen; *Ig*, immunoglobulin; *IM*, infectious mononucleosis.

Useful laboratory evaluations in patients with IM include hematologic and hepatic panels and serologic analysis. Complete blood cell counts often reveal an absolute lymphocytosis, often with more than 10% atypical lymphocytes (representing activated T cells). Other aberrations may include anemia, thrombocytopenia, and neutropenia, the latter developing 1 to 2 weeks into the illness. Autoimmune hemolytic anemia is uncommon, occurring in around 3% of cases.[244] Mild hepatitis may be manifested by elevations in the hepatic transaminases, alkaline phosphatase, and L-lactate dehydrogenase (LDH). Coagulopathy is usually absent. The most useful confirmatory examination is the serologic assay for heterophile antibodies. These IgM antibodies can be readily measured with a variety of rapid test kits (e.g., Monospot) and have high specificity. Although up to 15% of patients with IM may initially be negative for heterophile antibodies, many become positive on repeat testing performed during the second or third week of the illness.

Virus-specific serologies can help confirm a definitive diagnosis of EBV infection and should be used to diagnose IM in children under 4 years of age (who are often heterophile-antibody negative), patients with atypical presentations, or those with severe or prolonged illness.[240] EBV serology interpretations are shown in Table 16.5. Detection methods for EBV-related proteins or DNA are also available. Real-time PCR and measurements of EBV viral load seem particularly useful in diagnosing acute IM when the serologic studies are inconclusive.[245]

Complications of IM include splenic rupture, upper airway obstruction, hematologic issues (hemolytic anemia, thrombocytopenia, aplastic anemia, thrombotic thrombocytopenic purpura, hemolytic-uremic syndrome, and disseminated intravascular coagulation), chronic fatigue, and neurologic findings. Subcapsular splenic hemorrhage with rupture is fortunately quite rare (<0.5% of cases in adults). It presents as an abrupt onset of left upper quadrant abdominal pain and may be treated by splenectomy or nonoperative management. Upper airway obstruction may result from tonsillar hypertrophy and is treated as an inpatient with close observation, maintenance of the airway, hydration, and, occasionally, systemic corticosteroids.[244] Neurologic complications include cranial nerve palsies, Guillain–Barré syndrome, meningoencephalitis, aseptic meningitis, optic neuritis, and seizures. Other less common complications include pneumonia (which is often related to coinfection with a bacterial or another viral agent), electrocardiographic abnormalities, rhabdomyolysis, and chronic liver disease.[240,244] EBV is the most common infectious trigger of hemophagocytic lymphohistiocytosis (see Chapter 10).

Chronic fatigue syndrome (CFS) may follow IM in both adolescents and adults, with 13% of adolescents (mainly females) meeting criteria 6 months after IM in one study.[246] CFS is defined as at least 6 months of severe fatigue and disabling musculoskeletal and cognitive symptoms without any other explanation. In the aforementioned cohort, the figures for CFS in this group decreased to 7% at 12 months and 4% at 24 months after IM. It appears that female gender and greater fatigue severity are predictors for the development of CFS in adolescents with IM.[247] Some experts believe that CFS is not related to EBV infection, but that fatigue lasting weeks to months may occur in up to 10% of patients with classic IM.[248]

The management of IM is primarily supportive. Adequate rest, fluids, and analgesics (acetaminophen, nonsteroidal antiinflammatory agents) are commonly recommended. Patients with splenomegaly are counseled to avoid strenuous exercise and contact sports to prevent the complication of splenic rupture for 21 days after the onset of symptoms. After this time, limited noncontact aerobic exercise is permitted if the patient is asymptomatic, and contact sports can generally be resumed 4 to 6 weeks after the onset of symptoms if asymptomatic and no obvious splenomegaly.[248] Most splenic ruptures occur within 3 weeks of the diagnosis, but it has been reported as late as 7 weeks after the diagnosis.[249] Amoxicillin and ampicillin should be avoided in patients with suspected IM. Corticosteroids are generally recommended only for patients with complications such as marked tonsillar hypertrophy with the potential for airway obstruction, massive splenomegaly, myocarditis, hemolytic anemia, or hemophagocytic lymphohistiocytosis.[248] Acyclovir, which may show *in vitro* activity against EBV, is of no proven value in the treatment of EBV-associated IM or lymphoproliferative syndromes, although antiviral agents may benefit immunocompetent patients when used in conjunction with corticosteroids.[238,245,248]

Acute genital ulceration (AGU; ulcus vulvae acutum; Lipschütz ulcer) is another potential presentation of primary EBV infection, presenting most commonly in teenaged girls. The initial report of this observation is credited to Lipschütz, who in 1913 proposed a classification of AGU into three categories, the third type being the sudden onset of genital ulcers in nonsexually active girls and young women.[250] This presentation may be associated with several possible infectious agents, but one of the most common appears to be EBV. Other reported agents may include CMV, *Mycoplasma pneumonia*, *T. gondii*, adenovirus, and influenza A and B viruses. This is an important entity to recognize, given the potential misdiagnosis of sexual abuse.[251] The

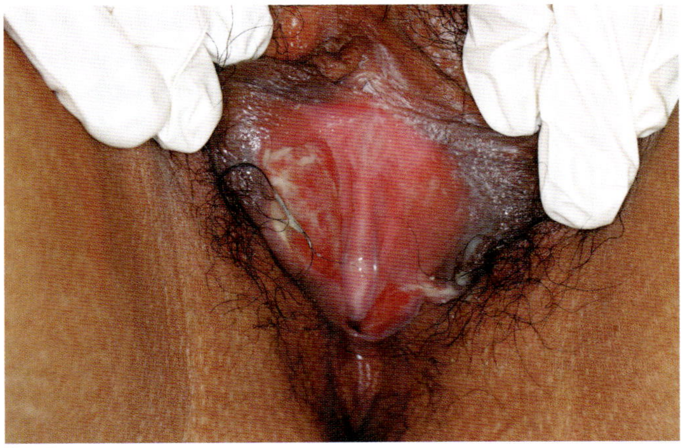

Fig. 16.39 Acute genital ulceration (Lipschütz ulcer). This 13-year-old nonsexually active girl presented with the acute onset of fever, chills, and dysuria. Clinical examination revealed well-demarcated ulcers with a fibrinous base, involving the bilateral labiae minorae. She healed completely over 4 weeks without scarring.

differential diagnosis may include sexually transmitted infections, genital aphthosis, Behçet syndrome, pyoderma gangrenosum, and extraintestinal Crohn's disease.

AGU associated with EBV infection presents with painful genital ulcers (Fig. 16.39), often bilateral (and occasionally in a "kissing pattern") and involving the labia minorae or majorae (or both). Edema is often present and may at times be severe. Tissue necrosis may occur, rarely necessitating surgical debridement. Other clinical features may include pharyngitis, lymphadenopathy, fever, and fatigue, but these classic symptoms of IM may not develop until later in the course (and in some patients may not develop at all).[252] The primary differential diagnosis is infection with HSV, and viral culture or PCR studies are often necessary, as are serologic studies for EBV. Seroconversion for EBV may be observed weeks after the initial presentation, with initially negative testing. EBV PCR testing on blood or genital tissue (when biopsy is performed) may be positive, although *in situ* hybridization and EBV RNA and protein staining in tissue samples suggests that AGU is most likely related to inflammatory events rather than direct viral cytopathic effects.[250,253] AGU caused by EBV infection is usually treated supportively, and the lesions tend to heal over 3 to 6 weeks. Topical and systemic corticosteroids have been recommended by some authors, and other reported options include doxycycline and colchicine.[250,254–256] This infectious cause of AGU is likely underrecognized and should be strongly considered in young females who have acute painful ulcers and who deny genital or oral sexual activity.[256]

Exanthems Associated with *Mycoplasma pneumoniae* Infection

Mycoplasmas are a distinct class of bacteria that lack rigid cell walls and are thus insensitive to antibiotics that inhibit cell wall synthesis such as penicillins. The best-recognized agent in this class is *M. pneumoniae*, a prominent etiology of atypical pneumonia in school-aged children, adolescents, and adults. This infection generally presents with the insidious onset of fever, malaise, headache, and cough, and may be associated with skin findings in up to one-third of patients. A variety of cutaneous eruptions have been potentially linked to *M. pneumoniae* infection. Some of these include nonspecific erythematous macular and papular eruptions,[257–259] erythema nodosum, urticaria, erythema multiforme minor,[260] GCS,[261] leukocytoclastic vasculitis,[262] bullous PPGSS,[263] Stevens–Johnson syndrome,[264,265] Henoch–Schonlein purpura,[266] and subcorneal pustular dermatosis.[267,268] Stevens–Johnson syndrome is the most significant cutaneous association with *M. pneumoniae* infection and is discussed in detail in Chapter 20. *Mycoplasma*-induced rash and mucositis (MIRM; see Chapter 20) is a newer term used to describe *M. pneumoniae*–associated mucocutaneous disease, which presents in younger patients (average age around 12 years) with prominent mucositis, typically sparse vesiculobullous or targetoid skin lesions, a milder course, infrequent sequelae, and very rare mortality.[269]

Table 16.6 Some Rickettsial Organisms and Their Disease Associations

Organism	Disease Association(s)	Vector
BARTONELLA		
Bartonella henselae	Bacillary angiomatosis, CSD, endocarditis, bacillary peliosis	?Cat flea
Bartonella quintana	Trench fever, bacillary angiomatosis, endocarditis, bacillary peliosis	Human body louse
COXIELLA		
Coxiella burnetii	Q fever, endocarditis	Tick
EHRLICHIA		
Ehrlichia chaffeensis	Human monocytic ehrlichiosis	Lone Star tick
Anaplasma phagocytophilum	Human granulocytic ehrlichiosis (anaplasmosis)	Deer (black-legged) tick, dog tick
RICKETTSIA		
Rickettsia akari	Rickettsialpox	House-mouse mite
Rickettsia conorii	Mediterranean spotted fever	Dog tick
Rickettsia prowazekii	Epidemic typhus	Human body louse
Rickettsia rickettsii	RMSF	Wood tick, dog tick, brown dog tick, Cayenne tick
Rickettsia parkeri	Spotted fever similar to RMSF	Gulf Coast tick
Rickettsia typhi	Endemic (murine) typhus	Rat flea
Rickettsia tsutsugamushi	Scrub typhus	Trombiculid mite

CSD, Cat-scratch disease; *RMSF*, Rocky Mountain spotted fever.

Rickettsial Diseases

Although the use of molecular technology has resulted in some reclassifications of agents included in the order Rickettsiales, these organisms are all included in this section. These genus groups include *Bartonella*, *Coxiella*, *Ehrlichia*, *Anaplasma*, and *Rickettsia*. Table 16.6 is a summary of several rickettsial organisms and their disease associations. Bacillary angiomatosis caused by *Bartonella henselae* and *Bartonella quintana* is discussed in Chapter 12. Cat-scratch disease, caused by *B. henselae*, is discussed in Chapter 14. Some other rickettsial disorders are discussed here.

Rickettsial infections are arthropod-borne diseases caused by microorganisms that occupy an intermediate position between bacteria and viruses. Spread by blood-sucking insects such as the body louse, fleas, and ticks, the various rickettsial diseases that occur in the United States include endemic or murine typhus, rickettsialpox, RMSF, and Q fever. Human granulocytic ehrlichiosis (HGE) (now also known as *anaplasmosis*) and human monocytic ehrlichiosis (HME) cases have also been reported with an expanding geographic distribution.

ENDEMIC TYPHUS

Endemic (murine) typhus is caused by *Rickettsia typhi* and is transmitted by the rat flea *Xenopsylla cheopis*. It occurs worldwide, especially in warm climates with heavy populations of rats or opossums.[270] Although endemic typhus occurs most often in developing nations, it continues to occur in the United States, especially in Gulf Coast areas and Texas.[271] Adults are most often affected, but children have constituted up to 75% of infections in some outbreaks.[270] Clinical manifestations most commonly include fever and headache (often frontal), with rash occurring in up to two-thirds of patients. The eruption is variably characterized as macular, papular, and occasionally petechial; in one systematic review, it was noted that the rash often spares the palms and soles.[272] Other features may include nausea, vomiting, malaise, myalgias, chills, diarrhea, anorexia, back pain, arthralgia, lymphadenopathy, conjunctivitis, and respiratory disease (pneumonia, effusion, respiratory failure). Central nervous system involvement, including altered level of consciousness, meningitis, meningoencephalitis, seizures, or ataxia, may also occur.[272] Chronic cognitive impairment may occur.[273] Effective treatments include doxycycline and chloramphenicol. Endemic typhus should be considered in the child with prolonged fever and a rash, especially those residing in Southern California, southern Texas, and Hawaii.[274]

RICKETTSIALPOX

Rickettsialpox, caused by *Rickettsia akari*, is transmitted to humans by the house-mouse mite *Liponyssoides sanguineus*. Although rickettsialpox is rarely reported or diagnosed, it remains endemic in certain regions of the United States, particularly New York City.[275] The disorder begins with the bite of an infected mite, which results in a black eschar and subsequently other symptoms. The classic triad of rickettsialpox consists of fever, eschar, and rash. The skin eruption presents as numerous monomorphous red papules with a small, central vesicular component. Although it may occasionally be confused with varicella, the rash of rickettsialpox is characterized by fewer lesions, less pruritus, monomorphous nature, and presence of an eschar at the site of the original bite of the mite.[275] Other features include myalgias, gastrointestinal symptoms, arthralgias, and lymphadenopathy. Although rickettsialpox is self-limited over 7 to 10 days, treatments of choice include doxycycline or chloramphenicol.

ROCKY MOUNTAIN SPOTTED FEVER

RMSF is caused by *Rickettsia rickettsii* and is the most common rickettsial illness in the United States. The spotted fever group (SFG) rickettsiae include *R. rickettsii*, *R. parkeri*, and *Rickettsia* species 364D, and importantly, epidemiologic surveillance in the United States may not distinguish between RMSF and other SFG rickettsioses.[276] In one 4-year period during the mid-1990s, the average annual RMSF incidence was 2.2 cases per million persons, with the highest incidence confirmed among children 5 to 9 years of age (3.7 per million).[277] Of 4800 cases reported to the CDC between 1990 and 1998, 20% of cases and 15% of reported deaths were in children under 10 years of age.[278] During 2000 through 2007, the annual reported incidence of RMSF increased to 7 cases per million persons, the highest rate ever recorded, and children ages 5 to 9 years appeared to have the highest risk of a fatal outcome.[279] Among children living in the southeastern and southcentral United States, 12% had positive *R. rickettsii* antibody titers in one serologic survey, and hence exposure to the agent may be more common than indicated by reports of disease.[280] Because of the rapid progression of disease and the high mortality rate that may be seen without appropriate therapy, prompt diagnosis and initiation of specific treatment are vital in children with RMSF. Despite the name of this disease, it has been reported throughout the continental United States except for in Maine and Vermont.[278,281] The highest incidence is in Oklahoma, Tennessee, Arkansas, and the South Atlantic region; the most important factor in transmission of the disease is the prevalence of infected ticks.[282,283] The majority of reported SFG rickettsiosis cases during 2008–2012 originated in five states: Oklahoma, Tennessee, Arkansas, Missouri, and North Carolina.[284]

RMSF is transmitted by the bite of the wood tick *(Dermacentor andersoni)* in the western United States and Canada and the dog tick *(Dermacentor variabilis)* in the eastern United States. Most cases occur during the spring and summer months. Even in areas considered to be highly endemic for the disease, only a small fraction of ticks are infected with *R. rickettsii*.[285] Up to 40% of individuals diagnosed with RMSF do not recall a history of tick bite.[285] Importantly, ticks may attach to any body site (some of which are difficult to observe), often have a painless bite, and commonly go unnoticed.[282]

Patients with RMSF usually report symptoms 3 to 12 days after the tick bite. The initial prodromal symptoms include the sudden onset of headache, gastrointestinal symptoms, malaise, and myalgias. These are followed by fever and rash (the latter typically presenting 2 to 4 days after the onset of fever). The classic triad of RMSF consists of fever, headache, and rash, but many patients with the disease do not show symptoms in this classic fashion. Headache is a very prominent feature, may be severe, and is usually accompanied by severe myalgias. Patients with gastrointestinal complaints may have nausea, vomiting, and generalized or focal abdominal pain, occasionally mimicking an acute abdomen.[285] Neurologic findings may include meningismus or impaired level of consciousness (which occurs in approximately one-third of cases),[286] encephalitis, seizures, and psychiatric complaints. Photophobia may also be present. An exanthem occurs in up to 90% of patients with RMSF and usually appears around day 3 to 5 of the illness. It begins as discrete erythematous blanching macules and papules, which begin in a peripheral fashion and spread centrally (centripetally). Common locations for early lesions include the ankles, wrists, palms, and soles. With time, the skin lesions evolve into petechial macules and papules (Fig. 16.40). Occasionally they become hemorrhagic, and focal areas of necrosis may occur. Larger areas of purpura may be present, and in some patients the skin eruption mimics that of meningococcemia. Skin necrosis and gangrene may occasionally result. Some patients have a delayed appearance of the rash, and in up to 10% the rash is completely absent ("spotless" RMSF).[285] These patients seem to have the same course as patients with a rash, and the index of suspicion must be higher in them, incorporating clinical and epidemiologic clues when present. Other mucocutaneous features may include hyperpigmentation, jaundice, and mucosal erosions. Late manifestations of RMSF may include renal failure, meningoencephalitis, adult respiratory distress syndrome, shock, arrhythmia, and seizures.

Laboratory findings in RMSF may include a left shift with a normal to low white blood cell count, thrombocytopenia, liver function abnormalities, and hyponatremia. A lymphocytic cerebrospinal fluid pleocytosis is often noted. The differential diagnosis of RMSF includes other rickettsial diseases, meningococcal disease, Kawasaki disease, drug reactions, measles, and other viral exanthems. The diagnosis is usually made on a clinical basis, and if the disease is even remotely suspected, prompt institution of a tetracycline-class antibiotic should occur. Biopsy of skin lesions reveals endothelial cell damage with a perivascular and interstitial mononuclear cell infiltrate and small vessel vasculitis, as well as extravasation of red blood cells and fibrin thrombi within vessels.[287,288] In patients with RMSF encephalitis, the "starry sky" pattern of multifocal punctate areas of diffusion restriction involving white matter may be seen on magnetic resonance imaging.[289]

The indirect fluorescent antibody (IFA) test is the most widely used diagnostic examination and detects anti–*R. rickettsii* IgM and IgG antibodies, which are usually present 10 to 14 days after acute infection.

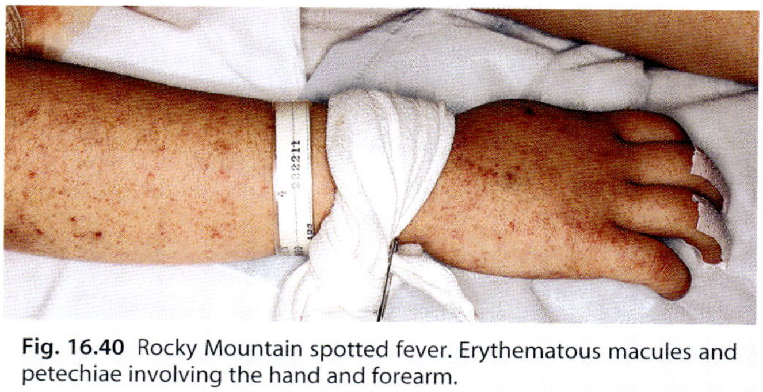

Fig. 16.40 Rocky Mountain spotted fever. Erythematous macules and petechiae involving the hand and forearm.

Enzyme-linked immunosorbent assay (ELISA) testing has also been utilized.[290] PCR-based diagnosis is typically available only in specialized laboratories. Skin biopsy with immunohistochemical staining is highly specific, but may not be available in all locales; when necessary, skin specimens can be submitted to the CDC via state health departments.

The treatment of choice for RMSF is doxycycline, which is preferable to other tetracycline agents because of its reliable absorption, twice-daily dosing schedule, and broader spectrum of coverage for other tick-borne diseases.[282,285] If RMSF is strongly suspected, treatment should be promptly initiated and not delayed while waiting for laboratory confirmation. Delay in diagnosis and in initiating treatment increases the risks for long-term morbidity and mortality.[291,292] Chloramphenicol is also effective but is generally used only for patients in whom a contraindication to doxycycline is present (e.g., pregnancy). In an analysis of risk factors for fatal RMSF, evidence for the superiority of tetracyclines was demonstrated even when compared with chloramphenicol therapy.[293] It should be noted that the risk of dental staining, which may be associated with doxycycline therapy in children under 8 years of age, is generally far outweighed by the risk of RMSF going untreated. Doxycycline therapy is recommended by the AAP and by the CDC as the treatment of choice in both RMSF and ehrlichiosis (see later).[294] Dental staining appears to be dose- and duration-related and is unlikely to occur in children treated with short courses of tetracyclines[283,295]; in one study of 58 children who received an average of 1.8 courses of doxycycline for RMSF before 8 years of age and were examined by licensed dentists after permanent teeth eruption, no tetracycline-like staining was observed.[296] Therapy should be continued until the patient demonstrates clinical improvement and is afebrile for at least 3 days. Most patients are treated for 7 to 10 days.

Useful measures in preventing RMSF include wearing long clothing when outdoors (especially when in high-risk areas for tick bites), use of insect repellents effective against ticks (see Chapter 18), and frequent inspection for ticks with tweezer removal when necessary. It seems that transmission of the organism probably cannot occur until after 24 hours of tick attachment.[297]

Q FEVER

Q fever, caused by the intracellular Gram-negative coccobacillus *Coxiella burnetii*, is a worldwide zoonosis affecting domestic animals, birds, and arthropods.[298] It is transmitted to humans through contact with infected domestic animals, including cattle, sheep, goats, or the products of these animals.[287] The primary route of human infection appears to be via inhalation of contaminated aerosols, and because the organism has a low respiratory infective dose, there has been some concern over its potential use as an agent of biologic warfare.[298] Tick bites, ingestion of unpasteurized milk or dairy products, and human-to-human spread are unusual sources of transmission of *C. burnetii* to humans.

The presentation of Q fever in humans is variable, and because the symptoms are so variable, it is likely underreported and underdiagnosed.[299] It may present as a nonspecific flu-like illness, atypical pneumonia, or hepatitis. In one retrospective series of over 1000 children with Q fever during an outbreak in the Netherlands, the most common presentations were respiratory tract infection and influenza-like illness. This series highlighted the nonspecific symptoms and their lack of any significant predictive value.[300] Other clinical manifestations may include fever, inflammatory heart disease (myocarditis, endocarditis, pericarditis), osteomyelitis, joint infection, and central nervous system infection.[301–303] Chronic recurrent multifocal Q fever osteomyelitis has been reported.[304] Malaise is common and may persist for months after the acute symptoms have disappeared. Rash is reported in up to 20% of patients overall but has a higher prevalence in children (up to 50%) and does not appear to have distinguishing features. Erythematous macules, petechiae, purpura, urticaria, vesicles, livedo reticularis, and erythema nodosum have been reported.[287] Subcutaneous nodules representing necrotizing granulomatous inflammation have also been observed.[305] The diagnosis of Q fever is confirmed by serologic studies or PCR, and treatment in children consists of doxycycline for 14 days, or if the disease is mild and uncomplicated, for 5 days followed by additional treatment with trimethoprim/sulfamethoxazole if fever persists.[299] In some patients, Q fever is a self-limited disease that is diagnosed retrospectively.[298] A history of recent contact with farm animals and pets in the presence of consistent clinical findings should prompt investigation for *C. burnetii*.[301]

EHRLICHIOSIS

Ehrlichia are obligate intracellular bacteria that belong to the family Rickettsiae. The two forms of disease of most concern in the United States are HME and HGE, both of which are transmitted by tick bites and have similar clinical manifestations.

HME (now often referred to simply as *ehrlichiosis*) is caused by *Ehrlichia chaffeensis* and occurs primarily in the southeastern and south-central United States. States with the highest reported incidences are Missouri, Delaware, Oklahoma, Tennessee, Arkansas, and Virginia.[306] The most common vector is the Lone Star tick *(Amblyomma americanum)*, and the distribution of disease closely parallels the endemic regions for this arthropod.[307] Most cases of HME occur during late spring and summer. *Ehrlichia ewingii* is a less commonly reported agent of human ehrlichiosis (occurring especially in immunocompromised individuals) and was initially identified as the etiologic agent of canine granulocytic ehrlichiosis. The overall rate for ehrlichiosis in the United States has increased fourfold since 2000.[306]

HGE, also known as *human granulocytic anaplasmosis (HGA)*, is caused by *Anaplasma phagocytophilum*, which was previously known as "the agent of human granulocytic ehrlichiosis."[308] This infection is caused by bites from an infected black-legged tick *(Ixodes scapularis)*, and in the western United States, the western black-legged tick *(Ixodes pacificus)*, and is seen with a broader geographic distribution in the United States. The recent highest annual incidence rates have been reported in Minnesota, Wisconsin, and Rhode Island.[309] Most cases of HGE occur between the months of May and August.

There may be considerable overlap of the clinical manifestations in patients with HME and HGE, although HME tends to be a more severe disease. Nonspecific symptoms of both disorders include fever, fatigue, headache, malaise, chills, myalgia, nausea, and rash (which is more common in pediatric patients). Hematologic aberrations may include progressive leukopenia, thrombocytopenia, and anemia, and hemophagocytic lymphohistiocytosis has been seen in the setting of *E. chaffeensis* infection.[310] Some patients have elevation of liver transaminases, alkaline phosphatase, and LDH, and hyponatremia may also be present. The clinical presentation of an acute abdomen has been rarely reported in affected children.[311] Hepatosplenomegaly and systolic murmur are common examination findings in patients with HME.[307] Shock necessitating pressor support and mechanical ventilation has been reported in patients with HME.[312] Neurologic features may include meningitis or meningoencephalitis (especially in HME) and peripheral nerve manifestations such as brachial plexopathy, cranial nerve palsies, facial nerve palsy, and demyelinating neuropathy (primarily in HGE).

The incidence of rash in patients with HME or HGE is not well established but seems to occur less often than that seen in patients with RMSF. It is estimated that around 60% of children infected with *E. chaffeensis* develop a rash.[306] It has been described as macular, papular, or petechial. Other less commonly reported patterns include vesicular, nodular, purpuric, vasculitic, erythrodermic, and ulcerated types.[287] The distribution is variable, although in the case of HME, it tends to spare the face, palms, and soles. The onset of the cutaneous eruption is most often within the first 3 to 10 days of the illness. The skin lesions seen in patients with HGE may predominate in the vicinity of the tick bite. The differential diagnosis of ehrlichiosis is broad, including septic shock, meningococcemia, thrombotic thrombocytopenic purpura, toxic shock syndrome, RMSF, Lyme disease, murine typhus, tularemia, babesiosis, and other tick-borne fevers.

Diagnostic options for ehrlichiosis include examination of peripheral blood smears (assessing for cytoplasmic clusters of organisms, or morulae), immunohistology, PCR assay, isolation of the organism, and serologic studies.[306,313] The most clinically relevant laboratory study is that of paired serologies (often via indirect IFA), which often need to be performed by a reference laboratory. Western blotting has also been utilized.[314] The treatment of choice for ehrlichiosis is doxycycline, and chloramphenicol is also a useful agent.[287,307,315] As with RMSF, treatment should be promptly initiated if there is a clinical suspicion for the diagnosis, and doxycycline is the treatment of choice even in children under 8 years of age. Rifampin has been successfully used in children with HGE and may be another option for patients with non-life-threatening disease.[134] Efforts to reduce contact with ticks are also useful in lowering the risk of ehrlichiosis.

The complete list of 315 references for this chapter is available online at http://expertconsult.inkling.com.

Key References

Wutzler P, Bonanni P, Burgess M, et al. Varicella vaccination—the global experience. Expert Rev Vaccines 2017;16(8):833–43.

Marin M, Meissner HC, Seward JF. Varicella prevention in the USA: a review of successes and challenges. Pediatrics 2008;122:e744–51.

American Academy of Pediatrics, Committee on Infectious Diseases. Policy statement: prevention of varicella: update of recommendations for use of quadrivalent and monovalent varicella vaccines in children. Pediatrics 2011;128:630–2.

Dabbagh A, Patel MK, Dumolard L, et al. Progress toward regional measles elimination—worldwide, 2000–2016. MMWR Morb Mortal Wkly Rep 2017;66(42):1148–53.

Bester JC. Measles and measles vaccination. JAMA Pediatr 2016;170(12):1209–15.

Remenyi B, Carapetis J, Wyber R, et al. Position statement of the World Heart Federation on the prevention and control of rheumatic heart disease. Nat Rev Cardiol 2013;10:284–92.

Lennon D, Stewart J, Anderson P. Primary prevention of rheumatic fever. Pediatr Infect Dis J 2016;35(7):820.

McCarthy M. Endemic rubella is eliminated from Americas, PAHO announces. BMJ 2015;350:h2348.

Bonvicini F, Bua G, Gallinella G. Parvovirus B19 infection in pregnancy—awareness and opportunities. Curr Opin Virol 2017;27:8–14.

Edmonson MB, Riedesel EL, Williams GP, et al. Generalized petechial rashes in children during a parvovirus B19 outbreak. Pediatrics 2010;125:e787–92.

Luzuriaga K, Sullivan JL. Infectious mononucleosis. N Engl J Med 2010;362(21):1993–2000.

Biggs HM, Behravesh CB, Bradley KK, et al. Diagnosis and management of tickborne rickettsial diseases: Rocky Mountain spotted fever and other spotted fever group rickettsioses, ehrlichioses, and anaplasmosis—United States. A practical guide for health care and public health professionals. MMWR Recomm Rep 2016;65(2):1–44.

17 Skin Disorders Caused by Fungi

CHAPTER OUTLINE

Fungi are a group of simple plants that lack flowers, leaves, and chlorophyll and get their nourishment from dead or living organic matter, thus depending on plants, animals, and humans for their existence. Fungal infections that affect humans may be superficial, deep, or systemic and can occasionally be fatal. Although they do not rank as pathogens with the bacteria or viruses, a number of species once thought to be ubiquitous and harmless have been implicated in various diseases, and with the increasing use of broad-spectrum antibiotics, corticosteroids, cytotoxic medications, and biologic agents, deep mycoses have become increasingly significant.

The pathogenic fungal diseases are divided into superficial and deep infections. The superficial infections are those limited to the epidermis, hair, nails, and mucous membranes. Deep fungal infections are those in which the organisms affect other organs of the body or invade the skin through direct extension or hematogenous spread.

Superficial Fungal Infections

There are three common types of superficial fungal infection: dermatophytosis, tinea versicolor, and candidiasis (moniliasis). Those caused by dermatophytes are termed *tinea, dermatophytosis*, or because of the annular appearance of the lesions, *ringworm*. In addition, tinea nigra, a superficial infection of the stratum corneum caused by a yeast-like fungus and often misdiagnosed as a melanocytic lesion, and piedra, an asymptomatic infection of the hair shaft, may be noted in both children and adults.

The dermatophytes are a group of related fungi that live in soil (geophilic), on animals (zoophilic), or on humans (anthropophilic). They digest keratin and invade the skin, hair, and nails, producing a diverse array of clinical lesions. Depending on the involved site, the infection may be termed *tinea capitis, tinea faciei, tinea barbae, tinea corporis, tinea manuum, tinea pedis, tinea cruris*, or *tinea unguium* (*onychomycosis*, tinea of the nails). The diagnosis and management of fungal diseases of childhood have become easier in the past decades due to the development of more effective diagnostic techniques and therapeutic agents.

DIAGNOSIS OF FUNGAL INFECTIONS

Tests for fungal infection are rewarding procedures readily available to all physicians, not merely those trained in dermatology. Diagnosis of ringworm of the scalp may be aided by the presence of fluorescence under a Wood light examination, although the changing epidemiology of this infection in the United States has made this examination clinically irrelevant in most cases. Other diagnostic studies that may be useful include direct microscopic examination of skin scrapings or infected hairs and fungal culture. These tests can be performed simply, inexpensively, and rapidly in the office. Laboratory confirmation of fungal infection is useful in confirming the diagnosis, in detecting the asymptomatic carrier state, and in the case of tinea capitis, in demonstrating a mycologic cure when clinical symptoms have resolved. Dermatophyte identification may also provide useful epidemiologic information (i.e., human-to-human vs. animal-to-human transmission) and may help guide the clinician's choice of antifungal therapy. Definitive proof of fungal infection should be considered when prolonged systemic therapy is being considered, in patients with some features but who lack lymphadenopathy (the most predictive clinical finding), and in patients who fail empiric therapy.[1]

Wood Light Examination

The discovery in 1925 that hair infected by certain dermatophytes would fluoresce when exposed to ultraviolet light filtered by a Wood filter led to a helpful but occasionally improperly used diagnostic tool. When a Wood light examination is performed, it must be remembered that infected hairs, not the skin, fluoresce when exposed to light rays emitted by this lamp. Although the nature and the source of the fluorescent substance in infected hairs are not fully understood, this phenomenon is believed to be the result of a substance, perhaps pteridine, emitted when the fungus invades the hair.

Optimally, a powerful Wood lamp should be used in a completely darkened room. The usefulness of Wood lamp examination depends on the pattern of arthroconidial formation and hair invasion. Organisms that result in ectothrix infection (i.e., *Microsporum audouinii* and *Microsporum canis*) result in brilliant green fluorescence with this examination. However, those organisms associated with endothrix infection (i.e., *Trichophyton tonsurans* and *Trichophyton violaceum*), where organisms are present within the hair shaft, show no fluorescence. *Trichophyton schoenleinii*, the cause of favus (see later), produces a pale green fluorescence on Wood lamp examination. Sources of error in Wood light examinations include an insufficiently darkened room; the blue or purple fluorescence produced by lint, scales, serum exudates, or ointments containing petrolatum; and failure to remember that it is the infected hair and not the skin that fluoresces.

Potassium Hydroxide Wet-Mount Preparations

Microscopic examination of skin scrapings is an important but commonly overlooked aid in the diagnosis of suspected fungal infection of the skin or hair. This examination will yield rapid results but requires considerable experience, because false-positive interpretations are common. Material for mycologic study should be taken by gently scraping outward from the active border of a suspected lesion with a number 15 scalpel blade or the edge of a glass slide. Moistening the skin with alcohol before performing the scraping may be useful in adhering the skin debris to the blade before it is smeared on a slide. Cut hairs, nail scrapings, subungual debris, and material from the edge of an affected nail may also be used for wet-mount examination. The material is placed on a glass microscope slide with care and spread out flat and evenly in a single layer. A coverslip is applied, and a few drops of 10% to 20% potassium hydroxide (KOH) are added at the side of the coverslip until the entire space between coverslip and slide is filled. Gentle heating of the preparation (with care to prevent boiling of the KOH, because this will cause crystallization) should be performed until the horny cells and debris are rendered translucent. If the KOH solution contains dimethylsulfoxide (DMSO), the slide should not be

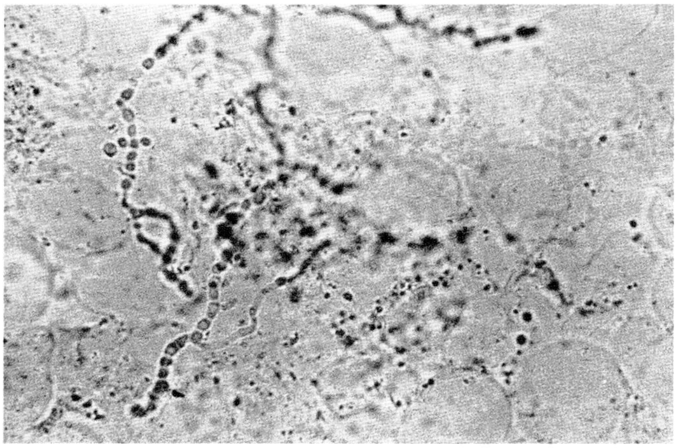

Fig. 17.1 KOH examination in tinea. Note the septated fungal elements (hyphae). (Courtesy Alfred W. Kopf, MD.)

heated, because heating a DMSO-KOH preparation will dissolve fungi as well as epidermal cells.[2]

After collection and preparation of the specimen, gentle pressure is applied to the coverslip. This will improve the preparation by forcing out trapped air and thinning the specimen, thus allowing better visualization of fungi. The light of the microscope condenser should be dimmed to enhance the contrast between the branched hyphae and epidermal elements, and the specimen should be viewed under low power. A positive KOH examination reveals branching fungal hyphae with septations (Fig. 17.1).

Fungal Culture

Although direct microscopic examination of skin scrapings will often confirm the suspicion of tinea, definitive identification rests on isolation of the fungus by the gold standard: fungal culture. There are several types of fungal culture media, but the most popular are Sabouraud dextrose agar or mycobiotic agar (Mycosel) containing cycloheximide and chloramphenicol, which suppress growth of common saprophytic and bacterial contaminants, respectively.[3] Dermatophyte test medium (DTM) agar is another commonly used media that also contains antibiotics (cycloheximide, gentamicin, and chlortetracycline) that inhibit saprophytic fungi and bacteria. DTM also contains a color indicator that changes from yellow to orange to red in the presence of dermatophytes. This medium is particularly useful for physicians who lack detailed knowledge of fungus-colony morphology and simply require confirmation of dermatophyte infection. However, one disadvantage of DTM is that the addition of the color indicator precludes laboratory identification of the exact dermatophyte because it may obscure some colonial features used to distinguish these organisms.

Specimens for fungal culture may be obtained via a variety of collection procedures. Traditional methods include plucking broken hairs or scraping scale, but these procedures may be frightening or painful for younger children. Other modalities include use of a sterile toothbrush, wet gauze, cytobrushes, and adhesive tape. Use of a cytobrush has demonstrated very high sensitivity when compared with the traditional method of scraping the scalp.[4] The simplicity and reliability of the cotton swab technique has also been confirmed.[5] In this method, a sterile cotton-tipped applicator moistened with tap water (or Culturette swab in transport medium) is rubbed vigorously and rotated over the affected area of the scalp and then inoculated onto the appropriate fungal medium. This technique is atraumatic, readily available, and both sensitive and specific, even with delays between collection and plating of the sample.[5]

Trichoscopy (which refers to dermoscopy of the hair) has been reported as a useful diagnostic modality in the diagnosis of various hair disorders, including tinea capitis.[6] A dermatoscope is a device composed of a magnifier attached to a nonpolarized light source utilized primarily by dermatologists. As such, this methodology is likely less applicable to the primary care provider. When utilized in tinea capitis, trichoscopy reveals comma-shaped and corkscrew hairs, black dots, and broken (not tapered) hairs.[6,7]

THE DERMATOPHYTOSES

Tinea Capitis

Tinea capitis, the most common dermatophytosis of childhood, is a fungal infection of the skin and hair of the scalp characterized by scaling and patchy alopecia. It is generally a disease of prepubertal children, especially those between the ages of 3 and 7 years, although infants and adults are occasionally affected. Neonatal tinea capitis has been reported.[8,9] In a prospective, cross-sectional surveillance study of children in kindergarten through fifth grade in a large US metropolitan area, 6.6% of children overall had positive cultures for *T. tonsurans*, and the infection rates at participating schools ranged from 0% to 19.4%, with Black children demonstrating the highest rates of infection (12.9%).

A variety of dermatophytes may cause tinea capitis, especially *T. tonsurans* (the most common etiology in the United States, where it causes >90% of infections), *T. violaceum*, *M. canis*, and *M. audouinii*. Across Europe, *M. canis* remains the most common organism, although shifts toward *T. tonsurans* are being observed, especially in the United Kingdom.[10,11] In Africa, Eastern Europe, and Asia, *T. violaceum*, *T. schoenleinii*, *M. ferrugineum*, and *M. audouinii* are the most common causes for tinea capitis.[11] These organisms may be anthropophilic (spread from humans, i.e., *T. tonsurans* and *T. violaceum*), zoophilic (spread from animals, i.e., *M. canis* and *M. audouinii*), or geophilic (spread from soil). Dermatophytes have a short incubation period (generally 1 to 3 weeks) and infect boys more commonly than girls. Predisposing factors for tinea capitis include large family size, crowded living conditions, and low socioeconomic class.[3] In addition to transmission from other humans or animals, dermatophyte spread via fomites (hairbrushes, combs, hats, and contaminated grooming instruments) is well documented. The reason for increased resistance to tinea capitis infection after puberty is unknown, but may be related to a higher content of fungistatic fatty acids in the sebum of postpubertal individuals. Hair care practices (styling, frequency of washing, use of oils or grease), traditionally believed to play a significant role in the acquisition of tinea capitis, appear to not play a major role.[12]

Asymptomatic scalp carriage of dermatophytes varies and tends to correlate with the amount of tinea capitis in a community.[13] Such carriers constitute a major reservoir for transmission of the organisms causing the disease. Asymptomatic carriage is most common with the anthropophilic organisms *T. tonsurans* and *T. violaceum*, and most carriers are Black, Afro-Caribbean, or Black children in Africa.[3] Household contacts may be a significant source of asymptomatic carriers, and cosleeping and comb sharing seem to be important factors in the spread of disease in this setting.[14] Varied treatment options have been suggested for the carrier state, although there is a paucity of well-designed clinical studies.

The clinical manifestations of tinea capitis are varied and are summarized in Table 17.1. It may present in a "seborrheic dermatitis" pattern, with diffuse scaling and minimal inflammation (Fig. 17.2), or with discrete scaly erythematous patches and plaques (Fig. 17.3). One or multiple patches of alopecia may be present (Fig. 17.4), and at times tinea capitis may present in a fashion similar to alopecia areata. "Black dot" tinea presents with alopecic areas with small black dots within them, representing the ends of broken-off hair shafts (Fig. 17.5). This form is most commonly seen with endothrix infections such as *T. tonsurans*. It should be noted that the black-dot sign is probably overemphasized and, although present, may often be relatively inconspicuous.

Scalp pustules may be present (Fig. 17.6) and need to be distinguished from bacterial or sterile folliculitis. Kerion (Figs. 17.7 and 17.8) is a markedly inflammatory presentation of tinea capitis and reveals a boggy plaque with alopecia, pustules, and often purulent drainage from the surface. These lesions represent a vigorous host immune response to the dermatophyte and are caused most often by *M. canis* and *T. tonsurans* (and in rural areas by *Trichophyton verrucosum*). Although kerions may heal spontaneously, aggressive therapy is desirable, because the severe inflammatory response may result in

Table 17.1 Clinical Manifestations of Tinea Capitis in Children

Clinical Feature	Comment
SCALP	
Alopecia	One or multiple patches; may simulate alopecia areata
Scaling	May be minimally inflammatory; may mimic seborrheic dermatitis
Erythema	Localized or widespread
Pustules	Differential diagnosis includes sterile folliculitis or bacterial folliculitis
"Black dots"	Alopecia with hair shafts broken off at surface of skin; may simulate trichotillomania
Kerion	Boggy, tender plaque with pustules and purulent discharge; represents a vigorous host immune response
Scarring	Rarely seen when untreated; usually follows kerion
Favus	Yellow, cup-shaped crusts around the hair
OTHER	
Lymphadenopathy	Common; cervical or occipital
Id reaction	Widespread, papular or papulovesicular eruption; extremity predominant; usually seen after initiation of therapy; must be recognized as distinct from true drug reaction

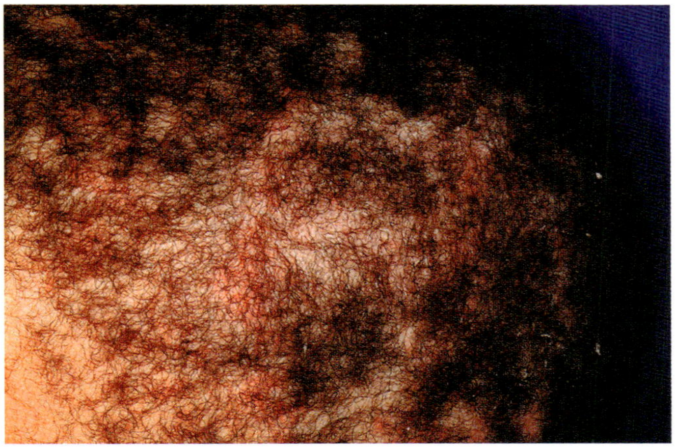

Fig. 17.2 Tinea capitis. Diffuse scaling with minimal erythema and patchy alopecia.

permanent scarring alopecia (Fig. 17.9). Kerion has also been observed in neonates.[15]

Lymphadenopathy, especially cervical or suboccipital, is common in patients showing symptoms of tinea capitis. In one study, the presence of lymphadenopathy was highly suggestive of a positive fungal culture in children who were suspected of having tinea capitis, especially those with the concomitant presence of alopecia or scaling.[16]

Favus, a severe chronic form of tinea capitis rarely seen in the United States, is caused by the fungus *T. schoenleinii*. This disorder is characterized by scaly erythematous patches with yellow crusts, or "scutula," representing hairs matted together with hyphae and keratin debris (Fig. 17.10). Such infections often result in scarring and permanent alopecia.[17]

A widespread papular hypersensitivity or dermatophytid (id) reaction may occur in patients with tinea capitis. This usually presents as

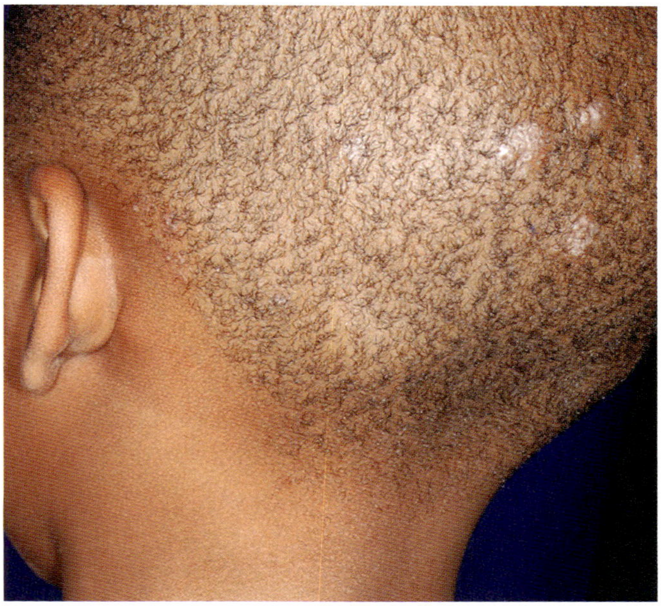

Fig. 17.3 Tinea capitis. Discrete scaly, erythematous plaques on the scalp of a 3-year-old boy with cervical lymphadenopathy and positive fungal culture.

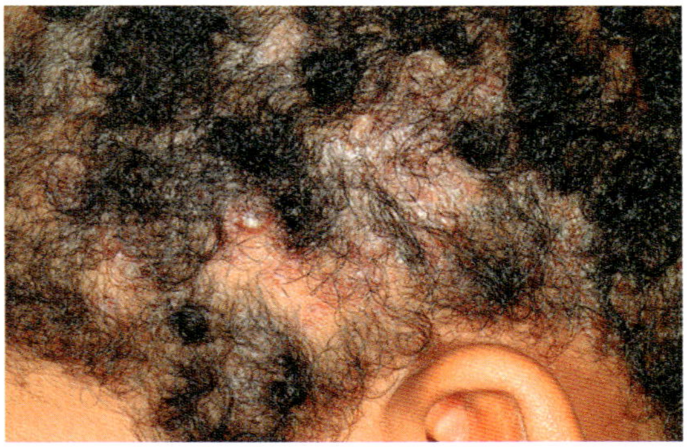

Fig. 17.4 Tinea capitis. Multiple patches of alopecia with erythema and scaling. Note the presence of pustules.

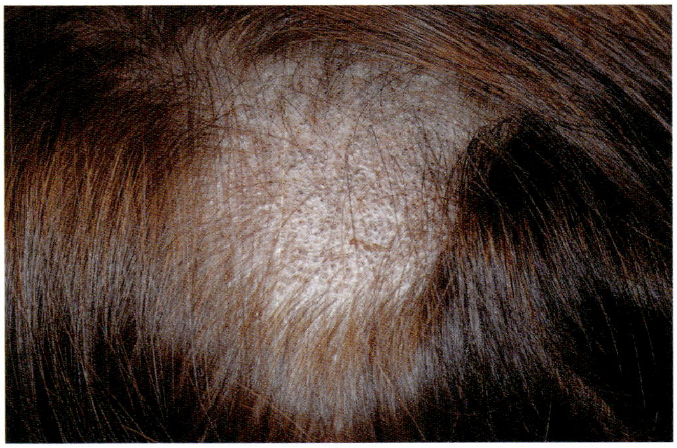

Fig. 17.5 "Black dot" tinea capitis. This well-demarcated patch of alopecia is composed of numerous broken-off hair shafts (black dots) in a 4-year-old girl with tinea capitis caused by *Trichophyton tonsurans*.

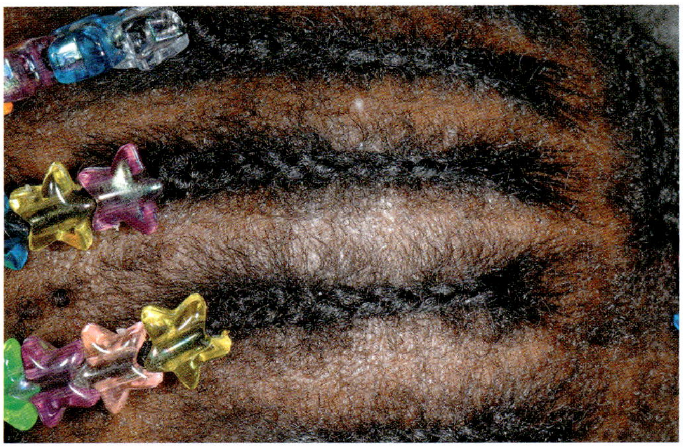

Fig. 17.6 Tinea capitis. This young girl had multiple pustules throughout her scalp with minimal inflammation, scaling, or alopecia. Culture revealed *Trichophyton tonsurans*.

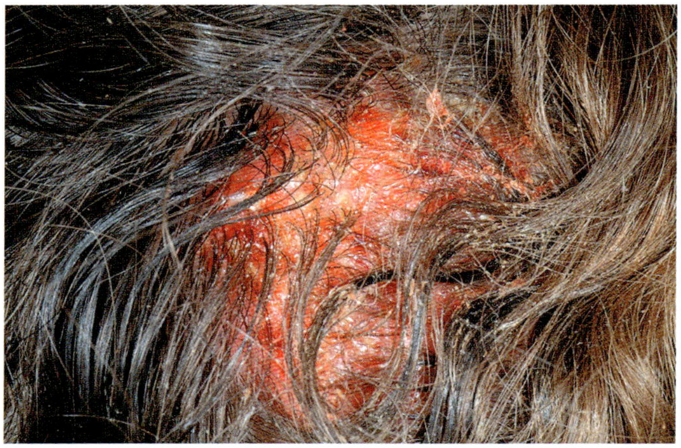

Fig. 17.7 Kerion. This fluctuant, erythematous, boggy, and crusted plaque was exquisitely tender to palpation. *Trichophyton tonsurans* was isolated in fungal culture.

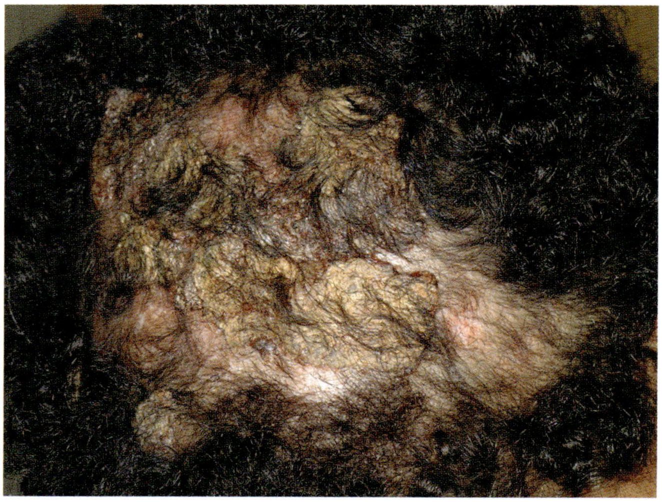

Fig. 17.8 Kerion. This 4-year-old boy presented with tender, fluctuant plaques with marked hyperkeratosis, underlying which were lakes of pus. Permanent alopecia was present after resolution of the infection.

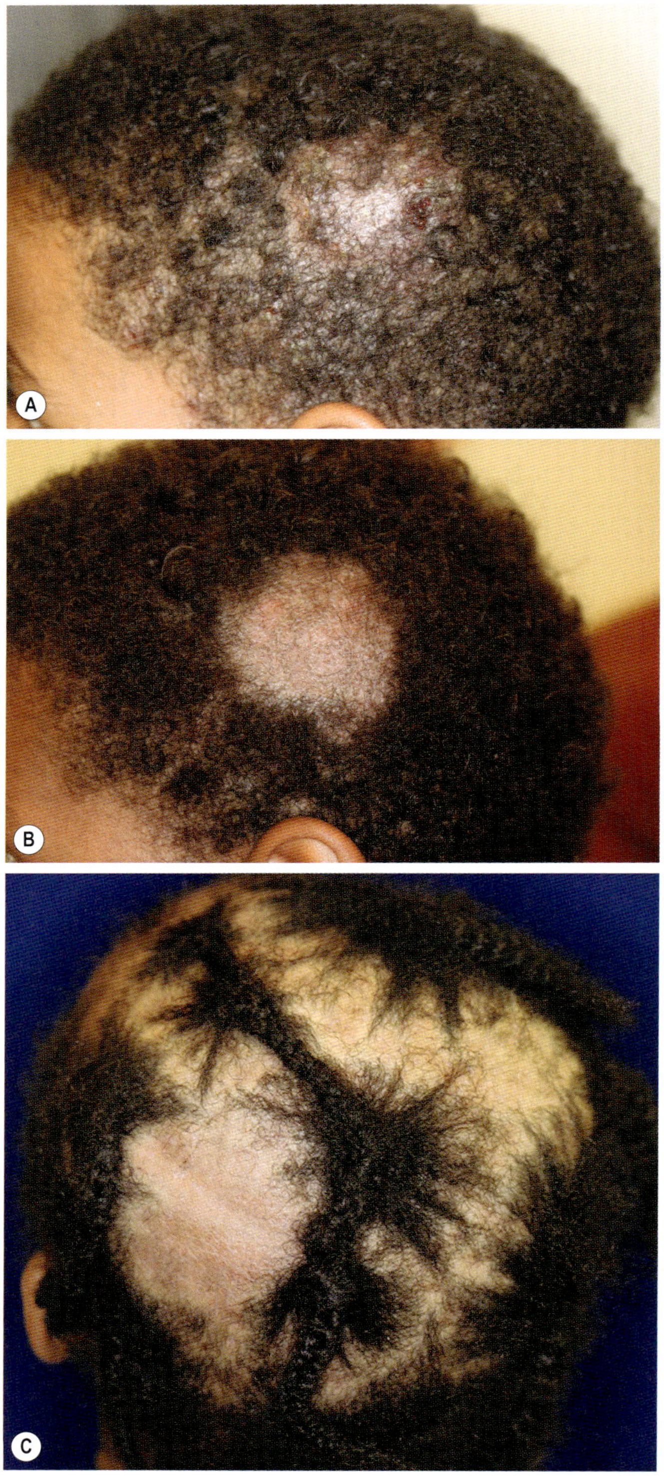

Fig. 17.9 Scarring alopecia after kerion. **(A)** Erythematous boggy plaque with pustules and crusting on the scalp of an 8-year-old boy. **(B)** Scarring alopecia after systemic antifungal therapy in the same patient as in **(A)**. **(C)** Marked scarring with alopecia in a 6-year-old girl after treatment for kerion.

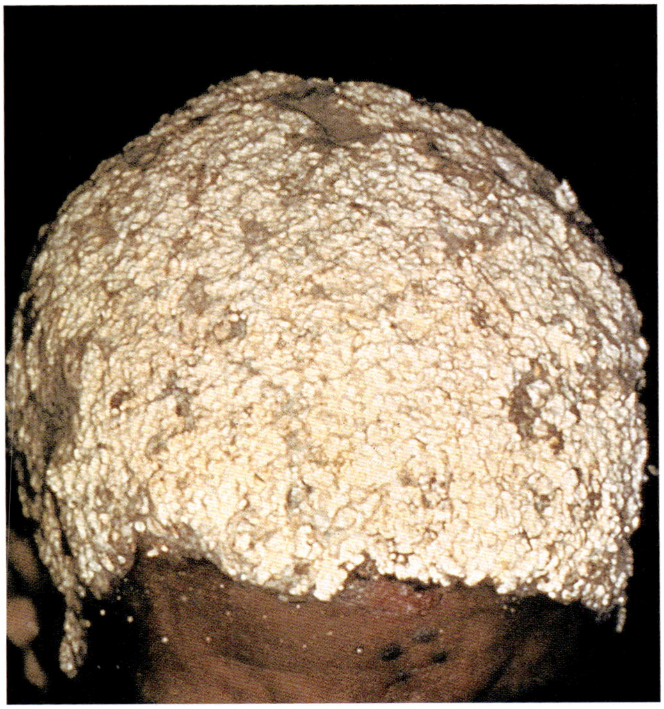

Fig. 17.10 Favus. This severe form of tinea capitis is caused most often by *Trichophyton schoenleinii.* (Courtesy Israel Dvoretzky, MD, and Benjamin K. Fisher, MD.)

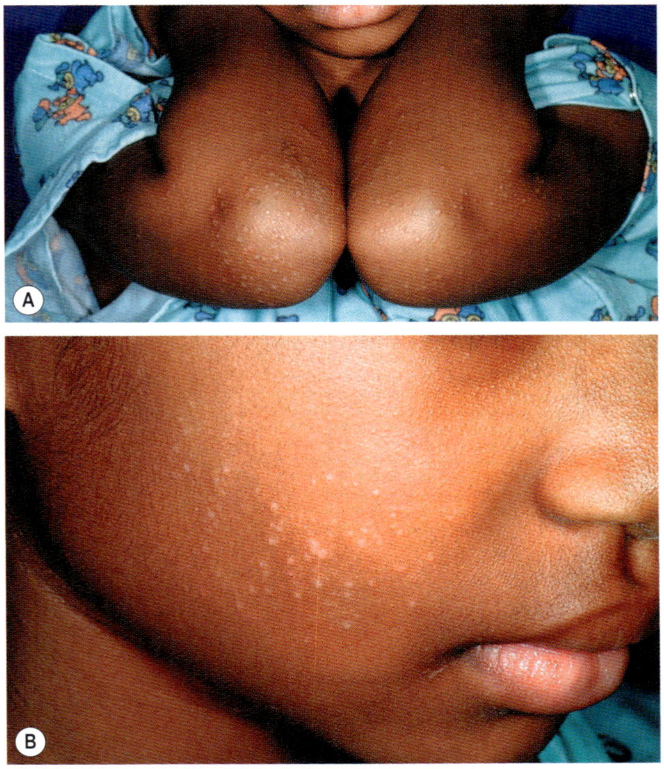

Fig. 17.11 Dermatophytid (id) reaction. These flesh-colored, pruritic papules developed on the extensor extremities **(A)** and face **(B)** after initiating oral therapy for tinea capitis.

tiny lichenoid papules on the scalp, trunk, and extremities (Fig. 17.11) that may be pruritic. This reaction is commonly seen after initiation of antifungal therapy and needs to be differentiated from a drug reaction so as to avoid the unnecessary discontinuation of therapy for the tinea. Although this distinction may not always be straightforward, drug reactions tend to be morbilliform, more widespread, and more erythematous. Id reactions represent an immune response to the dermatophyte and are best treated symptomatically with topical corticosteroid preparations and oral antihistamines as needed.

The differential diagnosis of tinea capitis includes seborrheic dermatitis, psoriasis, alopecia areata, trichotillomania, folliculitis, impetigo, lupus erythematosus, and a variety of less common scalp dermatoses. Confirmation of the diagnosis is desirable, and the gold standard is fungal culture, as discussed earlier. Wood light examination may be useful if the infection is caused by an ectothrix organism, but this is less common in the United States. Demonstration of the fungus by KOH wet-mount preparations of broken hairs or black dots collected with a forceps or of skin scrapings from scaly areas may be useful. Microscopic examination of an infected hair (Fig. 17.12) will reveal tiny arthrospores surrounding the hair shaft in *Microsporum* infection (ectothrix infection) and chains of arthrospores within the hair shaft (endothrix infection) in *T. tonsurans* and *T. violaceum infections*.

The color change in a DTM-plated fungal culture may begin within 24 to 48 hours for fast-growing dermatophytes and appears as a pinkish or red zone around the developing colony. The color will intensify as growth proceeds, with full color development for most cultures in 3 to 7 days (Fig. 17.13). When DTM medium is used, however, the culture should not be evaluated for color after 10 days, because contaminant fungal growth may cause color change by that time, thus leading to false-positive results. It must be remembered that fungi grow best at room temperature and require oxygen. Accordingly, the culture media should be left at room temperature, and the tops of the culture tubes or bottles should be left slightly unscrewed (or the tubes may be covered only with a cotton plug) to allow aeration of the preparation.

Tinea capitis requires systemic therapy because the drug needs to penetrate the hair follicle. For decades, the treatment of choice for tinea capitis has been griseofulvin, and this drug remained the only

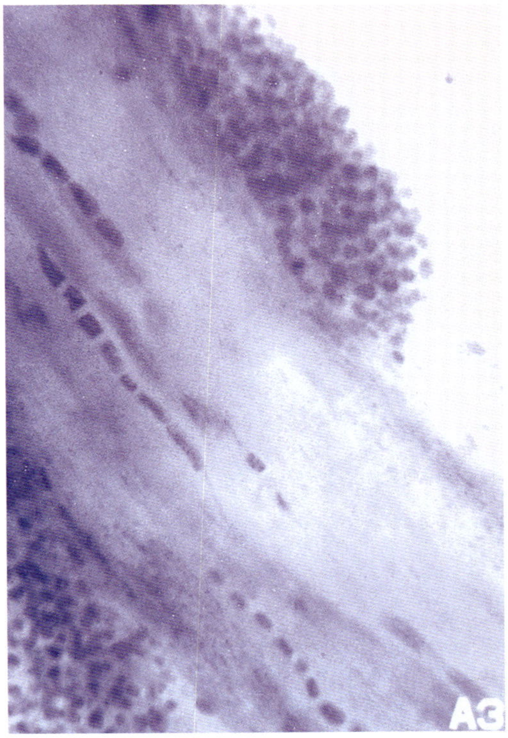

Fig. 17.12 KOH examination of hair. Note multiple spores surrounding the hair shaft (ectothrix) in this patient with *Microsporum* infection. (Courtesy Alfred W. Kopf, MD.)

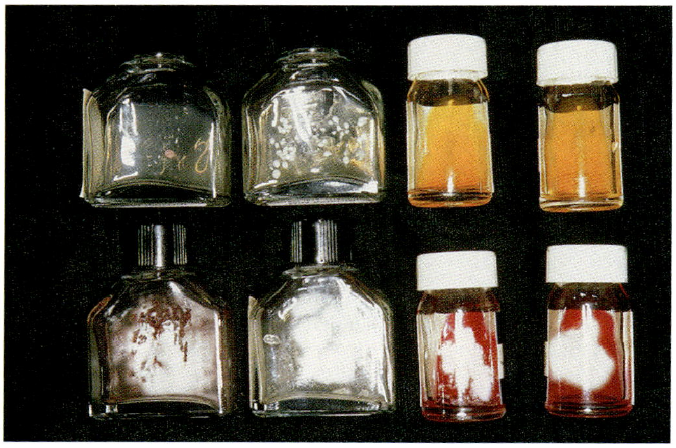

Fig. 17.13 Fungal cultures. Cultures plated on Sabouraud agar *(top row, two on left)* and dermatophyte test medium (DTM; *top row, two on right*) reveal fungal growth and color change (yellow to red on DTM), confirming the presence of a dermatophyte.

agent approved by the US Food and Drug Administration (FDA) for the treatment of this disorder in children for decades. Terbinafine oral granules are now also approved by the FDA for treatment of tinea capitis in children 4 years of age and older. Other agents, including the azole antifungals (most notably fluconazole and itraconazole), have been increasingly evaluated and used off-label as alternative approaches to therapy. Hence, although griseofulvin remains the gold standard, newer treatment options continue to be explored and may, in the near future, lead to a modification of the traditional approach to therapy. In some instances, these newer agents may be preferable, given similar efficacy to griseofulvin and shorter treatment durations.[18] A Cochrane review assessing the effects of systemic antifungal agents for tinea capitis in children reviewed 25 trials with nearly 4500 participants and found similar effects of griseofulvin and terbinafine in those with mixed *Trichophyton* and *Microsporum* infections, superiority of terbinafine over griseofulvin for complete cure of *T. tonsurans* infections, superiority of griseofulvin over terbinafine for complete cure of *Microsporum* species infections, and similar efficacy of fluconazole and itraconazole against *Trichophyton* infections.[19] Treatment of tinea capitis with these four oral antifungal agents in children under 2 years of age has been reported, with good efficacy in general and without significant side effects.[20]

Griseofulvin is a well-tolerated and safe drug that has been extensively used worldwide for this indication. Although in the past doses of 10 mg/kg per day were utilized, most experts currently recommend 20 to 25 mg/kg per day of microsize griseofulvin for 6 to 8 weeks (10 to 15 mg/kg per day if the ultramicrosize form is used). Absorption of griseofulvin is enhanced by a fatty meal, which should be recommended to the patient and parents. Treatment failures are reported and may represent increasing resistance of dermatophytes, although noncompliance with therapy or repeat exposure to infected contacts is probably a more common reason for treatment failure. Griseofulvin is approved for children ≥2 years, but has been used off-label by many experts in younger children.

Side effects of griseofulvin are rare and include headache, gastrointestinal (GI) disturbance, photosensitivity, and rare morbilliform drug reactions. Hematologic and hepatic toxicity is very uncommon, and routine laboratory monitoring is generally not recommended. Although potential cross allergy with penicillins or cephalosporins is often mentioned, in reality this risk is quite low. Concomitant therapy with an antifungal shampoo such as ketoconazole or selenium sulfide two to three times weekly is desirable, because these agents may aid in removing scales and eradicating viable spores, which may help decrease the potential spread of infection.[21,22] This recommendation should be made regardless of the choice of the systemic agent.

Contraindications to griseofulvin therapy include pregnancy, hepatic failure, and porphyria (especially acute intermittent, variegate, and porphyria cutanea tarda). The drug has rarely been implicated in causing exacerbations of lupus erythematosus or lupus-like syndromes.[23] Drug interactions include warfarin-type anticoagulants, barbiturates, and oral contraceptives, and in addition, a disulfiram-like reaction may occur with alcohol ingestion.

Terbinafine is an allylamine antifungal agent that has been demonstrated to be effective as therapy for tinea capitis. It is approved for onychomycosis and, as noted earlier, has been approved for treatment of tinea capitis in children 4 years of age and older (in the oral granule formulation). Comparative studies between terbinafine and griseofulvin have demonstrated that treatment with the former for 4 weeks is at least as effective as griseofulvin for 8 weeks.[24,25] In a comparison of terbinafine oral granules with griseofulvin oral suspension, the former resulted in greater rates of clinical cure and mycologic cure for patients infected with *T. tonsurans* (but not *M. canis*).[26] Meta-analyses of trials comparing griseofulvin to terbinafine have confirmed that the former is superior for infections caused by *M. canis*, whereas terbinafine may be superior for infections caused by *T. tonsurans*.[27,28] Studies have evaluated a variety of terbinafine treatment regimens and durations, including continuous therapy for 1 to 10 weeks (package recommendation for terbinafine granules: 6 weeks) and pulsed dosing, somewhat similar to that described for itraconazole (see later). Suggested dosing regimens for terbinafine include 3 to 6 mg/kg per day or a schedule based on patient weight. According to this schedule, the granules (which come in packets of either 125 mg or 187.5 mg) are dosed as follows: weight less than 25 kg: 125 mg/day; 25 to 35 kg: 187.5 mg/day; greater than 35 kg: 250 mg/day.[29] When the granules are used, they should be sprinkled onto nonacidic food such as mashed potatoes or pudding and swallowed without chewing.[30] Some authors have suggested that the weight-scheduled dosing may underdose individuals at the high end of the weight range. In a duration-finding study of terbinafine in the treatment of tinea capitis, a 2- or 4-week regimen was found to be clinically superior to a 1-week regimen.[31] If it is used, higher doses of terbinafine or a longer course of therapy may be necessary for *M. canis* infections.[32,33]

Oral terbinafine has an excellent safety profile overall and is the most commonly used systemic antifungal agent in Europe.[34] Side effects related to its use are rare and include GI symptoms, dizziness, headache, taste or smell disturbances, depression, and uncommonly, drug reactions (see Chapters 20 and 22). Elevated hepatic transaminases and cytopenias are occasionally seen, and some drugs, including cimetidine, terfenadine, and cyclosporine, may interact. Laboratory monitoring (complete blood cell count and liver enzymes) at baseline and during therapy is recommended by the FDA and some experts.

Ketoconazole, a broad-spectrum azole antifungal compound, has good activity against dermatophytes, especially *Trichophyton* species. However, given the potential risk of hepatotoxicity and the lack of a liquid formulation, this drug is not a favorable alternative to griseofulvin or terbinafine and is not recommended. Other azole antifungal agents such as fluconazole and itraconazole seem to offer more promise as alternative agents in the treatment of tinea capitis.

Fluconazole, which is approved for systemic mycoses as well as oral candidiasis in children ≥6 months, has been demonstrated effective in tinea capitis and may require a shorter treatment duration. It has an excellent safety profile, is usually well tolerated, and is available in a liquid suspension for children (10 and 40 mg/mL). Fluconazole has shown efficacy against both *Microsporum* and *Trichophyton* species. Most studies have evaluated dosing of 3 to 6 mg/kg per day for 2 to 4 weeks.[35–37] Once-weekly pulse dosing for 8 to 12 weeks has also been demonstrated effective.[38] In a prospective study of griseofulvin (25 mg/kg per day) versus fluconazole (6 mg/kg per day) for tinea capitis, clinical and mycologic cure rates were similar, and by day 21 of therapy, the majority of patients in both groups were deemed noncontagious via negative fungal culture.[39] Potential adverse effects of fluconazole include GI symptoms, headache, drug interactions, and drug reaction. Hematologic and hepatic toxicity may occasionally occur.

Itraconazole has been demonstrated to be effective in most tinea capitis studies. It is currently approved for onychomycosis and some systemic mycoses, and in studies has shown efficacy against both *Microsporum* and *Trichophyton* species. Itraconazole is available in a 100-mg capsule and a 10-mg/mL oral solution. Recommended dosing is 3 to 5 mg/kg per day, with the lower end of the dosing schedule utilized when the oral solution is used. Itraconazole is effective both in continuous dosing for 2 to 12 weeks and in a variety of pulsed dosing regimens. One such pulsed regimen consists of a daily dose for 1 week followed by repeat pulsing for 1 week given 2 weeks later, and a third pulse given 3 weeks after the second pulse.[40] In this regimen, the decision to administer the second or third pulse was determined by the response of the patient at that point in the therapy. Side effects of itraconazole therapy include headache, GI complaints, and occasional hepatic dysfunction. The oral solution seems to be associated with an increased incidence of GI side effects. Multiple drug interactions are possible, and hence all concomitantly ingested medications should be carefully referenced before considering itraconazole therapy.

An important consideration in the child with tinea capitis is school attendance and the issue of contagiousness. It is not practical to keep children with tinea capitis out of the classroom, because spore shedding may continue for months, even after adequate therapy.[41] Appropriate therapy should be instituted, and children receiving treatment should be allowed to attend school.[42] Measures should be taken, where feasible, to avoid transmission between susceptible hosts, including no sharing of combs, brushes, hats, or hooded jackets. Families should be questioned with regard to symptoms, with medical evaluation provided for suspected infection.[42] Haircuts, shaving of the head, or wearing a cap during treatment are unnecessary.

The treatment of kerion (also known as *kerion celsi*) deserves special mention. These markedly inflammatory reactions not uncommonly result in permanent scarring alopecia, and therefore rapid institution of aggressive therapy is indicated. In addition to antifungal therapy, systemic antibiotics should be considered, especially in the presence of significant crusting, because secondary bacterial infection may concomitantly occur. Skin swab for bacterial culture and sensitivity may be useful in this setting to guide the choice of antimicrobial. Oral corticosteroids are recommended by many in the treatment of kerions in a dose of 0.5 to 1 mg/kg per day for 2 to 4 weeks, although good controlled studies are lacking. Anecdotally, this approach seems to be associated with more rapid resolution of the inflammation and reduction of pain. However, some authors report excellent outcomes in patients with a kerion treated with antifungal therapy alone.[43]

Tinea Faciei

Dermatophyte infection of the face is referred to as *tinea faciei.* Although it often presents in a similar fashion to tinea corporis (see later) with annular, scaly plaques (Fig. 17.14), tinea faciei may sometimes be quite subtle clinically, especially if topical corticosteroids have been used. In some instances, when the classic annular configuration is absent or the changes are markedly inflammatory, it is referred to as *tinea incognito* (Figs. 17.15 and 17.16), which may also occur in nonfacial areas (Fig. 17.17). Tinea incognito typically occurs in patients who have received therapy with topical corticosteroids or calcineurin inhibitors.[44] Although localized mild tinea faciei may respond to topical antifungal therapy, systemic treatment (as described for tinea capitis) is often required to completely clear these lesions and minimize the rate of recurrence.

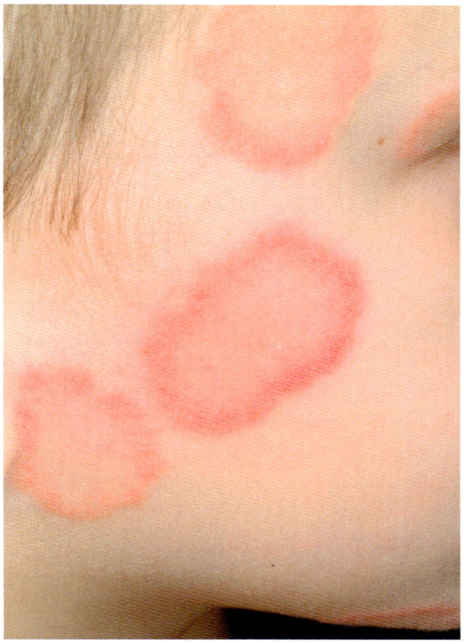

Fig. 17.14 Tinea faciei. Annular, erythematous scaly plaques of the face.

Tinea Barbae

Tinea barbae is an uncommon fungal infection of the bearded area and surrounding skin of adolescent and adult males. Because the most common etiologic agents are zoophilic species of *Trichophyton mentagrophytes* and *T. verrucosum* (occasionally *T. violaceum* and *Trichophyton rubrum*), it occurs primarily among individuals from rural areas in close contact with cattle or other domestic animals. Autoinoculation of *T. rubrum* from infected nails (onychomycosis) has been reported in association with tinea barbae.[45]

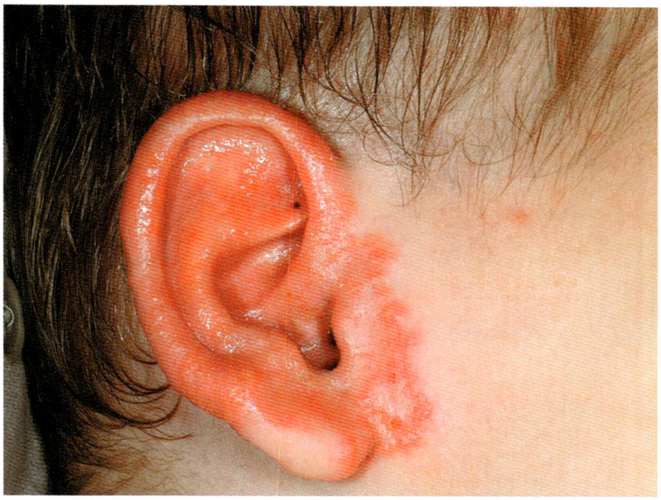

Fig. 17.15 Tinea faciei/incognito. This markedly inflamed ear had been treated with a variety of topical preparations (including topical corticosteroids, after which the annular border developed) before the diagnosis of tinea.

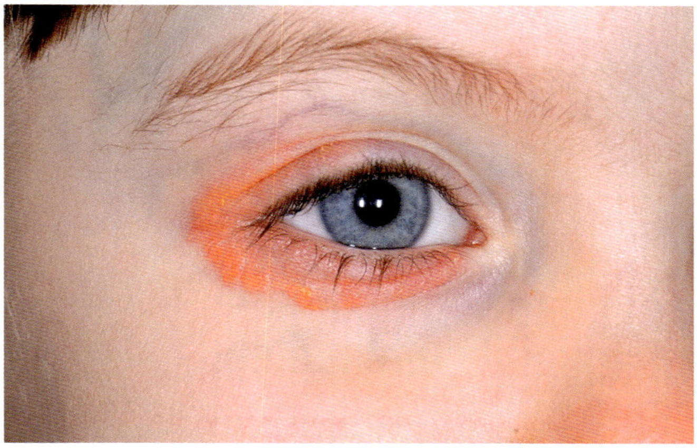

Fig. 17.16 Tinea faciei/incognito. This 2-year-old girl was treated with topical antibiotics and steroids before referral. Culture grew *Trichophyton tonsurans,* and the infection cleared with combined oral and topical antifungal therapy.

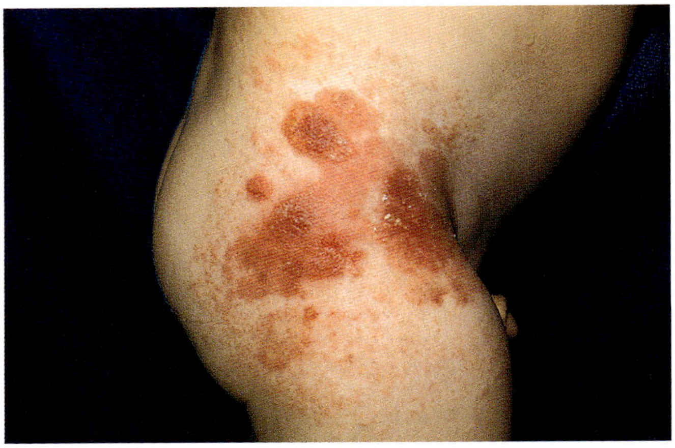

Fig. 17.17 Tinea incognito. This impressive dermatitis involving the diaper region ultimately cleared after systemic antifungal therapy. Fungal culture revealed *Trichophyton mentagrophytes*.

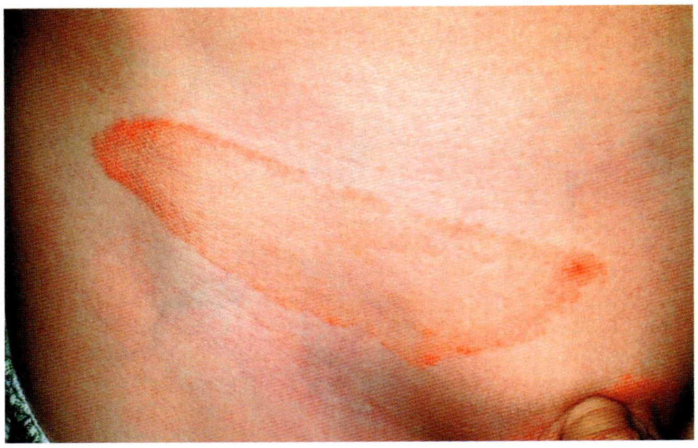

Fig. 17.18 Tinea corporis. An expanding, erythematous, annular plaque.

The infection is usually confined to one side of the face and may consist of a solitary lesion or multiple areas of involvement. The majority of infections are characterized by highly inflammatory purulent papules, pustules, exudate, crusting, and boggy nodules. The hairs within the infected areas are loose or absent, and pus may be expressed through the follicular openings. Spontaneous resolution may occur, or the lesions may persist for months with resultant alopecia and scar formation. Occasionally a less inflammatory superficial variety may occur, characterized by mild pustular folliculitis, erythematous patches with broken-off hairs, and a vesiculopustular border with central clearing similar to that seen in tinea corporis.

Tinea barbae must be differentiated from bacterial folliculitis of the bearded area (sycosis barbae), contact dermatitis, herpes zoster, or severe herpes simplex. Sycosis barbae is distinguished by the presence of papular and pustular lesions pierced in the center by a hair that is loose and easily extracted. Herpes simplex or herpes zoster usually presents with clusters of vesicles or erosions on an erythematous base, and the diagnosis is confirmed by polymerase chain reaction (PCR), direct fluorescent antibody examination, or viral culture. Tinea barbae can be confirmed by microscopic examination of a KOH wet mount of skin scrapings for fungal elements and/or fungal culture.

Treatment of tinea barbae consists of warm compresses (which help to remove crusts), topical or oral antibiotics for the common secondary bacterial infection, and the mainstay of therapy, an oral antifungal agent. With appropriate therapy, resolution occurs over 4 to 6 weeks.

Tinea Corporis

Superficial tinea infections of the skin are termed *tinea corporis*. Sites of predilection include the nonhairy areas of the face (particularly in children; see Tinea Faciei), the trunk, and extremities, with exclusion of ringworm of the scalp (tinea capitis), bearded areas (tinea barbae), groin (tinea cruris), hands (tinea manuum), feet (tinea pedis), and nails (onychomycosis). Contact with other individuals, such as is seen in high school and college wrestlers ("tinea corporis gladiatorum"), and domestic animals, particularly young kittens and puppies, is a common cause of the affliction in children. The causative organism in young children is often *M. canis* and occasionally *M. audouinii* or *T. mentagrophytes*. In older children and adults, *T. rubrum*, *T. verrucosum*, *T. mentagrophytes*, or *T. tonsurans* is more likely to be responsible. In children with infection caused by *T. rubrum* or *Epidermophyton floccosum*, parents with tinea infection (especially tinea pedis or onychomycosis) are commonly the source of infection. Tinea corporis caused by the zoophilic dermatophyte *T. equinum* has been reported after contact with horses during riding.[46]

Tinea corporis tends to be asymmetrically distributed and is characterized by one or more annular, sharply circumscribed scaly plaques with a clear center and a scaly, vesicular, papular, or pustular border (hence the term *ringworm*) (Figs. 17.18 and 17.19). When multiple

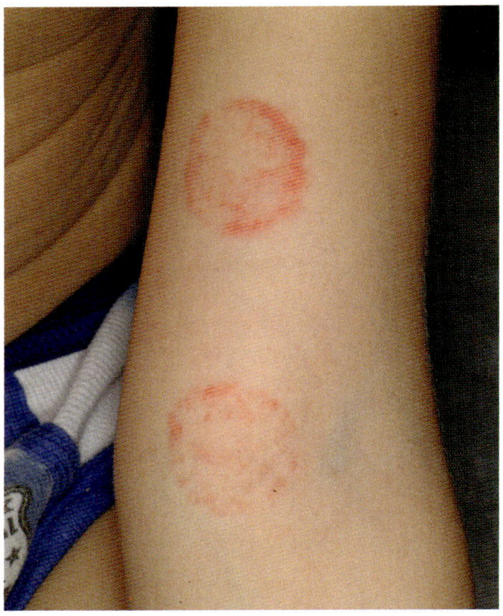

Fig. 17.19 Tinea corporis. Annular, erythematous, scaly plaques on the arm of a 4-year-old boy who also had tinea faciei.

lesions are present, they may become coalescent, resulting in bizarre polycyclic configurations (Fig. 17.20). Although tinea corporis may occur in people of all ages, it is most commonly seen in children, in individuals in warm humid climates, and in patients with systemic diseases such as diabetes mellitus, leukemia, or immunodeficiency. Although extensive tinea infection is considered a sign of possible immunodeficiency, it may also occur in otherwise-healthy, immunocompetent children (Fig. 17.21).

Tinea corporis commonly manifests as classic ringworm with annular, oval, or circinate lesions. The pattern, however, may be variable, and it may mimic a variety of other dermatoses, including the herald patch of pityriasis rosea, nummular eczema, psoriasis, contact dermatitis, seborrheic dermatitis, tinea versicolor, vitiligo, erythema migrans (Lyme disease), granuloma annulare, fixed drug eruption, and lupus erythematosus. The use of topical corticosteroids may mask the diagnosis by altering the presenting features while the infection persists. Presentations that may occur in this setting include tinea incognito (as described) and Majocchi granuloma. This perifollicular granulomatous disorder, which also occurs on the legs of women with tinea who shave, is a distinctive variant of ringworm and essentially represents a granulomatous folliculitis and perifolliculitis caused by *T. rubrum* or *T. mentagrophytes*. It presents with erythematous plaques or patches that reveal scattered papules, papulonodules, or pustules

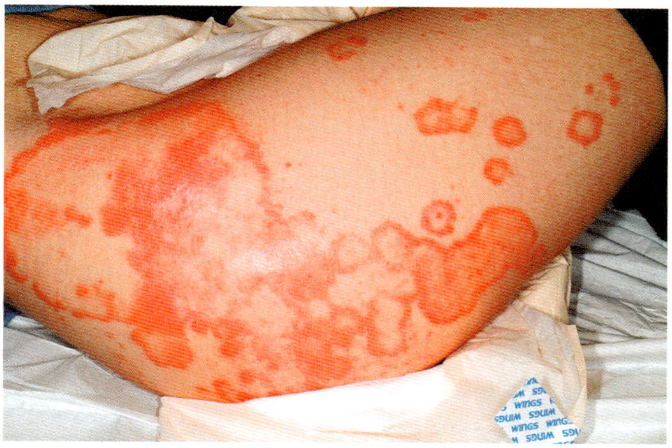

Fig. 17.20 Tinea corporis. Multiple annular erythematous plaques with confluence and a polycyclic configuration occurred in this immunocompromised patient.

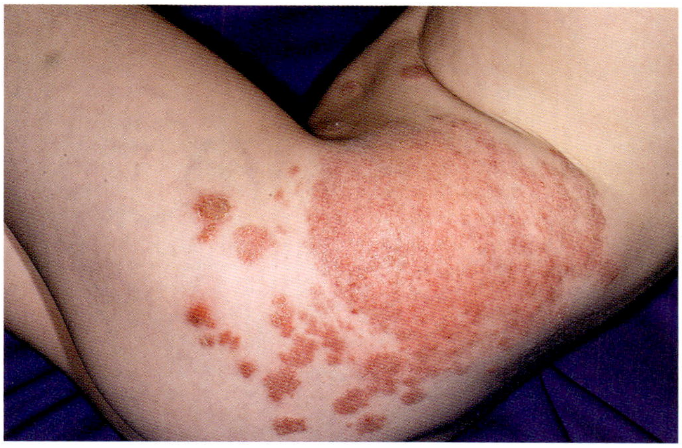

Fig. 17.21 Tinea corporis. Extensive involvement was noted in this otherwise healthy, immunocompetent 3-year-old girl. Culture revealed *Trichophyton mentagrophytes.*

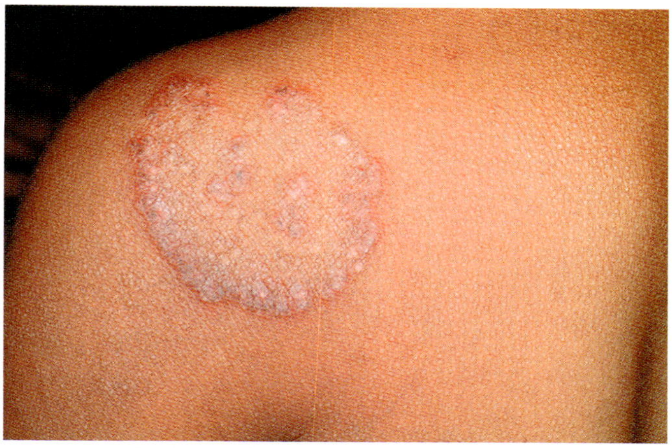

Fig. 17.22 Majocchi granuloma. This annular plaque developed follicular papules after treatment with topical corticosteroids.

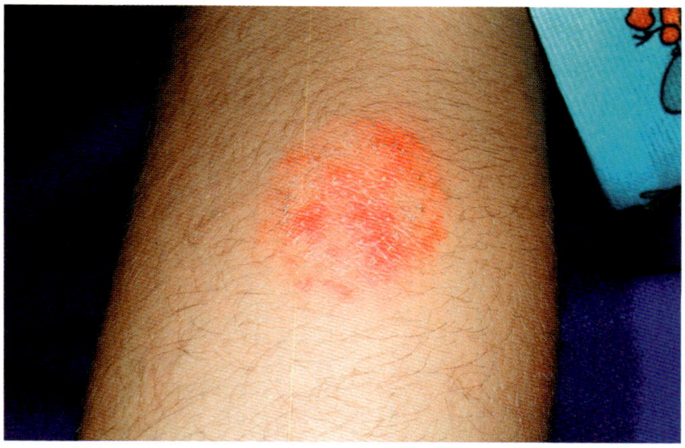

Fig. 17.23 Majocchi granuloma. An annular plaque studded with multiple small pustules. This lesion developed after treatment with topical corticosteroids.

studding the surface (Figs. 17.22, 17.23, and 17.24). If observed early in the course of the process, a hair may be noted in the center of the papular or pustular lesions.

Tinea corporis can often be diagnosed based upon the clinical presentation. Diagnostic examinations include KOH wet-mount examination of skin scrapings and fungal culture, as described earlier for tinea capitis. Wood lamp examination is usually not useful for diagnosing tinea corporis.

Confusion often exists among nondermatologists regarding the classification and management of cutaneous fungal infections. By definition, this term incorporates disorders caused by either dermatophytes or *Candida* infection. It must be recognized, however, that dermatophytes and *Candida* are not synonymous and that although nystatin is an effective agent against candidal infection, it is inappropriate and ineffective in the treatment of tinea (dermatophyte) infections. Conversely, some antifungal preparations that are active against dermatophytes, such as tolnaftate and terbinafine, seem to be minimally effective agents for treating candidal infections.

Topical antifungal therapy is generally effective for superficial or localized tinea corporis. These agents are usually applied twice daily, are well tolerated, and have very few side effects aside from occasional instances of irritant or allergic contact dermatitis. Table 17.2 lists some commonly used topical antifungal agents for dermatophyte infections.[47] Although clinical improvement and relief of pruritus may be seen within the first week of therapy, treatment should be continued for at least 2 to 3 weeks to ensure complete resolution.

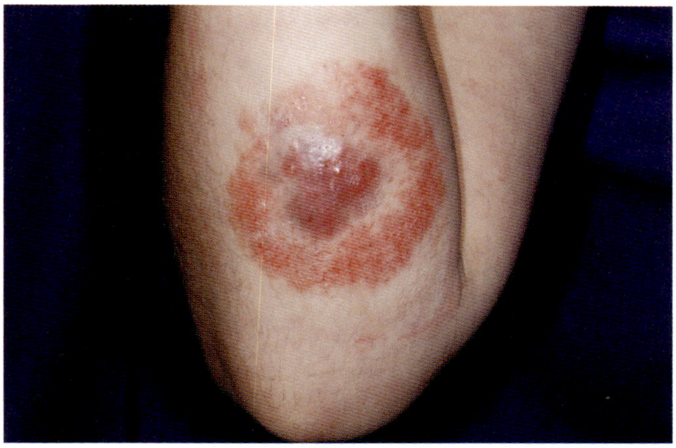

Fig. 17.24 Majocchi granuloma. This 7-year-old with type 1 diabetes mellitus developed this annular plaque with central fluctuance and pustules on his forearm, with progression after treatment with topical steroids. Culture revealed *Trichophyton mentagrophytes,* and the lesion cleared completely with topical and oral antifungal therapy.

Table 17.2 Some Commonly Used Topical Antifungal Agents for Tinea Infections

Generic Name	Trade Name (Select)	Type	OTC/Rx
Butenafine	Mentax, Lotrimin Ultra	C	Both
Ciclopirox	Loprox, Penlac	C, L, G, NL, Sh	Rx
Clotrimazole	Lotrimin, Mycelex, Desenex	C, L, S, P	Both
Econazole	Spectazole, Ecostatin	C	Rx
Efinaconazole	Jublia	S	Rx
Ketoconazole	Nizoral, Nizoral AD, Extina	C, Sh, F	Both
Miconazole	Monistat, Zeasorb AF, Micatin	C, L, P, S	OTC
Naftifine	Naftin	C, G	Rx
Oxiconazole	Oxistat, Oxizole	C, L	Rx
Sertaconazole	Ertaczo	C	Rx
Sulconazole	Exelderm	C, S	Rx
Tavaborole	Kerydin	S	Rx
Terbinafine	Lamisil	C, S	Both
Tolnaftate	Tinactin	C, G, P, S	OTC

Adapted from Carley C, Stratman EJ, Lesher JL, McConnell RC. Antimicrobial drugs. In: JL Bolognia, JV Schaffer, L Cerroni, et al., eds. Dermatology, 4th ed. London: Elsevier; 2018: 2215–41.

C, Cream; *F*, foam; *G*, gel; *L*, lotion; *NL*, nail lacquer; *OTC*, over-the-counter; *P*, powder; *Rx*, by prescription; *S*, solution; *Sh*, shampoo.

If a patient shows no clinical improvement after several weeks of therapy, the diagnosis should be reconsidered or, if confirmed and the patient has recalcitrant disease, a course of systemic therapy may be required. In certain situations, systemic antifungal therapy (similar to that described for tinea capitis) may be necessary from the start. These may include disseminated or severe disease, infection in an immunocompromised host, and Majocchi granuloma, in which case the depth of infection within the hair follicle requires the degree of penetration permitted only by a systemic agent.

Combination antifungal/corticosteroid preparations (i.e., 1% clotrimazole/0.05% betamethasone dipropionate) are widely used by nondermatologists in the treatment of superficial fungal infections, but care should be exercised with these products because their use may result in persistent or worsening infection.[48,49] In addition, some of these products contain a fairly potent corticosteroid, and hence their indiscriminate use can result in topical corticosteroid toxicities, including skin atrophy, telangiectasia, striae (Fig. 17.25), or systemic absorption. In some instances, such as severe tinea manuum or tinea pedis, such a combination product may be useful but should be applied for no longer than 2 to 4 weeks. This combination product should never be used in the diaper area, on the face, in fold areas, or under occlusion, and it is not recommended for children younger than 12 years of age.

Tinea corporis gladiatorum, which can affect an individual wrestler's ability to compete, as well as have an effect on entire wrestling squads, may require systemic therapy, especially when extensive. Many have advocated different approaches for prevention, although well-designed clinical trials have been minimal. In one study, 100 mg of oral fluconazole given once weekly resulted in a significantly decreased incidence of infection when compared with placebo.[50] In a prospective longitudinal study, 100 mg of fluconazole given once daily for 3 days before onset of the competitive wrestling season and again 6 weeks into the season led to a dramatic decrease in the incidence rate of tinea gladiatorum.[51]

Tinea Imbricata

Tinea imbricata (Tokelau), which is caused by *Trichophyton concentricum*, is a superficial dermatophyte infection seen primarily in tropical

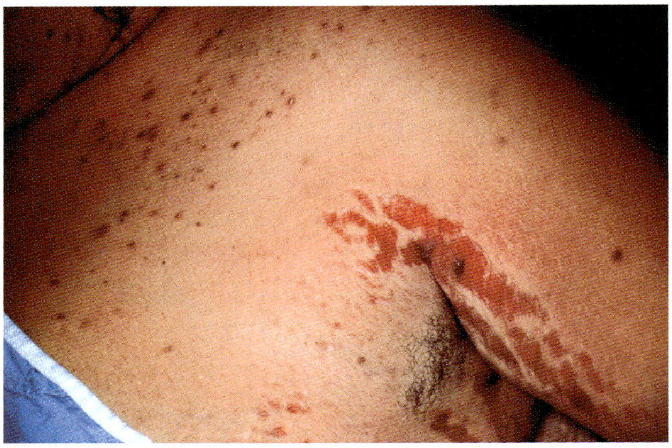

Fig. 17.25 Steroid-induced striae. These lesions developed in the axilla of this patient after long-term therapy with betamethasone dipropionate in combination with clotrimazole. (Courtesy Leonard Milstone, MD.)

regions of the Far East, South Pacific, South and Central America, and parts of Africa. It is characterized by concentric rings of scaling that form extensive patches with polycyclic borders (Fig. 17.26). With time, the lesions spread peripherally and form large plaques that may cover almost the entire skin surface, although the scalp, axillae, palms, and soles are usually spared. When fully developed, the concentric rings are seen as parallel lines of scales overlapping each other, resembling tiles or shingles (*imbrex* means "having overlapping edges," like a shingle) on a roof. Diagnosis is based on the characteristic clinical presentation, microscopic demonstration of interlacing septate hyphae, and identification of the organism by fungal culture. Although treatment with a systemic antifungal agent will usually clear the eruption within 2 to 4 weeks, there is a tendency for recurrence when treatment is discontinued. Susceptible individuals tend to carry the disease for their lifetime, given the difficulty in achieving a total cure.[52] Association with an underlying genetic or acquired immunodeficiency may be present in some affected individuals.[53]

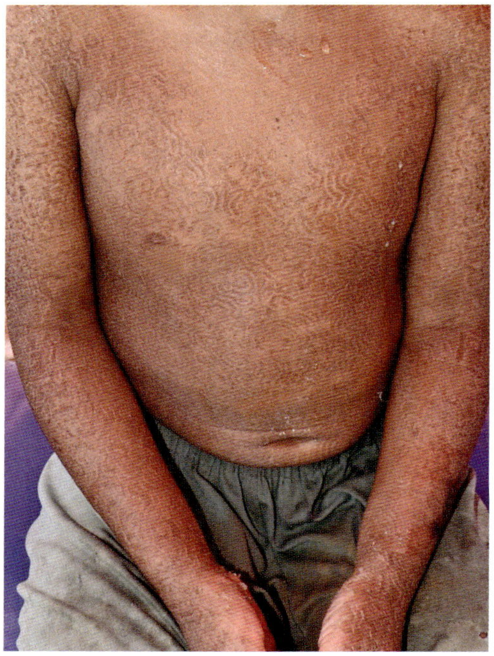

Fig. 17.26 Tinea imbricata. This 11-year-old boy from Malaysia presented with a 2-year history of generalized, concentric annular plaques on the anterior trunk and upper extremities. (Courtesy Leong Kin Fon, MBBS.)

Tinea Cruris

Tinea cruris ("jock itch") is an extremely common superficial fungal infection of the groin and upper thighs. It is seen primarily in male adolescents and adults and occurs less commonly in females. Tinea cruris is most symptomatic in hot, humid weather and is most commonly noted in obese individuals or those subject to vigorous physical activity and chafing. Tight-fitting clothing such as athletic supporters, jockey shorts, wet bathing suits, and panty hose may contribute to this condition as well. The three most common dermatophytes to result in tinea cruris are *E. floccosum*, *T. rubrum*, and *T. mentagrophytes*. Tinea pedis is a common coexisting condition, possibly related to autoinoculation of the dermatophyte with clothing that comes into contact with the feet.

Tinea cruris presents as sharply marginated, erythematous plaques with an elevated border of scaling, pustules, or vesicles. It is usually, but not always, bilaterally symmetric and involves the intertriginous folds near the scrotum, the upper inner thighs (Fig. 17.27), and occasionally the perianal regions, buttocks, and abdomen. The scrotum and labia majora are usually spared, and if they are involved or satellite papulopustules are present, the diagnosis of candidiasis (Fig. 17.28) should be considered. The lesions of tinea cruris may vary in color from red to brown, and central clearing may be present. In chronic infection, the redness and scaling may be slight, the active margin may be subtle or ill-defined, and lichenification may be present.

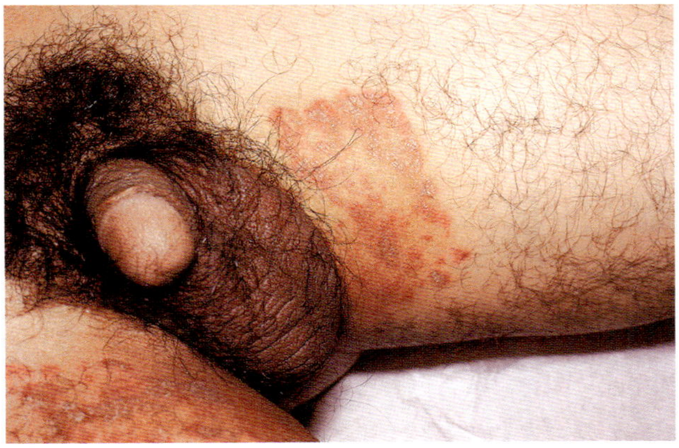

Fig. 17.27 Tinea cruris. Scaly, erythematous plaques involving the bilateral medial thighs.

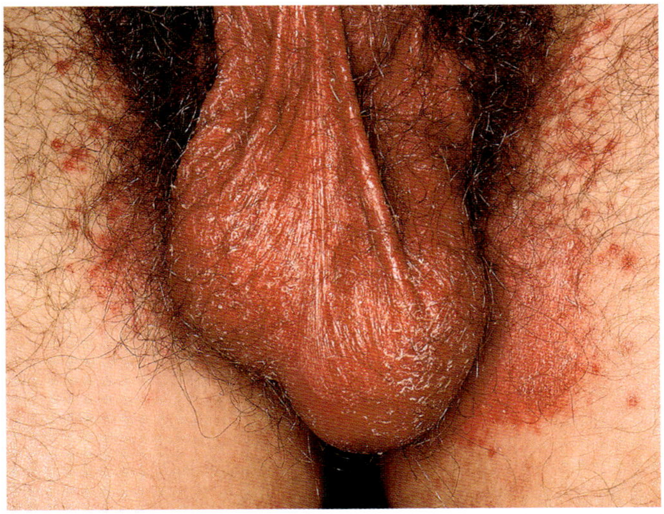

Fig. 17.28 Genital candidiasis. Erythema and scaling of the scrotum with involvement of the adjacent thigh regions. Note the associated satellite papules.

Tinea cruris must be differentiated from intertrigo, seborrheic dermatitis, psoriasis, irritant contact dermatitis, allergic contact dermatitis (generally resulting from therapy), or erythrasma (a superficial dermatosis caused by the diphtheroid *Corynebacterium minutissimum*). A characteristic coral-red fluorescence under Wood light examination is helpful in distinguishing erythrasma (see Chapter 14). The diagnosis of tinea cruris can be confirmed by a KOH wet-mount microscopic examination of cutaneous scrapings or by fungal culture.

Topical therapy (as discussed for tinea corporis) usually suffices for tinea cruris and is applied for 3 to 4 weeks. Other useful measures include reducing excessive chafing and irritation by the use of loose-fitting cotton underclothing, drying thoroughly after bathing or perspiration, and weight loss. The use of an absorbent antifungal powder (e.g., Micatin, Tinactin, or Zeasorb-AF) is sometimes helpful, and oral antifungal therapy is occasionally indicated for severe or recalcitrant disease. Tinea pedis, if present, should also be adequately treated as a preventive measure.

Tinea Pedis

Tinea pedis, or "athlete's foot," is relatively uncommon in young children but quite common in adolescents and adults, in whom it represents the most prevalent type of ringworm infection. Although children are not completely immune, most instances of athlete's foot in prepubertal individuals actually represent misdiagnosed cases of foot dermatitis, dyshidrotic eczema, contact dermatitis, or other dermatoses.[54,55] The differential diagnosis of tinea pedis also includes psoriasis, juvenile plantar dermatosis, erythrasma, and secondary syphilis. Associated conditions or complications include onychomycosis (see Tinea Unguium [Onychomycosis]), secondary bacterial superinfection, id reaction, and cellulitis. Untreated tinea pedis appears to be one of the most common risk factors for bacterial cellulitis of the lower extremities.[56] The three primary sources for acquisition of tinea pedis infections in children are families, schools, and swimming pools.[57]

The etiologic agents most often responsible for tinea pedis are *T. rubrum* and *T. mentagrophytes* and, less often, *E. floccosum* or (especially in children) *T. tonsurans*. The disorder may present clinically in a variety of different ways. The interdigital type, which is the most common presentation, reveals inflammation, scaling, and maceration in the toe-web spaces (Figs. 17.29 and 17.30), especially the lateral ones. The inflammatory or vesicular type shows inflammation with vesicles (Fig. 17.31) or larger bullae and usually results from *T. mentagrophytes* infection. This type occurs most often in summer, and an immune response to fungal elements may be reflected by a vesicular id eruption on the hands, extremities, and trunk. Moccasin-type tinea pedis presents with erythema, scaling, fissuring, and hyperkeratosis on the plantar surfaces, often extending to the lateral foot margins (Fig. 17.32). Contrary to the eruption seen in foot eczema, the dorsal aspects of the toes and feet are usually spared, although they may occasionally be involved (Fig. 17.33). This form may be more resistant to topical therapy, thus requiring an oral antifungal medication.

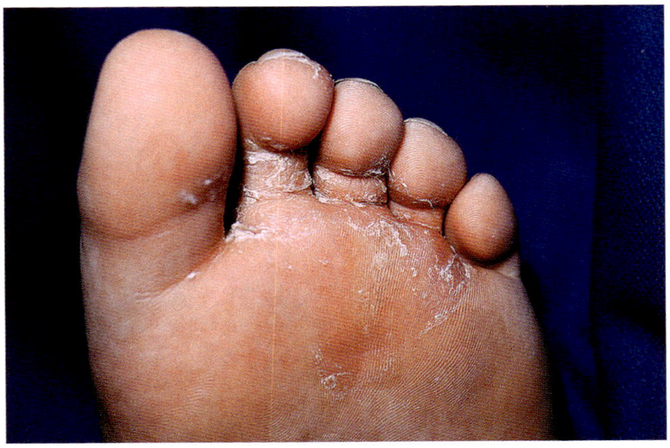

Fig. 17.29 Intertriginous tinea pedis. Scaling, erythema, and maceration of the plantar foot and toe-web spaces.

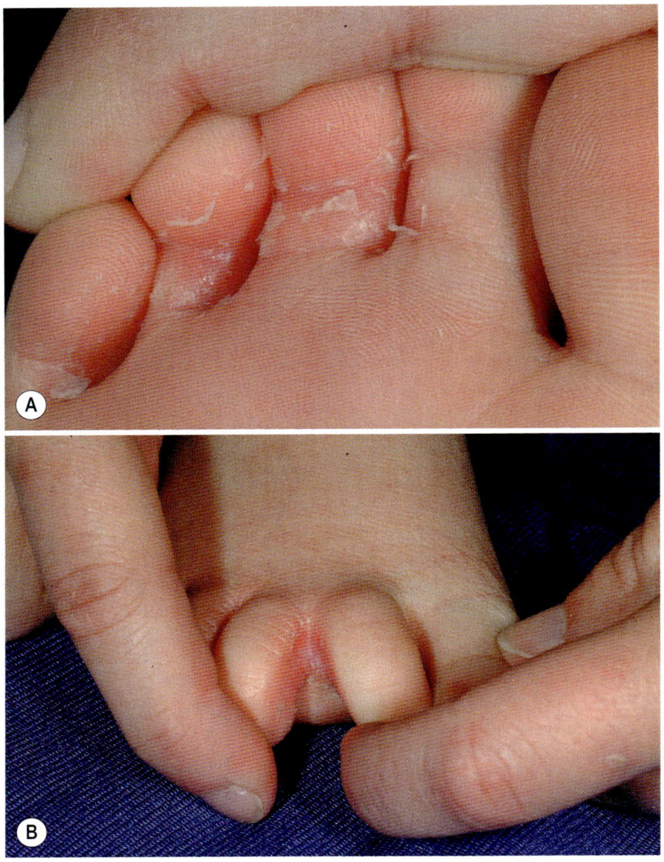

Fig. 17.30 Tinea pedis. This 6-year-old girl showed erythema and desquamation of the plantar foot and toes **(A)** and toe-web erythema and maceration **(B)**.

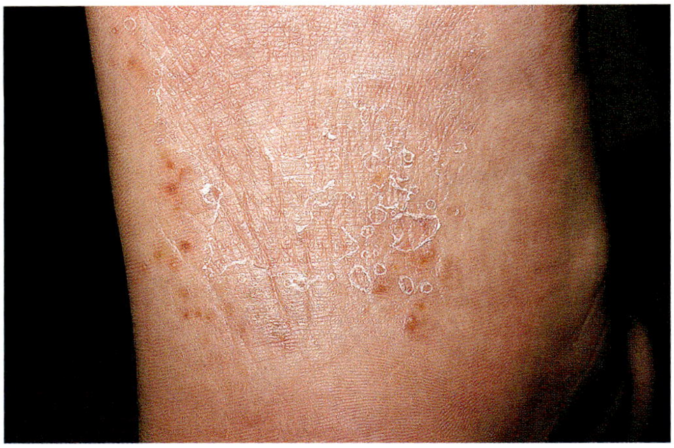

Fig. 17.31 Vesicular tinea pedis. Erythema and scaling are accompanied by intensely pruritic, deep-seated vesicles on the plantar surface.

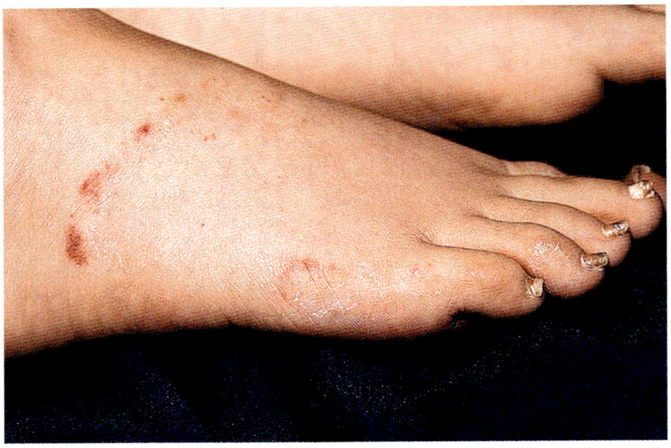

Fig. 17.32 Moccasin-type tinea pedis. Erythema and scaling with involvement of the lateral foot borders. Note the associated onychomycosis.

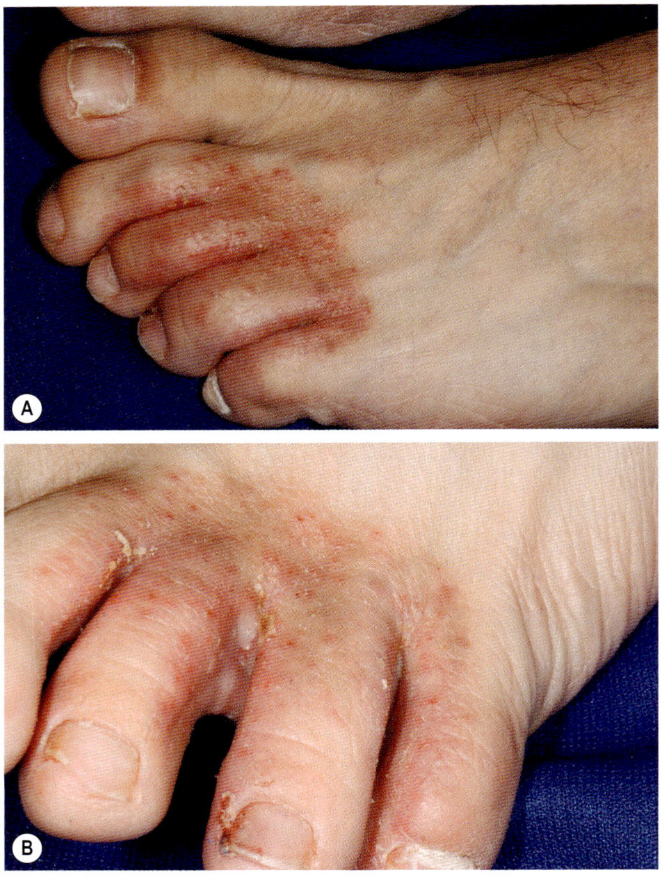

Fig. 17.33 Tinea pedis. Involvement of the dorsal surface of the foot **(A)** is occasionally noted, as shown in this 17-year-old male patient. Note the concomitant toe-web involvement **(B)**.

The diagnosis of tinea pedis is based upon the clinical picture, with confirmation by KOH examination and fungal culture when needed. Treatment may be challenging, and efforts to protect the feet from commonplace sites of exposure to the organisms (e.g., public showers, gyms, locker rooms, pool decking) and to keep the feet dry are both important. Such efforts might include thorough drying of the feet after bathing, avoidance of occlusive footwear or nonbreathable socks, and the use of sandals or other footwear in high-risk areas. Absorbent antifungal powders or sprays may be used once or twice daily in individuals prone to these infections, especially after physical exertion and bathing. Those prone to hyperhidrosis can use 6.25% to 20% aluminum chloride (i.e., Certain Dri, Drysol, Xerac AC), or in some cases oral anticholinergic agents such as glycopyrrolate (see Chapter 8), in an effort to decrease recurrent infection.

The usual treatment of choice for tinea pedis is a topical antifungal preparation applied twice daily. Acute vesicular lesions are best treated with wet compresses applied for 10 to 15 minutes two to four times daily in addition to the antifungal therapy. In patients with severely inflammatory disease or those with underlying chronic medical conditions such as diabetes or immunosuppression, oral antifungal therapy should be considered. The choices for oral therapy are similar to those discussed for tinea capitis, and a review of the literature suggests that terbinafine may be one of the more effective agents for this indication.[58]

In instances in which the diagnosis is indeterminate, a topical antifungal agent and a corticosteroid formulation may both be used for a short period (2 to 4 weeks), at which time a fungal culture performed at the initiation of therapy can generally confirm or refute the diagnosis of tinea. If the diagnosis of tinea pedis is confirmed, the topical corticosteroid can be discontinued. Moccasin-type tinea pedis may require the addition of a keratolytic agent (i.e., lactic acid or urea) in addition to the antifungal to treat the hyperkeratosis and accentuate penetration of the antimicrobial. Id reactions, when present, are best treated with topical corticosteroids and oral antihistamines (if needed) and generally improve with eradication of the primary infection.

Tinea Manuum

Ringworm infection of the palmar hand (tinea manuum) is uncommon in childhood and when present is generally seen in postpubertal individuals. When ringworm occurs on the dorsum of the hand, it is referred to as *tinea corporis* rather than *tinea manuum*. Tinea manuum is usually unilateral and is caused by the same fungi responsible for tinea pedis: *T. rubrum*, *T. mentagrophytes*, and *E. floccosum*. It may be seen in association with tinea pedis, and when occurring on only one hand presents in a fashion that has been termed *two-foot, one-hand syndrome*.

Clinical manifestations include a diffuse hyperkeratosis of the fingers and palm and a less common patchy inflammatory or vesicular reaction (Fig. 17.34). Involvement of the fingernails (onychomycosis, see later) commonly occurs and may be a clue to the diagnosis. When onychomycosis is present, it usually involves some, but not all, of the nails on the affected hand. Total nail involvement, if present, should suggest the possible diagnoses of psoriasis or lichen planus. The differential diagnosis of tinea manuum includes psoriasis, allergic or irritant contact dermatitis, dyshidrosis, and an id reaction. Unilateral involvement may be another clue to the diagnosis, which can be confirmed by KOH microscopic examination or fungal culture.

The management of tinea manuum is essentially the same as that recommended for tinea pedis, and when the latter infection is simultaneously present, it should be appropriately treated as well.

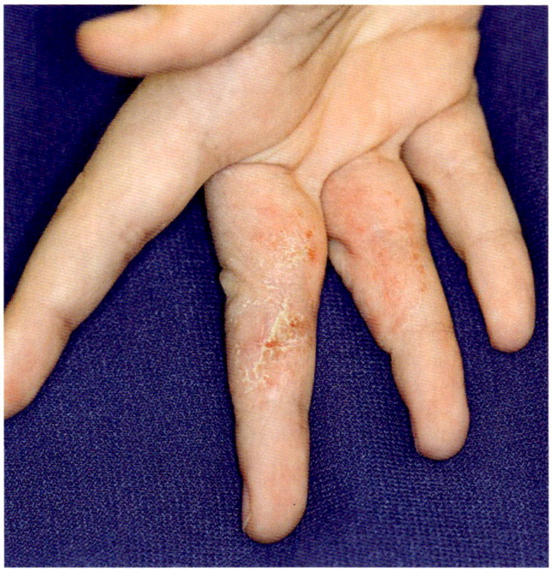

Fig. 17.34 Tinea manuum. Vesicles, erythema, and scaling on the palmar fingers of a 10-year-old girl who also had bilateral tinea pedis.

Tinea Unguium (Onychomycosis)

Onychomycosis is a general term that refers to a fungal infection of the fingernails or toenails. *Tinea unguium* is a term that specifically implies dermatophyte infection of the nails. However, the two terminologies are often used interchangeably in clinical practice, and for the purposes of the discussion, *onychomycosis* will refer to dermatophyte nail infections caused usually by *T. rubrum*, *T. mentagrophytes*, *T. tonsurans*, and *E. floccosum*. Periungual infection caused by *Candida albicans* is discussed in the section on candidiasis. Onychomycosis is more common in adults, although it does occur in children, often in association with tinea pedis or tinea manuum but also as a primary infection. The overall prevalence of onychomycosis in children has been estimated to be between 0% and 2.6%.[59,60] The lower incidence in children has been attributed to faster nail growth, smaller surface area for invasion, less nail trauma, lower incidence of tinea pedis, and less time spent in environments prone to infected fomites such as locker rooms.[61] The majority of prepubertal children with onychomycosis have a first-degree relative with onychomycosis and/or tinea pedis. Pediatric onychomycosis affects the toenails in two-thirds of patients and the fingernails in one-third[62]; it tends to be more common in children with Down syndrome (of whom >50% may have onychomycosis) and immunodeficiencies (e.g., human immunodeficiency virus [HIV] infection), although children being treated with chemotherapy for malignancy do not appear to have a higher frequency.[63–65]

Onychomycosis is classified into several different patterns, including distal lateral subungual, proximal subungual, white superficial, endonyx, and total dystrophic. The distal subungual type is the most common and is characterized by invasion of the underlying nailbed and inferior portion of the nail plate, which leads to onycholysis (detachment of the nail plate from the nailbed) and thickening of the subungual region, which takes on a discolored yellow-brown appearance[66] (Figs. 17.35 and 17.36). Proximal subungual onychomycosis is relatively uncommon and occurs when the invasion of the nail unit starts at the proximal nailfold (the area near the cuticle). Clinically, destruction of the proximal nail plate is seen along with similar changes to the distal subungual type (Fig. 17.37). This form of onychomycosis is most common in individuals infected with HIV, and it is considered by some to be an early marker for this infection. White superficial onychomycosis occurs with superficial infection of the nail plate and presents as well-delineated white plaques on the dorsal nail plate. Endonyx onychomycosis is notable for nail pigmentation, pitting, and transverse grooves, whereas the total dystrophic form is a severe and rare variant in children.

The diagnosis of onychomycosis is confirmed by direct microscopy of KOH wet-mount preparations and fungal culture. Material for examination should be taken from the subungual debris, underside of the nail plate, nail clippings, or nailbed when necessary. Confirmation of the diagnosis is important, because many cases of nail dystrophy

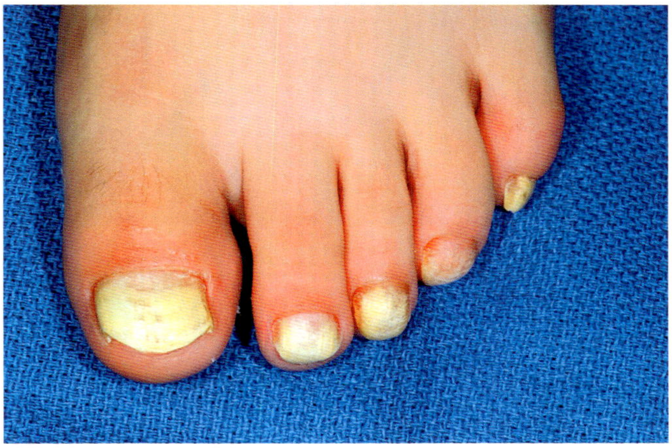

Fig. 17.35 Onychomycosis, distal subungual type. Yellow-white discoloration and thickening with the distal nail surfaces most involved.

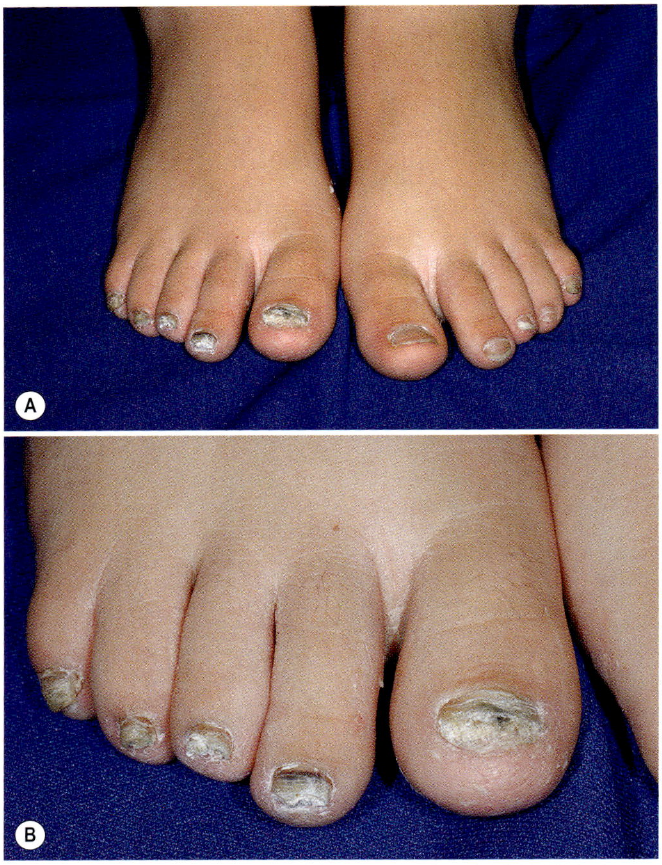

Fig. 17.36 Onychomycosis, distal subungual type. **(A)** Diffuse involvement of the right foot with partial involvement of the left foot was present in this 14-year-old girl with Down syndrome. **(B)** Note the marked subungual debris and nail plate destruction. Culture revealed *Trichophyton tonsurans*, a less common cause of onychomycosis.

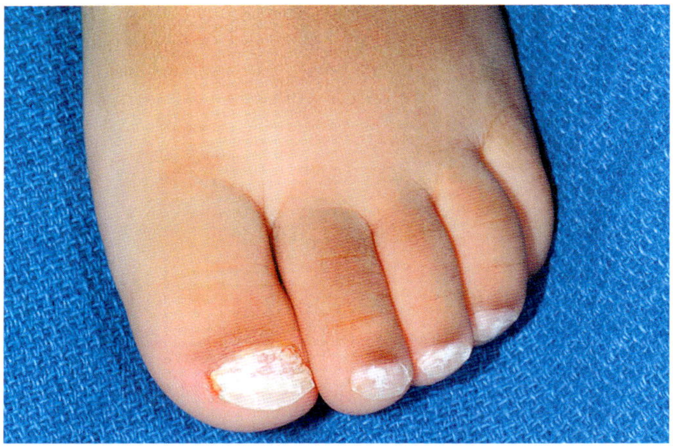

Fig. 17.37 Onychomycosis, proximal subungual type. White discoloration of the nail plate with the process originating at the proximal nailfold regions.

are not fungal in origin and are instead the result of another diagnosis such as psoriasis, postdermatitis onychodystrophy, chronic paronychia, trauma, drug-induced onycholysis, pachyonychia congenita, lichen planus, or a variety of other conditions (see Chapter 7). It must be remembered that onychomycosis is seldom symmetrical and that it is common to find involvement of only one, two, or three nails of only one hand or foot. In patients who have involvement of all nails, an alternative diagnosis should be highly suspected. In children diagnosed with onychomycosis, a search for other concomitant mycoses (especially tinea pedis and tinea capitis) should be completed.[67] Importantly, other close contacts with onychomycosis or tinea pedis should also be treated in an effort to end the cycle of transmission.

In general, topical agents have been traditionally viewed as minimally effective for the treatment of onychomycosis, in large part because of poor penetration through the nail plate. Topical antifungal therapy, however, is an important consideration as adjunctive therapy when tinea pedis is concomitantly present, in which case it may lower the relapse rate for onychomycosis, and may be an increasingly reasonable consideration for monotherapy of pediatric onychomycosis as newer medications and formulations become available. Ciclopirox 8% nail lacquer solution, approved for onychomycosis for 12 years of age and older, has shown promise as an effective topical agent, occasionally as monotherapy or more commonly as an adjunctive treatment.[68,69] In a randomized prospective study of 40 children with onychomycosis treated with ciclopirox monotherapy over 32 weeks, mycologic cure was achieved in 77%.[70] Tavaborole 5% solution has recently been approved for onychomycosis in children 6 years and older, and efinaconazole 10% solution is approved for adult onychomycosis and has been used by some in an off-label fashion for treating children with the infection. One drawback of topical antifungal therapy is the long treatment times required, often 6 to 12 months.

Definitive therapy for onychomycosis in many patients is best achieved with the use of oral antifungal agents. When considering therapy for this condition in children, many factors need to be incorporated into the equation, including the results of diagnostic studies, severity of the infection, age of the patient, and the risk-to-benefit ratios of the treatments being considered. Parents of younger children should be given the appropriate information regarding therapy and be allowed to make an informed decision. In many instances, a trial of topical therapy with further consideration of systemic therapy if needed down the road may be a desirable option for parents. A systematic review of published studies on systemic therapy for pediatric onychomycosis revealed cure rates of 70% to 80%, similar to that seen in adults, and good safety profiles.[71]

Griseofulvin was traditionally the treatment of choice for systemic therapy of onychomycosis. However, this agent requires long-term administration and is associated with low cure rates and high relapse rates. Newer antifungal agents, including fluconazole, itraconazole, and terbinafine, are effective therapies for this condition, and the latter two medications are FDA approved for this indication in adults. All of these agents have high affinity for keratin, another advantage over griseofulvin, and all remain concentrated in the nails for months after discontinuation of therapy.[66] In addition, they seem to result in much lower relapse rates.

The newer antifungal agents, none of which are FDA approved for pediatric onychomycosis, have been dosed in a variety of fashions in studies. Fluconazole has usually been given as a weekly dose (3 to 6 mg/kg) but may require 12 to 26 weeks (or longer) of treatment. It is not recommended as first-line therapy, given the better efficacy of itraconazole and terbinafine.[72] These agents appear to be quite effective with a more convenient dosing regimen. Itraconazole pulse therapy (given twice daily for 1 week/month for 3 to 4 months) is a preferred strategy in adults with onychomycosis, although it has also been used as continuous therapy for this indication. The pulsed dosing approach has been studied in pediatric patients and appears to be effective and relatively safe,[61,73] although adequately randomized trials are lacking. Terbinafine has demonstrated significant effectiveness in the treatment of onychomycosis. This agent is usually given as a daily dose for 6 (fingernails) to 12 (toenails) weeks, and several studies have suggested superior efficacy and cost-effectiveness over the other antifungal drugs.[74–76] The often-recommended weight-based daily dosing of terbinafine for children is 62.5 mg for those weighing less than 20 kg, 125 mg for those weighing 20 to 40 kg, and 250 mg (full tablet) for those weighing more than 40 kg. The low-end dose (62.5 mg) is most feasibly accomplished by giving one half-tablet every other day. Although there is no uniform recommendation regarding laboratory monitoring (i.e., complete blood cell counts and liver function studies) in pediatric patients treated for onychomycosis with terbinafine or itraconazole, many clinicians perform baseline evaluations (and occasionally intermittent tests during therapy). Teenagers who are being treated should be reminded to refrain from drinking alcohol during therapy.[72] In a retrospective study of 269 children treated with oral terbinafine for onychomycosis, grade 1 laboratory abnormalities were seen in just 4.2% (of those who had laboratory testing performed) during therapy.[77]

TINEA VERSICOLOR

Tinea versicolor (pityriasis versicolor) is an extremely common superficial fungal disorder of the skin characterized by multiple scaling, oval macules, patches, and thin plaques distributed over the upper portions of the trunk, proximal arms, and occasionally the neck or face. It is caused by the yeast forms of the dimorphic fungus *Malassezia furfur*, which are referred to as *Pityrosporum orbiculare* and *Pityrosporum ovale*. This organism is part of the normal cutaneous flora. The disorder occurs worldwide, and the majority of cases present in adolescents, possibly in relation to the lipophilic nature of the organism and the sebum-rich environment of the affected regions. Tinea versicolor only occasionally occurs in prepubertal children. Although *Malassezia* is part of the normal flora, in immunocompromised hosts this yeast may be associated with opportunistic infections, including catheter-related fungemia, peritonitis, septic arthritis, pulmonary infection, and sinusitis.[78]

The diagnosis is usually made clinically based on the characteristic presentation. Lesions may be most appreciated during summer months when sun exposure leads to increasing discrepancies in skin pigmentation between affected and unaffected areas. Examination reveals thin, scaly papules and plaques distributed on the chest, back (Fig. 17.38), and less commonly on the face and neck (Fig. 17.39). They may be hypopigmented or hyperpigmented (Fig. 17.40) depending on the patient's complexion and history of sun exposure, and sometimes mild erythema is present. Scalloping of the borders is common, and lesions may be so numerous that they coalesce into larger patches. Lower extremities and genitals are rare sites of involvement. A rare variant, termed *atrophying pityriasis versicolor*, presents with similar hyperpigmented or hypopigmented lesions with associated atrophy, which in most cases appears to be reversible.[79] Interestingly, azelaic acid is a dicarboxylic acid produced by *M. furfur* that inhibits the dopa–tyrosinase reaction, which may result in the hypopigmentation seen in this disorder. This acid is marketed as an acne therapy product for acne-induced hyperpigmentation (see Chapter 8).

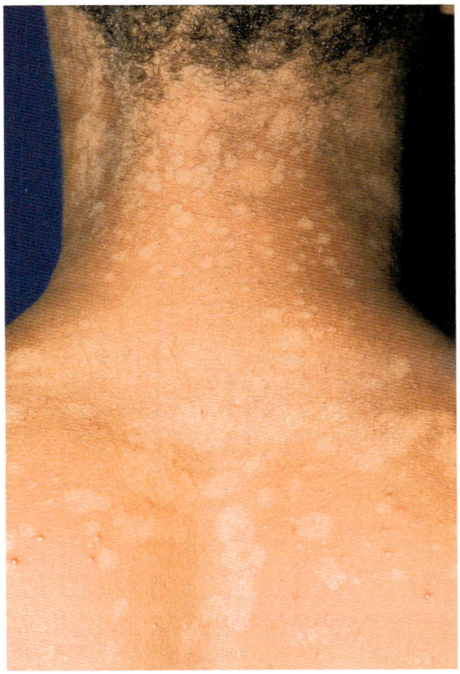

Fig. 17.38 Tinea versicolor. Hypopigmented, minimally scaly macules and patches of seborrheic areas of the trunk.

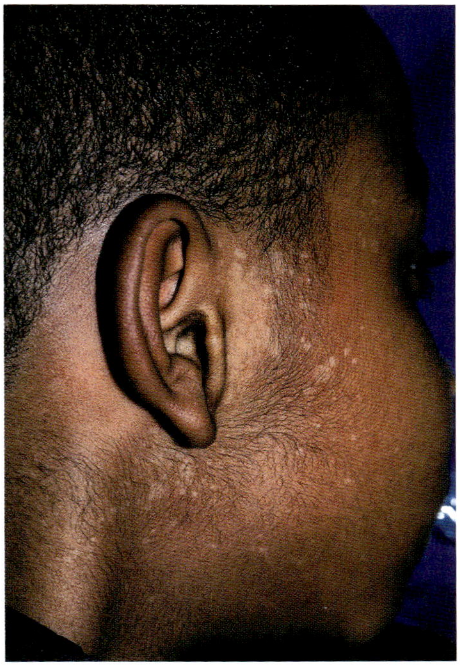

Fig. 17.39 Tinea versicolor. Occasional involvement of the face and/or neck is noted, especially in darkly pigmented individuals.

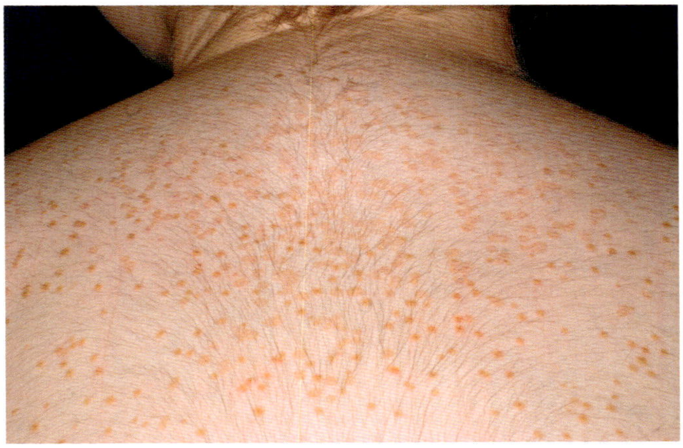

Fig. 17.40 Tinea versicolor. This immunosuppressed teenager with inflammatory bowel disease had hyperpigmented (rather than hypopigmented) scaly papules and plaques.

The differential diagnosis of tinea versicolor includes vitiligo, pityriasis alba, postinflammatory hypopigmentation or hyperpigmentation, pityriasis rosea, tinea, psoriasis, and confluent and reticulate papillomatosis of Gougerot and Carteaud (see Chapter 23). Distinguishing clinical features are usually sufficient to differentiate these various conditions. Vitiligo presents with depigmentation rather than hypopigmentation, with well-demarcated patches most often localized around orifices and bony prominences. Pityriasis alba presents with hypopigmented patches, but these lesions are usually limited to the face, occur in atopic individuals, and are only rarely as extensive as one would expect for tinea versicolor. The diagnosis can be confirmed by a KOH wet-mount of cutaneous scrapings, which reveals the highly characteristic short fungal hyphae and spores in grape-like clusters (the "spaghetti-and-meatballs" pattern) (Fig. 17.41) on microscopic examination. Fungal culture is generally not useful, because the organism is difficult to grow on culture media and *M. furfur* is part of the normal skin flora.

The treatment options for tinea versicolor are many, although better randomized, placebo-controlled prospective clinical trials investigating their efficacy and safety are needed.[80] Tinea versicolor may respond to a variety of topical preparations. However, because the course of the disorder is usually chronic, recurrences are common, and the pigmentary changes may take months to years to revert; adequate patient education and setting appropriate expectations are vital. Selenium sulfide 2.5% shampoo is a convenient, inexpensive, safe, and relatively effective mode of therapy, especially for younger patients. It is applied in a thin layer daily for 10 minutes before rinsing for 1 to 2 weeks. Less frequent intermittent applications (i.e., every other week or monthly) are then useful for maintenance. Ketoconazole 2% shampoo has also been recommended and was shown effective when applied as a single application or daily for 3 days.[81] Terbinafine 1% spray is applied once to twice daily for 1 to 2 weeks. Topical antifungal creams are also effective, but their use is often impractical, given the wide surface area of skin usually involved.

Oral therapy is desirable in patients with severe disease or recurrent disease or in those in whom topical therapies have failed. A variety of oral antifungal agents, including ketoconazole, fluconazole, itraconazole, and terbinafine, have been proposed for this condition. Multiple dosing regimens have been advocated, including continuous, intermittent, and single-dose approaches. A favorite systemic regimen for tinea versicolor is single-dose (400 mg) ketoconazole followed by physical activity to promote secretion of the drug onto the skin via sweating. The patient then delays showering or rinsing for 10 to 12 hours and repeats the therapy in 1 week. In recent years, however, the FDA has recommended against ketoconazole as a first-line antifungal therapy, given concerns over potentially severe liver toxicity.

Itraconazole single-dose therapy (400 mg) was compared with a 7-day continuous therapy (200 mg daily dose), and both regimens were found to be equally effective.[82,83] In another randomized prospective study, single- and multiple-dose regimens of ketoconazole and fluconazole were compared, and single-dose (400 mg) oral fluconazole provided the best clinical and mycologic cure rates with no relapse during 12 months of follow-up study.[84] In a study of extensive tinea versicolor, single-dose ketoconazole (400 mg) was compared with two doses of fluconazole (300 mg) with a 2-week interval between doses. Similar clinical response was noted in both groups (81.5% improvement for fluconazole, 87.9% for ketoconazole) with no significant adverse events in either group.[85] Based on a systematic review of systemic therapies for the condition, Gupta and colleagues recommended 200 mg/day of itraconazole for 5 to 7 days or 300 mg/week of fluconazole for 2 weeks.[86]

There is no current consensus or gold standard of care for systemic therapy of tinea versicolor. If an imidazole antifungal agent is used, however, the potential for drug interactions (especially with itraconazole and ketoconazole), liver toxicity (itraconazole and ketoconazole), congestive heart failure (itraconazole), and other side effects must always be considered and discussed with the patient and/or parent.

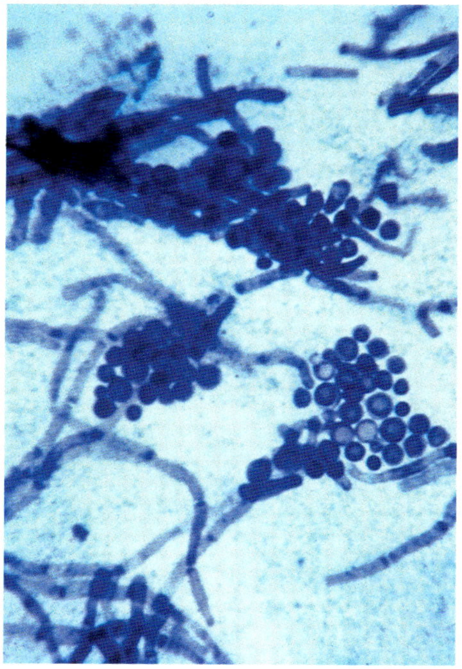

Fig. 17.41 KOH preparation of tinea versicolor. Short, blunt-ended hyphae and clusters of spores are present in the classic "spaghetti-and-meatballs" pattern in scrapings from a patient with tinea versicolor.

TINEA NIGRA

Tinea nigra is a superficial fungal infection of the stratum corneum caused by the black yeast-like mold *Phaeoannellomyces* or *Hortaea werneckii* (formerly called *Cladosporium* or *Exophiala werneckii*). Because it is not caused by a dermatophyte fungus, *tinea* (as with tinea versicolor) is a misnomer. This infection occurs most often in warm humid areas of Central or South America, Africa, Asia, and occasionally the coastal southern United States. It presents as an asymptomatic, light to dark brown or black, sharply marginated macule or patch, usually involving the palm and less likely the dorsal surface of the hand or plantar foot. Visible scaling is rare. The most important aspect of tinea nigra is the potential misdiagnosis as malignant melanoma. Other misdiagnoses may include postinflammatory hyperpigmentation, fixed drug eruption, or chemical stain.[87] Direct microscopic examination of a KOH wet-mount preparation of skin scrapings reveals gray-brown to green hyphae and budding yeast cells, and fungal culture is confirmatory. Dermoscopy, if performed, reveals a brown, fine-dotted granular appearance overlapping an amorphous light brown patch or spicules in a reticular linear pattern.[88,89] Tinea nigra is treated with a topical antifungal preparation such as miconazole, clotrimazole, or terbinafine cream. The application of keratolytic agents such as salicylic acid or Whitfield ointment (6% benzoic acid and 3% salicylic acid) or 10% thiabendazole solution are other therapeutic options.

PIEDRA

Piedra is an asymptomatic fungal infection of the hair shaft caused by *Piedraia hortae* (black piedra) or various *Trichosporon* species (formerly known as *Trichosporon beigelii*; white piedra). The species that most commonly cause white piedra are *Trichosporon inkin*, *Trichosporon cutaneum*, and *Trichosporon ovoides*.[90,91]

Black piedra is seen most commonly in tropical areas of South America, the Far East, and the Pacific Islands. It is characterized by small, hard, and adherent brown-black nodules on the hair shafts of the scalp, which on hair microscopy are composed of honeycomb-like masses of fungal asci and ascospores. These nodules contain phosphorus, sulfur, and calcium, which are all part of the extracellular material involved in the organization of the fungus.[92] Fungal culture usually confirms the diagnosis. Traditional therapy consists of hair removal by clipping or shaving, and oral terbinafine may be useful.[93]

White piedra is seen in temperate climates of South America, Europe, Asia, Australia, and the southern United States. It may affect the scalp as well as eyelash, eyebrow, beard, axillary, or pubic hair. Traditional burkha-clad Muslim women may be predisposed to this condition.[94] White piedra may be underreported in the United States, with recent reports in children from the northeastern states, several of whom were immigrants. This observation suggests that cases in the United States may be primarily imported and hence influenced by immigration trends.[95] It is characterized by asymptomatic, soft, white-tan elongated nodules on the hair shaft that may be mistaken for the nits of head louse infestation or hair casts. Additionally, the differential diagnosis may include monilethrix and trichorrhexis nodosa. Microscopic examination of a hair mount reveals yeast-like cells completely encircling the hair shaft and occasional hyphae perpendicular to the hair shaft. The organism can be recovered from a fungal culture. Again, clipping or shaving the hair is usually curative. Oral itraconazole and fluconazole have been demonstrated effective in open-label studies, but recurrence may be noted.[94,95] Concomitant use of an azole (i.e., ketoconazole) shampoo has been advocated as adjunctive therapy, and topical antifungal creams have also been used.

Although the etiologic agent of white piedra usually results in this benign hair condition, disseminated infection may occur in immunocompromised hosts, especially those with hematologic malignancies, history of organ transplantation, neutropenia, and HIV infection.[96–98] Low-birthweight neonates are another population at risk for fungal septicemia with this organism.[99] Cutaneous lesions may occur with disseminated disease and consist of purpuric papules, nodules, ulceration, and necrosis. Infection may also involve the lung, liver, heart, brain, and urinary tract. Therapy of *Trichosporon* sepsis/multiorgan dissemination is difficult, because many isolates are resistant to amphotericin B and echinocandins, and the mortality rate is high. Voriconazole has been suggested as the best treatment option.[100]

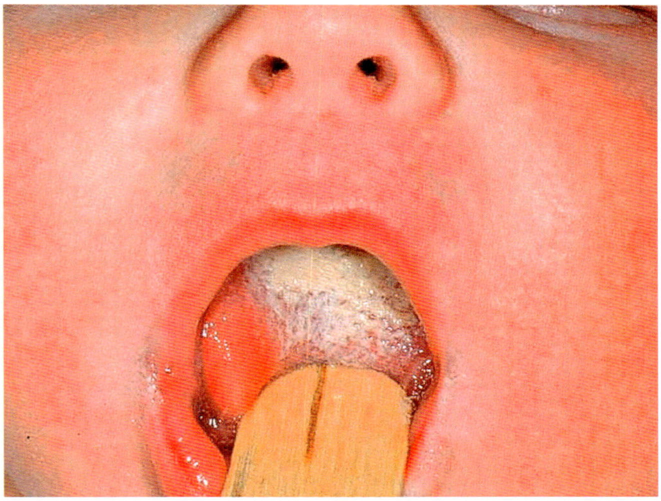

Fig. 17.42 Oral candidiasis. White, friable plaques on the dorsal tongue of an otherwise healthy infant girl.

Candidiasis

Candidiasis (moniliasis) is an acute or chronic infection of the skin, mucous membranes, and occasionally internal organs caused by yeast-like fungi of the *Candida* genus. Although several candidal species may be associated with human infection, *C. albicans* is by far the most common cause. *C. albicans* is not a normal cutaneous saprophyte but usually exists in the microflora of the oral cavity, GI tract, and vagina. It becomes a cutaneous pathogen when there is an alteration in host defenses, either localized or generalized, that allows the organism to become invasive.

Factors that predispose to candidiasis include endocrinologic disorders (e.g., diabetes mellitus, hypoparathyroidism, and Addison disease), genetic disorders (e.g., Down syndrome, acrodermatitis enteropathica, and chronic mucocutaneous candidiasis [CMC]), malignancy (especially leukemia or lymphoma), and certain systemic medications (e.g., antibiotics, corticosteroids, and immunosuppressive agents).

Newborns and infants are physiologically susceptible to candidal infection, which may be commonly manifested as oral candidiasis (thrush), diaper candidiasis, or intertrigo. Other presentations of candidal infection in childhood include vulvovaginitis, angular cheilitis (perlèche), and nail involvement (paronychia). Neonatal, congenital, systemic, and CMC are additional patterns of infection with *Candida*. Candidiasis in the infant is often traceable to an infected mother, who may be a vaginal or intestinal carrier of the organism. These infants may harbor *C. albicans* in the mouth or intestinal canal, and the infected saliva or stools constitute a focus for cutaneous infection. The presence of *Candida* species in the mouths of children has been proposed as a possible factor contributing to dental caries.[101] What follows is a review of several types of mucocutaneous candidiasis in children, including a discussion of congenital and neonatal candidiasis and risk factors for severe disease. Diaper candidiasis is discussed in detail in Chapter 2.

ORAL CANDIDIASIS (THRUSH)

Oral candidiasis (thrush) is a painless or painful *Candida* infection of the tongue, soft and hard palates, and buccal and gingival mucosae. It is characterized by white to gray, friable, pseudomembranous patches or plaques overlying a reddened mucosa (Fig. 17.42) (see Chapter 2, Fig. 2.31) and is most commonly seen in infants. Thrush may be acquired at the time of delivery during passage through an infected birth canal, during nursing from the skin of the mother's breast or hands, or from imperfect sterilization of feeding bottles.[102] Oral candidiasis also occurs at a greater rate in children with cystic fibrosis, diabetes, or immunodeficiency and in those who have undergone organ transplantation.[103,104] In some of these instances, the predisposition toward this infection may be related to therapies for the condition (e.g., inhaled or oral corticosteroids in patients with asthma). It has also been shown to be positively correlated with dental caries in children.[105]

The diagnosis of oral candidiasis is often clinical, and it can be confirmed by gentle attempts to remove the curd-like plaques that, in distinction to milk or formula residue, adhere to the underlying oral mucosa. Removal is accomplished by gently rubbing the area with a cotton applicator or tongue blade, which results in an underlying inflammatory mucosal erosion. The organism may be identified by microscopic evaluation of a KOH wet-mount preparation of these materials or by fungal culture. Although most infants with oral thrush do not experience impairment of appetite or feeding, severe disease may be associated with such complications, as well as significant pain. Immunocompromised infants often have a severe expression of oral candidiasis.

The usual approach to therapy, and one that is usually effective, is the administration of nystatin oral suspension, one dropperful in each cheek given four times daily. Massage of the suspension on the mucosa by the parent is useful after administration, and the medication is used for 7 to 14 days. Nystatin is unabsorbed from the GI tract, as are some other topical therapies that have been used, including gentian violet, amphotericin B, miconazole, and clotrimazole. Options for older children include nystatin and clotrimazole tablets or troches. Although it has been suggested that clotrimazole or nystatin troches or suppositories may be inserted into the tip of a slit pacifier or nipple for the treatment of infants with oral candidiasis, these approaches have not been evaluated in controlled studies, and the possibility of aspiration must be considered.[102,106] When treating infants with persistent or recurrent oral candidiasis, asymptomatic maternal vaginal candidiasis and candidal contamination of nipples or pacifiers should be considered as possible reservoirs for reinfection.[107] Oral antifungal agents, most notably fluconazole, have been demonstrated quite effective in the treatment of oral candidiasis in immunocompromised children.[108,109] In general, absorbable antifungal therapy should be used primarily if there is risk of dissemination or widespread disease is present.[110]

INTERTRIGO

The moist, warm conditions found in intertriginous areas favor the development of candidal infection. Intertrigo (see Chapter 3) refers to a condition marked by intense erythema in skin folds, including the axillary regions, the anterior neck fold (Fig. 17.43), posterior auricular regions, and inguinal creases. Although it does not always

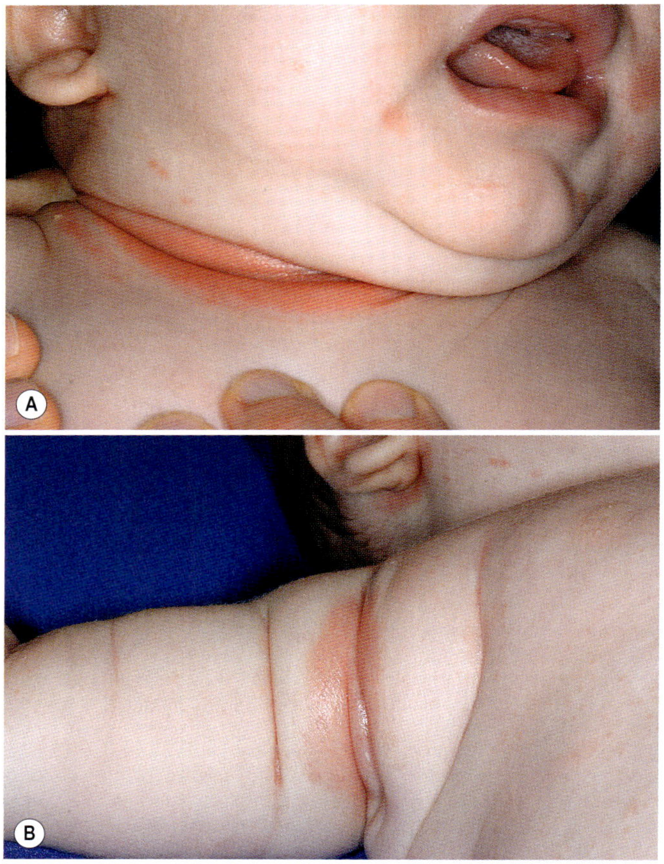

Fig. 17.43 Intertrigo. (A) Erythema and maceration of the anterior neck fold. Note the peripheral satellite papules and involvement of the auricular crease. (B) This infant also had involvement of the axillae. Skin swabs were positive for *Candida albicans*.

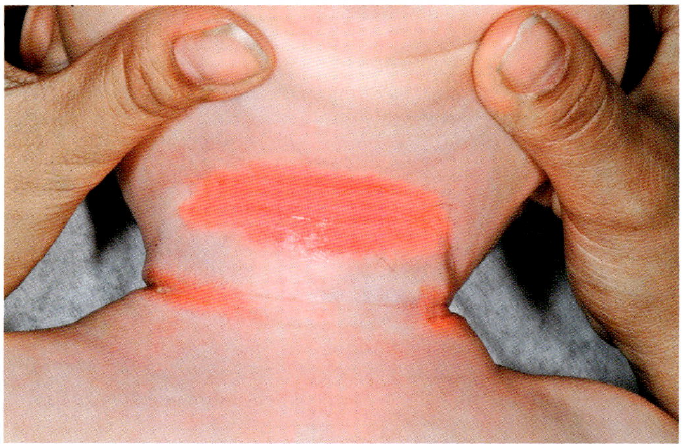

Fig. 17.44 Streptococcal intertrigo. This infant had well-demarcated erythema with erosive changes, weeping, and a foul odor. *Streptococcus pyogenes* was isolated on bacterial culture. Note the absence of satellite papules or pustules that are characteristic of candidal intertrigo.

represent a fungal process. *C. albicans* infection is common, and secondary bacterial (e.g., *Staphylococcus aureus*) infection may occasionally be present. *Streptococcal intertrigo* refers to intertrigo in association with group A β-hemolytic streptococcus (GABHS; *Streptococcus pyogenes*) infection.[111–113] It presents with intertriginous inflammation that is well demarcated, weeping, and superficially eroded (Figs. 17.44 and 17.45). It is often associated with a foul odor and lacks the satellite papules and papulopustules that are characteristic of candidal intertrigo. Surface swabs are helpful for confirming the diagnosis via streptococcal rapid antigen test and/or bacterial culture.[114]

Treatment of intertrigo with a topical antifungal agent (i.e., clotrimazole, econazole, or ketoconazole cream) applied two to three times daily is usually sufficient. More severe cases may require the addition of a low-strength topical corticosteroid or when bacterial infection is suspected, an appropriate oral antibiotic with activity against both *S. aureus* and GABHS.

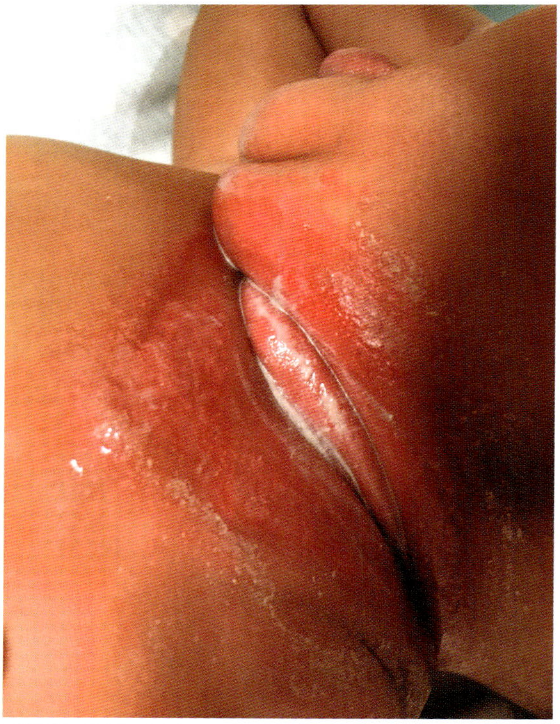

Fig. 17.45 Streptococcal intertrigo. This 4-month-old presented with irritability and these neck fold findings, which included erythema, erosive change, exudate, and foul odor. Culture was positive for both *Streptococcus pyogenes* and *Staphylococcus aureus*, and he responded rapidly to systemic antibiotics and topical care.

CANDIDAL VULVOVAGINITIS

C. albicans is a common inhabitant of the vaginal tract, and its incidence increases in diabetes and pregnancy and in females taking antibiotics or oral anovulatory preparations. When vulvovaginitis occurs, the labia become edematous and red, white patches appear on an erythematous mucosal surface, and leukorrhea (whitish discharge) develops. The resultant symptoms include itching, pain, burning, and dysuria. The infection may spread to the perineum, perianal region, gluteal folds, and upper inner aspects of the thighs as well. Although vulvovaginitis is more common in adults, it occurs in premenarchal as well as adolescent females, and in the latter, it may be a marker for type 2 diabetes; there also appears to be a link between hyperglycemia and development of candida vulvovaginitis.[115,116] Vulvovaginitis accounted for nearly 62% of all gynecologic problems seen during childhood and adolescence in one large study.[117] In premenarchal girls, psoriasis or atopic dermatitis may present with similar features and may be more common than candidiasis.[118] The differential considerations of candidal vulvovaginitis include bacterial infection, foreign body, contact dermatitis, poor hygiene, pinworm infestation, lichen sclerosus et atrophicus (typically quite distinguishable clinically), sexually transmitted infection (primarily in adolescents), and sexual abuse.[118–120] Importantly, many cases of vulvovaginitis in young girls are nonspecific without an identified infectious etiology. When there is an association with infection, in addition to possible *Candida*, the most common bacterial causes appear to be groups A and B β-hemolytic streptococci, *S. aureus*, *Proteus mirabilis*, *Escherichia coli*, *Haemophilus influenza*, *Branhamella catarrhalis*, and enterococci.[117,121–123] Anatomic and age-related factors that increase the chances of vulvovaginitis in young girls include the close proximity of the vagina to the anus (combined with tendency toward poor hygiene, which increases the risk of introduction of fecal flora), decreased estrogen levels (which lead to a thinned epithelium), alkaline pH, and lack of protection from pubic hair and labial fat pads.[120,124]

The diagnosis of candidal vulvovaginitis is established by the clinical signs and symptoms and by demonstration of the fungus by KOH wet-mount examination and/or fungal culture. Helpful approaches for vulvovaginitis in general include education on appropriate anogenital hygiene and correct wiping (front to back), avoidance of tight-fitting clothing, and avoidance of contact with known irritants. Treatment options for candida vulvovaginitis include antifungal vaginal tablets, cream, or suppositories (i.e., clotrimazole, miconazole, nystatin, terconazole) used daily for 3 to 7 days (up to 14 days for nystatin). A single-dose regimen using a 500-mg vaginal tablet of clotrimazole was also found to be clinically efficacious.[125] A single-dose regimen of fluconazole (150 mg) is quite effective in adolescents and adults.

PERLÈCHE

Perlèche (angular cheilitis) is a common disorder characterized by fissuring and inflammation of the corners of the mouth (Fig. 17.46) with associated maceration and exudate. This condition appears to be related to moisture collecting at the mouth angles and does not usually have any association with nutritional or vitamin deficiency. Whereas in adults it is often related to ill-fitting dentures, perlèche in children may be seen in conjunction with dental malocclusion, the presence of orthodontic appliances, and lip licking. Therapy is best accomplished by correction of the underlying predisposing factor; that is, the condition often improves after the completion of orthodontia or after modification of lip-licking behavior. Treatment consists of the application of a low-strength (i.e., class 6 or 7) topical corticosteroid ointment two to three times daily. A topical antifungal preparation (i.e., econazole or clotrimazole) should be added for more severe presentations, because *C. albicans* is often present. If secondary bacterial infection is present, topical or oral antibiotic therapy is also indicated. A favored treatment of the authors is the fixed formulation of nystatin (100,000 units/g) and triamcinolone acetonide 0.1% ointment, applied two to three times daily until resolved.

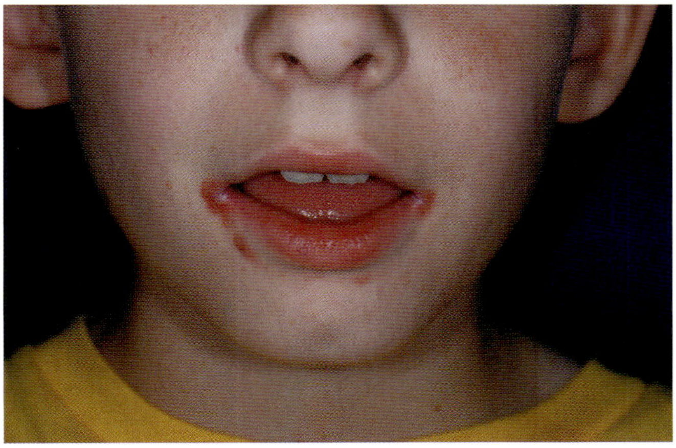

Fig. 17.46 Perlèche (angular cheilitis). Erythema, fissuring, and exudate of the mouth angles in a 10-year-old boy.

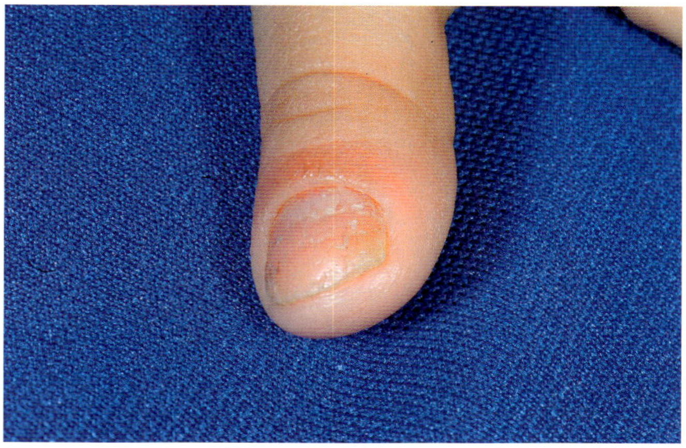

Fig. 17.47 Chronic paronychia. Nail plate ridging, periungual erythema, and cuticle loss are seen in this patient with chronic *Candida* infection.

CHRONIC PARONYCHIA

Chronic paronychia (see Chapter 7) is usually associated with *C. albicans* infection and presents with transverse ridging of the nail plate, loss of the cuticle, and mild proximal/lateral periungual erythema (Fig. 17.47). It is distinguished from acute paronychia not only by the natural history (acute paronychia is more sudden in onset) but also by lack of the marked edema, pain, and pustule formation, which are classically seen in the acute (bacterial) type. Chronic paronychia in children may be related to repeated finger or thumb sucking. Therapy with a topical antifungal cream applied twice daily is usually effective, although the nail plate may take several months to grow out normally. Oral fluconazole may also be effective for severe or resistant involvement. Attempts to decrease moisture of the affected digits will accentuate the response to therapy and help to minimize recurrences.

EROSIO INTERDIGITALIS BLASTOMYCETICA

Erosio interdigitalis blastomycetica (derived from Latin, meaning "an erosion between digits caused by a budding fungus") is a red, itchy, and occasionally slightly painful eruption of the web spaces between the fingers or toes. It is most common in individuals whose hands or feet are exposed to moisture often and most commonly involves the lateral two web spaces (i.e., between the third and fourth and between the fourth and fifth digits). Erosio interdigitalis blastomycetica presents with erythema, maceration, and peeling of the affected region (Fig. 17.48) with

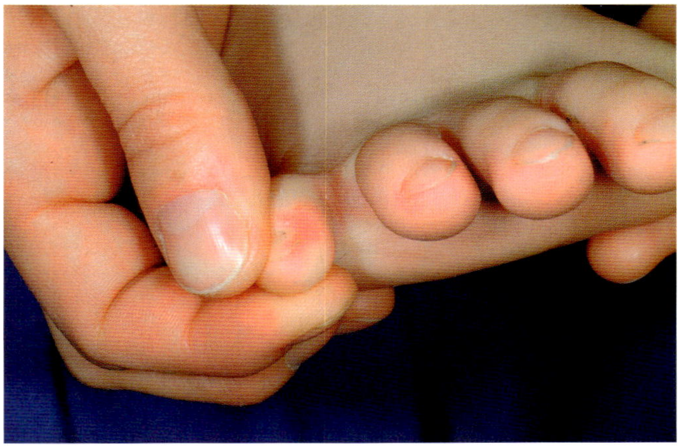

Fig. 17.48 Erosio interdigitalis blastomycetica. Erythema, maceration, and peeling of the fourth toe-web space. This eruption cleared rapidly with topical azole antifungal therapy.

a scaly and occasionally vesicular border. More severe presentations with marked inflammation and frank ulceration have been reported in adults and termed *interdigital ulcer.*[126] Erosio interdigitalis blastomycetica seems to be caused by infection with *C. albicans*, and occasionally there may be an associated Gram-negative infection (see Chapter 14). Treatment consists of keeping the hands and feet as dry as possible and the use of a topical antifungal and (when needed) antibacterial preparation.

BLACK HAIRY TONGUE

Black hairy tongue is a term used to describe a disorder primarily affecting adults and occasionally adolescents that is characterized by hypertrophic, elongated filiform papillae that form a dense black to blue-black surface on the midportion of the dorsal tongue. It occurs less often in young children but has been observed in an infant as young as 2 months of age, and was even reported in a 2-week-old baby.[127–129] The etiology is unknown, but it is frequently attributed to *C. albicans* or bacterial infection and is often associated with the prolonged use of antibiotics, including erythromycin and linezolid. Treatment consists primarily of improved oral hygiene, and gentle brushing of the dorsal tongue with a soft toothbrush and a small amount of toothpaste two to three times daily is usually effective.

NEONATAL AND SYSTEMIC CANDIDIASIS

Two types of candidiasis in the newborn period have been reported: a congenital form in which the skin lesions are present at birth or within the first 6 days of life and a neonatal form commonly seen after the first week of life. Neonatal candidiasis develops as a result of infection acquired by passage through an infected maternal birth canal. This perinatal or postnatal acquisition of *Candida* encompasses several clinical presentations, including localized disease (i.e., oral thrush and diaper dermatitis), systemic infection related to invasive procedures and infected indwelling devices, and invasive fungal dermatitis seen in extremely low-birthweight neonates. Although *C. albicans* is the primary pathogen, *Candida parapsilosis* has also become a significant pathogen in the neonatal setting (and in some reports has become the most commonly isolated species), and *Candida glabrata* has been reported after *in vitro* fertilization and embryo transfer.[130–135] Other species that may cause neonatal infections include *C. tropicalis, C. krusei*, and *C. lusitaniae.*[136]

Congenital candidiasis is acquired *in utero* and may be associated with premature labor, especially in instances where a foreign body (i.e., intrauterine device [IUD] or cervical sutures) is present. It may also be associated with *Candida*-associated chorioamnionitis.[137] A history of maternal candidal vulvovaginitis is common in infants with congenital candidiasis, although the former is present in a high percentage (up to 25%) of pregnant women and in most instances is not associated with this neonatal infection.[138] Congenital candidiasis tends to run a more benign course in full-term infants without risk factors but may result in serious systemic infection in premature neonates, especially those of extremely low birthweight. Other risk factors for invasive candidal infection include extensive instrumentation in the delivery room and invasive procedures utilized during the neonatal period. In patients with risk factors for dissemination, systemic antifungal therapy should be initiated.

Congenital cutaneous candidiasis (CCC) presents with multiple widespread erythematous macules, papules, and pustules (Fig. 17.49) and occasionally bullae. In full-term infants, this form of candidiasis is often limited to the skin and resolves over 1 to 2 weeks.[131] The most common locations of involvement are the back, extensor surfaces of the extremities, and skin folds, with relative sparing of the diaper area.[139] Pustules on the palms and soles (Fig. 17.50) are a common and useful diagnostic finding. Oral thrush is uncommon in this setting, but nail changes (yellow discoloration, thickening, paronychia) (Fig. 17.51) are occasionally present. Such nail changes may be the sole manifestation of congenital candidiasis, and onychomadesis (separation of the nail plate from the nailbed) with nail shedding may occur.[140] The clinical findings in CCC may resemble erythema toxicum neonatorum; bacterial folliculitis or pustulosis; bullous impetigo; and congenital herpes, varicella, enterovirus, or syphilis. The definitive

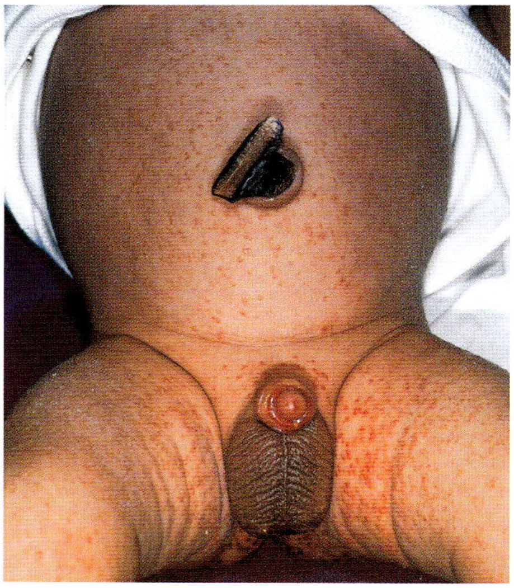

Fig. 17.49 Congenital cutaneous candidiasis. Widespread erythematous papules and pustules in a 10-day-old boy. This otherwise healthy child had involvement limited to the skin and no risk factors for dissemination. His mother reported a history of vulvovaginal candidiasis during the last trimester of pregnancy.

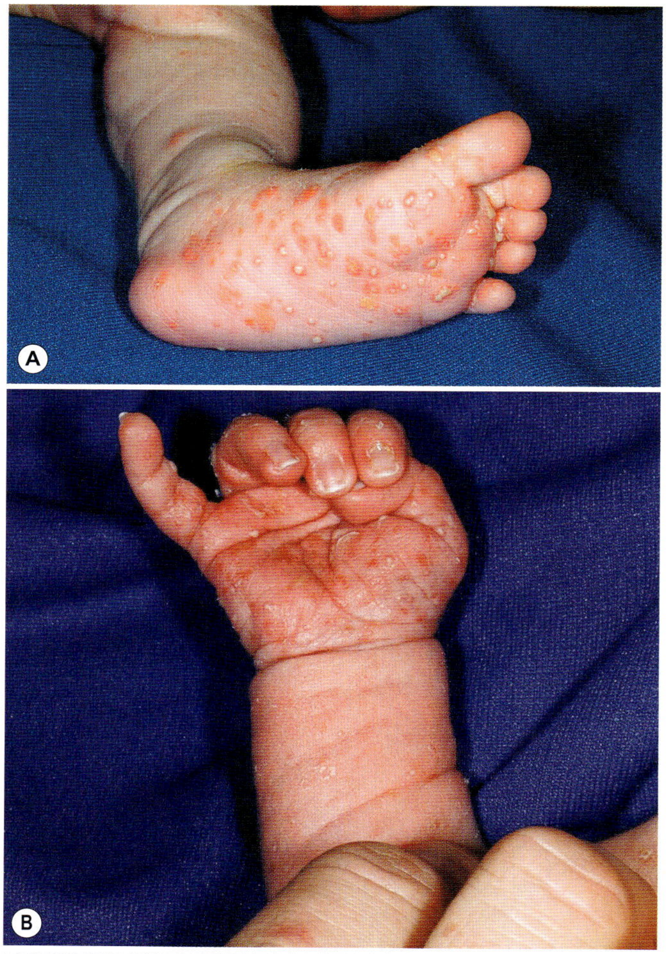

Fig. 17.50 Congenital cutaneous candidiasis. Erythematous papules, papulovesicles, and pustules were present at birth in this full-term infant male and were distributed on the trunk, extremities, soles **(A)**, and palms **(B)**. No extracutaneous involvement was noted.

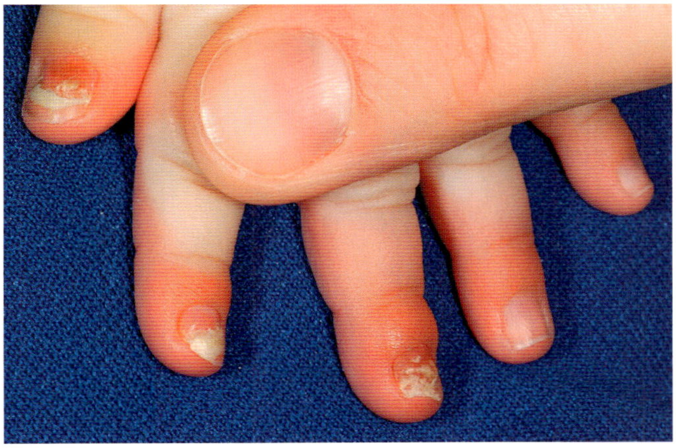

Fig. 17.51 Congenital candidiasis. Yellow discoloration with ridging and nail plate separation in a newborn male with no other manifestations of *Candida* infection.

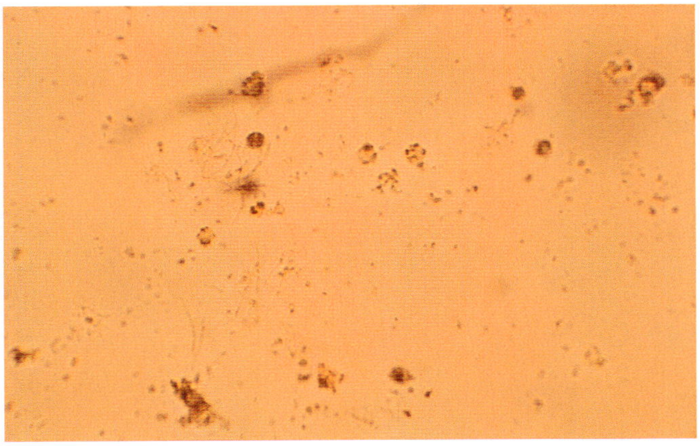

Fig. 17.52 KOH examination of candidiasis. Spores and pseudohyphae as noted on microscopic examination of skin scrapings from a patient with candidiasis.

diagnosis of CCC is made by the microscopic finding of spores and pseudohyphae on skin scrapings (Fig. 17.52) or culture of the organism. Another useful diagnostic modality is examination of the placenta, which may reveal typical changes of candidiasis (including funisitis or chorioamnionitis); subamniotic fungal abscesses or 1- to 2-cm yellow-white plaques may be noted on the placenta or umbilical cord.[139,141,142] In patients with CCC limited to the skin who are clinically stable and lack risk factors for disseminated disease, oral fluconazole therapy may be considered.[142]

Systemic candidiasis occurs primarily in very low-birthweight (<1500 g) infants and is typically seen between the second and sixth weeks of life. The immature immune defenses of this population contribute to this propensity toward systemic disease.[139] Predisposing factors, in addition to prematurity, include presence of a central catheter or endotracheal tube, receipt of intravenous lipid emulsion, administration of broad-spectrum antibiotics, and use of intrapartum antibiotics.[143] Systemic candidiasis is uncommon in infants of birthweight greater than 1500 g, but when it occurs, the greatest risk factors appear to be exposure to broad-spectrum antibiotics and thrombocytopenia (<50,000/mm^3).[144]

Common features of systemic candidiasis include apnea, hyperglycemia, temperature instability, lethargy, hypotension, and increasing respiratory requirements.[134] The skin surface may or may not be involved. These patients may have candidal septicemia, meningitis, urinary tract infection, or disseminated disease. Because the kidneys act as a filter for *Candida*, spores may be present on microscopic examination of urine samples.[141] Renal pelvis fungus balls may be seen in up to 42% of these infants, and endocarditis, septic arthritis, endophthalmitis, and osteomyelitis may also occur. The diagnosis is confirmed by isolation of *Candida* from blood, urine, cerebrospinal fluid, or other normally sterile sites. Other diagnostic methods garnering interest include detection of the fungal cell wall polysaccharide (1,3)-β-d-glucan (BDG) or mannan (a cell wall component of *Candida*) and PCR amplification from serum or plasma.[136,145] Systemic candidiasis requires parenteral antifungal therapy and may result in permanent neurodevelopmental deficits in long-term survivors. The mortality rate in extremely low-birthweight (<1000 g) infants is 20% to 34% and even higher when *Candida* is isolated from more than one sterile body fluid.[143,146] Fluconazole prophylaxis at a dose of 3 mg/kg at varying frequencies for 4 to 6 weeks has been advocated for neonates in nurseries with high rates of invasive candidiasis (>10%) and for very low- and extremely low-birthweight neonates.[147]

Invasive fungal dermatitis refers to a clinical entity seen in extremely low-birthweight infants and consists of a distinct cutaneous presentation of *Candida* infection in combination with a high risk for internal dissemination.[138] The affected infants develop lesions after several days of life. Skin involvement is characterized by erosive and ulcerative lesions (Fig. 17.53) with extensive crusting. Vesicles, bullae, and "burn-like" erythema may also be present, and desquamation and widespread denudation are common. A high index of suspicion should be maintained in extremely low-birthweight infants with any of these findings, because disseminated infection is common, including fungemia, meningitis, urinary tract infection, and other organ involvement. Extremely low-birthweight infants with disseminated *Candida* infection are at increased risk for neurodevelopmental impairment and death.[148] Potential risk factors for this form of candidiasis include vaginal birth, postnatal steroids, and prolonged hyperglycemia.[138] The immature skin barrier function seen in extremely premature infants is believed to be pathogenic, with skin serving as the portal of entry for this infection.[138,149]

CHRONIC MUCOCUTANEOUS CANDIDIASIS

Chronic mucocutaneous candidiasis (CMC) is characterized by recurrent infections of the skin; nails; and oral, esophageal, or genital mucosae with *Candida* species, usually *C. albicans*. This disorder appears to be a common phenotype for a variety of defects in the immune response, most notably in the cellular branch of the immune system and mainly the specific responses to antigens of *Candida* species.[150] CMC may be seen in the setting of primary immunodeficiencies, including severe combined immunodeficiency, dedicator of cytokinesis 8 *(DOCK8)* deficiency, signal transducer and activator

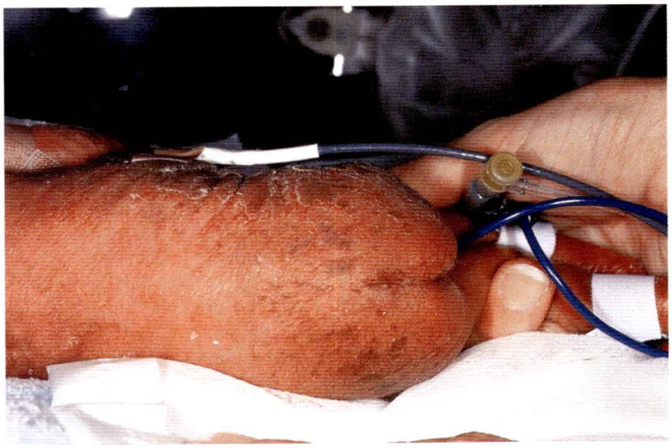

Fig. 17.53 Invasive fungal dermatitis. Erythema with maceration, crusting, and peeling in an extremely low-birthweight newborn with candidiasis. (Courtesy Moise Levy, MD.)

of transcription *(STAT)* 3 deficiency causing autosomal dominant hyperimmunoglobulin (Ig) E syndrome, and autosomal recessive autoimmune polyendocrinopathy-candidiasis-ectodermal dystrophy (APECED) associated with a mutation in *AIRE*. More recently, CMC has been associated with various inborn errors of interleukin (IL)-17–mediated immunity, shown in some autosomal dominant kindreds to be associated with gain-of-function *STAT1* mutations.[151–153] In patients with the *STAT1* mutation, reduced production of interferon-γ and IL-22 have also been demonstrated.[153] Pure CMC (without another syndrome association) has been reported in some families with mutations in the genes for the IL-17 receptor *(IL17RA)* and IL-17 ligand *(IL17F)*.[154] CMC has also been associated with *CARD9* deficiency, and in this setting may be associated with invasive fungal infections, including deep dermatophytosis, invasive infection with *Exophiala dermatitidis*, subcutaneous phaeohyphomycosis, and central nervous system (CNS) or GI infections with *Candida* species.[155]

The clinical features of CMC are marked by the mucocutaneous findings. Oral candidiasis (thrush), esophageal candidiasis, candidal diaper dermatitis, candidal intertrigo, and paronychia that are persistent and recalcitrant to therapy are all common. Angular cheilitis (perlèche) is also seen. Generalized, scaly, erythematous, and crusted papules and plaques may be present, especially on the scalp, where they may lead to scarring alopecia. Nail involvement is notable for nail plate thickening and discoloration, and chronic paronychia may be present. Systemic candidiasis does not usually occur in patients with CMC. Dental enamel dysplasia occurs in some patients with APECED syndrome (see later), and at times may be so severe that it leads to early loss of dentition. Other infections may occur with increased incidence in these patients as well, most commonly tinea, pyogenic skin infection, sinusitis, pneumonitis, and urinary tract infection. Severe complications that may occur in patients with CMC include squamous cell carcinoma, functional debilitation of the hands, esophageal strictures, and cerebral aneurysms.[156]

The most common endocrinopathies noted in association with CMC are hypoparathyroidism, hypoadrenalism (Addison disease), and gonadal failure. These endocrine abnormalities commonly do not appear until adolescence or adulthood, and therefore serial evaluations for endocrine function are indicated in patients with CMC, especially those with one endocrinopathy or with family members affected with APECED.[157] APECED, which is also known as *autoimmune polyendocrinopathy syndrome type I (APS1)*, is an autosomal recessive disorder caused by mutations in the autoimmune regulator *(AIRE)* gene.[158,159] The classic triad of this disorder is CMC, hypoparathyroidism, and primary adrenal insufficiency, and the diagnosis of APECED requires the presence of at least two of these components.[160] Besides the candidal infections and endocrine abnormalities, patients with APECED have ectodermal dystrophy manifested most commonly as alopecia areata (which may progress to alopecia universalis), as well as nail dystrophy (Fig. 17.54) and dental enamel defects. Other observed defects may include vitiligo, chronic active hepatitis, growth-hormone deficiency, thyroid disease, diabetes mellitus, pernicious anemia, keratopathy, ovarian failure, testicular failure, celiac disease, cerebellar ataxia, ptosis, retinitis pigmentosa, and iridocyclitis.[156,158,161,162] The three most common preceding features before presenting with the diagnostic dyad, as shown in one large series, included urticarial eruption, intestinal dysfunction, and enamel hypoplasia.[163] The autoimmune diathesis also is responsible for the candidal infections. Patients have been shown to have neutralizing autoantibodies directed against interferons (especially interferon-ω), IL-17, and IL-22, cytokines that are important in immune responses to the candidal organism, as well as an altered IL-23p19 response in monocytes.[154,163–166]

Treatment of CMC includes addressing the immunodeficiency status (and augmenting or correcting it when feasible) and administration of topical and/or oral antifungal medications. Topical antifungal creams are useful for treatment of localized cutaneous lesions. Oral or vaginal candidiasis may benefit from oral troches or suspensions and vaginal creams or suppositories, respectively. The mainstays of therapy for CMC, however, are the oral antifungal agents, including fluconazole and itraconazole. When these agents are used as ongoing therapy for this indication, the possible side effects, potential for drug interactions, and risk-to-benefit ratio must all be taken into consideration. Biologic therapies directed at the observed cytokine aberrations in these disorders are being studied.

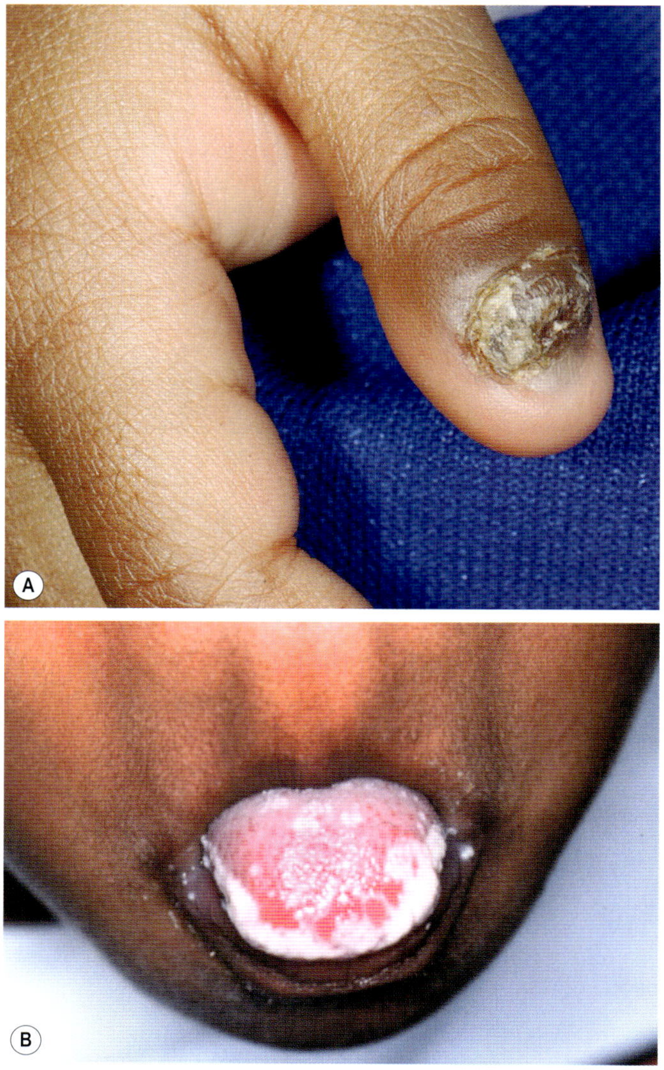

Fig. 17.54 Autoimmune polyendocrinopathy syndrome. This 18-month-old boy with a confirmed *AIRE* mutation had chronic mucocutaneous candidiasis, manifesting as treatment-resistant nail infection **(A)** and persistent oral thrush **(B)**.

Deep Fungal Disorders

In contrast to the superficial dermatophytes, which are confined to dead keratinous tissue, certain mycotic infections have the capacity for deep invasion of the skin or subcutaneous tissues, as well as the potential for systemic infection, especially of the lungs and reticuloendothelial system. There follows a review of several deep fungal infections, which have been divided into the subcutaneous, systemic, and opportunistic mycoses.

SUBCUTANEOUS MYCOSES

The subcutaneous mycoses are a group of disorders caused mainly by fungi that exist as soil saprophytes and are normally of low virulence but may result in infection involving the skin and subcutaneous tissues. Although these infections are found most often in adults with occupational exposure to soil and plants, all age groups are potentially susceptible. The primary subcutaneous mycoses are sporotrichosis, chromoblastomycosis, and mycetoma. Rhinosporidiosis, which has been classified variably as a fungus or a protozoan parasite, has been included in this category and usually affects the nasal, nasopharyngeal, and ocular mucosae. Others (not discussed here) include phaeohyphomycosis, entomophthoromycosis, and lobomycosis.

Sporotrichosis

Sporotrichosis is a granulomatous fungal infection of the skin and subcutaneous tissues caused by *Sporothrix schenckii*, a dimorphic fungus of worldwide distribution commonly isolated from soil and plants. It occurs in patients of all ages but is observed most commonly in adult males who, because of their occupation or leisure-time activities, are likely to be exposed to contaminated soil or vegetation (farmers, florists, gardeners, forestry workers, miners, and individuals who work with contaminated packing material). Childhood infection, although significantly less common, does occur and may go undiagnosed without a high index of suspicion.[167] Although human transmission can occur after close contact with suppurative wounds of sporotrichosis, the majority of clustered cases are most likely related to simultaneous inoculation from the same source.[168,169] Although disease is usually limited to the skin and subcutaneous tissues, disseminated sporotrichosis with fungemia may occur, especially in the setting of HIV infection.[170] Contact with infected cats was suggested as the predominant mode of transmission in a series of pediatric sporotrichosis from a hyperendemic region in Peru.[171]

The clinical presentation of sporotrichosis is variable, and several factors such as inoculum load, host immune status, virulence of the involved strain, and depth of the inciting trauma may influence the clinical presentation.[172] The lymphocutaneous form is the most common in adults and presents with a painless, erythematous papule or nodule that begins on exposed areas of skin, most commonly the upper extremity. The initial lesion often follows a penetrating injury such as that inflicted by a splinter, thorn, grain, rock, piece of glass, or cat scratch (cats are perhaps the only animals capable of transmitting this disorder[173]) contaminated with the organism. The lesions are often solitary and enlarge over several weeks. Secondary discrete lesions may develop and often progress toward more proximal sites, a pattern that has been referred to as *sporotrichoid*[174] (Fig. 17.55). Regional lymphadenopathy and lymphadenitis are common. The skin lesions may ulcerate centrally and heal with scarring, although spontaneous clearing is unusual. In a series of 25 children with sporotrichosis, 60% had lesions on an extremity (followed by the face as the next most common site), and the majority had the lymphocutaneous form of the infection.[175] Epidemic sporotrichosis related to transmission from infected cats was reported in 1998 through 2004 in Brazil and affected humans, cats, and dogs.[176]

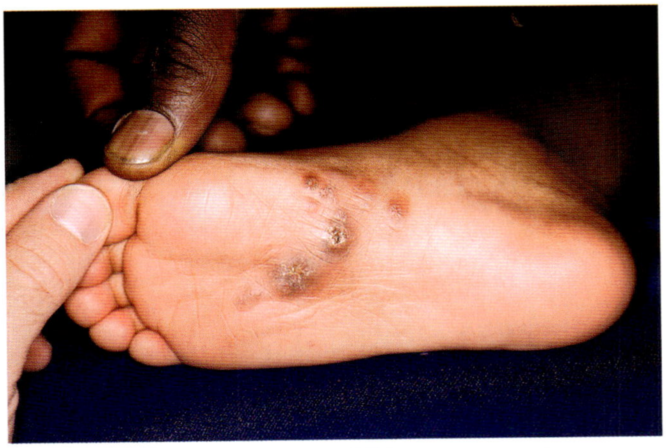

Fig. 17.55 Sporotrichosis. Erythematous papules and nodules on the plantar surface with early lymphangitic (sporotrichoid) spread.

The fixed cutaneous form of sporotrichosis is characterized by localized skin lesions without lymphatic involvement. The skin findings range from scaly papules to verrucous, ulcerated plaques or nodules with or without satellite lesions. This form seems more common in children, and there may be a delay in diagnosis, given the lack of a typical sporotrichoid distribution pattern.[167] It has been hypothesized that children manifesting fixed cutaneous forms may possess host factors that limit the infection to the inoculation site, even if the strain is capable of producing the more classic lymphocutaneous form commonly seen in adults.[177] This form of sporotrichosis was reported in a 3-week-old neonate in whom the source of infection was unknown.[178]

Disseminated cutaneous sporotrichosis is rare and usually occurs in individuals with immunologic defects or chronic disease. In these patients, the cutaneous lesions may be widespread and develop after hematogenous spread of the infection from a primary focus in the skin or an occult pulmonary focus. Multiple additional organs may be involved, including the bones, joints, and CNS. This form of sporotrichosis may mimic tuberculosis (especially with upper lung radiographic lesions) and is associated with significant morbidity and mortality. Multifocal cutaneous ulcers have also been reported in sporotrichosis in association with misuse of topical corticosteroids and self-inoculation.[179] Osteoarticular sporotrichosis has been used to describe involvement presenting as tenosynovitis, periostitis, or monoarticular arthritis, often in immunosuppressed individuals.[180]

The differential diagnosis of cutaneous sporotrichosis includes atypical mycobacterial infection, bacterial abscess or ecthyma, *Nocardia*, foreign-body granuloma, chromoblastomycosis, cutaneous manifestations of systemic mycoses, leishmaniasis, anthrax, and tularemia. The gold standard for diagnosis is fungal culture of a skin biopsy specimen. Direct examination of smears or biopsy material may be nonspecific. Histopathologic examination of skin biopsy specimens may reveal the organisms when enhanced via the application of special stains such as Gomori methenamine silver (GMS) or periodic acid–Schiff (PAS) stains. Molecular detection methods and serologic studies have also been utilized.[172]

The traditional treatment of choice for cutaneous sporotrichosis in adults has been orally administered saturated solution of potassium iodide (SSKI), 3 to 6 g/day for adults and half the dose for children. SSKI therapy may be associated with increased lacrimation or salivation, metallic taste, GI discomfort, diarrhea, and headache. Treatment is continued until 4 to 6 weeks after clinical resolution of lesions. This therapy is still the most commonly used treatment in resource-limited settings.[181]

The treatment of choice for sporotrichosis in developed countries is usually oral itraconazole for 3 to 6 months with a reported success rate of 90% to 100% for cutaneous or lymphocutaneous disease.[182] In children the recommended dose is 5 mg/kg daily, and in adults a range of 100 to 400 mg daily has been recommended. Fluconazole is another option, although it may be less effective. Terbinafine and local hyperthermia are other potential therapies for nondisseminated disease, and amphotericin B is indicated for patients with life-threatening, disseminated, or extensive infection. Electrosurgery and surgical excision have been occasionally utilized for small lesions.[183]

Chromoblastomycosis

Chromoblastomycosis (chromomycosis) is an uncommon chronic fungal infection of the skin and subcutaneous tissue caused by a variety of dematiaceous fungi (filamentous fungi with melanin-type pigment in the fungal wall). At least five organisms are implicated in the disease, including species of *Phialophora*, *Fonsecaea*, or *Cladophialophora*, all of which are common inhabitants of decaying wood and soil. Several cases have been reported after penetrating wounds of the skin, especially from splinters and thorns.[184] The disease is rare during childhood and is seen most commonly in tropical and subtropical climates; farmers and others involved in agricultural activities appear to be at highest risk.[185,186] The highest number of cases are diagnosed in Madagascar.[187] Other locations with high numbers of cases include Latin America, the Caribbean, Africa, and Asia.

Chromoblastomycosis is characterized initially by the formation of small scaly papules that may expand into nodules. The lesions, which are most often confined to the lower leg or foot, coalesce into larger nodules and plaques and characteristically develop a very verrucous (warty) surface. There may be purulent drainage, and the lesions may be painless or tender. The surface may be studded with multiple "black dots." Long-standing lesions may result in edema of the extremity and scarring. Potential complications include lymphedema (sometimes with elephantiasis), secondary bacterial infection, ankylosis, and malignancy (primarily squamous cell carcinoma, in long-standing cases).[188]

The differential diagnosis of chromoblastomycosis includes other deep fungal, mycobacterial, and bacterial infections, as well as cutaneous tuberculosis, leishmaniasis, leprosy, squamous cell carcinoma, psoriasis, cutaneous lymphoma, and tertiary syphilis. The diagnosis is confirmed by microscopic recognition of the organism in KOH wet-mount preparations or tissue biopsy specimens and by fungal culture. When the disease is localized, the treatment of choice is surgical excision of the affected tissue. Several destructive modalities, including cryotherapy/cryosurgery, heat therapy, electrodesiccation, CO_2 laser photocoagulation, photodynamic therapy, and radiation therapy, have been used. In more advanced cases, surgical or destructive approaches are not feasible and medical therapy is necessary. Systemic agents utilized for chromoblastomycosis include itraconazole (which appears to be the most effective[189]), terbinafine, voriconazole, thiabendazole, and possibly 5-flucytosine.[185,188] Amphotericin B tends to be less effective. Amputation of the affected limb is usually a last resort.[190]

Mycetoma

Mycetoma, also called *Madura foot*, is a chronic mutilating granulomatous infection of the subcutaneous tissues along with invasion of the fascia, muscles, and bone, and when an extremity is involved, enlargement of the affected area. Although the majority of lesions are seen on a lower extremity, they may also occur on the hand, shoulder, buttocks, knees, or other regions of the body. The organisms that cause mycetoma are usually introduced by skin trauma. Mycetoma is endemic in Latin America, the Indian subcontinent, Africa, and between the latitudes of 15° south and 30° north around the Tropic of Cancer (the so-called "mycetoma belt").[191] This belt includes Sudan, India, Mexico, Somalia, Senegal, Yemen, Venezuela, Colombia, and Argentina, with most cases reported in the former three (Sudan, India, and Mexico).[192,193]

Mycetoma may be caused by various species of true fungi (eumycotic mycetoma), including *Pseudallescheria boydii, Madurella mycetomatis, Madurella grisea,* and *Phialophora verrucosa*. It may also be caused by anaerobic fungus-like bacteria, the actinomycetes (actinomycotic mycetoma or actinomycetoma), usually by species of *Nocardia, Actinomadura,* or *Streptomyces*, including *Actinomadura madurae, Actinomadura pelletieri, Nocardia brasiliensis,* and *Streptomyces somaliensis*. These organisms exist as saprophytes in soil or on vegetable matter. The most common agent worldwide is *N. brasiliensis*. Mycetoma is uncommon in childhood and relatively rare in the United States, occurring most commonly in young adults (especially young men between 20 and 40 years) and workers in rural tropical and subtropical areas who walk barefoot and are thus more readily exposed to the organisms.

The infection begins as one or more small, firm papules that gradually evolve into subcutaneous nodules with sinus tracts, draining abscesses, edema, and enlargement of the affected extremity. Purulent drainage is common, and "grains" of various colors may be visible in the exudate, with the color depending on the infecting organism. Eventually, crusting and granulation tissue may develop, and the infection may extend to the deeper tissue levels and bone. Spread of the infection occurs locally and via lymphatics, akin to sporotrichosis. A preliminary diagnosis can be made by microscopic examination of the granules to identify their actinomycete or fungal nature, but tissue culture is generally necessary for confirmation. Molecular-based diagnostic techniques are also used.

Treatment of mycetoma depends on the causative agent. Therapeutic options for actinomycotic mycetoma include sulfonamides, streptomycin, tetracyclines, rifampicin, ciprofloxacin, amikacin, penicillin, amoxicillin-clavulanate, imipenem, and dapsone. Treatment of eumycotic mycetoma is more difficult and is usually a combined approach of medical and surgical therapy. Small lesions may be best treated with complete excision. Medical therapies include the azole antifungals (especially ketoconazole before the FDA warning regarding liver injury and now itraconazole), voriconazole, posaconazole, and amphotericin B (but poor activity *in vitro*).[193,194] Unfortunately, there is no single drug that gives consistently good results, and long-standing cases with extensive tissue destruction and fibrosis are often resistant to all forms of therapy.

Rhinosporidiosis

Rhinosporidiosis is a rare disorder caused by the organism *Rhinosporidium seeberi*. It occurs throughout the world but is most common in the tropics, especially in India and Sri Lanka. It has been occasionally reported in the United States, especially the southern portion. Although rare in children, a cluster of pediatric cases was reported in rural northeast Georgia between 1981 and 1994.[195] Studies have suggested a possible link to swimming or bathing in freshwater ponds, lakes, or rivers.[196] Although *R. seeberi* was originally thought to be a protozoan parasite, it has most consistently been classified as a fungus, given its microscopic appearance and identification with fungal stains. It has been classified more recently as a novel group of aquatic protistan parasites.[196]

Rhinosporidiosis is characterized by papules, nodules, and pedunculated vascular polypoid growths on the mucous membranes of the nose, nasopharynx, soft palate, and conjunctivae. Other potential sites of involvement include the upper respiratory passages, sinuses, lacrimal sacs, skin, larynx, genitalia, or rectum. Tracheal involvement has been rarely reported.[197] The surface often has a raspberry-like appearance and is studded with tiny white or yellow nodules. The lesions may become hyperplastic and may reach enormous size, and symptoms are often associated with physical obstruction. Diagnosis is confirmed by microscopic examination, and the organism is notoriously difficult to isolate in culture. Fine-needle aspiration cytology may reveal the sporangia and spores of *R. seeberi*.[198] Treatment generally consists of electrosurgical destruction or surgical removal of lesions when feasible. Antimicrobial agents, most notably dapsone, have been reportedly effective in some patients. Local injection of amphotericin B has also been reported as adjunctive therapy to help prevent relapse and spread of the infection.[199]

SYSTEMIC MYCOSES

The systemic mycoses comprise a group of fungal disorders that arise from internal foci, usually the lungs or upper respiratory tract. When the skin lesions result from dissemination of the infection, the prognosis is generally poor. Primary inoculation disease of the skin occasionally occurs with these infections. Disorders in this group include blastomycosis, coccidioidomycosis, paracoccidioidomycosis, and histoplasmosis. Actinomycosis and nocardiosis, although often included under the group of disorders because of true fungi, are actually caused by fungus-like Gram-positive bacteria and are discussed in the section on bacterial infections (see Chapter 14).

Blastomycosis

Blastomycosis (North American blastomycosis, Gilchrist disease, Chicago disease) is a systemic granulomatous infection caused by the dimorphic fungus *Blastomyces dermatitidis*. More recently, a second distinct species, *Blastomyces gilchristii*, has been identified and may be a more predominant etiology for pediatric blastomycosis.[200] This infection occurs most often in the southeastern and southcentral states that border the Mississippi and Ohio rivers and the Great Lakes states. It is considered endemic in several focal areas of northern Wisconsin and Michigan. Blastomycosis occurs in three forms: pulmonary, disseminated (systemic), and primary cutaneous inoculation, which is quite rare. Primary inoculation blastomycosis has been reported primarily in laboratory technicians working with the organism and in pathologists who perform autopsies on animals or humans with the disease.[201] The organism has been cultured from soil, which is believed to be the reservoir for infection in humans.[202] Blastomycosis is rare in children, especially those under 1 year of age, and when it occurs, extrapulmonary disease (including CNS involvement) is fairly common.[203,204] In one pediatric series, extrapulmonary disease occurred in 46% of infected children, with skin disease and bone involvement each occurring in 31%.[205] Infantile blastomycosis is notable for its difficulty in diagnosis and the potential severity of its course.[206] South American blastomycosis is a chronic granulomatous disease caused by *Paracoccidioides brasiliensis* and is also known as paracoccidioidomycosis. It is discussed briefly later in this chapter.

Primary infection usually involves the lungs, and patients may exhibit nonspecific flu-like symptoms, cough, low-grade fever, night sweats, hemoptysis, or minimal symptomatology. Chest radiography is often nonspecific during acute infection. Many patients with acute pulmonary blastomycosis may go undiagnosed and thus untreated. The disorder may heal spontaneously, progress to chronic pulmonary disease with or without cavitation, or disseminate, primarily to skin, subcutaneous tissues, bones, and joints. Acute respiratory distress syndrome (ARDS) may occasionally occur.[207] Other potential sites of dissemination are the GI tract, liver, spleen, genitourinary tract, and CNS.

Skin involvement in North American blastomycosis is most commonly associated with disseminated disease and only occasionally associated with primary inoculation. Primary cutaneous blastomycosis is extremely rare in children and often presents with a localized chancroid-like ulcer.[208] The primary types of skin changes noted in all forms of cutaneous blastomycosis are verrucous (warty) lesions and cutaneous ulcers.[209] Verrucous lesions present with heaped-up hyperkeratosis with a surrounding erythematous or violaceous color (Fig. 17.56). They may be confused with multiple other cutaneous infections or squamous cell carcinoma. The ulcerative lesions begin as papules or pustules and progress to superficial ulcers with granulation tissue (Fig. 17.57). Cutaneous lesions disseminated from a primary pulmonary focus are usually symmetrical and generally appear on the exposed areas of the body (the face, wrists, hands, and feet). Skin lesions may also occur over areas of osteomyelitis and present as draining sinus tracts. In patients with primary cutaneous inoculation blastomycosis, the skin lesions occur with focal lymphadenopathy or lymphangitis but without evidence for systemic involvement.[210] Sources for primary inoculation disease include clinical exposures as noted earlier (i.e., laboratory or morgue, primarily in adults), animal bite or scratch, and other forms of skin trauma. The skin lesions of blastomycosis heal eventually (even without therapy), often resulting in permanent scarring.

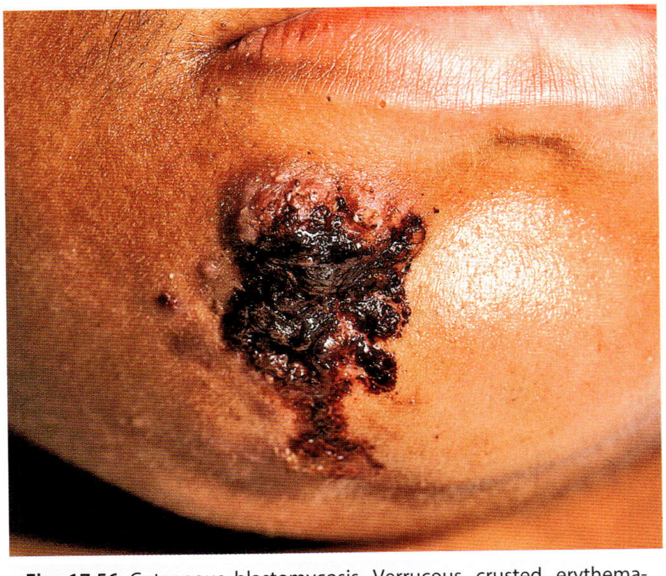

Fig. 17.56 Cutaneous blastomycosis. Verrucous, crusted, erythematous plaque on the chin in a 15-year-old male patient with respiratory symptoms and bone pain. (Reprinted with permission from Cummins RE, Romero RC, Mancini AJ. Disseminated North American blastomycosis in an adolescent male: A delay in diagnosis. Pediatrics 1998;102(4):977–979. © American Academy of Pediatrics. All rights reserved.)

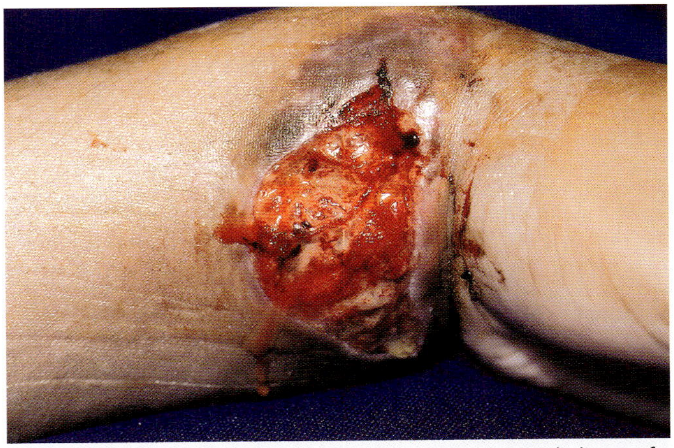

Fig. 17.57 Cutaneous blastomycosis. Vegetative, ulcerated plaque of the volar wrist in the same patient shown in Fig. 17.56. (Reprinted with permission from Cummins RE, Romero RC, Mancini AJ. Disseminated North American blastomycosis in an adolescent male: a delay in diagnosis. Pediatrics 1998;102(4):977–979. © American Academy of Pediatrics. All rights reserved.)

North American blastomycosis is diagnosed by identification of the thick-walled, broad-based budding yeast cells in tissue samples or growth in fungal culture. Serologic studies are not useful, and enzyme immunoassays are sensitive but not available on a widespread basis. Cytologic examination of specimens (i.e., sputum) may be useful.[211] Urine-antigen detection may be useful in children for both diagnosis and for monitoring response to therapy.[212] Deoxyribonucleic acid (DNA) probe and PCR assays have also been reported.[213] A high index of suspicion must be maintained in the patient with nonhealing cutaneous ulcers or verrucous skin lesions, especially if other symptoms of systemic disease are present, most notably those referable to the lungs or bones, and if the patient resides in (or has traveled to) an endemic area. Suspicion for this infection should also be high in children with these predisposing factors, especially when receiving immunosuppressive agents, including tumor necrosis factor alpha (TNF-α) inhibitors.[214] A delay in the diagnosis of blastomycosis is common, especially in children.[204,215,216]

Treatment depends upon the extent of disease and immune status of the patient. Whereas observation alone may be an option for mild pulmonary or primary inoculation skin disease, most patients require therapy, especially those with severe disease or immunocompromise or disseminated involvement. Local excision has been utilized for small lesions limited to skin. Systemic therapeutic options for blastomycosis include itraconazole, fluconazole, voriconazole, and amphotericin B. Azole antifungal therapy should be continued for at least 6 months and for at least 1 year in patients with blastomycotic osteomyelitis.[217,218] Life-threatening, CNS, or disseminated disease, as well as infection in the immunocompromised host, should be treated initially with amphotericin B (4 to 6 weeks), and therapy can be switched over to itraconazole after clinical stabilization.[217,218] Liposomal amphotericin B appears to have superior CNS penetration.

Coccidioidomycosis

Coccidioidomycosis is a deep fungal infection caused by *Coccidioides immitis*, a soil saprophyte endemic in the hot, arid desert areas of the southwestern United States (especially the San Joaquin Valley in California), Mexico, and parts of South America. Inhalation of airborne arthroconidia results in infection, which in many cases is asymptomatic. Rare fomite transmission has been reported.[219] Occasional epidemics of coccidioidomycosis have been seen, often after severe dust storms and even in 1994 after a California earthquake.[220] The incidence of coccidioidomycosis has been increasing in the United States, and in some highly endemic regions nearly 100% of the population has serologic evidence of past exposure.[201]

C. immitis infection is often asymptomatic or may present with influenza-like symptoms of fever, cough, chest pain, headache, sore throat, and fatigue.[221] Erythema nodosum or erythema multiforme may develop. Generalized arthralgias may accompany these acute symptoms, and this syndrome is referred to as *desert rheumatism* or *Valley fever.* Acute pulmonary infection, which accounts for 98% of cases, usually resolves without therapy over several weeks.[222] Around 5% of patients will have asymptomatic residual lesions in the lungs, usually nodules or thin-walled cavities.[222]

Extrapulmonary disease occurs in a minority of patients, and in this case the organism disseminates hematogenously to any of several organs, including the meninges, bones, joints, skin, and soft tissues. Disseminated disease is most common in Blacks, Filipinos, and Native Americans, as well as in patients with immunosuppression.[221] In one large series of pediatric coccidioidomycosis at a California children's hospital, Black children represented one-third of the group with extrapulmonary dissemination; this group also appears more likely, along with Hispanics, to require hospitalization.[223,224] In recent decades, *Coccidioides* species have become significant opportunistic pathogens in patients infected with HIV and in recipients of organ transplants.[225]

Skin involvement in coccidioidomycosis may be seen in the setting of acute disease or disseminated disease and, rarely, as a primary inoculation infection. During the acute phase of infection, a generalized erythematous macular exanthem may appear within the first 1 to 2 days of illness. As mentioned earlier, erythema multiforme or erythema nodosum lesions may also be present during this phase of the illness, as may Sweet syndrome (see Chapter 20) or an entity referred to as *interstitial granulomatous dermatitis.* The latter refers to a granulomatous dermatitis that may occur in the setting of a variety of infectious, inflammatory, or autoimmune disorders.[225] In addition to these "parainfectious" cutaneous stigmata, infectious skin lesions may present (primarily with disseminated disease) as single or multiple verrucous, granulomatous papules and plaques (Fig. 17.58); subcutaneous abscess; acneiform papules; and pustules. Although lesions may occur anywhere on the skin surface, they are most common on the head (particularly the nasolabial fold), neck, and chest.[226] Cutaneous findings in coccidioidomycosis are not specific, and as with many deep fungal disorders may suggest a variety of potential diagnoses in the differential. Primary cutaneous inoculation is relatively rare and occurs through injury by contaminated splinters or thorns or by accidental inoculation in laboratory or autopsy rooms. This form of coccidioidomycosis is usually characterized by a painless ulcerated plaque with lymphangitis and lymphadenopathy (similar to that seen in sporotrichosis or blastomycosis). Although healing usually takes place within a few months, there are rare reports of patients with primary cutaneous inoculation developing systemic dissemination.[227]

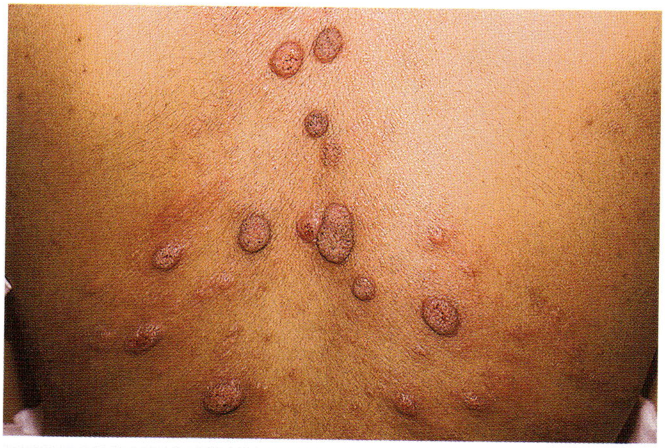

Fig. 17.58 Cutaneous coccidioidomycosis. Multiple verrucous papules and plaques in a patient with cutaneous coccidioidomycosis disseminated from a primary pulmonary infection.

The diagnosis of coccidioidomycosis can be confirmed by demonstration of the characteristic large, thick-walled mature spherules with endospores in tissue biopsy specimens. Fungal culture of materials such as pus, sputum, or aspirates will often grow *C. immitis*, but because the organism is highly infectious, special precautions are necessary to prevent laboratory accidents caused by airborne spread of arthrospores. Serologic and skin testing are also useful in making the diagnosis. The coccidioidin skin test usually becomes positive soon after the development of symptoms in patients with primary infection, although anergy may be present in progressive disease.[222] IgM and IgG (complement fixation) antibodies may be present, with the latter appearing between 4 and 12 weeks after infection and disappearing several months later if disease resolution occurs. Changes in the antibody titer may be useful for monitoring disease activity and response to therapy. A high titer of complement fixation antibody denotes severe extensive disease and a poorer prognosis; complement fixation antibodies in cerebrospinal fluid indicate the presence of CNS infection. Importantly, some serologic tests (complement fixation and immunodiffusion) can cross react with *Histoplasma* organisms.[228] *In situ* hybridization and PCR techniques may also be useful in confirming the diagnosis.[225]

The majority of infections with coccidioidomycosis are self-limiting, go undetected, and do not require specific therapy. Disseminated disease, however, may follow a fulminant course or persist for several years. The choice of the therapeutic agent and decisions regarding length of therapy depend on the immune status of the host, the seriousness of the infection, and the organs involved. Therapeutic options include fluconazole, itraconazole, and amphotericin B. Newer azole antifungals (e.g., voriconazole, posaconazole) have been reported but are not established for this indication in children. Amphotericin B is the recommended initial therapy for severe or progressive infection, and high-dose fluconazole is recommended for CNS infections.[228] Patients with CNS infection with *C. immitis* may require amphotericin B infusions into the cerebrospinal fluid (intrathecal administration). Pulmonary resection has a role in managing severe hemoptysis, sequestrations, or lung cavitations.

Paracoccidioidomycosis

South American blastomycosis (paracoccidioidomycosis) occurs almost exclusively in South and Central America and is caused by infection with the dimorphic fungus *Paracoccidioides brasiliensis*. The disorder is endemic in Brazil (where the majority of cases occur), Venezuela, Colombia, Ecuador, Argentina, and Peru. It may occur many years after relocation out of an endemic region.[229] It is most common in adults and uncommon in childhood, when it is referred to as the *acute juvenile form.* It is thought that the organism lives as a saprophyte on vegetation or in soil and that the infection is acquired by direct implantation into the skin or mucous membranes, possibly through the practice of cleaning the teeth with small pieces of infected vegetation or in pulmonary lesions by direct inhalation of the organism. An autosomal dominant mutation in *STAT4*, resulting in an error of IL-12–dependent interferon-γ immunity, may be associated with increased susceptibility to paracoccidioidomycosis.[230]

Paracoccidioidomycosis may present with a wide spectrum of involvement, ranging from asymptomatic pulmonary infection to symptomatic infection involving one or several organs that may progress in a fulminant fashion. The most common clinical manifestations in children are lymphadenopathy, weight loss, and fever.[231] The most common organs of involvement are the lungs, skin, mucosae, lymph nodes, and bone. Mucocutaneous involvement presents with infiltrative, ulcerative lesions on the lips and in the mouth, pharynx, or nasal cavity. The ulcerative and verrucous plaques may extend and ultimately progress to destroy the nose, lips, and facies. Pain and dental loss may occur. Hematogenous or lymphatic spread results in subcutaneous abscesses, and the lymph nodes draining the affected areas are palpable, painful, and adherent to the overlying skin, occasionally progressing to form chronic sinuses and suppurative plaques. Primary cutaneous infection is rarely reported.[232] The juvenile form tends to be more aggressive and involve primarily the reticuloendothelial system.[233]

Paracoccidioidomycosis is diagnosed by recognition of the typical yeast forms in tissue specimens, fungal culture, serologic studies (mainly in immunocompetent hosts), or newer molecular methodologies such as PCR, which may be useful in observing response to therapy.[229] Treatment usually consists of azole antifungals or amphotericin B.

Histoplasmosis

Histoplasmosis is another deep fungal infection caused by a thermally dimorphic fungus, in this case *Histoplasma capsulatum*. This organism (*H. capsulatum* var. *capsulatum*) is endemic in the Americas, especially in Ohio and the Mississippi river valleys and Latin America, and is more concentrated in places where the soil is enriched by bird excreta or bat guano.[233] The other variety, *H. capsulatum* var. *duboisii*, is endemic in some areas of Africa. Infection is usually acquired by inhalation of fungal microconidia and may result in various manifestations, from asymptomatic infection to disseminated, progressive disease. Transmission from fomites, direct inoculation, organ transplantation, and sexual contact have also been reported.[234] Histoplasmosis affects infants and children as well as adults. In developing countries, childhood malnutrition is the most frequent predisposing factor to infection.[235]

The manifestations of histoplasmosis are quite varied. The classically recognized forms are acute pulmonary, chronic cavitary, and disseminated. Primary infection is asymptomatic or produces very mild symptoms in up to 95% of patients. Many patients manifest pulmonary symptoms, including cough and chest pain along with fever and malaise. A chronic pulmonary form may resemble tuberculosis both clinically and radiographically. Involvement of the reticuloendothelial system may occur and accounts for most of the signs of progressive disseminated histoplasmosis (PDH). PDH tends to occur in patients with compromised cell-mediated immunity. Bone marrow involvement with pancytopenia is common, as are hepatosplenomegaly and lymphadenopathy.[236] GI bleeding, meningitis, adrenal gland involvement, and endocarditis may also occur with disseminated histoplasmosis. Disseminated disease occurs in less than 1% of those infected. Cardiac tamponade may develop in up to 25% of patients with pulmonary histoplasmosis.[234]

Skin involvement is uncommon in histoplasmosis but may be seen in the disseminated form and rarely in a primary inoculation form. The morphologic characteristics include papules, plaques, pustules, purpura, nodules, ulcers, abscesses, molluscum-like lesions, severe dermatitis, exfoliative erythroderma, and verrucous lesions. Erythema multiforme and erythema nodosum may both occur, usually in the setting of acute pulmonary infection. The characteristic ulcerative, mucocutaneous lesions of the nose, mouth, pharynx, larynx, genitals, and perianal region are seen in chronic disseminated disease and in patients with immunodeficiency. Lesions in these regions may present as superficial or deep ulcerations with heaped-up borders, nodular masses, or verrucous plaques.[237] Oral manifestations are seen in 25% to 75% of patients with disseminated disease.[238,239]

Children with histoplasmosis tend to have more disseminated disease. In fact, 20% of apparently immunocompetent patients with disseminated infection are children.[233] A disseminated form of histoplasmosis in infants may be associated with transient hyperglobulinemia and T-cell deficiency and when occurring after exposure to a large inoculum of the pathogen has a high mortality rate.[240] In children with histoplasmosis, the incidence of extensive ulcers along the GI mucosa that give rise to diarrhea and other GI disturbances suggests that organisms may be ingested rather than inhaled in these individuals.

The gold standard for diagnosing histoplasmosis is identification of the small intracellular yeast-like organisms in tissue specimens, sputum, or peripheral blood and fungal culture. Tissue biopsies from skin or mucosal lesions reveal necrotizing granulomas along with the yeast forms. Cytologic examination of tissue aspirates or fluids can provide presumptive evidence for the diagnosis. The usefulness of the histoplasmin skin test is quite low, given its nonspecificity, especially in endemic areas.[236] *Histoplasma* serologies (including complement fixation and immunodiffusion precipitin bands) are available but hampered by a delay in their detectability (for 4 to 8 weeks) and high rates of false-positive and false-negative responses. Antigen testing is considered the diagnostic modality of choice for histoplasmosis.[241] Detection of *Histoplasma* antigen in urine is useful and more sensitive than serum testing, but has the disadvantage of many potential causes for false-positive results, especially other endemic mycoses.[237,241] An enzyme-linked immunosorbent assay (ELISA) against *H. capsulatum* circulating antigens has good sensitivity and excellent specificity,[242] although it may not be readily available. PCR-based molecular assays have the advantages of high specificity and quick turnaround, but are not currently commercially available.

In mild cases of histoplasmosis, treatment may not be necessary, and the disorder runs a benign, self-limited course. For severe or disseminated disease, systemic antifungal therapy with amphotericin B is usually indicated. For more localized or less severe disease (e.g., chronic pulmonary histoplasmosis), oral azole antifungal therapy is an option. Various regimens have been reported in pediatric patients. Disseminated childhood histoplasmosis has been treated successfully with amphotericin B, itraconazole, ketoconazole (before the FDA warning), or voriconazole.[233,240,243] Amphotericin B is recommended for 1 to 2 weeks until there is clinical improvement in disseminated or severe infection, followed by itraconazole for an additional 12 weeks.[244] In patients with acquired immunodeficiency syndrome (AIDS) and severe histoplasmosis, amphotericin B is indicated, whereas itraconazole may be appropriate therapy for mild to moderate disseminated disease.[245] Fluconazole is less effective than the other azole antifungal agents, and clinical data on the newer azoles, voriconazole and posaconazole, are limited.[237,239]

OPPORTUNISTIC MYCOSES

With the spread of AIDS and advancements in cancer chemotherapy, bone marrow and solid organ transplantation, and both routine and intensive medical care, patient populations who are vulnerable to potentially fatal deep fungal infections have emerged. These organisms are generally nonpathogenic but in certain at-risk individuals who have an alteration or breakdown of host defenses may result in severe disseminated infection. The opportunistic mycoses to be discussed here include aspergillosis, cryptococcosis, fusarium, and mucormycosis. Risk factors for opportunistic mycoses are listed in Table 17.3.[246]

Aspergillosis

Aspergillosis is an uncommon opportunistic fungal disease of the respiratory tract and other sites caused by a variety of *Aspergillus* species. Although *Aspergillus fumigatus* is the most commonly identified pathogen, *Aspergillus niger, Aspergillus flavus, Aspergillus terreus, Aspergillus nidulans*, and other species have been reported in recent years. Invasive aspergillosis is most often seen in patients with prolonged neutropenia and in transplant recipients.[247]

Aspergillus species are ubiquitous and are normally nonpathogenic. When pathogenic, they primarily cause infection in the lung, although the skin, eyes, CNS, bones, GI tract, liver, spleen, lymph nodes, nasopharynx, and genitourinary tract may also be affected. In children, the highest-risk groups are those with AIDS, leukemia, corticosteroid or immunosuppressive therapy (including calcineurin inhibitors and TNF-α inhibitors), history of bone marrow or solid organ transplantation, chronic granulomatous disease, and severe combined immunodeficiency.[248–250] Neonates, especially premature ones, appear to be another population at risk for disseminated aspergillosis.[251] Other neonatal aspergillosis risk factors include corticosteroid use, prolonged hospitalization or use of antibiotics, hyperglycemia, and skin trauma from tape adhesive in relation to prolonged use of arm boards.[252,253] Despite aggressive therapy, invasive aspergillosis in children is associated with a mortality rate as high as 85%, although the pediatric survival rate appears to be improving with newer combination antifungal therapies.[254,255] Cutaneous aspergillosis has also been reported in immunocompetent adults and children, typically after intravenous catheter site occlusion or trauma.[256–258]

One of the most common characteristic manifestations of aspergillosis is the pulmonary intracavitary fungus ball. This is composed of colonies of *Aspergillus*, inflammatory exudate, cells, and fibrin in the form of a sphere that may measure from 1 to 5 cm in diameter. Although it occasionally causes hemoptysis, most patients with fungus

Table 17.3 Risk Factors for Opportunistic Mycoses/ Invasive Fungal Disease

Factor	Comment
Neutropenia	Usually prolonged, severe
Hematologic malignancy	And associated chemotherapy
Transplant recipient	Primarily BMT/HSCT
HIV infection/AIDS	Especially cryptococcosis
High-dose corticosteroids	Often in setting of GVHD therapy
Broad-spectrum antibiotics	
Alterations of oropharyngeal and gastrointestinal mucosae	Via chemotherapy
Altered skin integrity	Catheter sites, skin breakdown or occlusion, burns, wounds
Presence of catheters	Vascular, urinary
Extremes of age	Premature infants, elderly persons
Prolonged hospitalization	ICU
Diabetes mellitus	Specific to mucormycosis
Total parenteral nutrition	

Modified from Gutierrez Paredes EM, Gamez Perez L, Gonzalez Rodriguez AJ, et al. Disseminated fusariosis in immunocompromised patients. Eur J Dermatol 2011;21(5):753–735; and Pfaller MA, Pappas PG, Wingard JR. Invasive fungal pathogens: Current epidemiologic trends. Clin Infect Dis 2006;43:S3–14.

AIDS, Acquired immunodeficiency syndrome; *BMT,* bone marrow transplantation; *GVHD,* graft-versus-host disease; *HIV,* human immunodeficiency virus; *HSCT,* hematopoietic stem cell transplantation; *ICU,* intensive care unit.

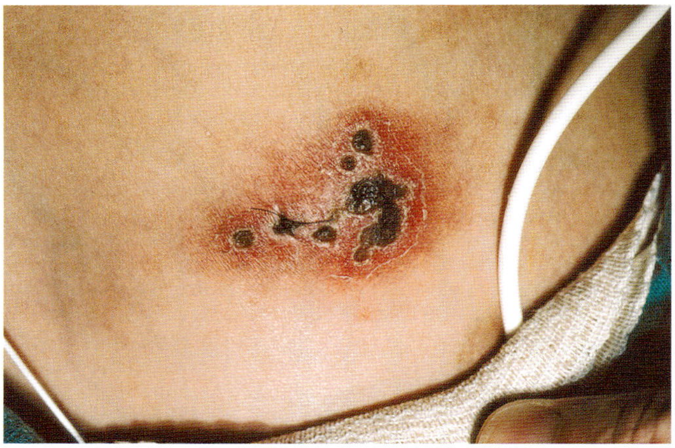

Fig. 17.59 Cutaneous aspergillosis. Erythematous plaque with necrosis and eschar formation in a young female with immunosuppression and disseminated *Aspergillus fumigatus* infection.

balls are asymptomatic. Another form of pulmonary disease is invasive pulmonary aspergillosis, which may be necrotizing and is often associated with multiorgan dissemination.

Cutaneous aspergillosis may occur in two forms: primary or secondary. Primary cutaneous aspergillosis usually occurs at sites of skin injury such as intravenous catheter insertion sites, burns, surgical wounds, or sites covered by various products including occlusive dressings and tape. Secondary cutaneous aspergillosis occurs with direct extension to the skin from underlying soft-tissue infection or hematogenous dissemination.[259] Less commonly, an opportunistic infection of the paranasal sinuses may result in mucopurulent or blood-tinged nasal discharge, headache, periorbital neuralgia, and rhinitis. With extension of this process, the face may become erythematous, swollen, warm, and tender, suggesting a diagnosis of cellulitis or erysipelas.

Cutaneous aspergillosis may initially present as nondescript erythematous macules, papules, or plaques. Common secondary findings include hemorrhagic bullae and necrosis (Fig. 17.59), which may extend rapidly. Eschar formation is often seen. In patients with hematogenous dissemination, embolic lesions present as widespread erythematous to purpuric macules and papules with ulceration and necrosis and may simulate the lesions of ecthyma gangrenosum (caused by *Pseudomonas aeruginosa*). Pustules overlying an erythematous patch are a common finding in the early cutaneous lesions of neonates and often progress to ulceration, necrosis, and eschar formation.[260]

The diagnosis of cutaneous aspergillus can be confirmed by tissue biopsy for histopathology and fungal culture. A deep skin biopsy is desirable to visualize the dermal and subcutaneous blood vessels, given the angiotropic nature of *Aspergillus* species. Fungal stains applied to the biopsy material will reveal large fungal hyphae with "acute-angle" branching, and this method will enable a more rapid diagnosis than awaiting results of the fungal culture. Blood cultures are rarely positive. ELISA and PCR testing are available in some centers and may offer a more rapid and reliable means of diagnosing disseminated aspergillosis, especially in immunocompromised children.[248] The galactomannan antigen assay appears to be sensitive in diagnosing invasive aspergillosis in children, although the cutoff thresholds for this population continue to be studied.[261–263]

The treatment of aspergillosis depends on the underlying immune status of the patient and risk factors for disseminated infection. In most cases, systemic therapy is indicated. Occasionally, surgical approaches may suffice (e.g., primary cutaneous aspergillosis in a burn patient without underlying risk factors for disseminated disease). Although amphotericin B has been the mainstay of systemic therapy for years, in some patients this agent is associated with untoward side effects and in others it may result in a suboptimal response.[247] Azole antifungal agents such as itraconazole have also been used with mixed results. The newer broad-spectrum triazole, voriconazole, has been evaluated and demonstrated effective in adults and children with invasive aspergillosis, although the numerous drug interactions may limit its usefulness in some patients.[247,264,265] Voriconazole is considered the drug of choice for all forms of invasive aspergillosis, the exception being in neonates, for whom amphotericin B is recommended.[250] Caspofungin has also been studied in salvage therapy for invasive aspergillosis, and a body surface area dosing calculation is preferred over a weight-based regimen for treating children with this agent.[266] Posaconazole is an option for resistant disease, and isavuconazole may be another option but has not been well studied in children.

Cryptococcosis

Cryptococcus neoformans is a ubiquitous encapsulated fungus capable of causing severe disease in immunocompromised individuals, especially those with AIDS. Disseminated disease has been rarely observed in immunocompetent children.[267] Whereas it is well established as the most common cause of life-threatening fungal infection in adults with HIV infection (an analysis of stored serum samples from HIV-infected adults with low CD4 counts enrolled in the United States between 1986 and 2012 found a prevalence of cryptococcal antigenemia of around 3%), infection in children with HIV may occur in up to 1% of those with AIDS.[268,269] The organism has been found in various fruits, soil, pigeon excreta, and cow's milk. It is believed to be acquired via inhalation of aerosolized particles from the environment, and recent data suggest that *C. neoformans* may infect many immunocompetent children early in life, resulting in either asymptomatic infection or nonspecific "viral" symptoms.[270] The incidence of cryptococcosis has declined in the past decade, largely because of the improvements in

HIV care and the use of combination antiretroviral therapy (cART).[271] However, it continues to be an important cause of morbidity and mortality in HIV-infected children who reside in areas with less access to antiretroviral therapy.[272] *Cryptococcus laurentii* is a rare species that may also result in cutaneous lesions, although it is most often implicated in pulmonary, ocular, and disseminated infections.[273] *Cryptococcus gattii* may result in a respiratory illness with neurologic findings and has been reported in the Pacific Northwest in the United States, British Columbia, Canada, Australia, and Papua New Guinea.[274]

Cryptococcal infection most commonly presents as meningitis, meningoencephalitis, or sepsis. Infection may be localized to the lungs, producing focal pneumonia, patchy infiltrates, solitary nodules, abscesses, or pleural effusion. Pulmonary symptoms, however, may be absent or minimal, and although pulmonary involvement may be progressive, in most instances CNS manifestations predominate and infection is detected only after dissemination, which may include the skin. Cutaneous lesions may present months before other signs of systemic infection.[275] They may occasionally occur after trauma or extension from bony involvement but are usually the result of hematogenous spread from a pulmonary focus.

Skin lesions, which occur in 6% to 15% of patients with systemic infection, present most commonly on the head and neck, where they may often mimic the lesions of molluscum contagiosum. They begin as painless, firm, pink to red papules, pustules, or acneiform lesions. The molluscum-like lesions may be umbilicated or contain a tiny central hemorrhagic crust and may be multiple.[275] Surrounding inflammation is usually absent. As the lesions enlarge they may form infiltrated plaques, nodules, abscesses, or ulcers, often with raised papillomatous borders. Subcutaneous nodules have also been reported as an initial presentation.[276] In patients with primary inoculation cutaneous cryptococcosis, the clinical findings most often observed are ulcers, abscesses, or cellulitis.[277]

The diagnosis of cryptococcosis is confirmed by demonstration of the characteristic organism (surrounded by a polysaccharide capsule and with characteristic budding seen in India ink preparations) in cerebrospinal fluid, skin lesions, sputum, or tissue sections. Definitive diagnosis relies on isolation of the organism from biopsy tissue or bodily fluids.[274] Serologic studies, immunoblotting, and ELISA or latex agglutination assays for the cryptococcal polysaccharide are other diagnostic modalities; PCR-based diagnosis remains investigational. The recommended therapy for meningeal or severe cryptococcosis is amphotericin B with 5-flucytosine, because combination therapy appears to be superior to amphotericin monotherapy.[278] Fluconazole or itraconazole suppression is recommended after completion of the primary therapy.[274]

Fusarium Infection

Fusarium species are molds that are normally found in soil and the air and may result in localized infections in the nail (fusarium onychomycosis or paronychia) or in burn sites or surgical wounds. However, invasive *Fusarium* infection (or fusariosis) is an increasingly prevalent, serious opportunistic fungal infection that occurs especially in patients with hematologic malignancy undergoing cytotoxic chemotherapy or bone marrow transplantation. Prolonged neutropenia seems to be the main risk factor for this infection. Skin lesions are common in patients with disseminated *Fusarium* infection and may serve as the portal of entry for more widespread involvement. Cutaneous involvement may be mistaken for aspergillosis, given the potential clinical overlap in presentation. Disseminated fusariosis is considered to be the second most common opportunistic infection in neutropenic patients after *Aspergillus* and appears to be the most common agent resulting in fungemia with cutaneous lesions.[279,280]

Immunocompromised patients with *Fusarium* infection may have refractory fever, skin lesions, sinusitis, myalgias, or pneumonia. Endophthalmitis may occur from hematogenous seeding as opposed to the fusarial endophthalmitis that occurs in immunocompetent hosts as a complication of advanced keratitis or after ophthalmologic surgery.[281] Fungemia with multiorgan involvement is possible, and the organism is more often cultured from the blood than is *Aspergillus*. Disseminated infection is often notable for skin lesions, which occur in up to 80% of these patients.[282] Skin lesions of fusariosis may include paronychia, tinea pedis, onychomycosis, digital ulcers, or widespread lesions most often involving the extremities. The disseminated lesions present most often as painful, red to gray macules or papules, with purpura, necrosis, and eschar formation.[283] They may mimic the lesions of ecthyma gangrenosum.[284,285] Pustules, cellulitis, abscesses, bullae, and subcutaneous nodules may also occur, and "target lesions" have been described.[285,286] Less common manifestations may include panniculitis, sporotrichoid lesions, and intertrigo.[280]

Fusariosis is usually diagnosed via microscopic examination of skin biopsy specimens with confirmation by fungal culture of tissues and/or blood. Treatment is difficult and includes regular or lipid formulations of amphotericin B, itraconazole, and correction of the neutropenia with granulocyte colony-stimulating factor (G-CSF)– or granulocyte-macrophage colony-stimulating factor (GM-CSF)–stimulated granulocyte transfusions.[285] Newer antifungal agents such as voriconazole or posaconazole may also have a role in the treatment of this serious infection.[286,287]

Mucormycosis

Mucormycosis (also known as *zygomycosis* or *phycomycosis*) is an opportunistic fungal infection caused by a group of organisms in the order Mucorales (of the class Zygomycetes). Infection of the immunocompetent host is extremely rare despite continual exposure to these organisms. Mucormycosis occurs mainly in immunocompromised individuals and in patients with debilitating diseases (e.g., diabetes mellitus, anemia, heart or liver disease, burns, leukemia, or lymphoma) and is among the most acute, fulminant, and fatal of all fungal infections.[288] It may also occur with increased incidence in patients exposed to hospital construction activity. It may involve any organ of the body but most commonly affects the skin, lungs, meninges, GI tract, and structures of the head and neck. Up to 10% of cases of mucormycosis may occur in immunocompetent individuals without identifiable predisposing factors.[289] In children, mucormycosis is associated with many of the risk factors outlined in Table 17.3; in addition, prematurity, low birthweight, malnutrition, and use of wooden tongue depressors and cotton stockinettes have also been reported in association with this infection.[290] Whereas the incidence of mucormycosis may be increasing in adults, a retrospective 7-year study at a large tertiary children's hospital suggested no such trend in pediatric patients.[291]

The causative fungi of mucormycosis include species of *Mucor, Rhizopus, Absidia, Cunninghamella*, and *Rhizomucor*. The most common cause of zygomycosis is *Rhizopus oryzae (arrhizus)*. These organisms are saprophytic and grow in soil and on decaying organic materials such as vegetation, fruit, and bread.[292] The portal of entry for these infections varies with the site of the disease. Rhinocerebral mucormycosis is the most common form and affects primarily patients with diabetes, as well as patients with immunocompromise. Importantly, dissemination of mucormycosis occurs in up to 38% of pediatric cases and more than half of infected neonates.[293]

Cutaneous or subcutaneous infections occur most often in diabetics with recurrent acidosis or in patients with a history of skin trauma or severe burns. This form of infection is characterized by hemorrhagic or necrotic papules and plaques, chronic indolent ulcers, and slowly enlarging dusky nodules. The initial lesion is often a small area of macular discoloration or dusky erythema that gradually enlarges and ulcerates. Necrosis may be marked, and there may be a foul-smelling purulent exudate. A gangrenous form results in rapid ulceration and necrotizing fasciitis–like tissue destruction. The skin lesions of cutaneous mucormycosis are not pathognomonic and may be confused with lesions of ecthyma gangrenosum, aspergillosis, deep fungal infections, other soft-tissue infections, pyoderma gangrenosum, or vasculitis.[288,294] The skin lesions may be primary or secondary, in which case they are related to hematogenous dissemination of the organism from a primary infection in another organ. Primary skin lesions often occur at sites of wound dressings, intravenous lines, and adhesive monitor leads.[295]

The rhinocerebral form is usually characterized by a suppurative necrotizing infection of the paranasal sinuses with periorbital pain, swelling, edema, proptosis, extraocular muscle paresis, and decreased visual acuity. This form is uniformly fatal within weeks when there is extensive involvement, and combined treatment with surgical debridement/resection and systemic antifungals is warranted.[296] Other reported forms of mucormycosis include GI, pulmonary, and disseminated. An angioinvasive form of mucormycosis has been described in neonates, usually those with the risk factors of prematurity, low birthweight, broad-spectrum antibiotic or corticosteroid therapy, and history of local skin trauma.[297] However, the most common types to occur in premature neonates appear to be the GI and cutaneous forms.[298]

The diagnosis of mucormycosis relies on tissue biopsy and histologic examination. Broad, nonseptated, thick-walled hyphae are seen and may be noted to be invading cutaneous blood vessels. Fungal culture is confirmatory. Therapy is difficult and often requires a combination of surgical debridement, treatment of the underlying disease process, removal of the source of infection (when possible), and intravenous amphotericin B. Lipid formulations of amphotericin B appear to be more efficacious in treating CNS mucormycosis.[299] Posaconazole may be a reasonable option for those who are resistant to or intolerant of amphotericin.[299]

The complete list of 299 references for this chapter is available online at http://expertconsult.inkling.com.

Key References

Feldstein S, Totri C, Friedlander SF. Antifungal therapy for onychomycosis in children. Clin Dermatol 2015;33:333–9.

Gupta AK, Lane D, Paquet M. Systematic review of systemic treatments for tinea versicolor and evidence-based dosing regimen recommendations. J Cutan Med Surg 2014;18(2):79–90.

Kaufman DA, Coggins SA, Zanelli SA, Weitkamp JH. Congenital cutaneous candidiasis: prompt systemic treatment is associated with improved outcomes in neonates. Clin Infect Dis 2017;64(10):1387–95.

Tragiannidis A, Tsoulas C, Groll AH. Invasive candidiasis and candidaemia in neonates and children: update on current guidelines. Mycoses 2015;58:10–21.

Adams-Chapman I, Bann CM, Das A, Goldberg RN, Stoll BJ, Walsh MC, et al. Neurodevelopmental outcome of extremely low birth weight infants with Candida infection. J Pediatr 2013;163(4):961–7.

Frost HM, Anderson J, Ivacic L, Meece J. Blastomycosis in children: an analysis of clinical, epidemiologic, and genetic features. J Pediatr Infect Dis Soc 2017;6(1):49–56.

Francis JR, Villanueva P, Bryant P, Blyth CC. Mucormycosis in children: review and recommendations for management. J Pediatr Infect Dis Soc 2018;7(2):159–64.

Kelly BP. Superficial fungal infections. Pediatr Rev 2012;33(4):e22–37.

Gupta AK, Paquet M. Systemic antifungals to treat onychomycosis in children: a systematic review. Pediatr Dermatol 2013;30(3):294–302.

Honig PJ, Frieden IJ, Kim HJ, Yan AC. Streptococcal intertrigo: an underrecognized condition in children. Pediatrics 2003;112:1427–9.

Benjamin DK, Stoll BJ, Gantz MG, et al. Neonatal candidiasis: epidemiology, risk factors, and clinical judgment. Pediatrics 2010;126(4):e865–73.

DiCaudo DJ. Coccidioidomycosis: a review and update. J Am Acad Dermatol 2006;55:929–42.

18 Infestations, Bites, and Stings

Parasites are a fascinating and important cause of skin disease in children. They produce their effects in various ways: mechanical trauma from bites or stings, injection of pharmacologically active substances that induce local or systemic effects, allergic reactions in a previously sensitized host, persistent granulomatous reactions to retained parts, direct invasion of the epidermis, or transmission of infectious disease by blood-sucking insects.

Arthropods

Arthropods are elongated invertebrate animals with segmented bodies, true appendages, and a chitinous exoskeleton. Those of dermatologic significance are the eight-legged arachnids (mites, ticks, spiders, and scorpions) and the six-legged insects (lice, flies, mosquitoes, fleas, bugs, bees, wasps, ants, caterpillars/moths, and beetles).

ARACHNIDS

The term *mite* refers to a large number of tiny arachnids, many of which live at least part of their lives as parasites upon animals or plants or in prepared foods. Of greatest clinical significance are itch mites *(Sarcoptes scabiei)*, grain mites, and harvest mites (chiggers). Avian mite–associated dermatitis is also well-recognized. Mites attack humans by burrowing under or attaching themselves to the skin, where they inflict trivial bites that result in associated dermatitides.

Scabies

Scabies is a common skin infestation caused by the mite *S. scabiei*. This mite is an obligate human parasite residing in burrowed tunnels within the human epidermis. Mites of all developmental stages may burrow into skin, depositing feces in their tracks. The female mite also lays eggs in these burrows, which serves to further propagate the infestation. The adult female mite has a lifespan of around 15 to 30 days, measures around 400 μm, and lays one to four eggs per day, which hatch in 3 to 4 days.[1,2] After hatching, the larvae mature into adult mites in 10 to 14 days, and the duration of the whole life cycle is 30 to 60 days.

Scabies is transmitted most often by direct contact with an infested individual, although acquisition from fomites such as bedding and clothing is also possible. The survival time for a mite separated from the human host is estimated at several days. It is estimated that 15 to 20 minutes of close contact time is required for the transmission of scabies from one person to another. Scabies disproportionately affects women and children, as well as individuals with certain predisposing conditions, including immunocompromise, severe mental or physical handicap, and human immunodeficiency virus (HIV) infection. Scabies is seen worldwide in infants and children, and in the United States there seems to be a fairly high incidence in foreign-born adoptees, especially those from Asia or Latin America.[3,4] It was also diagnosed in nearly 10% of international adoptees in a European cross-sectional cohort study.[5] The high incidence of scabies in internationally adopted children may be related to the high incidence of infestation seen in orphanages. Scabies continues to be a significant public health issue in the developing world, with a disproportionate burden of disease noted in children who live in overcrowded, lower socioeconomic tropical regions. A global burden of disease study revealed the greatest scabies burden in south, east, and southeast Asia; Oceania; and tropical Latin America.[6] High endemic rates of scabies are noted in closed communities and institutional environments.[7] In institutions, risk factors for scabies include institution type (with long-term care facilities and larger-sized institutions having a higher incidence), extensive physical contact between patients and care workers, movement of patients, delay in diagnosis, and poor implementation of infection control or treatment.[8]

The incubation period for classic scabies is around 3 weeks, with reinfestation resulting in more immediate symptoms.[9] The initial symptom of scabies is usually pruritus, which is often evident well before the clinical signs become apparent. Patients with scabies usually complain of worsening pruritus during nighttime hours. Infants and young children may also experience irritability and poor feeding. The skin findings include papules, nodules, burrows, and vesiculopustules (Figs. 18.1 through 18.5). The most common locations for scabies lesions are the interdigital spaces, wrists, ankles, axillae, waist, groin, palms, and soles. Burrows on the palms may reveal a pattern of scale reminiscent of the wake left on a water surface by a moving boat and has been termed the *wake sign*.[10] In infants, lesions may also be seen on the head (Fig. 18.6), which is rarely involved in older patients. Infants commonly have involvement of the palms, soles, dorsal feet, face, and axillae.[11] In older children and adolescents, the most common sites of involvement are the wrists, interdigital spaces, and waist. Although bullous lesions are uncommon in scabies, vesicles are often found in infants and young children,[12,13] probably due to the predisposition for blister formation in general that is seen in this age group. Occasionally the Darier sign may be positive, and hence the diagnosis of urticaria pigmentosa may be considered.[14] Genital involvement presenting as papules, crusted papules, or nodules (Figs. 18.7 and 18.8) and areolar lesions are other classic presentation patterns. Excoriations are commonly noted.

Scabies nodules are red-brown nodules (Figs. 18.9 and 18.10) that represent a vigorous hypersensitivity response of the host. They occur most commonly on the trunk, axillary regions, and genitalia and are seen primarily in infants. Although they eventually resolve, scabies nodules may be present for several months. They are occasionally misdiagnosed (both clinically and histologically) as signs of a neoplastic disorder (e.g., leukemia or lymphoma cutis).

Crusted, or Norwegian, scabies is a form of the disorder that presents as scaly, dermatitic papules or plaques. Crusted scabies may be localized or generalized and occurs primarily in immunocompromised patients (especially those with HIV infection) and in those who are mentally retarded or physically incapacitated.[9] The lesions of this disorder may mimic atopic dermatitis (Figs. 18.11 and 18.12), psoriasis, warts, or a drug reaction, and nail dystrophy may be present.

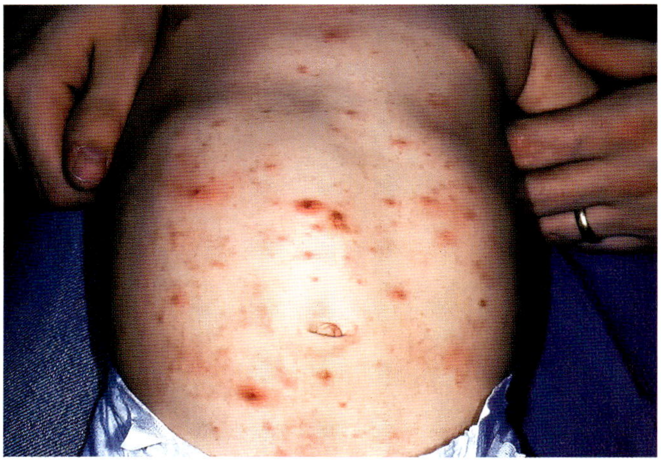

Fig. 18.1 Scabies. Erythematous papules with crusting in an infested male infant.

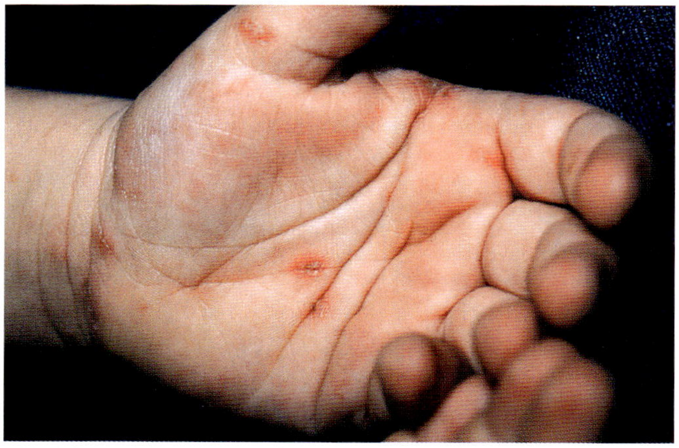

Fig. 18.2 Scabies. Erythematous papules and burrows involving the palm and wrist. Scrapings of lesions from the palmar creases have a high yield on microscopic examination.

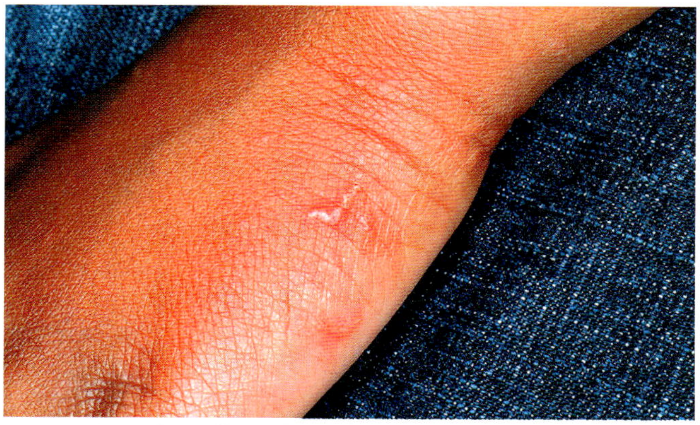

Fig. 18.3 Scabies. Curvilinear burrow of the lateral hand.

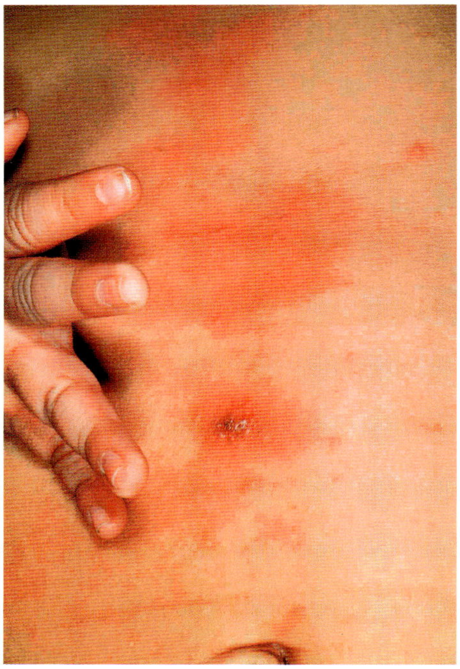

Fig. 18.4 Scabies. Crusted papule of the abdomen in an infant with scabies.

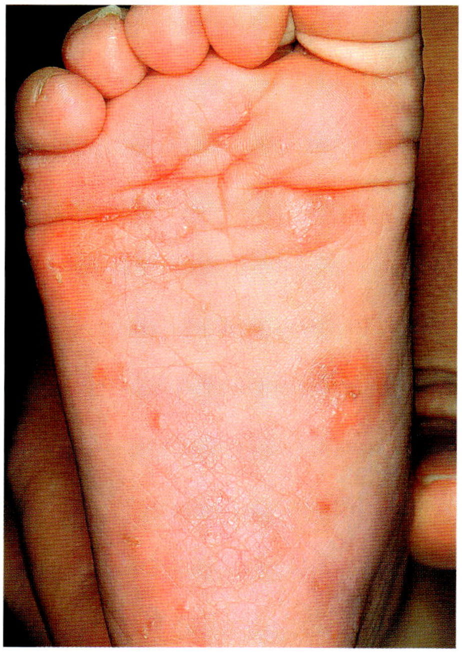

Fig. 18.5 Scabies. Erythematous papules and linear burrows of the plantar surface of the foot.

Crusted scabies is commonly misdiagnosed and mismanaged.[15] A delay in the diagnosis of crusted scabies may lead to the inadvertent exposure of multiple physical contacts. The lesions may become heavily crusted and hyperkeratotic and may be minimally pruritic in some patients. Crusted scabies is extremely contagious, given the large numbers of mites (often thousands) that may be present. In classic scabies, only around 12 mites on average are present. Patients with crusted scabies are often the source for large epidemics within hospitals, given the lack of recognition and subsequent diagnostic delay.

Complications of scabies are generally mild. They include secondary bacterial infection, impaired skin integrity, pain, and, rarely, debilitation related to limitations in movement secondary to pain. Secondary infection is most commonly the result of *Staphylococcus aureus* or group A β-hemolytic streptococci and presents as crusting, oozing, pustules or

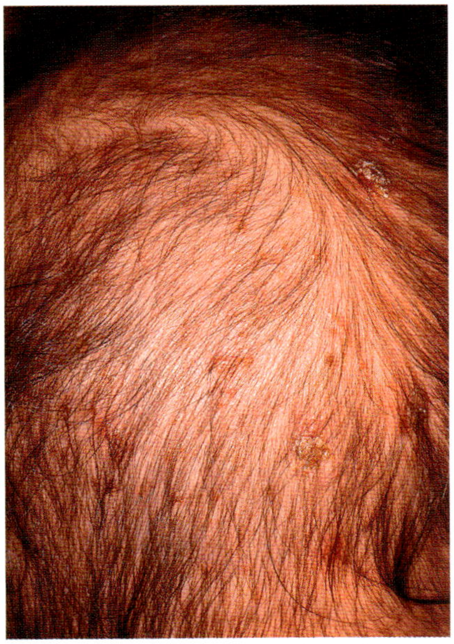

Fig. 18.6 Scabies. Erythematous papules and crusted papules of the scalp in an infant.

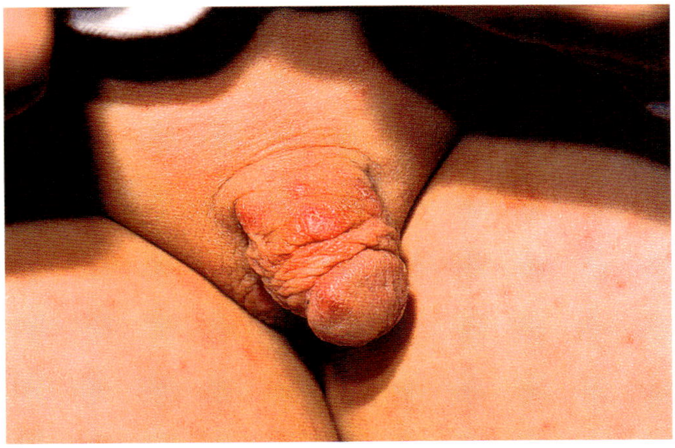

Fig. 18.7 Scabies. Erythematous papules of the penis with crusting of the glans penis. These findings are highly suggestive of scabies infestation.

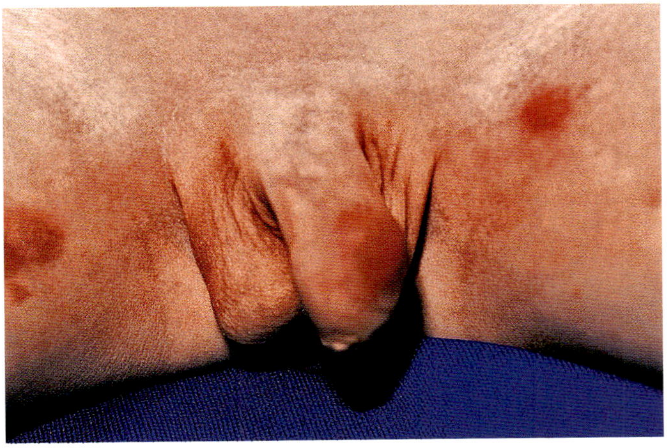

Fig. 18.8 Scabies. Nodules of the penis and inguinal regions in a young male recently treated for scabies.

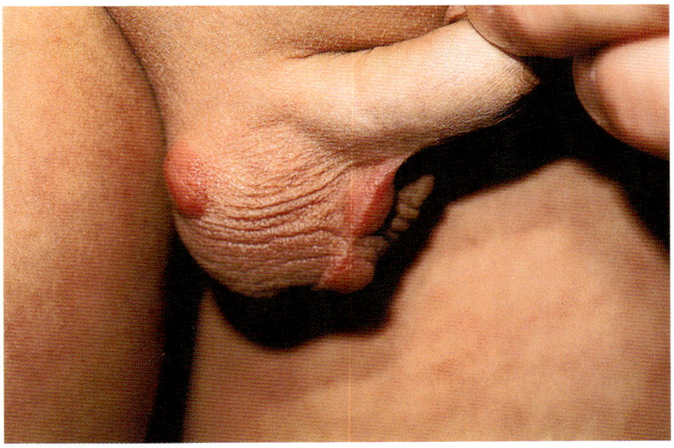

Fig. 18.9 Scabies nodules. These infiltrative nodules persisted for 6 months after effective treatment for scabies.

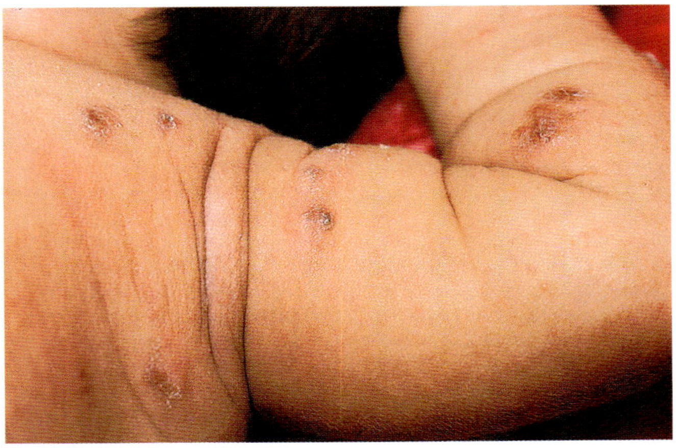

Fig. 18.10 Scabies nodules. Early scabies nodules developing at sites of crusting; these lesions persisted long after adequate therapy for the infestation.

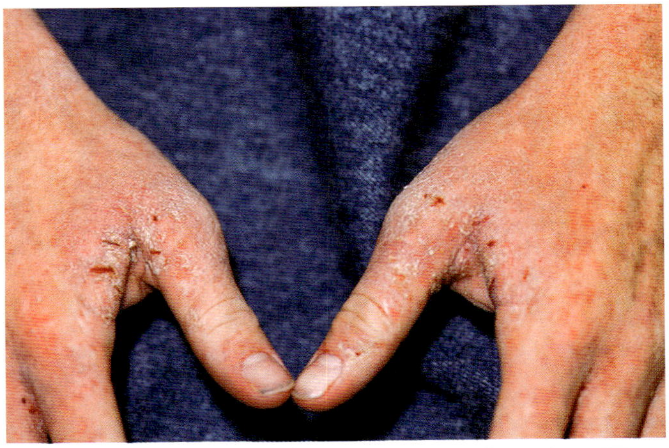

Fig. 18.11 Crusted scabies. This heart transplant recipient had eczematous, crusted plaques in a widespread distribution that was resistant to topical corticosteroid therapy. Mineral oil preparation revealed many live scabies mites.

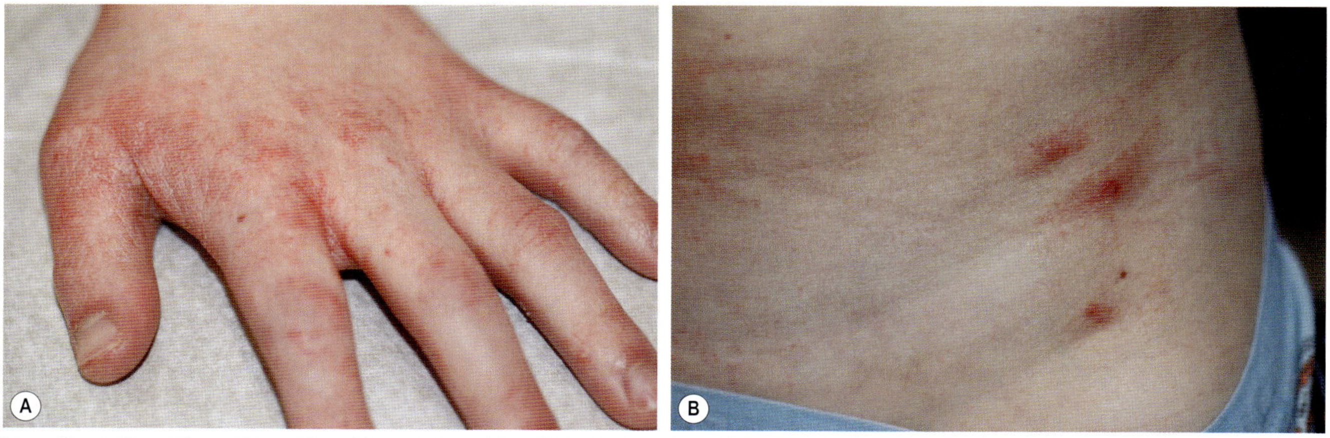

Fig. 18.12 Crusted scabies. This 10-year-old boy with Down syndrome and history of leukemia presented with a 4-month history of extreme pruritus and a dermatitis **(A)** resistant to topical corticosteroids and oral antihistamines, with scattered excoriated papules **(B)**. Scrapings of the skin rash revealed mites, eggs, and fecal pellets on mineral oil examination.

vesiculopustules. Bullous lesions have been described, especially in older adults, which on occasion may simulate (or possibly evolve into) the autoimmune blistering disorder bullous pemphigoid.[16,17] Necrotizing vasculitis in the presence of lupus anticoagulant has also been reported.[18]

Animal-transmitted scabies, which is *Sarcoptes* infestation transmitted from domestic animals, usually results in a short-lived infestation with spontaneous resolution in the human host. The close relationship of humans with dogs makes the canine form of animal scabies (*S. scabiei* var. *canis*) the most common type transmitted to humans.[19,20] Canine scabies, or sarcoptic mange, causes patchy loss of hair with scaling in the dog. It is seen most commonly in undernourished, heavily parasitized puppies, and a presumptive diagnosis can be made on the basis of exposure to a pet with a pruritic eruption, alopecia, and the characteristic mouse-like odor of animals with extensive sarcoptic infestation. In children with canine scabies, the papular eruption most commonly involves the forearms, lower region of the chest, abdomen, and thighs. The distribution differs from that of human scabies, in that it tends to spare the interdigital webs and the genitalia and burrows are absent. The mite of canine scabies does not reproduce on human skin, and therefore the infestation is usually self-limited, clearing spontaneously over several weeks.

The diagnosis of scabies is suggested in the child with pruritus, a papular or papulovesicular eruption with burrows, and the characteristic distribution pattern. However, the differential diagnosis may be broad and includes atopic dermatitis, contact dermatitis, seborrheic dermatitis, Langerhans cell histiocytosis, impetigo, pyoderma, viral exanthem, papular urticaria, arthropod bites, and acropustulosis of infancy. The latter, which may represent a postscabetic hypersensitivity response, is discussed in detail in Chapter 2. A definitive diagnosis of scabies is made via mineral oil examination (Box 18.1) with the microscopic identification of mites (Fig. 18.13) or their eggs or feces (scybala) (Fig. 18.14). Ideal skin lesions for sampling include burrows and fresh papules. In young patients in whom skin scrapings might be difficult, obtaining samples from adult contacts (i.e., parents) with lesions is a consideration. Skin biopsy is rarely necessary. A disposable skin curette (an instrument used for the destructive skin procedure called *curettage*) may be substituted for the scalpel blade if available and may be less frightening for young children and thereby minimize the risk of injury when performing the procedure in a very young or uncooperative child.[21] High-magnification video dermatoscopy is a noninvasive technique that has been reported for diagnosing scabies.[22]

Therapeutic options for scabies are listed in Table 18.1, and a few are discussed here in more detail. The treatment of choice for scabies is 5% permethrin cream, which is applied from the neck down and left on for 8 to 14 hours and followed by thorough rinsing. Permethrin, a synthetic pyrethroid, is a neurotoxin and an excellent scabicide with low potential for toxicity. There appears to be little, if any, resistance of scabies to permethrin, and overall the response rate to treatment is excellent. A second treatment with permethrin 1 week after the first is often recommended, although studies suggest a relatively high cure rate after a single application.[1,23] Treatment of all

Box 18.1 Performing a Mineral Oil Examination for Scabies

1. Apply a drop of mineral oil to the lesion(s) to be scraped.
2. Scrape through the lesion with a number 15 scalpel blade (a small amount of bleeding is expected with appropriately deep scrapings).
3. Smear contents of scraping on a clean glass slide.
4. Add a few more drops of mineral oil.
5. Place cover slip over oil and examine under microscope at low power.
   Criteria for a positive mineral oil examination:
   Scabies mite
   or
   Ova (eggs)
   or
   Scybala (feces)

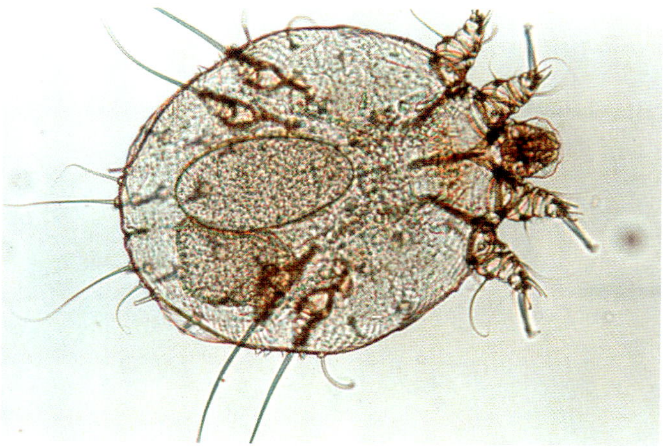

Fig. 18.13 Scabies mite. Note the eggs within the body of the mite. (Live scabies mite, ×40 magnification.)

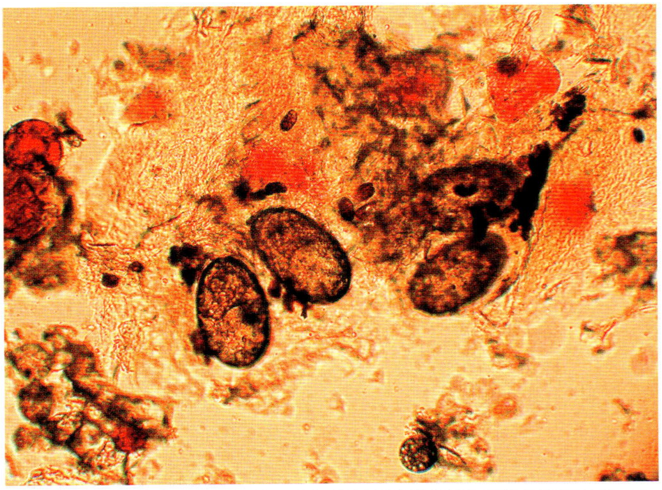

Fig. 18.14 Scabies preparation. This mineral oil preparation (performed on scrapings from the patient in Fig. 18.5) reveals multiple eggs *(larger, oval bodies)* and smaller fecal pellets ("scybala," *the dark brown circular concretions*).

close contacts is also recommended in an effort to minimize ongoing propagation of the infestation. In a systematic review and meta-analysis of scabies therapies, permethrin was demonstrated to be the most effective treatment.[24]

Permethrin should be applied in a thin, even coat and rubbed in well to all skin surfaces. In infants, application should include the scalp and face, with care to avoid the regions around the eyes and mouth. Special attention should be paid to applying the medication to web spaces, the umbilicus, the genitals, and the gluteal cleft. Fingernails and toenails should be trimmed short and the medication applied as well as possible to the region under the nail edge. Permethrin is not recommended for infants younger than 2 months of age or for pregnant (pregnancy class B) or nursing women. It is vital for patients and parents to understand that after appropriate therapy, signs and symptoms of scabies may not clear for 2 to 6 weeks after successful treatment because the hypersensitivity state does not cease immediately after eradication of the infection. The family should have this information before starting therapy, and it may be useful to provide a topical corticosteroid and oral antihistamine for symptomatic relief during this period.

Lindane (γ-hexachlorocyclohexane) 1% lotion was the primary therapy for scabies for years, before the development of permethrin and escalating reports of lindane-related toxicities. Lindane is applied to the skin for 8 to 12 hours with reapplication in 1 week. Although the majority of untoward effects attributed to the use of lindane have been associated with inappropriate, prolonged, or repetitive use, true toxicity potential does exist and becomes more relevant in infants and small children due to a relatively greater skin surface and possibly higher blood level accumulations in this age group. When *in vitro* percutaneous absorption of 5% permethrin was compared with 1% lindane, it was shown that human skin was 20-fold more permeable to lindane. In addition, *in vivo* guinea pig blood and brain levels of lindane were fourfold greater than permethrin levels after a single application.[25] Reactions attributed to the use of lindane have included eczema, urticaria, aplastic anemia, alopecia, muscular spasms, and central nervous system toxicity manifested by irritability, nausea, vomiting, amblyopia, headache, dizziness, and convulsions.[26–33] Lindane-resistant scabies has also been an increasing problem in the United States and Central America. This agent, which is recommended only as a second-line therapy, is banned in California. Other topical agents utilized in some areas for the treatment of scabies include 10% to 25% benzyl benzoate, 10% crotamiton, 0.5% malathion, and 8% to 10% sulfur ointment.

Ivermectin has been reported with increasing incidence as an off-label treatment option for scabies (it is not approved for this indication in the United States). This agent has been used extensively in veterinary medicine since 1981 for a wide variety of parasitic infestations in farm and domestic animals.[34] Oral ivermectin (Stromectol) is approved for the treatment of *Strongyloides* and onchocerciasis in adult humans. It is also effective for the treatment of loiasis and bancroftian filariasis.[35] Ivermectin acts by blocking chemical transmission across invertebrate nerve synapses that utilize glutamate or γ-aminobutyric acid (GABA), resulting in paralysis and death. It has selective activity against human parasites because of its high affinity for the channels found in the peripheral nervous system of invertebrates.[36] Several studies have evaluated the role of ivermectin in the treatment of scabies and found it highly effective in either a single- or two-dose regimen of 200 μg/kg per dose. Many recommend that this agent be given in two doses when used for classic scabies, separated by 1 to 2 weeks, because it is not ovicidal. Ivermectin is especially useful in immunocompromised patients with scabies and patients with crusted scabies, where it may be used alone or in combination with topical scabicides or keratolytic agents. When it is used in crusted scabies, ivermectin may need to be administered in three to seven doses, depending on the severity of the infection.[37,38] Topical 1% ivermectin, which is not readily available, has reportedly been effective as well, and may approach

Table 18.1 Treatment Options for Scabies

Name	Instructions for Use	Comment
Permethrin 5% cream (Elimite, Acticin)	Apply from neck down; rinse in 8–14 hours	Not for use under 2 months of age; may repeat in 1 week if necessary; treat scalp in infants
Lindane 1% lotion	Apply from neck down; rinse in 8–12 hours	Not recommended for infants; not first-line therapy; potential CNS toxicity
Sulfur 8%–10% ointment	Apply from neck down for 3 consecutive nights; rinse 24 hours after last application	Older therapy; malodorous; compounded in petrolatum; safe in infants, pregnant females
Crotamiton cream (Eurax)	Apply from neck down for 2 consecutive nights; rinse 48 hours after last application	High failure rate; may require up to five applications
Benzyl benzoate	Apply nightly or every other night for three applications	Not available in the United States
Ivermectin (Stromectol)	200 μg/kg per dose given orally for two doses, 1–2 weeks apart	Off-label use in United States; consider for severe infestations, crusted scabies, IC patients, scabies epidemics; should not be used under 5 years of age
Ivermectin 1% cream	Applied from neck down, rinsed in 8–12 hours	Off-label use in United States; second therapy recommended in 1 week; consider third application if no response
Malathion 0.5% lotion	Applied from neck down, rinsed in 24 hours	Off-label use in United States; considered second-line therapy in Europe; repeated in 7 days if necessary

CNS, Central nervous system; *IC*, immunocompromised.

the efficacy of topical permethrin.[39–41] Other experimental therapies for scabies include moxidectin (a macrocyclic lactone related to ivermectin), albendazole, and a variety of naturopathic approaches.[42]

Regardless of the treatment used for scabies, environmental decontamination is important, given the possibility of spread of scabies from fomites. Clothing, bed linens, and towels should be machine washed in hot water and dried using a high-heat setting. Clothing or other items (e.g., stuffed animals) that cannot be washed may be dry-cleaned or stored in bags for 3 days to 1 week, because the mite will die when separated from the human host. In addition, systemic antibiotic therapy should be given if secondary bacterial superinfection is present. Scabies nodules can be treated symptomatically with topical or intralesional corticosteroids.

Other Mites

Mites are small arachnids with mouthparts capable of puncturing and feeding on host tissue fluids. A variety of food and animal mites may result in pruritic dermatoses in exposed humans and may also be vectors of infectious diseases. Mite bites should be considered in the patient with an unexplained, itchy papular skin eruption.

Harvest mites (chiggers, jiggers, "red bugs") are a member of the American harvest mite family and are commonly found in the southern United States. Also known as *Trombicula alfreddugesi*, the chigger is distinct from other mites in that only the larva is parasitic to humans and animals. The eight-legged adult and nymphal stages are spent in a nonparasitic existence. Chiggers live in grain stems, in grasses, or in areas overgrown with briars or blackberry bushes, where they exist and feed on vegetable matter, minute arthropods, and insect eggs. The six-legged larva clings to vegetation awaiting the passage of an unsuspecting host and then attaches to the skin when the host brushes against the foliage.[43] The mite then injects an irritating secretion that causes itching and then drops to the ground to molt (or is scratched off) within a few days. The lesions of chigger bites present as urticarial, erythematous papules (Fig. 18.15). They occasionally reveal a hemorrhagic punctum, and in some patients there may be more diffuse erythema, vesicles, or bullae. Pruritus tends to be intense. The "summer penile syndrome" refers to a seasonal acute hypersensitivity reaction to chigger bites and presents with penile swelling, pruritus, and occasional dysuria.[44] Bites are often visible on the penis and scrotum.[45] Most patients have a history of recent exposure to woods, parks, or lawns.

Treatment of chigger bites consists of antihistamines, cool baths or compresses, and topical corticosteroids. Secondary infection should be treated with systemic antibiotics. Household vinegar (5% acetic acid) has been suggested as a useful measure for postexposure prophylaxis and treatment of pruritus.[43] Chiggers may be disease vectors for scrub typhus, hemorrhagic fever with renal syndrome, hantavirus pulmonary syndrome, and ehrlichiosis.[46]

Grain mites (straw itch mite, *Pyemotes ventricosus*) feed on the larvae of insects, seeds, grains, and plant stems. Persons coming into contact with infested straw and grain are particularly susceptible to this form of dermatitis.[47] This seasonal eruption presents as severely pruritic, pale pink to bright red macules, papulovesicles, or pustules followed by urticarial wheals. Occasionally, a purpuric eruption develops. In severe cases, constitutional symptoms and fever may be present, and the presentation may be mistaken for acute varicella. The eruption is self-limited, and treatment, as with chigger bite reactions, is supportive.

Avian mites (fowl mites, bird mites) are divided into two genera, *Dermanyssus* and *Ornithonyssus*. They are known to infest humans accidentally, resulting in a pruritic, widespread papular and urticarial dermatitis, often in covered areas of skin. *Gamasoidosis* is the term used to describe the human skin disorder resulting from nonburrowing, blood-sucking mites from birds and other animals.[48] The diagnosis of avian mite dermatitis is often overlooked because of a lack of awareness and the small size of the mites.[49] Common causes include *Dermanyssus gallinae* (chicken mite), *Dermanyssus americanus* (American bird mite), *Ornithonyssus sylviarum* (northern fowl mite), and *Ornithonyssus bursa* (tropical fowl mite). *D. gallinae*, the most common cause, infects various birds, including chickens, parakeets, pigeons, sparrows, swallows, canaries, and starlings.[50] Although the mite remains on the bird at night, during the day it may migrate to the nest and can survive without feeding for several months. When birds leave their nest in the spring or early summer, the mites search for other hosts, and human infestation may be the result. The mites may enter buildings via openings or crevices in walls and ceilings. Clinical examination reveals papules (Fig. 18.16), vesicles, and urticarial lesions without burrows because the mite does not burrow into the skin. The diagnosis of avian mite dermatitis is confirmed by identification of the mites found in pillows, bed sheets, clothing, nests, birds, and, rarely, humans. Special attention should be given to potential sites for nesting, such as porches, attics, eaves, air conditioning systems, and ventilation ducts. Pet gerbils were the source for *O. sylviarum* and *D. gallinae* in one report.[51] Treatment for avian mite dermatitis, as with other mite bites, is symptomatic.

Other mites may result in similar, nonspecific, pruritic papular eruptions in the human host. The rat mite, *Ornithonyssus bacoti*, is found in rats, and extermination of the rats is often necessary for eradication.[52] It has also been reported in pet hamsters.[53] *Cheyletiella* mites are large, animal-specific, nonburrowing mites that include *Cheyletiella blakei* (found on cats), *Cheyletiella yasguri* (found on dogs), and *Cheyletiella parasitovorax* (found on rabbits). When these mites are in close proximity to a human host, they bite quickly and run, returning to their animal host.[54] They are difficult to visualize with the human eye. Skin lesions include grouped pruritic papules, urticarial wheals, and, occasionally, bullous lesions.[55] Pets infested with *Cheyletiella* exhibit patches of fine, powdery scale ("walking dandruff"). Other mites of

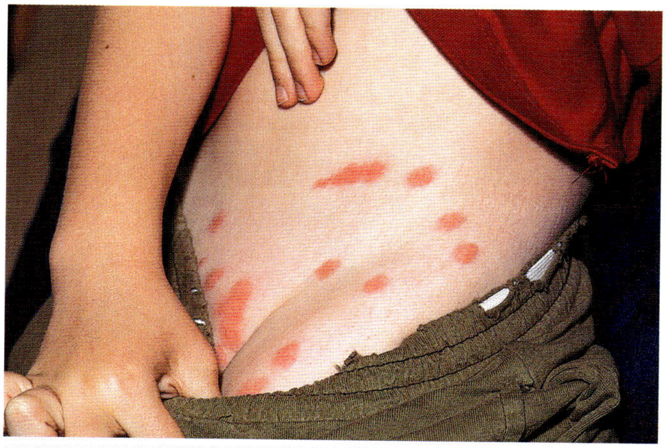

Fig. 18.15 Chigger bites. Multiple itchy, edematous, urticarial papules. Some revealed a small hemorrhagic punctum.

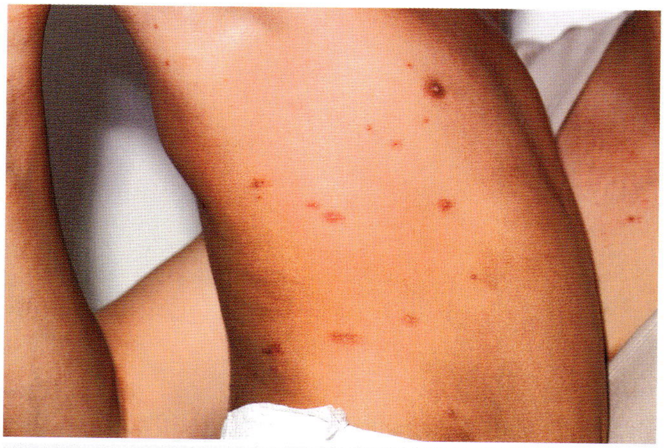

Fig. 18.16 Avian mite dermatitis. Multiple papules and papulovesicles were very pruritic. Upon investigation, a bird's nest was noted near the window in this patient's bedroom and was believed to be the source of the infestation.

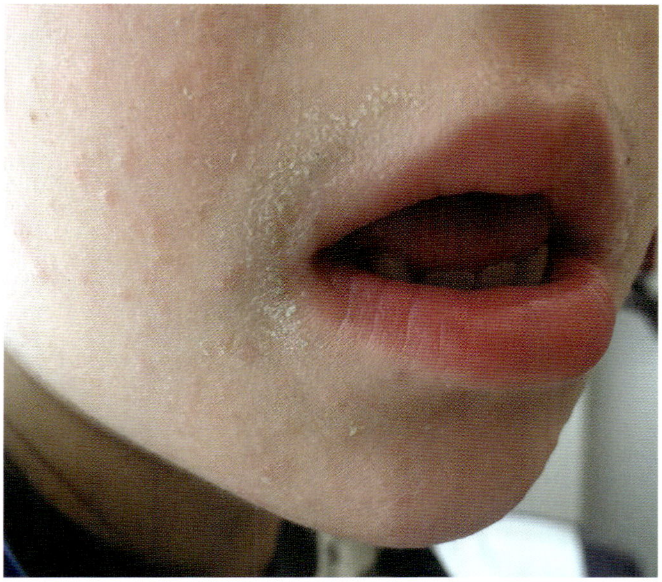

Fig. 18.17 Demodex folliculitis. Itchy erythematous papules and papulopustules on the cheeks and chin of an 8-year-old boy with acute lymphoblastic leukemia.

potential human concern include house-dust mites (*Dermatophagoides* species), the snake mite *(Ophionyssus natricis)*, and the house-mouse mite *(Liponyssoides sanguineus)*.

Demodex mites are present normally in adult human hair follicles and sebaceous glands of the face, where they are considered to be "commensal ectoparasites."[56] They are less commonly present in childhood skin. The two species are *Demodex folliculorum* and *Demodex brevis*. "*Demodex* folliculitis" presents as a very itchy, papular and pustular eruption on the face (Fig. 18.17), usually in children with leukemia or HIV infection.[56,57] There may be an accentuation in the perioral regions. Reported topical therapies have included 5% permethrin, metronidazole, sulfur, and sodium sulfacetamide.

Ticks

Ticks are large, globular arachnids with short legs, hard leathery skin, and mouthparts adaptable for sucking blood from mammals, birds, and reptiles. They are important vectors of diseases such as relapsing fever, rickettsial infections (Rocky Mountain spotted fever, Mediterranean spotted fever, Q fever, and ehrlichiosis; see Chapter 16), Lyme disease (see Chapter 14), babesiosis, Colorado tick fever, and tularemia. Although tick bites may be painful, the majority are painless and may go unnoticed.

Ticks are classified into three family groups: hard ticks (Ixodidae), soft ticks (Argasidae), and Nuttalliellidae.[58] They are found in grass, shrubs, vines, and bushes, from which they attach themselves to dogs, cattle, deer, and humans. Ticks penetrate the human epidermis with distal mouthparts called *chelicerae* (Fig. 18.18) and then insert another part called the *hypostome*, through which they feed on blood and deposit a variety of agents, including anticoagulant and antiinflammatory agents. Both acute and chronic dermatoses may result from tick bites. Acute changes include erythema, papules, nodules, bullae, ulceration, and necrosis. Multiple pruritic papules caused by infestation with tick larvae have also been reported.[59] Chronic changes include granulomas, alopecia, and secondary bacterial infection.[60] Localized foreign-body-type reactions may result from retained mouthparts or improper tick removal and occasionally persist for months to years. T- or B-cell cutaneous lymphoid hyperplasia may also be noted, often with copious numbers of eosinophils when tissue biopsies are analyzed histologically. The B-cell type may be difficult to distinguish from true B-cell lymphoma.[61]

Nondermatologic findings that may result from tick bites include anaphylaxis, fever, headache, flu-like symptoms, abdominal pain, and vomiting. Tick paralysis is a reversible disorder characterized by ascending motor weakness and flaccid paralysis. It is believed to be caused by a salivary neurotoxin injected into the victim while the tick is engorging, and it appears that the tick must feed for several days before paralysis occurs. Tick paralysis occurs more commonly in young girls, possibly due to their longer hair, which may augment tick attachment and hiding.[62] The classic clinical presentation includes an unsteady, ataxic gait followed by ascending symmetric paralysis, usually starting within 2 to 6 days of tick attachment. Upper extremity weakness and cranial nerve involvement (which may present as dysphagia, drooling, facial weakness, and dysphonia) may occur. If intervention does not occur, involvement may extend to the respiratory musculature, resulting in respiratory failure and subsequent death. Most cases of tick paralysis occur in children, and the mainstay of treatment is tick removal, which usually results in rapid resolution of the signs and symptoms.[62,63] An immunoglobulin E (IgE) antibody response against the oligosaccharide galactose-alpha-1,3-galactose (alpha-gal) has been linked to tick bites and may be associated with a delayed urticarial or anaphylactic response to the ingestion of red meat.[64–66]

Various methods of prevention for tick-borne diseases have been advocated. Avoidance of tick habitats may reduce risks, but this is not always feasible. Recommendations for clothing include wearing light-colored, long-sleeved clothes and footwear, tucking pants into socks,

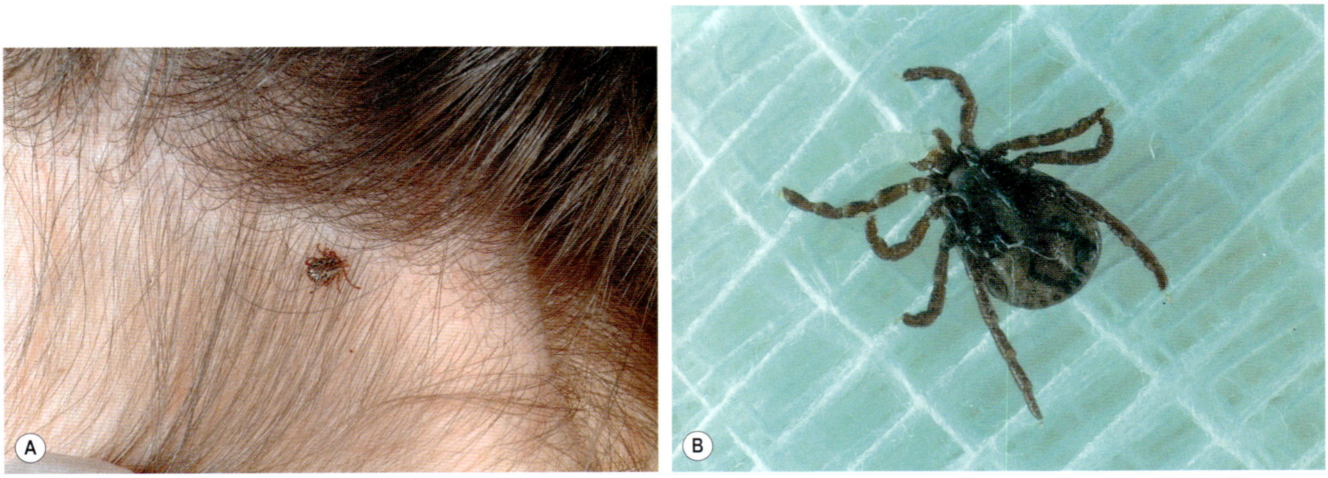

Fig. 18.18 Tick bite. **(A)** This tick was found on clinical examination of the scalp of this 9-year-old boy, who came to the office for an unrelated matter. He had been playing in a forested area in Michigan 3 days previously. **(B)** The tick after gentle manual removal.

and taping exposed edges.[58] Insect repellents containing N,N-diethyl-3-methylbenzamide (DEET) or picaridin applied to exposed areas of skin and permethrin applied to clothing are both effective parts of prevention (see later). Frequent examination of skin for ticks is also important in high-risk areas and during high-risk seasons.

Prompt tick removal is also important in reducing the transmission of disease. The entire tick must be removed completely, including the mouthpart and the cement the tick secretes to secure attachment.[67] A variety of commercial tick-removal devices are available and are quite successful. Manual extraction of a tick is performed with blunt, medium-tipped forceps. The tick is grasped as close to the skin as possible, and perpendicular traction is used to gradually extract the entire tick, taking care not to twist the forceps.[67] Should a portion of the tick be retained, a cutaneous punch biopsy will effectively remove it.

Spiders

Spiders, because of their menacing appearance, are often blamed for more damage than they actually create. Virtually all of the serious spider bites on the North American continent are caused by the black widow spider and the brown recluse spider. Bites of the former tend to have milder outcomes, whereas bites of the latter often result in more severe sequelae.[68] Children are more vulnerable to the effects of spider bites. Patients reporting spider bites are often diagnosed in emergency departments as actually having skin or soft-tissue infection.[69] The gold standard for diagnosing spider bites is collection and proper identification of the biting spider, although this rarely occurs.

The black widow spider, or *Latrodectus mactans*, is a potentially dangerous spider found mainly in southern Canada, the United States, Cuba, and Mexico. In the United States, widow spiders are considered indigenous in every state except Alaska.[70] The black widow spider is recognized by its coal-black color and globular body (1 cm in diameter) with a red or orange hourglass marking on the underside of its abdomen (Fig. 18.19). A web spinner (in contrast to burrowing spiders), it lives in cool, dark places in buildings and little-used structures, woodpiles, and garages, and often spins its web across outdoor furniture. Consequently, a significant number of bites in the southern United States occur around the genitalia and buttocks.

The black widow spider bites humans only in self-defense. The female spider is more dangerous than the male as a result of her larger size and more potent neurotoxin.[71] α-Latrotoxin, the potent black widow neurotoxin, triggers synaptic vesicle release from presynaptic nerve terminals, and its effects are the result of exocytosis of neurotransmitters.[72] Two red, punctate marks and local swelling are often seen, sometimes with the presence of a "target" lesion, and burning or stinging with intense pain develops at the site of the envenomation. This is followed, usually within 10 minutes to an hour, by severe cramping abdominal pain and spasmodic muscular contractions (referred to as *latrodectism*), which peak in around 3 hours. Rigidity of the abdominal musculature may mimic an acute abdomen. Irritability, sweating, anxiety, and agitation are also common. Priapism may occur. Hypertension within the initial hours after the bite occurs in 20% to 30% of patients,[71] and although it may be severe, it is often asymptomatic in children.[73] Although the bite may be fatal, most children recover spontaneously in 2 to 3 days.

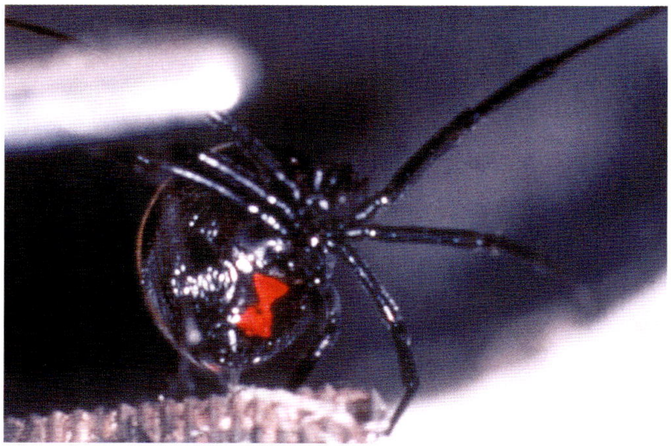

Fig. 18.19 Black widow spider. Note the classic red hourglass marking on the underside of the abdomen. (Courtesy Dirk M. Elston, MD.)

Treatment options for black widow spider bites include analgesics, benzodiazepines, calcium gluconate (controversial), and specific antivenin. Diazepam is the most commonly utilized benzodiazepine. Intravenous opioids are also utilized and seem very effective in providing symptomatic relief.[74] Antivenin therapy has been demonstrated useful, even when given as late as 90 hours after the bite.[75] Although specific antivenin may not be available in some parts of the world, redback-spider (*Latrodectus hasselti*) antivenin has also been shown to be effective in neutralizing *L. mactans* venom in mouse models.[76,77] Indications for the administration of *Latrodectus* antivenin are shown in Table 18.2, although use of this agent remains controversial in the United States. Potential reactions to antivenin include anaphylaxis and serum sickness.

Spiders of the *Loxosceles* genus cause cutaneous and subcutaneous injury primarily via the enzyme sphingomyelinase D (SMD) (see later). There are roughly 100 species of *Loxosceles* spiders, with 80% of them being found in the Western Hemisphere.[78] The brown recluse spider, or *Loxosceles reclusa*, is the one of the most dangerous spiders in the United States. This spider is indigenous to the area spanning eastward from southeastern Nebraska and the eastern half of Texas to the western part of Georgia.[79] The northern boundary includes southern Missouri, Illinois, Indiana, and Ohio, and the southern boundary is the Gulf of Mexico. In nonendemic areas, such as the western United States, physician overdiagnosis of brown recluse bites (also known as *loxoscelism*) is common.[80]

The brown recluse spider has an oval, tan to dark brown body, about 1 cm in length and 4 to 6 mm in width. A dark-brown violin-shaped marking extends dorsally from the eyes back to the distal cephalothorax (Fig. 18.20), and there are three pairs of eyes, rather than the four seen in other spiders. The brown recluse spider thrives in human-altered environments such as attics, basements, and boxes.[81] When in the house, the spider is often found in storage closets (among clothing, in boxes); when outdoors, it generally resides in grasses, rocky bluffs, woodpiles, and barns. Because of its normal shyness and predilection for dark recesses, it bites only in self-defense when approached.

The venom of *L. reclusa* contains numerous enzymes, most notably SMD2, as well as alkaline phosphatase, esterase, adenosinetriphosphatase (ATPase), and hyaluronidase. SMD may result in many effects, including lysis of red blood cells, complement activation, platelet activation, and thrombosis.[81] Activation of neutrophils results in the classic cutaneous necrosis seen and is a result of neutrophil secretion, with subsequent endothelial damage, thrombosis, and ischemia. The local effect on tissues seems to be directly related to the amount of venom injected.

The clinical presentation of loxoscelism begins within 6 hours of the bite, usually with pruritus, pain, and/or erythema at the site. These bites, however, may be relatively painless, and patients may be unaware of them occurring, which accounts for the rarity of spider identification in diagnosing these bites.[82] Within 24 hours, a red ring

Table 18.2 Indications for Administration of *Latrodectus* Antivenin

Indication	Comment
Hypertension	If uncontrolled
Pregnancy	
Comorbid conditions	Coronary artery disease, chronic obstructive pulmonary disease
Intractable pain	
Respiratory difficulty	
Priapism	

Adapted from Quan D. North American poisonous bites and stings. Crit Care Clin 2012;28:633–59 and Glatstein M, Carbell G, Scolnik D, et al. Treatment of pediatric black widow spider envenomation: a national poison center's experience. Am J Emerg Med 2018;36:998–1002.

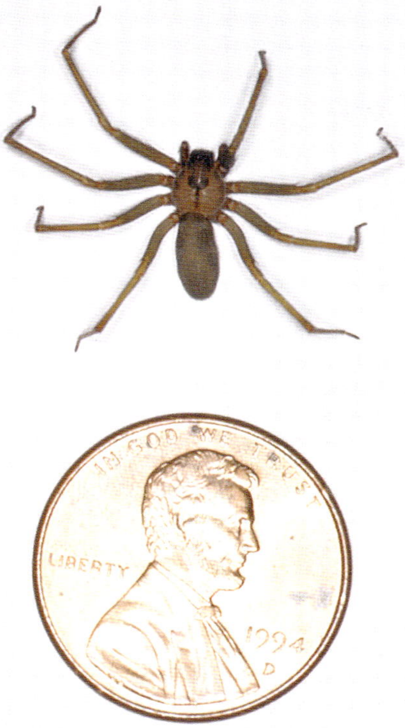

Fig. 18.20 Brown recluse spider. Note the brown, violin-shaped marking on the dorsal surface. The adjacent penny gives a size reference. (Courtesy Dirk M. Elson, MD.)

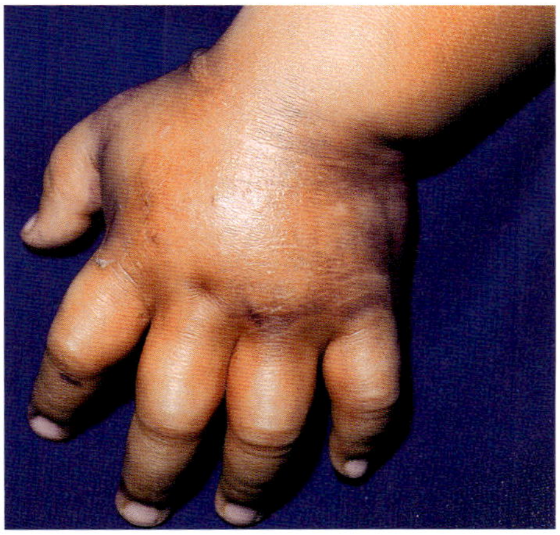

Fig. 18.21 Brown recluse spider bite reaction. Swelling and mild erythema are noted early in the course after a brown recluse spider bite.

develops around the bite site and is followed by blue-purple discoloration (Fig. 18.21), occasional hemorrhagic blisters, and an increase in pain. Ultimately, gangrenous ulceration with necrosis and eschar formation occurs (Fig. 18.22), occasionally with bulla formation. Anesthesia is often present in the center of the affected area. A generalized petechial or morbilliform eruption may also be present.[78] Systemic findings may include chills, fever, nausea, and joint pain. Rare findings include severe hemolysis, rhabdomyolysis, renal failure, and pulmonary edema. Necrotizing fasciitis has also been reported, and secondary hemophagocytic lymphohistiocytosis suspected.[83,84] Lymphangitis is not uncommon when the bite occurs on an extremity. In mild cases,

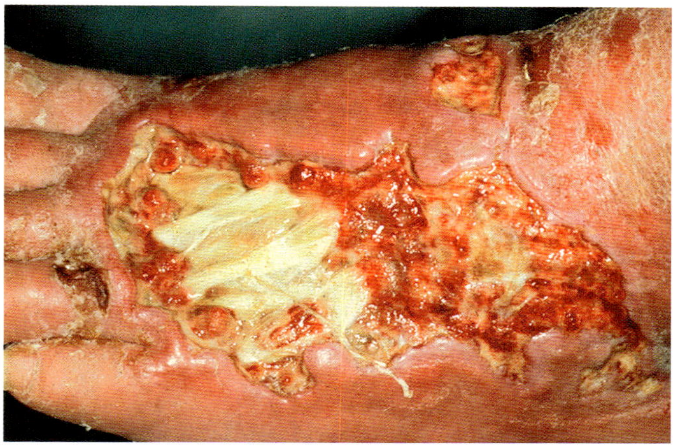

Fig. 18.22 Brown recluse spider bite reaction. Massive deep ulceration with eschar formation. (Courtesy Brooke Army Medical Center teaching file.)

L. reclusa bites may result only in a mild urticarial reaction. Systemic loxoscelism is uncommon overall (but when it occurs, it appears to be more common in children), and symptoms/findings may include fever, malaise, vomiting, headache, disseminated intravascular coagulopathy, and acute hemolytic anemia with jaundice. Thrombocytopenia, possibly related to IgG antiplatelet antibodies, may be present.[85] Renal failure rarely occurs.

Brown recluse spider bites heal very slowly, and scarring often results. Progression to pyoderma gangrenosum–like ulcers has been reported but is rare. For the majority of small, uncomplicated bite reactions, spontaneous healing is the rule. Conservative treatment measures for these patients include rest, ice, compression, and elevation (RICE) of the affected area. Antibiotics should be considered if secondary bacterial infection is suspected. Aspirin, antihistamines (most notably cyproheptadine), and tetanus vaccination may be considered, and dapsone therapy has been utilized but must be closely monitored, given the toxicity profile.[79] Dapsone is felt by some to be effective when administered early in the course of the bite reaction and may have its therapeutic effects via suppression of neutrophil chemotaxis. However, side effects, including dose-related hemolysis, agranulocytosis, cholestasis, and methemoglobinemia, limit its widespread use. When systemic signs and symptoms are present, fluid support should be given, and systemic corticosteroids may be considered. Other reported therapies have included hyperbaric oxygen, vasodilators, heparin, nitroglycerin, electric shock, curettage, and surgical excision.[78] Plasma exchange has been reported for severe hemolysis, which can hinder the ability to interpret optometric-based routine laboratory tests.[86] *Loxosceles* antivenin is available in some countries.

Scorpions

Scorpions are tropical photophobic arachnids that hide by day and hunt by night. They differ from other arachnids in that they have an elongated abdomen ending in a stinger (Fig. 18.23, *A*). Scorpions are found worldwide, particularly in the tropics, and in North America they are generally seen in the southwestern United States and Mexico. The Buthidae family are the most toxic of scorpions and are found mainly in India, Spain, the Middle East, and northern Africa.[71] The major scorpion offender in the United States is *Centruroides exilicauda* (also known as *Centruroides sculpturatus*, or the "bark scorpion"), which is found in the Southwest, especially Arizona.

Although the majority of scorpion stings in the United States are not severe and do not warrant significant medical therapy, children seem to be at greater risk of developing severe scorpion envenomation. Hence, children with a history of scorpion sting should be monitored carefully, particularly during the first 4 hours, to assess for a more serious reaction. Most symptoms have their onset within 15 minutes after envenomation. The venom apparatus of

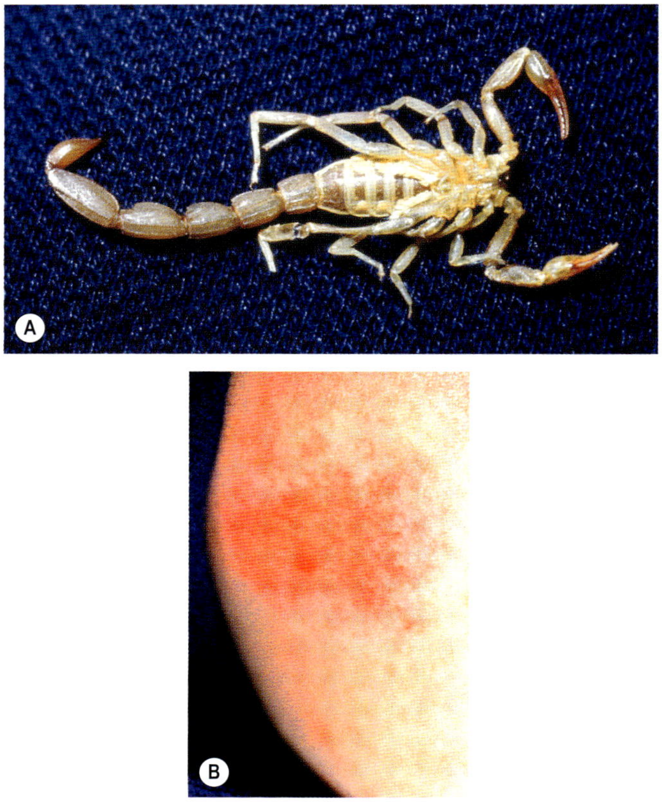

Fig. 18.23 Scorpion **(A)** and scorpion sting, early reaction **(B)**. Painful burning and erythema were present shortly after the sting.

the scorpion is carried in its curved stinger at the tip of the tail, which is swung over the scorpion's head to penetrate the victim's skin. During the day, scorpions hide in shoes, closets, clothing, and crevices. Some species of ground scorpions, however, may burrow and hide in gravel or children's sandboxes. They rarely attack humans, but will do so when accidentally disturbed, brushed against, or stepped upon. The effect of the sting depends on the amount of envenomation and the age and size of the individual. The majority of published reports of severe or fatal envenomation have been in children younger than 10 years of age.[87,88] Most pediatric scorpion stings occur on the lower extremity (between the knee and the foot) and the hand/fingers.[89]

During a sting, the scorpion releases two noxious agents: a localized hemolytic toxin and a dangerous neurotoxic venom. The hemolytic toxin may cause a painful burning sensation with pronounced redness (Fig. 18.23, *B*), swelling, discoloration, severe necrosis, lymphangitis, and, in some patients, disseminated intravascular coagulation or renal failure. The neurotoxic venom, which reaches the systemic circulation primarily via the lymphatics, may produce local numbness and a severe generalized reaction consisting of sweating, salivation, hyperthermia, tightness in the throat, abdominal cramps, cyanosis, muscle jerking, tongue fasciculations, convulsions, and, particularly in small children, respiratory paralysis and death. Tachycardia and hypertension are common and may persist for several hours. Priapism may be seen in up to 50% of males.[90] Pulmonary edema, with or without hemoptysis, and shock may develop. Local cutaneous reactions may vary and include erythema, petechiae, purpura, bullae, edema, induration, necrosis, and ulceration.[91] The diagnosis of scorpion sting is a clinical one, and experienced clinicians who practice in endemic regions can often recognize the clinical symptom pattern.[92]

Treatment for scorpion envenomation is difficult and without consensus on one gold standard of care. Immediate measures include application of a tourniquet above the area of the sting and the application of ice or cold water. *Serotherapy*, which refers to administration of scorpion antivenin, has been advocated by some but has been found ineffective by some investigators and may not prevent the development of cardiac problems.[71,93–95] Antivenin *Centruroides* (scorpion) equine immune $F(ab')_2$ (Anascorp) is approved by the US Food and Drug Administration (FDA) as an orphan drug and has been shown to be associated with more rapid resolution of envenomation symptoms, decreased use of sedative-hypnotics, and lower levels of plasma venom levels.[92,96] This product has been administered according to the FDA recommendation (three-vial initial dose) and in "off-label" fashion (one- to two-vial initial dose) in centers experienced in managing scorpion envenomation; this clinical decision appears to be influenced by envenomation grade, age, and presence or absence of respiratory distress.[97]

Fluid resuscitation, sedation, and treatment of hypertension may be indicated after scorpion stings. Prazosin therapy has been shown to decrease the development of acute pulmonary edema.[98] A large series of severe scorpion envenomation in children suggested that the beneficial effects of antivenin and/or prazosin is questionable when hospital admission is delayed.[88] Continuous intravenous midazolam infusion has been utilized to control agitation and involuntary motor activity.[99] Opioid analgesics may be required for pain relief. Although intravenous high-dose corticosteroid therapy was once recommended, it appears to offer no significant benefit in terms of mortality, duration of hospital stay, or cost.[100]

INSECTS

Insects are the class of arthropods characterized by division into three parts (a head, thorax, and abdomen). Noxious insects are ubiquitous, affecting all humans in some manner at one time or another. The insects of medical significance include lice, mosquitoes, flies, fleas, bed bugs, bees, wasps, ants, caterpillars/moths, and beetles.

Lice (Pediculosis)

Lice have plagued humans since ancient times. Infection is most common during times of stress, such as war, or in crowded environments, such as schools, camps, or institutions. After widespread use of dichlorodiphenyltrichloroethane (DDT) after the end of the Second World War, there were relatively few reports of pediculosis in the United States. Subsequent restrictions on the use of DDT in the United States since 1973, however, resulted in an increase in the number of cases, particularly pediculosis capitis and pediculosis pubis. Lice occur wherever there are humans. They spend their entire life as ectoparasites depending on human blood for sustenance. Their existence independent of humans is generally not possible. All lice feed by pressing their mouth against the host's skin, piercing the surface, and injecting an anticoagulant to facilitate the blood flow during feeding.

Lice are small, six-legged, wingless insects with translucent, gray-white bodies that become red when engorged with blood. They measure 1 to 4 mm in size and are visible to the naked eye on close inspection. Three species of lice infest humans:

1. *Pediculus humanus corporis* (the body louse)
2. *Pediculus humanus capitis* (the head louse)
3. *Phthirus pubis* (the pubic or "crab" louse).

Body lice and head lice (Fig. 18.24) are similar in appearance, with elongated bodies and three pairs of claw-like legs. Pubic lice, on the other hand, have short bodies and resemble crabs in appearance. The body louse is the only louse that can carry human disease, including louse-borne relapsing fever, trench fever, and epidemic typhus. Body and head lice are transmitted by close contact or occasionally via fomites, including clothing (body louse) and combs, brushes, and hats or other headgear (head louse). Pubic lice are transmitted by intimate physical contact and are considered in most cases to be a sexually transmitted disease. Nonsexual transmission of pubic lice may occur, though, and probably accounts for most cases of infestation involving the eyebrows and/or eyelashes in children, although the possibility of sexual abuse should always be considered in this setting.

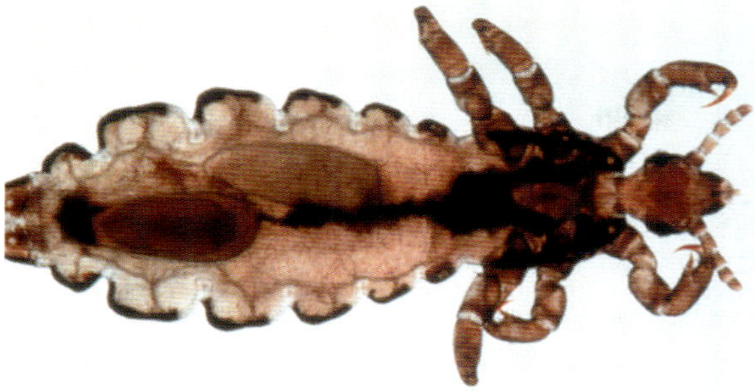

Fig. 18.24 Head louse. Note the elongated body, three pairs of legs, and nits (eggs) within the body of the louse.

Table 18.3 Differential Diagnosis of Nits

Diagnosis	Comment
Nits	Firmly adherent to hair shaft; not easily removed with fingers
Seborrheic dermatitis (dandruff)	Diffuse scalp scaling; scales occasionally adhere to hair but easy to remove; scalp erythema may be present
Hair casts	Keratin protein that encircles hair shaft; easily removed
Piedra	Fungal infection of hair; firm nodules attached to hair shafts, white or black in color
Psoriasis	Thick silvery scales, often present overlying red plaques on the scalp
Hair products	For example, hairspray, mousse, gel

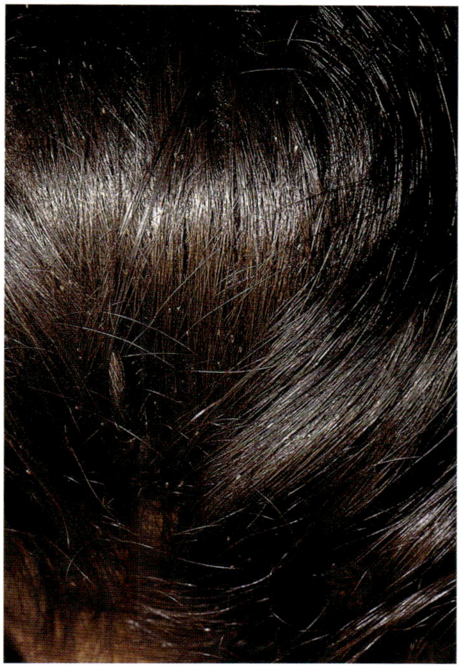

Fig. 18.25 Nits. These eggs are seen as tiny, gray-white specks attached firmly to hair shafts.

Louse egg cases are called *nits* and are firmly attached to the hair shaft with a cement that makes them difficult to remove. They are gray to yellow-white in color and are seen as tiny pinhead specks measuring 0.3 to 0.8 mm (Fig. 18.25). The nits of head lice are attached to the hair shaft at a more acute angle than those of pubic lice.[101] Head-lice nits are usually laid within 1 to 2 mm of the scalp, and, in general, attached nits farther from the scalp are more likely to be nonviable. Nits are usually easily distinguished from hair casts or dandruff by the inability to remove them from the hair shaft and, if necessary, microscopic evaluation. The differential diagnosis of nits is shown in Table 18.3. Nits incubate for about 1 week, and then young lice hatch, passing through several nymph stages and growing into adult lice over 1 to 2 weeks.

Pediculosis corporis (body lice) most commonly occurs in homeless individuals, refugees, victims of wars and natural disasters, and those living in crowded conditions.[102] The nits of the body louse attach firmly to clothing fibers, where they may remain viable for weeks. The louse itself is rarely observed on the skin. It obtains its nourishment by clinging to the patient's clothing and intermittently piercing the skin. The primary lesion is a small, red macule, papule, or urticarial wheal with a hemorrhagic central punctum. Primary lesions may be difficult to visualize due to excoriations related to scratching, and secondary impetiginization may be present. The diagnosis of body lice is confirmed by finding lice or nits in clothing, often in seams. Treatment consists primarily of thorough deinfestation of all clothing and bedding. Treatment of the patient with 5% permethrin cream or lindane 1% lotion may also be useful, because an occasional louse may remain and return to feed.

Pediculosis pubis (pubic lice, crab lice) involves primarily the pubic area but may also involve the scalp, eyebrows and eyelashes, beard, and other hairy areas. Blepharoconjunctivitis may be the presenting signs when eyelashes are involved, and this pattern has been reported in infants and children.[103] Live lice and nits are usually seen. Itching may be the initial symptom, but in persistent cases eczematization or secondary infection may occur. A characteristic skin finding is maculae ceruleae, which are gray-blue macules on the abdomen and thighs. They are felt to represent hemosiderin deposition in the deep dermis as a result of the bites. Treatment of pubic lice is generally similar to that used for head lice (see later), as well as laundering of all clothing and bed linens. Eyelash involvement is usually treated with an occlusive agent such as petroleum jelly.

Pediculosis capitis (head lice) is by far the most common form of lice to affect children and usually affects those between 3 and 12 years of age. As mentioned, it is spread primarily through head-to-head contact and less commonly via fomites, including headgear, combs, brushes, towels, and upholstery. Lice are capable of crawling, but not hopping or jumping. The transmission from fomites may contribute to the increasingly challenging cycle of head-lice infestation, although many of the lice found on combs are likely to be dead or injured.[104] Because most transmission occurs from direct contact with the head of an infested individual, the focus of control activities should be primarily on reducing the number of lice on the head and decreasing head-to-head contact. All socioeconomic groups are affected, although Blacks are less often infested with head lice, possibly related to the diameter, shape, or twisted nature of their hair shafts (which makes grasping of the shaft more difficult for the louse).[101,105–107] The clinical findings consist primarily of pruritus, with secondary excoriation and occasional secondary bacterial infection. Cervical and suboccipital lymphadenopathy may be present. Head lice do not transmit other infectious disease agents. The diagnosis is confirmed by finding live lice (Fig. 18.26) or viable nits on the scalp. In patients in whom the diagnosis is based only on nits, their viability can be confirmed by mounting them on a glass slide and performing microscopic evaluation at low power. Viable nits have an intact operculum (cap) on the nonattached end and a developing louse within the egg (Fig. 18.27).

Although the clinical syndrome of head lice infestation is not serious, it is a cause of significant psychosocial distress, embarrassment, and lost school and work days. The annual cost to society for head lice in the United States is extremely high and includes costs for prescription and over-the-counter therapies, clinical appointments, school

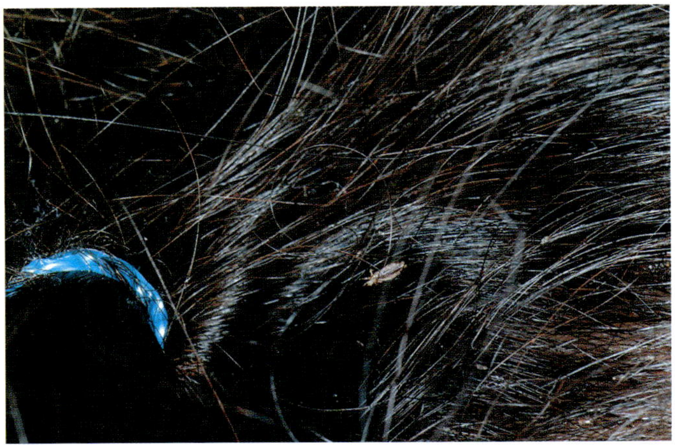

Fig. 18.26 Pediculosis capitis. Note the live head louse, easily seen with the naked eye.

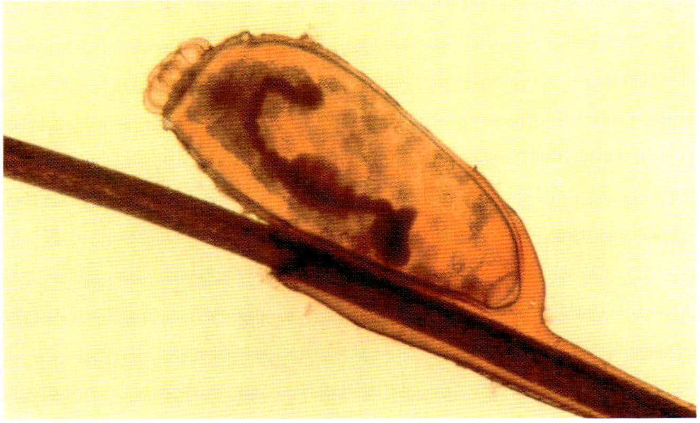

Fig. 18.27 Nit. This ×40-magnification light microscopy image shows a nit firmly attached to the hair shaft by a cement-like substance. Note the intact cap (operculum) and the developing louse within the egg.

nursing time, and time lost from work for caregivers.[108] Because nonviable nits may persist on hair shafts for several months, the potential exists for misdiagnosing active infestation when in fact there is none. It has been tradition in some communities for "no-nit" policies to be enforced, in which children with nits are excluded from school until they are adequately treated and all visible nits have been removed. Such policies may lead to unnecessary exposure to pediculicidal agents, missed school, and loss of parental work time.[109] The American Academy of Pediatrics (AAP) recommends against no-nit policies, because they have not been effective in controlling head-lice transmission.[110] In addition, the AAP discourages routine classroom or schoolwide screening for lice, suggesting that it is neither an accurate nor cost-effective means for lowering head lice incidences in schools.[110] Misidentification of nonlice, nonnit debris (such as dandruff, fibers, dirt, scabs, and hair casts) may also result in the overdiagnosis and consequent mismanagement of head lice.[111] Pediculicidal agents should be used only when viable nits or live lice are observed. In general, nits located close to the scalp are viable and unhatched, although in warmer climates, viable ones may be found several inches away from the scalp.

Treatment options for head lice are summarized in Table 18.4. Head-lice therapy is recommended for individuals diagnosed with an active infestation, and prophylactic therapy is recommended for bedmates and immediate members of the household of the infested index patient. The standard of care is application of 1% permethrin cream rinse to mildly damp hair, followed by rinsing 10 minutes later. Although permethrin is both pediculicidal and ovicidal, many physicians recommend a second treatment 7 to 10 days after the initial therapy; repeat therapy at day 9 may be optimal. This agent is FDA approved for children as young as 2 months of age and is recommended as first-line therapy by the AAP.[112] Increasing resistance concerns have been reported with permethrin (see later).

Lindane (or γ-benzene hexachloride) is a slow-acting pesticide that has been used often in the past. This agent is stored in fat and nerve tissues, and concerns regarding absorption and neurotoxicity have resulted in many recommending against its use, although most reported toxicities occurred with incorrect usage. Lindane use has been banned in the state of California since 2002, and is no longer recommended as a therapy option for pediatric lice infestation.[110,112] The synergized pyrethrins (i.e., pyrethrin + piperonyl butoxide) include extracts from the *Chrysanthemum* family. These agents are pediculicidal only, and resistance and treatment failures are more common.

Malathion is a weak organophosphate cholinesterase inhibitor that had been unavailable in the United States for several years. This agent was reintroduced in 1999 as a 0.5% lotion and approved for use in children 6 years of age and older. Some experts endorse its use as young as 2 years of age and older. It is not considered a first-line therapy. Malathion is both pediculicidal and ovicidal, and resistance is quite rare, although it is occurring in some parts of the world.[113] Resistance may be less likely in the United States, given the presence of terpineol, dipentene, and pine needle oil (which may possess pediculicidal activity) in the available formulation.[114] The isopropanol-containing vehicle contributes to its effectiveness but also its flammability.[101] Malathion 0.5% lotion is applied to dry hair and rinsed after 8 to 12 hours. A single application is sufficient for most patients, but repeat treatment in 7 to 10 days is recommended if live lice are again noted.

Benzyl alcohol 5% lotion is FDA approved in children 6 months of age and older. This agent is a nonneurotoxic product that kills lice via blockage of their respiratory mechanism. Although head lice have evolved the ability to temporarily close their breathing spiracles (holes), benzyl alcohol 5% lotion stuns the spiracles open while the mineral oil vehicle obstructs them, killing the lice via asphyxiation.[115] This product provides an alternative for parents who are concerned about the use of neurotoxic pediculicidal agents. Repeat therapy is necessary, and benzyl alcohol 5% lotion is not ovicidal.

Spinosad 0.9% suspension is a pediculicide approved in children 6 months of age and older. It originates from the fermentation of the *Saccharopolyspora spinosa* bacteria, which is normally found in soil, and it results in paralysis and death of the louse. It was found to have better efficacy than permethrin in one report.[116] Spinosad has pediculicidal and ovicidal activity and is applied to dry hair and rinsed off after 10 minutes. Therapy is repeated in 7 days if live lice are again noted. In a meta-analysis, spinosad therapy was associated with superior efficacy (defined as being free of lice 14 days after the last treatment) compared with permethrin.[117]

Ivermectin 0.5% lotion is approved in children 6 months of age and older and is derived from the fermentation of the bacteria *Streptomyces avermitilis*. The oral form (see later) is used to treat disorders such as onchocerciasis and strongyloidiasis (and off-label occasionally for head lice and scabies). It is applied to dry hair and rinsed after 10 minutes. The manufacturer recommends against repeat therapy without discussing this first with the healthcare provider. In a clinical trial of 78 patients with head lice, a single application of 0.5% ivermectin lotion was effective at eradicating lice in three-fourths of patients through day 15 after therapy.[118] A randomized comparison of single-application treatment with 0.5% ivermectin lotion to treatment with vehicle in 765 patients revealed statistical superiority of the former, with 85% and 74% of the ivermectin group lice-free at days 8 and 15, respectively.[119]

Other less conventional therapies have been used with variable success. These include 5% permethrin, oral trimethoprim-sulfamethoxazole, oral ivermectin, greasy preparations (i.e., olive oil, mayonnaise, and petroleum jelly, which are believed to work via occlusion of the respiratory spiracles of the adult louse), and styling gels.[101,107,120] None of these agents have been studied scientifically,

Table 18.4 Treatments for Pediculosis Capitis (Head Lice)

Name	Instructions for Use	Comment
Permethrin 1% cream rinse (Nix)	Apply to damp hair after shampooing; leave on for 10 minutes, then rinse	Pediculicidal and ovicidal; repeat treatment in 7–10 days; OTC
Pyrethrin + piperonyl butoxide (Rid, Pronto, A-200)	Apply to dry hair; leave on for 10 minutes, then rinse	Pediculicidal only; repeat treatment in 7–10 days; derived from chrysanthemum (do not use in patients with chrysanthemum or ragweed sensitivity); OTC
Malathion 0.5% lotion (Ovide)	Apply to dry hair; rinse after 8–12 hours	Approved for children 6 years and older (some endorse use in children down to 2 years of age); ovicidal and pediculicidal; not first-line therapy; flammable; repeat therapy in 7–10 days, if needed; Rx
Benzyl alcohol 5% lotion (Ulesfia)	Apply to dry hair; leave on for 10 minutes, rinse	Approved for children 6 months and older; pediculicidal only; kills lice by asphyxiation; contains no neurotoxic pesticide; repeat treatment in 7 days; Rx
Spinosad 0.9% suspension (Natroba)	Apply to dry hair; rinse after 10 minutes	Approved for children 6 months and older; pediculicidal and ovicidal; repeat therapy in 7 days, if needed; Rx
Ivermectin 0.5% lotion (Sklice)	Apply to dry hair; rinse after 10 minutes	Approved for children 6 months and older; pediculicidal only; Rx
Trimethoprim-sulfamethoxazole (Bactrim)	8–10 mg/kg per day, divided, twice daily for 10 days	Occasionally used off-label (not FDA-approved for lice); purportedly kills symbiotic bacteria in louse gut; risk of severe allergic reactions, including Stevens–Johnson syndrome and drug reaction with eosinophilia and systemic symptoms (DRESS); Rx
Ivermectin, oral (Stromectol, 3 or 6 mg tablets)	200 or 400 μg/kg single dose; repeat in 7–10 days	Occasionally used off-label for resistant cases or crusted scabies; FDA-approved for strongyloidiasis, onchocerciasis; side effects include headache, dizziness, nausea, vomiting; not recommended in children weighing <15 kg; Rx
Manual nit removal	Comb with fine-toothed nit-removal comb	Difficult, tedious (see text); recommended by some in conjunction with pediculicides
Permethrin 0.5% spray (Rid)	Spray on inanimate objects	For furniture and bedding; not for use on skin; OTC
Occlusive agents (petrolatum, olive oil, mayonnaise, liquid cleanser, others)	Applied and typically left on overnight, then rinsed out; blow-drying with handheld dryer reported as useful in conjunction with liquid cleanser	Therapeutic goal is suffocation of lice; potentially limited by ability of lice to temporarily close breathing spiracles; no evidence-based data to support efficacy; none are FDA-approved for this indication

CNS, Central nervous system; *FDA*, US Food and Drug Administration; *OTC*, over-the-counter; *Rx*, by prescription.

and their true effectiveness remains unclear. Trimethoprim-sulfamethoxazole is believed to kill symbiotic bacteria present in the louse gut and was shown in one study to work synergistically with 1% permethrin cream rinse when the two were used in combination.[121] The potential for severe allergic reaction to this agent makes it less desirable as a lice therapy. Ivermectin has been used as an off-label oral therapy and has typically been dosed at 200 μg/kg (single dose, followed by a second dose in 7 to 10 days if persistent infestation is present), similar to when it is used for scabies.[122] In a prospective randomized trial, oral ivermectin (at a higher dose of 400 μg/kg, repeated in 7 days) was found to be superior to 0.5% malathion lotion in children with difficult-to-treat infestations.[123] Thirty-minute applications of hot air have been studied as a potential therapy for head lice.[124]

Manual lice, and especially nit, removal is a tedious task that is unlikely to prevent spread of the infestation unless performed by professional nit-removing salons. Nits, given their firm adherence to the hair shaft, remain in place long after the viable louse has left the casing. It should be recalled that viable nits are deposited on hair close to the scalp (usually within 1 to 2 mm), and most nits that are farther out than 5 to 7 mm are no longer viable. However, in some instances nit removal is desirable, such as for esthetic purposes or in response to societal pressures. This is accomplished with manual removal and with fine-toothed nit combs, which are widely available and occasionally packaged with pediculicidal agents. Some lice comb products include LiceComb, Lockomb, and LiceMeister. *Wet combing* refers to use of the nit comb on damp hair, which is believed to slow down live lice and facilitate removal of nits. A variety of agents have been used in an effort to loosen the cement that attaches the nit to the hair shaft. These include vinegar, a variety of vinegar-based products, and 8% formic acid (Step 2). Multiple lice-removal salons are now open across the United States, offering manual nit removal and treatment with various nonpediculicidal topical agents; some also offer hot air therapy.

The issue of drug resistance has emerged over the years and clearly appears to be a significant consideration in certain communities. Before assuming true drug resistance, however, other reasons for therapeutic failure should be considered. These include misdiagnosis, repeat infestation, and nonadherence with therapy (which may include incorrect usage or nonusage of product). True resistance has been documented to permethrin, lindane, synergized natural pyrethrins, and malathion (primarily in the United Kingdom).[125–129] Malathion appears to be the agent with the least documented resistance, especially in the United States.[125,126] Lack of susceptibility to pyrethroid insecticides (permethrin, pyrethrins) is usually attributed to an amino acid substitution in a protein that confers "knockdown resistance" (termed the *kdr-like gene*), which subsequently desensitizes cholinergic nerves to the activity of these toxins.[130,131] However, the presence of this mutation has not correlated with clinical treatment failures with permethrin or pyrethrin in some series, suggesting the need for further study in identifying the exact mechanism(s) of resistance in these populations.[113,132]

Regardless of the method of therapy, other family members and close contacts should be examined, and those with evidence of infestation (or who share a bed with the index patient) should also be treated. Play areas and furniture can be vacuumed, and bedding, clothing, and headgear should be machine washed in hot water and dried on a high-heat setting. Items that cannot be washed may be dry-cleaned or placed in sealed plastic bags for 2 weeks. Hats, combs, brushes, grooming aids, towels, school lockers and hooks, and other items that come into contact with the head or head coverings should not be shared. Combs and brushes may be coated with the pediculicide for 15 minutes or soaked in rubbing alcohol for 1 hour followed by washing in hot soapy water. Alternatively, these items can be discarded and replaced with new ones.

Information for patients regarding management and control of head lice is available from the National Pediculosis Association at www.headlice.org.

Mosquitoes and Flies

Flies and mosquitoes belong to the order Diptera. One of the largest orders of insects, it includes the two-winged biting flies, gnats, and mosquitoes. Of these, mosquitoes are the most important from the standpoint of human health. They are seen worldwide and may be vectors of many important diseases such as encephalitis (including West Nile encephalitis), malaria, yellow fever, dengue, chikungunya, Zika virus, and filariasis. In the United States, the most common insect bites of infants and children are those of mosquitoes.

Mosquitoes are attracted to bright clothing, heat, humidity, and human odors, particularly those of young children. Carbon dioxide, released mainly in the breath but also from the skin, is a long-range attractant for mosquitos and can be detected from up to 36 meters away.[133] In unsensitized individuals, the ordinary mosquito bite produces only mild, local irritation. This manifests as a slight stinging sensation and a small, pruritic erythematous papule. In sensitized individuals, however, mosquito bites produce itching, urticarial wheals that may last for several hours to several days, or firm papules or nodules (Fig. 18.28) that may persist for longer periods. Occasionally, and particularly in the young, mosquito bites may produce blisters or hemorrhagic lesions. Excoriation of these lesions may result in secondary eczematization and impetiginization. Systemic Arthus-type reactions and anaphylaxis are rare but do occur. Hypersensitivity to mosquito bites has also been associated with Epstein–Barr virus–associated lymphoproliferative disorders, including natural killer (NK) cell leukemia/lymphoma.[134–136]

Although the diagnosis of insect bites is often obvious, differentiation from other papular, vesicular, and pruritic eruptions may also be suggested by the characteristic grouping of lesions, a central punctum when present, the acute nature of most reactions, as well as their seasonal incidence. Treatment of mosquito bites includes oral antihistamines, cool compresses, and topical antipruritic agents such as calamine lotion and topical corticosteroids. When topical corticosteroids are used, stronger preparations (i.e., class II through V) are most effective, with caution exercised not to apply these agents to the face, groin, or fold areas. Topical diphenhydramine should be avoided, given the risks of allergic contact sensitization. Cetirizine or loratadine taken prophylactically have both been shown to decrease immediate whealing and pruritus as well as delayed pruritus.[137,138]

Prevention is most effectively accomplished by the use of insect repellents (see later). Another important measure, especially during high-risk activities or exposure times, is the use of protective clothing (hats, socks and shoes, and long-sleeved shirts tucked into pants). Scented hairsprays, pomades, soaps, lotions, powders, colognes, and perfumes may attract all forms of stinging insects and should be avoided unless necessary. Although some have suggested that thiamine hydrochloride taken orally may help repel insects, this measure remains unproven. Efforts at reducing mosquito populations include ultrasonic electronic devices for use by the consumer and insecticide spraying programs, which have been adopted by several communities.

Various species of biting flies (sandflies, gnats, black flies, deerflies, horseflies) are known to attack the exposed areas of the face, neck, arms, and legs, with the production of painful or pruritic papules or nodules, often with vesiculation. Although lesions often disappear in a few hours, they may persist for several days and can be quite annoying, particularly in small children. Treatment consists of the prophylactic use of insect repellents and treatment of symptoms with acetaminophen, antihistamines, calamine lotion, or topical corticosteroids.

Nonbiting flies, including common houseflies, tend to feed at open wounds, exudates, and cutaneous ulcers and may produce myiasis, a far less common but significant skin disorder. Myiasis is usually a travel-associated dermatosis and is caused most often by infestation with *Dermatobia hominis* (human botfly). It is most common after travel to Central and South America.[139] Myiasis may present in several ways, including furuncular, migratory, and wound-associated myiasis, depending on the type of larvae.[140] The furuncular type is usually caused by *D. hominis.* In this disorder, the adult female lays eggs on other arthropods (flies, mosquitoes, ticks), and this vector then transmits the larvae to the skin of the human host. The larvae penetrate skin, mature in the dermis and subcutaneous tissues, and eventually reach such a size (Fig. 18.29) that they are unable to spontaneously emerge. Clinically, patients present with furuncular nodules (Fig. 18.30) that may drain (serosanguineous) and often have a central opening (sinus tract), which serves as a site for respiration and excretion. The patient may report a sensation of "crawling in the skin." The lesions occur most commonly on the head and other exposed areas of the body, and small black spiracles may be seen through the overlying skin punctum.[141] Oral myiasis resulting in oral and maxillofacial mutilation has been reported in children living in tropical regions.[142] Treatments for myiasis include extraction of the larvae through suffocation (petroleum jelly, butter, pork fat, paraffin, oil) or surgical extraction.[139,141,143]

Myiasis caused by *Cochliomyia hominivorax* (New World screwworm) may occur in persons living in Central and South America

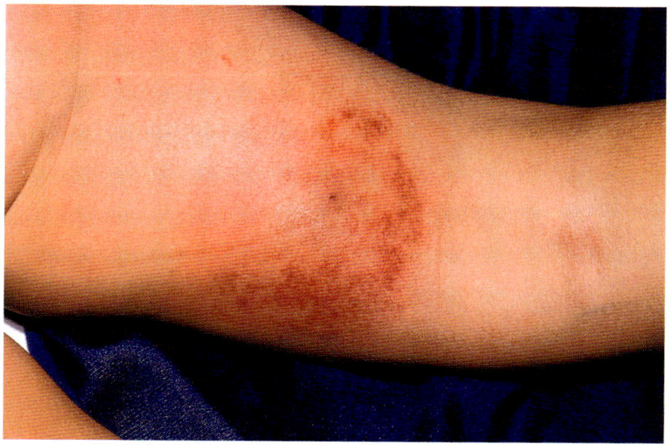

Fig. 18.28 Severe mosquito bite reaction. An indurated, firm, edematous plaque with secondary petechiae from rubbing.

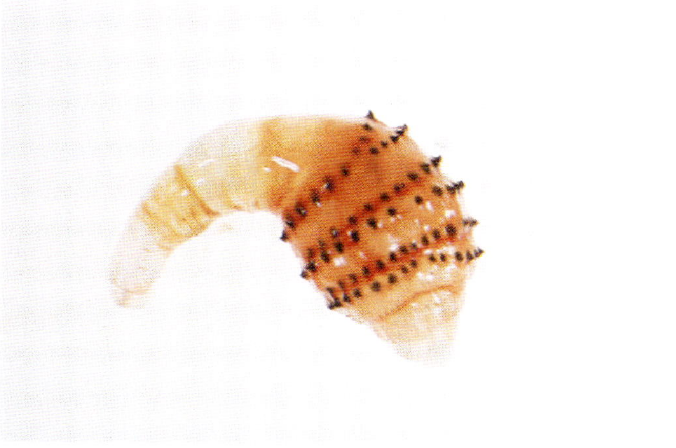

Fig. 18.29 Botfly larva. Note the posterior spines and odd shape of the second-stage larva, which makes it difficult to dislodge through the overlying tiny skin orifice.

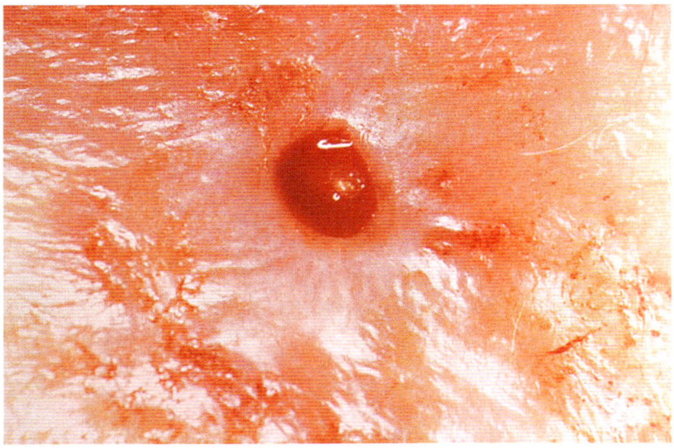

Fig. 18.30 Myiasis. A furuncular nodule with a small, central opening. Note the visible tip of the larva within the opening.

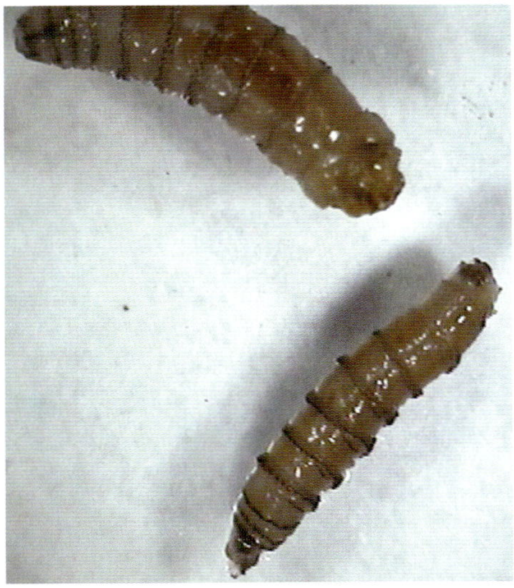

Fig. 18.31 Myiasis caused by *Cochliomyia hominivorax*. Almost 50 of these larvae were extracted from the small, well-demarcated scalp ulcer of a 13-year-old girl with Darier disease, who contracted the infestation while hiking in Peru.

or travelers to those regions and result in more tissue destruction. The third larval stage of these maggots contains powerful oral hooks at the forepart, which enable burrowing into deeper tissues and significant destruction (Fig. 18.31).[144,145] These screwworms have a predilection for the eyes and nasal and oral mucosae. Mechanical removal of maggots, tissue debridement, and treatment for secondary sequelae (i.e., bacterial infection) are the mainstays of treatment, and topical and oral forms of ivermectin have been utilized as adjunctive therapy.[146,147]

Fleas

Fleas (Siphonaptera) exist universally among animals and humans. Those that most commonly attack humans in the United States are the human flea *(Pulex irritans)*, the cat flea *(Ctenocephalides felis)*, and the dog flea *(Ctenocephalides canis)*. The eruption produced by a flea bite in a sensitized individual is an urticarial wheal or papule (Fig. 18.32), often with a centrally located hemorrhagic punctum. In highly susceptible individuals, particularly young children, wheals may progress and develop into tense bullae (Figs. 18.33 and 18.34). Flea bites are often multiple and grouped together in linear or irregular clusters on the arms, forearms, or legs or on areas where clothing fits snugly (thighs,

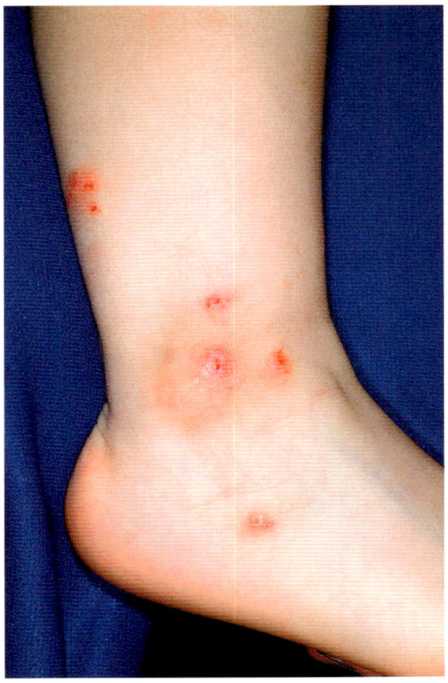

Fig. 18.32 Flea bites. Multiple excoriated, clustered red papules.

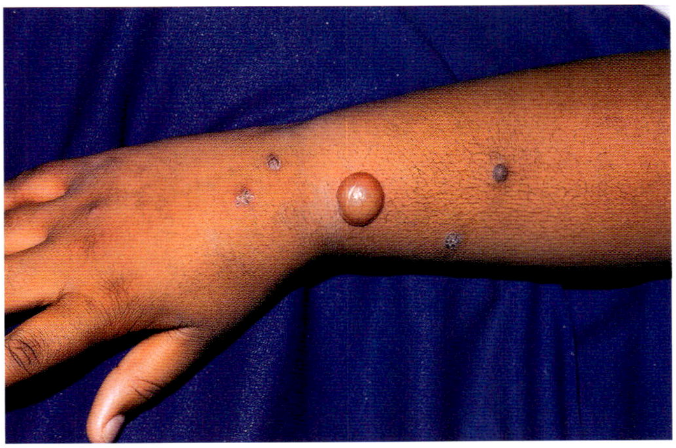

Fig. 18.33 Bullous flea bite reaction. Tense bulla and surrounding crusted papules in a patient with a hypersensitivity to flea bites.

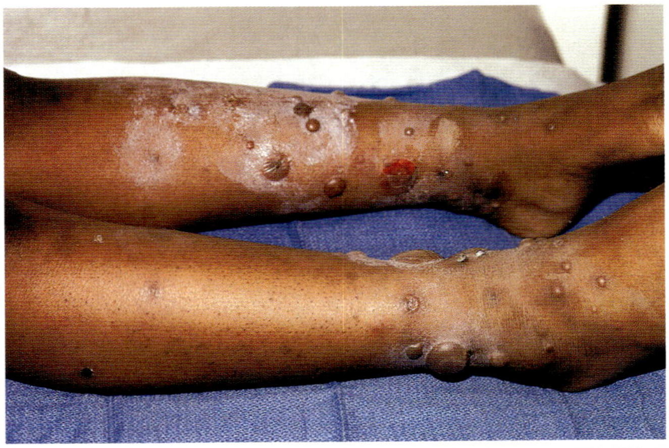

Fig. 18.34 Bullous flea bite reaction. Multiple tense bullae and secondary bacterial impetiginization in a patient with flea bite hypersensitivity.

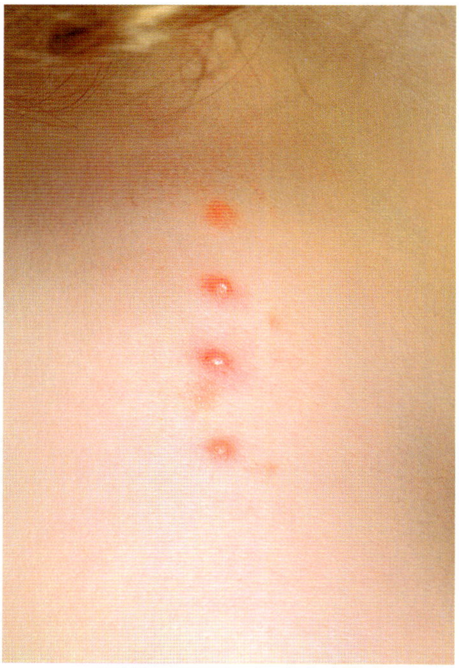

Fig. 18.35 Flea bites. The classic linear configuration of flea bites (the breakfast, lunch, and dinner sign) caused by the tendency of fleas to jump and crawl rather than fly.

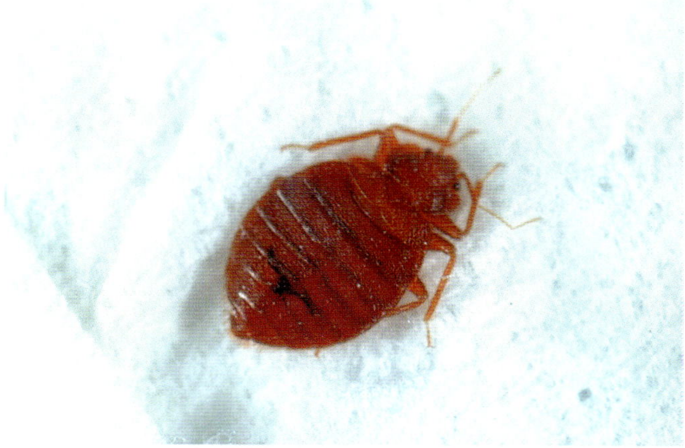

Fig. 18.36 Bed bug *(Cimex lectularius)*. Note the flattened, oval body and three pairs of legs. The family that brought it in had been complaining of itchy, red bite reactions for several months.

buttocks, waist, and lower abdomen). Bites in a linear configuration (the "breakfast, lunch, and dinner" sign; Fig. 18.35) are common and relate to their tendency to jump and crawl but not fly. Treatment is similar to that described for mosquito bites.

Elimination of fleas by treatment of suspected animal carriers and cleaning/spraying of carpets, floors, crevices, and other potentially infested areas should be considered. It should be noted that for every flea seen on the pet there are many more in the environment, that flea collars are not completely effective, and that animal flea sprays and powders, if used, must be repeated every 2 weeks during the summer months to be effective.[148]

Tungiasis is a skin infestation caused by the gravid sand flea, *Tunga penetrans* (chigoe flea, jigger flea). It is endemic in South and Central America, parts of Africa, India, the Caribbean, and Pakistan. Tungiasis is rare in the United States and usually seen in those who have traveled to an endemic region.[149] In endemic areas, it may be associated with long-term disability, immobility, and chronic pain.[150] In tungiasis, the female flea attaches herself to the warm-blooded host, burrows through the epidermis into the dermis, and gradually enlarges; her size may increase by 2000-fold during that time.[151] Clinical lesions are red nodules with a central punctum or ulceration, occasionally resembling an abscess. The favored sites are the toes and periungual skin. Treatment consists of flea removal (can be accomplished with a sterile needle or skin biopsy), wound care, tetanus prophylaxis (if not up to date on vaccinations), and, when necessary, treatment of secondary bacterial infection.[152]

Bed Bugs

Bed bugs are a member of the order Hemiptera, which also includes reduviid bugs. The most common species to parasitize humans is *Cimex lectularius*. Bed bugs are red-brown, blood-sucking, nocturnal insects that are 3 to 5 mm in size. They are wingless, with flattened oval bodies and three pairs of legs (Fig. 18.36). The female bug lives and deposits eggs on rough surfaces, cracks, and crevices, including mattress and wallpaper seams, box springs, linens, electrical outlets, and furniture seams; collections of their eggs and fecal matter typically allow for easy identification.[153] White sheets may also help in highlighting blood spots from the bugs.[153] Bed bugs avoid light, hiding out during the day in such locations and responding to warmth and carbon dioxide (which are both present in sleeping humans) at night. Bites present as erythematous papules, and the breakfast, lunch, and dinner sign may again be present. Bullous lesions may also occur.[154] Bed bug bites most commonly occur on exposed areas of the face, neck, arms, or hands. The actual lesions are not easily distinguished from other arthropod bite reactions.

Systemic reactions that may possibly be attributable to bed bug bites include urticaria, angioedema, asthma, and anaphylaxis. The bed bug is capable of traveling long distances in search of food, often from one house to another, and has been known to survive without food for up to 6 months to 1 year. It has been suggested that bed bugs may be vectors for hepatitis B, HIV, plague, yellow fever, tuberculosis, relapsing fever, leprosy, leishmania, filariasis, bartonellosis, or trypanosomiasis, although there is little evidence to support that they are vectors for any communicable diseases.[155–158] Methicillin-resistant *S. aureus* and vancomycin-resistant *Enterococcus faecium* were recovered from bed bugs collected from an impoverished community in Vancouver, British Columbia, suggesting that more studies are required to determine their potential at carrying pathogens and serving as vectors for transmission.[159] Since the late 20th century, bed bug infestations have been observed increasingly in homes, apartments, hotel rooms, bed and breakfasts, dormitories, hostels, trains, aircrafts, cruise ships, nursing homes, and hospitals.[159] An outbreak of the tropical bed bug *C. hemipterus* in a neonatal unit has been reported.[160] Although the exact basis for the increased bed bug resurgence is unclear, some have attributed it to increased worldwide travel, altered insecticide management, or increasing pesticide resistance.[158]

Treatment is directed at elimination of the bug from the environment with insecticides and eliminating potential hiding sites. Although individual lesions require no direct therapy, oral antihistamines, topical corticosteroids, or calamine lotion may be used for symptomatic relief. Systemic corticosteroids have occasionally been utilized. Preventive measures that have been advocated for bed bug bites include wearing pajamas that cover the majority of skin, covering bedposts with petrolatum, and manual inspection of hotel headboards and mattresses.[161] Once infestation has occurred, useful measures for eradication may include vacuuming of exposed hiding locations, washing all linens in hot water and drying on low heat, steam cleaning, use of mattress and box spring encasements, discarding of furniture, placement of insect-growth regulators, pesticide spraying, and use of commercial heat treatments.[152,161] Carbon dioxide fumigation has also been demonstrated effective against bed bugs.[162] The utilization of an experienced professional exterminator is highly recommended when dealing with a bed bug infestation.

Bees, Wasps, and Ants

Bees, wasps, and ants belong to the order Hymenoptera, a large order of insects that contains about 100,000 species. Like most other insects, they have three pairs of legs and four wings and are recognized by the narrow isthmus separating the abdomen from the thorax. These insects have stingers that can result in local or systemic reactions in susceptible individuals. Hymenoptera venom allergy can result in life-threatening anaphylactic reactions and is responsible for at least 40 deaths per year in the United States.[163,164] The three families of stinging insects in the order Hymenoptera include Vespidae (yellow jackets, wasps, and hornets), Apidae (honeybees and bumblebees), and Formicidae (stinging ants).

Bees, the only insects that produce food eaten by humans, live in almost every part of the world except the North and South Poles. Honeybees live and work together in large groups and do not sting unless frightened or injured. Africanized ("killer") honeybees are hybridized honeybees (from interbreeding of African and domestic honey bees in South America), originally introduced to increase efficiency in honey manufacturing. They tend to attack in swarms and have gradually been migrating into the United States. Although their venom is similar to that of other types of bees, the quantity of stings may result in a fatal reaction. Honeybees are only able to sting once, because the stinger is barbed (which keeps it attached to mammalian flesh) and attached to the abdomen; hence, disarticulation of the honeybee occurs with any attempt at removal.[70] Wasps, among the most interesting and intelligent of insects, may live together in cooperative fashion, as seen with the so-called "social wasps" (hornets and yellow jackets), or may live as solitary insects. Most wasps are beneficial to humans because they destroy large numbers of flies, caterpillars, and other insects that may be harmful. As with bees, wasps ordinarily do not sting humans unless they are bothered or frightened. However, yellow jackets and hornets tend to be quite aggressive, especially when near their nest or if disturbed.[164] Wasps are capable of multiple stings because their stingers are smooth and retractable; bees, on the other hand, usually eviscerate themselves after a single sting, given the barbed nature of their stingers.[165]

Symptoms of bee or wasp stings vary from mild local pruritus, pain, and edema to general anaphylactic reactions with associated difficulty in breathing and swallowing, hoarseness, slurred speech, gastrointestinal disturbances, abdominal pain, dizziness, weakness, confusion, generalized edema, cardiovascular collapse, and occasionally sudden death.

Ants, like bees and wasps, have large glands at the tip of the abdomen from which they introduce venom into wounds produced by their bites. The majority of ants are not aggressive and rarely sting large organisms.[166] However, two groups are considered medically important in the United States. The fire ant (*Solenopsis richteri* and *Solenopsis invicta*) is originally from South America and has spread rapidly in the southern United States, where it has become an agricultural pest and a health hazard.[167] It produces a venom more potent than that of other members of the order Hymenoptera. The fire ant was named for the extreme burning pain inflicted by its sting and tends to attack without warning.[168] During one bite cycle, the fire ant may inflict seven to eight stings in a circular pattern. The immediate reaction is characterized by a painful wheal and flare response, with vesicles developing over several hours. Pustular changes eventually occur, and some patients develop large, local erythematous reactions. Anaphylaxis is a common cause of significant morbidity and may be fatal. The harvester ant (*Pogonomyrmex* species), which also has a significant presence in the United States and is considered a stinging ant, is found primarily in the southwestern states.

The treatment of ordinary bee, wasp, or ant stings consists of local application of antipruritic shake lotions (i.e., calamine lotion), cool compresses or cool baths, and oral antihistamines. A papain solution made of one part meat tenderizer to four parts water may help relieve local symptoms of pain or discomfort. Severe allergic reactions are treated with epinephrine, antihistamines, oxygen, and systemic corticosteroids. Patients known to be at risk for severe systemic reactions to bee, wasp, hornet, yellow jacket, or fire ant stings should be given an epinephrine pen kit and be educated in its proper use in an emergency. Preventive techniques include education on practical avoidance measures and referral to an allergist for consideration of allergen testing and immunotherapy.

Allergen immunotherapy is an effective form of prevention for certain individuals at risk for severe insect-sting reactions. Commercial venoms for both skin testing and immunotherapy are available for yellow jackets, white-faced hornets, yellow hornets, wasps, and honeybees, and the complementary deoxyribonucleic acid (cDNA) of most major allergens of bee and vespid venoms has been cloned and is available in a recombinant form.[163,164] Sequential bee-sting challenge tests can be used as a diagnostic tool to assess the need for venom immunotherapy (VIT) in children who are allergic to bee venom.[169] Because the stinging insect cannot always be reliably identified, it is suggested that the testing physician include all geographically relevant insects when choosing the test panel.[170] VIT should be considered for any patient at risk for a systemic reaction to a Hymenoptera sting, especially those with anxiety or impairment in quality of life due to fears of future stings.[171] For fire ant immunotherapy, imported fire ant whole-body extract is the main reagent used.[168] The therapeutic goals of immunotherapy are to prevent life-threatening reactions, reduce morbidity from such stings, and decrease insect sting anxiety.

Blister Beetles

Blister beetles (*Cantharis vesicatoria*, order Coleoptera) contain cantharidin, a vesicant most concentrated in the beetles' genitalia and the active principle of the purported aphrodisiac Spanish fly.[172] The lesions produced accidentally by crushing blister beetles, by discharge of their body fluid on the skin, or by external therapeutic use of cantharidin (as in the treatment of molluscum contagiosum; see Chapter 15) consist of slowly forming blisters that involve the outer layers of the skin. Treatment depends on the extent and location of lesions. Simple aseptic drainage of large bullae and cool compresses generally give adequate relief of symptoms. If vesicles are not traumatized, they usually resolve in 3 to 4 days with subsequent desquamation and healing. Blister beetle ingestion, when reported, may result in oral mucosal blistering, abdominal pain, vomiting, hematuria, oliguria, and renal failure.[173] "Blister beetle dermatitis" may also occur after exposure to cantharidin (or another vesicant, pederin, found in the genus *Paederus*) and may mimic shingles, herpes infection, allergic contact dermatitis, or impetigo.[174]

Papular Urticaria

Papular urticaria is a common condition of childhood characterized by a chronic or recurrent papular eruption caused by hypersensitivity to a variety of bites, including those of mosquitoes, fleas, bed bugs, and mites. It is often pruritic and uncomfortable, and the resultant scratching may result in open erosions and secondary bacterial superinfection. One of the most challenging aspects of papular urticaria is convincing parents that the lesions are related to a bite reaction and identifying and eradicating the source of the offending insect.[175]

Papular urticaria presents with multiple urticarial, 3- to 10-mm papules (Figs. 18.37 and 18.38). Lesions are commonly grouped or clustered in a fashion similar to acute bite reactions. They may be excoriated or crusted, and a central punctum may be visible overlying each papule. Papular urticaria is most common in the summer and late spring, and flea bites are the most common cause. Individual lesions tend to resolve over 1 to 2 weeks and may heal with postinflammatory erythema or hyperpigmentation (Fig. 18.39). Recurrent episodes are common, especially if there is ongoing exposure to the offending insects.

The differential diagnosis of papular urticaria includes ordinary urticaria, pityriasis lichenoides et varioliformis acuta (PLEVA), papular acrodermatitis of childhood (Gianotti–Crosti syndrome), and lymphomatoid papulosis. Histopathologic examination of skin biopsy specimens reveals spongiosis (epidermal edema), subepidermal edema, and a mixed inflammatory infiltrate that often includes eosinophils.[176] Skin biopsy is useful both in confirming the diagnosis and in persuading the parents regarding the nature of the condition. Symptomatic treatment includes oral antihistamines and topical corticosteroids, as well as topical antipruritic preparations containing menthol, camphor, or pramoxine. Environmental control measures are also desirable when feasible.

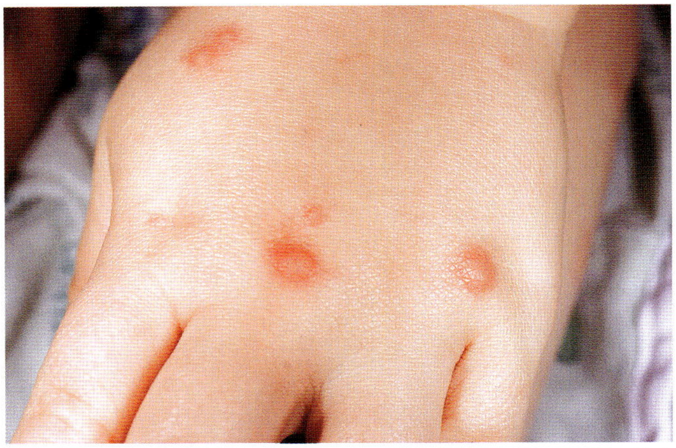

Fig. 18.37 Papular urticaria. These edematous, red papules would intermittently swell and become itchier.

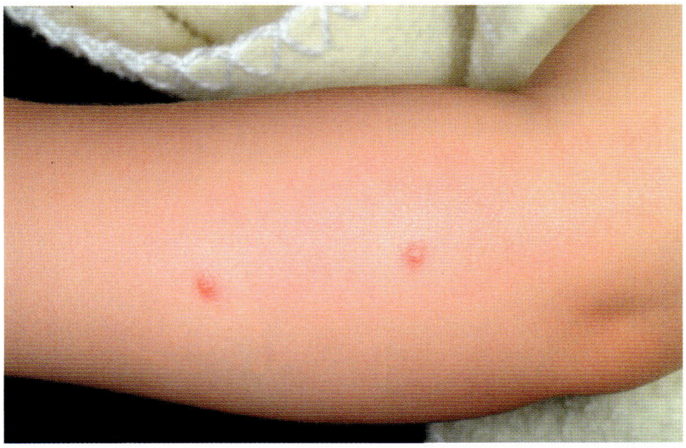

Fig. 18.38 Papular urticaria. These edematous, pruritic red papules continued to intermittently enlarge for many months.

Insect Repellents

Protection from insect bites includes several measures such as avoiding infested areas, wearing protective clothing, and controlling insect populations when possible. However, the most effective avoidance measure in most situations is the application of insect repellent to the skin. Several types of repellents are commercially available and include both synthetic chemicals and plant-derived essential oils.

DEET has traditionally been the most effective and most widely used repellent.[177] It is a broad-spectrum insect repellent that is effective against mosquitoes, biting flies, chiggers, fleas, and ticks.[178] Higher concentrations of DEET result in longer-lasting protection, although these effects seem to plateau at concentrations higher than 50%. In the United States, DEET is available in variable concentrations in multiple vehicles, including solutions, lotions, creams, gels, pump sprays, sticks, roll-ons, wristbands, and impregnated towelettes.[133,177] The mechanism of action of DEET is to provide a vapor barrier that deters the biting insect from coming into contact with human skin. Firm guidelines or recommendations for choosing an appropriate DEET concentration are not available. However, it is generally accepted that products with ≥20% DEET are most effective at providing adequate protection in most circumstances. Some general recommendations for the use of DEET-containing products are listed in Box 18.2. The Centers for Disease Control and Prevention (CDC) and the Environmental Protection Agency (EPA) recommend DEET as a first-line defense against mosquitoes.[179]

The use of DEET in young children has been a source of some concern, given rare reports of potential neurologic toxicity. Small amounts of DEET may be absorbed through the skin, yet seem to be completely eliminated (along with its metabolites) within 4 hours of application in adults.[180] Although the pharmacokinetics are not as well understood in children, reports of neurologic toxicity are rare, and, in fact, in one study of data collected by the American Association of Poison Control Centers, infants and children had lower rates of severe adverse events than did adults.[181] Many of the reports of DEET-related toxicity involved long-term, heavy, frequent, or whole-body application of DEET, and in some, the product was orally ingested.[178,182] In 1998 the EPA completed a reregistration eligibility decision for DEET, and in this process included a review of acute, subacute, and chronic toxicity data. The agency concluded that normal use of insect repellents containing DEET poses no significant risks to children or adults, that product labeling would be modified to include recommendations for safe use, and that child safety claims on labels were prohibited, given the lack of appropriate scientific data to

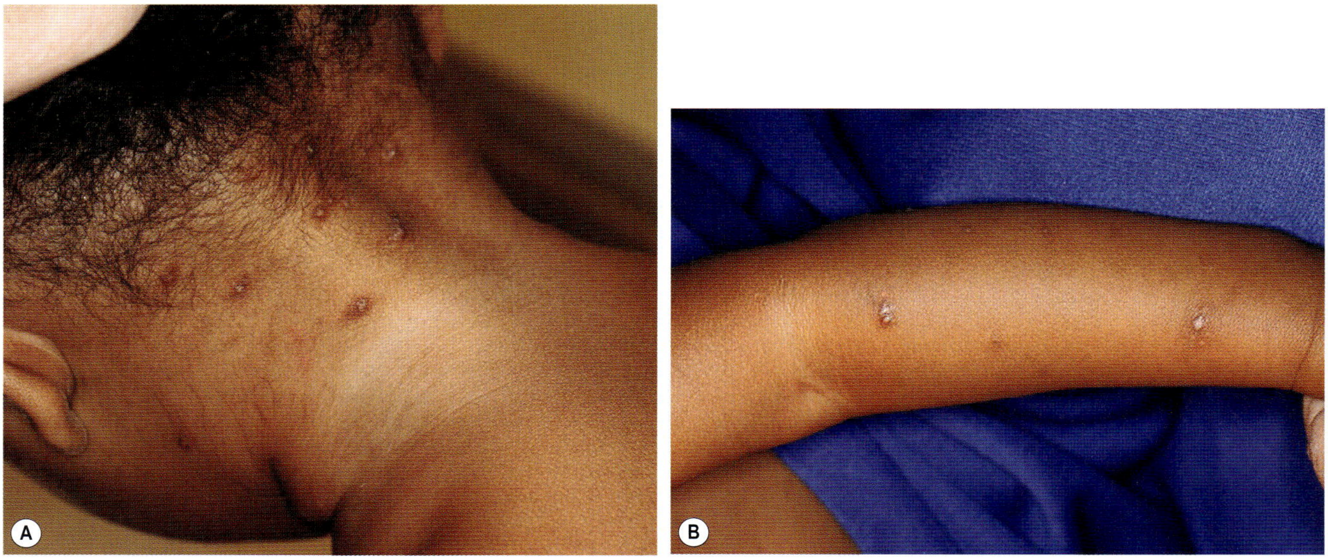

Fig. 18.39 Papular urticaria. These recurrent papules in a 2-year-old boy would heal with postinflammatory hyperpigmentation **(A and B)**, only to recur with erythema, edema, and marked pruritus in the same locations.

Box 18.2 Guidelines for the Safe Use of Insect Repellents in Children

Do not apply to infants under 2 months of age.
Read and follow all package directions and precautions.
Use just enough repellent to lightly cover the skin; do not saturate the skin.
Apply only to exposed skin; do not use on clothing or apply under clothing.
Apply sparingly to the face, and avoid contact with the eyes and mouth.
Do not apply to the hands of small children.
Do not allow young children to apply products themselves.
Do not use sprays in enclosed areas or near food.
If self-applied, rinse palms to avoid inadvertent contact with eyes and mouth.
Do not use on open skin, cuts, wounds, or inflamed areas.
Once inside, wash all treated areas with soap and water.
Keep repellents out of the reach of children.
Use a separate sunscreen; avoid using combined insect repellent–sunscreen products because clinical data are limited.

support such claims.[178,182,183] Human health risk assessments were conducted for DEET and picaridin (see later) and found no significant toxicologic risks from typical use of these repellents.[184] Over a 6-year period of data collection as part of the DEET Registry, seizures were the most common neurologic symptom reported with a possible temporal relationship to DEET exposure. However, children were not disproportionately represented, there was no apparent relationship between DEET concentration and the severity of outcome, and the reports of neurologic events (when considered relative to the number of annual DEET applications in the United States) were quite low overall.[185] The AAP, in the Red Book discussion of repellents for use on skin, recommends repellents with DEET concentrations not exceeding 30% (with concentrations between 20% and 30% recommended in infants and young children) and following such practical application guidelines as those outlined in Box 18.2.[186] The CDC recommends DEET at concentrations up to 50% for both adults and children over 2 months of age.

DEET-containing insect repellents should be carefully applied because they may damage plastics, rayon, leather, spandex, and other synthetic fabrics. They are not damaging, however, to cotton or wool. In addition, it should be remembered that DEET-containing products are flammable. Combination products containing DEET and sunscreen are not recommended, given the potentially decreased effectiveness of the sunscreen and the different recommended application frequencies of these two products. Questions about the safety of DEET can be addressed by the EPA-sponsored National Pesticide Telecommunications Network at www.ace.orst.edu/info/nptn.

Picaridin (KBR 3023) is an insect repellent that is effective against mosquitoes, biting flies, and ticks. It is usually used in a concentration of up to 20%. Picaridin is reportedly of similar efficacy to DEET, is odorless, and will not damage plastics or fabrics. Before its launch in the United States, picaridin was used fairly extensively in Europe and Australia. No serious adverse events have been reported to date. Other synthetic EPA-registered insect repellents available in the United States and Europe include IR3535, which fared poorly in an "arm-in-cage" study when compared with DEET, para-menthane-3, 8-diol (PMD, a synthetic version of oil of lemon eucalyptus), and 2-undecanone.[178,186] However, DEET and picaridin are the two most widely recommended insect repellents, with picaridin having the strongest data supporting its use as a second-line agent (after DEET) in one systematic review.[179]

Plant-derived repellents may have repellent activity, but none compare to the effectiveness and duration of action of DEET.[133] These products usually contain essential oils from any of several plants, including citronella, cedar, eucalyptus, lemongrass, and soybean. Citronella is the active ingredient in most "natural" repellents marketed in the United States. It has a lemony scent and is available in an oil and in candles. However, in areas with epidemics of mosquito-borne diseases (such as West Nile virus) or in high-risk settings, these products should not be relied upon as the sole protection from bites. When compared with DEET, a blend of the top three performing essential oils was found to offer some protection against various species of mosquitoes but significantly less so than the chemical repellent.[187]

Other approaches to mosquito repellency include ingested garlic or vitamin B_1 and treated or sound-emitting wristbands, each of which has less consistently demonstrated effectiveness. Permethrin, marketed in a 0.5% concentration (Permanone, Repel Permethrin Clothing and Gear, Sawyer Permethrin Clothing and Gear, Ben's Clothing and Gear) as a tick repellent, is also available and is sprayed on tents, clothing, and sleeping bags (but is not for use on skin). This product is also effective against mosquitoes, flies, and chiggers and works as a contact insecticide, resulting in central nervous system toxicity to the insect.

Caterpillars and Moths

Caterpillars represent the larval stage of butterflies and moths of the order Lepidoptera. The hairs of certain moths and caterpillars are known to produce dermatitis that can be severe and incapacitating to both children and adults. Dermatitis related to these insects has been known as *caterpillar dermatitis* and *lepidopterism*. In the United States, the most commonly seen and most irritating of these are those caused by the hairs of the brown-tail moth (usually seen in the northeastern part of the country) and the puss caterpillar (the larvae of the "flannel" moth, *Megalopyge opercularis*), seen from Virginia southward to the states bordering the Gulf of Mexico.[188–190] Contact with the oak processionary caterpillar *(Thaumetopoea processionea)*, found especially in oak forests in European countries, or the pine processionary moth *(Thaumetopoea pityocampa)*, found in Central Asia, North Africa, or southern Europe, may result in multiple symptoms, including pruritus, dermatitis, conjunctivitis, pharyngitis, and respiratory distress.[191,192] In some instances, affected individuals did not have direct contact with the caterpillar but only with another individual who had experienced contact, suggesting the possibility of human-to-human transmission of the relevant substance(s).[193]

Reactions produced by contact with the hairs and spines of these moths and caterpillars may be associated with the release of histamine and other vasoactive substances or from mechanical irritation by caterpillar hairs that become embedded in the pores of affected individuals. The precise mechanisms for these reactions are unclear, however, and may be related to irritant reactions, hypersensitivity reactions, or toxic envenomation.[194] They may be focal or more widespread. Examination typically reveals erythematous macules and papules, eczematous dermatitis, vesicles, urticaria, or even necrosis. Other reactions may include severe local pain, nausea, fever, swelling, numbness, muscle cramps, headache, seizures, and shock. The diagnosis of moth or caterpillar dermatitis can be confirmed by microscopic examination of tape strippings or scrapings of involved areas with demonstration of offending hairs. Although the disorder is self-limiting, relief can be obtained with the use of oral antihistamines, topical corticosteroids, ice packs, and topical antipruritic agents. In patients with severe reactions, fluid support, narcotics, and systemic corticosteroids may be necessary.

Other Cutaneous Parasites

CUTANEOUS LARVA MIGRANS (CREEPING ERUPTION)

Cutaneous larva migrans (CLM; creeping eruption) is a self-limited skin eruption caused by the larval stages of the dog and cat hookworms *Ancylostoma caninum* and *Ancylostoma braziliensis*, respectively. *Uncinaria stenocephala* has also been implicated. CLM is one of the most common skin diseases among travelers returning from tropical countries.[195] In the United States, most cases of CLM are contracted in the southeastern states, most notably Florida and Georgia.[196] Worldwide the disorder is most common in Mexico, Central and South America, Africa, Southeast Asia, and the Caribbean.[196,197] The adult hookworms release eggs while in the intestines of their definitive hosts (dogs or cats), and these eggs are passed along with stool onto sandy, warm soil. Humans become incidental hosts when larvae burrow through intact skin that comes into contact with the infested soil. The disorder is quite common in children because of high-risk behaviors (e.g., playing in the sand) seen in this age group. It occurs sporadically or in small epidemics in high-income countries and in tourists who have visited the tropics.[198] The most commonly involved areas are the extremities (especially feet), buttocks, and genitalia. The incubation period for CLM may be prolonged for weeks to months.[199] Preventive measures may include wearing shoes or sandals and sitting on a towel or chair while on sandy beaches.[200]

In the human host, the hookworm larvae are unable to complete their natural life cycle and remain confined to the upper levels of skin, wandering aimlessly and producing the characteristic cutaneous findings. Initially, skin findings may be limited to one or a few erythematous papules. Ultimately, serpiginous, raised, sharply demarcated plaques develop (Figs. 18.40 and 18.41) and may advance up to 1 to 2 mm/day. Follicular involvement with folliculitis (hookworm folliculitis) may also occur.[195,201] Vesicular or bullous lesions are rare. Without treatment, the larvae eventually die, but this may take several months.

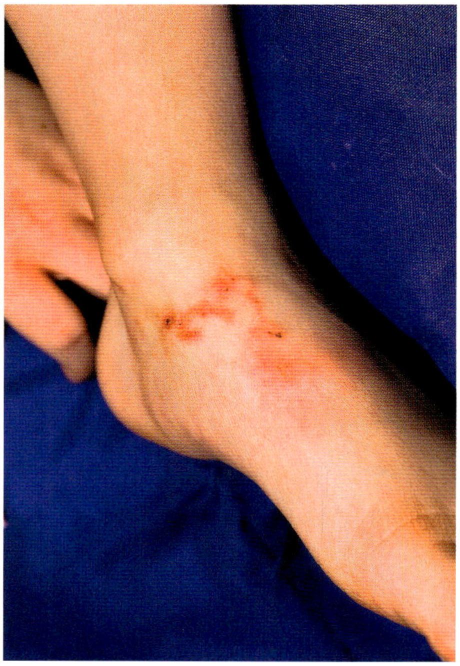

Fig. 18.40 Cutaneous larva migrans. A serpiginous, migratory plaque on the dorsal foot.

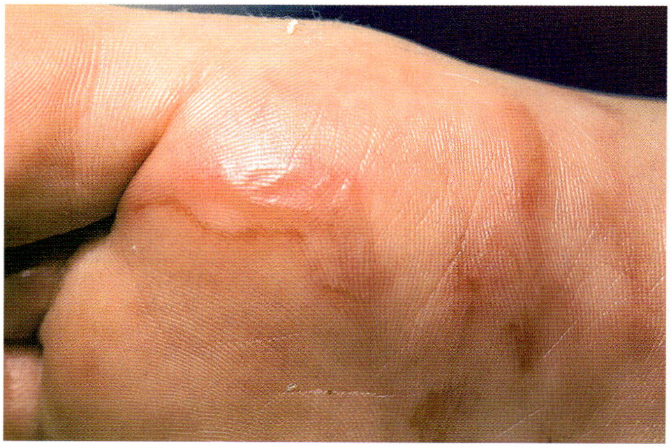

Fig. 18.41 Cutaneous larva migrans. The plantar surface of this young boy revealed a very itchy, linear plaque that was noted to continuously extend over the several days before diagnosis.

The lesions of CLM are extremely pruritic and may be complicated by pain and secondary bacterial infection. Although systemic dissemination of the parasite does not generally occur, eosinophilia is common, and pneumonitis (Löffler syndrome) may occasionally be present. Löffler syndrome is characterized by migratory pulmonary infiltrates, transient fever, malaise, and cough, and is believed to be caused by a type 1 hypersensitivity to larvae or, much less likely, migration of helminths to the lungs.[202]

The differential diagnosis of CLM may include other larval infestations such as *Strongyloides stercoralis* and *Gnathostoma spinigerum*. As opposed to CLM, the serpiginous rash of larva currens (a hypersensitivity reaction seen in some patients with strongyloidiasis) may progress at a rate of up to 10 cm/day.[203,204] Scabies, jellyfish stings, and phytophotodermatitis may also mimic CLM.[197] Treatment options for creeping eruption include liquid nitrogen cryotherapy (which was a traditional mainstay of treatment) and oral anthelminthic agents. Cryotherapy is rarely effective and is traumatic for most young children; hence it should be avoided for this indication. Oral agents demonstrated to be effective include thiabendazole, albendazole, and ivermectin. Thiabendazole is given at a dose of 25 mg/kg per day divided into two doses for 2 to 5 days. Potential side effects include headache, dizziness, and gastrointestinal upset. Alternatively, topical thiabendazole (500 mg/5 mL) can be applied four times daily and is often effective. Oral albendazole seems to be one of the most effective and well-tolerated therapies. The recommended pediatric dose according to the AAP is 15 mg/kg per day (up to 400 mg maximum) once daily for 3 days.[205] Side effects are rare with this agent, which has been used in nematode and cestode infestations. Use of these agents in young children has not been well studied. Ivermectin, an agent used primarily for onchocerciasis and other nematodes, has also been anecdotally reported as effective in open-label studies.[195] It is given as a single dose (200 μg/kg) and repeated in 1 to 2 weeks if necessary. The AAP suggests pediatric dosing of 200 μg/kg once daily for 1 to 2 days for children >15 kg.[205] In one series of 56 patients with CLM treated with single-dose ivermectin, the response rate was 98%.[206]

CERCARIAL DERMATITIS (SWIMMER'S ITCH)

Cercarial dermatitis (swimmer's itch, sawah itch, koganbyo) is an itchy, inflammatory dermatosis that results from penetration of human skin by nonhuman schistosome parasites. It occurs after swimming or wading in freshwater lakes, especially in the midwestern United States, and has also been demonstrated in the southwestern United States.[207] Cercarial dermatitis can also be acquired in the sea or brackish waters.[208] The most clinically relevant organisms are the *Trichobilharzia* species. The adult schistosomes reside in the mesenteric blood vessels of birds and mammals, and after passage from the blood to the intestine, eggs are deposited in water along with the host feces. Subsequently, miracidiae hatch and penetrate the intermediate host, usually snails.[209] Within the snail they develop into cercariae, which are multicellular larvae composed of an oblong body and a slender, bifurcated tail.[210] The cercariae leave the snails and reside in the upper levels of lakes until they can again infest the definitive host. However, they may also infest accidental hosts such as humans.

Swimmer's itch occurs on exposed areas of skin, which are the sites most readily available to the cercariae. Because humans are not the definitive host, the cercariae die within hours after skin penetration, and the host immune response results in the clinical eruption.[211] Often the initial infestation does not result in a reaction, but causes sensitization, which results in the clinical eruption after subsequent exposures.[209] Examination of the skin usually reveals nonspecific, erythematous papules and papulovesicles (Figs. 18.42 and 18.43). Excoriation may be present, and secondary bacterial superinfection is an occasional complication. Postinflammatory hyperpigmentation is common.

The distribution of the lesions combined with the history of exposure to a freshwater lake will combine to suggest the diagnosis of swimmer's itch. Activities that involve more extensive contact with lake water (e.g., wading, working on the dock, and swimming) are more likely to be associated with the disorder than other activities like boating, skiing, and tubing.[211] Cercarial dermatitis may be more common

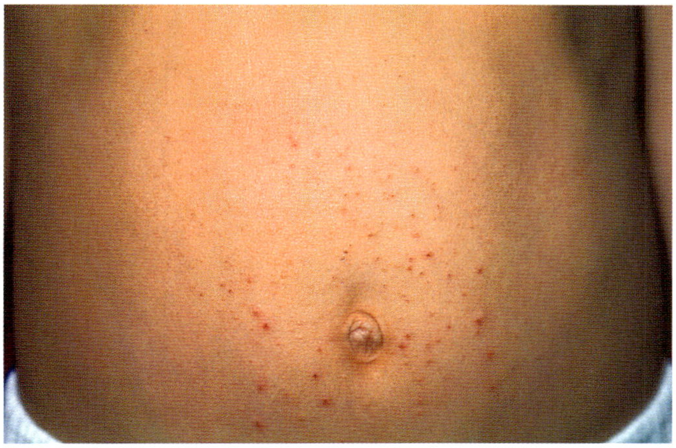

Fig. 18.42 Cercarial dermatitis. Multiple pruritic, excoriated papules and papulovesicles on exposed surfaces of the skin. The patient had been swimming in a freshwater lake along with family members, several of whom developed similar lesions.

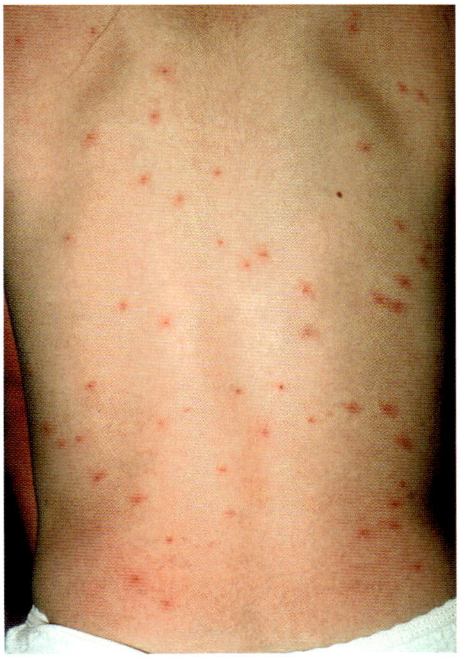

Fig. 18.43 Cercarial dermatitis. Itchy, excoriated papules and papulovesicles occurring on exposed areas of skin.

in children given their disproportionate time spent in shallow water.[210] Aquariums containing snails may also be a source of swimmer's itch.[209,212] Water analysis via filtration and polymerase chain reaction (PCR) detection may be useful if confirmation is required and snails cannot be found.[213] Treatment is supportive and consists of topical corticosteroids, topical antipruritic agents, oral antihistamines, and, rarely, systemic corticosteroids for severe cases.

Seabather's Eruption

Seabather's eruption, also known as *sea lice*, is not a true parasitic infestation but is commonly confused with cercarial dermatitis and is therefore included in this chapter. It results from a hypersensitivity reaction to the stinging nematocyst of a cnidarian (planula) larva, which includes jellyfish, Portuguese man-of-war, sea anemone, or fire coral (see later).[214] Most often it has been associated with exposure to the larval form of the thimble-sized jellyfish *Linuche unguiculata*.[214,215] Seabather's eruption occurs most commonly in marine saltwaters off of Florida, in the Gulf of Mexico, and in the Caribbean. (A discussion of traditional jellyfish stings can be found in the following section.)

The skin lesions of seabather's eruption tend to be limited to areas covered by the swimming garment; the swimwear tends to act as a filter, draining water and maintaining contact of the planulae against the skin.[216] Skin findings may include erythematous papules, pustules, and papulovesicles (Figs. 18.44 and 18.45). Urticarial plaques may also be present (Fig. 18.46), and pruritus is usually severe. Other symptoms may include fatigue, fever, chills, headache, abdominal pain, diarrhea, and nausea; these symptoms appear to be more common in children or in those who have severe envenomation.[217] Many patients recall having seen "thimble-sized" jellyfish in the waters, or

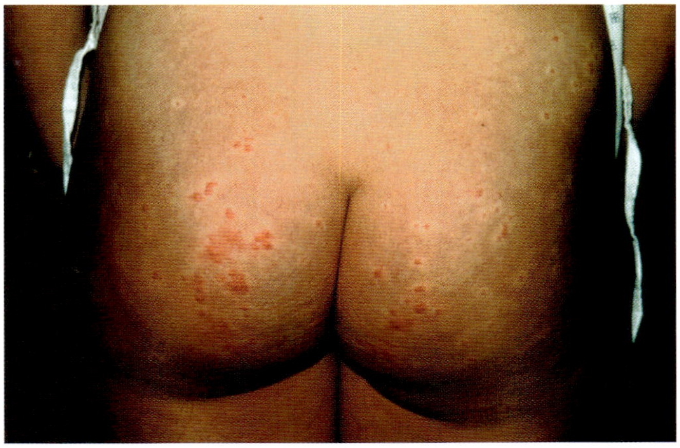

Fig. 18.44 Seabather's eruption. These edematous, erythematous papules were limited to sites covered by the swimming garment.

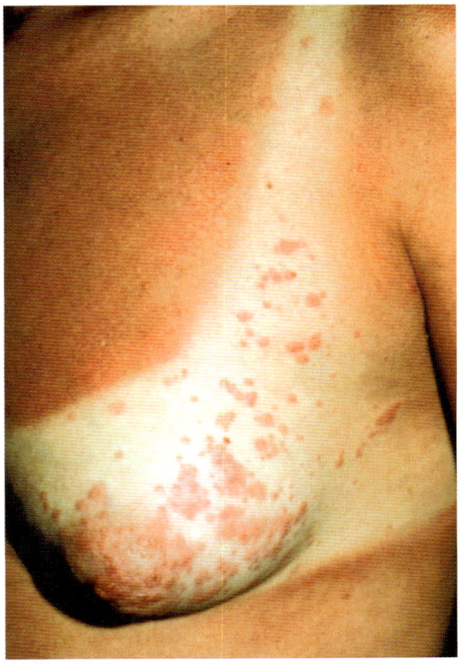

Fig. 18.45 Seabather's eruption. Erythematous papules and papulovesicles limited to sites covered by the swimming garment after a vacation in the Caribbean.

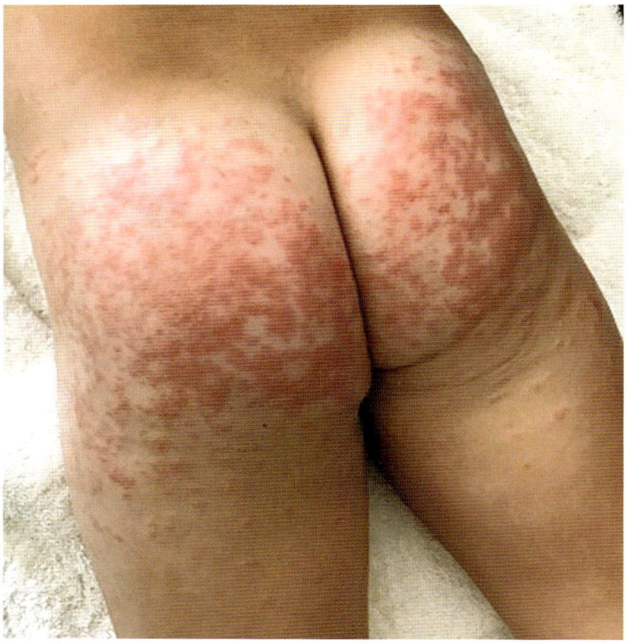

Fig. 18.46 Seabather's eruption. Urticarial papules and plaques appeared in this 7-year-old boy shortly after swimming in the ocean (and a freshwater pool immediately after) in the Bahamas. The lesions were intensely pruritic and accompanied by mild fever and abdominal pain.

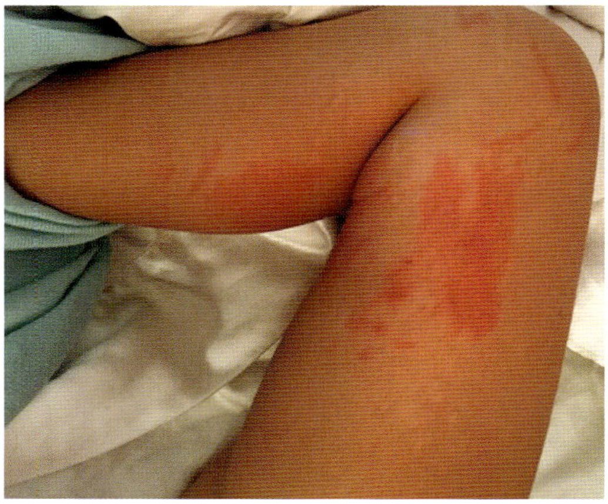

Fig. 18.47 Jellyfish sting. This 4-year-old girl developed linear and streaky, "whip-like" erythematous plaques with pain and pruritus on the extremities after a jellyfish sting while wading in the ocean in the southeastern United States. Recurrent dermatitis episodes lasted for several months.

tiny "black dots" along the water surface.[214] Symptoms may begin while in the water or when exiting, although in the majority of patients they begin several hours later. Longer swim times appear to increase the risk of seabather's eruption: in one report of 38 patients, the median duration of water exposure was 2.5 hours (range 1 to 8 hours).[217] In surfers, lesions may also develop in areas that make contact with the surfboard (abdomen, chest, and thighs).[218] Because freshwater is known to stimulate nematocyst discharge of toxins (via osmotic pressure change), removal of the bathing garment is recommended before rinsing, especially in areas where seabather's eruption warnings are posted.

The diagnosis of seabather's eruption is primarily a clinical one. It should be suspected in the patient with an itchy, papulovesicular eruption limited to covered areas of skin and occurring after exposure to saltwater. Skin biopsy[214] and serologic assays[214,219] have been used but are generally unnecessary. Treatment is symptomatic, as discussed earlier for swimmer's itch. An over-the-counter waterproof product, Safe Sea, contains sunscreens and several inactive ingredients that reportedly interfere with attachment (and hence injection of toxins) and the biochemical pathways that lead to symptoms. In a randomized, placebo-controlled side-by-side comparison field trial, jellyfish sting reactions were seen far less frequently on the side treated with active product (82% relative risk reduction).[220,221]

Jellyfish Stings

Cnidarians (phylum Cnidaria) are a group of aquatic animals that includes jellyfish, corals, sea anemones, and hydras. The cnidarian body consists of a gastrovascular cavity with a single opening through which food is ingested and waste is released. Cnidarians have tentacles encircling their mouth and bodies that are radially symmetrical. The phylum Cnidaria consists of four classes: Hydrozoa (Portuguese man-of-war), Scyphozoa (true jellyfish), Cubozoa (box jellyfish or sea wasps), and Anthozoa (sea anemones and corals).

Jellyfish are marine invertebrates that are found both in the ocean and in freshwater. They are responsible for the most common ocean-related envenomations acquired by humans, which may result in three types of responses, including immediate allergic, immediate toxic, and delayed allergic reactions.[222] The surface of jellyfish bodies and tentacles is covered in specialized cells called *cnidoblasts* that contain in their cytoplasm a nematocyst, or a capsule filled with a toxic fluid that is injected into human skin at the time of contact.[223] Cutaneous reactions to jellyfish stings may include urticarial wheals, burning, pruritus, and tenderness. Papules and papulovesicles often occur in linear and wispy patterns (Fig. 18.47), and more chronic postinflammatory pigmentary changes, scarring (including keloids), and lichenification may occur. Occasionally observed findings include thrombophlebitis, tender regional lymphadenopathy, angioedema, papular urticaria, and distant hypersensitivity-type skin reactions (i.e., an id reaction). Fatal anaphylactic reactions are rare but when they occur are more common in children.[224] Other reported sequelae include a persistent lichen planus–like eruption, Guillain–Barré syndrome, and recurrent dermal hypersensitivity (type IV allergic reaction), which may manifest as recurrent pruritic dermatitis for months or years.[222,225,226] *Seabather's eruption* refers to a papulovesicular eruption occurring in covered areas of skin in response to contact with nematocysts from thimble-sized jellyfish larvae (see previous section).

Treatment for jellyfish stings is supportive, and traditional considerations include pain control (nonsteroidal antiinflammatory agents, opioids), compression, application of vinegar (thought to help in deactivation of the nematocysts), avoidance of freshwater exposure (which may trigger firing of nematocysts), oral antihistamines, oral corticosteroids, and manual removal of tentacles when visible. Topical corticosteroids may be helpful. One systematic review of jellyfish sting therapy suggested that vinegar may cause pain exacerbation or further nematocyst discharge unless the envenomation is believed to be from the bluebottle *(Physalia)*, in which case it may be helpful; other authors, however, firmly believe in the benefit of topical vinegar in this setting.[227,228] Medical attention should be sought after a jellyfish sting, despite there being a lack of consensus on the most appropriate treatment regimen among emergency medicine physicians.[229] Hospitalization may be required for severe symptoms such as fever, chills, tachycardia, muscle spasms, cellulitis, or anaphylaxis.[230] Cardiopulmonary resuscitation and use of an epinephrine pen (when available) may be necessary if anaphylaxis occurs. Useful preventive measures include wearing protective swim or diving wear (such as a full-body Lycra stinger suit or equivalent) and avoidance of areas known to be infested with jellyfish.[231]

The complete list of 231 references for this chapter is available online at http://expertconsult.inkling.com.

Key References

Karimkhani C, Colombara DV, Drucker AM, et al. The global burden of scabies: a cross-sectional analysis from the Global Burden of Disease Study 2015. Lancet Infect Dis 2017;17(12):1247–54.

Levine M. Pediatric envenomations: don't get bitten by an unclear plan of care. Pediatr Emerg Med Pract 2014;11(8):1–12.

Dehghankhalili M, Mobaraki H, Akbarzadeh A, et al. Clinical and laboratory characteristics of pediatric scorpion stings. A report from Southern Iran. Pediatr Emerg Care 2017;33:405–8.

Devore CD, Schutze GE. Head lice. Pediatrics 2015;135(5):e1355–65.

Medical Letter on Drugs and Therapeutics. Drugs for head lice. JAMA 2017;317(19): 2010–11.

McMenaman KS, Gausche-Hill M. Cimex lectularius ("bed bugs"). Recognition, management and eradication. Pediatr Emerg Care 2016;32(11):801–4.

Patel RV, Shaeer KM, Patel P, et al. EPA-registered repellents for mosquitoes transmitting emerging viral disease. Pharmacotherapy 2016;36(12):1272–80.

Currie BJ, McCarthy JS. Permethrin and ivermectin for scabies. N Engl J Med 2010; 362(8):717–25.

McClain D, Dana AN, Goldenberg G. Mite infestations. Dermatol Ther 2009;22: 327–46.

Suchard JR. "Spider bite" lesions are usually diagnosed as skin and soft-tissue infections. J Emerg Med 2009;41(5):473–81.

Swanson DL, Vetter RS. Loxoscelism. Clin Dermatol 2006;24:213–21.

Skolnik AB, Ewald MB. Pediatric scorpion envenomation in the United States: morbidity, mortality and therapeutic innovations. Pediatr Emerg Care 2013; 29(1):98–103.

Chosidow O, Giraudeau B, Cottrell J, et al. Oral ivermectin versus malathion lotion for difficult-to-treat head lice. N Engl J Med 2010;362:896–905.

Hoffman DR. Ant venoms. Curr Opin Allergy Clin Immunol 2010;10:342–6.

19 Photosensitivity and Photoreactions

Sunlight emits a wide spectrum of radiation energy, extending from radio waves through infrared, visible, and ultraviolet (UV) light to X-rays.[1,2] The wavelength range of visible light is 400 to 800 nm and is relatively harmless, except for individuals with photosensitivity disorders, such as porphyria, solar urticaria, and polymorphous light eruption (PMLE). The infrared range is 800 to 1800 nm. The UVA and UVB wavelengths (280 to 400 nm) cause most cutaneous reactions, including in normal individuals who are exposed to sunlight, tanning booths, and an ever-expanding number of photosensitizers in the environment. Wavelengths less than 220 nm are absorbed by atmospheric gases, including oxygen and nitrogen, and those less than 280 nm are absorbed by the atmospheric ozone layer. The remaining middle wavelength (UVB, 280 to 320 nm) and long wavelength (UVA1, 340 to 400 nm; UVA2, 320 to 340 nm) UV radiation can reach the earth and be absorbed by biologic molecules. The skin is quite effective at protection from UV penetration, but the depth of penetration depends upon the wavelength. UVA easily reaches the deeper dermis, whereas UVB is absorbed in the epidermis and little reaches the upper dermis.

UV light also reaches the skin through reflection from snow (80% to 85%), sand (17% to 25%), water (5%, but up to 100% when the sun is directly overhead), sidewalks, and turf. UV light exposure also increases by 4% for every 1000-foot elevation above sea level. On a bright, cloudy day with thin cloud cover, it is possible to receive 60% to 85% of the amount of UV radiation present on a bright clear day. Hats and sun umbrellas provide only a moderate degree of protection, and surfaces with reflectivity greatly increase sunlight exposure.

Tanning and Sunburn Reactions

The visible short-term effects of UV light exposure are sunburn (Fig. 19.1; see Fig. 26.16) and tanning. The ability to cause sunburn markedly declines with increasing wavelength. UVA light at 360 nm is 1000-fold less effective in causing skin erythema (sunburn) than UVA light at 300 nm. UVB light is largely responsible for sunburn, with peak induction 6 to 24 hours after exposure. Sunburns gradually fade during the next 3 to 5 days, as the skin starts to desquamate. Reactivity to UVB light may range in severity from a mild asymptomatic erythema to a more intense reaction, with redness accompanied by tenderness, pain, edema, and, at times, vesiculation and bulla formation, particularly the day after the sunburn first appears. If the sunburned area is extensive, constitutional symptoms may include nausea, malaise, headache, fever, chills, and even delirium. Sunburn during childhood correlates with a higher risk of developing melanocytic nevi,[3] as well as UV light–induced skin cancers.

Tanning is also wavelength dependent and is biphasic. Immediate pigment darkening results primarily from exposure to UVA light, is caused by alteration and redistribution of melanin, and fades in 6 to 8 hours. Delayed tanning usually results from exposure to UVB and peaks at about 3 days after exposure. Fair skin is only able to tan with UVB dosages greater than the erythema threshold (i.e., a sunburn is required on type II skin; type I skin cannot tan; Table 19.1). In contrast, darker skin types (i.e., type III and higher) can tan significantly without burning (at suberythemogenic doses). Sunburn causes apoptosis (cell death) of keratinocytes ("sunburn cells") or, if the dosage is high enough, induces cell cycle arrest, allowing the cell to undergo repair of their deoxyribonucleic acid (DNA) template before proliferating. Sunburn also depletes the protective Langerhans cells, causes epidermal thickening (which reduces exposure of the basal keratinocytes to UV radiation) as a protective mechanism, stimulates release of inflammatory cytokines, and induces the formation of antioxidative enzymes (which reduce oxidative DNA damage). The tan induced by UVB involves increased melanin synthesis, increased numbers of melanocytes, and increased transfer of melanosomes to keratinocytes.

The long-term effects of chronic sun exposure include photoaging, photocarcinogenesis, and immunosuppression. Given its potential to penetrate more deeply into the dermis, UVA light is thought to play a particularly important role in photoaging. UVA light, but not UVB light, is able to penetrate through window glass, even if tinted.[4] Thus individuals who sit in offices exposed to UVA light through windows or drive cars extensively can show significant asymmetry in UVA damage on the face.[5] An exception is the laminated glass of windshields (as opposed to the nonlaminated glass on the sides of cars), which blocks most UVA light (up to 380 nm). Window films can be applied to block UVA radiation but allow vision.

UVA light is also the light used in indoor tanning, a practice prevalent particularly among older female adolescents.[6,7] This practice promotes skin damage, leading to an increased risk of both melanoma[8] and nonmelanoma skin cancer and photodamage, but no increased protection against sun exposure.[9,10] Indoor tanning has also led to psychological dependence and has been associated with a higher risk of other high-risk health behaviors.[11] The danger of using tanning facilities has led to legislation to control use by minors and limitations of exposure in almost every state and reclassification by the US Food and Drug Administration (FDA) of tanning beds as class II devices that require oversight and are subject to restrictions.[12] The prevalence of use of a tanning salon by college-aged students was 60.4% in 2009, with 33.1% using tanning salons more than five times a year.[13] From 2009 to 2017, however, indoor tanning declined (15.6% to 5.6%) across all age groups, and among White (37.4% to 10.1%) and Hispanic (10.5% to 3.0%) female adolescents, as well as White (7.0% to 2.8%) and Hispanic (5.8% to 3.4%) male adolescents.[11]

Many facilities now offer "safe" tanning, and these self-tanners are also available commercially. With all these self-tanners, an artificial tan is produced by dihydroxyacetone (DHA), a sugar that interacts with the stratum corneum proteins to produce a brown pigment made of polymers called *melanoidins,* which resist washing.[14] Higher concentrations and more applications of DHA increase the degree of tanning. The effect of DHA is seen within 1 to 3 hours of application, peaks 8 to 24 hours after application, and persists for 5 to 7 days.[15] Pigmentation is only lost with keratinocyte sloughing. Bronzers, which are often in tinted moisturizers or powders, sometimes contain

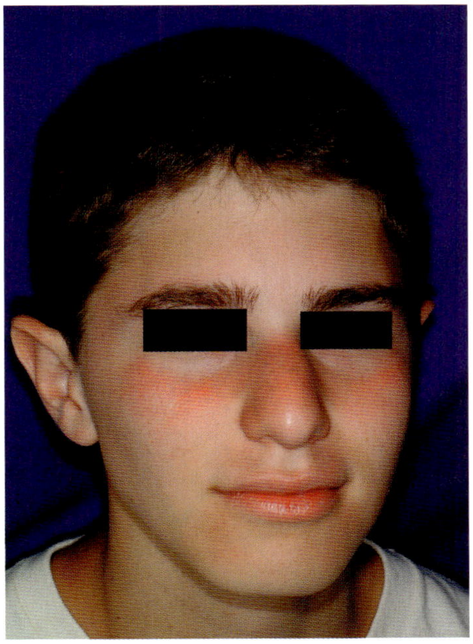

Fig. 19.1 Sunburn. This adolescent became more sensitive to ultraviolet light exposure while taking isotretinoin.

Table 19.1 Skin Types and Photosensitivity

Skin Type	Reactivity to Sun	Examples
I	Very sensitive: always burns easily and severely, tans little or not at all	Individuals with fair skin, blond or red hair, blue or brown eyes, and freckles
II	Very sensitive: usually burns easily, tans minimally or lightly	Individuals with fair skin; red, blond, or brown hair; and blue, hazel, or brown eyes
III	Moderately sensitive: burns moderately, tans gradually and uniformly	Average White individuals
IV	Moderately sensitive: burns minimally, tans easily	Individuals with dark brown hair, dark eyes, and white or light brown skin
V	Minimally sensitive: rarely burns, tans well and easily	Brown-skinned (Middle Eastern and Hispanic) individuals
VI	Deeply pigmented: almost never burns, tans profusely	Blacks and others with heavy pigmentation

DHA but often have other products that color skin temporarily, such as walnut shell extract, fig, or henna. Approximately 10.8% of adolescents have used a self-tanner, especially older White adolescents with a high to moderate level of sun sensitivity.[16] Self-tanners, unfortunately, provide minimal and transient sun protection, and their use is often in conjunction with tanning salon use rather than as a substitute.[17]

Prevention of sunburn depends primarily on the use of measures that reduce exposure to strong sunlight. This is especially important for fair-skinned individuals, particularly blue-eyed persons, redheads, blonds, and those with freckles who withstand actinic exposure poorly, burn easily, and, over the years, tend to suffer chronic effects of light exposure. The availability of sunscreens should not translate into increased sun exposure; using sensible sun protection practices beyond sunscreens should be encouraged. Prophylactic measures to reduce the impact of harmful UV rays include timing of outdoor activities to avoid peak UV light exposure between 10:00 AM and 3:00 PM in the warmer seasons of the year; wearing broad-rimmed hats, sun protective clothing, and sunglasses; and staying in the shade. Light-textured materials such as T-shirts (especially when wet) give only partial protection.[4] Clothes with a tighter weave are commercially available (e.g., www.coolibar.com; www.solumbra.com), or clothes can be laundered with a chemical (Tinosorb FD), which provides sun protection (e.g., SunGuard).

Sunscreens occupy an important position in the management of UV light exposure.[18–20] The lifetime use of sunscreen and sun avoidance has been calculated to reduce the lifetime risk of developing UV light–induced skin cancer by 78%,[21] although the issue of whether use of sunscreens reduces the development of nevi remains controversial.[22] Promoting routine sunscreen use in the pediatric population is important, including among adolescents whose behaviors escape parental influence.[23,24] However, sun safety practices (allowing teachers time for application, avoiding outdoor activities at times of peak sun intensity, making sunscreens available to students, or asking parents to apply sunscreens before school) are not routinely used in schools.[25] Personalized monitoring of UV radiation has been simplified by the commercial availability of devices in the forms of patches, nail art, and clip-ons that measure sun exposure through color change using photosensitive dyes and wirelessly send data to a smartphone.[26]

Sunscreens are available in a variety of formulations, but lotions and aerosol sprays are most often used.[27] Sunscreen labels reveal both the sun protection factor (SPF) and the capability of broad-spectrum UVA protection.[28] The designation *broad spectrum* provides information about the ability of the sunscreen to protect again nonerythema effects, especially from UVA light, including immune suppression, photoaging, and skin cancer. The SPF rating can be determined by dividing the least amount of time it takes to produce erythema on sunscreen-protected skin by the time it takes to produce the same erythema without sunscreen protection. Thus individuals using a sunscreen with an SPF of 15 who normally burn after unprotected sun exposure can theoretically stay out 15 times longer before getting the same degree of erythema. Therefore the SPF rating only informs about protection against sunburn from UVB light. The additional benefit from use of a sunscreen with an SPF greater than 30 is small compared with the incremental benefit at lower SPF numbers, but higher SPF may be important for individuals with high photosensitivity or exposure to intense sunlight. However, it should be recognized that the SPF is FDA tested with a concentration of 2 mg/cm^2, which is more than the majority of individuals apply (equivalent to 20 g applied to the entire body of an average 9-year-old). Applying half of the FDA test concentration only achieves half or less the labeled SPF,[29] suggesting that higher SPFs should be used unless a thick layer is applied.[30] In a recent split-face study that assessed actual use, even SPF 100 was more effective than SPF 50 at reducing sunburn after 6 hours of exposure. The current recommendation is reapplication every few hours, as well as after swimming, periods of excessive perspiration, and washing or showering. The term *waterproof* is no longer allowed on labels, and sunscreens must specify the water resistance period (e.g., for 40 or 80 minutes).

The most common sunscreen components and their absorbance capacity are listed in Table 19.2. Mineral (sometimes called *inorganic*) sunscreens (titanium dioxide and zinc oxide) in the form of nanoparticles protect skin by reflecting and scattering UV and visible light (280 to 700 nm); often, both of these agents are included in a mineral sunscreen. Both titanium dioxide and zinc oxide are considered GRASE (generally recognized as safe and effective). These mineral sunscreens are recommended for use in children but may leave a highly visible white residue, especially when used in adequate amounts.

Organic sunscreens are primarily aromatic compounds that absorb light at approximately 250 to 370 nm. The two organic FDA-approved UVA-absorbing sunscreens are avobenzone and Mexoryl SX (terephthalylidene dicamphor sulfonic acid). Avobenzone is not photostable but is often in sunscreens with stabilizing ingredients. Other

Table 19.2 Common Sunscreen Filters and Ultraviolet Protection

Sunscreen Filter	Wavelength Protection*
ORGANIC SUNSCREENS	
PABA derivatives	UVB
PABA and padimate O (octyl dimethyl PABA)	
Salicylates	UVB
Homosalate (homomethyl salicylate), octisalate (octyl salicylate), trolamine salicylate	
Cinnamates	UVB
Cinoxate (2-ethyoxyethyl p-methoxycinnamate), octinoxate (octyl methoxycinnamate, Parsol MCX)	
Benzophenones	
Dioxybenzone (benzophenone-8)	UVB, some UVA2
Oxybenzone (benzophenone-3)	UVB, UVA2
Sulisobenzone (benzophenone-4)	UVA2, some UVA1
Others	
Avobenzone (butyl methoxydibenzoylmethane, Parsol 1789)†	UVA2 and UVA1
Ensulizole (phenylbenzimidazole sulfonic acid)	UVB
Meradimate (menthyl anthranilate)	UVA2
Drometrizole trisiloxane (Mexoryl XL)	UVB, UVA2, UVA1
Ecamsule (terephthalylidene dicamphor sulfonic acid, Mexoryl SX)†	UVA2, UVA1
Octocrylene	UVB
Bisoctrizole (methylene bis-benzotriazolyl tetramethylbutylphenol. Tinosorb M)	UVB, UVA2, UVA1
Bemotrizinol (bis-ethylhexyloxyphenol methoxyphenyl triazine, Tinosorb S)	UVA2, UVA1
INORGANIC SUNSCREENS	
Titanium dioxide	UVA and UVB; if large enough particle, visible light
Zinc oxide	UVA and UVB; if large enough particle, visible light

PABA, Paraaminobenzoic acid; *UVA*, ultraviolet A; *UVB*, ultraviolet B.
*UVB = 290 to 320 nm, UVA2 = 320 to 340 nm, UVA1 = 340 to 400 nm, visible light = 400 to 800 nm.
†Only organic UVA blockers in the United States.

UVA-absorbing sunscreen ingredients are available outside of the United States, including in Europe, such as bis-ethylhexyloxyphenol methoxyphenol triazine (anisotriazine [Tinosorb S]), methylene-bis-benzotriazolyl tetramethylbutylphenol (Tinosorb M), and drometrizole trisiloxane (silatriazole [Mexoryl XL]), but the FDA has determined that insufficient evidence of safety is available to approve for US use.

Some sunscreens that were used in the past now are banned (PABA and trolamine salicylate). Oxybenzone (benzophenone-3) and octinoxate (octly methoxycinnamate) were banned in Hawaii in 2018 because of evidence of damage to coral reefs. Oxybenzone has been linked to hormone disruption, especially antiandrogenic effects, and has been found in human breast milk, amniotic fluid, urine, and plasma, attesting to its ability to penetrate skin.[31] However, oxybenzone is a component of many nonmineral sunscreens, including in conjunction with avobenzone, and eliminating it without resorting to mineral-containing sunscreens (including in noncomedogenic products for teenagers) can be difficult, given the limited repertoire of available, FDA-approved sunscreen ingredients.

Photoallergic and allergic (i.e., not requiring sun exposure) contact dermatitis from active and inactive sunscreen ingredients should be considered in children who present with photosensitivity. In a retrospective study of 157 children, 6.4% showed positive photopatch test results. Oxybenzone and octinoxate (largely phased out) were the most common active triggers.[32] Octocrylene is another ingredient commonly implicated. An ingredient in some sunscreens, alkyl glucoside (often listed in ingredients as arachidyl, cetearyl, cocoa, decyl, or lauryl glucoside), has experienced an increasing rate of contact allergies and was named the 2017 Allergen of the Year by the American Contact Dermatitis Society.[33] Allergic contact dermatitis, especially to decyl and lauryl glucoside, occurs more commonly in individuals with a history of atopy.[34] Tinosorb M (not available in the United States) contains decyl glucoside as a hidden ingredient and may be partly responsible for many cases of allergic contact dermatitis to sunscreens.

Although experts recommend that organic sunscreens be applied 30 minutes before the onset of sun exposure to enable adequate time to bind to the stratum corneum and show effectiveness, a 2018 study showed that 10 minutes before exposure may be adequate.[35] The inorganic sunscreens (with titanium dioxide/zinc oxide) can be applied immediately before sun exposure.[36]

Oral sunscreens containing antioxidants (e.g., lycopene, vitamins C and E) and botanicals (e.g., polyphenols such as green tea and flavonoids such as genistein) are now commercially available. They provide some protection against acute sun damage, but they are not effective in preventing sunburns or DNA damage, their long-term protective effects are not clear, and they should not replace other forms of photoprotection for children. Some of these antiinflammatory ingredients are added to topically applied sunscreens with the same issues.

The degree to which a person sunburns or tans depends on genetic factors and the natural protection of the skin. Skin types, accordingly, are ranked from skin type I, the most sensitive, to skin type VI, the least sensitive to sun damage (see Table 19.1). Because sun damage begins in children and is cumulative, it is strongly recommended that everyone adopt a program of sun protection and daily sunscreen use, preferably with an SPF of 15 or greater, from infancy on. Because increased melanin is not totally protective, even darker-skinned individuals can burn and should use sunscreen.

Considerable media attention has focused on the need for UV light–induced vitamin D synthesis in the skin as a rationale for sun exposure. Indeed, UVB light induces the synthesis of vitamin D_3 in epidermal cells, and this vitamin D_3 is then hydroxylated in the liver (to 25-OH-vitamin D_3) and kidney (to 1,25-OH-vitamin D_3).[37] However, the UV light exposure that stimulates vitamin D_3 production in the skin is inseparable from UV light exposure that is carcinogenic. Although vigorous sunscreen use may reduce the capacity of skin to produce vitamin D (and greater vitamin D deficiency has been linked to darker skin color), sunscreen use has not been linked with deficiency and oral administration of vitamin D likely suffices. The American Academy of Pediatrics recommends a minimum daily intake of vitamin D for infants, children, and adolescents to 400 IU/day, beginning shortly after birth.[38] Patients who require strict photoprotection as treatment should be monitored for possible vitamin D deficiency and provided dietary supplementation.[39] Evidence suggests that high doses of vitamin D_3 (200,000 IU), given 1 hour after experimental sunburn induction, block the sunburn response.[40–42]

Treatment of sunburn consists of cool compresses or cool tub baths in colloidal oatmeal (such as Aveeno), baking soda, or cornstarch; topical formulations with pramoxine or menthol; mild topical corticosteroid formulations; an emollient cream; and systemic preparations with analgesic and antiinflammatory properties, such as nonsteroidal antiinflammatory drugs (NSAIDs). When symptoms are severe, a short course of systemic corticosteroids (oral prednisone, or its equivalent, in dosages of 1 mg/kg per day, with tapering after a period of 4 to 8 days) will abort severe reactions and afford added relief.

Certain disorders predispose individuals to the adverse effects of UV light. For example, children with alopecia totalis (see Chapter 7), just as adults with androgenetic alopecia and balding at the vertex, have a higher risk of developing skin cancer at the exposed sites if not protected. Patients with diminished or absent melanin, as in oculocutaneous albinism (see Chapter 11), or with defective DNA-repair mechanisms, as in xeroderma pigmentosum, have an increased tendency to develop UV light–induced DNA damage and cutaneous malignancy. Individuals with nevoid basal cell carcinoma syndrome (see Chapter 9), which predisposes to the early onset of numerous basal cell carcinomas, usually have mutations in the *PTCH* gene, which can also be mutated by UV light exposure in sporadic basal cell carcinomas. Sunlight can also exacerbate or trigger certain dermatoses, among them acne (see Chapter 8); herpes simplex infection (see Chapter 15); lupus erythematosus, neonatal lupus, and dermatomyositis (see Chapter 22); Darier disease (see Chapter 5); pemphigus and bullous pemphigoid (see Chapter 13); and lichen planus and psoriasis (see Chapter 4).

Photodermatoses

Photosensitivity is a broad term used to describe abnormal or adverse reactions to sunlight energy in the skin.[43] Photodermatoses must be distinguished from reactions to sunlight from exaggerated exposure, which is a normal response. Photodermatoses have been classified into four groups: (1) immunologically mediated, (2) drug or chemical induced, (3) with defective DNA repair, and (4) photoaggravation of existing conditions.[44,45]

Photosensitivity in a child should be suspected if the child develops a sunburn reaction, swelling, or intense pruritus after limited exposure to sunlight or shows a rash or scarring predominantly in sun-exposed areas (face, V of the neck, and dorsal surface of the arms and hands).[46,47] The history in a patient with a photosensitivity disorder is of great importance in determining the cause (Table 19.3). Examination should focus on the distribution of lesions, including areas of sparing.[48] In a photosensitivity disorder, the upper eyelids, postauricular and submental areas, nasolabial and neck folds, volar aspect of the wrist, and antecubital fossae tend to be spared. The morphology of the lesions may be helpful as well (urticarial versus papular versus vesicular, and the presence of lichenification, which suggests chronicity).

Phototesting can be helpful in determining the cause of an acquired photodermatosis. Exposure to UV light of different wavelengths may replicate the lesions, offering the opportunity to see morphology that may not be present at the time of the examination, confirming the suspicion of photosensitivity, and determining the UV range that triggers the disorder.[49] Further laboratory investigations, such as antibody testing for suspected collagen vascular disease (e.g., antinuclear antibodies [ANAs], anti-ds DNA, anti-Ro, and anti-La antibodies), blood and 24-hour urine porphyrin levels, and photopatch testing in patients with suspected photoallergy, may be necessary. Performing a biopsy is rarely useful, except for suspected lupus erythematosus.

Table 19.3 Evaluation for Potential Photosensitivity Disorders

History	Age of onset; exposure to potential photosensitizers; season of the eruption; time of onset after exposure to the sun; duration of eruption; effect of window glass and exposure to other light sources, including tanning booths; history of atopy and other medical problems; response to medications and use of sunscreens; family history
Examination	Distribution and morphology
Phototesting	Action spectrum, time to onset, minimal urticarial dose, inhibition and augmentation spectra
Photopatch testing	If photoallergy is suspected
Laboratory	Complete blood cell count, metabolic panel, erythrocyte sedimentation rate, autoantibodies, esp. antinuclear antibody, porphyrins
Biopsy	Useful for lupus and possibly porphyrias, but not for other photodermatoses
	Fibroblast cultures for XP testing

XP, Xeroderma pigmentosum.

IMMUNOLOGICALLY MEDIATED PHOTODERMATOSES

Solar Urticaria

Solar urticaria accounts for less than 1% of type I (immunoglobulin [Ig] E–mediated) hypersensitivity reactions and is characterized by a sensation of pruritus or burning and erythema.[50–54] The arms, legs, and upper chest are most commonly affected. Areas with regular sun exposure, such as the hands and face, are less commonly involved. Onset typically is within 5 to 10 minutes of sunlight exposure and is followed almost immediately by a localized urticarial reaction confined to the exposed areas and an irregular flare reaction that may extend onto unexposed skin. Within 24 hours, lesions tend to resolve (usually in 1 to 3 hours); new lesions will not develop for 12 to 24 hours, even if subsequent exposure to sunlight occurs. Fixed solar urticaria, characterized by recurrent eruptions on the same body parts, is rare and less severe than typical solar urticaria.[55] Delayed fixed solar urticaria, occurring 6 hours after exposure, has been described.[56] Although the reaction is generally transient, scratching and rubbing may lead to secondary eczematization with persistent cutaneous changes. The disorder usually does not manifest until the third or fourth decade of life, and women are affected three times more often than men. It has been reported in infants and children,[57] however, and as early as 1 week of age.[58,59] The condition persists for more than a decade in most affected individuals and often for a lifetime. Angioedema[60] and systemic signs (headache, nausea, wheezing, dizziness, syncope, and, rarely, shock) have occasionally been reported in association.

The cause of solar urticaria is unclear, but the pathogenesis involves interaction of a cutaneous photoallergen with IgE-specific mast cells, leading to mast cell degranulation. Often phototesting can confirm the diagnosis and determine the wavelength range that causes the photosensitivity. If positive, whealing generally occurs within minutes. In some patients, the sensitivity involves the UVB range through the visible light range; most patients react within the range of 290 to 480 nm. A negative phototest occurs in many patients and does not exclude the diagnosis. In patients with mild forms of solar urticaria (those in whom the threshold is high), the disorder may be controlled simply by appropriate sunscreens and avoidance of prolonged unprotected sun exposure. Those individuals highly sensitive to sunlight, however, must completely avoid daytime exposure.

Nonsedating antihistamines (generally four times the recommended dose),[61] antimalarials, corticosteroids, intravenous Ig (IVIG), and plasmapheresis have been beneficial. Omalizumab may be an option for patients with high levels of IgE who fail antihistamine therapy.[60,62,63] In some individuals, sun tolerance may be established by carefully metered, increasing exposures ("hardening") to natural or artificial light or the oral administration of a psoralen followed by UVA (PUVA) light.

Polymorphous Light Eruption

Polymorphous light eruption (PMLE) is the most common of the immune-mediated disorders associated with photosensitivity, occurring in 10% to 15% of the US population.[64] Although predominantly a disorder of women in the second and third decades of life, PMLE is well recognized to occur in children[65] and more often in individuals with lighter skin types. Although its cause remains only partially understood,[66] PMLE has been hypothesized to involve resistance to UV light–induced immune suppression and subsequently cell-mediated immune reactivity to a cutaneous photoantigen. An autosomal dominant inherited form of PMLE has been described in Native Americans of both North and South America.[67] Onset of this hereditary form is in childhood, and female patients outnumber male patients 2:1.

Often referred to as *sun allergy* or *sun poisoning*, the clinical eruption consists of a group of polymorphic lesions that usually occur 1 to 2 days after intense sunlight exposure, often while on vacation. In some individuals the eruption is first seen in the spring and persists with continued sun exposure but may improve later in the summer as the skin "hardens" from UV light exposure. The lesions may range from small papular (Fig. 19.2), urticarial (Fig. 19.3), vesicular, or eczematous reactions to large papules, plaques,[68] or patterns resembling erythema multiforme. A "pinpoint" variant that resembles lichen nitidus clinically and histologically occurs more often in individuals with darker skin colors.[69,70] The face, sides of the neck, and sun-exposed areas of the arms and hands are most often affected. In children, PMLE usually begins on the face as an acute, erythematous, eczematous eruption with small papules. Pruritus may be severe. Lesions usually involute spontaneously in 1 to 2 weeks, provided no additional exposure to sunlight occurs.

Juvenile spring eruption is considered a subset of PMLE and is characterized by photo-induced, dull-red edematous papules and papulovesicles that are largely confined to the superior helices of the ears (Fig. 19.4).[71] Lesions may become vesicular and crusted and occasionally appear on the dorsal aspects of the hands and on the trunk.

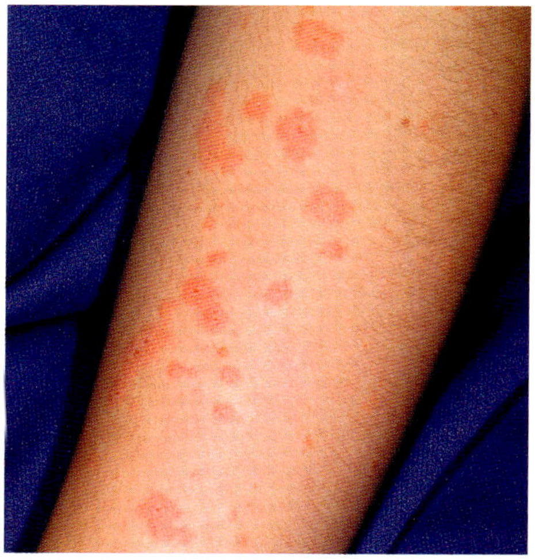

Fig. 19.3 Polymorphous light eruption. Urticarial form.

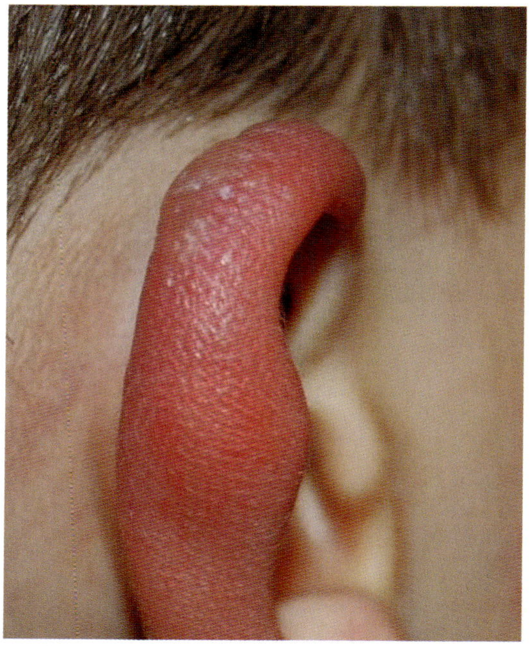

Fig. 19.4 Juvenile spring eruption. Tiny vesicles and erythema on the helix of the ears after sun exposure.

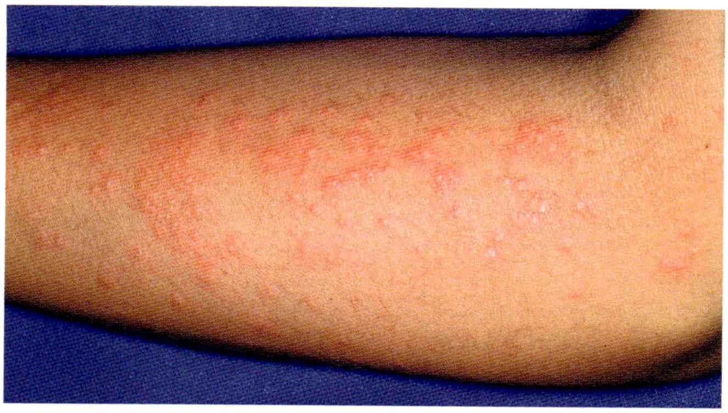

Fig. 19.2 Polymorphous light eruption. Papular lesions occurred 2 days after intense sun exposure.

Juvenile spring eruption occurs more commonly in boys than in girls and particularly between the ages of 5 and 12 years. Protuberant ears and lack of hair cover have been strongly associated,[72] but skin color and use of sunscreen have not. Lesions heal within a week, without scarring, unless secondary infection develops. Lesions are more difficult than PMLE to reproduce by exposure to UV light,[73] which has raised the question of whether the lesions, often appearing on a cool spring day, are more closely linked to pernio.[74]

The diagnosis of PMLE is suggested by the character of the lesions, their distribution, and their relationship to sun exposure.[75] Although often unnecessary, PMLE can be confirmed by provocative light testing with UVA and/or UVB[65] (minimal erythema dose [MED] tends to be normal), which is able to reproduce the spontaneous lesions in about 50% of patients. The testing involves exposing a site that has previously reacted repeatedly for about 4 consecutive days; testing should be performed in early spring before hardening has occurred. PMLE is distinguished clinically from solar urticaria based on the time course (within hours to days after exposure rather than minutes), duration (lasts for days rather than hours), and lack of urticaria. Some patients with systemic lupus erythematosus acquire sun-induced lesions indistinguishable from those of PMLE, and serologic testing should be performed (see Chapter 22). In addition, erythema multiforme may be photodistributed and thus confused with PMLE[76]; in contrast with erythema multiforme, PMLE skin samples have shown no evidence of herpes simplex virus.

Prevention of PMLE consists of sunscreens with good coverage of the UVA spectrum (when applied adequately with 2 mg/cm^2), sun-protective clothing, and the avoidance of midday sun exposure. Hardening or desensitization of skin by gradually increasing exposure two to three times weekly to narrowband UVB or PUVA light for 4 to 6 weeks before exposure helps the majority of treated patients. The addition of oral flavonoids (especially *Polypodium leucotomos* given for 12 weeks) or antioxidants in sunscreens has shown benefit in preventing PMLE.[77,78] If patients severely affected by this disorder anticipate temporary intense or prolonged sun exposure, a short course of systemic corticosteroids can be administered. Topical steroids may provide relief in mild cases. Topical vitamin D_3[79] or topical liposomal DNA-repair enzymes[80] may be of value. Antimalarials, β-carotene, and nicotinamide are of limited effectiveness.

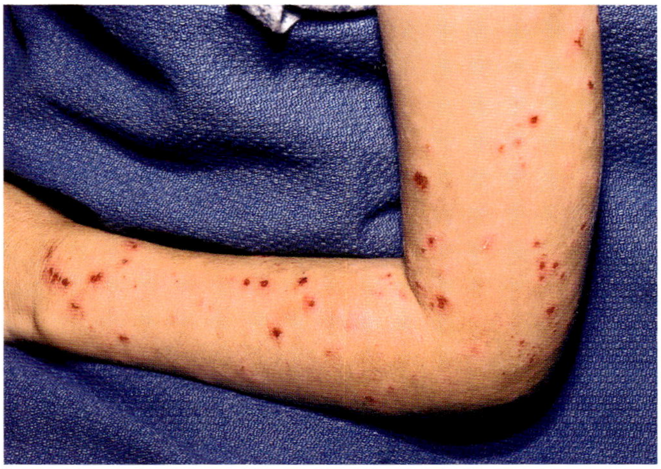

Fig. 19.6 Actinic prurigo. Note the excoriations and residual scars.

Actinic Prurigo

This photosensitivity disorder, also called *hydroa aestivale* and *Hutchinson summer prurigo*, is most commonly seen in the Indian and mestizo (mixed ancestry) populations of Mexico and other regions of Central and South America, although it has been described in the White and Asian populations.[81–83] It has been seen in many children in the United States and Canada but is rare in Europe. Most cases begin in childhood before puberty.[84] The condition is characterized by intensely itchy papules, plaques, and nodules in a symmetric distribution, along with excoriations and scars (Figs. 19.5 and 19.6). Some patients can be very uncomfortable and show secondary eczematization and lichenification. Although actinic prurigo predominantly affects exposed sites on the face and distal extremities, covered areas may be involved, particularly the sacrum and buttocks. Healed facial lesions leave minute linear or pitted scars. Seasonal exacerbation at the beginning of spring with improvement in the fall is common, although the lesions commonly do not clear during the winter; greater seasonal change occurs with higher latitudes. The oral or ocular mucosae are involved in 30% to 50% of cases. Cheilitis alone is seen in 28% of patients,[85] but 83% of patients experience pruritus, tingling, and pain of the vermilion.[86] Ocular findings most commonly include photophobia and conjunctivitis.[87]

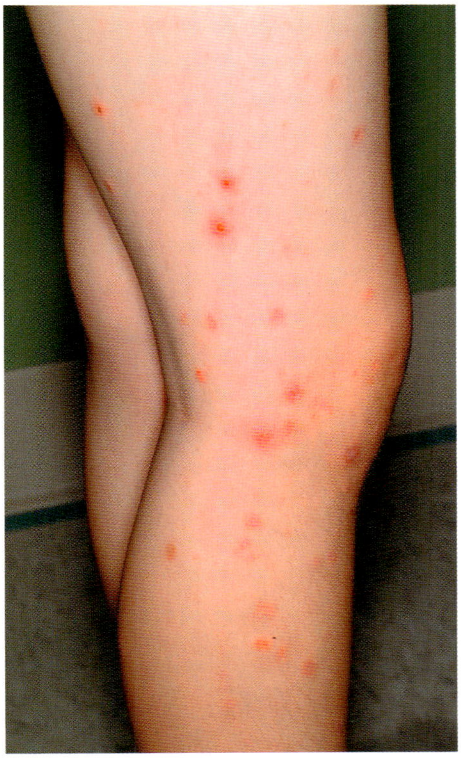

Fig. 19.5 Actinic prurigo. Intensely itchy papules with excoriations in this mild case with secondary eczematization.

The diagnosis is generally based on the clinical appearance. Biopsy of skin is generally not useful, although histologic evaluation of lip and conjunctival biopsy specimens shows the characteristic well-formed lymphoid follicles.[88] The presence of the eruption on both exposed and covered sites, its occurrence in winter, mucosal and conjunctival involvement, persistence beyond 4 weeks, and residual scarring of skin distinguish actinic prurigo from PMLE. Photosensitivity testing for MED is abnormal in up to two-thirds of patients. Human leukocyte antigen (HLA) DRB1*0407 is found in 60% to 70% of patients with actinic prurigo but only in 4% to 8% of DR41 controls)[89–91]; HLA DRB1*0401 is present in up to 20% of affected individuals with actinic prurigo. Although individuals with PMLE do not show these associations, 35% of patients with typical actinic prurigo have a history that suggests coexistence of actinic prurigo and PMLE or transition from one to the other.[92] Although the cause of actinic prurigo is unknown, the strong association with HLA markers suggests a role for major histocompatibility complex–restricted antigen presentation in the pathomechanism of the condition.

The disorder often has a chronic course that persists into adulthood; however, spontaneous resolution may occur during late adolescence. Vigorous sun protection and use of topical antiinflammatory agents for the pruritus lead to improvement in most patients. Short courses of systemic steroids can be helpful, but antimalarials have not had much effect. Complete resolution may require the addition of thalidomide (usually 50 to 100 mg/day),[93] which results in rapid clearing.[94] Oral cyclosporine and azathioprine have had some success in a few refractory cases.[95] The gradual introduction of exposure to narrowband UVB light has also helped some patients.

Hydroa Vacciniforme

Hydroa vacciniforme (HV) is a rare disorder known to result from chronic Epstein–Barr virus (EBV) infection.[96,97] Although it is considered a more benign photodermatosis in white children, a more persistent and severe form has been described primarily in children from Latin America and Asia. The classic lesions tend to appear each summer in children on uncovered parts of the body after exposure to sunlight. Boys are more often affected than girls. Rare familial cases have been described. The mean age of onset is 5 years in Whites[98] and 8 years in others.[99] The disease usually flares after sun exposure, and most patients show sensitivity to UVA light in monochromator phototesting, which may induce papulovesicular

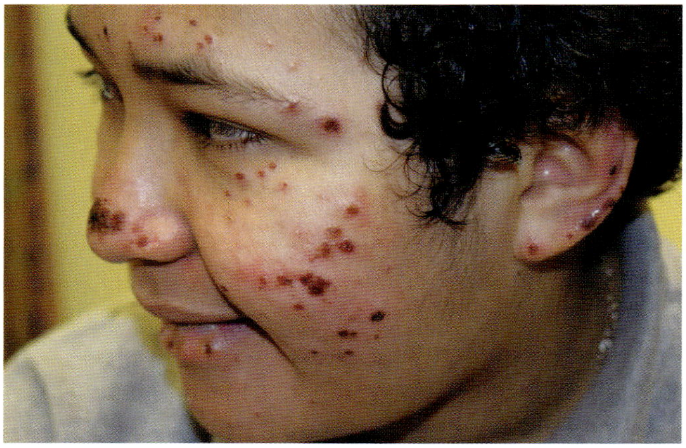

Fig. 19.7 Hydroa vacciniforme. Extensive hemorrhagic erosions and vesicles on sun-exposed areas. (Courtesy Dr. Aimee Smidt.)

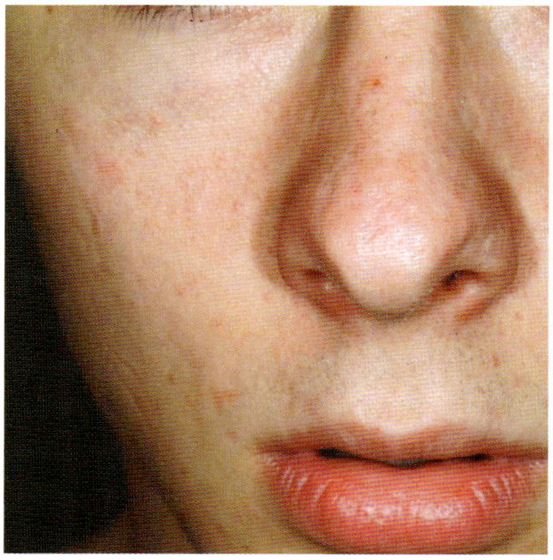

Fig. 19.8 Hydroa vacciniforme. Varioliform scarring on the nose in an adolescent who had severe episodes when younger.

lesions.[99] Biopsy of an active lesion showing reticular degeneration with EBV RNA in lymphocytes confirms the diagnosis. Detection of high levels of circulating EBV DNA (better in whole blood than in serum or plasma) also helps with the diagnosis.[100]

The primary lesion is a pruritic edematous papule, vesicle, or bulla that occurs within hours or days on uncovered surfaces exposed to sunlight.[53] Itching and burning, as well as mild constitutional symptoms, may occur a few hours before the outbreak of the cutaneous lesions. Lesions tend to appear on the face, the sides of the neck, and extensor surfaces of the extremities, and are arranged symmetrically over the nose, cheeks, ears, and dorsal surfaces of the hands (Fig. 19.7). The vesicles or bullae usually develop on an erythematous base and initially are rather tense. These are followed by central necrosis and umbilication that leads to healing with individual or confluent varioliform scarring within 1 to 2 weeks (Fig. 19.8). Mild conjunctivitis or keratitis, as well as corneal epithelial denudement, may be associated. In most, HV involutes spontaneously by the late teenage years with a mean duration of 9 years,[99] but persistence into adulthood has been described.[101]

The disorder can also be a more severe, persistent vesiculonecrotic eruption with frequent oral lesions and even cartilage or bone destruction, particularly in pediatric patients from Central and South America and Asia. Patients have marked facial edema, hemorrhagic bullae, atrophic scarring, and severe disfigurement in both sun-exposed and sun-protected sites. Patients often show an exaggerated hypersensitivity response to mosquito bites, in addition to the response to sunlight.[101,102] In some, systemic disease develops, with fever, hepatosplenomegaly, abnormal liver function testing, lymphadenopathy, leukopenia, and hemophagocytosis (now called HV-like T-cell lymphoproliferative disease).[103] This HV-like lymphoproliferative disorder is associated with higher-titer latent Epstein–Barr virus infection and monoclonal T-cell receptor gene rearrangements[104–107](see Chapter 10). However, there is no clinical or pathologic feature that predicts the progression.

Treatment of HV consists of strict sun protection, including broad-spectrum sunscreens (SPF at least 30), protective clothing, and avoidance of midday sun exposure. No intervention has been uniformly successful. Antivirals (acyclovir, valacyclovir), antimalarial drugs, thalidomide, β-carotene, oral fish oils,[108] and "hardening" by treatment in the spring with low-dose narrowband UVB light have been used with some therapeutic success.[109] Only stem cell transplantation is curative for those with more severe disease. The psychosocial and emotional impairment of HV on quality of life is significant, given the extensive disfigurement from scarring and the effect on daily life of strict sun avoidance.[110] Because of the potential risk of HV progression to HV-like lymphoproliferative disease, patients should be closely monitored for at least 10 years after diagnosis.

Photosensitivity Induced by Exogenous Sources

Photosensitivity reactions may be phototoxic (photoirritant) or photoallergic (Table 19.4).[111–114] Exogenous photosensitizers may reach the skin by topical or systemic routes. The clinical course is brief, and elimination of the offending drug or sunlight exposure usually results in improvement. In rare cases, however, the photosensitivity may persist for months after the last known exposure to the offending chemical. Such individuals are known as persistent light reactors, and the eruption (chronic actinic dermatitis) ranges from a chronic dermatitis initially restricted to sun-exposed surfaces to thickened hyperpigmented plaques. This rare disorder generally affects men and not pediatric patients.

PHOTOTOXICITY

Phototoxic reactions are common and can be likened to a primary irritant reaction. *Phototoxic reaction* refers to a nonimmunologic exaggerated sunburn or sunburn-like reaction characterized by erythema (and at times swelling and blistering), occurring within a few minutes to several hours (usually within a period of 2 to 6 hours) after exposure to UVA light and followed by hyperpigmentation and desquamation confined to the exposed areas. This type of sensitivity usually occurs with the first exposure to the photosensitizing substance, when the systemic or percutaneous absorption of the sensitizing substances is in high enough concentration to result in a photo-induced cutaneous reaction.

Plant-induced photosensitivity (phytophotodermatitis) is the most common phototoxic reaction of children.[115–118] The large majority are phototoxic reactions caused by the presence of furocoumarin compounds (psoralens) found widely in such plants as Rutaceae (e.g., limes and lemons), Umbelliferae (e.g., parsnips, carrots, dill, parsley, meadow grass, common rue, giant hogweed, and celery, most often celery infected with a fungus that causes pink rot disease), and Moraceae (e.g., fig). Psoralens can also reach the skin after ingestion, as has been noted after ingestion of contaminated celery and subsequent outdoor and tanning salon UV light exposure. With systemic ingestion, all sun-exposed areas are susceptible to reaction. Psoralens have also been used therapeutically in topical or oral formulations in combination with UVA light (PUVA therapy) as treatment of psoriasis and vitiligo; given the safety issues with PUVA, this intervention is rarely used in children. Furocoumarins can also be components in Chinese herbal medications.[119] Inhalation of traces of giant hogweed have been reported to cause obstructive pulmonary symptoms, and contact with the eye can lead to blindness.[120]

Table 19.4 Medications Most Commonly Associated with Phototoxic and Photoallergic Reactions

Phototoxic Medications	Photoallergic Medications
ANTIBIOTICS	**ANTIMICROBIALS (TOPICAL)**
Tetracyclines Sulfonamides Ciprofloxacin Nalidixic acid Isoniazid	Chlorhexidine Hexachlorophene Salicylanilides Sulfonamides
ANTIFUNGALS	**OTHER TOPICALS**
Griseofulvin Voriconazole	Sunscreens (especially benzophenones; see Table 19.2) Fragrances (sandalwood oil, musk ambrette, 6-methylcoumarin, oil of bergamot) Topical NSAIDs Promethazine hydrochloride
ANTIPSYCHOTICS	**SYSTEMIC AGENTS**
Phenothiazines Protriptyline	Sulfonamides Griseofulvin Quinolones NSAIDs (diclofenac, piroxicam, ketoprofen) Quinidine, quinine
CARDIAC MEDICATIONS AND DIURETICS	
Amiodarone Quinidine Furosemide Thiazides	
NSAIDS	
Naproxen, nabumetone, piroxicam, tiaprofenic acid, azapropazone	
CALCIUM CHANNEL BLOCKERS	
Amlodipine, diltiazem, nifedipine	
OTHERS	
Dyes (acridine, methylviolet, eosin) Furocoumarins Imatinib Lamotrigine Oral contraceptives Photodynamic therapy Psoralens Retinoids St. John's wort Sulfonylurea hypoglycemics Tar (topical) Vemurafenib	

NSAIDs, Nonsteroidal antiinflammatory drugs.

Phytophotodermatitis usually begins within a day after exposure to the furocoumarin and sunlight, ranges in severity from mild erythema with or without erosion to severe blistering (Fig. 19.9), and eventuates in a characteristic dense inflammatory hyperpigmentation. A bizarre linear streaking configuration of the dermatitis (Fig. 19.10), with subsequent hyperpigmentation, especially on the face, chest, hands, and lower legs of children, is characteristic. At times, only the hyperpigmented streak appears without prior erythema (Fig. 19.11). The purple coloration of skin and bizarre patterning can be mistaken for child abuse and the blistering for herpes simplex infection.[121–123] Extensive hand involvement can be noted from squeezing lime juice (Fig. 19.12). Streaks on the trunk have been

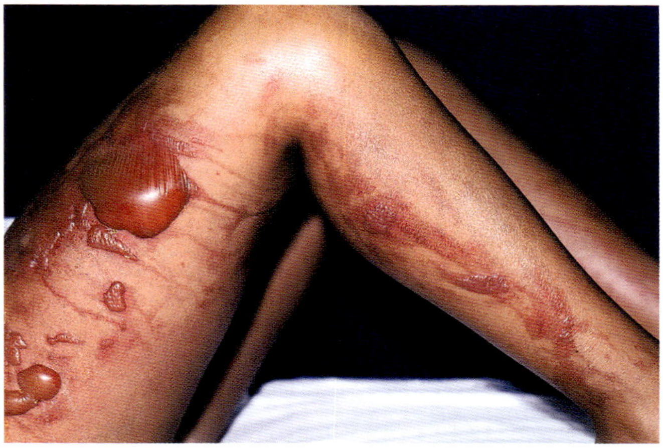

Fig. 19.9 Phytophotodermatitis. Severe blistering associated with linear patterns of erythema and hyperpigmentation in a girl who had rinsed her hair with lime juice and then had intense sun exposure.

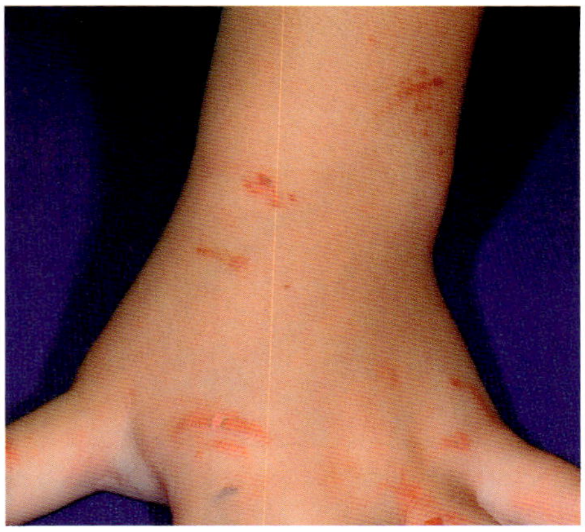

Fig. 19.10 Phytophotodermatitis. This child had been playing outside and was exposed to photosensitizing plants.

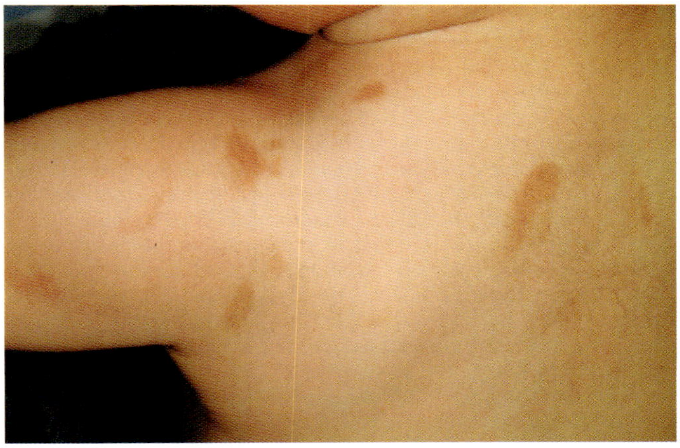

Fig. 19.11 Phytophotodermatitis. Intense hyperpigmentation in geometric patterns on the back of a young girl whose mother had been squeezing citrus fruit before picking her up while on vacation in the Caribbean.

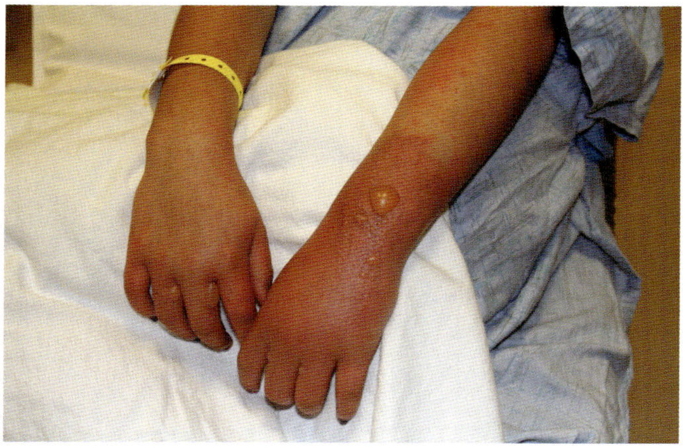

Fig. 19.12 Phytophotodermatitis. Extensive inflammation and bullae on the hands and distal arms after this girl squeezed limes to make ceviche and then had ultraviolet light exposure.

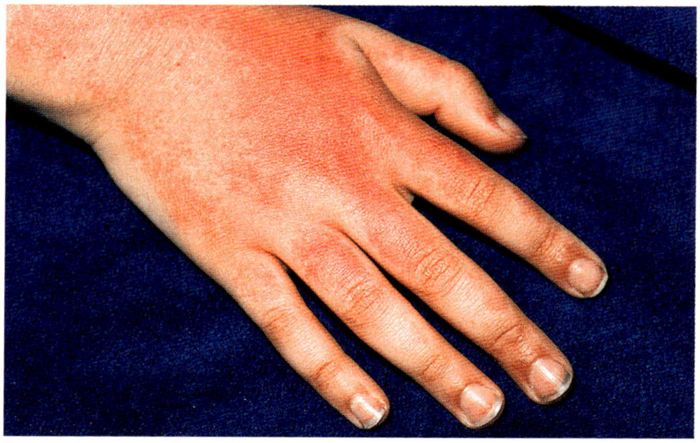

Fig. 19.13 Photosensitivity from medication. Severe sunburn reaction despite sunscreen application in a teenager taking doxycycline for acne.

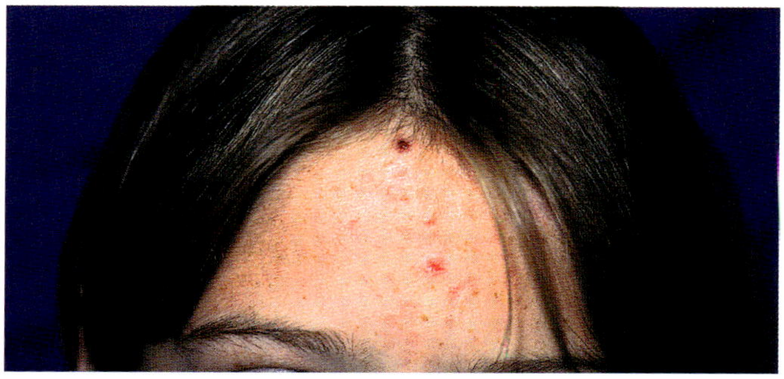

Fig. 19.14 Pseudoporphyria. Blisters and erosions on the face of a child with juvenile idiopathic arthritis taking celecoxib.

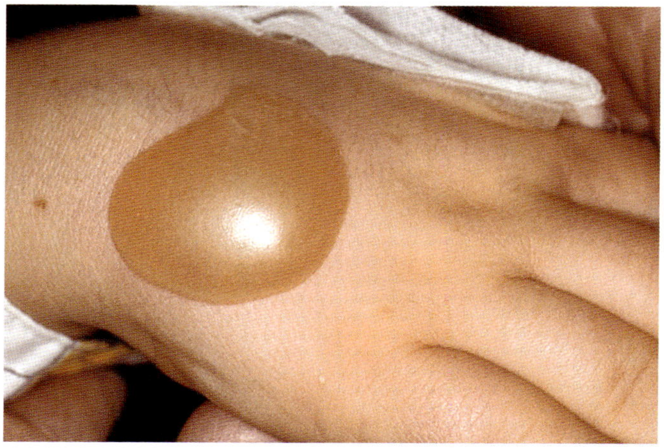

Fig. 19.15 Pseudoporphyria. Large bulla in a child receiving peritoneal hemodialysis.

noted after dripping of lime juice (sometimes used as a hair rinse or in drinks), and thumbprint-shaped macules on the lateral aspects of the trunk may be described after a parent with furocoumarins on the fingers picks up a child. Usually no treatment is necessary once the diagnosis is made, and the often-intense hyperpigmentation fades spontaneously over several weeks to months. However, severe burns have been induced in children by contact with phototoxins,[124] especially giant hogweed[125] and prolonged sunlight exposure, and have required debridement and surgical wound closure.[120,126,127]

Phototoxicity may present with a variety of manifestations. For example, exaggerated sunburn reactions can occur with thiazide diuretics, tetracyclines (Fig. 19.13), retinoids, vemurafenib, voriconazole, ciprofloxacin, and others, whereas skin fragility and blisters (pseudoporphyria) are the typical manifestation of exposure to NSAIDs, and telangiectasia results from calcium channel antagonists. Photoonycholysis most commonly occurs after administration of doxycycline[128] (see Chapter 8, Fig. 8.17). The phototoxicity from voriconazole, used to prevent fungal infections in transplant patients, occurs in 20% of treated children overall and in 47% of children treated for more at least 6 months[129,130]; a dosage of at least 6 mg/kg twice daily has also been associated with a higher risk of developing voriconazole-induced phototoxicity.[131] The eruption can be can be confused with graft-versus-host disease in these immunocompromised patients[132] and has been associated with a 4.6% risk of developing nonmelanoma skin cancer in areas that had a phototoxic reaction at a mean age of 15.5 years.[129]

Pseudoporphyria is a nonimmunologically mediated phototoxicity reaction characterized clinically by increased cutaneous fragility, vesiculobullae, and histopathologic features similar to those of patients with porphyria, but levels of porphyrins are normal.[133] It has been described in approximately 11% of children taking NSAIDs, especially naproxen sodium (Fig. 19.14, for juvenile idiopathic arthritis), and is especially common in patients with blue/gray eye color and fair skin.[134] The disorder has also been described in individuals receiving other NSAIDs,[135] dapsone, ciprofloxacin,[136] furosemide, imatinib,[137,138] metformin, nalidixic acid, tetracyclines, retinoids, amiodarone, pyridoxine/vitamin B6, and voriconazole.[130,139] A similar, if not identical, disorder has also been described in patients receiving hemodialysis (Fig. 19.15).[140]

A careful history and the presence of normal porphyrin levels in serum, erythrocytes, urine, and feces will generally establish the diagnosis. The cutaneous fragility tends to reverse rapidly on withdrawal of the causative medication but may only gradually reverse or even persist with new lesions for up to 1 month after discontinuation of the medication.[141] Pseudoporphyria associated with hemodialysis has responded to treatment with N-acetylcysteine or glutathione. Disfiguring facial scarring is a sequela in some affected children.

PHOTOALLERGY

Photoallergy is relatively uncommon and presumably is a form of cell-mediated delayed hypersensitivity.[142,143] The individual must first be sensitized to the allergen, which can require 7 to 10 days. When exposed to UV light, the light is absorbed by the photoantigen, which is thought to cause a change in the molecule. Instead of sunburn-type reactions, photoallergic responses are generally characterized by immediate urticarial or delayed papular or eczematous lesions that are not followed by hyperpigmentation. After the first sensitization,

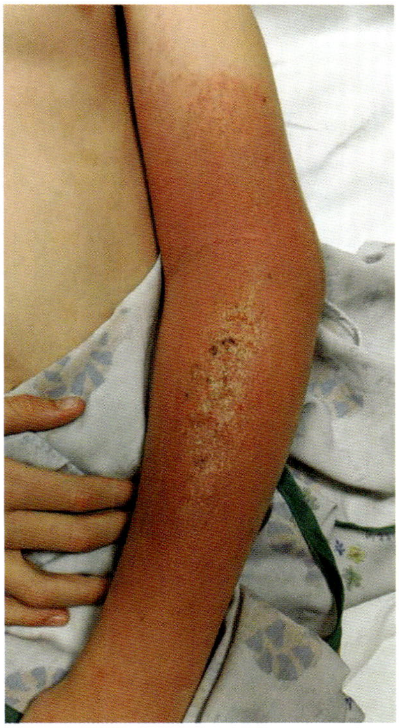

Fig. 19.16 Photoallergic reaction to sunscreen. This boy took a family vacation to Mexico and developed a photoallergic reaction to the benzophenone in his sunscreen.

subsequent photoallergic reactions generally appear within 24 hours, even after very brief periods of exposure. Sunscreens with chemical components (especially benzophenones) are the leading cause because of their extensive use (Fig. 19.16), although the risk of reaction with sunscreens containing these agents is less than 1% of that for allergic contact dermatitis.[144,145] In the past, children showed photoallergic reactions to salicylanilides (antimicrobial agents formerly in soaps but now only in industrial cleaners) and fragrances (musk ambrette, oil of bergamot). These chemicals are no longer used in personal products, but children or adolescents have been known to find a cologne with oil of bergamot, apply it to the skin, and develop berloque (berlock) dermatitis after UV exposure.[146] Promethazine hydrochloride cream and topical nonsteroidal antiinflammatory agents have caused photoreactions.

Suspected photoallergic contact dermatitis may be confirmed by photopatch testing. Photopatch testing is similar to traditional testing for contact dermatitis (see Chapter 3), except that two sets of patch tests are placed on the back. Twenty-four hours later, one set is uncovered and irradiated with UVA light. The following day a comparison is made of the covered and irradiated sites. A positive test reproduces the clinical eczematous lesion at the phototest site. Therapy is treatment with topical antiinflammatory agents and avoidance of exposure to the offending antigen.

Genetic Disorders Associated with Photosensitivity

Photosensitivity is a prominent feature of several genetic disorders, many of which are associated with defective DNA repair. Some of these are described elsewhere in this text, such as Kindler syndrome (see Chapter 13), trichothiodystrophy (see Chapter 7), and ataxia-telangiectasia (see Chapter 12).

XERODERMA PIGMENTOSUM

Xeroderma pigmentosum (XP) is a rare autosomal recessive disease characterized by cutaneous photosensitivity, a decreased ability to repair DNA damaged by UV radiation, and the early development of cutaneous and ocular malignancies.[147–149] The disorder is estimated to occur in one in a million individuals in the United States and Europe, with an incidence in Japan as high as one in 40,000 persons. The risk of developing cutaneous malignancy is slightly less in patients with darker skin types, but their risk of developing malignancy of the lips, tongue, and eyes is just as high as in light-skinned individuals. Historically, seven complementation groups (XPA through XPG) have been described based on *in vitro* cell fusion studies (Table 19.5), which are now recognized to correlated with mutations in specific genes whose products affect DNA repair.

The basic abnormality is absence of a component of the nucleotide excision repair complex, a multistep mechanism that includes recognition of the UV light–induced DNA lesion, unwinding of DNA, and then resynthesis and ligation of the DNA (transcription and transcription-coupled nucleotide excision repair [TC-NER]). XPA may help to assemble the DNA machinery around the damaged DNA site. This binding signals the XPB and XPD proteins to unwind the DNA in the damaged region and to allow DNA transcription. The XPF and XPG nucleases cut the DNA and allow excision of the UV light–induced pyrimidine dimers. DNA repair rates may range from 0% to 50% of normal levels. Alternatively, XP may result from DNA repair issues with preserved TC-NER with defects in XPC, XPE, and XPV. Complementation groups XPC and XPE recognize and bind to damaged DNA.[150–152] In the variant group (XPV), postreplication repair is defective but excision repair is normal. More than half of all cases in the

Table 19.5 Subtypes of Xeroderma Pigmentosum

Gene/Protein	Protein Function	Incidence	Skin Disease	Neoplasia	Neurologic Change	Comments
XPA	Confirms damage	Especially in Japan	+++	+++	+ to +++	Lowest repair activity
XPB/ERCC3	Helicase	Very rare	++ to +++	+++	+++	CS (two kindreds) One case of TTD
XPC	Detects damage	Most common	++ to +++	++; melanoma	Rare	
XPD/ERCC2	Helicase	20% of cases	++	+	Late onset or none	Tremendous variability in phenotype; TTD; XP/CS
XPE/DDB2	Detects damage	Rare	+	Rare	None or mild	Mild phenotype
XPF/ERCC4	Nuclease	Fairly rare	++	Few to none	Usually none	
XPG/ERCC5	Nuclease	Very rare	+++	Few or none	Cockayne type	CS has been associated
XPV/POLH	Polymerase	30% of cases	++ to +++	Later onset	++ in a few	

CS, Cockayne syndrome; *DDB*, DNA damage-binding protein; *ERCC*, excision repair cross-complementing genes; *TTD*, trichothiodystrophy; *XP*, xeroderma pigmentosum; *XP/CS*, xeroderma pigmentosum/Cockayne syndrome complex; *XPV*, xeroderma pigmentosum variant; +, mild; ++, moderate; +++, severe.

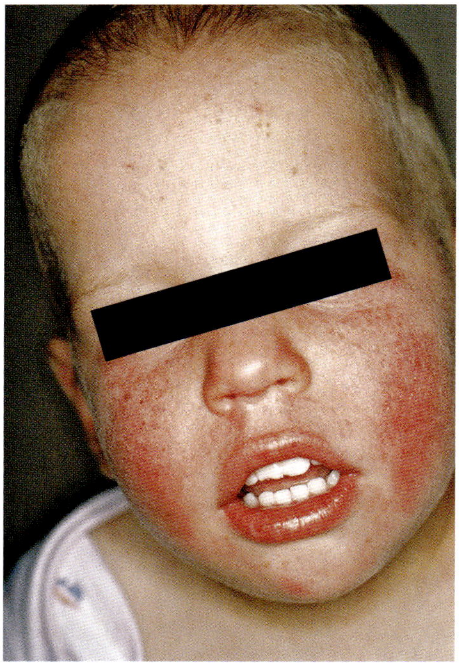

Fig. 19.17 Xeroderma pigmentosum. Sunburn after minimal sun exposure was the clue to diagnosis of xeroderma pigmentosum in a 9-month-old boy. Note the early freckling on the upper cheeks. This boy with XPA developed severe neurologic degeneration (DeSanctis–Cacchione syndrome) despite vigorous sun protection and no evidence of even a premalignant skin lesion by his mid-20s.

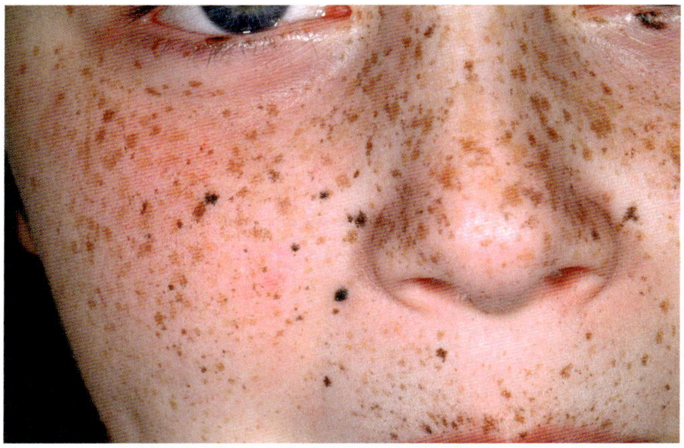

Fig. 19.18 Xeroderma pigmentosum. Note the many black-colored facial lentigines, which should raise concern about the possibility of xeroderma pigmentosum.

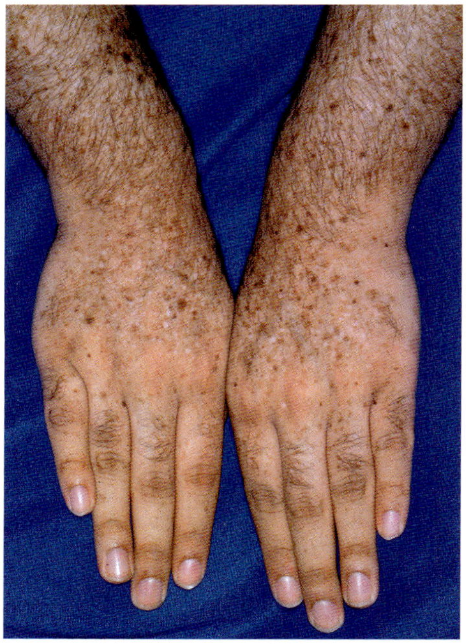

Fig. 19.19 Xeroderma pigmentosum. Despite total avoidance of ultraviolet light after diagnosis at 2 years of age, this adolescent boy showed extensive pigmentary changes.

United States are caused by mutations in the genes encoding XPC *(XPC)*, XPD *(ERCC2)*, or XPV *(POLH)*, although mutations in the genes encoding XPA and XPF are more common in Japan than in the United States and Europe.

In 75% of cases the first signs appear between 6 months and 3 years of age. The presenting feature of this disorder is photosensitivity to UV light, primarily at wavelengths 290 to 340 nm, but this sunburn after minimal UV light exposure only occurs in 50% to 64% of patients and is not a feature of XP patients with mutations in XPC, XPE, or XPV.[153,154] The sunburn may be severe with vesicles and bullae (Fig. 19.17) and is often accompanied by photophobia with chronic conjunctivitis during the first months of life.[155] Of those with ophthalmologic manifestations, 65% have photophobia, 44% interpalpebral conjunctival melanosis, and 43% conjunctival injection; malignancy occurs in 11% (periocular) and 2% (on the ocular surface).

The other 40% of cases do not show this sunburn reaction and instead tend to manifest initially with the lentigines (freckle-like pigmentation) that otherwise follow the early sunburns (Figs. 19.18 and 19.19). The skin ages prematurely with atrophy, telangiectasia, mottled hyper- and hypopigmentation, keratoses, and ulcerations, but not wrinkling; these observations likely reflect the sensitivity primarily to UVB rather than to UVA light, which is the primary cause of solar elastosis.[147] With continued exposure, the skin becomes xerotic, leading to the name XP. Areas of skin ordinarily protected by clothing remain relatively normal or may eventually show similar features, but to a lesser degree. Affected children resemble adults with severe actinic damage by early childhood.

Epithelial neoplasms, including malignancy, and progressive neurologic degeneration are major issues for many affected children.[156,157] Several tumors occur with increased incidence in XP (basal cell and squamous cell carcinomas, angiosarcoma, fibrosarcoma, atypical fibroxanthoma, keratoacanthoma, and melanoma) (Fig. 19.20).[158,159] In patients younger than 20 years of age with XP, the overall risk of developing basal cell and squamous cell carcinomas is 10,000 times that of the normal population (median age 9 years), and of melanoma 2000-fold greater (median age 22 years).[153,160] Interestingly, the melanomas in XP show a high rate of *PTEN* mutations (mammalian target of rapamycin [mTOR] pathway activation) rather than the typical RAS pathway activation, which may be important in considering choice of small molecule inhibitors.[161] The tendency to develop these neoplasms is a function of exposure to UV light and the subtype of XP (see Table 19.5). The lower risk of developing skin cancer in patients who show early sunburns[153] may reflect the earlier recognition of XP and intense early photoprotection. These tumors and their therapy cause considerable facial distortion. Patients with XP also have an approximately 10- to 20-fold increase in internal malignancies, including of the brain, lungs, hematopoietic system, kidney, and gastrointestinal tract, which may reflect concomitant sensitivity to physical and chemical carcinogens, such as cigarette smoke.[153,162] Although skin cancer is the most common cause of death (34%), internal cancer leads to death of 17% of patients.[153]

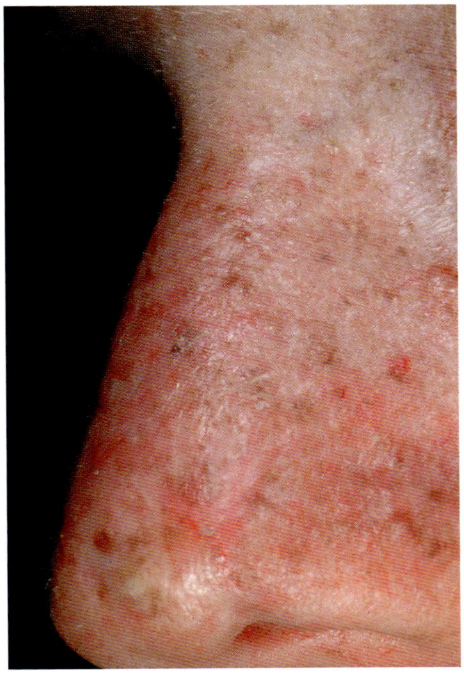

Fig. 19.20 Xeroderma pigmentosum. Severe actinic damage in an 18-year-old girl with inadequate sun protection. Note the scarring from removal of several basal cell carcinomas, beginning at 10 years of age.

Patients also have an increased risk of developing carcinomas of the anterior portion of the tongue[163] and may show leukoplakia.[162,164] The ocular manifestations largely involve the anterior part of the eye that is exposed to UV light.[165] By 3 years of age, most patients show blepharitis, symblepharon, and crusts of the palpebral margins. With continuing UV light exposure, affected individuals show conjunctival melanosis, scarring, atrophy, entropion or ectropion, trichiasis (irritation caused by the eyelashes), and at times loss of the lower lid. Ocular surface cancer develops in 10% of patients. Corneal opacities and ulcerations and choroidal melanomas have been described.[166]

Neurologic complications develop in approximately 30% of patients (termed the *DeSanctis–Cacchione syndrome*), most commonly in the XPA group[167] but also with XPB, XPD, and XPG. These may include microcephaly with developmental delay, poor growth and sexual development, choreoathetosis, hyporeflexia, cerebellar ataxia, and sensorineural deafness. These neurologic changes may have their onset in infancy but may not occur in some patients until the second decade of life. There is progressive loss of brain volume with advancing age in affected individuals. Testing of deep tendon reflexes and routine audiometry are good screening studies.[168] In this subset, it is the neurologic degeneration that leads to death of patients (cause of death in 31% of all patients with XP), and at an earlier age (median age of death with neurodegeneration is 37 years versus 29 years without neurodegeneration).[153]

The neurologic abnormalities and photosensitivity may be seen in individuals with the XP/Cockayne syndrome overlap (see Cockayne Syndrome section).[169,170] DNA excision repair defects and UV light hypersensitivity are also seen in a subset of patients with trichothiodystrophy (PIBIDS [photosensitivity, ichthyosis, brittle hair, intellectual impairment, decreased fertility, and short stature]; see Chapter 7).[147] Patients with trichothiodystrophy do not show an increased risk of developing skin cancer, although the reason for this distinguishing feature is unclear. XP and trichothiodystrophy may also coexist.[171]

Suspicion of the diagnosis of XP is made through clinical observation. In the past, confirmation involved UV light sensitivity and DNA repair assays, but genetic analysis is now the preferred testing for confirmation and subtyping, which cannot be determined by clinical features alone. Whole-exome sequencing has been performed[172] and has the advantage of analyzing the presence of mutation in all possible genes simultaneously. Immunohistochemistry of paraffin-embedded skin sections is a simple way to show absence of XPC.[173] Given the founder mutation in XPA in Japan, rapid genetic analysis for this mutation can easily be performed in individuals of Japanese descent.

All patients with XP require strict lifelong sun protection, including total sun avoidance, application of sunscreens that protect throughout the UVB and UVA spectrum, UV light shields over windows, sun-protective clothing (a sun suit designed by the National Aeronautics and Space Administration is also available), broad-brimmed hats, and sunglasses.[174] Methylcellulose eyedrops should be applied to keep the corneas moist, and soft contact lenses should be worn to protect against mechanical trauma in individuals whose eyelids are severely deformed. Corneal transplantation may be required for patients with severe keratitis and corneal opacity. All patients should be given vitamin D supplementation, given the sun avoidance.[175] Patients should avoid cigarette smoke and other environmental carcinogens. Surveillance for skin cancer by dermatologists and ocular complications by ophthalmologists is imperative.

Individual premalignant and malignant tumors should be treated by cryosurgery, application of topical 5-fluorouracil or imiquimod cream,[176,177] and use of these treatments for 3 weeks every 3 to 6 months starting during childhood has been advocated as prophylaxis.[174] Other interventions are intralesional interferon-α and surgical removal as appropriate for the neoplasm.[178] Four months of the oral hedgehog inhibitor vismodegib led to sustained complete clearance in a child with a nodular basal cell carcinoma of the nasal tip,[179] and one child responded to anti-PD-1 therapy (nivolumab) for sarcomatoid carcinoma of the scalp but developed melanoma and squamous cell carcinomas during therapy.[180]

Dermabrasion, laser resurfacing, and phenol-based peeling of skin with actinic damage have been helpful in reversing the pigmentary changes.[181,182] High-dose oral isotretinoin decreases the incidence of new skin cancers, but withdrawal of therapy results in reversal of its chemoprophylactic effect.[183]

"Readthrough" of premature termination codons by aminoglycosides to restore DNA repair[184] and targeted repair of XPC mutations using transcription activator-like effector (TALE) nucleases[175] have been shown as potential future interventions. XP has been diagnosed prenatally by showing DNA-repair defects in cultured amniotic fluid cells and by DNA analysis. Support groups for families with XP include the XP Society (www.xps.org), XP Family Support Group (www.xp-familysupport.org), and the XP Support Group (www.xpsupport-group.org.uk). A camp for families with XP (Camp Sundown) engages affected individuals and their families in daytime indoor activities and outdoor activities at night.

COCKAYNE SYNDROME

Cockayne syndrome (CS) is a recessively inherited disorder caused by defects in repair of actively transcribed DNA, either *ERCC8* (excision-repair cross complementing group 8; *CSA*) or, in 70% to 80% of patients, *ERCC6 (CSB)*.[185–191] The incidence in Western Europe is 2.7 per million births. A spectrum of severity for individuals with CS (classified as CS I, II, and III) or its variants (cerebrooculofacioskeletal syndrome [COFS] and UV-sensitive syndrome [UVSS]) has been described and modified criteria have been proposed (Box 19.1).[188,189] Arthrogryposis and congenital kyphosis are specific features of COFS (caused by *CSB*), within the CS spectrum. Affected individuals with COFS and CS II (usually CSB deficiency) more often show features from birth (e.g., weak cry, axial hypotonia, and peripheral hypertonia), whereas other children (especially with CSA) have no signs until infancy or even childhood and tend to be less severe. Early growth retardation, microcephaly, bilateral deafness (21% of neonates and 84% by 10 years of age), and loss of developmental progress are progressive.

The most common cutaneous changes are cold extremities (almost 90%; often with acral cyanosis and edema) and photosensitivity (almost 80%).[189] Photosensitivity manifests as sunburn after brief exposure and may occur even after exposure through a windshield. Within the spectrum, however, are patients without photosensitivity[192] or with photosensitivity but no other features (UVSS). Despite the photosensitivity, CS is not associated with sun-induced pigmentation

Box 19.1 Diagnostic Features and Subclassification in Order of Severity of Cockayne Syndrome and Its Variants

Major

Developmental delay
Progressive microcephaly
Progressive growth failure

Minor

Cutaneous photosensitivity
Progressive sensorineural hearing loss
Pigmentary retinopathy/cataracts
Enophthalmia
Enamel hypoplasia

Major criteria are required for diagnosis of CS I, CS II, and CS III in addition to at least three minor criteria.

COFS (subset of CSII)

Most severely affected
Death by infancy

CS II

Signs present at birth
Fulfills diagnostic criteria by infancy
Death usually 5 to 6 years of age

CS I

Signs first present by 2 years of age
Fulfills diagnostic criteria during childhood
Death usually in late teenage years

CS III

Signs first present at 3 to 4 years of age
Fulfills diagnostic criteria by early teens
Death usually at about 30 years of age

UVSS

Only presents with photosensitivity
Survival is likely normal

COFS, Cerebrooculofacioskeletal syndrome; *CS*, Cockayne syndrome; *UVSS*, UV-sensitive syndrome.

or malignancy. Although this light sensitivity eventually disappears, erythema with telangiectasias characteristic of photosensitivity, mottled pigmentation, scarring, and atrophy of these sites remain as prominent features. Nail dystrophy (often subtle), hair abnormalities (sparse, thin, dry, and/or pseudo–"tiger-tail" appearance), and hypohidrosis have also been described. Associated pruritus without skin inflammation is not uncommon and may be the presenting feature to a dermatologist. Approximately 30% have cutaneous hyperpigmentation. Loss of subcutaneous fat and cachectic wasting produces a "bird-like" facies with sunken eyes (Fig. 19.21, *A*). Patients show a tendency toward progressive ataxia, long limbs in proportion to body length, quick bird-like movements, disproportionately large hands and feet, progressive contractures of the joints, and large protruding ears. A characteristic "salt and pepper" pigmentary retinopathy has been described; optic atrophy and cataracts are not uncommon. Hearing loss (~75%) commonly starts in preschool years, and mental retardation can be severe. Affected individuals are generally below the third percentile for height and weight. Other abnormalities may include thickened skull bones and intracranial calcification, especially of the basal ganglia, elevated transglutaminases, and renal disease.

There is no effective treatment for patients with this disorder, and most patients die by the third decade of life as a result of arteriosclerotic vascular disease, profound neurologic deterioration, or both. In one study, early onset of cataracts (before 3 years of age) was associated with younger age of death (40% die by 5 years of age), early hearing loss, and contractures.[189] Patients with CS show defective DNA repair and hypersensitivity to UV light, which accounts for their photosensitivity.[170,193] Patients with CS show spasticity, ataxia, and peripheral neuropathy from demyelination, in contrast to neuronal degeneration in patients with XP. However, patients have been described with features of both XP and CS.[169,194,195] These patients usually have mutations in a different gene, *ERCC5 (XPG)*, but occasionally in *XPB*, *XPD*, or *XPF*. They show the short stature, sexual immaturity, and retinal pigmentation of CS; are sensitive to UV light; and develop the pigmentary abnormalities of XP. The risk of developing cutaneous malignancy is lower in XP-CS than in XP alone or XP with neurologic disease. Children with CS alone[195] have not been found to have an increased risk of malignancy during childhood, despite their recurrent sunburns (Fig. 19.21, *B*),[196] but the shortened lifespan precludes observation into the second decade for most

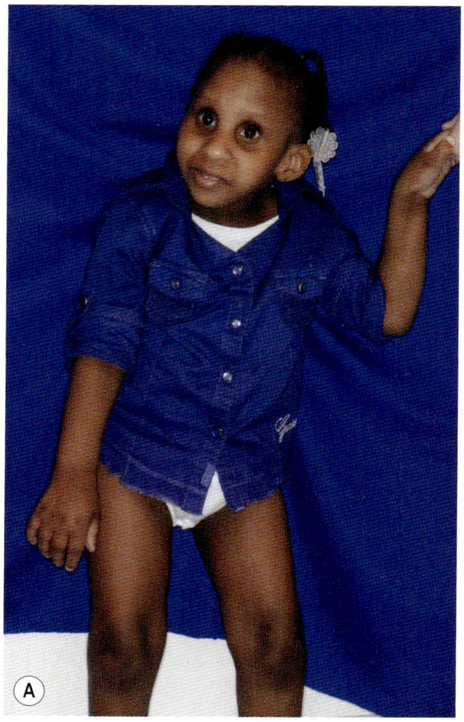

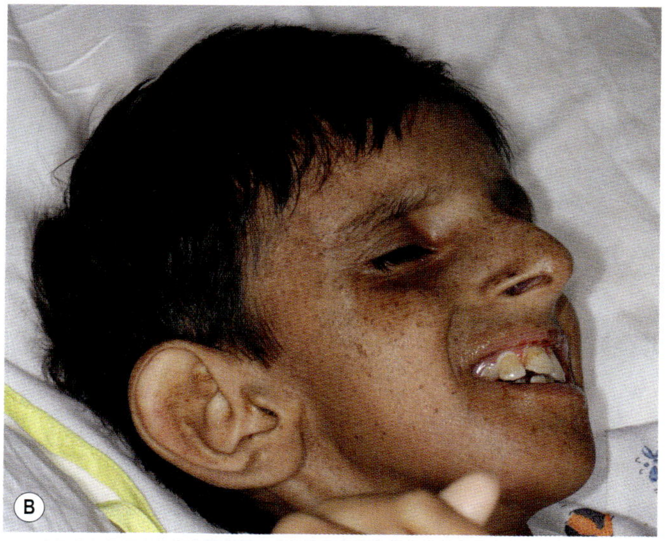

Fig. 19.21 (A) Cockayne syndrome II. Note the typical facial features with enophthalmia, microcephaly, and protruding ears as well as growth failure in this 7-year-old girl with mutations in *ERCC6 (CSB)*. **(B)** Xeroderma pigmentosum/Cockayne syndrome (CS) caused by mutations in *ERCC5 (XPG)*. Note the facial features of CS but the sun-induced lentigines and photophobia of XP.

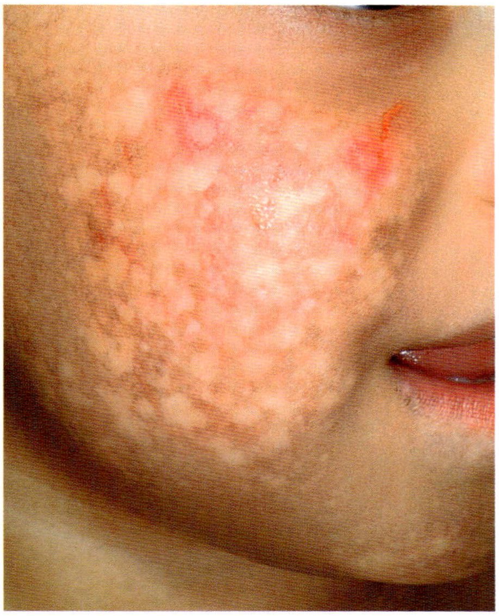

Fig. 19.22 Rothmund–Thomson syndrome. Reticulated pattern of telangiectasia and both hypopigmentation and hyperpigmentation on the cheek and ear. (Courtesy Sarah Chamlin, MD.)

affected individuals. Administration of daily niacin in a patient with XP/CS led to a dramatic photoprotective effect both clinically and in cultured fibroblasts, reminiscent of improvement in patients with pellagra.[197] Administration of metronidazole is contraindicated, because it may cause life-threatening acute hepatic failure in CS.

ROTHMUND–THOMSON SYNDROME

Rothmund–Thomson syndrome is an autosomal recessive disorder that occurs twice as often in boys than in girls.[149,198] Cutaneous features are seen in the first 2 years and often by 3 to 6 months of age. Most common are diffuse erythema and, at times, edema and vesiculation of the cheeks, forehead, chin, ears, buttocks, and extensor surfaces of the arms and legs, but sparing of the trunk. As the erythema resolves, the skin begins to show a reticulated pattern of telangiectasia, alterations in pigmentation (both hypopigmentation and hyperpigmentation), and areas of atrophy (poikiloderma) that progress until approximately 3 to 5 years of age (Fig. 19.22). Occasionally, affected individuals are born with poikiloderma or develop poikiloderma after the first year of life. Children may develop bullae after sun exposure or spontaneously; this tendency appears to subside as patients grow older. Approximately 30% of patients develop verrucous hyperkeratoses on the hands, feet, knees, and elbows later in childhood or during adolescence. Although photosensitivity is a feature of many cases and exposure to sunlight may extend the distribution of the eruption, UV light is unlikely to be the sole cause of the poikiloderma because it may be found before UV light exposure and can appear on unexposed areas. Adults with the disorder show an increased risk of development of squamous cell carcinomas at sites of the keratotic and atrophic lesions; melanoma and porokeratosis have also been associated.[199,200]

Patients are commonly short, and most show a history of low birthweight and short birth length as well as severe growth failure. Some have a characteristic facies with saddle nose, frontal bossing, wide forehead, and narrow chin, giving a triangular configuration to the face. Hypotrichosis with sparse or absent eyebrows or eyelashes (and sometimes involvement of the scalp, face, and body hair) occurs in 50% of patients, and premature graying has been reported. Nail dystrophy has been described in about 30% of patients, and dental abnormalities, caries, and periodontitis in almost 40%.[201]

Cataracts occur in about 6% to 40% of reported cases,[198] generally as bilateral anterior or posterior subcapsular opacities that evolve rapidly. Although they are first noted between 3 and 7 years of age in most patients, they have been described in an infant at 4 months of age and may appear as late as 40 years of age. Hypogonadism occurs in one-quarter of patients (female patients may be amenorrheic; male patients may have undescended testes).

Defective bone development is a common characteristic that occurs in up to two-thirds of affected individuals. Most common are absence or hypoplasia of the thumbs, radius, and occasionally the ulna; brachymetacarpophalangy; syndactyly; clinodactyly; and fusion or agenesis of carpal and tarsal bones.[202] Both hyperostosis and osteoporosis with fractures have been described.[203] Osteosarcoma has been described in 32% of patients, approximately half before 15 years of age, and most commonly affects the tibia or femur.[198,204,205] Surveillance for bone pain, swelling, or an enlarging lesion on a limb suggesting a tumor is important. Because of the risk of osteosarcoma, baseline radiologic evaluations of long bones are recommended by 3 years of age. Several other malignancies, aplastic anemia, and myelodysplasia have been described less commonly.[206]

Laboratory tests are usually normal, including assays of unscheduled DNA repair, increased sensitivity to alkylating agents such as mitomycin C, and chromosomes. Mutations in *RECQL4* have been found in 40% to 66% of affected patients[207] and have been associated with an increased risk of developing osteosarcoma.[208] *RECQL4* encodes a DNA helicase that is important for DNA replication, repair of UV light–induced DNA damage, and telomere maintenance.[209,210] Mutations in *RECQL4* also cause RAPADILINO and Baller–Gerold syndromes.[211] RAPADILINO (radial hypoplasia, patellar hypoplasia/aplasia, cleft or high-arched palate, diarrhea, dislocated joints, little size and limb malformations, slender nose, and normal intelligence) syndrome is associated with the osteosarcoma risk but not the poikilodermatous changes.[212] Baller–Gerold syndrome prominently features numerous bony defects and the risk of osteosarcoma, but the onset of poikiloderma is later and cataracts have not been described.

The early onset and noncutaneous features allow Rothmund–Thomson syndrome to be distinguished from other disorders with poikiloderma that are not related to *RECQL4* mutations (dyskeratosis congenita, Kindler syndrome, poikiloderma with neutropenia, hereditary sclerosing telangiectasia, Bloom syndrome, Fanconi anemia, XP, and nonhereditary disorders—chronic juvenile dermatomyositis and cutaneous T-cell lymphoma).[213] Any patient with poikiloderma deserves initial evaluation for neutropenia, which can distinguish patients with poikiloderma with neutropenia (Clericuzio type), another autosomal recessive genodermatosis resulting from mutations in *USB1* (formerly called *C16orf57*).[214–216]

Individuals with the Rothmund–Thomson syndrome have a normal life span, although the development of cancer may lead to premature death in some patients. The poikiloderma and facial telangiectasia have been treated successfully with laser. Cataract extraction may be necessary.

BLOOM SYNDROME

Bloom syndrome (congenital telangiectatic erythema) is a rare autosomal recessive disorder characterized by a triad of telangiectatic erythema, photosensitivity, and severe intrauterine and postnatal growth retardation.[149,217] Some 80% of affected children are male, and 50% are of Ashkenazi Jewish ancestry; the carrier rate among Ashkenazi Jews is 1 in 110 individuals. The disorder results from mutations in *BLM* (or *RECQL2*), a helicase of the RecQ family that participates in normal DNA replication.[218]

Affected patients are born at term with reduced body weight and size.[219] They have small, narrow faces with a prominent nose and ears, and the voice is high pitched. Although physical growth is stunted, intellectual and sexual development is normal. Erythema of the cheeks in a butterfly distribution, often resembling lesions of lupus erythematosus, appears between the second and third week of life, and typically spreads with exposure to sunlight to involve the nose, eyelids, forehead, ears, and lips. However, there is phenotypic variability, and some patients do not show the facial eruption.[220] The trunk, buttocks, and lower limbs tend to be spared. Although this light sensitivity eventually disappears, erythema, telangiectasia, mottled pigmentation, scarring, and atrophy of these sites remain as prominent features. Café-au-lait spots and areas of hypopigmentation have been described, especially on the trunk. Patients may show dolichocephaly, polydactyly, clinodactyly, syndactyly, cryptorchidism, shortened lower extremities, and clubbed feet.

Patients often have vomiting and diarrhea during infancy, which may be associated with gastrointestinal infections. The tendency toward recurrent respiratory infections increases the risk of chronic lung disease, the second most common cause of death in patients with Bloom syndrome. With increasing age, however, resistance to infection increases. Diabetes has been noted in 12% of patients[221]; men with Bloom syndrome are usually sterile, and women have reduced fertility.

Of the affected individuals, 20% develop malignancy, most commonly leukemia, at a mean age of 16 years. Lymphomas and leukemias occur 150 to 300 times more often than in normal individuals.[222] Solid tissue tumors of a wide variety of tissues, most commonly Wilms tumor, lymphosarcoma, and carcinomas of the oral mucosa and gastrointestinal tract, are seen at a mean age of 30 years in older, surviving individuals. Wilms tumor and osteosarcoma, however, have been described in the first decade of life. Decreased levels of IgG, IgM, and IgA, dysfunctional helper T cells, and abnormal delayed hypersensitivity have been described and may be related to defective lymphocyte maturation.

The diagnosis of Bloom syndrome can be confirmed by genotyping. In cytogenetic analysis, patients have a high incidence of chromosomal breakage, sister chromatid exchanges, and quadriradial configurations. Although there is no specific treatment, avoidance of sun exposure and protection by sunscreens can help prevent some of the cutaneous eruptions associated with photosensitivity. Appropriate antibiotics for gastrointestinal and respiratory tract bacterial infections are commonly helpful in the management of patients with this disorder. Because life expectancy is shortened by malignancy, periodic evaluation for possible neoplastic disease is advisable; however, exposure to ionizing radiation in screening tests should be minimized.[223,224]

SMITH–LEMLI–OPITZ SYNDROME

Photosensitivity is a feature of Smith–Lemli–Opitz syndrome, an autosomal recessive disorder that results from mutations in the sterol Δ-7-reductase gene, part of the pathway of cholesterol biosynthesis.[225] This syndrome occurs in 1:20,000 births in populations of northern and central European origin. Levels of vitamin D tend to be high because of increased precursor 7-dehydrocholesterol, but no evidence of toxicity has been associated.[226] Hedgehog pathway signaling is reduced as a result of the deficiency of cholesterol. Hypospadias is a prominent feature, so Smith–Lemli–Opitz syndrome is more easily recognized in males. Other features are mental retardation, abnormal sleep patterns, microcephaly, short or proximally placed thumbs, and congenital cardiac abnormalities, most commonly atrioventricular septal defect. Patients show a typical facies, and 80% show syndactyly of the second and third toes. Severe photosensitivity has been described in 57% of affected individuals[227] and typically occurs within minutes after exposure to UVA light.[228,229] Objective improvement in the photosensitivity has been demonstrated after supplementation with cholesterol,[230] and dietary cholesterol supplementation is now standard. Administration of simvastatin reduces irritability but does not otherwise improve the clinical features.[231]

HARTNUP DISEASE

Hartnup disease is a rare autosomal recessive, light-sensitive disorder characterized by a pellagra-like cutaneous eruption, neurologic abnormalities, and a specific aminoaciduria (caused by a defect in the cellular transport of a group of monoamino-monocarboxylic acids). The basic defects appear to be a failure in the absorption of tryptophan from the gastrointestinal tract and a renal tubular defect causing inadequate reabsorption of amino acids, including tryptophan. These result in reduced levels of available tryptophan and, accordingly, nicotinic acid, which in turn may be responsible for the pellagra-like photosensitivity. The condition results from mutations in *SLC6A19*,[232] which encodes the neutral amino acid transporter BOAT1.[233]

The biochemical defect (aminoaciduria) is a constant feature of Hartnup disease. Clinical manifestations, however, are intermittent, recurrent, and quite variable. The cutaneous eruption usually appears in the spring and summer. It may be present in early childhood, occasionally during early infancy, and, when present, is usually seen in children between 3 and 9 years of age. The cutaneous manifestations consist of a symmetric distribution of erythematous macules that tend to coalesce and eventuate in well-marginated red scaling lesions over light-exposed parts of the face, neck, uncovered areas of the arms, inframammary and perineal folds, elbows, knees, dorsal aspects of the hands, wrists, and lower legs. Once these lesions appear, they usually persist for weeks or months.

Acute dermatitis and blistering with secondary crusting and scarring often occur after sun exposure. These changes, together with marked postinflammatory hyperpigmentation, are similar to the findings seen in pellagra. Malnutrition and intercurrent infections often aggravate the dermatitis.[234] Glossitis, angular stomatitis, vulvovaginitis, diffuse hair loss and fragility, and nail abnormalities (longitudinal streaking) may also be seen. In many patients, the cutaneous manifestations become milder with advancing age and subsequent sun exposure. Hartnup disease with cutaneous manifestations resembling acrodermatitis enteropathica has also been described.[235]

Cerebellar ataxia is the predominant neurologic feature of Hartnup disease. Seen in more than two-thirds of those affected by this disorder, the ataxia seems to occur during periods when the rash is most prominent or after acute episodes of febrile illness. The gait is broad-based and unsteady, and patients have both nystagmus and an intention tremor. Ocular abnormalities include diplopia and ptosis, and some patients have mental retardation, emotional lability, or frank psychosis.

The diagnosis of Hartnup disease is based on the clinical picture and demonstration of specific amino acid and indole excretion patterns (not the total amino acid excretion). Treatment consists of avoidance of sunlight exposure and prolonged oral administration of high doses (40 to 200 mg) of nicotinic acid or nicotinamide. Because nicotinamide does not cause the flushing generally associated with administration of nicotinic acid, the former is generally the drug of choice. Although the eruption and ataxia seem to improve when patients are adhering to this regimen, assessment of therapy is difficult because the natural history of the disorder is one of spontaneous remission and exacerbation.

Pellagra

Pellagra is a systemic disturbance caused by a cellular deficiency of niacin resulting from inadequate dietary intake of nicotinic acid or its precursor (tryptophan) or the ingestion of certain antinicotinic substances, such as phenytoin, isoniazid, and ethionamide (also used for tuberculosis).[236–238] Niacin is required for the biosynthesis of ceramides and other stratum corneum lipids. Given the supplementation in foods and vitamins, pellagra rarely occurs except in countries where nutritional deficiency is common.[239] However, it has been described in adolescents with anorexia nervosa, children with malabsorption syndromes, and individuals maintained on diets high in corn[240]; it is more commonly seen in people with chronic alcoholism and malnourished homeless persons.

The disorder is characterized by seasonal recurrences and a classic triad of dermatitis, diarrhea, and dementia.[241] The onset of the disorder, however, may be heralded by weakness, loss of appetite, abdominal pain, mental depression, and photosensitivity. In later stages, nervous symptoms may predominate to such a degree that the cutaneous lesions may be overlooked. These include delirium, dementia, posterolateral spinal cord degeneration, and pyramidal and peripheral nerve involvement.

The most prominent cutaneous lesions of pellagra are precipitated by the sun and, although not always present, begin as asymptomatic or pruritic symmetric erythematous scaling macules on areas exposed to sunlight, heat, friction, or pressure. The usual sites of involvement include the face, neck, dorsal surface of the hands, arms, feet, inguinal region, and, particularly in infants and small children, the diaper area. The eruptions begin as well-marginated erythema and superficial scaling on sun-exposed areas resembling sunburn (with or without vesiculation or blister formation) that gradually subside, leaving a dusky brown-red discoloration. In acute cases, the lesions may progress to vesiculation, ulceration, exudation, cracking, and, at times, secondary infection. With chronicity, lesions become thicker, scalier, and ultimately fissured, atrophic, and deeply pigmented. On the lower neck, the eruption may appear as a broad collarette of dermatitis known as *Casal's necklace*. In cases in which the "necklace" is incomplete, the lesions maintain their symmetric and otherwise characteristic appearance. The nose has a distinctive appearance with a dull erythema of the nasal bridge, slight scaling, and a powdery appearance. Mucous membrane involvement, when present, consists of painful fissures and ulceration. The lips and cheeks are thin and pale; the mouth is dry; and the tongue is red, swollen, and at times darkened (the so-called *black tongue*). Aphthous ulcers, fissuring, and angular cheilitis are also common.

When the diagnosis is suspected, measurement of the urinary excretion of N_1-methylnicotinamide and/or pyridone (metabolites of niacin) is helpful. Treatment of pellagra consists of a high-protein diet and nicotinic acid or nicotinamide in dosages of 100 to 400 mg/day supplemented by vitamin B complex. If a good diet can be maintained, complete recovery is the rule. The disease tends to be progressive and, if untreated, may eventuate in death within several years.

The Porphyrias

The porphyrias comprise a group of disorders of porphyrin, the chemical precursor for hemoglobin synthesis[46,242–249] (Table 19.6). Porphyrins, the only well-established photosensitizers made by the human body, are excited by visible light at the wavelengths 400 to 410 nm (Soret band) and emit a red fluorescence. When exposed to this wavelength in the presence of oxygen, porphyrins release energy that reacts with the oxygen to generate free radicals and singlet oxygen that causes damage to cells and tissues. β-Carotene quenches free radicals and singlet oxygen and thus may lessen the damage.

Two phenotypic patterns of phototoxicity are seen in patients with porphyria: the immediate effects, characterized by pain, edema, erythema, and purpura; and the delayed effects, consisting of blistering and scarring. There are three main categories of porphyric disease in humans: erythropoietic, hepatic, and mixed, with mutations recognized in genes encoding 10 enzymes of the heme biosynthetic pathway (Table 19.7). The erythropoietic porphyrias are divided into erythropoietic porphyria (autosomal recessive) and erythropoietic protoporphyria (autosomal dominant and less often autosomal recessive or X-linked dominant); the hepatic porphyrias include acute intermittent porphyria (AIP), porphyria cutanea tarda, hereditary coproporphyria, and variegate porphyria. Hepatoerythropoietic porphyria is a mixed form. Cutaneous findings are not a feature of δ-aminolevulinate dehydratase deficiency porphyria or AIP.[46] A distinctive, transient purpuric eruption, limited to areas exposed to blue light, has been described in transfused neonates with hyperbilirubinemia[250]; elevated levels of protoporphyrins and coproporphyrins were detected in plasma (Fig. 19.23). The American Porphyria Foundation offers patients information and support (www.porphyriafoundation.com).

CONGENITAL ERYTHROPOIETIC PORPHYRIA

Erythropoietic porphyria (congenital erythropoietic porphyria [CEP], Günther disease) is very rare.[251–253] It is characterized by the appearance of red urine during infancy (Fig. 19.24), severe photosensitivity that occurs in the first 2 or 3 years of life, splenomegaly, and hemolytic anemia.[254] Hemolysis *in utero* may present as hydrops fetalis, but 76% show manifestations by 5 years of age and 41% have at least one manifestation at birth.[251]

Photosensitivity is commonly absent in the neonatal period but generally becomes apparent during the first years of life as exposure to the sun increases. Phototherapy during the neonatal period for hyperbilirubinemia may lead to generalized blistering.[255] Recurrent eruption of vesicles and bullae on sun-exposed areas of the skin (Fig. 19.25), filled with fluid that fluoresces pink, eventually results in mutilating ulceration, scarring, and loss of acral tissues, such as the ears, tip of the nose, eyelids, distal phalanges, and nails. Other common clinical features include hypertrichosis of the face and extremities and hyperpigmentation. The legendary werewolves of the Middle Ages, with fluorescent teeth and nails, mutilated and deformed ears, nose, and eyelids, and nocturnal habits caused by their sensitivity to

Table 19.6 Pathway of Porphyrin Heme Biosynthesis, Enzyme Defects, and Disease

Metabolites	Enzyme	Type of Porphyria
Glycine + succinyl-CoA		
g	δ-Aminolevulinic acid synthase (ALA synthase) 1 and 2	X-linked (ALAS2, erythroid-specific)
δ-Aminolevulinic acid		
g	ALA dehydratase	ALA dehydratase
Porphobilinogen (PBG)		
g	PBG deaminase	Acute intermittent
Hydroxymethylbilane		
g	Uroporphyrinogen III synthase	Congenital erythropoietic
Uroporphyrinogen III		
g	Uroporphyrinogen decarboxylase	Porphyria cutanea tarda/hepatoerythropoietic
Coproporphyrinogen III		
g	Coproporphyrinogen oxidase	Hereditary coproporphyria
Protoporphyrinogen IX		
g	Protoporphyrinogen oxidase	Variegate
Protoporphyrin IX		
g	Ferrochelatase	Erythropoietic protoporphyria
Heme		
g		
Cytochromes, hemoglobin, and myoglobin		

CoA, Coenzyme A.

Table 19.7 Types of Porphyria

Type of Porphyria	Inheritance	Enzyme Deficiency	Photosensitivity	Scarring	Hypertrichosis	Other
ERYTHROPOIETIC						
Congenital erythropoietic porphyria (CEP)	AR XLR	Uroporphyrinogen III synthase (UROS); GATA binding factor 1 (GATA1)	+++	+++	+	Erythrodontia, splenomegaly, hemolysis, bone fragility
Erythropoietic protoporphyria (EPP)	AD/AR XLD	Ferrochelatase; δ-Aminolevulinic acid synthase, erythroid-specific (ALAS2) Caseinolytic mitochondrial matrix peptidase chaperone subunit (CLPX)	++	+	±	Cholelithiasis, anemia, liver failure, marked skin burning or stinging
HEPATIC OR COMBINED						
Acute intermittent porphyria (AIP)	AD	Porphyrinogen deaminase	–	–	–	Acute abdomen and neuropsychiatric
Porphyria cutanea tarda (PCT)	AD	Uroporphyrinogen decarboxylase	++	++	+++	Milia
Hereditary coproporphyria (HCP)	AD	Coproporphyrinogen oxidase	+	+	+	Jaundice and anemia in the newborn (harderoporphyria) Acute abdomen and neuropathy
Variegate porphyria (VP)	AD	Protoporphyrinogen oxidase	+++	++	+	Acute abdomen
δ-Aminolevulinic acid dehydratase porphyria (ALAD porphyria)	AR	δ-Aminolevulinic acid dehydratase	–	–	–	Acute abdomen and neuropsychiatric
Hepatoerythropoietic porphyria (HEP)	AR	Uroporphyrinogen decarboxylase	+++	++	+	Erythrodontia, splenomegaly, anemia

AD, Autosomal dominant; *AR,* autosomal recessive; *XLD,* X-linked dominant; *XLR,* X-linked recessive.

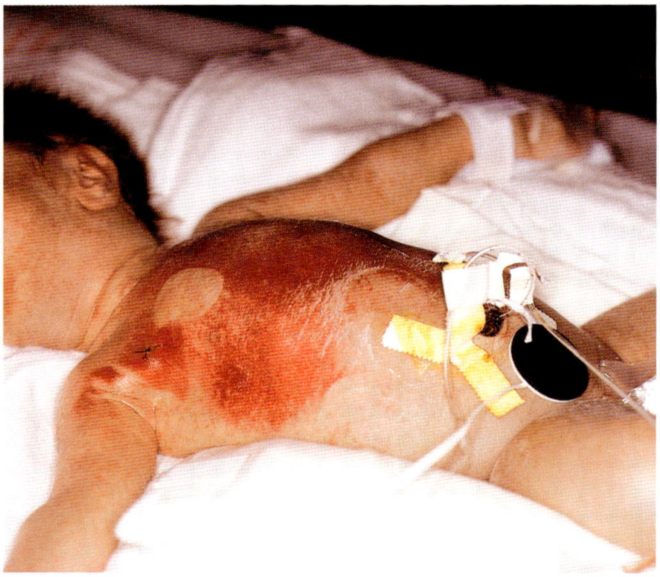

Fig. 19.23 Purpuric phototherapy-induced eruption. Dramatic purpuric eruption at the areas of maximal blue light exposure in a baby with elevated plasma levels of protoporphyrins and coproporphyrins. The baby had been transfused for Rh incompatibility and treated for hyperbilirubinemia. Note the sparing at the site of lead placement.

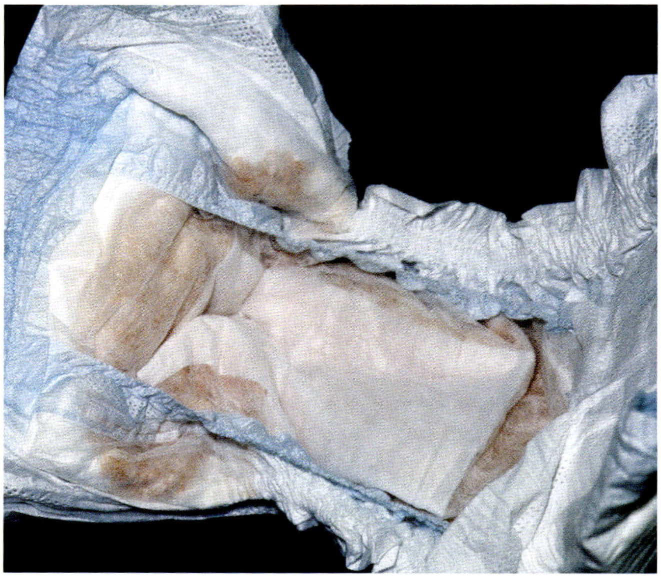

Fig. 19.24 Congenital erythropoietic porphyria. The diaper of an affected baby demonstrates the red color of urine.

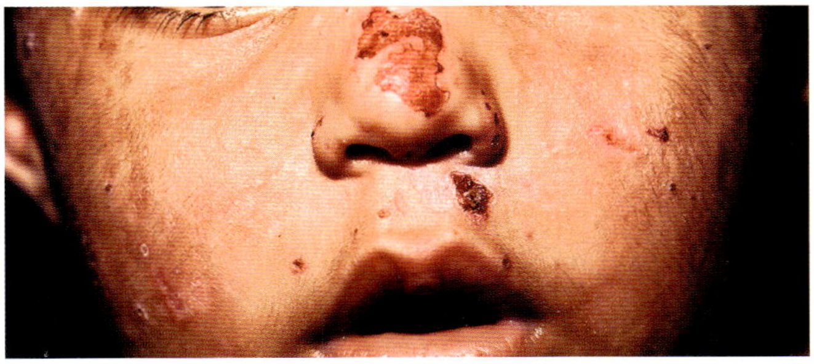

Fig. 19.25 Congenital erythropoietic porphyria. Vesicles, bullae, and crusts on sun-exposed areas.

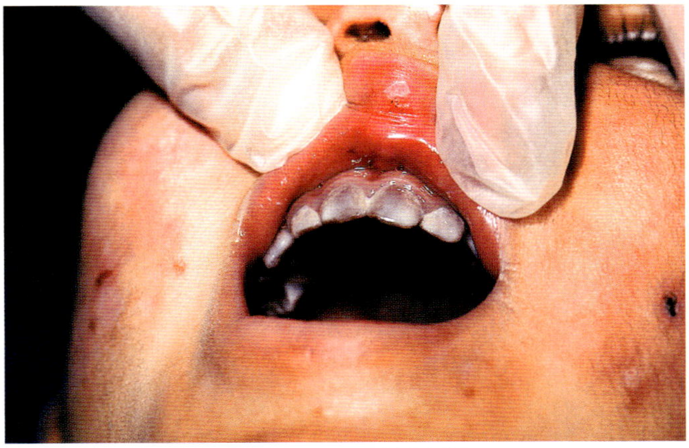

Fig. 19.26 Congenital erythropoietic porphyria. Brownish teeth that fluoresce under Wood lamp examination.

light, may have been persons afflicted with CEP. Asymptomatic pink hamartomatous papules of the perioral and perinasal area have been noted in several patients.[251]

The teeth are a pink to brown color (Fig. 19.26) and fluoresce under Wood lamp examination, because porphyrins bind to dental calcium phosphate. True erythrodontia of porphyria should not be confused with the pseudoerythrodontia of children with poor dental hygiene, which relates to overgrowth of fluorescent bacteria and can be removed. Microstomia, gingival recession, caries, and overcrowding of teeth are other features. Patients show a variety of ocular abnormalities that may lead to blindness, including photophobia, corneal scarring, ulceration, keratoconjunctivitis, and cataracts. Most patients have hemolytic anemia with associated splenomegaly. Neonatal jaundice, abnormal hepatic transaminases, and hepatomegaly are sometimes reported, and pancytopenia has been described. Bone fragility results from the expansion of the bone marrow, although porphyrins may also be directly toxic to bone. The color of the urine of patients may vary from faint pink to burgundy or port wine, depending on the concentration of uroporphyrin.

The biochemical disturbance is a deficiency of the enzyme uroporphyrinogen III synthetase (UROS), resulting in marked overproduction of uroporphyrin I and coproporphyrin I in circulating erythrocytes, bone marrow cells, plasma, urine, and feces. The cutaneous severity is proportional to porphyrin amounts in skin as well as light exposure. The severity of CEP is also influenced by concomitant mutation in *ALAS2* (erythroid-specific mitochondrial 5-aminolevulinate synthase), a modifier gene[256] (see Erythropoietic Protoporphyria section).

Although most patients have biallelic mutations in UROS, mutation in the gene encoding GATA binding factor 1 *(GATA1)* can also cause CEP as an X-linked recessive disorder.[257] *GATA1* is transcription factor that regulates the expression of UROS in developing erythrocytes but also is critical for normal erythropoiesis, globin gene expression, and megakaryocyte development. Affected children show thrombocytopenia, anemia that more closely resembles thalassemia, and dramatic increases in fetal hemoglobin (HbF). Milder disease with onset in early childhood has been described with *UROS* mutations in the erythrocyte-specific promoter region, which is adjacent to the GATA1 binding site.[258] A mild late-onset form has also been described in adult men with myeloid malignancy, especially myelodysplastic syndrome, leading to UROS deficiency.[259]

Wood light examination in patients with CEP may reveal reddish-orange porphyrin fluorescence in urine or aqueous suspensions of feces and thin smears of peripheral erythrocytes glow red under a fluorescent microscope. Patients (with UROS mutations) have normochromic anemia with elevated reticulocyte levels, circulating normoblasts, and normoblastic hyperplasia of the bone marrow.

Mild cases can be managed by avoiding sun exposure and trauma, as well as transfusions to suppress porphyrin overproduction. However, the prognosis of CEP is poor in severe cases, with few patients surviving into the fourth or fifth decade of life unless treated successfully by transplantation.[260–262] Death, when it occurs, is often associated with hemolytic anemia. Bone marrow and allogeneic stem-cell transplantation may correct all disease manifestations except the erythrodontia.[263] Avoidance of light at wavelengths less than 510 nm markedly diminishes the cutaneous manifestations, anemia, and splenomegaly. This includes protection from light through window glass (including blinds and window filters that decrease the relevant visible spectrum), wearing protective clothing, and use of opaque sunscreens that block a broader spectrum. Ophthalmologic intervention with eye lubricants and topical antibiotics, dental management, and administration of supplemental vitamin D and bisphosphonates as needed for osteoporosis is important. Splenectomy for the hemolysis and chronic transfusion regimens to suppress bone marrow activity and help with the hemolytic anemia are variably successful. Surgical reconstruction has decreased the progressive disfigurement from ectropion, microstomia, and nasal deformity.[261,264] Most *UROIIIS* missense mutations prevent efficient folding of proteins for proper function and stability, leading to proteasome degradation; the antifungal medication ciclopirox, a pharmacologic chaperone, has been found to stabilize the enzyme *in vitro* and in mouse models, reverting URO I levels in the blood and liver (thus increasing downstream protoporphyrin IX), and decreasing splenomegaly.[265]

ERYTHROPOIETIC PROTOPORPHYRIA

Erythropoietic protoporphyria (EPP), the most common form of porphyria in children, results most often from the combination of loss-of-function mutations of *FECH*, the gene encoding mitochondrial ferrochelatase and, on the other allele, a polymorphism carried by 10% of Western Europeans in the noncoding region (IVS3-48T>C) of *FECH*.[266–269] In EPP, levels of ferrochelatase, which accelerates the incorporation of iron into protoporphyrin, are only 15% to 25% of normal. Although the disorder is autosomal dominant, parent-to-child transmission of overt disease is uncommon. Having polymorphisms on both alleles does not cause disease; however, true autosomal recessive disease with loss-of-function mutations on both alleles of *FECH* occurs in about 3% to 5% of affected individuals and may be associated with EPP. Homozygous IVS3-48C polymorphism of *FECH* may be associated with a slight elevation in protoporphyrins and mild EPP.[270]

X-linked (dominant) protoporphyria (XLP) is a phenocopy of EPP and results from gain-of-function mutations in the C-terminal of the X-linked erythroid-specific 5-aminolevulinate synthase *(ALAS2)* gene, which is essential for hemoglobin formation.[271] The incidence of XLP is 10% of that of EPP from *FECH* mutations in North America and even less in Western Europe.[272] Males with XLP have twofold higher erythrocyte protoporphyrin levels than patients with EPP, increasing their risk of photosensitivity and liver disease. Based on the pattern of X-inactivation, females with XLP be clinically asymptomatic with normal protoporphyrins, be asymptomatic clinically with slightly elevated protoporphyrin levels, or have significant symptoms. A dominant mutation in *CLPX* was reported to cause an EPP-like disorder.[273] CLPX is part of a complex that mediates turnover of ALAS2, and its dysfunction leads to increased posttranslational stability of ALAS2 and abnormal accumulation of protoporphyrin IX (PPIX).[274]

The common subtlety of clinical signs and symptoms and the absence of increased levels of protoporphyrin in urine (because of the relative insolubility of PPIX in water) may lead to failure of recognition of EPP. Nevertheless, the disease usually becomes symptomatic between 1 and 6 years of age because of photosensitivity.[275] The condition may be detected during infancy because the baby cries after brief exposure to sunlight. It manifests acutely from early spring to late summer as burning, stinging, or itching of the exposed skin after 5 to 30 minutes of sunlight exposure.[276] The burning may be intensely painful and may occur in the absence of any skin change. This burning sensation[277] may be followed by pruritic reddened edematous plaques that return to normal within 1 to 2 days. Occasionally, papulovesicular (Fig. 19.27) and petechial eruptions occur and may persist for longer periods. Chronic skin manifestations are often mild, ranging from grossly undetectable lesions to shallow linear or elliptical pits on the face; linear furrows around the lips; thickened hyperkeratotic skin; dyspigmentation; and a weather-beaten, leathery, or pebbly appearance, particularly over the nose or knuckles (Fig. 19.28). Nails may be shed (photoonycholysis). Seasonal palmar keratoderma has been described as a sign of autosomal recessive EPP.[278]

Anemia has been reported in approximately 47% of patients. Rarely, hypersplenism (which responds favorably to splenectomy) is associated with the anemia. Cholecystitis and cholelithiasis have been reported in up to 12% of patients, with gallstones consisting of almost pure protoporphyrin IX. Overall 20% to 30% of patients have manifestations of hepatic abnormalities, most commonly a mild increase in hepatic aminotransferases. Progressive hepatic failure occurs in 2% to 4% of patients, usually after 30 years of age, from retention of protoporphyrins, cholestasis, and eventual cirrhosis. However, cholestatic liver disease has even been described in affected infants.[279] The severity of the disease correlates with the amount of circulating protoporphyrins. Liver function testing should be performed annually, and alcohol and drugs with potential hepatotoxicity or cholestatic effects should be avoided. Carriage of null allele mutations, autosomal recessive EPP, and XLP have a higher risk of hepatic complications.[271,280]

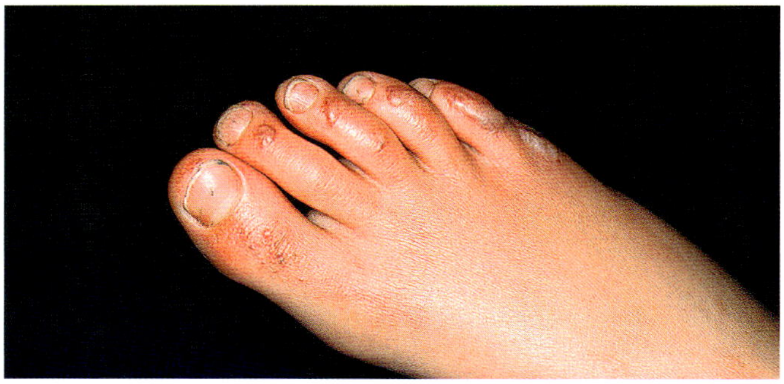

Fig. 19.27 Erythropoietic protoporphyria (EPP). Vesicular lesions are only occasionally seen in patients with EPP.

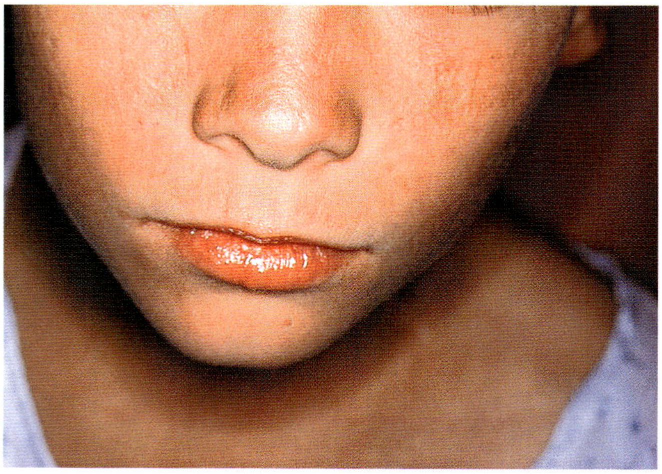

Fig. 19.28 Erythropoietic protoporphyria. Papular thickening of the skin after blistering is particularly common on the nose and overlying the knuckles.

Free protoporphyrin levels are high in circulating erythrocytes, plasma, bone marrow, liver, feces, and skin, but not in urine, so the best test is the free erythrocyte protoporphyrin level. Zinc-bound erythrocyte protoporphyrins are much higher in XLP (19% to 65% of erythrocyte protoporphyrins) but not in EPP (4% to 13%),[271] because ferrochelatase is needed to synthesize both iron protoporphyrin (heme) and zinc protoporphyrin. Although total protoporphyrins (which are primarily free erythrocyte protoporphyrin) are usually measured if the more easily obtained "zinc-protoporphyrin level" is ordered, ensuring that the test measures the free erythrocyte protoporphyrins is important. Fluorescence of the erythrocytes can be demonstrated by Wood light or fluorescence microscopy.[281] In contrast to erythropoietic porphyria, fluorescence of teeth and nails is not present and there is no increase in fecal or urinary levels of uroporphyrins, although fecal protoporphyrins and coproporphyrins are increased. Erythrocyte ferrochelatase levels are 10% to 50% of normal.

The management of EPP depends on limiting exposure to sunlight and use of sun-protective clothing and opaque sunscreens that block both UVA and visible, given the absorption spectrum of PPIX[282]. Some patients have had decreased photosensitivity after administration of β-carotene (Lumitene), which maximally absorbs in the visible spectrum at 450 to 475 nm and quenches free radicals in the skin. The usual dosage for children younger than 14 years of age is 30 to 150 mg and for adolescents is 120 to 180 mg (4 to 6 capsules a day). Skin yellowing, orange-colored stools, and occasional gastrointestinal upset may occur. Nevertheless, a systematic review did not confirm efficacy of β-carotene, vitamin C, or N-acetylcysteine.[283] Cimetidine inhibits heme biosynthesis and has been shown to reduce serum erythrocyte protoporphyrin levels, improve liver function, reduce photosensitivity, and improve or resolve photodamage in affected children.[284]

Narrowband UVB light using a PMLE protocol to harden skin (starting with 50% to 70% MED and increasing gradually) led to improvement in the majority of treated patients.[285] Subcutaneous implantation of 16 mg afamelanotide, an α-melanocyte–stimulating hormone analog to induce tanning, has markedly improved the quality of life in patients with EPP who have been treated chronically for up to 8 years[286] and in two clinical trials.[287] Transfusion may be required in patients with significant hemolytic anemia. Other therapeutic approaches that may be useful are cholestyramine, which helps prevent reabsorption of protoporphyrin excreted into the intestinal lumen, and chenodeoxycholic or ursodeoxycholic acid. For patients with progressively deteriorating liver function, liver transplantation can be lifesaving,[288,289] but the risk of biliary complications is high; disease recurrence may be delayed by administration intravenously of hemin (an iron-containing porphyrin) and plasmapheresis.

PORPHYRIA CUTANEA TARDA

Porphyria cutanea tarda (PCT) is the most common form of porphyria in adults and the second most common form of porphyria in children.[290–292] Estimated to have an incidence of 1 in 25,000, it usually presents during the third and fourth decades of life. Autosomal dominant cases result from a mutation in uroporphyrinogen decarboxylase *(UROD)*. UROD activity must be less than or equal to 20% of normal to manifest clinical signs, so other genetic and environmental factors are necessary to reduce levels beyond the 50% reduction from the primary genetic defect. In the familial form, the decreased UROD activity affects the liver, erythrocytes, and other tissues. Mutations in both *UROD* alleles usually lead to hepatoerythropoietic porphyria but may cause mild cutaneous disease.[293] About 80% of patients have the sporadic (type I) form in which the activity of UROD deficiency is inhibited specifically in the liver.

Skin lesions in PCT are vesicles or bullae on light-exposed cutaneous surfaces, especially the dorsal aspect of the hands, forearms, and face.[294] The blisters vary markedly in size from 1 mm to 3 cm across, with small blisters often being overlooked. They are most commonly filled by clear or slightly turbid liquid, but soon rupture, turn into erosions, and often become infected. On healing, the blister sites may scar or evolve into milia. These features may require differentiation from immunobullous disorders, especially epidermolysis bullosa acquisita (see Chapter 13). Other features include increased fragility of the skin, with erosions and ulcerations as a result of relatively minor trauma, hypertrichosis, and mottled hypopigmentation and hyperpigmentation of the face at sites of sun exposure. Sclerodermoid plaques (especially on the chest or temples) and dystrophic calcifications are rare in affected children.

PCT can be precipitated by iron overload[295] (including in the presence of thalassemia), hepatitis C, human immunodeficiency virus (HIV), alcoholic cirrhosis, Alagille syndrome,[295] hemodialysis, or administration of estrogens, hydantoins, griseofulvin, or chemotherapy drugs.[296] Accidental ingestion of the fungicide hexachlorobenzene was responsible for an epidemic of PCT in Turkey.[297] Mutations in *HFE*, associated with hemochromatosis. Certain polymorphisms in cytochromes,[298] and the transferrin receptor gene *(TFRC)* also increase the risk.[243] Diabetes mellitus is present in 25% of patients with PCT, and patients not uncommonly show hepatomegaly and abnormal hepatic transaminase levels. The development of cirrhosis is a precursor of the hepatocellular carcinoma, which eventually develops in about 3% of patients.

Confirmation of the clinical diagnosis of PCT can be made by increased levels of urinary and fecal uroporphyrins, slightly elevated fecal coproporphyrin and protoporphyrin levels, and positive fluorescence of the urine with a Wood light. As with other forms of porphyria, skin biopsy specimens of vesicular lesions show subepidermal bullae with dermal papillae arising irregularly from the floor of the bulla into its cavity ("festooning"). Periodic acid–Schiff (PAS)–positive material is deposited around blood vessels and sometimes at the dermal-epidermal junction, sites where immunofluorescent studies show deposition of IgG and complement. Familial and sporadic cases can be distinguished by erythrocyte uroporphyrinogen-decarboxylase activity and uroporphyrinogen-decarboxylase genotyping.

Treatment is dependent on the elimination of triggering factors (e.g., alcohol, estrogen, iron ingestion). Treatment with low doses of hydroxychloroquine (3 mg/kg twice weekly) leads to drug-uroporphyrin complexes that are excreted. Clinical remission ensues in about 3 months, and biochemical remission is achieved in about a year. If antimalarial treatment is ineffective, phlebotomy is used to remove iron stores and porphyrins. Once biochemical remission is achieved, treatment is stopped and the patient is monitored for relapse, which generally occurs within 3 years until spontaneous remission. Spontaneous remission has been reported, but 5% to 16% of adults with long-standing untreated disease and chronic hepatitis develop hepatocellular carcinoma.

HEPATOERYTHROPOIETIC PORPHYRIA

Hepatoerythropoietic porphyria, an extremely rare disorder, is considered to be a homozygous or heteroallelic form of PCT. The disease is usually manifest before 2 years of age.[299,300] Dark urine is the most commonly observed sign. Skin lesions appear in childhood, and the activity of UROD in all organs is usually decreased to less than 10% of normal. The disorder is characterized by excessive porphyrin production in the liver and bone marrow; increased erythrocyte porphyrin levels; and severe photosensitivity with vesicles, bullae, crusts, and erosions. Skin fragility, hypertrichosis (that begins in infancy and early childhood), mutilating scarring deformities similar to those of CEP, and scleroderma-like changes of sun-exposed skin also occur. The face and dorsal aspect of the hands are the most severely affected areas. Malar hypertrichosis may be striking, and patients have erythrodontia (reddish brown teeth) that fluoresces when exposed to a Wood lamp. In addition to clinical features similar to those of erythropoietic porphyria, hepatoerythropoietic porphyria has biochemical abnormalities suggestive of PCT and EPP. The diagnosis is confirmed by finding huge elevations of erythrocyte protoporphyrin, urinary uroporphyrin, and fecal coproporphyrin. Sun avoidance is critical; plasma iron concentrations are normal, and phlebotomy is ineffective.

HEREDITARY COPROPORPHYRIA

Hereditary coproporphyria has almost always been described in adults.[301] The few cases that have been documented in children were initially mistaken for HV.[302] Rare homozygous cases have been reported in neonates with hepatosplenomegaly, hemolytic anemia, jaundice, and photosensitivity (harderoporphyria)[303]; feces show marked elevations of coproporphyrins. Some 20% to 30% of patients are photosensitive, and the skin lesions resemble those of PCT, chronic and usually appearing many days after sun exposure. Most patients have acute attacks of abdominal pain identical to those seen in AIP and variegate porphyria. Abdominal pain progresses slowly over days with nausea progressing to vomiting. Occasionally, the pain is mostly in the back and extremities. Acute peripheral neuropathy and seizures have also been described. This condition, inherited as an autosomal dominant trait, is associated with heterozygous variants in *CPOX*, leading to defective coproporphyrinogen oxidase and accumulation of coproporphyrinogen III and its oxidized form, coproporphyrin III. Cutaneous eruptions occur concurrently with attacks of abdominal pain and psychiatric symptoms. The diagnosis is made by demonstration of elevated levels of coproporphyrin III in both urine and feces, and treatment is similar to that of patients with variegate porphyria, in addition to pain therapy for the acute abdominal attacks.

VARIEGATE PORPHYRIA

Variegate porphyria (congenital cutaneous hepatic porphyria, South African porphyria) is an autosomal dominant disorder that results from heterozygous mutations in *PPOX* and decreased activity of protoporphyrinogen oxidase. This disease has its onset after puberty and generally appears in the fourth to fifth decades of life; only a few cases in childhood have been described.[304] It has a high incidence in the Afrikaners of South Africa.[305] Individuals with homozygous or compound heterozygous mutations can show severe photosensitivity with blistering and scarring beginning in infancy.[306] Other features are developmental delay, mental retardation, nystagmus, seizures, and short stature.[307]

The features of variegate porphyria resemble those of PCT but tend to be milder and less easily provoked. Clinical manifestations include sun sensitivity with vesicles or blisters on light-exposed surfaces, hyperpigmentation, a weather-beaten or waxy complexion with excessive furrowing of the forehead (cutis rhomboidalis frontalis) and neck (cutis rhomboidalis nuchae), scars on the back of the neck and frontal hair margin, milia, and scleroderma-like plaques. The urinary findings overlap with those of both AIP and PCT, so diagnosis is based on the plasma porphyrin fluorescence (626 nM) and a more than twofold increase in excretion of fecal protoporphyrin. Treatment consists of avoidance of hepatotoxic agents and sun exposure, repeated phlebotomies, low-dose hydroxychloroquine therapy, and, in some patients, the administration of β-carotene.

ACUTE INTERMITTENT PORPHYRIA AND δ-AMINOLEVULINIC ACID DEHYDRATASE PORPHYRIA

AIP and δ-aminolevulinic acid dehydratase (ALAD) porphyria are rare disorders that share clinical features of episodes of acute abdominal pain associated with vomiting; constipation; peripheral paresis or paralysis; and psychological manifestations or psychoneuroses provoked by drugs that affect the liver, including barbiturates, sulfonamides, dapsone, griseofulvin, anticonvulsive agents, sulfonylurea compounds, and estrogens. Neither disorder tends to manifest before puberty or shows cutaneous features. AIP is an autosomal dominant disorder characterized by overproduction of porphyrin precursors (δ-aminolevulinic acid and porphobilinogen), which are excreted into the urine. ALAD porphyria, in contrast, is an even rarer autosomal recessive disorder with markedly deficient ALAD activity that results in overproduction of δ-aminolevulinic acid, but not porphobilinogen, in the urine.[308] False-positive urine porphyrin tests can be seen in children with heavy metal poisoning, including lead and mercury.[309]

The complete list of 309 references for this chapter is available online at http://expertconsult.inkling.com.

Key References

Quatrano NA, Dinulos JG. Current principles of sunscreen use in children. Curr Opin Pediatr 2013;25(1):122–9.

Christensen L, Suggs A, Baron E. Ultraviolet photobiology in dermatology. Adv Exp Med Biol 2017;996:89–104.

Chantorn R, Lim HW, Shwayder TA. Photosensitivity disorders in children. Part I. J Am Acad Dermatol 2012;67(6):1093.e1–18.

Chantorn R, Lim HW, Shwayder TA. Photosensitivity disorders in children. Part II. J Am Acad Dermatol 2012;67(6):1113.e1–15.

Naka F, Shwayder TA, Santoro FA. Photodermatoses: kids are not just little people. Clin Dermatol 2016;34(6):724–35.

Nitiyarom R, Wongpraparut C. Hydroa vacciniforme and solar urticaria. Dermatol Clin 2014;32(3):345–53.

Valbuena MC, Muvdi S, Lim HW. Actinic prurigo. Dermatol Clin 2014;32(3):335–44.

Guarrera M. Polymorphous light eruption. Adv Exp Med Biol 2017;996:61–70.

Sheu J, Hawryluk EB, Guo D, et al. Voriconazole phototoxicity in children: a retrospective review. J Am Acad Dermatol 2015;72(2):314–20.

DiGiovanna JJ, Kraemer KH. Shining a light on xeroderma pigmentosum. J Invest Dermatol 2012;132(3 Pt 2):785–96.

Giordano CN, Yew YW, Spivak G, et al. Understanding photodermatoses associated with defective DNA repair: syndromes with cancer predisposition. J Am Acad Dermatol 2016;75(5):855–70.

Yew YW, Giordano CN, Spivak G, et al. Understanding photodermatoses associated with defective DNA repair: photosensitive syndromes without associated cancer predisposition. J Am Acad Dermatol 2016;75(5):873–82.

Wilson BT, Stark Z, Sutton RE, et al. The Cockayne Syndrome Natural History (CoSyNH) study: clinical findings in 102 individuals and recommendations for care. Genet Med 2016;18(5):483–93.

Natale V, Raquer H. Xeroderma pigmentosum-Cockayne syndrome complex. Orphanet J Rare Dis 2017;12(1):65.

Wang LL, Levy ML, Lewis RA, et al. Clinical manifestations in a cohort of 41 Rothmund-Thomson syndrome patients. Am J Med Genet 2001;102(1):11–17.

Schulenburg-Brand D, Katugampola R, Anstey AV, et al. The cutaneous porphyrias. Dermatol Clin 2014;32(3):369–84.

Yasuda M, Chen B, Desnick RJ. Recent advances on porphyria genetics: inheritance, penetrance & molecular heterogeneity, including new modifying/causative genes. Mol Genet Metab 2019;128:230–31.

20 Urticarias and Other Hypersensitivity Disorders

CHAPTER OUTLINE

The hypersensitivity syndromes are a group of disorders mediated by immunologic or hypersensitivity reactions to foreign proteins such as food or drugs or to infectious agents, immunizations, and malignancies. Although diagnosis of these disorders is often relatively easy, difficulties commonly arise in determining the underlying cause. The most common hypersensitivity reactions are drug reactions,[1] and the skin is a common target. The overall incidence of drug reactions in hospitalized children is 9.5%,[2] and in outpatient children it is 2.5%, with reactivity to antibiotics occurring most often.[3] However, up to 10% of parents report suspected hypersensitivity to at least one drug,[4] most often β-lactam antibiotics.

The various types of drug reactions are summarized in Table 20.1.[5] Urticarial and exanthematous reactions are seen most often.[6,7] Some of these are life threatening and have been linked through the term *severe cutaneous adverse reactions* (SCARs)[8]: the Stevens–Johnson syndrome (SJS)/toxic epidermal necrolysis (TEN) spectrum, drug reaction with eosinophilia and systemic symptoms (DRESS), acute generalized exanthematous pustulosis, and generalized bullous fixed-drug eruptions. Other hypersensitivity disorders are lichenoid drug eruptions (Fig. 20.1) (see Chapter 4), nonbullous fixed drug eruptions, acneiform eruptions (see Chapter 8), pseudoporphyria (see Chapter 19), drug-induced vasculitis (see Chapter 21), and drug-induced lupus (see Chapter 22). Some children experience multiple antibiotic sensitivity, most commonly to penicillins, sulfonamides, cephalosporins, and macrolides.[9] In these children the manifestations of drug sensitivity can be different; for example, a child may show an exanthematous response to amoxicillin, DRESS after phenytoin, and erythroderma after ingestion of sulfamethoxazole within a period of a few months.[10] The general approach to a child with suspected drug reaction is outlined in Box 20.1.

Allergic Reactions

Allergy may be defined as a specific acquired alteration in the capacity of an individual to react to an antigen. Mediated by circulating or cellular antibodies, allergic reactions may be classified as immunoglobulin (Ig) E–mediated hypersensitivity (type I), cytotoxic (type II), Arthus-type toxic immune complex reactions (type III), and delayed-type hypersensitivity (type IV). Type I/anaphylactic reactions include local and systemic manifestations of the interaction between antigen and tissue cells previously sensitized with skin-sensitizing reaginic antibody, usually IgE. This interaction of antigen and antibody results in the release of pharmacologically active substances that produce urticaria, angioedema, anaphylaxis, hay fever, and asthma. Type II/cytotoxic reactions include those reactions initiated by antibody interacting with an antigenic component of the cell surface. The antigen may be a natural component of the cell or an unrelated antigen that has become associated with the cell. Examples include pemphigus (see Chapter 13), hemolytic disease of the newborn, transfusion reactions, hemolytic anemia, leukopenia, or thrombocytopenia caused by the reaction of antibody with drugs attached to blood cell surfaces. Type III/toxic immune complex reactions (Arthus-type reactions) are associated with the deposition of immune microprecipitates in or around blood vessels, which results in tissue damage through activation of complement or toxic products from leukocytes attracted to the areas. Examples include serum sickness, vasculitis, glomerulonephritis, and local Arthus reactions after injection of antigens into the skin, subcutaneous tissue, or muscle. Type IV/delayed-type hypersensitivity is the result of the interaction between antigen and specifically sensitized lymphocytic cells, which results in a mononuclear cell infiltration and the elaboration of toxic lymphoid cell products. Examples include

Table 20.1 Drug Eruptions in Pediatric Patients

Eruption	Key Drugs	Lesional Pattern	Mucosal Changes
Urticaria	Penicillins, cephalosporins, sulfonamides, minocycline, aspirin/ NSAIDs, antiepileptics, monoclonal antibodies, radiocontrast media	Pruritic erythematous wheals	None
Angioedema	Aspirin/NSAIDs, ACE inhibitors	Swelling of subcutaneous and deep dermal tissues	May be present
Serum sickness–like reaction	Cephalosporins, penicillins, minocycline, sulfonamides, macrolides, rifampin, ciprofloxacin, griseofulvin, itraconazole, bupropion, fluoxetine, rituximab, omalizumab, H1N1 vaccine	Urticarial or erythema multiforme–like	None
Exanthematous	Penicillins, sulfonamides, cephalosporins, antiepileptics	Erythematous macules and/ or papules	None
Drug hypersensitivity syndrome	Sulfonamides, phenytoin, phenobarbital, carbamazepine, lamotrigine, amoxicillin, allopurinol, sulfonamides, dapsone, minocycline, aspirin, vancomycin, azithromycin, abacavir, nevirapine, Chinese medicine	Edema (especially periorbital); erythematous macules and/or papules; sometimes vesicles or bullae	May be present
Lichenoid*	Captopril, enalapril, labetalol, nifedipine, propranolol, gold salts, hydrochlorothiazide, furosemide, spironolactone, hydroxychloroquine, ketoconazole, penicillamine, griseofulvin, tetracycline, carbamazepine, phenytoin, NSAIDs, hydroxyurea, imatinib, dapsone, sulfasalazine, allopurinol, iodides and radiocontrast media, IFN-γ, omeprazole, penicillamine, TNF inhibitors, sildenafil, leflunomide, human growth hormone	Discrete flat-topped reddish-purple papules and plaques	May be present
Fixed drug	Sulfonamides, ibuprofen, acetaminophen, salicylates, tetracyclines, pseudoephedrine, loratadine, teicoplanin, metronidazole, macrolides, barbiturates, lamotrigine, potassium iodide, quinine, phenolphthalein, foods and food flavorings (especially tartrazine)	Solitary to few erythematous, hyperpigmented plaques	Unusual
Pustular (AGEP)	β-Lactam antibiotics, cephalosporins, macrolides, clindamycin, terbinafine, paroxetine, hydroxychloroquine, contrast agents	Generalized small pustules and papules	None
Acneiform†	Corticosteroids, androgens, lithium, iodides, phenytoin, isoniazid, methotrexate	Follicular-based inflammatory papules and pustules predominate	None
Pseudoporphyria‡	NSAIDs, COX-2 inhibitors, tetracyclines, furosemide	Photodistributed blistering and skin fragility	None
Vasculitis§	Penicillins, NSAIDs, sulfonamides, cephalosporins	Purpuric papules, especially on the lower extremities; urticaria, hemorrhagic bullae, digital necrosis, pustules, ulcers	Rarely
Stevens–Johnson syndrome/toxic epidermal necrolysis	Sulfonamides, antiepileptics (especially phenytoin, carbamazepine, and lamotrigine), NSAIDs, penicillins, acetaminophen, allopurinol, dapsone, barbiturates	Target lesions, bullae, epidermal necrosis with detachment	Present
Drug-induced lupus‖	Minocycline, procainamide, hydralazine, isoniazid, penicillamine	Urticarial, vasculitic, erythematous	Rare

ACE, Angiotensin-converting enzyme; *AGEP,* acute generalized exanthematous pustulosis; *COX-2,* cyclooxygenase-2; *IFN,* interferon; *NSAID,* nonsteroidal antiinflammatory drug; *TNF,* tumor necrosis factor.
*See Chapter 4.
†See Chapter 8.
‡See Chapter 19.
§See Chapter 21.
‖See Chapter 22.

tuberculin and other skin test reactions, allergic contact dermatitis (see Chapter 3), lichenoid drug eruptions (see Fig. 20.1 and Chapter 4), fixed drug eruptions, TEN, and graft-versus-host-type reactions (see Chapter 25). Patch testing may be useful in determining the cause of allergic contact dermatitis (see Chapter 3).

Urticaria

Urticaria, a systemic disease with cutaneous manifestations, occurs at some time in the life of about 15% to 20% of all persons.[11] It is characterized by the appearance of transient well-circumscribed skin lesions that present as erythematous, intensely pruritic elevated swellings (wheals) of the skin or mucous membranes. More than 80% of cases of new-onset urticaria resolve in 2 weeks and more than 95% of new-onset cases within 3 months.[12] Urticaria may be spontaneous or inducible (e.g., contact urticaria and physical urticarias from cold, pressure, heat, sun, water, exercise/stress, stroking, and vibrations). Taking a thorough history is important in understanding potential triggers, subtype of urticaria, and choice of therapy (Box 20.2), and a physical examination will confirm the presence of urticaria and help to define its subtype. Several simple measures are available to track urticaria/angioedema activity, such as the Urticaria Activity Score, Angioedema Activity Score, and Urticaria Control Test[11]; none of these are currently validated in children.

Urticaria usually represents a type I (or immediate) hypersensitivity reaction in which the protein or its metabolite binds to IgE on the surface of cutaneous mast cells, leading to activation, degranulation,

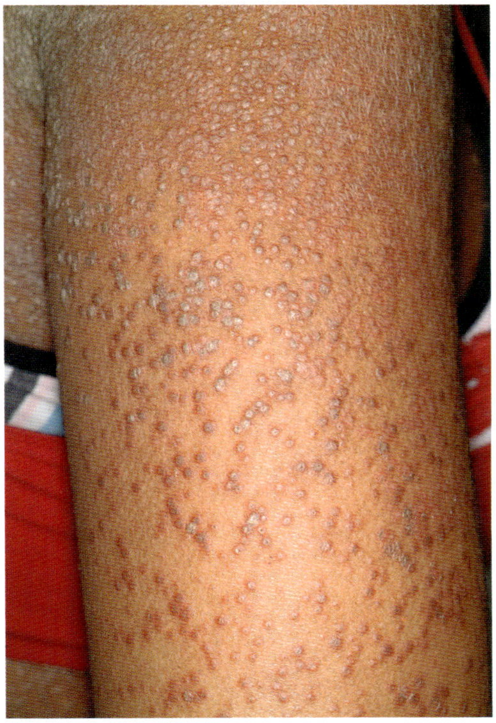

Fig. 20.1 Lichenoid drug eruption. Note the flat-topped character of these small papules.

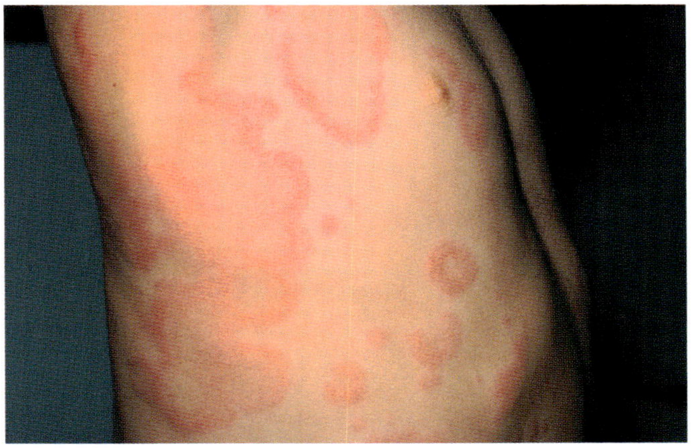

Fig. 20.2 Urticaria. Transient well-circumscribed erythematous wheals occurred in this girl as a reaction to administration of cefixime. Note the edematous center and halo of erythema. Circling a lesion and noting whether it is clear 24 hours later facilitates diagnosis.

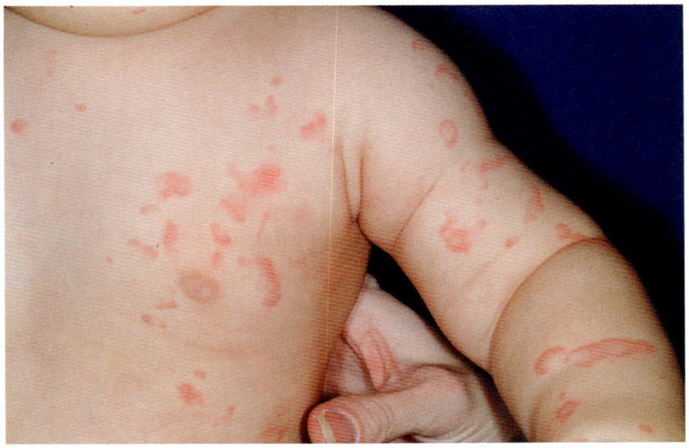

Fig. 20.3 Urticaria. Transient round and annular erythematous macules and slightly edematous plaques represent a reaction to cefdinir in this infant.

Box 20.1 Approach to the Patient with Suspected Drug Reaction

- Historical features
  - Drugs taken, date of initiation, and duration
  - Date of onset of eruption
  - Response to removal and rechallenge
- Clinical features
  - Lesional morphology
  - Number of lesions and distribution
  - Involvement of mucous membranes
  - Associated features: pruritus, fever, lymphadenopathy, visceral involvement
- Laboratory testing
  - Eosinophilia
  - Specific IgE levels
- Prick and intradermal tests for late-phase reactions (β-lactam allergy)
- Provocation testing

IgE, Immunoglobulin E.

Box 20.2 History to Gather in Assessing a Patient with Urticaria

- Duration of disease
- Frequency, duration of episodes, distribution, shape and size of wheals
- Association with angioedema
  - Triggering factors—exercise, physical agents (e.g., cold, heat, pressure, sun, water), foods, OTC and prescription medications, infection, stress
  - Relationship to travel, menstrual cycle, time of day, hobbies
  - Other medical history—allergies, infections, autoimmune disease, etc.
  - Associated noncutaneous manifestations—fever, joint pain, abdominal symptoms
  - Family history
  - Response to previous and current therapies (including duration and dose)
  - Past evaluations and results

OTC, Over the counter.

and release of vasoactive mediators such as histamine, leukotrienes, and prostaglandins. Examples of immunologically mediated urticaria are reactions to latex and reactions to peanuts (see later). Urticaria may also result from nonimmunologic triggering of mast cell release, such as from radiocontrast media, aspirin, many types of nonsteroidal antiinflammatory drugs (NSAIDs), or opiates.

Typical lesions of urticaria have an edematous center with a halo of erythema (Fig. 20.2). They vary from pinpoint-sized papules to large lesions several centimeters in diameter. Central clearing, peripheral extension, and coalescence of individual lesions result in a clinical picture of oval, annular, or sometimes bizarre serpiginous configurations (Figs. 20.3 and 20.4). When annular or serpiginous patterns of urticaria occur, they can be confused with erythema multiforme (EM) or serum sickness–like reactions, and the designation *urticaria multiforme* has been used (Fig. 20.5).[13,14]

Urticaria-like lesions may be part of a variety of other disorders, particularly maculopapular cutaneous mastocytosis/urticaria pigmentosa (see Chapter 8); bullous pemphigoid (prebullous stage; see Chapter 13); urticarial vasculitis (individual lesions persisting beyond 24 hours); Henoch–Schönlein purpura and acute hemorrhagic edema of infancy (see Chapter 21); systemic-onset juvenile idiopathic arthritis and systemic lupus erythematosus (see Chapter 22); autoinflammatory disorders, particularly the cryopyrin-associated periodic syndromes and Schnitzler's syndrome (especially with fever;

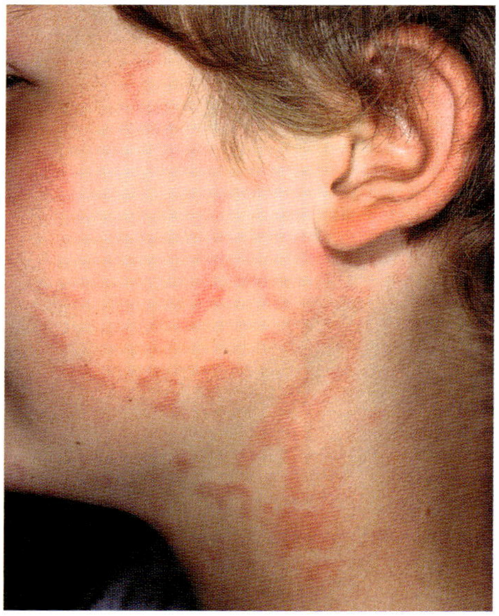

Fig. 20.4 Urticaria. These annular and serpiginous wheals developed within minutes of eating shrimp.

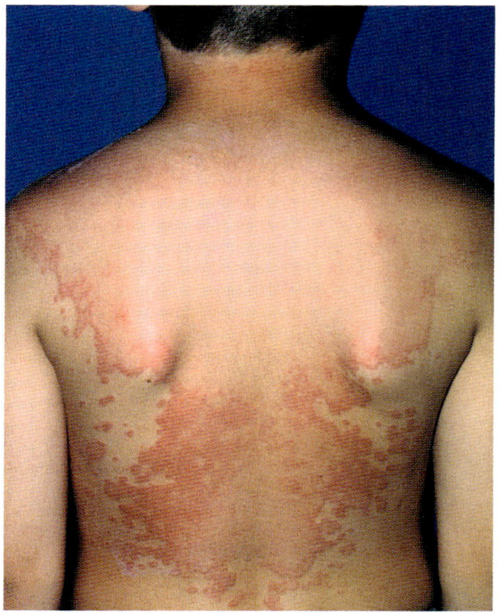

Fig. 20.6 Urticaria. Wheals may coalesce and cover large areas of the body.

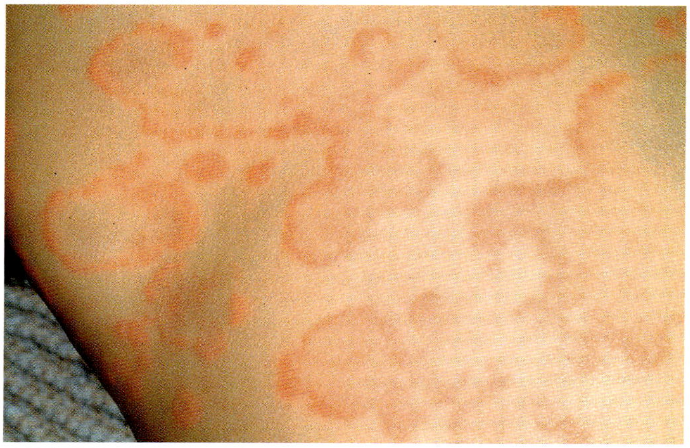

Fig. 20.5 Urticaria. Annular patterns of urticaria can be confused with erythema multiforme, and the term *urticaria multiforme* has been proposed.

see Chapter 25); and other hypersensitivity disorders (Wells' syndrome, hypereosinophilic syndrome).[15,16]

Urticaria may be localized to one small area or may become generalized (Fig. 20.6). Subcutaneous extension may result in giant wheals. In infants and young children, swelling of the distal extremities with acrocyanosis may be a prominent feature of the urticarial reaction. Occasionally, particularly in infants and young children, bullae may form in the center of the wheal, usually on the legs and buttocks. Individual wheals rarely persist longer than 12 to 24 hours. Parents can draw a circle around a few lesions to verify clearance of each individual lesion by approximately 24 hours or less. Those lasting longer than 24 to 36 hours are probably not true urticaria and may represent another vascular pattern such as urticarial vasculitis (see Chapter 21) or EM.

Urticaria of less than 6 weeks' duration is considered acute. In 80% of children, acute urticaria is the result of infection, often viral, whereas in adolescents food and drugs play a more significant role. Among foods, dairy products play a more common role in younger children, in contrast to nuts, seafood, berries, and grains in older children. Streptococcal infection, mycoplasma, histoplasmosis, and coccidioidomycosis in endemic areas are also well-known triggers, although almost every infectious agent has been associated with urticaria.

Overall, up to 10% of episodes of urticaria are related to drugs, and these are usually acute in nature. The penicillins are the most common drugs to trigger urticaria, but only 10% to 20% of individuals who report allergy to penicillin are really allergic when skin prick testing to penicilloyl-poly-lysine and then oral drug challenge (if negative) is performed.[17] Other drugs most likely to induce an urticarial drug reaction are cephalosporins, sulfonamides, tetracyclines (especially minocycline), antiepileptics, and monoclonal antibodies, including omalizumab. Although cross-intolerant reactions are more common than IgE-mediated reactions with NSAIDs,[18] selective immediate reactions to NSAIDs are becoming increasingly recognized with the widespread use of these medications in children (especially ibuprofen).[19] *In vitro* testing (immunoassays and basophil activation testing) can detect specific IgE antibodies for a limited number of drugs and complement prick testing but should be performed within 1 year after the occurrence of a reaction.[20] Anaphylactoid reactions (anaphylaxis without identifiable specific IgE antibodies) most commonly result from ingestion of acetylsalicylic acid. Nonimmunologically mediated urticaria may result from radiocontrast media and NSAIDs. Psychologic stress may exacerbate (but not cause) urticaria.

Urticaria that recurs often and lasts longer than 6 weeks is termed *chronic*. Chronic urticaria occurs in 0.1% to 0.3% of children and is much more common in adults[21]; it may be present continuously or nearly every day (chronic continuous urticaria) or as attacks separated by symptom-free periods of up to several weeks (chronic recurrent or intermittent urticaria).[22] Diagnosis and treatment of a patient with chronic urticaria demands a complete history and physical examination, appropriate laboratory evaluation, and an awareness of possible underlying disease.

Among children with chronic spontaneous (versus inducible) urticaria, 30% to 50% have autoimmune (also called *autoreactive*) urticaria,[23–25] caused by IgE antibodies to autoallergens (type I autoimmunity) or IgG autoantibodies recognizing the high-affinity IgE receptor ($Fc\varepsilon RI\alpha$) or, less commonly, IgE itself (type II autoimmunity).[26] Enzyme-linked immunosorbent assay and immunodot tests are in development to measure anti-$Fc\varepsilon RI\alpha$ antibodies directly.[27,28] Autoantibodies induce mast cell and basophil degranulation, so patients can be screened using the autologous serum skin test (ASST)[29] or the *in vitro* basophil activation test (BAT). The ASST is nonspecific; evaluates serum histamine-releasing factors in general,

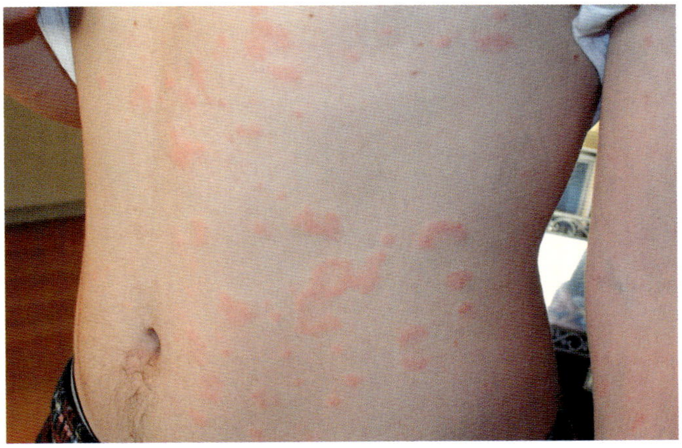

Fig. 20.7 Urticaria. Chronic urticaria in this teenager in association with autoimmune diseases type 1 diabetes and hypothyroidism. He failed to respond to treatment with antihistamines and required systemic corticosteroids and methotrexate for control.

not histamine-releasing autoantibodies; and is associated with a risk of infection. In the *in vitro* BAT, the demonstration of CD63 on the basophil surface by flow cytometry is a marker of histamine release[30,31] and distinguishes autoimmune from physical urticarias; it can also predict respond to cyclosporine versus omalizumab.[32,33] Patients may have autoimmune thyroid disease and, less commonly, celiac disease, type 1 diabetes, juvenile idiopathic arthritis, and systemic lupus erythematosus (Fig. 20.7).[34] Further investigation should be based on the known underlying causes, history, and examination and could include complete blood cell count, erythrocyte sedimentation rate, antinuclear antibody, CH50, free T4, thyroid-stimulating hormone, antithyroglobulin and antimicrosomal antibodies, and stool examination for parasites.

Reactions from food additives are unusual (overall in 9%), but elimination of an offending food or food additive leads to remission in 24 hours. Urticaria from food additives, artificial flavoring, or preservatives is not IgE mediated but rather is a pseudoallergic reaction and is often delayed (4 to 12 hours after ingestion).[35] Food avoidance correlates better with a positive history of food reactivity than with positive prick testing.[24] Among less common possible triggers of chronic urticaria are physical causes, drugs (especially aspirin and NSAIDs), immunizations, insect bites, inhalant or contact allergens, and infections (parasites,[36] *Helicobacter pylori*, *Chlamydia*, dental abscesses, sinus infections, low-grade urinary tract infection, and otitis).

In pediatric studies the rate of resolution of chronic urticaria is about 10% annually, with remission rates at 1, 3, and 5 years after the onset of chronic urticaria range from 16% to 18%, 39% to 54%, and 50% to 68%, respectively, regardless of whether the chronic urticaria is autoimmune.[25,37] In general, being female and older than 10 years of age are poorer prognostic signs. Time to remission is linked to disease activity, with high activity scores associated with longer time to remission.[38] In one study, chronic urticaria in children with positive BAT results (CD63 level $>$ 1.8) was twice as likely to resolve after 1 year versus in those with a negative BAT result,[39] suggesting that type 2 autoimmune urticaria (driven by IgG autoantibodies) resolves in children more quickly than type 1 autoimmune urticaria (driven by IgE autoantibodies).

Effective treatment of urticaria depends on identification of the causal factor and its elimination whenever possible.[40] First-line treatment in children is administration of a nonsedating histamine (H1) blocker such as cetirizine, loratadine, desloratadine, fexofenadine, levocetirizine, ebastine, rupatadine, or bilastine.[11,41–43] Dose escalation may then be required up to twofold to fourfold those used for management of allergic rhinitis, especially in children with chronic urticaria.[44,45] For chronic spontaneous urticaria, antihistamines are effective in about 50% of children. Addition of hydroxyzine, diphenhydramine, or another sedating H1 blocker at night may be considered but should not replace nonsedating antihistamines. Sedating antihistamines are best administered about 1 hour before bedtime to minimize daytime drowsiness. Paradoxical hyperactivity and irritability, which requires discontinuation of the medication, has occasionally been described in some infants and children with the administration of H1 blockers, especially diphenhydramine. Doxepin, a tricyclic antidepressant with H1- and H2-antagonistic effects, has also been used for the treatment of chronic urticaria but may lead to intolerable sleepiness. Approximately 80% of patients respond to antihistamines. Concomitant administration of an H2 blocker (such as famotidine or cimetidine) tends to be of limited value, but a leukotriene receptor antagonist (e.g., montelukast) can be considered if antihistamines are insufficient. Antihistamine administration should be continued for a few weeks after clearance of the urticaria with gradual tapering of the dosage to determine whether they are still needed for control. Avoidance of aspirin and NSAIDs may be helpful because these medications may exacerbate chronic urticaria.

Monthly administration of subcutaneous omalizumab (150 to 300 mg for adolescents, given every 4 weeks) is effective in 65% to 80% of those who do not respond to antihistamine.[46–50] Omalizumab is a monoclonal antibody that binds free serum IgE, inhibits IgE receptor activation, blocks antireceptor antibodies, and ultimately leads to unresponsiveness of cutaneous mast cells and basophils. Omalizumab has also been reported to be effective for physical urticarias, including cholinergic, cold, solar (see Chapter 19), heat, and delayed pressure types. Cyclosporine has a success rate of about 70% and is recommended as third-line care, given the potential side effects affecting blood pressure and renal function.[51] Cyclosporine inhibits both T cells and histamine release from basophils and mast cells.

Dapsone, methotrexate, mycophenolate mofetil, cyclophosphamide, hydroxychloroquine, sulfasalazine, intravenous immunoglobulin (IVIG), and plasmapheresis have all been used for resistant chronic urticaria but have less evidence than omalizumab and cyclosporine.[42,52–55] The subcutaneous administration of 0.1 to 0.5 mL of epinephrine 1:1000 is often effective for patients with angioedema and severe urticaria. Although often effective in patients with severe or persistent urticaria, administration of systemic corticosteroids should be reserved for acute reactivity in recalcitrant patients and should be limited to 10 days because of the many potential side effects.

Contact Urticaria

Urticaria may occur from skin exposure to antigen[56] rather than through ingestion or inhalation (Fig. 20.8). In this case the lesions tend to be localized to the site of contact, although rarely satellite lesions or even more generalized involvement has occurred. Infants and children with IgE-mediated food allergy may also have contact

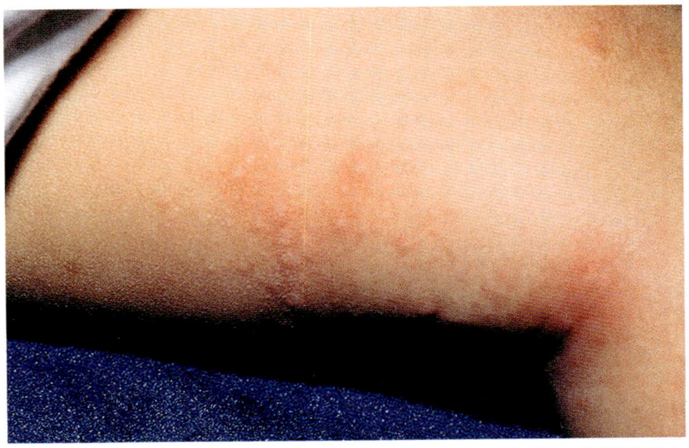

Fig. 20.8 Contact urticaria. Milk dripped on the thigh of this infant, leading to the rapid development of small wheals.

urticaria at sites of cutaneous exposure, such as on the face. In one study in which a drop of cow's milk was applied by the physician to the subject's healthy-appearing cheek ("finger test"), 45% of children with IgE-mediated cow's milk allergy developed a wheal and flare reaction within 20 minutes at the site of contact (37% of those without a history of atopic dermatitis and 71% of those with atopic dermatitis [AD]).[57] No child with non-IgE cow's milk allergy (i.e., with gastrointestinal symptoms, even with AD) or healthy controls developed contact urticaria.

Exposure to certain jellyfish, corals, caterpillars,[58] moths, and chemicals can lead to contact urticaria through pharmacologic means. Immunologic reactions can also result in contact urticaria, as often occurs with exposure to fish or latex. Localized small wheals have also been described after contact with the spines of pet hedgehogs.[59] Aquagenic urticaria is a variant of contact urticaria in which small urticarial papules arise at follicles after exposure to water.

Physical Urticarias

The physical urticarias are a group of disorders in which wheals occur in response to various physical stimuli.[60] These include dermographism and pressure, cholinergic, aquagenic, solar (see Chapter 19), and cold urticaria. Dermographism and cholinergic urticaria are quite common; cold urticaria is less common, and other patterns of physical urticaria are relatively rare. Challenge testing allows the diagnosis to be confirmed.[61]

Dermographism (dermatographism) is manifested by a sharply localized edematous or wheal reaction with a surrounding zone of erythema that occurs precisely at the site and within seconds of firm stroking of the skin (Fig. 20.9).[62] The wheal tends to be maximal in size and intensity at about 6 minutes after onset and persists for approximately 15 minutes. This common phenomenon, known as the *triple response of Lewis*, is often seen in infants, occurs in about 50% of children, and is noted in only about 1% of adolescents or adults. Nonsedating antihistamines and avoidance of triggers usually controls dermographism, but some patients require cyclosporine or narrow-band UVB.[63]

Pressure urticaria is a variant of dermographism, characterized by the development of hives or a deeper swelling simulating angioedema after local pressure, such as from clothing or jewelry, or weight bearing.[64] The reaction is often painful rather than pruritic and may occur immediately after the pressure or, more commonly, after a 4- to 6-hour delay ("delayed pressure urticaria").[64] Because of this delay in appearance, patients often fail to appreciate the cause of the disorder. The palms and soles are most commonly involved. Patients respond poorly to antihistamine therapy; some patients have responded to the leukotriene antagonist montelukast.[65]

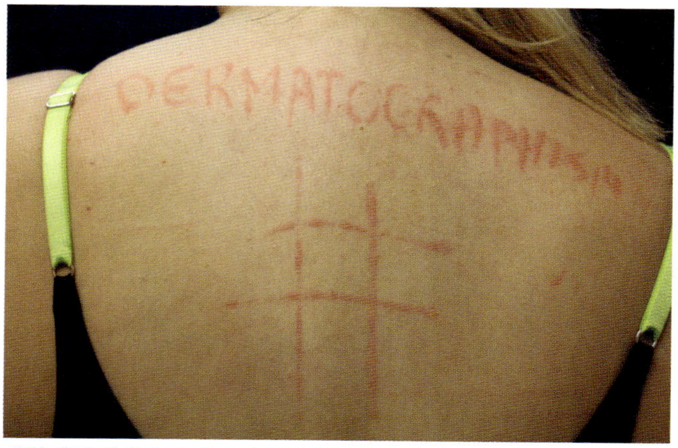

Fig. 20.9 Dermographism. Sharply localized edematous reaction with a surrounding zone of erythema that occurs precisely at the site and within seconds of firm stroking of the skin.

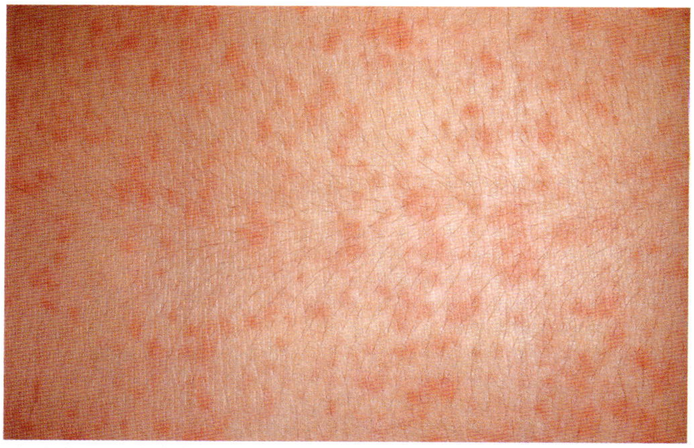

Fig. 20.10 Cholinergic urticaria. Discrete micropapular wheals are surrounded by a wide area of erythema and are induced by heat, exertion, or emotional stress.

Cholinergic urticaria (micropapular urticaria), which occurs in 5% to 7% of individuals with urticaria, is a very distinctive type.[66,67] It usually starts in adolescence and is associated with heat, exertion, or emotional stress. Cholinergic urticaria is characterized by a generalized eruption, especially on the trunk and arms, which consists of discrete, tiny wheals, 1 to 3 mm in diameter, with or without a surrounding area of erythema (Fig. 20.10). The wheals first appear within minutes after sweating begins and occasionally are accompanied by exercise-induced bronchospasm, headache, gastrointestinal discomfort, and faintness. The duration of the eruption varies from 30 minutes to several hours; after an episode, a refractory period of about 24 hours ensues. A subset of patients with cholinergic urticaria have hypohidrosis or anhidrosis.[68]

Acetylcholine is thought to participate in the pathomechanism of wheal formation, but immediate type skin responses to one's own sweat have been described. Once cholinergic urticaria occurs, the condition may recur for periods of months to years and then tends toward spontaneous improvement and resolution. Provocation tests for the diagnosis of cholinergic urticaria should be performed by increasing the body temperature through exercise (treadmill or stationary bicycle) or the use of a hot bath (42° C for 15 minutes). Treatment consists of H1 nonsedating antihistamines, which may need to be increased up to fourfold. Approximately 50% respond to this regimen. Addition of H2 blockade and/or montelukast may be helpful. Some patients have responded to omalizumab.[69] Other studies have demonstrated the efficacy of anticholinergic agents,[70] the addition of propranolol (β2-adrenergic blocker), and treatment and injection with botulinum toxin. Potential precipitating factors and avoidance of heat, excessive exertion, and excitement that leads to sweating should be avoided whenever feasible.

Aquagenic urticaria, a disorder that resembles cholinergic urticaria, occurs most often in adolescence and is characterized by small, intensely pruritic, perifollicular papular wheals with surrounding erythema (Fig. 20.11). The palms and soles are spared. The disorder is precipitated by contact with water or perspiration (irrespective of temperature). Exercise and other cholinergic factors do not precipitate this disorder. Patients can drink water without adverse reaction. Salt-dependent aquagenic urticaria is a subtype in which the children react primarily or exclusively when there is exposure to saltwater.[71] Antihistamines often improve reactivity but do not totally suppress it.

Cold urticaria accounts for approximately 3% of chronic urticaria and has been documented in infants as young as 6 months.[72] The urticarial reaction develops within a few minutes or hours after exposure to cold air or water, often on rewarming. It is classified as localized (type 1; 67% of patients), generalized (type 2; 14%), or with angioedema or anaphylaxis (type 3; 19%). Type 3 reactions usually occur with water immersion (swimming) but have also been reported with ingestion of cold food or beverages or exposure to cold air.

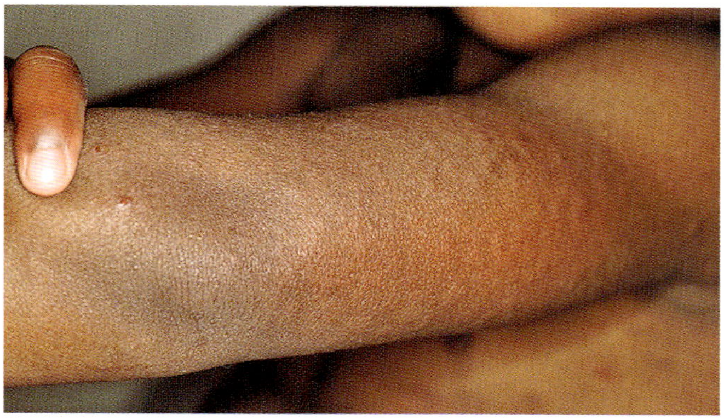

Fig. 20.11 Aquagenic urticaria. Small, intensely pruritic, perifollicular papular wheals with surrounding erythema that occur after contact with water or perspiration, regardless of temperature.

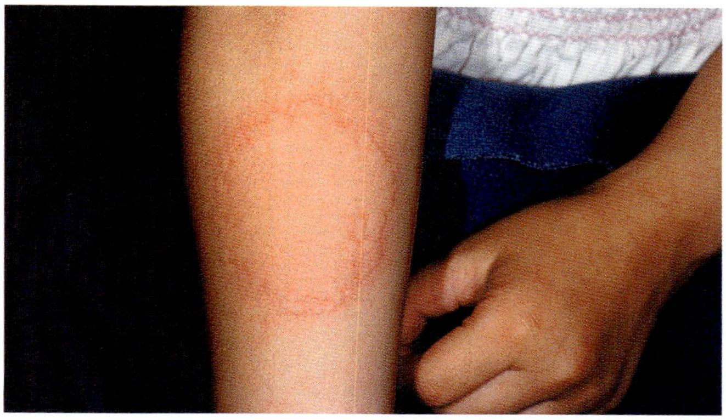

Fig. 20.12 Cold urticaria. Application of an ice pack to an extremity for 2 to 10 minutes can induce a wheal.

In highly sensitive individuals the urticarial reaction may be associated with respiratory or cardiovascular compromise, hypotension and, on occasion, syncope, loss of consciousness, and drowning.[73] Respiratory signs such as nasal stuffiness, cough, and dyspnea and oral or gastrointestinal symptoms such as swelling of the lips, swelling of the oral mucous membranes, dysphagia, and abdominal cramps may occur. Patients who experience oropharyngeal reactions to cool liquids or foods (especially lip swelling) are at increased risk for the development of systemic reactions.

Cold urticaria in children and adolescents is usually acquired, occurs more often in girls, and often appears suddenly. Anaphylaxis has been described in up to 30% at presentation.[74] Once symptoms develop, they are generally short-lived and recurrences usually disappear after a few months or years. Secondary forms of cold urticaria may also be associated with cold hemolysin and cold agglutinin syndromes. These forms, generally seen in adults, cause Raynaud phenomenon, acrocyanosis, and cutaneous ulcers. Some cases of cold urticaria manifested by itching, erythema, purpura, atypical Raynaud phenomenon, and ulceration are the result of cryoglobulins (see Chapter 21).

Cold urticaria can rarely be a manifestation of familial cold autoinflammatory syndrome (FCAS), an autosomal dominant disorder resulting from mutations in *CIAS1/NLRP3* (see Chapter 25). It is characterized by an urticarial or papular eruption, fever, chills, arthralgia, and sometimes headache, malaise, muscle tenderness, and significant leukocytosis. Patients more commonly complain of burning or stinging than of pruritus. Although the tendency to familial cold urticaria generally persists for life, the severity may decrease with advancing age. It generally develops after a latent period of several hours, and once it develops, it may persist for up to 48 hours. Familial atypical cold urticaria (FACU) is an autosomal dominant disorder with onset during childhood in which the urticaria and/or angioedema develop shortly after cold exposure (not delayed). Cold-stimulation testing is negative (no wheal), and in contrast with FCAS, patients do not have fever, chills, or joint complaints.[75] PLCG2 (phospholipase C gamma 2)–associated antibody deficiency and immune dysregulation (PLAID) is an autosomal dominant immunodeficiency syndrome associated with evaporative cold urticaria.[76,77] The cold urticaria presents within the first year in all patients and is characterized as pruritic blotchy macules but not true wheals; ice cube testing is negative. Patients may develop ulcerative lesions of the nasal tip, and occasionally fingers and toes, during the neonatal period that heal by infancy. They tend to develop granulomatous dermatitis, which may be widespread.[77] Recurrent sinopulmonary infections, common variable immunodeficiency (CVID), and autoantibodies (especially antinuclear and antithyroid antibodies) are commonly associated.

The diagnosis of cold urticaria requires a careful history and investigation for other possible causal factors. The diagnosis may be confirmed by reproducing signs through local application of an ice cube for periods of 2 to 10 minutes with observation after removal for at least 10 minutes. The best areas for this testing are the face, neck, and particularly the arms (Fig. 20.12). Results are positive, however, only in 70% of those tested. Although a positive test result is associated with an increased risk of anaphylaxis, in one study 12% of patients with anaphylaxis had a negative cold stimulation test.[72] Some patients fail to respond to ice but do respond to cold water or generalized cooling of the body. Critical temperature threshold testing shows an inverse relationship with disease severity and activity, which can be helpful for assessing both the severity and the impact of therapy.[78] Cold urticaria should be distinguished from cold-induced cholinergic urticaria, in which cholinergic urticaria occurs while exercising in the cold and is not induced by ice cube testing. Immediate ice cube tests also tend to be negative with FCAS, FACU, and PLAID syndromes.

Underlying disorders are rare in children. Cryoglobulinemia, cryofibrinogenemia, and cold agglutinins have all been reported, particularly in adults, and can reflect an underlying diagnosis of essential mixed cryoglobulinemia, hepatitis, autoimmune disease, or lymphoma. Cold urticaria can also be associated with infectious disorders (toxoplasmosis, Epstein–Barr virus [EBV], *H. pylori*, hepatitis C, and human immunodeficiency virus [HIV]) and autoimmune disease (particularly lupus erythematosus or celiac disease).

Patients with cold urticaria, and particularly with severe or widespread urticarial reactions, should carry epinephrine and be forewarned of the risk of drowning after loss of consciousness when swimming or bathing in cold water. The treatment of cold urticaria is aided by oral administration of antihistamines, particularly nonsedating H1 blockers, although the sedating antihistamine cyproheptadine is also particularly helpful for cold urticaria, and leukotriene receptor antagonists have been used adjunctively. Increases in doses of nonsedating antihistamine to four times the standard dosages have shown additional benefit (versus standard dosing) without increased adverse events.[79] For those patients who are unresponsive to systemic antihistamines, treatment with omalizumab appears to be helpful in almost 50%, suggesting a role for IgE.[80–83] Desensitization to cold is an alternative that is now rarely performed; an extremity is gradually cooled in cold water for 5 to 10 minutes per day with a gradual increase in the time of exposure and decrease of the temperature over a period of weeks or months. This treatment is not regularly effective and must be done cautiously to minimize the risk of systemic reaction. Patients with cold urticaria as a manifestation of an autoinflammatory syndrome often require interleukin (IL)–1 blockers (e.g., anakinra) for response.[84,85]

Anaphylaxis

Anaphylaxis is a life-threatening, immediate hypersensitivity reaction to the administration of an antigen that has previously produced a specific sensitization.[86] It is characterized within minutes to 1 hour after injection or ingestion of antigen by pruritus of the palms, soles, and scalp, urticaria, and/or angioedema with systemic signs (weakness, dyspnea, hypotension, and circulatory collapse). Mucosal involvement of the airway leads to acute respiratory distress, and swelling of the gastrointestinal mucosa can result in abdominal pain, vomiting, or diarrhea. The incidence in children and adolescents is 10.5 episodes per 100,000 person-years, and most children have a personal history of atopy. Anaphylaxis can occur during infancy,[87] although the risk peaks during early childhood and decreases thereafter.[88] A biphasic reaction may occur, with recurrence usually within 8 hours of the initial episode. Anaphylactic reactions most often occur after ingestion of foods,[89,90] especially peanuts, cow's milk, and hen's eggs in children (versus wheat and shellfish in adults), or in response to drugs or insect venom.[91,92] Anaphylactic reactions to latex and peanuts are particularly troublesome, because they are so ubiquitous in the environment. Having asthma as well as IgE-mediated food allergy increases the risk of developing food-induced anaphylaxis. Exercise-induced anaphylaxis may also occur and is commonly food dependent. Two subtypes have been described: nonspecific food-dependent exercise-induced anaphylaxis, in which filling the stomach before exercise is responsible, regardless of the kind of food ingested, and specific food-dependent exercise-induced anaphylaxis, an IgE-mediated food allergy in which anaphylaxis only occurs in combination with exercise. Several types of foods have been described to trigger exercise-induced anaphylaxis, but wheat appears to be most common.[93]

LATEX ALLERGY

Latex allergy is a reaction to a peptide in natural rubber and occurs most commonly in children with spina bifida, presumably as a result of the frequent exposure to catheters and latex gloves.[94] The use of latex-free or latex-safe equipment has markedly lowered the risk to children with spina bifida.[95,96] Atopic children also show an increased risk of latex allergy,[97] with up to 4% showing prick test reactivity.[98] Type I hypersensitivity reactions to latex may range from contact urticaria to life-threatening anaphylaxis. Severe anaphylactic shock without cutaneous erythema or urticaria has been described.[99] Type I reactions to latex differ from the type IV contact dermatitis reaction to antigens in rubber products (see Chapter 3). Children with type I hypersensitivity reactions often experience lip swelling after sucking on a pacifier or blowing up a balloon (Table 20.2). Aerosolized powder from latex gloves and inhalation may lead to runny nose, sneezing, itchy, swollen eyes, and wheezing in susceptible individuals. Approximately half of persons who react to latex show reactivity to certain foods, resulting in oral mucosal pruritus, urticaria, and wheezing; bananas, kiwis, avocados, and chestnuts contain proteins that cross-react with latex and are most commonly associated.[100]

Skin prick testing is most likely to yield positive responses to either latex or cross-reacting foods. Serum latex-specific IgE by ImmunoCAP can also be used to detect type I reactivity to latex, but the high rate of false positives should be taken into account when making a diagnosis of latex allergy in patients with pollen allergy (30%), especially in those sensitized to more than one pollen species.[101] Avoidance of latex and related triggers is critical, and nonlatex substitutes such as Mylar balloons and vinyl or neoprene gloves are generally available. Desensitization is the only effective way to resolve latex allergy; percutaneous and sublingual approaches appear to be safer than subcutaneous administration.[102]

Table 20.2 Examples of Latex Products in Household and Medical Use

Household	Medical
Balloons	Adhesive tape
Balls (basketball, Koosh, squash, tennis)	Bandages
Cell phone cases	Blood pressure cuffs
Computer mouse pads	Bulb syringes
Condoms	Catheters
Disposable diapers/rubber pants	Dental devices
Erasers	Electrode pads
Gloves for dishwashing	Face masks and their straps
Pacifiers, nipples	Gloves
Rubber bands	Injection ports
Rubber cement	Rubber syringe stoppers
Rubber raincoats and rubber boots	Stethoscope tubing
Shoe soles	Tourniquets
Socks with elastic	Vial stoppers
Sports equipment	Wound drains
Swimming masks and goggles	
Toys	
Underwear	

NUT ALLERGY

Nut-induced anaphylaxis is a risk in the 1.1% of individuals who are allergic to peanuts and tree nuts[103,104] and has resulted in 50 to 100 deaths annually in the United States. Screening tests such as prick tests and radioallergosorbent tests (RASTs) are suggestive, but only food challenge confirms reactivity. Avoidance of peanuts is extremely difficult, and there has been no means to protect against accidental ingestion, which often occurs despite reassurance from servers.[105] Allergic reactions through kissing are well documented, particularly in adolescents.[106] In one study, 13% of subjects still had detectable levels of peanut 1 hour after ingestion of 2 tablespoons of peanut butter on a sandwich.[107]

Although prenatal and postnatal avoidance of peanuts was encouraged for at-risk individuals in the past, current practices include early exposure to peanut to cause tolerance.[108,109] In a landmark trial of 500 infants at risk for peanut allergy, infants who avoided peanuts had a much higher risk of developing allergy than those who were given small numbers of peanuts regularly, regardless of whether they were sensitized to peanuts at baseline.[109,110] Guidelines recommend that infants with severe atopic dermatitis, egg allergy, or both be evaluated by specific IgE (sIgE) measurement and/or skin prick testing (SPT) and oral food challenge, if necessary)[111]; if peanut sIgE is less than 0.35 and/or SPT yields a 0- to 2-mm reaction, peanut can be introduced as early as 4 to 6 months of age (recommended is 6 to 7 g of peanut protein per week, divided into at least three feedings weekly; it should be introduced before 11 months of age). If the SPT measures 3 to 7 mm, peanut can be introduced in a supervised office setting or oral food challenge can be performed. For those with sIgE 0.35 or greater and/or SPT 8 mm or larger, referral to a specialist for continued evaluation and management is recommended. Infants with mild to moderate atopic dermatitis do not have to undergo this testing but should have peanut introduction as early as 6 months, whereas those without atopic dermatitis or food allergy can have peanut introduction that is age appropriate and according to family preferences.

For those with early evidence of peanut sensitization and allergy, immunotherapy has shown promise. Early oral immunotherapy (E-OIT), given for a median of 29 months in children 9 to 36 months of age with peanut allergy, led to sustained unresponsiveness to peanuts in oral food challenge at 4 weeks after stopping the E-OIT in 78% of those of those tested.[112] Other oral immunotherapy studies have similarly shown benefit in most children.

Omalizumab substantially increases the threshold of sensitivity to peanuts and may protect against unintended ingestion.[113] Oral immunotherapy with gradual increases in exposure to peanuts can decrease basophil activation, titrated skin prick tests, and peanut-specific IgE levels within 6 months.[114]

The treatment of anaphylaxis consists of the intravenous administration of antihistamines such as diphenhydramine (1.25 mg/kg), subcutaneous epinephrine (the adult-dose epinephrine autoinjector contains 0.3 mg of epinephrine as 0.3 mL of epinephrine 1:1000, and the pediatric-dose autoinjector contains 0.15 mg of epinephrine as

0.3 mL of epinephrine 1:2000) for grade 2 anaphylaxis or higher,[115] and sometimes intravenous corticosteroid.[116,117] Epinephrine is the only medication shown to be lifesaving when administered promptly, but it is underused.[118] Patients should have easy access to at least two doses of an epinephrine autoinjector, with thorough training regarding correct use of a given device and an emergency action plan. In addition to EpiPen, Auvi-Q is an autoinjector available that provides audio and visual cues regarding patient use and was found favorable to the traditional autoinjector for method of instruction, preference to carry, and device size.[119]

Because of the delay in onset of effectiveness, oral medications are not indicated. If hypotension is present, intravenous fluids should be initiated to permit the rapid administration of plasma volume expanders, fluids, and electrolytes. Once shock is overcome and oral fluids are well tolerated, oral corticosteroids may be initiated. Anyone at risk for anaphylaxis should wear a medical alert bracelet and carry epinephrine in case of emergency. Management of anaphylaxis in schools has recently received attention, especially because of its distinct challenges and the need to be able to urgently administer epinephrine.

Angioedema

The term *angioedema* (also called *giant urticaria* or *Quincke edema*) describes swelling of the eyelids, hands, feet, genitalia, the lips, tongue, airway, and gastrointestinal tract.[120,121] A 2018 classification included angioedema within the spectrum of urticaria.[11] Angioedema results from vasodilation, increased tissue permeability, and subsequent interstitial edema. These changes can occur because of mast cell or basophil degranulation with release of vasoactive molecules (histamine, leukotrienes, prostaglandin D2, platelet-activating factor) as an IgE-mediated type I hypersensitivity reaction or through direct cell degranulation. Alternatively, these changes can occur because of upregulated kinin pathway activation (increases in bradykinin) with loss of vascular endothelial cadherin in endothelial tight junctions and water movement to the extracellular space.

When it occurs in association with wheals, angioedema is a feature of urticaria. Fifty percent of patients with angioedema also show urticaria, and 10% of infants and children with urticaria show at least mild angioedema. Angioedema may also be a component of anaphylactic reactions. Angioedema with urticaria and/or pruritus is typically seen with IgE-mediated reactions, although urticaria is absent in 10% to 15% of patients with angioedema from an allergic cause. As with urticaria, chronic angioedema in children is often idiopathic and triggered by bacterial or viral infection. Most cases of idiopathic acquired angioedema are histamine responsive (histaminergic; termed *idiopathic histaminergic acquired angioedema* [IH-AAE]), and medications (especially aspirin and NSAIDs), allergens, and physical agents have also been implicated. Some patients with chronic angioedema may have IgG antibodies directed against the IgE receptor or IgE itself *(autoimmune angioedema)*.

In one retrospective study, NSAIDs were the trigger for angioedema in 21% of 16 to 21 year olds (versus only 2% in preschool years),[122] reminding of the need to inquire about use of over-the-counter products, including intermittently. In another study, 6% of children with angioedema unrelated to urticaria found NSAID use as the trigger,[123] and atopy increases the risk.[124] More than 80% of hypersensitive children may cross-react on challenge with another NSAID.

Angioedema without urticaria has been classified by the European Academy of Allergy and Clinical Immunology into four acquired and three autosomal dominant hereditary forms.[125] Two of the three acquired forms (induced by angiotensin-converting enzyme inhibitors and a nongenetic form of C1-INH deficiency) usually occur in adults.

Diagnostic evaluation should involve acquiring history of potential triggers (foods, recent infection, over-the-counter and prescription medications, exercise, response to heat and pressure, bites or stings, allergens, stress). Asking about occurrence of angioedema in the family, whether associated with wheals or pruritus, and response to antihistamine/steroid intervention is also important in considering hereditary angioneurotic edema. In most cases of angioedema, allergy testing and laboratory evaluation are not needed. The lip swelling of more chronic angioedema can be confused with the enlarged lips seen in children with inflammatory bowel disease, especially Crohn's disease, or that of granulomatous cheilitis (see Chapter 25). In addition, allergic contact dermatitis involving the face is sometimes mistaken for acute facial angioedema, although the associated dermatitis distinguishes the conditions. "Factitious" angioedema in children in association with psychiatric disease has also been described.[126]

Treatment of acute angioedema is focused on elimination of triggers (if possible) and administration of nonsedating H1 antihistamines,[127] which can be prescribed at up to four times standard dosing with minimal side effects. Next-step management is the addition of sedating first-generation antihistamines, H2 antihistamines, and leukotriene inhibitors. Immunomodulators are only considered if the child fails to respond to at least twice-daily dosing with nonsedating antihistamine plus a sedating antihistamine at night. Cyclosporine and omalizumab are most commonly used in children (especially as young as 9 and 12 years old, respectively). Alternatives are dapsone, methotrexate, sulfasalazine, and colchicine, but experience has largely been in adults. Systemic steroids are not used for chronic management.

C1 Inhibitor–Hereditary Angioneurotic Edema

Hereditary angioneurotic edema (HAE; hereditary angioedema), which occurs in approximately 1 in 50,000 to 1 in 10,000 persons,[128] is characterized by recurrent episodes of nonpruritic, nonerythematous edema of the subcutaneous tissue, particularly the hands, feet, and face, and of the gastrointestinal and/or upper respiratory tracts.[129,130] Most commonly, HAE results from a mutation in *SERPING1*, leading to haploinsufficiency of C1 inhibitor (C1-INH; type 1 HAE), the serine protease that inhibits proteases involved in the bradykinin pathway. Interestingly, levels are usually 5% to 30% of normal, despite having one normal allele. In about 15% of cases there is a mutation in *SERPING1* (usually a specific missense mutation in exon 8) that leads to C1-INH dysfunction (type 2 HAE). Deficiency or dysfunction of C1-INH leads to transient episodes of increased vascular permeability with increased cleavage of C4 by C1, depleting C4 levels. The major factor responsible for edema formation is now known to be bradykinin, which can induce leakage of postcapillary venules. Bradykinin is produced when high-molecular-weight kininogen is cleaved by plasma kallikrein, the activity of which is controlled by C1-INH. Less often, C1-INH function is normal (type 3 HAE). In most of these cases, heterozygous mutations are found in *F12*, encoding factor XII, a coagulation factor.[131] The clinical features of deficiency of C1-INH and deficiency of factor XII HAE) are similar,[132] and laboratory testing is required to distinguish these disorders. More recently, families with type 3 HAE have been found with a mutation in *PLG*,[132] encoding plasminogen, and an additional family with type 3 HAE had a mutation in *ANGPT1*,[133] encoding angiopoietin-1 protein, which maintains permeability of the vascular endothelial barrier.

The earliest symptoms of HAE often begin in infancy or early childhood, with 50% of cases manifesting before the age of 10 years. The frequency and severity of attacks are typically exacerbated during adolescence and subside in the fifth decade. Onset during the first decade is associated with greater severity.[134] Based on survey data, prodromes have been described in 82.5% to 95.7% of patients surveyed, most commonly involving the skin or gastrointestinal tract and hours to days before the onset of angioedema; fewer than 10% reported were rarely or never able to predict an attack.[135] Affected individuals are prone to sudden attacks of circumscribed subcutaneous edema (angioedema). In children the extremities (especially upper) and face are most often affected, and swelling may be severe enough to cause remarkable disfiguration of the affected parts. Areas of swelling may migrate, but the condition generally subsides 24 to 72 hours after onset. Several weeks of remission generally follow attacks. The skin and mucosal lesions may appear spontaneously or may be precipitated by minor trauma, especially dental work or surgery,[136] strenuous exercise, infection (especially of the airway), menses, pregnancy, administration of oral contraceptives or angiotensin-converting enzyme inhibitors, extremes of temperature, or emotional disturbances. There is no pitting, discoloration, pain, or itching associated with the edema. Urticaria is not associated, but up to 50% of affected children show a nonpruritic serpiginous or reticulated eruption that resembles erythema marginatum.[137] The erythema marginatum–like eruption may even be present in the neonatal period and should prompt evaluation of HAE if appropriate.

Gastrointestinal involvement is the presenting sign in 40% to 80% of affected children.[138] The recurrent colic and severe abdominal pain can simulate the acute abdominal pain of appendicitis. Nausea, vomiting, and diarrhea are additional complaints. Abdominal ultrasound may demonstrate edematous swelling of the intestinal wall and free peritoneal fluid. Involvement of the mucous membranes of the hypopharynx and larynx, although seen less often, may be particularly devastating; up to 25% of patients experience asphyxia, which is the leading cause of death and usually occurs during the third decade of life.

Diagnosis of HAE can be confirmed by the finding (at least twice and separated by 1 to 3 months) of reduced levels of C4 or C1-INH (quantitative and/or functional), or both. For those with C1-INH deficiency, levels tend to be 10% to 40% of normal, reflecting the haploinsufficiency.

Antihistamines and corticosteroids have not been effective in the management of HAE patients. Epinephrine is beneficial in the control of swelling in few patients. Tracheostomy commonly is lifesaving in patients with laryngeal obstruction. Management is classified as treating the acute attack (on-demand therapy), short-term prophylaxis (preprocedural), and long-term prophylaxis.[129] Treatment for on-demand therapy (which the most common need for pediatric patients) is focused on either replacement of C1-INH or inhibiting the synthesis or activity of bradykinin.[130,139]

In general, attacks tend to be less frequent and less severe in children, and most will not require long-term prophylaxis. However, prophylactic C1-INH administration with dosage escalation may be considered for children with more than two attacks per month, the need for acute treatment more than once annually, or more than one episode of severe abdominal pain in a year.[147,148]

As prevention, children and adolescents with HAE should not participate in contact sports, and toddlers should not attend daycare before kindergarten to minimize the risk of infection that could trigger attacks. Even the eruption of teeth and minor mechanical trauma can induce edema formation. If menstruation worsens HAE symptoms, long-term prophylactic doses can be increased, but oral contraceptives are triggers of the angioedema and should be avoided. Although use of angiotensin-converting enzyme inhibitor is unusual in children, these medications can exacerbate the signs of angioedema in affected individuals and should be avoided.[153]

Scombroid and Ciguatera Fish Poisoning

Scombroid fish poisoning (scombrotoxism) is a clinical syndrome that results from the ingestion of spoiled fish of the Scombridae family (tuna, mackerel, and bonito) and fish such as bluefish, mahi-mahi, amberjack, herring, sardines, and anchovies.[154,155] The disorder, thought to be related to high levels of histamine and saurine produced when these fish are improperly refrigerated, is characterized by pruritus; a diffuse erythema of the face and upper body,[156] somewhat resembling a sunburn; and, at times, giant hive-like lesions that develop within minutes to hours after ingestion of the toxic fish. Bacteria in the fish express a decarboxylase that converts histidine to histamine, which resists cooking and freezing. Symptoms resemble a histamine reaction and commonly include a hot, burning sensation rather than pruritus. The conjunctivae are often markedly injected, and many patients have a severe throbbing headache, tachycardia, palpitations, nausea, vomiting, abdominal cramps, diarrhea, dryness and a burning sensation or peppery taste in the mouth, urticaria, angioneurotic edema, oral blistering, hypotension, blurred vision, and asthma-like symptoms. Although superficially resembling an allergic reaction, patients with scombroid fish poisoning can be reassured that they do not have fish allergy and that scombroidosis will not occur when fish are handled properly. Symptoms are generally self-limiting and even if untreated tend to resolve within 8 to 10 hours. Treatment is supportive, and most patients treated with oral antihistamines become asymptomatic within 2 or 3 hours.

In contrast to scombroid fish poisoning, ciguatera fish poisoning is a common disorder endemic throughout the Caribbean and Indo-Pacific islands but has been reported in the United States. It is caused by the ingestion of ciguatoxin,[155] which originates from a dinoflagellate *(Gambierdiscus toxicus)*. Present in certain fish such as the red snapper, amberjack, and sturgeon, ingestion of affected fish (whether cooked, raw, or frozen) may result in this disorder. Clinical symptoms, which usually appear within 12 hours but sometimes within minutes after ingestion of ciguatoxin, include abdominal pain, cramping, diarrhea, nausea, vomiting, paresthesias, pain or burning when cold water is touched, arthralgia, myalgia, and, in severe cases, hypotension, shock, respiratory depression, paralysis, coma, and death. The duration of illness averages 8.5 days but may be prolonged. Treatment consists of supportive measures, and intravenous mannitol has been found to be extremely effective, lessening the neurologic and muscular dysfunction of affected patients within minutes of administration.[157]

Serum Sickness and Serum Sickness–Like Reactions

Serum sickness is an allergic reaction characterized by a cutaneous eruption (morbilliform, urticarial, or purpuric),[158,159] malaise, fever, lymphadenopathy splenomegaly, proteinuria, and arthralgias.[160] The skin rash (90%), arthritis (52%), and fever (41%) occur most often.[161] The syndrome, originally noted and most commonly seen after the administration of antiserum of horse or rabbit origin, is now rarely encountered. However, serum sickness–like reactions (SSLRs) occasionally occur in children, especially 1 to 3 weeks after exposure to cefaclor, which has been described in approximately 0.2% of treated children.[162,163] Penicillins (especially amoxicillin),[164] tetracyclines,[165] cefprozil, sulfonamides, macrolides,[166] ciprofloxacin, rifampin,[167] griseofulvin,[168] itraconazole, fluoxetine, bupropion,[169] rituximab,[170,171] omalizumab[172], and influenza vaccine[173] have also been implicated as triggers of SSLR.[3] SSLR more closely resembles urticaria (or urticaria multiforme) than true serum sickness (Figs. 20.13 and 20.14), and lesions commonly show large areas of lilac or violaceous discoloration, especially centrally (Fig. 20.15). This classic observation has led to use of the term *purple urticaria* to describe the skin lesions seen in SSLR. Noncutaneous features most commonly include fever, malaise, lymphadenopathy, and arthralgias with periarticular swelling, particularly symmetrically involving the knees and metacarpophalangeal joints (Fig. 20.16). True arthritis is uncommon and seen significantly less often than in patients with true serum sickness. Affected children may also demonstrate facial edema, eosinophilia, headache, myalgia, and gastrointestinal symptoms, but renal and neurologic disease is rarely associated. Histologic evaluation of biopsy section may reveal vasculitis associated with cutaneous deposition of immune complexes, but hypocomplementemia and circulating immune complexes, as seen in true serum sickness, are absent.

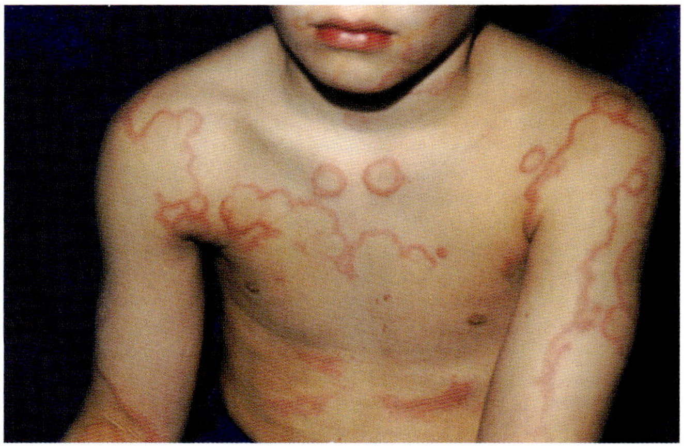

Fig. 20.13 Serum sickness–like reaction. Urticarial wheals occurred 2 weeks after exposure to cefaclor.

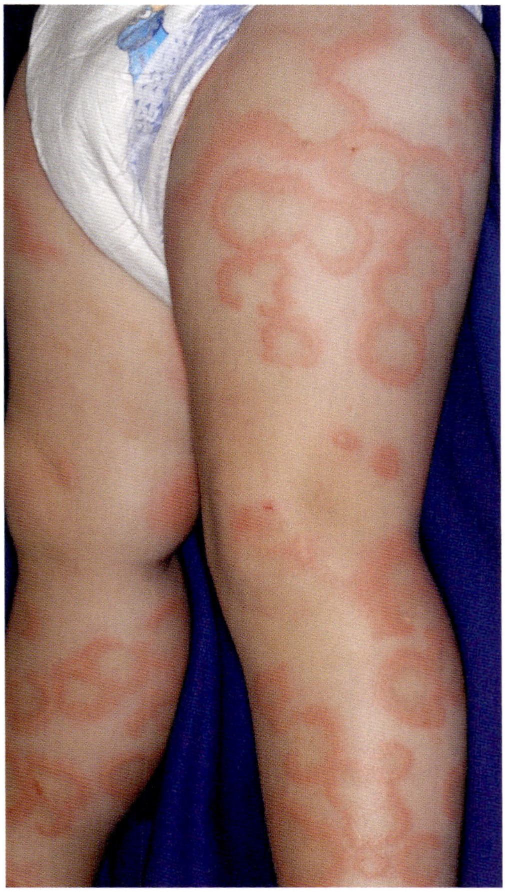

Fig. 20.14 Serum sickness–like reaction. Serpiginous and annular lesions that persisted more than 24 hours in a reaction to amoxicillin.

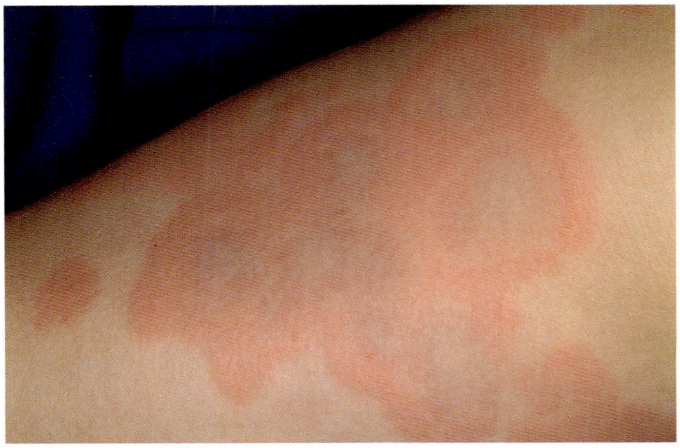

Fig. 20.15 Serum sickness–like reaction (SSLR). Note the central lilac discoloration, similar to that of erythema multiforme and typical of SSLR. This girl developed the reaction after 10 days of amoxicillin.

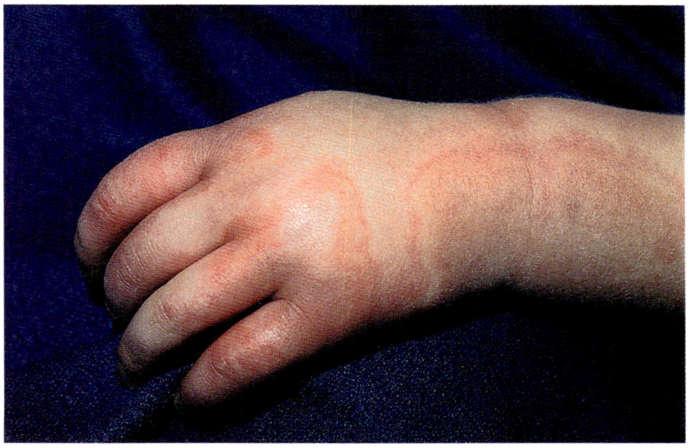

Fig. 20.16 Serum sickness–like reaction (SSLR). Note the swollen hand and large urticarial wheals in this girl with SSLR and arthralgias.

SSLR generally is a self-limiting disease that subsides within 2 to 3 weeks after discontinuation of the causative agent. In the case of cefaclor, biotransformation of the parent drug, genetic defects in metabolism of reactive intermediates, and increased *in vitro* lymphocyte cytotoxicity have been thought to participate.[174] SSLR has been described as well in association with other drugs,[160] infection with hepatitis B or C, and immunization against hepatitis B, rabies, and tetanus toxoid. Treatment with antihistamines, NSAIDs, and, if severe, a short course of systemic corticosteroids helps alleviate symptoms. In general, the risk of cross-reaction among β-lactam antibiotics is low, and patients who have reacted to cefaclor or cefprozil will usually tolerate other cephalosporins.

Exanthematous Eruptions

The most common drug eruptions are morbilliform or exanthematous eruptions, characterized by erythematous macules or papules (Figs. 20.17 and 20.18). The risk of this type of eruption is increased by viral infection, such as the near 100% incidence of an exanthematous reaction in patients taking penicillin who have EBV infection, or the increased risk of drug reactions in patients taking sulfonamides who have HIV infection.

Most commonly, an exanthematous eruption begins 7 to 14 days after initiation of a new medication and sometimes after drug discontinuation. If an individual is rechallenged after an initial course of taking a medication, the reaction may develop within a few days. Most commonly, the eruption is symmetric and begins initially on the trunk before becoming generalized. Mucous membranes are usually spared, but palms and soles are often involved. Patients may experience varying degrees of associated pruritus, and some have low-grade fever. Not uncommonly the eruption turns more of a brownish-red color in 7 to 14 days and may desquamate.

Penicillins, sulfonamides, cephalosporins, and antiepileptics are the most likely categories of drugs to cause exanthematous reactions. Viral exanthems tend to be indistinguishable from exanthematous drug eruptions and more commonly occur in pediatric patients. Eosinophilia favors a diagnosis of drug reaction; biopsy is generally not helpful. More severe drug reactions may be heralded by facial edema or marked eosinophilia, as in systemic hypersensitivity syndrome, or by mucous membrane lesions and dusky skin, as in SJS or toxic epidermal necrosis.

Treatment is largely supportive. The decision to discontinue a drug must be made based on the need for continuing the medication. Many patients will show clearance of the eruption despite continuation of medication (e.g., when an infant with otitis is treated with amoxicillin). However, patients may show progression to erythroderma. Desensitization has been used for reactions to sulfonamides in patients with HIV infection. Given the many nonallergic causes of morbilliform exanthematous reactions from use of β-lactams, oral drug provocation testing (with exposure to increasing amounts of the antibiotic) under direct physician supervision should be considered to exclude true allergy, especially for older children and adults with maculopapular and nonimmediate urticarial exanthems.

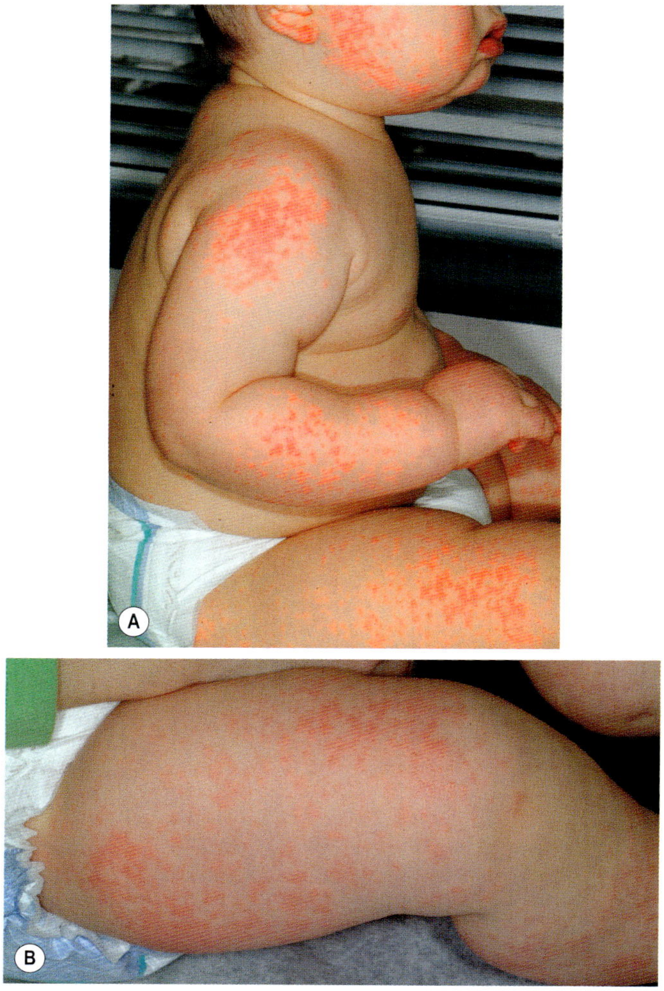

Fig. 20.17 Exanthematous drug reaction. (A, B) Erythematous papules in an infant administered amoxicillin for otitis media. Given the distribution, a viral exanthema (Gianotti–Crosti) would also be considered.

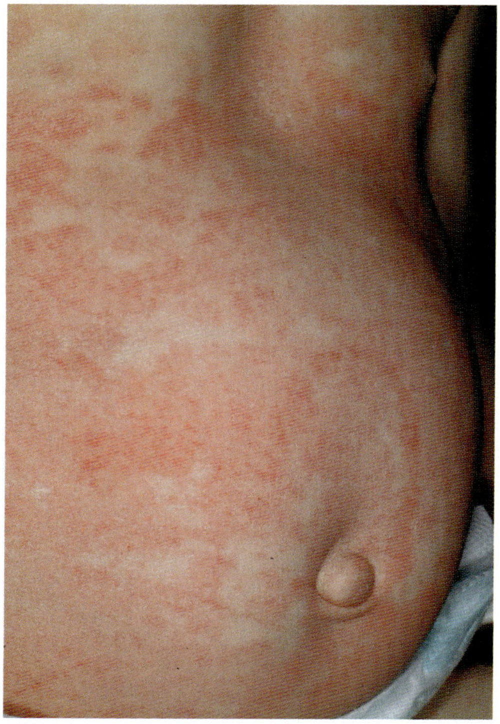

Fig. 20.18 Exanthematous drug reaction. Confluence of erythematous macules from administration of cefdinir.

Drug Reaction with Eosinophilia and Systemic Symptoms

DRESS syndrome, which is also called *drug hypersensitivity syndrome* (DHS), presents as an exanthematous drug reaction in association with fever, facial swelling, conjunctivitis, and often internal organ involvement that leads to mortality in 10% of patients.[175–177] The clinical manifestations of DRESS syndrome typically begin 1 to 6 weeks after initiation of a responsible medication.

Fever and malaise often appear first and may be seen in association with cervical lymphadenopathy and pharyngitis. The cutaneous eruption occurs in approximately 75% of patients. It often starts on the face with edema, especially periorbital, then erythema and pruritus (Fig. 20.19). The erythema then spreads caudally. The exanthematous eruption raises concern about SJS or TEN; the lack of mucosal involvement in DRESS can be a useful distinguishing feature.

Of visceral sites of involvement, the liver is most common (about 50%), and the hepatitis may be fulminant, leading to death. Lymphadenopathy is often seen, and patients may complain of joint pain. Inflammation of the kidney, central nervous system, heart, and lungs has often been described. Thyroiditis occurs in a subset of patients and may not be noted until 2 to 3 months after onset. Atypical lymphocytosis and eosinophilia are seen in most affected individuals early in the course.

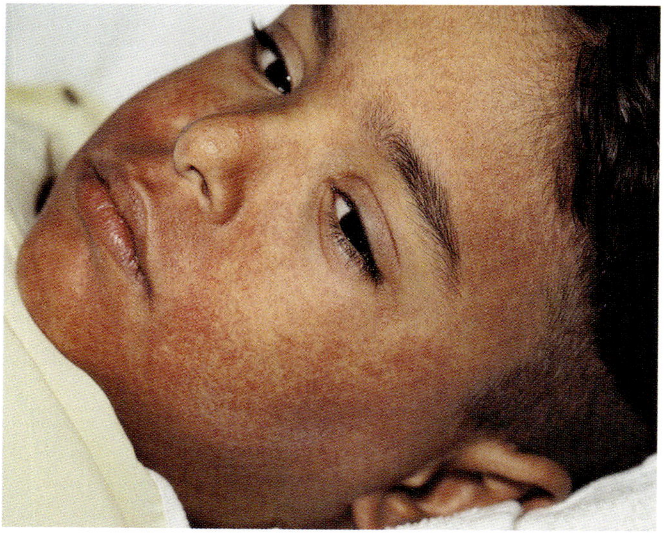

Fig. 20.19 Drug reaction with eosinophilia and systemic symptoms (DRESS). Three weeks after initiation of carbamazepine, this boy developed facial edema with dusky erythematous papules. The pruritic eruption subsequently spread caudally. Hepatic transaminase levels were noted to be significantly increased.

DRESS is most commonly caused by trimethoprim-sulfamethoxazole and the aromatic anticonvulsant agents, although viral infection has also been linked to DRESS. Sulfonamides are metabolized by acetylation to a nontoxic metabolite for renal excretion; slow acetylation has been associated with an increased risk of developing DRESS. Only aromatic amine forms of sulfonamides require this mechanism (e.g., these reactions do not occur with sulfonylureas and furosemide). Aromatic antiepileptics are metabolized by the cytochrome P450 system, and hereditary alterations in metabolism may lead to the accumulation of toxic arene oxide metabolites. Because these medications cross-react, affected individuals should avoid phenobarbital, phenytoin, carbamazepine, oxcarbazepine, and lamotrigine.[178] Alternative antiepileptics include valproic acid, benzodiazepines, gabapentin, zonisamide, topiramate, levetiracetam, and vigabatrin. Other drugs that less commonly cause this syndrome are minocycline, amoxicillin, dapsone, vancomycin,[179,180] abacavir, nevirapine,[181] aspirin,[182] allopurinol, and azithromycin,[183] as well as traditional Chinese medicine.[184] Reactions to doxycycline have not been described in patients who develop DRESS in response to minocycline. Clinical signs may vary dependent on the causative drug. For example, lamotrigine rarely causes eosinophilia, abacavir leads to primarily respiratory and gastrointestinal manifestations without eosinophilia or hepatitis, and allopurinol reactions often involve the kidney.[10,185]

The eruption of DRESS syndrome persists for weeks to months after medication withdrawal. After an initial period of improvement, the cutaneous and visceral manifestations of DRESS may flare 3 to 4 weeks after onset. Lymphocyte transformation tests may be useful in confirming the triggering medication but should be performed 5 to 8 weeks after onset in patients with DRESS.[186] Challenge with the offending drug after initial reaction leads to reactivation of the fever and erythroderma within hours after initiation.

A role for concurrent herpes family viral infections has been emphasized in adult DRESS, particularly with reactivation of EBV and human herpesvirus (HHV) type 6.[187,188] A pediatric study found concomitant evidence of HHV-6 infection in 50% of the children and in association with greater pulmonary involvement (50%) and longer duration of fever and hospital stay.[176]

Patients with suspected DRESS should have a variety of laboratory tests to consider visceral involvement. These include complete blood cell count, hepatic transaminases, serum creatinine level, urinalysis, and thyroid testing (which should be repeated after 2 to 3 months). Although topical corticosteroids and antihistamines may quell the pruritus in mild cases, patients with visceral involvement (especially for hepatitis, myocarditis, and interstitial pneumonitis) should be treated with systemic corticosteroids (1 to 2 mg/kg per day) for a few weeks, with gradual taper thereafter. Systemic corticosteroid treatment tends to shorten the hospital stay and reduce febrile days.[176] Anecdotal cases of successful treatment of DRESS with IVIG have been described.[189] Counseling of family members is important because first-degree relatives of individuals with DRESS have a higher risk of developing these drug reactions.

Stevens–Johnson Syndrome and Toxic Epidermal Necrolysis

Stevens–Johnson syndrome and toxic epidermal necrolysis are now considered to be variants of the same hypersensitivity disorder.[190–194] The incidence of these conditions is 6.3 to 7.5 per 100,000 children per year.[195] In a study of 708 patients, approximately 18% of those with SJS and TEN were children.[196] Classification has been based on the degree of epidermal detachment. Epidermal detachment of less than 10% of the total body surface area is considered SJS[197] (53 per 100,000 children); more than 30%, TEN (4 per million); and between 10% and 30%, a transitional SJS-TEN overlap condition (16 per million). In another study, 85% of pediatric cases had SJS, whereas 6% had SJS-TEN overlap and 9% had TEN.[198] Patients may appear to have SJS initially and typical TEN with disease progression (Table 20.3). At one time, SJS was lumped with EM (see Erythema Multiforme section and Table 20.3), which is now considered to be a distinct entity, primarily resulting from hypersensitivity to herpes simplex infection. Reactive infectious mucocutaneous or mucosal-predominant eruption (RIME), which includes mycoplasma-induced rash and mucositis (MIRM) and *Chlamydia pneumoniae*–induced rash with mucositis (CIRM), has also been separated from SJS (see Reactive Infectious Mucocutaneous or Mucosal-Predominant Eruption section and Table 20.3). Similarly, TEN was once confused with staphylococcal scalded skin syndrome (SSSS), a more superficial and crusted disorder in which the superficial blistering is caused by an exfoliatin produced by *Staphylococcus aureus* (see Chapter 14).

The SJS-TEN spectrum of SCARs is driven by cytotoxic T cells and features high levels of TNF, perforin/granzyme B, Fas/Fas ligand, and granulysin,[199] which promote keratinocyte apoptosis.[200] Microribonucleic acid (miR)–18a-5p, which targets an apoptosis gene *(BCL2L10)*, has been identified as a serum biomarker that can distinguish early TEN from other drug eruptions[201] Patients carrying *HLA-B*15:02*, which is common in the Asian population, are at strongly

Table 20.3 Classification of Epidermal Necrolysis and Comparison with Erythema Multiforme and RIME

	Erythema Multiforme	RIME	SJS	SJS-TEN	TEN
Lesional morphology	Fixed typical or atypical target lesions	Vesiculobullous; no typical papular targets	Targetoid lesions, dusky red macules, bullae	Targetoid lesions, dusky red macules, bullae	Targetoid lesions, dusky erythematous macules and plaques; detachment of epidermis
Localization of skin lesions	Acral distribution is characteristic; can be widespread	May be no skin involvement or limited	May be scattered and isolated; may be confluent, especially on the trunk and face	May be scattered and isolated; often confluent	Usually extensive involvement with widespread confluence
Involved skin	<2%	<10%	<10%	10% to 30%	>30%
Biopsy features	Individual apoptotic keratinocytes, but not large sheets of epidermal necrosis	Interface dermatitis with dyskeratosis	More interface dermatitis	Significant interface dermatitis + necrolysis	Predominantly necrolysis
Mucosal changes	Tends to be milder	Predominant erosive mucositis	Prominent	Prominent	May be less than in SJS
Systemic involvement	Minimal or absent	Often present (cough, fever, malaise, arthralgias)	Often present	Always present	Always present
Most common underlying cause	Typically HSV	Most often *Mycoplasma; Chlamydia* has been associated	Often drug-induced. Sometimes *Mycoplasma*	Usually drug	Most often drug; can be a feature of graft-vs.-host disease

HSV, Herpes simplex infection; *RIME*, reactive infectious mucucutaneous or mucosal-predominant eruption (includes *Mycoplasma* and *Chlamydia* induced); *SJS*, Stevens–Johnson syndrome; *TEN*, toxic epidermal necrolysis.

increased risk for carbamazepine-induced SJS/TEN, and this population should have human leukocyte antigens (HLAs) screened before initiating antiepileptic drugs.[202,203] Other HLA antigens are being recognized in non-Asian populations.[200] Lymphocyte transformation tests have helped to identify the causative agents in some affected children, but in contrast to those for children with DRESS syndrome, they need to be performed during the first week of the disorder.[186] The risk of developing SJS and TEN is significantly increased in patients with HIV infection and who have a decreased capacity to detoxify reactive intermediate drug metabolites (e.g., slow acetylators or individuals with defects in epoxide hydrolase–mediated detoxification).

The underlying triggers of SJS and TEN are similar, although drugs cause the majority of cases overall and in almost all cases of TEN (see Table 20.1).[204–208] In children, SJS is less commonly caused by medication than in adults,[209] and underlying mycoplasma[210] or herpetic infection should be considered. Although more than 200 medications have been implicated as potential triggers of SJS-TEN, sulfonamides, penicillins, phenobarbital, carbamazepine, and lamotrigine have been most strongly associated with SJS-TEN.[208] An algorithm for assessing drug causality in epidermal necrolysis (ALDEN) has been proposed and correlates well with case-control analysis results.[211]

Most patients show evidence of SJS or TEN 7 to 21 days after the first drug exposure. Occurrence is almost always within the first 8 weeks of drug use and rarely within the first few days of drug administration. Children with an earlier onset (mean 2 to 3 days) have been previously exposed to the drug or a cross-reacting analogue. Aromatic antiepileptics (phenobarbital, phenytoin, carbamazepine, lamotrigine) tend to cross-react and cannot be substituted for each other. Drugs with longer half-lives are associated with a higher incidence than those related but with shorter half-lives. NSAIDs, including ibuprofen, and acetaminophen[208] may also be triggers and possibly exacerbants with other drugs and are best avoided during hospitalization for SJS-TEN. Other infections,[205,206] neoplasia, autoimmune disorders, and vaccination[207] have also been implicated, particularly herpes simplex virus, which is more typically linked to EM.

Older children and adults are most likely to develop this spectrum of disorders, but the condition has been described in young infants and neonates.[212] High fever, pronounced constitutional symptoms, and varying degrees of generalized targetoid lesions, bullae, epidermal detachment, and mucosal erosions (of at least two sites) are characteristic (see Table 20.3).[213–215] Patients not uncommonly show a 1- to 14-day prodromal period before the abrupt eruption of the typical features. During this prodromal period, affected children may show fever, malaise, headache, cough, coryza, sore throat, vomiting, diarrhea, chest pain, myalgia, and arthralgias.

Cutaneous involvement most often appears initially on the face and upper trunk. Palms and soles are commonly involved (Figs. 20.20 and 20.21). Erythematous and purpuric macules may develop flaccid gray discoloration or bullae (Figs. 20.22 and 20.23), become confluent, and sometimes detach, leaving a raw, denuded base (Figs. 20.24 and 20.25). Some of the macular lesions may show a dusky center, which gives a target-like (targetoid) appearance; however, the characteristic concentric rings of EM are absent. Some patients show limited targetoid lesions and little detachment (more typical of SJS), and others show extensive detachment (more typical of TEN). The early

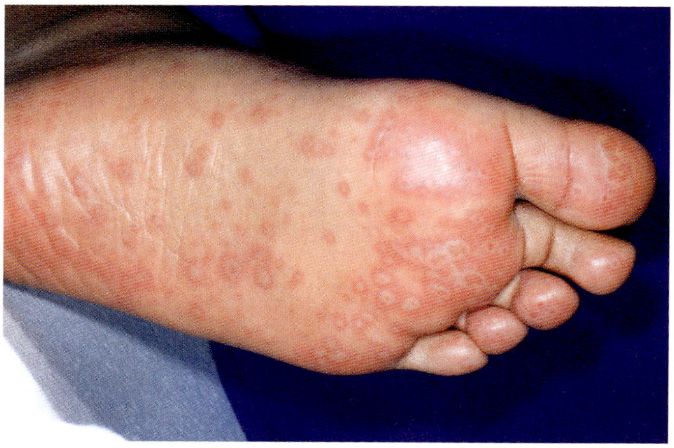

Fig. 20.20 Stevens–Johnson syndrome. Note the bullae on the sole in this girl who reacted to lamotrigine.

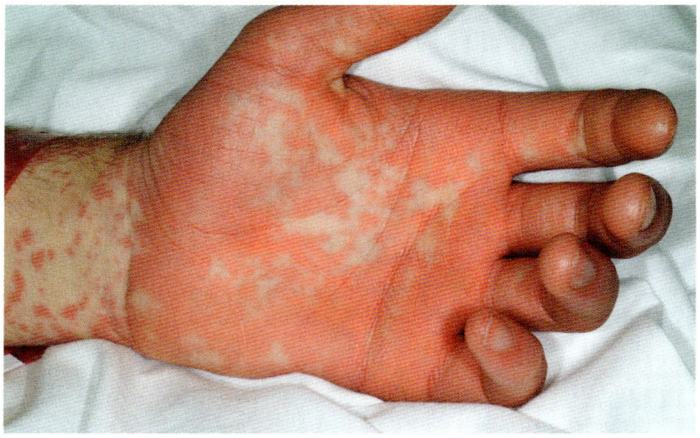

Fig. 20.21 Stevens–Johnson syndrome (SJS). Intensely erythematous macules are nearly confluent the palms of this boy with SJS from carbamazepine.

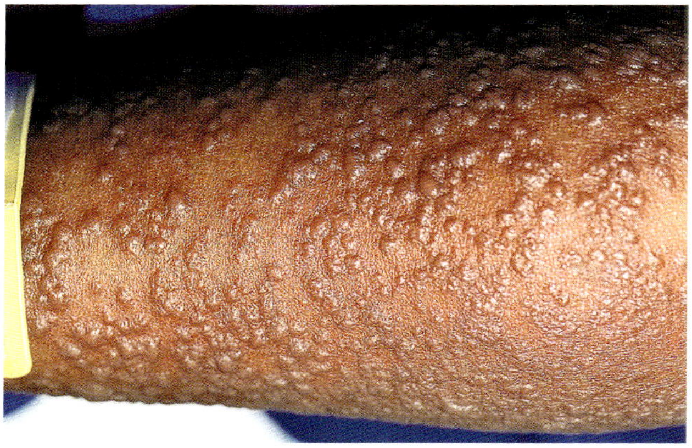

Fig. 20.22 Toxic epidermal necrolysis. Note the extensive small bullae that later coalesced and led to extensive denudation.

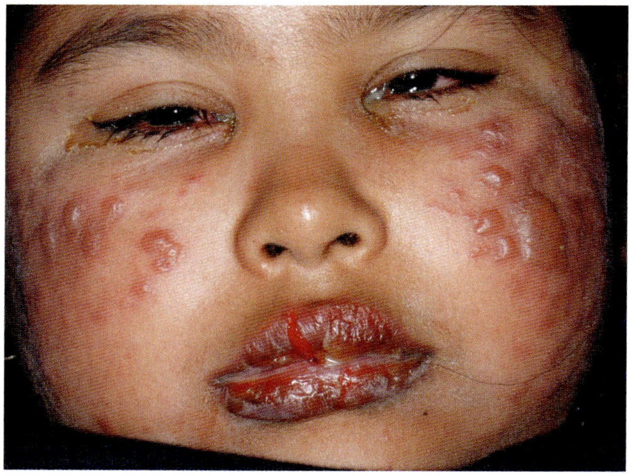

Fig. 20.23 Stevens–Johnson syndrome. Purpuric macules became bullous. Note the inflammation of the conjunctivae and lips.

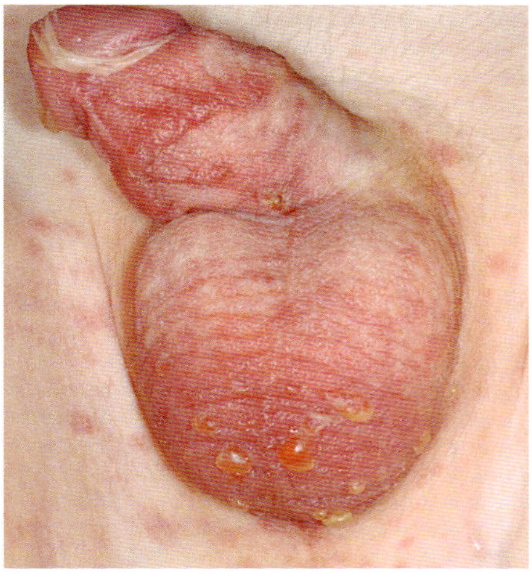

Fig. 20.24 Toxic epidermal necrolysis. Note the discrete bullae on the scrotum sloughing of mucosae at the glans. The sloughed skin resembles wrinkled, wet, tissue paper.

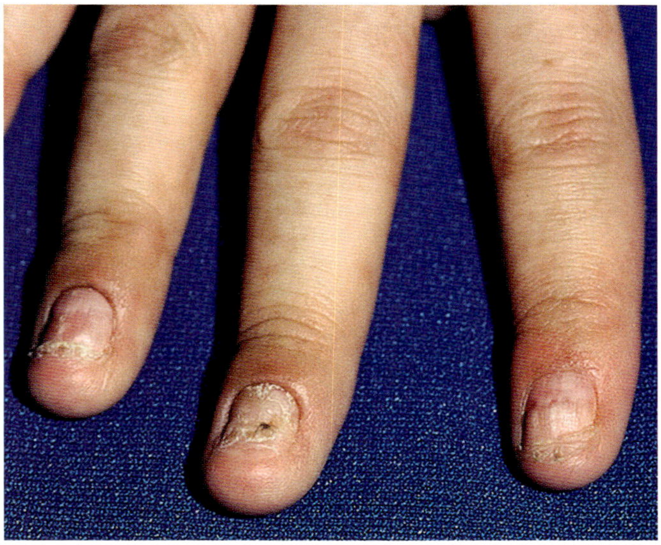

Fig. 20.26 Toxic epidermal necrolysis. Residual nail dystrophy in an adolescent girl who also had widespread postinflammatory hyperpigmentation.

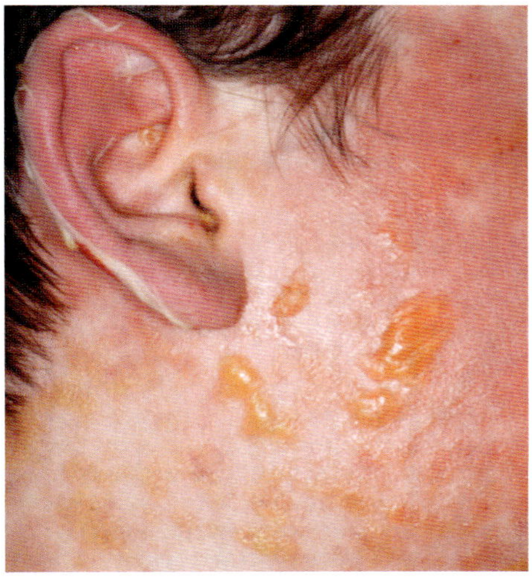

Fig. 20.25 Toxic epidermal necrolysis (TEN). Note the sloughing of skin on the ear, which is exacerbated by gentle stroking of the area (positive Nikolsky sign). The mucosal involvement in this boy originally was typical of Stevens–Johnson syndrome, but he progressed to the extensive denudement of TEN.

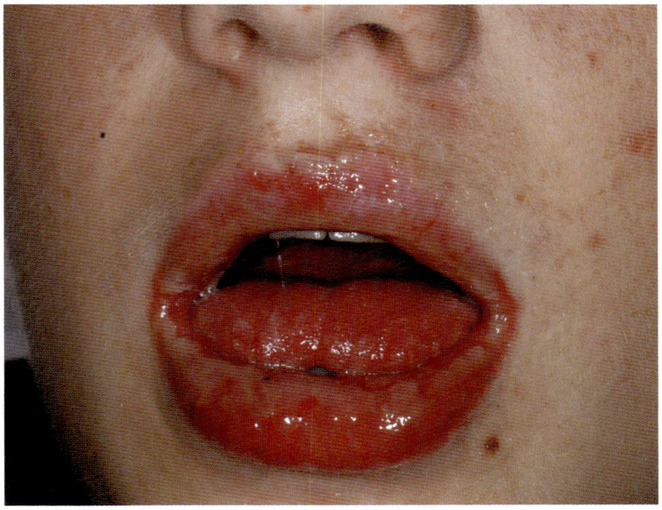

Fig. 20.27 Stevens–Johnson syndrome. Mucous membrane involvement with severe swelling and blistering of the lips and tongue. The reaction was to lamotrigine.

morbilliform eruption of TEN may be localized but more often is an extensive, painful erythroderma. After exerting light mechanical pressure with a finger to an area of erythema, the epidermis in patients with either SJS or TEN becomes wrinkled and peels off like wet tissue paper (see Fig. 20.25), the characteristic Nikolsky sign. The Nikolsky sign may be seen in patients without clinical evidence of epidermal detachment and can be a useful diagnostic tool. In addition to SJS and TEN, however, the Nikolsky sign may be seen in a variety of other bullous disorders (especially pemphigus, epidermolysis bullosa [see Chapter 13], and the SSSS [see Chapter 14]). Histopathologic examination of affected skin demonstrates necrosis of the lower epidermal cells with a sparse mononuclear cell infiltrate and, in the case of TEN, extensive necrosis with a subepidermal split. The epidermal necrosis correlates with the dusky blue coloration of lesions. The nails become dystrophic because of nailbed inflammation (Fig. 20.26).

Extensive mucosal involvement is more typical of SJS than TEN. The mucosal manifestations of SJS tend to occur 1 to 2 days before cutaneous manifestations. The mucous membranes of the lips, tongue, buccal mucosae, eyes, nose, genitalia, and rectum may show extensive bullae with grayish white membranes, characteristic hemorrhagic crusts, and painful superficial erosions and ulcerations (Figs. 20.27 and 20.28). Uncommonly, the esophageal and respiratory epithelial mucosae are affected. By definition, two or more mucosal surfaces are involved. The oral mucosa is always affected, resulting in inability to drink or eat and leading to a risk of dehydration. Genital area lesions lead to painful micturition and defecation. Although lesions of the oral mucosae tend to heal without scarring, strictures or stenosis of esophageal, vaginal, urethral, and anal mucosae have been described as sequelae.

Severe purulent conjunctivitis with photophobia is the typical ocular manifestation (see Fig. 20.28).[216] Corneal ulcerations, keratitis, uveitis, and panophthalmitis may also occur. Sequelae occur in 40% of patients[217] and may be grave, with a possibility of keratoconjunctivitis sicca, corneal ulceration or neovascularization, trichiasis, symblepharon, and partial or even complete blindness.[218] The severity of the acute ophthalmologic manifestations does not correlate with

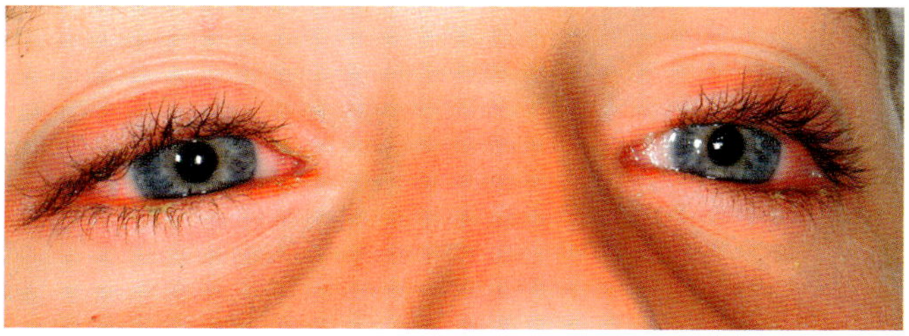

Fig. 20.28 Stevens–Johnson syndrome. This boy shows early ophthalmic involvement with conjunctival injection, eyelid edema, erythema, and exudative crusting.

long-term complications. Pulmonary involvement may occur as an extension from the oropharynx and tracheobronchial tree or may be the result of pneumonitis associated with an initiating viral infection or secondary infection. In extreme cases, renal involvement with hematuria, nephritis, and in some cases progressive renal failure may result. Esophageal or tracheal ulceration, pyoderma, lymphadenopathy, hepatosplenomegaly with elevated transaminase levels, myocarditis, arthritis and arthralgias, and/or septicemia may also complicate the disorder (Box 20.3).

SJS is most often confused with Kawasaki disease. However, the conjunctivitis of Kawasaki disease lacks exudation, and the mucosal erythema and dryness is not associated with hemorrhagic crust and mucosal denudation[219] (see Chapter 21). The targetoid cutaneous lesions of SJS may resemble the target lesions of EM (see Erythema Multiforme section), a disorder usually attributed to herpes simplex infection in children; EM may also show blistering of the lip and oral mucosae that resembles SJS, although the blisters of EM are usually fewer and less symptomatic.[220,221] The cutaneous lesions of EM are more often found on the extremities and/or face, whereas the atypical target or purpuric lesions of SJS are more commonly located on the trunk.[221] Children with the rare immunobullous disorder paraneoplastic pemphigus may exhibit the mucocutaneous manifestations of SJS or TEN; the presence of epidermal acantholysis in biopsy specimens and the demonstration of antibody deposition in indirect immunofluorescence testing or immunoblot evaluation of serum allows

Box 20.3 Features of Stevens–Johnson Syndrome and Toxic Epidermal Necrolysis

Constitutional

- Fever
- Dehydration

Mucocutaneous

- Stomatitis with hemorrhagic crusts
- Oral and genital erosions
- Dysphagia
- Purulent conjunctivitis with photophobia
- Occasionally, esophageal and pulmonary mucosal sloughing
- Dusky erythematous macules, targetoid lesions, bullae, and skin sloughing

Visceral

- Lymphadenopathy
- Hepatosplenomegaly with hepatitis
- Uncommonly: pneumonitis, arthritis, myocarditis, and nephritis

Laboratory Abnormalities

- Increased erythrocyte sedimentation rate (100%)
- Leukocytosis (60%)
- Eosinophilia (20%)
- Anemia (15%)
- Elevated hepatic transaminase levels (15%)
- Leukopenia (10%)
- Proteinuria, microscopic hematuria (5%)

paraneoplastic pemphigus to be distinguished (see Chapter 13). Other immunobullous disorders may also be confused with TEN (see Chapter 13). TEN and SSSS are usually easily distinguished; the blisters of TEN lead to denudement with keratinocyte apoptosis, whereas the desquamation of SSSS is superficial. In SSSS the staphylococcal exfoliatin targets desmoglein 1, a desmosome component; because desmoglein 3 in the lower epidermis is able to compensate for desmoglein 1, the blistering of SSSS is superficial rather than panepidermal. SSSS also shows a different distribution with periorificial predominance and not mucosal involvement. Features of TEN occur as a severe manifestation of acute graft-versus-host disease, which is otherwise distinguished by history, other clinical findings, and histologic findings (see Chapter 25).

Although mild cases of SJS may show significant improvement within 5 to 15 days, the course of SJS or TEN is often protracted and may last more than a month. Epidermal detachment may be extensive, leading to massive fluid loss similar to that of a patient with burns. Bacterial superinfection with sepsis, impairment of temperature regulation, severe dehydration, electrolyte imbalance, excessive energy expenditure, and alteration in immunologic function are the usual complications. End-organ failure can be severe despite adequate supportive therapy. In hospitalized children with the SJS-TEN spectrum, the mortality rate of SJS is 0%, SJS-TEN 4%, and TEN 16%.[197] A composite score (SCORTEN), developed to predict mortality in adults,[222] has been shown to be predictive in pediatric patients of mortality, length of hospital stay, and infectious complications, especially when scored on admission.[223] Predictors of mortality are renal failure, malignancy, septicemia, bacterial infection, and seizures.[197]

SJS and TEN are life-threatening disorders, and patients should be hospitalized. If damage to the epidermis is extensive, patients should be admitted to an intensive care unit or burn unit to allow special attention to fluid requirements, electrolyte balance, intravenous caloric replacement, and avoidance of secondary infection. If possible, all drugs administered within 2 months before onset of the eruption should be discontinued,[224] and infectious causes should be sought and treated. Severe oropharyngeal involvement often necessitates frequent mouthwashes and local application of a topical anesthetic. When ocular involvement is present, ophthalmologic consultation should be obtained. Short-term use of potent topical corticosteroids and application of amniotic membrane to the entire ocular surface have been advocated to preserve visual acuity and an intact ocular surface.[225–227] Patients should receive intravenous fluids and either a liquid diet, if tolerated, or parenteral nutrition; the measured resting energy requirement in pediatric SJS/TEN is increased by 30%.[228] A mouthwash containing aluminum-magnesium (Maalox), elixir of diphenhydramine, and viscous lidocaine (mixed 1 : 1 : 1) can be soothing and decrease pain. Oral histamines such as hydroxyzine or diphenhydramine can be beneficial, and more vigorous pain control is often necessary. Of note, TEN has also been associated rarely with acetaminophen ingestion in children.[229]

Manipulation should be avoided but if necessary should be performed in a sterile fashion. Intact areas of skin should be kept dry. Open wounds should be cleansed daily. Detached areas should be covered with nonadherent, moist dressings (such as petrolatum-impregnated gauze) until reepithelialization occurs. Periorificial areas can be treated with antibiotic ointment (such as bacitracin or mupirocin). Biological dressings or skin equivalents may be considered for patients with extensive denudation.[230]

The response to supportive care alone has been excellent in most children,[231] and the most important treatment remains identification and discontinuation of any potential triggering medication. Short-term administration of intravenous systemic corticosteroids (4 mg/kg per day) or pulsed intravenous steroids is sometimes advocated if started within the first 2 to 3 days of a drug-induced reaction.[232,233] A 2013 meta-analysis that collected studies from 1990 to 2012 found a trend toward survival[234] with use of systemic corticosteroids, and another meta-analysis suggested reduced recovery time (but not mortality) with the combination of steroids and IVIG.[199,235] In addition, some children with SJS or TEN have had shorter duration of fever and decreased development of new blisters with early administration (within 24 to 48 hours) of 2.5 to 3 g/kg per day IVIG for 3 days.[236–239] However, use of systemic steroids may increase morbidity and mortality from secondary infection, prolonging wound healing, masking early signs of sepsis, and triggering gastrointestinal bleeding. In addition, other studies and a meta-analysis have shown limited benefit in the use of IVIG,[240] including for pediatric disease,[241] and double-blind,[234] randomized, controlled trials have not been performed. As such, the administration of systemic steroids or IVIG as treatment is still controversial.

More recently, attention has focused on the use of TNF inhibitors, especially intravenous infliximab, for TEN.[199,242,243] In a trial of almost 100 affected adults, treatment with etanercept decreased predicted mortality, reduced healing time, and was associated with less gastrointestinal hemorrhage and lower levels of TNF and granulysin in blood and blister fluid than with systemic corticosteroids.[199] Cyclosporine[244–246] has also been used with good results. Thalidomide administration has been linked to increased mortality in a randomized, placebo-controlled trial.[247]

Long-term sequelae occur in 45% of affected children, including cutaneous dyschromia in 42%, which may persist for years.[198] Sun exposure should be avoided and sunscreens used liberally for at least a few months because of the potential for ultraviolet light–induced worsening of the residual dyspigmentation. Persistent nail dystrophy or anonychia is also commonly reported (see Fig. 20.26).[218] Late ocular complications include dry eye syndrome (59%), subjunctival fibrous scarring (33%), corneal erosions (29%), and, in fewer than 25%, trichiasis, symblepharon, and visual loss.[248] Artificial tears and lubricants may be required for several years after diagnosis, if not lifelong, because ocular disease tends to progress after hospital discharge.

Reactive Infectious Mucocutaneous or Mucosal-Predominant Eruption

RIME is the term for a disorder within the erythema multiforme to epidermal necrolysis spectrum that encompasses MIRM,[249] *Mycoplasma pneumoniae*–associated mucositis (MPAM), CIRM, and mucositis-predominant eruptions (see Table 20.3). RIME occurs more often in boys than girls, and the overall prognosis is favorable compared with SJS. Recurrences have been reported in 8% of cases.

Oral involvement can range from sloughing of the entire mucosae to localized erosions (Fig. 20.29). The most common ocular features are purulent bilateral conjunctivitis and photophobia, but conjunctival pseudomembrane formation and lid margin and conjunctival ulceration may also occur.[250]

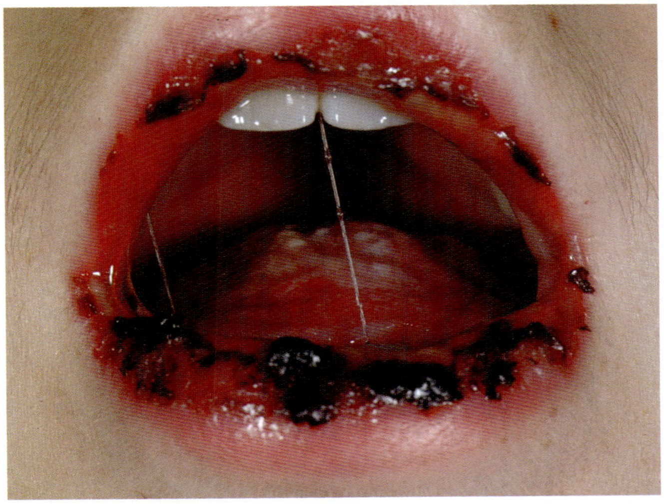

Fig. 20.29 Reactive infectious mucucutaneous or mucosal-predominant eruption from mycoplasma hypersensitivity. This boy had recurrent mucositis of the oral mucosae, eyes, and sometimes genital region with minimal skin involvement in association with mycoplasma infection.

Most cases result from mycoplasma infection, and characteristic features are cough, fever, malaise, and/or arthralgia with high levels of anti–*M. pneumoniae* IgM antibodies, serial cold agglutinins, or positive polymerase chain reaction (PCR) test for *M. pneumoniae* from the skin or oropharynx). Most patients with RIME have prodromal symptoms (fever, cough, malaise) about a week before the mucosal (and skin) eruptions. The mucositis typically occurs at two or more sites (oral in 94%, ocular in 82%, and urogenital in 63%).[249,251] By definition, less than 10% body surface area is detached, further distinguishing RIME from SJS.

Among affected patients with *Mycoplasma*-induced RIME, approximately half have polymorphic, usually sparse skin lesions and an additional one-third have no skin lesions at all, a transient morbilliform eruption, or few vesicles.[252] The remainder had more extensive skin involvement. Overall, skin lesions are vesiculobullous (77%), scattered target lesions (48%), and less often erythematous papules, macules, or pustules[253] or with a morbilliform appearance.[249] RIME has been reported in a father and son (at different times) with *Mycoplasma* infection, suggesting a genetic predisposition toward its development.[255]

Documentation of underlying infection is important because of the increasing reports of *Chlamydia* as the cause of RIME, now described in more than 20 cases and often clinically indistinguishable from *Mycoplasma*-induced RIME.[255] *Chlamydia*-induced RIME more often has cutaneous involvement (>90%), most often maculopapular (76%) or targetoid (35%), although vesiculobullous lesions have been described (6%). Oral erosions (86%), conjunctivitis (71%), and urogenital erosions (43%) have been described. Serologic detection of *Chlamydia pneumoniae* infection may be falsely negative and require real-time PCR for diagnosis. Both *Mycoplasma* and *Chlamydia* infections are treated with azithromycin, although the inflammation improves quickly with systemic steroid therapy.

Fixed Drug Eruption

Fixed drug eruption is a term used to describe a sharply localized, circumscribed round or oval dermatitis that characteristically recurs in the same site or sites each time the offending drug is administered.[256,257] The persistent residual hyperpigmentation leads to the name of the eruption, although occasionally lesions do not become pigmented.[258] In one series, fixed drug eruption was second in incidence to exanthematous reactions to drugs and occurred in 22% of children with cutaneous reactions to drug ingestion.[259] Lesions first occur 1 to 2 weeks after initial ingestion of the drug, but within 30 minutes to 8 hours after subsequent exposures. Fixed drug eruptions are type IV immune reactions and have been shown to result from $CD8^+$ memory T cells that persist intraepidermally at site of involvement and, on stimulation by drug, release interferon (IFN)–γ, leading to inflammation. Fas-Fas ligand interactions lead to the demonstrated basal keratinocyte apoptosis.

Lesions are solitary at first, but with repeated attacks, new lesions usually appear and existing lesions may tend to increase in size to more than 10 cm in diameter. Not uncommonly, lesions recur at the same sites. The lesions tend to be erythematous, edematous, and dusky at their onset, with well-defined borders. At times they may become bullous (Fig. 20.30), with subsequent desquamation or crusting and a residual hyperpigmentation that may persist for months (Fig. 20.31). Lesions can occur anywhere on the body but have a predilection for the perioral area, lips, hands, trunk, and genital region.[260,261] In a series of affected boys with genital involvement, the clinical presentation usually consisted of swelling and erythema of the penis and/or scrotum associated with pruritus or burning, restlessness, urinary retention, and painful micturition.[261]

By far the most common trigger of fixed drug eruptions in children is cotrimoxazole and other sulfa drugs.[262] Acetaminophen,[263,264] ibuprofen[265] and other NSAIDs,[266] and, less commonly, loratadine[267] and pseudoephedrine have also been causative, and a careful history of administration of over-the-counter products is of key importance. Although phenolphthalein was a common cause in the past, its elimination from over-the-counter laxatives has markedly diminished its culpability. Other causative preparations include phenytoin, cephalosporins,[268,269] ciprofloxacin, metronidazole, penicillins,[268,270] tetracyclines, erythromycin, teicoplanin,[271] quinine and its derivatives,

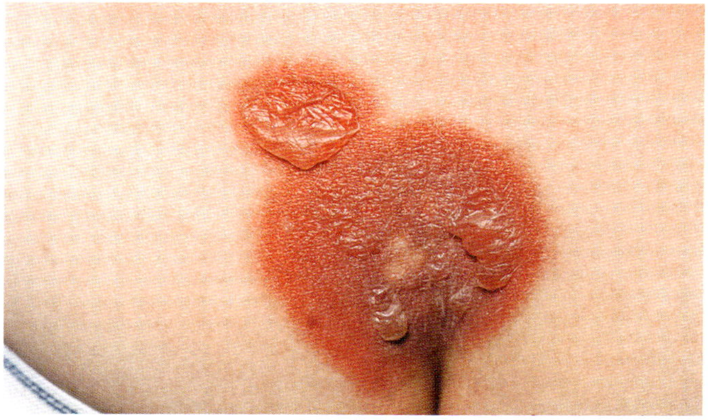

Fig. 20.30 Fixed drug eruption. Well-defined, dusky erythematous plaques that may be bullous.

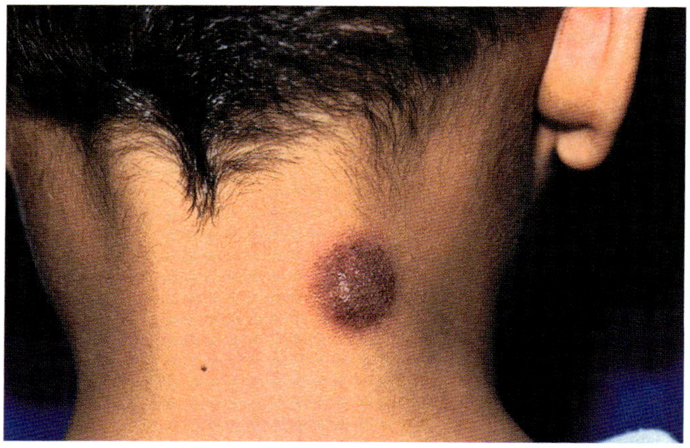

Fig. 20.31 Fixed drug eruption. The residual hyperpigmentation at the site of a fixed drug eruption may persist for months.

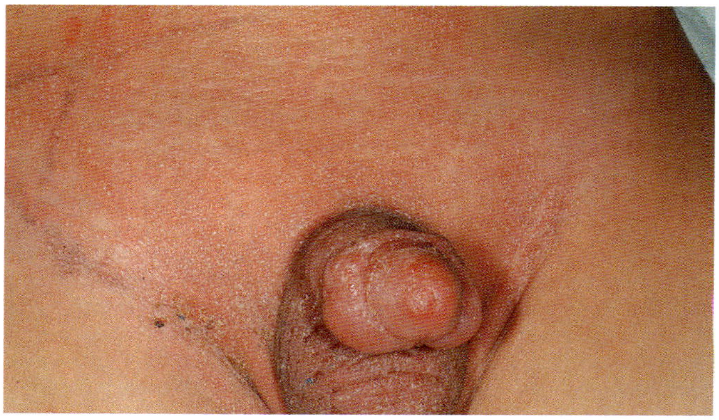

Fig. 20.32 Acute generalized exanthematous pustulosis. Affected individuals show large areas with erythroderma topped with nonfollicular, tiny, sterile pustules, usually in association with fever. Although often triggered by a virus or vaccination in children, this boy was taking an antiepileptic medication.

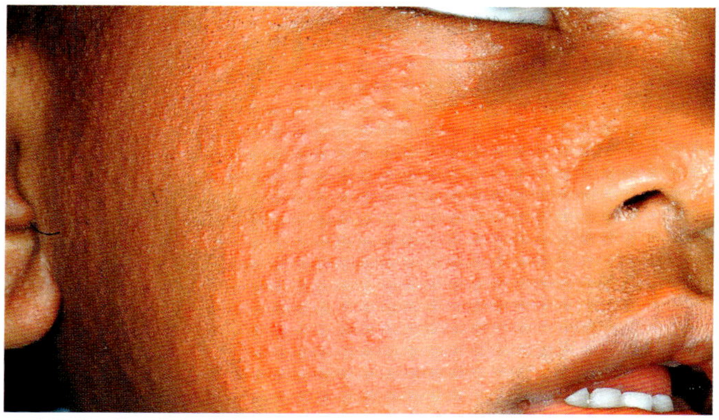

Fig. 20.33 Acute generalized exanthematous pustulosis. Pinpoint sterile papulopustules overlying erythroderma. No medication was associated, and the condition was attributed to a virus.

salicylates, potassium iodide, and metronidazole. Fixed food eruptions have been described after ingestion of various food substitutes and flavorings (especially tartrazine, as in artificially colored cheese crisps),[272] as well as licorice, cashews, lentils, and asparagus.

The diagnosis of fixed drug eruption is often missed, leading to repeated ingestion of the medication and recurrence. Lesions commonly may be mistaken for insect bites, urticaria, and, if more extensive, EM or in their stage of hyperpigmentation for erythema dyschromicum perstans. Biopsy can aid in the diagnosis of fixed drug eruption, especially in the early stage in which a lichenoid infiltrate with necrotic keratinocytes may be seen. Avoidance of the offending agent is key, but the associated pruritus can be controlled by application of medium-strength to potent topical corticosteroids. If necessary, challenge with the drug usually confirms the causative agent within 30 minutes to 8 hours but theoretically can trigger a more severe reaction. Patch testing at the site of a previous lesion can lead to a positive result in up to 30% of patients.[273]

Acute Generalized Exanthematous Pustulosis

Acute generalized exanthematous pustulosis (AGEP) affects 1 to 5 per million persons.[274] It has been described in several children,[275,276] although it is much more common in adults. AGEP is characterized by the acute onset of a generalized erythroderma topped with small, nonfollicular, sterile, pinpoint pustules, usually in association with fever (Figs. 20.32 and 20.33).[277] The eruption tends to be symmetric and accentuated in the antecubital and popliteal fossae, as well as the inguinal folds. The condition usually resolves spontaneously after 4 to 10 days with a characteristic pattern of desquamation.

Medication has been the usual trigger in adults and can cause AGEP in children.[278–280] Among implicated triggering agents have been antibiotics (amoxicillin-clavulanate, cephalosporins,[281] macrolides, clindamycin), terbinafine,[282] paroxetine, hydroxychloroquine,[283] and contrast agents.[284] Most affected children, however, are administered no medication, suggesting that the condition is often triggered in response to viral infection or possibly vaccine administration.[276] Pustular psoriasis is the key differential diagnosis.

Mutations in *IL36RN*, the gene encoding the IL-36 receptor antagonist, have been reported in AGEP (and pustular psoriasis; see Deficiency of IL-36 Receptor Antagonist [DITRA] section, Chapter 4).[285] The causative drug for AGEP has been shown to specifically induce IL-36γ release *in vitro*.[286] In addition, IL-36 cytokines, particularly IL-36γ, are highly expressed by keratinocytes and macrophages in AGEP skin (but not in drug-induced exanthematous eruptions), further suggesting a key role for IL-36γ secretion in AGEP. AGEP is also an unusual manifestation of *CARD14* activating mutations, which are associated with increased IL-36 expression.

Erythema Multiforme

Erythema multiforme is a specific self-limited hypersensitivity syndrome with a distinctive clinical pattern, the hallmark of which is the erythematous ring (the so-called *iris* or *target lesion*). The condition can occur at any age but is most commonly seen in young adults; 20% of cases occur in children. The majority of cases of EM in children are precipitated by herpes simplex virus (HSV) type 1 infection,[287,388] although HSV type 2 infection has been described in affected adolescents[289,290] and *Mycoplasma* has also been associated.[291] Approximately 50% of cases follow herpes labialis infection, usually by 3 to 14 days, although concurrent infection and EM have been noted. HSV DNA has been detected in the early erythematous papules or the peripheral area of target lesions in 80% of patients with EM[289] despite the low recovery of herpes simplex in cultures of lesions.[292] When associated with HSV, the disorder has been termed *herpes-associated EM (HAEM)*. Other viral disorders, including varicella,[293] orf, and EBV infection, have been implicated, and histoplasmosis has been associated in endemic areas. EM in association with high fever can be a sign of Kawasaki disease, especially in infants[294] (see Chapter 21).

The diagnosis of EM can generally be made by the clinical features and distribution of lesions (Box 20.4). The eruption is symmetric and may be noted on any part of the body, with a predilection for the palms and soles (Fig. 20.34), backs of the hands and feet, and extensor surfaces of the arms and legs. Lesions may be grouped, especially at the elbows and knees. As the disorder progresses over 72 hours (and occasionally as long as a week), lesions may extend to the trunk, face, and neck. Once present, lesions are fixed for at least 7 days.

The primary lesion of EM develops abruptly without a prodromal period (Figs. 20.35 and 20.36). The classic lesion is a "target" or "iris" lesion, in which there are three concentric zones: a central dusky cyanotic or violaceous region, a paler edematous zone, and a peripheral red ring, thus creating the multiformity of lesions. The central dusky clearing represents epidermal cell necrosis. Atypical papular lesions may have only two zones or poorly defined borders. Lesions may also become bullous (bullous EM) (Fig. 20.37), but in contrast to epidermal necrolytic disorders, less than 2% of the body surface area is generally involved (see Table 20.3). Careful inspection of the eruption in EM may disclose fine petechiae. Most lesions are asymptomatic, but itching or burning has been described. The isomorphic response (koebnerization) appears to participate in the development of lesions, with trauma and ultraviolet (UV) light injury as triggers.

Oral lesions are seen in 25% to 50% of children, usually in conjunction with cutaneous lesions. They initially appear as bullae that break soon after formation, accompanied by swelling and crusting of the lips and erosions of the buccal mucosa and tongue. Gingival involvement

Box 20.4 **Clinical Features of Erythema Multiforme**

Acute, self-limited, recurrent course
Duration of 1 to 4 weeks
Symmetrically distributed, fixed lesions
Concentric color changes in at least some lesions ("iris" or "target" lesions)
If present, mucosal involvement limited to the mouth
In children, most likely cause for recurrent disease is herpes simplex virus

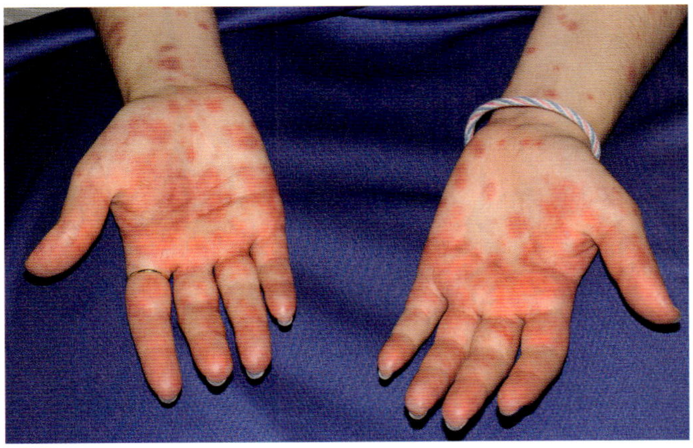

Fig. 20.34 Erythema multiforme (EM). Round erythematous swollen plaques and target lesions on the palms. This girl developed in EM in association with her systemic lupus erythematosus.

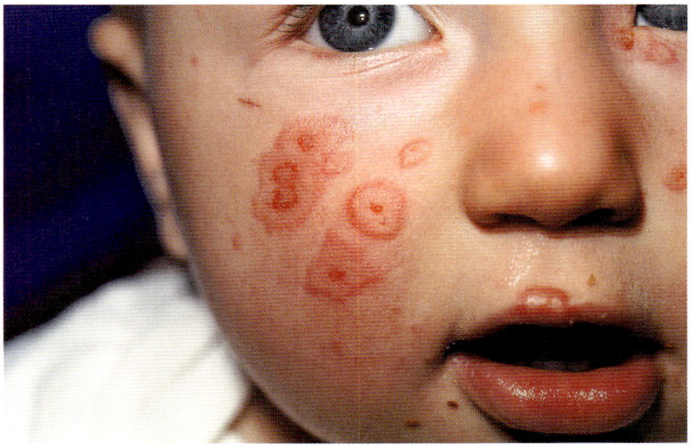

Fig. 20.35 Erythema multiforme. Classic target lesions and marginated wheals with central vesicles are characteristic.

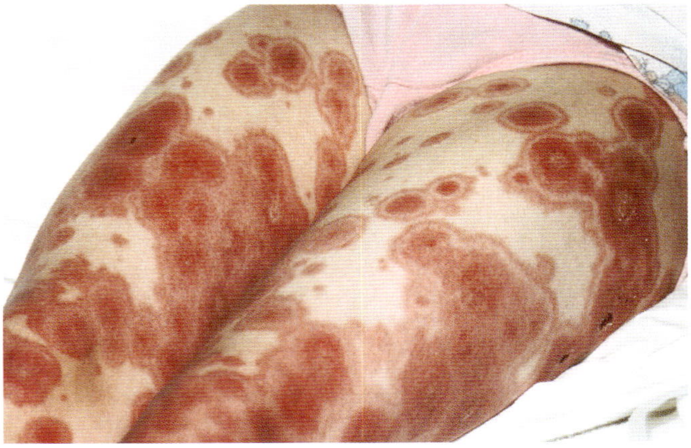

Fig. 20.36 Erythema multiforme. Extensive target lesions on the thighs of a 12-year-old girl. The recurrent reaction was suppressed by administration of oral acyclovir.

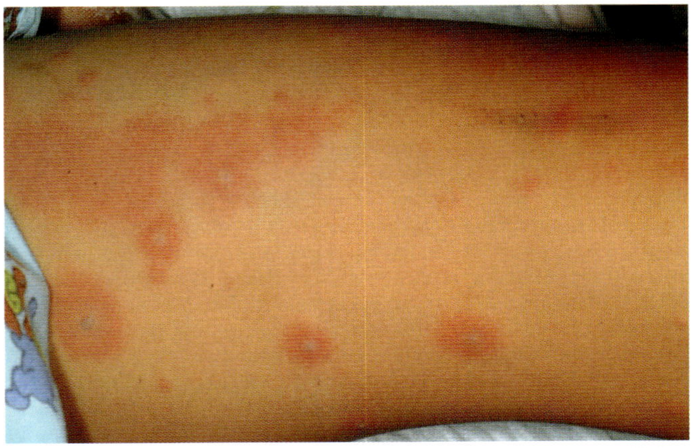

Fig. 20.37 Erythema multiforme, bullous. If central epidermal necrosis is extensive, the center of the lesion may become bullous.

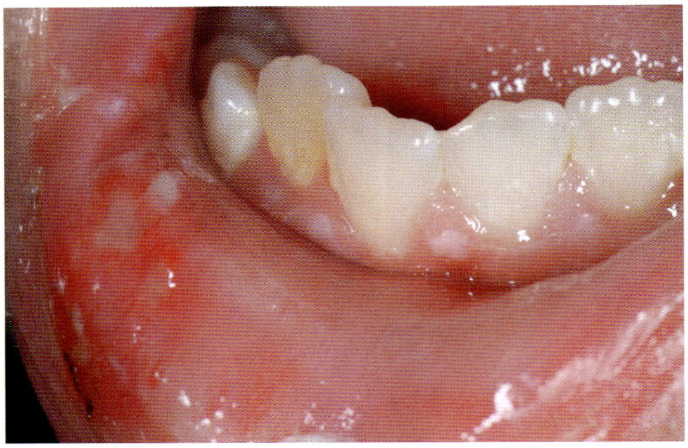

Fig. 20.38 Erythema multiforme (EM). The trigger for EM in children is commonly herpes simplex infection, which often precedes EM but may be detectable at the time when the EM is present.

is rare, which helps distinguish EM from primary herpes simplex infection of the mouth (Fig. 20.38). Most children with mucosal involvement have a few lesions and are mildly symptomatic; however, patients with extensively crusted lips and large bullous target lesions that may mimic SJS have been described and probably are better classified as RIME (see RIME earlier).[220,221] Systemic manifestations, when present, are mild and consist of low-grade fever, malaise, and, in rare cases, myalgia or arthralgia.

The major differential diagnosis for erythema multiforme is variants of urticaria ("urticaria multiforme") and viral exanthems. EM-like lesions can be a feature of Kawasaki disease and can be confused with acute hemorrhagic edema of infancy. Features that distinguish EM from SJS and TEN are described in Table 20.3. Biopsy of skin lesions is usually not needed to make the diagnosis and should be performed only to consider other conditions such as lupus erythematosus or vasculitis (including acute hemorrhagic edema of infancy).[295] Focal liquefaction degeneration of epidermal keratinocytes and exocytosis of mononuclear cells in the epidermis are seen.

Most episodes of EM heal within 2 to 3 weeks without sequelae. Recurrences a few times yearly, however, are common. Symptomatic treatment with oral antihistamines usually suffices. Given the association with HSV, however, prophylactic therapy with oral acyclovir (5 to 10 mg/kg per day) for 6 to 12 months should be considered for patients with recurrent disease.[288,289] Episodic therapy with acyclovir is not useful. Administration of immunosuppressive agents, such as oral corticosteroids, leads to longer and more frequent episodes.

Annular Erythemas

The annular erythemas (erythema marginatum, erythema annulare centrifugum [EAC], erythema migrans, and annular erythema of infancy) represent a group of reactive vascular dermatoses that are distinguished primarily by their oval, annular, arcuate, circinate, polycyclic, reticular, or serpiginous configurations with individual characteristics that allow differentiation into distinctive clinical categories.[296] They must be distinguished from other annular lesions seen in children, especially tinea, urticaria multiforme, EM and SSLR, annular pityriasis rosea, neonatal and subacute lupus erythematosus, granuloma annulare, and the annular lesions of erythrokeratodermia variabilis (see Chapter 5).

ERYTHEMA MARGINATUM AND RHEUMATIC FEVER

Erythema marginatum is a distinctive form of annular erythema that occurs on the trunk (especially on the abdomen) and the proximal extremities of patients with active rheumatic fever.[297,298] It is seen more commonly in children than in adults with rheumatic fever but still only occurs in 6% of affected children.[299] The occurrence of erythema marginatum often follows the onset of migratory arthritis by a few days but at times may also occur many months after the carditis.

Often easily overlooked, lesions are evanescent pink macules or papules that fade centrally in a few hours to several days, leaving a pale or sometimes pigmented center. They spread rapidly to form nonpruritic rings or segments of rings with elevated reticular, polycyclic, or serpiginous borders and may recur in crops in different areas. Lesions are commonly seen more easily in the afternoon, and coalescence of polycyclic lesions often results in a characteristic chicken wire–like appearance. Gentle warming of the skin tends to enhance visualization of pale or barely perceptible lesions. Although the eruption seldom lasts more than several weeks, occasionally it may recur at sporadic intervals for several months to years.

Erythema marginatum presents a clinical picture that characteristically resembles a variety of dermatoses, including urticaria, EM, and other transient figurate erythemas.[300] Unlike the characteristic rash of juvenile idiopathic arthritis (see Chapter 22), lesions of erythema marginatum are larger, spread centrifugally with central clearing, and are limited to the trunk and sometimes the proximal limbs. Histologic features of a neutrophilic perivascular infiltrate in the papillary dermis aid in diagnosis.

The most common associated features are carditis (76% to 93% of patients), fever (62%), congestive heart failure (44%), and arthritis (39% to 53%). Sydenham chorea is rarely seen. Approximately 2% of patients show urticarial lesions without annular rings,[301] and up to 2% have subcutaneous nodules, usually a late manifestation. The nodules of rheumatic fever are smaller than those seen in juvenile idiopathic arthritis and usually clear within a month. They tend to occur in crops, are symmetrically distributed, are nontender, and are more readily felt than seen, requiring a careful search. Differentiation of subcutaneous nodules of rheumatic fever from rheumatoid nodules and granuloma annulare is not possible on clinical or histologic grounds alone and requires the presence of other features.

Currently accepted criteria for the diagnosis of rheumatic fever include two major or one minor manifestation and evidence of recent group A streptococcal disease. The major manifestations include erythema marginatum, carditis, polyarthritis, chorea, and subcutaneous nodules. The minor manifestations include fever, arthralgias, previous rheumatic fever or rheumatic heart disease, leukocytosis, elevated erythrocyte sedimentation rate or positive C-reactive protein, and prolonged PR interval. Typical erythema marginatum has also been described in a patient with psittacosis.[302]

ERYTHEMA ANNULARE CENTRIFUGUM

Erythema annulare centrifugum (EAC) is an eruption characterized by persistent erythematous annular lesions, each with a clear center and a raised, thin, wall-like border that slowly enlarges centrifugally. Synonyms for EAC include *gyrate erythema* and *erythema perstans*.

Primary lesions of EAC tend to be single or multiple erythematous, edematous papules with a predilection for the trunk, buttocks, thighs, and legs (Figs. 20.39 and 20.40). They are asymptomatic except for occasional mild pruritus. The rings extend peripherally, usually slowly, 1 to 3 mm/day, sometimes up to 4 cm in a week. New lesions may form within the original circle. The resulting overall shape may be irregular, oval, circinate, semiannular, target-like, or polycyclic. The borders may eventually reach a size of 10 cm or more in diameter. The duration of the disease is extremely variable and may go on for weeks or months and, with new lesions appearing in successive crops, often for years.

At times the palpable border of the expanding ring may be topped by microvesicles or may show a fine collarette of scale on its trailing edge, suggesting a diagnosis of tinea corporis. Fungal infections can be distinguished by their more pronounced epidermal changes, with vesiculation or scaling or both at the edge of the lesions, by microscopic examination of skin scrapings, and by fungal culture. When the diagnosis is uncertain, histopathologic examination of cutaneous lesions showing focal infiltration of lymphocytes around the blood vessels and dermal appendages in a "coat sleeve" arrangement may help to establish the diagnosis.

The cause of EAC is unknown. Although it often occurs without apparent cause, most cases appear to be related to hypersensitivity to

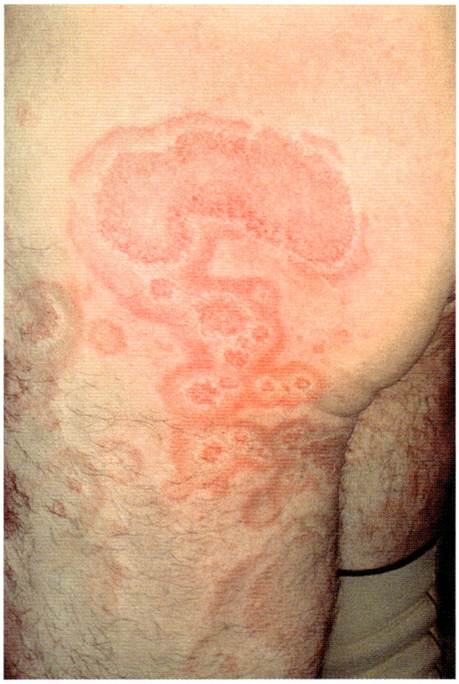

Fig. 20.39 Erythema annulare centrifugum (EAC). Slowly expanding annular lesions have dusky centers and palpable scaly erythematous borders. Although the annular rings showed no evidence of fungus, the EAC was thought to result from the patient's underlying tinea pedis.

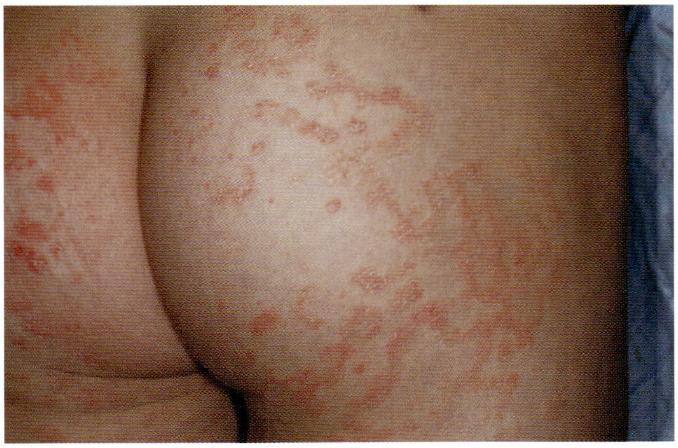

Fig. 20.40 Erythema annulare centrifugum. Although cultures did not show any evidence of fungal infection, the patient cleared completely with a course of fluconazole.

drugs, fungi, viruses (molluscum poxvirus[303,304] and herpes zoster),[305] certain foods, blood dyscrasia, autoimmune endocrinopathies or hepatitis,[306] or neoplastic disease (lymphomas). A neonate with EAC in association with pseudomonas sepsis infection has been described.[307]

Because EAC represents a hypersensitivity reaction, treatment depends on the determination and removal of the underlying cause. Antihistamines produce variable and usually incomplete relief; topical corticosteroids tend to be ineffective. Although systemic corticosteroids may aid the temporary resolution of lesions, unless the underlying cause is removed, the disorder commonly recurs as soon as medication is discontinued. Empiric treatment with oral fluconazole is often dramatically effective in those without a known cause (and negative fungal culture of the lesions), suggesting that fungal disorders are a common trigger[308] for the hypersensitivity. Cases with onset

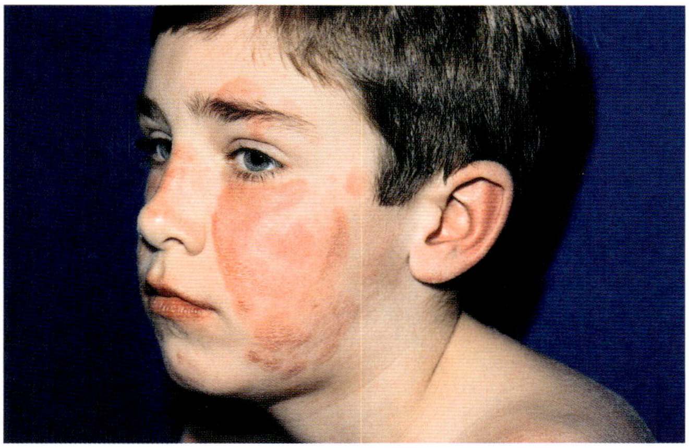

Fig. 20.41 Erythema annulare centrifugum. This 10-year-old boy has had chronic, transitory annular plaques on the face, trunk, and extremities since the first weeks of life. They only clear transiently with febrile episodes.

during the neonatal period or early infancy and persistence into adulthood have been described (Fig. 20.41).[309,310] The eruption in these cases clears with febrile episodes or subcutaneous administration of IFN-α.

Annular Erythema of Infancy

Annular erythema of infancy may be a subset of EAC or a distinct entity in which infants have cyclic eruptions of urticarial annular erythema without a demonstrable underlying cause.[311] Lesions of classic annular erythema of infancy last for only a few days, in contrast to the more persistent lesions of EAC. This benign disorder is asymptomatic. It may resolve spontaneously after 3 to 11 months.[311] Neonatal lupus (see Chapter 22) must be considered. Neutrophilic figurate erythema of infancy is considered a neutrophilic variant of annular erythema of infancy, although the recurrences of the annular erythema may continue beyond infancy.[312]

Eosinophilic Annular Erythema

Eosinophilic annular erythema (EAE) is characterized by persistent, nonscaly, erythematous annular and figurate papules and plaques in an annular or arcuate pattern. These lesions typically occur on the trunk and proximal extremities, have a chronic relapsing course, and histologically show abundant eosinophils amid the dense perivascular and interstitial infiltrates. EAE is challenging to treat, but responses to systemic steroids, antimalarials,[313] UVB light,[314] and dupilumab[315] have been described.

ERYTHEMA MIGRANS

Erythema migrans (erythema chronicum migrans), the earliest sign of Lyme disease, is a cutaneous eruption that occurs after a tick bite and is characterized by single or multiple erythematous expanding lesions with advancing indurated borders and central clearing (see Chapter 14). Erythema migrans is caused by the tick-borne spirochete *Borrelia burgdorferi* (see Figs. 14.43 and 14.44).

Panniculitis

Panniculitis is a term to describe a group of disorders in which the major focus of inflammation is the subcutaneous fat (Box 20.5).[316–319] The pathomechanism of most of these disorders is poorly understood. The most common subgroup is erythema nodosum (see later), which is often associated with streptococcal infection in children but is considered a hypersensitivity disorder seen with several systemic disorders. Other forms of panniculitis are also commonly linked to systemic disorders, particularly collagen vascular disorders

Box 20.5 Classification of the Subtypes of Panniculitis

Erythema nodosum
Infection
  Bacterial
  Mycobacterial (erythema induratum of Bazin)
  Fungal
Enzymatic disorders
  α1-Antitrypsin disease
  Pancreatic disease
Poststeroid
Malignant panniculitis
  Cytophagic histiocytic panniculitis
  Subcutaneous panniculitis-like T-cell lymphoma
  Edematous, scarring vasculitic panniculitis (hydroa-like lymphoma)
Drug reaction to BRAF V600E inhibition
Lipoatrophic panniculitis
  Associated with autoimmune disorders: systemic lupus erythematosus, deep morphea, juvenile dermatomyositis (usually subclinical), polyarteritis nodosa
  Lipophagic panniculitis of childhood
  Atrophic connective tissue panniculitis of the ankles
  Recurrent lobular panniculitis
Physical agents
  Cold panniculitis (popsicle, equestrian)
  Injections, including factitial
  Blunt trauma
Subcutaneous fat necrosis of the newborn
Sclerema neonatorum
Selected syndromes
  H syndrome
  CANDLE syndrome

CANDLE, Chronic atypical neutrophilic dermatosis with lipodystrophy and elevated temperature.

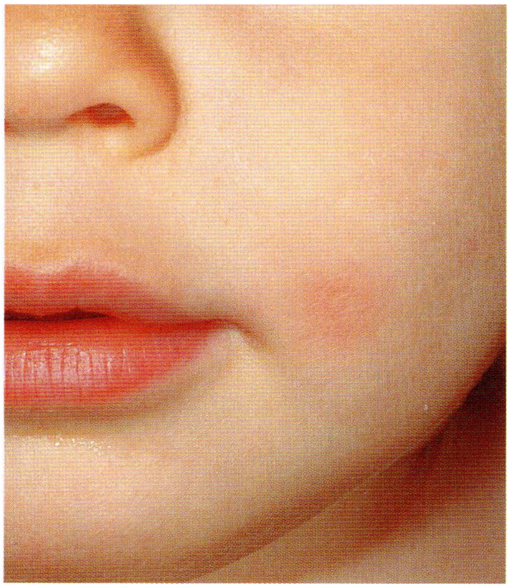

Fig. 20.42 Popsicle panniculitis. This subtle erythematous macule resulted from cold panniculitis of the cheek after sucking on a popsicle. At times, the erythema is much more intense.

(see Chapter 22), Behçet syndrome (see Chapter 25), lymphomas (see Chapter 10), diabetes (see Chapter 23), thyroid disease, and α1-antitrypsin or pancreatic enzyme deficiency and in association with generalized lipodystrophy. Disorders of the dermis, such as leukocytoclastic vasculitis and granuloma annulare, may show subcutaneous involvement but would not be considered primarily panniculitides. Infection may also lead to panniculitis, for example, especially with tuberculosis and erythema induratum of Bazin and less commonly with atypical mycobacterial infection[320–323] (see Chapter 14). Particularly in children who are immunocompromised, lobular panniculitis can be a feature of deep fungal infection (candidiasis, fusariosis,[324] aspergillosis, cryptococcosis, histoplasmosis, sporotrichosis, and chromomycosis) or bacterial infection (e.g., *Neisseria meningitidis, Streptococcus pyogenes, S. aureus, Klebsiella,* and *Pseudomonas* and *Nocardia* species).[325] Subcutaneous fat necrosis of the newborn[326] and sclerema neonatorum are discussed in Chapter 2.

Classification of the panniculitides may be difficult, and several previous subtypes, such as Weber–Christian disease and Rothman–Makai syndrome, are no longer considered to be separate entities. Histopathologic evaluation of a biopsy specimen large enough to include subcutaneous fat is often required to confirm the diagnosis of a specific form of panniculitis. Sections may show primarily septal involvement, as in erythema nodosum, or be lobular, as in the panniculitis associated with α1-antitrypsin disease. A largely lobular form with needle-shaped clefts within lipocytes is characteristic of subcutaneous fat necrosis of the newborn, sclerema neonatorum, and poststeroid panniculitis,[327] whereas necrosis is an early finding of the panniculitis induced by pancreatic enzymes.[328,329]

Cold panniculitis, which is most common in infants and children, is characterized by painful, poorly defined, erythematous plaques or subcutaneous nodules that develop in areas exposed to cold (Fig. 20.42).[330] Lesions appear several hours to 3 days after exposure and subside spontaneously, generally after a few weeks to a few months, leaving temporary residual pigmentation. The development of cold panniculitis in children appears to be related to the fact that subcutaneous fat solidifies more readily at lower temperatures in infants and young children than it does in adults. Cold panniculitis is often seen on the cheeks of toddlers and young children who suck popsicles ("popsicle panniculitis"),[331] at sites of contact with ice bags or cooling blankets before cardiac surgery or in treatment of arrhythmias,[332] and on the thighs and buttocks of young equestrians ("equestrian panniculitis"). These affected children are otherwise usually healthy, and no intervention is necessary. Cold panniculitis has also been described after ice therapy for supraventricular tachycardia.[333]

The red or purple-red nodules of factitial panniculitis result from the injection of foreign substances into the subcutaneous tissue. Diagnosis requires a high index of suspicion but can be confirmed if foreign material is found in biopsy sections. For example, polarized light microscopic examination may show birefringent particles or, as in the case of injected silicone, oily substances with a characteristic Swiss cheese–like picture of oil cysts surrounded by fibrosis and inflammation. Milk, feces, mineral oil, and paraffin are among other substances that may be injected, leading to factitial panniculitis. In young children, these factitial lesions raise the possibility of Munchausen syndrome by proxy[334] (see Chapter 26).

Poststeroid panniculitis, a rare entity of childhood, is characterized by small, sometimes pruritic or painful subcutaneous nodules on the cheeks, arms, trunk, and buttocks of young children. These generally develop within 2 to 4 weeks after the sudden discontinuation of systemic corticosteroid therapy.[335] Lesions tend to regress spontaneously without scarring.

Panniculitis can be a feature of malignancy, particularly lymphoma. Subcutaneous panniculitis-like T-cell lymphoma more commonly occurs in adolescents but has been described in infants[336–338] (see Chapter 10).[339,340] Patients develop skin-colored to erythematous, often painful, subcutaneous nodules or hemorrhagic plaques. Fever, mucosal ulcerations, hepatosplenomegaly with hepatic failure, pancytopenia, and intravascular coagulopathy are associated features. Biopsy sections show often atypical lymphocytes surrounding adipocytes (lobular panniculitis). The minority of affected children have associated hemophagocytosis, which portends a poor prognosis. In children, in contrast with adults, the face is commonly affected and systemic involvement is more common. Molecular genetic analysis and immunophenotyping should be performed; most results indicate clonal rearrangement. Suggested treatment includes initial administration of cyclosporine and prednisone for the inflammatory component, followed by combination chemotherapy for the lymphoma. Bexarotene has shown efficacy.[341]

Panniculitis has also been described as an adverse event in children administered BRAF V600E inhibitors, especially vemurafenib, for malignancy.[342] Children present with tender nodules, fever, and often arthralgias. Biopsy specimens show neutrophilic infiltration that is primarily lobular. The nodules clear with drug discontinuation and treatment with NSAIDs, but some have resolved without withdrawing the vemurafenib.[343] Tumor necrosis factor (TNF) inhibitors have been blamed for triggering lupus panniculitis in patients with other autoimmune disorders.[344]

Cytophagic histiocytic panniculitis is characterized by chronic panniculitis in association with fever, hepatosplenomegaly, and pancytopenia because of bone marrow hemocytophagocytosis. Histologically, the finding of cytophagic histiocytic panniculitis represents a reaction pattern that may be benign (in association with infection, especially EBV) or may prove to be associated with subcutaneous T-cell lymphoma. Panniculitis in association with vasculitis is a feature of hydroa-like lymphoma associated with EBV infection (see Chapter 19).

α1-Antitrypsin is a protease inhibitor made by the liver. Most normal individuals carry the MM genotype (i.e., both alleles are M) and have normal levels of α1-antitrypsin. Heterozygotes with one S or Z allele have a moderate deficiency of the inhibitor; individuals who are homozygous for the Z allele have a severe α1-antitrypsin deficiency. The clinical manifestations of α1-antitrypsin deficiency in children or adults may be cirrhosis, emphysema, pulmonary effusions, pulmonary embolism, membranous proliferative glomerulonephritis, pancreatitis, arthritis, vasculitis, angioedema, and panniculitis.[345] The panniculitis only occurs in 1 in 1000 patients with α1-antitrypsin deficiency,[346] usually homozygotes but rarely heterozygotic pediatric patients, including the MS phenotype.[347] It is characterized by erythematous to purple tender nodules or plaques most commonly seen on the lower trunk, buttocks, and proximal extremities after trauma. Deep necrotic ulcerations may develop and discharge an oily material. Lesions are often persistent and resistant to therapy but eventually heal with scarring and atrophy. Replacement of α1-antitrypsin by intravenous infusion is the most effective therapy and can lead to rapid clearance of the panniculitis, especially at higher doses (up to 90 mg/kg).[346]

Patients with *cutaneous polyarteritis nodosa* (PAN), a form of deep dermal and subcutaneous vasculitis, typically show painful oval or linear nodules on the lower extremities surrounded by livedo reticularis and often stellate necrosis (see Chapter 21, Figs. 21.17 and 21.18).[348] Raynaud phenomenon is rarely described, but digital lesions may progress to gangrene.[349] Streptococcal pharyngitis may precede the eruption.[350] Although the cutaneous features may manifest as an isolated benign form, the multisystemic form of PAN should be considered in children with distal livedo reticularis and distal ischemic necrosis in association with weight loss, fever, abdominal pain, musculoskeletal signs, renal disease, and peripheral neuropathy.[351–353] Mutations in *CECR1*, encoding adenosine deaminase 2, have recently been described as causative in families with systemic PAN; features of CECR1/ADA2 deficiency range from early-onset stroke to systemic vasculitis or vasculopathy and, in some patients, hypogammaglobulinemia.[354,355] Panniculitis during infancy and early childhood (without evidence of infection) can also be a feature of B-cell immunodeficiency with mutations in *TRNT1* (also associated with sideroblastic anemia, fevers, and developmental delay)[356] and *NFKB2* (also associated with common variable immunodeficiency and central adrenal insufficiency),[357] T-cell immunodeficiency with mutations in *LCK*,[358,359] and *GATA2*[360,361] mutations (also features genital and extragenital warts, myelodysplastic syndrome, vascular and/or lymphatic dysfunction, and pulmonary disease).

Other forms of panniculitis include *pancreatic panniculitis*, a disorder that probably results from breakdown of subcutaneous fat caused by enzymes released into the circulation from a nodular or neoplastic pancreatic disease[362] and may be associated with polyarthritis[363]; *erythema induratum*, a deep-seated subcutaneous infiltration of the lower legs, especially the posterior calves, that often ulcerates before healing and results in atrophic scars (see Chapter 14); and *traumatic panniculitis*, a disorder consisting of hard, indurated, inflamed nodules that occur after injury (Fig. 20.43). Lobular panniculitis may also lead to lipoatrophy (Fig. 20.44),[364–366] as occurs in some patients with systemic lupus erythematosus,[367,368] deep morphea, and juvenile dermatomyositis[369–372] (see Chapter 22). *Lipodystrophia centrifugalis abdominalis* is characterized by centrifugally expanding areas of lipoatrophy involving the lower abdomen, typically in preschool children and often in association with inguinal lymphadenopathy[373,374]; biopsy shows lobular panniculitis with fat necrosis. Most patients are Asian. The disorder may extend until teenage years, but response to topical corticosteroid or tacrolimus has been described. *Lipophagic panniculitis* (also called *annular lipoatrophic panniculitis of childhood*) begins with radially enlarging, tender erythematous nodules and plaques that are typically on the legs and ankles, sometimes in association with leg pain and fever. Biopsy specimens show a T-cell lobular inflammation.[375] Affected children may have evidence of thyroiditis or diabetes mellitus and may have autoimmune antibodies.[376–378] Oral corticosteroids and methotrexate are the treatment of choice,[379] but fat grafting may ameliorate cosmetically.[380] Panniculitis and lipoatrophy (particularly of the buttocks) are also features of *H syndrome*, an autosomal recessive disorder with panniculitis resulting from mutations in *SLC29A3*, a nucleoside transporter.[381–384] H syndrome is characterized by hyperpigmentation (often with induration) and hypertrichosis of the inner thigh that usually spreads to involve the middle and lower parts of the body with conspicuous sparing of the knees and buttocks. Patients also have hepatosplenomegaly, heart anomalies, and hypogonadism.

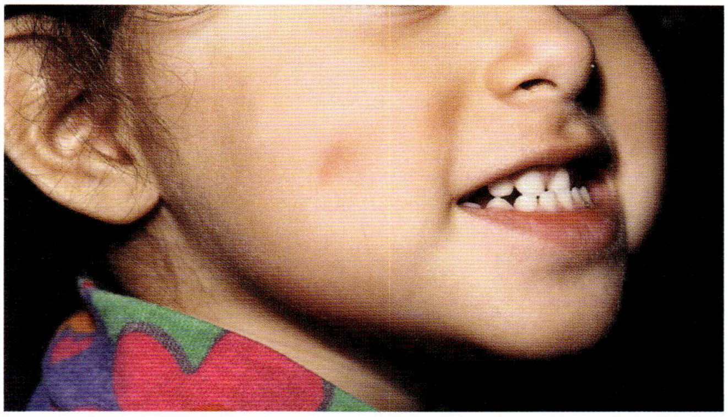

Fig. 20.43 Traumatic fat necrosis. The panniculitis occurred after blunt trauma to the cheek and led to lipoatrophy.

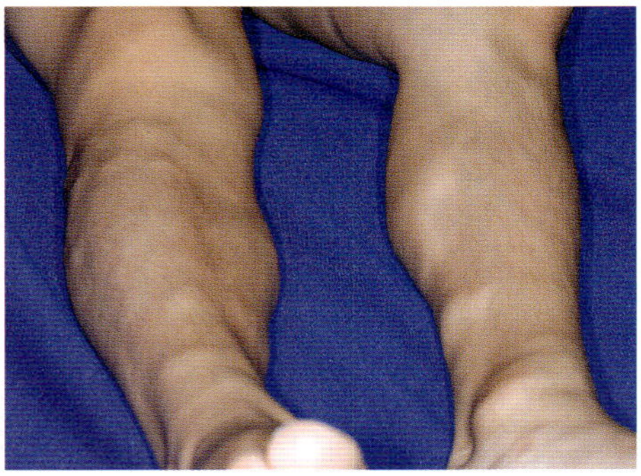

Fig. 20.44 Panniculitis and lipodystrophy. This teenager had autoimmune hepatitis and acanthosis nigricans in association.

Patients with a variety of autoinflammatory syndromes may also have panniculitis. Panniculitis with vasculitis and atypical cells is a feature of chronic atypical neutrophilic dermatosis with lipodystrophy and elevated temperature *(CANDLE) syndrome* (see Sweet Syndrome [Acute Febrile Neutrophilic Dermatosis] section).[385] OTULIN-related autoinflammatory syndrome (ORAS; also known as otulipenia or autoinflammation, panniculitis, and dermatosis syndrome [AIPDS]) is a potentially fatal, TNF-driven disease that features panniculitis in association with recurrent high fevers, diarrhea, arthritis, general failure to thrive, and signs of systemic inflammation.[386]

Erythema Nodosum

Erythema nodosum is a hypersensitivity reaction characterized by red, tender, nodular lesions.[387,388] Occurrence peaks during adolescence and is rare in children younger than 2 years of age. During childhood, girls are affected slightly more than boys, in contrast to adults, in which women are affected three to four times more often than men. The disease has its greatest incidence in the spring and fall and is less common in summer.

Lesions are most often is seen on the pretibial surfaces (Fig. 20.45) but occur more commonly in affected children on the thighs, arms, trunk, and face than in adults.[389] They are rarely found on the palms or soles (Fig. 20.46). They are most often 1 to 5 cm in diameter and symmetrically distributed, but unilateral involvement has been described.[390] Initially they appear as bright to deep red, warm, tender, oval, slightly elevated nodules. After a few days they develop a brownish red or purplish bruise-like appearance that is characteristic. Lesions do not ulcerate or leave scars.

Despite investigation, no underlying cause is found in most pediatric patients. Although possible causes are numerous (Box 20.6), the most common in the pediatric patient is β-hemolytic streptococcal infection. The list of other associated disorders is long, especially other infectious diseases (including tuberculosis, tularemia,[388] infection with *Yersinia*, *M. pneumoniae*,[391] or *Trichophyton mentagrophytes*[392] and infectious mononucleosis), administration of oral contraceptives, taking everolimus for tuberous sclerosis,[333] inflammatory bowel disease, celiac disease, and sarcoidosis.[393–398] In patients with coccidiomycosis, the presence of erythema nodosum suggests a positive prognostic sign and decreased risk of dissemination. Erythema nodosum leprosum shows panniculitis with leukocytoclastic vasculitis in biopsy sections.[399]

Box 20.6 Underlying Causes of Erythema Nodosum

Idiopathic (≈50%)
Infections
- β-Hemolytic streptococcal infection, especially pharyngitis (most common detectable cause)
- *Mycoplasma* infection, upper respiratory viruses (Epstein–Barr virus), mycobacteria (tuberculosis and atypical), coccidiomycosis in endemic areas
- Uncommon: *Trichophyton mentagrophytes, Yersinia, Shigella,* hepatitis B, brucellosis, meningococcosis, neisserial infection, cat-scratch disease, human immunodeficiency virus infection, *Chlamydia,* blastomycosis, histoplasmosis, sporotrichosis, syphilis, pertussis, *Escherichia coli,* leprosy

Inflammatory
- Sarcoidosis
- Inflammatory bowel disease
- Behçet disease

Malignancy (especially leukemia)
Drugs
- Oral contraceptives, sulfonamides, penicillins

Pregnancy

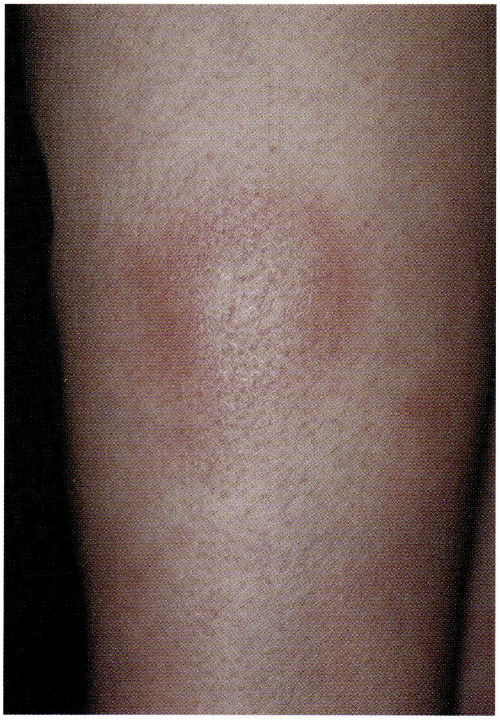

Fig. 20.45 Erythema nodosum. Tender, red, oval nodules are present on the extensor aspect of the legs.

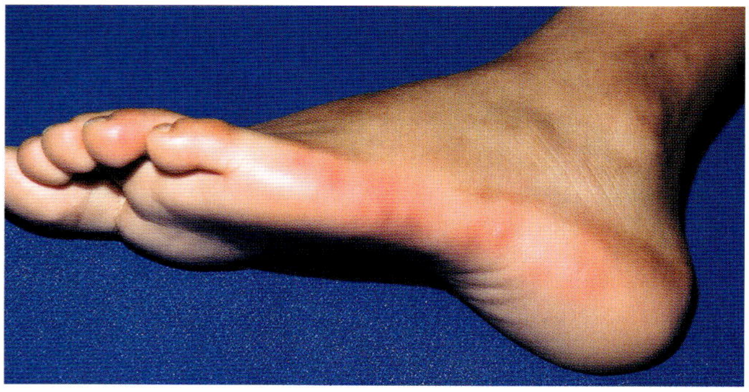

Fig. 20.46 Erythema nodosum. These inflamed nodules proved to be a hypersensitivity reaction to group A β-hemolytic streptococcal infection.

The eruption usually lasts 3 to 6 weeks but may recede earlier. Recrudescences may occur over a period of weeks to months, but attacks are seldom recurrent. Arthralgias may precede, coincide with, or follow the eruption in as many as 90% of cases. In the 10% of patients in whom the condition may present as a recurring disorder, recurrences are often associated with repeated streptococcal infection.

Erythema nodosum has a characteristic clinical picture, and diagnosis generally can be made on the basis of physical examination alone. Although diagnosis is usually not difficult, common bruises, cellulitis or erysipelas, deep fungal infections (such as Majocchi granuloma or sporotrichosis), insect bites, deep thrombophlebitis, angiitis, erythema induratum, and fat-destructive panniculitides can be confused with this disorder. Eccrine hidradenitis can resemble erythema nodosum on the palms or soles.[400] When the diagnosis is in doubt, bacterial and fungal cultures and histologic examination of skin biopsy specimens generally will help clarify the diagnosis.

The management of erythema nodosum is directed at identification and treatment of the underlying cause. Minimal evaluation usually involves obtaining a complete blood count (CBC), throat culture, an antistreptolysin O (ASO)/deoxyribonuclease (DNase) B titer, chest radiograph, and tuberculin testing. Bed rest with elevation of the patient's legs helps reduce pain and edema. When pain, inflammation, or arthralgia is prominent, NSAIDs can be prescribed. Salicylates, colchicine, potassium iodide (see Sweet syndrome), and, if severe, a short course of systemic corticosteroids are the most commonly used alternative therapies. In chronic or recurrent cases, detailed investigations must be performed to uncover the underlying cause. Intralesional corticosteroids commonly cause rapid involution of individual lesions and in persistent or recurrent eruptions oral corticosteroids may be beneficial.

Eccrine Hidradenitis

Idiopathic palmoplantar hidradenitis occurs suddenly in otherwise healthy children as erythematous painful nodules on the palms and soles (Fig. 20.47).[401,402] One case has been reported in a child with chronic granulomatous disease and palmoplantar hyperhidrosis.[403]

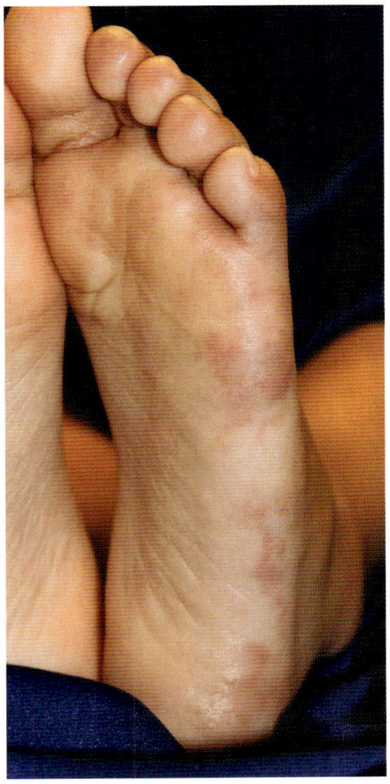

Fig. 20.47 Eccrine hidradenitis. This patient had tender erythematous nodules only on the feet. He was otherwise healthy and had not been exposed to chemotherapy. Note the resemblance to plantar erythema nodosum. Biopsy can distinguish.

The condition has been linked to vigorous physical activity, excessive sweating, and prolonged exposure to moisture. Lesional biopsies show neutrophilic perieccrine infiltrates, and the lesions are thought to result from mechanical rupture of the eccrine glands. Plantar surfaces are more commonly involved, leading to consideration of erythema nodosum, EM, bite reactions, chilblains, cellulitis, and embolic disease. In one affected infant, the eccrine hidradenitis delayed walking.[404] Although episodes recur in up to 50% of children, resolution typically occurs in 1 to 4 weeks, especially with rest. Therapy with topical and systemic corticosteroids is not clearly beneficial, although NSAIDs are often prescribed. Colchicine has also been used.[405]

Another form of eccrine hidradenitis is neutrophilic eccrine hidradenitis, a complication of cancer chemotherapy. Neutrophilic eccrine hidradenitis tends to develop 7 to 14 days after initiating chemotherapy, most commonly cytarabine. The disorder reflects the direct cytotoxicity of chemotherapy to the eccrine glands. Affected children are usually febrile, and the eruption is most commonly characterized by erythematous papules and plaques on the trunk, extremities, and face.[406]

Cutaneous Reactions to Cold

A variety of conditions can occur when one is exposed to cold. Frostbite is caused by exposure to extreme cold. Trench foot and immersion foot are caused by a combination of cold and wetness. Perniosis (chilblains) represents an exaggerated response to cold and dampness in a predisposed individual. Individuals may also develop cutaneous changes after exposure to cold with dysproteinemia, such as with cryofibrinogenemia or cryoglobulinemia.

FROSTBITE

Frostbite is a disorder caused by the actual freezing of tissue at temperatures of extreme cold (−19° C to −23° C [−2° F to −10° F]).[407,408] The duration of exposure, wind velocity, dependency of an extremity, application of emollients, and factors such as fatigue, injury, immobility, and general health potentiate the effects of the cold.[409] Frostbite is caused by direct cold injury to the cell, vascular insufficiency (constriction and vasoocclusion), and damage from inflammatory mediators. The vasoconstriction that occurs is an effort to conserve core body temperature at the expense of the distal extremities. Frostbite generally affects exposed areas such as the toes, feet, fingers, nose, cheeks, and ears. Rarely, frostbite has resulted elsewhere from application of an ice pack[410] or from improper use of commercially available cryotherapy devices for wart removal.[411] Adolescent intoxication and lack of parental supervision at the time of injury in younger children have been found to increase the risk of frostbite.[412]

Four degrees of severity have been described. Frostnip, or first-degree frostbite, shows redness, edema, and transient discomfort. In mild cases the affected area returns to normal within a period of a few hours with at most mild desquamation. Second-degree frostbite presents with marked erythema and swelling; the numbness is replaced by burning pain, and within 24 to 48 hours, vesicles and bullae appear. Although healing occurs, patients may show continuing sensory neuropathy and cold sensitivity. In third-degree frostbite, hemorrhagic bullae or waxy, mummified skin is seen, consistent with extensive tissue loss. Full-thickness involvement of the skin, muscle, tendon, and bone occurs in fourth-degree frostbite; although recovery is possible, amputation (either surgical or autoamputation) results for most patients.[413]

The goal of treatment is rapid rewarming to prevent further cold exposure and restore circulation.[414] The water bath temperature should be at least 40° C (104° F). Slow rewarming, use of dry heat, and rubbing with ice are all contraindicated. Pain during thawing and immediately after thawing should be treated with potent analgesics and sedatives. Core warming and fluid resuscitation are also important in patients with hypothermia. Other measures include wound care, administration of tetanus toxoid, avoidance of pressure and even light contact with the affected area, and vigorous treatment of infection when present. Thrombolytic therapy with intraarterial infusion of tissue plasminogen activator or iloprost (vasodilator) can improve perfusion.[414–416] If surgical measures are required, they should be delayed as long as possible. Because the prediction of tissue loss is difficult, amputation of necrotic tissue is best deferred for a period of at least 60 to 90 days to allow time for contracture, shrinkage, and the formation of a definitive line of demarcation between necrotic and viable tissue.

TRENCH FOOT (IMMERSION FOOT)

Trench foot is a cold-induced nonfreezing injury of the extremities that occurs in individuals constantly exposed to a wet and cold environment. The disorder resembles a mild to moderate frostbite, has predominantly been noted in the homeless,[417] and is uncommon in children, although ice skaters and ice-hockey players are at risk.[408]

During exposure there is usually an initial uncomfortable feeling of coldness followed by virtually no discomfort and at times a feeling of warmth as the nerves become sensitive. The limb becomes cold, numb, blue, swollen, and pulseless. The pain is aggravated by heat and relieved by cold. The ischemic tissue is prone to infection. In severe cases there is muscle weakness, joint stiffness, and gangrene that usually heals without tissue loss. A form of immersion foot has also been described in patients exposed to warm water for long periods. This disorder, characterized by a wrinkling, blanching, and maceration of the skin on the plantar and lateral aspects of the feet, has largely been reported in military personnel in tropical areas and in individuals who wear insulated boots for long periods. This form is generally reversible, leaving no residual disability.

Prevention is the best treatment. The skin should be rapidly dried should the condition occur. In the warm-water form of immersion foot, the application of silicone grease before water immersion may be helpful.

PERNIOSIS

Perniosis (chilblains) is an exaggerated response to cold in predisposed individuals.[418,419] In pediatric patients, it largely is seen in teenagers but has been described in younger children.[420] It has been noted in several adolescents with anorexia nervosa[421] and may relate to impaired thermoregulation. Wet linings in shoe boots have also been blamed. Characterized by the occurrence of localized cyanosis, erythematous nodules, or ulcerations on exposed extremities in cold and damp weather, the disorder is most common in Northern Europe and the northern United States.

Mild cases of perniosis are manifested by an initial blanching and then by ill-defined erythematous macules that become infiltrated and vary from a dark pink to a violaceous hue. In most cases the disorder is characterized by edematous patches of erythema or cyanosis that appear 12 to 24 hours after exposure to cold. Initially patients are usually unaware of the disorder. With time the areas become edematous and bluish red and eventually develop numbness, tingling, pruritus, burning, or pain.

Individual lesions tend to appear in a symmetric distribution, principally on the dorsal aspect of the phalanges of the fingers (Fig. 20.48) and toes (Fig. 20.49) and on the heels, lower legs, thighs, nose, and ears. The course is usually self-limiting and lasts 2 or 3 weeks. In young girls and adolescent women who wear skirts rather than slacks, the calves and shins are common sites of involvement. Chronic perniosis occurs repeatedly during cold weather and disappears during warm weather. Blistering and ulceration occasionally occur, and at times lesions may heal with residual areas of pigmentation.

Children with more persistent or atypical lesions should have laboratory testing to eliminate possible underlying causes. These include CBC, antinuclear antibodies (ANA), and cryoglobulin, cryofibrinogen, and cold agglutinin levels. Serum protein electrophoresis levels are usually assessed in affected adults, but the incidence of patients with monoclonal gammopathy is much lower in children. Pernio has been described as the presenting sign of blast crisis in acute lymphoblastic leukemia, with resolution after treatment of the leukemia.[422]

Perniotic lesions may also be seen in patients with lupus erythematosus (see Chapter 22), hemolytic anemia, and chronic myelomonocytic leukemia.[423] Painful chilblain-like lesions on the fingers, toes, and ears during infancy and early childhood may be the first manifestation (Fig. 20.50) and occur in 43% of patients with Aicardi–Goutières syndrome,[424] a disorder resulting from mutations in one of seven different genes. Aicardi–Goutières, which is sometimes called *familial chilblain lupus* when the pernio is a predominant feature, is associated with considerable phenotypic heterogeneity. In general, milder cases have heterozygous changes (autosomal dominant disorders) in *TREX1* (3′ repair exonuclease 1; AGS1), *ADAR* (double-stranded RNA-specific adenosine deaminase 1; AGS6), *IFIH1* (interferon-induced with helicase C domain 1; MDA5; AGS7),[425] or *SAMHD1* (SAM domain and HD domain-containing protein 1; AGS5)[424,426–428] and tend to have associated arthralgias, ANA, and sometimes cytopenias. Autosomal recessive forms of Aicardi–Goutières syndrome result from biallelic mutations in *TREX1*, *SAMHD1*, and *ADAR*, as well as *RNASEH2A*[429] (AGS4), *RNASEH2B* (AGS2), and *RNASEH2C* (AGS3).[430] The feet and hands are often cold, even without chilblain lesions. Affected children may have microcephaly, inflammatory encephalopathy and developmental delay, and arthritis. The early-onset encephalopathy and psychomotor delay are the presenting signs in many patients with more severe disease. Characteristic changes are noted on brain computed tomography (calcification of basal ganglia and white matter) and magnetic resonance imaging (leukodystrophic changes). Patients are often irritable, cry inconsolably, may have fevers without infection, and may lose motor skills. Biopsy results may resemble lupus erythematosus,[431] and autoimmune antibodies may be present. Upregulation of IFN-stimulated genes has been demonstrated, and the disorders are thought to result from accumulation of intracellular nucleic acids because of reduced nucleic acid degradation.

Pernio has also been described in a child with homozygous mutations in *IRAK4*, encoding IL-1 receptor-associated kinase[432]; the patient also had recurrent bacterial infections related to immunodeficiency. Lesions on the fingers, toes, and ears that resemble pernio can be an early manifestation of patients with an interferonopathy called *SAVI* (STING-associated vasculopathy with onset in infancy) *syndrome* and mutations in *TMEM173*, encoding STING.[433] A pernio-like disorder, primarily involving the toes, has been linked temporally with SARS-CoV-2 infection and may represent a mild manifestation, thought related to increased expression of interferon as an antiviral response.

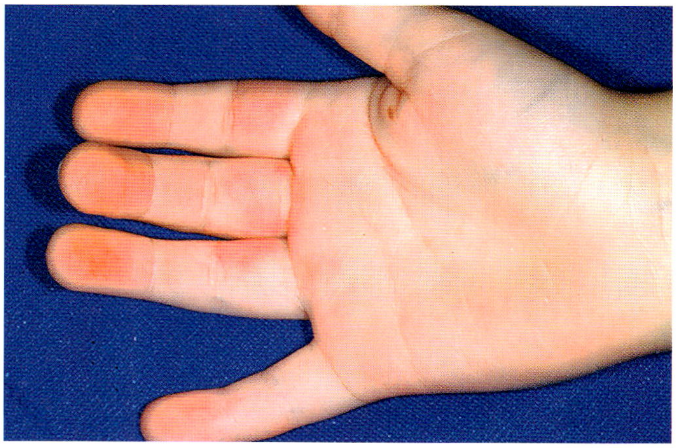

Fig. 20.48 Perniosis (chilblains). Edematous red, painful nodules appeared on the fingers after exposure to cold.

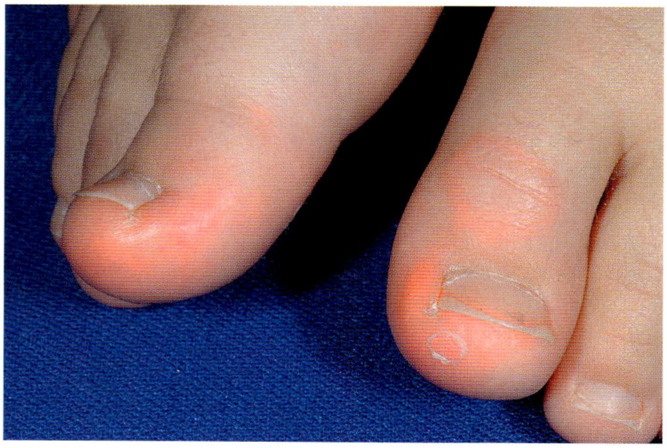

Fig. 20.49 Perniosis (chilblains). Note the inflamed nodules on the toes of this adolescent girl. Although nodules resolved, painful nodules continued to develop on an annual basis beginning in January and lasting until April. She was otherwise healthy.

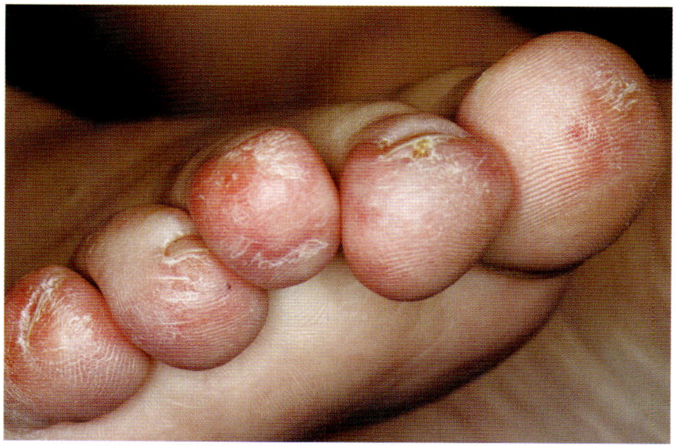

Fig. 20.50 Perniosis in association with Aicardi–Goutières syndrome. This patient presented at 20 months of age with erythematous nodules and erosions on the fingers that were not worse in cold weather. He later developed synovitis, speech issues, an abnormal gait, and small-fiber neuropathy. Aicardi–Goutières was suspected and *SAMHD1* mutation was detected at 8 years of age, the time of this picture.

Treatment of pernio consists of proper clothing to prevent undue exposure to cold, application of antipruritics, soothing lotions or ointments, and, in severe cases, administration of nifedipine[434,435] or pentoxifylline.[436] Hydroxychloroquine has also been reported to improve pernio.[437] For patients with pernio-like lesions as part of a type I interferonopathy, including Aicardi–Goutières syndrome[438] and SAVI syndrome,[439] baricitinib and ruxolitinib have been helpful, based on inhibition of the JAK/STAT pathway.[438,440]

COLD-SENSITIVE DYSPROTEINEMIAS

The cold-insoluble proteins that precipitate at low temperatures include cryoglobulins, cryofibrinogens, and cold agglutinins. Cryoglobulins are composed of immunoglobulins (see Chapter 21), often in association with hepatitis C virus RNA.[441,442] Cryofibrinogenemia involves increased circulating levels of fibrinogens (as well as fibrins and fibrin-split products) that gel in the cold.[443,444] In contrast to cryoglobulins, which may be found in serum samples, cryofibrinogens are consumed in clotting and thus are only present in plasma samples. Cold agglutinins are antibodies that promote aggregation of erythrocytes with cold exposure and are most commonly found in pediatric patients with mycoplasmal infection, although association with EBV has also been described.[445] Because cryoproteins may precipitate at a temperature as high as 35° C, the blood sample for testing must be maintained at 37° C until centrifugation. For testing, the sample is chilled to 4° C for 72 hours.

The most common manifestation of cold-induced dysproteinemia is palpable purpura that is often retiform (net-like) (see Chapter 21) and can progress to severe vasoocclusion (Fig. 20.51). Most individuals with cold-related occlusion syndromes have circulating cryoglobulins rather than cryofibrinogens or cold agglutinins. Other manifestations of increased levels of circulating cryoglobulins are urticaria, urticarial vasculitis, cold urticaria, livedo reticularis, pernio, Raynaud phenomenon, acral bullae, and digital ulcerations. In children, cryofibrinogenemia usually occurs as a secondary disorder related to infection or autoimmune disease,[446] but primary cryofibrinogenemia has been described.[447] The most common visceral manifestations of cryofibrinogenemia are arthralgias, weakness, neuropathy, and glomerulonephritis. Unexplained pain at sites with purpura or ecchymosis has been associated.[448] A rare autosomal dominant form has been described in children and is characterized by painful purpura, slow healing of small ulcerations, and pedal edema during the winter season.[449] If cold agglutinins cause clinical problems, the typical manifestation is hemolysis; acrocyanosis, Raynaud phenomenon, livedo reticularis, and necrosis rarely have been described. Identification and treatment of the underlying disorder, such as with immunosuppressant and B-cell depleting medication,[450] and cold avoidance are important in management.

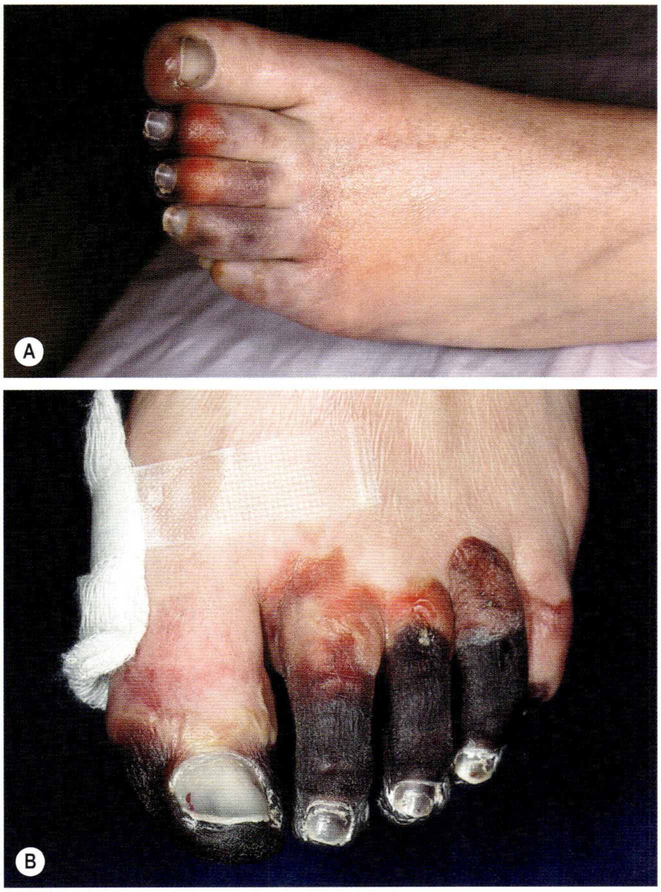

Fig. 20.51 Cryoglobulinemia. In this patient, palpable purpura and early vasoocclusion **(A)** progressed within 24 hours to severe vasoocclusion **(B)**, requiring digital amputation.

Cutaneous Reactions to Heat

Burns are the most common adverse reaction to heat (see Chapter 26). Erythema ab igne rarely occurs in the industrialized world with central heating.

ERYTHEMA AB IGNE

Erythema ab igne is an acquired, persistent reticulated erythematous and pigmented condition of the skin produced by prolonged or repeated exposure to moderately intense, but not burning, heat. It most commonly occurs from use of heating pads[451] but has been described after exposure to heat from fireplaces, hot water bottles, radiators,[452] heating elements in cars,[453] heating blankets in the intensive care unit,[454] and exposure to laptop computers (on the thighs).[455,456]

The disorder is characterized by a mottled appearance of the skin exposed to the heat and eventually is manifested by a reticulated, annular, or gyrate erythema that progresses to a pale-pink to purplish dark-brown color with superficial venular telangiectasia and hyperpigmentation (Fig. 20.52). As in burn scars, squamous cell carcinomas have been reported in plaques of erythema ab igne. When present, these carcinomas tend to be aggressive, with metastases occurring in more than 30% of cases.

Treatment of erythema ab igne consists of protection from further exposure to the offending heat source. Once exposure to heat is discontinued the erythema may fade, but the hyperpigmented changes are often permanent.

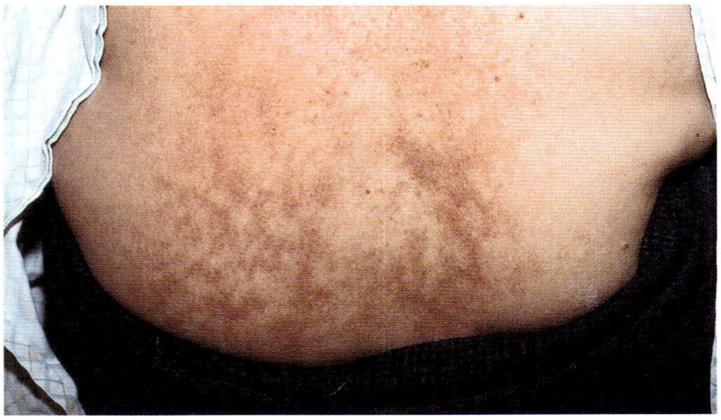

Fig. 20.52 Erythema ab igne. Reticulated brown pigmentation on the lower back after prolonged exposure to a heating appliance.

Sweet Syndrome (Acute Febrile Neutrophilic Dermatosis)

Acute febrile neutrophilic dermatosis (Sweet syndrome) is characterized by raised painful papules, nodules, plaques, or bullae on the limbs, face, and neck, accompanied by fever and leukocytosis.[457–459] Many children have a history of upper respiratory tract illness 1 to 3 weeks before the onset of lesions. The disorder has been described in an infant as young as the first weeks of life,[460] but only 5% of cases are in children. It is most common in women between 35 and 66 years of age.

Although commonly "idiopathic," 58% of children with Sweet syndrome have an associated underlying disease, which is usually uncovered by complete history and physical examination, as well as a CBC with smear evaluation. Most of these are "parainflammatory" conditions, with infection 1–3 weeks before the eruption. Upper respiratory tract infection is most common, but otitis media, viral meningitis, and HIV infection have also been associated.[461] Sweet syndrome has also been described with immunodeficiency[462] (T-cell deficiency,[463] CVID,[464] glycogen storage disease with neutropenia, and chronic granulomatous disease).[465,466] Other associated inflammatory disorders are inflammatory bowel disease,[467] systemic lupus erythematosus,[468,469] chronic multifocal osteomyelitis, vasculitis,[457] and Takayasu arteritis. Approximately 25% of children with Sweet syndrome have an underlying neoplastic or premalignant disorder (myelogenous leukemia, juvenile myelomonocytic leukemia,[461] myelodysplastic syndrome,[470] acute lymphoblastic leukemia, osteosarcoma, aplastic anemia, or Fanconi anemia[471,472]). Paraneoplastic Sweet syndrome more often presents on the face and oral mucosa. In such cases the Sweet syndrome manifests simultaneously with the malignancy, suggesting that the possibility of malignancy must be investigated upon presentation but is unlikely to develop after the initial evaluation. Drugs have been linked to Sweet syndrome, including granulocyte or granulocyte-macrophage colony-stimulating factor,[473] all-transretinoic acid,[474] trimethoprim-sulfamethoxazole, carbamazepine, imatinib, and minocycline, but in each case the patient had an underlying inflammatory or neoplastic disorder. A Sweet-like syndrome during the first 6 months of life has been associated with neonatal lupus and CANDLE syndrome, an autoinflammatory disorder caused by mutations in the *PSMB8* gene.[475,476] The lesions of CANDLE syndrome tend to be annular and show a characteristic mixed infiltrate with atypical myeloid cells, which aids in the diagnosis.

Patients with acute febrile neutrophilic dermatosis usually have spiking fevers early in the course associated with raised, brightly erythematous, painful papules, plaques, or nodules asymmetrically distributed on the face, neck, and limbs (particularly the upper arms) and sparing the areas between the upper chest and thighs. Lesions often occur in crops, and pathergy is common. Elevated plaques measure 1 cm or more in diameter, are distributed in an asymmetric pattern, and tend to develop partial clearing, resulting in an arcuate configuration as the border of the lesion advances (Fig. 20.53). They are indurated, red to plum colored, and heal without scarring, often leaving a residual reddish-brown color (Fig. 20.54). Larger plaques commonly have a mammillated surface from edema that simulates vesicles but is firm to palpation.

Leukocytosis ranging from 15,000 to 20,000 (with 80% to 90% polymorphonuclear leukocytes) is common, and myalgia, polyarthralgia, and polyarthritis of large joints have been reported in 15% to 25% of patients.[477] The fever precedes the cutaneous eruption by days to weeks in at least 50% of patients. Conjunctivitis and episcleritis may be present. Systemic inflammatory response syndrome with septic shock and multiorgan dysfunction has been associated in one child.[478] Rarely, postinflammatory slack skin with arterial laxity and aortic or mitral valve regurgitation has followed Sweet syndrome[479,480]; these children may develop potentially fatal coronary artery disease.[481,482]

Acute febrile neutrophilic dermatosis generally presents a characteristic clinical picture, which can be confirmed by cutaneous biopsy. To establish the diagnosis, it has been suggested that patients must fulfill both major criteria and at least two of the minor criteria (Box 20.7). Biopsy specimens show a dense dermal perivascular infiltration of polymorphonuclear leukocytes, sometimes with nuclear dust, but without vasculitis. A similar histologic picture can be seen in patients with neutrophilic urticarial dermatosis, usually related to underlying systemic lupus erythematosus in pediatric patients[483] but distinguishable clinically from Sweet syndrome by urticarial macules or plaques without edema and lasting less than 24 hours. A variant of Sweet syndrome with infiltration of myeloperoxidase-positive mononuclear cells *(histiocytoid Sweet syndrome)* has been described with clinical features and systemic disease associations similar to classic Sweet syndrome[484,485] but lacking the dermal neutrophilic infiltration and leukocytosis.

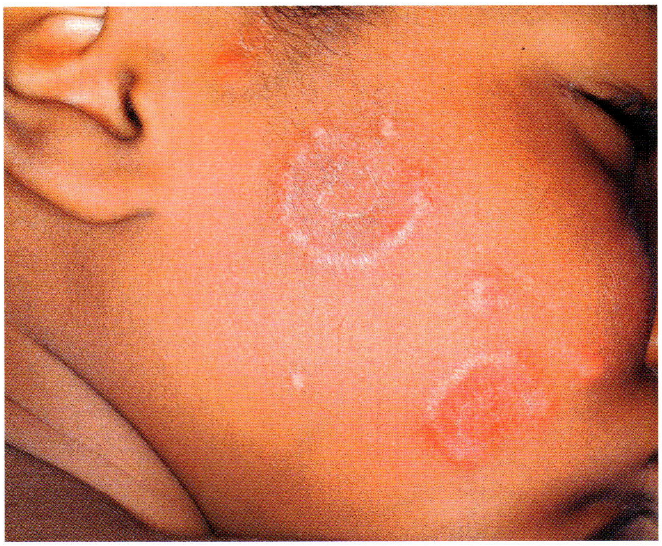

Fig. 20.53 Sweet syndrome. Asymmetric indurated annular plaques.

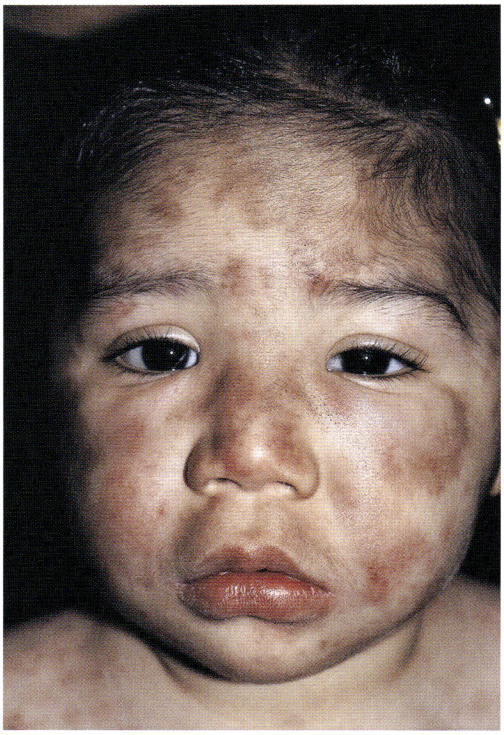

Fig. 20.54 Sweet syndrome. Asymmetrically distributed indurated plum-colored plaques and nodules are present. (Courtesy Dr. Sarah Chamlin.)

Box 20.7 **Major and Minor Criteria for Diagnosis of Sweet Syndrome**

Major Criteria

Abrupt onset of tender or painful erythematous or violaceous plaques or nodules
Predominantly neutrophilic infiltration of the dermis* without leukocytoclastic vasculitis

Minor Criteria

Illness preceded by fever or infection
Fever accompanied by arthralgia, conjunctivitis, or underlying malignancy
Leukocytosis >10,000/mm^3
Good response to systemic corticosteroids and lack of response to antibiotics

*Histiocytoid variant has a dermal infiltrate of myeloperoxidase-positive mononuclear cells and lacks associated leukocytosis.

If untreated, lesions of Sweet syndrome may extend and persist for up to a year, eventually resolving spontaneously without residual scarring. Patients generally respond to systemic corticosteroids (1 to 2 mg/kg per day) within a few days. Once the patient responds, the systemic corticosteroids should be tapered gradually over 2 to 3 months to prevent recurrences; some patients respond to corticosteroids but experience a flare with withdrawal. Potassium iodide, colchicine, dapsone, methotrexate, cyclosporine, chlorambucil, and anakinra (targeting the IL-1 receptor)[486] are treatment alternatives. The dosing of supersaturated potassium iodide is increased gradually as needed (50 mg iodide/drop with 0.2 to 0.75 drops/kg per day divided into three doses), continued for 6 weeks after clinical cure,[487,488] and then tapered as tolerated. Some recommend sipping with a straw to prevent tooth discoloration and mixing in juice to hide the taste. Because of potential suppression of thyroid function, thyroid function should be monitored every 6 to 12 months, including for 6 months after treatment discontinuation.

Bowel-Associated Dermatosis-Arthritis Syndrome

Bowel-associated dermatosis-arthritis syndrome (intestinal bypass disease, bowel bypass syndrome) was originally described as a complication of jejunoileal bypass surgery, which is only rarely performed in adolescents for obesity.[459,489] However, the disorder has also been described in individuals with gastrointestinal disorders, including inflammatory bowel disease.[490] The disorder is characterized by a flu-like illness (chills, malaise, and myalgia), asymmetric polyarthritis, tenosynovitis, thrombophlebitis, retinal vasculitis, and crops of skin lesions. Lesions are most often seen on the arms and hands and less often on the shoulders and flanks. They are generally asymptomatic or mildly pruritic. Lesions begin as 3- to 10-mm erythematous macules, which develop into purpuric vesiculopustules that undergo central necrosis and resemble insect bites. Lesions over acral areas may be painful and often mimic the pustulovesicular lesions of gonococcemia; lesions on the shins or ankles, which are generally erythematous, tender nodules, may be mistaken for erythema nodosum.

The eruption usually lasts for 2 to 6 days and recurs at varying intervals for weeks to months. It is thought to result from bacterial overgrowth in blind intestinal loops and production of circulating immune complexes directed against the bacterial peptidoglycans. Biopsy specimens of skin indicate a massive dermal infiltrate of neutrophils showing leukocytoclasia and occasionally a necrotizing vasculitis; some patients show lobular neutrophilic and septal panniculitis.

Short-term treatment of 1 mg/kg per day of prednisone markedly ameliorates the cutaneous and rheumatologic manifestations. Tetracycline, minocycline, metronidazole, clindamycin, sulfisoxazole, and dapsone have been suggested for both acute exacerbations and chronic prophylaxis. Surgical revision is curative.

Hypereosinophilic Syndrome

Hypereosinophilic syndrome is a multisystemic disorder characterized by peripheral blood eosinophilia of at least 1 500 eosinophils/μL without parasitic or allergic causes. Characteristically, the increase in eosinophils is present for 6 months or longer and is associated with infiltration of organs by eosinophils.[491–493] The condition is seen primarily in middle-aged men, but pediatric patients have been described.[494,495] The pathogenesis of the hypereosinophilic syndrome remains unknown, but many affected individuals have myeloproliferative disorders. The activated eosinophils are thought to cause the end-organ damage.

The manifestations can be variable, and almost any organ system can be involved. Approximately 50% of patients demonstrate cutaneous involvement. Pruritic erythematous or hyperpigmented macules, papules, serpiginous lesions with vesicles, purpuric papules (Fig. 20.55), splinter hemorrhages, nailfold infarcts, urticaria, Wells syndrome (see Wells Syndrome), erythema annulare, diffuse erythema, angioedema, livedo reticularis, and nodules, some of which are ulcerated, and mucosal ulcers have been described. These lesions may appear anywhere on the body but are generally present over the trunk and extremities.

Except for the blood and bone marrow involvement, cardiovascular disease is the major cause of morbidity and mortality. The heart often shows restrictive cardiomyopathy, endomyocarditis, and subendocardial fibrosis; myocardial infarction may result.[494,496] Pulmonary complications (seen in 40% of patients) include interstitial infiltrates, a persistent nonproductive cough, and pleural effusion. Neurologic findings include hemiparesis, dysesthesias or paresthesias, slurred speech, confusion, and, at times, coma. Affected individuals often show hepatosplenomegaly. Hepatic dysfunction, diarrhea with or without malabsorption, and renal involvement with persistent hematuria and hypouricemia have also been reported.

Hypereosinophilic syndrome is now classified based on underlying pathologic conditions as (1) myeloproliferative, (2) lymphoproliferative, (3) idiopathic/undefined, (4) overlapping, (5) associated, and (6) familial.[497] Treatment is now specific to the underlying disease. However, systemic corticosteroids are the treatment of choice for most pediatric patients. Mepolizumab, which inhibits IL-5, is another option and may be steroid sparing.[498,499] Myeloproliferative forms of the hypereosinophilic syndromes tend to respond to imatinib.[500] Other treatment modalities are hydroxyurea, vincristine, IFN-α2b, and fludarabine.[501]

Wells Syndrome

Wells syndrome (eosinophilic cellulitis) occasionally occurs in pediatric patients, including in neonates and young children.[502–505] The

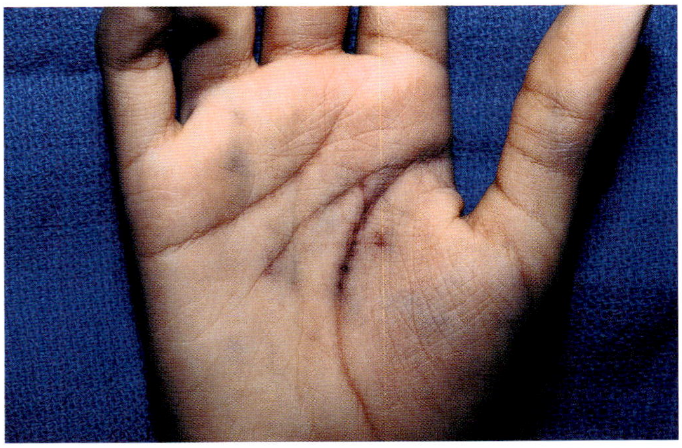

Fig. 20.55 Hypereosinophilic syndrome. This patient shows purpuric areas on the palms, but a wide variety of cutaneous manifestations occur in 50% of patients, ranging from pruritic erythematous or hyperpigmented macules and papules to serpiginous lesions with vesicles to purpuric papules, petechiae, and livedo reticularis.

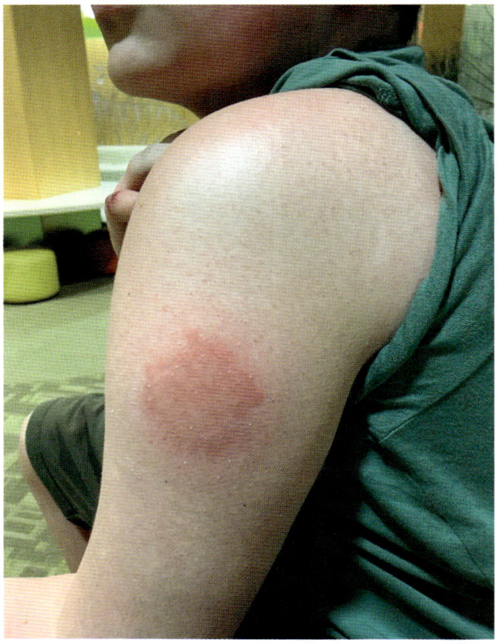

Fig. 20.56 Wells syndrome. An erythematous, edematous, cellulitis-like plaque is present in this patient. The diagnosis was confirmed by finding a dense eosinophilic infiltrate in the dermis with flame figures in biopsy sections. (Courtesy Dr. Brandi Kenner-Bell.)

condition starts with a prodromal burning sensation or itching (found overall in 82%) and spreads rapidly for 2 or 3 days. Patients most commonly show sudden outbreaks of erythematous, often painful or pruritic, edematous urticarial or cellulitis-like plaques, often with sharp pink or violaceous borders (Fig. 20.56). The morphology of lesions can vary. Although most children show plaque-type Wells lesions, granuloma annulare–like, papulovesicular, papulonodular, urticarial, bullous, and fixed drug–like lesions have all been described. Lesions most commonly affect the lower limbs, followed in incidence by the upper limbs, trunk, face, scalp, and neck. The disorder is associated with eosinophilia in 83% of patients.[506] The disorder gradually subsides over 2 to 8 weeks to be replaced by blue or slate-colored indurated patches that slowly fade. Recurrences are typical. The preceding history of insect bites, parvovirus B19 infection,[507,508] fungal infections, drug eruptions (particularly penicillin), reactions to vaccinations,[509,510] or underlying hematologic disease in some patients suggests that Wells syndrome represents a hypersensitivity reaction.

The clinical picture is striking, and the affected areas often resemble acute bacterial cellulitis, urticaria, insect bites, or a vesiculobullous contact dermatitis. Biopsy is usually necessary to confirm the diagnosis, and specimens show diffuse infiltration of eosinophils throughout the dermis with "flame figures," which can be seen in a variety of disorders of eosinophil activation. Peripheral eosinophilia is common. Although the prognosis of Wells' syndrome is generally excellent and most lesions tend to fade spontaneously, systemic corticosteroids hasten resolution. Dapsone, griseofulvin, minocycline, cyclosporine, and colchicine have sometimes been found to be effective.[511]

Pregnancy and Pregnancy-Related Dermatoses

Pregnant adolescents may experience a variety of physiologic changes during their pregnancy and postpartum periods (Box 20.8). In addition to these physiologic changes, a variety of pruritic dermatoses in association with pregnancy have been described. Although controversial, the specific dermatoses of pregnancy have recently been reclassified into pemphigoid gestationis (4.2%); pruritic urticarial papules and plaques of pregnancy (PUPPP) (21.6%); cholestasis of pregnancy (3%); a category of atopic eruption of pregnancy, which includes eczema during pregnancy (49.7%), prurigo of pregnancy (0.8%), and pruritic folliculitis of pregnancy (0.2%); and miscellaneous dermatoses (20.6%) (Table 20.4).[512–514] Pustular psoriasis (see Chapter 4) may be triggered by pregnancy as well and presents during the third trimester with erythematous patches studded with subcorneal pustules. Pustular psoriasis of pregnancy (also called *impetigo herpetiformis*) may lead to stillbirth or neonatal death because of placental insufficiency. Apart from pemphigoid gestationis, an intensely pruritic immune-mediated blistering eruption (reviewed in Chapter 13), the cause of pregnancy-related dermatoses is unknown.

PUPPP, also called *polymorphic eruption of pregnancy* (PEP), is the most common cutaneous disorder specifically related to pregnancy.[515,516] Intensely pruritic, the dermatitis occurs late in the third

Box 20.8 Most Common Physiologic Changes of Pregnancy and the Postpartum Period

Skin
- Striae
- Acrochordons

Vascular
- Palmar erythema
- Hemorrhoids
- Varicosities
- Edema, nonpitting
- Spider angiomas
- Pyogenic granulomas

Pigment
- Melasma
- Linea nigra
- Hyperpigmentation of the areolae

Hair
- Hirsutism
- Postpartum alopecia
- Telogen effluvium
- Androgenetic alopecia

Nail dystrophy

Table 20.4 Classification of Pruritic Dermatoses of Pregnancy

Name	Alternate Names	Risk to Fetus
Pemphigoid gestationis	Herpes gestationis, gestational pemphigoid	Increased risk of prematurity and small-for-gestational-age babies
Pruritic urticarial papules and plaques of pregnancy (PUPPP)	Toxic erythema of pregnancy, polymorphic eruption of pregnancy (PEP)	None
Atopic eruption of pregnancy, eczema in pregnancy, prurigo of pregnancy	Prurigo gestationis (of Besnier), papular dermatitis of pregnancy, early onset prurigo of pregnancy, pruritic folliculitis of pregnancy	None
Cholestasis of pregnancy	Obstetric cholestasis, intrahepatic cholestasis of pregnancy	Increased risk of premature labor, fetal distress, meconium staining, and fetal death

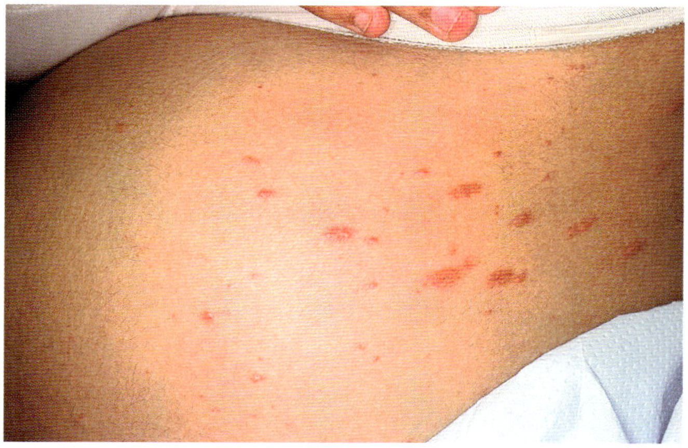

Fig. 20.57 Pruritic urticarial papules and plaques of pregnancy. Note the small erythematous papules and urticarial wheals on the distended abdomen of this pregnant adolescent.

trimester or in the immediate postpartum period. It occurs in approximately 1 in 160 pregnancies and 75% of the time affects a primigravida.[517] The disorder has only once been described in the neonate of an affected mother (in contrast to pemphigoid gestationis).[518] This is a disorder of exclusion, and no diagnostic test is available.

The condition usually begins as 1- to 2-mm urticarial papules on the abdomen (Fig. 20.57), often within the abdominal striae. These papules soon coalesce to form large erythematous plaques and then spread to involve the abdomen, buttocks, thighs, and, in some cases, the arms and legs. The upper chest, face, palms, soles, and mucous membranes tend to be spared. Although pruritus is commonly extreme, and patients are often unable to sleep, excoriations are rare. Topical application of corticosteroids usually provides symptomatic relief; if the condition is severe or unresponsive to topical medication, brief courses of systemic corticosteroids are often beneficial.

Intrahepatic cholestasis of pregnancy occurs in 1 in 1500 pregnancies (20% of cases of obstetrical jaundice) and is characterized by intense pruritus. The only skin lesions are excoriations. Affected women have generalized pruritus without history of exposure to hepatitis or hepatotoxic drugs, with appearance usually during the last trimester of pregnancy and disappearance within 2 to 4 weeks after delivery. The condition tends to recur during subsequent pregnancies in 65% of affected women and has been associated with risks to the fetus (see Table 20.4). The risk with twin pregnancies is higher, and a positive family history is seen in 50% of affected individuals.

Pruritus tends to be worse at night and on the trunk, palms, and soles. No primary skin lesions are seen. Approximately half of affected patients have jaundice, dark urine, or stools light in color. More severely affected women may have malabsorption, including that of vitamin K. The diagnosis can be confirmed by finding increased serum bile acids without evidence of viral hepatitis or another explanation. Treatments include rest and a low-fat diet, cholestyramine, oral guar gum (a dietary fiber that lowers bile acid levels), and ursodeoxycholic acid (which can substitute for more toxic bile acids).

Prurigo of pregnancy is a term used to describe a heterogeneous group of disorders that occurs earlier than PUPPP, usually in midtrimester, and is now included as part of atopic eruption of pregnancy (see Table 20.4). Cholestasis as a cause of pruritus must be eliminated through finding normal liver function tests. Pruritic folliculitis of pregnancy, a subset of prurigo of pregnancy, presents between the fourth and ninth months of pregnancy as a pruritic follicular papular and pustular eruption and generally resolves within a few weeks after delivery. Eczema in pregnancy presents, most commonly during the second trimester, as eczematous patches and plaques that can be generalized. Topical application of corticosteroids or narrowband UVB light have been helpful in the management of this subset of patients.

Autoimmune Progesterone Dermatitis

Autoimmune progesterone dermatitis is a rare disorder that most commonly begins at menarche and is thought to represent an autosensitivity reaction to progesterone.[519] In 73% of patients it is related to the menstrual cycle, with onset 3 to 10 days before menstrual flow begins and ending approximately 2 days into menses.[520] It may also be seen in individuals on anovulatory hormone therapy (9%) and in pregnant women during the first trimester of pregnancy (14%). The condition is characterized by urticaria, vesicles and bullae, papules, pustules, EM, and/or dyshidrotic eczema–like eruptions on the extensor surfaces of the thighs, forearms, hands, and buttocks.[521,522] Rarely the disorder may manifest with angioedema and laryngeal spasms requiring epinephrine administration.[523]

The diagnosis of autoimmune progesterone dermatitis can be confirmed by an urticarial wheal at the site of intradermal skin test to an aqueous progesterone suspension. Treatment is with oral contraceptives,[524] conjugated estrogens, or tamoxifen. Oophorectomy can be considered for patients unresponsive to other modes of therapy.

The complete list of 524 references for this chapter is available online at http://expertconsult.inkling.com.

Key References

Noguera-Morel L, Hernández-Martín Á, Torrelo A. Cutaneous drug reactions in the pediatric population. Pediatr Clin North Am 2014;61(2):403–26.

Waldman R, Whitaker-Worth D, Grant-Kels JM. Cutaneous adverse drug reactions: kids are not just little people. Clin Dermatol 2017;35(6):566–82.

Zuberbier T, Aberer W, Asero R, et al. The EAACI/GA(2)LEN/EDF/WAO guideline for the definition, classification, diagnosis and management of urticaria. Allergy 2018;73(7):1393–414.

Bernstein JA, Lang DM, Khan DA, et al. The diagnosis and management of acute and chronic urticaria: 2014 update. J Allergy Clin Immunol 2014;133(5):1270–7.

Zitelli KB, Cordoro KM. Evidence-based evaluation and management of chronic urticaria in children. Pediatr Dermatol 2011;28(6):629–39.

Anagnostou K. Anaphylaxis in children: epidemiology, risk factors and management. Curr Pediatr Rev 2018;14(3):180–6.

Pattanaik D, Lieberman JA. Pediatric angioedema. Curr Allergy Asthma Rep 2017;17(9):60.

Frank MM, Zuraw B, Banerji A, et al. Management of children with hereditary angioedema due to C1 inhibitor deficiency. Pediatrics 2016;138(5):e20160575.

Liotti L, Caimmi S, Bottau P, et al. Clinical features, outcomes and treatment in children with drug induced Stevens-Johnson syndrome and toxic epidermal necrolysis. Acta Biomed 2019;90(3-S):52–60.

Schwartz RA, McDonough PH, Lee BW. Toxic epidermal necrolysis. Part I. Introduction, history, classification, clinical features, systemic manifestations, etiology, and immunopathogenesis. J Am Acad Dermatol 2013;69(2):173, e1-13.

Schwartz RA, McDonough PH, Lee BW. Toxic epidermal necrolysis. Part II. Prognosis, sequelae, diagnosis, differential diagnosis, prevention, and treatment. J Am Acad Dermatol 2013;69(2):187, e1-16.

Polcari IC, Stein SL. Panniculitis in childhood. Dermatol Ther 2010;23(4):356–67.

Grassi S, Borroni RG, Brazzelli V. Panniculitis in children. G Ital Dermatol Venereol 2013;148(4):371–85.

Torrelo A, Hernandez A. Panniculitis in children. Dermatol Clin 2008;26:491–500, vii.

Uihlein LC, Brandling-Bennett HA, Lio PA, et al. Sweet syndrome in children. Pediatr Dermatol 2012;29(1):38–44.

Lee GL, Chen AY. Neutrophilic dermatoses: kids are not just little people. Clin Dermatol 2017;35(6):541–54.

21 *Vasculitic Disorders*

CHAPTER OUTLINE

- **Henoch–Schönlein (Anaphylactoid) Purpura**
- **Acute Hemorrhagic Edema of Infancy**
- **Hypersensitivity Vasculitis**
- **Urticarial Vasculitis**
- **Cryoglobulinemic Vasculitis**
- **Necrotizing Vasculitis with Granulomas**
- **Erythema Elevatum Diutinum**
- **Polyarteritis Nodosa**
- **Kawasaki Disease**

The term *vasculitis* refers to inflammation of blood vessels, a finding that can be seen in association with a variety of clinical manifestations and as either a primary or secondary phenomenon. Along with vessel inflammation there is deposition of fibrinoid material in vessel walls and the presence of nuclear fragments (nuclear dust) resulting from disintegration of neutrophilic nuclei (karyorrhexis) within the vessel wall and surrounding tissues (hence the terminology *leukocytoclastic vasculitis* [LCV]). The presence of vasculitis may result in tissue injury as a result of vascular stenosis, occlusion, aneurysm, or rupture. The incidence of childhood vasculitis has been estimated at 20 to 50 cases per 100,000 children per year, with geographic differences noted throughout the world.[1,2]

The vasculitic disorders are a heterogeneous group of conditions, many of which present with (or eventually result in) cutaneous manifestations. The range of clinical features is broad, from skin-limited changes to severe multiorgan involvement. Classification of the vasculitides is difficult and has most often been based on the gross and microscopic features of the disease process, primarily the vessel size involved (i.e., large, medium, or small). Large-vessel vasculitides, which will not be discussed here, include giant-cell (temporal) arteritis and Takayasu arteritis. Medium-sized vasculitides involve predominantly visceral arteries and include two of the most common forms of pediatric vasculitis syndromes, polyarteritis nodosa and Kawasaki disease (KD), both of which will be discussed. The other entities covered in this chapter all represent small-vessel disorders, which tend to involve primarily capillaries and venules; this category includes the most common form of pediatric vasculitis, Henoch–Schönlein purpura (immunoglobulin [Ig] A vasculitis), which in one retrospective study of LCV in children represented nearly 50% of all biopsy-proven cases.[3] It should be remembered that this classification of vasculitis based on vessel size is imprecise, and overlap in the size of involved vessels is common. A summary classification of pediatric vasculitides is shown in Table 21.1. The original patient groups used to develop vasculitis classification criteria by the American College of Rheumatology (ACR) did not include children. Subsequently the vasculitis working group of the Pediatric Rheumatology European Society (PRES), in conjunction with the European League Against Rheumatism (EULAR) and the Pediatric Rheumatology International Trials Organization (PRINTO), developed and validated criteria for some of the most common childhood vasculitides, a process that culminated in the 2008 Ankara Consensus Conference.[4,5] A summary of these criteria is shown in Table 21.2. Notably, Kawasaki disease, another one of the most common vasculitides in childhood, was not included in this classification; criteria set forth by the American Heart Association are typically used in this clinical setting.[6,7]

Henoch–Schönlein (Anaphylactoid) Purpura

Henoch–Schönlein purpura (HSP), also known as *anaphylactoid purpura* and *IgA vasculitis*, is a form of small-vessel vasculitis that occurs primarily in children (especially boys) between 2 and 11 years of age, most commonly occurring in children younger than 5 years. It is the most common type of childhood systemic vasculitis. The classic presentation is a combination of nonthrombocytopenic palpable purpura in dependent areas, arthritis, abdominal pain, and glomerulonephritis. HSP is an inflammatory disorder that has been linked hypothetically to several potential causal agents, although the exact etiology remains unclear; these agents include group A β-hemolytic streptococci (GABHS), *Helicobacter pylori, Haemophilus parainfluenza*, and other bacterial, mycobacterial or viral organisms; immunizations; and medications.[8,9] There are reports of patients with coexisting HSP and acute rheumatic fever, highlighting the potential association between GABHS and HSP.[10] *Bartonella henselae* has also been suggested as a potential causative infectious agent.[11] Although the nature of the immunologic reaction in HSP is not completely clear, the common history of antecedent upper respiratory tract infection preceding the onset of symptoms suggests a hypersensitivity phenomenon resulting in localized or widespread vascular damage. A fairly consistent immunologic observation is the deposition of IgA immune complexes in affected organs (i.e., skin, kidneys) when studied by immunofluorescence. IgA complexes, however, are not a necessary requirement for the development of HSP, and their absence should not exclude the diagnosis. Around one-third of patients have elevated serum IgA levels.[12] Several polymorphisms involving cytokines and cell-adhesion molecules that modulate inflammatory responses and endothelial cell activation have been observed and may correlate with disease susceptibility, extent of involvement, or severity of renal disease.[13] Mutations in the *MEFV* gene, which is classically associated with familial Mediterranean fever with homozygous or compound heterozygous mutation, have been described in some patients with HSP and may portend more common gastrointestinal and joint involvement and edema.[14]

The clinical picture of HSP is often, but not always, distinctive. Most patients with a rash present with an initial urticarial eruption of macules and papules (Fig. 21.1) that rapidly become purpuric and are distributed primarily on the lower extremities (Figs. 21.2 through 21.4) and buttocks (Fig. 21.5), in dependent locations. Lesions may also occur on the upper extremities, trunk, and face, and in some instances skin lesions may develop in patterns at pressure sites. In some patients, petechiae (Fig. 21.6) or ecchymoses ("bruises") (Fig. 21.7) may predominate over the typical palpable purpuric lesions. The cutaneous eruption is the presenting feature of HSP in 50% of cases.[8] Newer purpuric lesions develop and may result in a polymorphous appearance. Other skin lesion morphologies, including vesicular or bullous lesions (Fig. 21.8), erosions or ulcers, necrosis, gangrene, and even erythema multiforme–like lesions, may occur.[15,16] Marked edema of the hands, feet, scalp, or face may also be seen, especially in younger patients.[8,17] The disease often consists of a single episode that may last for several days to weeks, but in some cases recurrent attacks may occur at intervals for weeks to months.

Table 21.1 Classification of Pediatric Vasculitides

Predominant Vessel Size	Disorder
Large	Takayasu arteritis
Medium	Polyarteritis nodosa Kawasaki disease
Small	Hypersensitivity vasculitis (cutaneous leukocytoclastic vasculitis) Henoch–Schönlein purpura (IgA vasculitis) Acute hemorrhagic edema of infancy Hypocomplementemic urticarial vasculitis Cryoglobulinemic vasculitis Erythema elevatum diutinum (primarily adults) ANCA associated: Granulomatosis with polyangiitis (formerly known as Wegener granulomatosis) Churg–Strauss syndrome Microscopic polyangiitis
Other	Behçet syndrome Secondary vasculitides, including those related to infection, malignancy, medication, and autoimmune disorders

ANCA, Antineutrophil cytoplasmic antibody; *Ig*, immunoglobulin.

Table 21.2 Diagnostic Criteria for Some Childhood Vasculitides: Ankara Classification*

Disorder	Diagnostic Criteria
Henoch–Schönlein purpura	Purpura or petechiae (mandatory) with lower limb predominance† and at least one of following four criteria: Abdominal pain Histopathology (LCV with IgA deposits or proliferative GN with IgA deposits) Arthritis or arthralgia Renal involvement
Childhood polyarteritis nodosa	Histopathology (necrotizing vasculitis in medium- or small-sized arteries) or angiographic abnormalities‡ (mandatory) plus one of the following five criteria: Skin involvement§ Myalgia/muscle tenderness Hypertension Peripheral neuropathy Renal involvement
Granulomatosis with polyangiitis‖	At least three of the following six criteria: Histopathology (granulomatous inflammation within artery wall or perivascular area) Upper airway involvement¶ Laryngo-tracheo-bronchial stenosis Pulmonary involvement# ANCA positivity Renal involvement

Modified from Ozen S, Pistorio A, Iusan SM, et al. EULAR/PRINTO/PRES criteria for Henoch–Schönlein purpura, childhood polyarteritis nodosa, childhood Wegener granulomatosis and childhood Takayasu arteritis: Ankara 2008. Part II. Final classification criteria. Ann Rheum Dis 2010;69:798–806.

ANCA, Antineutrophilic cytoplasmic antibody; *GN*, glomerulonephritis; *Ig*, immunoglobulin; *LCV*, leukocytoclastic vasculitis.

*Also referred to as *EULAR/PRINTO/PRES criteria*.

†For purpura with atypical distribution, demonstration of IgA deposit in biopsy required.

‡Angiography: aneurysm, stenosis, or occlusion of medium- or small-sized artery.

§Livedo reticularis, nodules, infarctions.

‖Formerly known as *Wegener granulomatosis*.

¶Purulent/bloody nasal discharge, recurrent epistaxis/crusts/granulomas, septal perforation or saddle nose deformity, sinusitis.

#Nodules, cavities, or fixed infiltrates.

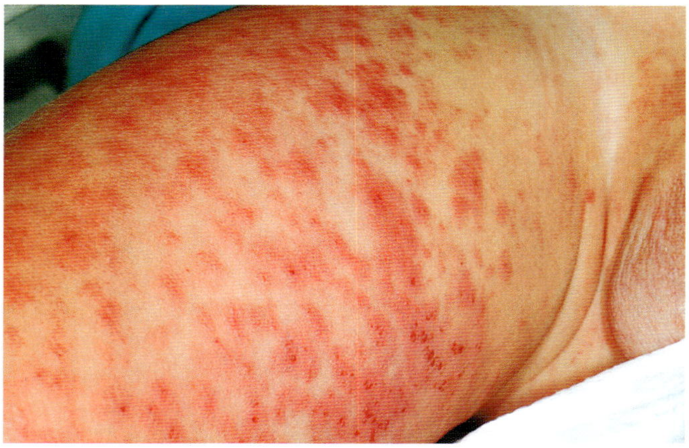

Fig. 21.1 Henoch–Schönlein purpura. These early lesions are urticarial in nature. Note associated central erosion/crusting in some of the plaques.

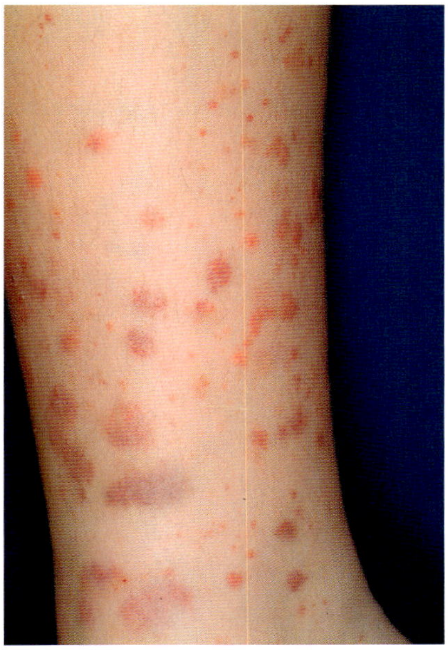

Fig. 21.2 Henoch–Schönlein purpura. Urticarial, purpuric papules and plaques on the lower extremity.

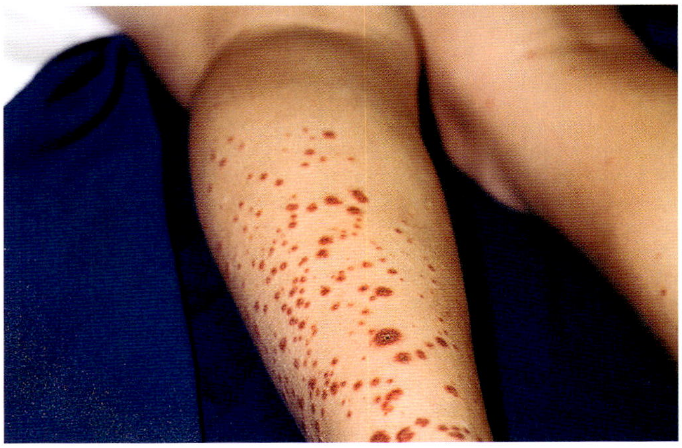

Fig. 21.3 Henoch–Schönlein purpura. Palpable purpuric papules and plaques.

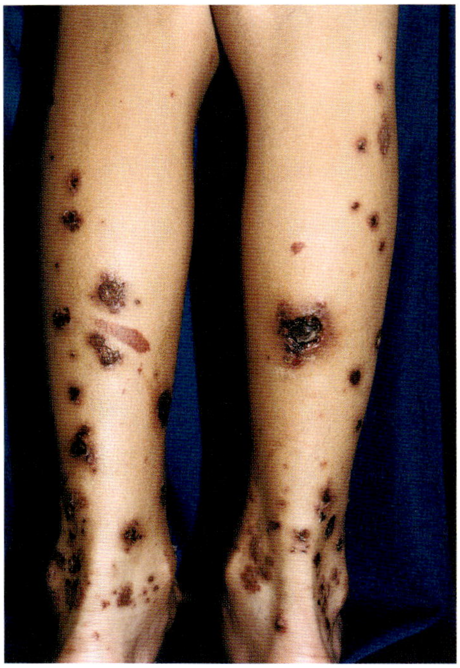

Fig. 21.4 Henoch–Schönlein purpura. These purpuric plaques became bullous with subsequent necrosis.

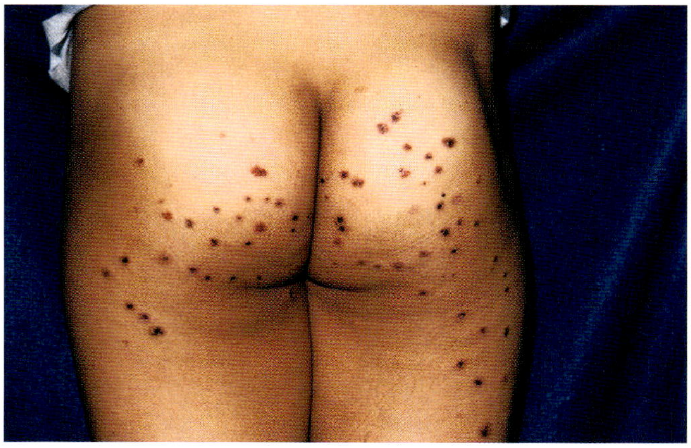

Fig. 21.5 Henoch–Schönlein purpura (HSP). Palpable purpura of the buttocks, a classic site of involvement in HSP.

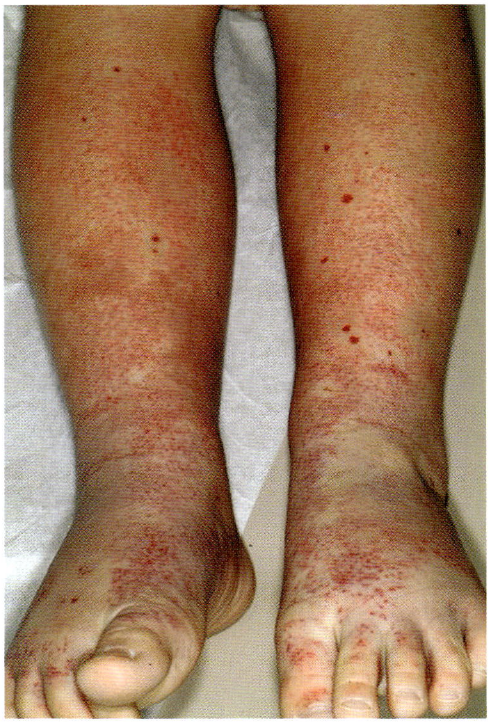

Fig. 21.6 Henoch–Schönlein purpura. This 4-year-old boy developed numerous petechiae with scattered purpuric nonblanchable papules on the feet, lower legs and buttocks 2 weeks after upper respiratory infection.

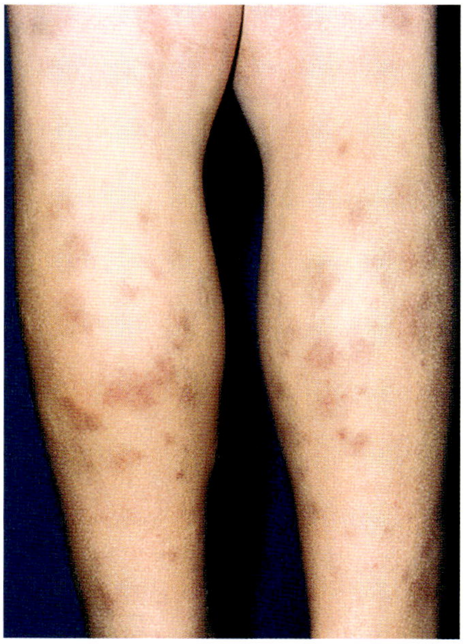

Fig. 21.7 Henoch–Schönlein purpura. Occasionally, patients have ecchymotic (bruise-like) lesions without classic purpura, as in this 9-year-old boy.

Individual lesions of HSP occur in crops, tend to fade after about 5 days, and eventually are replaced by areas of hyperpigmentation or ecchymoses. Although the differential diagnosis of the skin lesions may include drug reaction, erythema multiforme, or urticaria, the presence of palpable purpura (the hallmark of leukocytoclastic vasculitis) will usually clarify the true nature of the disorder. This characteristic finding, created by edema and extravasation of erythrocytes, gives individual lesions their diagnostic palpable and purpuric appearance as well as their nonblanching quality (i.e., individual lesions cannot be blanched when viewed through a glass slide exerting pressure over the surface, a technique called *diascopy*).

Occasionally the face, mucous membranes of the mouth and nose, and anogenital regions may show petechiae. In males, vasculitis of the scrotal vessels may lead to acute scrotal swelling with or without erythema or purpura (Fig. 21.9); penile swelling and purpura may also be present. Pain may be severe, and this presentation may mimic that of testicular torsion or other causes of "acute scrotum," necessitating ultrasonography and/or radionuclide scans to help differentiate between these disorders.[18] In one study, roughly 20% of males with HSP had scrotal involvement, and these patients were noted to have an association with headache, edema, and elevated C3 levels.[19]

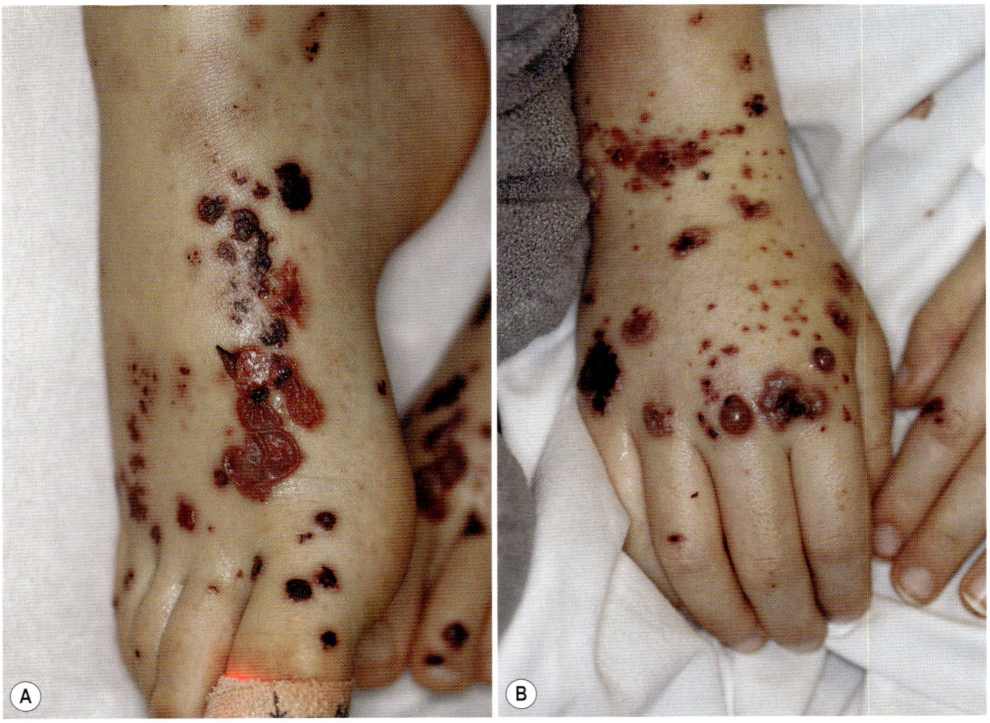

Fig. 21.8 Bullous Henoch-Schönlein purpura (HSP). This 6-year-old boy presented with palpable purpura with bullae and necrosis in a diffuse distribution (including the feet **(A)** and hands **(B)** as shown here), along with joint pain, abdominal pain with intussusception, nephritis, and hypertension.

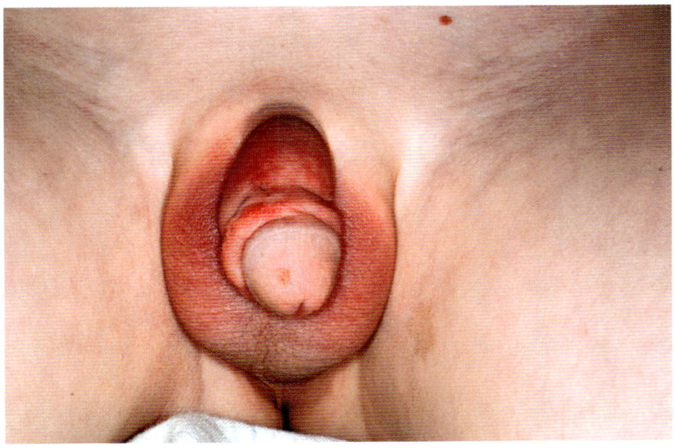

Fig. 21.9 Henoch–Schönlein purpura (HSP). This patient with HSP developed an acute onset of scrotal pain with edema and purpuric changes. Note associated swelling and purpura of the penis.

Systemic involvement in HSP, which is seen in up to 80% of cases, most commonly occurs in the kidneys, gastrointestinal tract, and joints. The degree of systemic involvement varies, with joint or gastrointestinal symptoms seen in as many as two-thirds of affected children. Renal disease occurs most often and is the most significant correlate of long-term prognosis.[12]

The clinical expression of HSP kidney involvement varies from transient microscopic hematuria to rapidly progressive glomerulonephritis. Glomerulonephritis is seen overall in 40% to 50% of children with HSP and is usually transient and benign.[20] The renal lesion in HSP is indistinguishable histopathologically from that of IgA nephropathy (Berger disease), although the latter tends to occur more often in older patients.[8] The renal involvement may not become apparent for several weeks; hence the importance of long-term follow-up monitoring for development of this complication. Most often, however, if kidney involvement is going to be seen, it will be found within 3 months of disease onset.[21] Microscopic hematuria is the most common clinical manifestation of HSP kidney involvement.[6] Potential correlates of kidney disease in HSP include age older than 4 years, persistent purpura, severe abdominal pain, and depressed coagulation factor XIII activity of less than 80%.[21] Initial renal insufficiency appears to be the single best predictor of the further clinical course in children with HSP nephritis.[22]

Gastrointestinal signs and symptoms result from edema and hemorrhage of the bowel wall as a result of vasculitis. They most often include colicky abdominal pain (which may be severe and associated with vomiting), hematochezia, and hematemesis. Visceral infarction or perforation, pancreatitis, cholecystitis, esophageal involvement, colitis, protein-losing enteropathy, intussusception, hemorrhage, or shock may also be associated. Intussusception, seen in up to 2% of patients, is more common in boys. Because non-HSP–associated intussusception generally occurs in children younger than 2 years of age, when intussusception is diagnosed in older children HSP must be strongly considered. Chronic intestinal obstruction with ileal stricture has also been reported, occurring months after resolution of the acute illness.[18,23] Gastrointestinal involvement with HSP is more likely when there are clinical findings of edema and cutaneous lesions above the waist.[24]

Joint involvement in HSP is characterized by tender and painful joints with primarily periarticular swelling. True arthritis is less common. Although the ankles and knees are most often affected, the elbows, hands, and feet may also be involved. HSP joint symptoms tend to be oligoarticular. Arthritic symptoms are usually transient and rarely result in permanent deformity.

In addition to the skin, genitourinary and gastrointestinal tracts, and joints, other organ involvement is occasionally seen in HSP. Central nervous system (CNS) involvement results most commonly in headache and, occasionally, behavioral alteration, hyperactivity, intracerebral bleeds, paresis, or seizures.[8,25] Status epilepticus has been rarely reported.[26] Respiratory involvement may range from an asymptomatic pulmonary infiltrate to recurrent episodes of pulmonary hemorrhage. Bleeding diathesis may occasionally occur.

The diagnosis of HSP is seldom difficult when patients exhibit the classic "tetrad" of organ involvement (skin, kidneys, gastrointestinal tract, and joints). However, many patients show only some of these findings, and the differential diagnosis depends on which organ-specific symptoms predominate. The differential diagnosis of palpable purpura may include hypersensitivity vasculitis (usually caused by drug reaction; see Hypersensitivity Vasculitis section), hemorrhagic diathesis (i.e., factor deficiency), or sepsis. In addition, the more "ecchymotic" lesions of HSP may be mistaken for child abuse[27] and must be evaluated within the context of the overall clinical presentation. When the diagnosis remains in doubt, histopathologic examination of a skin biopsy specimen is useful in confirming the presence of vasculitis. Direct immunofluorescence revealing IgA immune complexes is highly suggestive of but not pathognomonic for HSP. Other laboratory investigations to be considered include serum chemistry profile, blood cell counts, coagulation studies, abdominal radiographic studies, stool guaiac testing, urinalysis, and kidney biopsy. Early diagnosis of gastrointestinal HSP may be facilitated by high-spatial-resolution ultrasound and fecal calprotectin studies, both of which have been shown to have good sensitivity and specificity for abdominal disease.[28,29]

The overall prognosis for most patients with HSP is excellent, and full recovery without permanent residua is the norm. The disease tends to run its course over 4 to 6 weeks. In younger children, the disease is generally milder and of shorter duration with fewer renal and gastrointestinal manifestations and few recurrences. Renal disease is the most important prognostic indicator, and end-stage renal disease may occur in up to 5% of patients with nephritis. Long-term follow-up care is indicated in patients with kidney involvement. Recurrent flares of HSP may occur in up to 3% of patients and in one study had a lag period of 2 to 26 months after the initial presentation.[30]

Supportive care is sufficient for the majority of patients, and nonsteroidal antiinflammatory agents are useful for significant joint pain. The goals of HSP therapy are to minimize symptoms, decrease short-term morbidities, and prevent chronic renal insufficiency. Systemic corticosteroids have been advocated for patients with severe gastrointestinal, joint, or scrotal involvement, as well as for renal involvement. They are generally not recommended for rash, mild joint pain, or mild abdominal discomfort alone. Various regimens have been recommended for HSP nephritis, including oral methylprednisolone or prednisone, high-dose intravenous pulse methylprednisolone, urokinase, cyclophosphamide, mycophenolate mofetil (MMF), azathioprine, plasma exchange, dipyridamole, and heparin/warfarin.[22,31–36] Treatment with MMF may be helpful in achieving and maintaining long-term remission from HSP nephritis.[37] Severe gastrointestinal involvement may respond well to intravenous immunoglobulin therapy, but increasing proteinuria may be an associated limitation.[38]

The benefits of systemic steroid therapy for HSP remain somewhat controversial. A meta-analysis revealed that corticosteroids reduced the mean resolution time of abdominal pain, reduced the odds of developing persistent kidney disease, and reduced the odds of both surgical intervention and recurrence. However, in a long-term study assessing outcomes 8 years after a randomized placebo-controlled prednisone study in a cohort of 171 HSP patients, there were no differences between prednisone and placebo groups with regard to hematuria, proteinuria, or hypertension.[39] A retrospective cohort study of hospitalized children with HSP revealed an association between decreased hazard ratios for abdominal surgery, endoscopy and abdominal imaging, and early corticosteroid exposure.[40] Taken together, these and other reports suggest the need for more controlled studies of the effect of corticosteroids on HSP outcomes.

Acute Hemorrhagic Edema of Infancy

Acute hemorrhagic edema (AHE) of infancy (AHE of childhood, Finkelstein disease, Finkelstein–Seidlmayer syndrome) is a form of leukocytoclastic vasculitis characterized by fever, large purpuric skin lesions, and tender edema and reported most often in infants and children between the ages of 4 months and 3 years (and usually ≤24 months). The cutaneous lesions often have a "cockade" (medallion-like) pattern, with scalloped borders and central clearing (Fig. 21.10). They begin as edematous papules with petechiae and expand centrifugally with coalescence to result in the characteristic clinical pattern (Figs. 21.11 and 21.12).[41] Facial edema is common, and edema may also involve the ears and distal extremities. Scrotal and/or penile swelling may be present. Although the cutaneous eruption may be impressive, patients are typically otherwise well, and involvement of the gastrointestinal tract, kidneys, and joints is uncommon.[42] However, in one retrospective series of 26 patients with AHE, 50% had features of some systemic involvement, including arthralgias/arthritis, gastrointestinal hemorrhage, or microscopic hematuria.[43] Fever, present in around 50% of patients, is usually low grade.[44] Intussusception has been rarely observed.[45] The cause is unclear, although an infectious trigger (i.e., upper respiratory infection, conjunctivitis, pharyngitis, otitis media, or pneumonia) is hypothesized. Associations with vaccination have also been reported. Prodromal symptoms most often are limited to those of respiratory tract illness or diarrhea.[46]

Skin biopsy in AHE reveals leukocytoclastic vasculitis similar to HSP. Direct immunofluorescence studies, however, do not consistently reveal IgA deposition and in up to three-quarters of patients are entirely negative.[41,45–48] Laboratory findings may include leukocytosis and an elevated erythrocyte sedimentation rate, but hematuria,

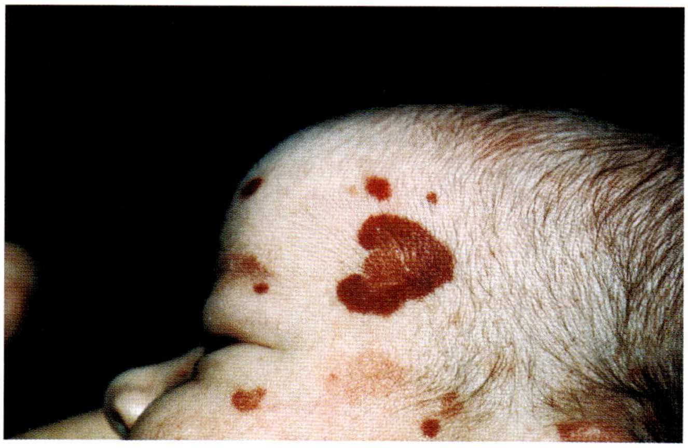

Fig. 21.10 Acute hemorrhagic edema of infancy. Medallion-like ("cockade") purpura in a newborn girl with congenital onset of the disease.

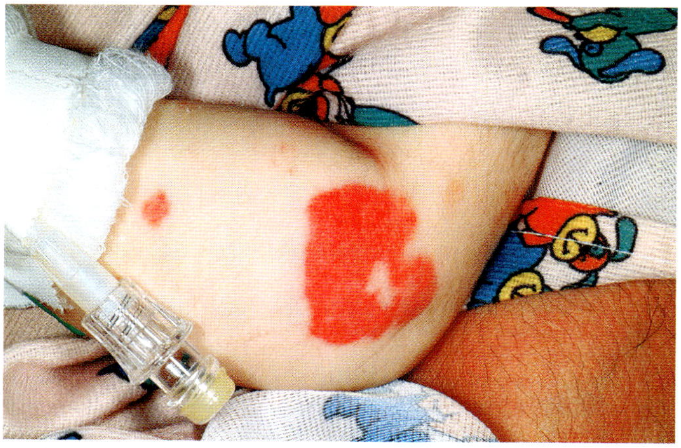

Fig. 21.11 Acute hemorrhagic edema of infancy. Purpuric patches with scalloped borders in an infant boy with the disorder.

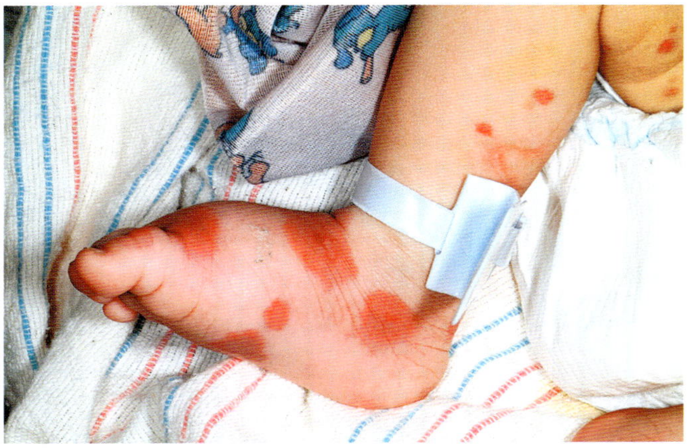

Fig. 21.12 Acute hemorrhagic edema of infancy. Multiple purpuric papules and plaques in the same patient shown in Fig. 21.11.

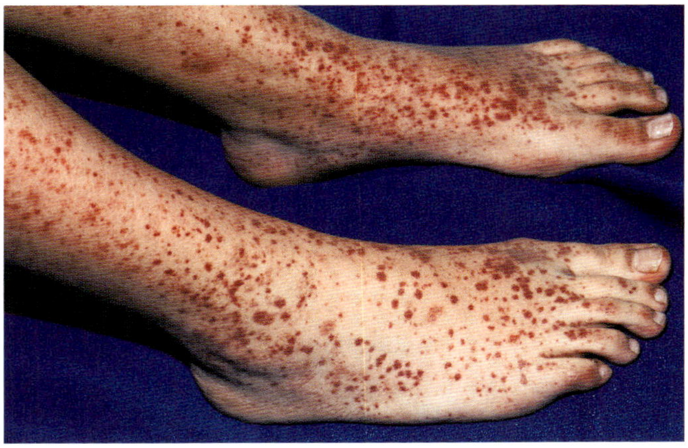

Fig. 21.13 Hypersensitivity vasculitis (HV). Multiple purpuric papules in an adolescent girl with a drug-induced HV.

proteinuria, and hematochezia are usually absent. The course of AHE is marked by a rapid onset with a short benign course followed by complete recovery, usually over 1 to 3 weeks.[49] No treatment is generally necessary, because AHE is typically a self-limited process (involuting in most patients within 3 weeks). Although the disorder resembles HSP, controversy exists over whether it represents an infantile form of HSP or whether it is a distinct and unrelated clinical entity. Arguments in favor of the latter include the usual lack of internal organ involvement, the absence of IgA immune deposits in most patients, and the overall benign course without a propensity toward recurrences.

Hypersensitivity Vasculitis

Hypersensitivity vasculitis (HV) (cutaneous small-vessel vasculitis, cutaneous leukocytoclastic vasculitis, cutaneous leukocytoclastic angiitis) is a term used to denote a leukocytoclastic vasculitis involving primarily the skin and in most cases is secondary to a drug ingestion or infectious process. It is most common in adults and significantly less common in children, in whom HSP is the most common form of cutaneous vasculitis. Potential infectious causes of HV include streptococci, hepatitis B and C, human immunodeficiency virus (HIV), nontyphoidal *Salmonella*, and *Mycobacteria* (both tuberculous and nontuberculous).[50,51] Other potential disease associations include autoimmune disorders and malignancy (hematologic and solid organ).

The diagnosis of HV is one of exclusion, and other causes of primary cutaneous vasculitis (i.e., HSP, cryoglobulinemic vasculitis [CV]) or secondary cutaneous vasculitis (i.e., urticarial vasculitis, connective tissue disorders, malignancy, endocarditis, Behçet disease) must be ruled out. The lesions of HV tend to occur in "crops" (groups of lesions of similar age) because of simultaneous exposure to the inciting antigen.[52]

Patients with HV most often present with palpable purpura (Fig. 21.13) and less often with urticaria, vesicles, pustules, superficial ulcers, or necrotic lesions. The lesions may be smaller and petechial in appearance in some patients (Fig. 21.14). Skin involvement is most notable in dependent areas and in areas of trauma or tight-fitting clothing.[53] Symptoms are usually absent, although pain or burning may be present, and systemic involvement is uncommon.

The list of potential drug causes of HV is extensive and includes multiple classes of antibiotics, nonsteroidal antiinflammatory agents, antiepileptic drugs, insulin, propylthiouracil, tumor necrosis factor-α (TNF-α) antagonists, levamisole, omeprazole, and oral contraceptives.[53–59] (For a more complete listing of potential drug etiologies, see Chapter 20.) Identification and withdrawal of the offending agent is vital in patients with HV, and in those with skin-limited disease no other specific therapy is usually necessary. For patients with either severe cutaneous or systemic involvement, therapeutic options

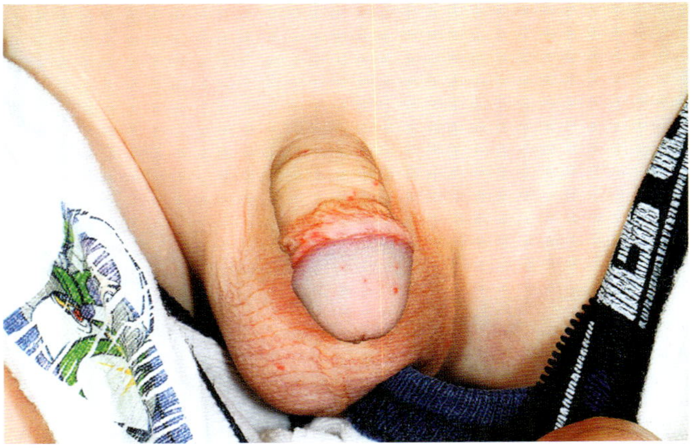

Fig. 21.14 Hypersensitivity vasculitis (HV). Petechial macules of the penile shaft, glans penis, and scrotum in a young boy with HV.

include corticosteroids, colchicine, dapsone, hydroxychloroquine, and other immunosuppressive agents, including mycophenolate mofetil, azathioprine, methotrexate, cyclosporine, and rituximab. The lesions of HV usually resolve over weeks to months with resultant postinflammatory hyperpigmentation.

Urticarial Vasculitis

Urticarial vasculitis (UV) refers to a type of cutaneous leukocytoclastic vasculitis that presents with urticarial features and is often associated with an underlying systemic disease. In contrast to common urticaria, the lesions of UV are distinct in that they last for longer than 24 to 48 hours, often have a dusky or purpuric appearance, are associated more often with burning than pruritus, and leave postinflammatory hyperpigmentation after resolution (Fig. 21.15).[52,60] Confirmation of the diagnosis of UV often requires skin biopsy given the potential overlap with other conditions, especially allergic urticaria.[61] Deposits of immunoglobulins, complement, or fibrin may be found around blood vessels in UV in up to 80% of patients.[62]

UV may be idiopathic or associated with other diseases including autoimmune disorders, infections, drug reactions, or paraneoplastic syndromes. Most patients can be characterized as having either normocomplementemic UV (in which case the majority represent idiopathic UV) or hypocomplementemic UV (see the following section). Patients with hypocomplementemic UV have a propensity toward more severe multiorgan involvement and systemic disease

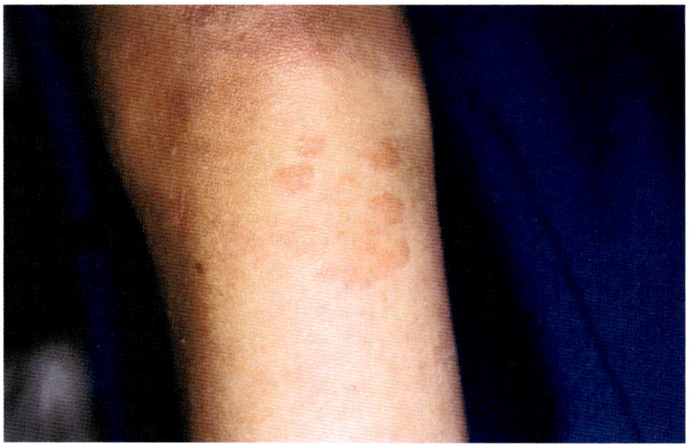

Fig. 21.15 Urticarial vasculitis. These urticarial plaques, which had been persistent and had a faint purpuric quality, revealed leukocytoclastic vasculitis on histologic evaluation. The patient was ultimately diagnosed with systemic lupus erythematosus.

associations.[52,60,61] The most commonly associated autoimmune disorders are systemic lupus erythematosus (SLE) and Sjögren syndrome (see Chapter 22). Serum sickness–like reactions to drugs, cryoglobulinemia, and hepatitis C virus (HCV) infection are also associated in some patients with UV, and it has been observed after some vaccinations.[63,64]

HYPOCOMPLEMENTEMIC URTICARIAL VASCULITIS SYNDROME

Hypocomplementemic urticarial vasculitis syndrome (HUVS) is the term used to describe patients with UV in association with angioedema and systemic symptoms, most often obstructive pulmonary disease and ocular inflammation (conjunctivitis, iritis, episcleritis, uveitis). Glomerulonephritis, gastrointestinal involvement, and arthritis may also be present, and the condition is relatively rare in pediatric patients.[65] Isolated microscopic hematuria may be the only sign of renal involvement, which may show features of systemic lupus erythematosus–associated kidney disease and can be progressive.[66] Decreased serum Clq levels are seen in most patients with HUVS, and autoantibodies against this factor are detectable in the serum.[60,67] Although antibodies to Clq are also found in some patients with SLE, HUVS appears to be a unique entity.

The cutaneous lesions of UV are urticarial in nature, favor the trunk and proximal extremities, and often have a purpuric quality. The primary distinguishing features are the persistence of lesions longer than is typical for allergic urticaria (2 to 6 hours), pain or burning, and associated hyperpigmentation as the lesions resolve. If the diagnosis of UV is confirmed, a thorough physical examination and laboratory investigation to assess for associated conditions are indicated. If an underlying disease is identified, specific therapy for that disorder is indicated. There is otherwise no specific therapy for UV. Various therapeutic modalities, including prednisone, hydroxychloroquine, indomethacin, azathioprine, colchicine, methotrexate, cyclophosphamide, mycophenolate mofetil, cyclosporine, intravenous Ig, rituximab, and dapsone, have been used but with an inconsistent response.[53,60–62,67–69]

Cryoglobulinemic Vasculitis

Cryoglobulins are circulating Igs that precipitate at temperatures less than 37°C and may be associated with any of several infectious, autoimmune, or malignant disorders. When these immune complexes deposit in blood vessel walls and activate complement, CV results. Cryoglobulins have been classified into three types based on the presence or absence of monoclonality and their association with rheumatoid factor. Type I (monoclonal cryoglobulinemia) is a monoclonal IgM or IgG antibody and is usually associated with a hematologic malignancy, most often B-cell lymphoproliferative diseases like Waldenstrom macroglobulinemia or multiple myeloma. Types II and III are composed of a mixed antibody response and hence are termed *mixed cryoglobulinemia*. The terminology *essential mixed cryoglobulinemia* is used to describe mixed cryoglobulinemia in the absence of other identified infectious, immunoblastic, or neoplastic disorders.[70] The most common infectious disease to be associated with CV is HCV, which is associated with mixed cryoglobulins.[71] Sjögren syndrome is also associated with mixed type cryoglobulins. In one large series of adults with SLE, cryoglobulins were detected in the sera of 25% of the patients and were associated with an increased incidence of HCV infection.[72] Patients with CV may experience a variety of skin manifestations, including purpura, papules, nodules, skin necrosis, urticaria, livedo reticularis, and bullous or ulcerated lesions.[53] The classic triad of CV is purpura, weakness, and arthralgias, along with possible multiorgan involvement.[70] Laboratory testing for cryoglobulins requires collection and transport of the blood sample at 37° C, storage at 4° C for 3 to 7 days, and subsequent determination of immunoglobulin composition via immunofixation or immunoelectrophoresis with quantification of the cryoglobulin fraction.[73] Treatment for CV should be directed toward the underlying systemic disease when one is identified. The main goals of therapy for mixed cryoglobulinemia are to eradicate HCV infection, delete the underlying B-cell clonal expansions that occur, and deplete the cryoproteins. A variety of antiinflammatory, antiviral, and immunosuppressive agents (including pegylated interferon-α, ribavirin, and rituximab) have been used to this end with variable success.[74]

Necrotizing Vasculitis with Granulomas

There are several systemic diseases in which necrotizing vasculitis is seen in association with granulomatous changes, including granulomatosis with polyangiitis (GPA), eosinophilic granulomatosis with polyangiitis (EGPA; formerly Churg–Strauss syndrome), and lymphomatoid granulomatosis. The first two will be discussed in this section. These disorders are primarily seen in adults but may also occasionally occur in children. They are often associated with antineutrophil cytoplasmic antibodies (ANCAs), which may play a pathogenic role and more importantly are useful in the diagnosis and management of (mainly small-vessel) vasculitides.[12] GPA and EGPA, along with the entity microscopic polyangiitis (MPA), have been collectively referred to as *ANCA-associated vasculitides* (AAV). AAV is defined as a necrotizing vasculitis predominantly affecting small blood vessels and associated with circulating ANCAs directed against myeloperoxidase (MPO) or proteinase 3.[75] Compared with adult-onset AAV, childhood-onset AAV is characterized by more tissue damage, higher relapse rates, and longer periods on maintenance therapy.[76] Constitutional symptoms including fever, anorexia, fatigue, and weight loss commonly precede other manifestations and, given their nonspecific nature, may result in a delay in diagnosis. Although a significant proportion of patients with pediatric AAV may not achieve remission, the majority respond to treatment with improvement in the Pediatric Vasculitis Activity Score.[77]

MPA, which is not discussed in detail here, is characterized by a necrotizing small-vessel vasculitis without granuloma formation and with a similar presentation to GPA with less common involvement of the ear, nose, and throat and occasional limitation to the kidneys.[78] Pulmonary capillaritis and necrotizing glomerulonephritis are seen, as are constitutional symptoms such as fever, malaise, arthralgias, myalgias, and weight loss.[79] Severe anemia may occasionally be the presenting symptom of MPA.[80,81]

GRANULOMATOSIS WITH POLYANGIITIS

GPA (formerly known as *Wegener granulomatosis*) is a necrotizing granulomatous vasculitis of small- to medium-sized arteries involving the upper and lower respiratory tract in association with kidney involvement and variable degrees of vasculitis in other organ systems. Although it is quite rare, among the primary systemic vasculitides in children GPA is one of the most common and has an annual incidence of 0.03 to 3.2 per 100,000 children. Classification criteria for GPA have been proposed by the ACR and the EULAR/PRES.[5] The latter diagnostic criteria, shown in Table 21.2, have been demonstrated more sensitive in classifying pediatric GPA than the ACR criteria.[82]

GPA usually presents with constitutional symptoms (malaise, fatigue, fever, and weight loss), and symptoms referable to the upper and/or lower respiratory tracts include cough, rhinorrhea, nasal stuffiness, nasal mucosal erosions or ulcers, earache, or sinusitis. Hemoptysis or pleurisy may be present, and nodular cavitary lesions in the lungs are a characteristic finding on radiographic studies. The nose, nasal sinuses, nasopharynx, glottis, trachea, bronchi, and lungs may all be affected by the necrotizing vasculitis, and subglottic stenosis and nasal deformity may result, the former occurring more commonly in children.[83] Conjunctival injection may be present, as may arthralgias, myalgias, and glomerulonephritis, although pediatric disease may present without renal involvement. End-stage renal failure may occasionally result.

Skin involvement occurs in up to 53% of pediatric patients with GPA.[83,84] The manifestations are variable but most commonly consist of palpable purpura. Necrotic papules and plaques (Fig. 21.16), subcutaneous nodules, vesicles, pustules, and even ulcers resembling pyoderma gangrenosum may occur.[85] Papulonecrotic lesions may favor the extremities (especially the elbows) but may also occur on the face and scalp.[53] Acneiform and folliculitis-like papules were present in 26% of patients in one retrospective review of pediatric GPA.[86] Purpura occurring on the lower extremities in conjunction with abdominal pain and hematuria may be the presenting feature of GPA, and this constellation may mimic HSP in the early stage.[87] Gingivitis can occur and presents as spongy, friable, and exuberant tissue with petechiae and preferential involvement of the interdental papillae. Ophthalmologic findings (which may occur in up to 50% of patients) include not only conjunctivitis but also dacryocystitis, episcleritis, corneoscleral ulceration, retinal artery thrombosis, uveitis, proptosis, cavernous sinus thrombosis, and pseudotumor of the orbits. Pericarditis, endocarditis, and coronary vasculitis have been reported, and peripheral neuropathy and cerebral vasculitis, with or without subarachnoid or intracerebral hemorrhage, have been noted in up to 25% of patients.

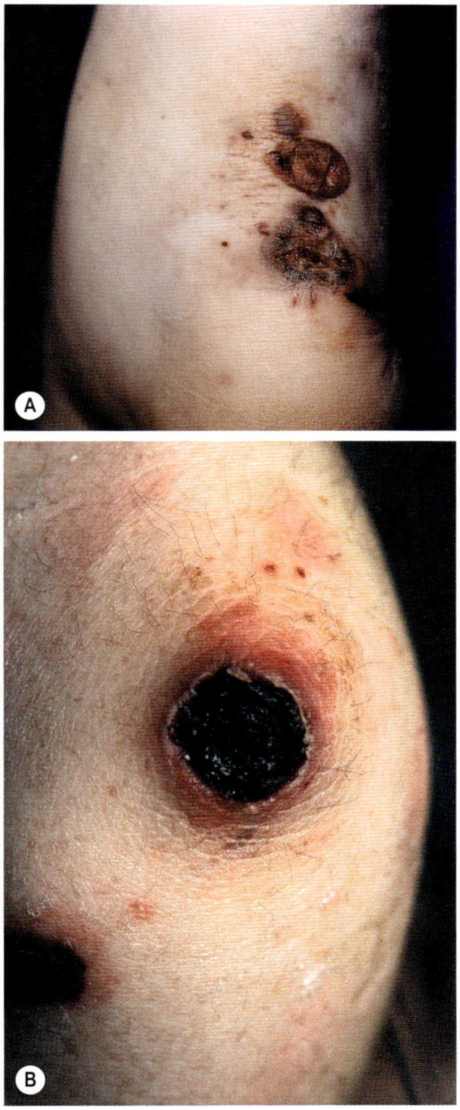

Fig. 21.16 Granulomatosis with polyangiitis (GPA; formerly known as Wegener granulomatosis). Painful, ulcerative, necrotic plaques on the ankle **(A)** and elbow **(B)** of a girl with GPA.

The diagnosis of GPA is suggested by the clinical presentation and confirmed by tissue biopsy examination in conjunction with laboratory findings. Histologic evaluation of tissues (especially skin, lung, or kidney) reveals the characteristic necrotizing granulomatous vasculitis picture, which is highly suggestive of (but not pathognomonic for) GPA within the appropriate clinical context. Up to 80% of patients with GPA have positive cytoplasmic ANCAs (c-ANCAs) and usually negative perinuclear ANCAs (p-ANCAs) on laboratory testing. In one series of pediatric patients with GPA, c-ANCA positivity correlated with kidney involvement.[83]

Before the advent of cytotoxic agents, GPA was nearly always a fatal disease, with a mean survival of 5 months. The most commonly used treatment is a combination of immunosuppressive agents, most often glucocorticoids and cyclophosphamide and occasionally azathioprine.[12,13] Less commonly used therapies include plasmapheresis, extracorporeal membrane oxygenation, intravenous immunoglobulin (IVIG), mycophenolate mofetil, methotrexate, and rituximab. Survival rates have improved with the addition of cytotoxic agents to the corticosteroids, but side effects and toxicities related to these drugs are a major source of morbidity. The use of methotrexate is advocated by some, and this agent has shown promise both in induction therapy in combination with glucocorticoids and in maintaining remission of the disease after induction with a cyclophosphamide and glucocorticoid regimen.[88,89] Cotrimoxazole is often used for treatment of GPA and may have benefit both in the prevention of opportunistic infection and in modifying disease activity.[13] Long-term morbidities related to GPA and its therapy may include infertility, skeletal complications (osteoporosis, avascular necrosis), renal failure, subglottic stenosis, hearing impairment, and nasal septal or upper airway deformities.[90,91]

EOSINOPHILIC GRANULOMATOSIS WITH POLYANGIITIS

EGPA, formerly known as *Churg–Strauss syndrome*, is a rare condition characterized by atopic manifestations and a granulomatous vasculitis involving small- and medium-sized arteries. It occurs primarily in men between 30 and 40 years of age and only rarely in children. A distinguishing feature of EGPA-associated asthma compared with typical allergic asthma is the late onset in the former, at a mean age of 35 years.

Patients with EGPA often experience a prodromal phase during which time they have allergic rhinitis and asthma, and occasionally sinusitis and nasal polyps. After several years, they develop peripheral eosinophilia, eosinophilic tissue infiltration, worsening of their asthma, gastroenteritis, and diffuse pulmonary infiltrates (second phase). The third, or vasculitic, phase presents with fever, weight loss, and widespread vasculitis and inflammation. If left untreated, this phase may result in death. Clinical manifestations may include arthralgias (often migratory), myositis, peripheral neuropathy, eosinophilic pneumonitis (Löffler syndrome), and occasional renal, cardiac, CNS, or ocular involvement. Cardiac involvement occurs in roughly half of the patients and may include pericarditis/pericardial effusion, myocarditis, dilated cardiomyopathy, valvular insufficiency, heart failure, and tamponade.[92,93] Skin involvement may occur in up to 70% of patients and includes palpable purpura, petechiae, subcutaneous nodules, urticaria, livedo reticularis, and papulonecrotic lesions similar to GPA.[53,94] Digital ischemic ulcers and Raynaud phenomenon have also been noted, as have areas with anetoderma (focal loss of elastic tissue).[95,96]

The ACR criteria for the diagnosis of EGPA support the diagnosis when four of the following six criteria are met: asthma, eosinophilia greater than 10%, mononeuropathy/polyneuropathy, nonfixed pulmonary infiltrates, paranasal sinus abnormality, and biopsy containing a blood vessel with extravascular eosinophils.[97] Laboratory studies may be useful because approximately 70% of adult patients with EGPA have a positive ANCAs, usually perinuclear with antimyeloperoxidase specificity (MPO-ANCA).[95] However, in contrast to adult patients, pediatric patients with EGPA may be negative for ANCA.[92,93,98,99] In adults, ANCA positivity appears to portend more common ear-nose-throat manifestations (rhinitis, sinusitis, polyps), peripheral nerve involvement, and renal disease, whereas ANCA negativity may predict more common cardiomyopathy.[100] Histopathologic evaluation of skin specimens is notable for extravascular eosinophils, granuloma formation, and necrotizing changes in small- and medium-sized vessels.

EGPA is treated with glucocorticoids with or without the addition of other immunosuppressive agents (i.e., cyclophosphamide, azathioprine), and the prognosis has traditionally been fairly favorable with a lower mortality rate compared with other systemic vasculitides. Combination therapy with other agents has been reported, including infliximab, mycophenolate mofetil, hydroxychloroquine, and methotrexate. Steroid-dependent asthma, however, is common and may persist even after the vasculitis is in remission.[101] In a large series of children with EGPA, more common cardiopulmonary manifestations, less common peripheral neuropathy, and higher mortality were noted when compared with the clinical experience in adults.[98] However, in other smaller series of children with EGPA, neurologic associations (especially mononeuritis multiplex) were present in a majority of patients.[93,99]

Erythema Elevatum Diutinum

Erythema elevatum diutinum (EED) is an uncommon dermatosis seen most often in middle-aged adults and characterized by violaceous papules, plaques, and nodules that have a predilection for acral and extensor surfaces. Common locations for the lesions of EED include the elbows, knees, dorsum of the hands and feet, pretibial surfaces, buttocks, and skin overlying the Achilles tendon.[102] The trunk and mucous membranes are usually spared. Histologically the lesions reveal a leukocytoclastic vasculitis.

EED presents with papules and plaques ranging in size from a few millimeters to several centimeters. They may be yellow and simulate xanthomas, but more often they are violaceous to brown, and less commonly erythema, vesicles, or bullae may be present. The differential diagnosis may include Sweet syndrome, pyoderma gangrenosum, granuloma annulare, Kaposi sarcoma, and bacillary angiomatosis.[103] Although the lesions are typically asymptomatic, they may be tender or painful and may be accompanied by systemic abnormalities such as arthralgias, fever, and malaise. A burning sensation within lesions has been reported by some patients and may worsen in the evening or after exposure to cold temperatures.[104] Spontaneous involution may occur after a period of years without scarring, but residual hypopigmentation or hyperpigmentation is common.

The pathogenesis of EED is unknown, although it is believed to be an immune complex–mediated vasculitis. It has been described in association with various conditions, including hematologic malignancies, infections (including streptococcal and both hepatitis B and C), autoimmune disease, and inflammatory bowel disease.[102,105] Rheumatoid arthritis–associated EED may present with the skin lesions in conjunction with peripheral ulcerative keratitis.[106] In recent decades, EED emerged as a dermatosis associated with HIV infection.[107] It has been reported in a young woman with juvenile idiopathic arthritis,[108] as well as in a school-aged boy with a history of recurrent streptococcal pharyngotonsillitis, in whom it abated after dapsone therapy and tonsillectomy.[109]

EED tends to run a chronic course and may be persistent or may occasionally spontaneously resolve. Although topical or intralesional corticosteroids may sometimes be useful, the response to these agents is generally unsatisfactory. Dapsone may be effective and to many is considered the treatment of choice, although the lesions often recur on discontinuation. Other reported therapies include colchicine, sulfapyridine, niacinamide, methotrexate, tetracycline, and cyclophosphamide. Surgical excision of large nodules is another therapeutic option.

Polyarteritis Nodosa

Polyarteritis nodosa (PAN), also known as *periarteritis nodosa*, is a relatively uncommon vasculitis in children that is characterized by inflammation of medium-sized (and in some cases, small-sized) arteries. Several subtypes of PAN have been identified, and the prognosis is variable and largely dependent on the extent of associated (extracutaneous) organ involvement. The two variants discussed in this section are cutaneous PAN (cPAN) and systemic PAN. An infantile type of PAN may occur in children younger than 2 years of age but is now considered by most to represent a severe form of KD. The clinical features of childhood PAN are briefly summarized in Table 21.3. The EULAR/PRINTO/PRES criteria for childhood PAN are shown in Table 21.2.

Patients with PAN often have constitutional symptoms, including fever, malaise, and weight loss, as well as myalgias and arthralgias. Painful skin nodules, purpura, ulcerations, and livedo reticularis (Fig. 21.17) are the most common cutaneous findings. The nodules vary from 0.5 to 1 cm, are tender to palpation, and are usually red-purple (Fig. 21.18). They may follow the course of superficial arteries and are especially common around the knee, anterior lower leg, and dorsum of the foot.[53] Healing of the ulcerative skin lesions of PAN may result in atrophic, ivory-colored, stellate-shaped scars and hyperpigmentation.[52] Oral manifestations may include ulceration of the hard palate, tongue, and buccal or gingival mucosae.[110] Peripheral ischemia with infarction or gangrene may occur (Fig. 21.19). Other manifestations include abdominal pain, hematochezia, neuropathy, Raynaud phenomenon, and cardiac and renal involvement, which may lead to renovascular hypertension. Pericarditis and valvular heart disease may occur. The lungs are usually spared in patients with PAN, although pleural effusions and pneumonitis have been reported.[111] Death, when it occurs, is usually attributable to renal failure, intracranial or intraabdominal hemorrhage, hypertensive heart failure, disseminated infection, or myocardial involvement.

Table 21.3 Clinical Features of Polyarteritis Nodosa in Childhood

	TYPE	
	Systemic PAN	**cPAN**
Presentation	Fever, CS	Fever, mild CS
Skin findings	Nodules, purpura, ulcers, livedo reticularis, infarction/gangrene, edema, Raynaud phenomenon	Nodules, purpura, ulcers, livedo reticularis, edema, gangrene
Extracutaneous involvement	Cardiac, renal, CNS/PNS, musculoskeletal, gastrointestinal, rarely pulmonary	Musculoskeletal, occasional PNS
Prognosis	Variable; relapse in around 35%	Good

Modified from Eleftheriou D, Dillon MJ, Tullus K, et al. Systemic polyarteritis nodosa in the young: a single-center experience over thirty-two years. Arthritis Rheum 2013;65(9):2476–85; and Bansal NK, Houghton KM. Cutaneous polyarteritis nodosa in childhood: a case report and review of the literature. Arthritis 2010;2010:687547.

CNS, Central nervous system; *cPAN*, cutaneous polyarteritis nodosa; *CS*, constitutional symptoms (fever, fatigue, weight loss); *PAN*, polyarteritis nodosa; *PNS*, peripheral nervous system.

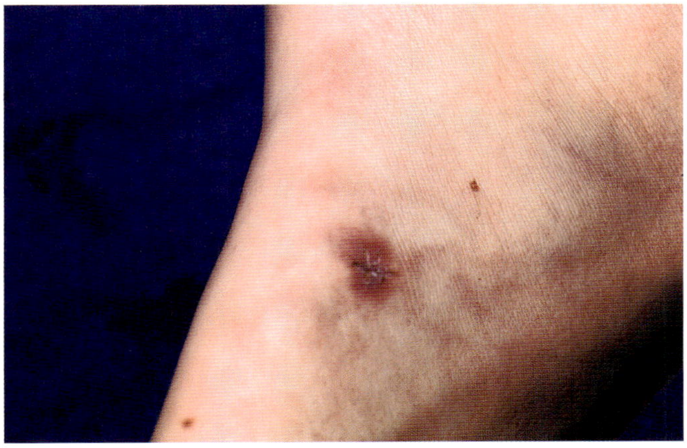

Fig. 21.17 Polyarteritis nodosa. Reticulate mottling (livedo reticularis) on the medial foot of a patient with polyarteritis nodosa.

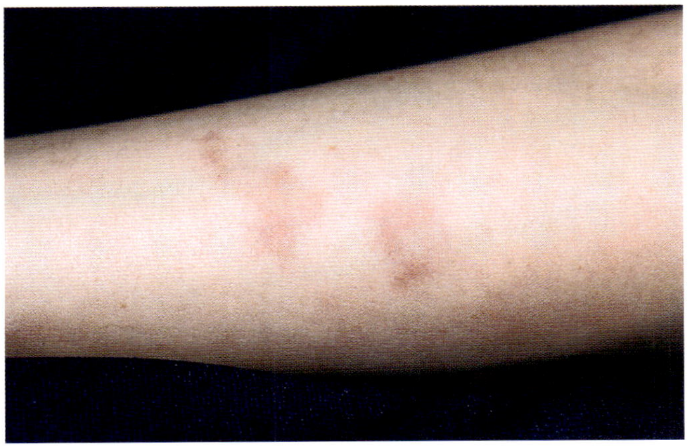

Fig. 21.18 Polyarteritis nodosa. These dusky red nodules were firm and tender to palpation.

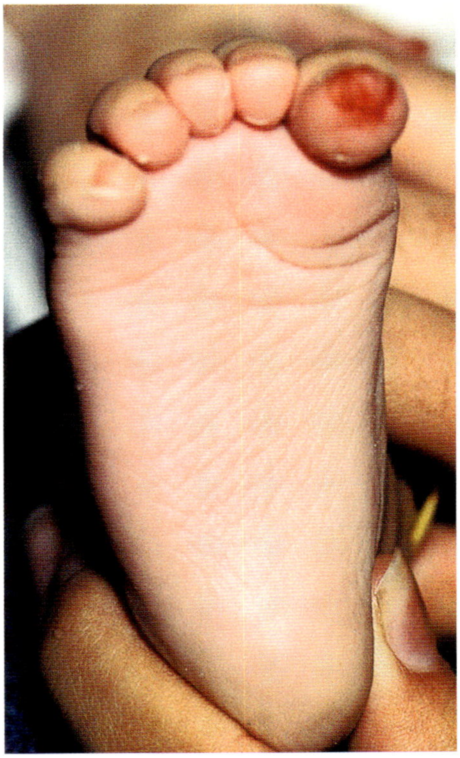

Fig. 21.19 Polyarteritis nodosa. This child with polyarteritis nodosa developed dusky red changes of the toes, followed by necrosis, as a manifestation of peripheral ischemia.

Although the cause of PAN is unknown, it is presumed to represent a hypersensitivity-type immune-complex vasculitis with deposits of IgM, C_3, or both in affected vessel walls.[112] Hepatitis B virus infection is associated in some cases, and group A streptococcal infection has been suggested as another potential infectious cause. Laboratory findings may reveal anemia, leukocytosis, thrombocytosis, and an elevation of acute-phase reactants.[113] Serologic markers may be useful because patients may have a positive ANCA (usually p-ANCA, although c-ANCA has also been observed). However, serologic studies alone are of limited use in the diagnosis of PAN given their lack of specificity or sensitivity. Skin biopsy examination is diagnostically valuable and reveals fibrinoid necrosis and inflammation of arteries in the deep dermis and subcutaneous layer and, in some cases, septal panniculitis. Direct immunofluorescence studies are variable, occasionally revealing IgM or C_3 deposition. Mutations in the gene for familial Mediterranean fever, *MEFV*, are found in some pediatric patients with PAN and may represent a susceptibility factor, especially in countries where familial Mediterranean fever and its carriers are more common.[114] Recessive loss-of-function mutations in *CECR1*, the gene that encodes adenosine deaminase 2 (ADA2), were demonstrated in six families who had multiple individuals with systemic and cutaneous PAN.[115]

cPAN (also known as *benign cPAN*) is the terminology used to describe a clinical variant of PAN in which cutaneous lesions predominate and there is no (or very limited) extracutaneous involvement. It is the most common form of PAN in children and tends to have a chronic course notable for remissions and relapses. The typical skin findings in cPAN are painful red nodules, especially on the lower extremities and malleoli with ulcers, purpura, and livedo reticularis. Peripheral gangrene and autoamputation occur with greater incidence in pediatric patients who have onset of cPAN in the first decade of life.[116] Constitutional symptoms including fever, arthralgias, myalgias, and peripheral nervous system involvement (mononeuritis multiplex, peripheral neuropathy, cranial nerve palsy) may occur, but visceral involvement is often absent. The most notable laboratory aberrations are leukocytosis and elevation of the erythrocyte sedimentation rate.[117] The definitive diagnosis of cPAN is established by histopathologic features in tissue biopsy specimens. The overall outcome of cPAN is traditionally believed to be favorable, although there are reports of cPAN evolving into systemic disease. In one retrospective series of 29 children with PAN, the ultimate clinical outcome was not predictable from the initial presentation (i.e., on the spectrum between cPAN and visceral PAN), and some patients with initial cPAN went on to develop severe complications and require immunosuppressant therapies.[118]

The mainstay of management for PAN is systemic corticosteroids. Cyclophosphamide, dipyridamole, azathioprine, mycophenolate mofetil, intravenous γ-globulin, methotrexate, and plasma exchange have also been used.[113,119–121] Refractory disease has been treated with TNF-α blockade (infliximab, etanercept, adalimumab), and rituximab has also been reported as effective.[122,123] In patients with skin-limited disease, therapy with aspirin or nonsteroidal antiinflammatory agents has also been advocated.[79,117,124] In a study comparing childhood- and adult-onset PAN, the former had a more benign course, with less renal and neurologic involvement and shorter duration of induction therapy compared with adult-onset disease.[121]

Kawasaki Disease

Kawasaki disease (KD; also acute febrile mucocutaneous lymph node syndrome) is an acute febrile disease of childhood that is one of the leading causes of acquired heart disease in the world. It was described initially in 1967 by Tomisaku Kawasaki. KD is most prevalent in Japan, and its incidence is much higher in Asian-American populations, possibly suggesting a unique genetic susceptibility. Pathologically, KD is a vasculitis involving the small and medium-sized muscular arteries with a predilection for involvement of the main coronary vessels.[125] As mentioned earlier in this chapter, many believe that the entity referred to in the past as infantile PAN in fact represents a severe phenotype of KD.

The majority of cases of KD occur in children younger than 5 years, with a peak incidence in those 2 years and younger. The disease tends to be more common in boys than girls, and the attack rate in siblings (1%) is 10-fold higher than in the general population.[126] The mean age of patients with KD is younger in Japan than in the United States. Regional epidemics of KD have been observed, and the disease may occur year round, although larger numbers occur during the winter and early spring. The incidence of KD in the United States and Europe is estimated at 4 to 25 per 100,000 children younger than 5 years.[127–129] In some regions throughout Asia, such as Japan, Korea and Taiwan, the incidence of KD may be up to 10 to 20 times higher than in the United States and Europe.[129]

The diagnosis of KD may be challenging, and misdiagnosis is common. In fact, missed diagnosis of KD is among the most common malpractice verdicts against child health practitioners.[130] Increasingly, atypical or "incomplete" presentations of KD are being diagnosed and tend to be more common in the youngest patients, in whom an extremely high level of suspicion must be maintained.[130] The diagnosis of KD should be considered in any infant with prolonged, unexplained fever. Delays in diagnosis and initiation of therapy may also occur more often in older children, who overall have a lower prevalence of disease.[131] In a large prospective study of patients with KD, common associated symptoms noted within 10 days before the diagnosis included irritability, vomiting, anorexia, cough, diarrhea, rhinorrhea, weakness, abdominal pain, and joint pain.[132]

The diagnostic criteria for KD are listed in Box 21.1. KD should be considered in the differential diagnosis of any infant or child with fever, rash, and red eyes.[126] The fevers in KD are usually of abrupt onset and are quite high (>39°C), and the response to antipyretics is usually minimal. The fever usually lasts 1 to 2 weeks in the absence of treatment but may last as long as 3 to 4 weeks.[133] Although the Centers for Disease Control and Prevention case definition of KD specifies fever persisting for 5 or more days, the diagnosis of KD is in some instances established before this time when other supporting features are present. The conjunctival injection (Fig. 21.20) is distinctive, with involvement of the bulbar conjunctivae more often than the palpebral conjunctivae and the absence of exudate (which may help in the differentiation from adenoviral infection). Perilimbal sparing (presenting as a white halo around the iris; Fig. 21.21) is characteristic and may be useful in differentiating KD eye involvement from other infectious or allergic processes.[126] Irritability is common in children with KD and may relate to cerebral vasculitis or aseptic meningitis.[134]

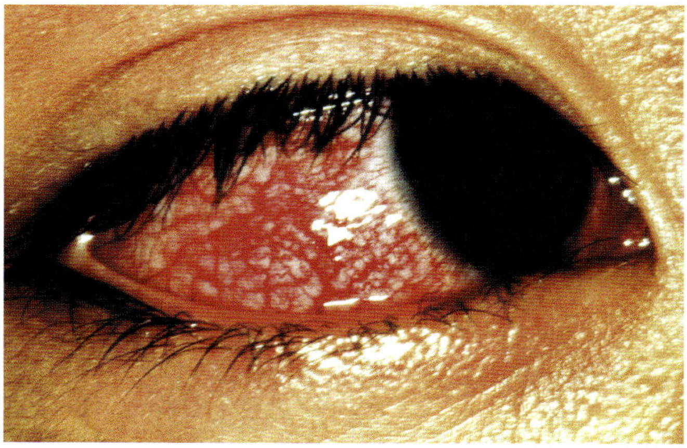

Fig. 21.20 Kawasaki disease. Nonexudative, bulbar conjunctival injection.

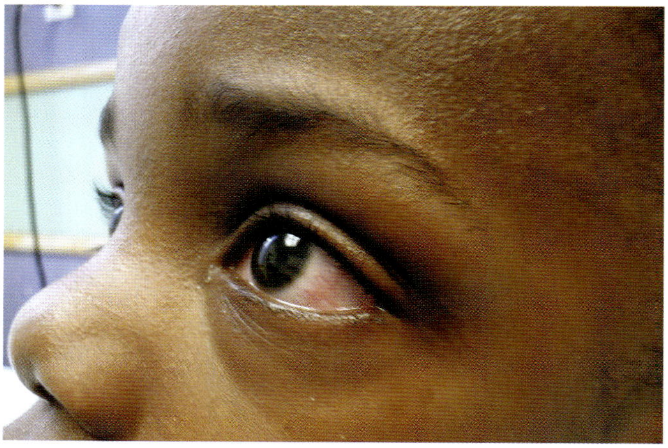

Fig. 21.21 Kawasaki disease. The conjunctivitis in this patient demonstrates the notable perilimbal sparing (halo of noninvolvement adjacent to the iris).

Box 21.1 Diagnostic Criteria for Kawasaki Disease

Classic Kawasaki Disease (KD)

Fever for 5 days or more,* plus at least four of the following five clinical signs:
- Bilateral nonexudative bulbar conjunctivitis
- Oral mucous membrane changes: erythema of the oropharyngeal mucosa, injected or fissured lips, strawberry tongue
- Peripheral extremity changes: erythema or edema of hands/feet (acute), periungual desquamation (convalescent)
- Polymorphous rash (maculopapular, diffuse erythroderma, or erythema multiforme-like)
- Cervical lymphadenopathy (at least 1.5 cm, often unilateral)

Incomplete KD

Fever for ≥5 days with two or three of the five clinical criteria for KD

Atypical KD

Patients who fulfill KD criteria but who have a clinical feature that is not typically seen with KD

Adapted from Rowley AH, Shulman ST. Kawasaki syndrome. Pediatr Clin N Am 1999;46(2):313–29; and McCrindle BW, Rowley AH, Newburger JW, et al. Diagnosis, treatment and long-term management of Kawasaki disease: A scientific statement for health professionals from the American Heart Association. Circulation 2017;135(17):e927–99.

*In the presence of fever and the other diagnostic criteria for KD, experienced physicians may make the diagnosis before the fifth day of fever.

Oropharyngeal changes in KD are most notable for dry, red, fissured, and crusted lips (Figs. 21.22 and 21.23). Hyperemia of the oral mucosa and a red strawberry tongue (Fig. 21.24) (similar to that seen in streptococcal scarlet fever) are also seen. The peripheral extremity changes include nonpitting edema of the dorsal hands (Fig. 21.25) and feet (Fig. 21.26) and erythema of the palms and soles (Fig. 21.27). The edema is characterized by flesh-colored or red-violaceous brawny swelling, along with fusiform swelling of the digits and taut skin noted on the dorsal surfaces. Patients may complain of pain or refuse to walk. Periungual desquamation (Fig. 21.28) is a later finding, generally seen in the subacute or convalescent stages of KD. It begins at the tips of the digits and over a period of days to weeks, gradually progresses to involve the fingers, toes, palms, and soles. Recurrent episodes of skin peeling after upper respiratory tract infection may occur in up to 11% of KD patients for several years after their recovery.[135] Transverse linear grooves in the nail plates (Beau lines; Fig. 21.29) may also be appreciated months into the course of disease.

Cervical lymphadenopathy is the least common feature seen in KD, occurring in approximately 50% to 75% of patients.[133] When present it is usually quite obvious on physical examination given the size of

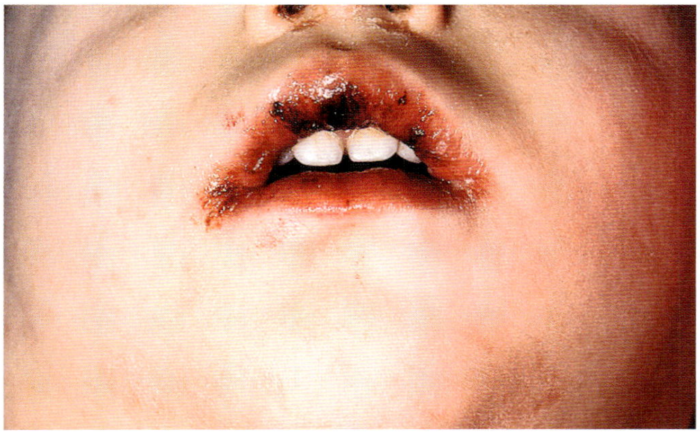

Fig. 21.22 Kawasaki disease. Lip hyperemia and crusting with fissures.

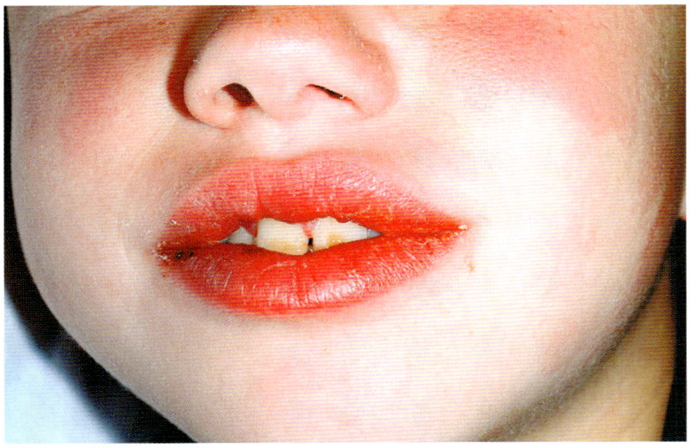

Fig. 21.23 Kawasaki disease. Lip hyperemia with mild crusting. Note the associated facial eruption.

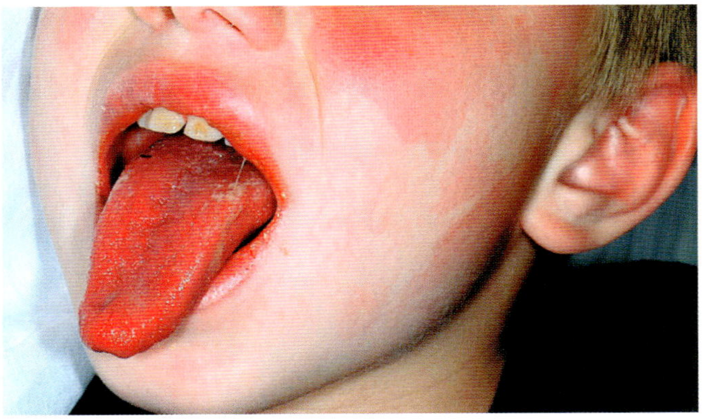

Fig. 21.24 Kawasaki disease. Hyperemia of the tongue with prominent lingual papillae ("red strawberry tongue").

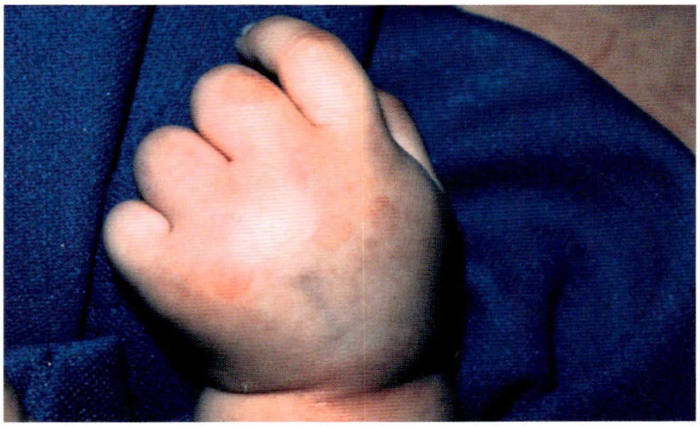

Fig. 21.25 Kawasaki disease. Nonpitting edema of the hand in a young boy with Kawasaki disease.

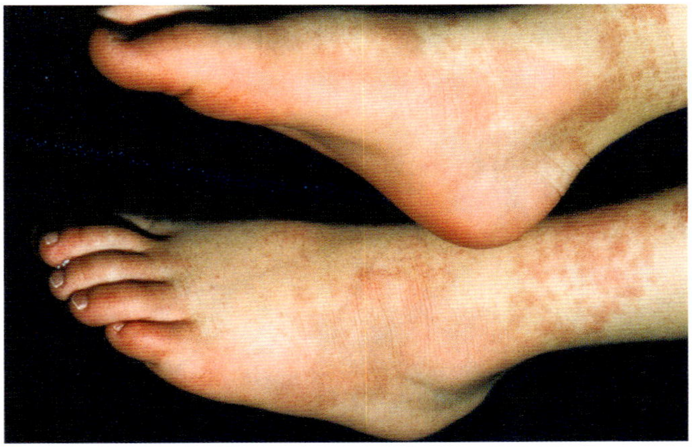

Fig. 21.26 Kawasaki disease. Mild edema of the feet accompanied by blanchable, erythematous macules and patches.

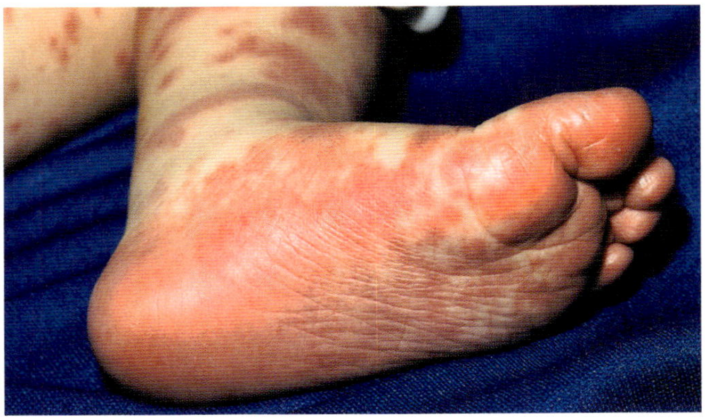

Fig. 21.27 Kawasaki disease. Confluent, erythematous patches and plaques of the sole in a young boy with Kawasaki disease.

the involved node(s). The diagnostic criterion specifies a size of at least 1.5 cm. Some patients with KD present with solely fever and unilateral enlargement of cervical lymph nodes. Generalized lymphadenopathy is not a feature of KD.

The cutaneous eruption of KD is polymorphous, and the majority of patients will have skin manifestations at some point during their illness. The most common presentations are that of a nonspecific, diffuse macular and papular erythematous eruption (Fig. 21.30) or a diffuse urticarial process (Fig. 21.31). A scarlet fever–like rash with "sandpapery" papules on a background of erythema, erythroderma, and erythema multiforme–like lesions (Fig. 21.32) may also occur. Small pustules superimposed on urticarial erythema have also been observed (Fig. 21.33).[136] An important finding on skin examination is accentuation of the eruption in fold areas, especially the groin

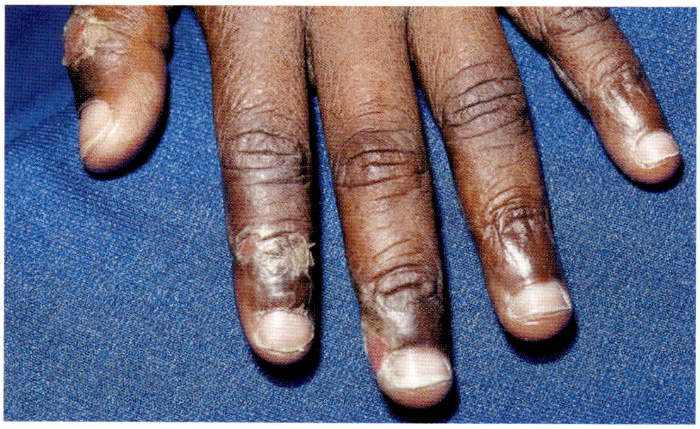

Fig. 21.28 Kawasaki disease. Digital and periungual desquamation occurred late in the course of the disease in this boy who had coronary arterial aneurysms.

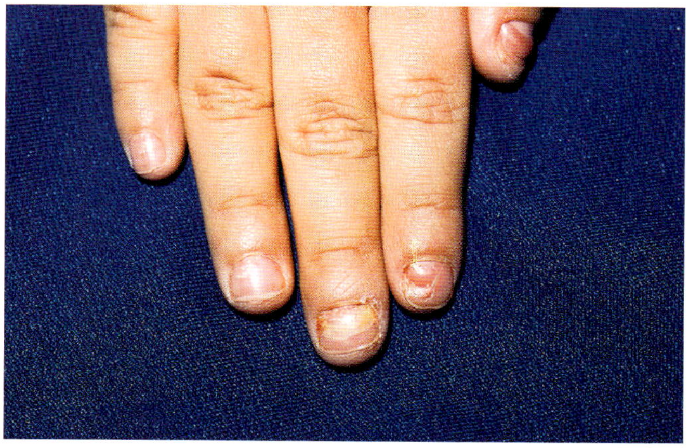

Fig. 21.29 Kawasaki disease. Transverse ridges (Beau lines) and nail-plate separation, which may occur several months after treatment for Kawasaki disease.

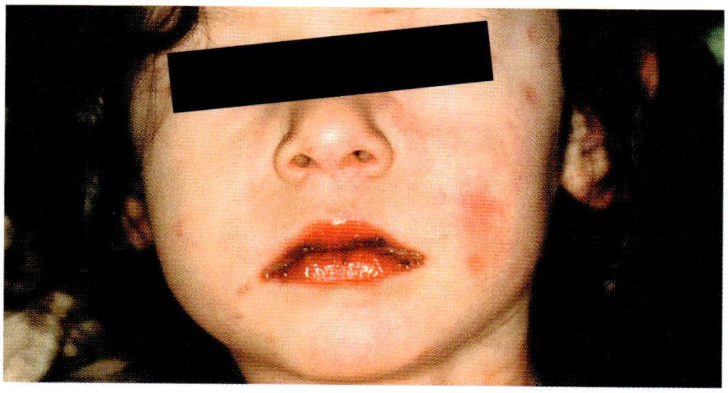

Fig. 21.30 Kawasaki disease. This young girl has hyperemic lips with crusting and a diffuse, confluent erythematous skin eruption.

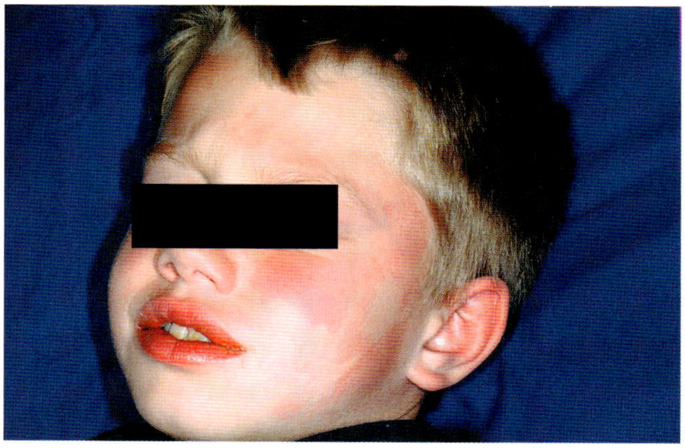

Fig. 21.31 Kawasaki disease. Urticarial patches are the prominent skin finding in this patient.

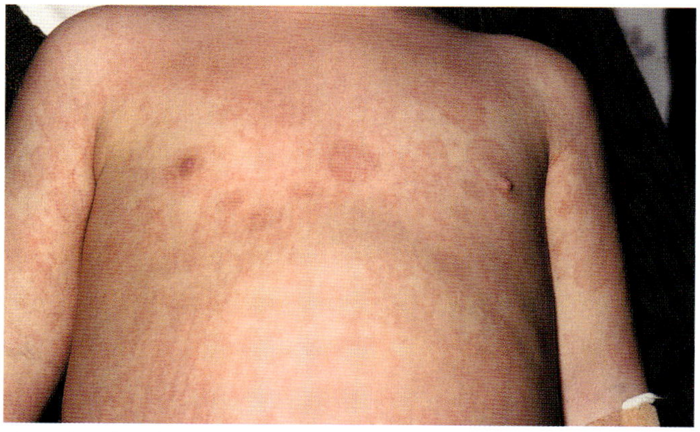

Fig. 21.32 Kawasaki disease. This child had a diffuse erythematous eruption with annular and targetoid (erythema multiforme–like) lesions.

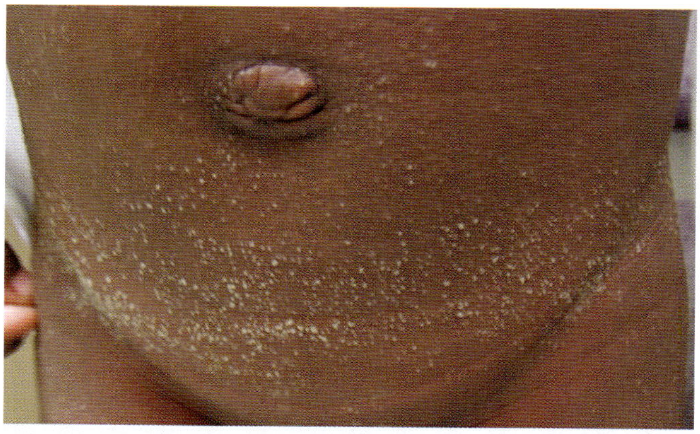

Fig. 21.33 Kawasaki disease. Diffuse erythroderma with multiple pustules were the presenting cutaneous features in this 5-year-old boy with high fevers, lip hyperemia and nonpurulent conjunctival injection.

(Figs. 21.34 and 21.35), which is quite common and should increase the practitioner's suspicion for KD in the presence of other suggestive clinical features. This erythematous, desquamating perineal eruption was found to occur in 67% of patients with KD in one series.[137] Erythema, induration, and ulceration at the bacillus Calmette–Guérin (BCG) vaccination site have been described during the course of KD.[138,139] Rarely, severe peripheral ischemia with resultant gangrene may occur (Fig. 21.36).[133] Although the cutaneous eruption of KD is quite polymorphous, vesicles, bullae, and purpura are virtually never seen. The histopathologic features of skin biopsy material from patients with KD are nonspecific.

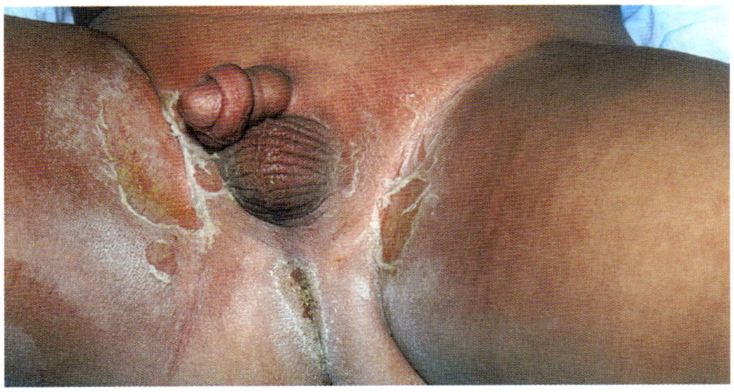

Fig. 21.34 Kawasaki disease. The classic perineal eruption of Kawasaki disease is notable for accentuation in folds and desquamation.

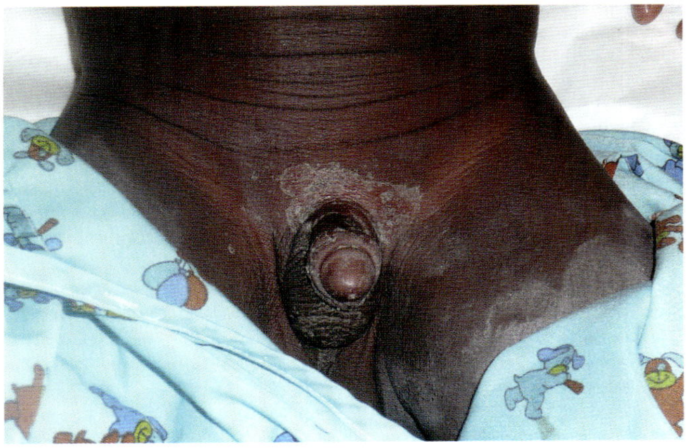

Fig. 21.35 Kawasaki disease. This perineal and genital desquamation was preceded by pustules and occurred in a 5-year-old boy with high fevers, conjunctival injection, oropharyngeal changes, lymphadenopathy, and markedly elevated inflammatory markers.

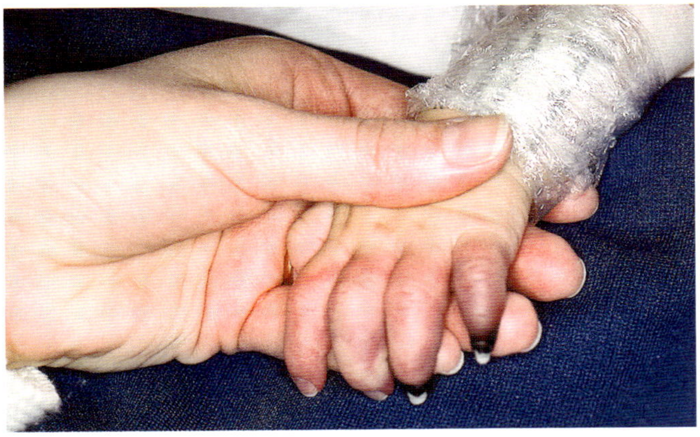

Fig. 21.36 Kawasaki disease. Peripheral ischemia with gangrene of the distal digits.

A psoriasis-like skin eruption, occasionally with a pustular psoriasis appearance, may also be seen in children during the acute or convalescent phases of KD.[140,141] In one series, two of nine patients had a family history of psoriasis, and in all of the patients the psoriasis resolved with therapy for the KD and did not recur.[140] Whether this observation reflects activation of "latent" psoriasis in genetically predisposed individuals or a common causative agent for both KD and psoriasis is unclear.

The differential diagnosis of children with fever, rash, and red eyes is broad and in addition to KD includes toxin-mediated bacterial infections (scarlet fever, toxic shock syndrome, staphylococcal scalded-skin syndrome), Rocky Mountain spotted fever, viral exanthematous illnesses (i.e., adenovirus, measles, enterovirus), drug reactions (including Stevens–Johnson syndrome and toxic epidermal necrolysis), and a variety of other infectious, inflammatory, or connective tissue disorders. The differentiation of KD from acute adenoviral infection can be challenging. Although the presentations of these two processes can be very similar, two potentially distinguishing features of adenovirus infection are a purulent (versus nonpurulent) conjunctivitis and the lack of a perineal accentuation of the rash.[142] A Kawasaki-like syndrome has also been observed in adults infected with HIV.[143] Because there exists no reliable diagnostic test to confirm KD, the diagnosis continues to rest on clinical vigilance, and the overall picture of the patient. Box 21.2 lists some useful clues to the diagnosis of KD.

Recurrent toxin-mediated perineal erythema (RTPE) is a benign, self-limited mucocutaneous disorder that may mimic some aspects of KD. The reported patients had perineal erythema, occasional involvement of the axillary and inguinal folds, and occasional desquamation of the fingers and feet.[144] Patients may report a recurrent history of such eruptions and are generally otherwise well. RTPE is believed to be caused by a unique clinical response to toxins elaborated by streptococci and staphylococci. Some patients have had positive pharyngeal or perianal cultures for GABHS.[144,145]

Other clinical features of KD include cardiac manifestations (see later), CNS and gastrointestinal involvement, extreme irritability, lethargy, urethritis with sterile pyuria, anterior uveitis, musculoskeletal complaints (arthritis and arthralgia), and peripheral gangrene. CNS involvement may include meningeal signs with cerebrospinal fluid (CSF) pleocytosis, cerebral infarction, sensorineural hearing loss, and cranial nerve palsies. Gastrointestinal manifestations include hepatomegaly, hepatitis, gallbladder hydrops, diarrhea, and jaundice. Laboratory findings of KD are listed in Table 21.4.

Cardiac sequelae represent the most serious complications of KD. Cardiac involvement may occur during the acute or later stages of the disease. Early manifestations include pericardial effusions/pericarditis and myocarditis, which may present with tachycardia and gallop rhythm.[125] Congestive heart failure, arrhythmias, and valvular regurgitation (especially mitral) may also occur. The most significant cardiac complication, though, is the development of dilation or aneurysms of the coronary arteries, which occur in up to 5% to 10% of patients despite the use of appropriate therapy (and in up to 20% of untreated children).[130,146,147] Changes in the coronary arteries may continue to evolve beyond the acute phase of the illness, but the development of aneurysms more than 8 weeks after the acute illness is quite unusual. Although death as a result of coronary occlusion has occasionally been noted after apparent recovery from the illness, most deaths occur suddenly between 3 and 8 weeks after the onset of the disease.

Kawasaki disease shock syndrome (KDSS) is a rare association, presenting during the acute phase of KD with hypotension and a shock-like state.[147] The shock in these patients may be distributive or cardiogenic, and KDSS is characterized by more coronary artery involvement,

Box 21.2 **Clinical Clues to the Diagnosis of Kawasaki Disease**

Persistent fever for more than 5 days
Fever unresponsive to antipyretics
Extreme irritability, inconsolable nature of child
Perilimbal sparing of conjunctival injection
Perineal accentuation of erythematous/desquamating rash
Erythema, induration, or ulceration of BCG vaccination site
Sterile pyuria
Gall bladder hydrops
Increasing ESR in light of clinical improvement/defervescence

BCG, Bacillus Calmette–Guérin; *ESR*, erythrocyte sedimentation rate.

Table 21.4 Laboratory Findings in Kawasaki Disease

Finding	Comment
Leukocytosis	Often neutrophilic; toxic granulations may be present
Anemia	Normocytic, normochromic
Thrombocytopenia	Associated with severe coronary disease, myocardial infarction
Thrombocytosis	In subacute stage (usually ≥10–14 days after onset of illness)
Increased ESR	Normalizes over 6–10 weeks
Increased CRP	Normalizes in 2–5 days with treatment
Low albumin	
Abnormal lipids	Decreased HDL, total cholesterol; increased triglycerides, LDL
Increased transaminases, bilirubin	Secondary to gallbladder hydrops
Sterile pyuria	Mild proteinuria occasionally
CSF pleocytosis	Mononuclear
Increased NT-proBNP	Associated with cardiomyocyte stress; may be a marker for those developing coronary artery disease

CRP, C-reactive protein; *CSF*, cerebrospinal fluid; *ESR*, erythrocyte sedimentation rate; *HDL*, high-density lipoprotein; *LDL*, low-density lipoprotein; *NT-proBNP*, *N*-terminal probrain natriuretic peptide.

resistance to IVIG, and a heightened inflammatory immune response.[148] Useful differentiating features between KDSS and toxic shock syndrome include echocardiographic abnormalities, more profound anemia and higher platelet counts seen in the former.[149]

The cause of KD remains a mystery. Hypothetical causes have included infectious agents (via conventional antigen), a toxin-mediated superantigen process, genetic predisposition, and immune activation. In support of an infectious etiology are the fact that KD presents in a similar fashion to some other self-limited exanthematous diseases, the seasonal predilection, the rare occurrence in infants younger than age 6 months (possibly suggesting protective maternal immunity), and the rarity of recurrences.[126] Many agents have been implicated but none proven definitively, including *Staphylococcus*, *Streptococcus* species, *Candida* species, *Rickettsia* species, herpesviruses, *Mycoplasma pneumoniae*, human adenoviruses, and Gram-negative bacteria.[125,150–152] Superantigen-secreting bacteria such as staphylococci and streptococci, specifically those that stimulate a Vβ2 T-lymphocyte response, have been postulated to be involved in the pathogenesis of KD.[153] IgA plasma cells have been identified in coronary vessel walls, pancreas, kidney, and respiratory tract in patients who succumbed to KD, suggesting entry of the KD causative agent through the upper respiratory tract with systemic spread to other organs.[154] An RNA virus that usually causes asymptomatic infection but KD in a subset of predisposed children has been suggested and is supported by CD8 T cells, oligoclonal IgA, and upregulation of cytotoxic T-cell and interferon pathway genes in the coronary arteries of fatal KD, as well as cytoplasmic inclusion bodies in ciliated bronchial epithelia.[155] The genetic predisposition hypothesis is appealing, given the disproportionately high attack rate among children of Japanese, Chinese, and Korean ethnicity, but the exact association remains unclear. Polymorphisms in the genes for C-reactive protein and TNF-α may be associated with a predisposition toward KD, with single-nucleotide polymorphisms occurring with greater frequencies in patients with KD compared with control subjects.[156] Other candidate genes in which polymorphisms may affect KD susceptibility include *ITPKC*, *FCGR2A*, *CAMK2D*, *CSMD1*, *LNX1*, *NAALADL2*, *TCP1*, *ACE*, *BLK*, *CASP3*, *CD40*, *FGβ*, *HLA-E*, *IL1A*, *IL6*, *LTA*, *MPO*, *PD1*, *SMAD3*, and *CCL17*.[157–162] A remarkable seasonality of KD has been observed, which is shared among extratropical areas (those north of the Tropic of Cancer) in the Northern Hemisphere.[163] A time series analysis of three geographically distinct regions with a high KD incidence (Japan, San Diego, and Hawaii) suggests that tropospheric wind currents may influence the development of disease via fluctuations in wind circulation (and possibly windborne transmission of the KD trigger).[164,165]

Treatment of KD is predicated on the ability to recognize the condition and rapidly render a diagnosis, which in some patients remains a challenge. The ultimate goals of therapy are to reduce inflammation and thus the potential for damage to the arterial wall.[126] The mainstays of therapy for KD are IVIG and aspirin, which should be initiated within the first 10 days of illness whenever possible.[131] In the United States, IVIG is generally given in one intravenous infusion of 2 g/kg infused over 12 hours, which was shown to be more effective than the more traditional 4-day course.[166] Issues surrounding IVIG therapy in KD include the expense of the preparation and the potential transmission of bloodborne pathogens, such as hepatitis C. Such transmission of infectious diseases is extremely rare since the institution of the current purification and processing practices in 1994.[130] A subgroup of patients with KD are resistant to IVIG therapy and seem to be at greatest risk for the development of coronary artery aneurysms and long-term sequelae.[125]

Aspirin is also started concurrently with IVIG, initially at a moderate (30 to 50 mg/kg per day) or high (80 to 100 mg/kg per day) dosage until the fever subsides (child is afebrile for 48 to 72 hours).[7] This higher-dose regimen of aspirin is useful for its antiinflammatory effect. Low-dose aspirin therapy (3 to 5 mg/kg per day) is then recommended, primarily for its antiplatelet effect. Unless the echocardiogram detects coronary artery abnormalities, aspirin therapy is discontinued once the laboratory studies normalize, which is usually within 4 to 6 weeks of the onset of disease. Risks of aspirin therapy include hepatitis, hearing loss, and Reye syndrome, the latter of which is mainly of significance in the setting of acute varicella or influenza. The moderate dosing of aspirin (i.e., 30 to 50 mg/kg per day) is often used in Japan given concerns in that population about potential hepatotoxicity.

Although the majority of patients with KD have an excellent response to these therapies, approximately 5% to 15% have a suboptimal response. In these patients a second dose of IVIG is often effective.[158] Other therapies that have been evaluated for KD (and for which there is no current consensus) include corticosteroids, pentoxifylline, and anti-TNF agents. A randomized prospective study failed to show any significant advantages of the addition of intravenous methylprednisolone to conventional primary KD therapy.[167] Other studies, however, have found that corticosteroids may in fact play a useful role as adjunctive initial therapy and that patients treated with steroids may have fewer coronary artery abnormalities.[168–170] Infliximab, a chimeric monoclonal antibody to TNF-α, has been used increasingly for IVIG-resistant disease in hospitalized patients in the United States[171] and has become the most commonly used third-line agent for KD.[172] It has been shown to be both efficacious and safe compared with a second infusion of IVIG in patients who had received initial IVIG therapy.[173,174] Etanercept, another TNF-α inhibitor, has also been demonstrated effective in smaller-scale studies.[175,176] Rituximab, cyclosporine, and cyclophosphamide may also be useful therapeutic agents for resistant KD.[177,178]

Long-term cardiac follow-up monitoring of patients with KD should include an echocardiogram twice during the first 2 months after illness onset (typically 1 to 2 weeks and 4 to 6 weeks) with further follow-up study depending on the individual patient's coronary artery status.[7] Children whose coronary arteries are normal at 2 months after the diagnosis of KD are considered free of cardiac disease, although several experts consider a history of KD to be a risk factor for the later development of coronary artery disease.[130] Some experts have recommended cardiac magnetic resonance imaging during adolescence for all KD patients to fully visualize the complete coronary arterial system.[179,180] Vascular lesions in adult survivors of KD may include coronary artery aneurysms, calcification, and stenosis, as well as valvular incompetence and myocardial fibrosis, either focal or diffuse.[181] The outcomes for patients with KD who are diagnosed at the extreme ends of the age spectrum (younger than 6 months or older than 9 years) appear to be suboptimal, with a greater incidence of coronary artery abnormalities.[182] "Recurrent fever syndrome," characterized by the reappearance of inflammatory symptoms after successful therapy for KD, has been observed in some patients; it may resemble the clinical entity known as periodic fever, aphthous stomatitis, pharyngitis, and adenitis (PFAPA) syndrome and suggests a possible genetic predisposition to autoinflammatory responses or environmental exposure susceptibility in these cohorts.[183]

The complete list of 183 references for this chapter is available online at http://expertconsult.inkling.com.

Key References

Johnson EF, Wetter DA, Lehman JS, et al. Leukocytoclastic vasculitis in children: clinical characteristics, subtypes, causes and direct immunofluorescence findings of 56 biopsy-confirmed cases. J Eur Acad Dermatol Venereol 2017;31:544–9.

McCrindle BW, Rowley AH, Newburger JW, et al. Diagnosis, treatment and long-term management of Kawasaki disease: a scientific statement for health professionals from the American Heart Association. Circulation 2017;135(17):e927–99.

Calatroni M, Oliva E, Gianfreda D, et al. ANCA-associated vasculitis in childhood: recent advances. Ital J Pediatr 2017;43:46.

Newburger JW, Takahashi M, Burns JC. Kawasaki disease. J Am Coll Cardiol 2016;67(14):1738–49.

Morishita KA, Moorthy LN, Lubieniecka JM, et al. Early outcomes in children with antineutrophil cytoplasmic antibody-associated vasculitis. Arthritis Rheumatol 2017;69(7):1470–9.

Wright AC, Gibson LE, Davis DMR. Cutaneous manifestations of pediatric granulomatosis with polyangiitis: a clinicopathologic and immunopathologic analysis. J Am Acad Dermatol 2015;72:859–67.

Eleftheriou D, Gale H, Pilkington C, et al. Eosinophilic granulomatosis with polyangiitis in childhood: retrospective experience from a tertiary referral centre in the UK. Rheumatology 2016;55:1263–72.

Batu ED, Ozen S. Pediatric vasculitis. Curr Rheumatol Rep 2012;14: 121–9.

Eleftheriou D, Dillon MJ, Brogan PA. Advances in childhood vasculitis. Curr Opin Rheumatol 2009;21:411–18.

Ferri C, Mascia MT. Cryoglobulinemic vasculitis. Curr Opin Rheumatol 2006;18:54–63.

Eleftheriou D, Dillon MJ, Tullus K, et al. Systemic polyarteritis nodosa in the young: a single-center experience over thirty-two years. Arth Rheum 2013;65(9):2476–85.

Holman RC, Belay ED, Christensen KY, et al. Hospitalizations for Kawasaki syndrome among children in the United States, 1997–2007. Pediatr Infect Dis J 2010;29:483–8.

Rowley AH, Shulman ST. Pathogenesis and management of Kawasaki disease. Expert Rev Anti Infect Ther 2010;8(2):197–203.

Burns JC, Herzog L, Fabri O, et al. Seasonality of Kawasaki disease: a global perspective. PLoS ONE 2013;8(9):e74529.

Son MB, Gauvreau K, Ma L, et al. Treatment of Kawasaki disease: analysis of 27 US pediatric hospitals from 2001 to 2006. Pediatrics 2009;124:1–8.

Dominguez SR, Anderson MS. Advances in the treatment of Kawasaki disease. Curr Opin Pediatr 2013;25:103–9.

22 Collagen Vascular Disorders

The connective tissue (collagen vascular, rheumatic) disorders represent a group of diseases characterized by inflammatory changes of the connective tissue of skin, muscle, joints,[1] and viscera. Among these, juvenile idiopathic arthritis, lupus erythematosus, juvenile dermatomyositis, systemic sclerosis (scleroderma), morphea, eosinophilic fasciitis, Sjögren syndrome, mixed connective tissue disease (MCTD), and antiphospholipid antibody syndrome (APS) exhibit specific cutaneous findings.

Juvenile Idiopathic Arthritis

Juvenile idiopathic arthritis (JIA) is a group of seven arthritides of children younger than age 16 years that last longer than 6 weeks and are of unknown cause.[2–4] JIA encompasses the former term *juvenile rheumatoid arthritis,* as well as other arthritides in children.[5] These include seven subtypes: systemic-onset arthritis (Still's disease; sJIA), oligoarthritis, seronegative (rheumatoid factor/RF-negative) polyarthritis, seropositive polyarticular arthritis, psoriatic arthritis (see Chapter 4), enthesitis-related arthritis, and undifferentiated JIA (Box 22.1).[5,6] Overall, juvenile arthritis has a prevalence of up to 1:1000 children younger than age 16 years.[7] Approximately 4% to 17% of these children have systemic-onset disease; 11% to 30%, rheumatoid factor (RF)–negative polyarticular arthritis; 2% to 7%, RF-positive polyarticular arthritis; 27% to 60%, oligoarthritis; 1% to 11%, enthesitis-related arthritis; 2% to 11%, psoriatic arthritis; and 11% to 21%, undifferentiated arthritis.[8] However, subtype distribution varies among countries; for example, although oligoarthritis is most common in Europe, polyarthritis is more common in New Zealand and India. RF, usually an immunoglobulin (Ig) M antibody against IgG, is unusual in children, especially children younger than 7 years of age, and is associated with greater synovial erosion with a poor prognosis. Antinuclear antibody (ANA) levels (which are positive in 10% of normal children, usually at a level of 1:40 to 1:80) are most commonly positive in children with oligoarticular disease (40% to 80%), especially in girls and with uveitis. The different subtypes of JIA are associated with human leukocyte antigen (HLA) types. Patients with JIA and coexisting atopy have been shown to have more active disease and worse outcomes, possibly because of ongoing immune dysregulation.[9,10]

Of the various forms of JIA other than psoriatic arthritis, systemic-onset disease (sJIA) is the only one with known cutaneous findings. sJIA affects boys and girls equally.[11] The eruption of sJIA is usually intermittent, occurring most often when patients have their characteristic daily or twice daily spiking fevers. The fevers generally reach 39° C or higher, and the children appear acutely ill with exacerbation of joint pain when fevers occur. The characteristic flat to slightly elevated macules or occasionally papules may resemble urticaria but are not pruritic. The eruption tends to be migratory, rarely persisting more than an hour in any location. Lesions typically measure 2 to 6 mm in diameter, vary from salmon-pink to red, and display a characteristic slightly irregular or serpiginous margin. The rash is often seen over pressure areas and can be associated with dermatographism. The blanching macules are often evanescent and commonly subside during periods of remission and a few hours after defervescence. Individual lesions may coalesce to form large plaques 8 to 9 cm in diameter. The eruption occurs predominantly on the trunk but often affects the extremities and occasionally the face (Fig. 22.1); it is accentuated by local heat or trauma. Seen in 25% to 50% of patients, it may precede fevers or visceral involvement by up to 3 years. In some patients the rash occurs during a period of only 1 week, and in others for a year or more. Biopsy helps confirm the diagnosis and shows dyskeratosis of the upper epidermis and sparse inflammation.[12] However, fever and rash often resolve after the polyarthritis emerges.

Many patients have extraarticular features, particularly hepatosplenomegaly, lymphadenopathy, pleuritis, and pericarditis, which may predate the joint manifestations by weeks to, rarely, years. A feature in pathogenesis is the increase in cytokines interleukin (IL)–1 and IL-6. Approximately 50% of affected individuals have a mild oligoarticular course with a good prognosis for remission; of the remaining 50%, approximately half will develop severe, recalcitrant, and destructive progressive polyarticular arthritis, although the increased availability of effective interventions is likely altering this high risk. Other complications of systemic-onset JIA include secondary amyloidosis, secondary infection, osteoporosis, and growth retardation. Macrophage activation syndrome (MAS), a life-threatening complication, affects 5% to 8% of patients (see later). In children with MAS, the evanescent skin rash is noted significantly less often than without MAS.[4,13]

Dysfunction in the innate immune system, its clinical features, and its poor response to therapies that ameliorate other forms of JIA have

Box 22.1 Subtypes of Juvenile Idiopathic Arthritis

Systemic-Onset Arthritis

Definition: Arthritis with or preceded by daily fever of at least 2 weeks' duration plus at least one of the following:
- Evanescent, nonfixed erythematous eruption
- Generalized lymphadenopathy
- Serositis
- Hepatosplenomegaly, splenomegaly, or both

Oligoarthritis

Definition: Arthritis that affects one to four joints during the first 6 months of disease. Two subtypes occur: (1) persistent oligoarthritis: never affects more than 4 joints; and (2) extended oligoarthritis: affects >4 joints after the first 6 months.

Exclusions:
- Family history of confirmed psoriasis in at least one first- or second-degree relative
- Family history of confirmed HLA-B27–associated disease in at least one first- or second-degree relative
- HLA-B27 positivity in a boy with the onset of arthritis after 8 years of age
- Positive RF testing
- Presence of systemic-onset arthritis as defined

Seronegative Polyarthritis (RF-negative)

Definition: Arthritis that affects >5 joints during the first 6 months with RF-negative testing at least twice and at least 3 months apart. Systemic-onset JIA must be excluded.

Seropositive Polyarthritis (RF-positive)

Definition: Arthritis that affects ≥5 joints during the first 6 months of disease, associated with a positive RF test twice and at least 3 months apart. Systemic-onset JIA must be excluded.

Psoriatic Arthritis

Definition: Must have arthritis and psoriasis, or arthritis and at least two of the following:
- Dactylitis
- Nail pitting or onycholysis
- Family history of confirmed psoriasis in at least one first-degree relative

Enthesitis-Related Arthritis

Definition: Arthritis and enthesitis, or arthritis or enthesitis and at least two of the following:
- Sacroiliac joint tenderness and/or inflammatory spinal pain
- HLA-27 positivity
- Family history of at least one first- or second-degree relative with confirmed HLA-B27–associated disease
- Anterior uveitis that is usually symptomatic (pain, redness, photophobia)
- Onset of arthritis in a boy after the age of 8 years

Systemic-onset JIA and confirmed psoriasis in at least one first- or second-degree relative must be excluded.

Undifferentiated Arthritis

Not fitting other subtypes

HLA, Human leukocyte antigen; *JIA*, juvenile idiopathic arthritis; *RF*, rheumatoid factor.

led several investigators to classify sJIA as an autoinflammatory, rather than autoimmune, disease (see Chapter 25).[14,15] In fact, an autosomal recessive subset of JIA was discovered, resulting from biallelic mutations in *FAMIN* (also called *LACC1*), which encodes laccase (multicopper oxidoreductase) domain-containing 1, an enzyme that is involved in regulation of inflammasome activation and promotion of reactive oxygen species (ROS) production.[16–18] Some patients have JIA that is more typical of sJIA, with the characteristic quotidian fever and associated eruption, symmetric polyarthritis affecting small and large joints, but lower frequencies or organomegaly, lymphadenopathy, and serositis. Others have been described with seronegative polyarthritis.

Oligoarticular JIA occurs more often in girls than in boys and peaks between the ages of 2 and 4 years. Children with oligoarticular JIA often complain of morning stiffness and may limp. Joints are warm and effused but not red, hot, or very painful. In about 50% of cases, the onset is monoarticular, with the knee, ankle, or elbow most commonly affected; the hip and small joints are usually spared. The acute onset of painful monoarthritis with refusal to bear weight is unlikely to be JIA, and infectious, traumatic, and malignant causes of joint pain should be considered. Approximately 20% to 30% of children with JIA have uveitis, which occurs most commonly in ANA-positive girls with early–onset oligoarthritis.[19,20] The classic picture is a chronic bilateral anterior uveitis, which is usually asymptomatic until significant, and sometimes irreversible damage to intraocular structures occurs. Patients with oligoarticular JIA and uveitis have worse ocular outcomes relative to patients with other causes of uveitis, necessitating regular screening examinations.[21] Treatment of the uveitis includes topical corticosteroids, mydriatics, systemic immunosuppressive agents, and surgical management of complications.

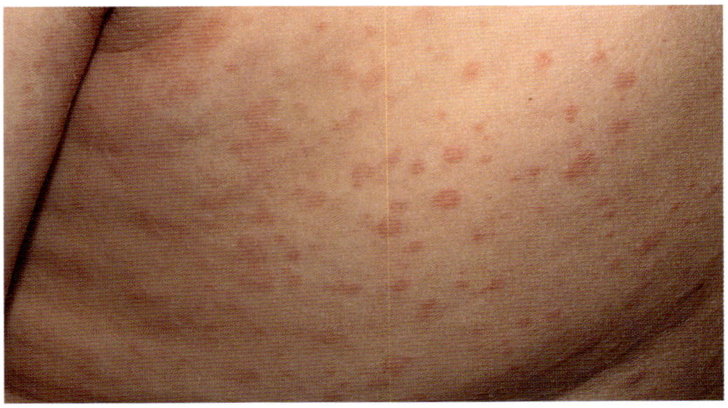

Fig. 22.1 Juvenile idiopathic arthritis (JIA). Evanescent macular eruption occurred with fever in this boy with systemic-onset JIA.

Polyarthritis (≥5 joints) usually has an insidious onset, although it may be acute. It often symmetrically involves the small joints (particularly of the hands and, less often, feet) and wrists. The temporomandibular and hip joints and cervical spine are often affected as well. Lymphadenopathy, hepatomegaly, and fevers may occur, although the fevers do not show the daily (quotidian) spikes seen in sJIA.

Children with enthesitis-related arthritis have characteristics of both JIA and juvenile spondyloarthropathies, with inflamed tendons (enthesopathy is inflammation of the attachment sites of tendons to bone), especially the Achilles tendons, in addition to asymmetric arthritis of one or more joints (typically of the lower extremities). Most affected individuals are boys older than age 6 years. Although children rarely show typical ankylosing spondylitis at onset, spondyloarthropathy not uncommonly develops by adulthood.[22] Arthritis associated with inflammatory bowel disease is a subset of this type. Acute anterior uveitis can occur in up to 27% of children and tends to present as an acutely painful, red, photophobic eye in contrast to the asymptomatic uveitis seen in oligoarticular JIA. RF and ANA are negative, and 65% to 80% are HLA-B27 positive.

Although more characteristic of SLE, scleroderma, and dermatomyositis, patients with JIA may also demonstrate cuticular telangiectasias. *Subcutaneous nodules* rarely are seen in children with JIA and occur most commonly in patients with RF-positive polyarthritis, particularly if the disease is recalcitrant to therapy. Barely palpable to several centimeters in size, they may be the first presenting sign of JIA. Their most common location is near the olecranon process on the ulnar border of the forearm. Less commonly, they may occur on the dorsal aspect of the hands, on the knees and ears, and over pressure areas such as the scapulae, sacrum, buttocks, and heels. In the areas of fingers and toes, subcutaneous nodules are only a few millimeters in size. Subcutaneous nodules are firm and nontender and may be attached to the periarticular capsules of the fingers. They can be easily confused with the subcutaneous form of granuloma annulare (see Chapter 9). Rheumatoid nodules and JIA must also be distinguished from fibroblastic rheumatism, a rare disorder characterized by the sudden but sometimes progressive onset of cutaneous nodules (Fig. 22.2), flexion contractures, and polyarthritis.[23,24] Some affected individuals respond to methotrexate. Although methotrexate[25] and

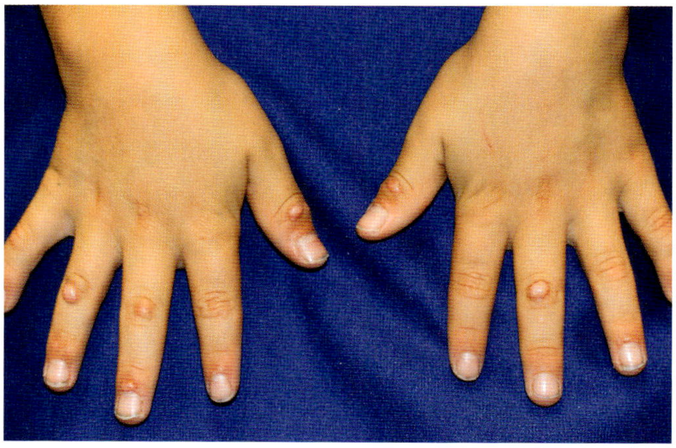

Fig. 22.2 Fibroblastic rheumatism. Firm skin-colored papules and nodules on the fingers of this young boy with juvenile idiopathic arthritis. With methotrexate, the lesions slowly cleared by early adolescence.

tumor necrosis factor (TNF) inhibitor[26] treatment have been linked to induction of subcutaneous nodules, particularly in rheumatoid arthritis, this nodulosis has only been described in adults.

Traditional nonsteroidal antiinflammatory drugs (NSAIDs) continue to be the first-line therapy in all but those with systemic JIA,[27,28] in addition to physical therapy and psychosocial support.[29] NSAIDs that preferentially inhibit the cyclooxygenase-2 (COX-2) enzymes have fewer gastrointestinal (GI) adverse effects and may be preferred in some patients. *Pseudoporphyria*, presenting with tense blisters in photodistributed sites, has most commonly been associated with the use of naproxen sodium but has been reported after administration of other NSAIDs as well, including COX-2 inhibitors (see Chapter 19).

Intraarticular injections of corticosteroids are used for children who do not respond to NSAID therapy or as initial therapy for oligoarthritis, but the use of steroids is otherwise limited because of low efficacy in preventing joint destruction and their many potential side effects.[30]

Disease modifying antirheumatic drugs (DMARDs) are nonsteroidal, non-NSAID drugs, and include biologics and nonbiologics. The DMARD methotrexate is usually the second line of treatment for persistent, active arthritis but is best initiated early in the disease course. Patients with oligoarticular arthritis tend to respond most favorably.[31,32] Blockade of TNF with biologics (etanercept, infliximab, adalimumab) in combination with methotrexate is particularly effective for children with polyarticular arthritis.[33] Others with efficacy are abatacept (fusion protein that downregulates T-cell stimulation) and rituximab (anti–B-cell antibody). Sulfasalazine has largely been used for enthesitis-related arthritis and oligoarthritis.

Systemic-onset JIA responds poorly to NSAIDs and TNF-α blockers (30% response). In addition to methotrexate[34,35] and abatacept (T-cell–activating agent/IgG1 fusion protein),[36] inhibitors of IL-1 (anakinra and canakinumab)[37,38] and IL-6 (tocilizumab, humanized anti–IL-6 receptor monoclonal antibody)[39–41] are increasingly being used for sJIA (with canakinumab preferred to anakinra because of its longer half-life and fewer injection site reactions). Moderate or high dosages of systemic corticosteroids, including pulse intravenous steroids to avoid long-term high-dose treatment, are occasionally used for short periods while awaiting the effects of other medications. As a chronic inflammatory disorder and in relation to use of systemic corticosteroids, JIA is associated with an increased risk of osteoporosis, which can be countered by treatment with calcium and vitamin D supplementation, bisphosphonates, and calcitonin.[42]

MACROPHAGE ACTIVATION SYNDROME

Macrophage activation syndrome, a severe, life-threatening complication of systemic-onset JIA, systemic lupus erythematosus (~9% of children with SLE),[43] and other connective tissue diseases,[44] is associated with hemophagocytosis of activated macrophages/histiocytes and multiorgan dysfunction. When observed in the absence of underlying connective tissue disease, this diagnosis is termed *hemophagocytic lymphohistiocytosis (HLH)* and can be primary (when familial) or secondary (typically in the setting of infection or malignancy) (see Chapter 10). The pathophysiology of both MAS and HLH are speculated to involve inability of natural killer (NK) or CD8 T cells to lyse infected antigen-presenting cells, leading to ongoing infection and resultant "cytokine storm." Patients with MAS and systemic JIA have been shown to harbor defects in NK-cell function and in genes that encode proteins crucial to lymphocytic cytolytic activity, including Munc 13-4 and perforin, which are also implicated in primary familial hemophagocytic lymphohistocytosis.[45] Clinical signs of MAS in sJIA are fever, hepatomegaly, splenomegaly, lymphadenopathy, central nervous system disease, hemorrhagic manifestations, and bone marrow hemophagocytosis. Patients often develop disseminated intravascular coagulation, which has a rapid course and may be lethal. Encephalopathy, respiratory distress, and renal failure have also been described.

The disease may present as pancytopenia with a falling erythrocyte sedimentation rate (ESR), in contrast to the increased ESR associated with flaring JIA. Formal diagnostic criteria for MAS in sJIA that have been used to develop a validated clinical score are hyperferritinemia (>684 ng/mL) and any two of the following characteristics: decreased platelet count (≤181 x 10^9/L), increased aspartate aminotransferase (>48 U/L), hypofibrinogenemia (≤360 mg/dL), and hypertriglyceridemia (>156 mg/dL).[46] Although macrophage hemophagocytosis in the bone marrow is a valuable sign, it is absent in >20% of patients, especially during the early stages. A scoring tool has been developed for diagnosing MAS with sJIA that includes age of onset, neutrophil count, fibrinogen level, splenomegaly, platelet count, and hemoglobin.[47] Serum soluble CD163 is a sensitive biomarker of MAS disease activity in sJIA.[48] Early recognition of MAS and treatment with high-dose corticosteroids with or without cyclosporine, etoposide, intravenous immunoglobulin (IVIG), and/or etanercept may be lifesaving.[49] Some patients with sJIA responding to tocilizumab[50] or canakinumab[51] have developed MAS, although some characteristic features (fever, high ferritin levels) may be masked by treatment.[52]

Systemic Lupus Erythematosus

Systemic lupus erythematosus (SLE) is a heterogeneous autoimmune disease characterized by autoantibody accumulation with immune complex deposition leading to end-organ damage. It often involves the skin but may affect almost any organ system. Autoantibodies are the hallmark of SLE, and activated B cells, T helper cells, and the cytokines that modulate inflammatory responses are thought to be the most appropriate targets for therapy. In cutaneous lupus, skin lesions show an antiepithelial cytotoxic immune response with release of cell debris and reactivation of epidermal innate immune pathways (via pattern recognition receptors), self-amplifying the proinflammatory response (especially with release of type I and III interferons and interferon-regulated proinflammatory cytokines and chemokines, particularly CXCR3 ligands CXCL9, CXCL10, and CXCL11).

Both genetic and environmental (especially ultraviolet light) factors are thought to play roles in its pathogenesis.[53] Reports of familial cases and a high concordance for clinical disease in monozygotic, but not dizygotic, twins support a strong genetic contribution to the development of SLE. SLE has been linked to at least 80 genetic susceptibility loci that encode protein products involved in innate and adaptive immunity, particularly in pathways of apoptosis and immune complex/cell debris clearance, activation of toll-like receptors (TLRs), and signaling of type I interferon (IFN) and nuclear factor (NF)–κB.[54–58] The availability of whole-exome sequencing has led to the discovery of pathogenic mutations in autosomal recessive juvenile-onset SLE (*PRKCD*, encoding protein kinase Cδ),[59] complement deficiency leading to SLE,[60] and autosomal recessive hypocomplementemic urticarial vasculitis (*DNASE1L3*).[61] Although most individuals with SLE do not have monogenic disease, these discoveries may increase understanding of the pathogenesis and lead to new ideas for therapy.

Table 22.1 Criteria for Classification of Systemic Lupus Erythematosus (SLICC)

Criterion*		Comments
CLINICAL CRITERIA		
1	Acute cutaneous lupus	Lupus malar rash (fixed erythema, flat or raised, over malar eminences, usually sparing nasolabial folds), bullous lupus, photosensitive lupus rash (not dermatomyositis), maculopapular lupus rash, or toxic epidermal necrolysis variant Subacute cutaneous lupus (nonindurated annular polycyclic or psoriasiform lesions that resolve without scarring)
2	Chronic cutaneous lupus	Classic discoid eruption (erythematous plaques with adherent keratotic scaling and follicular plugging, often atrophic scarring and dyspigmentation if older lesion; localized if only above the neck, otherwise generalized), lupus panniculitis (profundus), hypertrophic (verrucous) lupus, lupus tumidus, chilblains lupus, discoid lupus/lichen planus overlap, mucosal lupus
3	Oral ulcers	Palate, buccal, tongue, or nasal mucosa (no other cause identified)
4	Alopecia, nonscarring	Diffuse thinning or hair fragility in the absence of other causes (such as alopecia areata, iron deficiency, drugs, or androgenetic alopecia)
5	Synovitis	Must involve two or more joints with swelling or effusion or tenderness and at least 30 minutes of morning stiffness
6	Serositis	Pleuritis, pleural effusions or pleural rub; pericardial pain, effusion, rub or pericarditis without other cause
7	Renal	Persistent proteinuria >0.5 g/day or red blood cell casts
8	Neurologic	Seizures, psychosis, myelitis, mononeuritis multiplex, peripheral or cranial neuropathy, acute confusional state (all without other known cause)
9	Hemolytic anemia	
10	Leukopenia	<4000/mm^3 at least once or lymphopenia of <1000/mm^3 at least once without other cause
11	Thrombocytopenia	<100,000/ mm^3 at least once without other cause
IMMUNOLOGIC CRITERIA		
1	Positive ANA	Above laboratory reference range
2	Anti-ds DNA antibody	Above laboratory reference range (more than twofold if by ELISA)
3	Anti-Sm antibody +	
4	Antiphospholipid antibody +	+ Lupus coagulant or anti–β2-glycoprotein I, medium- or high-titer anticardiolipin antibody, or false positive
5	Low complement	C3, C4, CH50
6	Direct Coombs test	In the absence of hemolytic anemia

ANA, Antinuclear antibody; *DNA*, deoxyribonucleic acid; *ds*, double-stranded; *ELISA*, enzyme-linked immunosorbent assay; *SLICC*, Systemic Lupus International Collaborating Clinics; *Sm*, Smith.

*At least four criteria are required, including at least one clinical and one immunologic criterion. Biopsy-proven lupus nephritis plus a positive ANA or anti-ds DNA is also sufficient.

Environmental triggers, including ultraviolet (UV) light, medications, pesticides, heavy metals, tobacco, and infections, have all been linked to the development of SLE. In particular, exposure to UV light is a trigger, not only for cutaneous manifestations but also for flares of systemic disease.[62]

Approximately 15% to 20% of all cases of SLE occur within the first 2 decades of life. Of these, 60% occur between the ages of 11 and 15 years, 35% between 5 and 10 years, and 5% in children younger than 5 years of age. Other than neonatal lupus erythematosus (NLE), the disorder is rarely seen before the age of 3 years. Disease onset in the first decade of life is associated with a female to male ratio of 4:3, which increases to female predominance in the second decade (4:1), compared with a ratio of 9:1 in patients with adult-onset SLE. The overall incidence of childhood-onset SLE is 0.3 to 0.9 per 100,000 children, and prevalence is 5 to 10 (range, 1.89 to 25.7) per 100,000 children worldwide.[63] Both increased prevalence and severity are seen in Black and Hispanic children, especially because of the increased prevalence of nephritis.[64] Compared with SLE in adults, affected children have more severe disease in general, with an increased incidence of renal, neurologic, and hematologic involvement at the time of diagnosis.[65–67] In one study, 77% of pediatric patients required moderate to high dosages of corticosteroids, compared with 16% of adult patients.[68]

About 80% of patients with SLE have cutaneous involvement at some time, often as the presenting sign. Diagnosis of SLE requires Systemic Lupus International Collaborating Clinics (SLICC) criteria, which were established in 2012 (Table 22.1). These criteria are more sensitive (but less specific) at classification than the previous criteria established by the American College of Rheumatology in 1982.[69,70] The 1982 criteria included four mucocutaneous features: the malar eruption, discoid eruption, photosensitivity,[71] and oral ulcerations. In 2012, the dermatologic criteria for SLE were broadened to include the variety of subtypes of cutaneous lupus under either acute or chronic cutaneous lupus criteria. In addition, to prevent duplication of highly correlated terms related to cutaneous lupus, photosensitivity was replaced with diffuse, nonscarring alopecia.[72]

Cutaneous Lupus Erythematosus

Cutaneous lupus erythematosus (CLE) may occur as an isolated finding or in the setting of underlying SLE. Features of CLE may be classified as lupus specific or nonspecific, based on clinical and histopathologic characteristics. Lupus-specific subsets of cutaneous disease characteristically demonstrate lupus-specific features on histopathologic examination, including interface dermatitis and mucin deposition. These include acute CLE (ACLE), subacute CLE (SCLE), chronic cutaneous lupus erythematosus (CCLE), and intermittent CLE (ICLE; sometimes included under CCLE). Lupus-nonspecific cutaneous disease includes a variety of reactive phenomena that are not pathognomonic or specific for SLE but typically occur in active disease.

ACLE may present with a malar or butterfly rash or a more generalized morbilliform photodistributed eruption. In particular, the malar rash (Fig. 22.3), although seen in approximately 60% of patients with SLE,[71] is not specific but when present is often a sign of underlying systemic disease. This erythematous, mildly scaling eruption (Fig. 22.4) often appears over the cheeks and bridge of the nose, resembling the shape of a butterfly. It can be confused with the malar erythema of seborrheic dermatitis, erythematotelangiectatic acne rosacea, parvovirus infection, or cutaneous lichenoid graft-versus-host disease[73]; seborrheic dermatitis typically involves the nasolabial fold and shows scaling as well. Brightly erythematous papules and plaques can also be seen on the photo-exposed extremities and V-shaped region of the neck. When this eruption presents on the dorsal aspect of the hands in SLE, the areas overlying joints are typically spared (Fig. 22.5), in contrast to juvenile dermatomyositis.

SCLE, which represents 10% to 15% of all cases of CLE, only occasionally occurs in pediatric patients.[74,75] The cutaneous lesions of SCLE arise quite suddenly, mainly on the upper trunk, extensor surfaces of the arms, and dorsal aspect of the hands and fingers. The lesions may be annular and may enlarge and merge into psoriasiform or polycyclic lesions (Fig. 22.6) with thin and easily detached scales. UV light is usually associated with exacerbations, but lesions tend to be nonscarring. Although arthritis and fatigue are common, patients usually only have mild systemic manifestations. Most patients with SCLE have anti-Ro (SS-A) antibodies, and many have anti-La antibodies. Nonbullous annular lesions that clinically and histologically resemble Sweet syndrome (see Chapter 20) can also be seen as a manifestation of SLE; biopsy shows unique histologic features called the *histiocytoid form* of neutrophilic dermatosis.[76] Rowell syndrome was originally described as an erythema multiforme–like eruption in association with lupus (classically CLE), anti-La antibodies, and speckled ANAs; although controversy exists, most of these cases are probably SCLE or the concurrence of lupus and erythema multiforme.[77]

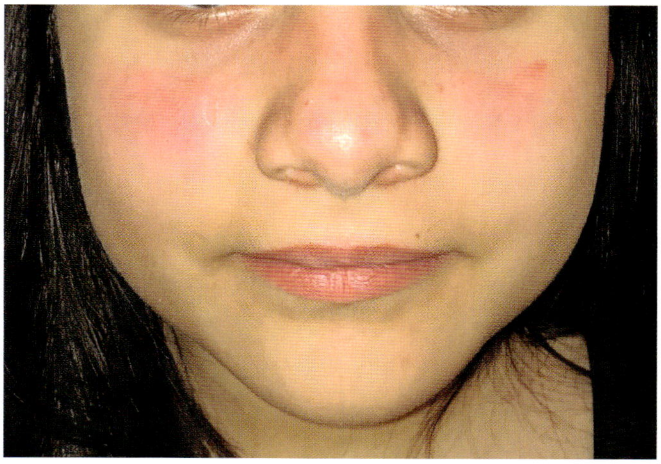

Fig. 22.3 Systemic lupus erythematosus (SLE). Distribution of the malar rash. This teenager with SLE had sun exposure and flared.

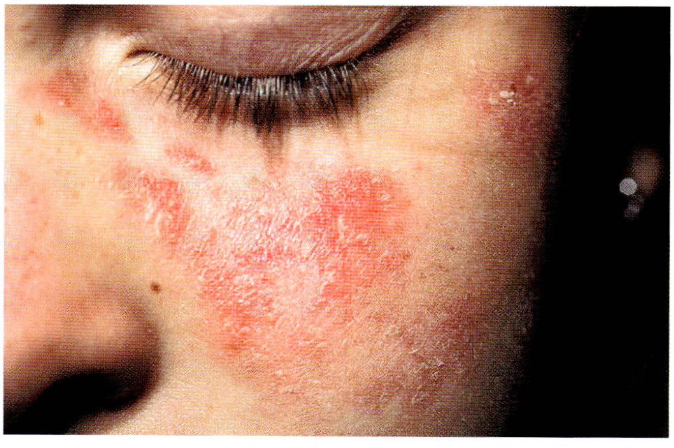

Fig. 22.4 Systemic lupus erythematosus. Mild scaling and erythema of the malar rash.

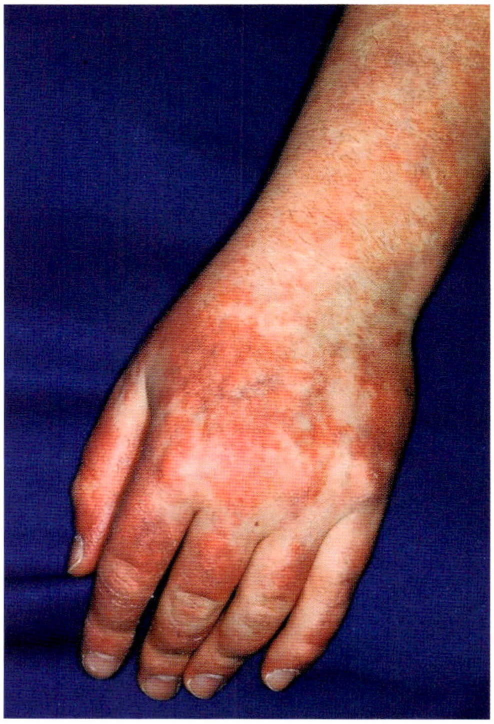

Fig. 22.5 Systemic lupus erythematosus. Bright erythema and scaling with relative sparing of skin overlying the joints, in contrast to the distribution of Gottron lesions in juvenile dermatomyositis. The periungual areas are involved.

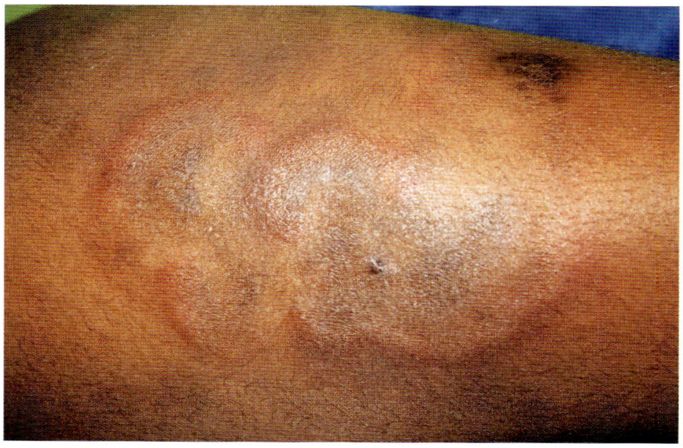

Fig. 22.6 Subacute cutaneous lupus erythematosus. The annular and polycyclic erythematous scaling lesions arose suddenly on this adolescent after sun exposure.

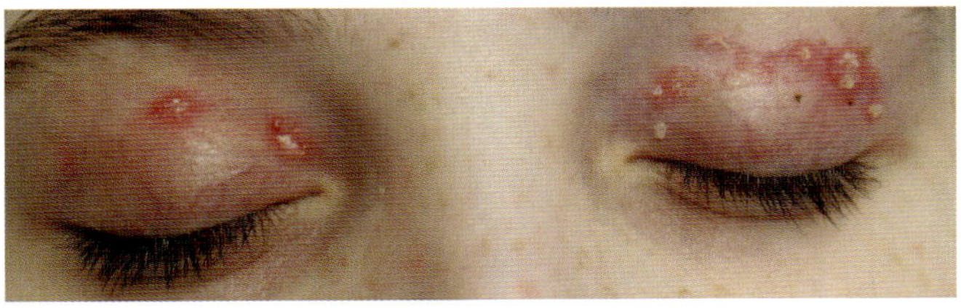

Fig. 22.7 Discoid lupus erythematosus. This teenager had erythematous scaling papules on the eyelids and eyelid margin telangiectasia.

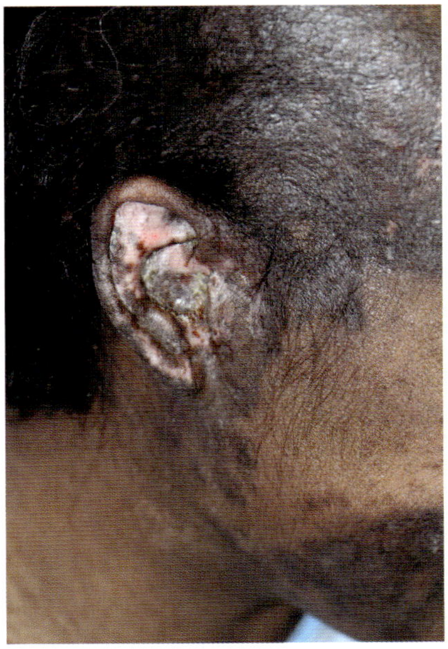

Fig. 22.8 Discoid lupus erythematosus (DLE). The ear is often involved with DLE. Note the well-defined plaques of purplish erythema, focal overlying scaling, and postinflammatory hyperpigmentation and depigmentation.

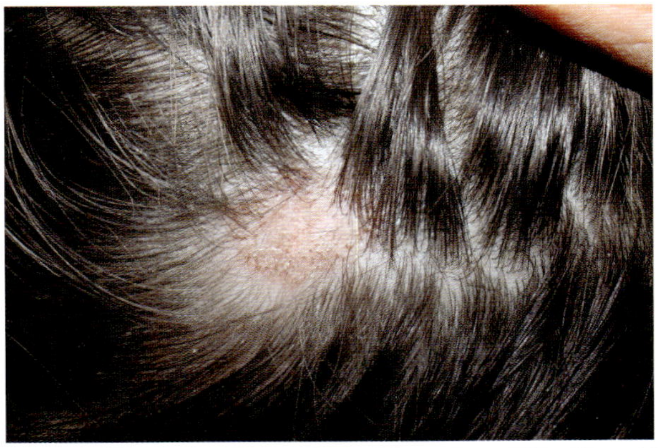

Fig. 22.9 Discoid lupus erythematosus (DLE). Alopecic plaque. Chronicity can lead to scarring alopecia.

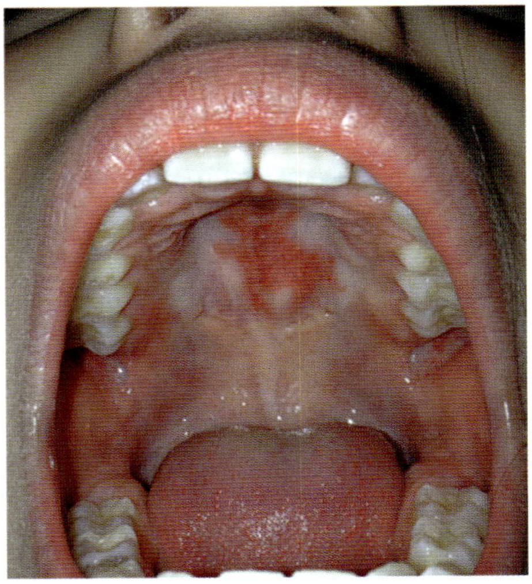

Fig. 22.10 Discoid lupus erythematosus. Dyspigmentation and atrophy of the hard palate.

SCLE is treated by strict sun protection, topical antiinflammatory agents, antimalarials, and occasionally systemic corticosteroids.

Tumid lupus (lupus erythematosus tumidus) is a form of ICLE. Red to purplish urticarial plaques that are relatively fixed in shape and do not undergo atrophy or scaling usually occur on the face or other exposed areas of the body as a sign of photosensitivity. The progression rate of lupus erythematosus tumidus to SLE is unknown.

CCLE is an umbrella term used to describe lesions of discoid lupus erythematosus (DLE), lupus panniculitis, and chilblain lupus. Individual lesions of DLE are well-circumscribed, elevated, indurated red to purplish plaques with adherent scale (Figs. 22.7 and 22.8) and fine telangiectasia. When untreated or as a sequela, discoid lesions may develop persistent areas of hyperpigmentation or hypopigmentation with atrophy. Discoid lesions can be asymmetric and are often exacerbated by exposure to UV light. Occasionally, discoid lesions are verrucous or hypertrophic.[78] DLE is most commonly found on the face, often with lesions on the ear helices and conchal bowls. Although the face is often the sole site of DLE without SLE, the scalp (Fig. 22.9), arms, legs, hands, fingers, back, chest, abdomen, and even mucosal areas (Fig. 22.10) may also be involved. At times the openings of hair follicles are dilated and plugged by an overlying scale. If the scale is thick enough, it can be lifted off in one piece. The undersurface then reveals follicular projections that resemble carpet tacks, a characteristic sign of LE. Discoid lesions have been described in a linear orientation that follows the lines of Blaschko[79,80] and are the most common subgroup of lupus to course along Blaschko lines.[81] Photosensitivity has been reported in only 12% with blaschkolinear lesions, and only 6.5% meet criteria for SLE.[81]

Fewer than 3% of patients with DLE develop disease before the age of 10 years. DLE may present as an isolated finding or as a manifestation of underlying SLE. Small studies in children have demonstrated an early rate of progression to SLE approaching 25% to 30% during a variable follow-up duration of months to years.[82–86] In one series of 40 patients, 15% presented as DLE with concurrent SLE but 26% eventually met criteria for SLE, with transition most common in the first year after DLE diagnosis,[87] mandating serial clinical and serologic evaluations for systemic disease. Both adults and children with generalized lesions (above/below the neck) are at higher risk for SLE.[82,88,89] However, children with DLE who develop SLE appear to follow a more benign course of systemic disease, with 89% of patients in one study meeting SLE classification criteria with mucocutaneous limited manifestations and no evidence of end-organ damage during 5 years of follow-up.[83] Based on consensus among pediatric dermatologists and pediatric rheumatologists, (1) screening laboratory testing should include complete blood cell counts with differential, urinalysis, complement levels, erythrocyte sedimentation rate, antinuclear antibody and other autoantibodies, hepatic function, and renal function/electrolytes; (2) the presence of arthritis or nephritis should increase concern about development of SLE; and (3) hydroxychloroquine is the first-line treatment for DLE in an attempt to slow potential progression.[90]

Intense inflammation of the fat (lupus panniculitis,[91] lupus profundus)[92] occurs in approximately 2% to 3% of patients with CLE and

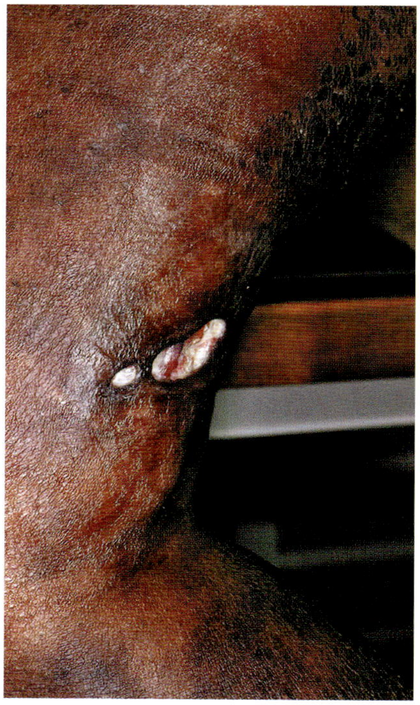

Fig. 22.11 Lupus panniculitis. This boy with systemic lupus erythematosus and lupus panniculitis (lupus profundus) developed tender nodules on the thighs that ulcerated.

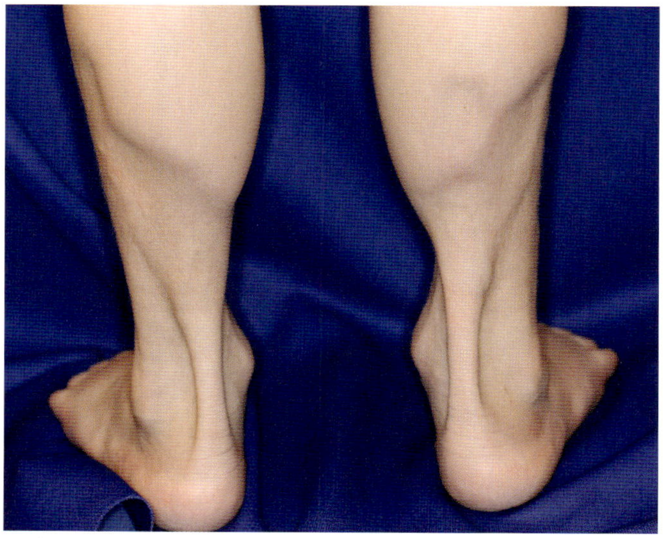

Fig. 22.12 Lipoatrophic panniculitis of the ankles. This 5-year-old boy developed erythematous plaques that resolves with marked atrophy of the ankles and lower calves. No systemic disorders were discovered, and his disease progression was slowed by administration of systemic corticosteroids and methotrexate.

may be associated with DLE or SLE or, not uncommonly, may occur as an isolated disorder.[93] Lesions are seen as firm, often asymptomatic, sharply defined, rubbery dermal and subcutaneous plaques or nodules with a predilection for the scalp, forehead, cheeks, upper arms, breasts, thighs, and buttocks. Linear lesions of lupus panniculitis along Blaschko lines have been described on the scalp, particularly in the parietal region, as well as in other locations.[94] Although the skin overlying the lesions usually appears normal, it often ulcerates (Fig. 22.11) or becomes depressed. Linear lupus may also be sclerotic,[95] suggesting overlap with linear morphea.

Biopsy of lupus erythematosus panniculitis shows a perivascular lymphocytic, plasma cell, and histiocytic infiltration in the deep dermis and subcutaneous fat without accompanying fat necrosis. The panniculitis may be lobular alone or involve both septae and lobules; most specimens show mucin deposition. Direct immunofluorescence often reveals Igs or C3 deposits at the basement membrane. Approximately 70% of patients with lupus panniculitis also have typical lesions of DLE, and 50% eventually develop systemic involvement or symptoms of SLE such as fever, arthralgia, and lymphadenopathy. Lesions of lupus profundus may persist for years and leave significant disfigurement. Although erythema nodosum (see Chapter 20) may occur in a patient with SLE, lupus panniculitis can often be distinguished from erythema nodosum by its relative lack of tenderness, greater chronicity, and lack of predilection for the lower legs. Lupus panniculitis must also be distinguished from subcutaneous lymphoma by histologic features and T-cell rearrangement studies.

Inflammatory panniculitis followed by lipoatrophy, likely autoimmune in mechanism but not associated with SLE or dermatomyositis, can involve localized areas, such as the ankles (Fig. 22.12) or abdomen.[96] Lipoatrophic panniculitis can also be seen in type 1 diabetes, Hashimoto thyroiditis, and JIA, which may manifest years after the onset of the panniculitis. The tender erythematous nodules demonstrate lobular panniculitis on histopathologic examination. With clearance, these nodules leave lipoatrophy that may progress to partial or even generalized lipodystrophy. Administration of systemic corticosteroids and/or steroid-sparing agents such as methotrexate can stop the development of nodules. Lipodystrophy and tender erythematous nodules are also a feature of chronic atypical neutrophilic dermatosis with lipodystrophy and elevated temperature (CANDLE syndrome),[97] a proteasome autoinflammatory disorder (see Chapters 20 and 25).

Nonspecific Clinical Manifestations of SLE

Nonspecific manifestations of SLE are distinguished by the absence of lupus-specific changes on histopathologic examination. These include a variety of reactive and inflammatory eruptions and are typically observed in active SLE. Livedo reticularis (Fig. 22.13, see also Fig. 12.90) blotchy bluish-red discoloration of the skin caused by vasospasm, is seen in several collagen vascular disorders, among them SLE, drug-induced SLE, APS, and scleroderma. Aggravated by exposure to cold, the reticulated erythema tends to be persistent and is most commonly found on the lower extremities. Vascular changes resembling livedo reticularis can be seen in a variety of genetic disorders with telangiectasia, such as Rothmund–Thomson syndrome (see Chapter 19) and FILS (facial dysmorphism, immunodeficiency, livedo, and short stature) syndrome, resulting from biallelic variants in *POLE1*.[98]

Raynaud phenomenon, seen in 10% to 30% of patients with SLE, may precede the onset of SLE by months or years. This phenomenon is described in more detail in the section on systemic sclerosis (SSc). Pernio (chilblains) are tender cyanotic to reddish-blue nodular swellings on the fingers or toes (see Chapter 20). Chilblain lupus manifests as cold-induced, reddish-blue, inflammatory acral lesions that may ulcerate (see Chapter 20).[99–102] Although sporadic chilblain lupus has been described in adolescents, most of the affected younger children have a familial form of chilblains, Aicardi–Goutières syndrome (see Chapter 20, Fig. 20.50). Chilblains must be distinguished from stimulator of interferon genes (STING)–associated vasculopathy with onset in infancy (SAVI) syndrome, an autoinflammatory disorder with acral vasculopathy that can be exacerbated by cold (see Chapter 25, Fig. 25.34).[103,104]

Chronic urticaria-like lesions (urticarial vasculitis) in children with SLE may be distinguished from classic urticaria by their tendency to persist longer than 24 hours and their lesser tendency to be pruritic (see Chapter 21, Fig. 21.15). A manifestation of immune complex deposition, urticarial vasculitis generally occurs in patients demonstrating clinical or serologic evidence of systemic disease activity, especially hypocomplementemia. Biopsy confirms the presence of leukocytoclastic vasculitis. Leukocytoclastic vasculitis can also be seen in biopsy specimens from purpuric lesions in patients with SLE.

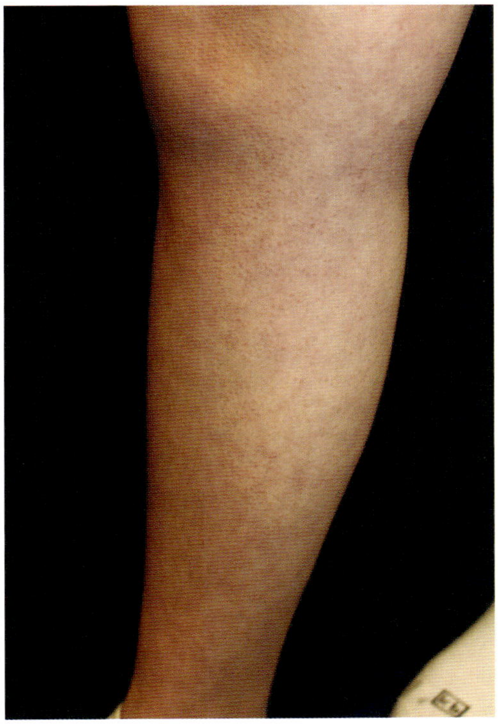

Fig. 22.13 Livedo reticularis. Bluish-red reticulated discoloration of the leg in a teenager with systemic lupus erythematosus.

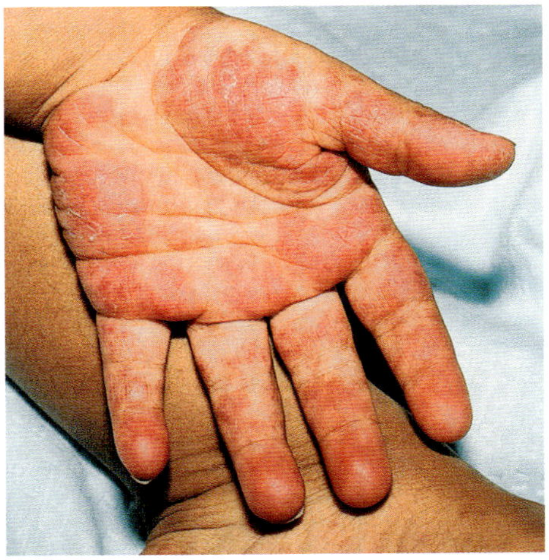

Fig. 22.14 Systemic lupus erythematosus. Erythema and papular telangiectasia on the palm and fingers of a child with lupus erythematosus.

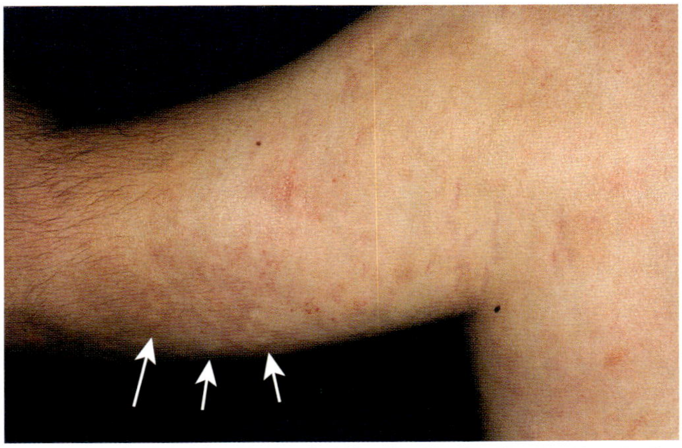

Fig. 22.15 Papulonodular dermal mucinosis in systemic lupus erythematosus (SLE). This teenager with long-term SLE in good control developed firm pruritic induration of the upper back and proximal arms with some palpable nodularity (indicated by *arrows*). Deposition of mucin, resembling that of scleredema, was noted in biopsy sections.

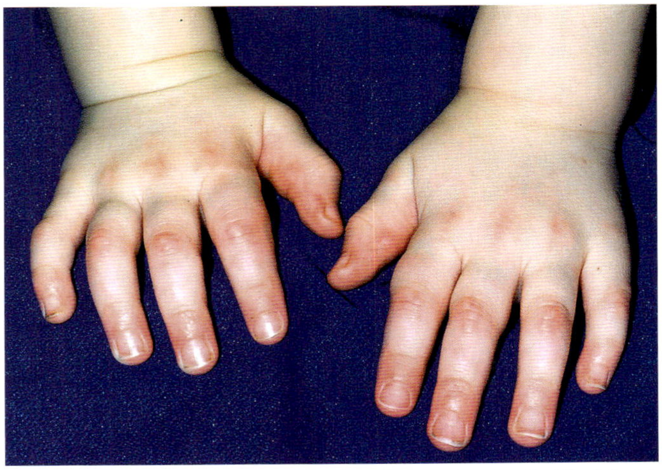

Fig. 22.16 Self-healing juvenile cutaneous mucinosis. The young girl developed numerous skin-colored to erythematous nodules and swelling on the fingers and also on the periorbital areas and trunk. She was otherwise well, and the lesions cleared during the subsequent years without intervention.

These purpuric lesions may ulcerate, leaving significant scarring. Erythema and papular telangiectasia of the palms and fingers (Fig. 22.14), linear telangiectasia of the cuticles and periungual skin (with or without thromboses), and periorbital or hand and feet edema[105] are other nonspecific cutaneous features of SLE.

Although bullous or crusted lesions of SLE may simply reflect fragility of skin because of liquefaction degeneration of basal keratinocytes, a distinctive (and rare) complication of SLE resembles bullous or epidermolysis bullosa acquisita (EBA) and has been called *bullous* (or *vesiculobullous*) *SLE* (*BSLE*; see Chapter 13, Fig. 13.41).[106–108] The treatment of choice is dapsone.[109] Indirect immunofluorescence on salt-split skin shows Ig and C3 deposits on the dermal side, and immunoblotting shows autoantibodies directed against type VII collagen, as in patients with EBA (see Chapter 13).[110,111] Subtle variations in IgG subtypes between EBA and BSLE have been shown by IgG subtyping. Other forms of immunobullous disorder, such as linear IgA disease, have also been described in association with SLE, emphasizing the need for immunofluorescence testing.[112]

Mucin deposition is a typical characteristic seen on skin biopsy sections of individuals with SLE. However, skin-colored, sometimes pruritic papules and nodules involving primarily the trunk, upper extremities, and occasionally the face are a clinical feature of SLE that reflects large amounts of mucin in the mid-dermis between collagen bundles[113,114] (Fig. 22.15). Papulonodular (dermal) mucinosis of SLE may occur any time during the course, including before onset of other features, and has a course that is independent of the course of the SLE. Mucinosis in children is also a histologic feature of self-healing juvenile cutaneous mucinosis, an unusual disorder characterized by the acute onset of multiple skin-colored to dusky erythematous asymptomatic papules and nodules.[115–117] Lesions mainly occur on the head and periarticular areas and can be a few centimeters in diameter (Fig. 22.16), in contrast to the more diffuse and, if discrete, papular lesions of the papulonodular mucinosis of SLE. Fever, muscle tenderness, arthralgias, and weakness may be associated.[118] Lesions spontaneously resolve during the subsequent months to a few years. Biopsy samples can be erroneously misdiagnosed

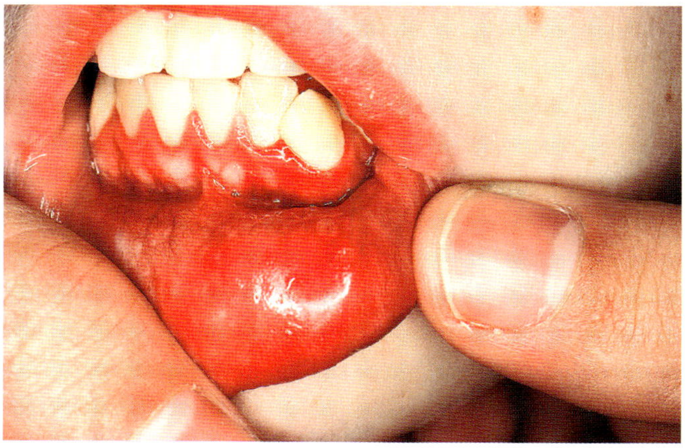

Fig. 22.17 Systemic lupus erythematosus. The gingival and buccal mucosae are red, edematous, and eroded, with subtle whitening. Note the roughness and erythema of the lips with the subtle whitening of the vermilion border.

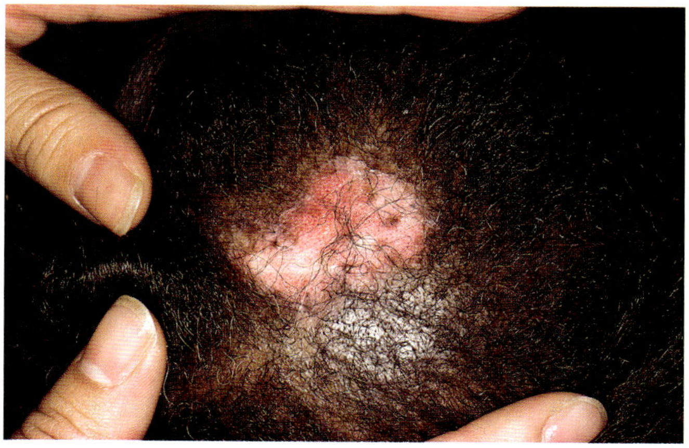

Fig. 22.18 Systemic lupus erythematosus (SLE). Discoid plaque associated with scarring alopecia of the scalp in a patient with SLE.

as panniculitis or proliferative fasciitis,[119] but mucin stains allow the characteristic deposition of large amounts of mucin to be identified so that the family can be reassured.

Mucosal membrane lesions (gingivitis, mucosal hemorrhage, erosions, and small ulcerations) are seen in 3% of patients with CLE and in up to 30% of pediatric patients with the systemic form of the disorder. A silvery whitening of the vermilion border of the lips is highly characteristic, and the lips may show slight thickening, roughness, and redness, with or without superficial ulceration and crusting (Fig. 22.17). The gingival, buccal, and nasal mucosae may also appear red, edematous, friable, and eroded or may exhibit silvery white changes.

Several forms of alopecia may occur in patients with SLE (overall in about 30% of patients). First, discoid lupus may present with scarring alopecia associated with multiple well-demarcated patches (Fig. 22.18) that exhibit erythema, scaling, telangiectasia, atrophy, and plugging (the classic changes of DLE). Second, patients with SLE may develop hair fragility, especially with acute exacerbations, that leads to hair breakage several millimeters from the roots, resulting in a receding hairline with a short, unruly, broken hairs ("lupus hair"), especially at the temple and forehead. Telogen effluvium may also occur in patients with SLE. Finally, there is an increased incidence of alopecia areata in patients with SLE, and these patients tend to have classic scalp dermoscopic findings including exclamation-mark hairs, black dots, broken hair, and yellow dots (see Chapter 7).[120,121]

The most common symptoms of SLE at presentation are constitutional (malaise, fever, and weight loss).[71] The arthritis, which occurs in up to 79% of pediatric patients,[71,122] is a symmetric polyarthritis involving both small and large joints.[1] It is commonly quite painful (in contrast to the arthritis of JIA), often out of proportion to the clinical findings, and tends to be nondeforming. Approximately 55% of pediatric patients develop renal involvement, most often during the first year of the SLE. Four types of nephritis have been described based on renal biopsy pattern: mesangial lupus nephritis, focal proliferative, diffuse proliferative, and membranous glomerulonephritis. Diffuse proliferative glomerulonephritis occurs most commonly (40% to 50%) but carries the worst prognosis, leading to end-stage renal disease in approximately 10% to 15% of patients with lupus nephritis.[123] The presence of anti–double-stranded (anti-ds) deoxyribonucleic acid (DNA) antibodies and hypocomplementemia is commonly associated with severe renal damage. Pulmonary involvement, particularly pleuritis, occurs in up to 30% of patients. Cardiac manifestations, including pericarditis, myocarditis, vasculitis affecting coronary arteries, and Libman–Sacks endocarditis, occur in approximately 15% of patients. A recognized issue, however, is the long-term risk of accelerated atherosclerosis[123]; the overall survival for SLE has improved for all causes except cardiovascular disease. Individuals with childhood-onset SLE can develop myocardial ischemia as early as 20 to 30 years of age.

Neuropsychiatric SLE (central nervous system [CNS] involvement) most commonly features headache, seizures, alterations in mental status, psychosis, and peripheral neuropathy and is seen in 20% to 30% of affected children[124]; most show evidence of neuropsychiatric involvement during the first year of the disease, but cognitive dysfunction occurs in almost 25%. Neuroimaging studies may show structural abnormalities, such as infarction; the addition of single-photon emission computed tomography (SPECT) scans may identify evidence of cerebral vasoconstriction and vasculitis as perfusion abnormalities and allow a diagnosis of lupus psychosis.

Lymphadenopathy, although it occurs more commonly in adults, is seen in up to 40% of children with SLE. Ocular findings are seen in 25% of patients (cotton-wool patches, optic neuropathy, perivasculitis, and edema of the optic disk). MAS occurs in approximately 9% of childhood-onset SLE, typically presents with high fever, and in some patients is associated with organ involvement (hepatomegaly, splenomegaly, neurologic signs, pancytopenia, coagulopathy, and high levels of liver enzymes, ferritin, and triglycerides [see Macrophage Activation Syndrome earlier this chapter]). The mortality rate of SLE is higher if MAS is associated.[43] In patients with suspected MAS, a bone marrow aspirate should be performed to consider cytopenia and possible hemophagocytosis. Ferritin levels will help to distinguish MAS from infection, in which hyperferritinemia tends to be less than in MAS.[63]

Laboratory Features in the Diagnosis of SLE

The diagnosis of SLE is chiefly clinical and is based on the presence of cutaneous lesions, systemic manifestations, and confirmatory laboratory tests (see Table 22.1). Biopsy of cutaneous lesions will confirm the diagnosis and shows (1) hyperkeratosis with keratotic plugging; (2) epidermal atrophy; (3) liquefactive degeneration of basal cells; and (4) a patchy, chiefly lymphoid cell infiltrate, especially around appendages and vessels.[125] Biopsy of lesional skin in DLE or SLE usually shows the deposition of immunoreactants at the epidermal–dermal border (the lupus band test). Sun-exposed areas should be avoided for this biopsy, if possible, because of the risk of a false-positive lupus band test at sun-exposed sites. Chest radiographs, electrocardiography, and echocardiography have been recommended as baseline screening components for any child with SLE.[63]

Serologic examination is the most important evaluation for children thought to have SLE, and ANA is the most valuable screening test. The serologic profiles in children with SLE are similar to those of adults, although some authors have reported a slightly increased incidence of positive antibody tests. The ANA test is almost always positive when a human substrate is used (e.g., Hep-2 cells); in contrast, 5% to 10% of patients with SLE have a negative ANA test when nonhuman tissues are used for testing. Having a positive ANA test does not make a diagnosis of lupus. It can be seen in patients with several other collagen vascular disorders and is present in 5% to 10% of the normal population.[126] However, an ANA level greater than 1:160 usually suggests an autoimmune disorder. Five patterns of ANA have been described: speckled (the most nonspecific), homogeneous, peripheral or shaggy (most patients with SLE and this pattern have anti-ds [also called *native*] DNA antibodies), nucleolar (often seen in patients with scleroderma), and centromere (largely associated with calcinosis, Raynaud, esophageal dysmotility, sclerodactyly, and telangiectasia [CREST]; see discussion on SSc).

Monitoring of serum complement is a critical test for determining lupus activity. The development of hypocomplementemia commonly signals the onset of renal disease. Total complement activity is monitored by functional hemolytic assay (CH50). Specific complement levels, particularly of C3 and C4, should be routinely checked by single radioimmunodiffusion assay. Not uncommonly, C4 levels may be depressed when C3 is normal, probably because patients with SLE are often missing one or more C4 allele.[127]

One risk factor for the development of SLE, especially with onset during childhood, is hereditary deficiency of the early complement components, C1 (C1q and less often C1r/s), C4, C2, and C3.[128] Screening for complement deficiency via CH50, AP50, C3, and C4 (or specific complement levels if appropriate) is important for younger children in particular. Virtually all children with C1q deficiency develop manifestations of lupus (Fig. 22.19).[129] The SLE that occurs in complete C1- or C4-deficient individuals typically presents early during childhood. C2-deficient individuals tend to have a lower risk and less severe disease with lower titers of antinuclear antibodies but increased anti-Ro antibodies. Lupus and other autoimmune disorders do not tend to occur in individuals with deficiency of the later components of complement, which instead are associated with an increased risk of developing infections, including neisserial infections. Lupus has also been seen in patients with chronic granulomatous disease, female carriers of the X-linked form of chronic granulomatous disease,[130] and patients with IgA deficiency.

Children who may have lupus should be tested for the presence of anti-ds DNA antibodies, which are found in about 50% of patients with SLE and have been associated with an increased risk of renal disease, particularly if complement levels are low. In contrast, anti-ribosomal P antibodies are inversely associated with renal involvement in juvenile-onset SLE.[65] Anti–single-stranded (ss) DNA antibodies are found in about 70% of patients and are nonspecific. However, complement-fixing anti-ss DNA antibodies are associated with renal disease, even without anti-dsDNA antibodies. Some patients with SLE have antibodies directed against nuclear ribonuclear proteins (nRNPs). Patients with anti-nRNP antibodies (30% to 40%) have a lower risk of renal disease and a better prognosis. Anti-nRNP antibodies and a speckled ANA pattern have also been described in patients with an overlap syndrome of lupus in association with sclerodactyly, esophageal dysmotility, Raynaud phenomenon, and pulmonary disease (MCTD). Raynaud phenomenon typically precedes the appearance of other signs and symptoms by several years in affected children. Fever, arthralgia, and myalgia are associated, and patients often have hypergammaglobulinemia, a positive RF, and normal complement levels.[131] The anti-Smith (Sm) antibody is specific for SLE, occurs in 20% to 35% of patients, and is associated with a higher risk of renal disease.

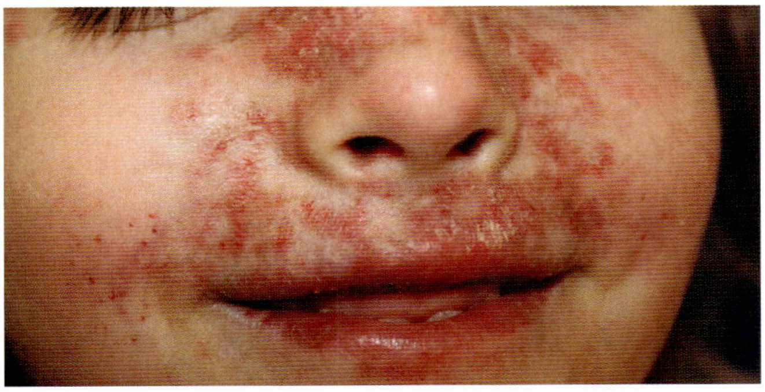

Fig. 22.19 C1q deficiency. During infancy, this girl started to develop scaling atrophic telangiectatic lesions on the face. Note the relative sparing of the perinasal area. Although not shown, the eyelids had severe telangiectasia.

Anti-Ro or anti-La antibodies are described in 32% and 16% of children with SLE, respectively (see Neonatal Lupus Erythematosus section). Compared with children with SLE without these antibodies, they are associated with a higher risk of photosensitivity, malar rash, cutaneous vasculitis, alopecia, and musculoskeletal involvement.[132] SCLE is unusual in children, but anti-Ro and anti-La antibodies can also be seen in children with SLE and complement deficiencies or Sjögren syndrome (see Sjögren Syndrome section).[133] Antiphospholipid (aPL) antibodies can occur in up to 65% of children with SLE and should be monitored annually; they portend for the development of irreversible organ damage, not just a higher risk of thrombosis (see Antiphospholipid Antibody Syndrome section).[134]

Other useful laboratory tests include the ESR as a measurement of inflammation; complete blood cell counts to detect leukopenia, thrombocytopenia, and a Coombs-positive hemolytic anemia; and routine urinalysis with blood urea nitrogen (BUN) and creatinine levels to detect renal abnormalities. Renal biopsy and serial blood pressure measurements are important tools for managing children with SLE and evidence of renal disease. As noted, if a patient with SLE has cytopenia and unexplained fever, the diagnosis of MAS, as described in the section on JIA, must be considered. The disease is best recognized by hyperferritinemia and subsequently hypertriglyceridemia and hypofibrinogenemia.[135]

Drug-Induced Lupus Erythematosus

Lupus may be triggered in pediatric patients by drugs, although the features tend to be milder and occurrence is considerably less than in adults, likely reflecting the more limited use of medications in children that are associated with the highest risk. These high-risk drugs are procainamide (occurrence 15% to 20%) and hydralazine (occurrence 5% to 8%).[136–138] The cutaneous features of drug-induced lupus can be divided into those of SLE, SCLE, and CCLE or DLE) (Table 22.2). More than 80 drugs can cause drug-induced lupus, especially with SLE-like manifestations.[138–141] In drug-induced SLE, the typical cutaneous features of classic SLE are often absent (e.g., malar rash, discoid lesions, Raynaud phenomenon, mucosal ulcers, alopecia). Rather, photosensitivity, lesions involving the skin vasculature (livedo reticularis, palpable purpura, ulcers, bullae, urticaria and urticaria vasculitis), and erythema nodosum are most often described. The exception is reactions caused by TNF-α antagonists; TNF inhibitors rarely cause drug-induced lupus but may manifest as the malar rash or discoid lesions and have been associated with a higher risk of developing renal disease than other forms of drug-induced lupus.[142–145]

The most common cause of drug-induced SLE in pediatric patients is minocycline, primarily used by adolescents with acne (see Chapter 8); overall, the risk is low. This reactivity to minocycline is specific and has not been described in patients who are administered tetracycline or doxycycline. Patients usually experience malaise in association with myalgia, arthralgia, or arthritis. Livedo reticularis, antineutrophil antibodies, and elevation of hepatic transaminase levels have been described, but evidence of vasculitis, renal disease, and neurologic involvement are unexpected. Drug-induced lupus from minocycline occurs most commonly in female patients and at an average of 2 years after starting the medication. Affected individuals usually show a symmetric polyarthralgia or polyarthritis involving the small joints of the wrists and hands. Isoniazid, hydralazine, and procainamides may lead to the polyserositis of lupus but rarely cause cutaneous or renal disease. Drug-induced lupus is usually associated with increased titers of antihistone antibodies (which can also be present in up to 50% of patient with SLE without a drug trigger), a positive ANA level, and often anti-ss DNA antibodies. Anti-ds DNA antibodies are usually absent, and complement levels tend to be normal.

Drug-induced SCLE shows the typical cutaneous features of SCLE, appearing at sun-exposed areas as annular polycyclic or papulosquamous

Table 22.2 Features of Drug-Induced Lupus Erythematosus

	Skin Features	Noncutaneous Signs	Laboratory Findings	Most Common Pediatric Trigger(s)
Drug-induced SLE	Photosensitivity, purpura, erythema nodosum, urticaria and urticarial vasculitis, necrotizing vasculitis Usually absent: malar or discoid rash (except TNF inhibitors), mucosal ulcers, alopecia, Raynaud phenomenon	Fever, arthralgias, myalgias, pericarditis, pleuritic, sometimes hepatitis Usually absent: CNS, renal, pulmonary involvement Hepatic changes from minocycline	ANA, antihistone antibodies, elevated ESR May be mild cytopenia	Minocycline, occasionally TNF-α inhibitors, and rarely carbamazepine
Drug-induced SCLE	Annular polycyclic lesions and/or papulosquamous lesions, including on legs Less commonly, erythema multiforme–like or vesiculobullous lesions, necrotizing vasculitis	Usually no arthritis, serositis, or major organ involvement	ANA, anti-Ro, anti-La	Terbinafine, griseofulvin NSAIDs (piroxicam, naproxen)
Drug-induced CCLE	Discoid lesions in photosensitive distribution	Usually no other signs	ANA	TNF-α inhibitors

ANA, Antinuclear antibody; *CCLE*, chronic cutaneous lupus erythematosus/discoid lupus; *CNS*, central nervous system; *ESR*, erythrocyte sedimentation rate; *NSAID*, nonsteroidal antiinflammatory drug; *SLE*, systemic lupus erythematosus; *SCLE*, subacute cutaneous lupus erythematosus; *TNF*, tumor necrosis factor.

lesions, but the legs are often involved, in contrast to classic SCLE. Disease usually develops 4 to 20 weeks after initiation of treatment. The most common drugs to trigger SCLE in children are antifungals (terbinafine and griseofulvin),[146] but other groups are antihypertensives, calcium channel blockers, angiotensin-converting enzyme (ACE) inhibitors, statins, and IFNs.[146,147] Drug-induced CCLE is very rare and usually results from use of TNF-α antagonists. Discontinuation of the offending agent is the most important intervention, with topical application of antiinflammatory medications if needed and systemic corticosteroids if a vasculitis is present. Cutaneous changes may improve within weeks after drug discontinuation, but complete resolution may be prolonged over several months.

Prognosis and Therapy for SLE

The prognosis for children with SLE has improved dramatically from nearly 100% mortality to a survival rate of greater than 90% because of earlier recognition and earlier and more aggressive therapy.[148,149] The main causes of death in children are renal failure, CNS lupus, myocardial infarction, cardiac failure, or infection. Sequelae of disease activity and administration of systemic medications, however, cause considerable morbidity in 88% of patients.[150] These include hypertension, growth retardation, chronic pulmonary impairment, premature atherosclerosis, ocular abnormalities, permanent renal damage, neuropsychiatric and neurocognitive impairment, osteoporosis, musculoskeletal damage, and gonadal impairment. Therapy for SLE depends on the extent of local and systemic involvement.[151–153]

Discoid lesions without SLE usually respond to topical antiinflammatory medications and sun protection. In addition, antimalarial therapy is considered first-line systemic therapy for cutaneous lupus and is beneficial for long-term suppression of the disease.[63,154,155] In adults, hydroxychloroquine has been shown to delay disease onset, prevent flares, retard renal damage, and reduce autoantibody accumulation.[156] For patients in whom hydroxychloroquine and topical therapy is insufficient, quinacrine can be added without increased risk of retinal toxicity. In a study of adults with cutaneous lupus who were not successfully treated with hydroxychloroquine monotherapy, the addition of quinacrine 100 mg once daily to hydroxychloroquine produced significant clinical improvement in 67% of patients, as measured by reduction in the cutaneous lupus activity scale.[157] Chloroquine can often be substituted for quinacrine if the latter is unavailable. Indeed, hydroxychloroquine and chloroquine may work by different mechanisms, with the former inhibiting antigen presentation by dendritic cells and direct binding of immunostimulatory nucleic acids, whereas the latter inhibits toll-like receptor-mediated cytokine production.[53] Systemically administered corticosteroid is uncommonly needed for control of discoid lupus.[158]

According to the recommendations of the American Academy of Ophthalmology, patients treated with an antimalarial should have a pretreatment ophthalmologic examination and annual screening after 5 years, or sooner if there is an unusual risk factor, to detect early retinopathy. In addition to standard testing of the parafoveal area (10-2 field evaluation), at least one form of more sensitive objective testing (multifocal electroretinogram, spectral domain optical coherence tomography, or fundus autofluorescence) should be performed.[159] The appropriate dosage of hydroxychloroquine for children is up to 6.5 mg/kg per day, with a maximum dosage of 400 mg/day. Several months of antimalarial therapy may be required before efficacy is seen.

Avoidance of exposure to sun and unshielded fluorescent light by wearing hats, sun-protective clothing, and appropriate broad-spectrum sunscreens with UVA as well as UVB protection is essential. These include sunscreens with a sun protection factor (SPF) of 30 or greater that contain good UVA blockers, such as titanium dioxide, zinc oxide, avobenzone, and/or the newer, more photostable UVA organic blockers (see Chapter 19). Cosmetic camouflage is an option for patients with residual dyspigmentation. Topical corticosteroids or calcineurin inhibitors (tacrolimus, pimecrolimus)[160] are effective for most inflamed cutaneous lesions, although relatively potent formulations may be required. Pulsed dye laser has reduced inflammation for facial lesions refractory to topical antiinflammatory medications and hydroxychloroquine.[161]

For patients with severe refractory disease, thalidomide has proven efficacy in cutaneous lupus, although its side effect profile often limits routine use.[162] Lenalidomide, a thalidomide analog, may also be used for severe scarring disease. A small study of patients with refractory CLE found that 86% achieved clinical remission with no influence on systemic disease. The drug is associated with fetal embryopathy, cytopenias, and an increased risk of thrombosis but, in contrast to thalidomide, not peripheral neuropathy.[163,164]

Patients with mild disease and arthralgias without nephritis may respond to NSAIDs, although GI irritation is a risk. Although aspirin is generally not a treatment of choice for the arthralgias, 1 to 3 mg/kg per day or an 81-mg tablet is the recommended dosage for individuals with higher levels of aPL antibodies (see Antiphospholipid Antibody Syndrome section).

In patients with more than mild disease, corticosteroids are the mainstay of therapy. In general, children are treated more aggressively than adults, with 97% receiving systemic steroids and 66% receiving other immunosuppressive drugs.[165] High dosages of systemic corticosteroids are usually given until complement and anti-ds DNA antibody levels normalize, with improvement noted in the clinical state. High-dosage pulsed intravenous methylprednisolone (30 mg/kg) is generally administered for significant acute flares. Corticosteroids can then be administered orally and tapered slowly to the lowest possible level that controls the disease. Both alternate-day and single-morning dose therapy may be effective for maintenance, although alternate-day dosing is preferable to lower the risk of growth retardation. Avascular necrosis occurs more commonly in children than in adults (10% to 15%) from steroid usage. Children with SLE and immunosuppressive medications are at increased risk of infection, including pneumococcal infection; the response to administration of pneumococcal vaccination, however, may be poor because of concomitant immunosuppressive medication. Patients should not receive live vaccinations during corticosteroid administration.

Given the association of chronic use of systemic corticosteroids with adverse effects on major organs (renal, cardiac, neurologic) and the recalcitrance of many patients to steroids alone, other immunosuppressive medications have also been administered to achieve or maintain disease control. The addition of an immunosuppressive agent, such as azathioprine, methotrexate, or mycophenolate mofetil,[166,167] is more beneficial for patients with nephritis than the corticosteroid alone and in general may reduce disease activity and/or allow lowering of the steroid dosage.[168] The recommended pediatric dosage for azathioprine is 2.5 to 3.5 mg/kg per day, for methotrexate is 0.4 to 0.6 mg/kg per week with folate given daily or the 6 days without methotrexate, and for mycophenolate mofetil is 40 to 50 mg/kg per day for children and 30 to 40 mg/kg per day for adolescents (or 600 to 1200 mg/m^2 per day). Cyclophosphamide use is most commonly reserved for patients with CNS disease or severe nephritis. The major potential side effects of these agents are hemorrhagic cystitis and sterility (cyclophosphamide); gastrointestinal discomfort (methotrexate), hepatitis (azathioprine); and aplastic anemia, infection, and malignancy (both cyclophosphamide and azathioprine). Mycophenolate mofetil has a better side effect profile. Oral Janus kinase (JAK) inhibitors are also being evaluated as steroid-sparing agents. Dapsone is of little value for SLE but can be quite effective for BSLE.

Autoantibodies and polyclonal B-cell activation are thought to be important in the pathomechanism of SLE. Targeting of specific B cells with rituximab (anti-CD20 chimeric mouse/human monoclonal antibody) has led to improvement, particularly for lupus nephritis and autoimmune cytopenia but also for cutaneous forms.[169] Use of higher daily dosages than used for lymphoma (e.g., 750 mg/m^2 rather than 350 mg/m^2), repeated therapy (days 1 and 15 or 375 mg/m^2 per dose once a week for four doses), and combination therapy (e.g., with cyclophosphamide and corticosteroids) have led to improved disease activity and decreased steroid burden without an increased risk of infection requiring hospitalization.[170] Belimumab, anti–B-cell activating factor (BAFF) antibody, is now approved by the US Food and Drug Administration (FDA) for intravenous administration to children 5 years of age and older with active, autoantibody-positive SLE who are receiving standard therapy. For end-stage renal disease, dialysis and transplantation are therapeutic options. Autologous stem-cell transplantation has been associated with significant morbidity and mortality, as well as high relapse rates in pediatric cases.[151]

Levels of 1,25-dihydroxy vitamin D and intact parathyroid are significantly lower in children with SLE, especially if they are overweight.[171] Preventive therapy for osteopenia in pediatric patients with SLE should include high dietary calcium intake with supplemental calcium and vitamin D as needed.[172] Maintenance of a good exercise program and minimizing steroid weight gain are also helpful. Although bisphosphonates are not routinely given to pediatric patients, their use in patients with pathologic fractures secondary to steroid-induced osteoporosis should be considered.

Neonatal Lupus Erythematosus

Neonatal lupus erythematosus (NLE) is a unique variant of lupus erythematosus found in neonates and infants (Box 22.2).[173–178] The diagnosis is most important as a marker for the mother, who may have autoimmune disease at the time of delivery (approximately half) or who are asymptomatic but at increased risk for developing SLE, Sjögren syndrome, overlap syndromes, or undifferentiated autoimmune syndrome within a median of 3 years.[179] Thus mothers of affected infants with NLE must be monitored and evaluated regularly.

Box 22.2 **Neonatal Lupus Erythematosus**

- Seen in infants born to mothers with a tendency for systemic lupus erythematosus, rheumatoid arthritis, Sjögren syndrome, or undifferentiated connective tissue disease
- May present as lupus-like rash, often in areas of sun exposure; facial erythema, especially periorbitally (raccoon eyes), annular lesions, discoid lesions, atrophic lesions, and/or telangiectasia
- Associated with anti-Ro (SS-A), anti-La (SS-B), and anti–U1 RNP (nRNP) antibodies
- Congenital atrioventricular heart block in 15% to 30%

nRNP, Nuclear ribonuclear protein; *RNP,* ribonuclear protein.

The occurrence of NLE is not related to titers and is not strictly genetic, based on its discordance in identical twins.[180] Nevertheless, developing the skin manifestations of NLE has been linked to carrying a polymorphism in the TNF-α receptor (308A; increases TNF-α expression in response to UV light) and the HLA genotypes *DRB1*03*.[181] Cardiac block has been increased with *DRB1*04* and *Cw*05*[182] haplotypes and a polymorphism in TGF-β (Leu10, associated with increased fibrosis).[183] *DRB1*13* and *Cw*06* are protective.[182]

Approximately 50% to 78% of babies with NLE show cutaneous manifestations at some point, with onset usually by a month of life.[184] However, up to 23% of affected babies show manifestations at birth, especially the cardiac manifestations and occasionally the cutaneous features.[185] Typically, new lesions do not occur after approximately 3 months of age. Lesions are most commonly localized to sun-exposed areas, particularly on the head and neck and the extensor surfaces of the arms, but they may occur anywhere on the skin surface. Lesions have been described in the genital area and on the palms and soles in 5% of patients.[186]

A variety of cutaneous manifestations have been described. Annular lesions or periorbital erythema (termed *raccoon eyes, owl eyes,* or *eye mask*) (Figs. 22.20 through 22.22) should always trigger consideration of the diagnosis in an infant. The annular lesions (Fig. 22.23; see Fig. 22.21) may be confused with annular erythema of infancy, Sweet syndrome,[187,188] or neonatal dermatophyte infection.[189] Discoid lesions (Fig. 22.24), scaly atrophic macules and patches, and telangiectasia[190] have also been described. Atrophic lesions may resemble round icepick scars, are often congenital, and commonly localize to the temporal areas of the forehead. The telangiectasia may be more petechial or may resemble the reticulated lesions of cutis marmorata telangiectatica congenita[191,192] or an extensive capillary malformation.[193] An infant with congenital varicelliform lesions has also been

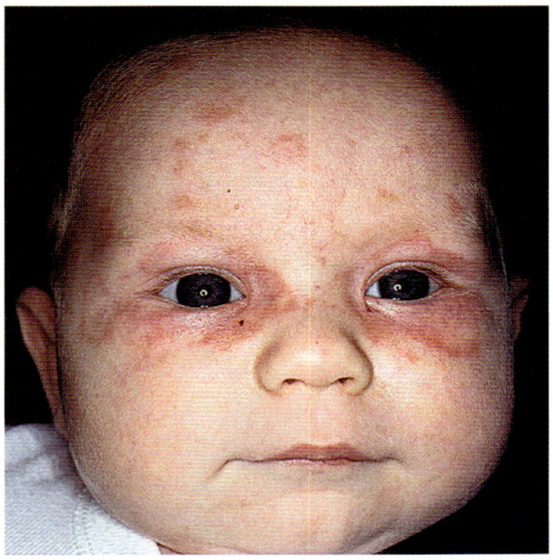

Fig. 22.20 Neonatal lupus erythematosus. Raccoon eyes and annular forehead plaques.

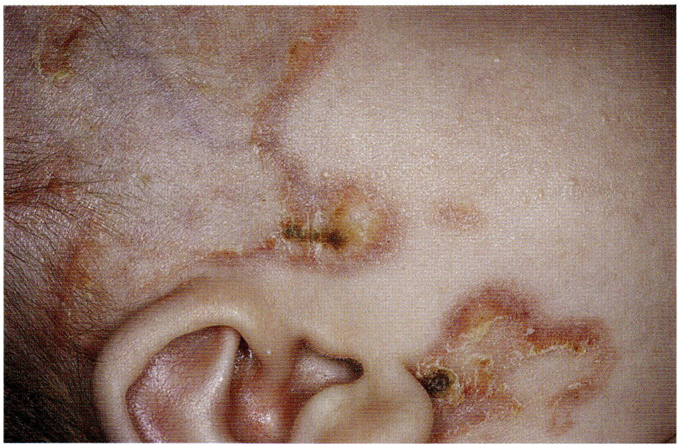

Fig. 22.21 Neonatal lupus erythematosus. Annular scaling plaques on the cheeks of this 6-week-old boy.

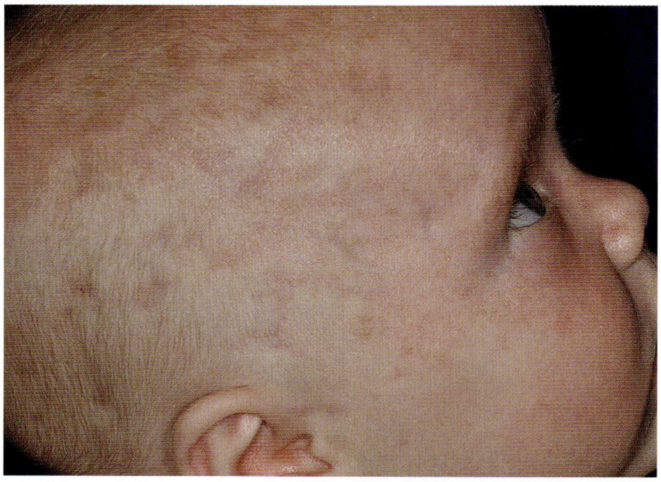

Fig. 22.22 Neonatal lupus erythematosus. Purplish erythema with focal atrophy in a reticular pattern on the face and scalp.

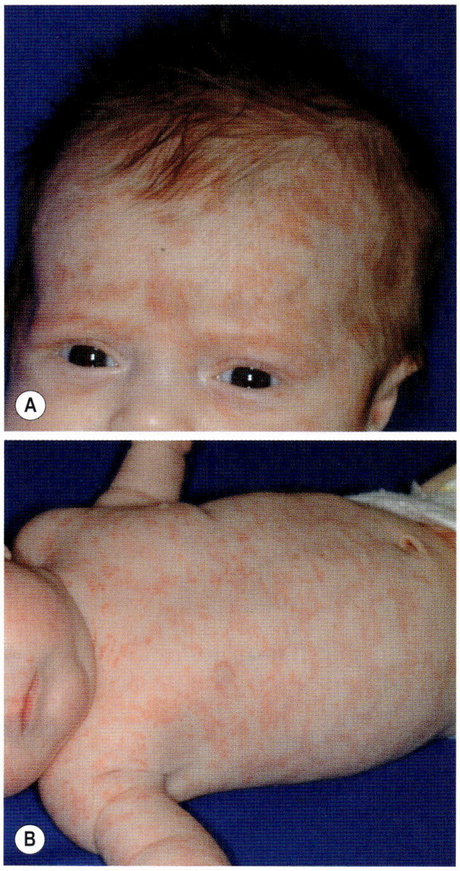

Fig. 22.23 Neonatal lupus erythematosus. **(A, B)** Annular plaques without detectable scale on the face, scalp, trunk, and extremities.

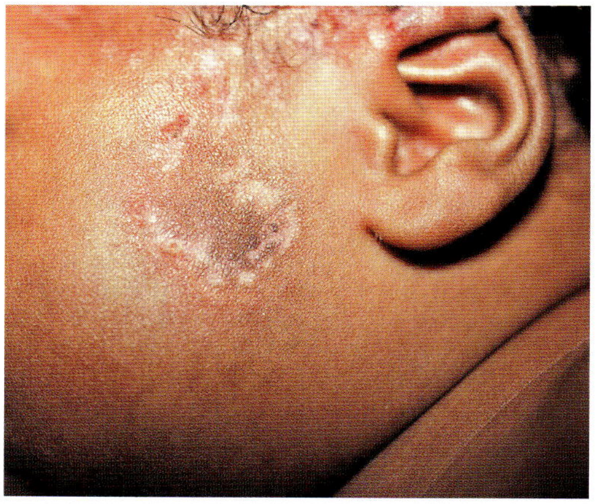

Fig. 22.24 Neonatal lupus erythematosus. Discoid lesions with atrophy and dyspigmentation on the face of a 2-month-old infant. His mother first showed signs of systemic lupus erythematosus 1 year after this baby was born.

described.[194] In addition to the cutaneous eruption, mucosal ulcerations have been noted in several affected babies.

NLE is the most common cause of congenital heart block. Congenital heart block occurs in 15% to 30% of affected patients as a result of *in utero* inflammation, fibrosis, and calcifications of the atrioventricular node and sometimes the sinoatrial node; 10% of patients with cardiac disease have cardiomyopathy.[180,195] Although the cardiomyopathy is usually apparent early, rarely it first manifests several months after birth.[196] Unlike the cutaneous complications of NLE, congenital heart block is usually irreversible. Some infants with first-degree and, rarely, with second-degree heart block have shown spontaneous resolution during the first few months of life, but most patients progress rapidly to third-degree block, including after birth. Two-thirds of infants with heart block require pacemakers.[197] Cardiac disease results in a 20% mortality,[198] not only from the heart block but also congestive heart failure or other associated complications such as transposition of the great vessels, patent ductus arteriosus, septal defects, and endocardial fibroelastosis.

Other systemic complications include liver involvement in 10% to 56% of patients (generally manifested by abnormal liver function tests and sometimes hepatomegaly, but occasionally cholestatic disease and liver failure).[180,195] The increase in liver function test levels is typically seen between 3 and 6 months of age. Splenomegaly, lymphadenopathy, and hematologic abnormalities (leukopenia, thrombocytopenia,[199] and both Coombs-positive and Coombs-negative anemia) affect 27% to 33% of infants with NLE. Subclinical evidence of CNS disease, including CNS vasculitis and stroke[200,201] as well as hydrocephalus,[202,203] has been seen on computed tomographic (CT) scans and ultrasounds in up to 18%.[178,204] Although clinical neurologic features are unusual, imaging studies for hydrocephalus are appropriate for NLE infants with a head circumference greater than the 95th percentile.[205] Pulmonary involvement is very rare.[206]

NLE results from the transplacental passage of maternal antibodies.[207] In 95% of cases, these antibodies are anti-Ro (SS-A) antibodies, often in association with anti-La (SS-B) antibodies. These antibodies have been found at sites of pathology in the epidermis and heart.[208] A subset of infants with neonatal lupus and their mothers have anti–U1 RNP (nRNP) antibodies, although cardiac disease is extremely rare in this subset.[194,209] Infants and mothers may also demonstrate a positive ANA titer and aPL antibodies.[208] Breastfeeding has not been shown to alter antibody levels or affect the development of cutaneous lesions.[210]

The anti-Ro antibodies have been shown to be causative for the cardiac block. Anti-Ro antibodies bind to fetal, but not to adult, cardiac myocytes and selectively injure the conducting system, a process that involves plasmin[211]; anti–U1 RNP antibodies do not bind to cardiac myocytes. When pregnant mice are injected with anti-Ro/La antibodies intraperitoneally, the antibody binds to the heart, epidermis, and liver, sites of inflammation in NLE, and is associated with tissue apoptosis.[212] Overall, 10% to 20% of babies of women with anti-Ro with and without anti-La antibodies develop cutaneous NLE; 1% to 2% develop heart block, and 27% have laboratory abnormalities.[213]

The diagnosis of NLE is aided by the presence of typical cutaneous lesions, systemic manifestations, and confirmatory laboratory studies (positive anti-Ro, anti-La, or anti–U1 RNP antibody tests of the infants and mothers). Because of the possibility of involvement of internal organs, a thorough physical examination, complete blood cell count with platelet count, and liver function tests are often recommended for infants suspected of having NLE. Infants with bradycardia or a murmur deserve an electrocardiogram and echocardiography. If any question regarding the diagnosis remains, cutaneous biopsy of a skin lesion can be performed and will show histopathologic features of lupus with injury to the basal epidermal cells as a prominent feature.[214]

Only 10% have persistent anti-Ro antibody at 9 months,[178] and clearance of cutaneous lesions generally occurs by 6 to 12 months of age. In a few patients, however, the cutaneous lesions disappeared within 1 month, and in others, the eruption has lasted up to the age of 26 months. Most cutaneous lesions clear without sequelae; however, cutaneous change may persist, especially on the face and scalp. In a retrospective study of more than 100 patients with a history of NLE, 34% had sequelae, including 17% with dyspigmentation, 13% with telangiectasia, and 9% with atrophic scarring that was associated with having skin lesions at birth.[176,215–217]

Appropriate treatment of NLE includes avoidance of sun exposure and treatment of visceral complications, which may necessitate administration of systemic corticosteroid therapy. Low- to mid-potency topical steroids or topical calcineurin inhibitors can be used to treat the cutaneous lesions, but lesions clear spontaneously and the use of topical antiinflammatory agents has not been shown to affect risk of residua.[216]

Patients with NLE do not show an increased risk of developing lupus and other autoimmune disorders beyond that of their siblings, suggesting that the small increased risk in this group of patients reflects their familial tendency, not the previous occurrence of NLE.[218] Mothers who have had a child with NLE, however, have a 36% overall risk of having a second affected child,[181] including a 23% risk of cutaneous manifestations and a 13% risk of cardiac issues (almost sixfold higher than the overall risk of congenital heart block in a first affected baby). A mother with a previous baby with NLE involving skin can have a subsequent baby with congenital heart block and vice versa. Fetal echocardiograms (weekly to every other week) between 16 and 26 weeks gestational age, the peak period of cardiac injury, are recommended for at-risk pregnancies. Systemic corticosteroids administered during pregnancy may decrease the risk of first- or second-degree heart block.[219] However, early studies with weekly monitoring have found that steroids do not prevent progression toward third-degree heart block, which can occur quickly *in utero*.[220–222] By introducing home monitoring for fetal heart block and rapid detection, treatment with dexamethasone with intravenous immunoglobulin in a small number of fetuses has reversed second-degree but not third-degree heart block.[223] Antimalarials, particularly hydroxychloroquine, are not teratogenic[224] and have been found to decrease the risk of cardiac, although not noncardiac, manifestations of NLE.[225–227] The combination of steroids with intravenous Ig and plasmapheresis is under investigation.[228]

Antiphospholipid Antibody Syndrome

Antiphospholipid antibody syndrome is an autoimmune thrombotic disorder characterized by venous and/or arterial thrombosis and the persistence of at least one circulating aPL antibody.[229] aPL antibodies in APS are thought to be pathogenic, rather than merely a serologic marker. aPLs are a heterogeneous group of autoantibodies reactive against either negatively charged phospholipids (e.g., phosphatidyl serine and cardiolipin) or proteins that are complexed with them (e.g., β2 glycoprotein I). When APS is suspected, screening should include lupus anticoagulant, anticardiolipin IgG and IgM, and anti–β2-glycoprotein I IgG and IgM.[230]

aPL antibodies are commonly found after bacterial and viral infections in children, leading to the requirement that two tests of aPL antibody levels be performed at least 12 weeks apart for diagnosis.[231,232]

In approximately half of affected pediatric patients, APS is a primary syndrome. The disorder can also occur secondarily, most commonly in children with SLE (38% of children overall).[231,232] Patients with SLE and APS may initially have primary APS, with a mean duration of 1.2 years before the onset of criteria to diagnose SLE.[231,232] All patients with possible SLE should be screened for aPLs.[230] ANAs and anti-ds DNA antibodies are detected much more commonly in children with secondary APS (86% versus 35% and 59% versus 6%, respectively).

Anticardiolipin, lupus anticoagulant, and anti–β2-glycoprotein I antibodies are found overall in 81%, 72%, and 67% of patients, respectively, without a significant difference between primary and secondary types of APS. Only 33% of pediatric patients have all three antibodies and 48% have two simultaneously, emphasizing the need to evaluate all three antibodies for diagnosis. Of note, having more than one aPL antibody does not increase the risk of thrombosis.

The age of onset is significantly younger in children with primary APS (8.7 versus 12.7 years), and 45% of tested children also have one or more inherited thrombophilic risk factors. These inherited prothrombotic disorders include methylenetetrahydrofolate reductase C677T polymorphism, factor V Leiden, protein S or protein C deficiency, prothrombin G20210A heterozygosity, and antithrombin III deficiency.

Manifestations may range from headache or livedo reticularis to stroke or severe tissue necrosis (Box 22.3).[233–236] The most common cutaneous manifestations of APS in children are livedo reticularis and Raynaud phenomenon, each occurring in approximately 6% of affected children. Livedo reticularis is characterized by prominent reticulated cutaneous vasculature, most commonly noted on the lower extremities (see Fig. 22.13 and Chapter 12, Fig. 12.90). Thrombosis is the most serious manifestation (see Box 22.3), and venous thromboses involving the lower extremities occur most commonly. Recurrent thromboses occur in approximately 20% of children,[231,232,237] especially with inadequate anticoagulant therapy and with an underlying inherited thrombophilia. The clinical triad of livedo reticularis, hypertension, and cerebrovascular disease, or Sneddon syndrome, is linked to aPL antibodies in individuals and has rarely been described in children.[238]

Five percent of children have life-threatening thrombotic disease with the rapid occurrence of thrombosis involving at least three organ systems developing simultaneously within a week *(catastrophic APS)*, which has a mortality of 27% to 50%.[239–241] Affected children are likely to be female and suffer from primary APS (each about 70%). The catastrophic event is often the first sign of APS in children (87%). Infections are often a precipitating factor (61%) and peripheral vessel thrombosis occurs in 52% of affected children.

aPL antibodies have been associated with a high risk of miscarriage in pregnant women. In successful pregnancy, transplacental passage of maternal aPL antibodies can rarely lead to neonatal thrombosis,[237] most commonly manifesting as stroke. The risk may be increased in aPL-positive neonates by acquired thrombic risk factors such as central lines, sepsis, prematurity, and heart disease or the hereditary prothrombic diseases previously mentioned. Neonates with stroke may have persistently elevated aPL titers for years that show no

Box 22.3 Antiphospholipid Antibody Syndrome in Children

Cutaneous and Subcutaneous Features

Livedo reticularis
Raynaud phenomenon
Palpable purpura/leukocytoclastic vasculitis
Superficial vein thrombosis
Deep venous thrombosis with ulceration
Pyoderma gangrenosum–like ulceration
Degos-like disease
Gangrene

Noncutaneous Features*

Thromboses*
- Pulmonary thromboembolism, hypertension
- Strokes, transient ischemic attacks
- Transverse myelopathy
- Cerebral venous sinus thrombosis
- Retinal vein thrombosis
- Renal artery thrombosis

Hematologic abnormalities (38%)
- Evans syndrome
- Thrombocytopenia
- Leukocytopenia
- Autoimmune hemolytic anemia

Neurologic abnormalities, nonthrombotic (16%)
- Migraine headaches
- Chorea
- Seizures

Hepatomegaly, enzyme elevation

*Venous thromboses occur in 60% of patients; arterial thromboses in 32% (45% of patients with primary antiphospholipid antibody syndrome [APS] and 18% with secondary APS); mixed thromboses in 3% of patients; and small vessel thromboses, particularly leading to digital infarctions in 6% of patients.

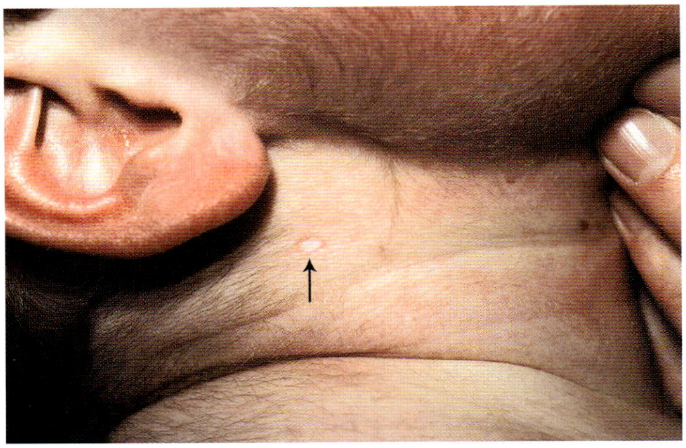

Fig. 22.25 Degos disease. Note the atrophic, porcelain-white center surrounded by telangiectasia. Note the hypertrichosis in this young boy from administration of prednisolone.

concordance with maternal aPL levels.[242] Neurocognitive abnormalities and epilepsy have also been reported in children born of mothers with APS.[243]

Despite the established association between aPL antibodies and thromboses, most individuals with circulating aPL antibodies do not show evidence of thrombosis. As such, it remains controversial whether to treat individuals prophylactically who show persistently positive aPL antibody levels but have no history of thromboses. There is no evidence to support the routine administration of low-dose aspirin in individuals with IgM or low titers of IgG antibodies; however, anticoagulants (e.g., aspirin at 1 to 3 mg/kg per day or an 81-mg tablet) should be considered in patients with higher levels of aPL antibodies, especially patients who will be immobilized or undergoing surgery. Administration of hydroxychloroquine may be protective against the development of thrombosis in aPL-positive children with SLE.[244] In addition, at-risk adolescents should be discouraged from smoking or treatment with estrogen-containing oral contraceptives. Children with aPL antibodies and thrombosis require anticoagulant therapy, but the use of these medications should be weighed in very active children and noncompliant adolescents because of the greater risk of hemorrhage. Children with catastrophic APS are treated with combination intravenous anticoagulation, corticosteroids, plasmapheresis, and sometimes intravenous gamma globulin or cyclophosphamide or rituximab.[240]

Degos Disease

Degos disease is rare in children but has been congenital in a few cases.[245,246] Typical lesions are asymptomatic 3- to 10-mm papules with an atrophic, porcelain-white center surrounded by an erythematous, telangiectatic border (Fig. 22.25). Lesions may appear in crops and typically involve the trunk and extremities; one adolescent with cutaneous Degos-like lesions has been described with localized unilateral involvement of the abdomen.[247] The disorder is characterized by multiple infarcts in the skin caused by a thrombotic vasculopathy that has been linked to complement C5b-9 deposition. Altered platelet function or fibrinolysis has been noted in some patients. Biopsy of lesional skin shows a characteristic acellular, ischemic wedge-shaped area of dermis underlying an atrophic but hyperkeratotic epidermis.

The disorder may involve only the skin ("benign atrophic papulosis") or may be a life-threatening systemic disease with infarcts in other organs ("malignant atrophic papulosis").[248] The GI tract[249] and CNS[250] are the most commonly affected organs. Although involvement of the GI tract is most typical, of the 25 reported pediatric cases of Degos disease, 56% showed CNS involvement and 48% had GI involvement. Acute hematemesis, abdominal pain, dyspepsia, abdominal distension, diarrhea, and constipation are signs of GI tract involvement, and patients may develop peritonitis, bowel infection, or perforation.[251] CNS manifestations include fatal hemorrhagic or ischemic strokes, polyradiculoneuropathy, and nonspecific neurologic symptoms, especially headache. In most cases, the skin lesions precede the occurrence of other manifestations by months to years. Most affected patients die within 2 to 3 years, particularly from sepsis from peritonitis, CNS bleeding, or pleural or pericardial involvement.

Approximately 36% of affected children have a more benign course without evidence of systemic involvement,[247] although patients who present with cutaneous lesions may progress to systemic disease.[252] Familial cases have been described.[253] Degos-like lesions have been described in patients with aPL antibodies and/or SLE and, less commonly, dermatomyositis,[235] suggesting that Degos disease is a distinctive disease pattern rather than a unique entity.[254] In patients with SLE and dermatomyositis, the lesions tend to be more telangiectatic and show more mucin deposition.

Administration of medications that inhibit increased platelet aggregation (especially aspirin and dipyridamole) may be helpful in some cases. Immunosuppression may worsen the skin lesions of Degos disease. Because Degos is linked to complement C5b-9 deposition, treatment of malignant atrophic papulosis may respond, including central nervous system disease, to treatment with eculizumab (humanized anti-C5 monoclonal antibody).[252]

Juvenile Dermatomyositis

Juvenile dermatomyositis (JDM) is an inflammatory disorder with an incidence of three per million children per year that primarily affects the skin, striated muscles, and occasionally other internal organs (Box 22.4).[255–260] In cases in which cutaneous changes are absent, the term *polymyositis* is used. Because the clinical and pathologic features of involved skin and muscles are similar, dermatomyositis and polymyositis are believed to be variants of the same disease process; however, 85% to 95% of children with an inflammatory myopathy have JDM.[261]

The criteria to make a diagnosis of JDM were originally described in 1975[262] but were revised in 2017 as the European League Against

Box 22.4 Clinical Features of Juvenile Dermatomyositis

General

Fever
Lethargy
Adenopathy

Skin, Subcutaneous, Mucosae

Heliotrope rash
Gottron papules, Gottron sign (erythema)
Nailfold capillary changes
Malar or facial eruption
Mouth ulcers
Gingival telangiectasia, bleeding gingivae
Skin ulcers
Limb edema
Xerosis and pruritus of skin, including scalp
Poikiloderma
Calcinosis
Lipodystrophy

Muscle

Muscle tenderness and myalgias
Muscle weakness

Joints

Arthralgia
Arthritis
Contractures

Gastrointestinal

Dysphagia/dysphonia
Gastrointestinal symptoms, especially pain

Pulmonary

Dyspnea from interstitial lung disease

Cardiac

Murmurs, cardiomegaly, pericarditis
Rarely, myocarditis, conduction abnormalities

Box 22.5 Features of Juvenile Dermatomyositis

- Progressive symmetric weakness of the proximal muscles (limb girdle and anterior neck flexors), with or without dysphagia or respiratory weakness
- Typical cutaneous findings of dermatomyositis: Heliotrope rash, Gottron sign and papules, periungual telangiectasia
- Elevation of muscle-derived serum enzyme levels (may be normal)
- Muscle biopsy evidence of myositis and necrosis
- Myositis-specific antibodies

Rheumatism/American College of Rheumatology (EULAR/ACR) classification for adult and juvenile inflammatory myopathies based on studies in 254 patients with JDM (and others with inflammatory myopathies)[263,264] (Box 22.5). Each item in the classification is assigned a weighted score and the total score provides a probability of having an inflammatory myopathy. Variables include age of onset, muscle weakness, skin manifestations (Gottron sign, Gottron papules, and heliotrope rash), other clinical manifestations, laboratory measurements, and, if performed, muscle biopsy features.[255] Patients with pathognomonic skin rashes of JDM are accurately classified without having a muscle biopsy. The new criteria improve the probability of classification as dermatomyositis[265] in adults, including in amyopathic cases.

JDM occurs more often in girls than boys (2.3:1) and has a bimodal age distribution, with one peak between 2 and 5 years of age and another at 12 to 13 years of age, giving a mean age of onset of 7 years of age; 35% of children have the onset of JDM before 5 years of age.[266] Overall, approximately 25% of all individuals afflicted with dermatomyositis are younger than 18 years of age at the time of onset. Malignancy is associated with adult dermatomyositis in about 20% of cases but is rare in pediatric patients.[267] In contrast to adults, children tend to have more inflammation and necrosis of muscle, calcinosis, periungual and gingival telangiectasias, ulceration, and small vessel vasculopathy but fewer myositis-associated antibodies, less interstitial lung disease and amyopathic disease, and a lower mortality rate.[258] The histologic features in muscle and IFN gene signature of JDM are similar in both adult and childhood disease.

The immune alterations that drive the small-vessel occlusive vasculopathy of JDM are still poorly understood, but environmental triggers, immune dysfunction, and specific tissue responses[268,269] are important. Although the onset shows seasonality and many children have preceding infectious features, no evidence of an associated infectious agent has been discovered. Maternal microchimerism has also been implicated in causing JDM and has been noted in 70% of peripheral blood T lymphocytes and 80% to 100% of muscle tissue samples from patients.[270,271] JDM is thought to be a disorder of both innate and adaptive immune systems, with immature regenerating muscle fibers expressing myositis-specific autoantigens at high levels, which induce toll-like receptor and dendritic cell stimulation, with lymphocyte activation toward production of type I IFNs, IL-6, CCL20, and autoantibodies. Children with active JDM are often lymphopenic but show a relative increase in the percentage of B cells, as defined by anti-CD19 monoclonal antibody binding. The major histocompatibility complex alleles HLAB8, HLADQA1*0501, HLADQA1*0301, HLADRB*0301, and HLADPB1*0101 confer increased risk. In addition, several other polymorphic gene loci have been shown to be risk factors.[255] A polymorphic variant of the TNF-α promoter that increases TNF-α expression (TNF-308A), including in response to UV light, is associated with a higher risk of calcinosis, ulcerations, and disease chronicity.[272,273] Polymorphisms in IL-1 and the IL-1 receptor antagonist also increase the risk of the development of calcinosis and JDM, respectively.[274,275]

Although myositis-associated antibodies (MAAs) were infrequently seen in children relative to adults, 70% of children with JDM have high titers of a single myositis-specific antibody (MSA).[255,276,277] Certain MSAs are found much more often in adults than in children, particularly anti-Jo-1 antibodies (against histidyl-tRNA synthetase; only 3% to 4% of patients with JDM) and anti-Mi-2 antibodies (against a DNA helicase; also only in 3% to 5% of children). However, more recently recognized autoantibodies targeting intracellular proteins (anti-TIF1-γ, anti-NXP2, and anti-MDA5) have been found in 60% to 75% of children with JDM (each child having a specific one) and are useful biomarkers for defining distinct clinical subsets and predicting prognosis.[259,260,278–280] Anti-TIF1-γ (also called *p155*) antibodies are detected in approximately 18% to 35% of children and are linked to more severe cutaneous involvement with generalized lipodystrophy. Anti-NXP2 (also called *anti-MJ* or *anti-p140*) antibodies, found in 15% to 22% of patients, are associated with a substantially increased risk of greater disease severity, calcinosis,[281] and contractures.[282] Anti-MDA5 (also called *anti-CADM*) antibodies, noted in 6% to 7% of JDM patients, predict a distinct phenotype that includes skin and oral ulcers, painful or asymptomatic palmar papules, alopecia, panniculitis, arthritis, milder and shorter duration muscle disease activity, and an increased risk of interstitial lung disease, which still occurs in a minority of children.[283–286]

Children with overlap disease may have anti–polymyositis-scleroderma (PM-Scl) antibodies (5% to 7%) or anti–U1 RNP (<6%) antibodies. ANAs are also present in 60% to 70% of newly diagnosed children, usually in a coarse speckled pattern, and are not useful in making the diagnosis or predicting course.

The onset of JDM is insidious in approximately 50% of affected children with subtle weakness, anorexia, malaise, abdominal pain, and the gradual development of a rash. In about 30% of children, the onset of the disorder is fulminant, with fever, profound weakness, and severe multisystemic involvement. The remainder have a subacute onset, often with the cutaneous eruption preceding the appearance of constitutional symptoms or evidence of myopathy by 3 to 6 months, although occasionally by as long as several years.

The amyopathic form, characterized by typical cutaneous manifestations without clinical or laboratory evidence of myositis, and a hypomyopathic form, with only cutaneous plus laboratory evidence of myositis, are less common in children (5% to 19%)[287] than in adults. Association of these forms with interstitial lung disease (with or without MDA5 autoantibody) has been reported but is unusual. In one study, 75% with clinically amyopathic JDM had anti-TIF1 antibody, 8% had MDA5 antibody, and 17% had no detectable antibody.[288]

The cutaneous features of JDM may be striking or so minor that they might be easily overlooked. A variety of cutaneous findings may be noted (see Box 22.4). Characteristic cutaneous lesions are inflammatory and telangiectatic and are found in 75% of affected children at presentation. A purplish-red erythema on the face and especially the eyelids is called the *heliotrope rash*, because it matches the color of reddish purple flower of the heliotrope plant (Fig. 22.26). Eyelid telangiectasia are found in more than 50% of children and persist longer than other sites of telangiectasia, despite therapy.[289] The telangiectatic, inflammatory eruption of JDM can also be seen on the upper cheeks, forehead, temples, and ears (Fig. 22.27). Sometimes the facial lesions are very edematous, leading to a periorbital and cheek edema. The facial edema and discoloration may be asymmetric, reflecting asymmetric disease activity; JDM has also first manifested in a Blaschkoid facial distribution with later involvement in a generalized distribution.[290] Violaceous, often confluent, telangiectatic erythema with fine scaling may also appear at the hairline of the scalp, nape of the neck, extensor surfaces of the arms and shoulders, elbows and knees, and the shoulder and center of the upper anterior trunk (the shawl sign) (Fig. 22.28). These telangiectatic eruptions are often accentuated when the affected area is dependent (e.g., with lowering the face for facial lesions). The distribution of the eruption and the common sparing of sun-protected areas suggest photosensitivity; UV light exposure is known to trigger both cutaneous and muscle signs.

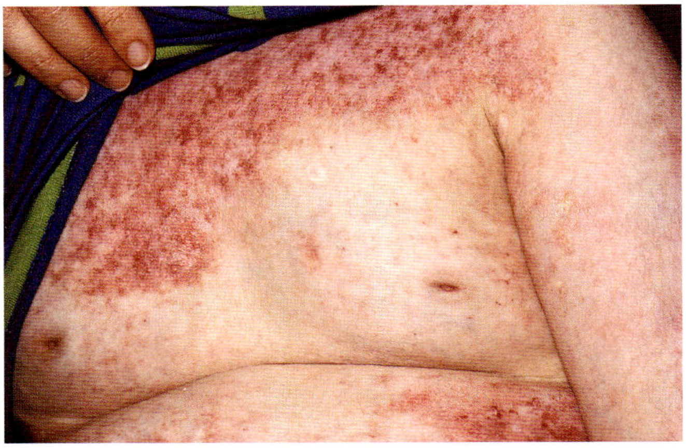

Fig. 22.28 Juvenile dermatomyositis. Telangiectasia and atrophy induced by sun exposure in this young girl, whose relatively uninvolved area was covered by her bathing suit.

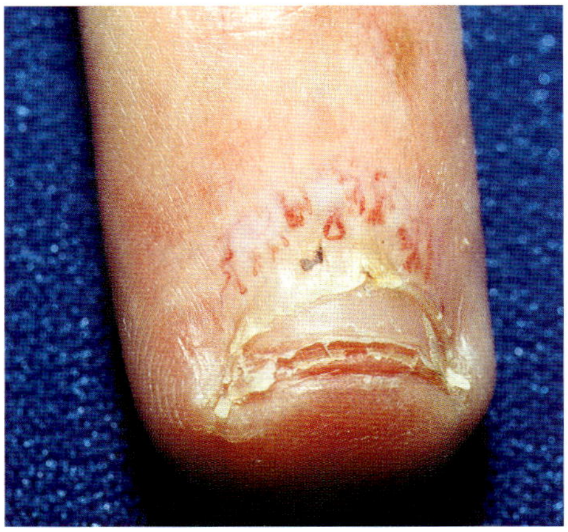

Fig. 22.29 Juvenile dermatomyositis. Periungual telangiectasia with cuticular hypertrophy.

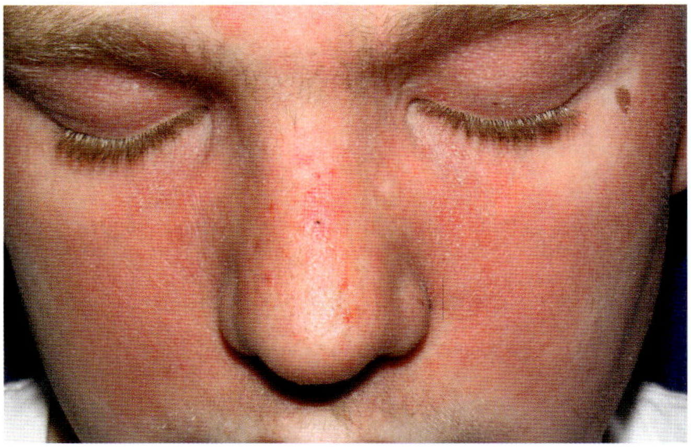

Fig. 22.26 Juvenile dermatomyositis. Telangiectasia and inflammation of the face. Note the sparing of the infraorbital, sun-shielded area.

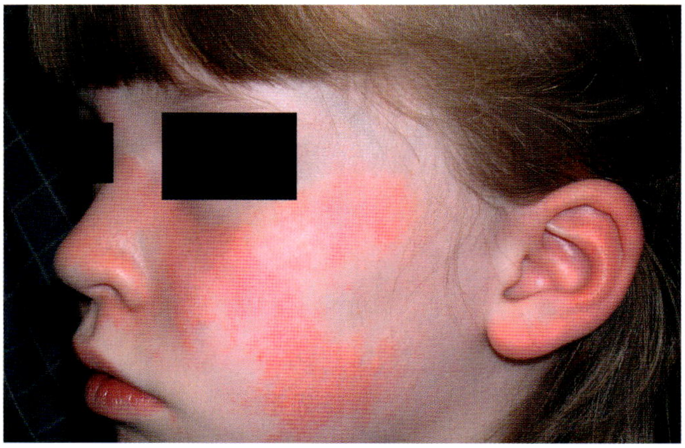

Fig. 22.27 Juvenile dermatomyositis. Facial inflammation and telangiectasia. Note the involvement of the ear.

Periungual telangiectasia (Fig. 22.29) is a characteristic feature of JDM and provides a good indication of cutaneous, rather than muscle, disease activity.[291] Viewing the nailfold area through a dermatoscope, ophthalmoscope, or otoscope to magnify the area after local application of mineral oil improves visualization and is considered important for monitoring cutaneous disease response. Nailfold capillary microscopy has shown that the periungual telangiectasia represents bushy capillary loops adjacent to avascular areas, perhaps a form of compensatory neovascularization. Erythema of the cuticle at the base of the nails commonly accompanies the periungual telangiectasia. At times the cuticles may also be thickened, hyperkeratotic, and irregular, giving an appearance of excessive picking or manicuring.

Pitted ulcerations of the fingertips, pressure points such as the elbows, lateral aspects of the trunk, axillae, genitalia,[292,293] and lateral ocular canthi are usually seen at presentation or with disease flares.[257] Thought to be a marker of severe disease, these ulcers leave residual atrophic scars.

Even though not exposed to sun, the mucous membranes often show telangiectatic involvement, with erythema of the palate and buccal mucosa, with or without ulceration, and telangiectasia of the gum margin (Fig. 22.30).

Telangiectatic erythema may overlie the dorsal interphalangeal joints (Gottron sign) and, when a component of a flat-topped papule,

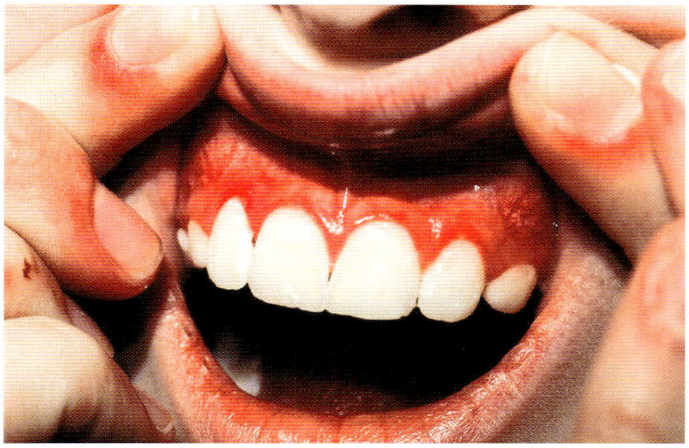

Fig. 22.30 Juvenile dermatomyositis. Telangiectasias of the gingivae are commonly associated. Note the periungual telangiectasia as well.

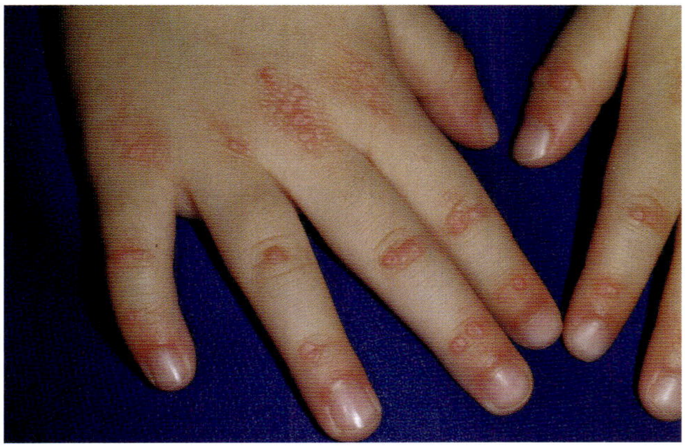

Fig. 22.31 Juvenile dermatomyositis. Gottron papules overlying the joints of the hands. Note the telangiectasia of the periungual areas.

is a pathognomonic sign of JDM (Gottron papule) (Fig. 22.31). Coupled with the facial eruption, these inflammatory lesions on the dorsum of the hand may be misdiagnosed as contact dermatitis. When the papule resolves, atrophy, telangiectasia, and hypopigmentation may persist (Fig. 22.32). Inverse Gottron papules have also been described with papules on the palmar surface (Fig. 22.33) and are associated with interstitial lung disease.[294–296]

Other cutaneous features include palmar erythema and thickening, which can be mistaken for dermatitis and sometimes includes so much hyperkeratosis and fissuring that it has been compared with a mechanic's hand.[297,298] A more generalized hyperkeratotic disorder that resembles pityriasis rubra pilaris and generalized erythroderma with scaling have also been described.[299,300]

Sclerodactyly may be seen in children with overlap syndrome that includes SSc. Panniculitis may manifest clinically as tender, indurated plaques and nodules, especially on the arms, thighs, and buttocks[301]; however, panniculitis is often observed in biopsy specimens and is not noted clinically. Limb edema is noted in some patients at presentation, but anasarca is rare and should prompt consideration of nephritic syndrome.[302]

Several cutaneous features of JDM are seen more commonly with disease chronicity. Many children and adolescents with chronic disease have intensely pruritic, xerotic skin that shows poikiloderma (Fig. 22.34), which is the combination of cutaneous atrophy, telangiectasia, and dyspigmentation (see Chapter 11). The scalp is dry, scaling, and pruritic as well.

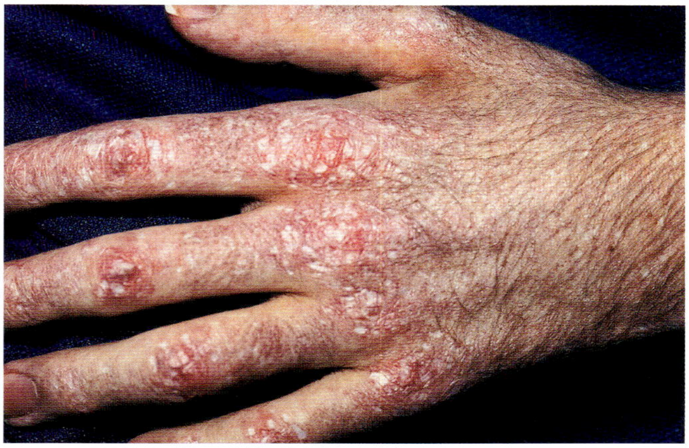

Fig. 22.32 Juvenile dermatomyositis. Atrophy telangiectasia and depigmentation are residual signs after clearance of the Gottron papules in this patient with chronic skin changes.

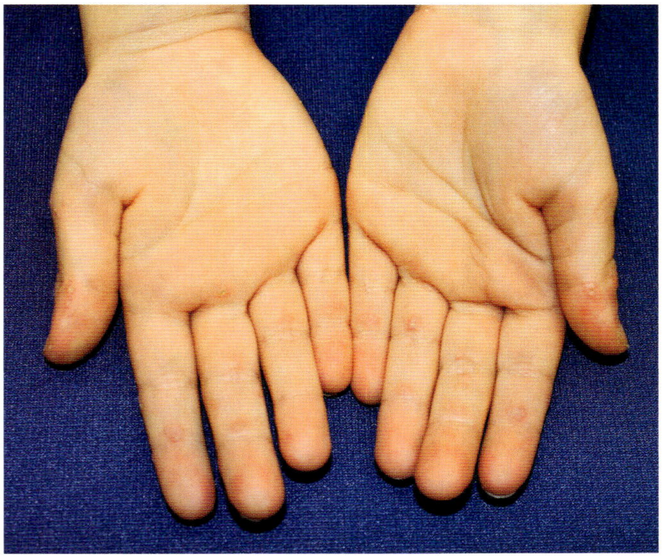

Fig. 22.33 Juvenile dermatomyositis. Inverse Gottron papules are seen on the palmar aspect of the hands and fingers and, less commonly, on the plantar aspect.

Cutaneous calcinosis develops in 18% to 24% of children,[261,303,304] in contrast to the up to 70% incidence of earlier reports. This decreased incidence of calcinosis can be attributed to both earlier diagnosis and to more aggressive, earlier treatment (see later). Nevertheless, calcinosis is a major cause of morbidity in JDM and is linked to younger age at disease onset, more persistent disease activity,[305] and the presence of anti-NXP2 (anti-p140) autoantibodies before the calcinosis develops, which are found overall in 20% of JDM patients.[281] Most commonly seen at sites of trauma, particularly on the buttocks, elbows, knees, and fingers, and around the shoulders, subcutaneous calcium deposits may produce local pain and can be extruded, leading to ulcers, sinuses, or cellulitis (Fig. 22.35). Ulcerations may also appear in children with dermatomyositis without calcifications, especially over joints (Fig. 22.36). Calcifications (see Chapters 9 and 23) appear as hard, irregular nodules that may drain a whitish, chalky material through their openings to the surface that resembles gritty toothpaste. The mean time to occurrence of calcinosis after onset is 2.5 to 3.4 years, although 3% of patients have calcinosis at diagnosis,[306] even without evidence of myositis. Sometimes patients have

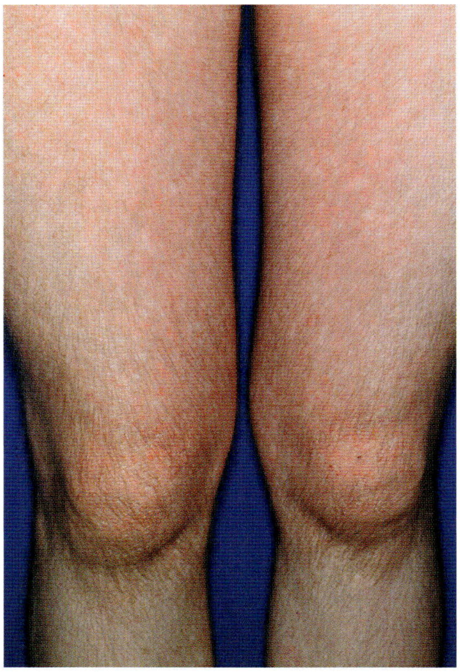

Fig. 22.34 Juvenile dermatomyositis. Poikilodermatous changes on the legs, characterized by telangiectasia, atrophy, and subtle reticulated hyperpigmentation.

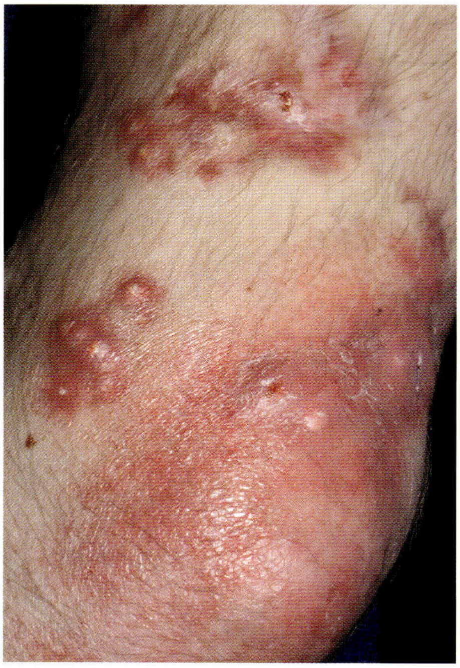

Fig. 22.35 Juvenile dermatomyositis with multiple calcifications. Even small calcifications over a joint may be exquisitely painful.

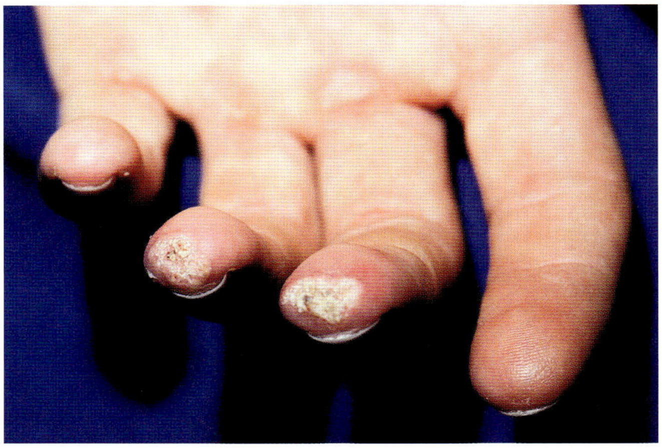

Fig. 22.36 Juvenile dermatomyositis. Note calcinosis on the fingertips.

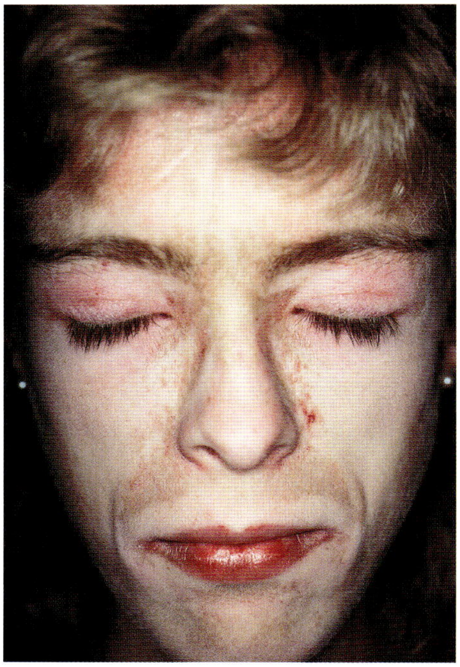

Fig. 22.37 Juvenile dermatomyositis (JDM). Facial lipoatrophy and persistent telangiectasia in an older adolescent. The onset of her JDM was 8 years earlier; although the myositis has been controlled, she had residual disfiguring cutaneous and subcutaneous manifestations with extensive, problematic calcifications.

widespread calcification along fascial planes, encasing muscles (universalis form) or even appearing as an exoskeleton on radiographic examination.

Contractures have been associated with the calcinosis and occur in 17% to 30% of patients with JDM. Lipodystrophy is a common feature in children with chronic disease, especially if poorly controlled and of longer duration, overall occurring in 9.7% of patients[303] (Figs. 22.37 and 22.38). The lipodystrophy may be generalized or partial and is characterized by a slowly progressive symmetric loss. The lipodystrophy is associated with insulin resistance and hyperlipidemia (hypertriglyceridemia and low levels of high-density lipoprotein [HDL]).[307] These cardiac risk factors can be present in patients with chronic disease, even without the lipodystrophy. Acanthosis nigricans has been described in 10% of patients later in the disease course (Fig. 22.39). The insulin resistance correlates with muscle atrophy, proinflammatory circulating cytokines, and a family history of diabetes but not with corticosteroid use.[308]

The myopathy of JDM affects primarily the proximal groups of muscles, especially the triceps and quadriceps, usually in a symmetric distribution. Muscle tenderness or stiffness is not uncommon but usually occurs later in the course rather than as a presenting sign. Affected children often complain of great fatigue and are unable to do

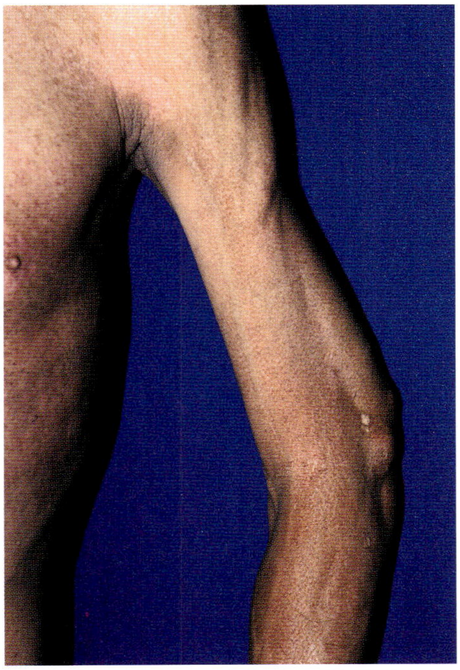

Fig. 22.38 Juvenile dermatomyositis (JDM). Profound lipoatrophy on the limbs of a young adult with a history since elementary school of JDM.

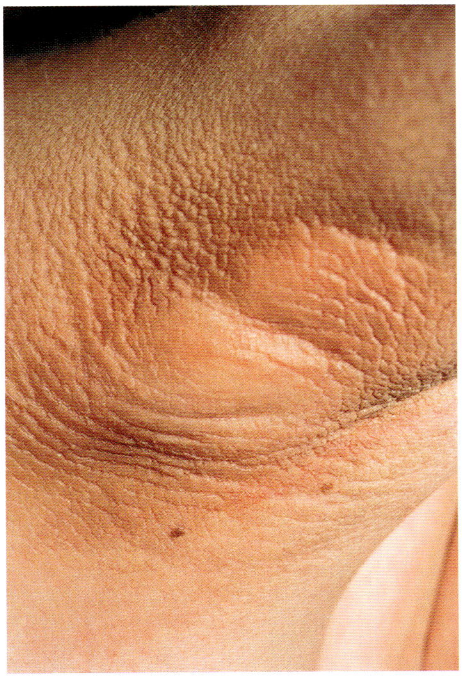

Fig. 22.39 Juvenile dermatomyositis. Acanthosis nigricans of the axillary area.

simple tasks, such as rising, squatting, walking, or reaching. In young children, muscle weakness may manifest as more demanding behavior. Physical therapists may be helpful as assessors of muscle strength, particularly in younger children. Speech may become nasal because of nasopharyngeal muscle weakness, and approximately 10% to 15% of patients complain of difficulty with swallowing.

A nondestructive, generally nondeforming arthritis occurs in approximately half of affected children at some time during the disorder, most commonly an asymptomatic arthritis of the knees; large and small joint polyarthritis has also been described.[306] Vasculopathy of the GI tract may lead to ulceration, perforation, pneumatosis intestinalis, or hemorrhage. D-xylose absorption has been decreased in patients with JDM, suggesting the decreased absorption of nutrients and medications, including oral corticosteroids, and leading to the suggestion that the disorder be treated with intravenous methylprednisolone for acute cases.[309] Dysphagia from impaired muscle function may lead to esophageal reflux and aspiration pneumonia, requiring intravenous feeding. Children with JDM have occasionally been described with hepatomegaly, cholestasis, or pancreatitis.

The majority of patients with JDM show a reduced ventilatory capacity without respiratory complaints, probably because of respiratory muscle weakness and poor chest wall compliance. Decreased diffusion capacity and evidence of interstitial lung disease is uncommon but may present with dyspnea on exertion. Cardiac disease is rare in children with JDM and mainly involves murmurs and cardiomegaly. Although pericarditis occurs, conduction defects and acute myocarditis are uncommon but severely damaging. Nevertheless, systolic dysfunction has recently been noted after long-term follow-up study (16.8 years) and is correlated with skin disease scores, not muscle disease activity.[310] Central or peripheral nervous system disease is very rare, in contrast with SLE. Similarly, other than conjunctival vessel tortuosity, eye disease is usually limited to cataracts from administration of systemic corticosteroids. IgA nephropathy has been described, but renal disease is not generally a feature of JDM.[311]

The presence of arthritis, significant dysphagia, renal disease, Raynaud phenomenon, or neuropathy should also prompt consideration of evaluation for overlap disease. Up to 10% of children with JDM show an overlap syndrome with features of SLE, SSc, or JIA.

The diagnosis of JDM is suspected on clinical grounds, based on the typical cutaneous manifestations and evidence of muscle weakness and/or tenderness. Increased levels of muscle enzymes and the demonstration of increased signal intensity on fat-suppressed T2-weighted magnetic resonance imaging (MRI) scans[312] provide evidence of muscle inflammation,[304] and whole-body MRIs have been advocated to estimate total inflammatory burden.[313] The increased signal intensity on MRI scans relates to accumulated extracellular water content. It is indistinguishable from other inflammatory myopathies or rhabdomyolysis but can be differentiated from muscular dystrophies. Several enzyme levels should be assessed concomitantly (serum aldolase, aspartate aminotransferase, lactic dehydrogenase, and serum creatine phosphokinase levels); aldolase is most commonly elevated and serum creatine phosphokinase is normal in about 35% of affected children with active disease.[304] Muscle biopsy of a site shown to be affected by clinical examination or MRI testing can be performed to confirm the presence of perifascicular and perivascular lymphocytic infiltration with atrophy, necrosis, and late fibrosis of the muscle fibers. Skin biopsy is usually not valuable in JDM.

Of JDM patients observed into adulthood (median time from diagnosis, 16.8 years), 90% of patients had persistent damage. This included damage to the skin (77%), muscle (65%), and skeletal (57%) systems.[314] Monitoring disease activity (versus inactivity) has been achieved through use of tools such as the Myositis Disease Activity Assessment Tool (MDAAT)[315,316] and, specifically for skin, the Cutaneous Dermatomyositis Disease Area and Severity Index (CDASI) and Cutaneous Assessment Tool-Binary Method (CAT-BM), which have been validated for use in JDM by pediatric dermatologists and rheumatologists.[317] These tools have allowed classification of the course of JDM. However, data are somewhat variable. In general, 50% to 73% of patients have continuing disease activity after a mean follow-up of 16.8 years, most commonly in the skin (59%).[318] In one study, this was further divided into the disease being monophasic (lasting remission within 1 or 2 years) in 37% to 47%, polyphasic in 3% to 18%, and chronic in 35% to -60%.[304,319] In contrast, a 20-year retrospective analysis found that 71% achieved a complete clinical response, but 73% of these subsequently had at least one flare despite intensive therapy.

Regardless of the variability in data regarding course, it is clear that inadequate treatment is a strong predictor of poor outcome.[289] A shorter duration of untreated disease and a lower JDM skin disease activity score at onset of disease are correlated with a monocyclic course.[291] The presence of persistent skin eruptions (especially Gottron papules) 3 months after initiation of treatment also predicts a longer time to remission, and if Gottron papules and nailfold capillaroscopy are both abnormal at 6 months after initiation, the outcome is particularly poor.[319] Organ damage 6 months after onset of treatment is also a predictor for poor prognosis.[314] By 36 weeks, persistent nailfold capillary changes, which correlate with skin disease rather than muscle disease, also predict a nonmonocyclic disease.[291]

During the active phase of dermatomyositis, children are particularly at risk for sepsis, sometimes masked by corticosteroids. Hospitalization may be advisable in the acute stage, especially if the disease involves palatal-respiratory muscles, to prevent aspiration and to ensure adequate respiration, including by feeding intravenously and using mechanical ventilation if necessary. Nevertheless, the mortality rate, formerly about 30% generally because of these complications and visceral perforation, has been markedly reduced by more aggressive intervention and most recently was found to be 3% to 5%.[261,288,303]

Most JDM is treated with high-dosage corticosteroid therapy, and many specialists now initiate pulsed intravenous steroids (30 mg/kg or up to 1.5 g), administered every 24 to 48 hours until laboratory values normalize.[320,321] Evidence-based algorithms for treatment have been proposed by several groups, including for tapering use of steroids. For example, one suggests three pulses of methylprednisolone and then tapering from 2 mg/kg per day to 1 mg/kg per day during the next 2 months based on reduction by at least 50% of various core set measures, some specific to myositis and some overall well-being, but not skin disease. Dosing is subsequently reduced to 0.2 mg/kg per day during the next 4 months and ultimately discontinued during the subsequent 18 months[322] with further improvement. Usage of pulse steroids, followed by oral corticosteroids or intermittent pulses if needed for continued control, has been shown to decrease the duration of rash, cause less functional impairment, and markedly reduce calcifications compared with those children treated with oral corticosteroids only. Side effects are not increased with pulse steroids, and the overall dosage of required corticosteroids tends to be less than that with oral treatment.

Methotrexate has been used most commonly as a steroid-sparing agent. Treatment of severe JDM early in the course with both intravenous methylprednisolone and methotrexate appears to be more useful than with either agent alone,[323] and patients with milder cases have responded to methotrexate (or intravenous immunoglobulin [IVIG]) alone.[324] Methotrexate can be administered orally or, preferably because of vasculopathic reduced intestinal absorption, by subcutaneous injection at a dosage of 1 mg/kg per week with a maximum of 40 mg/week. In a randomized trial, prednisone plus methotrexate led to better treatment responses in 6 months than prednisone alone or prednisone with cyclosporine; side effects were seen most often with steroid plus cyclosporine and infections were seen more often with either combination (including prednisone and methotrexate) than steroid alone.[325]

Intravenous γ-globulin has also been found to be an effective steroid-sparing agent, especially for cutaneous and pulmonary manifestations.[326,327] Mycophenolate mofetil is another option[328] and JAK inhibitors have been found useful in cases of adult dermatomyositis.[329] Other cytotoxic agents such as azathioprine in dosages of 1 to 3 mg/kg (up to 200 mg/day) or cyclosporine (5 mg/kg per day) may be used in severe life-threatening forms of dermatomyositis, or when the disease cannot be adequately managed with prednisone alone.

Biologic treatments, particularly rituximab, have shown promise.[330] Rituximab has been generally well tolerated, with infections and infusion reactions as the main adverse events. Although the onset of action can be slow, the response is good, including with more than one course.[259,331,332] TNF-α has been implicated in the pathogenesis and severity of JDM, and some patients have shown benefit, especially with administration of infliximab[333] and adalimumab[334]; however, other patients have not responded, particularly with etanercept, or have even worsened on a TNF-α antagonist. Abatacept and tocilizumab are other biologics that have been used by pediatric rheumatologists.[330] Disease that is refractory to immunosuppressants, including rituximab, can be treated with plasma exchange or autologous stem cell transplantation.[335,336]

The response of the cutaneous features of JDM to treatment may not correlate with the response of muscle[289]; skin manifestations may persist for years despite resolution of other signs of disease. Oral antimalarial agents, especially hydroxychloroquine (generally 5 to 6.5 mg/kg per day), are claimed to be helpful in controlling the cutaneous manifestations of JDM, but a recent paper showed no significant improvement from hydroxychloroquine specifically for skin disease activity.[289] Topical corticosteroids and calcineurin inhibitors do little to reverse the skin signs of JDM, although they may help with pruritus (e.g., topical fluocinolone 0.01% in oil for chronic scalp involvement). Counseling about sun protection is critical (see discussion for SLE).

The problematic calcinoses may gradually disappear but may be quite persistent and can cause considerable morbidity. Despite the long list of medications that have been used successfully in anecdotal reports in an effort to hasten clearance, no agent has been helpful in the majority of cases. Pediatric rheumatologists often increase systemic immunosuppression as first-line therapy but add targeted therapy for symptomatic patients. Bisphosphonates and IVIG are most often used (in addition to immunosuppression) and considered most successful.[305,337,338] Sodium thiosulfate can help clear calcinoses when given intravenously, orally, or even topically, but it is often poorly tolerated (e.g., oral administration may lead to severe diarrhea).[339] The combination of abatacept and sodium thiosulfate reduced the muscle and ulcerative skin disease activity, as well as calcifications.[340]

Surgical procedures may also be useful in selected situations.[341] Occlusive dressings (such as DuoDerm) over joint areas, particularly when areas are ulcerated and draining, have promoted healing. Physiotherapy is important for patients with or at risk for contractures to prevent deformity and increase muscle strength. MRI evaluations, myometry, and blood studies did not show increased muscle inflammation after exercise, suggesting that a moderate exercise program is acceptable with active myopathy.[342]

Management of amyopathic and hypomyopathic JDM is controversial. Some advocate aggressive management, given that calcinosis, skin ulcers, and muscle weakness may all occur months to years after the onset of cutaneous manifestations and given the known increased risk of calcinosis without early intervention.[288,343,344]

Systemic Sclerosis (Scleroderma)

The incidence of juvenile systemic sclerosis (jSSc) has been reported at 0.27 to 0.50 per million children per year, and fewer than 5% of patients with SSc have their onset before the age of 16 years.[345,346] jSSc has a mean age of onset of 8 years and is very rare before 5 years of age but has been observed in children as young as 5 months old. Disease in younger children has been associated with having the HLA DRB1*10 genotype. On average, it requires 1 to 4 years to make the diagnosis because the onset is often insidious.[347] As in adult-onset SSc, jSSc predominantly affects females (female/male ratio of 2.1 to 10.5:1), including in prepubertal patients.[348–352]

jSSc is classified into three major groups: (1) diffuse cutaneous (dc) SSc, (2) limited cutaneous (lc) SSc, and (3) overlap SSc. dcSSc is characterized by diffuse and rapidly progressive skin thickening of the proximal extremities, chest, or abdomen and skin distal to the elbows, knees, and neck. dcSSc is associated with early organ involvement (GI and lungs, with heart and kidneys to a lesser extent) and with antitopoisomerase (ATA) antibody. lcSSc is less common than dcSSc. It features limited and nonprogressive skin thickening of the distal extremities with prominent vasculopathy (Raynaud phenomenon, pulmonary arterial hypertension, risk of renal crisis), which can occur late; anticentromere antibody (ACA) is associated. Overlap SSc is much more common in children than in adults and includes dcSSc or lcSSc in association with another connective tissue disease, such as SLE, JDM,[353] Sjögren syndrome, or inflammatory arthritis.[354,355] Other scleroderma-like disorders include chronic graft-versus-host disease (see Chapter 25), eosinophilic fasciitis, scleroderma from toxins, nephrogenic systemic fibrosis, and sclerodermatous plaques in progeria, Werner syndrome (Chapter 6), and phenylketonuria (Chapter 24). In the neonate, stiff skin syndrome (Chapter 6) can be confused with SSc.

Box 22.6 Criteria for Diagnosis of Juvenile Systemic Sclerosis

Must be younger than 16 years at onset.

Major Criterion (Required)

Skin induration/thickening proximal to the MCP or MTP joints

Minor Criteria (Two Required) (Scleroderma-Specific Organ Involvement)

Cutaneous
- Sclerodactyly

Peripheral vascular
- Digital-tip ulcers
- Nailfold capillary changes (megacapillaries and avascular areas)
- Raynaud phenomenon

Gastrointestinal
- Dysphasia
- Gastroesophageal reflux

Cardiac
- Arrhythmias
- Cardiac failure

Renal
- Scleroderma renal crisis
- New arterial hypertension

Respiratory
- Decreased DLCO
- Pulmonary arterial hypertension (echocardiography; primary or secondary to interstitial lung disease)
- Pulmonary fibrosis (chest radiograph or high-resolution CT)

Neurologic
- Neuropathy
- Carpal tunnel syndrome

Musculoskeletal
- Tendon friction rubs
- Arthritis
- Myositis

Serologic
- Antinuclear antibody
- SSc-selective autoantibodies (antitopoisomerase 1 [Scl-70], anticentromere, anti-RNA polymerase I or III, anti-PM-Scl, antifibrillarin (U3-RNP), antifibrillin)

CT, Computed tomography; *DLCO*, diffusing capacity for carbon monoxide; *MCP*, metacarpophalangeal; *MTP*, metatarsophalangeal; *RNA*, ribonucleic acid; *SSc*, systemic sclerosis.

Major and minor criteria for jSSc[356] are shown in Box 22.6, with symmetric proximal skin sclerosis/induration being the major criterion for diagnosis. This classification distinguishes jSSc from overlap disease, which occurs more common in children than in adults (29% versus 9%).[357] dcSSc occurs in 90% to 100% of patients with jSSc. The organs involved (lung, kidney, joint, muscle, and heart) are similar in children and adults with SSc.[358] Compared with adults, jSSc has less visceral involvement but a greater prevalence of arthritis and myositis.[359] Some children have a rapidly progressive and fatal illness with cardiac involvement, but more commonly children have a chronic course with less overall mortality.[360]

Most often, the onset is insidious with Raynaud phenomenon the presenting sign (together with abnormal nailfold capillaries and elevated ANA titers). The Raynaud phenomenon is seen in 70% at onset and ultimately in virtually all affected children (Fig. 22.40). The condition may occur in children as young as 1 year of age. In jSSc, Raynaud phenomenon is associated with vascular intimal hyperplasia and fibrosis that manifests as dilated, sausage-shaped capillary loops and avascular areas (capillary dropout) that are not seen in patients with isolated Raynaud disease, acrocyanosis, or morphea. As in SLE and JDM, capillary microscopy of the nailfolds can be performed with an ophthalmoscope, otoscope, or dermatoscope and changes can be intensified by mineral oil placed on the nailfold area. The capillary changes are indistinguishable from those of patients with JDM, distinct from those of SLE. Raynaud phenomenon is precipitated by cold or emotional stress, and is characterized by pallor, cyanosis, and hyperemia with pain, burning, numbness, tingling, swelling, and hyperhidrosis of the affected fingers or toes. Rarely, Raynaud phenomenon

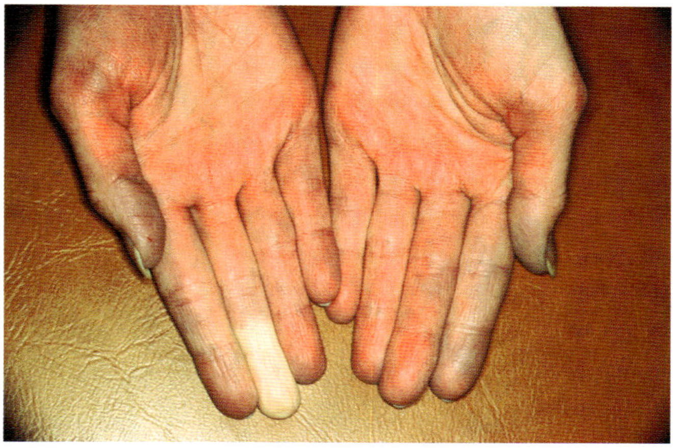

Fig. 22.40 Raynaud phenomenon. Note the blue discoloration of the thumbs and fingers with the sharply demarcated white coloration of the distal aspect of the third finger.

affects the nose, lips, cheeks, or ears. Nail changes in which the distal portion of the nailbeds adheres to the ventral surface of the nail plate and obliterates the space that normally separates these two structures have also been described. Digital pits or ischemic ulcers also reflect vascular insufficiency and affect 10% to 28% of children. Calcinosis is seen in up to 18%.

Overall, 69% of children with Raynaud phenomenon have primary disease (without an underlying collagen vascular disease).[361] In both primary and secondary forms of Raynaud phenomenon, girls predominate (80%). The age of onset, presence of livedo reticularis, and presence of aPL antibody cannot distinguish secondary from primary disease, but a positive ANA test and abnormal capillary pattern correlate strongly with the presence of an underlying disease[361]; as a result, the consensus of a group of European scleroderma experts was to test ANA, more specific antibodies for connective tissue disease, and nailfold capillaroscopy in all children with Raynaud phenomenon.[362] Primary Raynaud phenomenon is also not associated with digital tip pitting and ulceration. Raynaud phenomenon must be differentiated from acrocyanosis, which is common in thin adolescent girls as a purplish discoloration. The discoloration of acrocyanosis tends to affect the toes more than the fingers, to be mottled, and to largely persist with warming. Nailfold capillary changes are absent in acrocyanosis, but distal pulses may be faint. Raynaud phenomenon must also be distinguished from blue toe syndrome induced by mixed amphetamine salts, thought to be a reversible vasoconstrictive phenomenon.[363]

At onset, 60% of children have the characteristic early edema; although sometimes present at onset, skin tightening and eventually atrophy develop over months to years. The hands become shiny, with tapered fingertips and, ultimately, restricted movements as the tendons become shortened. Rarely, the more proximal extremities, trunk, or face are involved at onset. With time, however, the face may develop a characteristic appearance. The forehead becomes smooth and cannot be wrinkled, and atrophy and tightening of the skin give a characteristic appearance because of a fixed stare, pinched nose, prominent teeth, pursed lips, reduced oral aperture, and a perpetual grimace-like facies (Fig. 22.41). The smoothness of skin may also reflect loss of adnexal structures. Skin thickness is scored serially (modified Rodnan score), leading to a skin thickness progression rate. Calcification (Fig. 22.42), ulceration (Fig. 22.43), dyspigmentation, and telangiectasia may also be seen with chronic disease. The pigmentary changes in jSSc may be homogeneously hypopigmented or hyperpigmented, or may have a "salt and pepper"–like appearance because of retained perifollicular hyperpigmentation in areas of hypopigmentation (Fig. 22.44).

Early scleroderma is often associated with arthralgias and limited joint mobility. Patients may complain initially of weight loss, fatigue, GI symptoms, and exertional dyspnea. Muscle weakness is seen in up

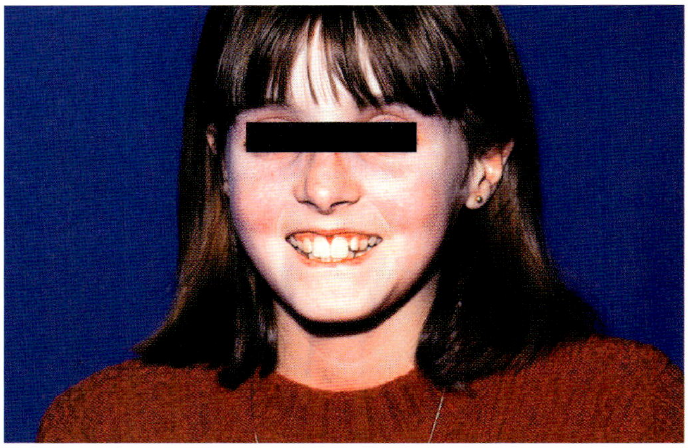

Fig. 22.41 Systemic scleroderma. Smooth atrophic skin, pinched nose, and fixed grimace are evident on the face of this adolescent.

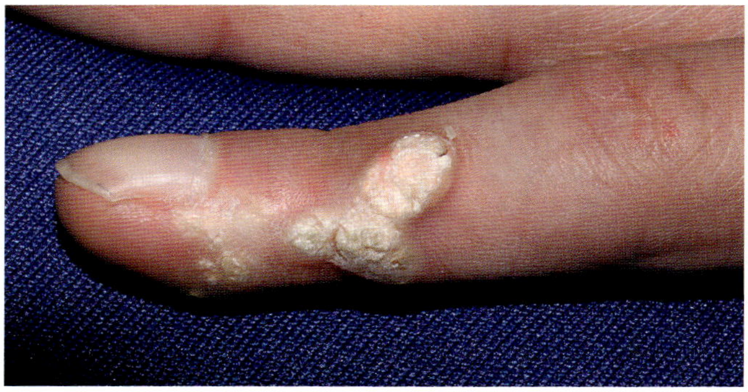

Fig. 22.42 Systemic scleroderma. Calcinosis on the finger. Note the tightness of the skin.

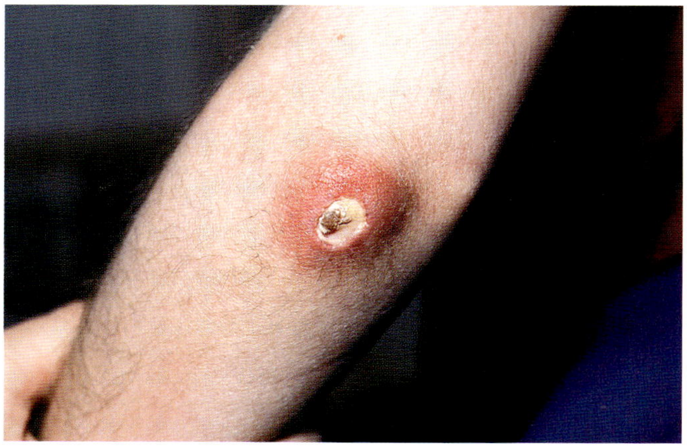

Fig. 22.43 Systemic scleroderma. Ulceration overlying a joint.

to 40% of children and often is associated with evidence of myositis (overlap syndrome). Arthritis and muscle inflammation in association are seen more commonly in children than in adults because of the higher prevalence of overlap syndromes.

Overall, GI manifestations have been described in up to 75% of children and have the greatest impact on quality of life.[364] In addition to the acid reflux[365] and decreased esophageal motility, patients have reported constipation, bloating, discomfort, regurgitation, weight loss, and malabsorption. Children are often asymptomatic, however, despite esophageal disease.

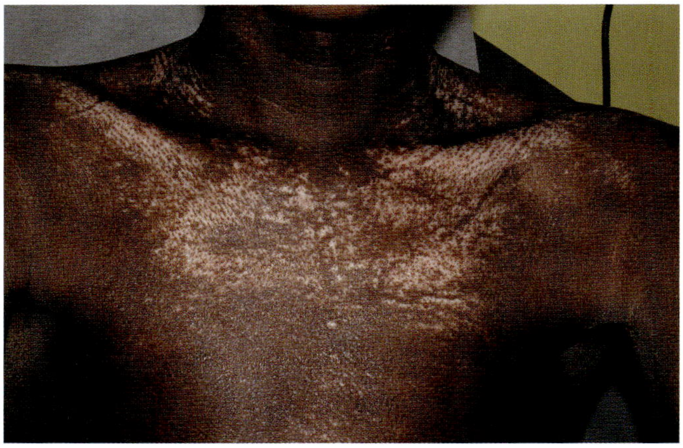

Fig. 22.44 Systemic scleroderma. Speckled depigmentation on the upper chest in this boy with systemic scleroderma.

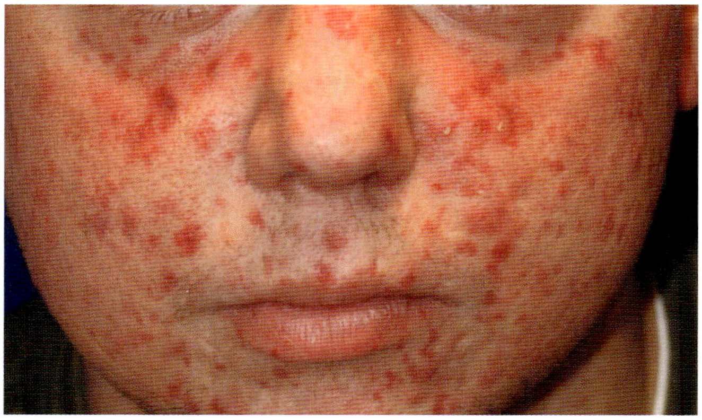

Fig. 22.45 Calcinosis, Raynaud, esophageal dysmotility, sclerodactyly, and telangiectasia (CREST) syndrome. Telangiectatic mats on the face. This adolescent boy had numerous calcifications, especially on the fingertips; Raynaud phenomenon; esophageal dysmotility; and sclerodactyly. He had an overlap syndrome with polymyositis.

Cardiac and pulmonary abnormalities are usually screened by chest radiograph, pulmonary function tests, and echocardiogram. Pulmonary function testing usually shows restrictive lung disease (54% of children), even if clinically silent.[366] High-resolution CT scanning can capture the early alveolitis that precedes pulmonary fibrosis. Pulmonary function testing reveals the decrease in forced air capacity and diffusing capacity for carbon monoxide that are particularly concerning.[367] Cardiac disease (occurring in 8% at onset but 24% during the course) is the major cause of pediatric mortality. It may be secondary to pulmonary hypertension (very uncommon) or may be primary (pericarditis, arrhythmia, cardiac failure). Severe cardiomyopathy has been described in children with SSc/myositis overlap.[368] Up to 60% of children have shown evidence of renal involvement, usually the result of renal vasculopathy and during the first 3 years of diffuse scleroderma. However, fewer than 5% develop renal failure and 0.7% experience scleroderma renal crisis (much less often than in adults). Regular monitoring of blood pressure is critical to identify rapid progression and hypertensive renal crisis. CNS involvement affects only 3% of affected children.

CREST syndrome (Fig. 22.45), a form of lcSSc, is quite rare in children. Patients generally have a more slowly progressive form of the disease and have anticentromere antibodies. Although some patients with the CREST syndrome may develop severe pulmonary hypertension, more extensive cutaneous lesions, and visceral involvement, the patients with this subset generally tend to have a relatively benign course.

The diagnosis of SSc is easily established when cutaneous sclerosis of the face and hands is present, particularly when it is associated with Raynaud phenomenon, nailfold telangiectasia, and visceral involvement. Laser Doppler imaging can help visualize the microvascular abnormalities.[369] Symptoms or signs of dysphagia or gastroesophageal reflux help confirm the diagnosis. A severity score (J4S) grades general, vascular, skin, osteoarticular, muscle, GI, respiratory, cardiac, and renal features as normal (0) to end stage (5).[370,371]

The presence of autoantibodies correlates with disease subset. Antitopoisomerase antibody (Scl70) is found in 20% to 46% of children and predicts rapid skin disease progression and interstitial lung disease, but not poorer survival in children. In contrast, ACA is found in only 2% to 16% of patients (versus 20% to 30% of adults) and is associated with lcSSc and pulmonary arterial hypertension. Anti–U1 RNP and PM-Scl antibodies are also each detected in about 15% of children and often described with overlap syndromes and in association with myositis and arthritis. RNA polymerase III (POL3) antibody, which portends the risk for scleroderma renal crisis, is rare in children but is found in up to 30% of adult-onset SSc. Most children with SSc have ANAs (78% to 97%), often of the speckled or nucleolar configuration; about 20% to 23% of children with SSc have a positive ANA test with a scleroderma-related autoantibody.

The 10-year survival rate for jSSc is 98%, considerably better than in adults with SSc (75%).[348,356,372] Most deaths result from cardiac (most common), pulmonary, or renal disease. Treatment of SSc in children is challenging and similar to that in adults. Early treatment before the occurrence of the irreversible fibrotic damage to tissue is ideal. General measures include avoidance of factors producing vasospasm (tension, fatigue, stress, cold weather, and smoking in adolescents) and minimizing trauma to the hands. Heated gloves are available, and emollients and dressings can be applied to ulcerated cutaneous sites. Calcium channel blockers such as nifedipine or nicardipine, which reduce smooth muscle contraction by reducing the uptake of calcium, are considered first-line therapy for Raynaud phenomenon. For those with an inadequate response, phosphodiesterase 5 inhibitors (sildenafil, tadalafil) are the next choice to improve[372] blood flow and reduce the severity of Raynaud phenomenon and digital ulcers. The endothelin receptor antagonist bosentan and nitropaste are other options. Intravenous infusion of iloprost or other prostanoids are used for severe jSSc at risk for digital infarct. Physiotherapy is important to limit contractures.

The arthritis may respond to NSAIDs or salicylates. Proton pump inhibitors (e.g., omeprazole and lansoprazole) are the treatment of choice for reflux esophagitis. General measures for treating reflux include elevating the head of the bed, staying upright after eating, a bland diet, and restricting the size of meals. Prokinetic drugs such as domperidone may improve motility, and antibiotics administered in rotation may decrease the risk of malabsorption from bacterial overgrowth. Intravenous pulse cyclophosphamide therapy has been recommended at a dosage of 0.5 to 1 g/m^2 every 4 weeks for at least 6 months for interstitial lung disease. Good hydration and frequent voiding are important to decrease the risk of cystitis. Endothelin receptor antagonists or phosphodiesterase 5 inhibitors, followed by intravenous infusions of prostacyclin analogues, have been used for the pulmonary artery hypertension.[373] Oxygen, antibiotics, and diuretics may also be required for lung disease, especially with congestive heart failure.

Immunosuppression with methotrexate or mycophenolate mofetil has been shown to improve the skin manifestations and has been particularly useful for children with overlap disorders. Corticosteroids do not appear to help the sclerodermatous process and may trigger renal crisis; however, systemic steroids may be used with caution to treat severe disabling arthritis or myositis. ACE inhibitors such as losartan and captopril are critical in controlling hypertension and stabilizing renal function. The renal disease may require dialysis. Several children who have not responded to other therapies have been treated with autologous stem cells with improvement in clinical signs and stabilization of pulmonary function.[374,375] Bosentan has been helpful for pulmonary hypertension in jSSc[376] and, in adults with SSc, for promotion of healing of cutaneous ulcerations.[377]

jSSc features pathologic thickening and tethering of skin, as well as visceral fibrosis and small vessel vasculopathy. Its pathogenesis involves alterations in the immune system,[378] vasculature, and connective tissue. Early disease has been associated with activation of macrophages and T helper (Th) 1/Th17 inflammatory pathways, whereas the late fibrotic disease has been associated with Th2 axis activation and improving T-regulatory (Treg) cell function. The cytokine imbalances stimulate fibroblasts and endothelial cells to produce cytokine mediators, such as transforming growth factor-β (TGF-β), platelet-derived growth factor (PDGF), and connective tissue growth factor (CTGF), which induce fibroblast activation and differentiation to myofibroblasts,[379] triggering collagen synthesis. An imbalance between matrix metalloproteinases (MMPs) and tissue inhibitors of MMPs may also play a role. Also of major importance are the presence of autoantibodies and the vasospastic phenomena with endothelial damage that precede digital, pulmonary, and renal fibrosis. Imatinib, which targets TGF-β/Smad[380] and PDGF[381] signaling, has shown some benefit. Support groups for patients with scleroderma are the Scleroderma Foundation (www.scleroderma.org), the Scleroderma Society (www.sclerodermasociety.co.uk), and Scleroderma Canada (www.scleroderma.ca).

Eosinophilic Fasciitis

Eosinophilic fasciitis (diffuse fasciitis with eosinophilia) is a sclerodermatous disease characterized by diffuse infiltration of the skin of the extremities, and less often the trunk, without visceral involvement or Raynaud phenomenon (Box 22.7).[382–384] Seen rarely in children, eosinophilic fasciitis occasionally evolves into generalized or localized morphea,[385–389] suggesting that the disorder is a deep variant within the spectrum of severe morphea.[390] In contrast to adults with eosinophilic fasciitis, the childhood form has a better prognosis; has a female predominance, more muscle involvement, and common involvement of the hands with painless contractures and sclerosis; and is associated with arthritis in only 25% of cases (versus 44% of adults).[391] The hematologic abnormalities that have been noted in adults (aplastic anemia, thrombocytopenic purpura) have not been described in children. However, renal involvement, especially IgA nephropathy, has been noted.

The disorder is characterized by a sudden onset of usually painful swelling, induration, and scleroderma-like changes of the skin with marked thickening of the subcutaneous fascia (Fig. 22.46). The skin

Box 22.7 Eosinophilic Fasciitis

- Scleroderma-like disease without Raynaud phenomenon or visceral involvement
- Painful swelling and induration of skin and subcutaneous tissue
- Usually acute onset after trauma, stress, or strenuous physical activity
- Cobblestone or puckered appearance; may resemble scleroderma later
- Eosinophilia and hypergammaglobulinemia common; occasional elevation in antinuclear antibodies or aldolase
- Usually good initial response to systemic corticosteroids

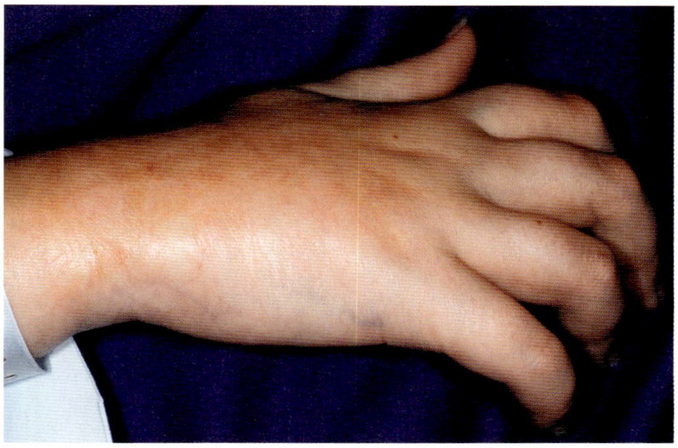

Fig. 22.46 Eosinophilic fasciitis. This girl has swelling, induration, and cobblestoning of the skin of the arms, hands, legs, and feet. Although many respond to systemic steroids, this girl required several other systemic immunosuppressants for response.

tends to have a cobblestone or puckered appearance and often has a yellowish or erythematous color. It is indurated, taut, and bound down without pigmentary change; the "groove sign," in which a vein is depressed, is seen in up to 50% of patients and is a clue to diagnosis, reflecting the depth of involved fascia. The hands, forearms, feet, and legs are most commonly affected initially, although the disease may progress to the trunk and face. When painless (which is unusual), the disorder has been mistaken for angioedema.[392] Although disease onset has been linked to trauma or excessive physical exertion, more recent studies have downplayed this potential association. Although systemic changes are usually absent in affected children, patients show peripheral eosinophilia early in the disease, hypergammaglobulinemia, and an elevated sedimentation rate. The ANA test may be positive during the course but is usually negative, especially at onset. A deep biopsy to include fascia may be necessary to confirm the diagnosis, but MRI is also helpful in demonstrating the depth of the inflammatory involvement. Sections show edema and infiltration of the lower subcutis and deep fascia by lymphocytes, plasma cells, and histiocytes. Eosinophils are often (but not always) detected, especially in early lesions; thick, sclerotic dermis is characteristically seen late in the disorder.

Patients usually have a good initial response to oral or pulse intravenous systemic corticosteroids, sometimes in combination with methotrexate, with resolution of soft tissue induration and correction of laboratory abnormalities.[393] High-dose intravenous pulse methotrexate has been administrated to affected adults (4 mg/kg monthly for 5 months) with significant resultant improvement 5 months after initiation.[394] Sirolimus has also been helpful for an affected adult.[395]

The majority of affected children experience gradual progression during 1 or more years to cutaneous fibrosis or painless flexion contractures, especially of the hands and feet.[385] Younger age at onset (younger than 7 years of age) and greater disease severity have been correlated with a higher risk of progression to residual fibrosis. Physiotherapy is important adjunctive therapy. In children who do not respond to systemic corticosteroids, other broadly immunosuppressive medications, IVIG,[396] dapsone,[397] infliximab,[392,398] rituximab,[399,400] retinoids, and UVA1 irradiation[390,401] may be considered.

Eosinophilic fasciitis must be distinguished from eosinophilia-myalgia syndrome, which has rarely been described in children and results from oral ingestion of contaminated L-tryptophan.[402] These patients show pronounced eosinophilia with myalgias, especially centrally, and vasculitis of the skin and other organs. The associated myopathy and sometimes elevated muscle enzymes can lead to confusion with an overlap autoimmune syndrome (of scleroderma and dermatomyositis).[393,403] Cutaneous lymphoma and hypereosinophilia syndrome must also be considered.

Nephrogenic Systemic Fibrosis

Nephrogenic systemic fibrosis (NSF; previously known as *nephrogenic fibrosing dermopathy*) has increasingly been recognized as a sclerosing disorder predominantly seen in patients with renal dysfunction who receive gadolinium-based contrast media as part of MRI testing. Although NSF was first described in 2000,[404] the first pediatric cases were reported in 2003[405]; in total, 23 pediatric cases have been described.[406] The signs of NSF may develop 2 to 75 days after exposure to the gadolinium.[407] Lesions are characterized by indurated papules and plaques, brawny thickening of skin with a *peau d'orange* appearance, and sometimes joint contractures. The extremities, buttocks, and trunk are usually involved, and the face is typically spared. Patients usually complain of associated pruritus, burning, and pain. Biopsy sections of skin show widened septae in with subcutaneous tissue with increased collagen and fibroblasts. Calcinosis cutis and perforating collagenosis may be seen concomitantly in biopsy sections. The disorder must be distinguished from scleroderma, scleromyxedema, and scleredema. The FDA warns against the use of all gadolinium agents in patients with glomerular filtration rates (GFRs) less than 30 mL/min, and the European guidelines specify a GFR of 30 to 60 mL/min.[408] The most successful treatment is renal transplantation or recovery of the acute renal injury to improve renal function.[409]

Scleredema

Scleredema (scleredema adultorum of Buschke) is a rare disorder of diffuse large areas of induration of skin that must be distinguished from scleroderma.[410,411] The condition most commonly occurs in adults with diabetes, but 29% of described cases are in children, half of these during the first decade of life.[412,413] Although scleredema may begin spontaneously, 65% to 95% of patients have the onset of their disorder within a few days to 10 weeks after an acute febrile illness. Of these, 58% of the infections are streptococcal; scleredema may also follow infections from influenza, measles, mumps, and varicella.[414,415]

The skin changes usually begin suddenly on the neck and then gradually spread to the upper trunk, and occasionally the arms and face, as nonpitting thickening. The abdomen and lower extremities, if involved, tend to show less thickening than the upper half of the body. The texture of skin has been described as brawny or woody, and children with facial involvement may show a mask-like facies. Although affected individuals are usually asymptomatic, some patients display a prodromal period with fever, malaise, and myalgias. In general, the condition is benign, although involvement of the skeletal and cardiac muscles has been reported. Tachycardia, arrhythmias, and pericardial effusions have been noted.[416] In addition, the tongue has been involved, making protrusion and mastication difficult. The thickening results from deposition of acid mucopolysaccharide, largely hyaluronic acid, which can easily be detected with colloidal iron or Alcian blue stains of lesional biopsies. The mechanism by which infection triggers scleredema in children is unclear. Therapy is generally unsuccessful, although high-dosage intravenous corticosteroids may have been helpful in one affected child.[417] Lesions usually resolve spontaneously within months to 2 years. Scleredema has rarely been described in a generalized form in sick neonates (sclerema neonatorum) and must be distinguished from subcutaneous fat necrosis of the newborn in this age group (see Chapter 2).

Morphea

Morphea is an autoimmune disorder characterized by localized areas of cutaneous sclerosis.[354,355,418–422] Although sometimes called *localized scleroderma*, use of the term *morphea* decreases the potential confusion with SSc, or scleroderma, a disorder with significantly greater morbidity that shares similar pathogenic features of immune activation and increased collagen production.[391,423,424] The presence of sclerodactyly or Raynaud phenomenon should alert the physician to consider the possibility of a systemic form of scleroderma, rather than morphea.

Morphea has been divided into five subgroups based on pattern and lesional depth: circumscribed, linear, generalized, mixed, and pansclerotic (Padua criteria[425]) (Box 22.8). In children, linear morphea (or linear scleroderma) is most common (42% to 65%), followed by the relatively localized circumscribed type (26% to 37%); in contrast, the

Box 22.8 Subsets of Morphea (Localized Scleroderma)

- Circumscribed morphea (round and oval lesions)
  - Plaque-type morphea
  - Guttate morphea
  - Atrophoderma of Pasini and Pierini
  - Lichen sclerosus–like
- Deep morphea (subcutaneous)
- Linear morphea/linear scleroderma (can be deep to muscle and bone)
  - *En coup de sabre*
  - Progressive hemifacial atrophy (Parry–Romberg)
- Generalized morphea (more than plaques, each >3 cm in diameter, involving at least two of seven anatomic areas: head/neck, right and left upper extremities, right and left lower extremities, anterior and posterior trunk)
- Mixed morphea (combination of two or more subtypes)
  - Pansclerotic morphea (circumferential limb involvement to all depths of skin, including muscle and bone)

circumscribed type of morphea is the most common form (60%) in adults.[426–428] Circumscribed morphea now includes deep morphea forms (morphea profunda, subcutaneous morphea). The development of bullae within lesions is very rare. Linear scleroderma includes the *en coup de sabre* and Parry–Romberg syndrome forms, in which facial involvement occurs. Morphea can be more extensive in distribution (generalized morphea, 7% to 11%) or depth (disabling pansclerotic morphea, extending from the dermis to the bone). Patients may show more than one type concurrently, most commonly linear and circumscribed types (mixed type, 8% to 15%).

The incidence of morphea is 0.4 to 1 in 100,000 individuals, occurring more often in White than other racial groups.[426,427] In children, morphea occurs at least 10 times more often than SSc.[366] The disorder occurs primarily in children and young adults with a 2 to 3:1 female-to-male ratio. The mean age in children is 5.2 to 8.2 years of age,[426,428,429] but morphea has been described in infants and even neonates. A family history of rheumatic or autoimmune disorders is reported in the first- or second-degree relatives of 12% to 24% of children, but only 2% of relatives have morphea. Of individuals with childhood-onset morphea, 5% developed a concomitant autoimmune disorder, including skin-localized disorders (psoriasis, alopecia areata, vitiligo).[427]

The unilateral nature of the disorder in most patients and the patterning of lesions have led investigators to hypothesize that affected patients have genetically susceptible cells in this distribution that are triggered by environmental exposure to develop morphea. Some patterns of morphea seem to follow lines of Blaschko, but others are clearly distinct. The potential link with *Borrelia* infection in European patients remains controversial, and no evidence for a potential link has been found in North American patients.[430] Administration of valproic acid was thought to trigger morphea in two patients.[431] Trauma, including from vaccination,[432,433] has also been postulated to trigger lesions of pediatric morphea, supported by recurrence of activation of morphea when corrective procedures are performed[434]; however, trauma is so common in children that controlled studies would be required to further consider its role.

The onset of circumscribed morphea is insidious, and superficial plaque-type lesions begin as flesh-colored, erythematous or lilac-colored patches that evolve during weeks to months into firm, hyperpigmented or ivory plaques, with or without a surrounding lilac or violaceous inflammatory zone. Signs of active disease include this violaceous rim, local warmth, raised borders and dermal thickening.[435] The ivory plaques may resemble lesions of lichen sclerosus et atrophicus (Fig. 22.47) but tend other evolve to develop hyperpigmentation (Fig. 22.48, A) and atrophy (see Fig. 22.48, *B*). Occasionally, patients have 1- to 3-mm papules of morphea (guttate morphea). Affected areas, in order of decreasing incidence, are the trunk, neck, extremities, and face. Morphea may also show localized areas of atrophy and resemble atrophoderma of Pasini and Pierini (Fig. 22.49), a disorder that many experts consider within the morphea spectrum[436] and may be isolated or associated with classic lesions of morphea.[437] The atrophoderma usually begins on the trunk during the late teens or early 20s but may even be congenital.[438–440] The atrophic patches extend very slowly with a depressed center and a "cliff-drop" border. Lesions of atrophoderma of Pasini and Pierini tend to increase in number for 10 years or more, primarily on the trunk, neck, and proximal extremities, and then generally persist without apparent change. Circumscribed morphea lesions typically vary from a few centimeters to several inches in diameter; fusion of many plaques may result in the more generalized form of morphea. Deep morphea feels indurated at a deep level; the skin surface may appear slightly puckered or hyperpigmented but often appears normal.

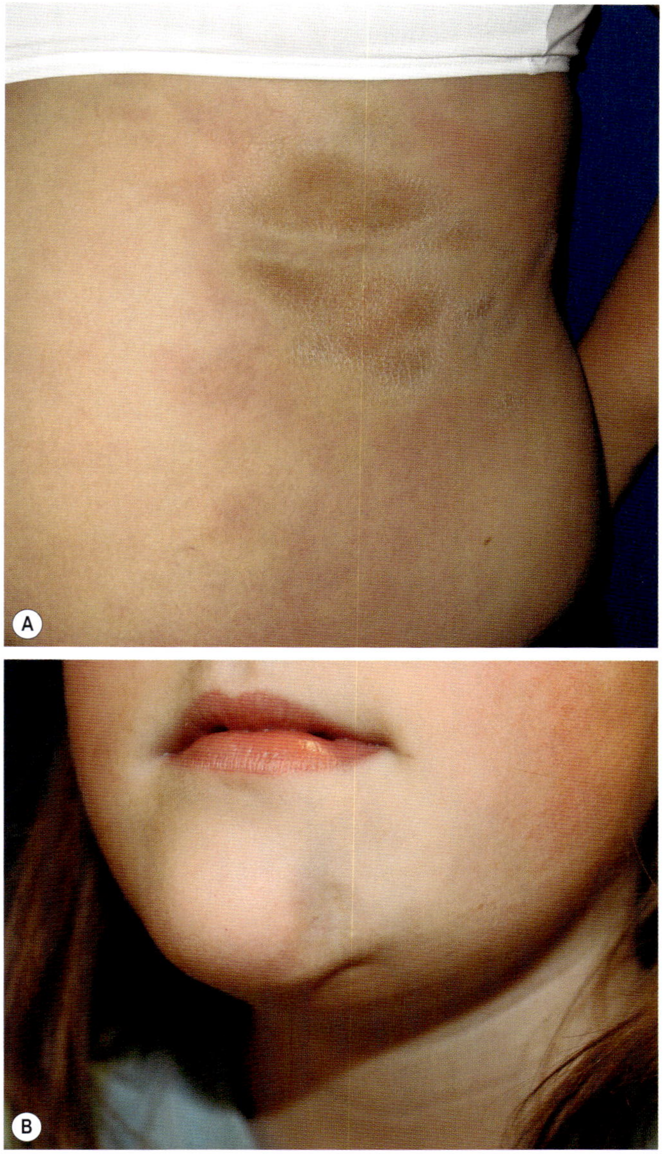

Fig. 22.48 Morphea. **(A)** Within this truncal lesion, one can see the central pale indurated area, the surrounding areas of dusky hyperpigmentation with atrophy and underlying induration, and the active violaceous border. **(B)** This linear morphea has resulted in facial asymmetry with residual localized dyspigmentation, telangiectasia, and dermal and fat atrophy.

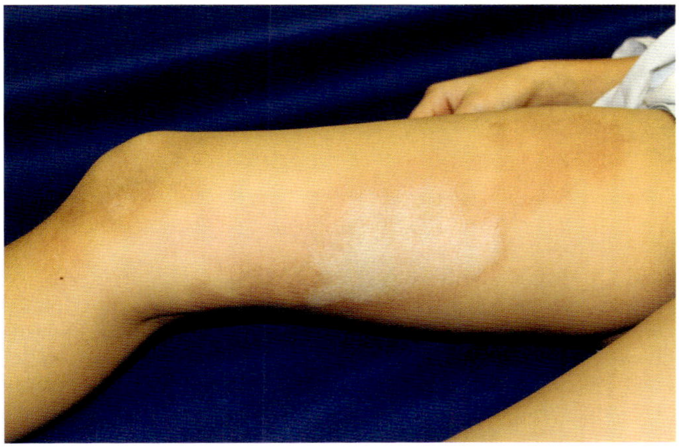

Fig. 22.47 Morphea. Ivory-colored atrophic plaques of morphea may resemble lesions extragenital lesions of lichen sclerosus et atrophicus.

Linear lesions (linear scleroderma) generally affect the limbs (occasionally the head or trunk). Their clinical appearance is similar to that of circumscribed plaque-like forms, but the violaceous peripheral ring

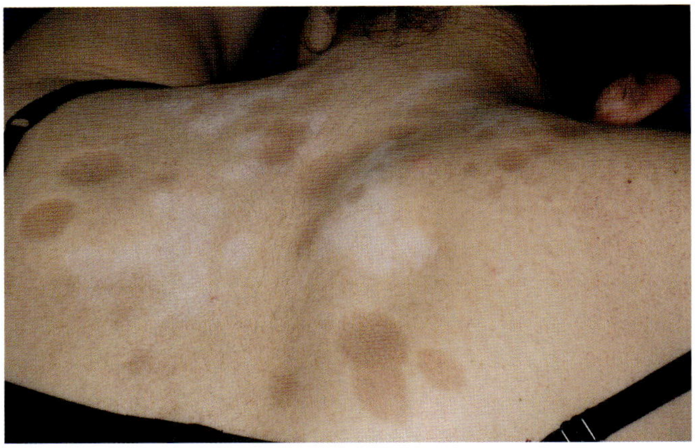

Fig. 22.49 Morphea. Atrophodermic patches in a girl with generalized morphea. Some of the lesions on the upper shoulders demonstrate the "cliff drop" depression of lesions.

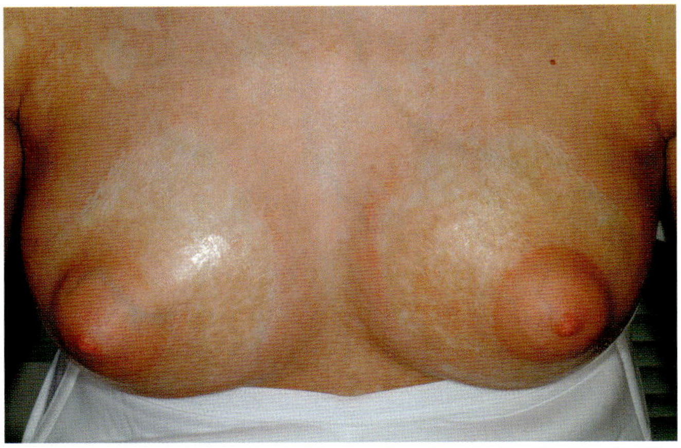

Fig. 22.51 This girl with generalized morphea and uncomfortable sclerosis of the chest had resultant deformity of the breasts. Note the taut breasts, areolar prominence, and shininess from skin atrophy.

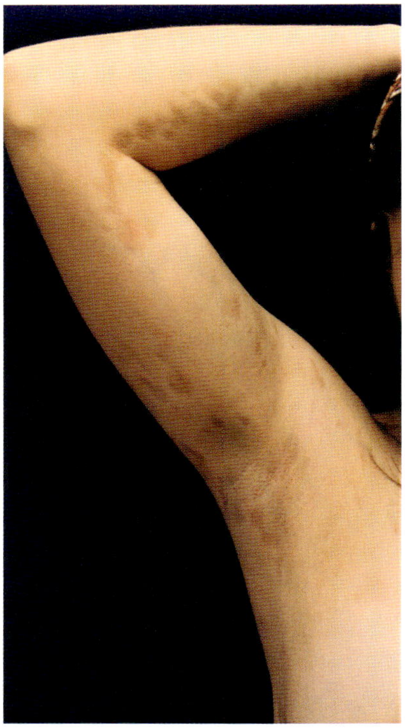

Fig. 22.50 Morphea. Note the linear collections of discrete oval plaques of induration and tissue loss, an arrangement that has been called *linear atrophoderma of Moulin*.

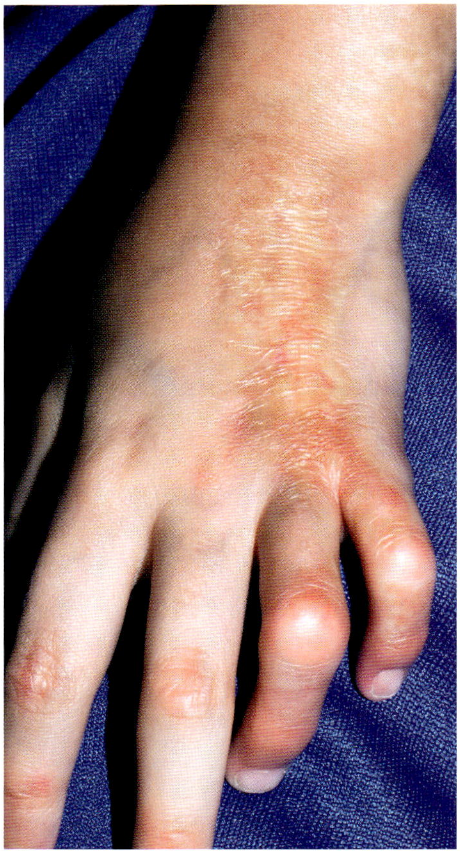

Fig. 22.52 Linear scleroderma. Flexion contraction of the hand in a girl with linear scleroderma. Note the limited extent to which she can straighten her fourth and fifth fingers.

is inconspicuous or only present at the advancing border. Lesions usually present as broad linear bands of induration with dyspigmentation (both hyperpigmentation and hypopigmentation). Much less commonly, a thin linear band of involvement with resultant atrophy and hyperpigmentation may occur *(linear atrophoderma of Moulin)* (Fig. 22.50). Associated atrophy of the skin and underlying subcutaneous tissue leads to a puckered or indented appearance with prominent veins; atrophy may also affect the underlying muscles, fascia, and bones. Linear scleroderma involving an extremity is associated with a risk of undergrowth, both linear and circumferential, of the affected limb, and involvement of the breast area can lead to undergrowth and severe deformity in female adolescents (Fig. 22.51). Impaired joint mobility and contractures (Fig. 22.52) are additional risks when the sclerodermatous area overlies a joint. Occasionally, roughening of one surface of the long bones underlying a linear area of morphea may be noted. This disorder, termed *melorheostosis*, is characterized radiographically by a picture suggesting that of wax flowing down the side of a candle. Linear morphea can also be associated with persistent neuropathy, with associated pain even when the underlying inflammation is controlled (Fig. 22.53). Calcinosis is occasionally present in plaques of linear scleroderma, and the underlying muscle may show an interstitial myositis.

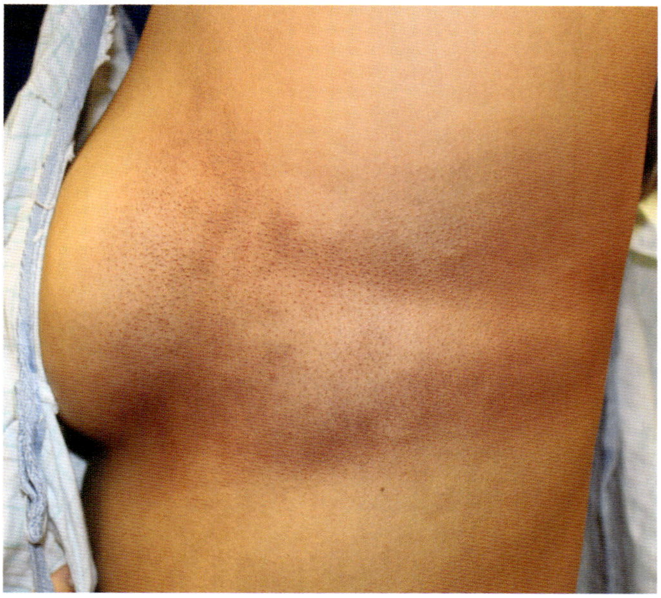

Fig. 22.53 Linear scleroderma. This band of intense inflammation and central induration coursed around the trunk in a bra distribution and was associated with intense neuropathic pain that persisted even when the inflammation was controlled.

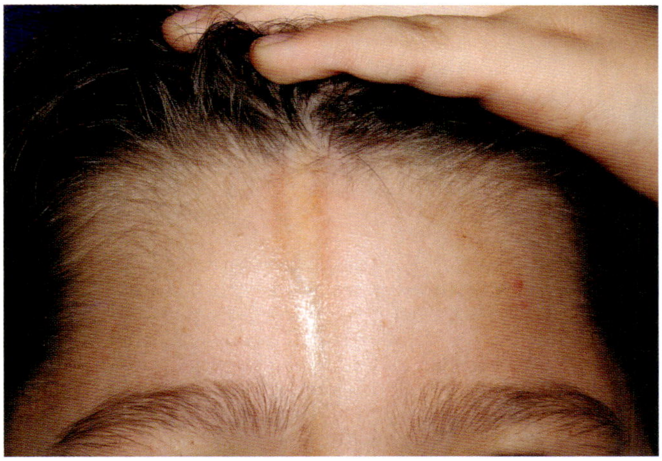

Fig. 22.54 *En coup de sabre* morphea. Extensive soft tissue atrophy and discoloration in a linear pattern on the forehead.

Linear scleroderma involving the frontal or frontoparietal region of the scalp (with or without associated facial hemiatrophy) is called *en coup de sabre* ("cut of a saber"). Although usually unilateral, bilateral cases of *en coup de sabre* have rarely been described.[441,442] This variant begins with a purplish to brown patch that becomes sclerotic and often progresses to a linear depressed groove. The initial presentation may be confused with a port wine stain if purplish in color without induration or depression,[443] but pulsed dye laser does not lead to improvement.[444] Lichen striatus of the forehead has also preceded *en coup de sabre* lesions.[445] With loss of subcutaneous tissue, it thus resembles a saber wound or cut on the frontoparietal scalp (Fig. 22.54). The groove may extend downward into the cheek, nose, and upper lip, and, at times, may involve the mouth, gum, chin, or neck. Extension to the scalp or periocular area leads to associated alopecia of the scalp in a linear distribution (Fig. 22.55) or local loss of eyebrow or eyelashes.

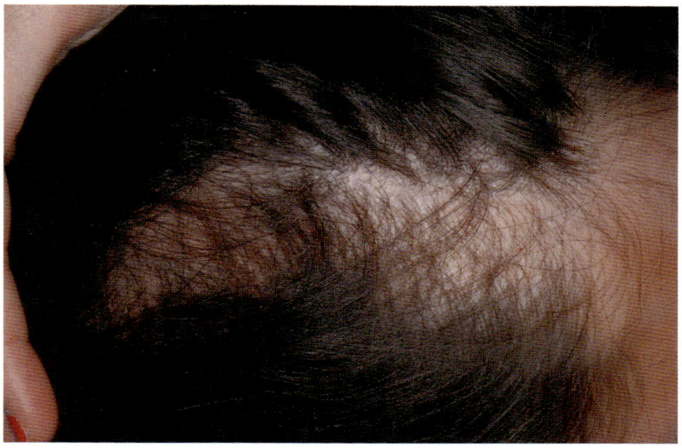

Fig. 22.55 *En coup de sabre* morphea. Note the extension into the scalp, leaving cicatricial alopecia.

Progressive facial hemiatrophy (Parry–Romberg syndrome) is a condition of slowly progressive atrophy of the soft tissue of half of the face. The disorder may be coupled with[446] (Fig. 22.56, *A*) or present without (see Fig. 22.56, *B*) associated dermal sclerosis; the latter raises the possibility that progressive facial hemiatrophy is a deep form of the *en coup de sabre* variety. Facial involvement with morphea has been particularly damaging to self-perception and subject to bullying.[447]

Both *en coup de sabre* and Parry–Romberg syndrome may be accompanied by alopecia, seizures, headaches, trigeminal neuralgia, enophthalmos, myopathy of external eye muscles, Adie pupil,[448] and atrophy of the ipsilateral half of the upper lip, gum, and tongue. Of these manifestations, headaches are most common, occurring in 67% of patients[449] and often meeting the criteria for migraines.[450] Intracerebral atrophy, white matter hyperintensity, and calcifications may be seen on MRI and CT evaluations of affected patients,[441,451–453] especially in patients with neurologic abnormalities.[449] The severity of *en coup de sabre* morphea does not correlate with neuroimaging changes.[449] Successful treatment of the morphea (e.g., with methotrexate) may reduce associated headaches and radiologic neurologic changes.[454] Botulinum toxin has also been used for associated headaches.[455]

Severe, generalized involvement involving the skin, fat, muscle and even bone has been termed *disabling pansclerotic morphea*.[456] This variant, usually affecting girls from 1 to 14 years, tends to have a relentless disabling course and may produce marked disability. Nonhealing ulcers (Fig. 22.57) and squamous cell carcinoma may develop at sites of involvement.[457,458] The disorder may be lethal in association with cachexia and sepsis.[459]

In most pediatric patients, the diagnosis of localized scleroderma is made clinically. However, histologic evaluation of lesional skin shows early inflammation with edema, subsequent sclerosis, and eventual atrophy. The dermis progressively thickens, and dermal appendages are lost. In contrast to SSc, there is more inflammation and more sclerosis of the papillary dermis. Although the development of the cutaneous sclerosis occurs in both morphea and SSc, the clinical features and prognosis of these two autoimmune disorders differs. Raynaud phenomenon and nailfold capillary dilation and dropout are seen in SSc, but rarely in morphea. Arthralgias occur in 15% to 24% of children affected by morphea[426,460,461] and have been described more commonly with linear scleroderma, generalized morphea, and circumscribed deep morphea. Dysphagia is not uncommon, and ocular (especially anterior segment inflammation)[462] and renal[463] abnormalities have also been described. However, the restrictive pulmonary and esophageal sclerosing complications of SSc very rarely arise in morphea.[426] Children with extracutaneous manifestations other than as noted for *en coup de sabre* morphea tend to have more severe skin disease (e.g., pansclerotic morphea, extensive linear scleroderma, generalized morphea). Morphea may also occur in patients

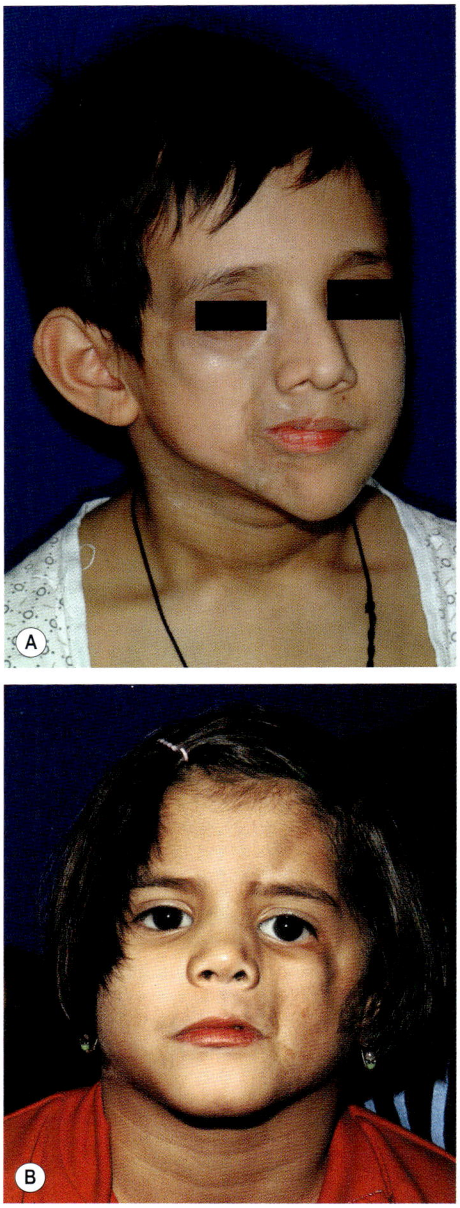

Fig. 22.56 Parry–Romberg syndrome. Hemifacial atrophy, with **(A)** or without **(B)** induration of the overlying skin. In **(A)**, the superficial sclerosis and atrophy is clearly visible.

with other collagen vascular disorders as part of an overlap syndrome (4.9%).[427]

Several laboratory tests may be abnormal in individuals with morphea, although to date they have no significant diagnostic or prognostic value. ESR may be increased, especially in children with linear and deep morphea.[428] Eosinophilia is seen in 15% overall, most often in the deep type.[428] ANA positivity, especially speckled and nucleolar patterns, occurs in 30% to 42% of affected children,[427,464] and RF is positive in 16% of patients. Autoantibodies (ANA, ssDNA, antihistone antibodies) are correlated with more extensive body surface area involvement, functional limitations, and higher skin scores in linear morphea.[464] Antitopoisomerase II antibodies have been detected in 76% of patients with localized scleroderma (and 85% in generalized morphea); these antibodies (in contrast to Scl70 antibodies) have been found in 14% of patients with SSc and are detectable in less than 10% of normal children and children with SLE or JDM.[465] Research has found that serum levels of B-cell activating factor (BAFF) are

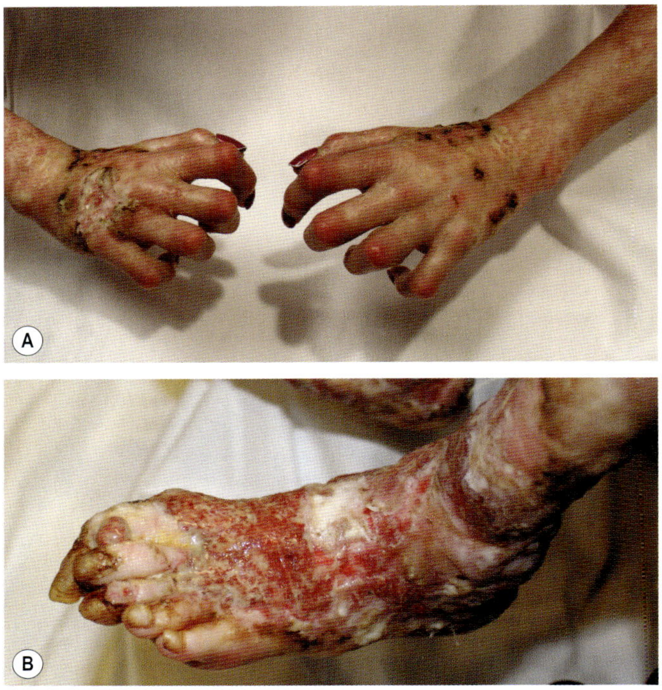

Fig. 22.57 Disabling pansclerotic morphea. This 13-year-old girl first developed indurated lesions of morphea on the trunk at 8 years of age, which rapidly progressed. Note the tight fingers, contractures, and cutaneous ulcerations on the hands **(A)** and the nonhealing ulcers with granulation tissue on her legs and feet **(B)**. She had no visceral involvement other than restrictive lung disease.

increased in morphea (as well as in SSc and SLE),[466] suggesting the potential value of belimumab (anti-BAFF monoclonal antibody). Although not linked to prognosis or therapeutic intervention, the research finding of increased anti–MMP-1 antibodies in about 50% of patients with morphea or SSc suggests a pathogenic role of decreased collagen I degradation.[467]

Morphea lesions can be subtle in their appearance and difficult to monitor for activity. Active lesions may show erythema, skin induration, and enlargement, but these characteristics can be subtle and difficult to appreciate. Skin thickening (especially centrally), atrophy, and dyspigmentation are part of the damage left behind. The Localized Scleroderma Cutaneous Assessment Tool (LoSCAT) and Localized Scleroderma Skin Damage Index (LoSDI) have been used to track clinical changes.[468,469] Thermography, laser Doppler flowmetry, and high-frequency ultrasound have been recommended as sensitive and noninvasive means for evaluating disease activity and risk of further tissue damage.[354,470–472]

Circumscribed type morphea lesions tend to improve within 3 to 5 years, but the residual hypopigmentation, hyperpigmentation, and occasional atrophy may persist indefinitely. Lesions of linear scleroderma tend to last longer, even having long periods of quiescence followed by reactivation.[473] Of patients with linear scleroderma, 24% to 31% report disease activity after 10 years of follow-up.[474,475] Patients with other types largely achieve complete remission either spontaneously or with therapy, although discontinuation or tapering of systemic medications has been associated with recurrence in 22%.[475] Virtually all patients show residual persistent atrophy and dyspigmentation, especially of the atrophy of the *en coup de sabre*/facial hemiatrophy variant.[474] Sequelae can be serious and range from moderate to severe cosmetic impairment (48%) to functional disability from joint contractures or limb length discrepancies (occurring in 38% to 51% of those with linear morphea)[476] (Fig. 22.58). Loss of skin adnexae, calcinosis in linear lesions, and ocular or CNS dysfunction may also occur.

Treatment for morphea depends on the extent of involvement, activity of the disease, and cosmetic or functional ramifications. Potent

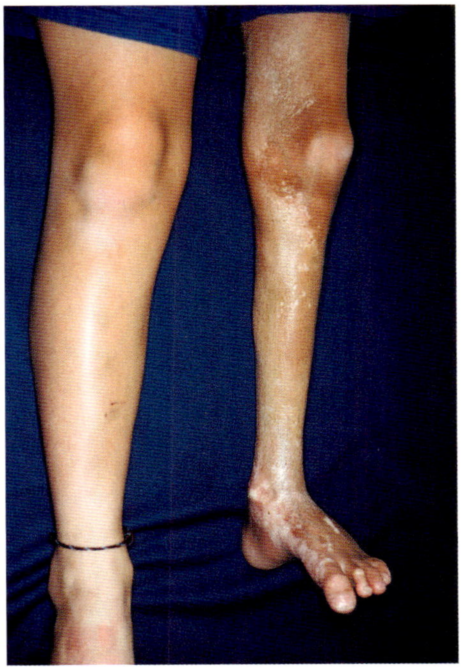

Fig. 22.58 Linear scleroderma with limb length discrepancy. Severe circumference and linear hypotrophy of the bone and soft tissue of the affected leg led to gait disturbance and compensatory scoliosis.

topical or intralesional corticosteroid therapy may hasten resolution of lesions but can result in localized atrophy. Calcipotriene ointment is the topical treatment of choice and has been shown to stop the progression of morphea and linear scleroderma when used early in the course, especially twice daily under occlusion,[477] but does not reverse tissue loss. Calcipotriol-betamethasone dipropionate[478] and imiquimod[479] have also shown benefit. The combination of physiotherapy, massage, warm baths, and exercise is often helpful for patients with linear morphea in whom the involvement overlies a joint because of the risk of contractures.

The first-line systemic therapy for disfiguring or disabling morphea/linear scleroderma is the combination of methotrexate and corticosteroids.[480,481] Systemic corticosteroids (1 mg/kg per day) are given (either orally or at higher dose as pulse intravenous) for the first 2 to 3 months, and methotrexate 0.3 to 0.6 mg/kg or 15 mg/m^2 per week (either orally or subcutaneously) is given initially and on a continuing basis. Approximately 75% of children show disease improvement that is usually maintained on medication for a mean of more than 2 years.[482–484] In one trial of 10 patients with localized scleroderma, all patients responded to this therapy and skin lesions became inactive.[480] The mean time to response was 3 months, and relapses were seen after the methotrexate was discontinued. Mycophenolate mofetil (600 to 1200 mg/m^2 per day) is an alternative for children who have failed to respond to steroids and methotrexate or in combination with methotrexate for greater effect.[485,486] There is also anecdotal evidence of improvement with rituximab,[487] IVIG,[488,489] and tocilizumab (anti–IL-6 receptor antibody)[490–492] for severe linear and pansclerotic morphea recalcitrant to other therapy. In one child, the addition of imatinib to steroids and methotrexate achieved control.[493] Oral calcitriol has also led to significant improvement in some children with linear scleroderma[494] but is limited by its risk of excessive urinary excretion of calcium, leading to renal calcium stones. Dietary calcium must be restricted, and serum calcium and phosphorus as well as the calcium/creatinine ratio in a 24-hour collection of urine must be monitored.

Psoralen plus UVA light (PUVA) has been shown to be efficacious for morphea, but its toxicity restricts its use in children. Medium-dose (70 J/cm^2) UVA1 (340 to 400 nm) significantly reduces the skin thickness of morphea.[495] Although UVA1 light has been thought to work best in lighter skin, good effects are seen as well in darker skin.[496] Home therapy may be an option in children without other UVA1 access. Twice-daily application of calcipotriol ointment combined with UVA1 phototherapy has led to significant softening and repigmentation of morphea lesions, but it is unclear whether these results are superior to topical calcipotriol or UVA1 therapy alone.[497] On the other hand, a comparative trial of UVA1 (30 sessions of 30 J/cm^2) versus fractional CO_2 laser (three sessions, 10,600 nm-power 25W) showed better clinical and patient satisfaction scores with the laser.[498]

Successful repair of contractures may be performed by release and coverage with grafts.[499] Leg shortening procedures to the normal leg may be performed after full growth is achieved, when the affected leg is significantly shortened by linear scleroderma. Orthodontic devices can assist in craniofacial development and minimize the progressive asymmetry of the lower face from Parry–Romberg syndrome.[500] For residual lesions with atrophy, excision can be considered if the affected area is small or the site can be hidden (such as the scalp). Facial lesions can be corrected by transplants of fat, bone, or cartilage, introduction of fillers, and pedicled or free flaps. Laser has been used to lighten the associated hyperpigmentation.[501] Fat transplants have been most successful for forehead lesions, with a mean of 51% to 75% improvement after at least a year, but have a poorer outcome on the chin, infraorbital, and nose areas.[501] In one study in adolescents with facial linear scleroderma (mean age, 15 years), 65% of whom had undergone multiple procedures, 90% were satisfied with their intervention and 100% would recommend surgical intervention to other patients.[502] Ideally, repair should be delayed until the lesion is inactive.

Lichen Sclerosus et Atrophicus

Lichen sclerosus et atrophicus (LSA; LS&A) is a disorder primarily of girls (85% to 90%), with a prevalence of greater than 1 in 900 girls.[503–506] It has its onset before 13 years of age in 10% to 15% of affected individuals; 70% of these childhood cases occur before 7 years of age, and the condition has been described during the first weeks of life. The mean age at development of symptoms is 5 years, with a mean age at diagnosis of 6.7 years. Delay in diagnosis can be associated with a greater risk of sequelae.[507]

Autoantibodies have been demonstrated against extracellular matrix protein-1 and BP180, but their role in pathogenesis is unclear.[508] Autoimmune disease in a parent or grandparent has been found in 65%[509,510]; LSA may also be reported in another family member.

The anogenital region is involved in 75% of affected children. Of those who have extragenital lesions, up to 42% have anogenital involvement as well. Extragenital lesions are asymptomatic and may begin asymmetrically but eventually become distributed in a symmetric manner, primarily on the trunk, neck, and extremities.[511] The extragenital eruption of LSA is characterized by sharply defined, small, pink to ivory white, slightly raised, flat-topped papules a few millimeters in diameter that aggregate and coalesce into plaques of various sizes (Fig. 22.59). The condition may be folliculocentric,[512] and as the condition progresses, atrophy and delling (fine follicular plugs on the surface of macules) may become highly diagnostic features of the disorder with white comedo-like openings that may be seen by dermoscopy.[513] Mosaic distribution of extragenital lichen sclerosus[514] has also been described. The Koebner phenomenon has been documented in cases of LSA in childhood; lesions may develop in surgical scars or sites of vaccination, and exacerbations of quiescent lesions may occur after local trauma or irritation. LSA (extragenital or genital region) occurs in 6% of patients with morphea[515] with 15% having another autoimmune disease.

In female patients, the anogenital lesions commonly tend to surround both the vulvar (Fig. 22.60) and perianal regions in an hourglass or figure-eight pattern. LSA in children most commonly presents in the genital area in girls with itching (70%), soreness (80%), pain with urination (43%), and bleeding (61%) from the vulvar and perianal areas; constipation occurs in more than 10%.[503,516] In studies of girls with vulvar disease or vulvar pruritus, 18% and 11% have lichen sclerosus, respectively.[517,518] A vaginal discharge from the lichen sclerosus may precede the vulvar lesions in about 20% of affected girls, but secondary bacterial vaginosis has also been described.[519]

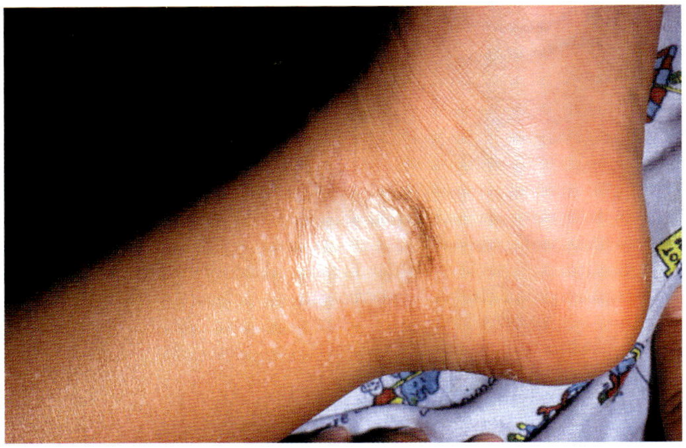

Fig. 22.59 Lichen sclerosus et atrophicus. Ivory atrophic plaque in a girl who also had genital involvement.

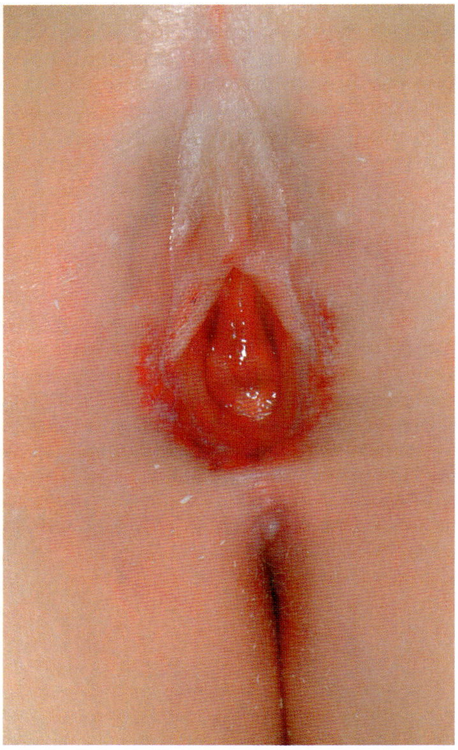

Fig. 22.60 Lichen sclerosus et atrophicus. Whitening, atrophy, inflammation, and purpura of the labia.

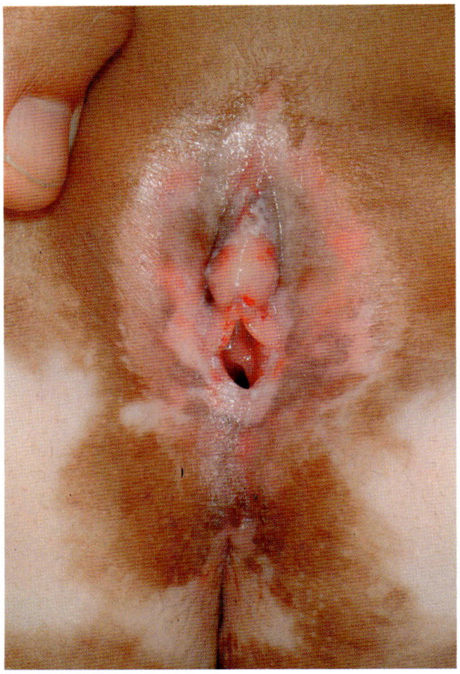

Fig. 22.61 Lichen sclerosus et atrophicus (LSA). This dark-skinned girl with advanced LSA shows partial obliteration of the clitoris. Note the associated purpura and depigmentation.

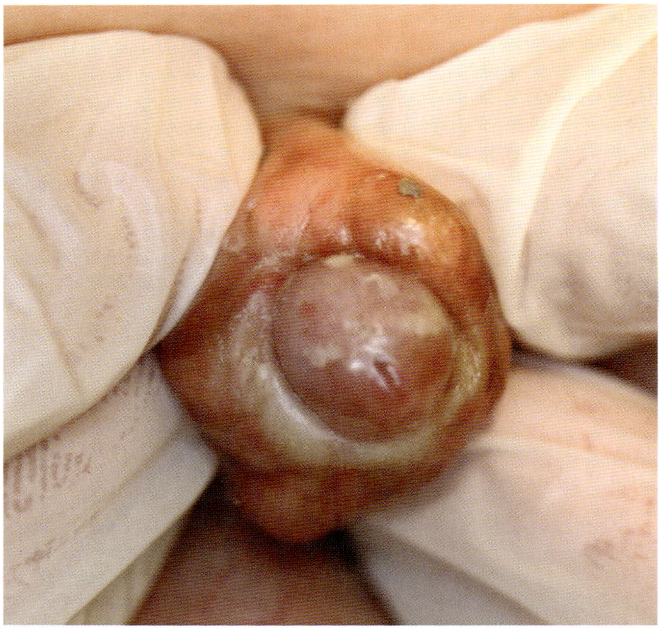

Fig. 22.62 Lichen sclerosus et atrophicus. Balanitis xerotica obliterans is seen on the glans.

Anogenital lesions uncommonly extend to include the skin on the inner aspect of the thighs. In many girls, erythema, purpuric areas (Fig. 22.61, see Fig. 22.60), blistering, and excoriations predominate, especially on the labia minora and clitoris. A vitiligoid form has been described, with depigmentation, with or without erythema or purpura, that tends to present with pain; symptoms and typical signs of LSA respond to potent topical steroids, but the depigmentation persists.[520]

When seen on the dorsum of the glans penis in males, the disorder has been termed *balanitis xerotica obliterans* (Fig. 22.62).[521,522] Clinical evidence of lichen sclerosus of the genital area in boys is less common than in girls, but lichen sclerosus is found in biopsy sections in 15% to 35% of circumcisions and has been blamed for 60% of cases of acquired phimosis.[523,524] Perianal involvement in boys is rare. Lichen sclerosus of the lips tends to be asymptomatic and less destructive, resembling vitiligo.[525]

Lichen sclerosus is often misdiagnosed when present in the genital area of girls as irritant dermatitis because of the associated itching and erythema, or as sexual abuse, owing to the purpura and bleeding. The associated white coloration may lead to confusion with vitiligo or postinflammatory hypopigmentation (see Fig. 22.61). The anal pruritus often raises the possibility of pinworm infestation, and the inflammation and discharge should cause one to consider candidiasis or bacterial vulvovaginitis.[519] The associated constipation or dysuria often leads to unnecessary GI or urinary tract investigations as well. Lichen sclerosus has been described in girls with an infantile perianal pyramidal protrusion (see Chapter 15, Fig. 15.38), a benign tag-like lesion that has been associated with constipation in many patients.[526–528] Although biopsy specimens of lesional skin show characteristic epidermal atrophy with subepidermal vacuolization, a hyalinized superficial dermis, and a band-like infiltration of lymphocytes beneath it, the diagnosis of lichen sclerosus is usually made on clinical grounds and confirmatory biopsy is both traumatic and unnecessary.

Application of clobetasol for 6 to 12 weeks is the treatment of choice to alleviate symptoms, followed by a taper in potency or frequency and intermittent use as needed, but there is considerable variability in recommendations.[529,530] Eighty-three percent of patients experience remission after initial treatment. In one study, however, relapses after initial treatment with clobetasol occurred in more than 40% and required an average of 3 years of intermittent maintenance therapy.[531] In prepubertal boys with phimosis, skin stretching and application of potent topical corticosteroids twice daily for 6 weeks led to a retractable prepuce, including in 67% of the boys with clinically detectable lichen sclerosus.[524] Topical tacrolimus 0.1% ointment has been used successfully to clear lichen sclerosus in girls, both as initial treatment and to promote continued remission.[532–534] Complete circumcision is the treatment of choice in boys with phimosis, but 7% to 19% require late surgery for meatal stenosis.[535] Precircumcision topical steroids[535] or topical tacrolimus ointment 0.1% ointment for 3 weeks after therapeutic circumcision may help decrease the rate of later meatal pathology and maintain control.[536] Plastic surgery may be required to correct labial fusion or clitoral obliteration from scarring. Treatment of extragenital lichen sclerosus is much more challenging than treatment of genital region disease. Although topical steroids and oral retinoids are occasionally helpful,[537] UVA light treatment (especially UVA1) and systemic medication used to treat morphea, such as methotrexate or mycophenolate mofetil (see Morphea section), may be required.[538,539]

Lichen sclerosus has been reported to improve or disappear at puberty in 60% of affected girls, although a study suggested that signs of the disease persisted in 75% postpubertally.[540] In female patients, atrophy of the clitoris and labia minora may occur, with fusion of the latter and stricture of the introitus. In patients in whom improvement has taken place, the disorder may be reactivated years later by trauma, pregnancy, or the administration of anovulatory drugs.

Although vulvar LSA in childhood does not predispose a patient to neoplasia, the incidence of lesional squamous cell carcinoma in adult cases has been estimated as 4.4%. Patients with cases persisting beyond puberty or having onset after puberty should be observed at intervals of 6 to 12 months for the possibility of leukoplakia or carcinoma. Newly arising nodules, erosions, or ulcers in lesions of LSA that persist for more than a few weeks require histologic examination. Development of genital carcinoma has been reported in an adult after clearance of lichen sclerosus during childhood.[541]

Anetoderma

Anetoderma (from the Greek, meaning "relaxed skin" describes an idiopathic atrophy of the skin characterized by oval lesions of thin, soft, loosely wrinkled, depigmented outpouchings of skin that result from weakening of the connective tissue of the dermis.[542] The disorder may be classified as primary macular anetoderma, which arises from apparently normal skin, or as secondary macular anetoderma, which follows previous inflammatory and infiltrative dermatoses. Some of these dermatoses include lupus erythematosus and other collagen vascular disorders, secondary syphilis, sarcoidosis, leprosy, tuberculosis, urticarial lesions, purpura, lichen planus, acne vulgaris, urticaria pigmentosa, molluscum contagiosum,[543] varicella,[544] juvenile xanthogranuloma,[545] and pilomatricomas.[546,547] A peculiar laxity of the eyelid (blepharosclerosis) may also follow chronic or recurrent dermatitis of the eyelids. When eyelid changes are seen in association with adenoma of the thyroid and progressive enlargement of the lips

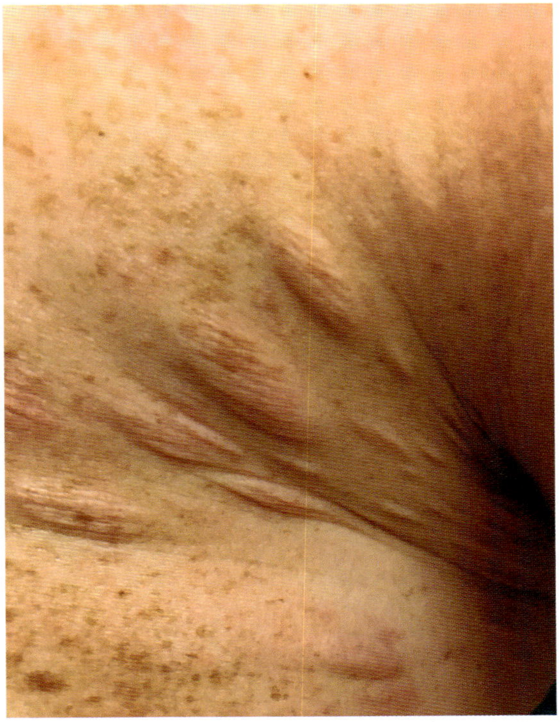

Fig. 22.63 Anetoderma. Well-demarcated circles of cutaneous atrophy on the anterior trunk and neck of a young boy progressively evolved into atrophic saccular outpouchings during the subsequent 8 years. Serial studies of antiphospholipid antibodies were negative.

resulting from inflammation of the labial salivary glands, the disorder is termed *Ascher syndrome*.

Based on whether an inflammatory reaction occurred before the appearance of the atrophy, two types of primary macular anetoderma have been described: anetoderma of Jadassohn–Pellizzari, in which the atrophic lesions are preceded by inflammation, and anetoderma of Schweninger–Buzzi, in which there is no evidence of inflammation. The underlying pathogenesis of primary anetoderma has not been established, but increases in MMP-2 and MMP-9[548] suggest a role of elastic fiber degradation. Serologic and direct immunofluorescent findings suggest that immunologically mediated mechanisms play a role in the elastolytic process.

Anetoderma of Jadassohn–Pellizzari is characterized by crops of round or oval pink 0.5- to 1-cm macules that develop on the trunk, shoulders, upper arms, thighs, sacral area, and occasionally face or scalp (Fig. 22.63). Usually seen in girls and women in their teens to 30s, and occasionally in children, the anetoderma begins with a sharply defined red spot that grows peripherally and becomes round or oval and slightly depressed. As the redness disappears, the characteristic atrophic, wrinkled, and pale herniation ensues. The herniation yields on pressure, admitting the finger through the surrounding ring of normal skin. Much like an umbilical hernia, the bulge reappears when the finger is released, and, at times, fatty tissue may infiltrate the lesions, giving them a more firm, soft, tumor-like appearance.

Anetoderma of Schweninger–Buzzi is manifested by the sudden appearance of large numbers of bluish-white macules, some of which are protuberant, without any preceding inflammatory eruption. Women are affected more commonly than men. Lesions are generally seen on the trunk, neck, face, shoulders, extremities, and back, and range from 10 to 20 mm in diameter. Seen during childhood or adult life, the disease is slowly progressive, and new lesions appear one by one or in groups, a few at a time, over several years. The essential difference in this form of anetoderma is a lack of inflammation and the relative absence of coalescence of lesions.

Anetoderma has also been described in premature infants after use of gel electrocardiographic electrodes, perhaps because of local hypoxemia from the pressure of the electrodes (see Chapter 2).[549,550] More widespread congenital anetoderma of unclear cause has also been described.[551] Drug-induced anetoderma has been described after administration of penicillamine, particularly in patients with Wilson disease. Prothrombotic abnormalities and aPL antibodies have been detected in the majority of patients in more than one investigation, and criteria for the diagnosis of APS have been fulfilled in some patie nts.[236,552,553] A hereditary form has rarely been described[554] and can manifest with skin lesions alone or in association with bony, neurologic, and ocular anomalies; the disorder most likely is autosomal dominant with incomplete penetrance, but the underlying pathogenesis is unclear. In all forms of macular anetoderma, the primary histopathologic feature is the destruction and loss of elastic fibers. No therapy is effective.

Relapsing Polychondritis

Relapsing polychondritis is an uncommon disorder in children characterized by inflammation of cartilage.[555–557] Most patients have demonstrated circulating antibodies against type II collagen and matrillin-1, both components of cartilage, suggesting an autoimmune pathomechanism with a strong IFN pathway component.[558] This concept is supported by the report of an infant with transient disease born to a woman with the condition.[559] Some patients have, or develop, concomitant collagen vascular disorders, especially lupus erythematosus.[560]

Typically, bilateral erythema, swelling, and pain of the ear is the most common manifestation (90%), with involvement of the auricle but sparing of the earlobe. Uncommonly, the disorder presents unilaterally. With chronic disease, the ear cartilage is destroyed, resulting in a scarred "cauliflower" ear; ulceration is rarely present at onset.[561] Nasal cartilage inflammation occurs in 70% of affected individuals and can eventuate in a saddle nose deformity. Nonerosive arthritis has been described in approximately 80% of patients, particularly involving the sternoclavicular, sternomanubrial, and costochondral joints. Approximately 65% of patients have ocular inflammation (conjunctivitis, episcleritis, uveitis, corneal ulceration, or inflammation of the optic nerve).

The most serious potential feature is respiratory tract involvement.[562] Patients may show hoarseness, dyspnea, cough, wheezing, or anterior neck tenderness with palpation of the trachea. Secondary pulmonary infection, airway collapse, or airway obstruction may ensue. Renal and cardiac manifestations have rarely been described. A variety of dermatologic features have been associated, among them aphthous ulcerations, palpable purpura, panniculitic nodules, pyoderma gangrenosum,[563] livedo reticularis, and neutrophilic disorders of skin, such as Sweet syndrome.

In children, the most commonly seen disorder to be considered in the differential is otomelalgia (red ear syndrome), a condition characterized by erythema, swelling, and pain of the entire ear that does not spare the earlobe. The condition is short-lived, responds to application of ice, and is episodic, rather than persistent (see Chapter 12; Fig. 12.92). Red ear syndrome can be associated with migraines.

The treatment of choice for relapsing polychondritis is systemic corticosteroids (1 mg/kg per day initially) and NSAIDs. TNF inhibitors, tofacitinib, dapsone, and methotrexate have been used as steroid-sparing agents.[564–566] Rituximab has been successful in treating resistant pediatric cases.[567] Emergency tracheostomy and/or airway stents may be required for upper respiratory tract involvement.[562,568] One child responded to oral ingestion of type II collagen as a tolerogen.[569]

Sjögren Syndrome

Sjögren syndrome is a chronic autoimmune disorder of unknown etiology that is uncommon in children.[570] Characteristic features are keratoconjunctivitis sicca (inflammation of the cornea and the conjunctiva with dryness and atrophy), xerostomia (dryness of the mouth from lack of normal secretion), and enlargement of the salivary and lacrimal glands (as a result of lymphocytic and plasma cell infiltration) (Box 22.9).[571] Sjögren syndrome can occur alone (primary)[572] or in association with virtually any other autoimmune disorder (secondary), although the most common are JIA and SLE. The manifestations of Sjögren syndrome may precede the onset of another autoimmune disorder by years.

In a review of 39 pediatric cases, the female/male ratio in children was greater than 3:1, with a mean age at onset of 8 years.[573] In children, the presenting sign is usually parotitis (62.5% versus 13% in adults) with parotid gland enlargement, which may be bilateral.[574–576] In addition, children with primary Sjögren syndrome report less dryness and have more lymphadenopathy and systemic symptoms compared with affected adults.[577]

Bacterial parotitis and lymphoproliferative disease must be included in the differential diagnosis. Almost 10% of the children have an extraglandular manifestation, and 51% experience at least one extraglandular manifestation during the course of the disease. The most common extraglandular feature is leukopenia (35%) with or without splenomegaly. Arthritis occurs in 15% of children (versus 38.5% of adults). Purpura and intense residual hyperpigmentation, especially on the lower extremities (hypergammaglobulinemic purpura), is the most common cutaneous manifestation (12% of children) (Fig. 22.64). Annular erythema, erythema nodosum, lipodystrophy, and multiple recurrent or persistent ranulas[571,578] (oral mucocele

Box 22.9 Sjögren Syndrome

Major Clinical Features

- Inflammation and chronic enlargement of salivary glands
- Keratoconjunctivitis sicca (dryness and atrophy of cornea and conjunctiva)
- Xerostomia (dryness of mouth)
- Fatigue
- May be associated with other autoimmune disorders, especially juvenile idiopathic arthritis

Cutaneous Features

- Dryness and scaling of skin (with partial or complete loss of perspiration)
- Sparse, dry, brittle hair
- Hypergammaglobulinemic purpura (usually lower extremities)
- Raynaud phenomenon

Laboratory Abnormalities

- Positive antinuclear antibodies; rheumatoid factor, anti-Ro, anti-La antibodies in majority
- Tests to show decreased tear formation and salivary flow

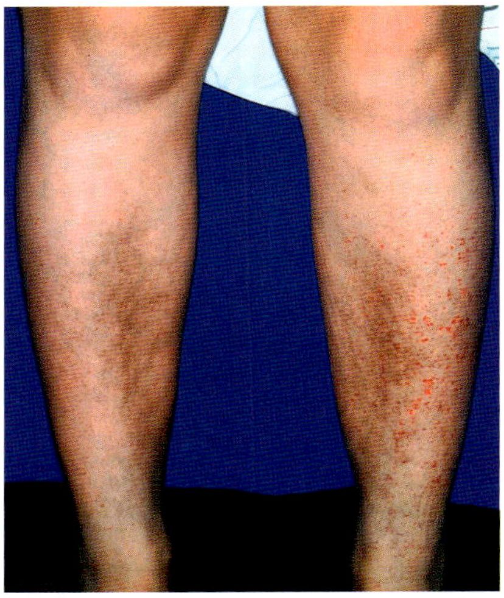

Fig. 22.64 Hypergammaglobulinemic purpura. Recurrent episodes of purpuric lesions on the lower extremities left darkly hyperpigmented macules that persisted. Joint pain and high levels of anti-Ro and anti-La antibodies as well as immunoglobulin G were associated. Administration of hydroxychloroquine eliminated joint pain and dramatically suppressed cutaneous flares, leading to gradual fading of the hyperpigmentation.

variant) may be seen on mucocutaneous evaluation. Mesangial proliferative glomerulonephritis[579] and extranodal marginal zone B-cell lymphoma[580] have also been described.

The most prominent mucosal manifestations are associated with dryness of the gingivae and other mucous membranes of the mouth and, at times, the conjunctivae, nose, pharynx, larynx, vagina, and respiratory tract.[581] The tongue may become smooth, red, and dry, and in severe cases, there may be difficulty in swallowing dry food. The lips may be cracked, fissured, or ulcerated, particularly at the corners of the mouth; the teeth commonly undergo rapid and severe decay; the eyes may be reddened and moist; and thick, tenacious secretions forming ropy mucous strands in the inner canthi may be noted (particularly when the patient first arises in the morning). Other ocular manifestations include a burning sensation, as if a foreign body is present in the eye, and the inability to produce tears in response to irritants or emotion.

A positive ANA test has been seen in 67% of children (versus 92% of adults) and RF in 71%. Positive anti-Ro and/or anti-La antibodies are detected in 73% of children with Sjögren syndrome, but the minority of children with these antibodies develop Sjögren syndrome.[582] Patients may show a decreased stimulated salivary flow rate and positive Schirmer (<5 mm wetting of a strip of filter paper inserted under the lower eyelid) and rose bengal (conjunctival staining) tests of the eyes. Sialography, ultrasound,[583] and CT scans of the parotid glands may show evidence of enlargement and inflammation.

Although no criteria for diagnosis have been established for pediatric Sjögren syndrome, which is more difficult to diagnose, in adults they include (1) positive serum anti-SSA/Ro and/or anti-SSB/La *or* positive RF and ANA titer at least 1:320; (2) labial salivary gland biopsy exhibiting focal lymphocytic sialadenitis; and (3) keratoconjunctivitis sicca, with specific criteria for the biopsy features and severity of the keratoconjunctivitis that may not be applicable to children.[584] The management of Sjögren syndrome includes treatment of the dry skin, keratoconjunctivitis, and xerostomia with lubricants, and therapy for the associated collagen vascular disorder if present. In a 12-week study of adults with Sjögren syndrome, pilocarpine (5 mg/dose three times daily) was more effective than artificial saliva at improving global assessment and salivary flow; side effects were nausea and sialorrhea.[585] Although systemic corticosteroids are capable of reducing the swelling of the salivary glands, they usually do not improve the function of affected glands, and their use is reserved for severely affected patients. Rituximab has shown benefit for the mucosal dryness and systemic manifestations in adults.[586]

Mixed Connective Tissue Disease

Only 0.6% of all pediatric patients with rheumatologic disease have MCTD (also called *overlap syndrome*), which begins before 16 years of age in 23% of individuals with MCTD.[587,588] At least 85% are female, and the earliest age of onset described has been 2 years of age (mean onset at age 9.5 to 12 years).[589] The disease is characterized by the combination of clinical features and laboratory data similar to those of SLE, scleroderma, and dermatomyositis (Box 22.10).

The distinguishing laboratory marker for this disease is the demonstration of serum antibody specific for nRNP (U1 RNP), a ribonuclease-sensitive component of extractable nuclear antigen (ENA). However, anti–U1 RNP is also seen in patients with SLE, systemic sclerosis, Sjögren syndrome, and undifferentiated connective tissue disease. In addition, most patients with MCTD have high serum titers of ANA in a speckled pattern. Up to 70% of patients have a high titer of RF. Anti-dsDNA (20%), anti-La (14%), anti-Ro (13%), and anti-Sm (10%) antibodies are also detected in children. High titers of anti–U1 RNP and also anti-Ro antibody are associated with lung fibrosis.

The most common presenting features of pediatric-onset MCTD are fatigue, pain (polyarthralgias, myalgias), and Raynaud phenomenon (mean, 73% of children).[590,591] In one study of 55 pediatric patients, all had Raynaud phenomenon, 94% had arthritis, 77% had puffy hands, and 58% had pulmonary manifestations. Features of SLE, systemic sclerosis (especially esophageal dysmotility/reflux), and polymyositis were seen in 98%, 77%, and 48%, respectively. The pulmonary disease can be insidious, especially early in the course, but leads to the greatest morbidity. Although some patients with MCTD have deforming arthritis, an evanescent nonerosive, nondeforming polyarthritis similar to that seen in patients with SLE is more common.

Approximately two-thirds of children with MCTD have cardiovascular involvement, including pericarditis, myocarditis, congestive heart failure, aortic insufficiency, and/or pulmonary arterial hypertension.[592] About 10% have clinical evidence of renal disease (more by biopsy evaluation),[593] and about 10% have neurologic abnormalities (trigeminal sensory neuropathy, vascular headaches, seizures, multiple peripheral neuropathies, and cerebral infarction or hemorrhage). The incidence of renal and cardiac involvement is higher in children than in adults with MCTD.[593] However, the course is more slowly progressive, overall has a lower risk of renal disease, and responds to lower doses of steroids than SLE or scleroderma. Progression toward scleroderma can be predicted by changes on capillaroscopy. High-resolution computed

Box 22.10 Mixed Connective Tissue Disease (Kasukawa Criteria)

Criteria: Must Meet All Three to Be Diagnosed with MCTD

- Raynaud phenomenon and/or swollen fingers or hands
- Must have at least one abnormal finding from two or more groups of findings:
  - SLE-like findings (facial eruption, polyarthritis, serositis, lymphadenopathy, leukopenia, thrombocytopenia)
  - Scleroderma-like findings (sclerodactyly, pulmonary fibrosis, vital capacity <80% of normal, carbon monoxide diffusion <70% of normal, decreased esophageal motility)
  - Polymyositis-like findings (muscle weakness, elevated serum levels of muscle enzymes, myogenic pattern on EMG)

Mucocutaneous Features

Alopecia
Heliotrope rash
Hypopigmentation and/or hyperpigmentation
Livedo reticularis
Lupus-like lesions, including malar telangiectasia and/or erythema
Mucosal dryness
Periungual telangiectasia
Photosensitivity
Raynaud phenomenon
Sclerodactyly

Musculoskeletal Features

Arthritis or arthralgia
Proximal muscle weakness
Tapered or sausage-shaped fingers

Gastrointestinal Features

Abnormal esophageal motility

Cardiac Features

Aortic insufficiency
Congestive heart failure
Pericarditis/myocarditis

Pulmonary Features

Abnormal pulmonary function tests
Pulmonary fibrosis

Neurologic Features

Headache
Peripheral neuropathy
Seizures

Renal Features

Glomerulonephritis

Laboratory Abnormalities

Elevated anti-RNP titer
Speckled ANA

ANA, Antinuclear antibody; *EMG,* electromyography; *MCTD,* mixed connective tissue disease; *RNP,* ribonuclear protein; *SLE,* systemic lupus erythematosus.

tomography is the preferred technique for serially assessing interstitial and parenchymal lung changes.[594] Hematologic complications, particularly severe thrombocytopenia, and autoimmune hepatitis are unusual but occur much more often in children than in adults.

The natural course tends to be an increase over time in the systemic sclerosis–like features, persistence of Raynaud phenomenon and arthritis, and diminution in features of SLE or polymyositis. After a mean follow-up of 16 years, 67% continue to have active disease, in association with higher titers of anti-RNP antibody and a positive RF.[591]

Immunosuppressive medications, particularly systemic corticosteroids, methotrexate, hydroxychloroquine, and nonsteroidal antiinflammatories, are most commonly used as therapy. Other interventions are based on manifestations (e.g., calcium channel blockers for Raynaud phenomenon). Rituximab has been used for the severe thrombocytopenia.[595] Long-lasting remission occurs in only 3% of patients; inflammatory manifestations (fever, arthritis, skin eruption) are most responsive to treatment, whereas the sclerodermatous features (sclerodactyly, esophageal disease) and vasculopathy (including Raynaud disease) tend to persist. In one study with 12 children, 92%, 79%, and 52% were free of organ involvement at 2, 5, and 10 years, respectively.[589] Tocilizumab (anti–IL-6 monoclonal antibody) dramatically improved the arthritis, but not other features, in 2 children with MCTD.[596] Immunoadsorption onto protein A in combination with low-dosage systemic steroids and bosentan led to remission in a recalcitrant patient.[597] Mortality is lower in children than in adults, especially if organ involvement can be detected and treated early.

The complete list of 597 references for this chapter is available online at http://expertconsult.inkling.com.

Key References

Rustad A, Nolan BE, Ollech A, et al. Incorporating joint pain screening into the pediatric dermatologic examination. Pediatr Dermatol 2020 Dec 4. doi: 10.1111/pde.14454.

Giancane G, Alongi A, Ravelli A. Update on the pathogenesis and treatment of juvenile idiopathic arthritis. Curr Opin Rheumatol 2017;29(5):523–9.

Borgia RE, Gerstein M, Levy DM, et al. Features, treatment, and outcomes of macrophage activation syndrome in childhood-onset systemic lupus erythematosus. Arthritis Rheumatol 2018;70(4):616–24.

Wenzel J. Cutaneous lupus erythematosus: new insights into pathogenesis and therapeutic strategies. Nat Rev Rheumatol 2019;15(9):519–32.

Groot N, de Graeff N, Avcin T, et al. European evidence-based recommendations for diagnosis and treatment of childhood-onset systemic lupus erythematosus: the SHARE initiative. Ann Rheum Dis 2017;76(11):1788–96.

Orbai A, Alarcón GS, Gordon C, et al. Derivation and validation of Systemic Lupus International Collaborating Clinics classification criteria for systemic lupus erythematosus. Arthritis Rheum 2012;64(8):2677–86.

Kuhn A, Ruland V, Bonsmann G. Cutaneous lupus erythematosus: update of therapeutic options. Part I. J Am Acad Dermatol 2011;65(6):e179–93.

Kuhn A, Ruland V, Bonsmann G. Cutaneous lupus erythematosus: update of therapeutic options. Part II. J Am Acad Dermatol 2011;65(6):e195–213.

Marmor MF, Kellner U, Lai TY, et al. Revised recommendations on screening for chloroquine and hydroxychloroquine retinopathy. Ophthalmology 2011;118(2):415–22.

Johnson B. Overview of neonatal lupus. J Pediatr Health Care 2014;28(4):331–41.

Vanoni F, Lava SAG, Fossali EF, et al. Neonatal systemic lupus erythematcsus syndrome: a comprehensive review. Clin Rev Allergy Immunol 2017;53(3):469–76.

Izmirly PM, Llanos C, Lee LA, et al. Cutaneous manifestations of neonatal lupus and risk of subsequent congenital heart block. Arthritis Rheum 2010;62:1153–7.

Rumsey DG, Myones B, Massicotte P. Diagnosis and treatment of antiphospholipid syndrome in childhood: a review. Blood Cells Mol Dis 2017;67:34–40.

Avcin T, Cimaz R, Rozman B. The Ped-APS registry: the antiphospholipid syndrome in childhood. Lupus 2009;18:894–9.

Robinson AB, Reed AM. Clinical features, pathogenesis and treatment of juvenile and adult dermatomyositis. Nat Rev Rheumatol 2011;7(11):664–75.

Chiu YE, Co DO. Juvenile dermatomyositis: immunopathogenesis, role of myositis-specific autoantibodies, and review of rituximab use. Pediatr Dermatol 2011;28(4):357–67.

Rider LG, Nistala K. The juvenile idiopathic inflammatory myopathies: pathogenesis, clinical and autoantibody phenotypes, and outcomes. J Intern Med 2016;280(1):24–38.

Pachman LM, Khojah AM. Advances in juvenile dermatomyositis: myositis specific antibodies aid in understanding disease heterogeneity. J Pediatr 2018;195:16–27.

Mamyrova G, Kishi T, Targoff IN, et al. Features distinguishing clinically amyopathic juvenile dermatomyositis from juvenile dermatomyositis. Rheumatology (Oxford) 2018;57(11):1956–63.

Ravelli A, Trail L, Ferrari C, et al. Long-term outcome and prognostic factors of juvenile dermatomyositis: a multinational, multicenter study of 490 patients. Arthritis Care Res (Hoboken) 2010;62:63–72.

Orandi AB, Baszis KW, Dharnidharka VR, et al. Assessment, classification and treatment of calcinosis as a complication of juvenile dermatomyositis: a survey of pediatric rheumatologists by the childhood arthritis and rheumatology research alliance (CARRA). Pediatr Rheumatol Online J. 2017;15(1):71.

Gowdie PJ, Allen RC, Kornberg AJ, et al. Clinical features and disease course of patients with juvenile dermatomyositis. Int J Rheum Dis 2013;16(5):561–7.

Consolaro A, Varnier GC, Martini A, et al. Advances in biomarkers for paediatric rheumatic diseases. Nat Rev Rheumatol 2015;11(5):265–75.

Zulian F, Cuffaro G, Sperotto F. Scleroderma in children: an update. Curr Opin Rheumatol 2013;25(5):643–50.

Li SC. Scleroderma in children and adolescents: localized scleroderma and systemic sclerosis. Pediatr Clin North Am 2018;65(4):757–81.

Torok KS. Pediatric scleroderma: systemic or localized forms. Pediatr Clin North Am 2012;59(2):381–405.

Fett N, Werth VP. Update on morphea. Part I. Epidemiology, clinical presentation, and pathogenesis. J Am Acad Dermatol 2011;64(2):217–28.

Fett N, Werth VP. Update on morphea. Part II. Outcome measures and treatment J Am Acad Dermatol 2011;64(2):231–42.

Pope E, Laxer RM. Diagnosis and management of morphea and lichen sclerosus and atrophicus in children. Pediatr Clin North Am 2014;61(2):309–19.

Laxer RM, Zulian F. Localized scleroderma. Curr Opin Rheumatol 2006;18(6):606–13.

Pequet MS, Holland KE, Zhao S, et al. Risk factors for morphoea disease severity: a retrospective review of 114 paediatric patients. Br J Dermatol 2014;170(4):895–900.

Zulian F, Martini G, Vallongo C, et al. Methotrexate treatment in juvenile localized scleroderma: a randomized, double-blind, placebo-controlled trial. Arthritis Rheum 2011;63(7):1998–2006.

Lewis FM, Tatnall FM, Velangi SS, et al. British Association of Dermatologists guidelines for the management of lichen sclerosus, 2018. Br J Dermatol 2018;178(4):839–53.

23 Endocrine Disorders and the Skin

Endocrinologic diseases often display cutaneous features that may provide diagnostic clues, and patients with these disorders may be more susceptible to a variety of mucocutaneous problems. Some of these conditions and their therapy, where applicable, are reviewed here. A thorough discussion of all endocrine disorders and their treatment is beyond the scope of this chapter.

Thyroid Disorders

Patients with hyperthyroidism or hypothyroidism may show a variety of skin findings. In some cases associated hair or nail defects may also be seen. Some of these findings are related to the imbalance in thyroid hormone, which may play a role in skin homeostasis via its influence on proteoglycan synthesis, epidermal differentiation, hair formation, and sebum production.[1]

HYPERTHYROIDISM

Box 23.1 summarizes the various cutaneous changes that may be seen in hyperthyroidism. This disorder is most often caused by an autoimmune thyroid condition: Graves disease. It may also be associated with a hyperfunctioning thyroid nodule, thyroid multinodular goiters, non-Graves thyroiditis, excessive thyroxine intake, or hypersecretion of thyroid-stimulating hormone (TSH). Cutaneous features occur most commonly in association with Graves disease, and these manifestations may more often be the result of autoimmune mediation rather than direct effects of thyroid hormones.[2]

The clinical features of hyperthyroidism include nervousness, emotional lability, tachycardia and palpitation, heat intolerance, weakness, fatigue, tremors, hyperactivity, increased appetite, weight loss, increased systolic and pulse pressure, accelerated growth, sleep disturbances, school problems, vomiting, diarrhea, and occasionally exophthalmos. An enlarged thyroid gland is often present. Specific findings that suggest Graves disease include thyroid ophthalmopathy, pretibial myxedema (PTM), and acropachy. The ophthalmopathy is secondary to periorbital deposition of glycosaminoglycans and may present with proptosis, ocular paralysis, or lid lag.

Pretibial Myxedema

PTM (also known as *thyroid dermopathy*) manifests as plaques on the anterior tibial surfaces and is related to localized accumulation of acid mucopolysaccharides. Other locations of involvement are occasionally reported, including the dorsal feet. The majority of patients with PTM have ophthalmopathy.[3,4] The onset of PTM usually follows the diagnosis of hyperthyroidism. Examination reveals nonpitting edema, nodules, and plaques with pink to purple to yellow-brown discoloration (Fig. 23.1). The overlying epidermis is thin with a waxy and sometimes translucent quality. Hypertrichosis with dilated hair follicles and a "*peau d'orange*" appearance may be noted. Polypoid or elephantiasis forms occur less commonly.[3] Although the pretibial surfaces are most commonly involved, other areas, including the face, scalp, upper extremities, and trunk, may reveal similar changes. The differential diagnosis may include cellulitis, trauma, erythema nodosum, or other mucinoses, and PTM can be confirmed by tissue examination of skin biopsy material in conjunction with laboratory findings. Histologic evaluation may reveal mucin deposition and reduced elastic fibers.

Thyroid Acropachy

Thyroid acropachy is more common in adults with hyperthyroidism; only occasionally occurs in children; and classically presents as the triad of digital clubbing, soft-tissue swelling of the hands and feet, and periosteal changes. Examination reveals thickening of the soft tissues over the distal extremities and (secondary to diaphyseal periosteal proliferation) of the distal bones. Drumstick-like clubbing, enlargement of the hands and feet, and radiographic changes (fluffy, spiculated, or homogeneous subperiosteal thickening with new bone formation) may be seen. Associated extremity and joint pain may be reported, and nail clubbing may also be seen. Thyroid acropachy and diabetic dermopathy (DD) are indicators of more severe Graves ophthalmopathy.[5,6]

Less specific cutaneous changes in hyperthyroidism include skin that is warm, velvety, moist, and smooth. Hair may be fine and thin. Facial flushing, increased sweating (particularly of the palms and soles), and palmar erythema are common, especially in the advanced state of the disease, called *thyrotoxicosis*. The nails grow rapidly, are shiny, and may reveal onycholysis (separation or loosening of the nail plate from the nailbed) with distal upward curvature (Plummer nails). Koilonychia (spoon-shaped nails; Fig. 23.2) and clubbing may also be noted. Chronic urticaria and generalized pruritus are uncommon manifestations of thyrotoxicosis, and chronic active hyperthyroidism can be complicated by Addison disease–like hyperpigmentation. However, the hyperpigmentation of hyperthyroidism is distributed differently, primarily on the shins (Fig. 23.3), posterior feet, and nailbeds.[7] Patients with hyperthyroidism may also have an increased incidence of alopecia areata and/or vitiligo.[8,9] Gynecomastia may be present in males and may be caused by increased conversion of testosterone to estradiol. Scleromyxedema, a condition marked by white-yellow papules, weight loss, monoclonal gammopathy, esophageal dysmotility, myopathy, and Raynaud phenomenon, has also been reported in patients (mainly adults) with hyperthyroidism.[10]

Box 23.1 Cutaneous Manifestations of Hyperthyroidism

Warm, velvety, moist, erythematous, smooth skin
Thin, fine hair; diffuse nonscarring alopecia
Hyperpigmentation (especially of palmar creases, soles, gingivae, buccal mucosa)
Facial flushing
Palmar erythema
Increased sweating
Nail changes (onycholysis, curvature, koilonychia, clubbing, yellow nails)
Pretibial myxedema
Periorbital edema
Chronic urticaria
Generalized pruritus
Thyroid acropachy (clubbing)
Increased incidence of vitiligo, alopecia areata
Gynecomastia (in men)

HYPOTHYROIDISM

Box 23.2 summarizes the various mucocutaneous changes that may be seen in hypothyroidism. Hypothyroidism in pediatric patients may be congenital or acquired. Clinical features of congenital hypothyroidism are shown in Box 23.3. Symptoms may be subtle in both forms of hypothyroidism, but decreased linear growth is an important indicator of both types of disease. Hypothermia, lethargy, and poor feeding are all characteristic of congenital disease, which is most often diagnosed on routine newborn screening examinations. Children with acquired hypothyroidism tend to be quiet and well behaved and as a result often receive high grades in school.

Congenital hypothyroidism may develop as a result of agenesis or dysgenesis of the thyroid gland (the most common cause), defective synthesis of thyroid hormone caused by an enzymatic defect, the presence of antithyroid antibodies in a pregnant mother, the lack of maternal iodine during pregnancy (endemic goiter), or the ingestion of antithyroid medications such as propylthiouracil or methimazole by a pregnant woman being treated for thyrotoxicosis. Iodine toxicity from iodine-containing skin antiseptic solutions has been implicated as a potential cause of transient hypothyroidism in newborn infants, although some studies refute this association.[11,12] Acquired hypothyroidism in children younger than 5 or 6 years of age may be caused by a delayed failure of thyroid remnants (with thyroid dysgenesis), by inborn defects of thyroid hormone synthesis, by ingestion of antithyroid agents, by thyroidectomy or ablation after radiation, or by chronic thyroiditis or hypothalamic-pituitary disease. After the age of 5 or 6 years, although the same etiologies may be involved, chronic lymphocytic thyroiditis (Hashimoto thyroiditis) is the most common cause. Although iodine deficiency is the most common cause of hypothyroidism worldwide, it is uncommon in the United States.

Cutaneous features of hypothyroidism reflect the hypometabolic state with reduced body temperature and reflex vasoconstriction. Patients often have dry, coarse, pale, and cool skin. Cutis marmorata (physiologic mottling) may be prominent. Hypohidrosis may lead to acquired palmoplantar keratoderma.[10] Myxedema may occur in hypothyroidism, again as a result of mucopolysaccharide deposition in skin. It most commonly occurs in the hands, feet, and periorbital locations and may also be deposited in the tongue, giving rise to macroglossia. Generalized puffiness may be present, and the skin may take on a yellow hue as a result of carotenemia (Fig. 23.4), especially on the palms, soles, and nasolabial folds. The hair is dull and brittle, and nails are ridged, brittle, and grow very slowly. Patients may have a dull, expressionless facies. Hypertrichosis of the back and shoulders may be seen, and alopecia may involve the lateral portions of the eyebrows (termed *madarosis*) or occur in a more diffuse pattern.[13] A collodion baby with concomitant congenital hypothyroidism has been reported.[14]

Parathyroid Disorders

Disorders of the parathyroid glands (hyperparathyroidism and hypoparathyroidism) may affect the skin in various ways and often present with cutaneous features that can assist the primary or consulting physician in diagnosis and management. Although primary parathyroid disease is uncommon in children, these glands play a major role in the regulation

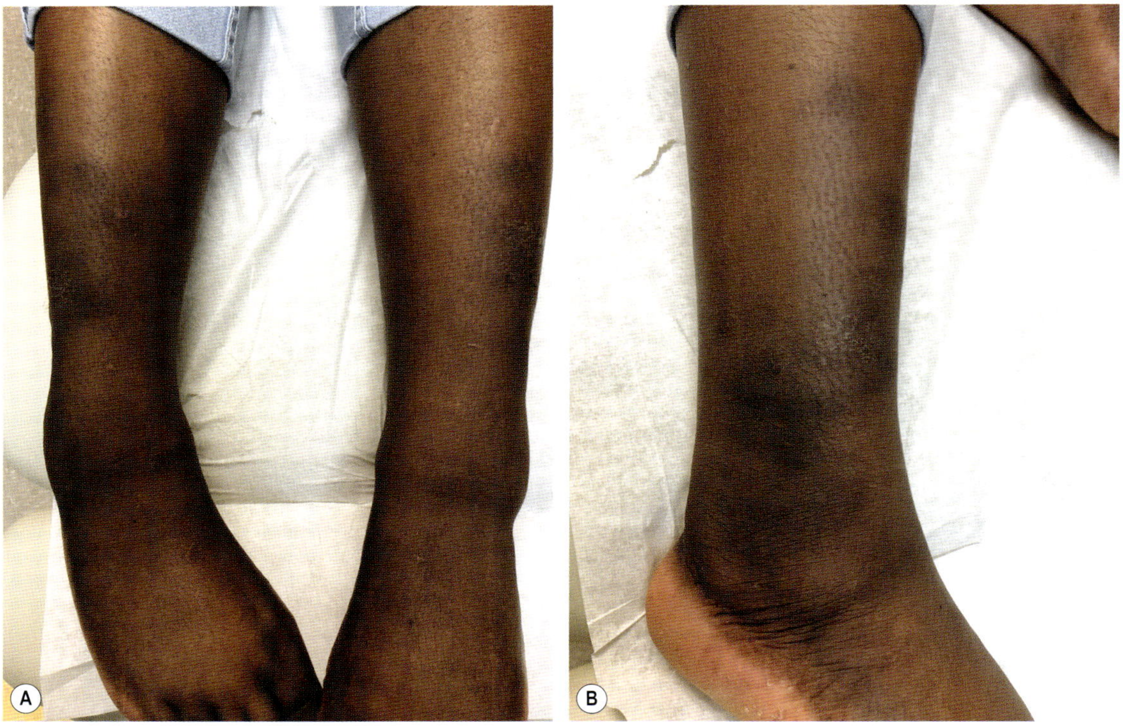

Fig. 23.1 Pretibial myxedema. Hyperpigmented, nodular plaques on the anterior and lateral tibial surfaces of a Black female with Graves disease **(A)**. Note the dilated hair follicles and peau d'orange appearance in some regions **(B)**. (Courtesy Sarah Adams, MD.)

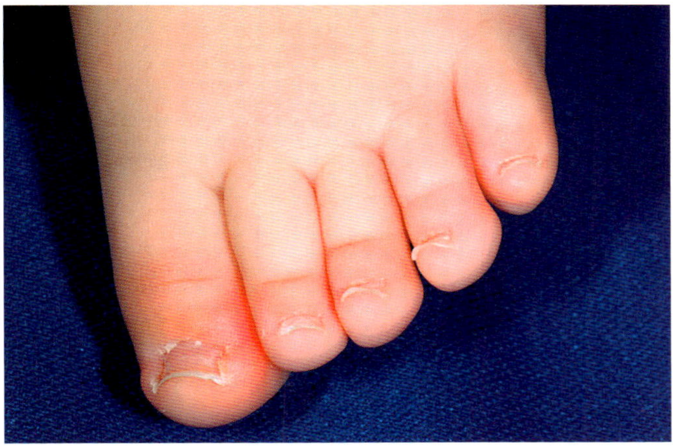

Fig. 23.2 Koilonychia. These spoon-shaped nails may occur in disease states (such as hyperthyroidism) or as a normal variant in young children, as in this infant.

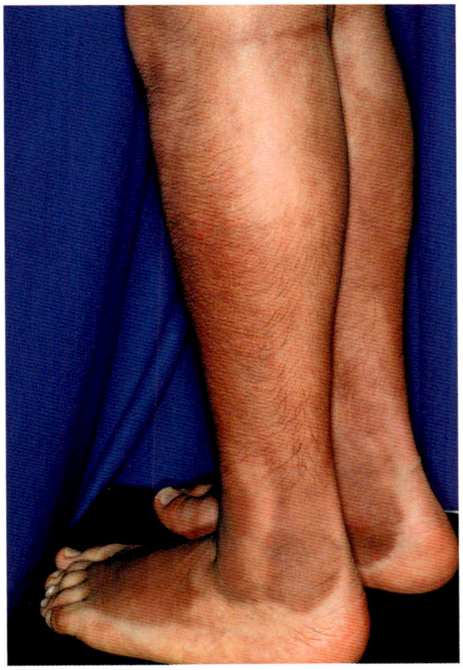

Fig. 23.3 Hyperpigmentation of hyperthyroidism. Diffuse hyperpigmentation of the lower extremities was present in this young Hispanic female with Graves disease.

of calcium and phosphorus metabolism, and associated abnormalities manifest distinctive clinical patterns. Parathyroid hormone (PTH) is one of the two main calciotropic hormones (the other one being calcitriol); these hormones regulate phosphate and calcium homeostasis.

HYPERPARATHYROIDISM

Primary hyperparathyroidism, one of the least common endocrine disorders of infancy and childhood, is rarely diagnosed in children younger than 16 years of age. When seen, it is usually the result of a familial, genetically determined hyperplasia of the parathyroid, which may present as an isolated hyperparathyroidism or as the hyperparathyroidism–jaw tumor syndrome, in which case ossifying tumors of the maxilla or mandible are present.[15] A malignant neoplasm of the parathyroid or an association with some other disease, such as is seen in patients with multiple endocrine adenomatosis (multiple endocrine

Box 23.2 **Mucocutaneous Manifestations of Hypothyroidism**

Dry, coarse, pale, cool skin
Dull, brittle hair with thinning
Cutis marmorata
Generalized myxedema (especially hands, feet, periorbital)
Carotenoderma
Nail changes (ridged, brittle, grow slowly)
Alopecia (diffuse, lateral eyebrows)
Hypertrichosis (back and shoulders usually)
Easy bruising
Ichthyosis
Eruptive or tuberous xanthomas
Livedo reticularis
Periorbital edema
Dermatitis herpetiformis (has been reported with Hashimoto thyroiditis, atrophic variant)
Protuberant lips
Macroglossia
Urticaria
Pruritus

Box 23.3 **Clinical Features of Congenital Hypothyroidism**

Puffy (myxedematous) facies
Sallow complexion
Wide anterior fontanel and sutures
Macroglossia and thick lips
Hypertelorism, depressed nasal bridge
Coarse, brittle hair
Hoarse cry
Translucent ("alabaster") ears
Umbilical hernia and abdominal distention
Heart murmur
Hypotonia and slow reflexes
Short stubby fingers and broad hands
Short lower extremities
Scalp seborrhea, purpura
Prolonged relaxation phase of tendon reflexes
Cold, mottled, or jaundiced skin
Sluggishness and inactivity
Delayed motor development, mental retardation
Lack of coordination and ataxia
Poor weight gain, stunted growth
Subnormal body temperature, poor circulation, and intolerance to cold
Delayed/defective dentition
Myxedema (some cases)

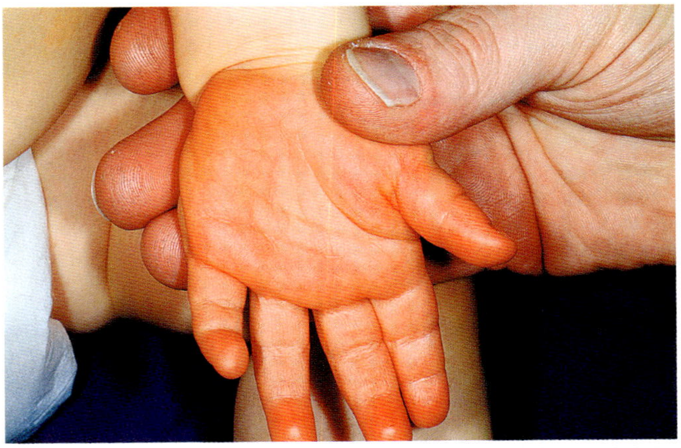

Fig. 23.4 Carotenemia. This yellow-orange skin coloration (carotenoderma) is especially prominent on the palms and soles. It may be seen in association with disease states (e.g., hypothyroidism) or with high intake of β-carotene-containing foods such as prepared baby foods containing orange vegetables, as in this healthy infant.

neoplasia [MEN]; see later) or chronic renal insufficiency, may also result in hyperparathyroidism.[16,17]

The majority of cases of hyperparathyroidism are sporadic, most often being caused by a single adenoma in the parathyroid gland. The clinical features of hyperparathyroidism include systemic effects of hypercalcemia: failure to thrive, muscular weakness, lethargy, anorexia, vomiting, fever, headache, constipation, weight loss, polydipsia, polyuria, mental retardation, metastatic calcification, and with marked hypercalcemia, stupor or death. Of these, metastatic calcification is the most common cutaneous manifestation, and in patients with sporadic hyperparathyroidism, this may be the only cutaneous finding. Hypercalcemia may also produce an ophthalmologic finding known as *band keratopathy*, which is the result of calcium and phosphate deposition beneath the Bowman capsule. Band keratopathy appears as a superficial corneal opacity resembling frosted or ground glass in a band-like configuration with white flecks or "holes" in the band resulting in a "Swiss cheese–like" appearance. It is not specific for hyperparathyroidism but may also be seen as a manifestation of hypercalcemia secondary to vitamin D intoxication, uremia, or sarcoidosis. It is not commonly found in patients with hyperparathyroidism when serum phosphorus levels are low and glomerular function is maintained.

Patients with chronic renal failure may experience several types of cutaneous manifestations. The skin of the patient with uremia may be pruritic, dry, scaly, sallow, and hyperpigmented; the sallow appearance is partially caused by anemia, and the hyperpigmentation appears to be the result of decreased renal clearance of melanocyte-stimulating hormone (MSH). Hyperparathyroidism secondary to chronic renal failure results from impaired synthesis of 1,25-dihydroxyvitamin D_3, which leads to hypocalcemia from impaired intestinal calcium absorption and, ultimately, increased levels of PTH. Hyperphosphatemia may result in a high serum calcium phosphate product and produce secondary calcification of the skin. This calcinosis cutis (see Chapter 9) manifests as hard calcium deposits in skin and subcutaneous tissues, especially in periarticular locations. These lesions may resolve spontaneously with correction of the serum calcium and phosphate levels. In addition to being seen in hyperparathyroidism, it may be noted in association with paraneoplastic hypercalcemia, milk alkali syndrome, sarcoidosis, and hypervitaminosis D. Calcinosis cutis has also been reported in the setting of *normocalcemic primary hyperparathyroidism*, in which case it represents preferential target organ deposition of calcium despite normal serum levels of calcium and phosphorus.[18]

When the calcification is more progressive and involves blood vessels, ischemic necrosis of skin and soft tissues occurs and is termed *calciphylaxis*. This rare (especially in children) and life-threatening condition results from vascular calcification and is most commonly reported in patients with end-stage renal disease. Clinically, it manifests as ecchymotic or infarcted areas of skin, bullous lesions, and plaques of calcinosis with periodic extrusion of calcium. Lesions of pediatric calciphylaxis are most commonly noted on the upper and lower extremities.[19] They are very painful, and mortality related to gangrene and sepsis is high. Extensive calcification in the heart and lungs may result in cardiorespiratory failure.[20] Parathyroidectomy is often, but not always, useful in this setting.[21–23] Histologically, calciphylaxis shows calcification of the walls of small and medium-sized blood vessels in the dermis and subcuticular regions.

The diagnosis of hyperparathyroidism is established by consistent elevations of total serum calcium above 12 mg/dL, the reduction of serum phosphorus concentrations below 4 mg/dL, and elevated levels of PTH. High alkaline–phosphatase levels usually indicate bone disease. This complication of hyperparathyroidism may be demonstrated radiographically by generalized demineralization of bones, destructive changes at the growing ends of long bones, subperiosteal erosions (particularly in the phalanges, metacarpals, and lateral portions of the clavicles), and in more advanced disease, generalized rarefaction, cysts, tumors, fractures, and deformities. Radiographs of the abdomen may reveal renal calculi or nephrocalcinosis, and ultrasonography and radioisotope scanning can confirm the diagnosis of primary hyperparathyroidism associated with an isolated parathyroid adenoma. In infants with parathyroid hyperplasia, cupping and fraying at the ends of long bones and ribs may suggest rickets, and severe demineralization and pathologic fractures are common.

HYPOPARATHYROIDISM/DIGEORGE SYNDROME

Hypoparathyroidism is characterized by hypocalcemia and inappropriate response of the parathyroid glands or, less often, with elevated PTH levels and lack of response to the hormone (see Pseudohypoparathyroidism/Albright Hereditary Osteodystrophy section). In childhood, hypoparathyroidism may develop as a congenital idiopathic disorder but usually appears in the neonatal period, in later infancy, or during childhood or as an acute condition after inadvertent removal or damage of the parathyroid glands during thyroid surgery. Congenital hypoparathyroidism may occur alone; may be seen as an autoimmune disorder, where it may occur alone or with other endocrine disorders; or may be a hereditary condition associated with an increased familial incidence of other endocrinologic disorders (Addison disease, pernicious anemia, and Hashimoto thyroiditis), candidiasis, and/or vitiligo. When associated with hypoplasia of the thymus and immunologic defects, the condition is known as *DiGeorge syndrome* (see later).

Idiopathic or congenital hypoparathyroidism usually first manifests with tetany or seizures and in 25% to 50% of patients, ectodermal defects. The skin of affected individuals is rough, dry, thick, and scaly; the hair and eyebrows are sparse; and the nails are short and thin with brittleness, crumbling, or longitudinal grooving. When hypoparathyroidism occurs during tooth development, pitting, ridging, absence of dental enamel, and absence or hypoplasia of the permanent teeth may result. Extensive calcification of skin and subcutaneous tissues has been reported in an infant with congenital primary hypoparathyroidism, although this is exceedingly rare.[24] Other clinical manifestations include convulsions, carpopedal spasm, muscle cramps and twitching, numbness or tingling of the extremities, laryngospasm or bronchospasm, exfoliative dermatitis, mental retardation, chronic diarrhea (especially in infants), photophobia, keratoconjunctivitis, blepharospasm, and cataracts. Mucocutaneous candidiasis is seen as a complication in 15% of patients with idiopathic hypoparathyroidism. Electrocardiography may reveal prolongation of the QT interval, and head imaging may show calcifications of the basal ganglia.[15] The combination of candidiasis, endocrinopathy, and ectodermal dysplasia has been termed *autoimmune polyendocrinopathy, candidiasis, and ectodermal dystrophy (APECED)* as well as *autoimmune polyglandular syndrome (APS) type 1* or *autoimmune polyendocrinopathy syndrome type 1* and is discussed in more detail in the section Autoimmune Polyglandular Syndromes (see also Chapter 17).

The cutaneous manifestations of hypoparathyroidism associated with surgical removal or injury of the parathyroid glands differ from those seen in patients with idiopathic or congenital hypoparathyroidism. These include thinning or loss of hair, the development of horizontal grooves (Beau lines) in the nails, or a complete loss of nails after episodes of tetany (these abnormalities revert to normal when hypocalcemia is controlled). Hyperpigmentation (predominantly on the face and distal extremities) may resemble melasma, pellagra, or Addison disease and also may occur in cases of postthyroidectomy hypoparathyroidism. Although cutaneous calcification has been noted, this complication is relatively uncommon. In a series of 21 patients with acquired hypoparathyroidism, the most common cutaneous manifestations were hair loss (especially axillary and pubic), coarsening of body hair, and dry skin.[25]

DiGeorge syndrome is a T-cell deficiency disorder that develops as a result of faulty embryologic development of the thymus and the parathyroid glands (a congenital malformation of the third and fourth pharyngeal pouches and the surrounding arches). The classic triad consists of cardiac malformation, hypocalcemia, and T-cell immunodeficiency. Defects of the great vessels may include truncus arteriosus, interrupted aortic arch, double aortic arch, or aberrant subclavian artery. Oral candidiasis is an almost constant finding in patients with this disorder, and overwhelming fungal, viral, or bacterial infection may lead to death early in infancy. Hypocalcemia and tetany may occur at an early age, and other features include chronic diarrhea, interstitial pneumonia, failure to thrive, micrognathia, hypertelorism, low-set ears, bifid uvula, shortened philtrum, bowed mouth, chronic purulent rhinitis, mental retardation, calcification of the central nervous system, and nephrocalcinosis.[26]

DiGeorge syndrome is associated with a deletion in the long arm of chromosome 22 and is also referred to as *22q11.2 deletion syndrome*

(22q11DS) or *velocardiofacial syndrome.*[27] The candidate gene for this disorder is termed *TBX1*, which encodes the T-box transcription factor 1. Approximately half of patients with DiGeorge syndrome are hemizygous for 22q11, and they have occasionally been found to have overlapping deletions in the 10p13/14 boundary.[28,29] These patients are at increased risk for developing psychiatric disorders, with one in four developing schizophrenia and one in six developing major depressive disorders.[30] Other reported psychiatric morbidities include attention-deficit/hyperactivity disorder, oppositional defiant disorder, and anxiety disorders.[31] Patients with 22q11DS may have varying rates of intellectual disability, especially with regard to visuospatial memory, face processing, and attention.[32] Camptodactyly (fixed flexion of the proximal interphalangeal joints) may be a feature.[33] When the immunodeficiency is severe, thymic or bone marrow transplantation should be considered.[34]

PSEUDOHYPOPARATHYROIDISM/ALBRIGHT HEREDITARY OSTEODYSTROPHY

Pseudohypoparathyroidism (PHP) is a hereditary disorder in which there is decreased target tissue responsiveness in the receptor tissues, particularly the kidneys and skeletal system, to PTH (rather than a true deficiency). PHP is subclassified into types Ia, Ib, Ic, and type II (which involves a different mechanism of resistance to PTH). *Albright hereditary osteodystrophy (AHO)* refers to PHP in conjunction with a clinical constellation of physical features, including short stature, central obesity, brachydactyly, ectopic ossification, and variable degrees of mental retardation.[35,36]

Pseudopseudohypoparathyroidism (PPHP) is a term used to describe individuals with AHO who have normal end-organ responsiveness to PTH. These patients do not develop hypocalcemia and tetany. PHP and PPHP are caused by different types of mutations in the *GNAS* gene, and the presence of genetic imprinting may lead to quite diverse clinical phenotypes.[35,37] Specifically, maternal inactivating mutations result in PHP-Ia, whereas paternal inactivating mutations result in PPHP and the disorder progressive osseous heteroplasia (POH), a disease of severe heterotopic ossifications of the subcutaneous tissues, skeletal muscles, and deep connective tissues (see Chapter 9).[36] This observation suggests that expression of the guanine nucleotide regulatory protein (Gsα) from the paternal and maternal alleles is not equivalent in the various tissues which depend on this hormonal mediation.[38]

Patients with PHP have hypocalcemia, hyperphosphatemia, and elevated serum levels of PTH. Hypothyroidism secondary to TSH resistance may be seen in PHP-Ia. Patients may also display resistance to other hormones, including gonadotropins and growth hormone (GH)–releasing hormone.[39] Ectopic calcification is common, and intracranial lesions usually involve the basal ganglia and occasionally other regions. Calcinosis cutis may occur and presents with multiple small papules, plaques, or nodules with a predilection for the scalp, hands and feet, periarticular regions, and chest wall.[40] Soft-tissue ossification (osteoma cutis) may be present at birth or develop during infancy or childhood (Fig. 23.5) and is often a presenting feature of the disease, along with hypothyroidism.[41] The subcutaneous calcifications or ossifications may occasionally present very early in life (even by 2 weeks of age) and in those patients (Fig. 23.6) may be vital to early recognition and diagnosis of PHP.[42] Dermal or subcutaneous hypoplasia may occasionally be noted in areas of cutaneous calcification.[43]

The characteristic features of AHO include short stature, obesity, and characteristic facial features, including round face, flat nasal bridge, and a short neck. Brachymetaphalangism refers to shortening of the fourth and fifth metacarpals and may be recognized by knuckle dimples when the patient makes a clenched fist.[40] In addition, the fourth and fifth fingers and toes may appear shortened (Fig. 23.7).[44] Plain radiography may confirm this feature when the clinical findings are subtle. Mental retardation may be present and may be less common with aggressive and early treatment for the hypocalcemia.

Disorders of the Adrenal Glands

Adrenal gland dysfunction may result in a variety of systemic effects with various cutaneous manifestations. Those of particular interest to the pediatrician, dermatologist, and pediatric dermatologist are

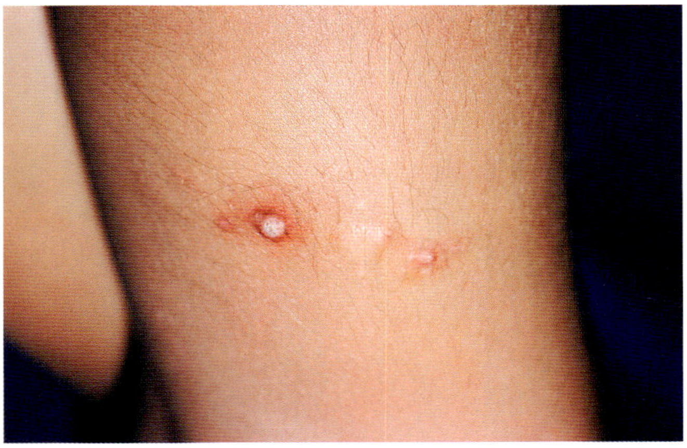

Fig. 23.5 Osteoma cutis. These rock-hard papulonodules revealed ectopic ossification microscopically.

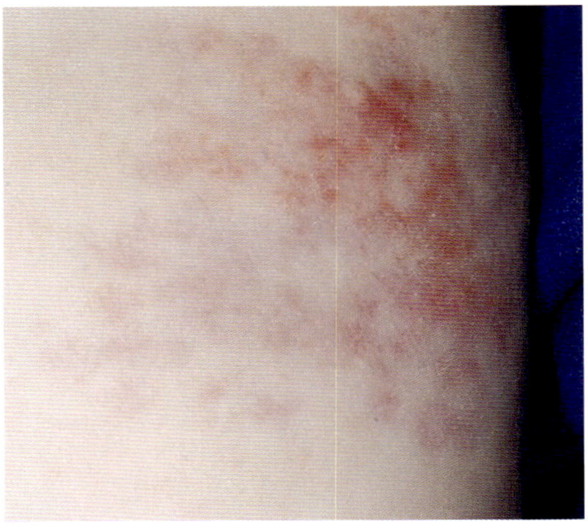

Fig. 23.6 Osteoma cutis. This red plaque developed at 2 months of age in this male infant. Several nodular firm areas were noted upon palpation, and skin biopsy revealed changes of osteoma cutis. He was subsequently found to have a mutation in *GNAS1* consistent with Albright hereditary osteodystrophy.

Addison disease, Cushing syndrome (CS), and adrenogenital syndrome (discussed under Disorders of Androgen Excess).

ADDISON DISEASE

Addison disease (primary adrenal insufficiency) is caused by the absence of glucocorticoids and mineralocorticoids despite an increased concentration of adrenocorticotropic hormone (ACTH) and is characterized by weakness, anorexia, weight loss, hypotension, decreased serum sodium and chloride, increased serum potassium, hypoglycemia, and hyperpigmentation of the skin and mucous membranes. Sporadic and recurrent "flu-like" episodes may provide a clinical clue to the diagnosis, especially in the setting of pigmentary alterations.[45] Hyperpigmentation in Addison disease is the result of increased production of proopiomelanocortin, which is cleaved to form MSH and ACTH.[46] This overproduction in the pituitary gland occurs as a compensatory phenomenon associated with decreased cortisol production by the adrenal glands. The hyperpigmentation of Addison disease occurs in the setting of primary adrenocortical failure, as opposed to secondary adrenal insufficiency, in which case ACTH levels are low and mineralocorticoid production remains relatively intact.[47]

The pigmentation of Addison disease is most intense in the flexures, at sites of pressure and friction, in the creases of the palms and soles

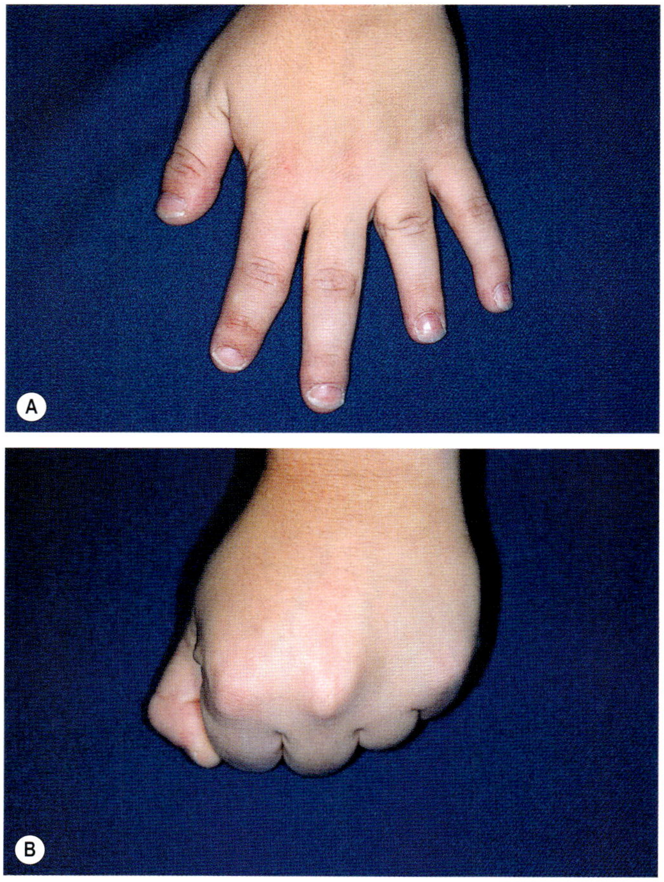

Fig. 23.7 (A) Brachymetaphalangism in a girl with pseudohypoparathyroidism, with shortened fourth and fifth metacarpals. **(B)** The "knuckle, knuckle, dimple, dimple" sign when she makes a fist. (Reprinted with permission from Schachner LA, Hansen RC, editors. *Pediatric Dermatology*. 3rd ed. Edinburgh, Scotland: Mosby; 2003.)

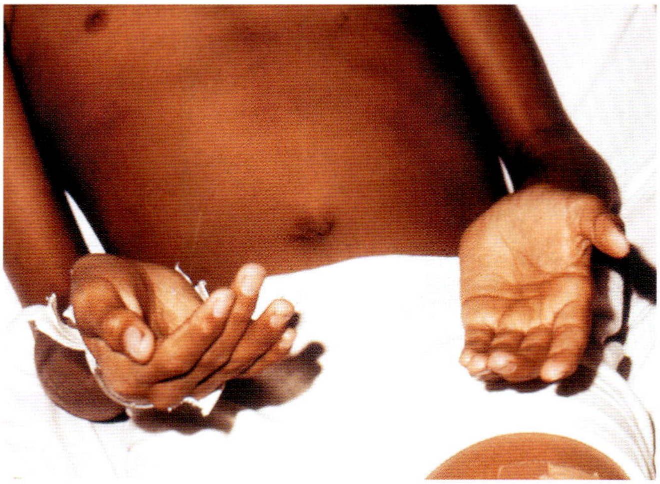

Fig. 23.8 Hyperpigmentation of Addison disease. Increased pigmentation of the palmar creases in this male with Addison disease. (Courtesy Anne Lucky, MD.)

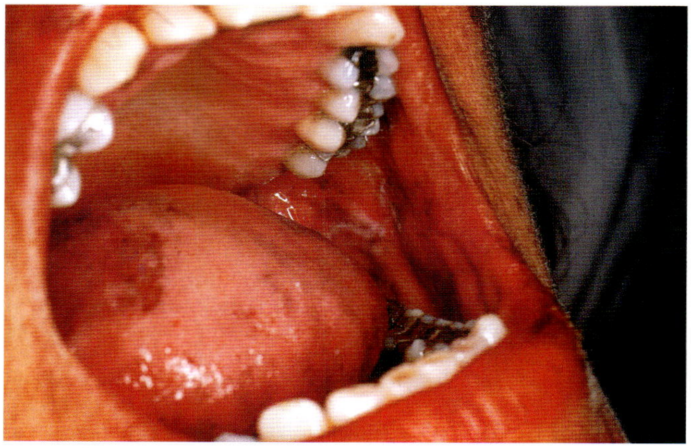

Fig. 23.9 Oral mucosa pigmentation of Addison disease. Note hyperpigmentation of the tongue and buccal mucosa in this patient with Addison disease.

(Fig. 23.8), in the nails, in sun-exposed areas, and in normally hyperpigmented areas such as the genitalia and areolae. Pigmentation of the conjunctivae and vaginal mucous membranes is common, and pigmentary changes of the oral mucosae (Fig. 23.9) include spotty or streaked blue-black to brown hyperpigmentation of the gingivae, tongue (Fig. 23.10), hard palate, and buccal mucosa. In addition, increased pigmentation may be noted in existing nevi.[48] The pigmentation may be quite diffuse in some children.[45] Labial pigmentation and longitudinal pigmentary streaks of the fingernails similar to those in Laugier–Hunziker syndrome have been observed.[49] Because the pigmentation may in some cases be subtle, comparison of the patient to other family members may be useful in highlighting the clinical findings.[47] In one series of 18 pediatric patients with primary adrenal insufficiency at one institution, 12 (67%) exhibited cutaneous hyperpigmentation.[50] Primary adrenal insufficiency without hyperpigmentation has been reported and may result in a delay in the diagnosis of Addison disease.[51] Loss of body hair may be another cutaneous finding in this disorder.

The diagnosis of chronic adrenocortical insufficiency is suggested by the clinical features and confirmed by serum electrolyte studies and cortisol level determinations after stimulation by ACTH (the ACTH stimulation test). A morning serum cortisol ("AM cortisol") level is a convenient and simple test but may be insensitive as a screening tool.[47] There are multiple potential causes of Addison disease, including adrenal dysgenesis (which may be related to a variety of genetic mutations), diseases resulting in adrenal destruction, or impaired steroidogenesis (disorders of cholesterol or steroid biosynthesis, including several forms of congenital adrenal hypoplasia). Although the majority of cases of Addison disease in the past century were attributed to tuberculosis, autoimmune disease currently accounts for most cases presenting outside of the newborn period.[52] APS types 1 and 2 may both present with this disorder as one component. Other nonautoimmune causes include infection, metabolic and infiltrative or metastatic diseases, and drug-induced damage.[53] The incidence of Addison disease is elevated in vitiligo probands and their first-degree relatives.[54] When these two disorders occur concurrently, patients may have a striking presentation of hypopigmentation and hyperpigmentation.

CUSHING SYNDROME

CS is a rare disorder caused by long-term glucocorticoid excess, which may be caused by a variety of different etiologies. It is divided into ACTH-dependent types (including pituitary-dependent Cushing disease, ectopic ACTH syndrome, and adrenal hyperplasia) and non-ACTH-dependent types (including adrenal adenoma, adrenal carcinoma, and adrenal hyperplasia).[55] The most common form is pituitary-dependent bilateral adrenal hyperplasia, termed *Cushing disease*. Endogenous CS is fairly uncommon in children, and the lack of classic features of hypercortisolism in pediatric patients may delay diagnosis and treatment. In all patients with CS, there is loss of diurnal variation of ACTH and cortisol secretion, which leads to sustained hypercortisolism.[56] Growth retardation to complete linear growth arrest is the hallmark of the disease in children and growing adolescents, although in a large review of children with CS, the majority had normal or advanced skeletal maturation.[57,58] CS may also result from the systemic administration of exogenous glucocorticoids (including oral, parenteral, or, rarely, topical) or ACTH and should be suspected by the findings of suppressed ACTH and cortisol with no response to corticotropin-releasing hormone (CRH) or ACTH, respectively.[55] CS has occurred after intralesional corticosteroid injections for keloids in a child.[59] The authors have observed CS in a few children after topical application of ultrapotent corticosteroids for extensive alopecia areata/totalis and severe atopic dermatitis. Neonatal CS is rare and may be associated with adrenocortical tumors or genetic syndromes, including Li–Fraumeni, McCune–Albright, or Beckwith–Wiedemann syndromes.[60] A variety of genetic causes of (and syndromic associations with) CS are being identified.[61]

The clinical findings in CS are multiple and usually suggest the presence of hypercortisolism. Noncutaneous signs and symptoms include truncal obesity, diminution of the linear growth rate, diabetes mellitus or glucose intolerance, gonadal dysfunction, hypertension (in around 50% of patients), muscle weakness, fatigue, mood disorders, sleep disturbances, menstrual irregularities, osteoporosis, delayed or accelerated bone age, edema, polydipsia, polyuria, and fungal infections.[55,62,63] The typical growth chart in a child with CS reveals a severely diminished linear growth curve, with continued weight gain across percentiles. This is in distinction to the growth chart in a child with exogenous obesity, which reveals increasing linear growth.[64,65]

The cutaneous features of CS are listed in Box 23.4. Addison disease–like pigmentation (particularly on the face and neck) has been noted in 6% to 10% of patients and is seen primarily in the ACTH-dependent forms of the disease. Other skin findings include a characteristic plethoric "moon" facies with telangiectasias over the cheeks; increased fine lanugo hair on the face and extremities; purplish striae (stretch marks, see later) at points of tension such as the lower abdomen, flanks, thighs, buttocks, upper arms, and breasts; fragility of dermal blood vessels with an increased tendency toward bruising at sites of minimal trauma; poor wound healing; and steroid acne. The latter usually presents as red papules or small pustules distributed primarily on the upper trunk (Fig. 23.11), arms, neck, and to a lesser degree, the face. Temporal scalp hair regression may be present.[66] There is a tendency to develop cutaneous fungal infections (e.g., tinea corporis, onychomycosis, candidiasis, pityriasis versicolor), and disseminated mycobacterial infection has been reported.[67] Patients with CS classically have fatty deposits over the back of the neck, termed the *buffalo hump* (Fig. 23.12).

CS is diagnosed based on suspicious clinical findings and the results of laboratory testing. A 24-hour urinary free-cortisol test is a widely used assay for diagnosing hypercortisolism and has a very high specificity and sensitivity.[55,56] Other diagnostic studies include plasma cortisol measurement (limited by diurnal variation), low-dose dexamethasone suppression test (excellent sensitivity but requires overnight hospitalization), high-dose dexamethasone suppression test, ACTH measurement (useful for discriminating between ACTH-dependent and ACTH-independent forms), late night salivary cortisol measurement, inferior petrosal sinus sampling, and the CRH stimulation test.[56,68,69] Radiographic imaging may be useful for assessing for pituitary or adrenal tumors. The treatment options for CS depend on the etiology and may include transsphenoidal pituitary surgery, external pituitary radiotherapy, excisional surgery (adrenal tumors), and mitotane (an adrenocytolytic agent). With the exception of striae, the cutaneous effects of CS most often completely heal after successful therapy.[70] After treatment, glucocorticoid replacement and stress dosing of cortisol are often required.

Box 23.4 Cutaneous Features of Cushing Syndrome

- Facial plethora and telangiectasias
- Hirsutism, fine lanugo hair growth
- Violaceous striae (especially over the abdomen, flanks, and upper arms)
- Acne
- Bruising
- Poor wound healing
- Skin atrophy
- Thin, translucent skin
- Hyperpigmentation (seen only in ACTH-dependent form)
- Acanthosis nigricans
- Frequent fungal infections (e.g., tinea corporis, pityriasis versicolor, candidiasis)
- Male-pattern alopecia (in females)

ACTH, Adrenocorticotropic hormone.

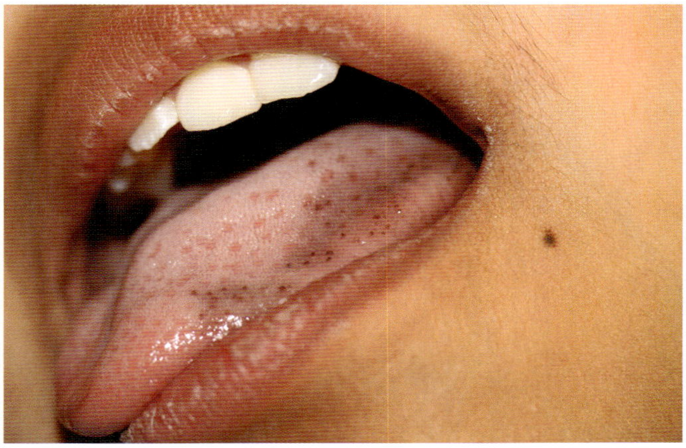

Fig. 23.10 Tongue pigmentation in adrenal insufficiency. Note the hyperpigmented papillae (and flattening of dorsal papillae) in this teenaged female with a history of adrenal insufficiency caused by familial glucocorticoid deficiency.

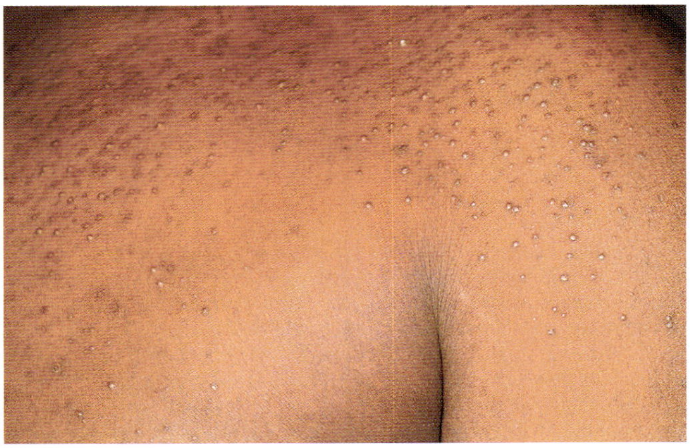

Fig. 23.11 Steroid acne. Erythematous papules and papulopustules on the chest and upper arms.

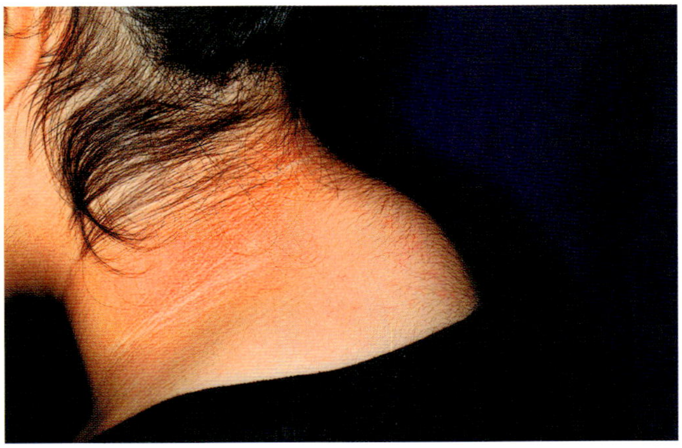

Fig. 23.12 Buffalo hump. This finding consisting of fatty deposits over the posterior neck and upper back may be associated with either endogenous or exogenous Cushing syndrome.

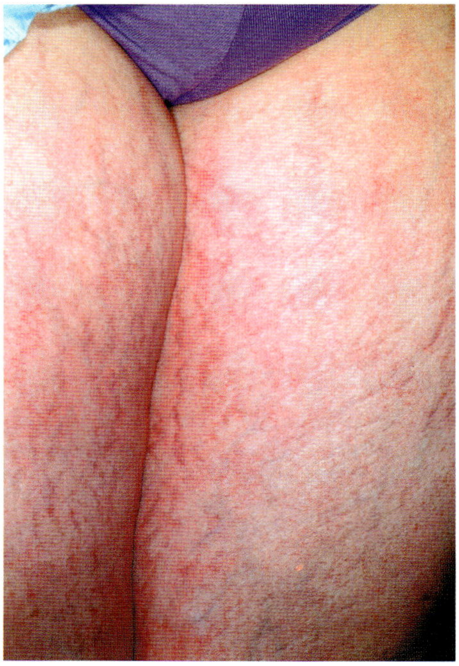

Fig. 23.13 Striae distensae. These early lesions appear as pink, linear depressions in the skin.

Striae distensae (stretch marks), mentioned earlier, are linear depressions of the skin that are initially pink (Fig. 23.13) or purple and later become more flesh-colored, translucent, and atrophic (Fig. 23.14). They are most commonly seen in areas subject to stretching such as the lower back, buttocks, thighs, breasts, abdomen, and shoulders. Striae may develop physiologically in up to 35% of girls and 15% of boys between the ages of 9 and 16 years. Causes of striae include stretching exercises, rapid growth, obesity, adolescence, pregnancy, CS, and prolonged use of systemic or potent topical corticosteroids. They may be seen in patients with anorexia nervosa, mainly the restrictive (vs. the bulimic) form.[71] They can occasionally be mistaken for nonaccidental injury or physical abuse.[72] Although the precise cause of striae is unknown, their formation appears to be related to stress-induced rupture of connective tissue, alteration of collagen and elastin, and dermal scarring in which glucocorticoids suppress fibroblastic activity and newly synthesized collagen fills the gaps between ruptured collagen fibers.[73] Elastic fibers are fine in early lesions and thickened in older lesions of striae.[74] Treatment of striae is challenging, and most therapies are generally unsatisfactory.

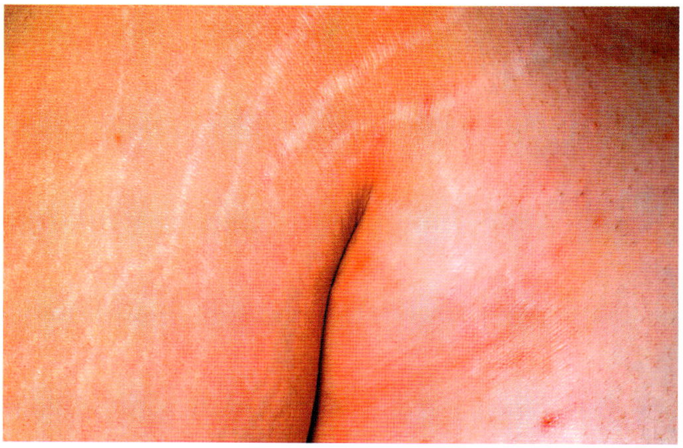

Fig. 23.14 Striae distensae. These older lesions appear as flesh-colored, linear, atrophic bands.

Many of the lesions that occur during adolescence tend to become less noticeable with time. It has been suggested that topical tretinoin cream may be helpful for some patients, although the results are mixed. Other topical agents reportedly effective in some patients include glycolic and trichloroacetic acid peels and topical hyaluronic acid preparations.[75] The flashlamp-pumped pulsed-dye laser has also been used for treating these lesions, but data suggest that this modality should be reserved for patients with the more fair skin phenotypes (types II to IV).[76–78] Other treatment modalities that have been reported for striae include intense pulsed light, excimer laser, copper–bromide laser, fractional photothermolysis, and microdermabrasion.[75,79,80]

Disorders of Androgen Excess

Patients with androgen excess may initially present with a variety of skin-related conditions, including hirsutism, acne, and alopecia. Hyperandrogenism may be related to benign or malignant ovarian, testicular, or adrenal tumors; functional overproduction of androgens by the adrenal glands or ovaries; or exogenous androgens. The clinical findings of hyperandrogenism may vary depending on the pubertal development of the child, and these are summarized in Box 23.5. The two disorders to be discussed in this section are congenital adrenal hyperplasia (CAH) and polycystic ovary syndrome (PCOS).

A brief mention of exogenous androgen excess is in order, in light of the expanding US market for testosterone-replacement therapies. These products are the standard of care for androgen deficiency and are available as depot injectables, subcutaneously implanted pellets, transdermal patches, topical gels, and buccal tablets.[81] Inadvertent drug transfer to spouses and/or children (secondary exposure) may occur in association with use of the topical agents and may present with precocious puberty in young children or virilization in exposed adult females.[81–83] Although skin-to-skin contact is presumed to be the primary mode of transfer, spread via shared linens may also be possible. These reports highlight the importance of adequate education in contact precautions when topical androgens are prescribed, as well as vigilance on the part of pediatric practitioners, with recognition of this potential cause for precocious puberty. The US Food and Drug Administration (FDA) added a boxed warning about the risks of secondary transfer to topical testosterone product labels in 2009.[84]

CONGENITAL ADRENAL HYPERPLASIA

CAH (also known as *adrenogenital syndrome*) is a term used to describe a constellation of diseases characterized by impaired steroid metabolism in the adrenal cortex, which is caused by mutations in genes that encode enzymes in pathways involved in cortisol biosynthesis. The most common cause of CAH is 21-hydroxylase (21OH) deficiency, and

Box 23.5 Clinical Features of Hyperandrogenism

Prepubertal

Precocious sexual development:
- Sex appropriate (males)
- Sex inappropriate (females)

Rapid linear growth
Accelerated bone age
Axillary and pubic hair development
Acne
Hirsutism
Neonate:
- Hyperpigmentation of the genitalia
- Ambiguous genitalia

Postpubertal

Acne
Hirsutism
Androgenetic alopecia
Amenorrhea or irregular menses
Infertility
Other virilizing signs (deep voice, increased muscle mass, male habitus)
Early cardiovascular disease

other enzymes that may be defective include 11 β-hydroxylase (11βOH), 17 α-hydroxylase (17OH), steroidogenic acute regulatory protein (StAR), P450 cholesterol side-chain cleavage enzyme (SCC), P450 oxidoreductase (POR), and 3 β-hydroxysteroid dehydrogenase type 2 (3βHSD2).[85,86] 21-hydroxylase deficiency occurs in about 1 in 10,000 to 1 in 15,000 live births worldwide.[87] It is inherited in an autosomal recessive fashion, and the gene *(CYP21A2)* is located in the human leukocyte antigen (HLA) class III region on the short arm of chromosome 6p.[88,89] Due to the defect in cortisol synthesis, the adrenal cortex in these disorders is stimulated by corticotropin, and overproduction of cortisol precursors occurs, some of which are diverted toward synthesis of sex hormones. This androgen excess leads to clinical signs of hyperandrogenism, and concomitant aldosterone deficiency may result in salt wasting, failure to thrive, hypovolemia, and in some cases, shock.[90]

One of the most classic presenting features of female children with CAH (21-hydroxylase deficiency) is ambiguous genitalia (Fig. 23.15). Because of exposure to high systemic levels of adrenal androgens during gestation, affected girls are born with a large clitoris, rugated and partially fused labia majora, and a common urogenital sinus in place of a separate urethra and vagina.[90] The degree of virilization is variable and may range from simple clitoromegaly to the appearance of a penile urethra. In severe forms, important features in distinguishing the virilized female genitalia from true male genitalia include the absence of testicles and the presence of normal internal sex organs.[91]

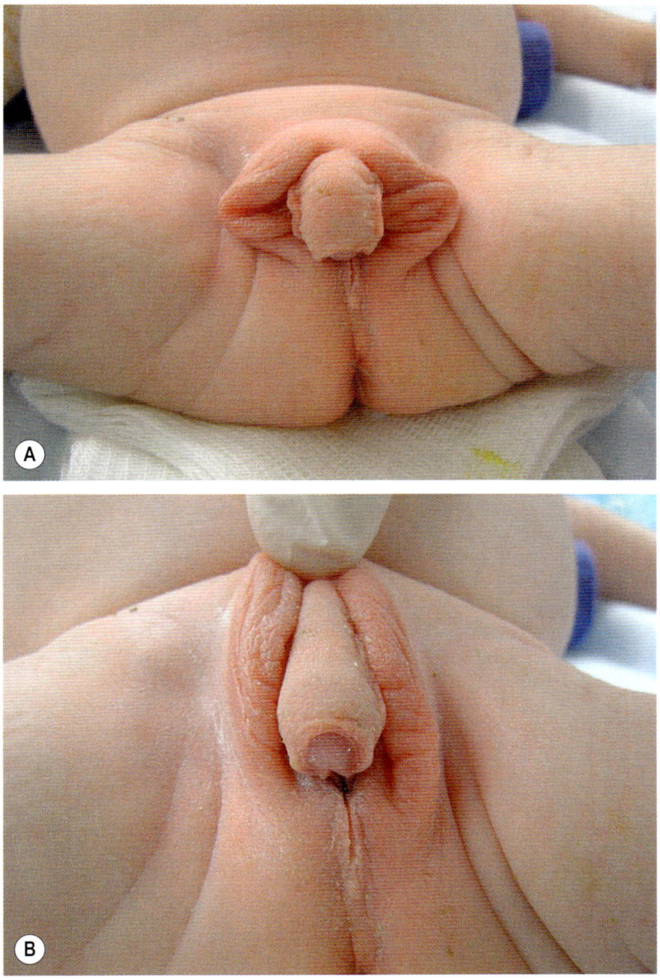

Fig. 23.15 Congenital adrenal hyperplasia. This newborn has ambiguous genitalia. Note the marked clitoral enlargement (resembling a penis), the rugated and partially fused labia majorae **(A)**, and the common opening between the vagina and the urethra (urogenital sinus) **(B)**. (Courtesy Marleta Reynolds, MD.)

Affected boys may have no obvious physical signs of the disorder, although subtle hyperpigmentation and/or penile enlargement may be present. Some forms of CAH, such as 17 α-hydroxylase/17,20-lyase deficiency, may result in ambiguous or female-appearing external genitalia in males, identical to androgen insensitivity syndrome.[92]

In patients who are not treated or in whom therapy is inadequate, long-term exposure to these androgens results in rapid somatic growth, advanced skeletal age, and premature development of secondary sexual characteristics, including development of pubic and axillary hair, clitoral growth, and penile growth in males. Although linear growth may be accelerated during childhood, these patients often ultimately have short stature because of premature epiphyseal closure. Centrally mediated precocious puberty may occur. Hirsutism is a common feature in patients with nonclassic (partial) 21-hydroxylase deficiency, and when menstrual irregularity and acne also occur, the presentation may simulate that of PCOS (see later). Patients with nonclassic CAH do not have ambiguous genitalia at birth and usually have premature adrenarche and advanced skeletal maturation.[93]

Abnormalities of reproductive function are common in CAH, and infertility is often present. Affected males have fewer problems with reproductive function. Salt wasting is seen in up to 75% of patients with classic 21-hydroxylase deficiency due to decreased synthesis of aldosterone. These patients are prone to hyponatremia, hyperkalemia, hypovolemia, dehydration, and shock. Hyperpigmentation, most notably of skin creases and the genitalia, may occur as an early sign of adrenal insufficiency. Classic 21-hydroxylase deficiency is diagnosed by the finding of markedly elevated levels of serum 17-hydroxyprogesterone, the main substrate for the enzyme; this is the measurement utilized in newborn screening protocols. Second-tier screening with liquid chromatography–mass spectrometry/mass spectrometry (LC-MS/MS) can be used to measure a panel of steroids.[86] The cosyntropin (corticotropin) stimulation test is useful for differentiating this disorder from other steroidogenic enzyme defects. Molecular-based genetic testing is available for CAH, and prenatal diagnosis is possible using chorionic villus and amniotic fluid cells for deoxyribonucleic acid (DNA) analysis.[94] Fetal DNA harvested from maternal plasma has also been investigated as a noninvasive approach to prenatal diagnosis. Management for CAH consists of glucocorticoid (with stress dosing during times of intercurrent illness) and mineralocorticoid replacement, supplemental sodium chloride, and surgical management of ambiguous genitalia, which is traditionally recommended between 2 and 6 months of life.[90] However, in recent years, some advocacy groups and physicians have recommended delaying surgery for patients with disorders of sex development (DSD), so that the patients themselves can be involved in medical decision-making when older. There appears to be no consensus regarding the indications, timing, and postsurgical evaluations for DSD surgery, suggesting a need for further collaborative prospective studies and multidisciplinary centers of expertise.[95] When the diagnosis is known, dexamethasone administered to the mother before the ninth week of gestation may prevent the development of genital ambiguity.[96]

POLYCYSTIC OVARY SYNDROME

PCOS (also called *Stein–Leventhal syndrome*) is the most common androgen disorder of ovarian function[97] and among the most common endocrine disorders in women.[98] It is estimated to affect between 6% and 15% of women, depending on the diagnostic criteria utilized. Patients with PCOS have increased androgen production and disordered gonadotropin secretion, resulting in amenorrhea or severe oligomenorrhea, increased testosterone levels, and enlarged polycystic ovaries on ultrasound examination. Women with PCOS also have metabolic derangements related to insulin resistance and an increased risk of type 2 diabetes mellitus. The hormonal dysregulation seen in PCOS usually begins during adolescence.[99] The pathophysiology of PCOS is multifactorial, and it has been found to cluster in families with a history of PCOS, non–insulin-dependent diabetes mellitus (NIDDM), cardiovascular disease, and breast cancer.[100]

Three sets of diagnostic criteria have been utilized for adult women, including the 1990 National Institutes of Health criteria (which requires chronic oligoovulation plus clinical or biochemical signs of hyperandrogenism); the 2003 Rotterdam criteria (which requires two of three criteria: chronic oligoovulation or anovulation, clinical or biochemical signs of hyperandrogenism, and polycystic ovaries); and the criteria of the Androgen Excess-PCOS Society (which defines PCOS as hyperandrogenism manifested as hirsutism and hyperandrogenemia, and ovarian dysfunction based on chronic oligoovulation or anovulation and polycystic ovaries).[101,102] There have traditionally been no formal diagnostic criteria in adolescents, but consensus was recently reached by invited representatives of international subspecialty societies on the criteria shown in Box 23.6.[103,104] It should be remembered that for many females, PCOS typically begins during adolescence with activation of the hypothalamic-pituitary-adrenal (HPG) axis.[105]

Hirsutism and acne vulgaris are two common manifestations of PCOS, and in fact, the leading cause of hirsutism in adolescence is PCOS (see Chapter 7).[106] Hair growth occurs in androgen-dependent areas, including the face, neck (Fig. 23.16), chest, back, and lower abdomen, and may be most severe on the trunk.[107] It may be less noticeable in adolescents (given their shorter duration of hyperandrogenism) and is less common in some ethnic backgrounds such as Asians.[99] Although hirsutism has been considered a clinical marker for hyperandrogenism, its diagnosis can be subjective and there is interobserver variability; in addition, its severity may correlate little or not at all with the severity of androgen excess.[108] Acne is a common finding, and in one study of 119 women with acne but without menstrual disorders, obesity, or hirsutism, PCOS was found on ultrasound in 45%.[109] These findings suggest that PCOS is common in women with acne even in the absence of other suggestive clinical findings. Alopecia can also be seen in association with the hyperandrogenism of PCOS, but appears to be a relatively infrequent finding in this population. When present, it may present as female pattern loss (hair loss primarily over the central scalp) or as male pattern loss (with frontotemporal and vertex recession).[110]

Acanthosis nigricans (AN) (see later) is another common cutaneous finding in patients with PCOS. It presents with hyperpigmented, velvety plaques of the neck folds, axillae, and other intertriginous areas. AN is a marker for insulin resistance, although the latter appears to be only one factor leading to its development.[111] Other important components of PCOS include menstrual irregularity and obesity. Anovulation or oligoovulation commonly occur, although women with PCOS can ovulate spontaneously. Secondary amenorrhea, oligomenorrhea, and dysfunctional uterine bleeding may all occur, and delayed menarche may be seen in girls.[112] Adolescent females with oligomenorrhea secondary to PCOS may be difficult to distinguish from those with physiologic anovulation. Obesity is often present, with a centripetal weight distribution and increased waist-to-hip ratio of greater than 0.85.[112] Some patients with PCOS display a metabolic pattern of atherogenic lipid profile, glucose intolerance, and increased fasting insulin level, with an increased incidence of type 2 diabetes mellitus and cardiovascular disease.[97] Studies of adult women with type 2 diabetes mellitus show a prevalence of PCOS higher than that reported in the general population.[113]

Box 23.6 Diagnostic Criteria for Polycystic Ovary Syndrome (PCOS) in Adolescents

PCOS should be diagnosed in adolescent females when there is unexplained persistent hyperandrogenic anovulation using age- and stage-appropriate standards

Caveats:

Abnormal uterine bleeding pattern should be present for ≥2 years
- If <2 years, these girls can be considered to be "at risk" for PCOS

Hyperandrogenism:
- Best diagnosed by persistent serum total and/or free testosterone elevation above adult norms
- Moderate to severe hirsutism is suggestive of hyperandrogenism; mild isolated hirsutism is not considered evidence of hyperandrogenism
- Moderate to severe acne, especially when persistent and poorly responsive to topical therapies, should prompt evaluation for hyperandrogenism

Adapted from Witchel SF, Oberfield S, Rosenfield RL, et al. The diagnosis of polycystic ovary syndrome during adolescence. *Horm Res Paediatr.* 2015;83:376–89 and Rosenfield RL. The diagnosis of polycystic ovary syndrome in adolescents. *Pediatrics.* 2015;136(6):1154–65.

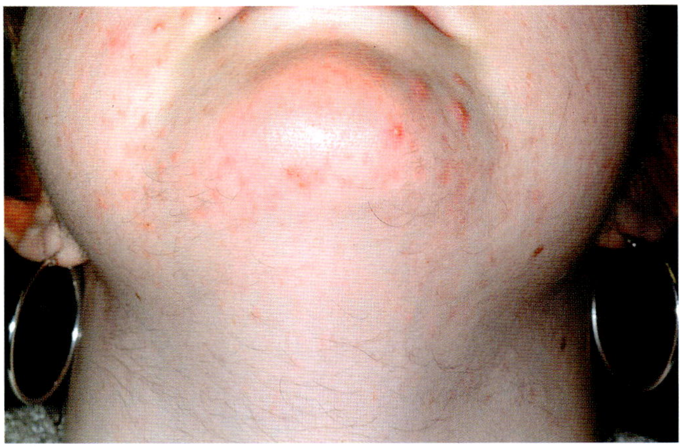

Fig. 23.16 Hirsutism. The hair growth in this adolescent female with polycystic ovary syndrome occurs in androgen-dependent areas and is accompanied by acne.

The clinical presentation of PCOS and its associated features have overlap with other entities described in the literature. The association of hyperandrogenism, insulin resistance, and AN has been called *HAIR-AN syndrome*. Although the potential causes of hyperandrogenism in this syndrome are multiple, PCOS may be present in many patients. It is possible that the etiology of insulin resistance (and resultant hyperinsulinemia) could produce both polycystic ovaries and hyperandrogenism.[114] *Syndrome X* is a term that has been used to describe a systemic disease notable for hyperinsulinemia and hyperandrogenism. *Metabolic syndrome* has been the terminology used to describe patients with abdominal obesity, dyslipidemia, glucose intolerance, and often, PCOS.[115] These patients are also prone to hypertension, hyperuricemia, fatty liver disease, chronic inflammation, endothelial dysfunction, and coagulopathy.[115] Importantly, there is a threefold increase in the risk of coronary heart disease and stroke. Sleep disorders such as obstructive sleep apnea and excessive daytime sleepiness have been increasingly recognized in patients with PCOS.

The diagnosis of PCOS is suggested by the clinical features of hyperandrogenism and prolonged menstrual irregularity and confirmed by finding elevated serum androgens and excluding other potential causes. The ultrasound finding of polycystic changes is common, but such changes may also be seen in normally menstruating adolescents or in other conditions, and so this must be kept in appropriate context during the evaluation. In addition, some adolescents with PCOS may not have polycystic ovaries. Screening for glucose intolerance and diabetes mellitus should be performed in all patients with PCOS, as should fasting lipid levels. Box 23.7 lists the recommended diagnostic testing for adolescents suspected of having PCOS.[116]

Treatments for the condition are primarily directed at symptoms and lifestyle modifications and include hormonal regulation, weight reduction via nutritional changes and physical exercise, and treatment for hirsutism and acne. A serious attempt at weight loss and increased physical activity should be first-line therapy; weight loss itself has been associated with decreased testosterone, increased sex hormone–binding globulin, normalization of menses, and improved fertility in females with PCOS.[117] Combined estrogen–progestin contraceptives provide regular withdrawal bleeds, contraception, and improvement in hirsutism and acne. Antiandrogen medications such as spironolactone may also be of benefit. The use of insulin-sensitizing drugs such as metformin may be effective for anovulation and may benefit the associated metabolic derangements.[118] Metformin may result in a lower body mass index (BMI) and more improvement in menstrual irregularity when used in combination with lifestyle modification (compared with the latter alone).[119] Other options for treatment of hirsutism include mechanical hair removal (i.e., plucking,

Box 23.7 Recommended Testing for Adolescents Suspected of Having Polycystic Ovary Syndrome

Laboratory

Human chorionic gonadotropin (HCG) (urine or serum)
Follicle-stimulating hormone (FSH)
Luteinizing hormone (LH)
Estradiol
Thyroid-stimulating hormone (TSH)
Prolactin
Testosterone (total and free)
Dehydroepiandrosterone sulfate (DHEA-S)
Sex hormone–binding globulin (SHBG)
Androstenedione
17-hydroxyprogesterone
ACTH stimulation testing (if indicated)

Radiologic

Pelvic ultrasonography (transabdominal if virginal, or transvaginal)

If PCOS Confirmed:

Fasting glucose and insulin
2-hour oral glucose tolerance test
Fasting lipid panel

ACTH, Adrenocorticotropic hormone; *PCOS*, polycystic ovary syndrome.
Modified from Rackow BW. Polycystic ovary syndrome in adolescents. *Curr Opin Obstet Gynecol*. 2012;24:281–287; Nicandri KF, Hoeger K. Diagnosis and treatment of polycystic ovarian syndrome in adolescents. *Curr Opin Endocrinol Diabetes Obes*. 2012;19:497–504 and Witchel SF, Oberfield S, Rosenfield RL, et al. The diagnosis of polycystic ovary syndrome during adolescence. *Horm Res Paediatr*. 2015;83:376–389.

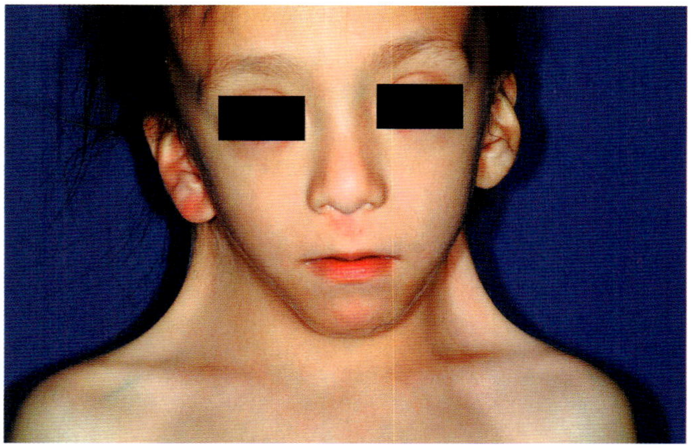

Fig. 23.17 Pterygium colli in Turner syndrome. This neck webbing is likely the result of *in utero* cystic hygroma.

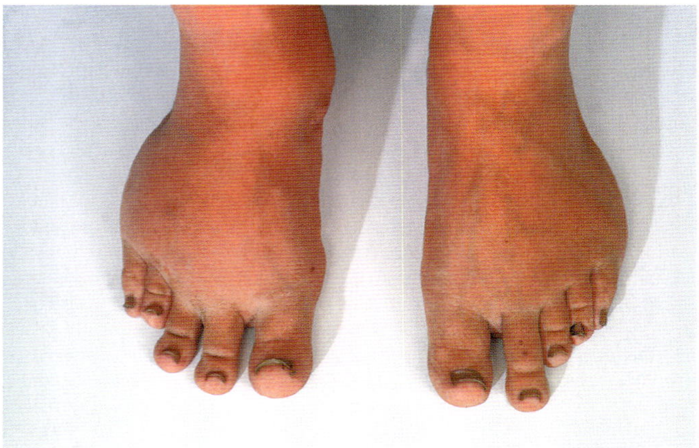

Fig. 23.18 Nail changes in Turner syndrome. Note the hypoplastic, hyperconvex toenails and hypoplasia of the fourth and fifth metatarsals in this girl with gonadal dysgenesis. (Reprinted with permission from Schachner LA, Hansen RC, editors. *Pediatric Dermatology*. 3rd ed. Edinburgh, Scotland: Mosby; 2003.)

waxing, shaving, chemical depilatories, and laser therapy), topical inhibitors of ornithine decarboxylase (eflornithine), and gonadotropin-releasing hormone agonists.

Gonadal Dysgenesis/Turner Syndrome

Gonadal dysgenesis, or Turner syndrome (TS), is a condition characterized by short stature and ovarian dysgenesis. Patients are females with either a missing X chromosome (45,X) or an abnormality of one of the X chromosomes. It occurs in 1 in 2000 to 1 in 5000 female live births.[120] Genomic imprinting, whereby allelic genes or chromosomes are expressed differently depending on the parent of origin, has been implicated in TS in which up to 80% of patients have retained the maternal X chromosome.[121] The rate of spontaneous fetal loss for 45,X fetuses is high; TS may occur in up to 3% of all fetuses and may cause up to 10% of all spontaneous fetal loss (the majority terminating during the first and second trimesters).[122]

In addition to short stature and ovarian failure, patients with TS may have lymphatic abnormalities, skeletal abnormalities (micrognathia, broad "shield" chest, kyphoscoliosis, Madelung wrist deformity, high-arched palate, short limbs), hearing and cardiac defects, renal abnormalities, and endocrinopathies (most notably involving the thyroid and glucose metabolism). Patients with TS are at increased risk for metabolic syndrome, low-grade inflammation, and hepatic and muscle dysfunction.[123] Congenital cardiovascular disease is present in approximately 50% of girls with TS, the most common being bicuspid aortic valve; aortic coarctation (10%) and hypertension (25% of adolescents and 50% of adults) may also occur.[124] Characteristic physical findings also include a low posterior hairline, cubitus valgus, unusual rotation of the ears, downward displacement of the lateral canthus, epicanthal folds, inverted or hypoplastic nipples, and shortened fourth and fifth metacarpals and metatarsals. Learning deficits occur in the majority of patients with TS, and psychiatric conditions may be more common.

Abnormalities of the lymphatic system include cystic hygroma (macrocystic lymphatic malformation), which when occurring *in utero*, may result in neck webbing or pterygium colli (Fig. 23.17). Transient lymphedema of the distal extremities, mainly the hands and the feet, may occur, and nail dysplasia may be seen as a result of intrauterine peripheral lymphedema.[125] This lymphedema usually resolves by 2 years of age; however, it may recur later in life. Deep furrows of the scalp, similar to what has been termed *cutis verticis gyrata*, may also be the result of preceding lymphedema.[126] Treatment for TS-associated lymphedema depends on its severity and may range from no active therapy to compression stockings, manual lymph drainage, or decongestive lymphatic therapy.[127]

The nails in patients with TS are characteristic, revealing hypoplasia and hyperconvexity (Fig. 23.18).[44] Increased numbers of melanocytic nevi are commonly noted, although clinical atypia is not necessarily more prominent.[128] Despite the increased numbers of melanocytic nevi, there appears to be a lower-than-expected incidence of malignant melanoma in patients with TS, possibly reflecting the relationship between sex hormones and melanoma development.[129,130] Multiple pilomatricomas, including giant lesions, have been reported in girls with TS.[131,132]

Pituitary Disorders

HYPERPITUITARISM

The pituitary gland, an endocrine organ located in a bony cavity (the sella turcica) at the brain base, is divided into anterior and posterior portions. Both portions secrete a variety of hormones under the influence of the hypothalamus. These hormones include GH, TSH, ACTH, luteinizing hormone (LH), follicle-stimulating hormone (FSH), prolactin, antidiuretic hormone (ADH, vasopressin), and oxytocin. Skin manifestations of hyperpituitarism include those related to excess GH, glucocorticoids (see Cushing Syndrome section), and prolactin (not discussed here). Most GH-secreting pituitary tumors are eosinophilic adenomas. Disorders that can be associated with GH-secreting pituitary tumors include McCune–Albright syndrome (MAS; see later); Carney complex (see Chapter 11); MEN types 1 and 4 (see later); familial isolated pituitary adenoma; and the paraganglioma, pheochromocytoma, and pituitary adenoma association (3PA).[133] Early-onset gigantism may also be caused by an Xq26.3 genomic microduplication, likely associated with a *GPR101* genetic mutation, and has been termed *X-linked acrogigantism* (X-LAG).[134] Excessive secretion of GH by pituitary-gland tumors or pituitary hyperplasia produces gigantism in children whose epiphyses have not yet closed and acromegaly in individuals whose normal bone growth has ceased. Acromegaly is rare in children, but transitional acromegalic features at times may be seen in affected adolescents. Soft-tissue overgrowth of the hands, feet, face, and nasal tip occur. Patients may have a large furrowed tongue, thick lips, lantern jaw, broad spade-like hands with squatty fingers, hypertrichosis, and hyperpigmentation in a pattern similar to that observed in patients with Addison disease. Although the cause of the hypertrichosis is not well understood, the hyperpigmentation is related to increased secretion of MSH. Other cutaneous manifestations of acromegaly include excessive sweating, oily skin, acrochordons (skin tags), heel-pad thickening, eyelid swelling, and AN.[135] Early noncutaneous complaints in patients with acromegaly may include headache, visual disturbances, weakness, and paresthesias, and impaired glucose tolerance may be present.[136]

Cutis verticis gyrata (coarse furrowing of the skin on the posterior aspect of the neck and the vertex of the scalp; Fig. 23.19) is caused by an increase in dermal collagen; as a result, excessive skin buckles and forms furrows and ridges that resemble gyri of the cerebral cortex (hence the terminology). In addition to being an occasional manifestation of hyperpituitarism, cutis verticis gyrata may occasionally occur as a primary disorder without other associated abnormalities (termed *primary essential cutis verticis gyrata*). It has been reported in association with TS (see earlier) and Noonan syndrome, and similar changes have also been seen in patients receiving vemurafenib and whole-brain radiotherapy for malignant melanoma.[137–141] Treatment options for cutis verticis gyrata are limited and primarily surgical.[142] It may also be seen as part of a disorder called *pachydermoperiostosis*, which manifests in thickening of the skin of the face and scalp, clubbing of the fingers, and periostosis of the long bones. Severe progressive arthritis has rarely been reported in association with this syndrome.[143]

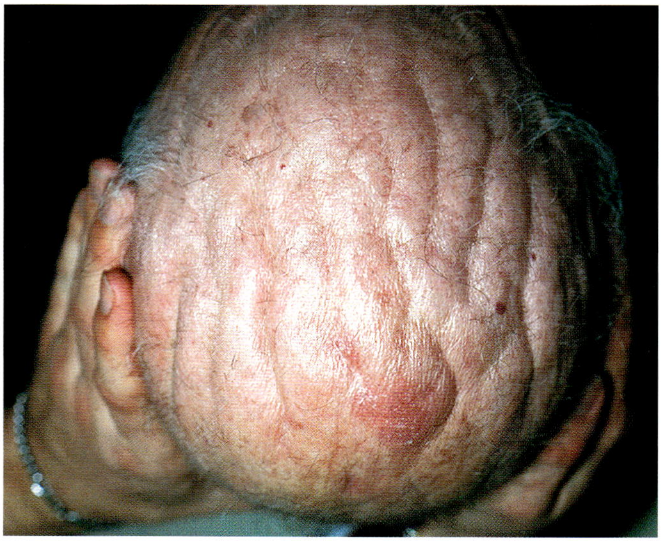

Fig. 23.19 Cutis verticis gyrata. This coarse furrowing of the skin on the scalp may be associated with hyperpituitarism or as part of a disorder called *pachydermoperiostosis*.

HYPOPITUITARISM

Pituitary insufficiency (hypopituitarism) refers to a group of disorders resulting from a deficiency in secretion of one or more hormones derived from the pituitary gland. These include idiopathic hypopituitarism (panhypopituitarism, Simmonds disease), Sheehan syndrome (pituitary deficiency usually arising as a result of hemorrhage or infarct), pituitary tumors (especially craniopharyngioma, Langerhans cell histiocytosis), autoimmune disorders, trauma, infections (e.g., tuberculosis), congenital abnormalities, or ablation of the pituitary gland by surgery or radiation used for the treatment of local tumors. Systemic manifestations of hypopituitarism may include those related to mineralocorticoid and glucocorticoid deficiencies (see Addison Disease section), hypothyroidism, GH and gonadotropin deficiency, and diabetes insipidus secondary to ADH deficiency.

The most obvious skin manifestations of pituitary insufficiency are pallor secondary to anemia and decreased cutaneous blood flow, and a predisposition toward sunburn with decreased ability to tan (because of a decrease in melanin pigmentation secondary to diminished or absent secretion of MSH). Other features (and proposed causes) include smooth, fine skin (GH deficiency) or myxedematous, coarse, dry skin (hypothyroidism and GH deficiency). The face may be slightly puffy and pale or yellowish (secondary to carotenoderma from hypothyroidism). Hair is thin and sparse with alopecia (hypothyroidism and androgen deficiency), and the nails grow slowly. Adolescent males may have a smooth scrotum with absence of hair and rugae (androgen deficiency).[144] Gonadotropin deficiency may result in loss of axillary, pubic, and body hair and micropenis in males.

Multiple Endocrine Neoplasia Syndromes

The MEN syndromes are familial disorders characterized by benign and malignant tumors of multiple endocrine glands. Cutaneous manifestations may also be found in these disorders. The clinical manifestations of MEN syndromes are inconsistent and reflect the variable involvement of hormone-producing tissues. These disorders are inherited in an autosomal dominant fashion. The endocrine and cutaneous manifestations of the MEN syndromes are summarized in Table 23.1.

MEN 1 (Werner syndrome) is characterized by tumors of the parathyroid glands, endocrine pancreas, and anterior pituitary. Thyroid and adrenal gland tumors may also be seen, as may foregut carcinoid tumors.[145] Clinical manifestations may be related to primary hyperparathyroidism, gastrinoma, tumors secreting neuroendocrine peptides, and prolactinomas. There is an increased risk of malignant endocrine tumors, including parathyroid, thymic, bronchial (carcinoid), and enteropancreatic neuroendocrine tumors.[146] The gene for MEN 1 (*MEN1*) was initially mapped to chromosome llql3, and genetic testing is available.[146,147] This gene encodes a protein called *menin*, which functions as a tumor suppressor protein and in whose absence cellular replication, hyperplasia, and tumorigenesis are increased.

Cutaneous manifestations of MEN 1 include lipomas, angiofibromas, collagenomas, confetti-like hypopigmented macules, and gingival papules.[145] Café-au-lait macules may also occur, although not in the high numbers usually associated with neurofibromatosis. The multiple facial angiofibromas (Fig. 23.20) are clinically and histologically indistinguishable from those that occur in the setting of tuberous sclerosis, although they tend to present later in life in MEN 1, usually during the third or fourth decade.[145,148] In addition, they may involve the upper lip and vermilion border. Nonetheless, facial angiofibromas, which were once felt to be pathognomonic for tuberous sclerosis (and traditionally referred to as *adenoma sebaceum*), are no longer considered a specific marker for that disorder. In one series of patients with MEN 1, 88% had facial angiofibromas.[145] Collagenomas, which are hamartomas of connective tissue, tend to be more discrete and papular in MEN 1 than the histologically similar lesions ("shagreen patch") seen in patients with tuberous sclerosis.[145] Protuberant collagenomas have been reported, with rapid growth after surgery to remove an

Table 23.1 Endocrine and Mucocutaneous Manifestations of Multiple Endocrine Neoplasia Syndromes

Syndrome *(Gene)*	Endocrine*	Mucocutaneous
MEN 1 *(MEN-1)*	Parathyroid Anterior pituitary NET – pancreatic, lung, gastric Thyroid Adrenal glands PPGL	Angiofibromas (facial) Collagenomas Hypopigmentation (confetti-like) Gingival papules Lipomas Café-au-lait macules Melanoma
MEN 2 (2A) *(RET)*	Thyroid Parathyroid PPGL Adrenal glands	Lichen amyloidosis Dermal hyperneury† Sclerotic fibromas‡
MEN 3 (2B) *(RET)*	Thyroid PPGL Parathyroid (extremely rare) Adrenal glands	Mucosal neuromas (lips, eyelids, tongue) Café-au-lait macules Lichen nitidus
MEN 4 *(CDKN1B)*	Parathyroid Anterior pituitary Adrenal glands NET – pancreatic, lung, gastric	None

MEN, Multiple endocrine neoplasia; *NET*, neuroendocrine tumors; *PPGL*, pheochromocytoma and paraganglioma
*May be hyperplasia, benign tumors, malignant tumors.
†Hyperplastic proliferation and increased number of cutaneous nerve fibers.
‡Reported in one patient.

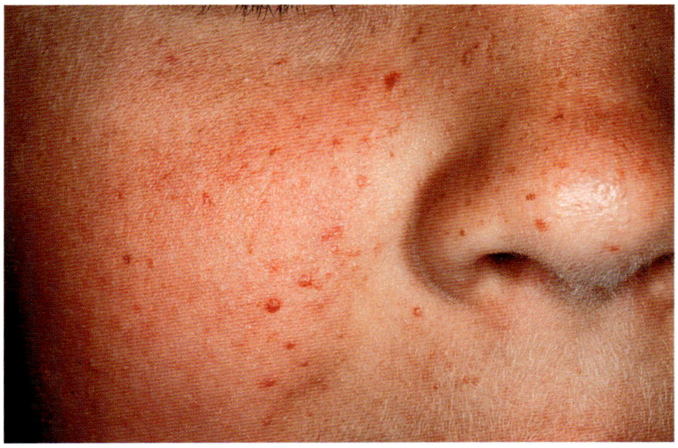

Fig. 23.20 Facial angiofibromas. These pink to red, dome-shaped smooth papules occur most commonly on the cheeks, nasolabial folds, and chin and may be seen in the setting of MEN 1 or tuberous sclerosis. They may occasionally be confused with lesions of acne vulgaris.

endocrine tumor.[149] Melanoma may occur with increased incidence in patients with MEN 1.[150] Patients who have a cluster of tumors suggestive of the syndrome or with single proliferative disorders with a high correlation, such as prolactinoma or multigland parathyroid hyperplasia, or with facial angiofibromas in the absence of stigmata of tuberous sclerosis, should be screened for MEN 1.[151]

MEN 2 (MEN 2A, Sipple syndrome) is a rare autosomal dominant disorder caused by a point mutation in the *RET* protooncogene. Clinical findings include medullary thyroid carcinoma, pheochromocytoma, and parathyroid hyperplasia. Hirschsprung disease may also occur with increased incidence. Cutaneous manifestations are not a significant feature of MEN 2A. The one that has received the most attention is lichen amyloidosis, which presents as multiple infiltrated papules overlying a well-demarcated plaque on the upper back (especially the interscapular region) or extensor surfaces of the extremities.[152,153] These lesions often begin with intense pruritus, with the subsequent development of brown-colored papules on the skin[154] and the histologic finding of amorphous material in the papillary dermis that stains as amyloid.[155,156] Dermal hyperneury (hyperplastic proliferation and increased number of cutaneous nerve fibers) and sclerotic fibromas (typically seen in patients with *PTEN* hamartoma tumor syndrome; see Chapter 9) have also been reported.[157]

MEN 3 (MEN 2B, mucosal neuroma syndrome) is characterized by medullary thyroid carcinoma, pheochromocytoma, ganglioneuromatosis, a Marfanoid body habitus, and only very occasional parathyroid hyperplasia. Medullary thyroid carcinoma is the initial presentation in most patients with MEN 3/2B (as well as those with MEN 2/2A) and remains the major cause of morbidity.[158] This disorder is also caused by an activating mutation in the *RET* protooncogene.

Mucocutaneous manifestations of MEN 3 include multiple mucosal neuromas that are often present by the preschool years. These ganglioneuromas involve the anterolateral tongue and lips and may also be located on the conjunctiva and eyelids.[159,160] Lip involvement results in diffusely enlarged lips with a fleshy, bubbled appearance. The upper lip is usually more involved than the lower lip. The tongue lesions are usually limited to the anterior third of the surface and appear as pink-white, somewhat translucent papules and nodules (Fig. 23.21). They may be congenital or noted during the first few years of life and are an important feature, because they may be the initial marker of the syndrome. Although multiple mucosal neuromas are nearly pathognomonic for this disorder, they may rarely occur without other clinical, biochemical, or molecular evidence of MEN 3.[161] Multiple lesions of lichen nitidus have also been observed.[162]

Ocular involvement may involve the limbus of the conjunctivae and the eyelids, in which case it results in thickening of the lid margin and distortion or displacement of the eyelashes (Fig. 23.22). Nasal, laryngeal, and gingival neuromas may also be present, and skin lesions are occasionally seen. Café-au-lait macules may also be a cutaneous component of the syndrome. Intestinal ganglioneuromatosis (distinct from Hirschsprung disease) is another feature of MEN 3, presenting with intermittent intestinal obstruction, gas formation, diarrhea, and failure to thrive.[159] Musculoskeletal features of Marfan syndrome are common, including tall stature, elongated limbs, pes cavum, and pectus excavatum, but cardiac or ocular abnormalities typical of that disorder are absent.

Genetic testing for *RET* mutations should be performed early in life for individuals with a known family history of MEN 2/2A or 3/2B and can identify young carriers at an early stage, often before the development of cancer.[153] In primary relatives of patients affected by medullary thyroid carcinoma with no identified *RET* mutation, linkage

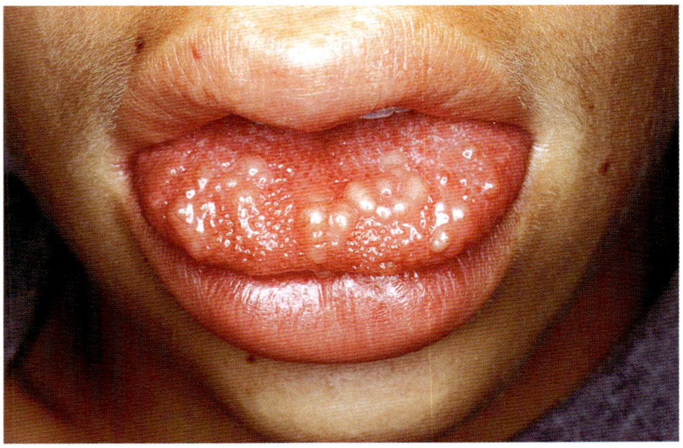

Fig. 23.21 Mucosal neuromas in multiple endocrine neoplasia 2B. Characteristic lingual neuromas and protuberant fleshy lips are present in this 16-year-old male with mucosal neuroma syndrome.

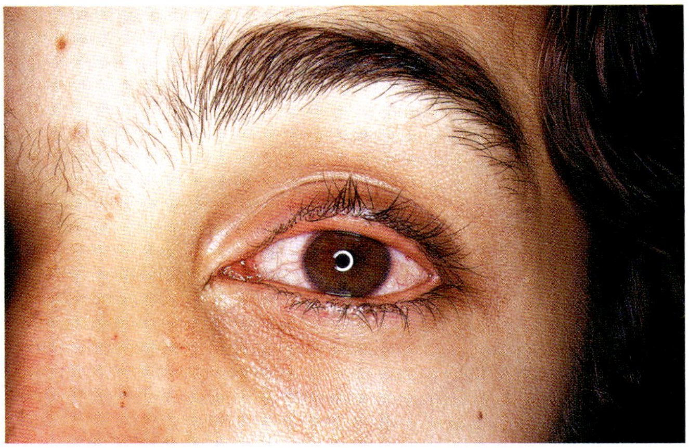

Fig. 23.22 Eyelid changes in multiple endocrine neoplasia 2B. Neuromas of the eyelid margins result in thickening and displacement of the lashes.

analysis and biochemical testing for MEN should be performed. Total thyroidectomy is recommended for all patients at risk.[159,163]

MEN 4 is a more recently described subtype of MEN and is caused by mutations in the *CDKN1B* gene.[164] Clinical manifestations include those related to parathyroid neoplasia; adenomas of the anterior pituitary; neuroendocrine tumors of the pancreas, lung, and stomach; and adrenal neoplasia. Cutaneous features have not been reported to date.[165]

Patients and families carrying the diagnosis of MEN are best cared for by a multidisciplinary program that provides access to endocrinologists, geneticists, endocrine surgeons, clinical psychologists, and gastroenterologists.[166] Biochemical and genetic screening of family members is recommended to facilitate prophylactic surgery (where indicated) and early tumor detection.[167] Support is available at www.amensupport.org.

Autoimmune Polyglandular Syndromes

APSs are a group of disorders in which multiple endocrine and nonendocrine defects occur together. The best characterized of these syndromes is APS1, also known as *APECED syndrome*. This autosomal recessive condition is defined by the presence of two of three conditions: adrenocortical failure (Addison disease), hypoparathyroidism, and mucocutaneous candidiasis.[168] It occurs with increased incidence in Finnish, Iranian, Jewish, and Sardinian populations.[169] APS2, the most common APS, is characterized by Addison disease in conjunction with thyroiditis and/or diabetes mellitus. APS3 has been defined as autoimmune thyroid disease in conjunction with other autoimmune endocrinopathy, excluding adrenal disease. More recently, immune dysregulation, polyendocrinopathy, enteropathy, and X-linked (IPEX) syndrome has been recognized as a rare disorder caused by mutations in the *FOXP3* gene and resulting in overwhelming autoimmunity and absence or dysfunction of regulatory T cells (see Chapter 3). Children with this syndrome often die early in life without prompt diagnosis and bone marrow transplantation.

The symptoms of APS1 commonly begin in infancy, although studies of affected individuals reveal marked heterogeneity in clinical features and age of onset of manifestations.[170] In addition to hypoparathyroidism and adrenal failure, other associations may include insulin-dependent diabetes mellitus, gonadal failure, autoimmune thyroiditis, chronic active hepatitis, malabsorption, and parietal-cell atrophy.[171,172] Autoimmune hepatitis may occur and can be one of the presenting features.[173] Cerebellar ataxia with pseudotumor, ptosis, and retinitis pigmentosa were also noted in a large series from Russia.[174] Candidiasis is seen in nearly all patients, and in the majority of patients it appears first before the endocrinologic manifestations.[175]

Oral candidiasis (thrush; Fig. 23.23) tends to be chronic and has a peak incidence during the first 2 years of life.[176] Candidal infection may also take the form of angular cheilitis (perlèche; Fig. 23.24), hyperplastic or atrophic oral candidiasis, candidal esophagitis, diaper or perianal candidiasis, scalp infection, intertrigo, or nail infection. These changes, taken together, are also referred to as *chronic mucocutaneous candidiasis* (see Chapter 17). When chronic candidal infection occurs in the esophagus or larynx, stricture formation may result. Nail involvement leads to thickening (Fig. 23.25), brittleness, and discoloration with associated inflammation of the periungual areas (paronychia). Many postpubertal female patients may experience candidal vulvovaginitis.[176] Generalized candidiasis in these patients is rare, but serious lung infection may occasionally occur. Mucocutaneous candidal infections that are unresponsive to topical therapy should be considered an alerting sign for possible APS1.[170]

Alopecia areata occurs in around one-third of patients with APS1,[172] often presents in childhood, and may progress to alopecia universalis. It tends to begin around the peripubertal years. Vitiligo occurs in some patients and is quite variable in extent. Urticarial

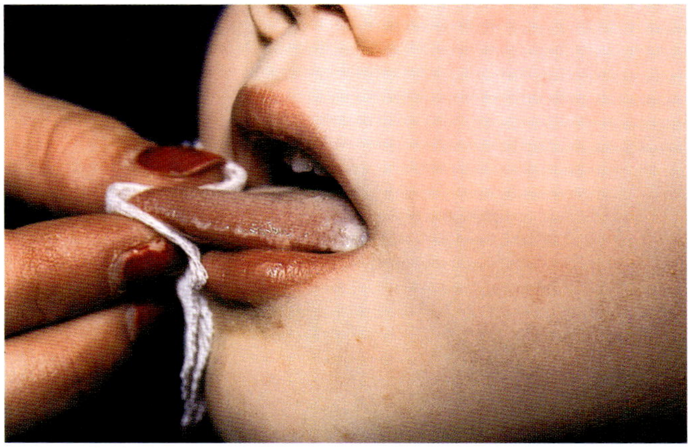

Fig. 23.23 Oral candidiasis. White plaques of the lateral tongue (thrush) in a young female with chronic mucocutaneous candidiasis and diabetes mellitus.

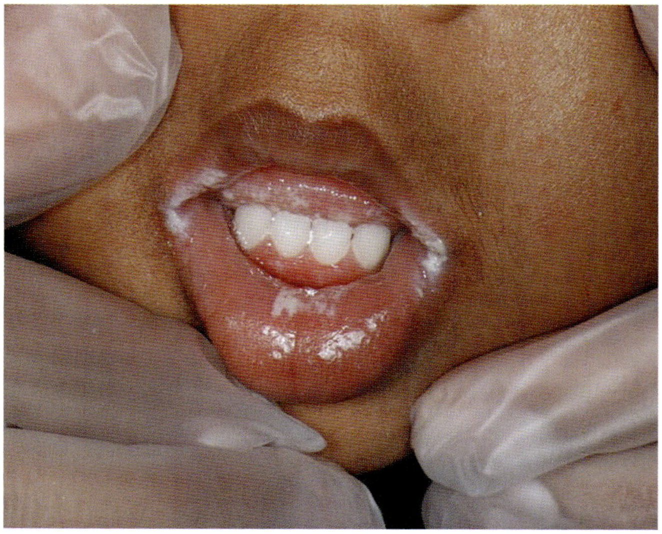

Fig. 23.24 Perlèche (angular cheilitis). In this condition, which can occur as a component of chronic mucocutaneous candidiasis, as shown in this 18-month-old male with autoimmune polyendocrinopathy, candidiasis, ectodermal dystrophy (APECED) syndrome, candidal infection presents as erythema, fissures, and maceration at the mouth angles.

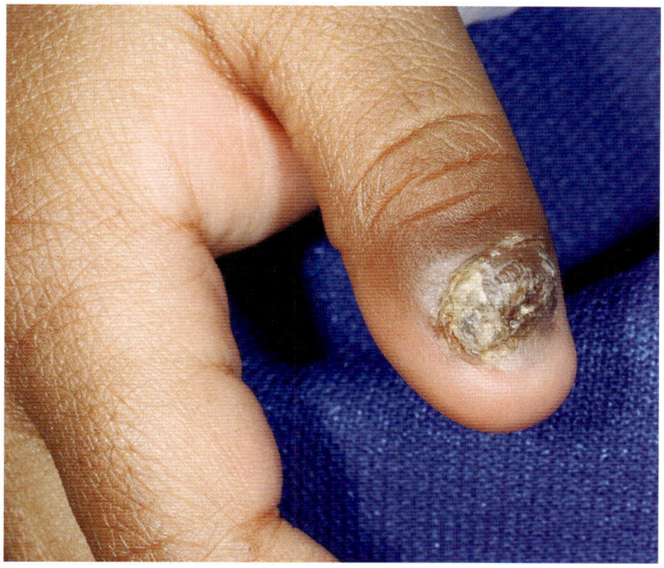

Fig. 23.25 Nail candidiasis. Nail plate thickening with hyperkeratosis and yellow discoloration, along with mild periungal erythema, were present in the same patient as in Fig. 23.24.

eruptions occurred in 66% of patients in one large series.[177] The most consistent cutaneous features are those representing ectodermal dystrophy. APS1 patients often have enamel hypoplasia of permanent teeth, and nail dystrophy with pitting affects around half of the patients.[176] They are more prone to dental caries, abscesses, and tooth loss.[178] In a series of 52 Norwegian patients with APS1, the most frequent presenting features were enamel hypoplasia, hypoparathyroidism, and mucocutaneous candidiasis.[179]

The gene mutated in patients with APS1 is termed *AIRE*, for "autoimmune regulator." It is localized to the short arm of chromosome 21 and may act as a transcriptional regulator.[169,171] Mutations in *AIRE*, of which over 100 have been documented in the Human Gene Mutation Database, result in loss of central tolerance to a number of self-antigens, with impaired clonal deletion of self-reactive thymocytes, which may subsequently attack a variety of host organs.[180,181] Patients with APS1 produce autoantibodies to various cytokines, including interleukin (IL)-17A, IL-17F, IL-22, and type 1 interferons; altered IL-23 signaling has also been described.[182,183] *AIRE* mutations may also be associated with rheumatoid arthritis, systemic sclerosis, and sporadic alopecia areata and vitiligo.[184] Treatments for APS1 include hormone replacement, aggressive treatment for mucocutaneous candidiasis, and close surveillance for the development of additional autoimmune conditions.

McCune–Albright Syndrome

MAS is defined clinically as the triad of fibrous dysplasia of bones (polyostotic fibrous dysplasia), patchy cutaneous pigmentation, and various endocrinopathies, most notably precocious puberty. Other associated endocrine disorders include pituitary adenomas (resulting in GH excess), hyperthyroid goiters, and adrenal hyperplasia.[185] Renal phosphate wasting with or without rickets/osteomalacia, as well as hepatic and cardiac involvement, have also been reported.[186] The endocrinopathies of MAS are all characterized by autonomous excessive hyperfunction of hormonally responsive cells, which respond to signals through activation of the adenylate cyclase system.[187] Activating mutations in the guanine nucleotide–binding (G) protein gene *GNAS*, which encodes a subunit of the G protein that stimulates adenylate cyclase, have been identified in patients with MAS.[188] A postzygotic somatic mutation leads to a mosaic distribution of cells bearing the defect.[185] As mentioned earlier in this chapter, germline inactivating mutations of this same gene are present in patients with AHO (PHP).

The pigmentary lesions of MAS, which are seen in approximately 50% of patients, present as one or more café-au-lait macules or patches with a distinct distribution pattern: they rarely extend beyond the midline, and the majority are on the same side of the body as the skeletal lesions.[188] The most common sites of involvement are the buttocks and lumbosacral regions, and lesions may follow the lines of Blaschko. These café-au-lait lesions have irregularly ragged or serrated borders (Fig. 23.26) that are described as resembling the "coast of Maine," in contrast to the café-au-lait spots of neurofibromatosis, where the smooth borders are said to resemble the "coast of California." They are usually present early in life and often are the first sign of this disorder. Bilateral involvement and lack of respect for the midline may occasionally be observed.[189] Oral mucosal hyperpigmentation, resembling the lesions more typically seen in lentiginosis syndromes, has been reported.[190] Diffuse scalp alopecia with histologic features of fibrous dysplasia has been reported.[191]

Fibrous dysplasia is a rare bone disorder that results in bone pain, fractures, bony deformity, and occasionally neurologic compression. It occurs most often as a bone-limited process, and less than 5% of patients have concomitant endocrine dysfunction.[192] Most patients with MAS have either solitary or multiple fibrous dysplasia lesions of bone, which tend to develop during the first decade. Although any bone can be involved, the proximal femurs, pelvis, and skull base are most common, and progressive deformity with fractures may occur. Radiographic studies reveal lytic lesions with scalloped borders and a "ground-glass" pattern. Computed tomographic imaging or bone biopsy may be required to confirm the diagnosis in questionable cases. Precocious puberty is a common initial manifestation in girls with MAS (much less common in boys) and is recognized by the development of secondary sexual characteristics before 9 years of age.[188] Affected girls have ovarian cysts that function autonomously and produce high serum levels of estradiol, with suppression of gonadotropins.[193] In males, testicular tumors associated with penile enlargement may be present, and Leydig- and/or Sertoli-cell tumors or hyperplasia are common.[186] In addition, growth hormone excess appears to occur more frequently in males (versus females) with MAS.[194]

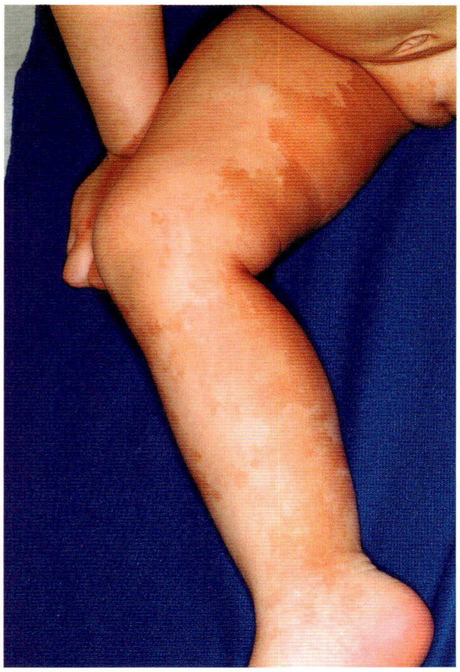

Fig. 23.26 Café-au-lait lesions in McCune–Albright syndrome. Well-demarcated tan patches with a ragged border involving the labia majora, thigh, leg, and foot in this 18-month-old female.

Disorders Associated with Diabetes Mellitus

Diabetes mellitus is a common chronic disease, and up to 30% of patients with diabetes mellitus may have some form of cutaneous disorder. The exact influences of plasma glucose homeostasis, insulin resistance, elevated BMI, and/or components of metabolic syndrome on these cutaneous findings are, in many instances, unclear. Some skin findings associated with diabetes mellitus include poor wound healing, necrobiosis lipoidica (NL), diabetic dermopathy, diabetic bullae, acrochordons, acanthosis nigricans, and the syndrome of limited joint mobility and waxy skin.[195–197] For some skin conditions, the exact association between the disorder and diabetes mellitus is uncertain, and for many, the pathogenesis remains unproven. Box 23.8 lists some potential cutaneous associations with diabetes mellitus. A select number of these disorders will be discussed here. Glucagonoma syndrome, which may be associated with mild diabetes mellitus and cutaneous manifestations, is discussed separately in the next section.

NECROBIOSIS LIPOIDICA DIABETICORUM

NL (also known as *necrobiosis lipoidica diabeticorum*) is a fairly distinct clinical entity that, although not the most common, is the best recognized cutaneous marker of diabetes mellitus.[195] It may be seen outside of the setting of diabetes mellitus, although up to three-quarters of patients with NL have or will have diabetes mellitus; among patients with diabetes mellitus, it occurs in less than 1% of patients.[198,199] NL is predominantly seen in females and has an average age of onset of 34 years.[195,200] However, it may occur in children, and its presence may suggest a higher risk for diabetic nephropathy and retinopathy.[201] In up to one-third of patients with NL, these cutaneous lesions may precede the diagnosis by up to several years or present simultaneously with diabetes mellitus. NL is most commonly seen in patients who are insulin dependent. The etiology is unclear but may relate to microangiopathy resulting from glycoprotein deposition in the vasculature. Poorer glycemic control, longer duration of disease, and higher insulin requirements have been positively correlated with the development of NL.[202]

Lesions of NL typically occur in the pretibial areas and are usually asymptomatic. They present as slowly enlarging, irregularly bordered, red to yellow-brown to violaceous plaques (Fig. 23.27). The center often becomes atrophic and more yellow, and there may be superficial telangiectasias, especially later in the course. Older lesions may be primarily brown in color. Multiple lesions are usually present, and ulceration may occur in up to one-third of patients with NL. Skin biopsy can be useful for diagnosis, revealing degeneration of collagen with inflammation and granuloma formation. However, it is preferable to avoid surgical procedures in this location in patients who have

Box 23.8 Some Cutaneous Associations with Diabetes Mellitus

Established or probable association

Necrobiosis lipoidica (NL) diabeticorum
Diabetic dermopathy
Diabetic bullae
Acanthosis nigricans
Acrochordons (skin tags)
Scleredema diabeticorum
Limited joint mobility and waxy skin syndrome
Partial lipodystrophy
Malignant otitis externa
Neuropathic leg ulcers
Perforating disorders
Eruptive xanthomas
Hemochromatosis
Carotenemia
Pruritus, especially anogenital or generalized
Xerosis and anhidrosis
Yellow nails, koilonychias
Psoriasis (and psoriatic arthritis)
Increased susceptibility to infections:
Candida albicans
Staphylococcus aureus
Group A β-hemolytic streptococcus
Pseudomonas aeruginosa
Dermatophytes (tinea pedis, onychomycosis)
Corynebacterium minutissimum (erythrasma)

Possible association

Disseminated granuloma annulare
Vitiligo

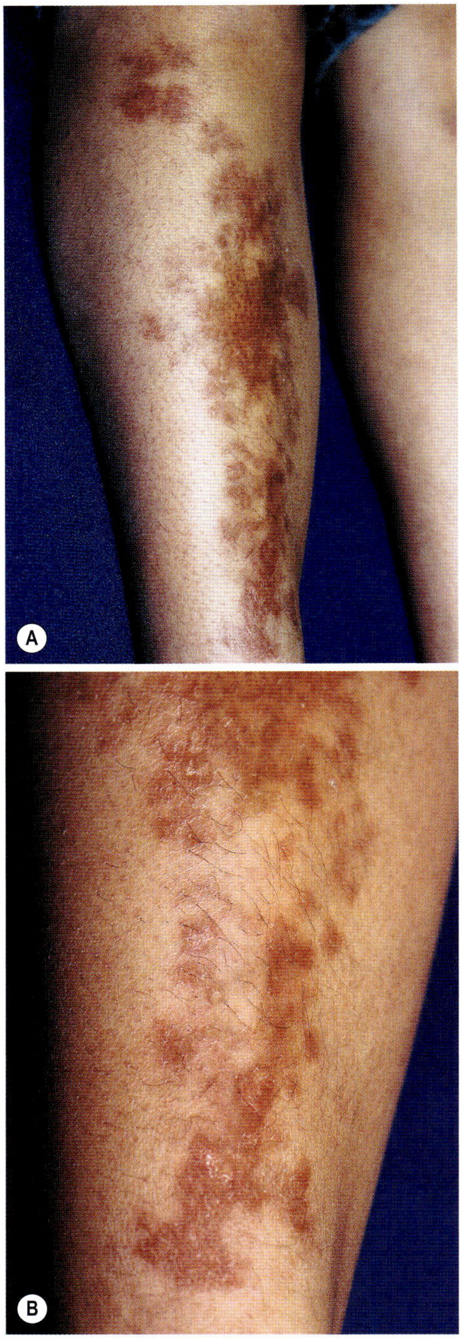

Fig. 23.27 Necrobiosis lipoidica diabeticorum. Waxy, yellow-brown plaques **(A)** were present in this young girl with diabetes mellitus, with subtle atrophy present on closer inspection **(B)**.

diabetes mellitus when possible. The diagnosis is usually strongly suggested in the presence of sharply demarcated, waxy plaques with a red or violaceous border on the anterior tibial surfaces of a patient with diabetes mellitus. The cause of NL is unclear but may relate to microangiopathy, endarteritis, vasculitis, or delayed hypersensitivity. Squamous cell carcinoma in long-standing lesions has been reported in adults, mainly in the setting of superimposed nonhealing ulceration.[203,204]

The treatment of NL is challenging, and there is no established gold standard of care, because the clinical response to various treatments is quite variable. When there is no ulceration and lesions are relatively asymptomatic, watchful waiting and protection from injury are appropriate.[129] The influence of strict diabetic control on the lesions of NL is controversial. Many have suggested that glucose control has no effect on the appearance or clinical course of NL, whereas others support the opposite hypothesis.[130,198,205] Cosmetic cover-ups are useful for patients in whom the appearance of lesions is bothersome. Active therapy of lesions has included topical and intralesional corticosteroids, aspirin, dipyridamole, pentoxifylline, clofazimine, cyclosporine, mycophenolate mofetil, systemic corticosteroids, chloroquine, topical tretinoin, hyperbaric oxygen, anti–tumor necrosis factor alpha (TNF-α) agents (infliximab, etanercept), and topical psoralen plus ultraviolet A (PUVA) light therapy.[200,206–213] Local corticosteroid products should be used with caution because they may contribute to further atrophy or ulceration. Antiplatelet therapy with aspirin is reportedly quite effective and well tolerated, although this observation has not been confirmed by randomized clinical trials.[205] Pulsed-dye laser has been used and may benefit the telangiectatic and erythematous components.[214] Ulcerated lesions of NL are treated with local wound care, semipermeable wound dressings, and topical or systemic antibiotics. Surgical excision with split-thickness skin grafting may be useful.[215]

DIABETIC DERMOPATHY

DD (also called *spotted leg syndrome* and *shin spots*) is the most common cutaneous marker for diabetes mellitus. It is considered by some to be a pathognomonic sign of the disease.[216] DD is seen most often in older patients with diabetes mellitus and only occasionally in children. It presents as multiple well-circumscribed, brown macules and patches with a tendency toward bilateral involvement of the pretibial surfaces. The lesions often become atrophic and take on the appearance of scars. They are occasionally scaly and measure from several millimeters up to 2 cm. Lesions of DD may occasionally occur on the scalp, forearms, or trunk, but the pretibial surfaces are the most common site of involvement in the majority of patients. The etiology of these lesions is unclear, but some have suggested that their presence may be a clinical sign of an increased likelihood of retinopathy, nephropathy, and neuropathy.[217] It may also be associated with large vessel (coronary artery) disease.[216] In a histopathologic study of 14 skin biopsies from DD taken at the time of autopsy in patients with diabetes mellitus, the most common findings were melanin and hemosiderin deposition with arterial or arteriolar wall thickening seen in a minority of specimens.[218]

Lesions of DD are in large part uninfluenced by treatment. Because the condition is asymptomatic, it requires no therapy aside from protection from trauma and supportive wound care should lesions become inflamed or infected. Although lesions may resolve spontaneously, others may appear individually or in asymmetric crops.[200]

DIABETIC BULLAE

Diabetic bullae are an uncommon association with diabetes mellitus and present as spontaneously arising large blisters with a predilection for the distal extremities. Diabetic bullae are felt to be a distinct marker for diabetes mellitus. The condition is seen primarily in adult men with long-standing poorly controlled diabetes and peripheral neuropathy, but has been observed rarely in children.[219] The most common location for these bullae is the dorsal and lateral surfaces of the lower legs and feet (Fig. 23.28). Occasionally, patients may have lesions on the hands or forearms.[195] They range in size from less than 1 cm to several centimeters. There is usually no history of trauma, and the lesions usually have no surrounding erythema. These lesions are generally asymptomatic, and healing occurs over several weeks with supportive wound care. They often heal without scarring, although in some patients, atrophy and scarring typical of dystrophic epidermolysis bullosa may result.[200,220]

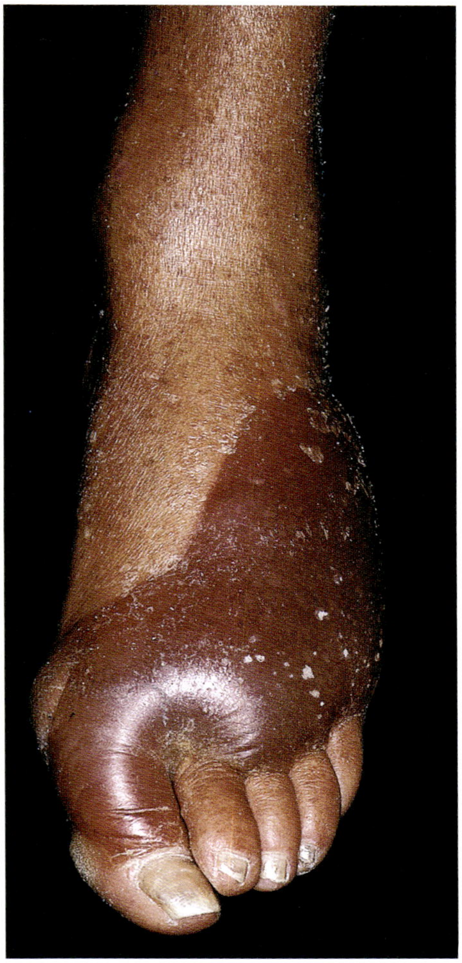

Fig. 23.28 Diabetic bullae. These large, painless, tense bullae may occur in the setting of diabetes mellitus, often with no history of preceding trauma.

ACANTHOSIS NIGRICANS

AN is a symmetric cutaneous eruption consisting of brown, velvety plaques that involve primarily the skin folds. It may be associated with several different clinical settings, including obesity, insulin resistance, various syndromes, malignancy, and medications, as well as occurring as "benign" and mixed types.[221] Table 23.2 summarizes the various clinical associations with AN. The discussion here will focus primarily on AN associated with obesity, insulin resistance, and diabetes mellitus.

AN presents as dark brown, velvety thickening of the skin involving the axillae (Fig. 23.29) and the neck, especially the posterior and lateral neck folds (Fig. 23.30). The initial change is hyperpigmentation followed by eventual thickening with intensification of skin markings.[222] In addition to the characteristic areas of involvement, there may be velvety hyperpigmentation and/or verrucous hyperkeratosis of the knuckles (Fig. 23.31), genitalia, perineum, face, thighs, breasts, and flexural regions of the elbows and knees. Occasionally the eruption of AN may become generalized[223,224] (Fig. 23.32), and mucosal involvement may occur, manifested as thickening and papillomatosis of eyelids, conjunctivae, lips, and oral mucosa. The differential diagnosis of AN may include epidermal nevi, lichen simplex chronicus,

Table 23.2 Clinical Associations with and Variants of Acanthosis Nigricans

Association	Comments
"Benign"	Form of epidermal nevus; may be autosomal dominant; associated with multiple nevi
Obesity	Most common type; insulin resistance common; increased incidence of type 2 diabetes mellitus
Malignancy	Usually adults, rarely observed in children; sudden onset and rapid spread; especially abdominal adenocarcinoma
Syndromes	Multiple syndrome associations, including Bloom, Prader–Willi, Lawrence–Seip, PCOS, Beare–Stevenson, and syndromes related to *FGFR3* mutations (including Crouzon syndrome, hypochondroplasia, achondroplasia, SADDAN syndrome); also lupus erythematosus, dermatomyositis, scleroderma
Medications	Niacin, corticosteroids, oral contraceptives, diethylstilbestrol, others
Acral type	Dorsal hands, fingers, feet
Unilateral type	Unilateral distribution or "nevoid"; may persist unchanged or progress to bilateral involvement
Mixed type	Two of the earlier types occurring together

Adapted from Schwartz RA. Acanthosis nigricans. *J Am Acad Dermatol.* 1994;31(1):1–19 and Mustafa M, Moghrabi N, Bin-Abbas B. Hypochondroplasia, acanthosis nigricans, and insulin resistance in a child with FGFR3 mutation: Is it just an association? *Case Rep Endocrinol.* 2014;840492.

FGFR3, Fibroblast growth factor receptor 3; *PCOS,* polycystic ovary syndrome; *SADDAN,* severe achondroplasia with developmental delay and acanthosis nigricans.

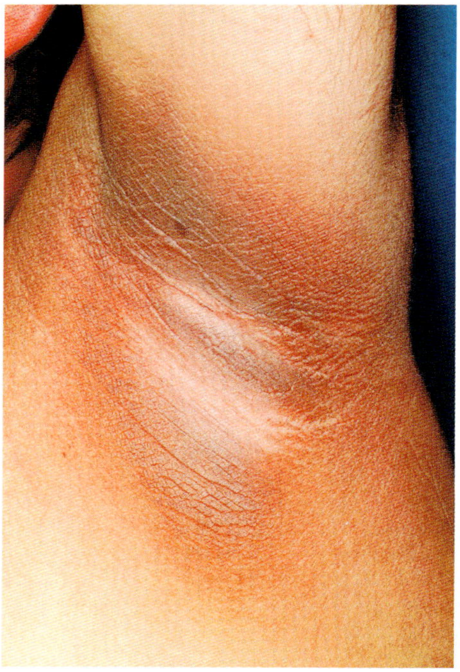

Fig. 23.29 Acanthosis nigricans. Velvety hyperpigmentation involves the axillae in this patient.

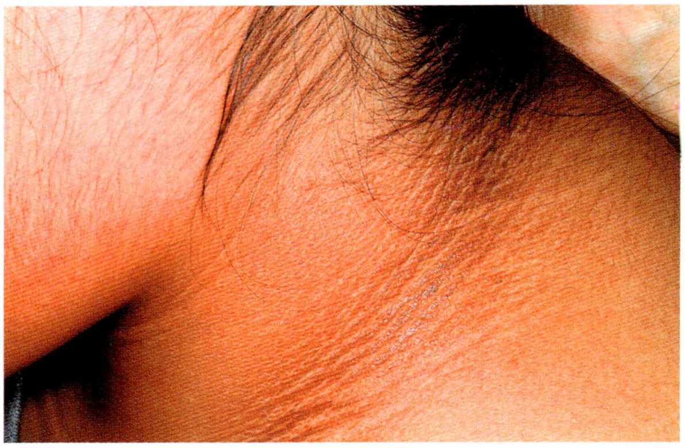

Fig. 23.30 Acanthosis nigricans. Velvety hyperpigmentation is present on the lateral and posterior neck folds of this obese teenaged female.

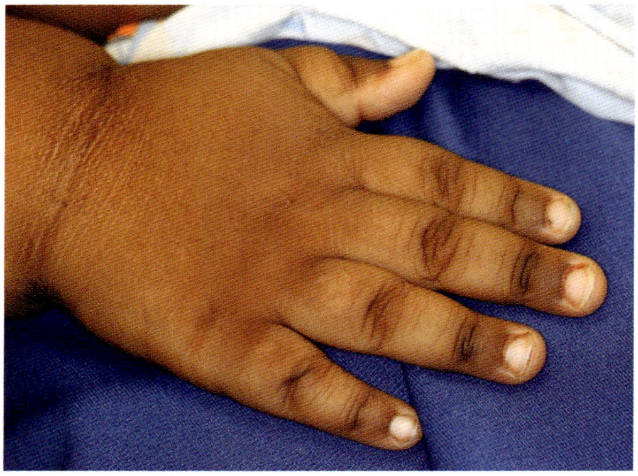

Fig. 23.31 Acanthosis nigricans. Hyperpigmentation with velvety changes may occasionally occur overlying the knuckles. Note involvement over the dorsal wrist fold as well.

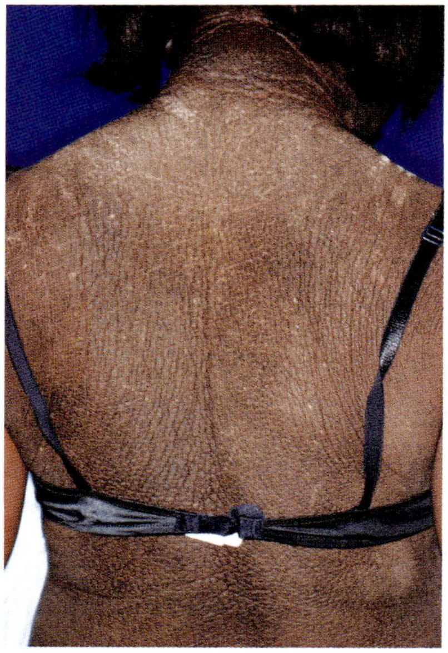

Fig. 23.32 Diffuse acanthosis nigricans. This 12-year-old girl with diffuse acanthosis nigricans had developmental delay and a confirmed mutation in fibroblast growth factor receptor 3 *(FGFR3).*

postinflammatory hyperpigmentation, confluent and reticulated papillomatosis (see later), erythrasma, and endocrine disorders with hyperpigmentation (Addison disease).

Hyperinsulinemia appears to predispose individuals to AN, and patients with inactivating insulin receptor mutations often have severe involvement.[225] Children with AN often have greater body weight and body fat mass, greater basal and glucose-stimulated insulin levels during oral glucose tolerance testing, and lower insulin sensitivity. Importantly, after adjusting for body-fat mass and age, the differences in glucose metabolism and insulin studies were less significant in some studies, indicating that increased BMI should still suggest the possibility of hyperinsulinemia whether or not AN is present.[225] However, other studies have disputed this finding, showing that AN is associated with hyperinsulinemia and impaired glucose metabolism independent of BMI.[226,227] In a study of 149 overweight white children, those with AN had greater BMI, waist circumference, and total body fat, but after correcting for age and BMI, there was no evidence for increased abdominal fat.[228] Among Blacks, AN is strongly associated with obesity and insulin resistance and identifies a subset with a much higher prevalence of NIDDM than is present in Blacks in the general population.[229] AN is associated with obesity in every ethnic group but occurs with greatest incidence (within the obese population) in Native Americans, followed by Blacks, Hispanics, and Whites.[230] It should be considered a clinical surrogate for laboratory-determined hyperinsulinemia and indicates a high risk for NIDDM.[230,231] In one study comparing obese pediatric patients with and without AN, insulin resistance was noted to worsen with increasing AN severity.[232] As mentioned earlier in this chapter, AN and insulin resistance may also be associated with hyperandrogenism as part of the HAIR-AN syndrome, which may also have PCOS as a feature.

The pathogenesis of AN is unclear. In patients with hyperinsulinemia, insulin may bind to insulin-like growth factor receptors in the epidermis, resulting in papillomatosis (thickening with folding). There are no successful therapies for AN, and the primary focus should be on treatment for the underlying condition. In obesity-associated disease, weight reduction itself seems to reduce the findings of AN. Screening for associated comorbidities should be considered, using an individualized approach that incorporates race and family history along with physical findings to decide on further laboratory testing.[233] Topical or oral retinoids may benefit some patients, and lactic acid–containing emollients (e.g., LactiCare, AmLactin, Lac-Hydrin) or other keratolytic agents (salicylic acid, urea) may also be useful.

Confluent and Reticulated Papillomatosis

Confluent and reticulated papillomatosis (CARP) of Gougerot and Carteaud is briefly discussed here because of its clinical overlap with AN. CARP is a rare disorder characterized by hyperpigmented papules confluent in the center and reticulated at the periphery. They have a characteristic distribution involving the intermammary region (Fig. 23.33) most commonly, as well as the epigastric area (Fig. 23.34) and upper back. Less commonly, the neck, axillae (Fig. 23.35), face, and shoulders may be involved. This disorder is seen primarily in adolescents and young adults, is typically asymptomatic, and occurs in females twice as often as males. The differential diagnosis for CARP may include AN, tinea versicolor (see Chapter 17), and *prurigo pigmentosa (PP)*. The latter presents with erythematous papules in a reticulated pattern (Fig. 23.36) and marked pruritus, with a predilection for the trunk and proximal extremities. Histologically, spongiosis and dyskeratosis are noted in distinction to the hyperkeratosis, papillomatosis, and basilar pigmentation seen in CARP, and it tends to respond well to the same oral therapy (minocycline or doxycycline, see later) with subsequent postinflammatory hyperpigmentation.[234]

The cause of CARP remains unknown, although there are several speculative theories. An association with insulin resistance has been hypothesized, and the condition has been reported in patients with concomitant AN, obesity, and hyperinsulinemia.[235] However, in most patients, no such association exists. An abnormal host immune response to *Pityrosporum orbiculare (Malassezia furfur)* has also been suggested, given clinical resemblance to tinea versicolor and the occasional response of patients to treatment with topical or oral antifungal agents, although this association remains controversial.[236,237]

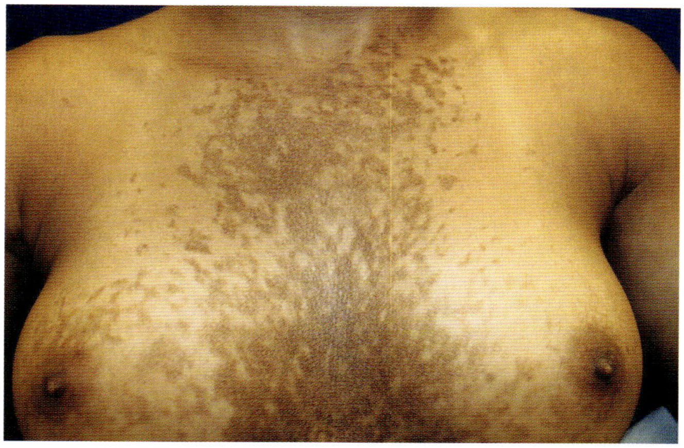

Fig. 23.33 Confluent and reticulated papillomatosis. Hyperpigmented papules and plaques with a reticulate appearance around the periphery involving the intermammary regions of a 16-year-old female patient.

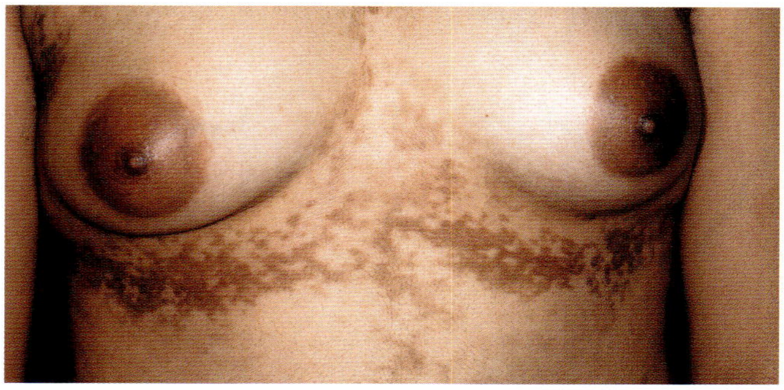

Fig. 23.34 Confluent and reticulated papillomatosis. Reticulate tan papules, patches, and plaques involving the epigastrium, inframammary areas, and sternum.

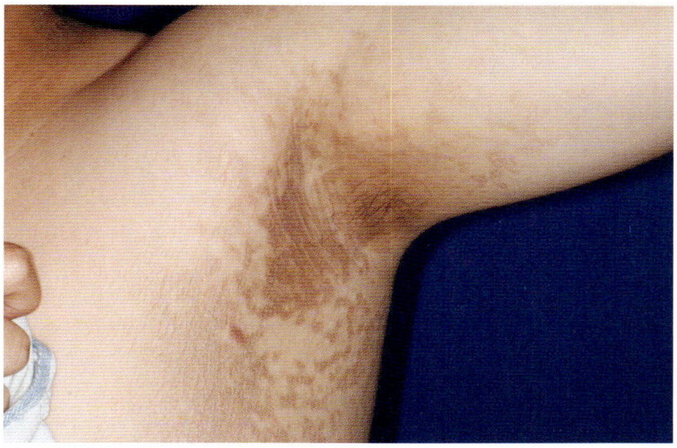

Fig. 23.35 Confluent and reticulated papillomatosis. Hyperpigmented thin plaques, which were confluent centrally and reticulated at the periphery, were present in the bilateral axillae of this 16-year-old male patient who also had classic acanthosis nigricans affecting the neck folds. These axillary changes resolved completely with oral minocycline and lactic acid–containing emollients.

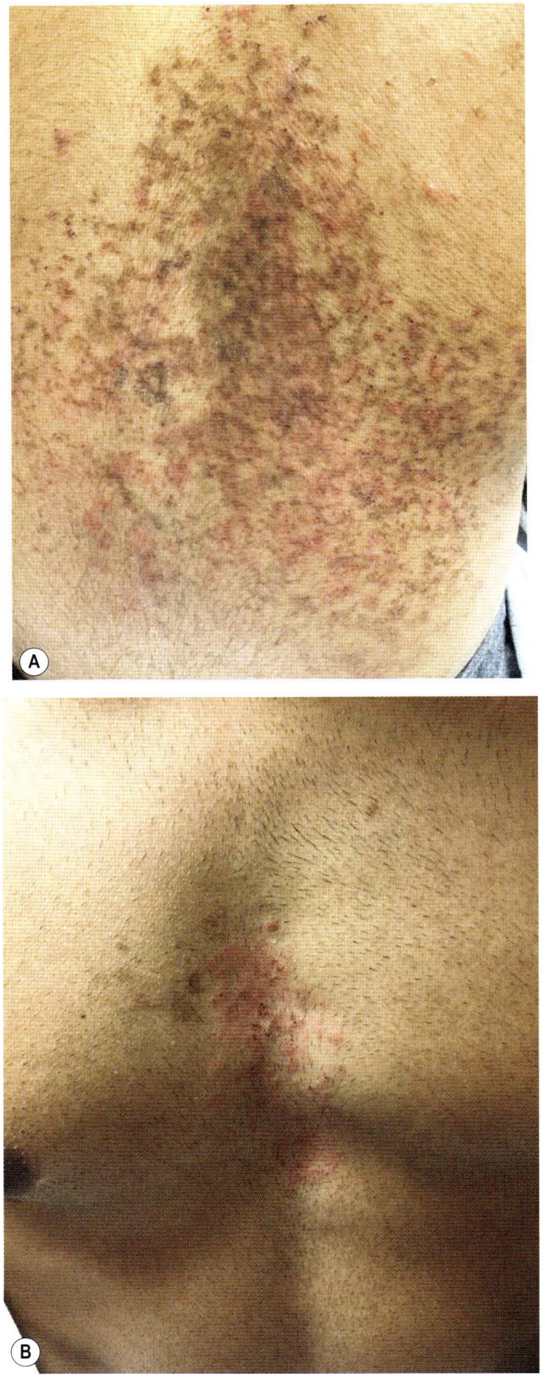

Fig. 23.36 Prurigo pigmentosa. This 17-year-old male patient presented with coalescing erythematous papules and plaques overlying reticulated hyperpigmented patches on his back **(A)** and central chest **(B)**. Skin biopsy revealed changes consistent with prurigo pigmentosa, and the erythematous components cleared rapidly with oral minocycline. (Courtesy Sarah Stein, MD.)

Potassium hydroxide examinations on skin scrapings for fungal elements are negative in the majority of patients.[238] A hypopigmented variant of CARP has been described and may be challenging to differentiate clinically from tinea versicolor.[239]

Treatment of CARP is often, but not always, successful. A significant proportion of patients seem to respond to minocycline or doxycycline,[240–243] although the mechanism of action is unclear. Minocycline in conjunction with a topical lactic acid–containing emollient is often useful. Other reported therapies of variable effectiveness include topical selenium sulfide shampoo, oral or topical retinoids, oral and topical antifungal agents, topical tacrolimus, topical vitamin D analogues, topical salicylic acid, and topical urea.

Scleredema Diabeticorum

Scleredema (see Chapter 22) is a rare disorder characterized by diffuse and symmetric induration of the skin. There are two forms: scleredema of Buschke (which tends to occur after upper respiratory infection, especially streptococcal) and the diabetes mellitus–associated form. Scleredema diabeticorum occurs most often in middle-aged, obese men, although it has been reported in childhood and even in a congenital form.[244] The most common sites are the neck and upper back, but eventual extension to other areas may occur, including the face, scalp, chest, and arms. The skin in affected areas is firm and indurated without pitting and cannot be wrinkled or pressed into folds.[195] The surface appears taut and shiny with loss of normal surface markings. Scleredema is painless but may be uncomfortable for patients, given the textural changes and limitation of movement. Occasionally, involvement of the tongue, pharynx, and esophagus may result in dysarthria and dysphagia. Rare associations include pleural, pericardial, or peritoneal effusion; skeletal muscle dysfunction; and paraproteinemia. Histologic evaluation of biopsy tissue characteristically reveals collagen bundles separated by mucin deposits. The course of scleredema diabeticorum is variable. It may improve with control of the diabetes mellitus,[245] although this is inconsistent; in some patients, it persists for many years. Therapy is challenging, and the results are often disappointing. Treatments reported include antibiotics, corticosteroids, steroid-sparing immunosuppressant agents, chemotherapy, cyclosporine, radiation, light therapy (including UVA1 and PUVA therapy), physiotherapy, and attention to glycemic control.[246–248]

Glucagonoma Syndrome

Patients with glucagon-secreting, pancreatic islet α-cell neuroendocrine tumors may have a distinctive dermatosis termed *necrolytic migratory erythema (NME)*. Glucagonoma syndrome is characterized by the triad of this cutaneous eruption, a glucagon-secreting tumor, and diabetes mellitus.[249] Weight loss, anemia, and stomatitis are common. Patients with this syndrome are generally middle-aged to elderly, with only rare reports of affected adolescents or young adults.[250]

The cutaneous findings of NME are a hallmark of this syndrome. These skin changes may be present for several years before the diagnosis is made. Characteristic features include eroded erythematous plaques that most often begin in the groin, perineum, and buttocks, with eventual extension to the extremities and perioral areas. The plaques are often well demarcated and annular and reveal scaling, vesicles, and bullae. Erosions and pustules may develop (the latter occasionally studding the periphery of the plaques), and crusting is common. Induration, psoriasiform changes, lichenification, and bronze pigmentation may occur. The skin lesions of NME evolve sequentially from erythema to blistering to crusting to resolution and are characterized by a pattern of spontaneous remissions and exacerbations.[249] Secondary superinfection with *Staphylococcus aureus* or *Candida* (especially at perineal sites) is common. In addition, glossitis, stomatitis, angular cheilitis, alopecia, and nail dystrophy may be present.[251] Patients often appear ill and may have venous thromboses. The average 5-year survival rate is less than 50%.[252] The differential diagnosis of NME may include several nutritional deficiency–related dermatoses, staphylococcal scalded skin syndrome, psoriasis, and toxic epidermal necrolysis. A more localized variant, *necrolytic acral erythema*, presents as erythematous eroded and blistering plaques on the lower extremities and is associated with hepatitis C infection.[253]

The diagnosis of NME is suggested by the histologic findings of necrosis and/or pallor of the upper layers of the epidermis, confluent parakeratosis, and spongiosis. The diagnosis of glucagonoma syndrome is confirmed by finding an elevated serum glucagon level or identifying the neuroendocrine tumor radiographically or histologically. Complete surgical resection of the tumor, when feasible, is the treatment of choice and is usually associated with complete to near-complete resolution of the cutaneous eruption.

The complete list of 253 references for this chapter is available online at http://expertconsult.inkling.com.

Key References

Baldauff H, Witchel SF. Polycystic ovary syndrome in adolescent girls. Curr Opin Endocrinol Diabetes Obes 2017;24:56–66.

Tafaj O, Juppner H. Pseudohypoparathyroidism: one gene, several syndromes. J Endocrinol Invest 2017;40:347–56.

Lodish M. Cushing's syndrome in childhood: update on genetics, treatment, and outcomes. Curr Opin Endocrinol Diabetes Obes 2015;22:48–54.

El-Maouche D, Arlt W, Merke DP. Congenital adrenal hyperplasia. Lancet 2017;390(10108):2194–2210.

Rosenfield RL. The diagnosis of polycystic ovary syndrome in adolescents. Pediatrics 2015;136(6):1154–65.

Schmidt TH, Khanijow K, Cedars MI, et al. Cutaneous findings and systemic associations in women with polycystic ovary syndrome. JAMA Dermatol 2016; 152(4):391–8.

Orlova EM, Sozaeva LS, Kareva MA, et al. Expanding the phenotypic and genotypic landscape of autoimmune polyendocrine syndrome type 1. J Clin Endocrinol Metab 2017;102:3546–56.

Bruserud O, Oftedal BE, Wolff AB,et al. *AIRE*-mutations and autoimmune disease. Curr Opin Immunol 2016;43:8–15.

Song X, Zheng S, Yang G, et al. Glucagonoma and the glucagonoma syndrome (review). Oncol Lett 2018;15(3):2749–55.

Doshi DN, Blyumin ML, Kimball AB. Cutaneous manifestations of thyroid disease. Clin Dermatol 2008;26:283–7.

Antal Z, Zhou P. Addison disease. Pediatr Rev 2009;30(12):491–3.

Antal Z, Zhou P. Congenital adrenal hyperplasia: diagnosis, evaluation and management. Pediatr Rev 2009;30:e49–57.

New MI, Abraham M, Yuen T,et al. An update on prenatal diagnosis and treatment of congenital adrenal hyperplasia. Semin Reprod Med 2012;30(5):396–9.

Davidovici BB, Orion E, Wolf R. Cutaneous manifestations of pituitary gland diseases. Clin Dermatol 2008;26:288–95.

Salpea P, Stratakis CA. Carney complex and McCune Albright syndrome: an overview of clinical manifestations and human molecular genetics. Mol Cell Endocrinol 2014;386(1–2):85–91.

Reid SD, Ladizinski B, Lee K, et al. Update on necrobiosis lipoidica: a review of etiology, diagnosis and treatment options. J Am Acad Dermatol 2013;69(5):783–91.

Brickman WJ, Huang J, Silverman BL, Metzger BE. Acanthosis nigricans identifies youth at high risk for metabolic abnormalities. J Pediatr 2010;156:87–92.

24 Inborn Errors of Metabolism

The inborn disorders of metabolism are a group of primarily autosomal recessive hereditary disorders that result in metabolic and clinical defects. (More comprehensive discussion of some of these topics is covered elsewhere: disorders of tyrosine metabolism [Richner–Hanhart syndrome], Gaucher syndrome, and multiple sulfatase deficiency are mentioned in Chapter 5; Menkes syndrome in Chapter 7; alkaptonuria in Chapter 11; Fabry disease and fucosidosis in Chapter 12; and Hartnup disease in Chapter 19.) Most developed countries have instituted comprehensive screening programs during the first week of life that allow detection of many of these defects, among them biotinidase deficiency, aminoacidopathies, urea cycle defects, and organic acid disorders.[1]

Phenylketonuria

Phenylketonuria (PKU; phenylpyruvic oligophrenia) is an autosomal recessive disorder of amino acid metabolism characterized by mental retardation, diffuse hypopigmentation, seizures, dermatitis, and photosensitivity (Table 24.1).[2–4] The classic form is caused by a deficiency of phenylalanine hydroxylase or its cofactor, tetrahydrobiopterin. Its incidence is estimated to be 1 in 10,000 births. Because of mandatory screening in the neonatal period, the disorder is detected early in developed countries, and the clinical features do not appear if early dietary control is achieved. Screening is achieved by a variety of different tests ranging from a semiquantitative bacterial inhibition assay (Guthrie test) to mass spectrometry assays. If missed in the neonatal period by screening, the diagnosis depends on the demonstration of elevated serum levels of phenylalanine (20 mg/dL or higher, 10 to 50 times that of normal), normal or elevated levels of plasma tyrosine (normal is approximately 1 mg/dL), or elevated urinary levels of phenylpyruvic acid. The latter can be detected by a characteristic green or blue color that results when a few drops of urine are added to a 10% solution of ferric chloride. The normal phenylalanine/tyrosine ratio is 1:1; in PKU it is greater than 3:1. The observed pigmentary dilution is thought to result from the inhibitory effect of phenylalanine on tyrosinase. Carriers of PKU have a twofold greater risk of developing melanoma.[5]

Most commonly seen in individuals of northern European ancestry, 90% of affected individuals are blond, blue-eyed, and fair-skinned, given the important role of phenylalanine and its derivative, tyrosine, in pigment formation. A peculiar musty odor, attributable to decomposition products (phenylacetic acid or phenylacetaldehyde) in the urine and sweat, and early intractable vomiting are characteristic. Infants appear to be normal at birth and, if untreated, develop manifestations of delayed intellectual development sometime between 4 and 24 months of age. Seizures, attention-deficit/hyperactivity disorder, hypertonicity, hyperreflexia, a peculiar gait, speech delay, and self-destructive behavior have been described. Skeletal changes include microcephaly, short stature, pes planus, and syndactyly. The dermatitis appears in 10% to 50% of untreated patients and resembles atopic dermatitis; sclerodermoid changes of the proximal extremities, sparing the hands and feet, may present during the first 2 years of life.[6,7] These changes regress with appropriate treatment.

Management consists of a diet low in phenylalanine content, starting at as early an age as possible.[8] This can be initiated by the use of formula from which most of the phenylalanine has been removed or a synthetic amino acid preparation devoid of phenylalanine. Restriction of phenylalanine leads to reversal of the seizures, dermatitis, and pigmentary dilution, but the effect on intellectual function depends on the age at which therapy is initiated. Little benefit for intellectual function can be achieved if therapy is initiated after 2.5 years of age, and optimal benefit is achieved if it is initiated by 2 months of age. It should be remembered that phenylalanine is high in many foods and is a metabolite of the sweetener aspartame. Children and adolescents with PKU who achieve dietary control early in life are well adjusted and have an excellent quality of life.[9] These diets, however, are also higher in carbohydrates and have been linked to higher basal insulin levels, insulin resistance, and high body mass index (BMI) and waist circumference[10] percentiles. Tetrahydrobiopterin (BH4) may reduce phenylalanine levels in some patients who do not adequately adhere to the prescribed diet[11] and has been shown to significantly improve within 4 weeks the attention-deficit/hyperactivity disorder and executive function of patients.[12]

Although there is some controversy about continuation of phenylalanine restriction in later childhood and adults, lack of dietary control during the first trimester of pregnancy of affected mothers (>600 μM or 10 mg/dL phenylalanine) has led to cardiac defects in 15% of offspring, particularly coarctation of the aorta and hypoplastic left heart.[13] Optimal levels during pregnancy of 120 to 360 μM/L are recommended. Some patients maintain low levels of phenylalanine as adults without dietary manipulation, including with use of phenylalanine ammonia lyase (pegvaliase; pegylated PAL), an enzyme substitute therapy that converts phenylalanine to trans-cinnamic acid and ammonia.[14]

Disorders of Tyrosine Metabolism

Clinical disorders of tyrosine metabolism include neonatal tyrosinemia, tyrosinemia I, and tyrosinemia II (Richner–Hanhart syndrome). Of these, only Richner–Hanhart syndrome exhibits cutaneous manifestations and is described in Chapter 5. These include palmoplantar keratoderma with painful erosions and photophobia with corneal erosions.

Table 24.1 Errors of Protein Metabolism

Disorder	Inheritance	Defect	Clinical Features	Diagnosis	Treatment
Phenylketonuria	AR	Phenylalanine hydroxylase (Phe)	90% are blond, blue-eyed, and fair-skinned; musty odor; sclerodermatous plaques; eczematous dermatitis; photosensitivity; retardation; microcephaly; short stature	Guthrie test, ferric chloride test	Low phenylalanine diet; tetrahydrobiopterin (BH4) and phenylalanine ammonia lyase (pegvaliase) are other ways to lower Phe levels
Homocystinuria	AR	Cystathionine synthetase	Ectopia lentis, myopia, arachnodactyly, seizures, mental retardation, cerebrovascular accidents, sparse light or blond easily friable hair, malar flush, wide-pored facies, livedoid rash, "Charlie Chaplin–like" gait and "rocker-bottom" feet	Cyanide nitroprusside test	Low methionine diet with pyridoxine (vitamin B_6)
Alkaptonuria (ochronosis)	AR	Homogentisic acid oxidase	Dark urine; blue to brownish-black pigment on nose, malar region, sclerae, ears, axillae, genitalia; staining of clothing ("beads of ink" perspiration); arthritis; contractures; rupture of Achilles tendon; mitral and aortic valvulitis and/or calcific aortic stenosis	Ferric cyanide reduction	Nitisinone
Trimethylaminuria	AR	Flavin mono-oxygenase type 3	Odor of rotting fish	Trimethylamine in urine	Dietary avoidance of choline
Wilson disease (hepatolenticular degeneration)	AR	*ATP7B*; ceruloplasmin metabolism	Kayser–Fleischer rings, hyperpigmentation, azure lunulae, neurologic and liver dysfunction	Aminoaciduria, decreased ceruloplasmin	Chelating agents (BAL, versenate, or D-penicillamine; trientine has fewer side effects, but is weaker and more expensive); zinc to sequester copper; liver transplantation if liver failure
Lesch–Nyhan syndrome	X-LR	HPRT deficiency	Mental retardation, spastic cerebral palsy, choreoathetosis, self-mutilation	Increased uric acid, orange uric acid crystals in diaper	Allopurinol; purine nucleoside phosphorylase inhibition

AR, Autosomal recessive; *BAL,* British antilewisite or dimercaprol; *HPRT,* hypoxanthine–guanine phosphoribosyl transferase; *X-LR,* X-linked recessive.

Cobalamin Deficiency

Hereditary disorders of intracellular cobalamin metabolism are a group of autosomal recessive disorders that can result from mutations in several genes (*Mut*, *cblA-cblG*, *CblJ*, and *CblX*). Cobalamin deficiency leads to accumulation of methylmalonic acid and homocysteine in the blood and urine from reduced activity of methylmalonyl-CoA mutase and methionine synthase. Hematologic and neurologic abnormalities are most common. Biallelic mutations in *ABCD4*, which encodes an ABC transporter involved in the intracellular processing of cobalamin, led to diffuse progressive skin hyperpigmentation but hair lightening, macrocytic anemia, and cobalamin deficiency in a 12-year-old child.[15] Treatment with oral cobalamin (3 mg daily) led to metabolic correction and some reduction in the skin hyperpigmentation. Cobalamin deficiency during the neonatal and infantile period may result from severe vitamin B_{12} deficiency in the pregnant or breastfeeding mother,[16] which may be asymptomatic. Features in the affected baby are localized skin hyperpigmentation (genital), macrocytic anemia, lethargy, and cobalamin deficiency.

Homocystinuria

Homocystinuria is an autosomal recessive disorder of methionine metabolism that results from an absence or deficiency of cystathionine β-synthase, the pyridoxine-dependent hepatic enzyme that catalyzes the formation of cystathionine from homocysteine and serine.[17] Based on biochemical testing, the disorder is most common in Ireland (1 in 65,000 births) and has a worldwide incidence of 1 in 344,000.[18] However, a study in Norway using genotyping showed an estimated birth prevalence of 1 in 6400.[19]

The disorder affects predominantly the eyes, central nervous system, blood vessels, and bones (see Table 24.1). Subluxation of the ocular lenses (ectopia lentis) occurs in 82% of patients by 15 years of age[20] and is usually present by 10 years of age. Developmental delay is evident during infancy, and most untreated patients develop seizures and significant retardation. Bony abnormalities include a body habitus similar to that seen in Marfan syndrome (see Chapter 6) and generalized osteoporosis, which is seen radiographically in 50% of affected individuals by 15 years of age. Platyspondylia (congenital flattening of the vertebral bodies) and hollowing out of the vertebral bodies by pressure of the vertebral disks are also seen radiographically, and kyphoscoliosis, pectus carinatum, and genu valgum are common. Some patients have rocker-bottom feet, and most have a shuffling toe-out "Charlie Chaplin–like" gait. Megaloblastic anemia has also been described.[21]

The vascular complications can be life threatening; the chance of a vascular event during childhood is 25% to 30% and increases to 50% by 30 years of age. These include pulmonary embolism, myocardial infarction, transient ischemic attacks, cerebrovascular accidents, abdominal aortic aneurysm, and venous thromboses. Cutaneous features include sparse, light or blond, coarse hair that can darken and become softer with treatment; a malar flush[22]; coarse, wide pores on facial skin; and a reticulated livedoid vasculopathy (cutis reticulata) on the face and extremities.

The presence of homocystinuria is suggested by clinical features and can be confirmed by a urinary cyanide or sodium nitroprusside testing (turns a beet-red color) and by amino acid chromatography of the serum and urine. The presence of homocysteine in the urine establishes the diagnosis. In the blood, homocysteine and methionine are elevated, whereas cysteine levels are decreased. Unfortunately, there are no neonatal manifestations of homocystinuria, and not all newborns with this disorder have increased blood methionine levels.

In at least 50% of patients, the disease is responsive to pyridoxine and can be controlled with the combination of pyridoxine (vitamin B_6: 150 mg/day for an infant to 500 mg/day for an adolescent), folic acid, and vitamin B_{12} (cobalamin). For those who do not respond to vitamins alone, a methionine-restricted, cystine-supplemented diet is required as well.[23] Betaine, a methyl donor that remethylates homocysteine to methionine, has been used as an adjunct to treatment, especially in patients who do not respond to vitamin therapy. As with PKU, early institution of therapy dramatically reduces the risk of complications. Enzyme replacement therapy has been shown to reduce symptoms in mouse models[24] and has moved to human trials.[25]

Trimethylaminuria

Trimethylaminuria (the fish odor syndrome) is a metabolic disorder in which accumulation of trimethylamine in the sweat, saliva, and urine gives rise to an unpleasant "rotting fish" odor.[26] There are no visible cutaneous changes, but one-third of patients with an unexplained intermittent malodor were shown to be positive for the disorder using a standard choline challenge.[27] The odor is episodic and thus may not be detected during examination, although chronic halitosis is common.[26]

Trimethylaminuria usually results from mutations in the flavin-containing monooxygenase type 3 (*FMO3*) gene,[28] although variants in other oxidoreductase genes have recently been found.[26] The liver is unable to convert the trimethylamine generated in the intestinal tract by bacterial degradation of choline- and lecithin-containing foods such as saltwater fish and seafood, egg yolk, liver, kidney, soy beans, meat, broccoli, cauliflower, cabbage, Brussel sprouts, wheat germ, milk (from wheat-fed cows), and yeast to the nonodorous oxide metabolite.[29] The psychosocial effects of the condition can be devastating, including disruption of schooling, clinical depression, and attempted suicide. Treatment is best accomplished by avoidance and limitation of choline-containing foods,[23,30] although organ damage can develop if choline levels are too low. Administration of metronidazole has also led to a clinical and biochemical response.[31]

Wilson Disease (Hepatolenticular Degeneration)

Wilson disease is an autosomal recessive disorder that results from mutations in *ATP7B*, which encodes a copper-transporting adenosine triphosphatase (ATPase).[32] Deficiency leads to an inability to synthesize normal amounts of ceruloplasmin.[33,34] Patients show abnormal hepatic excretion of copper and toxic accumulations of copper in the liver, brain, and other organs. The clinical triad that results consists of progressive neurologic dysfunction, hepatic cirrhosis, and pathognomonic pigmentation of the corneal margins (Kayser–Fleischer ring) (see Table 24.1).

The disorder can be detected as early as 4 years of age but usually manifests during adolescence. The clinical signs at presentation can be quite varied. Although initial signs of the disorder are often neurologic (intention tremors, dysarthria, ataxia, incoordination, personality changes, psychiatric problems,[35] and worsening school performance and handwriting), signs of liver insufficiency[36] (jaundice, ascites, hepatomegaly, hematemesis, and cutaneous spider angiomas) are present at onset in 40% to 50% of affected individuals.[37]

Hyperpigmentation of the anterior lower legs, genital region, or even in a generalized distribution[38] may be the presenting sign and may be misinterpreted as Addison disease. In addition, patients may manifest a vague greenish discoloration on the skin of the face, neck, and genitalia. Increased deposition of melanin, but not copper or iron, is seen in cutaneous biopsy specimens. Blue or azure lunulae of the nails have been reported in individuals with this disorder, but also have been observed in normal individuals as a complication of phenolphthalein or quinacrine ingestion, and in argyria. White discoloration of the nails has also been noted.[39] Xerosis has been described in almost half of affected children.[39]

Kayser–Fleischer rings are seen as dense golden-brown or greenish-brown pigmentation localized near the limbus of the cornea. Occurring in about 95% of patients with this disorder and best visualized by side lighting and slit-lamp examination, this discoloration is produced by the deposition of copper in the Descemet membrane at the periphery of the cornea. In younger children, anterior segment optical coherence tomography has been suggested as a substitute for slit-lamp examination[40] because of limited cooperation. Kayser–Fleischer rings may also be seen in other copper overload states such as primary cirrhosis, intrahepatic cholestasis of childhood (Byler syndrome), and chronic active hepatitis. Wilson disease is progressive and, if untreated, is inevitably fatal. Death usually results from infection, hepatic disease, or liver failure.

Elevation of blood and urine copper levels is typical of Wilson disease. A ceruloplasmin level of <150 mg/L has higher diagnostic accuracy than the conventional cutoff of <200 mg/L, which can then include some infants and patients with liver failure or nephrotic syndrome.[41] Liver biopsy and molecular genetic testing can also be used for diagnosis.[42]

Treatment depends on removal of accumulated copper depositions in the body. Chelating agents such as D-penicillamine or trientine (triethylene tetramine dihydrochloride)[43] increase urinary excretion of copper. An alternative or maintenance medication is elemental zinc (1 to 3 mg/kg per day divided three times daily), which some propose should be the treatment of choice.[44] Because discontinuation of therapy can result in rapid deterioration, treatment is lifelong. Penicillamine can produce allergic or toxic reactions, fever, cutaneous rashes, leukopenia, thrombocytopenia, elastosis perforans serpiginosa[45,46] (see Chapter 6; Fig. 6.15), other dermal disorders,[47] and immunobullous skin disease.[48] Because penicillamine inhibits pyridoxine-dependent enzymes, patients should also be given daily supplements of pyridoxine (12.5 to 50 mg/day). In an effort to minimize copper deposition, patients should be encouraged to limit their ingestion of copper-rich foods such as liver, nuts, chocolate, cocoa, mushrooms, brain, shellfish, dried foods, and broccoli. Liver transplantation can be lifesaving for patients with hepatic failure.[42,49,50]

Lesch–Nyhan Syndrome

Lesch–Nyhan syndrome, an X-linked recessive disorder of purine metabolism, is characterized by mental retardation, choreoathetoid movements, and self-mutilation.[51] The condition is caused by a deficiency of hypoxanthine–guanine phosphoribosyl transferase (HPRT),[52] which leads to an overproduction of uric acid and the clinical features associated with this disorder (see Table 24.1). Patients appear normal at birth and may develop normally for 6 to 8 months. The first recognizable sign of the disease is often orange uric acid crystals (resembling grains of sand) in the diaper or as hematuria during the early months of life.

The onset of cerebral manifestations may be subtle, with difficulty in sitting or standing without help, involuntary movements, dystonia, spasticity, and increased deep tendon reflexes. Although mental retardation may vary in degree, it usually is severe, and abnormal behavior remains a striking characteristic of the disease. The main clinical feature of this disorder is a loss of tissue about the mouth or fingers that occurs, not because of an inability to feel pain but rather due to the child's habit of compulsive self-destructive biting of these areas. In time, without adequate restraints, all of the lower lip accessible to the teeth may be chewed away. The face, fingers, and wrists may also be mutilated, and because young children commonly bite others, caution should be exercised when handling children with this disorder. Other destructive behaviors include head banging, extension of arms when being wheeled through doorways, tipping of wheelchairs, eye-poking, fingers in wheelchair spokes, and rubbing behaviors. Other manifestations of hyperuricemia, such as tophaceous deposits, nephropathy, and gouty arthritis, occur later. Reticulated pigment changes in a variant form have been described.[53]

Not to be confused with familial dysautonomia (Riley–Day syndrome) and congenital insensitivity to pain with anhidrosis (see Chapter 8), other conditions characterized by biting and self-mutilating behavior, Lesch–Nyhan syndrome can be confirmed by the clinical presentation and laboratory demonstration of increased levels of uric acid in the blood and urine.[54] Heterozygous females are asymptomatic. Management includes the use of xanthine oxidoreductase inhibitors, particularly allopurinol (10 mg/kg per day or, if >10 years of age, 600 to 800 mg/day divided twice daily), in an effort to control uric acid levels. Inhibition of purine nucleoside phosphorylase, which catalyzes the cleavage of purine ribonucleosides, allows lowering of the dose of oxidoreductase inhibitors.[55] Physical restraints (hand bandages and elbow splints) may be used to help control the self-mutilating behavior of patients.[51] Lip biting may require extraction of deciduous teeth, but permanent teeth should be spared, because lip biting usually diminishes with age.

Dermatitis from Nutritional Abnormalities

ACRODERMATITIS ENTEROPATHICA

Acrodermatitis enteropathica is an autosomal recessive disorder that generally appears in early infancy and is characterized by a triad of acral and periorificial skin lesions, diarrhea, and alopecia (Table 24.2).[56–58] The condition first manifests days to weeks after birth if an infant is bottle-fed and shortly after weaning if breastfed. The disorder results from mutations in *SLC39A4 (ZIP4)*, which encodes an intestinal zinc transporter *ZIP4*[59] that is a cofactor for many metalloenzymes and a component of DNA-regulatory proteins. This zinc transporter is also expressed in epidermis and regulates the activity of ΔNp63, which is important for epidermal homeostasis.[60]

The basic cutaneous lesion of acrodermatitis enteropathica is an erythematous, scaling, crusted, psoriasiform, eczematous, or vesiculobullous[61] eruption (see Fig. 2.35). Lesions tend to be localized around the body orifices (mouth, nose, ears, eyes, and perineum; Figs. 24.1 and 24.2) and symmetrically located on the buttocks (Fig. 24.3) and extensor surface of major joints (elbows, knees, hands, and feet), the scalp, and the fingers and toes (hence the term *acrodermatitis*). On the face, the eroded and crusted peribuccal plaques may appear impetiginized, and secondary infection with *Candida albicans* is common. When the fingers and toes are involved, there is marked erythema and swelling of the paronychial tissues, often with subsequent nail deformity. If unrecognized or untreated, acrodermatitis enteropathica follows an intermittent but relentlessly progressive course, and, as a consequence of general disability, infection, or both, commonly ends in death.

Typically, infants with acrodermatitis enteropathica are listless, anorexic, and apathetic. Many infants show frequent crying, irritability, and restlessness. Tissue wasting may be present, with an associated failure to thrive. During periods of exacerbation, frothy, bulky, foul-smelling diarrheal stools are often present. Other findings may

Table 24.2 Genetic and Acquired Nutritional Disorders

Disorder	Cause	Features	Evaluation	Therapy
Zinc deficiency	Acrodermatitis enteropathica Decreased zinc in breast milk Poor zinc diet Malabsorption Zinc-poor IV hyperalimentation	Periorificial dermatitis, stomatitis, glossitis, alopecia, irritability, diarrhea, failure to thrive, candidal infections, photophobia	Zinc levels, serum alkaline phosphatase; zinc levels in maternal breast milk	Zinc supplementation
Biotin deficiency	Holocarboxylase deficiency Biotinidase deficiency Malabsorption Ingestion of egg whites Biotin-poor IV hyperalimentation	Periorificial dermatitis, conjunctivitis, blepharitis, alopecia, candidal infections, metabolic acidosis, vomiting, lethargy, developmental delay, seizures, ataxia, optic atrophy, hearing loss	Urinary organic acids, plasma ammonia and lactate, serum biotin, specific enzyme activity	Biotin supplementation
Deficiency of vitamin B_{12} or isoleucine from restrictive diets	Organic acidurias Citrullinemia Maple syrup urine disease Methylmalonic acidemia Propionic acidemia	Periorificial dermatitis, alopecia, candidal infections, metabolic acidosis, vomiting, failure to thrive, lethargy, developmental delay, hypotonia, pancytopenia	Urinary organic acids; plasma ammonia and glycine levels, plasma isoleucine levels	Dietary manipulation (results from effects of low-protein diet; some respond to vitamin B_{12} supplementation)
Cystic fibrosis	Deficiency of CFTR	Periorificial and truncal dermatitis, occasionally alopecia, failure to thrive, diarrhea, irritability, edema	Sweat test, serum albumin, gene analysis, mutational analysis of *CFTR* gene	Pancreatic enzymes, vitamin and zinc supplementation
Essential fatty acid deficiency	Inadequate dietary intake	Generalized scaling with underlying erythema, intertriginous erosions, alopecia, decreased pigmentation of hair, failure to thrive, thrombocytopenia, and anemia	Plasma linoleic, linolenic, arachidonic and eicosatrienoic acid levels; check for other deficiencies	Supplementation of essential fatty acids
Kwashiorkor	Inadequate protein; often infants taken off milk protein for allergies or dietary fads without adequate replacement	Superficial desquamation with erosion (flaky paint), edema with moon facies and pallor, hyperpigmentation and hypopigmentation, ecchymoses, sparse, dry lusterless hair with decreased pigmentation and "flag sign," cheilitis, dry mucosae, irritability and failure to thrive, irritability and apathy, secondary skin infections, diarrhea, hepatomegaly	Serum albumin, good dietary history	Slow supplementation with protein, correction of electrolyte imbalances

CFTR, Cystic fibrosis transmembrane conductance regulator; *IV*, intravenous.

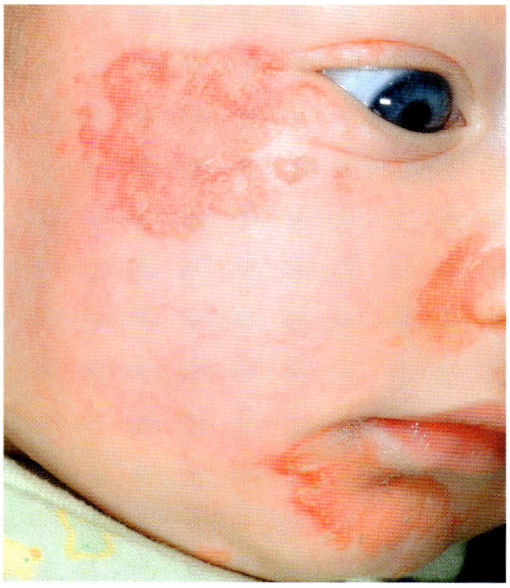

Fig. 24.1 Acrodermatitis enteropathica. Moist, sharply marginated psoriasiform plaques around the mouth, nose, and eyes of an infant.

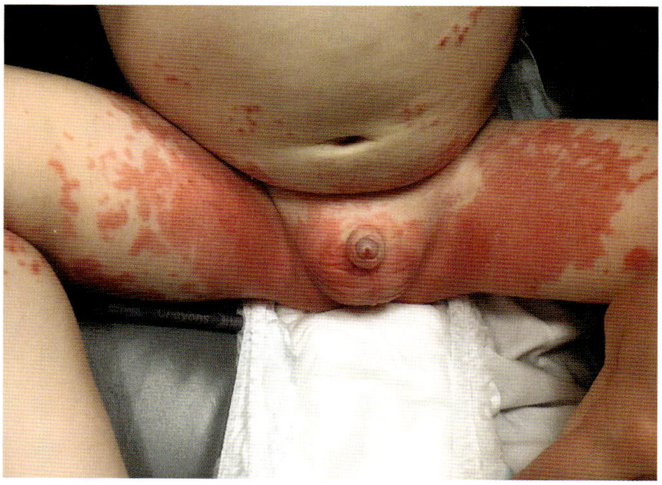

Fig. 24.2 Acrodermatitis enteropathica. Psoriasiform plaques of the groin, inner thighs, and lower abdomen.

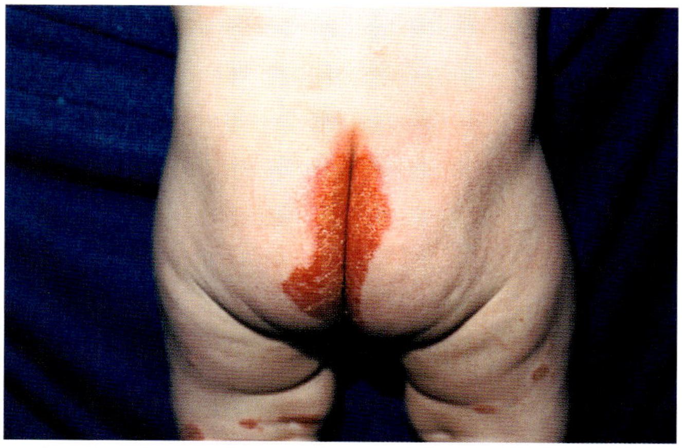

Fig. 24.3 Acrodermatitis enteropathica. Sharply marginated psoriasiform plaques of the perianal area and buttock.

include conjunctivitis; photophobia; stomatitis; perlèche; nail dystrophy; recurring candidal or bacterial infection; and alopecia of the scalp, eyelashes, and/or eyebrows.[62] Children suffering from this disorder exhibit a striking uniformity of appearance, mainly because of the alopecia and periorificial lesions.

In addition to the classic inherited disease, zinc deficiency with signs mimicking acrodermatitis enteropathica may occur in babies who are breastfed by mothers with inadequate secretion of zinc in the maternal milk.[63] Maternal mutations in *SLC30A2 (ZnT-2)*, which encodes a protein required for zinc secretion, have been found.[64] Zinc deficiency with clinical manifestations may also be seen in individuals receiving long-term parenteral nutrition with inadequate zinc supplementation[65]; patients who have had intestinal bypass procedures; premature infants with low zinc storage (particularly those fed exclusively with human milk); patients with Crohn's disease[66]; infants with human immunodeficiency virus (HIV) infection and diarrhea (causing inadequate absorption of zinc); patients with cystic fibrosis with poor zinc absorption[67–69]; patients with celiac disease[70,71]; adolescents with anorexia nervosa[72,73]; individuals on zinc-deficient vegetarian diets; and patients with low pancreatic enzyme levels resulting in poor intestinal absorption of zinc.[58,74] In babies with cystic fibrosis, the manifestations of zinc deficiency are often noted at 3 to 5 months of age, before any evidence of pulmonary disease. The low serum albumin level and abnormal sweat test can confirm the diagnosis. Mothers with extremely poor nutrition and zinc deficiency may also have a baby with zinc deficiency if breastfeeding. An acrodermatitis enteropathica–like eruption can be seen with biotin deficiency and kwashiorkor (see later).

The diagnosis of acrodermatitis enteropathica is based on the clinical features and low serum zinc levels (50 mcg/dL or lower). It should be noted, however, that zinc contamination of glass tubes and rubber stoppers often occurs; blood samples should be collected in acid-washed sterile plastic tubes with the use of acid-washed plastic syringes. Low serum alkaline phosphatase levels (even when the serum zinc level is normal), low serum lipid levels, and defective chemotaxis may be found. Skin biopsy is not diagnostic but may be useful in some patients. In breastfed babies with zinc deficiency, zinc levels can be measured in maternal milk.

Zinc sulfate supplementation (5 to 10 mg/kg per day) usually provides approximately 1 to 2 mg/kg per day elemental zinc; the dosage of other formulations necessary to provide sufficient elemental zinc may require adjustment if zinc sulfate is not used. When given in divided doses two or three times a day, improvement in temperament and decrease in irritability can generally be noted within 1 or 2 days; the appetite improves in a few days, and diarrhea and skin lesions begin to respond within 2 or 3 days after the initiation of therapy. Hair growth begins after 2 to 3 weeks of therapy, and increase in the growth of the infant generally occurs within approximately 2 weeks. After the patient's condition appears to be stabilized, zinc levels should be monitored at periodic (6-month) intervals, followed by the adjustment of continuing supplemental zinc[75] to the lowest effective dosage schedule. Because foods may have an effect on the absorption of zinc, zinc supplementation should be administered 1 or 2 hours before meals. If zinc supplementation causes gastrointestinal upset (nausea, vomiting, gastric hemorrhage), zinc gluconate can be substituted and tends to cause fewer gastrointestinal problems. Less zinc supplementation may be required for acquired or dietary zinc deficiency. In infants who have zinc deficiency because of defective maternal mammary zinc secretion, zinc supplementation can be discontinued after weaning.

Disorders That Resemble Acrodermatitis Enteropathica

BIOTIN DEFICIENCY/ORGANIC ACID DISORDERS

Dermatitis resembling acrodermatitis enteropathica, often in association with alopecia and changes in hair texture, has been described in patients with biotin deficiency and in certain organic acid disorders.[76,77] Cutaneous features resembling acrodermatitis enteropathica have been described in methylmalonic acidemia,[78,79] propionic acidemia,[78] glutaric aciduria type I,[80] maple syrup urine disease,[81]

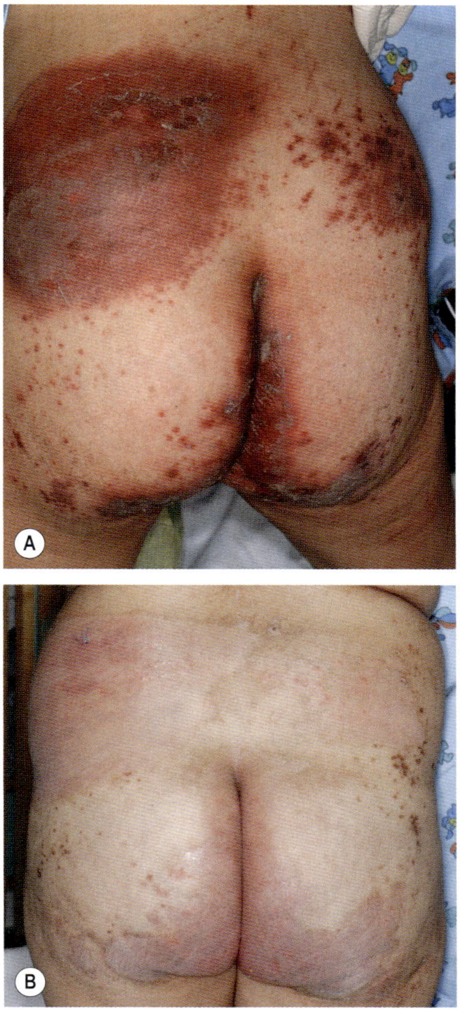

Fig. 24.4 Methylmalonic acidemia. **(A)** This patient developed the typical erosive and desquamative eruption while on a restricted diet. **(B)** Isoleucine deficiency was discovered, and the eruption cleared within a week when isoleucine was added to the diet.

ornithine transcarbamylase deficiency,[82] and citrullinemia[83] because of dietary restriction and deficiency of amino acids, especially isoleucine (Fig. 24.4).[84,85] Acrodermatitis enteropathica–like eruptions have also been reported in children with Hartnup disease (see Chapter 19).[86,87] Staphylococcal scalded skin syndrome is sometimes considered in the differential diagnosis because of the periorificial location of lesions. Biotin deficiency activates innate, Th1, and Th17 proinflammatory responses,[88,89] which has been linked to the inflammatory skin lesions.

Biotin, part of the vitamin B complex, is required for the function of four carboxylase enzymes[74]:

1. 3-Methyl crotonyl-CoA carboxylase, essential for the catabolism of leucine
2. Propionyl CoA carboxylase, essential for the catabolism of isoleucine, threonine, valine, and methionine
3. Pyruvic acid carboxylase, required for the gluconeogenesis and regulation of carbohydrate metabolism
4. Acetyl CoA carboxylase, an enzyme of long-chain fatty acid synthesis that contains biotin

Biotin deficiency may be induced by a biotin-deficient diet, such as with ingestion of large quantities of raw egg white (which contains avidin, a protein that binds to biotin and prevents its absorption in the

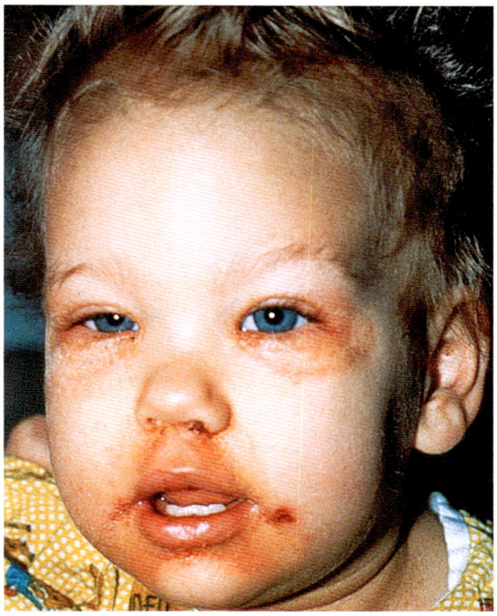

Fig. 24.5 **Biotin deficiency. Scaly, periorificial dermatitis in a child with biotin-responsive carboxylase deficiency.** (From Williams ML, Packman S, Cowan MJ. Alopecia and periorificial dermatitis in biotin-responsive multiple carboxylase deficiency. J Am Acad Dermatol 1983;9(1):97–103.)

intestine) and/or prolonged parenteral nutrition to which biotin has not been added (see Table 24.2). The resulting deficiency is manifested by anorexia, lassitude, a pale tongue, grayish pallor of the skin, atrophy of the lingual papillae, hair loss, anemia, muscle pains, dryness of the skin, and a scaly dermatitis, all of which disappear after biotin administration or by cooking, boiling, or steaming the egg white, which causes avidin to lose its biotin-binding capacity. Decreased biotin levels have also been noted in patients who have been administered antiepileptics (phenytoin, carbamazepine) and may result in seborrheic dermatitis–like lesions and alopecia.[90,91]

Several autosomal recessive disorders may manifest as an acrodermatitis enteropathica–like eruption, because they require biotin as a cofactor. Cheilitis and diffuse erythema with erosions and desquamation are features of methylmalonic acidemia before therapeutic amino acid restriction.[79,92,93] Inherited biotin deficiency also occurs in two forms of multiple carboxylase deficiency, one of which presents acutely during the neonatal period (neonatal form) and the other during early infancy (juvenile form).[94] These disorders occur in up to 1:40,000 births. Both forms usually show a sharply marginated, brightly erythematous scaling eruption of the periorificial areas, scalp, eyebrows, and eyelashes (Fig. 24.5).[95] Alopecia can manifest as hair thinning or total alopecia. Secondary candidiasis is not uncommon.[96] The neonatal form, which results from deficiency of holocarboxylase synthetase, appears in the first few weeks of life with metabolic acidosis, ketosis, and, rarely, cutaneous manifestations. Patients show feeding and breathing difficulties, seizures, hypotonia, and lethargy; without early diagnosis and treatment, they usually die. The juvenile form of the disorder, which first manifests at 2 months of age or older, is the result of deficiency of biotinidase, which is required for recycling of endogenous biotin.[97] Patients have low levels of biotin in the blood and urine and impaired biotin absorption and/or transport. In addition to the cutaneous features, the juvenile form is characterized by seizures (especially myoclonic spasms that respond partially to antiepileptics), hyperventilation or apnea, recurrent infections (including candidal skin infections), keratoconjunctivitis, ataxia, hypotonia, glossitis, and life-threatening acidosis and massive ketosis. Biotin deficiency has also been described from dietary deficiency (low-biotin formulas in infants).[98,99]

The diagnosis of biotin deficiency can be established by a decreased concentration of plasma biotin. Deficiencies of biotinidase or holocarboxylase synthetase also show an increase in the urinary metabolites 3-hydroxyisovaleric acid, 3-methylcrotonyl-glycine, 3-hydroxypropionic acid, methylcitric acid, and lactic acid. Biotin deficiency can be treated by intravenous multivitamins containing 60 mcg of biotin or by the oral administration of 5 to 10 mg of biotin daily. Higher concentrations of biotin may be required for holocarboxylase synthetase deficiency.[100] Skin and neurologic signs tend to improve within a few weeks, although neurologic dysfunction can be permanent if treatment is delayed. More than 50% of patients whose disease is not recognized early have hearing loss that does not improve with biotin therapy.

KWASHIORKOR

Kwashiorkor is a severe form of protein deficiency in which edema, hypoalbuminemia, and dermatosis predominate.[101] Seen primarily in underdeveloped countries, several cases of kwashiorkor have been described in developed countries as well.[102,103] In underdeveloped locations, kwashiorkor is associated with poor food intake, recurrent infections, poor sanitation, and disturbance of the microbiota.

Cases in developed countries have been described because of nutritional ignorance, food allergen avoidance, food fads, and child abuse.[104] Particularly common is the substitution of rice "milk," which has only a miniscule content of protein and is not a milk substitute.[105] In children with chronic protein and caloric malnutrition, particularly from Africa, signs usually present during the second or third year of life with the onset of weaning from breastfeeding. In contrast, patients in developed countries most commonly show features during the first year of life with a rapid onset of edema. Kwashiorkor has also been described with malabsorption disorders, including infantile Crohn's disease,[106] pancreatic insufficiency,[107] and cystic fibrosis.[108,109]

The clinical picture consists of a blanching erythema with an overlying reddish-brown scale that shows a sharply marginated raised edge. This edge resembles paint that is lifting up and about to peel off, leading to the term *flaky paint dermatosis* (Figs. 24.6 and 24.7). In contrast to lesions of pellagra, the dermatosis seldom appears on areas exposed to sunlight and tends to spare the feet and dorsal areas of the hands. Photosensitivity, purpura, and excessive bruisability may also be present. Other associated features include changes in mental behavior, anorexia, apathy, irritability, growth retardation, and fatty infiltration of the liver with hypoproteinemia. As a result of the hypoalbuminemia, affected children show edema of the face (moon facies) (Fig. 24.8), feet, and abdomen (potbelly appearance).

In mild cases the cutaneous eruption is associated with a superficial desquamation; in severe cases there are large areas of erosion that have been mistaken for Stevens–Johnson syndrome and/or toxic epidermal necrolysis.[110] As the disease progresses, the entire cutaneous surface develops a reddish or coffee-colored hue. Other associated features include circumoral pallor, loss of pigmentation (especially after minor trauma), and depigmentation of the hair. In darker-haired children, the hair color can change to a reddish-brown hue or even gray or straw color (Fig. 24.9). The dyschromia

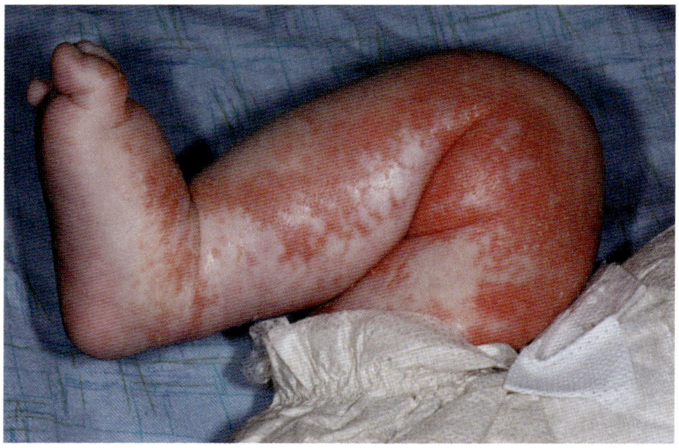

Fig. 24.6 Kwashiorkor. Sharply marginated dermatitis with irregular borders on the leg of an infant with severe hypoalbuminemia from dietary deficiency. Note the desquamation and edema.

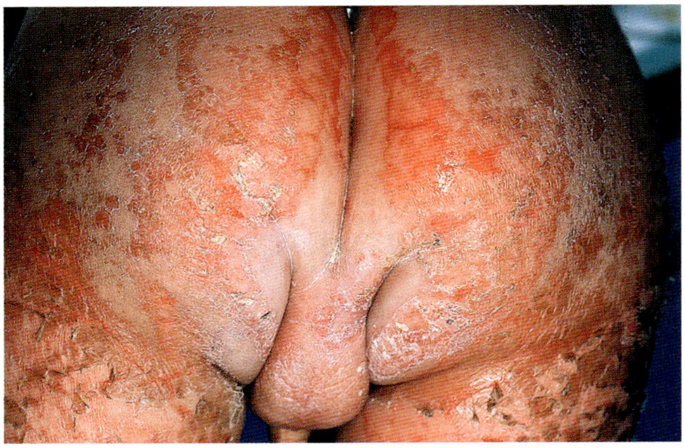

Fig. 24.7 Kwashiorkor. Note the brown, peeling, "flaky paint" appearance of the posterior aspect of the upper thighs.

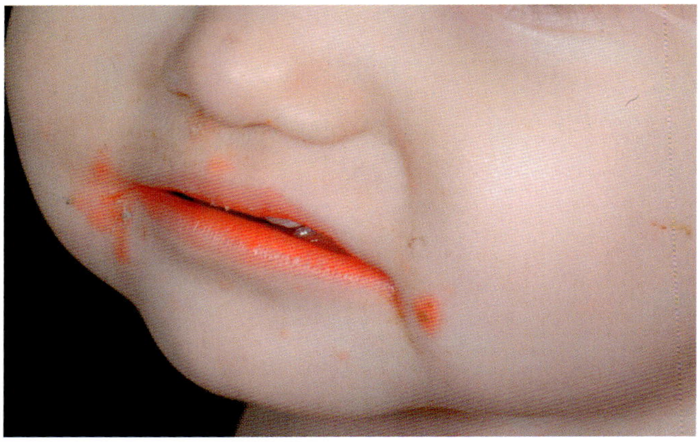

Fig. 24.8 Kwashiorkor. Moon facies and generalized dermatosis.

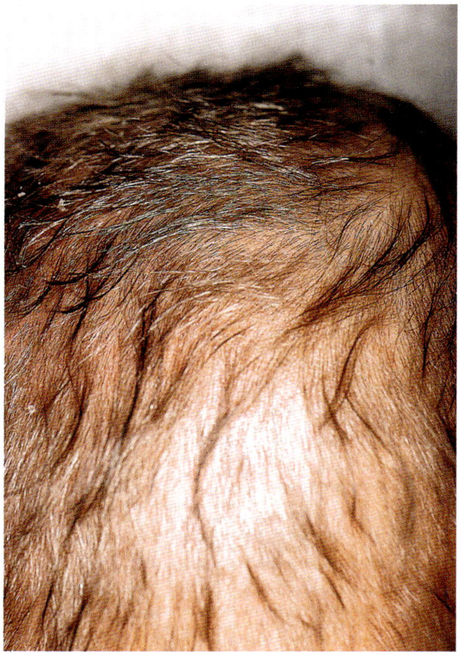

Fig. 24.9 Kwashiorkor. The hair often loses its coloration and may become gray or straw-colored.

with hypopigmentation has been attributed to a deficiency of tyrosine, which is critical for melanin synthesis. When periods of malnutrition alternate with intervals of adequate dietary intake, alternating bands of light and dark color (the flag sign) are produced in the hair.

The condition may be difficult to distinguish from acrodermatitis enteropathica, and in fact, children may have concomitant zinc deficiency as well. The hypoalbuminemia and edema are helpful signs to distinguish kwashiorkor from acrodermatitis enteropathica and other disorders of nutritional deficiency. Children with marasmus have both protein and caloric deficiency. They appear emaciated (vs. the edematous appearance of children with kwashiorkor); have dry, scaling skin that may show follicular hyperkeratosis; and often have thin, sparse hair. In the setting of a child with atopic dermatitis and restricted diet, the concurrence of kwashiorkor may mistakenly be thought to be part of the dermatitis.

Children afflicted with kwashiorkor may become extremely ill, and if they are not treated, the mortality rate can be 30% or more, primarily resulting from infection (impairment of immunity) and electrolyte imbalance with diarrhea. In underdeveloped countries where the disorder is common, breastfeeding should be continued for as long as possible to prevent the protein malnutrition. However, refeeding is complicated and involves provision of fluid, electrolytes (especially potassium and phosphate), and other micronutrients, such as folate. The World Health Organization (WHO) has developed formulations to slowly refeed in the hospital, such as F-75 (75 calories and 0.9 g of protein per 100 mL)[111] and F-100 (100 calories and 2.9 g of protein per 100 mL), but inexpensive ready-to-use-therapeutic foods, milk-, and peanut butter-based preparations similar in composition to F-100 have facilitated home-based refeeding[112] in underdeveloped countries.

ESSENTIAL FATTY ACID DEFICIENCY

Essential fatty acid (EFA) deficiency can also be manifested by periorificial dermatitis and a generalized xerotic or eczematous dermatitis (see Table 24.2).[113] Failure to thrive, alopecia with lightly colored hair, and thrombocytopenia are other signs that may occur. The condition usually occurs in patients receiving parenteral nutrition without lipid supplementation,[114] in association with severe fat malabsorption from gastrointestinal disorders, or with surgery of the gastrointestinal tract. EFA has also been described in patients with cystic fibrosis, anorexia nervosa, and acrodermatitis enteropathica. Decreased plasma levels of linoleic, linolenic, arachidonic, and eicosatrienoic acid, as well as an icosatrienoic/arachidonic acid ratio of greater than 0.4 confirms the diagnosis. The treatment consists of oral or parenteral fat emulsions. Home parenteral nutrition with lipid emulsions that contain a mixture of olive oil and soybean oil has not led to clinical or biochemical evidence of EFA[115] deficiency. If these cannot be administered, topical application of 2 to 3 mg/kg soybean or safflower oil may be sufficient to restore plasma levels of linoleic acids but may not maintain stores in the liver or other tissues.[116]

The Hyperlipidemias

The hyperlipidemias (hyperlipoproteinemias) represent a group of metabolic diseases characterized by persistent elevation of plasma cholesterol levels, triglyceride (TG) levels, or both. Because plasma lipids circulate in the form of high-molecular-weight complexes bound to protein, the term *hyperlipidemia* also indicates an elevation of lipoproteins, hence justification for the term *hyperlipoproteinemia* for this group of disorders. The dermatologic manifestation is the xanthoma, which may also be seen in metabolic disorders with normal levels of lipids (sitosterolemia and cerebrotendinous xanthomatosis) and disorders with deficiencies in high-density lipoproteins. Xanthomas can provide a clue that a child has a serious lipid abnormality and is at risk for other abnormalities, particularly vascular disease.

Lipid levels can be assayed in blood samples taken after a 12-hour fast. Plasma lipoproteins differ significantly in electrostatic charges, thus permitting their separation by electrophoretic mobility techniques into four major fractions: chylomicrons and β-, pre-β-, and α-lipoproteins. By means of ultracentrifugation it is also possible to separate the plasma lipoproteins into four major groups: chylomicrons and very low-density lipoproteins (VLDL; including the pre-β-mobility lipoproteins), low-density lipoproteins (LDL or LDL-C, the β-mobility lipoprotein), and high-density lipoprotein (HDL; the α-mobility lipoprotein), which correlate well with those separated by electrophoresis. TGs are the major core lipids of chylomicrons and VLDLs. Cholesterol esters predominate in the core of LDLs, HDLs, remnants of VLDLs (also known as *intermediate-density lipoproteins* or *IDLs*), and chylomicrons. Apolipoproteins mediate the binding of lipoproteins to their receptors in target organs and activate enzymes that metabolize lipoproteins (Table 24.3). The levels of lipoproteins allow classification of the familial hyperlipidemias into five groups, designated as hyperlipoproteinemias I through V (WHO/Frederickson classification system), each with its own specific clinicopathologic, prognostic, and therapeutic features (Tables 24.4 and 24.5). Of these, types I and II most commonly present during childhood.

Lipoproteins can be synthesized from dietary intake or made endogenously in the liver. Dietary TG are degraded by pancreatic lipase and bile acids to fatty acids and monoglycerides, but they are repackaged after intestinal absorption with cholesterol esters to form the central core of a chylomicron. This core is surrounded by free cholesterol, phospholipids, and apolipoproteins (see Table 24.3). In the circulation, this TG core is hydrolyzed by lipoprotein lipase (LPL), leaving a chylomicron remnant of predominantly cholesterol ester and releasing fatty acids to peripheral tissues; LPL is activated by apolipoprotein C-II and requires hormones such as insulin. The endogenous pathway of lipid synthesis begins in the liver with the formation of VLDLs from hepatic TGs and circulating free fatty acids.

Xanthomas are lipid-containing papules, plaques, nodules, or tumors that may be found anywhere on the skin and mucous membranes.[117,118] Although the mechanism of their formation is not completely understood, it appears that serum lipids infiltrate tissues,

Table 24.3 Apolipoproteins and Their Function

Apolipoprotein	Association with Lipoprotein	Function
ApoA1	HDL, chylomicrons	Main protein of HDL; activates lecithin/cholesterol acyltransferase
ApoA3	VLDL, HDL, chylomicrons	Interacts with LDL receptor and affects lipoprotein metabolism
ApoB48	Chylomicrons	Only in chylomicrons; ApoB100 without LDL receptor-binding domain
ApoB100	LDL, VLDL	Main protein of LDL; binds to LDL receptor
ApoC2	HDL, VLDL, chylomicrons	Activates lipoprotein lipase
ApoC3	VLDL	Inhibits lipoprotein lipase and hepatic lipase to delay catabolism of triglyceride-rich particles
ApoE2, E3, E4	HDL, VLDL, chylomicron remnants	Binds to LDL receptor

HDL, High-density lipoprotein; *LDL*, low-density lipoprotein, *VLDL*, very low-density lipoprotein.

Table 24.4 Laboratory Findings in Lipid Disorders

Disorder	Inheritance	OMIM No.	Prevalence	Cholesterol	Triglycerides	VLDL	Chylomicrons	LDL	HDL	Serum	Cause
Type I	AR		1/million	↑	↑↑↑	↑	↑↑↑	↓	↓↓↓	Creamy top	
a: Familial hyperchylomicronemia		239600, 246650, 615947									a: Deficiency from mutations in lipoprotein lipase; *LMF1*; *GPIHBP1*
b: Familial apoprotein C2 or A-V deficiency		207750, 133650									b. Deficient ApoC2 or ApoA5 (see Type 5)
c: —		118830									c. LP lipase inhibitor in blood
Type II			1 in 500 for heterozygotes	↑	Nl or ↑	↑	Nl	↓	↓	Clear	
a: Familial hypercholesterolemia	AD	143890, 144010, 603776									LDL receptor defect in 60%–80%; *APOB, PCSK9,* each <5%
	AR	603813									*LDLRAP1*
b: Familial combined hyperlipidemia	AD, AR	144250	1 in 100							Clear	Polygenic Decreased LDL receptor and ApoB100 dysfunction
Type III Familial dysbetalipoproteinemia	AR	107741	1 in 10,000	↑	↑	↑	↑	↓	Nl	Turbid	ApoE2 synthesis
Type IV Familial hypertriglyceridemia	AD	144600	1 in 100	↑	Nl ↑	↑	Nl	↓	↓↓	Turbid	Renal disease, diabetes
Type V	AR	144650	Very rare	↑	↑↑↑	↑	↑	↓	↓↓↓	Creamy top, turbid bottom	Apo A-V (ApoA5) deficiency

AD, Autosomal dominant; *AR,* autosomal recessive; *HDL,* high-density lipoprotein; *LDL,* low-density lipoprotein; *LP,* lipoprotein; *Nl,* normal; *OMIM,* Online Mendelian Inheritance in Man; *VLDL,* very low-density lipoprotein; ↑ increased; ↓ decreased.

Table 24.5 Disorders of Lipids: Clinical Findings and Management

Disorder	Xanthomas	Cardiovascular	Gastrointestinal	Neurologic	Ophthalmologic	Other Findings	Management
Type I	Eruptive, tendinous, xanthelasmas	None	Acute abdomen, hepatosplenomegaly, pancreatitis	None	Lipemia retinalis, retinal vein occlusion	Diabetes, lipemic plasma	Diet, statins, fibrates, ezetimibe (may not control) PCSK9 inhibitors Mipomersen and lomitapide through restricted distribution; Plasmapheresis
Type II	Planar, especially intertriginous, tendinous, tuberous	Generalized atherosclerosis	None	None	Arcus cornea	None	Type IIa: bile acid sequestrants, statins, niacin Type IIb: statins, niacin, fibrate, fish oil
Type III	Planar, especially palmar, tuberous	Atherosclerosis	None	None	None	Abnormal glucose tolerance, hyperuricemia	Statins, fibrate
Type IV	Eruptive, tuberous	Atherosclerosis	Acute abdomen, hepatosplenomegaly, pancreatitis	None	Lipemia retinalis	Obesity	Statins, fibrate, niacin
Type V	Eruptive, tuberous	Atherosclerosis	Acute abdomen, hepatosplenomegaly, pancreatitis	None	Lipemia retinalis	Obesity, hyperinsulinemia	Niacin, fibrate
Tangier	Macular rash, foam cells in biopsies	Atherosclerosis	Acute abdomen, hepatosplenomegaly	Peripheral neuropathy	Corneal infiltration	Enlarged orange tonsils, lymphadenopathy	
Apolipoprotein A-I and C-III deficiency	Planar and tendon xanthomas, foam cells in biopsies	Atherosclerosis	Normal	Normal	Corneal clouding	None	
HDL deficiency with planar xanthomas	Planar xanthomas, foam cells in biopsies	Atherosclerosis	Hepatomegaly	Normal	Corneal opacity	None	

HDL, High-density lipoprotein.

where they are phagocytized by macrophages to form lipid-laden foam cells. They are then deposited, particularly in areas subjected to stress and pressure. Depending on their morphology, anatomic location, and mode of development, xanthomas can be categorized as *plane, eruptive or papuloeruptive, tendinous*, or *tuberous*. Recognition of these types of lesions, in addition to biochemical testing and physical examination, provides clues to possible metabolic abnormalities and diagnosis of specific metabolic diseases. Of note, juvenile xanthogranuloma (JXG; see Chapter 10), the most common xanthomatous skin lesion seen in children, does not have an association with systemic hyperlipidemias or other metabolic abnormalities.

PLANE (PLANAR) XANTHOMAS

Plane (planar) xanthomas range from soft, yellow-orange, and brown-yellow macules to slightly elevated plaques (Fig. 24.10). They are generally seen on the face, sides of the neck, upper trunk, buttocks, elbows, and knees, but they may occur anywhere on the body and have a marked predilection for surgical or acne scars and the palmar creases.[119,120] Commonly seen plane xanthomas are xanthelasmas, which occur on or near the eyelids and are rarely seen in children or adolescents. Xanthelasmas in pediatric patients, in contrast with those in adults, are almost always associated with an underlying lipid abnormality. Intertriginous plane xanthomas, as in the antecubital fossae or the web spaces of the fingers, are usually associated with homozygous familial hypercholesterolemia.[95] Plane xanthomas of the palmar creases (xanthoma striatum palmare) suggest the diagnosis of dysbetalipoproteinemia, especially when the child also has tuberous xanthomas. Plane xanthomas also occur in children with cholestasis from biliary obstruction, including after liver transplant,[120] biliary atresia, or primary biliary cirrhosis (Box 24.1), because of the accumulation of circulating unesterified cholesterol and in patients with an underlying monoclonal gammopathy, such as in Castleman disease.

ERUPTIVE (PAPULOERUPTIVE) XANTHOMAS

Eruptive (papuloeruptive) xanthomas appear in crops of multiple 1- to 4-mm, red to yellow-orange papules (Fig. 24.11) and are often surrounded by an erythematous base. Although they may involve the trunk and oral mucosa, they have a predilection for sites subjected to pressure or trauma, particularly the extensor surfaces of the arms, legs, and buttocks. Papuloeruptive xanthomas are almost always associated with hypertriglyceridemia (often to levels of >3000 mg/dL).[121,122] They can result from deficiency of LPL activity, as in patients with LPL deficiency (type I hyperlipoproteinemia); dysfunctional apolipoprotein C-II, (impaired insulin activity); overproduction by the liver of TG-rich lipoproteins (as in endogenous familial hypertriglyceridemia [type IV hyperlipoproteinemia]; or elevation of both chylomicrons and VLDLs of type V hyperlipoproteinemia). Environmental factors and underlying diseases can also significantly elevate TG levels. Among these are obesity, alcohol abuse, diabetes, nephrotic syndrome, therapy with estrogens or retinoids, and metabolic syndrome associated with antipsychotic drugs[123] (see Box 24.1). The mechanism for retinoid-induced hypertriglyceridemia is elevation of hepatic VLDL production. Severe hypertriglyceridemia has also been described with pediatric systemic lupus erythematosus in association with anti–apolipoprotein C-II antibody[124] and in association with post–stem cell transplant metabolic disease.[125]

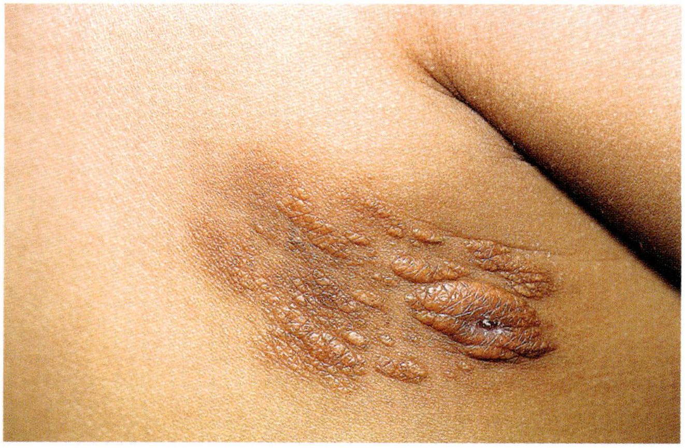

Fig. 24.10 Plane xanthomas in a girl with homozygous type II hyperlipoproteinemia.

Box 24.1 Potential Causes of Secondary Hyperlipidemia in Pediatric Patients

- Endocrine
  - Anorexia nervosa
  - Diabetes mellitus
  - Hypercortisolism
  - Hypopituitarism
  - Hypothyroidism
  - Lipodystrophy
  - Metabolic syndrome
  - Obesity
- Hepatic
  - Cholestasis
  - Biliary atresia
  - Biliary cirrhosis
  - Posttransplantation
  - Hepatitis
- Pregnancy
- Renal
  - Chronic renal failure
  - Hemolytic-uremic syndrome
  - Nephrotic syndrome
- Storage disease
  - Cystine storage disease
  - Gaucher disease
  - Glycogen storage disease
  - Niemann–Pick disease
  - Tay–Sachs disease
- Medications
  - Alcohol
  - Anabolic steroids
  - Antidepressants
  - Antipsychotics (second generation)
  - Antiretroviral therapy
  - Bile acid sequestrants
  - Oral contraceptives/estrogens
  - Corticosteroids
- Retinoids
- Sirolimus
- Others
  - Burns
  - Common variable immunodeficiency
  - Klinefelter syndrome
  - Progeria
  - Werner syndrome

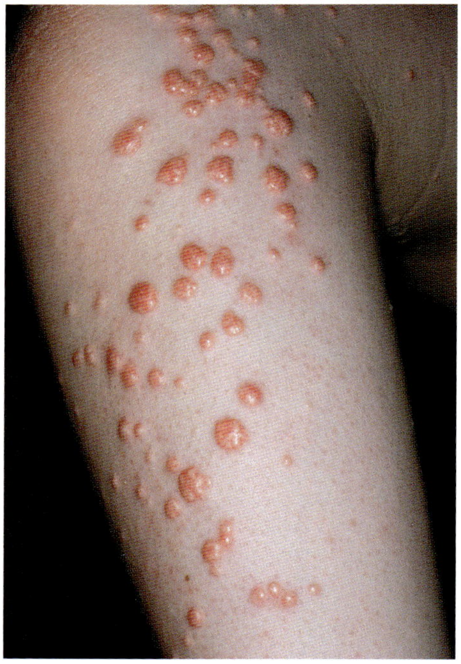

Fig. 24.11 Xanthomas in hyperlipidemia. Eruptive xanthomas in a boy with nephritic syndrome. More commonly, eruptive xanthomas are grouped. Biopsy confirmed the diagnosis of xanthoma.

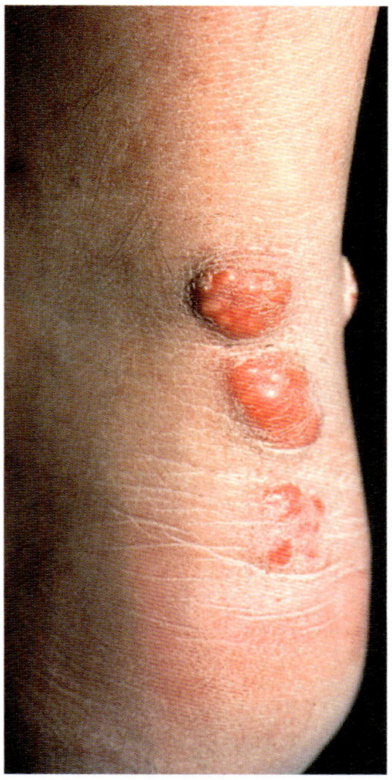

Fig. 24.12 Xanthomas in hyperlipidemia. Tendinous xanthomas in an adolescent with type II hyperlipoproteinemia.

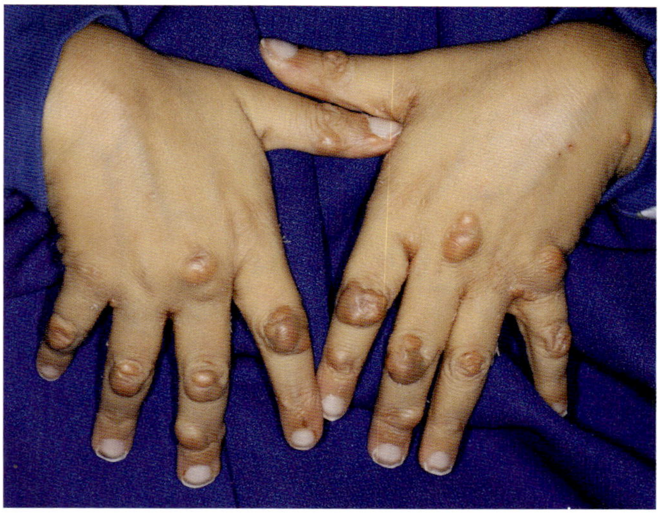

Fig. 24.13 Xanthomas in hyperlipidemia. Tuberous xanthomas in a boy with Alagille syndrome.

TENDINOUS XANTHOMAS

Tendinous xanthomas are skin-colored or yellowish, smooth, freely movable subcutaneous nodules and tumors.[126] They have a predilection for the extensor tendons of the elbows, knees, heels (Fig. 24.12), hands, and feet. These nontender, firm nodules measure 1 cm or more in diameter. They usually are seen or palpated on the Achilles tendon and the tendons on the dorsal aspect of the hands. They are most commonly seen in either heterozygotes or homozygotes with familial hypercholesterolemia (type II hyperlipidemia) but may also be seen in individuals with familial defective apolipoprotein B-100, cerebrotendinous xanthomatosis, and sitosterolemia.[127] Xanthomas involving tendons of the hand and feet may present with soft tissue swelling and morning stiffness that is confused clinically with arthralgias, but improves when lipid levels are lowered.[128,129]

TUBEROUS (TUBEROERUPTIVE) XANTHOMAS

Tuberous (tuberoeruptive) xanthomas are large, firm, nodular, sessile, or pedunculated; flesh-colored; or yellowish to red xanthomas (Fig. 24.13).[130] They occur on the palms and extensor surfaces subject to stress or trauma, particularly the elbows, knees, hands, and buttocks. Located in the dermis and subcutaneous layers, they can enlarge to 5 cm or more in diameter, and in contrast to tendon xanthomas, are not attached to underlying structures. These lesions are found in patients with hypercholesterolemia, particularly with familial hypercholesterolemia (type II hyperlipoproteinemia),[131] hepatic cholestasis, or dysbetalipoproteinemia (type III hyperlipoproteinemia). Some 80% of individuals with dysbetalipoproteinemia have tuberous xanthomas. Tuberous xanthomas are also found in sitosterolemia.[132]

OTHER XANTHOMAS

Other xanthomas not part of the hyperlipoproteinemia spectrum include *xanthoma disseminatum*, an uncommon clinical entity characterized by red-yellow or mahogany-colored papular and nodular lesions with a predilection for the flexural creases[133] (see Chapter 10), and *verruciform xanthomas*, a rare disorder manifested by solitary, 0.2- to 2-cm, verrucous papillary or flat to lichenoid, gray to reddish-pink, sessile, occasionally pedunculated lesions. These lesions are most commonly seen on the oral mucosa and lips and occasionally on the penis, scrotum, vulva, groin, digits, nostrils, and areas of epidermal hyperplasia, such as in congenital hemidysplasia with ichthyosiform nevus and limb defects (CHILD syndrome; see Chapter 5), lymphedema,[134] or epidermolysis bullosa (see Chapter 13).

The five major types of hyperlipoproteinemias are summarized in Tables 24.4 and 24.6.[135] Type I hyperlipoproteinemia (Bürger–Grütz disease, familial LPL deficiency, and familial hyperchylomicronemia syndrome) is a rare disorder, which occurs in 1:500,000 to 1:1,000,000 persons, but most cases present during childhood. It typically results biallelic mutations in LPL, but may occasionally be due to deficiency of apolipoprotein C-II (apoC-II), apolipoprotein A-V (apoAV), lipase maturation factor 1 (LMF1, which aids LPL transport and folding), or glycosylphosphatidylinositol-anchored high-density lipoprotein-binding protein (GPIHBP1),[136] which binds LPL and transports it to capillary lumens where LPL acts. The presence of an LPL inhibitor or low plasma levels of LPL from GPIHBP1 autoantibodies (including in children with hyperchylomicronemia or from transplacental passage of antibodies from an affected mother)[137] can also lead to the disorder. The LPL enzyme and its cofactor, apoC-II, cleave free fatty acids from TG in dietary-derived chylomicrons and hepatic VLDL. Without LPL, chylomicrons massively accumulate in the blood, liver, spleen, and pancreas. TG levels are also very high (typically 1000 to >10,000 mg/dL; heterozygous carriers can have fasting TG levels of 200 to 750 mg/dL).

The disorder is usually discovered because of lactescence (manifested by a creamy or chocolate appearance) of whole blood[138] in an infant or child with bouts of abdominal pain. The pain usually relates to pancreatitis, but may be caused by lipid accumulations in the liver and spleen or a splenic infarct. The lactescence results from TG accumulation because of decreased clearance of plasma chylomicrons. Other complications are steatorrhea, diabetes, and pancreatic calcification, especially if patients do not comply with the low-fat diet, but the risk of atherosclerosis is not increased. About two-thirds of children with type I disease have eruptive xanthomas, primarily localized to the buttocks, shoulders, and extensor surfaces of the extremities.[139] Eruptive xanthomas occur when the serum TG level exceeds approximately 2000 mg/dL. Other clinical signs are hepatosplenomegaly and lipemia retinalis. Increased levels of chylomicrons can also be found in familial hypertriglyceridemia or in patients with diabetes or hypothyroidism, or in those undergoing therapy with retinoids, glucocorticoids, or estrogens.

Type II hyperlipoproteinemia (now divided into 2A, familial hypercholesterolemia[140] and 2B, familial combined hyperlipidemia) is the most common and best-understood disorder of the lipoprotein disorders in pediatric patients.[141–145] Generally, the diagnosis of these disorders is made by the high fasting lipid levels and family history of cardiovascular disease and hyperlipidemia.

Familial hypercholesterolemia has been linked in 60% to 80% of affected families to mutations or copy number variants[146] in *LDLR* (low-density lipoprotein receptor) or mutations in *ApoB100* or *PCSK9*, encoding proprotein convertase sutilisin/kexin type 9 (see Table 24.3[147]). The disorder is codominant, in that manifestations can occur, albeit milder, in heterozygotes. Heterozygotes (1/250 persons) have plasma concentrations of total cholesterol and LDL cholesterol that are increased by twofold to threefold.[148] Homozygotes (1/250,000) have levels five to six times normal values from birth to early childhood. Mutations in genes encoding the LDL receptor adapter protein 1, APOE, or lysosomal acid lipase may mimic familial hypercholesterolemia. Having high LDL-C and a known mutation is associated with a 22-fold increase in cardiovascular disease.[149]

In contrast, familial combined hyperlipoproteinemia is a complex genetic disorder for which at least 35 genetic loci of susceptibility have been found and environment influences play a major role in manifestation, but the disorder has not been linked to specific genetic mutations. Although the disorder typically presents in adulthood, obesity unmasks the disorder during adolescence, and, as a result, combined hyperlipidemia is three times more prevalent in children than familial hypercholesterolemia. The disorder results from excessive production of hepatic VLDL and apoB-100, reduced fatty acid uptake in adipose tissue, and reduced clearance of chylomicron remnants, leading to high TG levels, normal or elevated LDL cholesterol, and low HDL cholesterol levels.

Children with homozygous disease may have planar xanthomas at birth or by the first decade (including intertriginous xanthomas) and tendon and tuberous xanthomas by 15 years of age.[150–153] Rarely, tuberous xanthomas are the first manifestation.[154] Arcus cornea (lipid deposits around the edge of the cornea), angina pectoris, and myocardial infarction often present during the second decade. Carotid plaque has been noted as early as 4 years of age,[155] and coronary artery bypass or aortic valve replacement may be required during childhood.[156–158] Ten percent to 15% of heterozygous individuals develop tendon xanthomas during the second decade of life, particularly involving the Achilles tendon and the extensor tendons of the hands, but only rarely show angina pectoris during late teenage years.

Type III hyperlipoproteinemia (also known as *dysbetalipoproteinemia or broad β disease*) is usually first diagnosed in adulthood, but sometimes first manifests during childhood.[159–161] Most affected individuals are homozygotes for the *ApoE2* allele (allele found in 1% of individuals, and homozygosity occurs in 1 in 5000 to 10,000 individuals), although dominant negative (heterozygous) mutations in ApoE can also be causative. The *apoE* gene is a ligand for chylomicrons, IDL, and VLDL receptors in the liver. Having the genetic mutation and exposure to medication or environmental triggers (obesity, hormonal abnormalities, such as hypothyroidism) leads to abnormal uptake and metabolism, with resultant accumulation of these lipoproteins ("remnant lipoproteins") in the blood. A clue is the relatively equivalent levels of cholesterol and TGs (300 to 1000 mg/dL). Approximately 75% of patients have plane xanthomas of the palms and/or tuberous xanthomas. Some patients have eruptive xanthomas on areas subject to pressure (elbows, knees, buttocks). Affected individuals are at risk for cardiovascular and peripheral vascular disease because of the high levels of remnant lipoproteins.

Type IV disease (familial hypertriglyceridemia) has typically manifested in adulthood but is now being diagnosed during adolescence because of the increase in obesity. Severe hypertriglyceridemia is typically linked to secondary causes, particularly renal disease, diabetes and insulin resistance, total parenteral nutrition, and defective regulation of bile acid synthesis (with abnormally high production of bile acids[135,162]). The familial form occurs in 1/500 individuals and is a complex genetic disorder without any recognized monogenic variants. The primary issues are overproduction of hepatic VLDL and impaired catabolism of TG-rich lipoproteins, resulting in markedly increased secretion of TG-enriched VLDL particles. There is no increase in apoB-100 or LDL, and mortality from cardiovascular disease is only increased after decades. However, familial hypertriglyceridemia is the most common cause of pancreatitis not due to gallstones or alcohol abuse, which tends to occur when TG levels exceed 1000 to 1500 mg/dL, although early stages can be seen with TGs as low as 500 mg/dL. Pancreatitis usually presents as abdominal pain, vomiting, and ileus.

Type V disease (seen in familial hyperchylomicronemia with hyperprebetalipoproteinemia or occasionally ApoC2 deficiency) occasionally presents in preadolescent children. Patients are usually obese and have acute abdominal pain. Eruptive xanthomas are most common. Diabetes, glycogen storage disease, ingestion of contraceptives, and alcohol abuse may trigger manifestations.

Treatment of hyperlipidemias is type specific but most commonly includes dietary modification and statins (hydroxymethylglutaryl [HMG]-CoA reductase inhibitors),[163,164] which decrease LDL levels by increasing LDL receptor expression and thus hepatic reuptake of LDL.[165] Based on a recent recommendation of the American Academy of Pediatrics, initial management of children ≤10 years of age with an LDL of >130 mg/dL should be lifestyle changes, but if LDL remains >190 mg/dL after 6 months of nonpharmacologic management, treatment with statins should be considered.[166] Statins have been shown to reduce carotid intima media thickness in children and adolescents with heterozygous familial hypercholesterolemia.[167] However, most with familial forms of hyperlipidemia do not achieve sufficient reduction in LDL without additional intervention. Addition of cholesterol-lowering agents (fibrates, which act on *PPARα* to decrease free fatty acid production; cholestyramine or colestipol, which are ion exchange resins for sequestration of bile acids; and niacin) and/or ezetimibe (which selectively inhibits the absorption of cholesterol)[168–170] may also be insufficient and/or poorly tolerated. In some of these individuals, PCSK9 inhibitors (such as subcutaneously administered evolocumab or alirocumab)[171] may further reduce LDL levels by 60% through preventing degradation of the LDL receptor, thus reducing cardiovascular risk. However, most individuals with homozygous forms of familiar hypercholesterolemia have only a partial reduction in LDL. Drugs that act independently of LDL receptors, mipomersen (an antisense oligonucleotide that inhibits messenger RNA [mRNA] expression of *apoB*) and lomitapide (inhibitor of microsomal TG transfer protein) are now approved for homozygous familial hypercholesterolemia but have several potential adverse events, particularly hepatotoxicity, and their use is only through a highly restricted monitoring program. Another agent in development is evinacumab, which inhibits angiopoietin-like 3 (ANGPTL3). ANGPTL3 increases levels of TG, LDL, and HDL cholesterol. Evinacumab has been shown to further lower cholesterol by 50% in patients only partially responsive to other agents[172] and is also able to lower TGs by 80%.[173] Omega-3 fatty acids may provide benefit as well in lowering TGs. Other drugs in development target high levels of lipoprotein Lp(a) or apolipoprotein C-III.[174] Apheresis[175,176] and even liver transplantation[177] are still not infrequently required for recalcitrant cases of homozygous hypercholesterolemia. Successful therapy can lead to dramatic shrinkage or clearance of xanthomas.

ALAGILLE DISEASE

Hyperlipidemia with hypercholesterolemia and xanthomas is also a feature of Alagille syndrome (arteriohepatic dysplasia, Watson–Alagille syndrome),[178–180] an autosomal dominant disorder caused by mutations in *JAG1*, which encodes a ligand for the Notch receptor and is critical for determination of cell fates in early development.[181] The most characteristic feature is congenital intrahepatic biliary hypoplasia with cholestasis and pruritus. Most patients show an unusual facies with a prominent forehead; hypertelorism; eyes deeply set in the orbits; atrophy of the iris; a pointed, bulbous, or saddle-shaped nose; and a sharply pointed chin, even in relatives without other features.[182] Other features may include vertebral anomalies, cardiovascular disease (generally pulmonic stenosis or aneurysms), renal abnormalities, hypogonadism, and physical and mental retardation.[183] The xanthomas have been described in approximately 30% of affected children, may appear as early as the first year of life, and are associated with high cholesterol levels.[179] The xanthomas are most often tuberous (see Fig. 24.13) and are often widespread, especially over extensor surfaces and fold areas. They may form confluent plaques, especially on the elbows and knees. Secondary eczematization is common, given the intense pruritus from cholestasis. Early photosensitivity with sunburn and residual facial scars resembling erythropoietic protoporphyria have rarely been described.[184,185] Death before 5 years of age as a result of cardiac failure, renal failure, or both has occurred, but the prognosis of children with Alagille syndrome is generally better than that of patients with congenital biliary atresia, in whom survival to 2 years of age is unusual. Transplantation, partial biliary diversion,[186] and other means to lower cholesterol result in clearance of the xanthomas.[179] Although the combination of intense pruritus and xanthomas in a young child should prompt consideration of Alagille syndrome, the differential diagnosis includes other obstructive biliary tract disorders and Joubert/COACH syndrome with congenital hepatic fibrosis; Joubert/COACH syndrome features distinctive cerebellar and brain stem malformations, oligophrenia, congenital ataxia, and coloboma, in addition to hepatic fibrosis and hypotonia.[187]

SITOSTEROLEMIA

Individuals with this autosomal recessive disorder have 30- to 100-fold elevations in plasma levels of plant sterols[188] and often have highly increased cholesterol levels[189,190] due to mutations in two adjacent sterol adenosine triphosphate (ATP)–binding cassette transporters: *ABCG5* (encoding sterolin-1) or *ABCG8* (encoding sterolin-2).[191] Deficiency of these proteins leads to increased intestinal absorption and decreased biliary excretion of sterols. Although a rare disorder, the condition may be underdiagnosed. In a recent study of a large population undergoing advanced lipid testing, about 4% of patients with a fasting serum LDL-C concentration >190 mg/dL also had significantly elevated β-sitosterol concentrations (>8.0 mg/L), and 27.5% of those with high enough β-sitosterol levels to be diagnostic of sitosterolemia (>15 mg/L) had LDL-C concentrations >190 mg/dL.[192]

Affected children show tuberous and tendinous xanthomas during the first decade of life,[193] as well as arthritis, premature vascular disease,[194] and a high risk of fatal cardiac events during the teenage years and early adulthood.[195] Hematologic features can include hemolytic anemia with stomatocytosis, macrothrombocytopenia, splenomegaly, and abnormal bleeding.[32,196,197] The mainstay of therapy includes dietary restriction of both cholesterol and plant sterols. Foods rich in plant sterols include vegetable oils, wheat germs, nuts, seeds, avocado, shortening, margarine, and chocolate.[198] Treatment with ezetimibe, which inhibits cholesterol absorption, also reduces the plasma concentrations of plant sterols in patients.[199,200] The combination of ezetimibe and cholestyramine has also been used successfully to clear the xanthomas.[197,201,202]

CEREBROTENDINOUS XANTHOMATOSIS

Cerebrotendinous xanthomatosis is an autosomal recessive disorder caused by mutations in *CYP27A1* (sterol 27-hydroxylase).[203,204] As a result, large amounts of cholestanol, the 5-α-dihydro derivative of cholesterol, accumulate in virtually every tissue, leading to diarrhea in infancy, juvenile cataracts in childhood, tendinous xanthomas in the second to third decades of life with atherosclerosis, and progressive neurologic dysfunction in adulthood.[205] These neurologic signs include dementia, psychiatric disturbances, seizures, progressive paresthesias, mental retardation, and cerebellar problems.[206] Neonatal cholestasis[207] and autism spectrum disorder[208] have also been associated. Replacement therapy with chenodeoxycholic acid (750 mg/day) reduces cholestanol synthesis and concentrations, can clear the xanthomas, and, if started early enough (in one study by 15 years after the onset of neurologic manifestations[209]; in another study by 24 years of age),[210] can improve neurologic function.[203]

DEFICIENCIES IN HIGH-DENSITY LIPOPROTEIN

Low levels of HDL cholesterol are most commonly seen in disorders of TG metabolism but may occur in the presence of otherwise normal levels of lipids and be associated with xanthomas. These disorders are Tangier disease, apolipoprotein A-I and C-III deficiency, and HDL deficiency with planar xanthomas (with decreased levels of ApoC3).

TANGIER DISEASE

Tangier disease (familial HDL deficiency) is an autosomal recessive disorder characterized by hypocholesterolemia (50 to 125 mg/dL), an almost complete absence of plasma HDL, and massive deposition of cholesterol esters in tissues. The disorder results from homozygous mutations in the ATP-binding cassette *(ABCA1)* transport protein, which mediates the efflux of cellular cholesterol to the HDL particle in plasma for transport to the liver.[211,212] TG levels may be normal or slightly elevated (150 to 250 mg/dL), and plasma ApoA1 levels are less than 3% of normal. The disorder commonly manifests during childhood. The tonsils are enlarged and show distinctive alternating bands of red, orange, or yellowish-white striations overlying the normal red mucosa.[213] Lipid deposits in the skin and other organs may be accompanied by a persistent maculopapular eruption over the trunk and abdomen, hepatosplenomegaly, lymph node enlargement, infiltration of the cornea in adults, and alterations in the intestinal and rectal mucosa. Several patients have had recurrent peripheral neuropathy.[214]

The Mucopolysaccharidoses

The mucopolysaccharidoses (MPSs) are inherited disorders of lysosomal hydrolases that catabolize glycosaminoglycan (GAG), a sulfated component of connective tissue.[215,216] As a result, dermatan sulfate, heparin sulfate, and/or keratan sulfate accumulate within cells and are excreted in excess amounts in the urine. First described by Hunter in 1917 (and labeled *gargoylism* in 1936), these disorders can now be divided into at least seven subtypes that share clinical features, mode of inheritance, and nature of the accumulated mucopolysaccharide. Affected individuals are normal in appearance at birth but, as with all lysosomal storage disorders, progressively show features with advancing age, beginning during infancy. Patients with any of the MPSs can show hypertrichosis, especially over the back and extremities, and thickened, roughened, taut inelastic skin, especially over the fingers because of the accumulation of GAG. Only individuals with Hunter syndrome (MPS type II, iduronate-2-sulfatase deficiency) have specific cutaneous features (papulonodules), although extensive, persistent congenital dermal melanocytosis (formerly called *Mongolian spots*) have been described in children with MPS I/ Hurler[217–219] and MPS II/ Hunter[220,221] syndromes.

The disorders tend to present because of dysmorphic features or psychological and learning difficulties, or as severe bony dysplasia. Considerable heterogeneity within subgroups has been described. Urinary screening tests for GAG should be followed by specific enzyme assays. Hunter syndrome (MPS II) is an X-linked recessive disorder; all others are autosomal recessive. Hurler syndrome, or MPS I, is presented as the prototype MPS; Hunter syndrome is also discussed in detail because it is the one form of MPS that shows a distinctive cutaneous feature: dermal papules and nodules. Table 24.6 summarizes the clinical and biochemical features of all of the MPSs.

HURLER SYNDROME

Hurler syndrome (MPS I-H, MPS I in McKusick's original classification) is the most common of this group of disorders.[222–224] Seen in approximately 1 in 100,000 births, it appears in the first year of life. MPS I is a particularly grave disorder, with death occurring in almost all cases before the age of 10 years, usually from cardiac failure or respiratory infection.

Patients are usually diagnosed toward the end of the first year of life because of their coarse facial features (Fig. 24.14). Many have umbilical and inguinal hernias at presentation and recurrent respiratory infections before diagnosis. Other cardinal features of Hurler syndrome include coarse hair; macrocephaly with frontal bulging; premature closure of the sutures with hyperostosis, commonly leading to

Table 24.6 The Mucopolysaccharidoses

Disorder	Inheritance	Enzyme	Storage	Clinical Features
MPS I-H Hurler	AR	α-Iduronidase	DS, HS	Severe retardation, corneal clouding, hepatosplenomegaly, chondrodystrophic dwarfism, generalized Mongolian spots; early death
MPS I-S Scheie	AR	α-Iduronidase	DS, HS	Bone and joint involvement, retinopathy, corneal clouding, sometimes cardiac abnormalities; normal intelligence
MPS II Hunter	X-LR	Iduronate 2-sulfatase	DS, HS	Cutaneous papules and nodules on scapula, posterior axillae, thigh, buttocks, atypical retinitis pigmentosa; normal cornea
MPS III Sanfilippo	AR	Several subtypes*	HS	Aggressive behavior, severe neurologic involvement, mild somatic changes
MPS IV Morquio	AR	A: Galactose-6-sulfatase B: β-galactosidase	KS	Striking dwarfism but not dysmorphic, corneal opacity, severe osteoporosis, extreme short stature; atlantoaxial dislocation leads to chronic cervical myelopathy and progressive paresis; restrictive respiratory disease usually leads to death; normal intelligence
MPS VI Maroteaux–Lamy	AR	Galactosamine-4-sulfatase	DS	Dwarfism, severe corneal, and bony lesions; cardiac involvement, respiratory obstruction; normal intelligence
MPS VII Sly	AR	β-glucuronidase	HS, DS	Often born with hydrops fetalis, severe Hurler-like phenotype if survive
MPS IX	AR	Hyaluronidase	HA	One patient; short stature, periarticular soft-tissue masses

AR, Autosomal recessive; *DS*, dermatan sulfate; *HA*, hyaluronic acid; *HS*, heparan sulfate; *KS*, keratan sulfate; *MPS*, mucopolysaccharidosis; *X-LR*, X-linked recessive.
*A: heparan N-sulfatase; B: N-acetylglucosaminidase; C: acetyl-CoA: glucosamine N-acetyltransferase; D: N-acetylglucosamine-6-sulfatase.

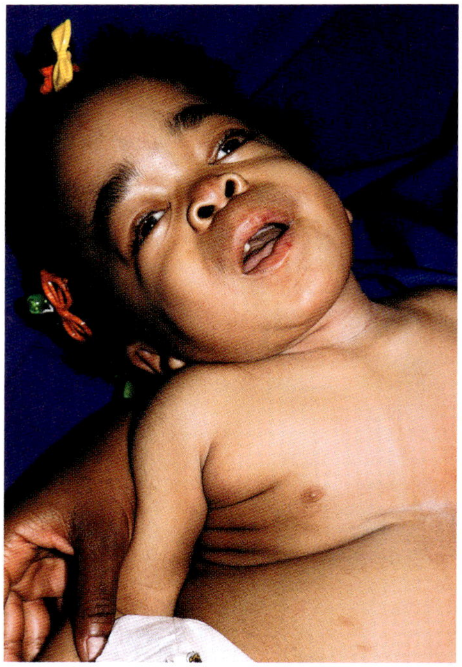

Fig. 24.14 Hurler syndrome. Coarse facial features, macrocephaly, scaphocephalic skull, flattened nasal bridge, hypertelorism, short neck, chest deformity, and protuberant abdomen in a girl with Hurler syndrome (MPS I).

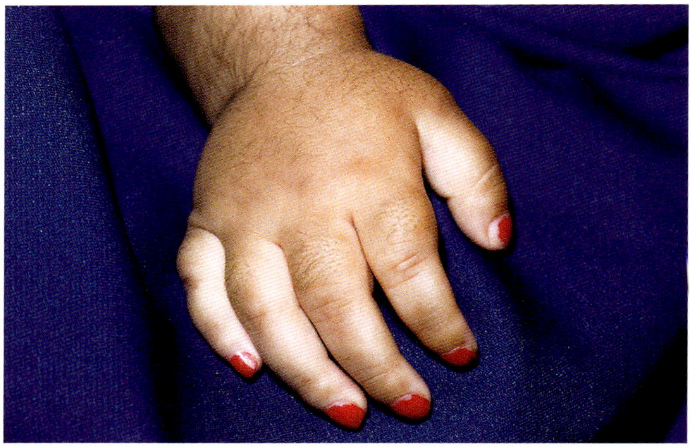

Fig. 24.15 Hurler syndrome. Broad hands with stubby fingers and limited joint extension. Note the hypertrichosis.

a scaphocephalic skull; flattened nasal bridge with a saddle-shaped appearance; hypertelorism; protuberant tongue; short neck; protuberant abdomen because of hepatic and splenic enlargement; deformity of the chest; shortness of the spine; laxity of the abdominal wall with inguinal and umbilical hernias; broad hands with stubby fingers; a claw hand due to stiffening of the phalangeal joints (Fig. 24.15); limitation of extensibility of the joints; severe, progressive mental retardation; and marked retardation of growth. Although most affected infants are normal or above normal in length during the first year of life, the growth rate starts to decrease by 2 years of age. By age 3, almost all patients are below the third percentile for stature. Clouding of the cornea develops in all patients with Hurler syndrome and is best seen by side-lighting of the cornea; if severe visual loss occurs, however, it is usually related to retinal involvement. Deafness is almost always a feature, and cardiac involvement may range from severe early life-threatening cardiomyopathy to progressive valve disease. Approximately 40% of affected individuals develop hydrocephalus, and a large head circumference, even without hydrocephalus, is often noted. Dysplasia of the odontoid process increases the risk of atlantoaxial subluxation and acute spinal cord damage. Upper respiratory tract obstruction and sleep apnea related to the large tongue and midfacial hypoplasia may require corrective surgery.[225]

There is a wide range of heterogeneity in severity and manifestations of Hurler syndrome. At the other end of the spectrum is Scheie syndrome (MPS I-S, formerly MPS V), which also results from mutations in the gene encoding (α)-L-iduronidase. Patients with Scheie syndrome have normal intelligence and may have a normal lifespan,

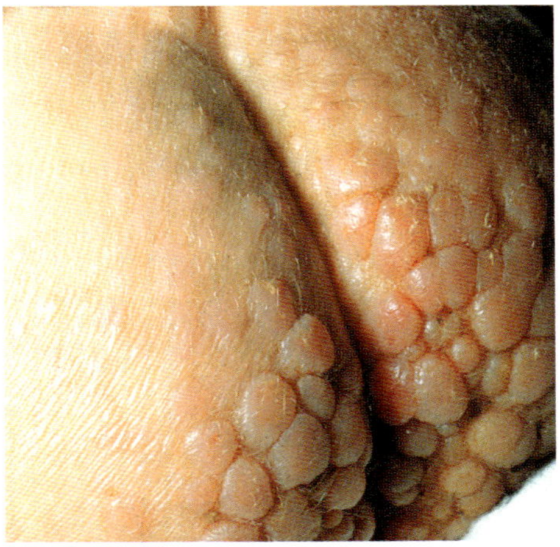

Fig. 24.16 Hunter syndrome. Distinctive, firm, flesh-colored papules and nodules on the buttocks (a cutaneous marker of Hunter syndrome, or MPS II).

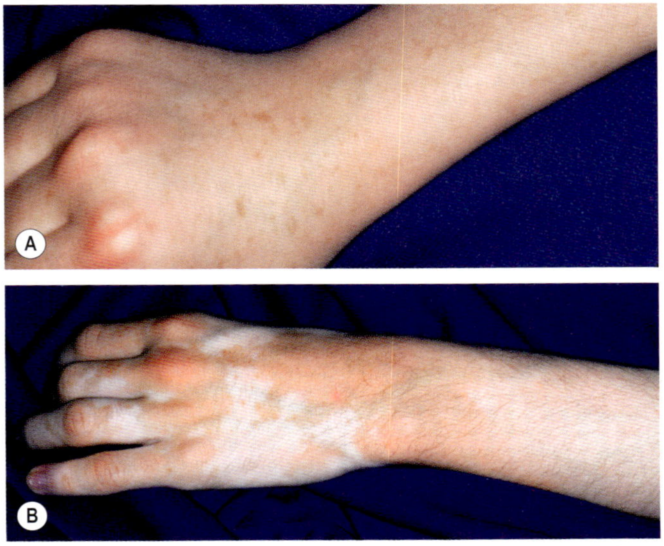

Fig. 24.17 Dyspigmentation with GM3 synthase deficiency. **(A)** Hyperpigmented macules, especially acrally, begin late in childhood and give GM3 synthase deficiency the name *salt and pepper syndrome.* **(B)** Vitiliginous lesions tend to appear in late adolescence and can become extensive.

with predominantly bone and joint problems. Carpal tunnel syndrome occurs commonly, and corneal transplantation may be considered for corneal clouding (assuming lack of concurrent retinopathy as a cause of visual loss). Cardiac valvular insufficiency may develop and require surgery.

HUNTER SYNDROME

Hunter syndrome (MPS II) is distinguished from Hurler syndrome by an X-linked recessive inheritance, longer survival, lack of corneal clouding, and the different biochemical defect with deficiency of the lysosomal enzyme iduronate-2-sulfatase.[226–228] The earliest signs are hernia, the coarse facial features, and claw hands, all presenting at a mean age of 3 to 4 years.[229] As with Hurler syndrome, patients show coarse, straight scalp hair. Mental retardation progresses at a slower rate, and humping of the lumbar area (gibbus) does not occur. Progressive deafness is a feature of 50% of patients and can impair speech development. A mild form of MPS II (type IIB) may show only mild skeletal abnormalities,[230] and skin lesions may be the presenting feature.[231]

The distinctive cutaneous changes are found in the minority of affected boys.[232,233] They consist of firm flesh-colored to ivory-white papules and nodules that often coalesce to form ridges or a reticular pattern in symmetric areas between the angles of the scapulae and posterior axillary lines, the pectoral ridges, the nape of the neck, buttocks (Fig. 24.16), and/or the lateral aspects of the upper arms and thighs. They appear before age 10 years and can spontaneously disappear.

THERAPY FOR MUCOPOLYSACCHARIDOSES

Palliative therapy for the hydrocephalus and joint stiffness and pain are appropriate, but surgical correction of the skeletal or cardiac abnormalities is not, given the limited life expectancy. Hematopoietic stem cell transplantation is standard treatment and can stabilize cognitive improvement when performed before 9 to 24 months of age.[234,235] Other effects are unpredictable but can include softening of coarse hair and facial features and improvement in corneal clouding, hepatomegaly, upper airway obstruction, and cardiomyopathy (but not the constellation of bony defects [dysostosis multiplex] or cervical instability). Enzyme replacement therapy with α-L-iduronidase (laronidase) can also reduce GAGs and improve respiratory and cardiac function, as well as the hepatomegaly and joint mobility in patients with MPS I.[222,236,237] Enzyme replacement therapy (ERT) with idursulfase, recombinant lysosomal iduronate-2-sulfatase, has been noted to improve the skin texture, as well as the hepatosplenomegaly, bronchitis, and physical activity of Hunter syndrome.[238,239] However, ERT cannot pass the blood–brain barrier to improve neurocognitive function.[236,240–242] In general, outcomes from transplantation have been superior to enzyme replacement, but both have better outcomes than lack of treatment.[243] The combination of ERT and transplantation may benefit patients with more severe manifestations.[222]

Other Storage Disorders

Several other storage disorders may show cutaneous features, particularly angiokeratomas and pigmentary changes. Among these are the mucolipidoses (mucolipidosis I [also called *sialidosis II*], mucolipidosis II, and mucolipidosis III);[244] the sphingolipidoses (Fabry disease, Farber lipogranulomatosis,[245] Gaucher disease,[246] GM1 gangliosidosis,[247] salt and pepper syndrome/GM3 synthase deficiency[248] [Fig. 24.17],[248–250] and multiple sulfatase deficiency); and other storage disorders of carbohydrate metabolism (aspartylglycosaminuria, fucosidosis, galactosialidosis,[251] α-mannosidosis, Salla disease, and Schindler disease).[252–258] The features of these storage disorders, their cutaneous manifestations, and their underlying causes are summarized in Table 24.7. (Fabry disease and fucosidosis are discussed in more detail in Chapter 12.) The neonatal form of Gaucher disease, type II, may present as a collodion baby, whereas multiple sulfatase deficiency (mucosulfatidosis) is phenotypically identical to recessive X-linked ichthyosis (see Chapter 5). All of these conditions are inherited in an autosomal recessive fashion, except for Fabry disease, which is X-linked recessive.

The complete list of 258 references for this chapter is available online at http://expertconsult.inkling.com.

Table 24.7 Other Storage Disorders with Cutaneous Manifestations During Childhood

Disorder	Inheritance	Enzyme	Cutaneous Features	Clinical Features
Aspartylglycosaminuria	AR	Aspartylglycosaminidase	Angiokeratomas	Speech delay, otitis media, behavioral change resembling MPS III
Fabry	X-LR	α-Galactosidase	Angiokeratomas, hypohidrosis	Acroparesthesias, progressive renal disease (see Chapter 12)
Farber lipogranulomatosis	AR	Ceramidase	Painful subcutaneous nodules, especially over joints	Hydrops fetalis, chronic pulmonary disease with granulomatous infiltration of the lungs, hepatosplenomegaly neurodegeneration; granulomatous infiltration of the mucosae with hoarse cry, recurrent vomiting, dysphagia
Fucosidosis	AR	α-Fucosidase	Angiokeratomas, sweating abnormalities, purple nail bands	Neurodegeneration, dysostosis, respiratory infections, hepatosplenomegaly, growth retardation, resembles MPS (see Chapter 12)
Galactosialidosis	AR	Defective protective protein/cathepsin A; proteolysis of both β-galactosidase and neuraminidase	Angiokeratomas	Hydrops fetalis, skeletal abnormalities, myoclonus, cherry-red macular spots, ataxia, mild mental retardation
Gaucher, type II	AR	β-Glucocerebrosidase	Collodion baby	Severe neurologic involvement, marked hepatosplenomegaly (see Chapter 5)
GM1 gangliosidosis	AR	β-Galactosidase	Angiokeratomas, extensive congenital dermal melanocytosis	Dysostosis multiplex, hepatosplenomegaly, early neurologic degeneration, corneal clouding
Mannosidosis	AR	α-Mannosidase	Angiokeratomas	Middle ear and respiratory infections; may have mild learning difficulties to severe MPS I-like phenotype and seizures
Multiple sulfatase deficiency	AR	Posttranslational processing of multiple sulfatases	Ichthyosis (recessive X-linked)	Hepatosplenomegaly, dysostosis, progressive neurologic deterioration (see Chapter 5)
Mucolipidosis I (sialidosis type II)	AR	Neuraminidase I	Angiokeratomas	MPS I phenotype; dysostoses multiplex, progressive retardation
Mucolipidosis II (I-cell disease)	AR	N-acetylglucosaminyl-1-phosphotransferase	Malar telangiectasia, puffy eyelids, prominent periorbital veins; thick, rigid skin	MPS I phenotype; gingival hypertrophy, dysostosis multiplex, stiff joints, respiratory tract infections, cardiac failure
Mucolipidosis III (pseudo-Hurler's polydystrophy)	AR	UDP-N-acetylglucosamine 1-phosphotransferase	Can have scleroderma-like features with dry, indurated, dyspigmented skin	Milder than other mucolipidoses; onset usually at ≈3 years with coarsening of face, growth deficiency, progressive joint stiffness, claw hand deformity, gait impairment, scoliosis, dysostosis multiplex; may have mild intellectual disability
Salla disease (infantile sialic acid storage)	AR	Sialic acid transporter	Hypopigmentation	Hydrops fetalis, recurrent infections, failure to thrive, dysostosis multiplex, cardiac disease, coarse facies, learning disabilities
Salt and pepper syndrome	AR	GM3 synthase	Small acral pigmented macules; vitiliginous lesions	Severe intellectual disability, seizures, choreoathetosis, spasticity, scoliosis, dysmorphic facies
Schindler	AR	α-N-acetylgalactosaminidase	Angiokeratomas	Variable; may have myoclonus, spasticity, progressive dementia

AR, Autosomal recessive; *MPS*, mucopolysaccharidosis; *X-LR*, X-linked recessive.

Key References

Seyhan M, Erdem T, Selimoglu MA, et al. Dermatological signs in Wilson's disease. Pediatr Int 2009;51:395–8.

Corbo MD, Lam J. Zinc deficiency and its management in the pediatric population: a literature review and proposed etiologic classification. J Am Acad Dermatol 2013;69(4):616–24.

Gehrig KA, Dinulos JG. Acrodermatitis due to nutritional deficiency. Curr Opin Pediatr 2010;22:107–12.

Ozturk Y. Acrodermatitis enteropathica-like syndrome secondary to branched-chain amino acid deficiency in inborn errors of metabolism. Pediatr Dermatol 2008;25:415.

Bhutta ZA, Berkley JA, Bandsma RHJ, et al. Severe childhood malnutrition. Nat Rev Dis Primers. 2017;3:17067.

Alvares M, Kao L, Mittal V, et al. Misdiagnosed food allergy resulting in severe malnutrition in an infant. Pediatrics 2013;132(1):e229–32.

O'Regan GM, Canny G, Irvine AD. "Peeling paint" dermatitis as a presenting sign of cystic fibrosis. J Cyst Fibros 2006;5:257–9.

Youngblom E, Pariani M, Knowles JW. Familial hypercholesterolemia. In: Adam MP, et al., editors. GeneReviews® [Internet]. Seattle (WA): University of Washington, Seattle; 1993--2020. 2014 Jan 2 [updated 2016 Dec 8].

Harada-Shiba M, Arai H, Oikawa S, et al. Guidelines for the management of familial hypercholesterolemia. J Atheroscler Thromb 2012;19(12):1043–60.

Shah AS, Wilson DP. Primary hypertriglyceridemia in children and adolescents. J Clin Lipidol 2015;9(5 Suppl.):S20–8.
Defesche JC, Gidding SS, Harada-Shiba M, et al. Familial hypercholesterolaemia. Nat Rev Dis Primers 2017;3:17093.
Wiegman A. Lipid screening, action, and follow-up in children and adolescents. Curr Cardiol Rep 2018;20(9):80.
Wraith JE, Jones S. Mucopolysaccharidosis type I. Pediatr Endocrinol Rev 2014;12(Suppl. 1):102–6.
Ashrafi MR, Shabanian R, Mohammadi M, et al. Extensive Mongolian spots: a clinical sign merits special attention. Pediatr Neurol 2006;34:143–5.
Tran MC, Lam JM. Cutaneous manifestations of mucopolysaccharidoses. Pediatr Dermatol 2016;33(6):594–601.
Mimouni-Bloch A, Finezilber Y, Rothschild M, et al. Extensive Mongolian spots and lysosomal storage diseases. J Pediatr 2016;170:333–e1.
Scarpa M, Almássy Z, Beck M, et al. Mucopolysaccharidosis type II: European recommendations for the diagnosis and multidisciplinary management of a rare disease. Orphanet J Rare Dis 2011;6:72.
Tylki-Szymańska A. Mucopolysaccharidosis type II: Hunter's syndrome. Pediatr Endocrinol Rev 2014;12(Suppl. 1):107–13.

25 Skin Signs of Other Systemic Diseases

CHAPTER OUTLINE

Primary Immunodeficiency Disorders

Recurrent infections, including those involving the skin, raise the possibility that a child has an immune deficiency. The most common cause of immunodeficiency in children is acquired immunodeficiency resulting from human immunodeficiency virus (HIV) infection (see Chapter 15). Less commonly, children with evidence of an immunodeficiency have an inherited disorder.[1–6] Genetic immunodeficiency disorders may show a variety of cutaneous abnormalities, some of which are unique and characteristic of the disorder, and others, such as dermatitis, that are shared by other immunodeficiencies and other disorders.

It is beyond the scope of this chapter to review all immunodeficiencies, or even all that may manifest with mucocutaneous features. In addition, primary immunodeficiency disorders are frequently reclassified, with a major update most recently in 2015.[7] Some of these immunodeficiencies are discussed elsewhere because of their manifestations. Wiskott–Aldrich syndrome and hyperimmunoglobulinemia E (hyper-Ig) syndrome are discussed in Chapter 3 due to the common presence of dermatitis. Chediak–Higashi and Griscelli syndromes, the silvery hair syndromes associated with immunodeficiency, are reviewed in Chapter 11 with the disorders of pigmentation. The telangiectasias that allow ataxia–telangiectasia to be distinguished from other forms of ataxia are described in Chapter 12. Complement deficiencies are mentioned in Chapter 14 because individuals with a deficiency of a late complement component have an increased risk of neisserial infection, in Chapter 20 because hereditary angioedema (HAE) can be confused with angioedema, and in Chapter 22 because deficiency of the early components of complement may lead to a lupus-like disorder. Given its characteristic recurrent and recalcitrant candidal infections, chronic mucocutaneous candidiasis is reviewed in Chapter 17.

Signs that should raise the suspicion of acquired or hereditary immunodeficiency are listed in Box 25.1. Screening laboratory tests for a patient with recurrent cutaneous infections suspected of having an immunodeficiency are suggested in Table 25.1. Although flow cytometry is increasingly used to identify immune cell deficiencies and diagnose specific subtypes of immunodeficiency, multicolor flow cytometry has recently been shown to reveal distinct populations among patients with a wide variety of immunodeficiencies, allowing early diagnostic screening beyond seeking cellular deficiencies.[8]

IMMUNOGLOBULIN DEFICIENCIES

Children with deficiencies of immunoglobulins (Igs) primarily manifest with bacterial infections beginning at 3 to 6 months of age, at a time when transplacentally derived maternal Igs wane.[9,10] In general, the treatment of hypogammaglobulinemia is antibody replacement by intravenous infusions of immune serum globulin and vigorous antibiotic therapy.[11]

The most common Ig deficiency is selective IgA deficiency, found in 1 in 500 individuals, of whom 10% to 15% show clinical manifestations. About 5% of patients with IgA deficiency have mutations in *TACI*, which encodes a tumor necrosis factor (TNF) receptor family member. B cells in individuals with *TACI* mutations have impaired isotype switching and do not produce IgA, and often IgG, in response to *TACI* ligand. The most common features are sinopulmonary bacterial infections and *Giardia* gastroenteritis. Approximately one-third of patients with clinical manifestations develop immune-mediated disorders, some of which involve the skin. These include an atopic-like dermatitis, lupus erythematosus with selective IgA deficiency linked to mutations in *IFIH1*,[12] vitiligo, recurrent candidal infections, lipodystrophy, and idiopathic thrombocytopenic purpura. Two percent of individuals with celiac disease have full or partial selective IgA deficiency; this subgroup of patients has more concomitant autoimmune disorders and may have persistent elevation of IgG serologies, even with disease improvement.[13] The risk of allergy is also increased with selective IgA deficiency, including asthma, cow's milk allergy, and allergic rhinoconjunctivitis.

In addition to their decreased levels of IgA, 30% to 50% of affected individuals have serum anti-IgA IgG antibodies, leading to a risk of fatal anaphylactic reactions upon administration of blood products with IgA-bearing lymphocytes; if intravenous immunoglobulin (IVIG) is necessary, only IVIG with low IgA content should be administered.[14]

IgA deficiency may transition into (and is seen with increased incidence in families with) combined variable immunodeficiency (CVID),[15] a heterogeneous group of disorders with decreased Ig levels (IgG, IgA, and sometimes IgM) and variable functional T-cell abnormalities.[16,17] Patients with CVID most commonly show pyodermas, extensive warts, widespread dermatophyte infections, and dermatitis. They are predisposed to pyogenic infections of the upper and lower respiratory tract, as well as gastrointestinal infections, particularly those caused by *Giardia*. Noncaseating granulomas of the lungs, liver, spleen, and/or skin have been described and are not associated with microorganisms. These granulomas have recently been shown to result from emergence of immunodeficiency-related viruses with altered immune, replication, and persistence properties from the live attenuated rubella vaccine, often persistent for decades subclinically.[18,19] Individuals with CVID also have an increased risk of autoimmune diseases, including vitiligo (Fig. 25.1), alopecia areata, and vasculitis. The incidence of lymphoma is increased 400-fold and that of cancer overall 8- to 13-fold. CVID is primarily a disorder of adults, with the mean age of onset 23 to 33 years[20]; however, 25% of

Box 25.1 Signs of Immunodeficiency

- History of infections
  - Increased frequency, severity, and duration
  - Unusual manifestations
  - Unusual infecting agents
  - Chronic infections, incomplete clearing
  - Poor response to appropriate agents
  - Severe viral infections
  - Recurrent osteomyelitis
- Failure to thrive
- Diarrhea, vomiting, malabsorption
- Clues to specific types of immunodeficiency
  - Hematologic abnormalities (e.g., Wiskott–Aldrich syndrome)
  - Arthritis (e.g., Wiskott–Aldrich syndrome or early complement deficiency)
  - Paucity of lymph nodes (e.g., SCID) or lymphadenopathy (e.g., CGD)
  - Follicular-based pustules in a neonate (e.g., hyper-IgE syndrome)
  - Hepatosplenomegaly (e.g., CGD, Omenn syndrome, or Wiskott–Aldrich syndrome)
  - Oral ulcers (e.g., chronic granulomatous disease or hyper-IgM syndrome)
  - Poor wound healing (e.g., leukocyte adhesion deficiency)
  - Silvery hair (e.g., Chediak–Higashi or Griscelli syndromes)
  - Telangiectasia (e.g., ataxia-telangiectasia)

CGD, Chronic granulomatous disease; *IgE*, immunoglobulin E; *SCID*, severe combined immunodeficiency.

cases are diagnosed before 21 years of age, with a peak incidence in children aged 5 to 10 years and a minimum age of 4 years used to exclude patients with other primary immunodeficiency disorders.[21] Death in patients with CVID usually results from lymphoma, hepatitis, respiratory insufficiency, or gastrointestinal disease.

Most cases of panhypogammaglobulinemia in children represent X-linked hypogammaglobulinemia (also called *X-linked agammaglobulinemia*), a disorder caused by mutations in *BTK*, which encodes a tyrosine kinase that regulates the conversion of pre-B cells to B cells able to differentiate and produce Igs.[22] Less commonly, pediatric patients may have a transient form during infancy with early failure to thrive, protracted diarrhea, sinopulmonary infections, pyodermas, and cutaneous abscesses, but with reversal when Ig is produced at 18 to 30 months of age. Approximately 10% have an autosomal recessive form of panhypogammaglobulinemia.

Boys with X-linked hypogammaglobulinemia develop recurrent bacterial infections in the first year of life and have an increased susceptibility to hepatitis B and enteroviral infections. Furuncles and cellulitis are the most common infections. An atopic-like dermatitis is common, and noninfectious cutaneous granulomas have been described. There is an increased predisposition to the development of pyoderma gangrenosum,[23] which has been linked to Warthin–Starry-positive *Helicobacter bilis* infection; although difficult to grow, the *Helicobacter* organisms are detectable by polymerase chain reaction (PCR) and electrospray ionization time-of-flight mass spectrometry.[24] A small percentage of patients develop a dermatomyositis-like disorder with slowly progressive neurologic involvement, usually related to echoviral meningoencephalitis. Up to 6% of patients develop lymphomas.

Patients with X-linked hypogammaglobulinemia with hyper-IgM (HIM) tend to have neutropenia and deficiencies of IgA, IgE, and IgG, but increased levels of IgM and isohemagglutinins.[25] Rather than a primary B-cell defect, affected individuals have a primary T-cell defect. Cross-linking of CD40 on B cells induces switching of Ig classes from IgM to IgG, IgA, or IgE. Mutations in X-linked HIM lead to a dysfunction of the ligand for CD40 (CD40L). B cells from patients with HIM express functional CD40, but the T cells express the defective CD40 ligand and cannot bind CD40.[26,27] Three other forms of HIM are autosomal recessive; these result from deficiency of CD40 itself,[28] activation-induced cytidine deaminase (AICD), or uracil-N-glycosylase (UNG),[29] the latter two being signaling components downstream of the CD40 receptor that are critical to B-cell differentiation and class switching. A rare form of X-linked immunodeficiency sometimes associated with HIM is linked to hypohidrotic ectodermal dysplasia (see Chapter 7) and has been linked to mutations in the *NEMO (IKBKG)* gene, the same gene that is mutated in incontinentia pigmenti (see Chapter 11).

Table 25.1 Screening Laboratory Testing for the Child with Recurrent Infections

Test	Primary Immunodeficiency
Complete blood count with differential, platelet count, examination of smear	Giant leukocyte granules (Chédiak–Higashi syndrome) Thrombocytopenia (Wiskott–Aldrich syndrome) Leukocytosis (chronic granulomatous disease and leukocyte adhesion deficiency)
Quantitative immunoglobulins	X-linked hypogammaglobulinemia (all Igs ↓) Transient hypogammaglobulinemia (all Igs ↓) PLAID* and APLAID syndromes (all Igs ↓) Common variable immunodeficiency (IgG↓, IgA↓ ±IgM↓) Selective IgA deficiency (IgA↓) Selective IgM deficiency (↓gM↓) Hypohidrotic ectodermal dysplasia with immunodeficiency (HED-ID) (±IgG↓ ±IgA↓ IgM↓) Hypogammaglobulinemia with hyper-IgM (Igs↓ IgM↑) Ataxia–telangiectasia (IgG2↓ IgG4↓ ↓IgA IgE↓) Wiskott–Aldrich syndrome (IgM↓, ±IgG↓ IgA↑ IgE↑) Hyperimmunoglobulin E (↑↑IgE)
Flow cytometry (T and B cells)	Severe combined immunodeficiency (lack of T cells ± B cells); specific subtypes have markers, such as γc chain in X-linked SCID Leukocyte adhesion defect (CD18 deficiency) Chronic granulomatous disease (deficient $gp91^{phox}$, $p22^{phox}$, $p40^{phox}$, $p47^{phox}$, $p67^{phox}$)
Total hemolytic complement (CH50)	Complement deficiencies (marked reduction)
Quantitative dihydrorhodamine flow cytometry	Usually <10% (but can be up to 30%) of normal reduction in chronic granulomatous disease
Hair shaft examination	Small, regular melanin aggregations in Chediak–Higashi syndrome Large, irregular aggregations in Griscelli syndrome

Ig, Immunoglobulin.
*PLAID: Phospholipase Cc2-associated antibody deficiency and immune dysregulation; APLAID: Autoinflammation and PLAID.

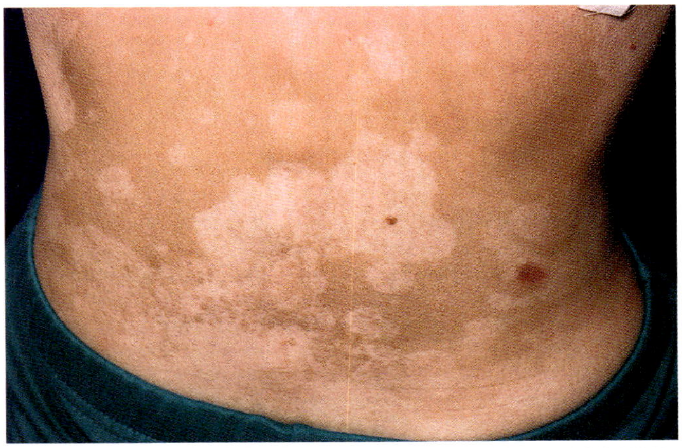

Fig. 25.1 Common variable immunodeficiency (CVID). Individuals with CVID or IgA deficiency have an increased incidence of autoimmune disorders, as evidenced in this adolescent with CVID and vitiligo.

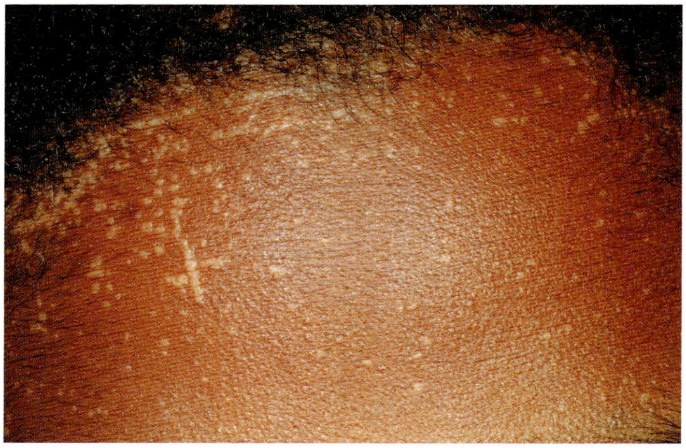

Fig. 25.2 X-linked hypogammaglobulinemia with hyper-IgM. Extensive warts are a commonly observed cutaneous manifestation of boys with this form of immunodeficiency. Note the numerous flat warts studding the forehead.

Patients with HIM often seek treatment during infancy with bacterial and sometimes fungal or opportunistic sinopulmonary infections (most common feature), pyodermas, and gastrointestinal infections (especially with opportunistic infections such as *Cryptosporidium*), hepatosplenomegaly, cervical adenitis, autoimmune disorders (especially thyroiditis and hemolytic anemia),[30] and an increased risk of lymphoma.[28,31] Numerous widespread warts (Fig. 25.2), oral and perianal area ulcerations, and sclerosing cholangitis are additional features.[32] Extensive warts are also a feature of warts, hypogammaglobulinemia, infections, and myelokathexis (WHIM) syndrome, which results from gain-of-function mutations in the chemokine receptor *CXCR4*[33] and has been treated with plerixafor, a selective antagonist of CXCR4.[34] Additional disorders with T-cell impairment, including EVER1 and EVER2 deficiency, DOC8 deficiency (see Chapter 3), Netherton syndrome (Chapter 5), GATA2 deficiency,[35] TAOK2 deficiency,[36] and STK4 deficiency,[37,38] also feature an increased risk of warts.

X-linked lymphoproliferative disease (XLP) is characterized by an abnormal response to Epstein–Barr virus infection because of mutations in either *SH2DIA*, which encodes signaling lymphocytic activation molecule (SLAM)-associated protein (SAP) (XLP-1) or XIAP (XLP-2), critical proteins for cytotoxic T-cell function.[39–41] Affected boys are healthy until they first develop infectious mononucleosis during childhood or adolescence. Fever, pharyngitis, maculopapular rash, lymphadenopathy, hepatosplenomegaly, purpura, jaundice, and hemorrhagic colitis, and often hypogammaglobulinemia as well, are typical features. The virus stimulates a rapidly progressive B-cell lymphoma, often with superimposed bacterial sepsis, which leads to death in 70% of affected boys, especially with hemophagocytic lymphohistiocytosis and without transplantation.[42]

CHRONIC GRANULOMATOUS DISEASE

Chronic granulomatous disease (CGD) is a group of disorders characterized by severe recurrent infections. These infections result from an inability of phagocytic leukocytes to generate oxidative metabolites and activate neutrophil granule elastase and cathepsin G, with the resultant inability to kill certain intracellular bacteria and fungi.[43,44] The estimated incidence is 1 in 200,000 births, approximately half of that of SCID. In all forms of CGD, the function of the nicotinamide dinucleotide phosphate (NADPH) oxidase complex is reduced. The disorder usually presents with acute bacterial infections, particularly suppurative lymphadenitis (classically from *Serratia marcescens*) and recurrent pneumonias. Hepatosplenomegaly and lymphadenopathy may be associated. Some affected children present with inflammation, particularly with very early-onset inflammatory bowel disease.[45] Patients develop granulomas, primarily of the lungs, liver, skin, and genitourinary and gastrointestinal tracts, as an abnormal immune response.[46–49]

The most common form of CGD is X-linked recessive (two-thirds of cases)[50] and results from mutations in *CYBB*, which encodes the membrane-bound component of NADPH oxidase cytochrome b-245 beta-chain or gp91^{phox} (*phox* is short for *phagocyte oxidase*); 90% of affected individuals are male. Autosomal recessive forms (25% to 30% of patients) are due to mutations in other components of phagocyte NADPH oxidase. The most common cause is mutations in *NCF4*, encoding the cytoplasmic component p47^{phox}, but mutations in *CYBA* (encoding p22^{phox}, also called *neutrophil cytochrome b light chain*) and *NCF2* (also called *NOXA2*; encoding p67^{phox}) have also been described. Patients with CGD commonly show leukocytosis, anemia, elevated erythrocyte sedimentation rate (ESR), and hypergammaglobulinemia. Skin tests for delayed hypersensitivity, phagocytosis, and chemotaxis are normal. Carrier and affected patients are often detected by quantitative dihydrorhodamine flow cytometry to measure dihydrorhodamine 123 (DHR) oxidase activity.[51] The nitroblue tetrazolium (NBT) screening assay is now rarely performed (in which the oxidized yellow form of NBT is reduced to a blue formazan precipitate). Flow cytometry[52,53] and immunoblots can detect the selective loss of membrane phagocyte oxidase components. However, mutations that lead to deficiency of gp91^{phox} or p22^{phox} cannot be differentiated by these techniques because both are components of cytochrome b_{558} and the entire cytochrome is absent if one component is deficient; thus gene sequencing is required.

The skin, lungs, and perianal area are most often the sites of infection. Early lesions are usually cutaneous staphylococcal pyodermas and abscesses of the face and perianal area, sometimes associated with purulent dermatitis and regional lymphadenopathy. Cutaneous lesions can resemble seborrheic dermatitis, Sweet syndrome, and scalp folliculitis; perioral and intraoral ulcerations may resemble aphthous stomatitis.

The organisms associated with CGD are usually catalase-positive and include *Staphylococcus aureus* and opportunistic gram-negative bacteria (especially Enterobacteriaceae *Serratia*[54] and *Klebsiella*, as well as *Pseudomonas*). These organisms all require oxidative metabolism (generation of superoxide anion and other reactive oxygen species) for intracellular killing by neutrophils, monocytes, macrophages, and eosinophils. Other organisms that may cause infection in patients with CGD with increased incidence are *Aspergillus*, *Candida*, *Cryptococcus*, *Fusarium*, and *Nocardia*.[55] Bronchopneumonia and suppurative lymphadenitis are the most prevalent noncutaneous infections. These infections respond to appropriate antibacterial therapy and, in some cases, surgical drainage. The extracutaneous organs most commonly involved in CGD are the lymph nodes, lungs, liver, spleen, and gastrointestinal tract (Box 25.2). Female carriers are at increased risk of infection if DHR activity is $<20\%$[56] and particularly $<10\%$, leading to the suggestion that antimicrobial prophylaxis be used in these individuals as well.[57]

Noninfectious inflammation is a common complication, especially in those with *CYBB* mutations. Approximately 40% of patients with X-linked CGD develop some form of inflammatory bowel disease.[50] CGD has been misdiagnosed as Crohn's disease because of the overlap in features (failure to thrive, diarrhea, abdominal pain, weight loss, perianal abscesses, ulcers and fistulas, bowel obstruction, anemia, hypoalbuminemia, and granulomatous colitis).[58,59] At least 50% of patients have noninfectious lung issues, especially during adulthood. Although lung infections are most common, inflammatory complications are also described (interstitial lung disease, chronic obstructive pulmonary diseases, lung nodules, and pleural effusions) and may be difficult to diagnosis without tissue evaluation. Granulomas are a classic noninfectious finding, particularly of the colon, stomach, and bladder. Chorioretinitis, uveitis, and ocular granulomas occasionally occur. In a recent study of patients who reached adulthood, 13% developed skin issues.[60] These included granulomatous acne, inflammatory nodules, photosensitivity, cutaneous lymphocytic infiltration, and aphthous stomatitis. In fact, development of systemic or discoid lupus erythematosus is the most commonly seen autoimmune complication in affected individuals,[61] including in those with a recessive form. Female carriers of *CYBB* mutations even more commonly show aphthous stomatitis, lupus-like eruptions, arthralgias, and

Box 25.2 Signs and Symptoms in Patients with Chronic Granulomatous Disease

Seen in more than 50% of patients
- Lymphadenopathy, lymphadenitis
- Hepatosplenomegaly
- Bronchopneumonia
- Failure to thrive

Seen in 25% of patients or less
- Persistent diarrhea
- Pleuritis or empyema
- Septicemia or meningitis
- Hepatic or perihepatic abscess
- Osteomyelitis

Seen in less than 25% of patients
- Perianal abscess
- Periorificial dermatitis, folliculitis
- Aphthous stomatitis
- Cutaneous signs of systemic and discoid lupus
- Ocular inflammation
- Lung abscess
- Peritonitis
- Obstructive granulomas

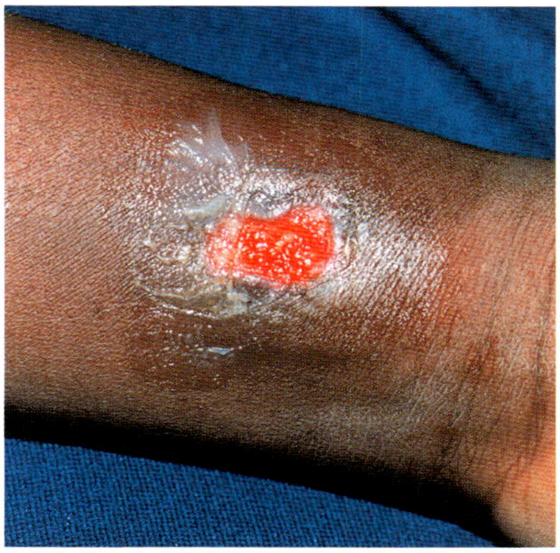

Fig. 25.3 Leukocyte adhesion deficiency. Small wounds can lead to large ulcerations that may resemble pyoderma gangrenosum. The ulceration on this boy's leg, initiated by a scratch from his sister, eventually extended to several centimeters in diameter and required a graft. (Reprinted with permission from Schachner LA, Hansen R, eds. *Pediatric Dermatology*. London, UK: Churchill Livingstone; 1995.)

photosensitivity.[62,63] In contrast to infection, these features have not been correlated with baseline oxidative burst function in carriers. Photosensitivity reactions have been described in patients administered voriconazole, and poor wound healing, including the development of pyoderma gangrenosum, has occurred postoperatively.

Antibiotic treatment of infection with surgical intervention as needed, as well as prophylactic trimethoprim–sulfamethoxazole and itraconazole therapy,[64] have been used in most affected individuals.[65] Short courses of systemic corticosteroids have been helpful for patients with obstructive visceral granulomas. Restoration of normal oxidase activity in ≥20% of circulating neutrophils markedly reduces the risk of infection.[57] Stem cell therapy with replacement of defective neutrophils is better than conventional antimicrobial therapy with respect to fewer serious infections and surgeries, better growth, and improved quality of life[66,67] in patients with X-linked CGD.[68–70] Transplantation should be performed as early as possible, given better outcomes, especially before the occurrence of CGD-related organ damage. The estimated survival of nontransplanted patients has been 88% at 10 years of age and 55% at 30 years old. In a recent study, the survival with unrelated donors was equivalent in outcome to parental (carrier) donors,[71] suggesting that X-linked carrier donors should be avoided, given their increased risk of autoimmune and inflammatory issues.[57] Targeted gene-editing technologies are under investigation preclinically, especially for patients with autosomal recessive CGD.[72]

LEUKOCYTE ADHESION DEFICIENCIES

The leukocyte adhesion deficiencies (LADs) are a group of three autosomal recessive disorders that affect the ability of neutrophils, cytolytic T lymphocytes, and monocytes to be mobilized into extravascular sites of inflammation.[73] LAD1 is most common and results from mutations in CD18, leading to deficiency or dysfunction of the β_2 subunit of integrins. The principal ligand for these integrins is *ICAM1*, which participates actively in neutrophil and monocyte chemotaxis and phagocytosis.

Patients with LAD have frequent skin infections (especially facial cellulitis and perianal infection), mucositis, and otitis, with a 5- to 20-fold increase in peripheral blood leukocytes. Poor wound healing is characteristic and leads to paper-thin or dysplastic cutaneous scars. Minor skin wounds may become large ulcerations that resemble pyoderma gangrenosum (Fig. 25.3), especially if secondarily infected. Periodontitis is a typical feature and if, severe, may lead to loss of teeth. Bacterial and fungal infections may be life threatening. Delayed separation of the umbilical cord is a common historic clue to the diagnosis. Psoriasis has been described in affected individuals with mild disease.[74] More than 75% of patients with severe disease die by 5 years of age; more than half of the patients with moderate deficiency die between the ages of 10 and 30 years.

A second form of LAD (LAD2) is an autosomal recessive disorder caused by mutations in *FUCT1*. *FUCT1* encodes a GFP-fucose transporter that is required for formation of sialyl-Lewis X, a ligand for selectins on the surface of neutrophils.[75] In addition to their elevated leukocyte counts and recurrent bacterial infections, patients have short stature, a distinctive facies, and developmental delay. A third type of LAD (LAD3), which features a bleeding tendency, is caused by a mutation in *FERMT3*, which encodes kindlin-3 and prevents activation of β1, β2, and β3 integrins.[76] Dermal hematopoiesis, leading to the "blueberry muffin" presentation, has been described in affected infants and children.[77] Petechiae and mucosal hemorrhage are common, and mucosal bleeding is the presenting sign in more than 70% of patients.[78]

Therapy of the soft-tissue infections includes antimicrobial agents and, as appropriate, debridement of wounds. Scrupulous dental hygiene reduces the severity of the periodontitis. Death usually occurs by 2 years of age in patients with severe LAD unless successful bone marrow transplantation or cord blood transplantation is performed.[79] Oral fucose has been helpful for some patients with LAD2.

SEVERE COMBINED IMMUNODEFICIENCY

SCID is a group of disorders with similar clinical manifestations and immune dysfunction but different biochemical, cellular, and molecular features (Table 25.2).[7,80–84] Newborn screening for SCID using the T-cell receptor excision circle (TREC) assay to detect neonatal T-cell lymphopenia has allowed much earlier detection[85] and is now the most common means of detecting SCID in the United States.[86–88] TREC assays also allow detection of "leaky" SCID in which some T cells are present with limited function.

Based on newborn screening, the prevalence of SCID is now estimated to be 1 in 50,000 births and the percentage with the X-linked recessive form has decreased from approximately 50% to only 19%,[89] although it still the most common form. This X-linked recessive form results from mutations in the gene that encodes the γ_c chain,[90] a component of several interleukin receptors, which is critical for T-cell and natural killer (NK)-cell function. Recombination activating gene (RAG) proteins RAG1 or RAG2 mediate deoxyribonucleic acid (DNA) double-strand breaks that allow variable (diversity) joining (V[D]J) recombination and Ig diversity, and their deficiency results in Omenn syndrome (15% of SCID).[91–93] Mutations in adenosine deaminase

Table 25.2 Classification of Selected Forms of Severe Combined Immunodeficiency^

Disorder	Gene	Diagnostic Tests	Cells
ADA deficiency	*ADA*	Red cell ADA levels and accumulation of toxic metabolites	$T^-/B^-/NK^-$
AK2 deficiency	*AK2*	Defective survival of hematopoietic precursors	$T^+/B^+/NK^-$
Artemis deficiency	*Artemis*	Defects in V(D)J recombination; increased sensitivity to radiation	$T^-/B^-/NK^+$
CD8 deficiency	*CD8*	CD8 expression deficiency	$T^+/B^+/NK^+$ ($CD8^-$)
CARD11 deficiency	*CARD11*	CARD11 expression; abnormal IL-12 production, Treg-cell deficiency	$T^+/B^+/NK^+$
CD45 deficiency	*CD45*	CD45 expression	$T^-/B^+/NK^+$
IL-7 receptor deficiency	*IL-7 receptor α*	IL-7 receptor α expression	$T^-/B^+/NK^+$
JAK3 deficiency	*JAK3*	*JAK3* expression/signaling	$T^-/B^+/N^{--}$
MHC class I deficiency	*TAP1* and *TAP2; TAPBP; B2M*	MHC class I expression	$T^+/B^+/NK^+$ ($CD8^-$)
MHC class II deficiency	*CIITA* *RFX5* *RFXAP*	HLA-DR expression	$T^+/B^+/NK^+$ (fewer $CD4^+$)
Moesin deficiency	*MSN*	Deficient moesin expression	$T^-/B^-/NK^-$
PNP deficiency	*PNP*	Red cell PNP levels and metabolites	$T^-/B^-/NK^-$
RAG deficiency* Omenn syndrome	*RAG1* and *RAG2*	Defects in V(D)J recombination; T- and B-cell clonal analysis	$T^-/B^-/NK^+$
T-cell receptor deficiency	*CD3g*	*CD3* expression	$T^-/B^+/NK^+$
X-linked SCID†	Common γ chain	γ_c expression by FACS	$T^-/B^+/NK^-$
ZAP70 deficiency	*ZAP-70*	*ZAP-70* expression	$T^-/B^+/NK^-$

ADA, Adenosine deaminase; *AK2*, adenylate kinase 2; *HLA-DR*, human leukocyte antigen DR; *IL*, interleukin; *MHC*, major histocompatibility complex; *PNP*, purine nucleoside phosphorylase; *RAG*, recombinase activating gene; *SCID*, severe combined immunodeficiency; *V(D)J*, variable (diversity) joining.
^For current classification (2015), see Picard C, Al-Herz W, Bousfiha A, et al. Primary immunodeficiency diseases: An update on the classification from the International Union of Immunological Societies Expert Committee for Primary Immunodeficiency 2015. *J Clin Immunol* 2015;35:696–726.
*Most common autosomal recessive form (15% of autosomal recessive types have biallelic RAG1 mutations).
†Most common X-linked recessive form (19% overall).

(ADA1) occur in 10% of neonates and lead to accumulation of adenosine, which is toxic to lymphocytes.

Infants may present with a generalized seborrheic-like dermatosis, a morbilliform eruption, or exfoliative erythroderma with alopecia. Extensive cutaneous inflammation is a characteristic of 98% of infants with Omenn syndrome,[94] a subset of SCID with reticuloendothelial cell proliferation. Patients with Omenn syndrome typically show hepatosplenomegaly (88%), lymphadenopathy (80%), alopecia (57%), eosinophilia, and a high serum IgE level.[91] Oral and genital ulcers are characteristic of defects in patients with an *Artemis* mutation, especially in Athabaskan-speaking American Indian children.[95] Multicentric dermatofibrosarcoma protuberans (DFSP)[96] and pulmonary alveolar proteinosis[97] have been described in association with ADA deficiency.[98] Recurrent varicella and bacterial infections are seen in the recently described form related to deficiency of moesin.[99] Profound T-cell deficiency has also more recently been related to biallelic loss-of-function mutations in CARD11 (or its signaling partners BCL10 and MALT1), leading to recurrent and severe infections; monoallelic missense mutations in CARD11 lead to abnormal T-cell responses with susceptibility to infection, multiorgan atopy (including atopic dermatitis and urticaria), and autoimmunity (lichen sclerosis, cutaneous necrotizing granulomatous inflammation).[100–106] Major histocompatibility complex (MCH) class I deficiency may manifest with vasculitis and/or pyoderma gangrenosum.

Acute graft-versus-host disease (GVHD) from maternal cell engraftment or nonirradiated transfusions should also be considered in an infant with an extensive cutaneous eruption.[107] Biopsy will allow differentiation. A more chronic form of GVHD (often with the acute form *in utero*) may also present as lesions that resemble lichen planus, lamellar ichthyosis, or scleroderma (see Graft-Versus-Host Disease section).

Recurrent infections, diarrhea, and failure to thrive are apparent by 3 to 6 months of age. The most common early infections are candidal infections and pneumonia caused by bacteria, viruses, or *Pneumocystis jiroveci*. Patients with SCID usually lack tonsillar buds, a thymus, and palpable lymphoid tissue despite recurrent infections. Nearly all patients with SCID have a profound deficiency of T lymphocytes and a low absolute lymphocyte count. Patients are further classified by the results of fluorescent activated cell sorter (FACS) analysis into those with B lymphocytes (T^-/B^+ SCID) and those without B lymphocytes (T^-/B^- SCID). Further subclassification can be made according to the presence or absence of NK cells (see Table 25.2). However, it is now clear that many immunodeficiency disorders have cells that are differentiated into these subtypes but do not function normally, leading to immune dysregulation, infection, and sometimes cancer.[84] The specific diagnosis is confirmed primarily by direct genetic analysis and flow cytometric analysis of peripheral blood mononuclear cells with antibodies directed against specific proteins missing from the cell surface, such as *JAK3* or γ_c.

Early diagnosis of SCID is critical, preferably before the administration of live vaccines, nonirradiated blood products, and, in countries where applicable, bacille Calmette–Guérin (BCG). Patients with SCID have a high risk of BCG-associated complications[108] (34% disseminated and 17% localized) and subsequent death, especially if they are given the vaccination at 1 month of age or younger and with T-cell numbers of 250/mcL or less at diagnosis.[109] The natural outcome for SCID is poor, and most patients die by 2 years of age without intervention.

Hematopoietic stem cell transplantation in infants is the treatment of choice[110] and leads to 5-year survival of 95% of infants if performed in the first 3 months of life, regardless of donor or conditioning regimen. Most deaths after transplantation occur during the first

2 to 5 years after transplantation and result from infections. Bone marrow–derived CD34+ cells transduced with the SIN-γ_c modified γ-retrovirus vector without preparative conditioning has led to T-cell recovery without evidence of leukemia after up to 3 years of follow-up in boys with X-linked SCID.[111] Enzyme replacement therapy (ERT) is available for ADA SCID,[112] both as a bridge to definitive treatment and in addition to stem cell transplantation; however, it is costly, requires weekly to biweekly intramuscular injections, and has a decreasing effect on lymphocyte counts with time, likely due to the development of anti-ADA antibodies.[88] Even definitive therapy with transplantation does not prevent late complications or comorbidities, including the continued need for immunoglobulin injections (up to 58%), chronic human papillomavirus infections (up to 25%), chronic gastrointestinal issues (especially poor feeding and diarrhea, 20%), sinopulmonary infections (20%), growth retardation (≈15%), and neurocognitive issues, especially attention-deficit/hyperactivity disorder. There is a high risk of autoimmunity (especially hemolytic anemia) and GVHD.

Graft-Versus-Host Disease

Children who undergo transplantation are at risk for several cutaneous complications.[113] Most common among these are infections, drug reactions (given the large number of prescribed medications), GVHD,[114] and the increased risk after transplantation of skin cancer.

GVHD should be distinguished from *host-versus-graft reaction*, which occurs when a graft or transplant (e.g., skin, heart, or kidney) is placed in a normal individual and the host's circulating immune cells react to the foreign tissue, causing graft or transplanted tissue destruction. In GVHD, the reverse happens.[115,116] GVHD most commonly occurs in children with malignancy who receive hematopoietic stem cell transplantation after radiation and chemotherapy or in immunodeficient children who receive nonirradiated blood products. Reactions to transfusions often occur 7 to 10 days after the transfusion.[117] Nevertheless, GVHD may be advantageous in patients with hematologic malignancies, helping to clear host neoplastic cells (e.g., graft-vs.-leukemia). *In utero* GVHD may occur in immunodeficient babies exposed to maternal antigens.[107] GVHD also uncommonly occurs in recipients of solid organ transplants[118] (most often small bowel and liver transplants) and can be fatal.[119–121] In these patients, 87% have skin involvement, typically described as a "maculopapular rash."[122] Although poorly described morphologically, the eruption occurs an average of 48 days after transplantation, is rarely pruritic, and is associated with a mortality rate of 72% from sepsis and multiorgan failure.[123] Patients who receive autologous transplants may have a mild cutaneous form of aGVHD that occurs 1 to 3 weeks after transplantation and resolves spontaneously.

GVHD was previously classified as acute (aGVHD) or chronic (cGVHD) based on the threshold of before or after 100 days posttransplant. However, specific clinical features that define acute vs. chronic disease do not necessarily agree with the timing after transplantation. In addition, changing practices that affect recipient immune status, among them the introduction of reduced-intensity conditioning, donor lymphocyte infusions, and second allogeneic stem cell transplants, have contributed to the changes in GVHD presentation. Classification now includes (1) classic aGVHD; (2) persistent, recurrent, or late-onset aGVHD (beyond 100 days after transplantation); (3) classic cGVHD; and (4) an overlap syndrome with features of both aGVHD and cGVHD. The latter two types can present any time, including before 100 days after transplantation (Table 25.3).[124] It is recognized that the pathomechanism of aGVHD vs. cGVHD is distinct. In aGVHD, the immune dysregulation results from stimulation of the host's antigen-presenting cells by activated donor mature T cells (especially Th1 lymphocytes) in host target organs,[125] amplifying T-cell activation and expansion, and culminating in target organ apoptosis and dysfunction. cGVHD, however, occurs by a complex mechanism that includes activation initially of innate immune responses, followed by more chronic inflammation mediated by adaptive immune activation (T and B cells) and ultimately the production of profibrotic cytokines by activated T cells. The risk of GVHD is greater in patients given a transplant from a partially matched family donor or an unrelated volunteer than an allogeneic transplant from a human leukocyte antigen (HLA)-identical donor.[126]

Table 25.3 Classification of Graft-Versus-Host Disease

Type of GVHD	Time after Transplantation	Features
Acute GVHD (aGVHD)		
Classic	≤100 days	aGVHD only
Persistent, recurrent, or late onset	>100 days	aGVHD only
Chronic GVHD (cGVHD)		
Classic	Any	cGVHD only
Overlap syndrome	Any	aGVHD + cGVHD

The most common cutaneous manifestation of aGVHD is an erythematous to violaceous macular or papular (morbilliform) eruption, which often begins on the ears, face, neck, palms, and soles and then becomes generalized (Figs. 25.4 to 25.6). The cutaneous eruption may become confluent and desquamate. Variants are ichthyotic, eczematous,[127] psoriatic,[128] pityriasis rubra pilaris–like, or diffuse and perifollicular. Distribution along Blaschko lines has been

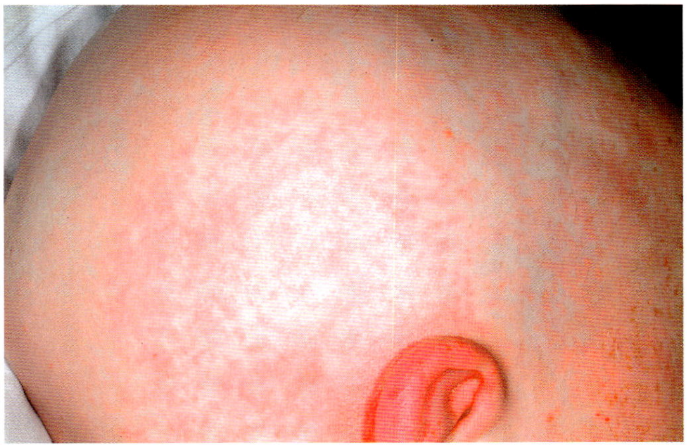

Fig. 25.4 Acute graft-versus-host disease. Involvement of the scalp, ears, palms, and soles is common.

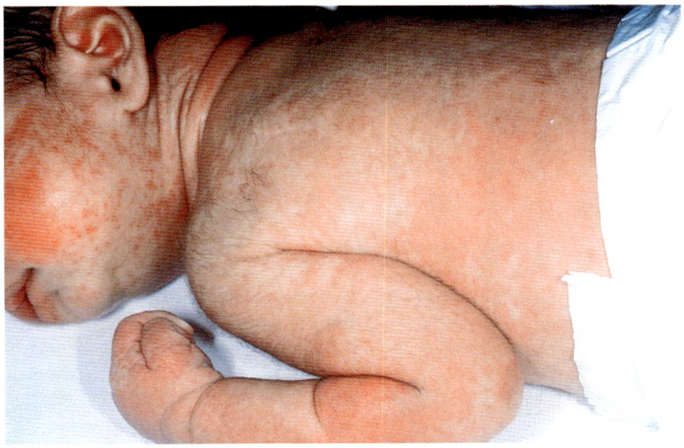

Fig. 25.5 Acute graft-versus-host disease. Almost confluent eruption of erythematous macules and papules in an immunodeficient neonate treated with extracorporeal membrane oxygenation (ECMO) and transfusion of nonirradiated blood.

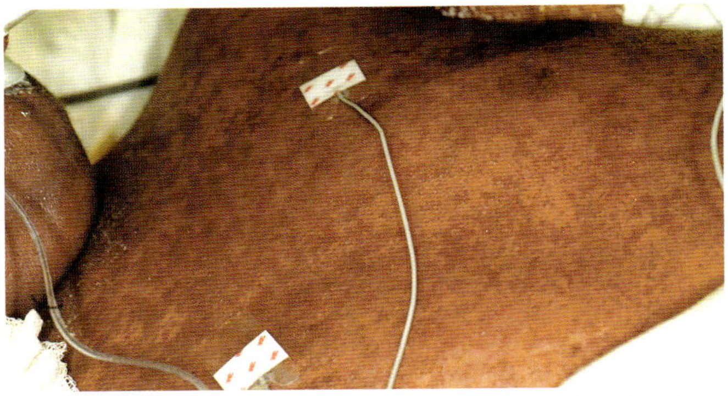

Fig. 25.6 Acute graft-versus-host disease. Note the generalized erythematous macules but also the jaundice, reflecting liver disease. This boy died after transplantation.

reported.[129,130] Mild to moderate aGVHD most often presents with a nonspecific cutaneous eruption and thus can be confused with infection (especially viral), drug reaction,[131] and reactions related to the transplant (e.g., the self-limited eruption of lymphocyte recovery; engraftment syndrome, characterized by associated fever and vascular leak with weight gain, edema, ascites, pulmonary infiltrates, and hypotension[132]; and toxic erythema of chemotherapy, which is painful and usually localized to the palms, soles, and intertriginous areas). Severe aGVHD may resemble exfoliative erythroderma or toxic epidermal necrolysis (TEN). The TEN associated with aGVHD must be differentiated from TEN associated with a drug eruption[133] based on time course and drug exposure. Eosinophilic pustular folliculitis has recently been described as another posttransplantation eruption, which can be confused with aGVHD but occurs 2 to 3 months after transplantation and responds well to topical corticosteroids.[134]

aGVHD usually involves the skin, gastrointestinal tract, and liver (in that order of incidence).[135] Patients with aGVHD may complain of nausea or crampy abdominal pain and have watery or bloody diarrhea, hepatomegaly, and hepatic function abnormalities. Many patients are anorexic and have fever. Staging depends on the extent of specific organ involvement (of skin, liver, and gut), and grading reflects the staging of each organ collectively. Staging of skin in aGVHD is based on extent (stage 1: <25%; 2: 25% to 50%; 3: >50%; and 4: generalized erythroderma, usually with bulla formation). Grade 1 aGVHD involves stage 1 or 2 skin involvement and no organ involvement, whereas grade 4 aGVHD requires stage 4 skin and liver involvement.

Abnormalities seen in biopsy specimens reflect the clinical severity of the cutaneous manifestations and range from nonspecific changes, to basal keratinocyte vacuolization with scattered necrotic keratinocytes surrounded by lymphocytes (the characteristic "satellite cell necrosis"), to severe epidermal necrosis. As such, biopsies are not helpful for patients with milder disease and do not tend to affect treatment decisions.[136] Laboratory tests may show eosinophilia and elevation of bilirubin and hepatic transaminase levels. aGVHD grading predicts prognosis and is based on extent and degree of organ system involvement, as well as percentage of body surface area involved by the aGVHD.[137]

cGVHD often resembles autoimmune disorders and, in contrast to aGVHD, can affect virtually any organ, leading to significant morbidity with decreased quality of life and overall survival[138] (Table 25.4). Early lesions of cGVHD most commonly resemble lichen planus with flat-topped violaceous papules and plaques (including mucosal changes of lichen planus) (Figs. 25.7 and 25.8), which is the most common manifestation[139] (see Chapter 4). Lichenoid lesions may be localized to Blaschko lines or to the site of previous herpes zoster infection.[140] Some patients with cGVHD manifest lichen sclerosus (Fig. 25.9). Early features may also be nonspecific, manifesting as xerosis with or without follicular prominence or ichthyotic (Fig. 25.10). Eczematous and psoriatic variants of cGVHD are rarely seen.[127,139] Later changes of cGVHD[141] include generalized xerosis,

Table 25.4 Features of Chronic Graft-Versus-Host Disease

Location	Characteristic Features	Other Features
Skin	Lichen planus–like Poikilodermatous Lichen sclerosis–like, including vaginal scarring, stenosis Sclerotic (or lichen sclerosus–like)	Depigmentation Hypopigmentation and hyperpigmentation Ichthyotic changes Genital erosions, ulcers, fissures Erythema, maculopapular rash Pruritus Hypohidrosis Keratosis pilaris
Hair		Alopecia, nonscarring or cicatricial; can be diffuse Premature graying
Nails		Ridging, onycholysis, loss, pterygium
Oral	Lichen planus–like	Mucosal atrophy Xerostomia Ulceration Mucocele Keratotic plaques Sclerosis with restricted opening
Eyes		Dry eyes Cicatricial conjunctivitis Keratoconjunctivitis sicca Punctate keratopathy
Joints/muscle	Contracture from sclerosis Fasciitis, arthritis	Myositis
Gastrointestinal	Chronic diarrhea Upper esophageal strictures, stenosis, webbing Hepatomegaly	
Lungs	Bronchiolitis obliterans Interstitial fibrosis	

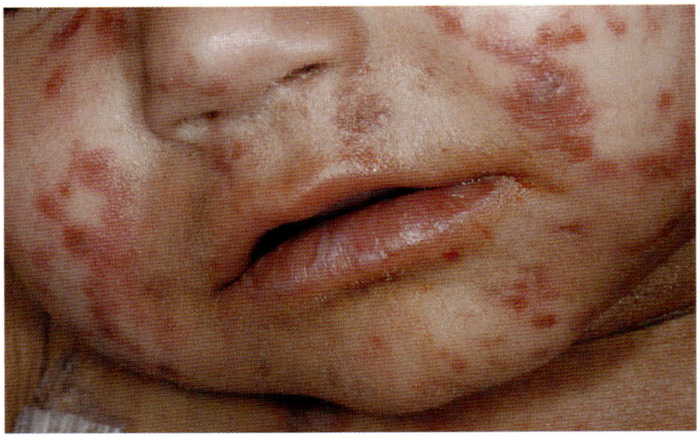

Fig. 25.7 Chronic graft-versus-host disease (GVHD), lichenoid. After bone marrow transplantation, this boy had acute GVHD and subsequently developed violaceous lichenoid papules of the face, trunk, and extremities. Note the white plaque of lichen planus on the lower lip.

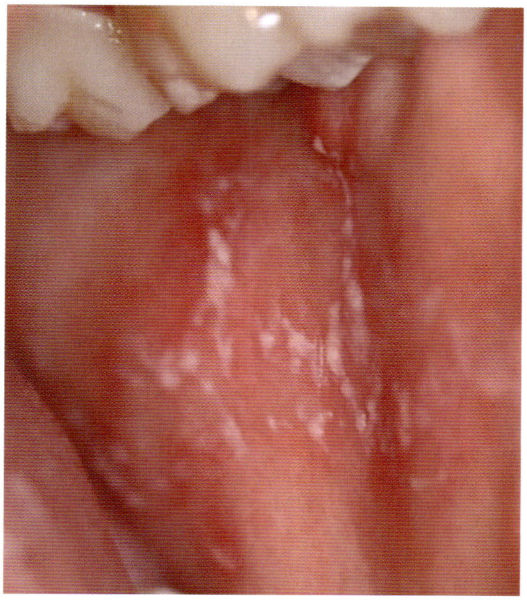

Fig. 25.8 Chronic graft-versus-host disease (GVHD), lichenoid. Note the white flat-topped papules on the buccal mucosa of this girl with early chronic GVHD. (Courtesy Dr. K. Vivar.)

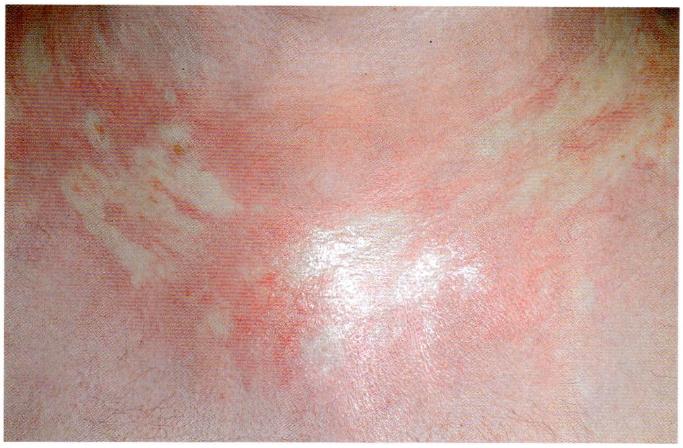

Fig. 25.9 Chronic graft-versus-host disease (GVHD). The changes of chronic GVHD can resemble those of other autoimmune skin disorders. In this case, the cutaneous plaques resembled those of morphea/lichen sclerosus et atrophicus.

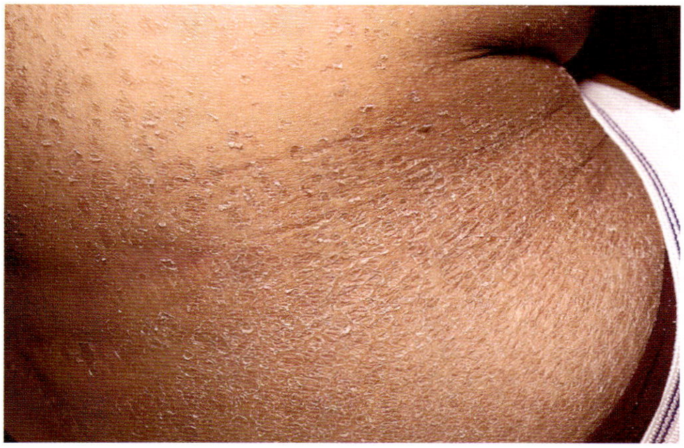

Fig. 25.10 Chronic graft-versus-host disease (GVHD), ichthyotic. The ichthyotic changes of chronic GVHD resemble those of ichthyosis vulgaris.

patchy dyspigmentation, and sclerodermatous changes[136,142,143] (Fig. 25.11); joint contracture (Figs. 25.12 and 25.13); vitiligo[144] (Fig. 25.14); progressive poikiloderma (characterized by reticulated hypopigmentation and hyperpigmentation, atrophy, and telangiectasia); ulcerations[145]; keratoderma (see Fig. 25.13); and nail dystrophy, sometimes with pterygium formation (Fig. 25.15; see Fig. 25.14) resembling that of dyskeratosis congenita (see Chapter 7, Fig. 7.69).[146] Alopecia that may be diffuse (and sometimes permanent), localized (areata),[144] androgenetic, or cicatricial (Fig. 25.16) has been noted, and permanent alopecia often relates to the use of a conditioning regimen with busulphan.[147] Disseminated porokeratosis has also been described after stem cell transplantation and may respond to acitretin.[148] The many autoimmune changes associated with cGVHD likely reflect reduced Treg cells.

Affected individuals may have dry eyes (as in Sjögren syndrome; see Chapter 22), conjunctivitis/keratitis, and desquamative esophagitis with stricture formation. Weight loss can result from dysphagia and mucositis. Other manifestations are chronic diarrhea, hepatomegaly, lymphadenopathy, myositis, arthritis, pleural and pericardial effusions, and pulmonary fibrosis. cGVHD is subclassified as *mild, moderate*, or *severe* based on the number of organs involved, the presence of pulmonary involvement, and resultant disability.[124,149]

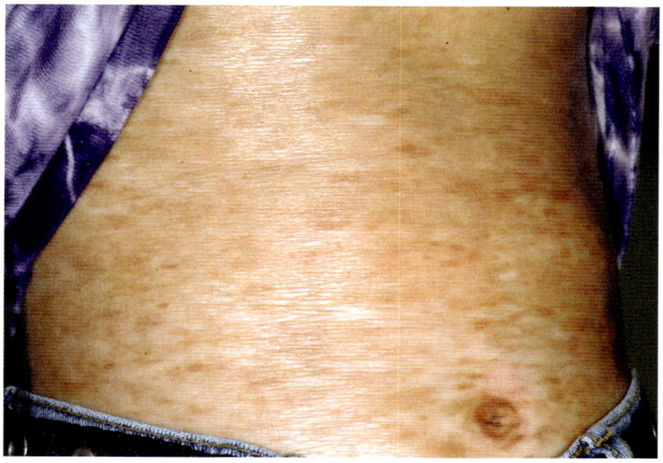

Fig. 25.11 Chronic graft-versus-host disease. Hypopigmented and hyperpigmented indurated plaques in a generalized distribution, seen here on her abdomen; 15 years later, the dyschromia persisted.

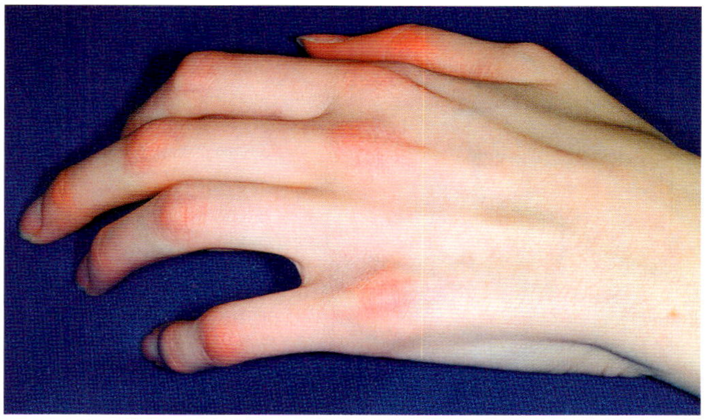

Fig. 25.12 Chronic graft-versus-host disease. Sclerodactyly and subtle telangiectasia overlying the knuckles, as seen in patients with systemic scleroderma and juvenile dermatomyositis.

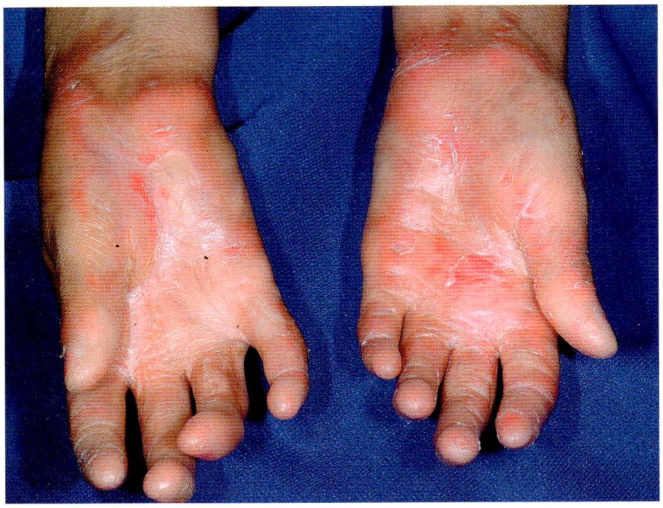

Fig. 25.13 Chronic graft-versus-host disease (GVHD). Sclerodactyly and generalized scaling were noted at birth in this girl with immunodeficiency and *in utero* GVHD.

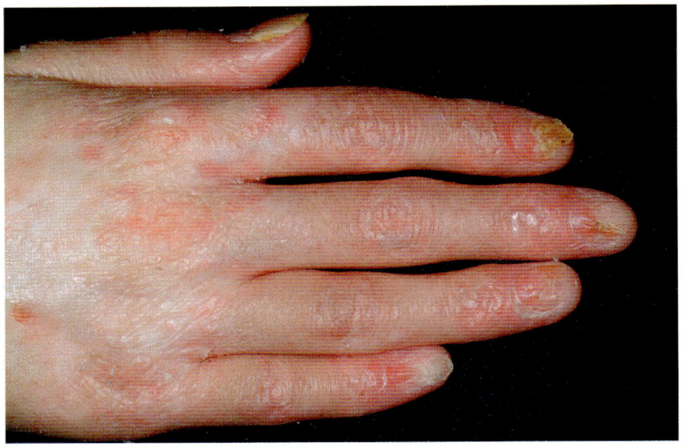

Fig. 25.15 Chronic graft-versus-host disease. Note the cutaneous atrophy and nail dystrophy, including onycholysis and pterygium formation, resembling the nails of lichen planus.

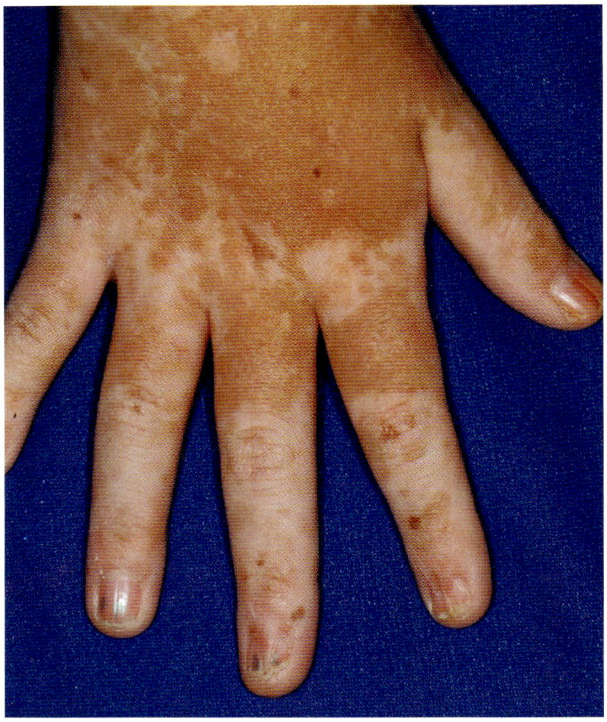

Fig. 25.14 Chronic graft-versus-host disease. Vitiligo on the dorsal aspect of the hands. Note the pterygium formation of the fingernails.

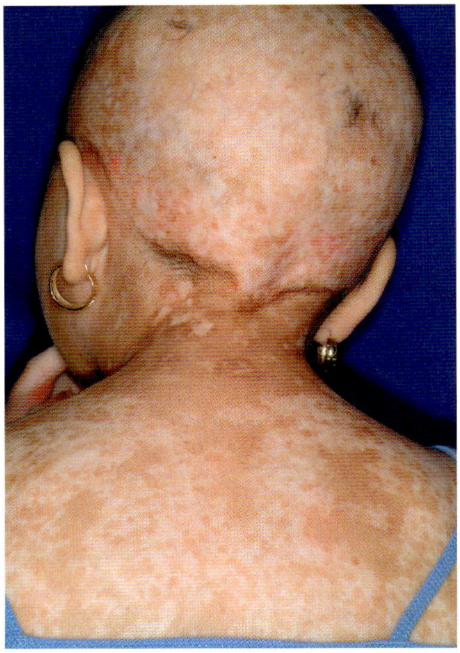

Fig. 25.16 Chronic graft-versus-host disease. Note the extensive alopecia of the scalp with dyschromia and numerous sclerodermatous plaques of the scalp and back.

Patients with cGVHD show evidence of immune dysfunction and have recurrent infections. The majority of patients with cGVHD have eosinophilia and hypergammaglobulinemia. Many have thrombocytopenia and increased titers of a wide variety of autoimmune antibodies, especially antinuclear antibodies (ANAs).[136] Liver function testing may show evidence of cholestasis. Pulmonary function tests are abnormal in approximately 50% of patients, and chest radiographs may reveal interstitial fibrosis. Biopsies of skin lesions show changes consistent with the clinical picture. For example, patients with lichenoid lesions have the histologic changes of lichen planus (see Chapter 4), often with satellite cell necrosis. Patients with sclerosis tend to show band-like inflammation at the dermal–epidermal junction and dermal sclerosis with obliteration of adnexae. Direct immunofluorescence analysis of skin specimens often shows the linear deposition of immunoreactants at the dermal–epidermal junction.

cGVHD occurs in 6% (matched sibling cord blood) to 65% (matched unrelated donor peripheral blood stem cell transplants) of pediatric patients; in one recent study, cGVHD occurred in 18% of all transplanted children, with 90% showing lichenoid lesions and 30% developing sclerosis.[150] Although patients may develop cGVHD without preceding aGVHD, having aGVHD that resolves or progresses directly is a major risk factor for development of cGVHD (11-fold increased risk), emphasizing the importance of preventing aGVHD. Other risk factors are an unrelated or mismatched donor, use of peripheral blood stem cells, older age of donor or recipient, use of total body irradiation, male recipient with a female donor, and malignant disease.[151] For patients with myeloablation (full-intensity conditioning, which eliminates all malignant and marrow hematopoietic cells), prophylaxis usually involves 2 to 12 months of tacrolimus (or cyclosporine), with or without a short course (about 1 month) of methotrexate. With reduced-intensity conditioning before transplant, which does not fully eradicate malignant and hematopoietic cells and instead relies on immunologic antihost and antitumor effects, prophylaxis often involves administration of oral tacrolimus and mycophenolate mofetil (MMF) (or corticosteroid). In both situations, anti–T-cell serotherapy with either antithymocyte globulin or alemtuzumab (Campath) is usually added for unrelated donor transplants and also reduces graft rejection; for haploidentical donors, T-cell depletion or CD34 selection is often performed. Environmental isolation, bowel rest through hyperalimentation, irradiation of blood products, and prevention of infection are other protective measures.

The mortality rate of aGVHD ranges from 12% for mild disease to 55% for severe aGVHD, usually because of infection.[152] The mortality of cGVHD is 25%, usually from infection, hepatic failure, and malnutrition. Decreased survival of patients with cGVHD has been associated with thrombocytopenia, progressive onset, extensive cutaneous involvement, gastrointestinal involvement, and a low Karnofsky performance status at diagnosis.[136]

Topical corticosteroids, with or without topical calcineurin inhibitors, are used for grade I disease. Ultraviolet (UV) light (preferably, nbUVB and UVA1) may also be helpful for skin-predominant aGVHD. If grade II through IV aGVHD develops, the first-line therapy is continuing prophylactic immunosuppression (optimizing calcineurin inhibitor levels) and adding intravenous methylprednisolone at 2 mg/kg per day.[149] Steroids are tapered when there is a clinical response, given the high risk of adverse events with continued use of high doses. For skin GVHD, topical steroid and/or tacrolimus may be added, with oral administration of budesonide for gastrointestinal GVHD. Patients who fail to respond to corticosteroid alone after 5 to 7 days (60% to 70% of patients) can be treated with salvage therapy, such as MMF,[153–155] anti-TNF antibodies (e.g., infliximab), mammalian target of rapamycin (mTOR) inhibitors (e.g., sirolimus/rapamycin),[156–158] anti-interleukin (IL)-2 antibodies (e.g., daclizumab or basiliximab),[159,160] antithymoglobulin, the combination of an anti-IL2 and an anti-TNF antibody,[161] or extracorporeal photopheresis (ECP).[162–165] Responses in general are poor if initial steroid treatment is not successful and the risk of infection is high. If at least two second-line treatments fail, alternatives are alemtuzumab,[166] methotrexate, pentostatin,[167,168] and mesenchymal stem cells.[135,169–172]

Similar regimens have been used to treat cGVHD, although there is no proven standard. Prednisone and calcineurin inhibitors are the most commonly used first-line therapies.[136] The mean duration of therapy for patients with cGVHD is 3 years, with about 50% of patients able to discontinue therapy 5 years after transplantation. Second-line treatment (steroid resistant or steroid sparing) includes one of more of the following: ECP, rituximab,[173] imatinib mesylate (may increase range of motion with sclerotic cGVHD),[174–177] MMF, mTOR inhibitors, and low-dose methotrexate. ECP has been associated with cutaneous response rates of 60% to 80% and the ability to reduce the dose of systemic corticosteroid.[165,178] ECP works by collecting white blood cells, exposing them to 8-methoxypsoralen, and treating with UV light before reinfusing in an effort to apoptose cells but activate regulatory T cells. Disadvantages of ECP are the time required for each treatment, the frequency of required therapy, and the potential for large volume shifts in small children.[168] Overall, the 5-year survival rate is 50% for those who respond to therapy for GVHD and 30% for those with an incomplete or no response.

Anecdotal reports of responses in pediatric patients with cGVHD to systemic ruxolitinib have also been described.[179] However, responses are variable (31% failure rate) and toxicity is high. Targeting concurrently the IFNγ and IL-6 receptors by JAK inhibition (baricitinib more than ruxolitinib) has been shown to both prevent and reverse established GVHD in a mouse model while enhancing graft-versus-leukemia, a therapeutic benefit of GVHD.[180] Ibrutinib, an inhibitor of Bruton tyrosine kinase that prevents and treats cGVHD in mouse models,[181,182] was recently shown to treat cGVHD in an early phase human trial.[183]

In addition to use of topical antiinflammatory agents, mucocutaneous manifestations of GVHD may improve from administration of thalidomide or acitretin.[184–187] Although nbUVB has been used[188] for cutaneous sclerotic GVHD, UVA1 phototherapy is a favored intervention, because its longer wavelength penetrates more deeply. Phototherapy is not immunosuppressive, but its long-term effects are unknown. Supportive intervention for cGVHD includes supplemental nutrition (usually parenteral), scrupulous care of wounds, physical therapy to prevent joint contractures and disability, artificial tears, cutaneous emollients and sunscreens, and prophylaxis against *Pneumocystis* infection with trimethoprim–sulfamethoxazole. Routine skin surveillance is important for transplanted patients, not only to monitor for GVHD but also for the potential later development of mucocutaneous squamous cell carcinomas, which occurs more frequently in individuals who have had cGVHD.[189,190] Education about the risk of skin cancer and self-examination is also of importance.[191] Overall, 13% to 55% of cancers after organ transplantation involve the skin. Squamous cell carcinomas and basal cell carcinomas occur more often than Merkel cell carcinoma and melanoma. In one study, 20% of transplanted pediatric patients developed nonmelanoma skin cancer at an average of 17.2 years after renal transplantation.[192]

Anorexia Nervosa and Bulimia

Anorexia nervosa and bulimia nervosa are severe disorders associated with potentially serious medical complications (Box 25.3).[193–196] Anorexia nervosa occurs in up to 3% of pubertal females and less commonly in prepubertal females or males. In both disorders, patients have an intense preoccupation with food and an irrational concern about gaining weight. Bulimic patients tend to binge eat and attempt to lose weight by vomiting[197] and abusing laxatives, diuretics, diet pills, or emetics. The cutaneous features, which reflect endocrinologic changes and malnutrition, usually occur when the body mass index drops to less than 16 kg/m^2.[198,199] Affected individuals often show self-induced lesions as well, particularly the characteristic superficial ulcerations and hyperpigmented calluses or scars on the dorsal aspect of the second and third fingers (Russell sign), the result of repeated

Box 25.3 Cutaneous Signs of Anorexia Nervosa and Bulimia Nervosa

- Xerosis
- Generalized pruritus
- Loss of subcutaneous fat
- Carotenemia
- Acne
- Petechiae and purpura
- Edema, especially pretibial and pedal
- Calluses on the dorsum of the hand (Russell sign)
- Other self-inflicted injuries
- Poor wound healing
- Pellagra
- Scurvy
- Acrodermatitis enteropathica
- Seborrheic dermatitis
- Acral changes
  - Periungual erythema
  - Acrocyanosis
  - Acral coldness
  - Perniosis
- Oral changes
  - Cheilitis/perlèche
  - Aphthous stomatitis
  - Gum recession
  - Enamel erosion and dental caries
- Hair changes
  - Telogen effluvium
  - Increased lanugo-like body hair
  - Dry hair
- Brittle, dystrophic nails
- Enlarged parotid and salivary glands (full cheeks despite malnutrition)
- Heating pad–induced erythema ab igne

abrasion of the skin against the maxillary incisors during forced emesis.[200,201] Other emesis-associated complications include recurrent sore throat, hoarse voice, and dental erosions. Nutritional deficiency, such as zinc deficiency,[202] scurvy, and pellagra,[203] have occurred, as has erythema ab igne from chronic use of a heating pad for warmth.[204,205] Because of the potential severity of these disorders, it is important that physicians recognize the early signs and symptoms, particularly in view of the fact that patients tend to deny their illness or minimize the severity of their symptoms. The cutaneous manifestations are reversible when weight is gained. Many patients respond well to the combination of antidepressant and cognitive behavioral therapy.

Autoinflammatory Disorders

Innate immunity is activated in response to infection or tissue injury, including in skin. Neutrophils, mast cells, macrophages, and NK cells are key effectors of the innate immune system, although T and B lymphocytes, which are more typically associated with adaptive immunity, may contribute. Autoinflammatory disorders are characterized by recurrent episodes of inflammation in affected organs because of excessive antigen-independent innate immune activation. These bouts of inflammation are not associated with infection, high-titer autoantibodies or antigen-specific T cells, or allergy.[206–209] Many of these disorders have recurrent fevers, and the originally characterized autoinflammatory disorders were called *periodic fever syndromes.*

Monogenic autoinflammatory disorders are the best characterized forms and have been classified as inflammasomopathies, interferonopathies, ubiquitinopathies/relopathies, or others[210–212] (Table 25.5). In general, these disorders first manifest during childhood, although the onset may be in adults with milder or atypical forms. Cutaneous features may include urticaria,[213] pustules, papulosquamous lesions (psoriatic- or pityriasis rubra pilaris–like), neutrophilic dermatosis, acne, hidradenitis suppurativa/sterile abscesses, pyoderma gangrenosum, eczematous lesions, granulomatous lesions, purpura with vasculitis,

Table 25.5 Autoinflammatory Disorders

Disorder	Inheritance	Genetic Defect	Gene Product	Associated Features
Inflammasomopathies				
Familial Mediterranean fever	AR	*MEFV*	Pyrin (marenostrin)	Recurrent fever of short duration (2–3 days) Serositis with abdominal pain, pleuritis, and chest pain Pericarditis, scrotal swelling, splenomegaly, erysipelas-like eruption in minority of patients High risk of renal amyloidosis if untreated Good response to colchicine, IL-1 blockade
TNF receptor–associated periodic syndrome (TRAPS)	AD	*TNFRSF1A*	P55 TNF receptor	Recurrent fevers that are prolonged (1–3 weeks) Serositis, rash, conjunctivitis, periorbital edema, arthritis 10%–25% incidence of renal amyloidosis Response to etanercept and IL-1 blockade
Mevalonate kinase deficiency (MVK)/ hyper-IgD syndrome (HIDS)	AR	*MVK*	Mevalonate kinase	Early onset (usually first year) Periodic fever lasting 4–5 days Urticarial eruption (>90%), abdominal pain with vomiting and diarrhea, arthritis Headache, hepatosplenomegaly, painful cervical adenopathy, aphthous stomatitis, leukocytosis, high levels of IgD Response to steroids, NSAIDs, simvastatin, IL-1 blockade Often improves by adulthood Amyloidosis rare[+]
Familial cold autoinflammatory syndrome (familial cold urticaria)[*]	AD	*NLRP3/CIAS1*	Cryopyrin	Cold-induced nonpruritic urticaria, arthritis, fever and chills, leukocytosis Responds to IL-1 blockade
Muckle–Wells syndrome[*]	*AD*	*NLRP3/CIAS1*	Cryopyrin	Recurrent urticaria, sensorineural hearing loss, amyloidosis Responds to IL-1 blockade
Neonatal onset multisystem disease (NOMID)[*†]	AD	*NLRP3/CIAS1*	Cryopyrin	Neonatal onset urticaria, chronic aseptic meningitis, arthropathy and bone deformities, fever, ocular changes and hearing loss Responds to IL-1 blockade
NLRC4-activating mutations	AD	*NLRC4*	NLRC4	Fevers, macrophage activating syndrome or erythematous plaques, and arthritis
NLRP1-activating mutations	AD	*NLRP1*	NLRP1	Fevers, spiky hyperkeratoses or keratosis lichenoides chronica–like lesions, arthritis, autoimmune disorders
NLRP12-activating mutations	AD	*NLRP12*	NLRP12	Cold urticaria (FCAS2), aphthous stomatitis, abdominal discomfort, and diarrhea
Periodic fever, aphthous stomatitis, pharyngitis, and cervical adenitis (PFAPA) syndrome	Likely polygenic inheritance	Unknown	Unknown	Periodic fevers, aphthous stomatitis, pharyngitis, and cervical adenitis, malaise, headache
Pyogenic sterile arthritis, pyoderma gangrenosum, and acne (PAPA) syndrome	AD	*PSTPIP1/C2BP1*	PSTPIP1/C2BP1	Pyogenic (sterile, destructive) arthritis, pyoderma gangrenosum, acne, myositis
PASH, PAPASH, PsAPASH (see column at right for definitions)	AD	PSTPIP1 or NCSTN in some cases of PASH	PSTPIP1/C2BP1 or nicastrin	PASH combines PG, acne, hidradenitis suppurativa/HS; PAPASH either combines PAPA and PASH or adds psoriasis; PsAPASH combines psoriatic arthritis

Table 25.5 Autoinflammatory Disorders—cont'd

Disorder	Inheritance	Genetic Defect	Gene Product	Associated Features
Interferonopathies				
STING-associated vasculopathy with onset in infancy (SAVI) syndrome	AD	*TMEM173*	STING	Acral telangiectatic vasculopathy with soft-tissue loss, sometimes large pustules Fevers, adenopathy, interstitial lung fibrosis May respond to JAK inhibitor
Chronic atypical neutrophilic dermatosis with lipodystrophy and elevated temperature (CANDLE) syndrome; also called *proteasome-related autoinflammatory syndrome* (PRAAS) (see Chapter 20)	AR	*PSMB8* Less often *PSMB4, PSMB9, PSMA3*	Proteasome subunit β type	Chronic atypical neutrophilic dermatosis with lipodystrophy and elevated temperature (fever), lymphadenopathy, purpuric patches and nodules, arthralgias Same as Nakajo–Nishimura syndrome May respond to JAK inhibitor
Aicardi–Goutieres syndrome	AD, AR	7 genes; see Chapter 20	7 gene products; see Chapter 20	Pernio, arthralgias, positive antinuclear antibodies, fevers, neurologic issues vary in severity but often result in profound intellectual disability and/or encephalopathy, developmental regression, dystonia, and spasticity
Ubiquitinopathies/ relopathies				
LUBAC component deficiency	AR	*HOIL-1L, SHARPIN, HOIP*	HOIL-1L, SHARPIN, HOIP	Autoinflammation, immunodeficiency, myopathy; lymphangiectasia in HOIP deficiency
Otulipenia (otulin-related auto-inflammatory syndrome [ORAS])	AR	*OTULIN*	Otulin	Fever, diarrhea, panniculitis, arthritis, failure to thrive
Haploinsufficiency A20	AD	*TNFAIP3*	A20	Familial Behçet disease; mucosal ulcers, arthritis, vasculitis
Others				
Blau syndrome	AD	*NOD2/CARD15*	CARD15	Onset usually <5 years old Granulomatous dermatitis, uveitis, synovitis Good response to TNF inhibitors; skin eruption responds to macrolides, especially erythromycin
Majeed syndrome	AR	*LPIN2*	Lipin-2	Multifocal osteomyelitis, congenital dyserythropoietic anemia, inflammatory dermatosis Responds to IL-1 blockade
Deficiency of the IL-1 receptor antagonist (DIRA)	AR	*IL1RN*	IL-1 receptor antagonist	Fetal distress, joint swelling with periosteal inflammation, severe osteopenia, lytic bone lesions, respiratory involvement, thromboses, aphthae, pyoderma gangrenosum, pustulosis Responds to IL-1 blockade
Deficiency of the IL-36 receptor antagonist (DITRA)	AR	*IL36RN*	IL-36 receptor antagonist	Usually generalized pustules, fever and malaise May have palmoplantar pustulosis or AGEP-like disorder Nail dystrophy, arthritis, cholangitis
CARD14-mediated pustular psoriasis (see Chapter 4)	AD	*CARD14*	CARD14	Pityriasis rubra pilaris, plaque psoriasis, erythroderma with pustular psoriasis; AGEP Usually responds to ustekinumab or Th17 inhibition May respond partially to methotrexate TNF inhibition
PLAID syndrome (phospholipase Cγ2-associated antibody deficiency and immune dysregulation)	AD	*PLCG2*	Phospholipase Cγ2	Evaporative cold urticaria, acral ulcerations, granulomatous plaques, hypogammaglobulinemia, infections, sometimes allergic and autoimmune disorders
APLAID syndrome (Autoimmunity + PLAID)	AD	*PLCG2*	Phospholipase Cγ2	Neonatal-onset vesiculopustules, cutaneous granulomas, acral hemorrhagic blisters; immunodeficiency with recurrent infections; enterocolitis; arthralgias; deafness
Deficiency of adenosine deaminase 2 (DADA2)	AR	*ADA2*	Adenosine deaminase 2	Livedo reticularis to PAN-like systemic vasculopathy, early-onset fevers; vasculitis of CNS (strokes), intestine, liver, kidneys; hypogammaglobulinemia; blood cell deficiencies

AD, Autosomal dominant; *AGEP,* acute generalized exanthematous pustulosis; *AR,* autosomal recessive; *CAPS,* cryopyrin-associated periodic fever syndrome; *Ig,* immunoglobulin; *IL,* interleukin; *NLRC4,* Nod-like receptor family, caspase recruitment domain–containing 4; *NSAID,* nonsteroidal antiinflammatory drug; *PAN,* polyarteritis nodosa; *STING,* stimulator of interferon genes; *TNF,* tumor necrosis factor.

*One of the cryopyrin-associated periodic syndromes (CAPS).

+Amyloidosis is unusual in Blau, HIDS, PAPA, and PFAPA syndromes.

†Also called chronic infantile neurologic cutaneous and articular (CINCA) syndrome.

livedo, lipodystrophy, nonspecific cutaneous inflammatory eruptions, and aphthous ulcers (Table 25.6). Systemic inflammatory manifestations include fever, arthritis, uveitis, serositis (peritonitis, pleuritic), and/or meningitis. Some patients may have organ enlargement (lymphadenopathy, splenomegaly) and amyloidosis with chronic, long-term disease.

Autoinflammatory disorders reflect abnormalities in innate immunity, often with increases in proinflammatory cytokines (e.g., IL-1β, IL-17, IL-18, IL-36, TNF). These cytokines are also increased and involved in the pathogenesis of several polygenic autoinflammatory disorders, such as psoriasis, neutrophilic disorders, and granulomatous disorders, suggesting common pathogenic mechanisms. In addition, features typical of polygenic disorders (e.g., pyoderma gangrenosum, pustular psoriasis, Behçet disease, and sarcoidosis) are seen in monogenic autoinflammatory disorders, which have led to classification of these polygenic disorders as autoinflammatory. As such, many of these disorders are described in this chapter, before the presentation of the monogenic disorders. Some autoinflammatory disorders are described in other chapters (e.g., see Chapter 4 for psoriasis and chronic recurrent multifocal osteomyelitis [CRMO]; Chapters 4 and 8 for synovitis, acne, palmoplantar pustulosis and psoriasis, hyperostosis, and osteitis syndrome [SAPHO]; Chapter 20 for Sweet syndrome; and Chapter 22 for systemic juvenile idiopathic arthritis [JIA]).

Polygenic Forms of Autoinflammatory Disorders

PYODERMA GANGRENOSUM

Pyoderma gangrenosum (PG) is a severe, chronic, ulcerative autoinflammatory disorder of the skin.[214–216] Although much more commonly described in adults, 4% of cases have occurred in infants and children.[217,218] PG has an incidence of 0.26 per 100,000 per year in children 10 to 19 years of age and 0.06 per 100,000 per year in children under 10 years.[219] PG has been described in siblings.[220] It is a feature of some rare forms of inflammasomopathies.

Although PG commonly occurs in children without associated disease, it often develops in pediatric patients before, concurrently, or after onset of a systemic disorder. Most common associations in children are inflammatory bowel disease (more in Crohn's disease—see Crohn's Disease section—than in ulcerative colitis), but immunodeficiency (especially HIV infection, leukocyte adhesion defect,[221,222] SCID,[223] CVID,[224] chronic granulomatous disease, hyper-IgE syndrome,[225] and selective IgA deficiency),[226] hematologic disorders (especially leukemia),[227,228] Takayasu disease with or without airway or pulmonary disease,[229–231] and rheumatic disorders (especially JIA, systemic lupus erythematosus, Henoch–Schönlein purpura, and in association with antiphospholipid antibodies)[232,233] have all been reported. PG can also be seen in patients with PAPA (see Fig. 25.33, *B*), PASH, PAPASH, and PsAPASH syndromes (see The Inflammasomopathies section); chronic recurrent multifocal osteomyelitis[234]; Majeed syndrome[235]; and SAPHO syndrome.[236] PG tends to occur during adolescence in most pediatric patients with inflammatory bowel disease and inflammasomopathies. In children with onset during infancy, Takayasu disease is the most common association and may occur years after the onset of PG. PG can occur as a drug reaction, particularly with use of TNF inhibitors,[237,238] despite their use as therapy (see Chapter 4 for the paradoxical occurrence of psoriasis-like lesions with the use of TNF inhibitors); in adults, PG has been associated with pegfilgrastim (granulocyte-stimulating factor) and gefitinib (epidermal growth factor [EGF] receptor inhibitor).[239] PG-like ulcerations have been described as well in granulomatosis with polyangiitis,[240] a systemic, necrotizing, small vessel vasculitis associated with circulating antineutrophil cytoplasmic antibodies (ANCAs).

The diagnosis is considered based on clinical features. PG is characterized by a painful sloughing ulceration with purulent or vegetative base and an elevated dusky blue or reddish purple undermined border surrounded by a rim of inflammation (Figs. 25.17 and 25.18).[241] The lesion usually begins as a tender papulopustule or erythematous nodule that undergoes necrosis and ulcerates. Ulcer extension is variable

Table 25.6 Skin Manifestations of Hereditary Autoinflammatory Disorders

Mucocutaneous Feature	Autoinflammatory Disorder/Gene
Urticaria	FMF/*MEFV* NOMID/CINCA (CAPS)/*NLRP3* Muckle-Wells (CAPS)/*NLRP3* Mevalonate kinase disorders/*MVK* TRAPS/*TNFRSF1A*
Cold urticaria	FCAS/*NLRP3* FCAS2 (NLRP12-AD)/*NLRP12* PLAID and APLAID/*PLCG2*
Pustulosis, papulosquamous features (psoriasis- or PRP-like)	DIRA/*IL1RN* DITRA/*IL36RN* CAMPS/*CARD14* PAPASH syndrome/*PSTPIP1*
Neutrophilic dermatosis or vasculitis	FMF/*MEFV* NOMID/CINCA (CAPS) *NLRP3* Familial Behçet syndrome/*TNFAIP3* PAPA syndrome/*PSTPIP1* SAVI syndrome/*TMEM173* CANDLE (PRAAS)/*PSMB8* ORAS syndrome/*OTULIN* Majeed syndrome/*LPIN2* ADA2 deficiency/*ADA2* Blau syndrome/*NOD2*
Macrophage activation syndrome	NLRC4-MAS/*NLRC4*
Panniculitis	CANDLE (PRAAS)/*PSMB8* ORAS syndrome/*OTULIN* Blau syndrome/*NOD2*
Acne, hidradenitis suppurativa, sterile abscesses, and/or pyoderma gangrenosum	PAPA, PASH, PAPASH, PsAPASH syndromes/*PSTPIP1*
Eczematous	PLAID and APLAID/*PLCG2*
Granulomatous	Blau syndrome/*NOD2* PLAID and APLAID/*PLCG2* ADA2 deficiency/*ADA2*
Erysipelas-like eruption	FMF/*MEFV*
Livedo	Aicardi–Goutieres/many genes (Chapter 20) SAVI syndrome/*TMEM173* ADA2 deficiency/*ADA2*
Lipodystrophy	CANDLE/PRAAS/*PSMB8* ORAS syndrome/*OTULIN*
Aphthous stomatitis	Familial Behçet/*TNFAIP3* FCAS2 (NLRP12-AD)/*NLRP12* Majeed syndrome/*LPIN2* PAPA-like/*PSTPIP1* PFAPA/polygenic

ADA2, Adenosine deaminase 2; *APLAID*, autoinflammation and PLCγ2-associated antibody deficiency and immune dysregulation; *CAMPS*, CARD14-mediated pustular psoriasis or CARD14-associated psoriasis; *CANDLE*, chronic atypical neutrophilic dermatosis with lipodystrophy and elevated temperature syndrome; *CAPS*, cryopyrin-associated periodic fever syndrome (also called *NLPR3-associated autoinflammatory disease* [NLRP3-AID]); *CINCA*, chronic infantile neurologic cutaneous and articular; *DIRA*, deficiency of the IL-1 receptor antagonist; *DITRA*, deficiency of the IL-36 receptor antagonist; *FCAS*, familial cold autoinflammatory syndrome; *FMF*, familial Mediterranean fever; *MVK*, mevalonate kinase; *NLRC4-MAS*, NLRC4-associated macrophage activation syndrome; *NOMID*, neonatal-onset multisystemic inflammatory disease; *ORAS*, otulin-related autoinflammatory syndrome; *PAPA*, pyogenic arthritis, pyoderma gangrenosum, and acne; *PASH*, pyoderma gangrenosum, acne, and suppurative hidradenitis; PAPASH, psoriasis (or arthritis) + PASH; *PsAPASH*, psoriatic arthritis + PASH; PFAPA, periodic fever, aphthous stomatitis, pharyngitis, and adenitis; *PLAID*, PLCγ2-associated antibody deficiency and immune dysregulation; *PRAAS*, proteasome-related autoinflammatory syndrome; *PRP*, pityriasis rubra pilaris; *SAVI*, STING-associated vasculopathy with onset in infancy; *TRAPS*, TNF receptor–associated periodic syndrome.

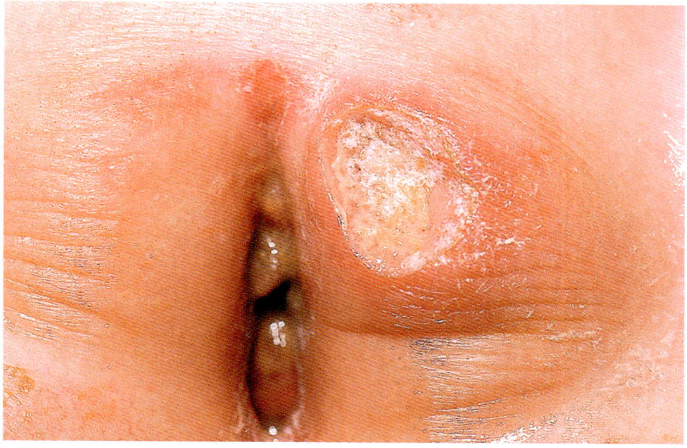

Fig. 25.17 Pyoderma gangrenosum. Painful ulcer on the vulva of a girl with Crohn's disease.

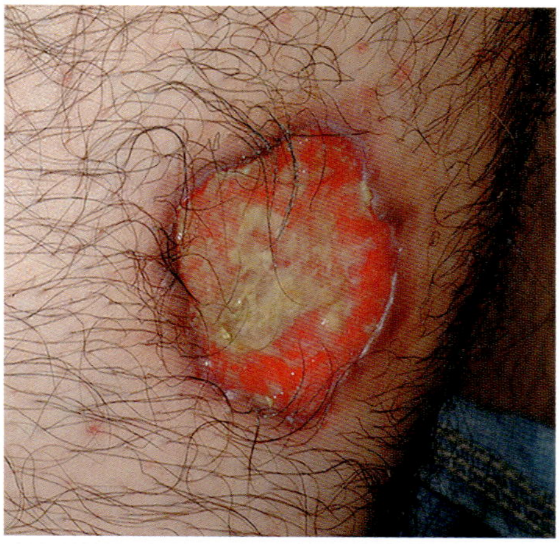

Fig. 25.18 Pyoderma gangrenosum. Painful leg ulceration with an inflamed, undermined border. Note the pustule distal to the ulceration, often the earliest sign of a new site of involvement. The most common underlying condition in affected children is inflammatory bowel disease, although no underlying abnormality may be discovered.

but can be rapid, with rates of up to 1 cm in a day. Cultures yield no organisms. During healing, the border collapses and epithelial projections extend into the ulcer (*Gulliver sign*). The ulceration heals with cribriform scarring (Fig. 25.19). Pathergy, the development of lesions at sites of minor trauma due to release of proinflammatory cytokines and chemokines that recruit and activate neutrophils, occurs in 20% of patients with PG and may be more common in childhood cases. PG developed at multiple sites of physical abuse in one child.[242] Pathergy is also thought to contribute to the tendency for PG to occur around peristomal sites[243,244] in children with associated inflammatory bowel disease, as well as in postoperative PG.[245,246] Consensus-based diagnostic criteria have recently been described that require the major criterion of biopsy of the ulcer edge (ideally when not on immunosuppressive medication or when flared) showing neutrophilic infiltration, as well as having at least four of eight minor criteria.[247] These include exclusion of infection; pathergy; history of inflammatory bowel disease or inflammatory arthritis; history of papule, pustule, or vesicle ulcerating within 4 days of appearing; peripheral erythema, undermined border, and tenderness at ulceration site; multiple ulcerations, at least one on an anterior lower leg; cribriform or "wrinkled paper" scar(s) at healed ulcer sites; and decreased ulcer size within 1 month of initiating immunosuppressive medication(s). Having many of these minor criteria may allow diagnosis without biopsy in children. If a biopsy is performed, however, an elliptic specimen of a well-developed edge (not a fresh area of extension) that includes the margin and ulcer

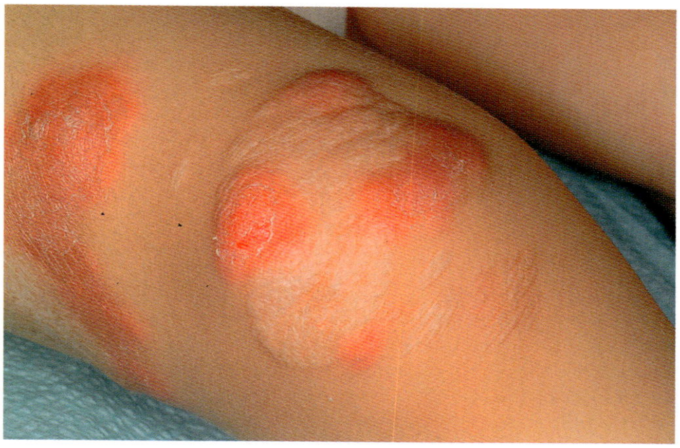

Fig. 25.19 Pyoderma gangrenosum. Partial response to treatment with cyclosporine. Note the persistent inflammation and evidence of healing ulcerations with residual cribriform scarring. The pyoderma gangrenosum healed fully and remained quiescent while the child was given etanercept, but this young boy developed Takayasu disease several years after onset of the pyoderma gangrenosum despite ongoing inhibition of TNF-α activity.

floor is recommended; sections show massive infiltration with neutrophils, as well as hemorrhage and vessel necrosis.

Lesions in older children and adolescents (as in adults) are most often found on the lower extremities (especially the anterior tibial surface) but can be seen anywhere on the body, including mucosal and peristomal sites.[248] In one pediatric study, lesions were found as commonly on the trunk as on the lower extremities (both 77%).[215] The head, airway, and anogenital areas are more common sites of involvement in neonates, infants, and younger children.[249–252] Pustular, bullous, vegetative, and superficial[253,254] variants have been described. The bullous form[255] may be difficult to distinguish from bullous Sweet syndrome (see Chapter 20). Biopsy findings are nonspecific, but special stains and cultures of biopsy specimens may help distinguish PG from other disorders, including vasculitis and infectious causes of ulceration.

Affected individuals may experience fever, malaise, myalgias, and arthralgias that range from monoarthritis to destructive polyarthritis. Pulmonary[256] and splenic lesions have also been described.[257]

Treatment of PG involves use of systemic and topical antiinflammatory medications to promote wound healing and decrease pain, as well as a vigorous attempt to control the underlying disease. Debridement and other mechanical trauma may worsen the ulcerations by increasing pathergy and should be avoided. Systemic corticosteroids are usually the initial drug of choice. Cyclosporine or systemic tacrolimus,[258] TNF-α inhibitors (etanercept, adalimumab,[259] infliximab),[260–266] ustekinumab,[267] IL-1β/IL-1 receptor inhibitors (canakinumab and anakinra), dapsone, clofazimine, MMF, and IVIG[268,269] have been used successfully as steroid-sparing agents. Although IL-17 inhibitors may be useful for treating PG, some patients have developed PG during IL-17 inhibitor therapy.[270,271] Topical tacrolimus ointment applied a few times daily has improved ulcer healing[272]; intralesional steroid injections may be appropriate for adolescents. Stoma closure and resection of affected bowel in patients with inflammatory bowel disease have been advocated for peristomal involvement.[243]

Amicrobial Pustulosis of the Folds

Although occurring primarily in adults, amicrobial pustulosis of the folds (APF) has been described in children,[273] especially in the second decade of life. Three major criteria are required to make this diagnosis: (1) pustulosis involving one or more major folds, one or more minor folds (e.g., perinasal, retroauricular, and external auditory canals), and the anogenital area; (2) histologic pattern consisting of intraepidermal spongiform pustules and a mainly neutrophilic dermal infiltrate; and (3) negative culture from an unopened pustule. One additional minor criterion is required for diagnosis from among the following: (1) association with one or more autoimmune or autoinflammatory disorders, (2) positive ANAs at a titer of 1/160 or higher, or (3) presence of one or more serum autoantibodies. Pustules tend to be symmetrically in the folds and often involve the scalp and nails. APF has a chronic, relapsing course and typically responds to corticosteroids. However, dapsone, cyclosporine, and TNF inhibition has been used effectively as well. The condition has been associated with several autoimmune disorders and inflammatory bowel disease, including in patients treated with anti-TNF agents, as a paradoxical reaction.

Behçet Disease

Behçet disease is a chronic multisystemic autoinflammatory disorder characterized by recurrent oral and genital ulcerations and inflammatory disease of the eye.[274–277] Overall, the prevalence globally is 10.3 per 100,000 persons,[278] with the highest prevalence rates in Turkey. Although even neonatal onset without maternal Behçet disease has been noted,[279] Behçet disease usually begins in patients between 10 and 45 years of age, with approximately 17% of cases beginning before 17 years of age.[280] Neonatal Behçet disease usually occurs in infants born to mothers with the disease and generally disappears spontaneously by the time the infants reach the age of 6 months. Characterized by aphthous stomatitis and skin lesions, affected neonates rarely have severe, life-threatening complications.[281,282]

Although most studies have suggested that Behçet disease has a predilection for males,[283] including in pediatric patients, an international registry enrolled equal numbers of boys and girls.[284] Only 2% to 5% of cases are in children.[285] In general, the disease is less severe and more delayed in its full manifestation in pediatric patients.[286]

Behçet disease is thought to be an autoinflammatory disorder influenced by genetics and environment, with Th1/Th17 skewing and decreased Treg cells. Most patients carry HLA-B*5 and particularly its subset Bw51 alleles, the strongest-known risk factor.[287,288] Some 15% to 45% of children have an affected family member, in contrast to 8% of adults.[280,289] Dominantly inherited Behçet disease is now recognized to result from haploinsufficiency of A20, encoded by *TNFAIP3* (see the A20 Haploinsufficiency section). Loss-of-function mutations lead to activation of the NF-κB pathway.

Cutaneous and oral ulcerations are the most common clinical features of pediatric Behçet disease.[289–291] Oral lesions, noted at some point in 95% of affected children, are the initial manifestation in 83% of pediatric patients[290] and occur approximately 8 years before other signs.[292] The ulcerations begin as erythema and within 1 to 2 days become superficial erosions that range from smaller ulcerations, indistinguishable from aphthous stomatitis, to deeply punched-out necrotic ulcers on the lips, buccal mucosa (Fig. 25.20), tongue (Fig. 25.21), and, less commonly, the gingivae. They have regular sharp edges and vary from a few millimeters to a centimeter in diameter. Minor aphthae have a diameter of less than 1 cm, resolve in 7 to 10 days, do not scar, and are most common, whereas major aphthae are larger, deep, more painful, and tend to scar. Sometimes aphthae are grouped (herpetiform aphthae). The ulcer base is covered with a yellowish-gray exudate, and the margin is surrounded by a red halo. Oral lesions recur at intervals varying from weeks to months; by definition, aphthae must recur at least three times yearly. Features of Behçet disease and relapsing polychondritis have also been described as mouth and genital ulcers with inflamed cartilage (MAGIC) syndrome.

Genital ulcerations are seen in 34% to 60% of children with Behçet disease and occur more often in girls than in boys. They are found on the vulva and vagina of females (Fig. 25.22) and the scrotum or base of the penis in males. They are similar in appearance to the oral ulcerations but less painful and may be overlooked. Perianal ulcerations are less common but have been noted more often in children than in adults (up to 30%). Genital ulcerations are usually deeper than oral ulcerations (Fig. 25.23) and may scar. As with oral ulcerations, they remit in 1 to 2 weeks and tend to recur. Epididymo-orchitis has also been described, characterized as scrotal pain and swelling.[293]

Other cutaneous lesions of Behçet disease present a varied picture. Seen in approximately 80% of affected children, they consist of folliculitis, pustules, pyoderma, acneiform lesions, furuncles, abscesses, ulcerations, erythema nodosum–like lesions, and palpable purpura (Fig. 25.24). Pathergy (the formation of an ulceration at an area of trauma, skin prick, or venipuncture) is a common feature.

Ocular lesions are seen in approximately 50% of boys but only 15% to 20% of affected girls. They usually occur after 10 years of age, are

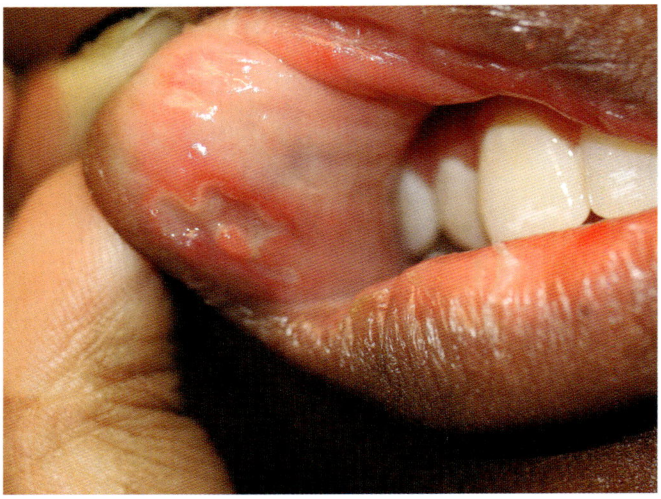

Fig. 25.20 Behçet disease. Large, painful ulceration on the buccal mucosa.

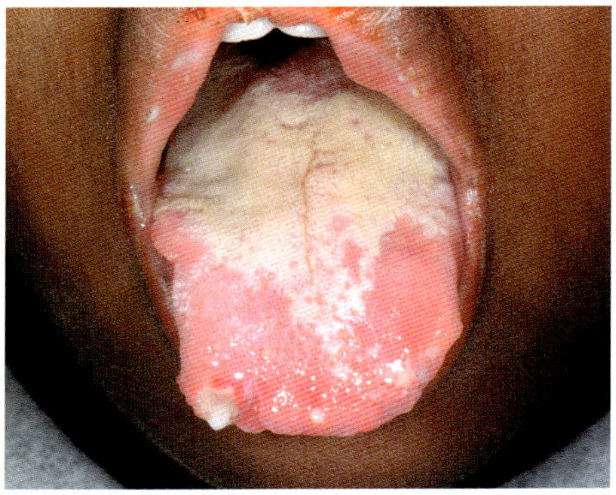

Fig. 25.21 Behçet disease. Major and minor aphthae on the tongue. Note the scalloping of the tongue border from past scarring lesions.

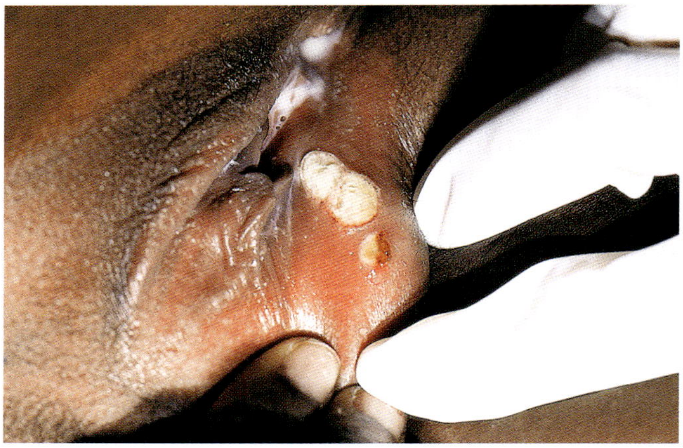

Fig. 25.22 Behçet disease. Vulvar ulcerations.

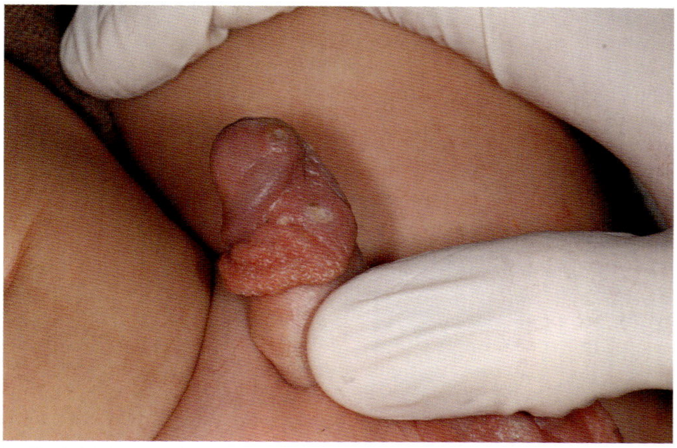

Fig. 25.23 Behçet disease. Genital region ulcers on the glans penis and foreskin in a boy with a positive family history of Behçet disease and HLA-B51 positivity.

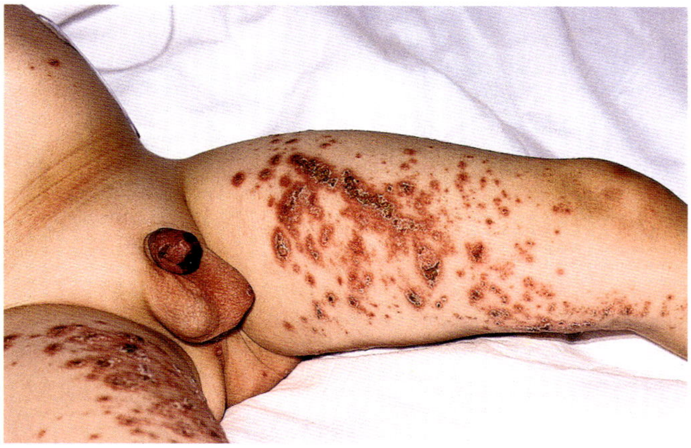

Fig. 25.24 Behçet disease. Palpable purpura on the inner thighs and glans penis of this boy with Behçet disease. Superficial ulcerations were also noted on the penile shaft. Biopsy of affected areas showed leukocytoclastic vasculitis.

Box 25.4 International Criteria for Behçet Disease in Adult vs. Pediatric Patients

CRITERION	ADULT†	PEDIATRIC*
Recurrent oral aphthous stomatitis (≥3 attacks/year)	2 points	1 point
Genital ulcers (typically with residual scarring)	2 points	1 point
Other skin involvement (acneiform lesions, necrotic folliculitis, erythema nodosum)	1 point	1 point
Ocular manifestations (anterior or posterior uveitis, retinal vasculitis)	2 points	1 point
Neurologic signs (beyond isolated headaches)	1 point	1 point
Vascular signs (venous thrombosis, arterial thrombosis, arterial aneurysm)	1 point	1 point
Positive pathergy test	1 point	0 points

†≥4 points are required for diagnosis of adult Behçet disease. Pathergy testing is optional, but if positive adds 1 point toward the score.
*≥3 points are required to classify as pediatric Behçet disease.

less common than in adults, and are associated with a worse prognosis. Conjunctivitis and photophobia may be early ocular findings, but bilateral panuveitis is the most common manifestation (more than 80% of children with eye findings)[294]; posterior uveitis is found more often than anterior uveitis. Retinal vasculitis and retinitis occur in the majority of children with ocular features, and cataracts, maculopathy, and optic atrophy have been described.

Fever and constitutional symptoms are variable. Musculoskeletal complaints, especially arthralgia and arthritis, are found in up to 75% of affected children. Gastrointestinal complaints are more common in children than in adults[295] and may warrant endoscopic evaluation, especially in children under 10 years of age. They range from vague abdominal pain (up to 50%) and anorexia to diarrhea and hemorrhagic colitis. Just as in inflammatory bowel disease, fecal calprotectin has been found to be a noninvasive marker for intestinal involvement.[296] Central nervous system (CNS) involvement is often the most severe prognostic feature of this disorder.[297] Seen in 20% to 50% of patients, it often manifests as headache and most commonly reflects cerebral venous sinus thrombosis.[283,298] Arterial or venous thrombosis can also affect the lower extremities and can be recurrent.[299–301] Renal involvement, an uncommon complication, may be seen, with a spectrum ranging from asymptomatic abnormalities detected on urinalysis to a rapidly progressive glomerulonephritis and nephrosis. Other unusual findings in children include pericarditis, orchitis, and epididymitis.

The diagnosis of Behçet disease is based on the constellation of typical clinical manifestations. Diagnosis in a patient with the full triad of oral and genital ulcers and ocular inflammation is not difficult, but many show partial manifestations. Criteria to diagnose Behçet disease include the International Study Group (ISG),[302] the International Criteria for Behçet Disease (ICBD),[303] and the Paediatric Behçet's Disease (pediatric specific; PEDBD)[304] criteria. ISG criteria, established in 1990, had low sensitivity and required the presence of oral aphthae at least three times yearly, despite the fact that not all patients met this criterion. ISG criteria diagnosed only 29% to 53% of the pediatric Behçet disease patients,[275,305] whereas the ICBD criteria have been met in 80%. The ICBD were proposed in 2014 for adults,[303] and the PEDBD represent a 2015 adaptation for pediatric patients (Box 25.4). In a cohort of Turkish and Israeli children, PEDBD criteria were 73.5% sensitive and 98.9% specific.[305] However, the PEDBD criteria only classified 46% and 26% of affected children from Italy and the UK, respectively. This modification for pediatric patients[304,306] eliminated potential points for pathergy and gave equal weight to all clinical signs, including giving the cutaneous (particularly folliculitis, acneiform lesions, and erythema nodosum), neurologic, and vascular signs vs. the oral and genital ulcerations. Although pathergy is common, a negative pathergy test does not rule out the diagnosis. Pathergy can also be a feature of pediatric PG, leukemia, and bowel bypass syndrome (see Chapter 20). Biopsy is usually not helpful, but having HLA-B51 positivity can be useful supporting evidence of the diagnosis.

Treatment of the aphthous ulcers with potent topical or intralesional corticosteroids, topical application of tacrolimus, oral rinses with elixir of diphenhydramine, or application of 2% viscous lidocaine can give symptomatic relief. For mucocutaneous ulcerations, colchicine is often helpful. Therapy is begun with a dosage of 0.6 mg twice daily for the first week. If the patient has no nausea, vomiting, or diarrhea, the dosage can be increased to three times a day, but colchicine is poorly tolerated by pediatric patients. Dapsone can also be helpful, especially in children with recurrent oral ulcerations. In severe cases, corticosteroids, alone or in combination with immunosuppressive agents such as methotrexate and azathioprine, are usually successful and are still the recommendation for management of thromboses.[307] However, the demonstrated activation of inflammatory cytokines TNF-α, IL-1β, and IL-6 has led to new therapeutic approaches. Inhibitors of TNF,[308–310] IL-1[311] (anakinra, canakinumab), IL-6 (tocilizumab),[312] and IL-12/IL-23 (ustekinumab),[313] as well as rituximab, have been used successfully.[314] Thalidomide 50 to 100 mg once weekly to once daily has also led to improvement, but its use is limited by constipation, fatigue, and peripheral neuropathy, which may be irreversible, and it is now rarely used. The overall mortality rate of Behçet disease in children is 3%; death usually results from large-vessel vasculopathy (aneurysm, thrombosis), intestinal perforation, CNS involvement, or as a complication of therapy.

Orofacial Granulomatosis

Orofacial granulomatosis (OFG; also called *cheilitis granulomatosa* or *granulomatous cheilitis*) (Fig. 25.25) is characterized by face and lip swelling (macrocheilitis). It is the most common manifestation (93% with facial swelling and 66% with lip swelling) of Melkersson–Rosenthal syndrome, which also includes recurrent facial paralysis (30%) and a furrowed or "scrotal" tongue (lingua plicata, 30%) (Fig. 25.26).[315,316] No prodrome warns of attacks, and patients experience no associated erythema, pain, or pruritus. The disorder is more prevalent in males and has a mean age of onset of 11 years.[317] The swelling can increase the size of the lip by twofold to threefold, leading to chapping from exposure of the mucosa. Both lips may be involved, and the swelling may be bilateral or unilateral. In addition to the swelling of the lips and other oral mucosal structures, the eyelids may be swollen. The attacks usually disappear within days or weeks but commonly tend to persist after several recurrences. Facial palsy usually occurs on the side of the facial swelling and tends to resolve spontaneously.[318]

The cause is unknown. Attacks usually start during adolescence with paralysis of a facial nerve; repeated severe headaches; edema of the circumoral tissue of the upper lip or cheeks; and occasionally edema of the gingivae, sublingual area, and lower lip. The edema is usually asymmetric, but the whole face may be involved. Associated signs include hyperhidrosis, loss of taste, and visual impairment. Biopsy specimens show noncaseating granulomas in an edematous stroma that may be indistinguishable from the granulomas of Crohn's disease,[319] and the relationship between Crohn's disease and OFG remains controversial. In one systematic review, gastrointestinal signs were present in 26% at the time of OFG diagnosis, 40% of children were diagnosed with Crohn's disease, and OFG preceded signs of Crohn's disease in more than 50%.[317] Concomitant perianal disease and a family history of Crohn's disease are associated with a higher risk of Crohn's disease.

Intralesional injections of triamcinolone or systemic administration of corticosteroids can control the facial and mucosal swelling; intermittent application of topical clobetasol gel may also lead to improvement. Minocycline (or macrolides in younger children), with or without corticosteroids, has been helpful.[320,321] Other therapies include thalidomide, dapsone, azathioprine, clofazimine, and TNF-α inhibitors, particularly infliximab.[322–324]

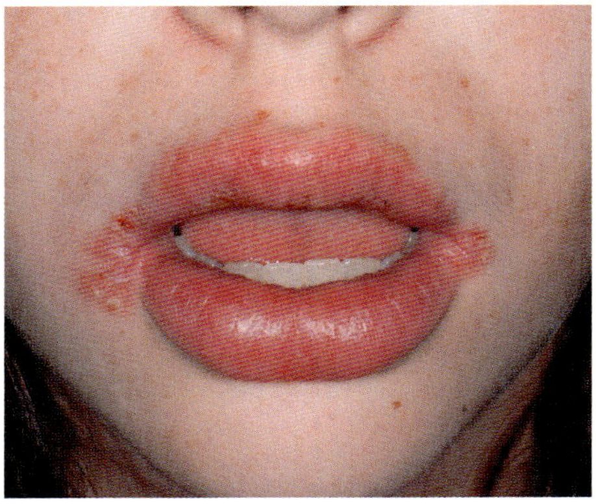

Fig. 25.25 Orofacial granulomatosis. Granulomatous infiltration limited to the lip(s) is called *cheilitis granulomatosa*.

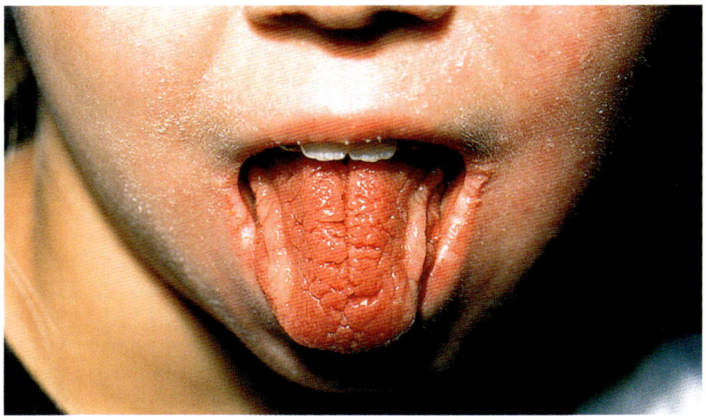

Fig. 25.26 Orofacial granulomatosis as part of Melkersson–Rosenthal syndrome. Scrotal tongue.

Crohn's Disease

Crohn's disease is a granulomatous disorder of the intestinal tract that usually has its onset between 15 and 30 years of age but has been described in young children.[325–327] It is more prevalent than ulcerative colitis in children and has a more aggressive and rapidly progressive disease compared with adult onset. Disease in children younger than 6 years tends to be more aggressive than disease in older children and adolescents. Approximately[328] one-third of pediatric patients have small intestinal disease, one-third have ileocolitis, and one-third have colitis. Total colitis is more common than segmental or isolated proctitis.[326] Growth failure,[329,330] delayed pubertal development, and osteopenia[331] are important complications of Crohn's disease.

The pathogenesis of Crohn's disease is complex. The disorder is thought to occur in genetically predisposed individuals when the intestinal mucosal immune function is altered by exogenous agents, such as infectious organisms, or host factors, such as stress or disruption of intestinal barrier function or vascular supply.[332] The disorder occurs twofold to fourfold more often in Ashkenazi Jews and has been linked to certain HLA alleles (DR3, DQ2, DR103), as well as sequence variants in *NOD2/CARD15*. The CARD15 protein senses bacterial peptidoglycan and plays a central role in the NF-κB activation response to microbial products.[333,334] Granulomatous colitis is also a feature of a subset of individuals with Hermansky–Pudlak syndrome (see Chapter 11).[335]

Skin manifestations may occur before, concomitantly, or after other evidence of disease.[336–338] Perianal skin tags are found in 75% to 80% of patients with Crohn's disease (Fig. 25.27) and occur before gastrointestinal manifestations in 25% of patients. Other skin and mucosal findings are noted in 22% to 44% of patients (Table 25.7) and occur more often in patients with colonic vs. small intestinal disease. Erythema nodosum (see Chapter 20) occurs in up to 15% of patients with Crohn's disease and has been shown to correlate with the presence of arthritis.[339] PG[340] (see Fig. 25.17) occasionally precedes the development of bowel symptoms and has a course unrelated to the activity of the bowel disease. Oral aphthous ulcers have been described in greater than 50% of pediatric patients with Crohn's disease.[341] Pyostomatitis vegetans—erythematous pustular lesions associated with erosions and ulcerations—is considered a marker for inflammatory bowel disease. Leukocytoclastic vasculitis occasionally occurs (Fig. 25.28). Cutaneous changes related to nutritional deficits (particularly acrodermatitis enteropathica caused by zinc deficiency) can occur as well.

Cobblestoning of the buccal mucosa[326] is seen in up to 20% of affected individuals. Painless swelling of the lips, resembling OFG, may be the initial presentation of Crohn's disease in a child or adolescent[342] and may precede the gastrointestinal symptoms by several years (Fig. 25.29).[343–347] Similarly, the vulva, scrotum, and penis may show erythema, swelling, and fissuring.[348–352] Perianal lesions may extend onto the adjacent perineum, abdomen, or buttocks with

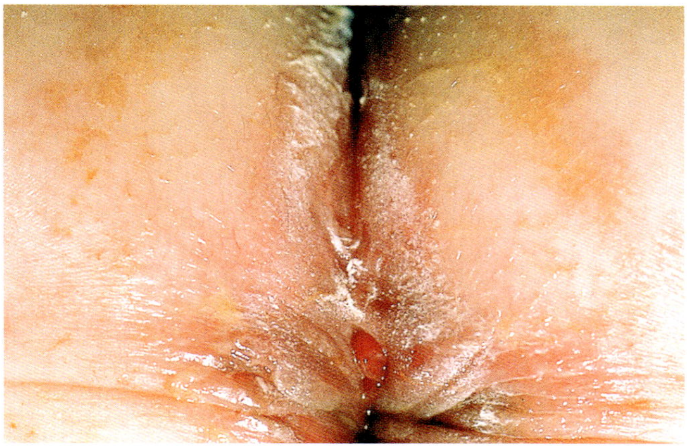

Fig. 25.27 Crohn's disease. Perianal tags are an early manifestation and seen in most affected children.

Table 25.7 Mucocutaneous Manifestations of Crohn's Disease

	Specific	Nonspecific
Cutaneous	Extraintestinal cutaneous Crohn's disease	Erythema nodosum Pyoderma gangrenosum Polyarteritis nodosa Erythema multiforme Leukocytoclastic vasculitis Sweet syndrome Epidermolysis bullosa acquisita
Anogenital	Perianal fissures and tags Sinus tracts Labial or scrotal edema Vulvoperineal Crohn's disease	
Oral	Orofacial granulomatosis Cobblestoning Mucosal tags	Aphthous stomatitis Angular cheilitis Pyostomatitis vegetans

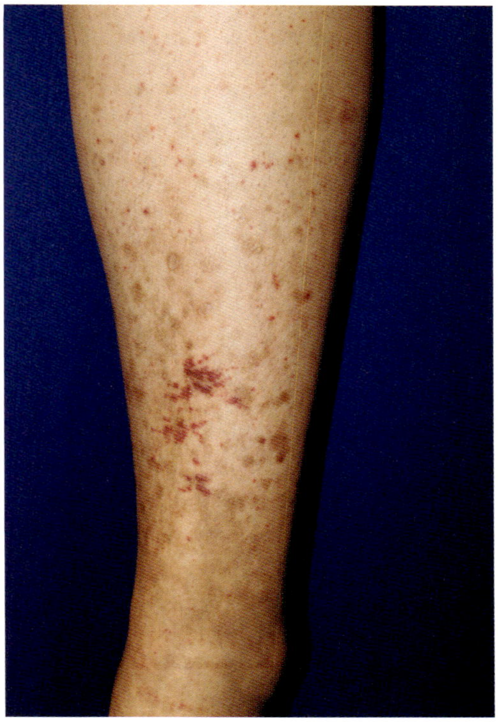

Fig. 25.28 Crohn's disease. Associated leukocytoclastic vasculitis on the legs.

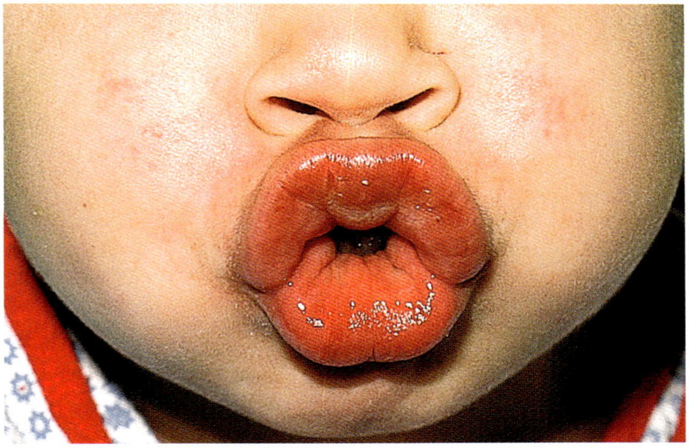

Fig. 25.29 Crohn's disease. Note the infiltration of the lips, which showed noncaseating granulomas in biopsy sections.

fissures. Sinus tracts are common.[353,354] Nasal perforation[355] and chronic granulomatous otitis externa[356] have been described. Abdominal surgical sites may also be loci for cutaneous involvement. Biopsy provides the clue to diagnosis, although the noncaseating granulomas resemble those of Melkersson–Rosenthal/cheilitis granulomatosa and sarcoidosis. Special stains (periodic acid–Schiff, Ziehl–Nielsen, and Gram) are important to consider infectious causes of granulomas. These granulomatous lesions of the lips and anogenital area are considered "contiguous" Crohn's disease because of their proximity to the gastrointestinal tract. Granulomatous lesions elsewhere are considered extraintestinal (sometimes called *metastatic*) cutaneous Crohn's disease.[357,358] These lesions typically are dusky red, swollen/indurated plaques, most commonly found on the genital region of children, lower extremities, abdomen, or trunk; lesions less commonly show no erythema or are ulcerating.[359]

Barium contrast studies are particularly important for investigating small bowel disease, but endoscopy and colonoscopy are important tools for upper and lower bowel disease, respectively. Exclusive enteral nutrition has been advocated by many experts as first-line therapy. Otherwise, initial treatment involves administration of systemic corticosteroids (including budesonide) and aminosalicylates, with the early addition of azathioprine or 6-mercaptopurine as steroid-sparing alternatives for maintenance therapy.[360] TNF-α inhibitors (especially infliximab and adalimumab) are very helpful as well and reduce the need for surgery.[361–365] However, up to 40% do not respond to induction with TNF inhibitors, and therapy with ustekinumab (anti-IL-12/IL-23) or vedolizumab (anti-$\alpha_4\beta_7$ integrin) is a newer approach.[366] Calprotectin is a commonly used marker of disease activity and is most useful for monitoring large intestinal disease.[367]

The development of psoriasiform dermatitis is common in patients with Crohn's disease treated with TNF-α inhibitors and often manifests in the periorificial and genital areas, scalp, hands, and feet[368–370] (see Chapter 4; Fig. 4.34). The mechanism for the common occurrence of psoriasiform dermatitis is unclear but has been linked to IL-23 receptor polymorphism.[371] Azathioprine-induced Sweet syndrome has also been described in association with Crohn's disease.[372] Oral metronidazole has been used for extraintestinal cutaneous Crohn's disease[373,374]; intralesional or topical applications of potent topical corticosteroids or tacrolimus[375] have helped clear the ulcerations of PG. Colectomy in Crohn's disease does not prevent recurrence (which is common) and should be used selectively.[376,377]

Sarcoidosis

Sarcoidosis is a systemic granulomatous disorder of unknown etiology with CD4+ Th1 cell and monocyte activation, leading to hypergammaglobulinemia, sarcoidal granulomas (predominantly affecting the lungs, eyes, skin, and reticuloendothelial system), and ultimately fibrosis. The condition presents most often in adults between the ages of 20 and 40 years. In pediatric patients, it is most commonly seen in adolescents between 9 and 15 years of age, in which manifestations resemble those of adult patients.[378] In a US series of pediatric sarcoidosis, 72% to 81% of older children were Black (vs. only 7% to 28% of young children).[379]

There is no single reliable test for sarcoidosis. Because the clinical picture may be mimicked by other diseases, histologic confirmation is advisable. In typical lesions, the characteristic histopathologic finding consists of islands of large, pale-staining epithelioid cells containing few, if any, giant cells intermingled with histiocytes and lymphocytes. Sarcoidosis must also be distinguished from infectious granulomatous conditions, particularly mycobacterial and fungal infections, but cultures and special stains of biopsy sections are negative. Cutaneous anergy is common, but children should be tested for reactivity to tuberculin.

SARCOIDOSIS IN OLDER CHILDREN AND ADOLESCENTS

Adolescents and older children may have fever and weight loss.[380] Cutaneous involvement occurs in 15% to 25% of pediatric patients and in older children.[381] Several specific and nonspecific lesions have been described, although no lesion is pathognomonic.[382] Most typical are yellow-brown to red, flat-topped papules, infiltrated plaques, and nodules that show an apple-jelly color when diascopy (pressure applied with a glass slide) is performed, a characteristic sign of granulomas. Scaling is sometimes apparent as well. These granulomatous lesions are most commonly localized to the face, and an annular configuration of lesions around the nares, lips, and eyelids is highly characteristic, although any site, including the mucosae,[383] palms, and soles, may be involved. Lesions often occur in areas of trauma or scarification. Other cutaneous manifestations of sarcoidosis include subcutaneous, often painful, nodules (Darier–Roussy sarcoidosis), ichthyosis (ichthyosiform sarcoidosis, usually most prominent on the lower extremities), generalized erythroderma with scaling, livedo[384] reticularis–like changes, and hypopigmentation. More than 20% of affected children have erythema nodosum (see Chapter 20), which often manifests at onset and is a good prognostic sign[379] that usually portends clearance of the adenopathy. The combination of erythema nodosum, bilateral hilar adenopathy, uveitis, and fever has been called *Löfgren syndrome*. Lupus pernio is a variant of sarcoidosis in which soft, infiltrated, violaceous plaques are located on the nose; cheeks; ears; forehead; and the dorsal aspects of the hands, fingers, and toes (Fig. 25.30). This variant can cause significant scarring and deformity and is a marker for upper respiratory involvement, including the larynx.

The lung is the most commonly involved site in older children and adolescents, as in adults. A dry, hacking cough is the most common complaint, but patients may have dyspnea and develop parenchymal lung disease. Lymphadenopathy may be generalized but typically involves the hilar nodes and is symmetric. More than 90% show an abnormal chest X-ray at onset. Clinical evidence of liver involvement is detected in approximately one-third of patients, although more than half show granulomas when the liver is biopsied. Splenic enlargement has been associated with extensive visceral fibrosis and a poor prognosis. Granulomatous infiltration of the heart may lead to arrhythmias and infiltration of the lung to congestive heart failure.

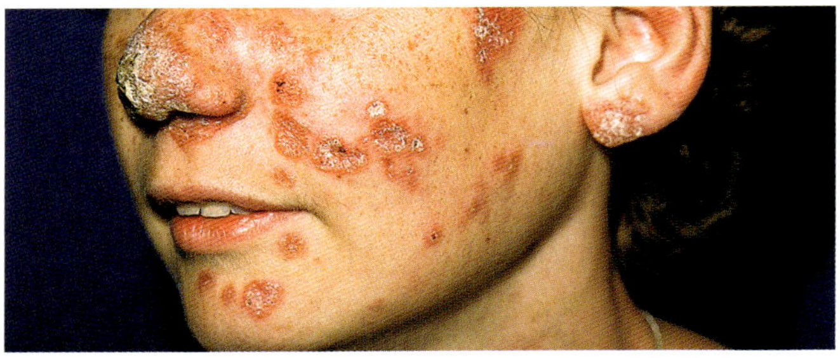

Fig. 25.30 Sarcoidosis. The lupus pernio form of sarcoidosis shows infiltrated violaceous plaques on the nose, cheeks, and ears. This girl had hoarseness due to her laryngeal involvement with sarcoidosis and was left with severe scarring after treatment.

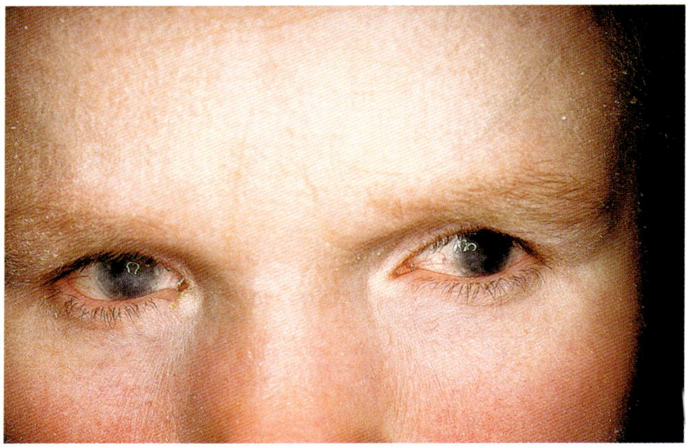

Fig. 25.31 Sarcoidosis. Uveitis in a teenager with sarcoidosis since early childhood. She had ichthyosiform scaling overlying granulomatous papules and arthritis.

Some patients with renal involvement will show hypercalciuria, renal stones, and ultimately renal failure from excessive production of 1,25-dihydroxyvitamin D_3, with or without hypercalcemia[385]; calciphylaxis has also been reported in association with end-stage renal disease, manifesting as painful violaceous plaques, retiform purpura, or subcutaneous nodules, which can progress to nonhealing ulcers and cutaneous gangrene.[386]

Although more common in young children, arthritis is a component of sarcoidosis in older children and can be the presenting feature in more than 10%. Overall, up to 74% of pediatric patients have eye involvement, particularly anterior segment uveitis (Fig. 25.31). Conjunctival granulomas are often seen on biopsy, and lacrimal gland inflammation is not uncommon. Chorioretinitis, keratitis, and glaucoma may occur as well, resulting in blindness. Neurologic manifestations are associated with a poorer prognosis and overall affect 5% to 10% of older patients, most commonly with facial nerve paralysis. Facial palsy may be the presenting sign.[387] The combination of uveitis, facial nerve palsy, parotid gland enlargement, and fever has been called *uveoparotid fever* or *Heerfordt syndrome*. Lytic lesions of the distal bones rarely occur and are asymptomatic.

Thorough evaluation includes ophthalmologic examination with slit-lamp testing, chest radiographs (with chest computed tomography [CT] scanning if needed), pulmonary function testing, electrocardiogram, and 24-hour urine calcium measurements. Many affected patients have hyperglobulinemia, especially Blacks. Patients may show hypercalcemia (7% to 24% and usually transient), leukopenia, eosinophilia (>50% of children), and usually an increased ESR. The angiotensin-converting enzyme (ACE) level is often elevated but may be increased in other granulomatous disorders as well and has a 40% false-negative rate.

The natural course of sarcoidosis in childhood is insidious, and the condition often regresses completely after many years, especially in those with an acute onset. Chronic, progressive sarcoidosis has a poorer prognosis and rarely involutes. Features that portend a worse prognosis include chronicity; lupus pernio; symptoms lasting longer than 6 months; Black race; involvement of more than three organ systems; and later-stage pulmonary disease.[388] The overall mortality rate is 1% to 5%.

Corticosteroids (1 mg/kg per day initially with tapering as possible) can suppress the acute manifestations of the disorder.[389] However, given the hazards of prolonged systemic corticosteroid therapy and the common spontaneous resolution of sarcoidosis, the administration of systemic corticosteroids is best reserved for rapidly progressive and disfiguring skin lesions, ocular disease, and significant visceral abnormalities (persistent hypercalcemia; joint involvement; lesions of the nasal, laryngeal, and bronchial mucosa; severe, debilitating, or rapidly progressing lung disease; CNS lesions; persistent facial palsy; myocardial involvement; and hypersplenism). Methotrexate is the most commonly used steroid-sparing systemic agent for pediatric sarcoidosis, and MMF and TNF-α inhibitors (particularly infliximab) have also been used successfully.[390] Ophthalmic steroid preparations may be used adjunctively for eye disease. Nonsteroidal antiinflammatory drugs (NSAIDs) can be used for the arthritis, and hydroxychloroquine and allopurinol have been used successfully for skin lesions.

SARCOIDOSIS IN PRESCHOOL CHILDREN (see Blau Syndrome in the Other Monogenic Forms of Autoinflammatory Disorders Section)

Sarcoidosis in preschool-aged children differs from that of older children, adolescents, and adults,[379,391,392] and is characterized by exuberant, boggy polyarthritis and severe panuveitis (commonly suggesting a diagnosis of JIA),[393] cutaneous manifestations, and a conspicuous absence of pulmonary abnormalities (Table 25.8).[394,395] The majority of young children with this presentation (also called *early-onset sarcoidosis* [EOS]) have been found to have heterozygous mutations in *CARD15* and thus have Blau syndrome, an autosomal dominant disorder with the cutaneous granulomas and other features of EOS (see Blau Syndrome section).[396–398] Blau syndrome/EOS is associated with increased flaring and morbidity and has a poorer prognosis than sarcoidosis in older children and adults.

Skin manifestations are present in more than 75% of affected individuals and tend to be the presenting manifestation in more than 90% of patients. Granulomatous skin changes tend to have the earliest age of onset (median in one study of 21 patients, 2.25 years [range 3 months to 20 years] vs. joint involvement [mean 4 years] and uveitis [mean 9.5 years]).[399] Over time, the skin-colored to hyperpigmented granulomatous papular lesions may evolve to appear livedoid, vasculitic,[400] urticarial,[401] ichthyotic, poikilodermatous, or ulcerated.[399] Additional clinical features may be fever, erythema nodosum, sialadenitis, lymphadenopathies, transient neuropathies, nephritis, interstitial lung disease, vitamin D–mediated hypercalcemia with generalized osteosclerosis,[402] and visceral granulomas (especially hepatic).[403–406] Treatment is primarily with TNF inhibitors,[407] particularly infliximab, although the skin lesions tend to respond well to erythromycin and other oral macrolides.[408]

Table 25.8 Common Features of Sarcoidosis in Older vs. Younger Children

Older Children and Adolescents	Preschool-Aged Children
Fever, weight loss	Low-grade fever
Skin lesions	Polyarthritis
Cough, dyspnea	Skin lesions
Lymphadenopathy	Iridocyclitis with uveitis
Hepatomegaly	Parotid gland enlargement
Splenomegaly	Lymphadenopathy, especially peripheral
Arrhythmias	Splenomegaly
Congestive heart failure	
Renal stones (hypercalciuria)	
Uveitis	
Facial paralysis	

THE INFLAMMASOMOPATHIES

Inflammasomopathies[409,410] result from abnormalities of the inflammasome, a macromolecular intracellular complex that senses microbial products and endogenous "danger signals." Inflammasomes contain a pattern recognition receptor, most often nucleotide-binding oligomerization domain-like receptor (NLR).[411] NLRP3 (also called *NALP3* or *cryopyrin*) is the best characterized and is central to inflammasomopathies. In addition to NLRP3, NLPR1 and NLRC4 (NLR containing a caspase recruitment domain) are components of inflammasomes. Activation of the inflammasome requires two signals. The priming signal, which is from toll-like receptors (TLRs) or cytokines (particularly TNF), activates NF-κB signaling and upregulates expression of NLRP3 (as well as pro-IL-1β and pyrin). The second signal is mediated by stimulation of pathogen-associated molecular patterns (PAMPs) or damage-associated molecular patterns (DAMPs), which promotes formation and activation of the NLRP3 inflammasome complex. In addition to NLRP3, this complex includes an adaptor protein (ASC) and caspase-1. Activated caspase-1 cleaves the inactive proinflammatory cytokines pro-IL-1 and pro-IL-18 to their active forms (IL-1 and IL-18), which leads to inflammatory responses in patients with inflammasomopathies.

NLRP1 and NLRC4 are components of other inflammasomes that play critical roles in innate immunity by directly assembling in inflammasomes and regulating inflammation. Similar to NLRP3, NLRP1 and (Nod-like receptor family, caspase recruitment domain-containing 4) activate caspase 1 and thus increase production of IL-1 family cytokines. Mutations in inflammasomes NLRP3, NLRP1, and NLRC4 are linked to a variety of autoinflammatory disorders, most of which are autosomal dominant.

Inflammasomopathies include the cryopyrinopathies or cryopyrin-associated periodic syndromes (CAPS). Among these disorders related to defective cryopyrin are familial cold autoinflammatory syndrome (FCAS), Muckle–Wells syndrome (MWS), and neonatal-onset multisystemic inflammatory disorder (NOMID).[412] Others result from abnormalities or deficits in proteins that interact directly or indirectly with the inflammasome and are activated by TNF receptor signaling, such as pyrin (as in hereditary periodic fever syndromes, especially familial Mediterranean fever [FMF]) and PSTPIP1 (pyogenic sterile arthritis, pyoderma gangrenosum, and acne [PAPA] and related syndromes). The duration and periodicity of fevers, as well as other clinical features, allow clinical diagnosis among the hereditary periodic fever syndromes.[413] Fever is shortest in FMF (mean 2 to 3 days) and longest in TNF-α receptor–1 associated syndrome (TRAPS) (mean, 5 to 9 days in milder disease and up to 21 days in more severe disease). Among clinical features, vomiting and splenomegaly may be features of hyperimmunoglobulin D syndrome (HIDS). In addition, having ethnicity from Mediterranean areas may suggest FMF, given that FMF-associated mutations occur in more than 10% of some populations of Turks, Armenians, and Ashkenazi Jews. The diagnosis of periodic fever syndromes is often delayed. In an international retrospective chart review, TRAPS and mevalonate kinase deficiency (MKD)/HIDS were diagnosed at 5.8 and 7.1 years after onset, in contrast to 1.8 years for FMF.[414] Clinical criteria for considering diagnosis, including genetic testing, have recently been proposed based on data from the Eurofever Registry and consensus of the Paediatric Rheumatology International Trials Organisation (PRINTO) group[211] (Box 25.5).

FAMILIAL MEDITERRANEAN FEVER

FMF (benign paroxysmal peritonitis, familial paroxysmal polyserositis, familial recurrent polyserositis, Armenian disease) is the prototype of the hereditary autoinflammatory disorders.[415–417] It results from mutations in *MEFV* (Mediterranean fever gene), which encodes for

Box 25.5 Clinical Criteria for Classifying Hereditary Periodic Fevers and PFAPA

FMF: At least six of the nine following criteria:
Present: (1) Eastern Mediterranean ethnicity, (2) episodes last 1–3 days, (3) abdominal pain, (4) chest pain, (5) arthritis
Absent: (6) Aphthous stomatitis, (7) urticarial eruption, (8) maculopapular eruption, (9) painful adenopathy
TRAPS: Must score ≥5 points
Present: (1) Fever ≥7 days (2 points) or fever for 5–6 days (1 point), (2) migratory rash (1 point), (3) periorbital edema (1 point), (4) myalgia (1 point), (5) positive family history
Absent: (6) Aphthous stomatitis (1 point), (7) pharyngitis/tonsillitis (1 point)
MKD: Must have at least three of the six following criteria:
(1) Age of onset <1 year), (2) painful adenopathy, (3) gastrointestinal symptoms, (4) aphthous stomatitis, (5) maculopapular rash, (6) recognized triggers
CAPS: At least two of the five following criteria must be present:
(1) Urticaria eruption, (2) cold-/stress-induced episodes, (3) sensorineural hearing loss, (4) chronic aseptic meningitis, (5) skeletal abnormalities (frontal bossing/epiphyseal overgrowth)
PFAPA: Must have at least seven of the eight following criteria:
Present: (1) Episodes that last 3–6 days, (2) pharyngitis/tonsillitis, (3) cervical lymphadenitis, (4) periodicity
Absent: (5) Diarrhea, (6) chest pain, (7) skin rash, (8) arthritis

Criteria suggested by Gattorno M, Hofer M, Federici S, et al. Classification criteria for autoinflammatory recurrent fevers. Ann Rheum Dis 2019;78(8):1025–32.

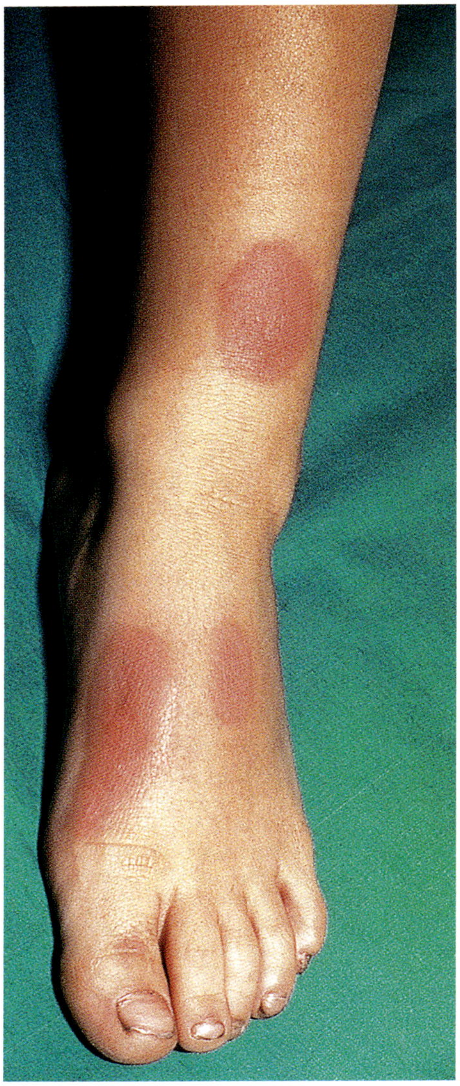

Fig. 25.32 Familial Mediterranean fever. Erythematous nodules on the dorsal aspect of the foot and pretibial area of an affected child. (Courtesy James E. Rasmussen, MD; reprinted from Hurwitz S. *The Skin and Systemic Disease in Children*. Chicago, IL: Year Book Medical Publishers; 1985.)

pyrin (also called *marenostrin*), an inflammasome sensor.[413,418] Autosomal dominant and autosomal recessive forms have been described. Heterozygous gain-of-function mutations in MEFV lead to increased sensing of stimuli by pyrin, with increased secretion of proinflammatory cytokines IL-1β and IL-18 and heightened cell sensitivity to toxic agents.[419] Cellular responses to NLRP3 and NLRC4 are not altered, suggesting that the decrease in threshold activation of the pyrin inflammasome does not affect other inflammasomes. MEFV mutations leading to autosomal recessive disease are thought to reduce the negative regulation by pyrin on the NLRP3 inflammasome.[420] The disorder is most commonly seen in individuals of Arabic, Turkish, or non-Ashkenazi Jewish descent, in whom one in five persons carries a pathogenic genetic variant.

Abdominal pain and fever are the most common features.[421,422] The acute attacks of high fever and serositis (peritonitis, pleuritis, and synovitis, with abdominal, chest, and articular pain) begin during the first decade in 67% of cases and by the second decade in 90%. The attacks typically last 1 to 3 days. The erysipelas- or cellulitis-like lesions, the most common cutaneous manifestations, occur in about 10% of patients (range, 5% to 30%) (Fig. 25.32).[423,424] Of importance, these painful, warm, swollen, erythematous, and well-defined plaques can occur in children without a history of fevers, although acute-phase reactants are increased.[425] Both the skin signs and the arthritis may be precipitated by trauma. Other cutaneous manifestations include urticaria, erythematous papules, vesicles, bullae, and subcutaneous nodules that histologically resemble periarteritis nodosa or vasculitis. The most common form of vasculitis in FMF is Henoch–Schönlein purpura (IgA-associated vasculitis, 1% to 7% of patients).[426] Skin lesions usually appear on the calves, around the ankles, and on the dorsal aspects of the feet but can affect unusual sites, such as the face and trunk, and tend to be recurrent. Vasculitis of the CNS, large vessels, and coronary arteries may also occur. Heterozygotes may manifest signs of FMF, although the mechanism is unclear.[418]

Usually a single organ is affected during an attack. Attacks last from a few hours to 4 days and recur throughout life with variable periodicity. Asymptomatic intervals may last as long as several years. Although symptoms of the monoarticular joint inflammation persist longer than episodes of peritonitis, sometimes for several months, chronic residual manifestations are rare.

Amyloidosis occurs in about 25% of untreated patients and causes death in 90% of individuals affected with amyloid-induced renal dysfunction before the age of 40. The risk of developing amyloidosis is a function of the duration between disease onset and diagnosis and of the frequency of episodes of chest pain, arthritis, and erysipelas-like erythema.[427] In one study of 600 affected children, 13% of children with FMF developed a concomitant disease: 5% developed vasculitis, 3.5% JIA, 2% sacroiliitis, and 1.2% inflammatory bowel disease.[428] In general, these manifestations developed when not taking colchicine.

The diagnosis of FMF is dependent on clinical features and, as needed, genetic testing. Colchicine (1 to 2 mg per day) prevents the recurrence of attacks and the amyloidosis[429,430]; once-daily usage may be as effective and safe as two to three divided daily doses.[431] The dosage of colchicine required for control has been shown to depend on genotype, body surface areas, and expression of biomarkers, particularly S100.[432] Symptomatic heterozygotes should also be treated with colchicine, although long periods of remission have been described in these symptomatic carriers.[418] Anakinra or canakinumab[433] (directed against IL-1), interferon (IFN)-α, corticosteroids, and cyclophosphamide have been used in rare patients who are unresponsive to colchicine.[434,435] FMF has variable expressivity in its phenotypic manifestations, suggesting a role for modifier genes. Indeed, FMF patients carrying a *CARD15/NOD2* mutation have a higher rate of erysipelas-like erythema and acute scrotum attacks, a trend for a higher rate of colchicine resistance, and more severe disease compared with patients without this additional mutation.[436] Specific point mutations in *MEFV* (encoding pyrin) in exon 2 have recently been described to cause pyrin-associated autoinflammation with neutrophilic dermatosis (PAAND), an autosomal dominant disorder with recurrent fevers, neutrophilic dermatosis, arthralgias, myositis with myalgias, and increased acute-phase reactants.[437] In addition, one family with such a point mutation had PG, severe pustular acne, suppurative hidradenitis, and neutrophilic panniculitis in association with polyarthralgias and oligoarthritis (PAPASH syndrome, see Inflammasomopathies with Pyoderma Gangrenosum section).[438]

TNF Receptor–Associated Periodic Syndrome

TRAPS is an autosomal dominant disorder caused by mutations in the p55 TNF receptor (TNFR1), encoded by *TNFRSF1A*,[439] or defects in shedding of the receptor.[440–443] The febrile attacks tend to last longer than those of FMF—at least 5 days and sometimes up to 3 weeks (mean, 11 days with 70 symptomatic days per year).[444] They usually have no periodicity, despite the name, but are recurrent rather than continuous, with flares in almost 90% of affected individuals.[443] Fever always occurs in children but is sometimes absent in adults. Only 25% of patients can identify triggers, and a minority have prodromal symptoms (periorbital edema, malaise, headache). Manifestations usually begin during childhood in more than 90% of patients (median age of symptom onset, 3 to 4 years old); somatic mosaicism of *TNFRSF1A* has been described in TRAPS with adult onset.[445] More than 75% of patients have cutaneous involvement.[446] Most typical is the erythematous swollen plaque with indistinct margins that is warm and tender to palpation. It is most commonly located on the extremities, where it may begin distally and migrate proximally during the attack. The eruption is described as maculopapular or urticarial, each in approximately 25% of patients. Localized or generalized serpiginous erythematous patches and plaques and pseudofolliculitis have also been described. Painful myalgias accompany the eruption in 70% of patients and may precede the appearance of cutaneous signs. Severe abdominal pain and arthralgias or occasionally arthritis occur in most patients, but thoracic and scrotal pain, orbital edema, and conjunctivitis are also common complaints. Amyloid deposition, especially in the kidneys and liver, is described in 10% to 25% of individuals with TRAPS at a median age of 43 years.

The diagnosis of TRAPS can be confirmed by genetic testing. Corticosteroids are the most effective treatment, but daily administration has been required; NSAIDs provide symptomatic relief. Etanercept,[447] anakinra,[448] and tocilizumab have been efficacious in some patients, but infliximab and adalimumab may induce paradoxical inflammatory reactions,[449,450] which may be mutation dependent.

Periodic Fever Associated with Mevalonate Kinase Deficiency (Hyperimmunoglobulin D Syndrome)

Periodic fever associated with MKD, or HIDS, is an autosomal recessive disorder that presents during the first 6 months of life in 60% of patients and by 5 years of age in 92%.[451] More than 90% of patients show the cutaneous eruption of erythematous macules and/or papules. Fever is also often associated with lymphadenopathy (71%), diarrhea (69%), joint pain (67%), abdominal pain (63%), and splenomegaly (63%). Inflammatory attacks typically last approximately 1 week and recur every 4 to 8 weeks. Renal deposition of amyloid is rare.[452]

Mutations in *MVK* lead to deficient mevalonate kinase,[453,454] disruption of cholesterol biosynthesis, and a shortage of isoprenoid end products, leading to inflammasome activation and IL-1 mediated inflammation.[455,456] Complete deficiency of mevalonate kinase (vs. the 1% to 8% residual activity in MKD) results in mevalonic aciduria, which is associated with growth and mental retardation and morphologic abnormalities, in addition to recurrent fevers, rash, lymphadenopathy, and inflammation of the joints and gastrointestinal tract. High serum levels of IgD are characteristic of HIDS[457] but have now been shown in some patients with FMF and TRAPS.

Fevers respond dramatically to steroids, but the frequent recurrence of fevers makes steroid therapy untenable. IL-1 inhibitors are the treatment of choice.[458] However, other cytokines are activated as well,[459] and in patients in whom IL-1 inhibition is insufficient, TNF inhibitors[460,461] and tocilizumab may decrease the inflammation. Administration of simvastatin improves inflammatory attacks; simvastatin inhibits 3-hydroxy-3-methylglutaryl-coenzyme A (HMG-CoA) reductase, which precedes mevalonate kinase in the isoprenoid pathway.[462]

THE CRYOPYRINOPATHIES OR CAPS: FAMILIAL COLD AUTOINFLAMMATORY, MUCKLE–WELLS, AND CINCA/NOMID SYNDROMES

Although originally described as separate disorders, these three autosomal dominant syndromes are all caused by mutations in the gene *NLRP3/CIAS1* (cold-induced autoinflammatory syndrome[463] 1),[464,465] encoding cryopyrin (or NALP3). Gain-of-function mutations in *NLRP3* activate the NLRP3 inflammasome and increase IL-1β. The mutations that result in the different syndromes are largely distinct. Somatic NLRP3 mosaicism is now recognized in some CAPS patients and may explain features of CAPS without detection of the NLRP3 mutation in blood. In one series, 8% of CAPS patients were found to be mosaic, with the clinical features consistent with CAPS but a median age of onset of 50 years.[466] Mosaicism has also been detected in patients with features of NOMID and MWS.[467] Use of next-generation sequencing (rather than Sanger sequencing) increases the change of detection of low-level mosaicism.

Recurrent urticaria-like eruptions are common to all three syndromes. In FCAS (FCAS1; familial cold urticaria), the mildest condition of the group, the urticaria is delayed in its onset, usually a few hours after exposure to cold, and persists for less than 24 hours. Fever, conjunctivitis, and arthritis are also seen.[468] FCAS must be distinguished from FCAS2, a newly described autosomal dominant disorder caused by mutations in *NLRP12* (component of NLRP12 inflammasomes) and responsive to IL-1 inhibition as well as glucocorticoids (see Other Inflammasomopathies section). Cold-induced autoinflammation is also a feature of PLAID syndrome, caused by dominant mutations in *PLCG2*, encoding phospholipase Cγ2 (see PLAID and APLAID Syndromes section).

MWS is an autosomal dominant autoinflammatory disorder characterized by recurrent urticarial eruption, arthralgias, conjunctivitis, sensorineural hearing loss,[469] and risk of reactive AA amyloidosis (with increases in the fragment AA protein of Serum Amyloid A), resulting from the progressive visceral accumulation of amyloid fibrils. Proteinuria or renal insufficiency from renal amyloidosis can be observed in up to 25% of patients. Female sex and hearing loss are risk factors for more severe disease.[470] In milder cases, fever is not a feature.[471]

Chronic infantile neurologic cutaneous and articular (CINCA), or NOMID, syndrome typically presents as fever and nonpruritic urticarial erythema during the first week of life.[472,473] The urticarial rash usually begins on the extremities and tends to migrate, even during examination. It has a waxing and waning course but never tends to resolve entirely.[474] Arthralgias and arthritis develop early during the first weeks of life and are thereafter persistent, leading to disabling destructive arthropathy during infancy. Bony deformities, especially of the knees, are characteristic, with distinctive radiographic findings of patellar and long bone ossification with overgrowth. Chronic aseptic meningitis has been associated with headaches in older children, and patients may have seizures, spasticity, and motor defects. Some affected children have developed brain atrophy during the neonatal period, which has been linked to developmental delay and retardation. Papillitis with optic atrophy and anterior uveitis are the most common ocular manifestations, with a mean age of onset of 4.5 years; severe visual loss occurs in 26% of patients with ocular disease.[475] Bilateral sensorineural progressive hearing loss is commonly associated as well. Most patients show typical angelic facies with frontal bossing, a saddleback nose, and midfacial hypoplasia. Lymphadenopathy, splenomegaly, premature atherosclerosis,[476] increased ESR, eosinophilia, leukocytosis, and hyperglobulinemia are features of chronic inflammation. Early death has been linked to infection, vasculitis, and amyloidosis.

Other than for NOMID syndrome, the diagnosis is often delayed, especially in milder cases (median diagnostic delay in one study for MWS/FCAS was 20.6 years vs. 2.1 for NOMID).[477] Given the need for early diagnosis and rapid initiation of therapy, diagnostic criteria have been suggested. A recent model found that seven clinical features helped to make the diagnosis: urticaria-like rash, episodes triggered by cold, sensorineural hearing loss, musculoskeletal symptoms, arthralgia, chronic aseptic meningitis, and skeletal abnormalities; having at least two of these features plus elevated inflammatory markers (C-reactive protein/serum amyloid A) was diagnostic for NLRP3 mutation, regardless of subtype, with a sensitivity of 81% and specificity of 94%.[478]

IL-1 inhibitors, such as anakinra[479] and canakinumab, usually lead to rapid resolution of inflammation in CAPS.[480–483] Canakinumab administration every 4 to 8 weeks is well tolerated and leads to a complete response in most patients, even with colchicine-resistant FMF.[479,484,485] Canakinumab has also been shown to improve kidney function[486] in MWS with overt renal amyloidosis.[487] Although most patients respond well to anti-IL-1 therapy, only 50% with the sensorineural hearing loss have restoration of hearing with therapy.[477] TNF inhibitors and stem cell transplantation have been used for severely affected patients who fail to respond to IL-1 inhibition. MCC950, a small molecule inhibitor of *NLRP3*, reduced IL-1β and showed promise in a mouse model and *ex vivo* samples from individuals with MWS.[488] The recent demonstration of IL-17-associated neutrophil recruitment suggests IL-1-induced activation of Th 17 cells and that IL-17/IL-17RA inhibitors may be new therapeutic targets.[468]

Other Inflammasomopathies

NLRC4-activating (gain-of-function) mutations lead to a recently described form of inflammasomopathy.[489,490] Affected individuals have variably presented during the neonatal period with fever, recurrent fevers, and features of macrophage activation syndrome (see Chapter 22) or stress-triggered erythematous plaques and joint pain in affected older children and adults. IL-1 inhibition is the treatment of choice. An activating NLRC4 mutation has also been linked to FCAS.[491]

Polymorphisms in *NLRP1* have been linked with autoimmune disorders (vitiligo, systemic lupus erythematosus, type 1 diabetes, and rheumatoid arthritis). *NLRP1* mutations cause NLRP1-associated autoinflammation with arthritis and dyskeratosis (NAIAD), an autosomal recessive disorder that combines features of autoimmune and autoinflammatory disorders.[492] Affected patients presented during infancy with recurrent fevers and filiform follicular hyperkeratosis, sometimes generalized and reminiscent of the spicule-like cornified plugs seen in IFAP syndrome (see Chapter 5) or trichostasis spinulosa (see Chapter 7).[492] Biopsies show epidermal dyskeratosis and inflammation. Additional features that have developed with progressing age are arthritis, autoimmune hemolytic anemia and thyroiditis, photophobia and uveitis, variably high ANA levels, and infections. As with other inflammasomopathies, serum levels of IL-18 and caspase 1 are high. Responses to retinoids and IL-1β inhibition have been described. Given the keratotic lesions, siblings with biallelic mutations in *NRLP1* have been classified as a form of keratosis lichenoides chronica (see Chapter 4).[493] An autosomal dominant form has been linked to a heterozygous missense mutation in the pyrin domain of NLRP1 with clinical characteristics of palmoplantar keratoderma, corneal opacities and intraepithelial dyskeratosis, and laryngeal dyskeratosis.[494] Mutations in *NLRP12* (a component of NLRP12 inflammasomes) cause FCAS2, characterized by recurrent cold-induced episodes of fever, urticarial eruption, aphthous stomatitis, adenopathy, abdominal discomfort and diarrhea, failure to thrive, arthralgias, myalgias, and headache.[495]

PERIODIC FEVER, APHTHOUS STOMATITIS, PHARYNGITIS, AND CERVICAL ADENITIS SYNDROME

Periodic fever, aphthous stomatitis, pharyngitis, and cervical adenitis (PFAPA) syndrome (or Marshall syndrome) is the most common periodic fever syndrome and occurs primarily in children under 5 years of age.[496,497] The incidence in Europe is 2.3 cases per 10,000 children per year.[209]

IL-1β monocyte production is dysregulated in patients with PFAPA syndrome, with elevated CXCL10 chemokine. These laboratory features, together with the periodic fever, has suggested classification of PFAPA as an inflammasomopathy. Familial cases are often described (both autosomal recessive and autosomal dominant patterns), with parents of children with PFAPA having more episodes of recurrent pharyngitis and aphthous stomatitis and more siblings having these signs of PFAPA than in the control population.[498] Although the role of genetic vs. environmental factors remains unknown, genetic susceptibility loci now link recurrent aphthous stomatitis, PFAPA syndrome, and Behçet's disease (in order of increasing severity), placing these disorders on a common spectrum.[496,499–501] Nevertheless, approximately 20% of affected individuals have variants in *NLRP3* (encoding nucleotide-binding oligomerization domain-like receptor/NLR containing a pyrin domain 3),[502] and affected individuals have a fourfold increase in a frameshift variant in CARD8, which negatively regulates the NLRP3 inflammasome through its interaction with NALP3 or caspase 1.[503]

Affected children have fever greater than 39° C with a mean duration of 4 to 5 days and regular recurrence every 3 to 8 weeks. Pharyngitis has been described in almost 90% of patients, cervical adenitis in 78%, and aphthous stomatitis in 38% to 71%[504–506] Clinical features tend to be most pronounced at days 2 and 3 of the febrile course. Attacks of mild abdominal pain, vomiting, headache, and malaise are common; arthralgias, genital ulceration,[507,508] erythematous cutaneous eruptions, and neurologic signs are uncommon. Children are well between flares.

Other inflammatory disorders with fever, including infectious disorders, must be considered, especially if the fever lasts longer than the typical 4- to 5-day duration. The fever tends to be poorly responsive to acetaminophen and/or ibuprofen. Given the associated aphthous stomatitis, cyclic neutropenia must be considered in the differential diagnosis. The periodicity of fever, as well as the well-being and normal levels of acute-phase reactants between episodes, helps distinguish from other autoinflammatory syndromes. Short courses (one or two doses) of corticosteroids can be highly effective in controlling symptoms but may shorten the duration of remission[509]; in one study of 32 children, symptoms remitted in 81% within 24 hours of steroid administration.[510] Patients have been shown to respond to IL-1 inhibition.[511] Tonsillectomy has also been associated with improvement.[512–514] Tonsils of patients with PFAPA syndrome have shown significant increases in *Candida albicans* and biofilm formation compared with controls, but less *S. aureus*, *Varicella zoster*, and herpes simplex virus, and no difference in group A β-hemolytic *Streptococcus*.[515] In most patients, episodes tend to occur less often or disappear with advancing age (before adulthood), without any long-term sequelae.[516] PFAPA can occur in adults, who tend to have less frequent recurrent pharyngitis and fever.[517]

Inflammasomopathies with Pyoderma Gangrenosum

PYOGENIC STERILE ARTHRITIS, PYODERMA GANGRENOSUM, ACNE (PAPA) SYNDROME

This autosomal dominant disorder is characterized by PG-like ulcerative lesions, usually in the second decade of life; severe cystic acne; and episodes of inflammatory arthritis that lead to significant joint destruction.[518–520] PG lesions are usually seen on the leg but may occur at acne sites (Fig. 25.33). Sterile abscesses have been described at sites of parenteral injections. Nonulcerated erysipelas-like lesions (more typical for the presentation of FMF) have been described in association with arthritis during childhood.[520]

Affected family members may show variable expressivity. Mutations occur in *PSTPIP1/CD2BP1*, which encodes CD2-binding protein 1, a

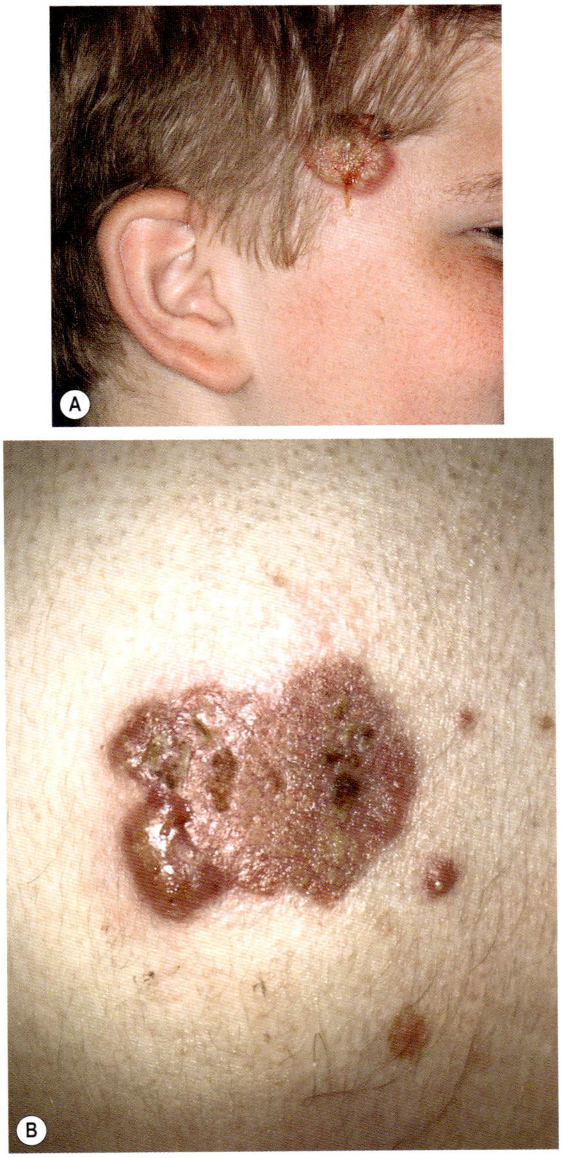

Fig. 25.33 Pyogenic sterile arthritis, pyoderma gangrenosum, and acne (PAPA) syndrome. This 11-year-old boy had small inflammatory papules of acne on the face, which rapidly became purulent plaques **(A)** and then ulcerated to form pyoderma gangrenosum, leaving residual scars. He also had arthritis. His disease was brought under control with golimumab (TNF inhibitor) and isotretinoin throughout adolescence, but in his early twenties (without isotretinoin) he developed mild truncal acne and recurrence of the pyoderma gangrenosum **(B)**.

protein that interacts with pyrin.[521] Disease activity has been shown to correlate with increased NLRP3-mediated IL-1β secretion, although patients with a history of flares involving the joints release more cytokines (IL-1β, Il-6, and TNF) than those with mostly skin involvement.[522]

PAPA syndrome is treated with oral corticosteroids, and marked improvement has been noted with TNF inhibitors, abatacept (inhibits T-cell activation), and anti–IL-1 treatment.[523] Even mild inflammatory acne risks becoming ulcerated PG, so administration of isotretinoin should be considered to prevent acne altogether.[524]

PG and acne have also been associated with suppurative hidradenitis, thus comprising PASH syndrome.[525–527] Some cases have also had mutations in PSTPIP1 and NCSTN (the latter encoding nicastrin and known to be mutated in familial hidradenitis suppurativa), but in others no candidate genes have shown variants.[528] PASH syndrome is not associated with arthritis, but PAPASH syndrome combines the two syndromes and has been described in association with mutations in *MEFV* exon 2 (encoding pyrin).[438] PAPASH has also been used to describe PASH plus psoriasis, and PsAPASH to include psoriatic arthritis with PASH syndrome.[529] PG with acne and ulcerative colitis has also been described.[530,531]

INTERFERONOPATHIES

In contrast to most autoinflammatory diseases, the inflammation in the interferonopathies are not highly responsive to IL-1 blockade and, instead, leads to excessive IFN signaling[47,48] and response to JAK inhibitors, such as baricitinib.[532–535] Aicardi–Goutieres is an interferonopathy characterized by chilblain-like lesions (pernio), acrocyanosis, and sometimes livedo reticularis. Lesions may begin in the neonatal period. CNS abnormalities are the predominant extracutaneous features (see Chapter 20 and Table 25.5). The disorder is primarily autosomal recessive and results from mutations in a variety of genes with products that metabolize DNA and ribonucleic acid (RNA) molecules, thus preventing their recognition as foreign by innate immune sensors and limiting IFN-driven immune activation (see Chapter 20).

STING-Associated Vasculopathy with Onset in Infancy (SAVI) Syndrome

The pathway toward activation of type I IFN after sensing the presence of cytosolic DNA (either from a foreign source, such as a virus, or from endogenous cells, as in autoimmune disease) involves activation of STING (stimulator of interferon genes), leading to initiation of the expression of IFN-inducible genes. STING-associated vasculopathy with onset in infancy (SAVI) syndrome is a recently described disorder that results from heterozygous mutations in *TMEM173*, encoding STING. The disorder is characterized by the onset by 6 months of age of telangiectatic vasculopathy (Fig. 25.34) with pustules and residual scarring and soft-tissue loss.[536] Lesions are characteristically localized to acral sites: hands, feet, nose, cheeks, and ears with exacerbations in cold weather. Patients have systemic inflammation (increased ESR and C-reactive protein) with intermittent low-grade fevers, hilar or paratracheal adenopathy, and sometimes interstitial lung fibrosis, which may lead to death. Widespread vasculopathy has been described. The treatment of choice is JAK inhibition (baricitinib, ruxolitinib).

CANDLE Syndrome

Ubiquitination involves the attachment of specific molecules to proteins that target them toward their fate related to cell localization, interaction with other proteins, signal activation, or degradation. The proteasome is a cellular structure that has proteolytic sites responsible for protein degradation, primarily for removing intracellular waste after ubiquitination.

Immunoproteasomes are induced by IFNs in cells undergoing stress. Chronic atypical neutrophilic dermatosis with lipodystrophy and elevated temperature (CANDLE) syndrome was originally described as resulting from biallelic mutations in the proteasome subunit beta type-8 (PSMB8)[537] but has more recently been reported in association with dominantly inherited mutations in PSMB8 or with digenic mutations of PSMB8, together with one of the related components of the immunoproteasome PSMB4, PSMB9, or PSMA3.[538] Another name for these disorders that affect immunoproteasomes is *proteasome-related autoinflammatory syndrome* (PRAAS). The result is insufficient catalytic activity by the proteasome; inadequate clearance of ubiquitinated and oxidated proteins, causing stress; and excessive synthesis of type I IFN. Patients typically present during infancy with recurrent skin eruptions (usually violaceous nodules) on predominantly the trunk and extremities (Fig. 25.35), hepatomegaly, and recurrent fever. They characteristically progress to show periorbital and digital swelling and panniculitis-associated lipodystrophy with metabolic syndrome (Fig. 25.36) (see Chapter 20).[539,540] Although patients may respond to corticosteroids, systemic immunosuppressives, and

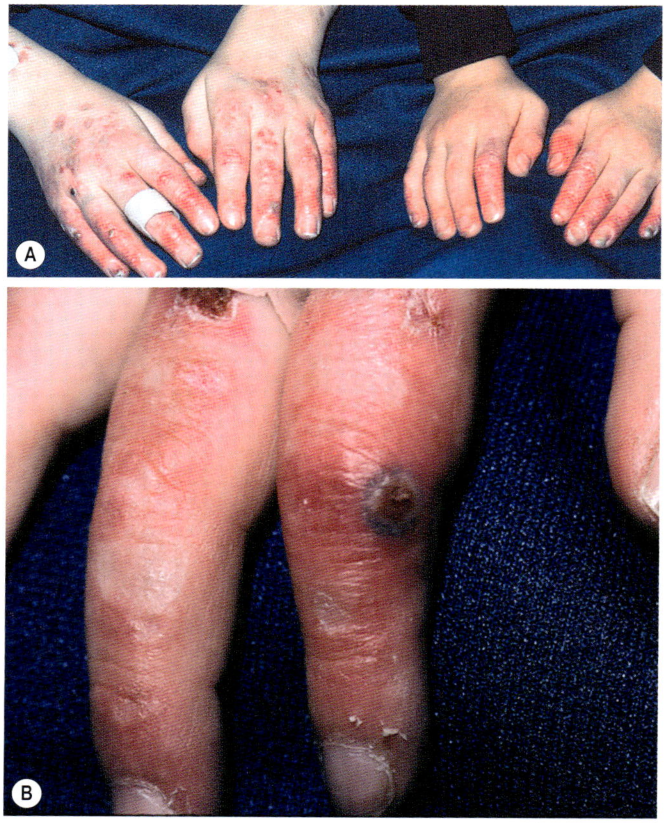

Fig. 25.34 Stimulator of interferon genes (STING)-associated vasculopathy with onset in infancy (SAVI) syndrome. (**A**) These two unrelated boys both show the acral telangiectatic vasculopathy of SAVI syndrome. One of these boys died at 14 years of age because of his pulmonary disease. (**B**) Closer image of the vasculopathic changes of the fingers in one of these affected boys.

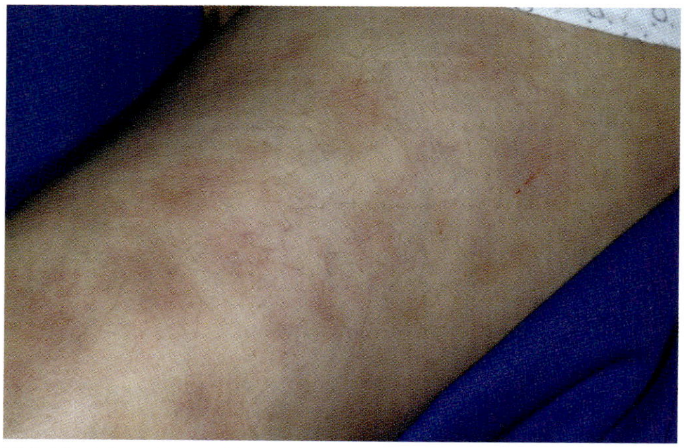

Fig. 25.35 CANDLE syndrome (PRAAS). Vasculopathic nodules on the thighs of a young affected girl; the first lesion began at 9 months of age.

anti-TNF antibodies, JAK inhibitors (baricitinib), which block IFN signaling, have led to the best results in controlling disease.

The Ubiquitinopathies (Relopathies)

The ubiquitinopathies are NF-κB-related autoinflammatory disorders due to alterations in ubiquitination of signaling pathway components.[541,542]

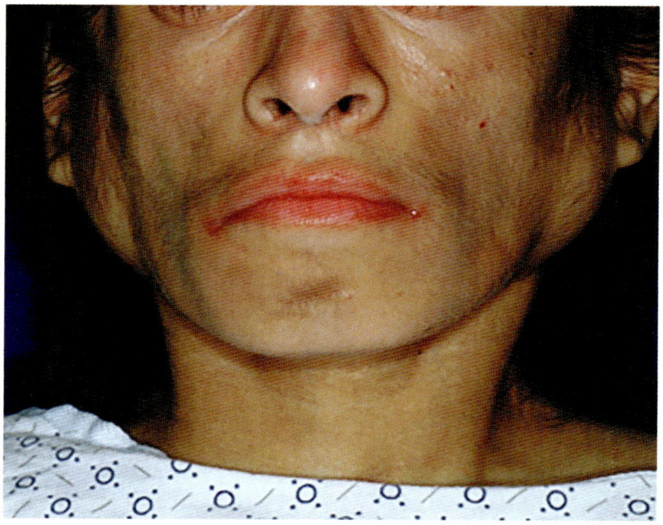

Fig. 25.36 CANDLE syndrome (PRAAS). By teenage years, an affected girl experienced profound metabolic syndrome with lipodystrophy (note the cheeks), hirsuitism (lateral cheeks), central obesity, and acanthosis nigricans.

LUBAC Component Deficiency

A complex called *linear ubiquitin chain assembly complex* (LUBAC) regulates innate and adaptive immune responses, as well as cell death, through maintaining the stability of several receptors, among them the TNF receptor (TNFR1), TLRs, the IL-1 receptor, and inflammatosome receptor signaling complexes. The attachment of linear ubiquitinated chains is required for assembly of the receptor signaling complexes. LUBAC is composed of three proteins (HOIL-1L, SHARPIN, and HOIP). Biallelic loss-of-function mutations in the LUBAC proteins HOIL-1L or HOIP are associated with diminished or absent LUBAC formation, reduced linear ubiquitination, and decreased NF-κB pathway activation.[543–546] LUBAC activity is counterregulated by otulin and A20. The disorder is characterized by multiorgan autoinflammation with high levels of proinflammatory cytokines, immunodeficiency (especially T-cell lymphopenia and poor antibody production with recurrent infections), and myopathy. Lymphangiectasis has been described in HOIP deficiency.[544] Amylopectinosis (glycogen accumulation) is another feature.

OTULIN-RELATED AUTOINFLAMMATORY SYNDROME

Deubiquitinating enzymes limit the proinflammatory signaling by removal of activating (otulin) and/or conjugating (A20) degradative ubiquitin signals. Otulipenia, or otulin-related autoinflammatory syndrome (ORAS), is the result of mutations in the deubiquitinase and loss-of-protein function.[541,547] Lower levels of otulin are associated with accumulation of polyubiquitinated proteins of the NF-κB pathway; elevated levels of secreted proinflammatory cytokines, such as IL-6 and TNF; and activation of the NF-κB, JAK/STAT, and TNF signaling pathways. Clinical features include onset during the first months of life of fevers lasting 2 to 3 weeks, joint swelling, gastrointestinal inflammation with diarrhea, poor growth, erythematous patches, nodules and sometimes pustules, sterile neutrophilia, autoimmunity with the presence of autoantibodies, lipodystrophy with neutrophilic panniculitis, medium-sized vasculitis and vascular occlusion, and systemic inflammation. Patients have not had evidence of primary immunodeficiency. Patients typically respond to TNF inhibition[547] and, if necessary, stem cell transplantation.

A20 HAPLOINSUFFICIENCY

Loss-of-function heterozygous missense mutations in *TNFAIP3* lead to haploinsufficiency of A20 and familial Behçet disease. Affected individuals have the onset before 2 years of age of fevers, early-onset systemic inflammation, erythematous papules, folliculitis, skin abscesses, oral pustules with ulceration, CNS vasculitis, arthralgia, and/or arthritis.[541,548] In contrast, heterozygous frameshift mutations in *TNFAIP3* cause an autoimmune lymphoproliferative syndrome (ALPS)-like phenotype.[549–551] More commonly, ALPS results from mutations in proteins of the FAS-dependent apoptosis pathway (FAS, FAS ligand [FasL], and caspase 10). Clinical features of ALPS are persistent fever; lymphadenopathy; hepatomegaly; thrombocytopenia; hypergammaglobulinemia; presence of autoantibodies; elevated levels of soluble FAS ligand, IL-10, and IL-18; and increased lymphoproliferation.

OTHER MONOGENIC FORMS OF AUTOINFLAMMATORY DISORDERS

Blau Syndrome

Blau syndrome is an autosomal dominant disorder with the cutaneous granulomas and other features of early-onset sarcoidosis (see Sarcoidosis section).[396–398] The complete classic triad (skin eruption, arthritis, and recurrent uveitis) occurs in 42% of patients with Blau syndrome,[552,553] and cutaneous features are usually the first to appear.[554] Generalized asymptomatic, small, erythematous papules on the trunk and extremities are most commonly seen (Figs. 25.37 and 25.38), often leaving small pitted scars as sequelae. However, the cutaneous lesions have variably been described as eczematous, ichthyosiform (misdiagnosed as ichthyosis vulgaris), or lichenoid.[555,556] Relapses and remission are common. Erythema nodosum is the second most common skin manifestations of Blau syndrome, and leukocytoclastic vasculitis involving skin has also been described.

Boggy synovitis and tenosynovitis of the wrists, fingers, knees, and ankles are characteristic and show symmetric, nonerosive arthritis radiographically.[557] Despite the chronicity, joint destruction is uncommon, and range of motion is usually not reduced, in contrast to the arthritis of JIA. However, the proximal interphalangeal joints disproportionately develop contractures, leading to camptodactyly (usually congenital flexion contracture of a finger).[558] Bone dysplasia can also be seen.

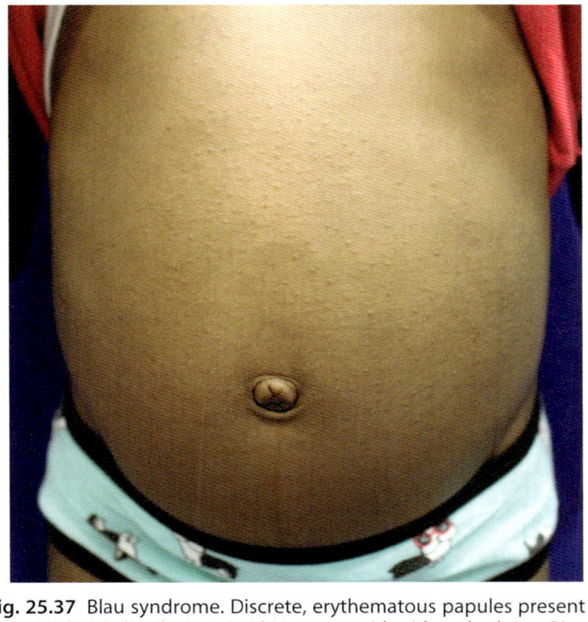

Fig. 25.37 Blau syndrome. Discrete, erythematous papules present in a generalized distribution in this young girl with arthralgias. Biopsy showed noncaseating granulomas.

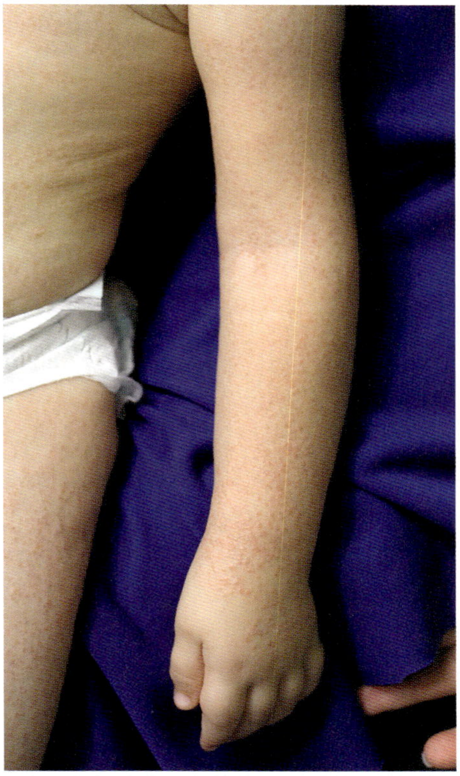

Fig. 25.38 Blau syndrome/early-onset sarcoidosis. Erythematous granulomatous papules on the arm, trunk, and thigh of a 5-year-old boy with a *CARD15* mutation.

Ocular involvement is extremely common in children,[559] especially an insidious bilateral granulomatous iridocyclitis with uveitis that involves not just the anterior uveitis (as in JIA) but also posterior uveitis. The mean age of onset of ocular disease is 4 years, and it ultimately develops in 80% of patients.[396] Keratitis, retinitis, optic atrophy, glaucoma, cataracts, retinal detachment, and involvement of the eyelids and lacrimal glands may also occur. Of those with ocular involvement, 11% show moderate visual impairment and 16% become blind.

Other manifestations are noted in about one-third of patients. In addition to the erythema nodosum, low-grade fever, and sialadenitis with parotid gland enlargement, splenomegaly and lymphadenopathy are relatively common. Other signs are large-vessel vasculitis, cranial (but not central) neuropathy, interstitial lung disease, interstitial nephritis, pericarditis, and hepatomegaly without abnormal hepatic function.

The cutaneous granulomatous papules may respond to chronic administration of macrolides, especially erythromycin,[408] but may leave tiny atrophic macules. Methotrexate and TNF-α inhibitors are most often used for extracutaneous manifestations; thalidomide and IL-1 inhibition have also been reported to be effective.[560,561]

Deficiency of the Interleukin-1 Receptor Antagonist

In autosomal recessive deficiency of the IL-1 receptor antagonist (DIRA),[562,563] IL-1 activity is markedly increased because of deficiency of an antagonist that also binds to the IL-1 receptor and prevents IL-1 activity.[564] Affected infants and young children show fetal distress, joint swelling with periosteal inflammation, severe osteopenia with lytic bone lesions, respiratory involvement, thrombotic episodes, oral mucosal and cutaneous PG-like ulcerations, and a localized to generalized pustular eruption that resembles pustular psoriasis (Fig. 25.39). Fever occurs occasionally (not periodically) and only in a few patients. DIRA must be also be distinguished from *Majeed syndrome*, an autosomal recessive disorder that also features

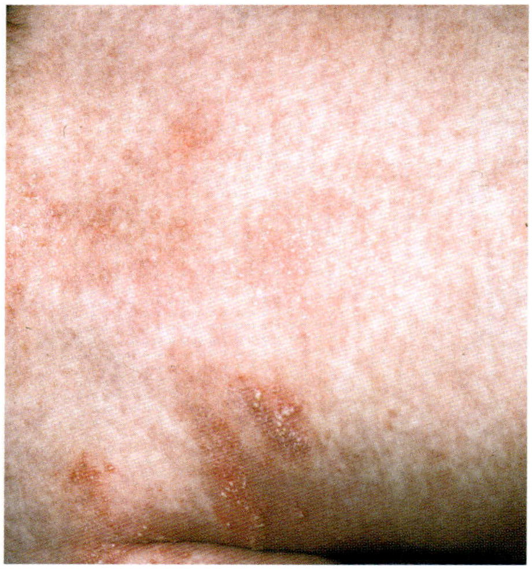

Fig. 25.39 Deficiency of IL-1 receptor antagonist. This Puerto Rican boy with failure to thrive and multifocal lytic lesions of bone showed numerous plaques of erythematous pustules.

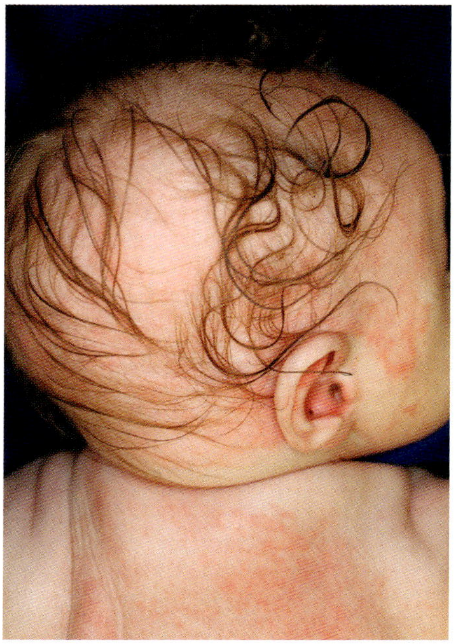

Fig. 25.40 Phospholipase Cγ2-associated antibody deficiency and immune dysregulation (PLAID) syndrome This young girl with hypogammaglobulinemia had atopic dermatitis, pruritus, and intermittent urticaria that was exacerbated by sweat-induced evaporative cooling.

chronic recurrent multifocal osteomyelitis and an inflammatory dermatosis that can vary from a Sweet syndrome–like eruption to chronic pustulosis; Majeed syndrome features congenital dyserythropoietic anemia, results from mutations in *LPIN2* (encoding lipin-2), and responds well to IL-1 inhibition.[565] Administration of anakinra (2 mg/kg per day) dramatically reverses the inflammatory manifestations, whereas other systemic immunomodulators have largely failed to cause improvement.

Deficiency of the Interleukin-36 Receptor Antagonist

Another rare autosomal recessive autoinflammatory disorder associated with a pustular psoriasis–like eruption is deficiency of the IL-36 receptor antagonist (DITRA), caused by mutations in *IL36RN*, encoding the IL-36 receptor antagonist.[206,566,567] The IL-36 receptor antagonist inhibits NF-κB activation by IL-36α, β, and γ. The disorder may have its onset during infancy or childhood or, less commonly, during adulthood and should be considered in adult patients with generalized pustular psoriasis without a history of plaque psoriasis.[568] Some affected individuals have pustules localized to the palms and soles or disease that resembles acute generalized eruptive pustulosis (AGEP) (see Chapter 20). Nail dystrophy, arthritis, and/or cholangitis have been noted in the minority of patients.[567] Bacterial or viral infections and menstruation may be triggers. Patients often respond to systemic retinoids,[569] but steroids, methotrexate, cyclosporine, etanercept, infliximab,[570] secukinumab,[571,572] ustekinumab,[573] and anakinra[574] have also been used. Most recently, intravenous administration of an inhibitor of the Il-36 receptor has been shown to clear the pustular psoriasis of adults with DITRA. DIRA[575] and DITRA need to be distinguished from *CARD14-mediated pustular psoriasis* (CAMPS), an autosomal dominant disorder in which affected children may manifest symptoms of pityriasis rubra pilaris, plaque psoriasis, erythrodermic psoriasis, pustular psoriasis, AGEP, or an overlap disorder (see Chapter 4). Mutations in *AP1S3* also cause pustular psoriasis, particularly palmoplantar (see Chapter 4). Lesions resembling generalized pustular psoriasis have been described in adults with mutations in *LDHA*, encoding the M (muscle) subunit of lactate dehydrogenase. Erythmatous papulosquamous eruptions[576] begin during childhood.[577]

PLAID AND APLAID SYNDROMES

Mutations in *PLCG2*, encoding phospholipase Cγ2, are the cause of phospholipase Cγ2-associated antibody deficiency and immune dysregulation (PLAID) syndrome (typically in-frame deletions; also called *familial cold autoinflammatory syndrome 3* [FCAS3]) and APLAID syndrome (autoimmunity with PLAID syndrome; typically missense mutations). *PLAID syndrome* is characterized by evaporative cold urticaria; the neonatal onset of ulcerating lesions in acral regions, especially the nose and fingers; recurrent cutaneous granulomatous plaques; mild immunodeficiency (especially hypogammaglobulinemia), atopic (atopic dermatitis [Fig. 25.40], asthma, food allergy) and autoimmune (thyroiditis and vitiligo) disorders; infections (especially interstitial pneumonitis and bronchiolitis); and positive ANAs.[578,579] Severe pruritus is a common complication and is exacerbated by sweating with evaporative cooling of the sweat; oral glycopyrrolate has been used to reduce sweating and improve the associated pruritus.[580] *APLAID syndrome* is characterized by a neonatal-onset vesiculopustular eruption, cutaneous granulomas, recurrent acral hemorrhagic blisters, recurrent cellulitis, enterocolitis, conjunctivitis, sensorineural deafness, arthralgias, and immunodeficiency with recurrent infections.[581]

DEFICIENCY OF ADENOSINE DEAMINASE 2

In contrast to deficiency of ADA1, which leads to SCID (see Severe Combined Immunodeficiency section), deficiency of adenosine deaminase 2 (DADA2) from biallelic mutations in *ADA2* leads to a vasculitis syndrome.[582–584] Characteristics are early-onset fevers and vasculopathy that can manifest as livedo to polyarteritis nodosa (PAN). Vasculitis can lead to ischemic and/or hemorrhagic strokes but can affect several other organs (especially the intestines, liver, and kidneys) and is also associated with hematologic manifestations (most often hypogammaglobulinemia but also red cell aplasia, thrombocytopenia, and neutropenia). First-line treatment is TNF inhibition, although bone marrow failure and severe immune deficiency may require stem cell transplantation.

The complete list of 584 references for this chapter is available online at http://expertconsult.inkling.com.

Key References

Picard C, Al-Herz W, Bousfiha A, et al. Primary immunodeficiency diseases: an update on the classification from the International Union of Immunological Societies Expert Committee for Primary Immunodeficiency 2015. J Clin Immunol 2015; 35:696–726.

Subbarayan A, Colarusso G, Hughes SM, et al. Clinical features that identify children with primary immunodeficiency diseases. Pediatrics 2011;127:810–16.

Rivers L, Gaspar HB. Severe combined immunodeficiency: recent developments and guidance on clinical management. Arch Dis Child 2015;100(7):667–72.

Cirillo E, Giardino G, Gallo V, et al. Severe combined immunodeficiency—an update. Ann N Y Acad Sci 2015;1356:90–106.

Baird K, Cooke K, Schultz KR. Chronic graft-versus-host disease (GVHD) in children. Pediatr Clin North Am 2010;57:297–322.

Shi CR, Huang JT, Nambudiri VE. Pediatric cutaneous graft versus host disease: a review. Curr Pediatr Rev 2017;13(2):100–10.

Bhat T, Coughlin CC. Dermatologic considerations in pediatric transplant recipients. Curr Opin Pediatr 2018;30(4):520–5.

Dhir S, Slatter M, Skinner R. Recent advances in the management of graft-versus-host disease. Arch Dis Child 2014;99(12):1150–7.

Kechichian E, Haber R, Mourad N, et al. Pediatric pyoderma gangrenosum: a systematic review and update. Int J Dermatol 2017;56(5):486–95.

Schoch JJ, Tolkachjov SN, Cappel JA, et al. Pediatric pyoderma gangrenosum: a retrospective review of clinical features, etiologic associations, and treatment. Pediatr Dermatol 2017;34(1):39–45.

Kone-Paut I. Behcet's disease in children, an overview. Pediatr Rheumatol Online J 2016;14(1):10.

Bulur I, Onder M. Behcet disease: New aspects. Clin Dermatol 2017;35(5): 421–34.

Lazzerini M, Bramuzzo M, Ventura A. Association between orofacial granulomatosis and Crohn disease in children: systematic review. World J Gastroenterol 2014; 20(23):7497–504.

Vaid RM, Cohen BA. Cutaneous Crohn disease in the pediatric population. Pediatr Dermatol 2010;27(3):279–81.

Mälkönen T, Wikström A, Heiskanen K, et al. Skin reactions during anti-TNFα therapy for pediatric inflammatory bowel disease: a 2-year prospective study. Inflamm Bowel Dis 2014;20(8):1309–15.

Strumia R. Eating disorders and the skin. Clin Dermatol 2013;31(1):80–5.

Shetty AK, Gedalia A. Childhood sarcoidosis: a rare but fascinating disorder. Pediatr Rheumatol Online J 2008;6:16.

Wouters CH, Maes A, Foley KP, et al. Blau syndrome: the prototypic autoinflammatory granulomatous disease. Pediatr Rheumatol Online J 2014;12:33.

Pathak S, McDermott MF, Savic S. Autoinflammatory diseases: update on classification diagnosis and management. J Clin Pathol 2017;70(1):1–8.

Gattorno M, Hofer M, Federici S, et al. Classification criteria for autoinflammatory recurrent fevers. Ann Rheum Dis 2019;78(8):1025–32.

Georgin-Lavialle S, Fayand A, Rodrigues F, et al. Autoinflammatory diseases: state of the art. Presse Med 2019;48(1 Pt 2):e25–48.

Lachmann HJ, Papa R, Gerhold K, et al. The phenotype of TNF receptor-associated autoinflammatory syndrome (TRAPS) at presentation: a series of 158 cases from the Eurofever/EUROTRAPS international registry. Ann Rheum Dis 2014;73(12):2160–7.

Hofer M, Pillet P, Cochard MM, et al. International periodic fever, aphthous stomatitis, pharyngitis, cervical adenitis syndrome cohort: description of distinct phenotypes in 301 patients. Rheumatology (Oxford) 2014;53(6):1125–9.

Wekell P. Periodic fever, aphthous stomatitis, pharyngitis, and cervical adenitis syndrome—PFAPA syndrome. Presse Med 2019;48(1 Pt 2):e77–87.

Marrakchi S, Guigue P, Renshaw BR, et al. Interleukin-36-receptor antagonist deficiency and generalized pustular psoriasis. N Engl J Med 2011;365(7):620–8.

26 Abuse and Factitial Disorders

Child Abuse

Child abuse is a broad term used to describe a spectrum of nonaccidental trauma inflicted upon children. Kempe et al. are generally credited with emphasizing the prevalence and importance of this entity when they coined the term *battered child syndrome* in 1962.[1] This "syndrome" has subsequently been expanded to include an array of childhood abuses, including physical abuse, sexual abuse, and neglect. Child abuse continues to be one of the most significant causes of childhood morbidity and mortality in the United States.[2] In federal fiscal year 2016, 676,000 US children (a rate of 9.1 victims per 1000 children in the population) were victims of abuse and neglect; the highest rate of victimization was in the birth to 1-year age group (24.8 per 1000 children).[3] In one 10-year study of medical records submitted to the National Pediatric Trauma Registry, child abuse accounted for 10.6% of all blunt trauma to patients under 5 years of age.[2] Children who are abused tend to be younger, with the highest incidence seen in those under 3 years of age. High-risk groups include children with a history of prematurity, physical handicap, and behavioral problems and children who are American Indian/Alaskan Native or Black.[4] Factors that appear to be associated with an increased risk of abuse are summarized in Table 26.1.[5–7] Up to 75% of abuse may be missed in the acute care setting because of failure of recognition by medical professionals, and this may lead to lost opportunities to intervene.[8]

Various patterns may be evident in families where abuse is an issue. These include parents who were the victims of abuse themselves, parents with emotional disturbances, stressful crises within the family unit (e.g., loss of job or financial distress), and lack of a close support network for the family (see Table 26.1).[9] Recognition of abuse is vital, because the trauma tends to be repeated (an abused child has up to a 50% chance of being abused again), and the risk of future injury or death is high. Instances in which there is a delay in reporting the injury, in which the degree and type of injury are at variance with the history offered, or in which the parents are evasive or vague as to the cause of injury are all suspicious and should lead to consideration for an abuse investigation. In evaluating the child with possible abuse, a detailed history is the most important component of the assessment.[10] Vital details include the alleged mechanism of the injury, developmental history of the child, past medical history (especially of any disorders that may mimic abuse, such as coagulopathy or skin disorders), history of prior injuries, social history, and family history. A complete physical examination should be performed and should include high-quality photography of cutaneous lesions. A *sentinel injury* is a visible minor injury (often bruising or intraoral injury) in the precruising infant that cannot be rationally explained and is concerning for abuse. These injuries are rarely seen in nonabused infants, and their identification, followed by appropriate reporting and intervention, may prevent further abuse to the baby.[11]

Radiographic findings in child physical abuse are often useful in the evaluation and are not discussed in great detail here. Findings that may increase suspicion for abuse include the classic metaphyseal lesion (also known as *corner fracture* or *bucket-handle fracture*), skull and femur fractures, and healing fractures, although each of these findings must be considered in the appropriate context of the medical history and physical examination findings.[12,13]

Although abused children may exhibit multiple abnormalities on physical and radiographic examination, this section will focus primarily on the cutaneous stigmata.

PHYSICAL ABUSE

Nonaccidental injuries in children may take many forms, and often the skin reveals pathologic findings. Cutaneous trauma may be seen in the form of ecchymoses, burns, lacerations, bite marks, abrasions, choke marks, thermal injuries from scalds, underlying hematomas, pigmentary changes, and scars.

Ecchymoses (bruises) are the most common type of skin injury seen in children who have been abused. Lesions on the hands and face; adult human bites; and lesions on the cheeks, mouth, lips, lower back, buttocks, or inner thighs are particularly suspect. Ecchymoses in various stages of healing are more suggestive of abuse and have been referred to as *repeated injuries*.[14] Ecchymoses on padded areas such as the buttocks, torso, face, and genitalia (Fig. 26.1, *A*) or uncommonly injured areas (earlobe, neck, lip, philtrum) are more concerning for possible abuse.[5] In a study of discriminating bruising characteristics in children who have been abused, characteristics that were more predictive of abuse included bruising on the torso (see Fig. 26.1, *B*), ear (see Fig. 26.1, *C*), or neck (in a child ≤4 years of age, termed the *TEN-4* clinical decision rule) and bruising in any region in an infant younger than 4 months of age.[8] Abuse-associated bruising should be differentiated from accidental bruising, which is more common in ambulatory children and occurs most commonly over bony prominences such as the forehead and shins.[5] Any bruising in the noncruising infant under 9 months of age should raise significant suspicion for abuse. There are many potential mimics and non-abuse-related causes of ecchymoses, including congenital dermal melanocytosis, hypersensitivity vasculitis (Henoch–Schönlein purpura or acute hemorrhagic edema of infancy), Ehlers–Danlos syndrome, vascular malformations, infantile hemangiomas, inks or dyes, and bleeding disorders.

The configurations of lesions in battered children are morphologically similar to the items or methods used to inflict the trauma and may be useful in the abuse investigation. Multiple evenly spaced markings (Fig. 26.2) or curvilinear loops and arcuate lesions (Figs. 26.3 and 26.4) such as those that may be induced by lashing with a doubled-over belt or electric cord are typical of these trauma-induced lesions. They are usually ecchymotic, but they may also present as abrasions (Fig. 26.4), lacerations, or hyperpigmentation.

Belt-buckle imprints (ecchymotic or hyperpigmented) may result from intentional trauma with these items. Adjacent, small, ecchymotic macules (Fig. 26.5) are typical of pinch marks. Shackles on the wrists, ankles, or neck leave easily identifiable rings that are red if fresh and hyperpigmented if long-standing. Ligature marks on the neck (see Fig. 26.6) or extremities and grab or slap marks (fingertip bruises; Fig. 26.7) on the shoulders, hands, or legs are particularly suspicious and highly suggestive of deliberate trauma. Slapping

Table 26.1 Factors Associated with an Increased Risk of Child Abuse

Child	Parent	Both
Prematurity, age under 1 year	Partner violence within the family	Neighborhood factors
Intellectual disability	History of past abuse or neglect	Crime
Physical disability	Substance abuse	Poor recreational activities
Congenital anomalies	Mental health disorders	Low socioeconomic status
Clinging	Unemployment	Poor parent–child relationships
Excessive or inconsolable crying	Lack of external support	Substandard housing
Expectations inconsistent with normal child development	Black child in single-parent household	Poor impulse control
Toilet training or toilet accidents (preschoolers)	Adolescent in age/young parental age	Rely on children for emotional support

Modified from Swerdlin A, Berkowitz C, Craft N. Cutaneous signs of child abuse. *J Am Acad Dermatol.* 2007;57:371–92; Peck MD, Priolo-Kapel D. Child abuse by burning: a review of the literature and an algorithm for medical investigations. *J Trauma.* 2002;53:1013–22; Dubowitz H, Bennett S. Physical abuse and neglect of children. *Lancet.* 2007;369:1891–99; Petska HW, Sheets LK. Sentinel injuries. Subtle findings of physical abuse. *Pediatr Clin N Am.* 2014;61:923–35.

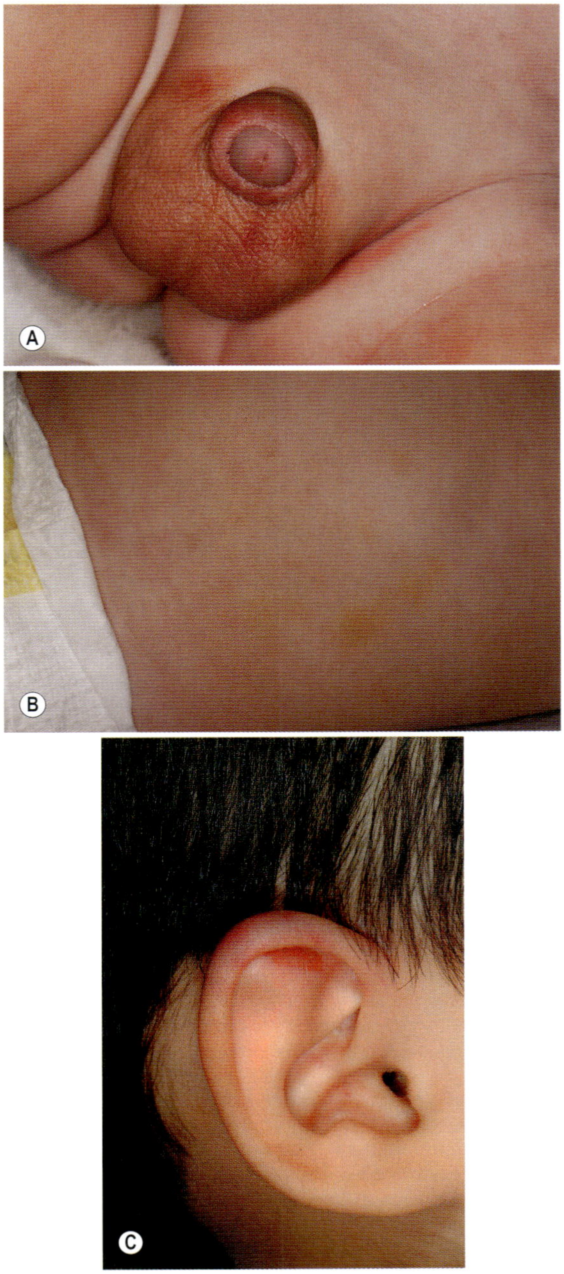

Fig. 26.1 Child abuse. Ecchymoses in certain locations, such these lesions noted on the genitalia **(A)**, abdomen **(B)**, and superior ear **(C)**, are more suggestive of nonaccidental trauma. Of ear ecchymoses, the most concerning location for abuse-associated bruising is the earlobe.

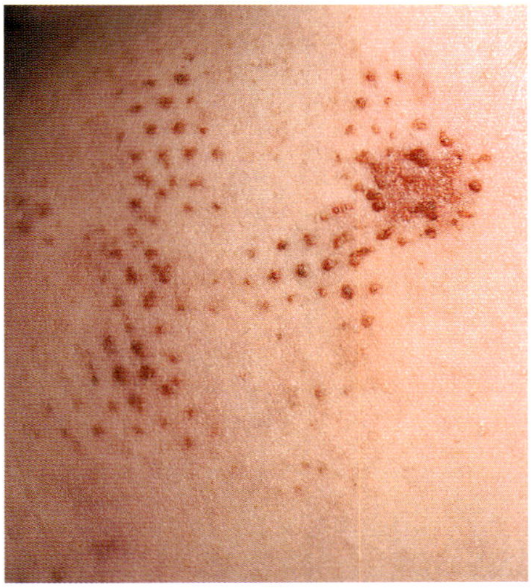

Fig. 26.2 Child abuse. The evenly spaced nature of these markings should arouse suspicion for an outside source of these skin findings.

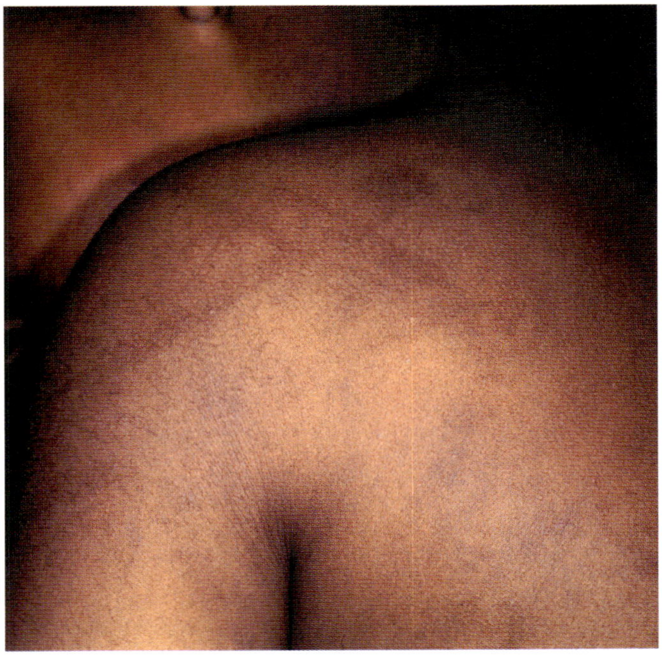

Fig. 26.3 Child abuse. These multiple overlapping, linear, and hyperpigmented patches were the result of postinflammatory changes at sites of whipping.

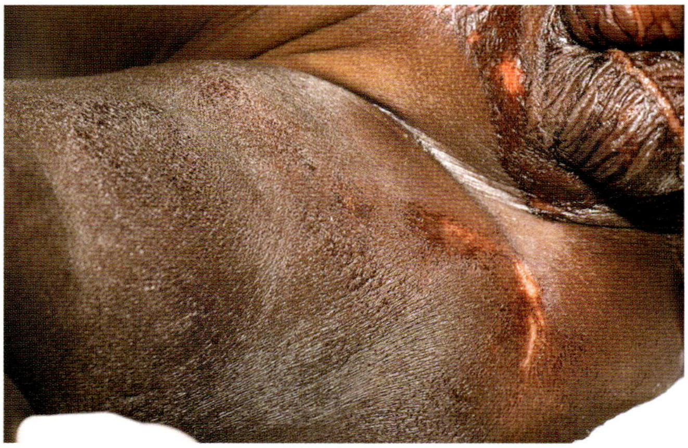

Fig. 26.4 Child abuse. These burns, the result of intentional contact with a hot wire, presented as curvilinear erosions.

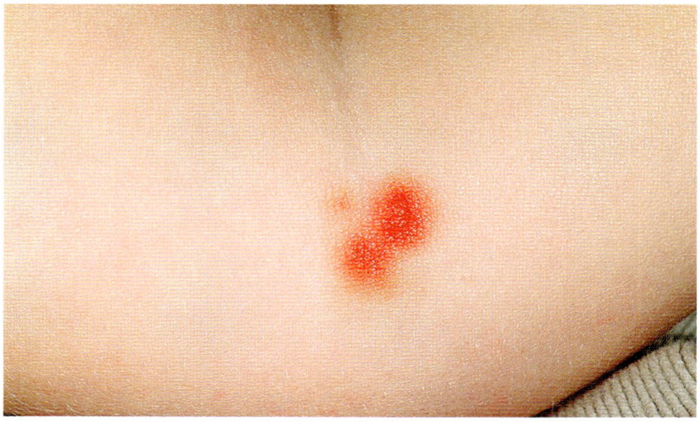

Fig. 26.5 Child abuse. Adjacent ecchymotic macules are typical of pinch marks.

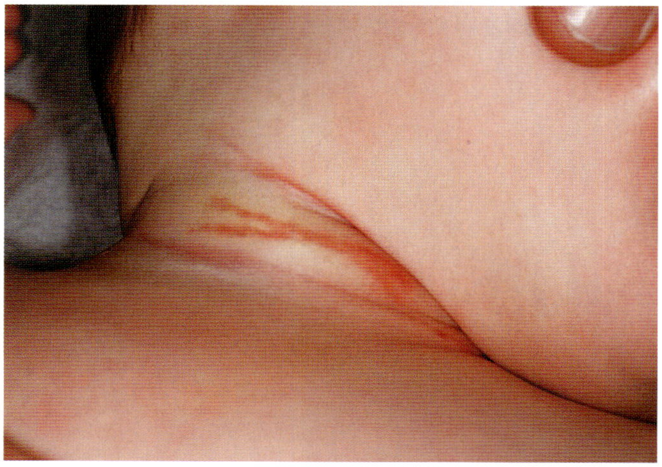

Fig. 26.6 Child abuse. These petechial linear abrasions were believed to be the result of a strangulation attempt in a child who had numerous other skin manifestations of abuse.

injuries result in linear bruising that outlines the blunt objects (fingers) because of the breakage of superficial skin capillaries. *Çao gio* ("coining") and cupping, Asian customs believed to treat a variety of ailments, may be confused with ecchymotic lesions of abuse and must be appropriately recognized (see Cutaneous Mimickers of Abuse and Factitial Disorders section).

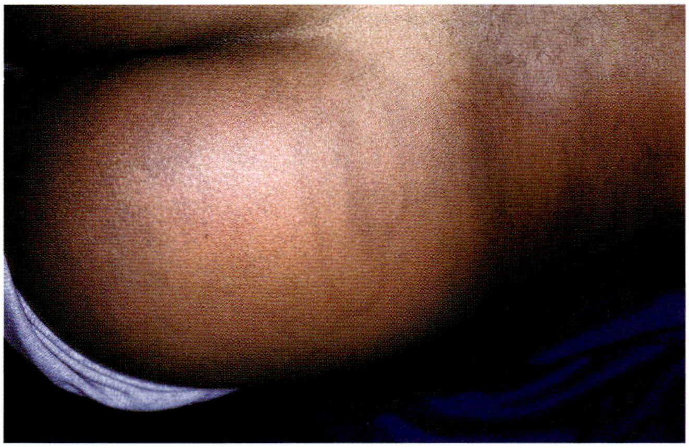

Fig. 26.7 Child abuse. Fingertip bruises present as hyperpigmented patches in the shape of fingers at sites of excessive slapping or spanking.

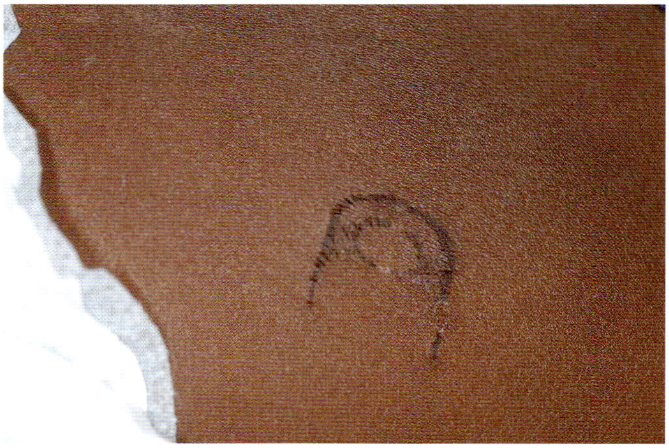

Fig. 26.8 Child abuse. This geographically shaped burn was believed to have been inflicted with the heated metal end of a disposable cigarette lighter.

Burns are a very common type of injury seen in abused children and result from thermal injury to the skin and subcutaneous tissues. Burns can also be electrical, chemical, or radiant in nature. Thermal burns may be inflicted with cigarettes, matches, scalding liquid, or other heated objects (Fig. 26.8) and are often mistaken for lesions of impetigo. Cigarette burns present as 8- to 10-mm, deep, round, crusted ulcers that heal with scars and pigmentary changes (Figs. 26.9 and 26.10). Although they may be accidental, multiple lesions with deeper involvement and significant scarring are highly indicative of abuse, because this pattern is usually suggestive of prolonged contact. The differential diagnosis of cigarette burns includes ecthyma, cellulitis, herpes, and bullous impetigo. Burns inflicted with cigarette lighters are nearly always intentional, given that a minimal sustained flame time of 50 seconds is required for a typical cigarette lighter to reach a temperature capable of inflicting such thermal damage.[15]

Branding injuries occur after prolonged contact with a heated object, and they may take on the shape of the object used to inflict them. Burns inflicted with a hot iron (Figs. 26.11 and 26.12) reveal differing pigmentary changes between the heated metal surface and the steam vent openings. Figs. 26.13 and 26.14 demonstrate burns inflicted by a heated metal spoon, with the shape of the spoon readily visible in the resultant skin markings. Dunking scald injuries are most commonly seen in infants and toddlers and present with a characteristic "stocking and glove" distribution on the extremities or with "doughnut-type sparing" that occurs when the child's buttocks are held against the cooler tub or basin.[9] These patients have erythema and blistering indicative of a second-degree burn. It should be remembered that children will not

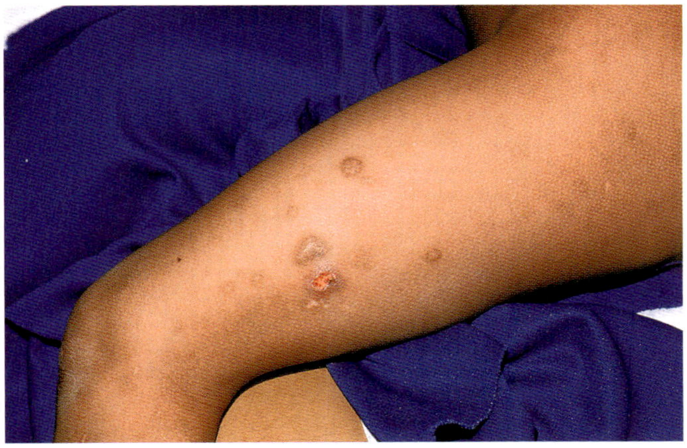

Fig. 26.9 Cigarette burns. This patient has evidence of fresh lesions (erythematous, eroded plaque) and older lesions in the forms of hyperpigmentation and scars.

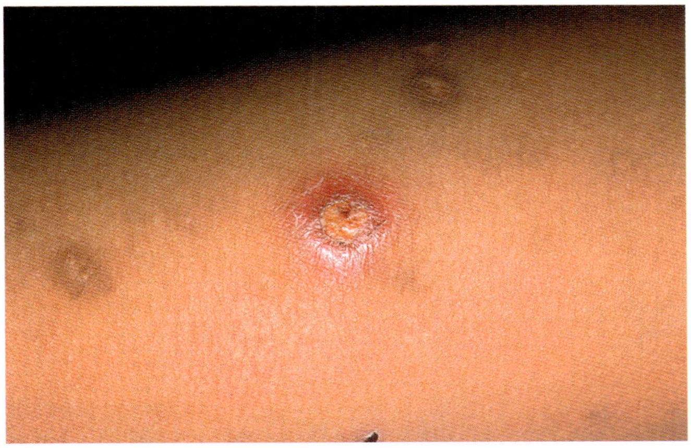

Fig. 26.10 Cigarette burns. These burns demonstrate the classic abuse finding of lesions in various stages of healing.

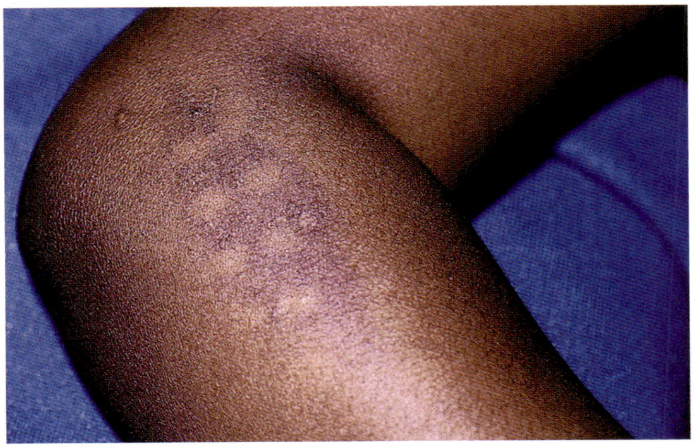

Fig. 26.11 Iron burn. This hyperpigmented patch is studded with evenly spaced, normally pigmented regions that correlate with sites of steam vent openings.

stay in contact with a hot surface or scalding hot water. They normally test the heat of the water and step into the bath with one foot at a time. Accordingly, symmetric burns on the feet, the buttocks, or the hands require careful investigation and evaluation. Stun-gun injuries have been observed in the setting of physical abuse and present as evenly

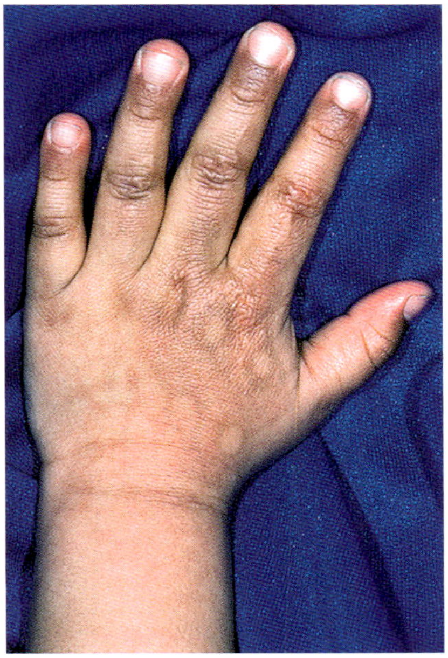

Fig. 26.12 Iron burn. This child's hand reveals the classic hyperpigmentation with evenly spaced macules of sparing that occur at sites of steam vent openings.

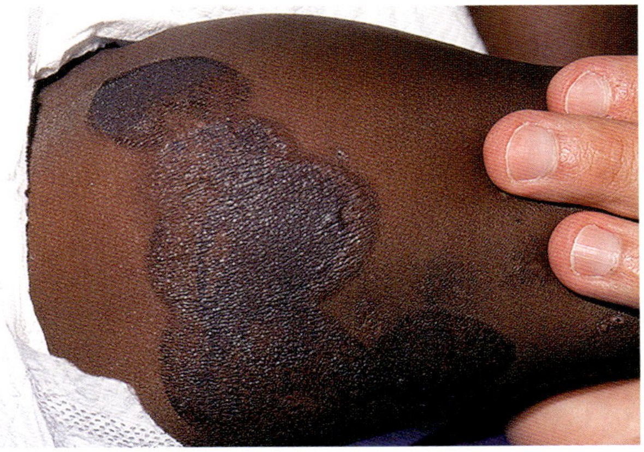

Fig. 26.13 Child abuse. This infant had burns inflicted with a heated metal spoon. Note the overlapping oval-shaped patches of pigmentation and crusting.

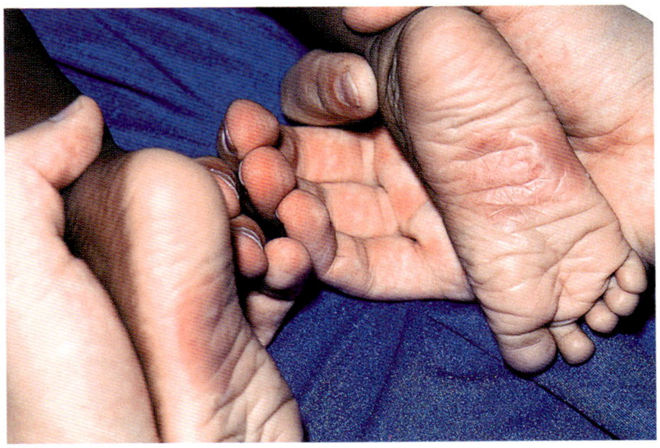

Fig. 26.14 Child abuse. The same infant as that shown in Fig. 26.13 had these blistering burns on the plantar surfaces. They were inflicted with a heated metal spoon.

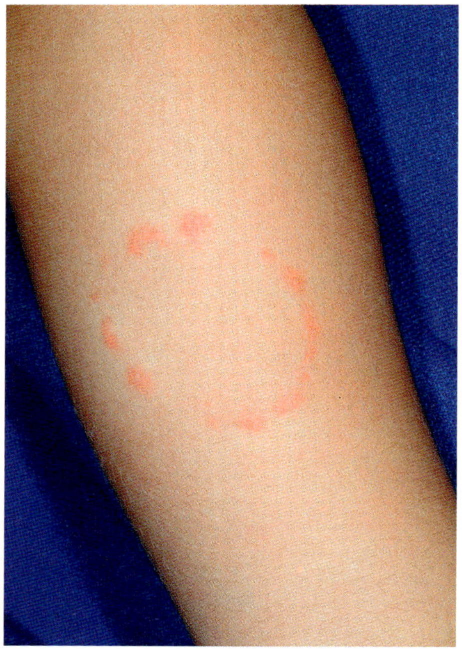

Fig. 26.15 Bite marks. These erythematous, petechial macules and papules revealed a dental arch width of 2.5 cm, more consistent with a child's bite. There were no other clinical features of (or concerns for) child abuse in this 2-year-old girl.

spaced (4 to 5 cm apart), erythematous to hypopigmented papules and macules, usually occurring in multiples.[16]

Bite marks are another pathognomonic sign of nonaccidental trauma. The human bite is differentiated easily from the dog bite by the contusing and crushing characteristics of the latter; dog bites rip and tear the flesh. It is important to distinguish adult from child bite marks because the former is more likely to be seen in an abusive setting. Adult bites are characterized by a dental arch width greater than 3 cm, whereas the markings of a child's bite tend to be significantly narrower than 3 cm (Fig. 26.15). The discovery of one bite mark necessitates a thorough examination of the child's entire body for further evidence of bites or other findings of abuse.[17] Traumatic alopecia may occur when the parent pulls the child's hair because the hair provides a readily accessible "handle" that can be used to grab or jerk at the child. The resultant alopecia is an irregularly bordered area that may reveal hemorrhage, hair breakage, and scalp tenderness.

Oral injuries are another common feature in abused children. Findings may include tears of the labial or lingual frenulum caused by a blow to the mouth, forced feeding, or forced oral sex.[17] Other manifestations include burns or lacerations of the gingivae, tongue, or palate from overly hot food or utensils. Teeth may also be involved, including fracture, displacement, or avulsion.

A difficult situation arises when the physician observes recent skin injuries in the child who does not seek treatment for trauma. In one large series, 76% of children between 9 months and 17 years of age seen in a clinic for a reason other than trauma were found to have at least one recent skin injury. Injuries were more prevalent in the summer (in regions with a temperate climate) and were most commonly observed on the shins and knees.[18] The authors offered certain unusual characteristics that may suggest a greater risk of physical abuse (or bleeding disorder), and these include uncommon location; more than 15 injuries; bruises in a child younger than 9 months of age; numerous injuries elsewhere than the lower limbs; numerous injuries in cold seasons in a temperate climate; and injuries other than bruises, abrasions, or scratches.[18] In another series of infants aged 6 to 12 months, bruises were noted to be generally limited to the face, head, or shins, and there was a direct correlation between the number of bruises and increases in mobility.[19] In this group, the prevalence rate of bruises was 12%, and they were most often solitary.

SEXUAL ABUSE

Sexual abuse has been defined in many ways, including "any exploitative sexual activity between a child and an adult"; "any sexual activity that a child cannot comprehend or give consent to, or that violates the law"; or "when a child is engaged in sexual activities that he/she cannot comprehend, for which he/she is developmentally unprepared and cannot give consent, and/or that violates the law or social taboos of society."[9,20,21] Studies have suggested that between 5% and 25% of adults report having been sexually abused as a child, and in 2006, the Fourth National Incidence Study on Child Abuse and Neglect found an estimated 1.8 children per 1000 population were victims of sexual abuse.[22] It is important to realize that boys may be the victims of sexual abuse as well as girls, although the former tend to be less likely to disclose abuse, and thus it is likely underreported, underrecognized, and undertreated.[23] Adolescents are the perpetrators in up to 20% of reported cases of sexual abuse, and although women may be perpetrators, these allegations are significantly less likely than those involving males.[21] Up to one-fifth of adolescents who regularly use the Internet have been solicited by strangers for sex through the Internet. Childhood sexual abuse may lead to a variety of physical and mental symptoms and disorders, including depression, suicidal ideation, eating disorders, low self-esteem, and posttraumatic stress disorder.[24] In one large meta-analysis, sexual abuse early in life was a significant risk factor for suicide attempts, with a pooled odds ratio of 1.89 when compared with the baseline population.[25]

The perpetrator of childhood sexual abuse is often well known or related to the victim. Activities involved in sexual abuse may include oral–genital, genital, or anal contact by or to the child, as well as nonphysical abuses such as voyeurism, exhibitionism, or involvement of the child in pornography.[21] Sexual abuse should be differentiated from "sexual play" or age-appropriate exploratory behavior. The child who has been sexually abused may exhibit a variety of features, including behavioral changes, school difficulties, regression, depression, eating disturbance, sexual acting out, symptoms referable to the genitourinary or gastrointestinal tracts, pregnancy, various somatic complaints, or a sexually transmitted infection (STI).[20]

Mucocutaneous findings suggestive of sexual abuse are listed in Table 26.2. However, it should be noted that many children who have been sexually abused in the past may have a relatively normal physical examination. Many prepubescent patients seen in emergency departments for a sexual abuse evaluation have not experienced recent

Table 26.2 Mucocutaneous Findings in Childhood Sexual Abuse

Finding	Comment
Hymenal changes	Attenuated hymenal tissue, disruption of hymenal contour; acute laceration or ecchymosis, petechiae
Anal area changes	Boys and girls; changes in anal tone, hematomas, abrasions, lacerations; scarring, skin tags; dilation
Fossa navicularis or posterior fourchette scarring	Lacerations
Inner thigh changes	Abrasions, ecchymosis (concerning but not diagnostic)
Labia minora changes	Scarring or tears (concerning but not diagnostic)
Other genital injuries	Circumferential injuries to penile shaft or glans penis; lacerations of penis, scrotum, perineum, labia, vagina
Oral injuries or diseases	Unexplained erythema or petechiae of the palate; oral or perioral gonorrhea or syphilis (pathognomonic for sexual abuse in the prepubertal child)

Table 26.3 Implications of Sexually Transmitted Diseases and Clinical Findings for the Diagnosis of Childhood Sexual Abuse

STD or Finding	Implication for Abuse	Suggested Action
Gonorrhea*	Diagnostic	Report
Syphilis*	Diagnostic	Report
HIV infection*,†	Diagnostic	Report
Chlamydia*	Diagnostic	Report
Trichomoniasis	Highly suspicious	Report
Anogenital warts*,‡	Suspicious	Report
Genital herpes§	Suspicious	Report
Bacterial vaginosis	Inconclusive	Clinical follow-up care
Presence of sperm, semen, or acid phosphatase	Diagnostic	Report
Pregnancy	Diagnostic	Report

Modified from Swerdlin A, Berkowitz C, Craft N. Cutaneous signs of child abuse. *J Am Acad Dermatol.* 2007;57:371–92 and Kellogg N, American Academy of Pediatrics Committee on Child Abuse and Neglect. The evaluation of sexual abuse in children. *Pediatrics.* 2005;116(2):506–12.
HIV, Human immunodeficiency virus; *STD,* sexually transmitted disease.
*If not perinatally acquired.
†If not transfusion acquired.
‡Not uncommonly transmitted via benign mode; see discussion in Chapter 15.
§Unless caused by autoinoculation.

abuse, in distinction to adolescents, who often come after the acute assault.[26] A normal anogenital examination therefore does not preclude prior sexual abuse. The physical examination should be most focused on areas involved in sexual activity, including the mouth, breasts, genitals, perineum, buttocks, and anus. In females, a more thorough examination of the medial thighs, labia majora and minora, clitoris, urethra, hymen and hymenal opening, fossa navicularis, and posterior fourchette should be included.[21] In males, the thighs, penis, and scrotum should be closely examined.

Examinations for STIs should be performed when indicated. Factors to be considered include the possibility of oral, genital, or rectal contact and the child's symptomatology. Table 26.3 summarizes the implications of various STIs and clinical findings for reporting childhood sexual abuse. Anogenital warts, which may be sexually transmitted in children, are often the result of benign, nonsexual transmission, especially in infants and young toddlers (see Chapter 15). Nonsexual modes of transmission include perinatal transmission, autoinoculation (child with common warts spreads them via skin-to-skin contact to his or her own anogenital region), heteroinoculation (caregiver with common warts spreads them via skin-to-skin contact to anogenital region of child), and possibly indirect spread from fomites. Importantly, molluscum contagiosum lesions involving the anogenital region in children are nearly always a result of benign transmission or autoinoculation and should not be considered indicative of childhood sexual abuse. The details of the evaluation, treatment, and reporting of childhood sexual abuse are beyond the scope of this chapter but are well documented elsewhere. Importantly, however, when the diagnosis of childhood sexual abuse is being considered, review of the case with an expert in such evaluations (such as a child abuse pediatrician) is advisable. In the primary care office, five issues should be addressed: the child's imminent safety, reporting to child protective authorities, the child's mental health, the need for a thorough physical examination, and the need to collect forensic evidence (in a specialized clinic or qualified emergency department).[22] Recent data suggest that five or more examinations per month may be required for ongoing competency in the interpretation of medical and laboratory findings in children in whom sexual abuse is suspected.[27] Although the medical history is the most important piece of evidence in the evaluation for childhood sexual abuse, physical examination findings are extremely important to the subsequent investigation and potential legal action, and findings must be exquisitely documented, with photographic documentation recommended.[28]

NEGLECT

Neglect may be either physical, emotional, or both. The former results when a parent or caretaker fails to provide necessities of life such as food, appropriate supervision, shelter, clothing, or medical care.[9] General findings in the neglected child may include lack of immunizations, poor nutrition and growth, and developmental or behavioral problems. Potential cutaneous findings include poor hygiene, untreated injuries, infections, and infestations. Severe or extensive sunburns (Fig. 26.16) may be a sign of parental neglect, although several conditions and medications may make children more sensitive to ultraviolet light. It is important to bear these in mind whenever the possibility of neglect or abuse is being considered.

Physical neglect may also present as dental neglect, which is defined as the "willful failure of parent or guardian, despite adequate access to care, to seek and follow through with treatment necessary to ensure a level of oral health essential for adequate function and freedom from pain and infection."[29] Findings may include dental caries, periodontal disease (Fig. 26.17), and other oral conditions. When left untreated, these conditions can lead to significant pain, infection, and loss of function, and these outcomes can adversely affect learning, nutrition, normal growth and development, and communication ability.[29]

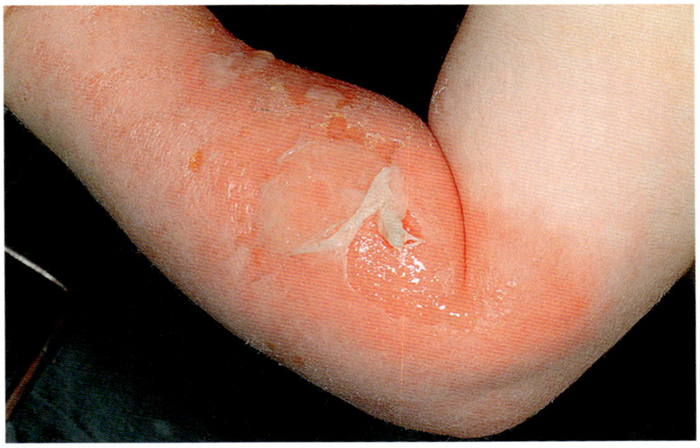

Fig. 26.16 Neglect. This toddler came to the clinic for a routine follow-up examination for eczema and was noted to have this blistering sunburn.

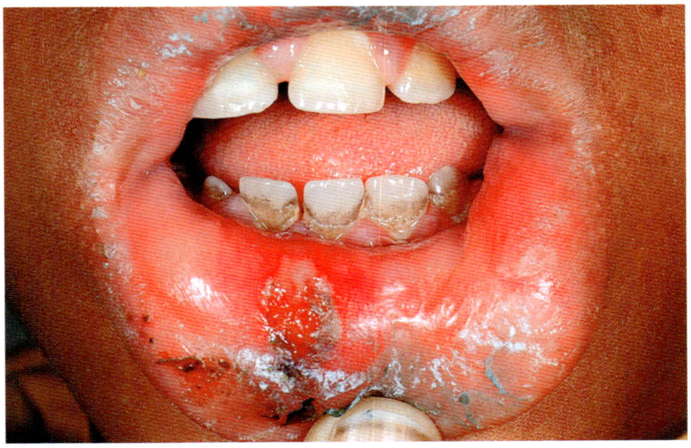

Fig. 26.17 Neglect. Dental neglect in this young boy presented as dental caries, periodontal disease, and aphthous ulcerations of the labial surfaces. This lesion was also culture-positive for herpes simplex virus.

Factitial Skin Disorders

Factitial skin disorders (also called *self-inflicted skin lesions*) are a group of disorders characterized by self-inflicted lesions or artifacts on the skin. The individual cases vary in terms of the visible lesions and the underlying motive that causes the patient to act. These disorders may be associated with a variety of psychopathologic conditions, and comanagement with a psychologist or psychiatrist is often necessary. Factitial skin disorders fall under the rubric of psychodermatologic conditions or psychocutaneous disorders, although these two classifications also include dermatologic conditions with secondary psychiatric sequelae (alopecia areata or albinism) and dermatologic conditions that may be aggravated by psychological factors (acne, atopic dermatitis, psoriasis).[30] Diagnosis of factitial skin disorders is often delayed, and management is challenging, requiring the development of a therapeutic alliance between the physician and patient and treatment of any underlying psychiatric comorbid conditions. The diagnosis of factitial skin disorders largely remains a diagnosis of exclusion.[31] Treatment often requires a multidisciplinary approach that may include the pediatrician, dermatologist, psychologist, and/or psychiatrist.

FACTITIOUS DERMATITIS/DERMATITIS ARTEFACTA

Factitious dermatitis is one type of factitious disorder that is caused by a conscious or subconscious behavior driven in response to internal psychological stressors and not associated with secondary gain.[31] *Dermatitis artefacta (DA)* is often the terminology used to describe a disorder in which the skin is the purposeful target of self-inflicted injuries. In DA, the patient creates the lesions on the skin in order to satisfy a psychological need (of which he or she is often not consciously aware) and in the pursuit of secondary gain.[31,32] There appears to be the need to satisfy an internal emotional necessity—the need to be cared for.[33,34] The desired gain may be obvious or may not be readily evident. DA occurs predominantly among women, with a wide range in the quoted ratios of women to men, from 3:1 to 20:1.[33] It may have its onset at any time, although it most commonly occurs in teenagers and young adults. When it occurs in children, DA may be related to various stressors, including school examinations, bullying, and discord in the home.[35] Several comorbid conditions may be present, including borderline personality disorder, disorders of impulse control, depression, anxiety, obsessive-compulsive disorder (OCD), and psychotic disorders.[30,32,34,36] It may also result from a transient maladaptive response to a recent psychosocial stressor(s). A past and/or current history of sexual abuse is common.[33,37] Patients with DA often have a close connection (either personally or through a close family member) with the health care field, and many have an "encyclopedic" grasp of medical knowledge and/or terminology. Some have suggested abandoning the terms *factitial dermatitis* and *DA* in favor of the terminology *factitious disorders in dermatology*.[38] Management of these disorders can be extremely challenging and frustrating and requires establishment of a trusting relationship between the patient, family, and clinician; many families decline psychiatric referral, given denial of a psychological component.[39]

DA has a variety of presentation patterns. Importantly, the cutaneous features are often only one facet of the entire picture because these patients often have involvement of other organ systems and have visited numerous medical specialists for other bizarre or unexplained symptoms. The skin lesions themselves may consist of purpura, excoriations, abrasions, crusting, necrosis, blisters, ulcers, erythema, nodules, hematomas, or scarring. When blisters are present (bullous DA), modes of injury often include thermal, electrical, or chemical injury.[40] The lesions of DA usually lack features of recognizable dermatoses. Notable features often include linearity, geometric arrangements, and sharp demarcation from the surrounding normal skin. The face, upper trunk, and upper extremities are the sites most often involved, and there is notable sparing of areas outside of the patient's reach (e.g., the middle back). There is often a prominence on one side, depending on the handedness of the patient. The lips may also be involved, presenting usually as persistent bleeding and crusting.[41] Presentation as recurrent atypical periorbital cellulitis has been reported.[42] The lesions are often fully formed and are all in a similar stage of development. The inability of the patient to give details of evolutionary change has been termed *hollow history* and is quite typical of DA.[32,33,43] Although skin biopsies are not routinely performed, the presence of multinucleated epithelial cells appears to be a common finding in DA and may provide a clue to the diagnosis.[44] Reported modes of injury include rubbing; scratching; picking; cutting; gouging; pinching; puncturing; biting; sucking; applying suction; applying heat, dye, or caustic substances; and injecting caustic materials or bodily secretions.[30,32] The differential diagnosis may be broad and depends on the nature of the inflicted injury. A clue to the diagnosis of DA is indifference or lack of concern on the part of the patient, who will often deny pain or discomfort despite the impressive physical findings.[31] Bullous DA caused by thermal injury may result after the "salt and ice challenge," a dare contest in which participants sprinkle salt on the skin followed by compression with an ice cube.[45]

Box 26.1 Entities Which May Be Considered Before Reaching the Diagnosis of Factitious Purpura

- Coagulopathies
- Vasculitides including Henoch–Schönlein purpura, Takayasu arteritis
- Infections
  - Meningococcemia
  - Rickettsial disorders
- Leukemia, other malignancy
- Child abuse/caregiver-fabricated illness
- Connective tissue disorders (e.g., Ehlers–Danlos syndrome)
- Hereditary hemorrhagic telangiectasia
- Cultural folk remedies (e.g., coining, cupping)

Adapted from Ring HC, Miller IM, Benfeldt E, Jemec GBE. Artefactual skin lesions in children and adolescents: review of the literature and two cases of factitious purpura. *Int J Dermatol*. 2015;54:e27–32.

Factitious purpura, which is a form of mechanical purpura, may result in a detailed, lengthy investigation for other medical causes before the diagnosis is entertained (Box 26.1). Patients may be entirely unaware that they are causing the skin lesions. A common form of factitious purpura is that caused by sucking air from a drinking glass placed over the chin and lower lip, resulting in a well-demarcated, circular area of purpura (Fig. 26.18).[46] Other forms may be caused by a variety of instruments or objects, with the purpuric lesions corresponding to the patterns of those objects. Figs. 26.19 through 26.31 depict some various presentations of DA.

Malingering may present with lesions similar to DA, but in this setting the patient self-inflicts injury consciously, often with a secondary gain. These patients may exhibit "*la belle indifference*," which refers to an apparent lack of frustration, despite the recurrent nature of their symptomatology.

Neurotic (psychogenic) excoriations are lesions self-inflicted by patients who have an irresistible urge to manipulate their skin.[34] It is

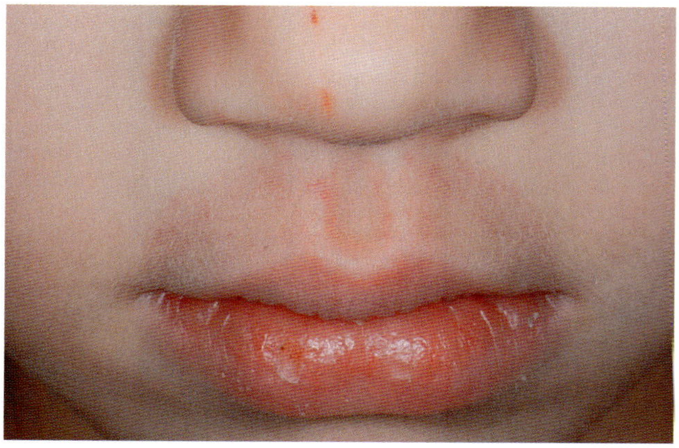

Fig. 26.18 Suction purpura. This well-demarcated, petechial patch over the upper lip and philtrum area arose after this young girl repeatedly sucked air from a cup placed over her lips and upper chin.

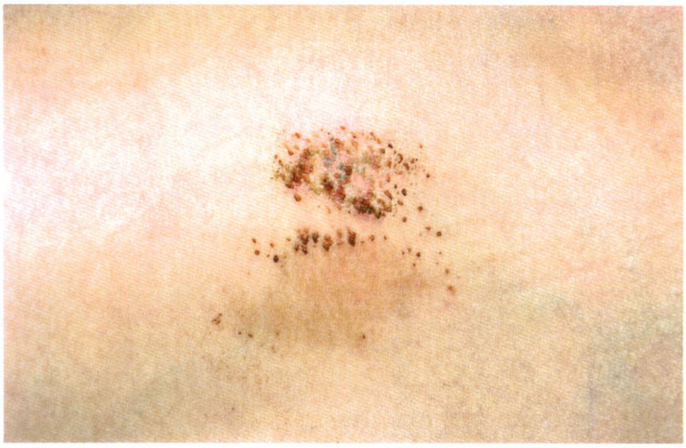

Fig. 26.19 Dermatitis artefacta. Well-demarcated abrasions and hyperpigmentation in a 10-year-old boy.

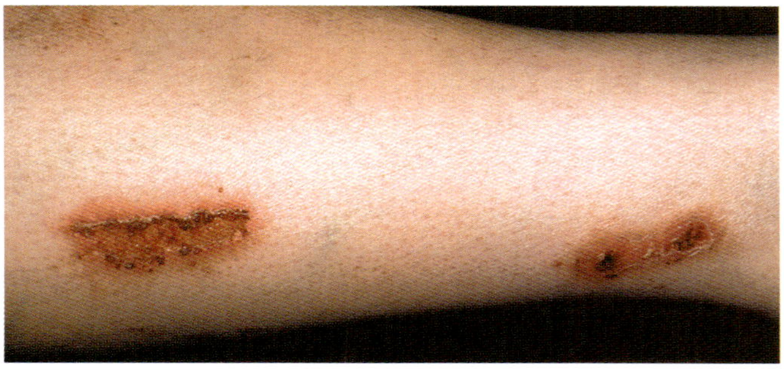

Fig. 26.20 Dermatitis artefacta. Sharply demarcated, eroded, erythematous plaques from chronic rubbing.

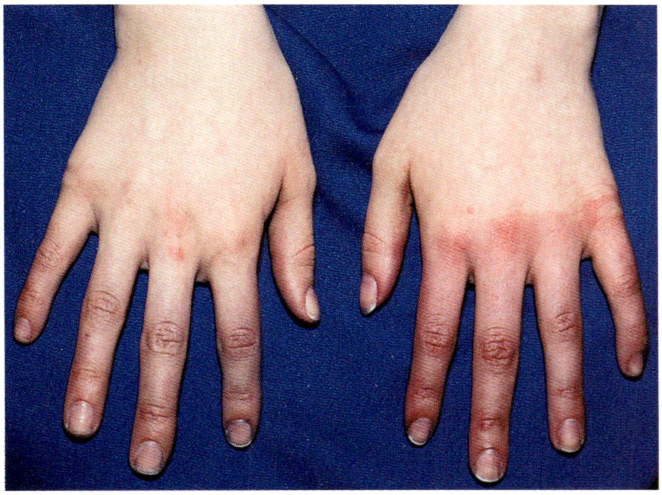

Fig. 26.21 Dermatitis artefacta. This localized discoloration of the hand had been caused by intentional exposure to fabric dye.

often related to mood disorders, anxiety disorder, drug abuse, or OCD.[47] The cycle of neurotic excoriations may begin with a true physical stimulus, such as pruritus, or a skin lesion or irregularity, such as an acne papule. The latter is referred to as *acne excoriée des jeunes filles* and occurs when even mild acne lesions (especially

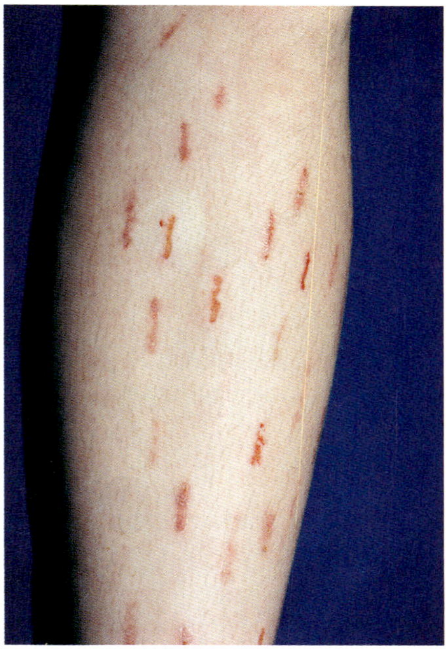

Fig. 26.22 Dermatitis artefacta. These evenly spaced, linear, hemorrhagic markings were self-induced.

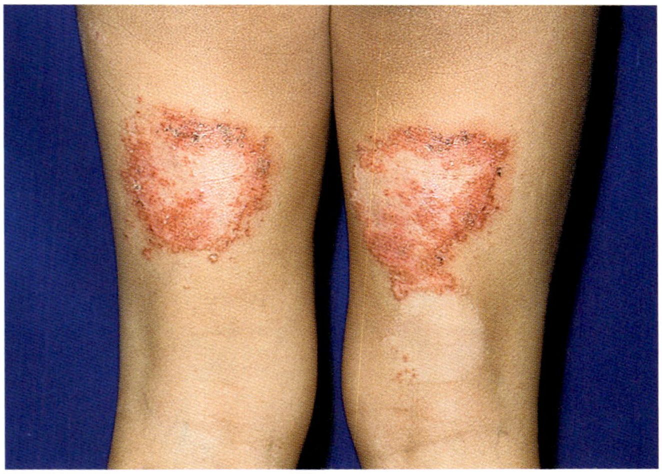

Fig. 26.23 Dermatitis artefacta. This patient with underlying atopic dermatitis had acute worsening in these areas, which ultimately was found to be self-inflicted.

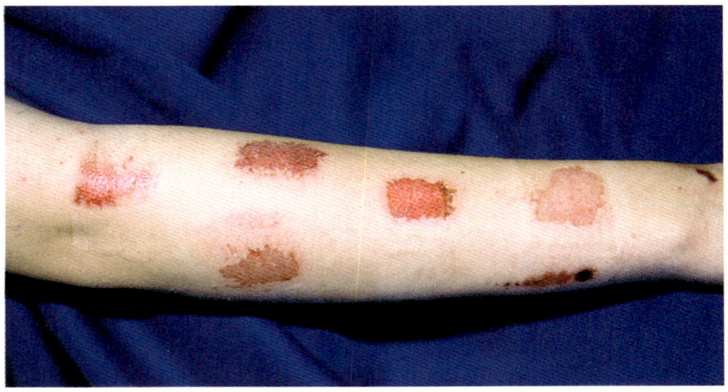

Fig. 26.24 Dermatitis artefacta. These well-demarcated erosions are notable for their even spacing and sharp, linear borders.

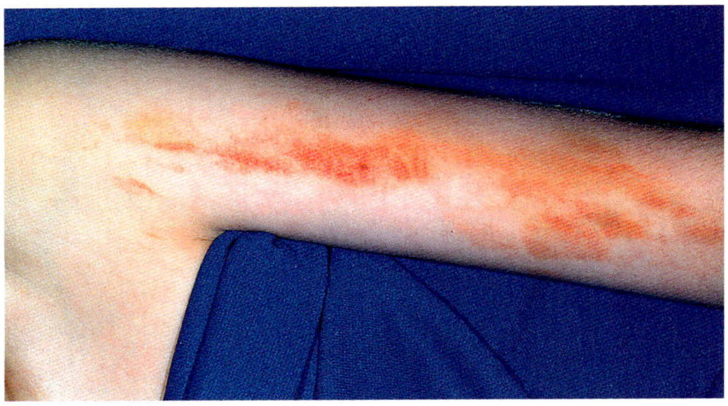

Fig. 26.25 Dermatitis artefacta. Linear purpura is a common finding in factitial skin disease.

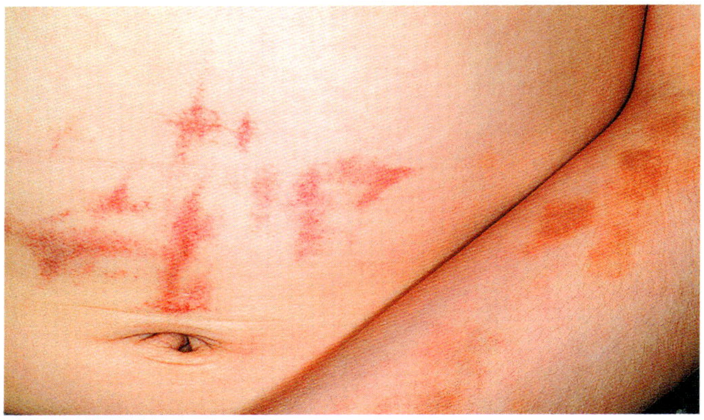

Fig. 26.26 Dermatitis artefacta. These linear and stellate purpuric patches were present in the same patient shown in Fig. 26.25. Note the associated resolving purpuric areas located on the arm.

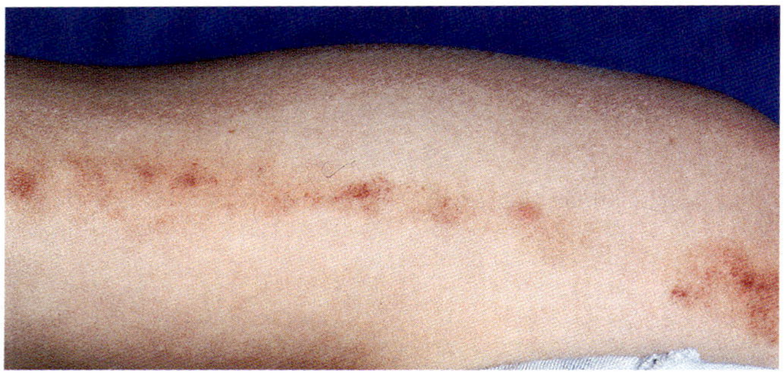

Fig. 26.27 Dermatitis artefacta. Linear purpura was present on both arms of this school-age boy.

those on the forehead) are squeezed or excoriated (Fig. 26.32). This behavior may result in permanent scarring, and although some patients may fulfill diagnostic criteria for OCD, many do not. Patients with neurotic excoriations usually acknowledge the behavior and may have any of several comorbid conditions, including OCD, a personality disorder, anxiety, or depression. The picking activity is performed most often with the fingernails, although some patients may use an auxiliary tool such as the point of a knife.[24] The resultant skin lesions reveal erythema, erosions, weeping, crusting (Fig. 26.33), pigmentation, or scarring. There is often a notable sparing of the

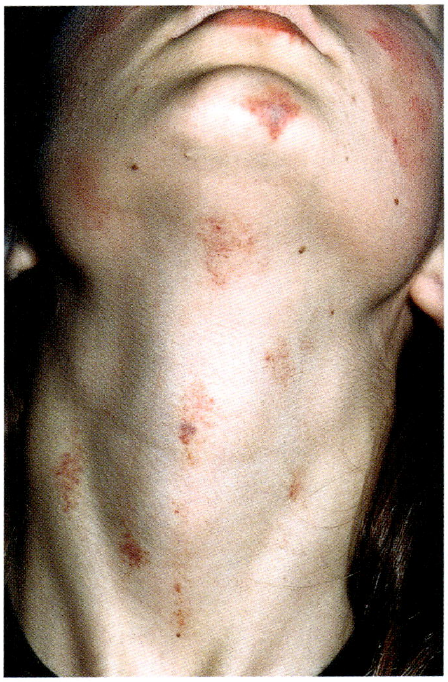

Fig. 26.28 Dermatitis artefacta. Irregularly shaped, purpuric patches of the neck and face.

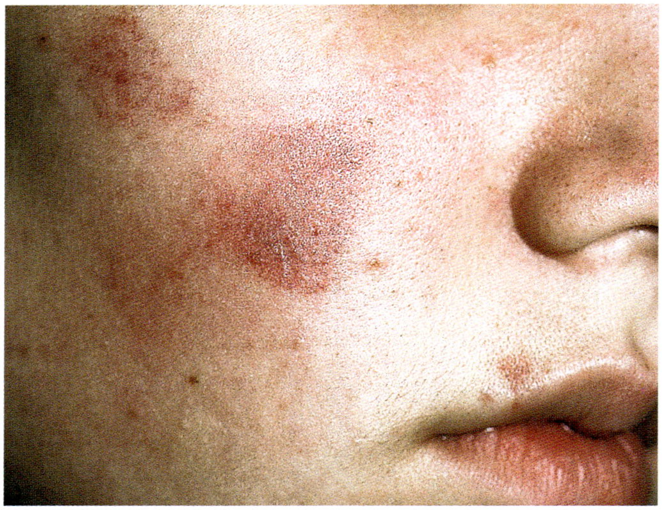

Fig. 26.29 Dermatitis artefacta. Purpuric patches with geometric and linear borders in the same patient shown in Fig. 26.28.

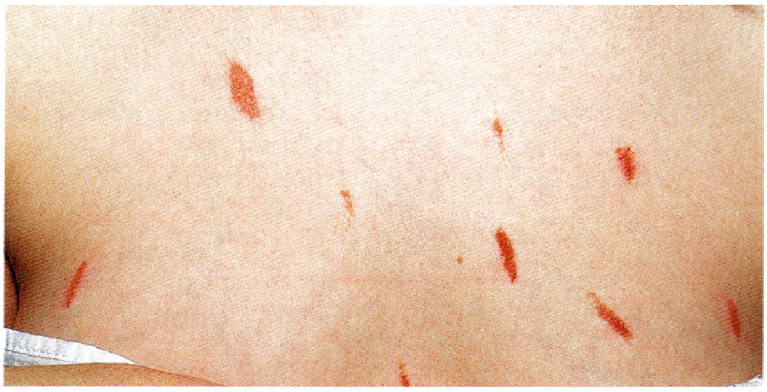

Fig. 26.30 Dermatitis artefacta. Well-demarcated, linear, purpuric macules.

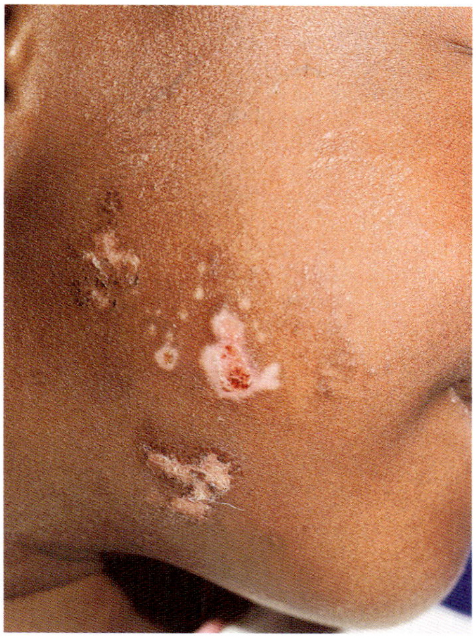

Fig. 26.31 Dermatitis artefacta. These eroded and scarred plaques reveal irregular borders consistent with self-manipulation.

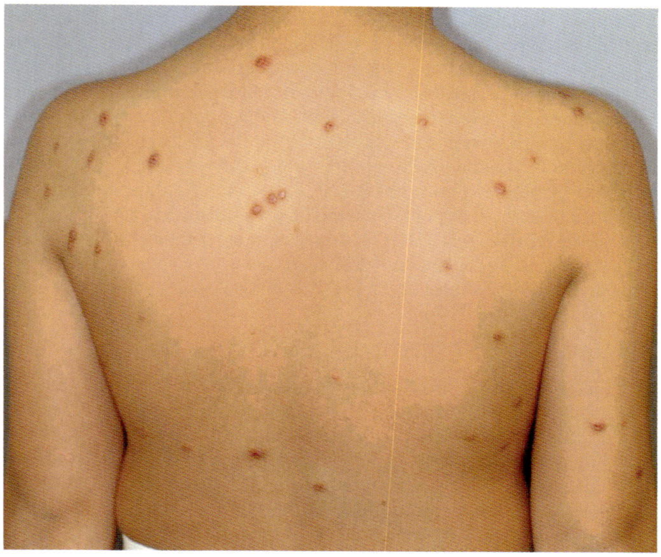

Fig. 26.34 Prurigo nodularis. This boy had numerous discrete, lichenified firm papules on his upper and lower back, forearms, and lower extremities. Note the zone of sparing over the middle back, an area that was difficult for him to reach.

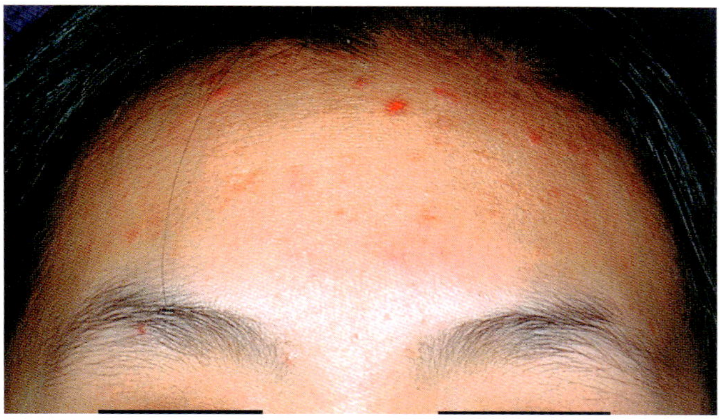

Fig. 26.32 Acne excoriée. Acne papules with erosions, scarring, and hyperpigmentation are typical of this condition.

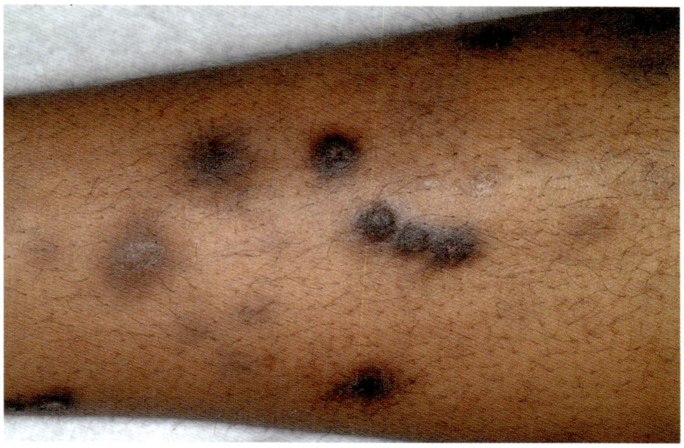

Fig. 26.35 Prurigo nodularis. Firm, lichenified, hyperpigmented papules were present on the arms and legs of this 9-year-old girl.

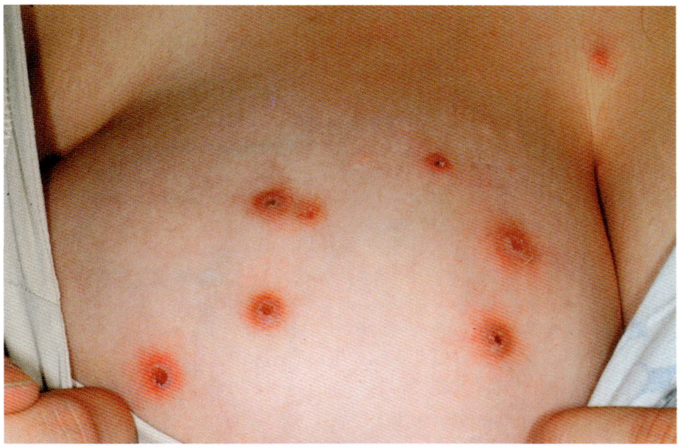

Fig. 26.33 Neurotic excoriation. This adolescent girl acknowledged her repeated picking and scratching, which resulted in these erythematous eroded and crusted papules on her bilateral breasts.

upper lateral back areas. Self-inflicted facial excoriations in toddlers may represent *midface toddler excoriation syndrome (MiTES)*, which may be associated with neurologic deficits or congenital insensitivity to pain; parents of the reported children with this condition acknowledge the self-induced nature.[48]

Prurigo nodularis (PN) is a condition characterized by firm papules and nodules with pruritus. It most typically presents with discrete, 2- to 10-mm, firm, lichenified hyperkeratotic papules that may reveal some central excoriation or crusting (Figs. 26.34 and 26.35). Common locations include the extremities and the upper and lower back, often with a zone of sparing noted in the middle back, which is a difficult location for the patient to reach. The cause of PN is unknown. It has been seen in a variety of settings, including bite reactions, atopic dermatitis (see Fig. 3.17), allergic contact dermatitis, folliculitis, psychosocial disorders, thyroid disease, malignancy, iron-deficiency anemia, kidney failure, gluten sensitivity, obstructive biliary disease, and infections (including hepatitis, human immunodeficiency virus [HIV], and mycobacteria).[49,50] If generalized pruritus is reported by the patient, a laboratory investigation (including blood counts, kidney and liver function tests, and thyroid and parathyroid screening) may be warranted.[50] Skin biopsy may be useful if infection is included in the differential diagnosis, but PN is most often a clinical diagnosis. Treatment for PN is notoriously difficult and may include topical corticosteroids or calcineurin inhibitors (tacrolimus and pimecrolimus), topical capsaicin, ultraviolet phototherapy, and antihistamines. In severe cases, systemic agents such as cyclosporine, methotrexate, thalidomide, naltrexone, and etretinate have been used.[49–52] Treatment with the interleukin-4 receptor alpha antagonist dupilumab has been reported useful for patients with generalized and/or treatment-resistant PN.[53–55] Psychological intervention is often necessary, and there appears to be an association between PN and both depression and anxiety.[56]

DELUSIONAL INFESTATION

A delusional disorder is characterized by adherence to a possible, yet implausible, belief for which there is no supportive objective evidence.[57] Monosymptomatic hypochondriacal psychosis (MHP) is characterized by a delusional ideation that revolves around one concern, in contrast to schizophrenia, in which case patients have multifunctional deficits in mental functioning.[58] The most common type of MHP with dermatologic relevance is delusional infestation (DI). This disorder, also known as *delusions of parasitosis*, is characterized by the conviction of an individual that he or she is infested with pathogens in the absence of any objective evidence. The pathogens of concern may be parasites (the most frequently reported concern, hence the prior terminology), insects, worms, bacteria, or fungi. Patients with DI, most often older adult females, complain of having the sensation of crawling, burrowing, and biting insects or worms on their skin. They may complain of stinging or pins-and-needles sensations. They may use pesticides (on themselves, their pets, or household items), hire exterminators, move to an alternative residence, or resort to self-mutilation (using fingernails, tweezers, or other instruments) in an attempt to remove the offending arthropods.[59] A history of psychiatric illness can be elicited in most patients with this disorder.[60] This discussion is focused on primary DI; a secondary form may arise from certain medical conditions such as stroke, cardiovascular disease, vitamin (especially B_{12}) deficiency, diabetes, or psychiatric diagnoses such as schizophrenia or depression.[61]

Patients with DI often attend the clinic with spurious samples of the "parasite" that when microscopically examined turn out to be lint, skin cells, scabs, or other debris. Skin findings may include excoriations, erosions, ulcerations, hair loss, lichenification, pigmentary alteration, secondary infection, and scarring. The delusional beliefs of DI can sometimes be induced upon family members or close friends, and in psychiatric terminology this shared psychosis has been termed *folie a deux* or, when more than two family members are involved, *folie a famille*.[62–63] Treatment of the disorder is challenging, with the antipsychotic medication pimozide being the most often utilized pharmacologic agent. Other utilized agents have included aripiprazole, haloperidol, olanzapine, quetiapine, and risperidone.[59,61,64,65] Before therapy, however, exclusion of true skin disorders (scabies, dermatitis herpetiformis, or insect bite reactions) should be considered.[66] Expertise in interactions with DI patients is valuable and includes strategies to build a trusting alliance, set emotional boundaries, acknowledge the patient's misery, and establish therapeutic rapport.[59,65]

Morgellons disease is a term that initially began to surface in 2002 and whose name was taken from the label, given in 1674 in France by Sir Thomas Browne, to children who had hair-like skin extrusions and sensations of movement.[67] This terminology provides an alternative to the decades-old nomenclature of delusions of parasitosis (DI), although many consider the two disorders to be part of the same spectrum.[68–72] Alternatively, some have reported an association between Morgellons disease and infection with *Borrelia burgdorferi* (the agent of Lyme disease), based on polymerase chain reaction and/or *in situ* DNA hybridization studies, as well as skin cultures, histology, and immunohistochemistry.[73]

Patients with Morgellons disease complain of cutaneous dysesthesias, resulting in skin manipulations in an effort to extract the "organisms," thin fibers, filaments, or other foreign materials. They may experience itching or crawling sensations, and many report the sense that bugs or worms are stinging or biting them. The examination findings may include excoriations, ulcers, lichenification, and prurigo nodules. Patients with Morgellons disease, much like those with DI, may bring samples or debris in bottles, jars, or bags to the appointment. Examination of these contents often reveals lint, hair, debris, fuzz, dead skin, material fibers, or bugs.[69] Others have suggested that the filaments represent biofilaments of human origin composed of collagen and keratin.[73] Management of the condition is difficult and includes establishing good rapport, excluding skin or other organic conditions, consideration for the use of psychotropic medications, and treatment of secondary skin infection when necessary. Low-dose trifluoperazine, a high-potency typical antipsychotic, was shown in one series to be effective in patients with Morgellons disease, with limited adverse events.[74] Long-term antibiotic therapy has reportedly been useful.[70,75] Collaborative care with a psychiatrist or a psychodermatology clinic is strongly encouraged for both Morgellons disease and patients with DI.

OBSESSIVE-COMPULSIVE DISORDERS

OCD is characterized by the presence of obsessions (recurrent thoughts or images experienced as intrusive or senseless) or compulsions (repetitive, intentional behaviors performed to diminish discomfort or future harm and felt to be unreasonable or excessive).[76] The essential features required for diagnosis in the *Diagnostic and Statistical Manual of Mental Disorders (DSM)* 5 is that the obsessions or compulsions are severe enough to significantly affect the daily routine and social or work functioning and the patient does not realize that they are excessive or unreasonable.

The expression of OCD may take the form of a dermatologic disorder. Entities that may fall into this spectrum are listed in Table 26.4. Clinical features that may suggest an OCD-related spectrum disorder include a heightened concern for cleanliness, fear of contamination, excessive worry about life-threatening illnesses or STIs, inappropriate concerns about body odor, and worries regarding an unattractive appearance or hair loss.[30,77]

OCD often begins in childhood or early adulthood, and most patients have a waxing and waning course. Comorbid conditions are common, including depression and anxiety disorders. Childhood OCD may be associated with Tourette syndrome, tics, family history of OCD, developmental delay, and hyperactivity.[78] The most common cutaneous presentations are trichotillomania (see Chapter 7), onychophagia, onychotillomania (Fig. 26.36) (see Chapter 7), excoriation (skin picking) disorder, and acne excoriée (see Chapter 8).[77,79] *Onychophagia* refers to the compulsive habit of nail biting, which becomes pathologic when excessively time consuming or associated with social avoidance.[38] *Onychotillomania*, also known as *nail picking disorder*, refers to repetitive picking or pulling of the fingernails or toenails, resulting in atypical morphologies, which may include grooves,

Table 26.4 Obsessive-Compulsive Disorder and Some Possibly Associated Dermatologic Conditions

Disorder	See Chapter Number for Details
Acne excoriée	8
Body dysmorphic disorder	Current
Irritant dermatitis (handwashing)	3
Lichen simplex chronicus	3
Lip-licker dermatitis	3
Neurotic excoriations/skin picking disorder	Current
Onychophagia/onychotillomania	Current
Rhinotillexomania (pathologic nose picking)	Current
Prurigo nodularis	3
Trichotillomania	7

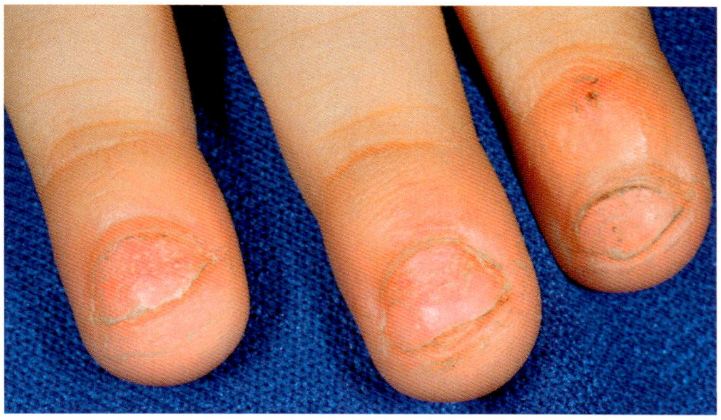

Fig. 26.36 Obsessive-compulsive disorder. This 6-year-old boy has features of onychophagia (nail biting; note shaggy, uneven, and short distal nail plates) and onychotillomania (nail picking; note damage to cuticles). The associated nail pitting was felt to be related to underlying 20-nail dystrophy of childhood.

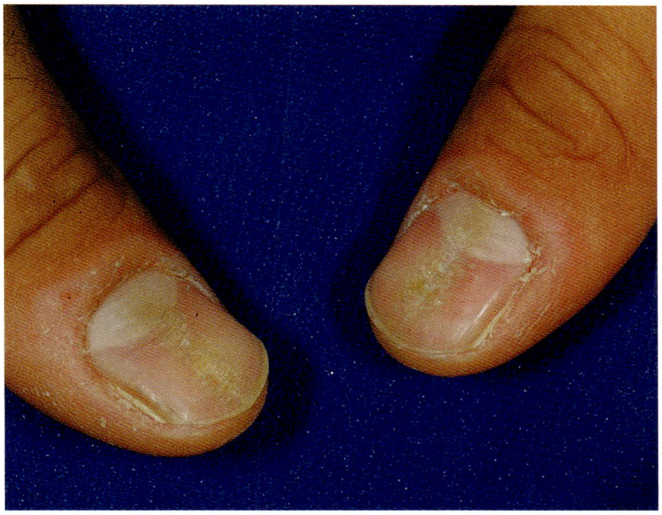

Fig. 26.37 Habit tic deformity. Multiple central nail plate transverse grooves in a boy who admitted to frequently picking at this cuticles and nails.

dystrophy, roughness or atrophy of the nail, and typically with asymmetric involvement; the periungual skin and cuticle are often inflamed, eroded, edematous, or crusted.[80] A related disorder, termed *habit tic deformity* (see Chapter 7), is related to repetitive manipulation of the cuticle and proximal nail fold and presents with central nail plate depression and multiple transverse grooves (Fig. 26.37). *Rhinotillexomania* (compulsive nose picking) has been recognized as a potential manifestation of OCD when it becomes socially compromising or physically harmful. Nasal septum perforation has been reported in some patients. *Excoriation (skin picking) disorder,* which is also known as *neurotic excoriation* (see earlier this chapter), is characterized by recurrent picking of the skin with resultant tissue damage; acne excoriée is one subtype of this disorder. In severe types, patients may use instruments such as tweezers or pins to pick and dig into their skin.[81] Importantly, patients with pediatric OCD experience chronicity and intractability of the disorder despite multiple interventions.[82]

Body dysmorphic disorder (BDD) is defined as preoccupation with an imagined defect in appearance. BDD, which falls into the OCD spectrum of disorders, may present with dermatologic symptoms or concerns. These include concerns about an unattractive appearance, acne scarring, wrinkles, hair thinning, early skin aging, hirsutism, greasy skin, body odor, large or misshapen nose, small genitalia, or blushing.[77,79,83,84] Patients with BDD may spend many hours a day worrying about their obsession and visually inspecting the "abnormality," which may affect social and professional functioning. BDD occurs at high rates in patients with eating disorders. Tanning addiction has been classified as one subtype of BDD.[85] In adolescents, BDD may be unrecognized, given overlap with "normal concerns for teenagers," and hence, its diagnosis and therapy may be delayed.[84]

Treatment of OCD spectrum disorders includes both behavioral and pharmacologic therapies, most notably the tricyclic antidepressants and selective serotonin reuptake inhibitors. N-acetylcysteine was demonstrated to be effective in reducing symptoms of excoriation disorder in one randomized controlled trial.[86] Cognitive behavioral therapy is considered the first-line therapy for BDD.

PSYCHOGENIC PURPURA/GARDNER–DIAMOND SYNDROME

Psychogenic purpura (autoerythrocyte sensitization syndrome, Gardner–Diamond syndrome) is a rare disorder characterized by recurrent episodes of painful ecchymoses (Fig. 26.38) in various locations. The patients are most often young adult females with emotional disturbances, and the lesions commonly occur after trauma, surgery, or severe emotional stress.[87,88] The individual lesions resolve over 2 weeks. Psychiatric associations include depression, OCD, hypochondriasis, hysterical and borderline personality disorders, and anxiety.[87–89] In one large series, underlying psychiatric diagnoses were present in 54% of patients.[90] In 1955 Gardner and Diamond suggested that the disorder was associated with autosensitization of patients to their own blood.[91] Traditionally the diagnosis was confirmed by intradermal injection of the patient's own erythrocytes, which may result in reproduction of the clinical lesions. The exact pathophysiology of this disorder remains poorly understood, with some proposed mechanisms including emotion-stimulated activation of the kallikrein–kinin system, immunologic dysregulation, platelet defects, and dysregulation of fibrinolytic pathways.[90]

The skin lesions of Gardner–Diamond syndrome are often consistent with a factitial dermatosis, given their purpuric nature, irregular distribution, peculiar morphology, and erratic onset. However, confirmation

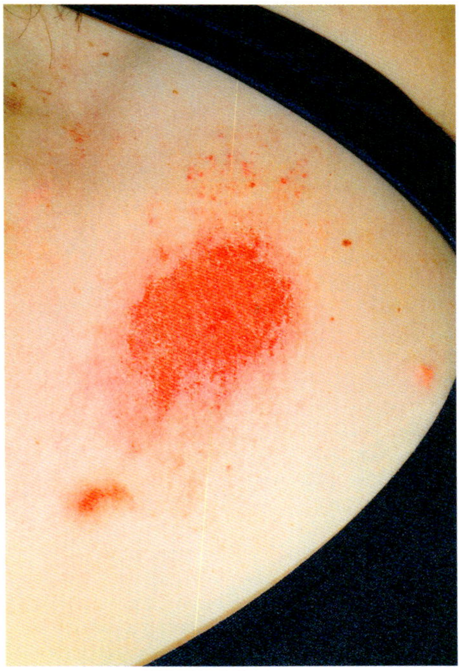

Fig. 26.38 Psychogenic purpura. This young female with a history of anxiety disorder complained of recurrent, spontaneous ecchymoses. Examination revealed ecchymotic patches with superimposed abrasions.

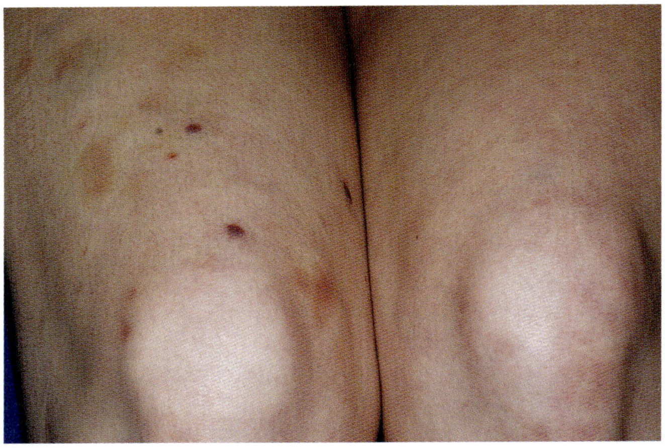

Fig. 26.39 Psychogenic purpura. This 16-year-old female patient with a history of anxiety and attention-deficit disorder presented with a 1-year history of spontaneous, recurrent bruises, which were tender to touch and associated with "burning." She improved dramatically after combined psychotherapy and pharmacotherapy.

of a self-inflicted process is often difficult, if not impossible. During the prodromal stage, nonspecific symptoms such as malaise and fatigue may be reported. The skin lesions develop rapidly after sensations of burning and stinging and evolve over 1 or 2 days from erythematous to ecchymotic (Fig. 26.39) . They resolve over 7 to 10 days. Associated findings such as hematuria, epistaxis, or menorrhagia are occasionally noted. Histologic evaluation of skin biopsy samples reveals nonspecific features, including perivascular inflammation (without frank vasculitis), erythrocyte extravasation, and pigment deposition.[92] Avoidance of confrontation with the patient, establishment of rapport, and psychiatric evaluation and therapy are indicated. Psychotropic medications (especially selective serotonin reuptake inhibitors and tricyclic antidepressants) and hypnotherapy have been utilized.[92,93]

CAREGIVER-FABRICATED ILLNESS

Caregiver-fabricated illness (also known as Munchausen syndrome by proxy, pediatric condition falsification, factitious disorder by proxy, child abuse in the medical setting, and medical child abuse) is a form of child maltreatment caused by a caregiver who falsifies and/or induces a child's illness, leading to unnecessary and potentially harmful medical investigations and/or treatment.[94] Munchausen syndrome is the traditional designation for a form of factitious disorder characterized by dramatic presentations with factitious complaints, exaggerated lying, and "physician shopping." Patients have recurrent feigned symptoms and often have borderline or antisocial personality types. Caregiver-fabricated illness occurs when a parent or caregiver creates an illness in a child and is a form of child abuse inflicted most often by the mother. The stereotype of a mother involved in caregiver-fabricated illness is one who works in the health care field, is estranged from the child's father, is quite friendly with the medical staff, and seems relatively unconcerned when the physician is unable to render a diagnosis.[95] The perpetrators are often quite familiar with medical terminology and diseases and usually have pathologic attachments to their children.[96] A history of working in a day care setting is also common.[95] Somatoform and factitious disorders are common among perpetrators, as are personality disorders, especially antisocial, histrionic, borderline, avoidant, and narcissistic types.[97]

The classic four criteria set forth for caregiver-fabricated illness are medical illness in a child that is fabricated by a parent; the child is brought for repeated medical evaluation or treatment and often undergoes multiple medical procedures; the perpetrator denies the actions; and acute symptoms and signs resolve when the child and caregiver are separated.[43] Two circumstances should be present for this diagnosis to be confirmed: harm or potential harm to the child involving medical care and a caregiver who is causing it to happen.[98]

Box 26.2 Potential Red Flags for Caregiver-Fabricated Illness in a Child

Persistent symptoms that defy medical explanation
Unusual signs or symptoms (case often considered "atypical")
Symptoms out of proportion to physical findings
Caregiver is neither satisfied nor reassured when informed of positive progress
History is inconsistent
Caregiver encourages additional investigations or consultations
Signs and symptoms consistently occur in presence of same caregiver
Lack of response (or unusual response) to established therapies
Caregiver with history of somatization disorders

Modified from Flaherty EG, MacMillan HL. Caregiver-fabricated illness in a child: A manifestation of child maltreatment. *Pediatrics.* 2013;132:590–97 and Squires JE, Squires RH. A review of Munchausen syndrome by proxy. *Pediatr Ann.* 2013;42(4):e67–71.

Features of the clinical scenario usually include persistent symptoms that defy medical explanation, involvement of an adult caregiver (usually the biologic mother), and an involved physician who is eager to piece together the presentation and ameliorate the patient's confusing symptoms.[99] Inconsistent results of consecutive diagnostic testing is one clue to the diagnosis.[100] Potential indicators of caregiver-fabricated illness in a child are listed in Box 26.2.

A variety of clinical symptoms or features may be seen in the child victim of caregiver-fabricated illness. These include infant or sleep apnea, factitious coagulopathy, bruising, failure to thrive, hypoglycemia, abnormal urinalysis, seizures and other neurologic symptoms, cyanosis, vomiting and diarrhea, recurrent infections, sepsis, lethargy, behavior problems, fever, melena or hematochezia, electrolyte abnormalities, and bone and joint problems.[43,94–96,68,101] The dermatologic aspects of this disorder may invariably be referred to as *factitious dermatitis by proxy* or *DA by proxy*. Skin findings have been reported in 3% to 9% of cases.[101] These lesions may present with any of the morphologies discussed earlier for factitious dermatitis/DA, including erythema, blistering, burns, lacerations, puncture wounds, and dermatitis.

The diagnosis of caregiver-fabricated illness can be challenging. The three forms of presenting signs or symptoms include covert injury induced in secret by the caregiver, fabrication of symptoms by the perpetrator, and symptoms neither induced nor fabricated but exaggerated by the caregiver.[102] The former is rendered when there is unquestionable evidence of commission, such as capturing the act during covert videotape surveillance (CVS) in the hospital setting.[103] Some experts believe that such CVS is required in order to make a definitive and timely diagnosis in most cases of caregiver-fabricated illness.[95] When used, adequate safeguards including continuous surveillance and an agreed-upon plan of action must exist in order to prevent further injury to the child.[98] The use of CVS remains controversial, with some arguing that it is an invasion of a parent's right to privacy or constitutes entrapment. If utilized, hospital-implemented protocols that guide its use are encouraged.[94] A diagnosis of exclusion is occasionally rendered when all other possible explanations for the child's condition have been considered and excluded.[103] Consultation with all colleagues who have cared for the child and a "separation test," in which the child is demonstrated to be free of disease outside the care of the mother, are useful.[104] Child protective services should be involved and the perpetrator referred to a professional with significant experience in caregiver-fabricated illness. Long-term morbidity or permanent disability is common in survivors.

Cutaneous Mimickers of Abuse and Factitial Disorders

Although child abuse or factitial disorders should always be considered in the child with unusual skin marks or injuries, several potential mimickers must be kept in mind. These are summarized in Table 26.5.[105–109] Although they are not discussed in detail here, it is important to recognize potential cutaneous mimickers in order to reduce the erroneous diagnosis of child abuse.[110]

Table 26.5 Potential Mimickers of Abuse or Factitial Disorders

Disorder	Chapter/Comment
Accidental burns	Various, including enuresis blanket, acetic acid, objects heated by sun (e.g., bike seats, car upholstery)
Allergic contact dermatitis	Chapter 3; may be confused with abuse, especially when vesicular or bullous
Anal fissures	Most commonly associated with constipation, passage of hard stools; however, occasionally associated with sexual abuse
Autoimmune bullous disease	Chapter 13; vulvar pemphigoid, linear IgA bullous disease of childhood
Behçet syndrome	Chapter 25
Berloque dermatitis	Chapter 19; phototoxic reaction to fragrance products
Bullous impetigo	Chapter 14; may be confused with cigarette burns
Crohn's disease	Chapter 25; may present with perianal erythema, fissures, skin tags, bleeding, scarring, swelling
Ecthyma	Chapter 14; confused with cigarette burns; usually caused by GABHS
Ehlers–Danlos syndrome	Chapter 6; may have poor wound healing, scarring, easy bruising
Enlarged hymenal opening	Important reassuring features include intact hymenal tissue at posterior rim, lack of laceration/ deep notching/bruising/bleeding[105]
Epidermal nevus	Chapter 9; perianal lesions may be confused with anogenital condylomata[106]
Epidermolysis bullosa	Chapter 13; especially dominant dystrophic or simplex varieties
Fixed drug eruption	Chapter 20
Folk remedies	Current chapter; includes coining, cupping, moxibustion, neonatal salting; see text
Hematologic disorders	Various, including hemophilia, von Willebrand disease, leukemia, ITP
Henoch–Schönlein purpura	Chapter 21; may be confused with ecchymoses, although other features (distribution, joint/scrotal swelling, kidney/GI involvement) help to differentiate
Herpes zoster	Chapter 15; may be confused with abuse when involves genital (S2, S3) dermatomes
Incontinentia pigmenti	Chapter 11; vesicular and pigmentary lesions with bizarre patterning
Labial adhesions	
Lichen sclerosus et atrophicus	Chapter 22; genital variant confused with sexual abuse; may be bullous
Congenital dermal melanocytosis (formerly known as Mongolian spots)	Chapter 11
Netherton syndrome	Chapter 5; dermatitis, ichthyosis, failure to thrive, and alopecia may be confused for abuse
Neuroblastoma	Chapter 10; orbital metastases may present with periorbital ecchymoses ("raccoon eyes")
Nevus of Ota or Ito	Chapter 11
Normal bruising	Most commonly children 2–5 years of age; consider distribution, developmental status, history; see discussion in text
Osteogenesis imperfecta	Chapter 6; frequent fractures, osteoporosis, short stature, frontal bossing, blue sclerae
Perianal pyramidal protrusion	Chapter 15
Perianal streptococcal dermatitis	Chapter 14
Phytophotodermatitis	Chapter 19; phototoxic reaction to psoralens (lemons, limes, celery, parsley, dill)
Straddle injury	Can be mistaken for sexual abuse; accidental injuries rarely bilaterally symmetric, often involve bruising of inner thighs and/or labia majora
Vaginal foreign body	May result in vaginal discharge, bleeding
Xeroderma pigmentosum	Chapter 19; severe sunburn may be confused with neglect

GABHS, Group A β-hemolytic streptococci; *GI*, gastrointestinal; *IgA*, immunoglobulin A; *ITP*, idiopathic thrombocytopenic purpura.

A number of cultural practices may be confused with abuse, given the trauma-induced skin lesions that result. With the increasing influx of Asian immigrants entering the United States, traditional East Asian medicine methods are being practiced with increasing incidence. The philosophy of East Asian medicine is to achieve a state of balance and equilibrium, including proper flow of energies within "channels" or "meridians."[111] The goal of traditional folk remedies is to facilitate this energy balance. It is important for the pediatric practitioner to be familiar with these culturally based therapies, which include coining/spooning, cupping, moxibustion, neonatal salting, traditional pinching therapy ("*ba sha*"), gridding, bloodletting, and warm-needle acupuncture.[111–118] The former four entities will be briefly discussed here.

Coining is also known as *spooning, coin rubbing, skin scraping*, or *çao gio*. It is an ancient Vietnamese folk remedy performed by applying heated, mentholated oil to the back, chest, and shoulders and then vigorously rubbing a coin on selected parts of the body in order to produce linear petechiae or ecchymoses (Fig. 26.40).[116] Other items that may be used include a ceramic Chinese soup spoon, water buffalo horn, piece of jade or ginger root, or edge of a jar cap. Whereas a coin is traditionally used by the Vietnamese, a spoon is commonly the instrument used by the Chinese, in which case the practice is referred to as *quat sha*.[117] Those who utilize coining believe it to be useful for a variety of complaints, including headache, fever, pain, and inflammation. Although serious injury is rare, minor and even major burns (resulting from ignition of the oil in the skin) have been reported.[116]

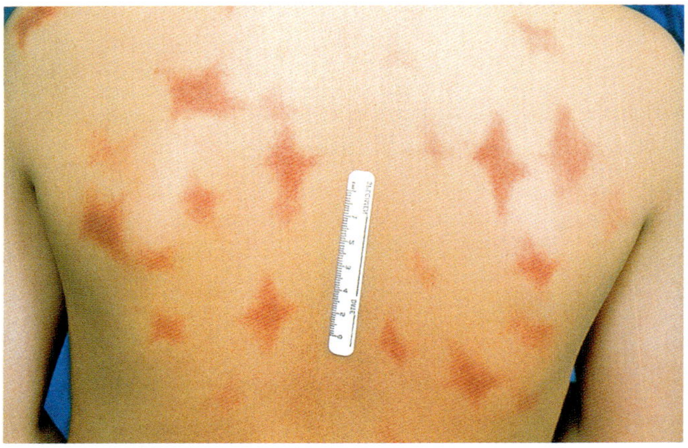

Fig. 26.40 Coining. These linear and stellate purpuric patches were caused by the vigorous rubbing of a coin on the skin, termed *coining*, or *çao gio*. (Courtesy Jean Hlady, MD.)

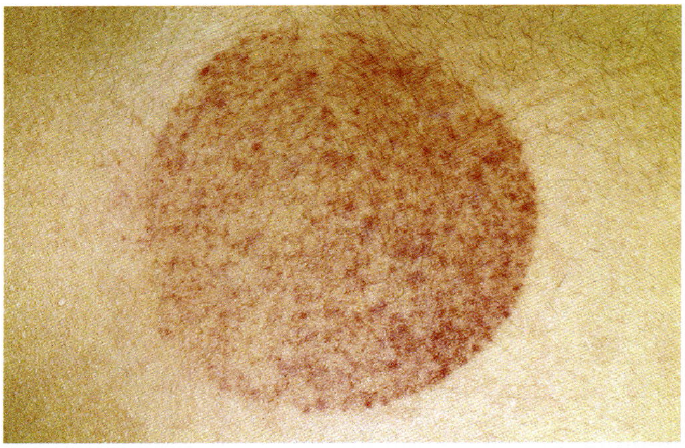

Fig. 26.42 Cupping. Close-up image of the ecchymotic lesion seen in the female patient in Fig. 26.41.

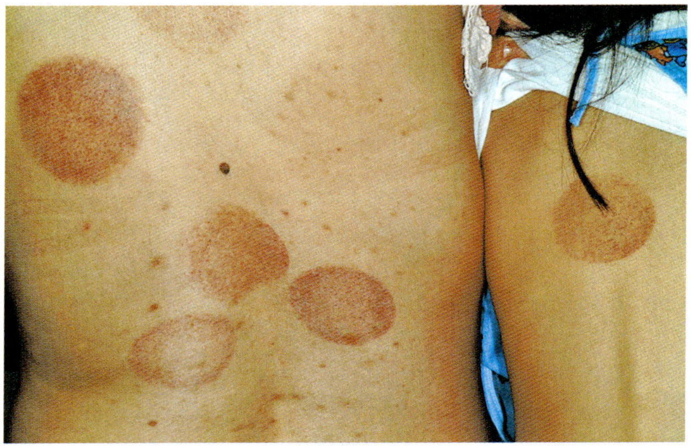

Fig. 26.41 Cupping. This 7-year-old girl *(right)* who was brought to the clinic for an unrelated skin complaint was noted to have this round, ecchymotic lesion on her back. Examination of her mother *(left)* revealed multiple such lesions that were being induced by cupping in hopes of treating her rheumatoid arthritis. The family performed the procedure on the girl at her request.

Cupping is an ancient technique dating back to the fourth century BC in Egypt.[118] It is practiced in the United States most often by Russian immigrants but is also utilized within Asian and Mexican-American cultures (where it is referred to as *ventosas*).[117] It is used to relieve such symptoms as abdominal pain, abscesses, stroke paralysis, lower back pain, indigestion, menstrual irregularities, fever, congestion, and poor appetite. With this remedy, a cup or jar is immediately placed on the skin after a cotton ball soaked with alcohol has been ignited within the cup to create a suction vacuum. The procedure results in circular ecchymotic lesions (Figs. 26.41 and 26.42) with eventual hyperpigmentation. In Middle Eastern cultures, the skin may be initially lanced, with some blood drawn into the cup during the procedure. This has been referred to as *wet cupping*.

Moxibustion is another folk remedy utilized primarily in Asian cultures for a variety of complaints, including enuresis, behavioral disorders, asthma, and pain.[111,117] It has also been utilized for correction of breech presentation[119] and for treatment of tennis elbow.[120] In moxibustion, the moxa herb (mugwort herb, *Artemisia vulgaris*) is rolled into a cone or cigar, ignited, and placed on the appropriate body part (either directly or indirectly with a medium separating the moxa from the skin). It is allowed to burn to the point of pain, and the resulting skin lesions vary from transient redness to second-degree burns that resemble cigarette burns on acupuncture sites and may scar. As with all folk remedies, these lesions may be confused with intentional child abuse. Indirect moxibustion, in which the lit moxa stick is held near (not on) the skin until it turns red, is less painful and less often results in scarring.[121]

Neonatal salting is a custom in Turkey, typically performed in the first days of life. This procedure, which consists of application of salt to the newborn's skin (ranging from localized to widespread application), is believed to prevent excessive sweating and body odor as an adult.[114] The most frequently reported complication of this practice is hypernatremia, which can be fatal.[122,123] However, salting can also lead to skin damage, as was reported in a 1-week-old infant who had been subjected to this custom for 3 days and presented with hypernatremia and severe scrotal ulcerations; such a presentation could also be mistaken for child abuse.[114]

The complete list of 123 references for this chapter is available online at http://expertconsult.inkling.com.

Key References

Child Maltreatment 2016: Summary of key findings. Child Welfare Information Gateway, July 2018. At www.childwelfare.gov/pubPDFs/canstats.pdf. Accessed April 30, 2019

Zeanah CH, Humphreys KL. Child abuse and neglect. J Am Acad Child Adolesc Psychiatry 2018;57(9):637–44

Jenny C, Crawford-Jakubiak JE, and Committee on Child Abuse and Neglect. The evaluation of children in the primary care setting when sexual abuse is suspected. Pediatrics 2013;132:e558–67

Adams JA, Kellogg ND, Farst KJ, Harper NS, Palusci VJ, Frasier LD, et al. Updated guidelines for the medical assessment and care of children who may have been sexually abused. J Pediatr Adolesc Gynecol 2016;29:81–7

Kuhn H, Mennella C, Magid M, Stamu-O'Brien C, Kroumpouzos G. Psychocutaneous disease. Clinical perspectives. J Am Acad Dermatol 2017;76:779–91

Sridharan M, Ali U, Hook CC, Nichols WL, Pruthi RK. The Mayo clinic experience with psychogenic purpura (Gardner-Diamond syndrome). Am J Med Sci 2019; 357(5):411–20

Dubowitz H, Bennett S. Physical abuse and neglect of children. Lancet 2007;369:1891–9.

Pierce MC, Kaczor K, Aldridge S, et al. Bruising characteristics discriminating physical child abuse from accidental trauma. Pediatrics 2010;125(1):67–74.

Preer G, Sorrentino D, Newton AW. Child abuse pediatrics: prevention, evaluation, and treatment. Curr Opin Pediatr 2012;24:266–73.

Adams JA, Starling SP, Frasier LD, et al. Diagnostic accuracy in child sexual abuse medical evaluation: role of experience, training, and expert case review. Child Abuse Negl 2012;36:383–92.

Shah KN, Fried RG. Factitial dermatoses in children. Curr Opin Pediatr 2006;18:403–9.

Foster AA, Hylwa SA, Bury JE, et al. Delusional infestation: clinical presentation in 147 patients seen at Mayo Clinic. J Am Acad Dermatol 2012;67:673.e1–10.

Flaherty EG, MacMillan HL. Caregiver-fabricated illness in a child: a manifestation of child maltreatment. Pediatrics 2013;132:590–7.

Stirling J, the Committee on Child Abuse and Neglect. Beyond Munchausen syndrome by proxy: identification and treatment of child abuse in the medical setting. Pediatrics 2007;119(5):1026–30.

Ravanfar P, Dinulos JG. Cultural practices affecting the skin of children. Curr Opin Pediatr 2010;22:423–31.

Index

Page numbers followed by "f" indicate figures, "t" indicate tables, and "b" indicate boxes.

D

E

F